Clinical Magnetic Resonance Imaging

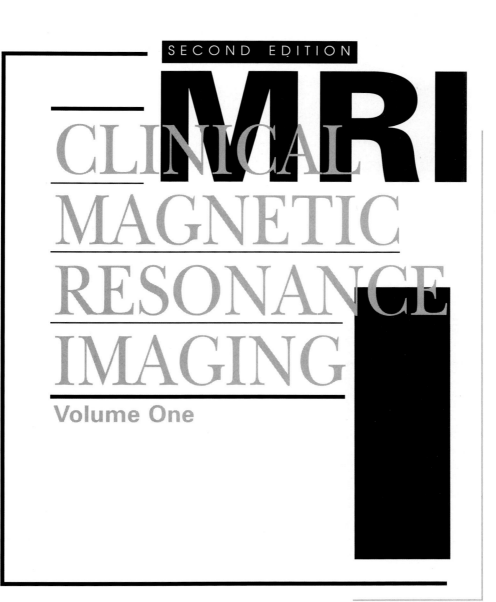

SECOND EDITION

MRI

CLINICAL MAGNETIC RESONANCE IMAGING

Volume One

Robert R. Edelman, MD
Professor of Radiology
Harvard Medical School;
Director of Magnetic Resonance Imaging
Department of Radiology
Beth Israel Hospital
Boston, Massachusetts

Michael B. Zlatkin, MD
Director of Musculoskeletal Imaging and
   Magnetic Resonance Imaging
Radiology Associates of Hollywood, Florida;
Director of Sports Medicine Imaging
Health South Doctors' Hospital
Coral Gables, Florida;
Clinical Associate Professor of Radiology
University of Miami School of Medicine
Miami, Florida

John R. Hesselink, MD, FACR
Professor of Radiology and Neurosciences
University of California, San Diego,
   School of Medicine;
Chief of Neuroradiology and Magnetic
   Resonance
Department of Radiology
University of California,
   San Diego, Medical Center
San Diego, California

W.B. SAUNDERS COMPANY

A Division of Harcourt Brace & Company
Philadelphia   London   Toronto   Montreal   Sydney   Tokyo

W.B. SAUNDERS COMPANY
A Division of Harcourt Brace & Company

The Curtis Center
Independence Square West
Philadelphia, Pennsylvania 19106

Library of Congress Cataloging-in-Publication Data

Clinical magnetic resonance imaging / [edited by] Robert R. Edelman,
John R. Hesselink, Michael B. Zlatkin.—2nd ed.

p.   cm.

Includes bibliographical references.

ISBN 0–7216–5221–2

1. Magnetic resonance imaging.   I. Edelman, Robert R.   II. Hesselink,
   John R.   III. Zlatkin, Michael B.   [DNLM: 1. Magnetic Resonance
   Imaging.   WN 185 C641 1996]

RC78.7.N83C56 1996   616.07′548—dc20

DNLM/DLC   95–20424

Volume One ISBN 0–7216–6978–6
Volume Two ISBN 0–7216–6979–4
Set ISBN 0–7216–5221–2

Clinical Magnetic Resonance Imaging, second edition

Printed in the United States of America

Last digit is the print number: 9   8   7   6   5   4   3   2   1

To
Daniel and Laura
Kay and André
Marilyn, Nancy, and Robert

CONTRIBUTORS

MARY K. ADAMIS, MD
Staff Radiologist, Beth Israel Hospital, and Instructor in Radiology, Harvard Medical School, Boston, Massachusetts
Artifacts in MRI: Description, Causes, and Solutions; MR Angiography of the Body; Glossary of MR Terms

CHARLES M. ANDERSON, MD, PhD
Associate Professor of Radiology, University of California, San Francisco; Chief of MRI, San Francisco Veterans Administration Medical Center, San Francisco, California
MR Angiography: Basic Principles

SUSAN M. ASCHER, MD
Assistant Professor of Radiology, Georgetown University School of Medicine; Associate Director, MR Services, Georgetown University Medical Center, Washington, DC
Pancreas, Spleen, Bowel, and Peritoneum

WILLIAM S. BALL, JR., MD
Professor of Radiology and Pediatrics, University of Cincinnati; Chief, Section of Pediatric Neuroradiology, and Director, Imaging Research Center, Children's Hospital Medical Center, Cincinnati, Ohio
Metabolic, Congenital Neurodegenerative, and Toxic Disorders

A. JAMES BARKOVICH, MD
Professor of Radiology, Neurology, Pediatrics and Neurological Surgery, University of California, San Francisco, San Francisco, California
Pediatric Spine: Congenital and Developmental Disorders

CARLOS BAZAN, III, MD
Clinical Associate Professor, University of Texas Health Science Center at San Antonio; Staff Radiologist, University Hospital and Audie Murphy Veterans Administration Hospital, San Antonio, Texas
Spinal Cord and Intradural Disease

JAVIER BELTRAN, MD
Professor of Radiology, New York University School of Medicine; Chairman, Department of Radiology, Hospital for Joint Diseases, New York, New York
Ankle and Foot

GEORGE S. BISSET, III, MD
Professor of Radiology and Pediatrics, Duke University Medical Center; Vice-Chairman, Department of Radiology, and Director, Section for Pediatric Radiology, Duke University Medical Center, Durham, North Carolina
Pediatric Orthopedics

JUDY S. BLEBEA, MD
Assistant Professor of Radiology, Department of Radiology, University of Cincinnati, Cincinnati, Ohio
Bone and Soft Tissue Tumors

LIZANN BOLINGER, PhD
Assistant Professor, Department of Radiology, University of Pennsylvania, Philadelphia, Pennsylvania
Spectroscopy: Basic Principles and Techniques

THOMAS J. BRADY, MD
Professor of Radiology, Harvard Medical School; Director, MGH-NMR Center, Department of Radiology, Massachusetts General Hospital, Boston, Massachusetts
Biochemical Basis of the MRI Appearance of Cerebral Hemorrhage

SUSAN E. BRALEY, MD
Assistant Professor of Radiology, Department of Radiology, University of Cincinnati; Attending Physician, University Hospital, Cincinnati, Ohio
Bone and Soft Tissue Tumors

RICHARD A. BRONEN, MD
Associate Professor of Diagnostic Radiology and Neurosurgery, Yale University School of Medicine, New Haven, Connecticut
Epilepsy

ELIZABETH D. BROWN, MD
Resident in Radiology, University of North Carolina Hospitals, Chapel Hill, North Carolina
Kidneys, Adrenal Glands, and Retroperitoneum

JEFFREY J. BROWN, MD
Associate Professor of Radiology and Director, Magnetic Resonance Imaging, Mallinckrodt Institute of Radiology, Washington University Medical Center, St. Louis, Missouri
Pancreas, Spleen, Bowel, and Peritoneum

STEPHEN M. BROWN, MD
Clinical Assistant Professor, Department of Radiology, University of Miami School of Medicine, Miami, Florida; Director of Musculoskeletal MRI and MRI Research, University Community Hospital, Tampa, Florida
Kinematic MRI of Joints

JAMES A. BRUNBERG, MD
Associate Professor of Radiology, Neurology, and Neurosurgery, University of Michigan; Director, Division of Neuroradiology, and Co-Director, Division of Magnetic Resonance Imaging, University of Michigan Hospitals, Ann Arbor, Michigan
Pituitary Gland and Parasellar Region

CARL V. BUNDSCHUH, MD
Associate Professor of Radiology, Eastern Virginia Medical School; Director of Neuroradiology and MRI, Medical Center Radiologists and Sentara Hospitals, Norfolk, Virginia
Postoperative Lumbosacral Spine

RICHARD B. BUXTON, PhD
Associate Professor of Radiology and Director of Magnetic Resonance Research, University of California, San Diego Medical Center, San Diego, California
Principles of Diffusion and Perfusion MRI

J. JEFFREY CARR, MD
Assistant Professor of Radiology, Department of Radiology, Bowman Gray School of Medicine, Wake Forest University, Winston-Salem, North Carolina
Thorax

DAVID CHENG, MD
Clinical Fellow in Radiology, Harvard Medical School; Clinical Diagnostic Resident in Radiology, Brigham and Women's Hospital, Boston, Massachusetts
Functional Cardiac Imaging

DAISY CHIEN, PhD
Applications Scientist, Siemens Medical Systems, Inc., Erlangen, Germany
MR Angiography: Basic Principles

BRIAN W. CHONG, MD, FRCP(C)
Assistant Professor of Radiology, Department of Radiology, Section of Neuroradiology, University of California, Davis, School of Medicine, Davis, California
Pituitary Gland and Parasellar Region

MERVYN D. COHEN, MB, ChB, BSc, DCH, FRCR, MD
Professor of Radiology and Director of Pediatric Radiology, Indiana University School of Medicine, Indiana University Medical Center, and Riley Hospital for Children, Indianapolis, Indiana
Pediatric Body

ANTONIUS DEGRAUW, MD, PhD
Associate Professor of Pediatrics and Neurology, University of Cincinnati Medical Center and Children's Hospital Medical Center, Cincinnati, Ohio
Metabolic, Congenital Neurodegenerative, and Toxic Disorders

MONY J. DE LEON
Professor of Psychiatry and Director of Neuroimaging Research Lab, Departments of Psychiatry and Radiology, New York University Medical Center, New York, New York
Neurodegenerative Disorders

KATHLEEN DUPUIS, RT, BS
MRI Chief Technologist, Beth Israel Hospital, Boston, Massachusetts
Practical MRI for the Technologist and Imaging Specialist

ROBERT R. EDELMAN, MD
Professor of Radiology, Harvard Medical School; Director of Magnetic Resonance Imaging, Department of Radiology, Beth Israel Hospital, Boston, Massachusetts
Basic Principles of MRI; Practical MRI for the Technologist and Imaging Specialist; Artifacts in MRI: Description, Causes, and Solutions; Fast MRI; Spontaneous and Traumatic Hemorrhage; MR Angiography of the Body; Functional Cardiac Imaging; MRI Scan Protocols

W. SCOTT ENOCHS, MD, PhD
Clinical Fellow in Diagnostic Radiology, Harvard Medical School and Massachusetts General Hospital, Boston, Massachusetts
Organ- and Tissue-Directed MRI Contrast Agents

JULIA R. FIELDING, MD
Instructor in Radiology, Harvard Medical School; Associate Radiologist, Brigham and Women's Hospital, Boston, Massachusetts
Female Pelvis

J. PAUL FINN, MD
Director of MR Research and Development, Siemens Medical Systems, Inc, Iselin, New Jersey
Pulse Sequence Design in MRI

DUANE P. FLAMIG, PhD
Director of Research, Department of Magnetic Resonance, Baylor University Medical Center, Dallas, Texas
Breast

LAWRENCE R. FRANK, PhD
Assistant Professor, Department of Radiology, University of California, San Diego; Physicist, Department of Radiology, Veterans Administration Medical Center, San Diego, California
Principles of Diffusion and Perfusion MRI

RICHARD J. FRIEDLAND, MD
Attending Physician, Dutchess Radiology Associates and Vassar Brothers Hospital, READE, Poughkeepsie, New York
Epilepsy

RUSSELL C. FRITZ, MD
Assistant Clinical Professor of Radiology, University of California, San Francisco, San Francisco; National Orthopaedic Imaging Associates, Greenbrae, California
Elbow

WARREN B. GEFTER, MD
Professor of Radiology, University of Pennsylvania Medical Center, Philadelphia, Pennsylvania
Thorax

AJAX E. GEORGE, MD
Professor of Radiology and Medical Director of Neuroimaging Research, New York University Medical School, New York, New York
Neurodegenerative Disorders

SEBASTIAN GLOBITS, MD
Cardiology Fellow, University of Vienna, Vienna, Austria
Adult Heart Disease

JAMES GOLOMB, MD
Clinical Instructor, Department of Neurology, New York University Medical Center, New York, New York
Neurodegenerative Disorders

MITHAT HALILOGLU, MD
Assistant Professor of Radiology, Hacettepe University, Hacettepe, Ankara, Turkey
Pediatric Body

STEVEN E. HARMS, MD
Medical Director, Department of Magnetic Resonance, Baylor University Medical Center, Dallas, Texas
Breast

HIROTO HATABU, MD
Instructor in Radiology, Harvard Medical School; Clinical Fellow, MR Section, Beth Israel Hospital, Boston, Massachusetts
Thorax

JOHN F. HEALY, MD
Clinical Professor of Radiology, University of California, San Diego; Chief of Radiology, Veterans Administration Hospital, San Diego, California
Brain Stem, Posterior Fossa, and Cranial Nerves

JOHN R. HESSELINK, MD, FACR
Professor of Radiology and Neurosciences, University of California, San Diego, School of Medicine; Chief of Neuroradiology and Magnetic Resonance, Department of Radiology, University of California, San Diego, Medical Center, San Diego, California
Brain: Indications, Techniques, and Atlas; Infectious and Inflammatory Diseases; White Matter Disease; An Atlas and an Approach to Spine Imaging; Degenerative Disease; Pediatric Spine: Congenital and Developmental Disorders; MRI Scan Protocols

RICHARD J. HICKS, MD
Assistant Professor in Diagnostic Radiology, Tufts University School of Medicine, Boston, Massachusetts; Director of Magnetic Resonance Imaging, Baystate Medical Center, Springfield, Massachusetts
Supratentorial Brain Tumors

CHARLES B. HIGGINS, MD
Professor of Radiology and Vice Chairman of Radiology, University of California, San Francisco, Medical School, San Francisco, California
Adult Heart Disease

MARY HOCHMAN, MD
Instructor in Radiology, Harvard University and Beth Israel Hospital, Boston, Massachusetts
MR Angiography of the Body

ANDRE I. HOLODNY, MD
Assistant Professor of Radiology, UMDNJ–New Jersey Medical School, Newark, New Jersey
Neurodegenerative Disorders

ERIK K. INSKO, MD, PhD
Department of Radiology, Hospital of the University of Pennsylvania, Philadelphia, Pennsylvania
Spectroscopy: Basic Principles and Techniques

J. RANDY JINKINS, MD
Director of Neuroradiology, University of Texas Health Science Center, San Antonio, Texas
Postoperative Lumbosacral Spine

FERENC A. JOLESZ, MD
Associate Professor of Radiology, Harvard Medical School; Director, Division of MRI, and Director, Image-Guided Therapy Program, Brigham and Women's Hospital, Boston, Massachusetts
MRI-Guided Interventions

EMANUEL KANAL, MD
Associate Professor, University of Pittsburgh School of Medicine; Director of Clinical and Educational MR, Department of Radiology, University of Pittsburgh Medical Center, Pittsburgh, Pennsylvania
Bioeffects and Safety of MR Procedures

SPYROS K. KARAMPEKIOS, MD
Lecturer in Radiology, School of Medicine, University of Crete; Attending Physician, Departments of Neuroradiology and Interventional Radiology, University Hospital of Crete, Heraklion, Crete, Greece
Infectious and Inflammatory Diseases

RICHARD W. KATZBERG, MD, MBA
Professor, Department of Radiology, School of Medicine, University of California, Davis; Chair, Department of Radiology, University of California, Davis, Medical Center, Sacramento, California
Temporomandibular Joint

CHARLES W. KERBER, MD
Professor of Radiology and Neurosurgery, School of Medicine, University of California, San Diego; Director of Interventional Neuroradiology, University of California, San Diego, Medical Center, San Diego, California
An Atlas and an Approach to Spine Imaging

UTE KETTRITZ, MD
Clinical Research Fellow, University of North Carolina, Chapel Hill, North Carolina
Kidneys, Adrenal Glands, and Retroperitoneum

MICHAEL V. KLEIN, MD
Clinical Instructor, Department of Radiology, University of California, San Diego, Medical Center, San Diego, California
Brain: Indications, Techniques, and Atlas

KIM KNOX
Consultant, MR Research, University of California, San Diego, Medical Center/Magnetic Resonance Institute, San Diego, California
An Atlas and an Approach to Spine Imaging

CHARLES F. LANZIERI, MD, MBA
Associate Professor of Radiology, Case Western Reserve University School of Medicine; Director of Neuroradiology, University Hospitals of Cleveland, Cleveland, Ohio
Paranasal Sinuses and Nasal Cavity

RANDALL B. LAUFFER, PhD
Assistant Professor, Department of Radiology, Harvard Medical School, Boston, Massachusetts; Chairman and Chief Scientific Officer, Metasyn, Inc., Cambridge, Massachusetts
MRI Contrast Agents: Basic Principles

NATHAN H. LEBWOHL, MD
Associate Professor of Clinical Orthopedics and Rehabilitation, University of Miami School of Medicine; Attending Physician, Jackson Memorial Medical Center, Miami, Florida
Vertebral and Paravertebral Abnormalities

RALPH E. LEE, MA, RT
Research Associate, University of California, San Francisco, San Francisco, California
MR Angiography: Basic Principles

NADJA M. LESKO, MD
President of Surry Radiological Associates, Mt. Airy, North Carolina
Congenital Heart Disease

KERRY M. LINK, MD
Associate Professor of Radiology, Codirector of MRI, Bowman Gray School of Medicine, Winston-Salem, North Carolina
Congenital Heart Disease

MAHMOOD F. MAFEE, MD
Professor of Radiology, MRI Center/Eye and Ear Infirmary, University of Illinois at Chicago Medical Center; Director, MRI Center, and Director, Radiology Section, Eye and Ear Infirmary, University of Illinois Hospital, Chicago, Illinois
Orbital and Intraocular Lesions

WARREN J. MANNING, MD
Assistant Professor of Medicine and Radiology, Harvard Medical School; Associate Director, Non-invasive Imaging, and Co-Director, Cardiac MR Center, Beth Israel Hospital, Boston, Massachusetts
Functional Cardiac Imaging

THOMAS J. MASARYK, MD
Head, Section of Neuroradiology, Department of Radiology, The Cleveland Clinic Foundation, Cleveland, Ohio
Aneurysms and Vascular Malformations

HEINRICH P. MATTLE, PD, DR MED
Privatdozent, Universitaet Bern; Chefarzt-Stellvertreter, Neurologische Universitaets-klinik, Inselspital, Bern, Switzerland
Spontaneous and Traumatic Hemorrhage

ROBERT F. MATTREY, MD
Professor of Radiology, University of California, San Diego, San Diego, California
Scrotum and Testes

THOMAS MICHAELIS, MD
Senior Spectroscopist, Huntington Medical Research Institutes; Boswell Fellow, California Institute of Technology, Pasadena, California; Biomedical NMR Group, Max Planck Institute, Göttingen, Germany
MR Spectroscopy of the Brain: Neurospectroscopy

SCOTT A. MIROWITZ, MD
Associate Professor of Radiology, Washington University School of Medicine; Radiologist-in-Chief, Jewish Hospital of St. Louis; Co-director of Body MR, Mallinckrodt Institute of Radiology, St. Louis, Missouri
Musculoskeletal MRI Techniques

DONALD G. MITCHELL, MD
Professor and Director, MR Services, Department of Radiology, Thomas Jefferson University Hospital, Philadelphia, Pennsylvania
Liver and Biliary System

WILLIAM A. MIZE, MD
Assistant Professor of Pediatric Radiology, University of Minnesota Medical School; Assistant Professor of Pediatric Radiology, University of Minnesota Hospital, Minneapolis, Minnesota
Pediatric Orthopedics

JONATHAN S. MOULTON, MD
Associate Professor of Radiology, Department of Radiology, University of Cincinnati Medical Center, Cincinnati, Ohio
Bone and Soft Tissue Tumors

MARCUS MÜLLER, MD
Director, Body MRI, Inselspital, University of Bern, Bern, Switzerland
MR Angiography of the Body

MICHAEL A. NISSENBAUM, MD, FRCP(C)
Chief, MRI Clinical Services, MRI Scan Center, Fort Lauderdale, Florida
Bone Marrow

ALEXANDER M. NORBASH, MD
Assistant Professor of Radiology, Stanford University, Stanford, California
Nasopharynx and Deep Facial Compartments

GERALD V. O'REILLY, MD
Clinical Director, CHEM Center for MRI, Stoneham, Massachusetts
Spontaneous and Traumatic Hemorrhage

WALLACE W. PECK, MD
Assistant Clinical Professor in Radiology, University of California, San Diego, San Diego; Director of MRI and Chief of Neuroimaging and Head and Neck Radiology, St. Joseph Hospital and Children's Hospital of Orange County, Orange, California
Pediatric Spine: Congenital and Developmental Disorders

JOHN PERL, II, MD
Associate Staff, Neuroradiology, Department of Radiology, The Cleveland Clinic Foundation, Cleveland, Ohio
Aneurysms and Vascular Malformations

M. LOREN PERLMUTTER, MD, PhD
Clinical Fellow, Beth Israel Hospital, Boston, Massachusetts
Male Pelvis

M. JUDITH DONOVAN POST, MD
Professor of Radiology, Ophthalmology, and Neurological Surgery, University of Miami School of Medicine; Attending Physician, Jackson Memorial Medical Center, Miami, Florida
Vertebral and Paravertebral Abnormalities

POTTUMARTHI V. PRASAD, PhD
Instructor of Radiology, Harvard Medical School; MR Physicist, Beth Israel Hospital, Boston, Massachusetts
Principles of Diffusion and Perfusion MRI

GARY A. PRESS, MD
Chief of Neuroradiology and Director of Magnetic Resonance, Kaiser-Permanente Medical Center, San Diego, California
Developmental Disorders

KENT B. REMLEY, MD
Assistant Professor of Radiology and Otolaryngology, University of Minnesota School of Medicine, Minneapolis, Minnesota
Skull Base and Temporal Bone

DAVID ROSENBACH, MD
Director, Center For Sports Medicine, Carrolwood Radiology and MRI, Tampa, Florida
Kinematic MRI of Joints

BRIAN ROSS, MD
Director, Clinical Magnetic Resonance Spectroscopy Unit, Huntington Medical Research Institutes, Pasadena; Professor of Clinical Medicine and Professor of Radiology, University of Southern California, Los Angeles, School of Medicine, Los Angeles; Visiting Associate, Division of Chemistry and Chemical Engineering, California Institute of Technology, Pasadena, California
MR Spectroscopy of the Brain; Neurospectroscopy

ARMANDO RUIZ, MD
Assistant Professor of Clinical Radiology and Neurological Surgery, University of Miami School of Medicine; Attending Physician, Jackson Memorial Medical Center, Miami, Florida
Vertebral and Paravertebral Abnormalities

MITCHELL D. SCHNALL, MD, PhD
Associate Professor of Radiology, University of Pennsylvania School of Medicine; Chief, MRI Section, Hospital of the University of Pennsylvania, Philadelphia, Pennsylvania
Male Pelvis

GERHARD SCHROTH, MD
Professor of Neuroradiology and Chief, Neuroradiology Section, Inselspital, Bern, Switzerland
Spontaneous and Traumatic Hemorrhage

RICHARD C. SEMELKA, MD
Associate Professor of Radiology, University of North Carolina School of Medicine; Director of Magnetic Resonance Services, University of North Carolina Hospital, Chapel Hill, North Carolina
Liver and Biliary System; Kidneys, Adrenal Glands, and Retroperitoneum; Pancreas, Spleen, Bowel, and Peritoneum

FARID F. SHAFAIE, MS, MD
Senior Resident, Department of Radiology, Eastern Virginia Medical School, Norfolk, Virginia
Postoperative Lumbosacral Spine

FRANK G. SHELLOCK, PhD
Associate Professor of Radiological Science, University of California, Los Angeles, School of Medicine, Los Angeles; Director, Research and Quality Assurance, Future Diagnostics, Inc., Los Angeles; Director, Research and Technology Advancement, American Health Services Corporation, Newport Beach, California
Bioeffects and Safety of MR Procedures

ORLANDO P. SIMONETTI, PhD
Senior Research Scientist, Siemens Medical Systems, MR Research and Development, Iselin, New Jersey
Pulse Sequence Design in MRI

TEREASA M. SIMONSON, MD
Former Assistant Professor, University of Iowa College of Medicine, Iowa City, Iowa; Staff Neuroradiologist, St. Cloud Hospital, St. Cloud, Minnesota
Stroke and Cerebral Ischemia

EVELYN M. L. SKLAR, MD
Associate Professor of Clinical Radiology and Neurological Surgery, University of Miami School of Medicine; Attending Physician, Jackson Memorial Medical Center, Miami, Florida
Vertebral and Paravertebral Abnormalities

ECKART STETTER, PhD
Manager, MR Physics, Siemens Medical Systems, Erlangen, Germany
Instrumentation

DAVID W. STOLLER, MD
Assistant Clinical Professor of Radiology, University of California, San Francisco; Director, California Advanced Imaging, San Francisco, California
Knee

RICHARD E. STRAIN, JR., MD
Clinical Assistant Professor of Radiology, University of Miami School of Medicine, Miami; Department of Orthopedics, Memorial Regional Hospital, Hollywood, Florida
Orthopedics

CLARE M. C. TEMPANY, MD
Assistant Professor of Radiology, Harvard Medical School; Director of Body MRI, Brigham and Women's Hospital, Boston, Massachusetts
Female Pelvis

VENKATESAN THANGARAJ, BS
Systems Analyst/Programmer, Magnetic Resonance Imaging Department, Beth Israel Hospital, Boston, Massachusetts
Practical MRI for the Technologist and Imaging Specialist

KEITH R. THULBORN, MD, PhD
Associate Professor of Radiology and Psychiatry, University of Pittsburgh Medical School; Chief, Magnetic Resonance Research, University of Pittsburgh Medical Center, Pittsburgh, Pennsylvania
Biochemical Basis of the MRI Appearance of Cerebral Hemorrhage

WILLIAM G. TOTTY, MD
Professor of Radiology, Washington University School of Medicine; Radiologist, Barnes Hospital, St. Louis, Missouri
Hip

PATRICK A. TURSKI, MD
Professor of Radiology, Neurology, and Neurosurgery, University of Wisconsin Medical School; Chief, Section of Neuroradiology, University of Wisconsin Hospital, Madison, Wisconsin
Aneurysms and Vascular Malformations; Basic Principles of MR Angiography and Flow Analysis: Cerebrovascular Applications

RICHARD J. WAITE, MD
Assistant Professor, University of Massachusetts Medical Center, University of Massachusetts Medical School, Worcester, Massachusetts
Injuries to the Musculotendinous Unit

STEVEN WARACH, MD, PhD
Assistant Professor of Neurology and Radiology, Harvard Medical School; Associate Neurologist and Director, Division of Cerebrovascular Diseases, Beth Israel Hospital, Boston, Massachusetts
Diffusion and Perfusion MRI: Functional Brain Imaging

ROBERT M. WEISSKOFF, PhD
Assistant Professor of Radiology, Harvard Medical School, and Director of NMR Physics Research, MGH-NMR Center, Massachusetts General Hospital, Charlestown, Massachusetts
Basic Principles of MRI

RALPH WEISSLEDER, MD, PhD
Assistant Professor, Harvard Medical School; Director, MR Pharmaceutical Program, Massachusetts General Hospital, Boston, Massachusetts
Organ- and Tissue-Directed MRI Contrast Agents

JANE L. WEISSMAN, MD
Assistant Professor, University of Pittsburgh School of Medicine; Assistant Professor of Radiology and Otolaryngology and Director of Head and Neck Imaging, University of Pittsburgh Medical Center, Pittsburgh, Pennsylvania
Neck

GEORGE WESBEY, MD
Director, Magnetic Resonance Imaging, Scripps Memorial Hospitals, LaJolla and Encinitas, Encinitas, California
Artifacts in MRI: Description, Causes, and Solutions

MICHELLE L. HANSMAN WHITEMAN, MD
Assistant Professor of Clinical Radiology, Otolaryngology, and Neurological Surgery, University of Miami School of Medicine and Jackson Memorial Medical Center, Miami, Florida
Vertebral and Paravertebral Abnormalities

PIOTR A. WIELOPOLSKI, PhD
Research Scientist, Dr. Daniel den Hoed Kliniek, The Netherlands
Fast MRI

WADE WONG, DO
Associate Clinical Professor of Radiology, University of California, San Diego, School of Medicine; Associate Clinical Professor of Radiology and Staff Neuroradiologist, University of California, San Diego, Medical Center; San Diego Veterans Administration Medical Center; and the John M. and Sally B. Thornton Hospital, San Diego, California
Lower Face and Salivary Glands

WILLIAM T. C. YUH, MD, MSEE
Professor, University of Iowa College of Medicine; Director of MRI and Neuroradiology, University of Iowa Hospital, Iowa City, Iowa
Stroke and Cerebral Ischemia

GARY P. ZIENTARA, PhD
Assistant Professor, Department of Radiology, Harvard Medical School; Senior Research Physicist, Division of Magnetic Resonance, Department of Radiology, Brigham and Women's Hospital, Boston, Massachusetts
MRI-Guided Interventions

MICHAEL B. ZLATKIN, MD
Director of Musculoskeletal Imaging and Magnetic Resonance Imaging, Radiology Associates of Hollywood, Florida; Director of Sports Medicine Imaging, Health South Doctors' Hospital, Coral Gables, Florida; Clinical Associate Professor of Radiology, University of Miami School of Medicine, Miami, Florida
Shoulder; Wrist; Kinematic MRI of Joints; Orthopedics; MRI Scan Protocols

FOREWORD

In the 15 years since the clinical introduction of magnetic resonance imaging (MRI), tremendous strides have been taken. The modality is firmly established as a core diagnostic tool in the fields of neuroradiology and musculoskeletal imaging. In addition, there is increasingly widespread use of MRI for disorders affecting the abdomen, pelvis, and cardiovascular system. Despite the already profound impact on treatment of patients and the remarkable pace of technical innovation that has occurred to date, there continues to be an expansion of clinical applications and the brisk pace of technical development shows no sign of abating. In the 5 years since the first edition of *Clinical Magnetic Resonance Imaging* was published, diffusion imaging, perfusion imaging, MR angiography, and MR cholangiopancreatography are just a few areas in which basic innovations in pulse sequence design and system hardware have led to major clinical applications. In an era of managed care and stringent cost containment, fast imaging techniques offer to reduce the expense of an MRI study substantially. Functional MRI is giving profound insights into the relationship between structure and function in the brain and is also being applied to other organs such as the heart and kidney. MRI-guided therapy could provide a minimally invasive alternative to conventional neurosurgical techniques.

The book begins with an extensive review of the basic principles, technical issues, and image artifacts involved in using MRI. Issues with the most clinical relevance are emphasized. These include fast imaging, contrast agents, diffusion and perfusion imaging, MR angiography, and spectroscopy. Next follows a section on neuroradiologic applications for the brain, head and neck, and spine. Detailed atlases of the brain and spine are provided, using images obtained with state-of-the-art high-field systems. There follows a survey of the features of a variety of commonly and uncommonly encountered clinical entities. Other sections consider the applications of MRI in the chest, breast, abdomen, pelvis, and cardiovascular and musculoskeletal systems. The editors have authored or coauthored a large number of chapters in the book, which enriches the text, and have solicited the assistance of recognized experts in the field for the others. The editors and their contributors should be commended for their successful efforts in achieving a clear synthesis of the technical and clinical issues involved in the practice of MRI. This edition represents an important new contribution to the field and is a worthy successor to their popular first edition.

HERBERT Y. KRESSEL, MD

PREFACE

In the 6 years since the publication of the first edition of *Clinical Magnetic Resonance Imaging*, the initial promise of MRI has come to fruition to an extent that could hardly have been anticipated. For instance, the early skepticism of orthopedic surgeons has been so thoroughly overcome that musculoskeletal MRI has become a mainstay of orthopedic diagnosis. Standard pulse sequences for brain and spine imaging that in the past lasted 10 minutes or longer can now be completed in a fraction of the time with better image quality. MR angiography, in conjunction with duplex sonography, has proved capable of replacing the more expensive and invasive procedure of contrast angiography for evaluation of the extracranial carotid arteries. An MR angiogram of the abdominal aorta and iliac vessels can be completed within a single breath-hold.

This second edition has been completely rewritten and greatly expanded from the highly popular first edition. It provides a comprehensive guide to the use of MRI in the body, central nervous system, and musculoskeletal system. Basic principles and practical applications of the latest technologies are provided, including the newest pulse sequences such as fast spin-echo and echo-planar imaging, radiofrequency coil configurations including multicoil arrays, MR angiography including high-resolution neurovascular imaging, and the latest breath-hold contrast-enhanced methods for imaging of the aorta and peripheral vessels, coronary artery imaging, diffusion and perfusion imaging of stroke, spectroscopy, and interventional MRI. As in the first edition, we have attempted to present the entire range of clinical and scientific topics in a clear, understandable manner that can be easily assimilated by both the novice and the advanced MRI practitioner.

Concomitant with rapid progress has been maturation of the technical and clinical aspects of many MRI applications. One can now make rather firm recommendations for pulse sequences and major clinical indications of MRI in the brain, spine, and musculoskeletal system without much risk that these recommendations will become obsolete in the near future. However, these recommendations must be tempered by the reality that MRI practitioners operate using various levels of software and hardware. For instance, the use of breath-hold three-dimensional MR angiography would be applicable only on systems with the software and gradient systems needed for extremely short repetition and echo times. Another example would be the use of fat suppression, which can be a problem on low-field systems if chemical-shift–selective methods are attempted. Nonetheless, approaches to the technical and clinical challenges of MRI are presented that should help guide practitioners to the optimal strategies for the particular system configuration and clinical needs.

The editors are privileged to have been involved from the early stages in the development of MRI as a clinical entity. We hope with this textbook to share our immense enthusiasm for this exciting, clinically invaluable, and ever-changing field.

We would like to thank our assistants Amy Dowd and Eve Elly; our MRI technologists; the staff of W.B. Saunders Company, including Denise LeMelledo, Dolores Meloni, Judith Gandy, and Lisette Bralow; and the entire group of outstanding authors who contributed to this textbook, as well as our families for their endless patience and understanding during the course of this project.

ROBERT R. EDELMAN, MD
JOHN R. HESSELINK, MD
MICHAEL B. ZLATKIN, MD

CONTENTS

VOLUME ONE

PART III   HEAD AND NECK

VOLUME TWO

PART IV   SPINE

PART V BODY

PART VI CARDIOVASCULAR SYSTEM

PART I

PHYSICS INSTRUMENTATION AND ADVANCED CLINICAL APPLICATIONS

Basic Principles of MRI

ROBERT M. WEISSKOFF ■ ROBERT R. EDELMAN

Magnetic resonance imaging (MRI) represents a continuing revolution in medical technology. MRI provides detailed images of the human body with unprecedented soft tissue contrast. Because of the innate versatility of this modality, tissue anatomy, pathology, metabolism, and flow are all amenable to noninvasive evaluation. After its discovery in the 1940s, the phenomenon of nuclear magnetic resonance was applied primarily as a tool in physical chemistry. Nearly four decades passed before MR was successfully employed in medical imaging.

In this chapter, we review the basic principles of medical MRI. This chapter is written for the novice who is interested in a simplified approach to the field and provides introductory material for the later chapters of this book. Those interested in more detailed discussions are referred to other chapters in this text and to other references.[1–5]

Nuclear magnetic resonance is defined as the enhanced absorption of energy that occurs when the nuclei of atoms within an external magnetic field are exposed to radiofrequency (RF) energy at a specific frequency, called the *Larmor* or *resonance frequency*. The phenomenon was first seen in particle beams by Rabi and coworkers in 1939[6] but was made observable practically in liquids and solids by several groups in the middle 1940s. Bloch, in 1946, placed his own finger within the probe of an early MR spectrometer and observed a strong signal from hydrogen nuclei. In a sense, this experiment marked the first biologic application of MR. Bloch and Purcell shared the Nobel Prize for elucidating the phenomenon of MR in solids and liquids.[7, 8]

Although the observed MR signal comes from the nuclei, the characteristics of this signal depend on the specific chemical environment of those nuclei. This signal dependence proved ideal for both qualitative and quantitative chemical analysis. Furthermore, the energies involved in MR are nonionizing (Fig. 1–1) and can easily penetrate the human body. These features suggested an enormous biomedical potential for MR, because it might provide a means for studying the biochemistry of human subjects in vivo. However, the clinical potential of the method was limited by its inability to provide spatial localization of the MR signal, so that it could not be applied as an imaging technique. Lauterbur solved this localization problem by using magnetic field gradients and by 1973 was able to produce the first images of water samples.[9] However, it was not until 1977 that Damadian and colleagues[10] acquired the first human images using a prototype superconducting magnet. Concurrently, British investigators, including Andrew, Mansfield, and Hinshaw, developed point and line scanning signal localization techniques.[11, 12] Many significant technical innovations followed, such as three-dimensional (3D) data acquisition, two-dimensional (2D) single-slice acquisition using selective irradiation, 2D multislice acquisition fast scanning with gradient-echo and echo-planar techniques, and the integration of MRI and MR spectroscopy.

In this chapter, we introduce the basic concepts of MRI: fundamental phenomenology of magnetic resonance, how an MR image is constructed, and how its contrast can be manipulated. The chapter ends with a brief description of the instrumentation used in commercial MRI scanners.

OVERVIEW OF THE MRI PROCESS

Several steps are involved in the production of an MR image (Fig. 1–2). These are discussed in greater detail later but may be summarized as follows:

1. Randomly oriented tissue nuclei are aligned by a powerful, uniform magnetic field, producing an equilibrium "magnetization" of the tissue.

2. This magnetization is then disrupted by properly tuned RF pulses. As the nuclei recover ("relax") to equilibrium, they produce RF signals that are proportional to the magnitude of the initial alignment. Tissue contrast (i.e., differences in signal) develops as a result of the different rates at which nuclei relax with the magnetic field.

3. The positions of the nuclei are localized during this process by purposely distorting the magnetic field with spatially dependent magnetic fields, called *gradients*.

4. The signals are measured, or read out, after a user-determined time has elapsed from the initial RF excitation.

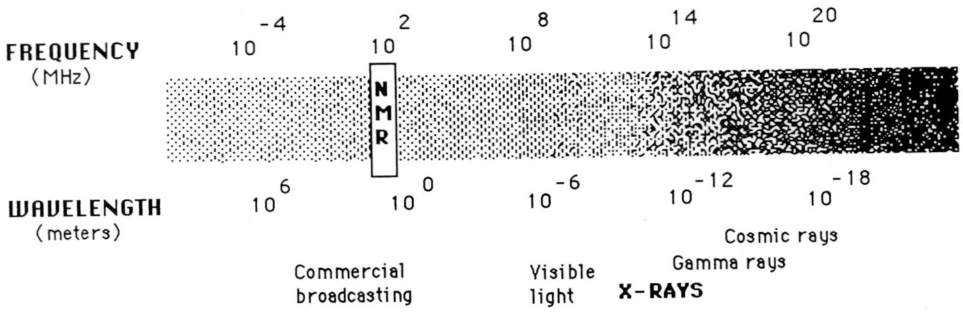

FREQUENCY
(MHz)
10^-4
10^2
10^8
10^14
10^20
NMR
WAVELENGTH
(meters)
10^6
10^0
10^-6
10^-12
10^-18
Commercial broadcasting
Visible light
X-RAYS
Gamma rays
Cosmic rays

FIGURE 1–1. Electromagnetic spectrum. Unlike conventional radiography, MR uses nonionizing RF energy.

5. The signal is transformed by the computer into an image using a mathematic process called the *Fourier transform* (FT).

We now discuss the basic physical principles that underlie the MRI process.

BASIS OF MAGNETIC RESONANCE

ROLE OF MAGNETS IN MR: "MAGNETIZING" NUCLEI

A hydrogen nucleus, being a solitary proton, behaves in certain respects like a tiny bar magnet. This magnetism is an intrinsic property of the proton and can be thought of in analogy with a fundamental physical law: moving electrical charges produce magnetic fields. Although no charges are actually spinning in the nucleus, this intrinsic property is called *spin*. The major effect of this spin is that it lets the nuclei interact with applied magnetic fields: the spins have a tendency to line up with an applied field. Different nuclei have different spins: hydrogen has spin ½; sodium has spin 3/2; helium has no spin at all. Although some forms of MR can be performed using any nuclei with spin, the nuclei with spin ½ are particularly easy to observe.

When the hydrogen atom is placed within an external magnetic field, its nucleus behaves much like the needle of a compass. That is, when placed in the external field, the nucleus aligns itself parallel to the north-south axis of this field, with the north pole of the dipole opposite the south pole of the external field (Fig. 1–3*A*). In actuality, according to quantum mechanical principles, if we measure this spin ½ dipole, we can find it aligned only exactly with (parallel) or against (antiparallel) the applied field (Fig. 1–3*B*). The two alignments correspond, respectively, to lower and higher energy states of the dipole. The energy difference between these two states, ΔE, is proportional to the magnetic field, B, and to a factor related to the intrinsic spin of the nucleus:

$$\Delta E = h\gamma B \qquad (1a)$$

This factor γ is called the gyromagnetic ratio and is characteristic of each nucleus. (The factor h is Planck's constant and relates energy to frequency in quantum mechanics.) It is an interesting fact that despite our

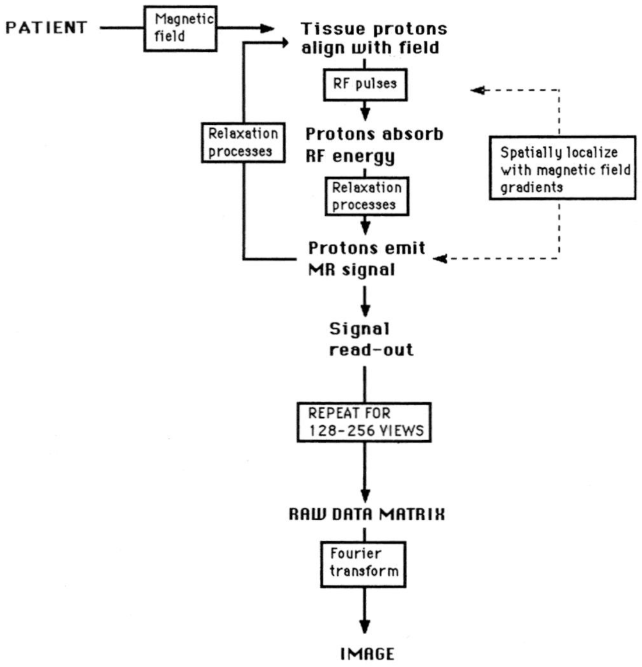

PATIENT
Magnetic field
Tissue protons align with field
RF pulses
Relaxation processes
Protons absorb RF energy
Spatially localize with magnetic field gradients
Relaxation processes
Protons emit MR signal
Signal read-out
REPEAT FOR 128-256 VIEWS
RAW DATA MATRIX
Fourier transform
IMAGE

FIGURE 1–2. Summary of steps involved in the formation of the MR image, starting with the patient entering the magnetic field.

S
N
S
N
A
B
Parallel
Anti-parallel

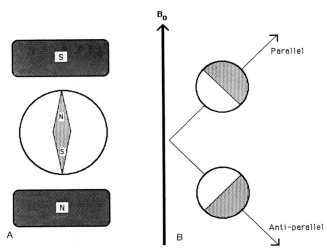

FIGURE 1–3. Comparison of the magnetic properties of a compass and a proton. *A*, The compass always points in one direction. S = south; N = north. *B*, The proton may be aligned in either of two directions: parallel to the applied magnetic field (B_0) or antiparallel to the field.

ability to calculate from first principles γ for electrons (which also have spin ½) to 11 significant digits, the theoretic understanding of γ for the most simple nucleus still eludes us.

Because of this energy difference, an externally applied magnetic field tends to create a net excess of nuclei aligned in the lower energy, parallel direction compared with the antiparallel orientation. This excess population is represented by a vector called the *net magnetization* (**M**). For all nuclei, this energy difference is much smaller than the average thermal energy of the system (kT, where k is Boltzmann's constant and T is the absolute temperature in kelvins). In this case, we can estimate the population difference easily: it is simply the ratio of the MR energy difference ΔE to kT:

$$\mathbf{M} \propto \Delta E / kT$$

The main reason for using powerful magnets in MRI and MR spectroscopy is to make **M** large enough to observe. For example, the difference in energy (ΔE) between the parallel and antiparallel alignments in the earth's small magnetic field (~ 0.5 G or 5×10^{-5} T) causes fewer than one proton per billion extra to line up with rather than against the field (Fig. 1–4A). However, because ΔE increases in direct proportion to the external magnetic field strength, many more spins occupy the lower energy (parallel) state (Fig. 1–4B) at higher field. Thus, at 1.5 T, the magnetization is 30,000 times larger or roughly 10 ppm. Although this might seem like a small imbalance, all the useful medical imaging proceeds from observing this tiny population difference.

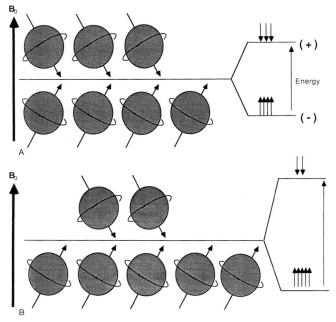

FIGURE 1–4. The degree of alignment of protons with an applied magnetic field depends on the strength of the field. *A*, With a weak field, the energy difference between the parallel and antiparallel states is small, so protons tend to distribute nearly equally between the two alignments. *B*, With a stronger field, more protons tend to align in the lower energy parallel orientation, resulting in a larger net magnetization **M**.

TABLE 1–1. MR CHARACTERISTICS OF VARIOUS ELEMENTS

NUCLEUS	γ (MHz/T)	NATURAL ISOTOPIC ABUNDANCE (%)	RELATIVE SENSITIVITY*	SPIN
^{1}H	42.576	99.985	1	½
^{2}H	6.536	0.015	0.0096	1
^{13}C	10.705	1.108	0.016	½
^{14}N	3.076	99.635	0.001	1
^{15}N	4.315	0.365	0.001	½
^{17}O	5.772	0.037	0.029	³⁄₂
^{19}F	40.055	100	0.834	½
^{23}Na	11.262	100	0.093	³⁄₂
^{31}P	17.236	100	0.066	½
^{33}S	3.266	0.74	0.0023	³⁄₂
^{39}K	1.987	93.08	0.0005	³⁄₂

*At constant field, with sensitivity of the ^{1}H nucleus = 1; 1 g of material compared with 1 g of hydrogen.

WHY HYDROGEN IS THE ELEMENT OF CHOICE FOR MRI

Many elements could, in theory, be imaged by MR. Any nucleus with an odd number of either protons or neutrons can produce an MR signal. However, MR is primarily applied to the imaging of hydrogen, for two reasons: 1) high sensitivity for the hydrogen MR signal and 2) high natural abundance of hydrogen.

The high sensitivity for the signal from the hydrogen nucleus comes from the *gyromagnetic ratio* γ. The larger this value, the larger ΔE is for a given B, and thus more net magnetization is produced in a given magnet. In addition, as we will see, this gyromagnetic ratio specifies the resonance frequency of that nucleus in a 1-T magnetic field. The efficiency with which the MR signal is detected (i.e., the sensitivity) improves with increasing signal (resonance) frequency. Simple hydrogen (^{1}H) has the highest gyromagnetic ratio of any element, and thus hydrogen produces the greatest signal per nucleus.

Perhaps even more important, hydrogen is by far the most prevalent atom in most living systems (Table 1–1). Thus, although other elements can be imaged, the combination of sensitivity and abundance has limited the usefulness of images from elements other than hydrogen.

ROLE OF RADIOFREQUENCY PULSES IN THE MR SIGNAL: DETECTING SIGNAL

The strong, static magnetic field aligns the protons, establishing an equilibrium magnetization, **M**. To observe this magnetization (i.e., to image the body), we must disrupt the equilibrium. The RF pulse represents the first step of a process by which **M** is transformed into a usable MR signal. There are two ways to look at this process: 1) at the level of an individual atom and 2) at the level of the group behavior of large numbers of atoms.

Single Nucleus (Quantum Mechanical View)

How does the effect of a strong magnetic field tie in with the effect of an RF pulse? First, as discussed earlier, a magnetic field creates an energy difference (ΔE) between protons aligned with and against the magnetic field. Second, an RF pulse consists of packets of energy, called *photons;* the amount of energy in each packet depends on the frequency of the RF pulse. (That is what Planck's constant determines: $\Delta E = hf_{photon}$.) If the amount of energy in the photon, as determined by its frequency, precisely matches ΔE, then, and only then, a proton absorbs energy from the RF pulse and flips from the lower energy to the higher energy state (Fig. 1–5). This special frequency is called the Larmor or resonance frequency. It is a function of field strength and the type of nucleus, as expressed by

$$f_L = \gamma B_0 \qquad (1b)$$

where f_L = resonance frequency (megahertz), B_0 = applied magnetic field strength (tesla), and γ = gyromagnetic ratio, which can be defined in megahertz per tesla or radians per tesla. (f_L is also commonly expressed as $\omega_0 = \gamma B_0$, where ω_0 is the angular frequency in radians per second, equal to $2\pi f_L$. Note that in Equation 1b, the 2π factor has been incorporated into the value for the gyromagnetic ratio.) The resonance frequency of the hydrogen nucleus ($\gamma = 42.58$ MHz/T) at a field strength of 1 T is approximately 42.6 MHz and at 1.5 T is 63.9 MHz. What happens if the spins are irradiated with photons of a frequency different from the Larmor frequency? To first order, absolutely nothing. This is why the phenomenon is called magnetic *resonance*. It occurs only for a specific frequency, which originates from the basic interaction of the spins with the applied magnetic field.

Group Behavior of Atoms (Classic View)

Although the foregoing view makes clear why only one frequency affects the protons, it does not help clarify what we actually detect in the scanner. Unlike any individual spin, which, when measured, can have only two alignments, the *net* magnetization of a group of protons, **M**, may be oriented in any direction. By convention, the direction of the main field (B_0) is called the *z axis* or the *longitudinal axis*. The plane perpendicular to the main field is called the *x-y* or

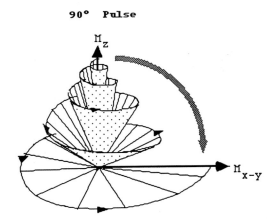

90° Pulse

FIGURE 1–6. Effect of a 90° pulse on the net magnetization **M** is to tilt **M** into the transverse plane. The combination of the tilt produced by the RF pulse with the precession of the spins results in a complex spiraling motion. Note that as **M** is rotated by 90°, the M_z component is reduced to zero and M_{x-y} becomes equal to **M**.

transverse plane. Spins can be detected only when their magnetization is in the transverse plane. Before the application of an RF pulse, the net magnetization is aligned along B_0; that is, the protons are aligned along the z axis. To be detected, they must be rotated into the transverse plane.

The dynamics of spins are fairly simple: spins rotate, or *precess,* precisely at the Larmor frequency of the applied magnetic field. In the classic view, the spins are tipped out of equilibrium by applying a second, oscillating, RF magnetic field. This magnetic field, called B_1, is produced by a set of wires called the *transmitter coil*. In an MR system, this coil is designed and physically oriented so that its B_1 field is in the transverse plane, that is, perpendicular to M_0. When the RF pulse is applied, the effect of its B_1 field is to cause **M** to rotate away from its equilibrium alignment along the z axis (Fig. 1–6).

The angle by which the RF pulse rotates **M** off the z axis is called the *flip angle*. The flip angle increases with the amplitude and duration of the RF pulse. Any flip angle can be applied. The choice of flip angle depends on the particular imaging method. For instance, in spin-echo pulse sequences, described later, a 90° RF pulse is used to excite the protons. How large a B_1 field is required to produce this 90° tip? If we use a 1-ms-long RF pulse, the spins must be precessing at 250 Hz to make one fourth of a rotation (90°) in 1 ms. Because the Larmor constant is 42.58 MHz/T, we find $B_1 = 6 \times 10^{-6}$ T or 6 μT. Thus, a much smaller magnetic field is required to tip the spins into the transverse plane than to create useful magnetization. This is another property of resonance.

Provided that **M** is initially oriented along the z axis, a 90° RF pulse rotates **M** completely into the transverse plane (Fig. 1–7). Small flip angles, used for gradient-echo pulse sequences (see Chapter 10) rotate only a portion of **M** into the transverse plane. As already described, this transverse component of **M** is responsible for the production of the MR signal.

One concept that physicists find helpful for describing the motion of the protons is that of a rotating reference frame. When viewed from the outside (e.g.,

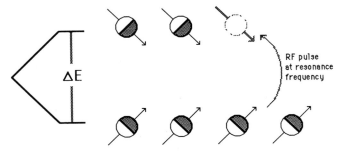

FIGURE 1–5. The application of an RF pulse at the resonance frequency causes some spins to flip from the parallel to the antiparallel orientation.

RF Pulses

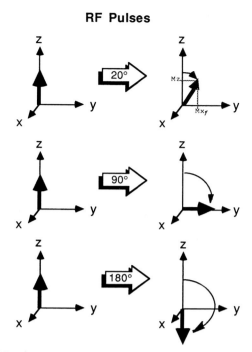

FIGURE 1–7. An RF pulse can be applied to produce any flip angle, depending on the strength and duration of the pulse. Note that in the rotating frame, as shown here, the effect of the RF pulse is to produce a simple tilt of the net magnetization **M**, unlike the situation depicted in Figure 1–6.

see Fig. 1–6), the motion of the magnetization vectors may appear complex because, as the protons tilt into the transverse plane, they continue to wobble, or precess, around the z axis. To simplify the motion, one can imagine that the viewer is standing at the origin of the coordinate system and rotates at the same rate as the magnetization vector as it precesses about the z axis. (Thus, this frame rotates at the Larmor frequency.) In this rotating reference frame, the precession appears frozen. As a result, the application of an RF pulse is seen to produce a simple tilt of the magnetization into the transverse plane or beyond (see Fig. 1–7) rather than a spiraling motion. In this frame, rotating along with the protons, after excitation the magnetization stays in the transverse plane. However, even though the magnetization is static in this reference frame, if we view the same magnetization back in the laboratory frame, the protons are seen to rotate around in the transverse plane at f_L.

Once the magnetization is in the transverse plane, **M** precesses about the direction of the main field, analogous to the precession of a spinning top that results when it is tilted from the vertical axis. The precession of the component of **M** in the transverse plane induces a voltage across the ends of a properly designed coil, called a *receiver coil* (see later) (Fig. 1–8). This voltage constitutes the MR signal.

The concept of *transverse magnetization* introduces an apparent paradox. If an individual proton can be found to be aligned in only one of two directions, either with or against the applied magnetic field, how can a 90° RF pulse tilt the proton magnetization so

that it is perpendicular to the magnetic field? This paradox results from attempting to describe the behavior of the macroscopic quantity (**M**) in terms of concepts that apply only to submicroscopic structures (individual protons). The paradox can be resolved only by considering the average behavior of a large number of protons. Let us consider the effect of a 90° RF pulse. As discussed previously, the RF pulse equalizes the number of spins in the parallel and antiparallel alignment. However, the RF pulse has an additional effect. Like the transaxle of a car, which locks the relative rotational positions of the right and left wheels, the RF pulse locks the phases of the magnetic moments into a coherent relationship. As a result, on the average, the *transverse* components of the individual magnetic moments have the same phase angle and add together to produce an **M** in the x-y plane. Therefore, even though no individual proton is ever aligned in

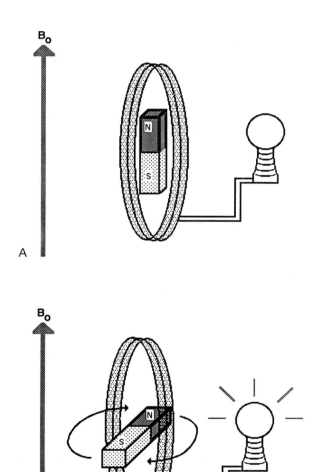

FIGURE 1–8. Production of an MR signal by the proton is analogous to the generation of electricity in a dynamo. *A*, With the net magnetization **M** aligned with B_0, there is no precession and therefore no signal. *B*, After a 90° RF pulse, **M** is aligned in the transverse plane. Precession of **M** induces an electrical voltage (MR signal) in a properly oriented antenna.

the transverse plane, the **M** of large groups of protons can be.

SPATIAL LOCALIZATION OF THE MR SIGNAL: IMAGING NUCLEI

Up to this point, we have assumed that all the protons in the body are equivalent, with identical Larmor frequencies, and affected equally by the applied RF pulses. To *image* the body, however, we must make these protons somehow different, so that spins from one part of the body can be distinguished from those from another. Although MRI can be thought of in similar ways to other diagnostic modalities, its image generation techniques are unique. One way to appreciate this uniqueness is to consider the "radiation" used in the imaging.

With current MR systems, images can be obtained with a spatial resolution competitive with that of computed tomography (CT) and ultrasonography. However, it is impossible to collimate radio waves as one can collimate x-rays and sound waves. Furthermore, these other modalities use wavelengths in the submillimeter range, whereas MRI uses RFs whose radiation would have wavelengths on the order of several meters. Indeed, with most imaging techniques, image resolution is limited by the wavelength of the radiation. (This is why electron microscopes have better resolution than optical microscopes.) How, then, is submillimeter resolution achieved by MRI when its wavelength is greater than 1 meter?

This simple answer is that MRI entirely avoids using the "wave" properties of the radio. In fact, it is a misnomer to call the energy used by MRI radio waves at all. Instead, MRI uses the precision of the Larmor relationship to encode signals "parametrically," that is, to make them depend spatially on some parameter of the resonance. One may consider the uniform B_0 field, in which all nuclei resonate at the same frequency, to be analogous to an untuned harp with all its strings identical in pitch (Fig. 1–9). In listening to such an instrument, one could not tell which harp string was plucked to produce a particular pitch. How-

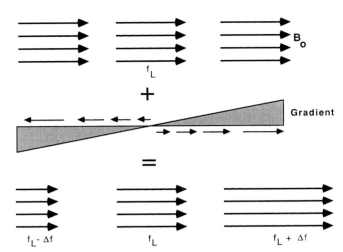

FIGURE 1–10. Gradient magnetic field superimposed on the main field (B_0) produces a positional variation in the local magnetic field strength and resonance frequencies (Δf). As a result, the resonance frequencies of the tissue nuclei depend on position. f_L = resonance frequency without gradient.

ever, the situation is different for a properly tuned harp: by making the pitch depend on the location of the string along the harp, one can easily tell which string is plucked. Just as middle C and concert A have unique, well-defined positions on a harp, so, too, the application of a position-dependent magnetic field perturbation, called a gradient, tunes the resonance frequencies according to position along that gradient.

EFFECT OF A MAGNETIC FIELD GRADIENT

A magnetic field gradient is a weak magnetic field that is produced by additional coils positioned within the magnet bore. This field is much smaller than the main magnetic field. For instance, a typical gradient might produce a peak magnetic field difference of 10 to 15 mT across a distance of 1 m. Even newer high speed–capable MR scanners, with much stronger peak gradients up to 25 mT/m, produce fields that are small perturbations of the main field strengths of 300 to 1500 mT. The magnetic field produced by the gradient coils differs in another important respect from the main field. Unlike the highly uniform main field, the magnetic fields produced by the gradient coils are spatially dependent.

The gradient (G) produces a change in the magnetic field, ΔB, that depends on the precise location of the proton:

$$\Delta B = Gx \qquad (2a)$$

where x = the proton's position along the gradient. When the gradient is superimposed on the main field (Fig. 1–10), the resonance frequencies assume unique values, depending on the position along the gradient, as expressed by

$$f_L = \gamma B_0 + \gamma Gx \qquad (2b)$$

Equation 2b shows that the gradient makes the

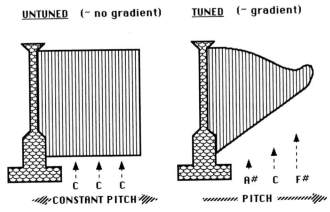

FIGURE 1–9. Application of a magnetic field gradient has a function analogous to the tuning of a harp.

protons' frequency depend on their position, just like the strings on the harp. This frequency dependence is exploited in several different ways in MRI, both for selecting a volume of nuclei to image and for imaging the nuclei within that volume. There are many ways to make this image; the most common method uses the 2D Fourier transform (2DFT) and 3D Fourier transform (3DFT) to transform spin-warp–encoded data. We consider 2D methods first, because 3D methods are merely an elaboration of 2D techniques.

TWO-DIMENSIONAL IMAGING METHODS

In 2DFT imaging, different methods are employed to localize nuclei along the three orthogonal axes (Fig. 1–11A): 1) one gradient is applied with the RF pulse to selectively excite the spins from a single slice, 2) a second gradient encodes location along one in-plane dimension in the frequency of the MR signal, and 3)

a third gradient encodes location along the other in-plane dimension in the phase of the MR signal. Because of the alteration or "twisting" of phase used for spatial localization in this method, it is also called *spin warp.*

For convenience (and by habit), we sometimes refer to the slice-selection direction as z, the frequency-encoding direction as x, and the phase-encoding direction as y. However, this designation is arbitrary and is unrelated to the physical orientation of the x, y, and z gradient coils. The x, y, z coordinate system is oriented differently for different planes of section (i.e., axial, sagittal, coronal, and oblique).

Slice Selection

When the slice-selection gradient is applied, the resonance frequencies of the tissue protons become linearly related to position along the z axis (Fig. 1–12). Individual resonance frequencies correspond to indi-

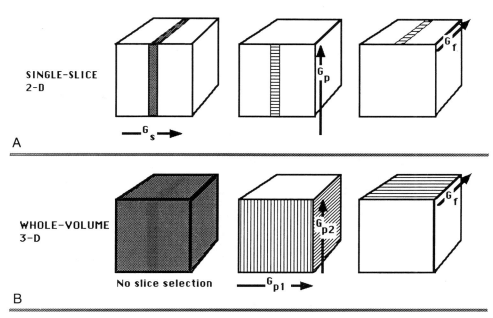

FIGURE 1–11. *A* to *C,* Comparison of spatial localization methods for 2DFT and 3DFT imaging.

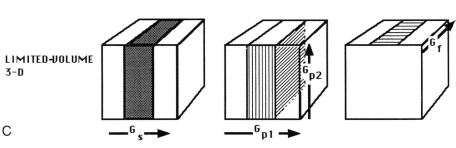

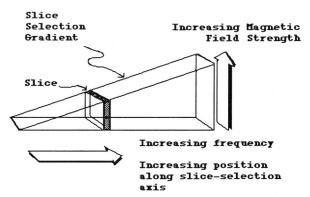

FIGURE 1–12. In the presence of the slice-selection gradient, the application of an RF pulse at a specific frequency excites tissue nuclei in a single slice.

vidual planes of nuclei; these planes are oriented perpendicular to the z axis. If an RF pulse of a specific frequency is applied while the slice-selection gradient is activated, only nuclei in the plane corresponding to that frequency resonate. The location of those excited protons depends on the frequency of the slice-selecting RF pulse. The location of the excited plane can be shifted by increasing or decreasing the frequency of the RF pulse.

A short RF pulse is actually made up from a spread of frequencies, called the pulse *bandwidth*. Thus, an RF pulse excites all spins whose Larmor frequency falls within the RF pulse's bandwidth. As a result, in the presence of the slice-selection gradient, the RF pulse excites a slice of tissue having a finite thickness. The slice thickness depends on the ratio of two factors: 1) the strength of the slice-selection gradient and 2) the bandwidth of the RF pulse.

As the slice-selection gradient strength is increased, the range of frequencies across a given distance is increased. As a result, an RF pulse with a fixed bandwidth excites fewer spins and the slice thickness is decreased. Conversely, a weak slice-selection gradient and the same RF pulse produce a thick slice. Thus, the amplitude of the slice-selection gradient is the primary means of adjusting the slice thickness in most scanners. (Another way to alter the slice thickness would be to modify the bandwidth of the RF pulse. Although this can be done, in most systems the slice thickness is adjusted primarily by changing the strength of the slice-selection gradient.) Thus, the result of the slice-selection process is that only the spins within the desired slab are tipped into the transverse plane. All other spins in the body are left alone.

Frequency Encoding

Once a plane of protons is excited, spatial localization is performed in one of the two in-plane dimensions perpendicular to slice selection. Whereas slice selection is performed during *excitation*, this next level of encoding occurs during the *detection* of the MR signal. During the detection period, spatial position along the x axis is encoded into the frequency content

of the signal by applying the frequency-encoding gradient. The effect of this gradient is to tune the resonance frequencies of the nuclei like the previously mentioned harp strings, and therefore the frequencies of the signals they produce, according to spatial position. Because the number of protons at each spatial position is encoded into the strength of the resonance signal at a given frequency, this type of encoding is referred to as *frequency encoding* and the axis encoded this way as the *frequency-encoded direction*. Because the scanner records the data from the excited protons during this period (using its analog-to-digital converter) and the protons' signal is "read" by the computer at this time, this gradient is also called the readout gradient.

During readout, the signal is measured as a series of brief samples; the number of samples (typically 256) determines the number of pixels along the x direction. The readout period, or *sampling time,* has a duration that can vary widely but typically assumes values from 5 to 30 ms.

What types of signals are present in these sampled data? Typical frequency-encoded gradients are of order 5 mT/m. Across a 20-cm field of view (FOV), this gradient produces a 40-kHz modulation ($\approx$5 mT/m $\times$ 0.2 m $\times$ 42.58 MHz/T). That is, protons at the far right and far left of the FOV have resonance frequencies that differ by 40 kHz. This is just a small perturbation of the main MR signal, which is tens of megahertz. Thus, an MR scanner operates somewhat like a frequency modulation radio. The main signal is actually quite near the U.S. frequency modulation radio band, but the proton signal causes an audio frequency modulation of this signal. To convert the MR signal into spatial information, it must be demodulated into the proper frequency range: the center frequency of the MR system (e.g., 64 MHz at 1.5 T) is essentially subtracted from the MR signal before signal analysis.

Fourier Transform

The measured MR signal represents the sum of the signals from the innumerable individual nuclei within a single slice. This composite signal varies continuously in amplitude as a function of *time*. However, the positions of nuclei are encoded in the *frequency* content of the signal. To extract the individual frequency components (frequency domain) from the time-varying signal (temporal domain), the computer employs a mathematic operation, the FT (Fig. 1–13). The FT performs an operation for the computer in decoding MR signals analogous to that of the basilar membrane of the human cochlea in processing sound. Somewhat like the human ear deciphering the individual notes of a chord played on a harp, the FT isolates the number of spins at each frequency during the readout period; that is, the FT tells us what frequencies are simultaneously present in the signal.

The FT is applied to each frequency-encoded line of data to extract the frequency content of the signal and thereby determine the density of spins along the x axis.

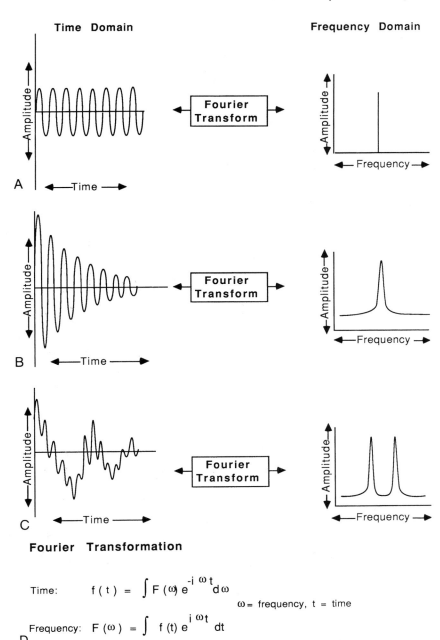

FIGURE 1–13. Fourier transform. *A*, FT of a sine wave yields a single frequency. *B*, FT of an MR signal from a single proton. *C*, FT of an MR signal from two spins in different positions. *D*, Mathematic notation for the FT.

Phase Encoding

The combination of slice selection for excitation plus frequency encoding for readout explains two of the three dimensions required to produce a tomographic image. However, in any cross-sectional imaging modality such as CT or MRI, multiple spatial projections of an object are required to reconstruct an image of that object. In CT, projections are acquired by physically rotating an x-ray fan beam. In MRI we could perform a similar process, rotating the direction of the frequency-encoding gradient throughout the plane perpendicular to the slice-selection gradient. In fact, this is the way the original MR image was produced by Lautebur. However, the bulk of clinical scanning uses a different method, called spin-warp im-

aging, that simultaneously makes use of the frequency and the phase of the MR data. It does this by adding yet another gradient in the final, perpendicular direction, after the excitation of the slice but before the frequency-encoded readout.

As with frequency encoding, the phase-encoding gradient imposes a linear relationship between precessional frequency and position (Fig. 1–14). In this case, however, all that matters is the net phase shift (θ) accumulated by the protons at the *end* of the phase-encoded pulse:

$$\theta = \gamma G y T \qquad (3)$$

where G = magnitude of phase-encoding gradient, y = position along the phase-encoding axis, and T =

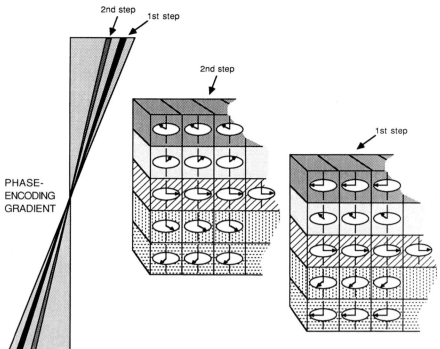

FIGURE 1–14. Principle of phase encoding. The application of a phase-encoding gradient imposes a spatial dependence on proton phase. Different phase-encoding steps use different gradient amplitudes. Note that protons at the center of the gradient experience no phase change.

duration of the gradient. This encoding pulse occurs after the excitation but before the frequency-encoded readout. That is, to encode the final orthogonal direction, the initial phase of the readout is made spatially dependent. (In many ways, phase encoding is formally identical to frequency encoding: frequency encoding is simply continuous phase encoding. That is, while the readout gradient is on, the protons' phase advances $\theta = \gamma GxT$, just as in the preceding equation, except that T is the duration between the time samples during the readout. In the frequency-encoded direction, T continues to evolve with constant G to increase θ. In the phase-encoded direction, T is constant and G changes [Fig. 1–15].)

Phase encoding requires multiple readouts in the perpendicular direction. These additional readouts usually require additional excitations, and these multiple excitations are why MRI generally takes so long. However, as we will see, the multiple excitations are also an opportunity to add contrast to the MR images. Because the time between excitations is such an important determinant of contrast, it has its own name, TR, or time between repetitions. After all the phase-encoding steps have been performed (i.e., after a number of TR periods), the FT is again applied, this time in the phase-encoded direction, thus determining the position along the y axis.

The use of the three orthogonal gradients is summarized in Figure 1–16.

Multislice Imaging

The technique described in the previous section produces an image from a single, cross-sectional slice of the body. If only a single slice could be excited during each TR interval, the scan time for a complete examination would be prohibitively long. Fortunately, there is usually considerable dead time between each readout period and the next excitation, during which time the system is idle. Within this idle period, excitation and readout of additional slices can be performed (Fig. 1–17), so the time required to image many slices is essentially the same as the time required to image one.

Scan Times and Signal Averaging

Commonly, it is necessary to average data measured during multiple data acquisitions or excitations to improve the signal-to-noise (S/N) ratio. The S/N ratio improves with $\sqrt{NEX}$, where NEX is the number of excitations. Background noise caused by certain types of artifacts, such as those resulting from periodic motion, also improves approximately in proportion to $\sqrt{NEX}$.

A penalty must be paid for signal averaging: increased scan time. This is expressed as

$$\text{Scan time} = TR \times N_y \times NEX \qquad (4)$$

where N_y = number of phase-encoding steps. For instance, the scan time for an image with a TR of 500 ms, 128 phase-encoding steps, and two excitations is 128 seconds; with four excitations, the scan time would be 256 seconds. The expression for scan time assumes that only one phase-encoding line is acquired during each TR interval. However, many pulse sequences in common use, such as fast spin echo, acquire multiple phase-encoding lines during each TR interval. In this case, the scan time is expressed as

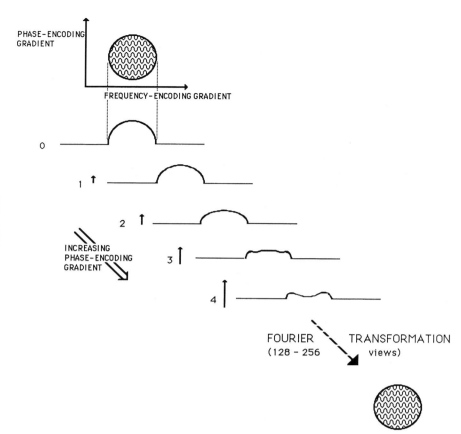

FIGURE 1–15. Increasing amplitudes of the phase-encoding gradient produce successively larger amounts of signal distortion. The signals from all the phase-encoding steps are then Fourier transformed to produce an image.

$$\text{Scan time} = \text{TR} \times N_y \times \text{NEX/ETL} \qquad (5)$$

where ETL is the *echo train length* (or *turbo factor*), that is, the number of phase-encoding lines acquired in each TR interval. If TR is short (e.g., <10 ms), the entire image can be acquired in less than 1 second, which is helpful in reducing motion artifacts. An example of such a technique is the turbo fast low-angle shot, or turboFLASH, sequence. The TR factor is entirely eliminated for *single-shot echo-planar imaging*, in which all the phase-encoding lines are acquired after a single RF excitation.

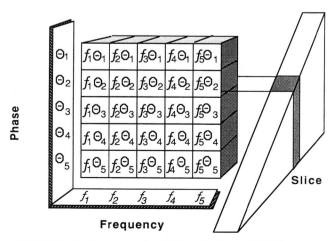

FIGURE 1–16. Summary of spatial localization in 2DFT imaging.

Projection Reconstruction

FT imaging has the drawback that a compensation gradient and phase-encoding gradient must be applied before readout, delaying measurement of the signal for several milliseconds. Although this delay is of minor significance in most cases, a few tissues, in particular lung, have T2 relaxation times (see later) on the order of a few milliseconds or less. In this case, it may be useful to encode the data by using projection reconstruction.[13] The data can be encoded directly after RF excitation by a readout gradient without first applying a compensation gradient. The orientation of the gradient is electronically rotated after each readout. As in CT, a projection reconstruction algorithm is used to reconstruct the data. Submillisecond echo time (TE) and reduced motion artifacts can be obtained by this approach. Drawbacks include longer scan times, lower S/N ratio, and artifacts related to oversampling the low-frequency samples. A short TE can also be obtained with FT imaging if strong magnetic field gradients (like those used for echo-planar imaging) are available.

Three-Dimensional Imaging

For most clinical applications, data are acquired by using multislice 2DFT methods. In certain applications, it is advantageous to perform a 3D data acquisition. The 3D methods involve excitation and acquisition of data simultaneously from a large volume or

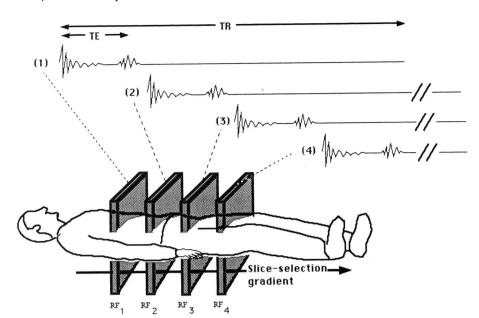

FIGURE 1–17. Sequential application of multiple RF pulses (RF₁, RF₂, and so on) at different frequencies results in excitation of multiple slices. The number of slices that can be acquired depends on TR, TE, and other factors.

slab (see Fig. 1–11*B* and *C*), whereas 2D methods acquire data from individual slices. To do this, 3D methods phase encode spatial information along the slice-selection (z) direction, as well as in the y direction. As with 2DFT imaging, spatial localization along the x direction is obtained by frequency encoding during the readout period. Reconstruction of 3D data requires a 3DFT algorithm rather than the usual 2DFT method.

Because they use a weaker slice-selection gradient for a given slice thickness, 3DFT methods have the advantage, compared with 2DFT, that they allow thin (e.g., <1 mm) sections to be acquired. In addition, 3D acquisitions produce essentially contiguous slices, which is often not the case with 2DFT methods because of imperfect slice profiles. Because the images are thin and contiguous, 3D data allow high-quality images to be reconstructed along any arbitrary plane of section.

The relatively long imaging times for 3D scans generally preclude using conventional spin-echo pulse sequences. However, in conjunction with reduced excitation flip angles, gradient-echo pulse sequences permit a much shorter TR to be used (e.g., <30 ms), which reduces the imaging time for 3D data to just a few minutes. The 3D gradient-echo acquisitions are finding increasing use in high-resolution imaging of the musculoskeletal system and in MR angiography. With an inversion prepulse, strongly T1-weighted 3D acquisitions can be obtained, called 3D *magnetization-prepared rapid gradient echo*.[14] T2-weighted 3D volumes can be acquired using a multiple-slab fast spin-echo acquisition.[15]

There are two types of 3DFT acquisitions: 1) *isotropic,* meaning equal spatial resolution along all three dimensions of the volume element *(voxel),* and 2) *anisotropic,* meaning lower spatial resolution along the slice-selection dimension. In both types of 3D methods, a relatively thick slab is initially excited. This slab is then subdivided into a number of thin slices, or *partitions,*

by phase encoding along the z direction. The number of partitions is equal to the number of phase-encoding steps. The scan time for a 3D data set increases with the number of partitions, as expressed by

$$\text{Scan time} = \text{TR} \times N_y \times N_z \times \text{NEX} \qquad (6)$$

where N_z = number of z phase–encoding steps.

FACTORS THAT AFFECT THE MR SIGNAL: IMAGE CONTRAST

One of the features that make MR so attractive for biomedical imaging is that the image contrast can depend on a combination of physical (e.g., density of protons), chemical (types of molecules with which those protons interact), and biologic (intact membranes, tissue orientation, flow) properties. To exploit these interactions, the MR scanner has, perhaps, the most "knobs" of any of the diagnostic modalities. In this section, we describe the underlying factors and illustrate how these factors affect MR image contrast.

DENSITY, T1, AND T2

The two most important properties that describe this interaction of the physics, chemistry, and biology are spin density and relaxation. Spin density is, quite simply, the number of MR-visible spins per volume. Relaxation is a bit more complex and is a simplified way to describe the reestablishment of equilibrium after excitation. As we will see, relaxation is the most biologically variable process and thus is the predominant source of useful contrast on MR images.

There are two types of relaxation, longitudinal (T1, or spin-lattice) relaxation and transverse (T2, or spin-spin) relaxation. These describe the way in which the longitudinal (z) magnetization recovers and the way in

TABLE 1–2. PROTON DENSITY, T1, AND T2 AS A FUNCTION OF MAGNETIC FIELD STRENGTH

TISSUE	T1						T2	PROTON DENSITY (%)
	0.02T*	0.2 T†	0.3 T‡	1.5 T§	2.4 T‖	4.0 T¶		
Fat	—	240	—	—	279	—	60	9.6
Gray matter	239	—	—	998	—	1250	91	10.6
White matter	200	—	380	718	—	1070	76	10.6
Cerebrospinal fluid	—	—	1155	—	—	—	140	10.8
Liver	—	380	—	—	570	—	40	9.7
Muscle	—	400	—	—	1023	—	50	9.3
Spleen	—	420	—	—	701	—	20	9.8
Pancreas	—	290	—	—	605	—	60	9.8
Bone marrow	—	—	320	—	554	—	—	—

*From Agartz I, Saaf J, Wahlund L-O, Wetterberg L: T1 and T2 relaxation time estimates in the normal human brain. Radiology 181:537–543, 1991.
†From Rupp N, Reiser M, Stetter E: The diagnostic value of morphology and relaxation times in NMR-imaging of the body. Eur J Radiol 3:68–76, 1983.
‡From Wehrli FW, MacFall JR, Newton TH: Parameters determining the appearance of NMR images. In: Newton TH, Potts DG, eds. Advanced Imaging Techniques, Volume II. San Anselmo, CA, Clavadel Press, 1983.
§From Breger RK, Rimm AA, Fischer ME, et al: T1 and T2 measurements on a 1.5-T commercial imager. Radiology 71:273–276, 1989.
‖From Damadian R, Zaner K, Hor D, DiMaio T: Human tumors detected by nuclear magnetic resonance. Proc Natl Acad Sci USA 71:1471–1473, 1974.
¶From Barfuss H, Fischer ME, Hentschel D, et al: Whole-body MR imaging and spectroscopy with a 4-T system. Radiology 169:811–816, 1988.

which the (detectable) transverse magnetization disappears, respectively. T1 and T2 relaxation times may vary among tissues by a factor of 10. On the other hand, proton density, like electron density in CT images, varies among different tissues by only a few percent (Table 1–2).

T1 Relaxation

As we described in the beginning of this chapter, MR depends on the slight energy difference between the aligned and antialigned orientations of the nuclei to the magnetic field. However, even though it is energetically favorable for the nuclei to line up with the field, they cannot do so instantaneously; there must be some process by which the spins either give up or absorb energy to reach their "flip" orientation. For example, in the vacuum of outer space, it would take longer than the lifetime of the universe for an isolated proton to line up with a 1.5-T field! This is because there is no energy that can "tickle" the spins to cause them to reorient. In the body, on the other hand, it takes between 0.1 and 10 seconds for the protons to align with the field. This orientation time is called the

spin-lattice relaxation time, or T1. (The "lattice" in this name comes from the general tendency of physicists to describe the thermal reservoir to which a select population is coupled as the bath or the lattice. It can also refer more specifically to the 3D lattice of nuclei in a solid.)

The T1 time also describes the time it takes the spins to regain equilibrium after they have been excited by a 90° pulse in an imaging sequence. Right after excitation there is no longitudinal magnetization; it has all been tipped into the transverse plane. The magnetization then begins to relax back to equilibrium. This recovery of longitudinal magnetization (i.e., M_z) can be described mathematically:

$$M_z(t) = M_0[1 - \exp(-t/T1)] \qquad (7)$$

Thus, T1 is an exponential time constant that is related to the period required for the longitudinal component to recover to 63% of its equilibrium alignment (86% after $2 \times T1$, 95% after $3 \times T1$, and 99% after $5 \times T1$; Fig. 1–18).

As described earlier, MR images are not produced from a single excitation of the protons. The protons must be excited multiple times to produce enough

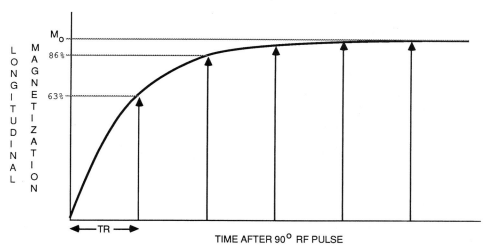

FIGURE 1–18. Longitudinal magnetization versus time after a 90° RF pulse. The longitudinal magnetization regrows toward the maximal value (M_0) at a rate determined by the T1 relaxation time.

TIME AFTER 90° RF PULSE

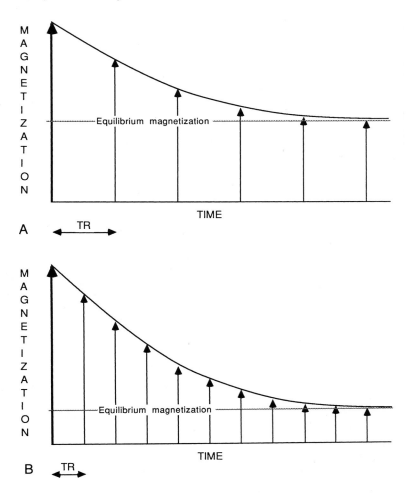

A

B

FIGURE 1–19. Effect of TR on longitudinal magnetization. After several RF pulses, an equilibrium is attained between TR and T1 relaxation. *A*, With long TR, equilibrium magnetization is large. *B*, With short TR, equilibrium magnetization is smaller.

data for the image, with a period TR between excitations. As shown in Figure 1–19, after several excitations, a balance is reached between the rate of T1 relaxation and TR, resulting in an equilibrium value for the longitudinal magnetization. This value is reduced from the maximal value (determined by the proton density), depending on the ratio of TR to T1. Because the excitation pulse tips the longitudinal magnetization into the transverse plane to be detected, the strength of the MR signal is proportional to the value of the longitudinal magnetization that existed at the instant before the RF pulse. If the TR is long, the protons can fully realign between excitations and produce a strong signal (Fig. 1–20*A*). However, if the TR is short with respect to T1, there is only partial realignment. Because protons must realign with the magnetic field before they can produce a signal, the signal strength is reduced (Fig. 1–20*B*). As a result, differences in T1 relaxation times translate into differences in tissue signal (i.e., contrast). Protons that relax

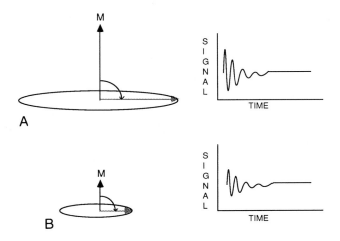

A

B

FIGURE 1–20. Longitudinal magnetization is translated by an RF pulse into signal strength. *A*, With a large longitudinal magnetization, signal strength is large. *B*, With a small longitudinal magnetization, signal strength is reduced.

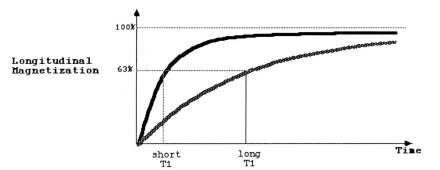

FIGURE 1–21. For two tissues, the longitudinal magnetization of the tissue with the shorter T1 relaxation times regrows more quickly.

quickly (short T1) have large longitudinal magnetization and produce a high signal intensity; protons that relax more slowly (long T1) have less recovered magnetization and thus produce less signal (Fig. 1–21).

For instance, fat has a shorter T1 (200 to 300 ms) than gray or white matter (600 to 800 ms). The protons therefore realign quickly after an RF pulse and the signal appears brighter. Tumors have longer T1 relaxation times (>1000 ms). The protons therefore recover more slowly and the signal appears darker. When a TR is chosen that is comparable to or shorter than the T1 values in the tissue, the resulting image contrast depends inversely on T1. This type of pulse sequence is called *T1 weighted.*

T2 Relaxation

Once they have been excited (i.e., tipped into the transverse plane), the coherent, precessing protons produce the detectable MR signal. This signal disappears at a higher rate than the T1 signal. The process is called T2 *relaxation* and includes the exchange of energy among neighboring spins; because of this, it is also called *spin-spin relaxation.* To understand T2 relaxation, we must first reintroduce the concept of phase. For this purpose, let us consider a simple analogy between the precession of transverse magnetization and the outcome of a track meet (Fig. 1–22).

The protons can be thought of as individual runners on a track. At the instant immediately after the firing of the starter's gun, the runners are in identical positions at the starting line. As each runner moves around a circular tract, his or her position can be represented by the angle between him or her and the starting line. This angle is the phase. If all the contestants run at precisely the same speed, they maintain identical phase angles as they move around the track. That is, their

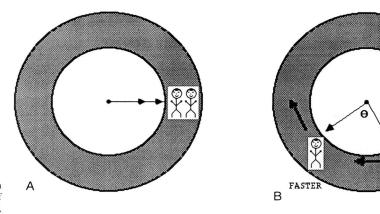

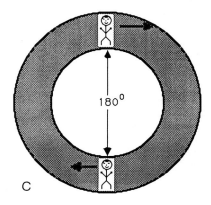

FIGURE 1–22. Analogy between proton phase and a track meet. *A,* At the start of the race, runners have the same phase. *B,* Because one runner is faster than the other, a phase angle (θ) develops over time (i.e., partial dephasing). *C,* Eventually, the runners are at opposite ends of the track (i.e., complete dephasing).

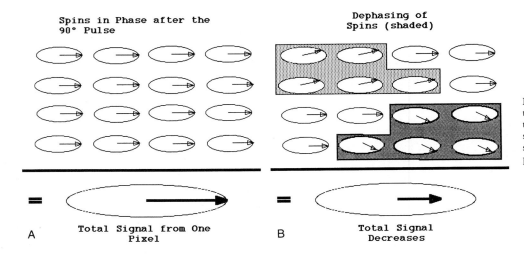

Spins in Phase after the 90° Pulse

Dephasing of Spins (shaded)

Total Signal from One Pixel

Total Signal Decreases

A

B

FIGURE 1–23. Relationship between proton phase and signal intensity. *A*, With all spins in phase, signals add to produce a large net signal. *B*, With some spins out of phase, net signal decreases.

phases remain *coherent*. However, some runners inevitably move faster than others, and the phase angles of the faster runners increase more rapidly than those of the other contestants. This difference in phase increases as the race progresses. The loss of phase coherence is called *phase dispersion* or *dephasing*.

If we liken the firing of the starter's gun to the application of a 90° RF pulse, then immediately after the RF pulse the transverse magnetization vectors from different protons have identical phases, resulting in a strong MR signal. We know from Equation 1b that each spin precesses precisely at a frequency given by its local magnetic field. If all protons saw exactly the same magnetic field, they would remain phase coherent indefinitely. However, local magnetic field inhomogeneities cause some nuclei to experience a slightly stronger magnetic field and others to experience a weaker field. As a result, the protons dephase, reducing the net transverse magnetization. The reduction in net transverse magnetization causes signal loss (Figs. 1–23 and 1–24).

The local magnetic field inhomogeneities are produced by two factors: 1) microscopic effects related to magnetic interactions among neighboring molecules (chemistry) and 2) macroscopic effects related to spatial variation of the external magnetic field (physics). As we will see, dephasing caused by molecular interactions alone is related to T2. Dephasing produced by both factors taken together is related to T2*. T2* is always shorter than T2, resulting in more rapid loss of signal (Fig. 1–25). Right after the excitation pulse, the MR signal decays through both processes (the spin cannot tell if its field inhomogeneity is caused by some nearby molecule passing by or by a macroscopic, non-uniform magnetic field caused by the presence of a nearby aneurysm clip!). This rapid decay of signal is called the *free induction decay* (FID) and falls more or less exponentially as T2*. There is a 63% decrease after one T2* interval, 86% after two T2* intervals, and so on.

The knob on the MR scanner that provides image contrast that depends on transverse relaxation corresponds to the TE. It is simply the time between the middle of the excitation and the middle of the readout used for frequency encoding. By moving the readout period farther from the excitation (i.e., making TE longer) we increase the signal loss caused by transverse relaxation.

So far, we have described how to get contrast that depends on the total transverse relaxation, T2*. How-

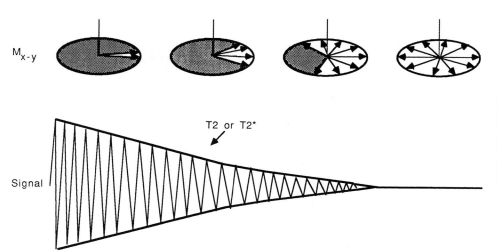

M_{x-y}

T2 or T2*

Signal

FIGURE 1–24. Relationship between signal decay and proton phase. Immediately after an RF pulse, all protons precess in phase, resulting in a strong signal. Over time, the protons dephase, and signal is lost at a rate characterized by T2* or, if a spin echo is used, T2.

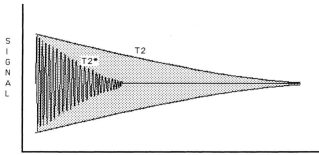

FIGURE 1–25. Signal loss caused by T2* decay is much more rapid than that caused by T2 decay.

ever, in most cases, we care far more about the "chemical" part of this relaxation, T2. To observe T2 alone, we need a trick. It turns out that MRI has a good one, called the spin echo, that eliminates the static magnetic field effects and leaves only fluctuating fields that come from chemical interactions. This spin echo is essentially a time reversal pulse and can be understood using the track analogy of Figure 1–22.

Imagine that the runners, who all have different speeds, are told to turn back when they hear a second shot from the starter's gun. How does the race proceed? At the starting gun, the runners are all in phase, but because they run at different speeds they quickly generate phase dispersion, getting out of phase (T2* decay). After some time T, the starter fires the gun again. The runners who ran the fastest (and got the farthest) start racing back; the slow runners (who got

the least far) about-face and return as well. As long as they run at exactly the same speed in the second half of the race as in the first, at time 2T all the runners return exactly to the starting line. That is, all the runners are once again in phase. In MRI, at time 2T, the spins are once more aligned and an echo of the original FID is produced (Fig. 1–26).

What about true T2 relaxation during this time? In the simplest sense, the time reversal pulse cannot do anything about these phase inhomogeneities. Because the fluctuating magnetic fields caused by chemical interactions are essentially random, they are not the same before and after T, the time of occurrence of the time reversal pulse. As a result, they are not rephased by this pulse. Hahn's great discovery was that a 180° pulse can act as a nearly perfect time reversal pulse to eliminate the static dephasing and leave just the T2 part of transverse relaxation.

MR sequences that use this 180° pulse are called spin-echo sequences, because it is this echo at time TE that is encoded. (The 180° pulse thus occurs at time TE/2.) For a given TE, the intensity of the signal from a tissue having a long T2 decreases less than that from a tissue having a short T2 (Fig. 1–27). For instance, the measured signal intensity of water, with T2 greater than 2 seconds, changes negligibly as the TE is lengthened from 15 to 30 ms. On the other hand, the signal intensity of liver, with T2 less than 50 ms, decreases by nearly 50%. Differences in T2 relaxation times can be translated into image contrast by using pulse sequence timing parameters that emphasize T2 effects. This type of pulse sequence is called *T2 weighted.* Sequences that

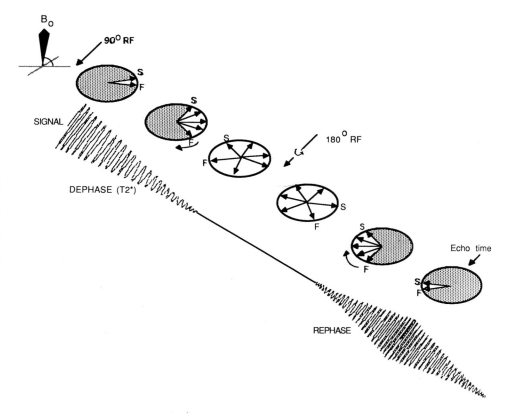

FIGURE 1–26. The spin echo. After a 90° RF pulse, spins dephase rapidly. The application of a 180° refocusing pulse eliminates the effects of static magnetic field inhomogeneities, so that most spins are in phase at TE. Some residual dephasing is present at the echo owing to T2 effects, which are irreversible. F = spins with faster precession; S = spins with slower precession.

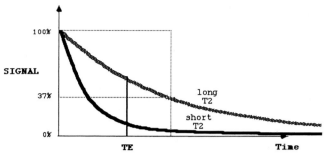

FIGURE 1–27. Signal strength versus time for two tissues with different T2 relaxation times. Signal decays more slowly for the tissue with the longer T2. Note that T2 contrast initially increases and then decreases as TE is lengthened.

do not use the 180° pulse are usually called *gradient-echo sequences* and are sensitive to full T2* effects.

PROTON DENSITY

The number of protons in a given volume contributes to all images. That is, if no protons are present, there is no image intensity regardless of whether we use T1 or T2 weighting. However, we can also create images that have minimal T1 and T2 weighting (e.g., long TR, short TE); the contrast that remains is based on the visible *proton density* (r or N[H]) (Fig. 1–28).

It is important to understand the difference between MR proton density and the true number of hydrogen nuclei per unit volume. The latter hardly varies at all in most tissues; the former, although weaker than relaxation, is at least occasionally important. The difference between the two is that some protons, because of their physicochemical environment, are difficult to see with MR. For example, many of the protons in tissue are bound up in large macromolecular complexes that can be thought of as quasi-solid (e.g., in cell membranes, connective cellular structures). These protons can have a short T2 (<0.1 ms) and thus dephase even with short (<5 ms) TE imaging sequences. Other protons are in regions of the body with such profound magnetic field inhomogeneity that T2* is so

short that imaging sequences have difficulty resolving them (e.g., in the lungs). Finally, protons in truly solid materials, such as cortical bone and dense calcifications, also produce no signal or MR images. These protons have both short T2 and long T1 (>10 seconds), so that both T1 and T2 weighting eliminates their signal in imaging studies.

Although it is generally true that cortical bone and calcifications are not directly observed, they may produce a visible signal when the calcium is hydrated owing to the presence of associated free water. The fact that cortical bone fails to produce an MR signal does not preclude its being imaged by MRI. For example, within a vertebral body, a low signal from cortical bone is outlined by a contiguous higher signal from medullary bone and adjacent disk material. Many types of bone pathology, including fractures and tumor invasion, are clearly demonstrated by increased signal from soft tissue hemorrhage or edema, which replaces the low signal of normal cortical bone. However, the fine detail of cortical bone is often inferior to that demonstrated by plain films and CT. Calcifications are also poorly shown by conventional MRI methods, although it has been demonstrated that the use of gradient-echo pulse sequences can enhance the detection of soft tissue calcification by virtue of magnetic susceptibility effects (see Chapter 10).

MORE ABOUT MECHANISMS OF RELAXATION

Molecular Mechanisms for Relaxation

T1 relaxation and T2 relaxation are complex processes that are enhanced by certain magnetic interactions among nuclei and molecules. There are several pathways by which T1 and T2 relaxation can occur. Most of these processes depend on close interactions between water and other molecules. All molecules, large and small, are in a constant state of motion, tumbling and colliding with other molecules. Each of these molecules has its own minute magnetic field. Intramolecular motion and interactions with nearby molecules produce fluctuations in the local magnetic field experienced by a proton. A small molecule such as water moves quickly, so it produces rapid magnetic fluctuations. A large molecule such as a protein moves more slowly and produces magnetic fluctuations at a correspondingly lower rate.

It turns out that these magnetic interactions can promote both T1 and T2 relaxation, but the extent to which they do so depends on the rate at which the magnetic fields fluctuate. One way to simplify expressing this concept is in terms of the *correlation time* (t_c), which represents the time scale at which the fluctuations occur. With rapid molecular motion, the correlation times are short; conversely, with slow motion the correlation times are longer (Fig. 1–29). Ultimately, relaxation occurs because the fluctuating fields have a correlation time that allows them to cause spin flips or magnetization exchange between two spins.

One of the most powerful heuristic ways of thinking about spin-spin or spin-lattice relaxation is to consider

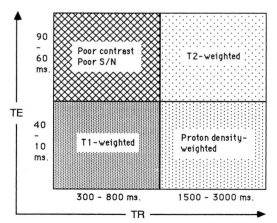

FIGURE 1–28. Simplified representation of image contrast as a function of TR and TE.

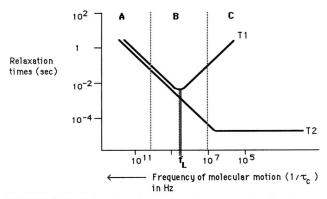

FIGURE 1–29. Relaxation time versus frequency of molecular motion $(1/\tau_c)$. Free water has rapid diffusion and long T1 and T2 times *(region A)*. Bound water associated with restricted motion has shorter T1 and T2 times *(region B)*. Very restricted motion results in very short T2 times *(region C)*.

two coupled spins and their energy levels in the magnetic field (Fig. 1–30). These two spins can be aligned with the field (spin up, state A in Fig. 1–30), antialigned with the field (spin down, state D), or in either of two superpositions with one up and one down (states B and C). Relaxation (making a transition) requires a photon with precisely the right energy. The Larmor frequency f_L represents the frequency corresponding to that energy.

Consider first T1 relaxation, which involves changes in the total magnetization (i.e., the number of spin up and spin down nuclei). To make a transition from A to B or C or from B or C to D requires energy at f_L. We can also make a transition from A to D with energy at $2f_L$. (Because transitions between B and C cause no net change in magnetization, they do not matter for T1.) Thus, the degree of T1 relaxation depends precisely on the amount of fluctuating energy (the source of the photons) present in the system at both f_L and $2f_L$.

Now consider T2 relaxation. Although it is not obvi-

ous from the diagram, it is reasonable to assume that any transition in Figure 1–30 would disrupt the phase coherence of the system. That is, not only energy at f_L and $2f_L$ but also transitions between B and C (low-frequency fluctuations near DC [direct current]) enhance T2 relaxation.

Thus, the magnetic fluctuations in the tissue at DC, f_L, and $2f_L$ are responsible for relaxation. The τ_c tells us two things about the spectrum of the fluctuating magnetic fields (Fig. 1–31). First, $1/(2\pi\tau_c)$ is the uppermost frequency limit of fluctuations with correlation time τ_c. Thus, a tumbling protein with $\tau_c \sim 1.6 \times 10^{-8}$ second, would have an upper limit in its field fluctuations around 10 MHz. Second, all other things being equal, the total energy at any given frequency is proportional to τ_c. This is because the total energy (i.e., the area under the spectra in Fig. 1–31) associated with the fluctuations is roughly constant ($\sim kT$). Thus, because the frequencies spread up to $1/(2\pi\tau_c)$ and their area is constant, the amplitude must be proportional to τ_c. We can therefore make the following generalizations about τ_c and relaxation:

1. If the rate of fluctuation $(1/\tau_c)$ is much higher than the resonance frequency of the water protons, there is only mild enhancement of T1 and T2 relaxation. Although there are fluctuations at DC, f_L, and $2f_L$, they are spread so thinly throughout the spectrum (τ_c is so small) that the energy at any given frequency is small. This situation exists, for example, in pure water, in which the molecules are moving rapidly. As a result, both T1 and T2 are extremely long (seconds) (see Fig. 1–29A).

2. If the rate of fluctuation is lower, on the same order of magnitude as the f_L, both T1 relaxation and T2 relaxation are strongly promoted (see Fig. 1–29B). This situation exists in certain proteinaceous solutions, in which the bulky protein molecules move slowly and restrict the motion of nearby water molecules (Fig. 1–32).

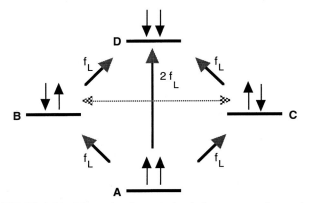

FIGURE 1–30. Schematic of energy levels between two interacting spins. Transitions from A to B or C require one packet of energy at the Larmor frequency f_L, as do transitions from B or C to D. Transitions from A to D require energy at twice the f_L; those between B and C require low-frequency fluctuations. All the transitions cause T2 relaxation; only those between different net spin states cause T1 relaxation.

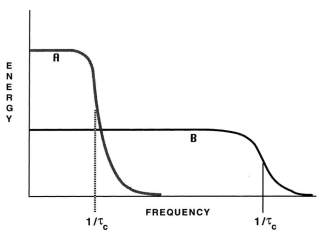

FIGURE 1–31. Density of energy available to cause relaxation. For interactions with lower $1/\tau_c$ (A), the spectrum is more limited at higher frequencies than for interactions with higher $1/\tau_c$ (B). In this case, if f_L was between these two $1/\tau_c$ values, more dramatic T1 relaxation would be seen at B.

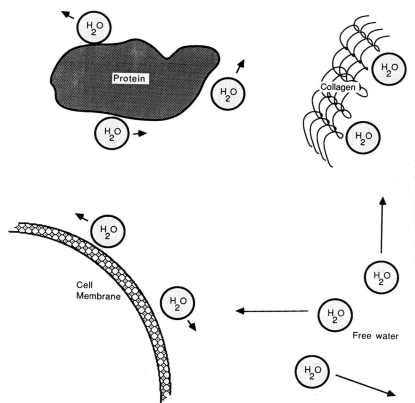

FIGURE 1–32. Effect of molecular motion on relaxation times. "Free" water (H_2O) molecules diffuse rapidly: T1 and T2 relaxation times are both long. The motion of "bound" water molecules associated with proteins and cell membranes is restricted; T1 and T2 relaxation times are shorter than those of free water. With restricted motion, as, for example, with water molecules bound to collagen, T2 relaxation times are quite short.

3. If the rate of fluctuation is much lower than the resonance frequency, only T2 relaxation is promoted (see Fig. 1–29C). This is because there is still considerable energy at DC (which is useful for T2 relaxation) but none at the higher f_L and $2f_L$. This situation exists in tendons and chronic scar tissue, in which the motion of water molecules is severely restricted by the highly organized collagen fibrils and other substances.

Both T2 and T1 relaxations occur simultaneously, and T2 relaxation is always faster than T1 relaxation (Fig. 1–33). How much faster depends on the physical and chemical structure of the tissue. In pure water, relatively few molecules move slowly. As a result, relaxation effects associated with slow molecular motions are minimal, and T2 relaxation times are nearly as long as T1 relaxation times. However, in most tissues, which contain proteins as well as other components that restrict molecular motion, T2 is much shorter than T1 (typically tens of milliseconds versus hundreds of milliseconds) (see Table 1–2).

Certain tissues have unique properties that may help to determine their relaxation properties. For instance, melanotic melanoma lesions may have a short T1 because of the presence of paramagnetic melanin. Liver may have a relatively short T1 because of both the high density of endoplasmic reticulum, which provides a large surface area for binding intracellular water,

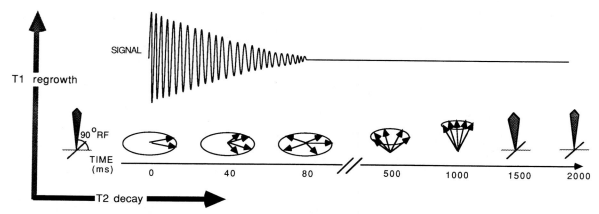

FIGURE 1–33. T1 relaxation and T2 relaxation are simultaneous processes. Note that T2 relaxation is completed much more rapidly than T1 relaxation.

and its content of paramagnetic substances.[16, 17] Water motion is restricted in mucinous lesions, such as mucoceles, and in fibrosis, accounting for the short T2 and low signal intensity of these lesions.

Finally, one should remember that the description of T1 and T2 for biologic tissues is by necessity an oversimplification. Most imaging voxels contain heterogeneous relaxation environments either microscopically (e.g., intracellular and extracellular, intravascular and extravascular) or macroscopically (e.g., partial volume effects between cerebrospinal fluid and cortical gray matter, local variation in edema), and thus several relaxation times may be present. Signal decay from such a tissue may therefore not fit a simple exponential. However, disease processes change the local chemistry or biology and thus change the relaxation environment of the voxels that include the disease. As a result, there is often some change in T1 or T2, and we can produce some change on our MR images.

Dependence of T1 Relaxation Times on Field Strength

As just discussed, T1 relaxation depends on the presence of magnetic field fluctuations near f_L or $2f_L$. Because this frequency is proportional to the strength of the magnet (whereas the intrinsic molecular motions obviously are not), relaxation rates tend to depend on the magnetic field strength. As a rule, most of the important fluctuations for water protons are relatively low in frequency (related to the tumbling proteins), and thus T1 tends to decrease at higher field strengths.

Because T2 relaxation includes the DC fluctuations, increases in resonance frequency have a much less dramatic effect on this relaxation pathway. As a result, T2 relaxation times tend to be relatively independent of field strength.

For imaging, the field strength dependence of T1 relaxation times has an important bearing on choice of pulse sequence and image contrast. Pulse sequences that produce high-contrast images at one field strength may produce images with poor contrast at another field strength. However, if one takes into account the differences in T1 relaxation times and adjusts the scan parameters accordingly, high-contrast images can be obtained at almost any field strength.

Although the T1 relaxation times of all tissues increase with field strength, the T1 increase depends on the type of tissue.[18] It is interesting to note that the T1 relaxation time of fat does not increase as much as that of other tissues, because of the different molecular composition of fat (see Table 1–2). Because signal intensity is inversely related to the T1 relaxation time, fat appears brighter than other tissues as the field strength increases. This observation would be of little practical importance, except that motion produces certain types of artifacts, called *ghosts,* that degrade image quality. Because the motion of a bright structure typically produces worse artifacts than the motion of a dark one (see Chapter 3), the motion of fat produces worse ghost artifacts at high field strengths than it does at lower field strengths. This observation is particularly relevant for imaging the abdomen.

Correlation of T1 and T2 Relaxation Times

As a rule, most MR-visible materials that have long T1 also have long T2. That is, the absence of fluctuating fields is more relevant than the precise frequency of the fluctuations. In addition, many types of disease are associated with an increase in the free water content (long T1 and T2) and thus increases in T1 and T2. These changes result in signal changes that often permit the ready distinction of pathologic from normal tissues (Table 1–3).

Although T1 and T2 relaxation times change in the same direction in response to changes in free water content, their effects on image signal intensity are opposite, as discussed further later. As T1 increases, signal intensity decreases; however, as T2 increases, signal intensity also increases. If a pulse sequence were selected that produced equal T1 and T2 weighting, then, for pathologic tissues, the signal decrease produced by the long T1 would be opposed by the signal increase produced by the long T2, resulting in an intermediate signal that might be difficult to distinguish from the signal for normal tissue (see Fig. 1–28).

For this reason, we choose pulse sequences that are weighted toward either T1 or T2, but not both, to maximize the image contrast between normal and pathologic tissues. With spin-echo imaging methods, a rule of thumb for image interpretation is that T1-weighted images generally depict pathologic tissues as less bright than normal tissues, whereas on T2-weighted images diseased tissue usually appears brighter than normal tissue. Which type of contrast proves most clinically useful depends on both the organ system and the specific pathologic process being evaluated. (One exception to this rule is short-tau inversion recovery [STIR] imaging, discussed later, with which one can obtain additive T1 and T2 contrast, although often at the expense of increased imaging time.)

OTHER SOURCES OF CONTRAST FOR THE MR IMAGE

T1, T2, and proton density are the predominant sources of MR image contrast. However, several others are clinically important and, via the flexibility of the MR scanner, can be exploited for diagnostic imaging.

MAGNETIC SUSCEPTIBILITY

Nearly all materials have some interaction with a magnetic field. The nuclear interaction, although critical for MR, is actually one of the weakest. The more important interactions tend to be due to the electrons. The general term for the magnetizability of a material is its *magnetic susceptibility,* which can be thought of as the material's tendency to distort an applied field. The

TABLE 1–3. APPEARANCES OF TISSUE ON MR IMAGES

TISSUE	T1-WEIGHTED IMAGE	T2-WEIGHTED IMAGE
Fat*	Very bright	Intermediate to dark
Cysts		
Watery fluid	Very dark	Very bright
Proteinaceous fluid	Intermediate to bright	Very bright
Brain		
White matter	Bright	Dark
Gray matter	Dark	Bright
Cerebrospinal fluid	Very dark	Very bright
Bone marrow		
Yellow*	Very bright	Intermediate to dark
Red†	Intermediate	Dark
Cortical bone	Very dark	Very dark
Cartilage		
Fibrocartilage	Very dark	Very dark
Tear of fibrocartilage‡	Intermediate	Intermediate to bright
Hyaline‡	Intermediate	Intermediate
Intervertebral disk		
Normal‡	Intermediate	Bright
Degenerated	Intermediate to dark	Dark
Osteophyte		
Marrow containing	Bright	Intermediate to dark
Calcified only	Dark	Dark
Tendons/ligaments§	Very dark	Very dark
Muscle	Dark	Dark
Lung‖	Very dark	Very dark
Liver		
Normal parenchyma	Bright	Dark
Metastasis¶	Dark	Usually bright, may have dark center
Hemangioma	Dark	Bright
Fatty infiltration†	Bright	Dark
Iron overload	Intermediate to dark	Very dark
Pancreas	Bright	Dark
Spleen	Dark	Bright
Contrast-enhanced tissue		
Gadolinium chelate		
Low concentration	Very bright	Bright
High concentration	Intermediate to dark	Very dark
SPIO	Dark	Very dark
Ultrasmall SPIO	Bright	Very dark
Fluosol	Very dark	Very dark
Hematoma**		
Hyperacute (<6 h)	Intermediate	Intermediate
Acute (6–24 h)	Intermediate to dark	Dark
Subacute (1 d–1 mo)	Bright rim	Bright
Chronic (>1 m)	Dark rim ± bright center	Dark rim ± bright center

*Bright on T2-weighted images acquired using fast spin-echo sequence with short interecho interval.
†Dark on out-of-phase image.
‡Bright on proton density–weighted image.
§Increased signal, particularly on proton density–weighted images, when tissue is oriented at 55° to B_0 (magic angle effect).
‖Increased parenchymal signal with TE <2 ms or fast spin-echo sequence with very short interecho interval.
¶Hepatocellular carcinoma, melanoma, hemorrhagic lesion may appear bright on T1-weighted image.
**Low signal because of magnetic susceptibility effects predominantly seen on high-field images, more pronounced on gradient-echo than spin-echo images. Time frames indicated for hematoma evolution are approximations; in reality the time frames may vary widely from the values shown.

net induced magnetization is usually proportional to the applied field: M = χB, where χ, the volume magnetic susceptibility of the tissue, summarizes its magnetic properties. All materials have a tendency to counteract the presence of the magnetic field (diamagnetism), decreasing its effect inside them. In some materials, however, some of the electrons tend to line up with the magnetic field, producing additive fields. These materials are called *paramagnetic*. (If this sounds suspiciously like the phenomena underlying MR, it is; sometimes MR is referred to as nuclear paramagnetism.) The effect of diamagnetic or paramagnetic materials on the internal magnetic field of a tissue is approximately given by

$$B_{eff} \text{ (tissue)} \sim B_0 + B_0\chi \qquad (8)$$

This expression has an ~ sign because the exact field shifts depend strongly on the geometry of the perturber. For example, a sphere (like a head) distorts the field in a much different way than a leg (a cylinder). The shift in the magnetic field is proportional to χ and the strength of the external magnetic field. Most proteinaceous materials have comparable degrees of diamagnetism, but there are some important exceptions. For example, deoxygenated hemoglobin is strongly paramagnetic. In addition to the diamagnetic and paramagnetic materials, some rarer types are encountered in MR:

1. *Superparamagnetic substances* more strongly attract magnetic lines of force. These substances have more potent magnetic effects than do paramagnetic substances, primarily because multiple coupled electrons are acting in concert, behaving as a giant dipole. This is basically a solid-state effect, requiring some degree of crystallization. Examples of superparamagnetic substances are hemosiderin and superparamagnetic iron oxide (SPIO).

2. *Ferromagnetic substances* remain permanently magnetized after being removed from a magnetic field, because of the alignment of multiple magnetic domains. Ferromagnetic substances include a number of iron- and cobalt-containing metal alloys and are often used in common refrigerator magnets.

Variations in magnetic susceptibilities within a voxel, such as those related to air-tissue or bone-tissue interfaces, produce local inhomogeneities in the magnetic field. In addition, the shape of the body itself (water surrounded by air) produces field nonuniformity. These field inhomogeneities produce dephasing, which in turn results in T2* signal loss (see Chapter 3). Although a source of artifacts, magnetic susceptibility effects can also be useful in delineating certain types of pathologic conditions, such as hemorrhage and calcification. Because gradient-echo images are more sensitive to these susceptibility effects than are spin-echo images (the spin echo eliminates static field inhomogeneity), T2*-weighted scans are often used to see these effects.

CONTRAST AGENTS

In addition to biologic sources of contrast, several common exogenous materials are used clinically to enhance contrast. The contrast agents in clinical use or under development include 1) nonselective contrast agents (e.g., gadolinium diethylenetriaminepentaacetic acid [Gd-DTPA], 2) targeted agents (e.g., SPIO), and 3) negative-contrast agents (i.e., agents that contain no mobile hydrogen). The first two types work by adding an exogenous source of field fluctuation that enhances relaxation. The latter work by eliminating the source of proton signal altogether. These agents, summarized in the following, are considered in more depth in Chapters 5 and 6.

Nonselective Contrast Agents

Most contrast agents in clinical use or under investigation are paramagnetic and exploit the lanthanide elements, which, because of their large number of unpaired electrons, have large susceptibility (see Chapter 5). The most potent of these for MRI is gadolinium, a rare earth element, which contains seven unpaired electrons in its native state. The gadolinium is chelated with DTPA or other ligands to reduce the toxicity of the heavy metal ion.[19] Examples of other paramagnetic substances are manganese, iron, and free radicals. The magnetic fields associated with unpaired electrons in paramagnetic substances have a potent effect on proton relaxation in nearby water molecules. Gadolinium chelates distribute interstitially like the iodinated contrast agents used in CT.[20] They are used for many of the same applications, including screening and characterization of brain tumors[21, 22] and differentiation of postoperative scar from recurrent disk herniation.[23] Compared with iodinated contrast agents, gadolinium chelates are used in much lower concentrations, hence are far safer,[24] and produce larger changes in tissue contrast. Although the dominant effect of paramagnetic substances on MR images is T1 shortening, these substances actually shorten both T1 and T2 relaxation times. The effectiveness of a paramagnetic contrast agent can be expressed in terms of its *relaxivity,* which is the slope of the linear relationship between relaxation rate (1/T1 or 1/T2) and the concentration of the agent.[25] The relaxivity is dependent on magnetic field strength and temperature. These agents usually change T1 by a much larger fraction of its unenhanced value than T2, so enhancement by paramagnetic contrast agents is usually best seen on T1-weighted images. Fat saturation[26] or magnetization transfer pulses[27] can be applied to reduce background signal intensity and thus make enhanced lesions even more conspicuous.

Although paramagnetic contrast agents generally increase the signal intensity of enhanced tissues, there are exceptions. For instance, highly concentrated gadolinium in the renal collecting system has such a short T2 that it appears dark. A hemorrhagic lesion may have such a short T1 that the tissue is almost fully relaxed, so that the additional T1 shortening caused by a contrast agent may not result in detectable increase in signal.

Other agents work by eliminating signal by replacing water-bearing tissue with material devoid of mobile protons. As a result, the material appears dark no matter which pulse sequence is used. An example of such a substance is perfluorooctylbromide, a fluorine-containing molecule that can be used as a contrast agent for the intestine. Some oral contrast agents occur naturally or can be derived from over-the-counter medications. For instance, blueberry juice has a high manganese content[28] and Geritol solutions contain paramagnetic iron[29]; both can be used to enhance the upper gastrointestinal tract. Clays such as kaolinate are diamagnetic; they shorten the T2 relaxation time of the bowel contents by adsorbing water to their surfaces and thus act as negative-contrast agents.

Still another approach is to use hyperpolarized noble gases such as helium 3 or xenon 129.[29a] Such agents could be used for lung or perfusion imaging. However, preparation of such agents requires special equipment such as a high-power diode laser. The remarkably long T1 of hyperpolarized noble gases and high diffusivity necessitate particular care in pulse sequence choice.

Targeted Agents

It is possible to synthesize compounds containing paramagnetic moieties that are taken up by various transport systems. For instance, manganese is chelated to the active form of vitamin B_6 in the compound Mn(II)-*N,N'*-dipyridoxylethylenediamine-*N,N'*-diacetate-5,5'-bis(phosphate).[30] The manganese chelate is taken up by the hepatocyte and is excreted into the biliary system and thus is a hepatobiliary-specific agent. Another approach is to coat a paramagnetic iron core with a substance such as dextran to change the pharmacokinetic properties of the contrast agent.[31, 32] An example of such an agent is SPIO, a particle that is selectively taken up by the reticuloendothelial system including the liver, spleen, bone marrow, and lymph nodes. Unlike normal liver tissue, most liver tumors do not take up SPIO, although uptake does occur in cavernous hemangiomas and some hepatocellular carcinomas. SPIOs predominantly shorten T2 rather than T1, so the main effect is signal loss on T2-weighted images. If the particle size is reduced further, both T1 and T2 are shortened. Such ultrasmall particles have a long half-life in the blood (up to hours), so they can be used as blood-pool contrast agents for MR angiography. Further modifications to increase tissue specificity are also possible. For instance, an antibody fragment can be covalently linked to the particle coat to confer immunologic selectivity or the particle can be otherwise modified for receptor selectivity (e.g., by using asialoglycoprotein in the coat, hepatic receptors for this molecule are targeted).

BLOOD AND FLOW

Blood, which is a fairly complex fluid, has several properties that make its behavior, as a tissue, quite different from that of its surroundings. The most important of these properties for MR are that 1) its flow affects image intensity on T1-weighted scans and 2) its oxygenation state affects image intensity on T2- and T2*-weighted scans. These properties are discussed extensively in later chapters of this book (Chapters 7 to 9), and we briefly summarize the behaviors here.

Blood has a variety of cellular and proteinaceous components. It is a non-newtonian fluid, in that the viscosity decreases as the velocity of flow increases. Because of its high water content, blood has a high proton density (0.81 to 0.86) and a long T1 relaxation time that is dependent on hematocrit.[33, 34] Its T1 at 1.5 T is normally of the order of 1.2 seconds. Its magnetic state depends on the degree of oxygenation: deoxyhemoglobin is strongly paramagnetic, and thus the T2 relaxation time depends on oxygenation state. At 1.5 T, T2 can vary between 30 and 250 ms as the oxygen saturation of the blood varies from 30% to 96%.[35] Arterial blood has a T2 of the order of 200 ms; the T2 of venous blood is much lower. This property has several useful consequences. For instance, the T2 relaxation time can be used for noninvasive determination of oxygen tension in vivo. It is also the basis of the blood oxygen level–dependent contrast used in functional neuroimaging for task activation studies.[36]

Based on its relaxation properties, arterial blood can look bright on T2-weighted images. However, this is true only when the signal is not modulated by flow effects. With the exception of sluggish flow (e.g., in leg veins or large aneurysms), flow causes the observed intravascular signal to diverge in a complex manner from the expected appearance.

The ability of MRI to depict flowing blood noninvasively has been recognized for many years. Flow imaging is covered in detail in Chapter 9 and is discussed only briefly here. Flow can produce either an increase or decrease in signal intensity. There are two sources of decrease. First, a spread of velocities within a voxel can cause a spread of phases in the transverse magnetization after excitation and thus cause flow-related dephasing of the transverse magnetization. Second, in a spin-echo sequence, if the spins move between the 90° pulse and the 180° pulse, they are not completely refocused. As the distance moved by the spins depends on TE, this effect, too, causes the flow-related signal to decrease with TE. On the other hand, the flow of blood can bring "fresh," unsaturated spins into the plane, apparently counteracting the saturation of magnetization that one might expect from the relatively long T1 of the blood. The latter effect (sometimes called paradoxical enhancement) makes the blood act as if it had a shorter T1 than the surrounding tissue and thus appear bright on T1-weighted scans (see Chapter 9). Thus, the appearance of flowing blood depends strongly on the particular imaging technique used.

Flow void (loss of signal) is emphasized by rapid flow, use of a thin section, or long TE. Large vessels such as the aorta are reasonably well evaluated with spin-echo sequences, but smaller vessels such as the renal or peripheral arteries are more readily studied by gradient-echo sequences.[37] Flowing blood usually appears bright in gradient-echo images, and the brightness increases with velocity (flow-related enhancement). Multiple electrocardiogram-gated gradient-echo images spanning the various phases of the cardiac cycle can be obtained to show dynamic flow patterns, which is of value for measuring flow and for evaluating flow patterns, such as in the true and false lumens of a dissection. A series of images acquired by using 2D or 3D gradient-echo sequences can be processed into a projection angiogram using the maximal intensity projection algorithm.[38] This algorithm extracts the brightest pixels along a user-selected orientation into a projection image similar in appearance to a digital subtraction angiogram.

Most work with MR angiography has to date been concentrated on the head and neck, with promising results. Study times for evaluation of the carotid bifurcation are practical, on the order of 5 to 15 minutes. The sensitivity of MR angiography for carotid bifurcation disease is in excess of 90%; the specificity varies depending on the particular pulse sequence.[39] In many centers, MR angiography is routinely used to confirm findings at duplex sonography or in conjunction with MRI of the brain in patients with suspected cerebrovascular disease. At some institutions, MR angiography has partly replaced contrast angiography for presurgical evaluation of the carotid bifurcation. In the brain, MR angiography is commonly used to screen the circle of Willis for aneurysms, particularly in asymptomatic patients.[40] In the body, it is used for imaging of portal and systemic veins and larger arteries such as the aorta. The technical challenges of imaging blood vessels in the body are substantially greater than in the head and neck, and one must contend with the problem of respiratory motion of the chest and abdomen.[41] A persistent limitation of MR angiography is that abnormal flow patterns cause artifacts, which tend to exaggerate the severity of stenoses. However, the accuracy of MR angiography has improved with the introduction of extremely short TE and other sequence modifications.

HEMORRHAGE

The complexity of the biochemistry of blood and the sensitivity of MRI to this biochemistry make MR detection of the natural history of hemorrhage possible. The biochemistry and MR appearance of hemorrhage are reviewed in detail in Chapters 7 and 21. On CT scans, the appearance of hemorrhage is related only to tissue density, which ultimately, in blood, is related to the iron concentration in the hemoglobin. However, on MR images, the appearance of hemorrhage is affected by a number of different factors, including the magnetic properties of hemoglobin and its breakdown products as well as the intactness of the red blood cells. In brief, fresh, arterial blood filling a hemorrhage has a long T1 and T2 and thus appears bright on T2 images and dark or isointense with brain on T1 images. As this hemorrhage ages and the blood is deoxygenated, the increased paramagnetism of the deoxyhemoglobin shortens T2 and especially T2* in the hemorrhage and in the brain surrounding it, making the hemorrhage appear dark on T2 and especially gradient-echo images. Eventually the cells lyse, and this T2* effect goes away. At this stage, the hemoglobin begins to be converted to methemoglobin, which, because of a configurational change of the protein, allows much better water access to the (large dipole) iron groups in the molecule. As a result, T1 relaxation is enhanced, just as it is with an exogenous dipole relaxation agent like Gd-DTPA. At this stage, the hemorrhage appears bright on T1-weighted scans. Finally, the iron is broken down and sequestered to prevent its toxic release into the body. At this stage, it has been postulated to be a nearly superparamagnetic crystal and thus appears dark on T2-weighted scans.

CHEMICAL SHIFT

In addition to relaxivity, the local chemical environment can subtly modify a proton's resonance frequency. The electron cloud surrounding the nucleus of an atom shields the nucleus from the applied magnetic field. As a result, the effective local magnetic field experienced by the nucleus (B_{eff}) is altered, and the nuclear resonance frequency is shifted, according to Equation 1b. This shift of the resonance frequency is called the *chemical shift*. The reduction in the local magnetic field caused by the chemical shift (σ) can be expressed as

$$B_{eff} = (1 - \sigma)B_0 \qquad (9)$$

For protons, these shifts tend to be small. For instance, the difference between a proton in a water molecule and one on a CH_2 group in fat is only about 3.5 ppm. Chemical-shift effects are the basis of MR spectroscopy, which attempts to exploit the wealth of information that is particularly available from looking at the metabolites present in the cells. In MR images, however, for which the vast bulk of the signal simply comes from either free tissue water or protons in fatty chains, this chemical shift is mostly apparent in the mispositioning of fat signals compared with water. This effect, called *chemical-shift artifact,* is described in detail in Chapter 3. More positively, the chemical shift can be exploited to image or suppress one moiety. These techniques are described in greater detail in the following section on pulse sequences.

DIFFUSION

Another property of biologic water is its brownian motion. This motion, or "diffusion," is the random, translational motion of molecules caused by their thermal energy and associated with the viscosity of the medium. The ability to detect diffusional effects in vivo is unique to MR. Some of this is already implicitly included in normal (i.e., T1 and T2) relaxation: the water diffusion dictates some of the correlation times relevant for relaxation (see earlier discussion of relaxation). In addition, diffusion of water protons through the inhomogeneous magnetic field caused by paramagnetic iron in acute hemorrhage causes the dephasing that is responsible for signal loss in T2-weighted spin-echo images. However, for the most part, diffusion is not directly apparent in MR images acquired with conventional pulse sequences. Special sequences using strong magnetic field gradients can be used to detect diffusional effects (see Chapter 8). Because certain tissue properties can be seen only via their diffusional change, this diffusion weighting can be diagnostically useful. For instance, in acute ischemia, diffusion is reduced well before relaxation changes can be observed. This change can be detected within minutes of the onset of ischemia and hours before changes are apparent in T2-weighted images (see Chapter 26). In addition, whereas in most tissues diffusion is isotropic (i.e., equal in all directions), the hydrophobic myelin sheath of axons slows diffusion perpendicular to the sheaths. As a result, in white matter tracts and in nerves, diffusion is anisotropic (i.e., greater in some directions than others) and diffusion weighting causes greater increases in signal loss along the direction of the tracts. Diffusion in several other tissues with highly ordered structures, notably skeletal muscle and myocardium, is also anisotropic.

MAGNETIZATION TRANSFER CONTRAST

As discussed earlier, proton density refers to the concentration of MR-visible protons. In many tissues, there can be a substantial amount of "hidden" water. This water, although not directly visible, can affect the visible protons. For example, if an RF pulse is applied at a frequency substantially different (e.g., >1 kHz) from f_L, one would not expect there to be much effect on tissue signal. In practice, however, one finds a reduction (which can be greater than a factor of 2) in the signals from many tissues. The primary cause for this reduction is that the "invisible" protons are not MR insensitive; rather they simply have such a short T2 (<0.1 ms) that they cannot be seen at any reasonable TE. Such protons may be associated with large immobile proteins, membranes, and so forth. However, once excited they can have a visible effect: they can transfer their saturation to the mobile (visible) protons, thus increasing the saturation of the visible protons.

Because this restricted pool continually exchanges magnetization with the mobile pool, there is a reduction in the signal intensity of tissues that contain both mobile and restricted protons (Fig. 1–34). Such tissues include brain, liver, and muscle, among others (Table 1–4). The effect is called *magnetization transfer* (MT) contrast.[42] Tissues that have a paucity of restricted protons, such as cerebrospinal fluid, urine, and blood, show minimal if any signal change. In addition, as this effect is essentially an additional path of T1 relaxation, MT pulses only minimally affect tissues with short T1. Thus, MT pulses have a minor effect on the signal intensity of fat or that of gadolinium-enhanced tissue.

MT pulses are implemented similarly to chemical-shift–selective pulses used for fat suppression, but with a larger frequency offset. In commercial MR systems, MT pulses are applied nonselectively at a frequency approximately 1.5 kHz away from the f_L. If applied much closer to the f_L, the MT pulse causes direct saturation of the tissue signal. If it is applied much farther away, substantially more RF power is required to cause sufficient saturation of the tissue signal. MT pulses must be applied repeatedly for a substantial

effect. There is a great amount of RF power deposition, particularly at higher field strengths such as 1.5 T, because power deposition increases approximately with the square of the RF frequency. This power deposition is more of a limitation in the body than in the head, because so much more tissue is exposed to RF when the body coil is used as a transmitter.

There are several potential clinical applications for MT contrast.[43] MT pulses have proved clinically useful for intracranial MR angiography.[44] They reduce the signal from brain but only slightly reduce the signal intensity of blood, so that blood-brain contrast is improved, making small vessels better delineated. MT pulses are also helpful for contrast-enhanced T1-weighted imaging, because they only slightly reduce the signal intensity of tissues with short T1 relaxation times, such as contrast-enhanced tumors.[45] As with MT MR angiography, the signal intensity of brain tissue is reduced, so that the conspicuity of contrast-enhanced lesions is improved. The amount of MT is affected by the physical and chemical state of the tissue. Thus, the MT rate is apparently lowered in multiple sclerosis and thus may be of value in characterizing the degree of demyelination in plaques.[46] MT effects can cause substantial alterations of tissue contrast even in routine imaging,[47] especially when pulse sequences (see later), such as fast spin echo and multislice spin echo, are used in which large number of 180° pulses are applied.

TISSUE ORIENTATION

There are several cases in MRI in which the tissue orientation (i.e., the angle the tissue makes to the static magnetic field) can have a substantial effect on signal intensity. These are most typically found when the tissues themselves have oriented fiber structures. The two most important effects are an angular dependence of T2 and diffusional signal loss.

Changes in T2 with angle are usually the result of the "magic angle" effect.[48, 49] Dipolar interactions between two spins, which cause the magnetic field fluctuations responsible for T2 relaxation, are proportional to $(3 \cos^2 \theta - 1)$. The rapid rotation of mobile spins quickly averages away these fluctuations (i.e., none near DC; see earlier discussion of relaxation mechanisms), but in crystalline solids the lack of motion eliminates the averaging. As a result, the T2 in solids is short. However, this dipolar interaction goes to zero when the angle with B_0 is approximately 55°. (This trick is used by solid-state MR spectroscopists: they actually spin their crystalline samples at this magic angle to narrow the resonance line.) When a tissue with a highly ordered structure, such as a tendon, is oriented at a 55° angle to B_0, the signal "magically" increases compared with orientations at other angles. This causes bright areas to appear in portions of curved tendons and ligaments, such as the rotator cuff (Fig. 1–35) and knee ligaments, that can simulate pathologic characteristics, particularly on proton density–weighted images.

TABLE 1–4. MAGNETIZATION TRANSFER RATES FOR VARIOUS TISSUES*

TISSUE	M_s/M_0
Fat	1.0
Blood (ventricular cavity)	1.0
Heart muscle	0.3
Skeletal muscle	0.2
Gray matter	0.61
White matter	0.58
Cerebrospinal fluid	1.0
Skin	0.2
Bone marrow	0.9
Articular cartilage	0.25

*M_s and M_0 represent the longitudinal magnetization of a tissue with and without MT saturation, respectively. A large M_s/M_0 ratio implies a small MT effect, and conversely a small ratio implies a strong effect. Although a value of 1.0 has been reported for blood, implying no MT effect, our clinical experience has been that there is a 10% to 15% reduction of vascular signal for intracranial MR angiography using MT pulses.

Adapted from Balaban RS, Ceckler TL: Magnetization transfer contrast in magnetic resonance imaging. Magn Reson Q 8:116–137, 1992. © Raven Press, New York.

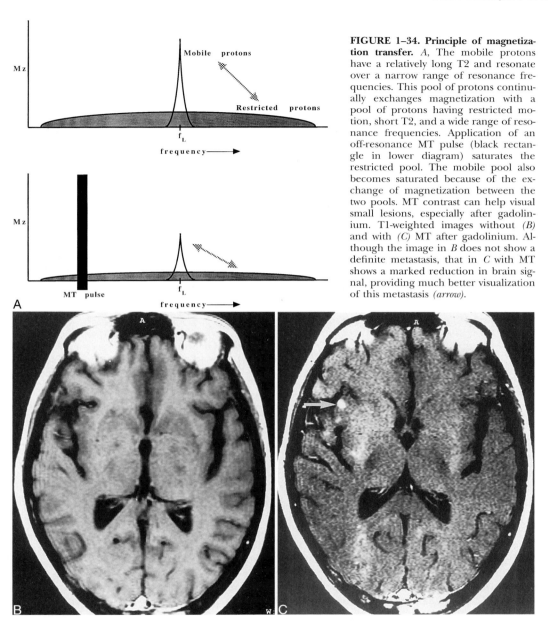

FIGURE 1–34. Principle of magnetization transfer. *A,* The mobile protons have a relatively long T2 and resonate over a narrow range of resonance frequencies. This pool of protons continually exchanges magnetization with a pool of protons having restricted motion, short T2, and a wide range of resonance frequencies. Application of an off-resonance MT pulse (black rectangle in lower diagram) saturates the restricted pool. The mobile pool also becomes saturated because of the exchange of magnetization between the two pools. MT contrast can help visual small lesions, especially after gadolinium. T1-weighted images without *(B)* and with *(C)* MT after gadolinium. Although the image in *B* does not show a definite metastasis, that in *C* with MT shows a marked reduction in brain signal, providing much better visualization of this metastasis *(arrow).*

MANIPULATING THE MR SIGNAL: PULSE SEQUENCES

T1, T2, and proton density are intrinsic tissue parameters over which the user has no control. However, the operator can alter tissue contrast and S/N ratio by the choice of pulse sequence. *Pulse sequence* refers to the time sequence of commands the MR scanner uses to create its images. It includes the temporal placement of the gradient, RF pulses, and data acquisition. The pulse sequence completely controls the desired contrast in the MR image, and much of the power of MRI comes from the flexibility of these sequences. In the past decade, increasingly complex or special-purpose sequences have been developed to optimize the diagnostic value of the MR scans. Pulse sequence design is considered in depth in Chapter 4. As an

introduction, however, in this section we describe the various families of pulse sequences and explain their underlying physical principles and clinical applications.

A pulse sequence represents a series of RF and gradient pulses used to produce a spatially localized signal. Pulse sequences must be repeated multiple times to obtain enough data to form an image. The TR is usually defined as the time from the center of the first RF pulse in one repetition of the sequence to the center of the first RF pulse in the next repetition of the sequence. The signal is measured over a time interval called the *readout period.* The time at which the signal is measured is the TE. The TE is typically defined as the time that elapses between the center of the first RF pulse and the center of the echo. As discussed in the section on contrast, TE controls the

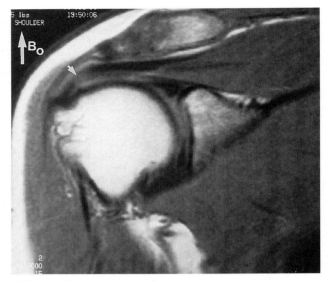

FIGURE 1–35. Coronal oblique proton density–weighted spin-echo image of the right shoulder of a healthy subject shows a focal elevated signal in the supraspinatus tendon *(arrow)*, probably caused by a magic angle effect at 55° obliquity to B_0.

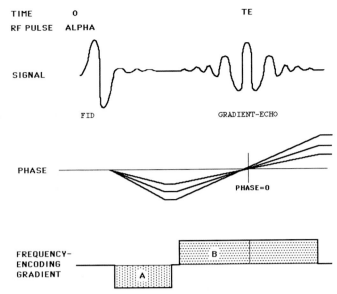

FIGURE 1–36. Principle of the gradient echo. Simplified diagram of pulse sequence showing frequency-encoding gradient. Dephasing gradient pulse (A) produces negative phase shift. Rephasing gradient (B) produces compensatory positive phase shift. At the TE, phase shifts are precisely canceled.

amount of T2 weighting and TR controls the amount of T1 relaxation introduced into the image.

Types of MR Signals

Different combinations of RF pulses and gradient pulses can be used to produce different types of MR images. Although an oversimplification, it is sometimes useful to think of the RF pulses as the controller of contrast and the gradient pulses as the controller of tomography. Many possible signals can be produced, but only a few of these are routinely used for imaging. We have already described these, but we summarize them here in Table 1–5.

The FID represents the signal that is produced immediately after an RF pulse. This signal decays away like T2*. When a second RF pulse is applied, the combination of pulses produces a spin echo, whose amplitude decays like T2. Occasionally more than these two RF pulses are used for images. Often the third pulse precedes the spin echo or FID and is used to prepare the magnetization before the imaging sequence to add additional contrast.

Whereas theoretically any part of the echoes could

be used to make an MR image, the most robust imaging (and really all imaging that is performed on commercial imagers currently) requires complete refocusing of the imaging gradients at some time during the data acquisition. That is, it is important to acquire the data both before and after the instant when the imaging gradients (which cause the MR signal to dephase based on position) have no net effect. Because the application of the gradients causes the signal to dephase immediately, the trick used to acquire data *before* dephasing is to include a reversal of the gradient before the data acquisition (Fig. 1–36). That is, if a gradient G is to be used to image the spins, then a gradient −G is applied for a duration T before the data acquisition. As a result, at a time T into the readout, there is no net cumulative effect of these imaging gradients; all the spins are in phase. This maximum of signal intensity is called an "echo." Unlike the spin echo, which is elicited by the RF pulses, the gradient echo occurs because of the gradient reversal. All imaging sequences, regardless of whether they encode the spin echo (T2) or FID (T2*), use a gradient echo to read out the spins. The resulting terminol-

TABLE 1–5. TYPES OF SIGNALS MEASURED IN MRI

SIGNAL	NUMBER OF RF PULSES	HOW SIGNAL IS PRODUCED	COMMENTS
Free induction decay	1 (90°)	Magnetization rotated into x-y plane	Very short TE Poorly suited for imaging
Gradient echo	1 (α)	Same as above + gradient reversal	Fast imaging Flow imaging Bad artifacts resulting from B_0 inhomogeneity
Spin echo	2 (90°, 180°)	Same as above + gradient reversal + RF refocusing	Routine clinical use Insensitive to B_0 inhomogeneity

ogy, however, is a little convoluted. A spin-echo image is one that encodes the spin echo; a gradient-echo image forgoes this spin echo and simply encodes the FID.

Methods for producing these signals, as well as their clinical applications, are now reviewed.

SPIN ECHO

In its most basic form, the *spin-echo pulse sequence* (Fig. 1–37) consists of two RF pulses, 90° and 180°, separated in time by equal intervals of TE/2:

$$90°\text{-TE/2-}180°\text{-TE/2-(spin echo)}$$

The 90° RF pulse excites the protons and produces an FID signal. The 180° RF pulse refocuses the transverse magnetization so that dephasing effects resulting from static magnetic field inhomogeneities, caused by the magnet or local differences in magnetic susceptibility, are canceled at the echo at time TE. As a result, the image is T2 weighted rather than T2* weighted.

Spin-echo scans are usually performed as multislice acquisitions. The maximal number of slices that can be acquired practically depends on several variables and can be summarized by

$$\text{Number of slices} = \text{TR}/(\text{TE} + \Delta) \quad (10)$$

where Δ is a lumped, system-dependent factor that is related to the pulse sequence structure and performance constraints of the gradients, RF, and measurement systems. For a given TR, more slices can be acquired if TE is short than long.

In a spin-echo pulse sequence, additional 180° RF pulses can be applied to generate multiple echoes (Fig. 1–38), with no increase in scanning time unless the TR must be lengthened to accommodate the additional echoes, as expressed by Equation 10. The benefit of multiecho sequences is that the additional echoes provide better image display of T2 tissue characteristics. For example, a tissue such as liver, which appears bright with an early echo but dark with later echoes, can be inferred to have a short T2. Conversely, a tissue such as cerebrospinal fluid, which appears bright with late as well as early echoes, must have a long T2. Images obtained with a long TE can help discriminate between tumor and surrounding edema. More commonly, multiecho imaging is used to acquire a short-TE image "for free" when acquiring long-TE, T2-weighted

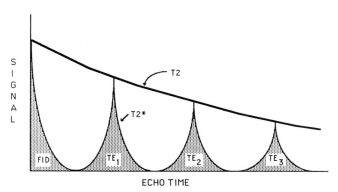

FIGURE 1–38. Signal decay in multiecho spin-echo acquisition.

images. In this case, one obtains a short-TE, density-weighted scan along with the T2-weighted image in essentially the same time.

Spin-echo images have, as already described, contrast that is manipulated primarily through adjusting TE and TR (see Fig. 1–28):

1. Images acquired with short TR (TR ~ T1) and short TE (TE << T2) are *T1 weighted* (Fig. 1–39A).

2. Images acquired with long TR (TR >> T1) and short TE (TE < T2) are called *proton density–weighted* or *balanced images* (Fig. 1–39B).

3. Images acquired with long TR and long TE (TE ~ T2) are *T2 weighted* (Fig. 1–39C).

On T1-weighted images, tissues that have short T1, such as fat, appear bright, whereas tissues that have long T1, such as tumors and edema, appear dark. On T2-weighted images, tissues with long T2, such as tumors, edema, and cysts, appear bright, whereas tissues that have short T2, such as muscle and liver, appear dark. On proton density–weighted images, tissues with increased proton density appear moderately bright. Both T1- and T2-weighted images are always partly weighted toward proton density as well.

The fourth option (short TR and long TE) is routinely avoided in practice. Because T1 contrast and T2 contrast are in opposite directions (i.e., long T1 corresponds to dark images on T1-weighted scans; long T2 corresponds to bright images on T2-weighted scans) and because T1 and T2 in soft tissues are often correlated (i.e., tissues with long T1 usually have long T2), the resulting image tends to have nearly no contrast.

FAST SPIN ECHO

Fast spin-echo images have tissue contrast that is similar to that of conventional spin-echo images but can be acquired in a fraction of the time.[50–53] The basic idea is to use a multiecho spin-echo sequence. Instead of reconstructing a separate image from each echo, the echoes are individually phase encoded, thus acquiring from each 90° pulse more of the data needed to generate an image. To first order, the image contrast resulting from this scheme is determined by the TE of

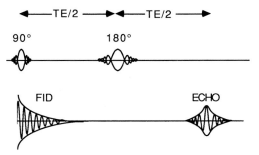

FIGURE 1–37. Simplified diagram of spin-echo pulse sequence.

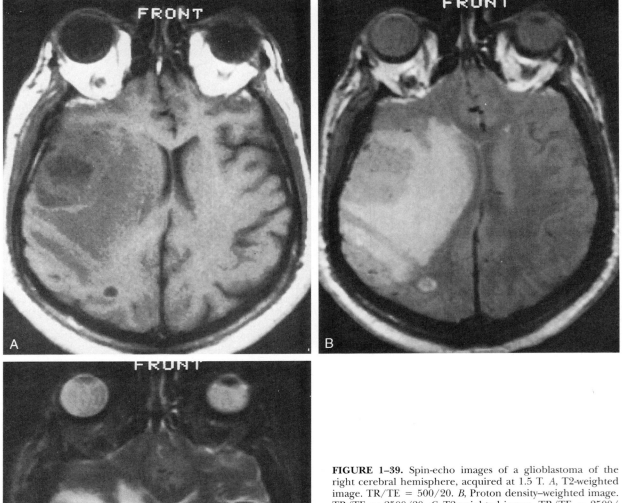

FIGURE 1–39. Spin-echo images of a glioblastoma of the right cerebral hemisphere, acquired at 1.5 T. *A*, T2-weighted image. TR/TE = 500/20. *B*, Proton density–weighted image. TR/TE = 2500/20. *C*, T2-weighted image. TR/TE = 2500/80. Note signal changes of fat, cerebrospinal fluid, normal brain, cystic tumor, and surrounding edema. Also note that signal is absent from the cortical bone in the inner and outer tables of the skull but that signal is present in the marrow-containing diploic space.

the echoes acquired with the weakest phase-encoding gradients. Scan times are reduced by a factor equal to the number of encoded echoes. Typically, from 4 to 16 echoes are encoded, giving a reduction in scan time by a factor of 4 to 16. The reduction in scan time is half as much if both proton density– and T2-weighted images are reconstructed from the same data. Fast spin-echo images are typically acquired in just a few minutes, compared with 10 minutes or longer using conventional spin echo. In many applications, particularly for head, spine, and pelvic imaging, fast spin-echo sequences have replaced their conventional counterpart.

However, there can be significant contrast differences between conventional and fast spin-echo techniques. For instance, fat often appears brighter with fast spin echo than with conventional spin echo (particularly with short interecho spacing), and susceptibility effects in hemorrhage may be more difficult to detect. Fast spin-echo and other fast imaging sequences are considered further in Chapters 4 and 10.

GRADIENT ECHO

Gradient-echo pulse sequences bearing abbreviations such as FLASH, GRASS, and FISP* use only a single RF pulse, as represented by

$$\alpha\text{-TE-(gradient echo)}$$

where α is an RF pulse with a flip angle that is usually less than 90°. Despite their simple structure, gradient-echo pulse sequences produce images with complex contrast behavior, a phenomenon considered in depth in Chapter 10. We consider only a few of the major features here—those related to the use of a reduced excitation flip angle and the absence of a 180° refocusing RF pulse:

1. Unlike conventional spin-echo pulse sequences, which use a 90° flip angle for excitation, for gradient-echo imaging the flip angle may be freely varied. By using an extremely small flip angle, the longitudinal magnetization is only slightly perturbed (see Fig. 1–7), so spins can almost fully remagnetize between RF pulses, even with short TR. As a result, faster imaging is possible than with spin-echo sequences. The flip angle controls the degree of T1 contrast in these studies: lowering the flip angle reduces the amount of longitudinal magnetization that must recover and thus decreases any differences that might be due to tissues having different T1 values. Increasing the flip angle tends to increase this difference. Thus, low flip angle studies tend to use density weighting, whereas higher flip angle studies tend to use T1 weighting.

Although the reduced flip angle provides less signal per measurement than a 90° RF pulse, when short TR values are used, this is more than compensated for by the larger number of signals that are measured per second. With gradient-echo techniques, high-quality scans can be obtained in as little as 1 second. This feature can be useful for the imaging of dynamic processes, such as cardiac motion, contrast enhancement, and blood flow, and for the reduction of motion artifact.

2. Because gradient-echo sequences lack a refocusing RF pulse, images generated with these sequences are sensitive to effects of static magnetic field inhomogeneities (i.e., T2* effects). This increases both artifacts and potentially useful biologic information. Hemorrhage and calcification produce variations in local magnetic field homogeneity (magnetic susceptibility effects), leading to localized signal loss on gradient-echo scans. This signal behavior often improves the detectability of these lesions. It has been proposed that phase-sensitive gradient-echo imaging can distinguish calcified from iron-containing lesions, because calcium is diamagnetic and produces a negative phase shift whereas iron is paramagnetic and produces a positive phase shift.[54] On the other hand, air-tissue and tissue-bone interfaces decrease T2* as well, so that T2* imaging tends to be used in only special cases.

3. The signal from flowing blood is increased compared with that of conventional spin-echo sequences (see Chapter 9). This property is utilized for the production of cardiac cineangiograms and MR angiograms.

INVERSION RECOVERY

One way to produce images with dramatic differences associated with T1 is to prepare the magnetization before the spin-echo portion of the sequence with an additional, 180° pulse. Because this pulse acts when the spins are predominantly longitudinal, it rotates the spins from the $+z$ axis all the way to the $-z$ axis. This "inversion" of the magnetization and its subsequent recovery dictates the contrast in these *inversion recovery* (IR) images:

$$180°\text{-TI-}90°\text{-TE/2-}180°\text{-TE/2-(spin echo)}$$

The waiting period, called the *inversion time* (TI) allows the protons to remagnetize, which they do at rates that depend on T1. After this waiting period, an MR signal is produced using a spin-echo pulse sequence, although more commonly using a fast spin-echo readout for reduced scan times.

Unlike T1-weighted spin-echo sequences, the IR sequence usually uses a long TR to allow tissue to remagnetize fully between RF pulses. T1 contrast thus develops during the interval TI. Tissues with short T1 remagnetize quickly and produce a strong signal when the 90° RF pulse is applied. However, tissues with long T1 remagnetize less during the TI interval and, unless TI is quite short, produce a weak signal (Fig. 1–40).

Magnitude Reconstruction Versus Phase-Sensitive Reconstruction

The level of T1 contrast obtained with IR images also depends on whether the images are sensitive to the phase of the MR signal (Fig. 1–41). Most MR systems generate IR images that are insensitive to the phase of the signal. On these *magnitude images*, information about whether the longitudinal component of **M** is positive or negative is lost. As a result, M_z can vary between 0 and 1. Some systems actually produce *phase-sensitive images*, which can depict whether M_z is positive or negative. As a result, M_z can vary from -1 to 0 to 1; that is, the dynamic range for T1 contrast is doubled (Fig. 1–42). However, these phase-sensitive images are more sensitive to image distortions produced by motion or magnetic field inhomogeneity. This problem can be partially eliminated by phase correction algorithms, which are available on some MR systems.

Short-Tau Inversion Recovery for Fat Suppression and Additive T1 and T2 Contrast

The IR sequence with the greatest clinical use is the STIR sequence. STIR offers two general benefits that

---

*FLASH = fast low-angle shot; GRASS = gradient-recalled acquisition in the steady state; FISP = fast-imaging with steady-state precession.

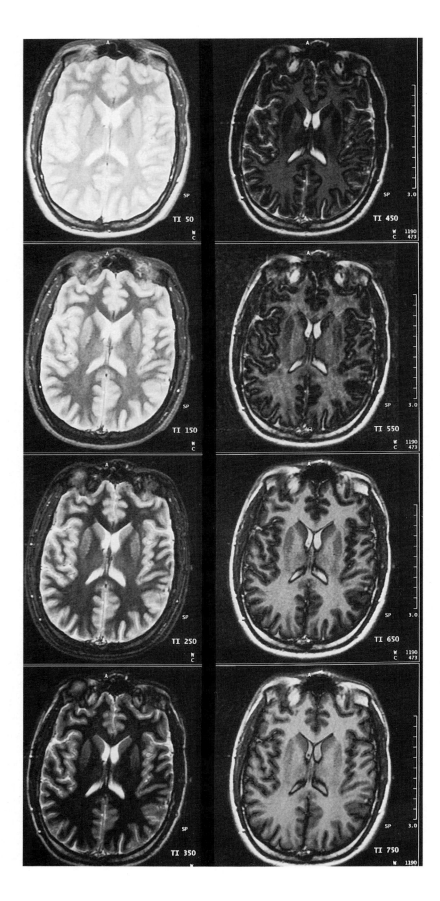

FIGURE 1–40. Inversion recovery images. By progressively increasing the inversion time TI, signals from increasingly long T1 are first attenuated (null) and then recover. (Courtesy of D. Kaufman, Siemens Medical Systems, Iselin, NJ.)

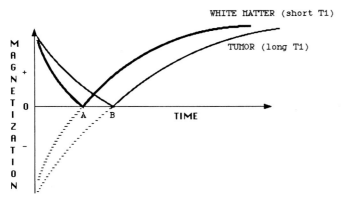

FIGURE 1–41. Longitudinal magnetization versus time after 180° RF pulse in an inversion recovery pulse sequence. For each tissue, there is an inversion time (A and B), which results in negligible signal from that tissue. Phase-sensitive image *(dashed line)* retains sign of magnetization and may result in improved tissue contrast.

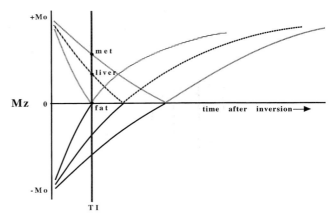

FIGURE 1–43. Illustration of STIR contrast for fat, liver, and a metastasis (met). Immediately after the 180° pulse in an IR sequence, M_z for all tissues is negative. The longitudinal magnetization recovers according to the T1 of each tissue. If a short T1 is used (e.g., 150 ms), then M_z of fat is near zero and its signal is nulled. M_z for other tissues is still negative. However, a magnitude reconstruction displays only positive signals, so the curves are reflected above the zero line. As a result, the contrast relationships are reversed and the metastasis appears brighter than the liver. The lesion-liver signal difference is further improved by the addition of T2 weighting.

are described in the following: 1) fat suppression and 2) positive T1 and T2 contrast.

The fat suppression aspect relies on the principle that the longitudinal magnetization of any tissue, in crossing from a negative to a positive value, must pass through zero (Fig. 1–43). If the MR signal is read out when the magnetization is near zero, little or no signal should be produced. This condition allows signal from a selected tissue to be eliminated based on its T1 relaxation time. The appropriate choice of TI depends on TR and T1. If a tissue is fully magnetized (i.e., TR is long), the null occurs at TI = 0.69 × T1. For fat, which has the shortest T1 of any commonly imaged tissue constituent, this TI is quite short, on the order of 150 ms, although the precise value depends on the

choice of TR and the field strength–dependent value of T1. By suppressing the normally intense signal from fat, STIR greatly increases the conspicuity of lesions that are embedded in fat, such as lymph nodes, edema in the bone marrow, breast parenchyma, and multiple sclerosis plaques in the optic nerve. In the abdomen, the method reduces artifacts caused by respiratory motion by eliminating the bright band of abdominal fat that is usually responsible for these artifacts. Because of the short TI, on STIR images, tissues with long T1 relaxation times (e.g., metastases) appear brighter than tissues with shorter T1 relaxation times (e.g., liver) (see Fig. 1–43). Unlike other fat suppression techniques in which frequency-selective pulses are applied (see later), STIR is not dependent on a high degree of B_0 homogeneity for effective fat suppression. On the other hand, STIR cannot necessarily distinguish the short T1 of fat from the short T1 of a subacute hemorrhage (e.g., to distinguish fat in a teratoma from blood in an endometrioma), as they are both equally suppressed. This distinction is trivial with chemical-shift–selective pulses.

The contrast relationships seen in T1-weighted spin-echo imaging are reversed with STIR. The reversal arises from the fact that using the magnitude reconstruction (the norm), large negative values of M_z appear as positive signals (see Fig. 1–43). Thus, for any tissue that remains inverted at TI (i.e., below $M_z = 0$), shortening T1 decreases signal intensity. Thus, a lesion with a long T1, such as a metastasis, remagnetizes less in the TI interval than does normal tissue, such as liver. When the magnitude of the signals is reconstructed, the more negative M_z from the metastasis translates into a more positive (and hence brighter) signal in the final image. If one also uses a long TE, this further increases the signal intensity of the lesion

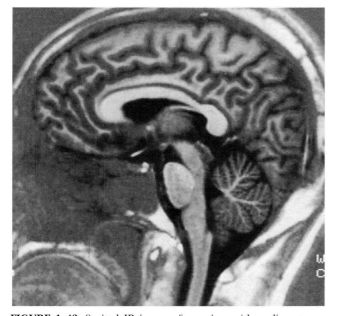

FIGURE 1–42. Sagittal IR image of a patient with a clivus tumor, using phase-sensitive reconstruction. Note excellent T1 contrast, as seen in differentiation of gray and white matter. Also note that background (signal near zero) appears gray. Cerebrospinal fluid (long T1) appears black, and fat (short T1) appears bright.

compared with that of normal tissue. Thus, T1 contrast and T2 contrast are additive with STIR imaging. However, STIR is not necessarily a good sequence for detecting contrast enhancement, because the decreased T1 caused by the agent actually decreases signal intensity rather than increasing it and thus does not necessarily improve lesion conspicuity.

Fluid-Attenuated Inversion Recovery

A second application of IR is at the other end of the T1 spectrum, choosing a TI to null fluids, which tend to have the longest T1 values of the visible tissue constituents. For example, the T1 of cerebrospinal fluid is several seconds, and thus to null its signal a long TI (e.g., 1.5 to 2 seconds) must be used. Because the T1 of most lesions is much shorter than that of cerebrospinal fluid, M_z recovers well past the null point over the long TI interval. Therefore, lesions appear bright against a background of dark cerebrospinal fluid. This variant of IR is called fluid-attenuated IR (FLAIR). Because the signal from cerebrospinal fluid can mask the signal from lesions adjoining the cerebral ventricles or the spinal cord, the fluid-attenuated IR sequence can increase lesion sensitivity. This feature may be particularly useful for detection of multiple sclerosis plaques. Because all other tissues have shorter T1, when fluid is at the null point, the other tissues are not inverted (i.e., $M_z > 0$). Thus, unlike the situation in STIR imaging, T1 contrast behaves like a conventional spin echo: shorter T1 corresponds to brighter images than long T1.

Fat-, Water-, and Silicone-Selective Imaging

In some cases, one chemical species is clinically more interesting and the elimination of other moieties would improve the diagnostic image quality. Because the protons have slightly different frequencies, it is possible to image selectively (or suppress selectively) one chemical species. Alternatively, the relaxation property of one species relative to another may also be exploited, as done with fat.[55] These techniques are generally selective based on either the T1 relaxation time (STIR) or the chemical shift (chemical-shift–selective imaging, phase contrast, two- and three-point Dixon techniques).

STIR, which was just described, can provide robust fat suppression. However, there are several limitations to the use of IR for fat suppression. First, image contrast is substantially altered compared with that for typical sequences, and the S/N ratio tends to be lower for the same imaging time. Second, because of the reversal of the normal contrast relationships with STIR sequences, contrast enhancement with gadolinium chelates may actually cause a decrease rather than an increase in tissue signal. Finally, the technique does not readily distinguish between fat and tissues with short T1 associated with subacute hemorrhage or melanin.

The other techniques are based on the chemical shift differences between moieties. For example, fat protons and water protons have different resonance frequencies. There is a dominant fat peak associated with methylene ($-CH_2-$) protons at a frequency approximately 3.5 ppm lower than that of water protons, corresponding to a frequency shift of 220 Hz at 1.5 T. ("Fat" actually has a complex spectrum, with contributions from methyl, vinyl, and other lipid constituents.[56]) As another example, frequencies of the dimethylsiloxy units $[-Si(CH_3)_2-O-]_n$ of silicone breast implants are shifted even lower, approximately 80 Hz lower than that of fat at 1.5 T.

There are two general ways to generate chemical selectivity based on these frequency shifts: 1) selective excitation or saturation and 2) phase-sensitive reconstruction.

By using an appropriate pulse sequence,[57] one can selectively image or suppress the signals from water, fat, or silicone. The signal intensity of fat, water, or silicone can be selectively suppressed by applying an RF pulse, called a chemical-shift–selective pulse, tuned to the proper frequency. For instance, a narrow-band RF pulse at 220 Hz below the water frequency will, at 1.5 T, excite the fat resonance without exciting the water resonance. By dephasing these spins before the regular frequency-selective slice selection, one generates a fat-suppressed image. (At 1 T the pulse would be at 140 Hz below the resonance frequency.) Long RF pulses are used to keep the bandwidth of the RF pulse narrow enough (e.g., ≤ 100 Hz) to avoid overlapping the water resonance. These pulses can have complex, computer-optimized shapes or be as simple as a series of RF pulses, called binomial pulses, with an amplitude ratio that follows Pascal's triangle. In all cases, the net effect of this RF pulse is to tilt the fat magnetization into the transverse plane, where it can be eliminated by a spoiler gradient, while keeping the water magnetization along the longitudinal axis, where it is unaffected by the spoiler gradient.

The main limitations of fat suppression are related to B_0 and B_1 field inhomogeneities. Because the chemical-shift difference simply makes the spins resonate at the slightly different magnetic field, imperfections in the static field (B_0) can mimic the frequency shifts caused by chemistry. That is, nonuniformity of the order of 3.5 ppm will cause the fat suppression pulses to saturate fat protons in some regions and water protons in other regions. This is especially a problem away from the isocenter of the magnet (e.g., for shoulder imaging or for body imaging with large slice shifts) or near air-tissue or bone-tissue interfaces (e.g., skull base, near paranasal sinuses).[58] "Shimming" (deliberate adjustment of the magnetic field to make it more uniform) on a patient-by-patient basis is helpful, although it may not be possible to shim adequately across the entire volume of interest. For example, perfect shimming across the entire abdomen or across the entire head is not likely. As a result, the tradeoff of improved conspicuity in some regions for (variable) suppression of desired signal can be a complex one. For instance, in MR angiography fat suppression may be effective locally but may cause water suppression elsewhere, thus saturating inflowing blood.

In addition to static field inhomogeneity, nonuniformity of the RF excitation field (B_1) causes the flip angle of the fat saturation pulse to vary across the image, resulting in variable degrees of fat suppression. Even modest B_1 inhomogeneity can dramatically limit the effectiveness of fat suppression; for example, a 20% variation in B_1 limits fat suppression to about a factor of 3.

Instead of trying to suppress the signal intensity of fat, one can selectively excite water protons. Selective water excitation often gives more uniform results than fat suppression, because the fat signal is absent regardless of the B_1 field inhomogeneities. (This happens because the water excitation pulse acts as a 0° pulse for fat. Zero multiplied by anything is still zero.) For whole-volume 3D imaging, a nonselective RF pulse can be applied at the f_L to selectively excite water protons. For slice-selective imaging, the situation is more complex. The difficulty is that slice selection is performed by using a selective excitation RF pulse as well; the slice-selection gradient translates the band of frequencies into a slice. One proposed solution is to generate a different kind of slice-select pulse, called a *spatial-spectral* pulse, that excites a narrow band of chemical species within a spatial slice. These are composite RF pulses, applied with a time-varying slice-selection gradient, that are selective in both position and frequency[59] (Fig. 1–44).

Instead of selectively suppressing or exciting the spins of interest, it is also possible to use phase information to distinguish species. Phase-contrast gradient-echo imaging is an example of this strategy. To understand these methods, imagine first that one is imaging with a gradient-echo pulse sequence and the signal is measured immediately after the RF excitation (i.e., TE = 0); the transverse magnetization vectors of fat and water signals would then be precessing coherently, that is, in phase. In this case, the fat and water signals from protons residing in the same voxel would be additive. Because water protons precess 3.5 ppm more rapidly than fat protons, over time the phase of the water protons would advance with respect to the fat protons. At a certain time after excitation, the transverse magnetization vectors of the water and fat protons would be 180° out of phase, resulting in signal cancellation and an out-of-phase or opposed image. (At 1.0 T this time = $1/(3.5 \times 42.6 \text{ Hz})/2 = 3.4$ ms.) The water and fat signals thus oscillate in and out of phase with a periodicity (ΔTE) determined by the magnetic field strength according to

$$\Delta TE = 3.4 \text{ ms}/B_0 \text{ (in tesla)} \qquad (11)$$

When TE is equal to an even multiple of ΔTE, the fat and water signals are in phase, whereas images acquired at odd multiples of ΔTE show signal loss caused by fat-water phase contrast. For instance, at 1.5 T a TE of 2.2 ms gives an opposed image and a TE of 4.5 ms an in-phase image. At 1.0 T the corresponding out-of-phase and in-phase TE values are 3.4 and 6.8 ms. Fat-water signal modulation does not occur with spin-echo pulse sequences because of the refocusing effect of the 180° pulse.

Opposed images are readily identified by dark borders surrounding organs at fat-water interfaces. This artifact is not limited to the frequency-encoding direction, as is the case for the usual chemical-shift artifact seen with both spin-echo and in-phase gradient-echo sequences.

Phase-contrast gradient-echo images (not to be confused with the entirely different phase-contrast imaging used for flow quantification or angiography) can be acquired in just a few seconds. Use of phase-contrast imaging is helpful for detection of fat-water mixtures, as in fatty infiltration of the liver, fat in an adrenal adenoma, and differentiation of normal red bone marrow (fat-water mixture) from infiltrated marrow (mostly water). Phase-contrast imaging would not be useful for detection of fat occupying an entire voxel, such as fat in a lipoma or teratoma, because the modulation comes from the destructive interference of the fat and water in the same voxel (Fig. 1–45).

The phase-contrast method is at the heart of the more quantitative two- and three-point Dixon techniques. In these methods, the goal is to create completely separate fat and water images.[60] Both of these methods depend on using a spin-echo sequence in which the 180° pulse is moved slightly. This makes the spin echo shift relative to the center of the readout. As a result, the spins acquire some net phase because of their frequency differences. That is, when the 180° pulse is moved from TE/2 to (TE − Δ)/2 (i.e., by a time Δ/2), the spin echo shifts earlier by a time Δ. The net effect is to add gradient echo–like contrast during the extra Δ. Fat and water become out of phase by ($\Delta\sigma\gamma B_0$) radians, where σ is the chemical shift of 3.5 ppm.

For the two-point method, one acquires two spin-echo images with different offsets to produce a phase shift of 180° between the fat and water signals. The offset Δ is determined by the main field strength according to

$$\Delta = 3.4 \text{ ms}/B_0 \text{ (T)} \qquad (12)$$

where, as before, Δ is half the time the 180° is shifted. The similarity of this equation to the one given previously for phase-contrast gradient-echo imaging is no coincidence; the whole idea of the Dixon technique is to add gradient-echo contrast into the spin echo, and the physics is the same.

Complex addition and subtraction of these two images ideally give pure fat and water images. Unfortunately, local magnetic field variations cause errors in fat-water separation, particularly because of the inability to discern, in any given voxel, which species is fat and which is water. To help eliminate this problem, a three-point Dixon technique was proposed in which an additional image with a 360° phase shift is acquired. In this image, fat and water are again in phase, so that any phase accumulation comes from the net voxel frequency shift related to B_0 field inhomogeneities. This technique produces three images—a fat image, a water image, and a B_0 field map—and largely elimi-

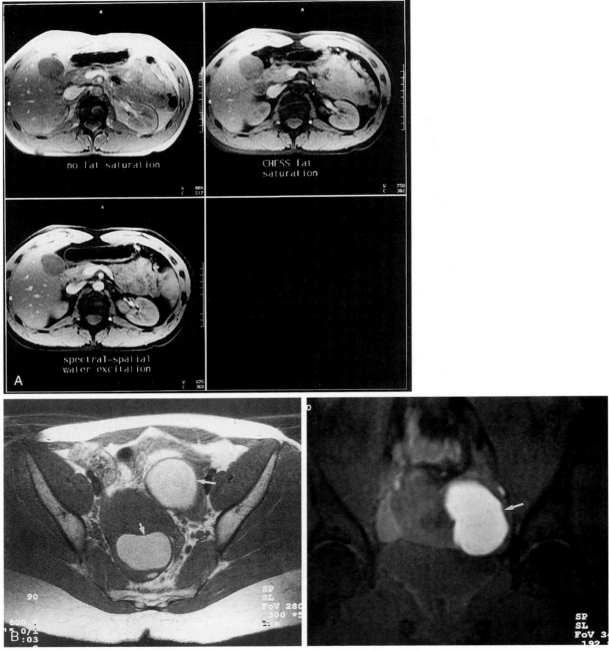

FIGURE 1–44. Fat suppression. *A,* Abdominal MR image without (upper left, gradient echo, TR/TE/FA = 40/8/30°) and with (upper right) fat saturation, both in body phased-array coil. In an unsuppressed image, the aortic signal is bright because of rapid inflow of unsaturated blood. For the image at the upper right binomial fat suppression was used. Suppression in plane is effective, but fat saturation behaves like water saturation in some other planes. For example, inadvertent water saturation near the heart due to field inhomogeneity causes the aortic signal to be suppressed, which is undesirable for MR angiography. The image at the lower left shows the improvement obtained by selectively exciting water (rather than fat suppression), in this case using a spatial-spectral excitation for slice selection, improving in-plane fat suppression and preserving the inflow signal in the aorta. *B,* Use of fat suppression to differentiate blood products from fat, both of which can be bright on T1-weighted images. *Left,* T1-weighted axial image showing two hemorrhagic endometriomas *(arrows)* that appear bright. *Right,* On a fat-suppressed coronal image, the hemorrhagic lesion appears bright *(arrow).* In contrast, the fatty signal from a dermoid cyst would have been suppressed.

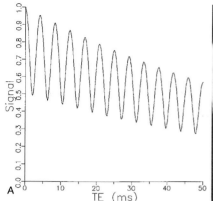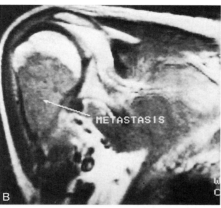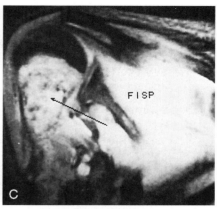

FIGURE 1–45. *A,* Calculated signal intensity versus TE at 1.5 T in a gradient-echo image of simulated marrow consisting of 75% fat and 25% water. The oscillations in the signal intensity are due to a slight difference between the resonance frequencies of fat and water (i.e., chemical shift). *B* and *C,* Patient with oat cell metastasis to right humeral shaft. Gradient-echo images are sensitive to bone marrow abnormalities such as metastatic lesions. On T1-weighted SE image *(B),* normal marrow appears bright and metastasis appears dark. On proton density–weighted gradient-echo image *(C),* marrow appears dark and metastasis appears bright.

nates errors in fat-water separation. It is also an effective technique for making silicone-only images in patients with breast implants.[61]

STIMULATED ECHOES

Although they are rarely used in current clinical practice, there is more to spin echoes than the simple echo produced from two RF pulses. For instance, when three RF pulses are applied, there is the potential for a signal to be created, called a *stimulated echo*. The first RF pulse tilts a component of the longitudinal magnetization into the transverse plane. The second RF pulse drives the transverse magnetization into a longitudinal orientation along the negative z axis, storing in the amplitude of the longitudinal magnetization the result of the dephasing. The third RF pulse tilts the longitudinal magnetization from the z axis back into the transverse plane again and generates the stimulated echo signal. If the time between the first two pulses is TE/2, the echo occurs at a time TE/2 after the third pulse. (Note that there is an echo that comes from the first two pulses, but that is the "standard" spin echo.) The stimulated echo has some interesting properties: 1) The magnetization is stored along the z axis after the first two RF pulses, where it is subject to T1, but not T2, relaxation. Therefore, one can wait for hundreds of milliseconds before applying the third RF pulse and still obtain a measurable signal (except for tissues with short T1, such as fat). 2) The phase of the FID after the first RF pulse is preserved in the stimulated echo, even if the echo is acquired hundreds of milliseconds later. 3) Only a maximum of half of the original longitudinal magnetization comes back in the echo, so the S/N ratio is lower than for a gradient or spin echo.

Stimulated echoes are not for general clinical use; more often, they are a source of image artifacts (see Chapter 3). Because many RF pulses are applied in the course of acquiring an image, there is always the potential for generating stimulated echoes. In fact, stimulated echoes are largely unavoidable and routinely alter image contrast in fast spin-echo sequences (see Chapter 4). However, stimulated echoes do have their applications. For instance, the stimulated echo acquisition method is used for single-voxel proton spectroscopy (see Chapter 30) and diffusion-weighted imaging (see Chapter 8) and may be the only way to generate certain quantitative images of moving organs.

SUMMARY OF PULSE SEQUENCES

Because of the simple contrast behavior of spin-echo pulse sequences and the relative insensitivity to various sources of image artifacts, spin-echo methods are routinely used in clinical practice. Particularly for T2-weighted acquisitions, fast spin-echo sequences have, for many sites, replaced conventional spin echo because of the severalfold reduction in scan time. Fast spin echo has also allowed a resurgence of IR methods that previously seemed too costly in time (long TR) for clinical practice. However, with the advent of fast spin-echo imaging, IR acquisitions can be completed in just a few minutes. STIR has proved especially useful for showing bone marrow edema and for detecting lymphadenopathy, and fluid-attenuated inversion recovery improves detection of demyelinating lesions in the brain and spinal cord. Finally, gradient-echo methods have proved invaluable for specific applications, such as fast imaging and imaging of calcifications and hemorrhage, and for high-resolution 3D applications (MR angiography, joint studies, morphologic studies).

INTRODUCTION TO MR IMAGE QUALITY

In this section, we introduce some of the concepts important for understanding MR image quality. Because of the vast flexibility of the MR scanner, it is simple to ask for combinations of scanning parameters that are guaranteed to produce poor image quality. The goal of this section is to discuss some of the MR imaging parameters and how they affect image quality.

BASIC CONCEPTS

Spatial resolution, contrast-to-noise (C/N) ratio, and S/N ratio are all critical parameters that determine the likelihood of detecting pathologic changes on MR images. All these parameters also interact with each other and with the total examination time.

Spatial resolution, which seems intuitively a simple concept, is actually quite difficult to define in general in diagnostic imaging (e.g., is it the size of the smallest lesion one would confidently identify? Is it the size of the smallest pixel on the displayed image? How do imaging artifacts like Gibb's ringing or motion of the patient affect it?). In MRI, for simplicity we usually define the spatial resolution simply in terms of the FOV and the matrix size:

$$\text{Pixel} = \text{FOV}/\text{matrix} \qquad (13)$$

For a long-T2 object that is perfectly stationary, this pixel size is pretty close to the more rigorous definitions of resolution as well.

The ease with which a signal can be detected in a voxel is often measured in terms of the ratio of the proton signal in the voxel to its noise. The noise, in this case, means approximately what you would see on the image if there were no protons in the voxel. (A better definition is that if you imaged the same object many times, the noise would be the fluctuation in the measurements in that voxel). The ratio of the signal to these fluctuations is the S/N ratio. To first order, the lower the S/N ratio the grainier the image appears.

In MRI, just about everything affects the S/N ratio. However, a useful (and not too oversimplified) expression for S/N is

$$\text{S/N} = k(\text{proton density})(\text{voxel volume}) \\ (\text{magnetization})\sqrt{\text{time}} \qquad (14)$$

where k is a sensitivity constant related to the coil (see later section on instrumentation). The next two terms represent the number of imageable protons in the volume; the total signal depends on the presence of these protons. The term "magnetization" depends strongly on the pulse sequence and the underlying biology (e.g., T2, T1, and flow) and includes nearly all of the important effects that produce image contrast. It is the fraction of the total magnetization that the given sequence elicits. (A spin-echo sequence with extremely short TE and extremely long TR elicits nearly 100% of the total magnetization; shallow flip angle, short-TR sequences would elicit far less.) The product of the first three terms is thus the amount of magnetization produced by the sequence within the voxel: the signal.

The last term represents the noise. The primary source of noise in nearly all clinical scanners is the patient's body itself. The random, thermal motion of the conductive ions in the body produces this noise. For all practical purposes, this noise is "white"; that is, it is uniformly distributed throughout the image, causing the same absolute amount of graininess across all objects in the same image. For many kinds of noise, the amount of noise relative to the signal decreases as the square root of the averaging time. That is, quadrupling the time during which the signal is measured doubles the resulting S/N ratio. Thus, this last term, which deals more with the noise part of the S/N ratio, is increased by increasing the number of averages (NEX) as well as by decreasing the bandwidth of the receiver. (Figure 1–46 gives an example of the increase in S/N ratio resulting from increasing the number of averages.)

Perhaps more important for diagnostic imaging than the S/N ratio is the related concept of C/N ratio. Whereas the S/N ratio is related to the ease of detection of some signal, the C/N ratio is related to the detectability of differences between the voxels of different tissues. It is this difference (i.e., the contrast) that is at the heart of diagnostic imaging. For simplicity, we can define the C/N ratio as the difference between the S/N ratios of two different tissues under the same imaging sequence. Thus, it is possible to increase the C/N ratio between two tissues even if their respective S/N ratios are lower. In fact, this is the general case in MRI: it usually costs signal to gain contrast.

We now discuss in greater depth S/N ratio, resolution, and C/N ratio.

INTERACTION OF SPATIAL RESOLUTION AND SIGNAL-TO-NOISE RATIO

In this section we discuss the factors that determine spatial resolution. As described earlier, the resolution is the FOV divided by the matrix size. For instance, with a 25 × 25-cm FOV and 256 × 256 matrix, the pixel dimensions would be 1 × 1 mm. The FOV represents the horizontal or vertical distance from one side of the image to the opposite side. For body imaging, the typical FOV might be 32 to 50 cm, whereas for head imaging the FOV would be smaller, on the order of 16 to 24 cm. In some applications, such as imaging of the temporomandibular joint (TMJ), FOV less than 12 cm is preferred. The FOV is typically reduced by increasing the strengths of the phase-encoding and frequency-encoding gradients.

As we see from our master S/N equation, the resolution directly affects S/N ratio. For instance, imagine comparing a TMJ image with an abdominal one—for example, a body with a 36-cm FOV and 6-mm slices and TMJ with a 12-cm FOV and 3-mm slices, both with 256×256 matrices. The voxel size of the body image is thus 18 times larger, and if we used the same coil the S/N ratio would be 18 times lower for the TMJ image. The primary reason in MRI (as opposed to CT, for instance) for the complication of the abundance of special-purpose coils is that there is insufficient S/N ratio to image the TMJ at the required resolution

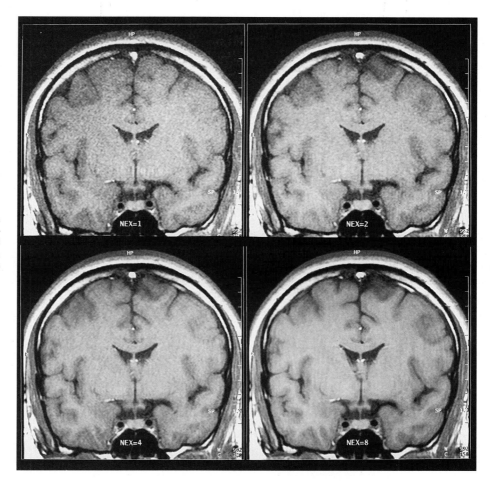

FIGURE 1–46. Effect of averaging on image S/N and C/N ratios. NEX (number of averages) increases from 1 to 8 going from upper left to lower right. (Courtesy of D. Kaufman, Siemens Medical Systems, Iselin, NJ.)

using the body coil. We could use averaging, but because the S/N ratio goes as the square root of the time, it would require $18 \times 18 = 324$ NEX (i.e., forever!) to achieve the same S/N ratio as the large voxels.

In many MR systems, an asymmetric (rectangular) FOV can be selected. The FOV is reduced asymmetrically by increasing the amplitude of the phase-encoding gradient without changing the amplitude of the frequency-encoding gradient. The distance across the image is then smaller in the y direction than in the x direction. Compared with a symmetric FOV, the asymmetric FOV provides greater spatial resolution along one direction, because the same number of pixels now spans a smaller distance. The main drawbacks of an asymmetric FOV are reduced S/N ratio (smaller voxel) and more risk of wraparound artifact along the phase-encoding direction.

The matrix size represents the number of pixels in the x and y directions. A variety of matrix sizes are available on commercial systems. If the FOV is symmetric in x and y, then equal resolution in both directions is provided by a 256×256 matrix. For the same FOV, spatial resolution can be improved by increasing the matrix size (e.g., to 512×512), but this is at the expense of longer scan times and lower S/N ratios. How much lower? The pixel volume is reduced by a factor of 4, but the scan time is increased by a factor of 2, so the net reduction in S/N ratio is $4/\sqrt{2} \approx 2.8$.

Conversely, to reduce scan time, the number of phase-encoded projections can be decreased. An image can be acquired with a rectangular 256×128 (x, y) matrix in half as much time as with a 256×256 matrix; however, the spatial resolution in the y direction is reduced by half; the S/N ratio in each voxel is increased by $\sqrt{2}$: the voxel size is increased by 2, but the scan time is reduced by a factor of 2.

It is important not to confuse the acquisition matrix with the display matrix. For instance, images may be interpolated for display onto a 512×512 or 1024×1024 pixel matrix, whether the image is acquired using a 256×256, 256×128, or other size matrix. It is the true acquisition matrix in MRI that determines the S/N ratio and resolution.

Theoretically, the ultimate in-plane spatial resolution that can be obtained on an MR image is high (<0.01 mm). For human imaging, however, pulse sequence design, gradient limitations, S/N ratio, and considerations related to the patient place the practical lower limit of spatial resolution at a few tenths of a millimeter.

CONTRAST AND SIGNAL-TO-NOISE RATIO ON SPIN-ECHO IMAGES

As noted previously, a tissue's image brightness is directly proportional to the strength of the MR signal arising from that tissue. Consequently, for different tissues to be distinguished on an MR image, they must have different image brightnesses. This concept is expressed in the term *contrast*, which represents the difference in signal intensities between two or more tissues. As already mentioned, it is not the contrast but the contrast compared with the noise that is generally important for lesion detection. (In reality, the complexities of visual recognition can make it difficult to quantify the relative importance of contrast, S/N ratio, and spatial resolution.[62] For instance, one study has suggested that, in some situations, S/N ratio improvements beyond a certain level may not help in lesion detection, and a reduction in pixel size may become more important.[63] However, for simplicity, we generally talk about the C/N ratio achievable between two tissues.)

A number of factors affect MR image contrast. They can be divided into two basic groups: 1) factors intrinsic to tissue and 2) extrinsic, operator-dependent factors. Principal intrinsic factors include proton density, T1, and T2. Extrinsic factors include the two principal pulse sequence variables: TR and TE. Manipulation of these extrinsic parameters is necessary to maximize image contrast.

The strength of the signal from a given tissue is proportional to the product of three weighting terms: 1) the proton density (ρ); 2) a T1-weighting term, which is a function of T1 and TR; and 3) a T2-weighting term, which is a function of T2 and TE. By weighting we mean the influence of a given term on image contrast, attributable to differences in ρ, T1, or T2. For spin-echo imaging, this relationship is expressed approximately by the following equation:

$$\text{Signal} = \rho[1 - \exp(-TR/T1)] \times [\exp(-TE/T2)] \qquad (15)$$

Many other terms "tweak" this expression, several of which are subjects of entire chapters in this book: flow, diffusions, and so forth. However, for simplicity here, we consider only ρ, T1, and T2.)

Proton Density–Weighted Images

As previously mentioned, the proton densities of various tissues tend to differ far less than T1 or T2. The best way to produce a proton density–weighted image is thus to minimize T1 and T2 weighting by using a spin-echo sequence with long TR and short TE or a gradient-echo sequence with a low flip angle. It should be noted that, because of the slightly greater ρ of tumors and other lesions, differences in ρ tend to oppose contrast on T1-weighted images and enhance contrast on T2-weighted images.

T1-Weighted Images

Contrast resulting from T1 differences (T1 weighting) is increased as TR is reduced because T1 differences then have a greater effect on signal intensity (Fig. 1–47; see Fig. 1–21). For T1-weighted images, the choice of TR is not critical for most tissue compari-

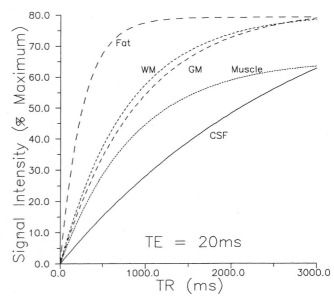

FIGURE 1–47. Calculated signal intensity versus TR for spin-echo pulse sequence. WM = white matter; GM = gray matter.

sons as long as TR is on the order of T1. For most tissues, a choice of TR in the range 300 to 800 ms provides some degree of useful T1 weighting (Fig. 1–48; see Fig. 1–28). However, the difference between contrast and C/N ratio can be illustrated by considering what TR gives the "best" behavior. Figure 1–49*A* shows the MR signal as a function of TR for two hypothetic tissues, one with T1 = 600 ms and one with T1 = 800 ms, with the same ρ. Figure 1–49*B* shows the difference (i.e., contrast) between them. We see that the contrast is maximum at 700 ms, although it is just about the same everywhere between 450 and 1150 ms. The fairly general conclusion is that peak contrast is obtained with TR around the average of the T1 values that we are trying to distinguish.

Is this a fair comparison? For example, it takes twice as long to make a 1000-ms image as a 500-ms one; that is, in the same time, we could perform a scan with two NEX for TR = 500. What happens if we include the effects of this total imaging time? The result for the "equal-time" C/N question is plotted in Figure 1–49*B*. The peak is now closer to 350 ms, although it is fairly flat from 200 to 800 ms. In general, the peak C/N ratio for constant scanning time occurs at about one half the average T1. Thus, we see that the best T1 contrast is obtained by choosing TR somewhat less than the T1 values of the tissues involved. In the brain at 1.5 T this usually means setting TR to approximately 400 to 600 ms. Shorter TR provides relatively little signal; longer TR provides a high signal but no contrast between tissues of different T1 values.

The choice of TE is also important in maintaining T1 contrast: TE should be minimized to reduce the effects of T2 weighting, that is, to minimize the effects of the $\exp(-TE/T2)$ term in the signal equation. However, TE = 0 ms is nearly impossible in a spin-echo image. Therefore, all so-called T1-weighted im-

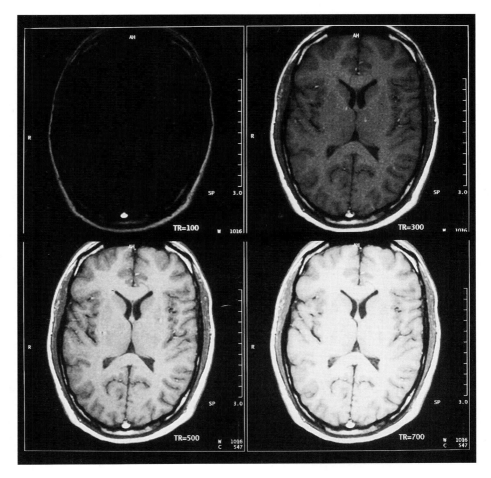

FIGURE 1–48. T1 contrast between gray and white matter and TR. At short TR, there is little signal except from short-T1 species (fat). Increasing TR to 300 and 500 ms increases both signal and contrast. As TR increases further, however, even though the signal increases, contrast between gray and white does not. (Courtesy of D. Kaufman, Siemens Medical Systems, Iselin, NJ.)

ages contain some degree of T2 weighting, which increases as the TE is lengthened. (Furthermore, low-bandwidth techniques are commonly used to improve the S/N ratio, especially on lower field systems. Although the use of low-bandwidth techniques lengthens the minimal TE, the resultant loss of image contrast may be justified by the improvement in image quality.)

T2-Weighted Images

If we eliminate the effects of T1 (e.g., by choosing TR >> T1 for spin-echo sequences), the image contrast is determined solely by the proton-density and T2-weighting terms (Fig. 1–50). The relationship of tissue signal and contrast to TE is depicted in Figure 1–51, which shows the signals as a function of TE for two hypothetic tissues with the same proton density and T2 = 60 and 80 ms. We see that although the tissue signal is highest for both tissues at short TE, the tissue contrast is poor. As the TE is lengthened, differences in T2 produce differences in tissue signal intensities. Therefore, tissue contrast improves as TE is lengthened. However, after a certain point, lengthening TE actually worsens tissue contrast, because all tissue signals become small and their differences may be masked by background noise. In general, the best T2 contrast is obtained when TE is intermediate between the T2 relaxation times of the tissues.

It is impractical with most MRI systems to obtain a purely T2-weighted image, because the TR is then so long that imaging times are unacceptable (unless special techniques, such as echo-planar techniques, are used; see Chapter 10). In practice, to obtain a T2-weighted image, a TR is chosen that gives small amounts of T1 contamination but practical scan times. The choice of TR depends on field strength, because T1 relaxation times increase at higher field strengths. Typical values of TR for a T2-weighted scan at 0.35 T are 2.0 to 2.5 seconds and at 1.5 T are 2.5 to 3.0 seconds.

T1 contamination in T2-weighted scans is particularly problematic because in most tissues changes in T1 and T2 tend to go the same way. That is, if pathologic change lengthens T1, it also lengthens T2. Because T1 weighting makes long-T1 species appear darker and T2 weighting makes long-T2 species appear brighter, adding T1 contrast to the T2 images tends to wash out useful contrast. For this reason, T1 contrast caused by noninfinite TR is often referred to as T1 contamination.

Crossover

When practical values for TR and TE are used in double-echo spin-echo sequences, the type of contrast changes or "crosses over" from the first to the second

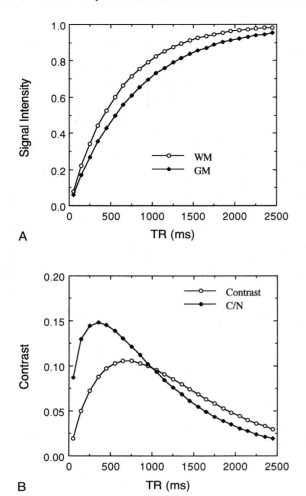

A

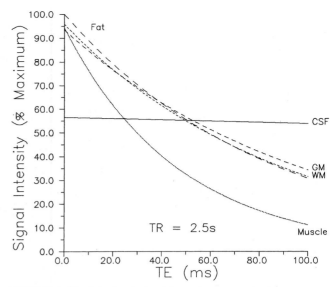

FIGURE 1–50. Calculated signal intensity versus TE for spin-echo pulse sequence. Note that even with long TR not all tissues start with the same signal intensity, owing primarily to residual T1 weighting and, to a lesser extent, differences in proton density.

B

FIGURE 1–49. *A*, Signal (normalized to 1.0) for tissues with T1 = 600 ms (WM) and T1 = 800 ms (GM). *B*, Contrast and C/N ratio for fixed total imaging time. Maximal contrast per image occurs at TR ~ 700 ms, but maximal contrast per time occurs at TR ~ 350 ms.

image contrast, S/N ratio, scan time, the patient's motion, and so on. Many standard protocols have been developed through experience. Examples are presented throughout the clinical chapters of this text and in Appendix I.

OVERVIEW OF HARDWARE

We now present a basic overview of the hardware involved in producing the MR image (Fig. 1–54). Instrumentation is discussed in greater detail in Chapter 14.

echo. Crossover occurs because the long TR used in T2-weighted imaging results in contrast curves that are still partly T1 weighted. At long TE values, T2 contrast becomes the dominant mechanism (Fig. 1–52).

Crossover can be useful for image interpretation because two tissues may have similar signal intensities and be difficult to distinguish at one TE but may have quite different intensities at another TE. For instance, on the first echo of a double-echo spin-echo acquisition, a periventricular multiple sclerosis plaque might be readily distinguished from darker cerebrospinal fluid (Fig. 1–53*A*). However, cerebrospinal fluid appears bright on the more T2-weighted second echo and may obscure the plaque (Fig. 1–53*B*). On the other hand, the second echo may improve the characterization of cystic lesions. Although the optimal choice of TE is seldom known a priori, if one selects a relatively short first TE (e.g., 20 to 30 ms) and a relatively long second TE (e.g., 80 to 90 ms), one can be reasonably assured that one or other of the images will show satisfactory contrast between two tissues.

In summary, MR scanning protocols are usually a compromise among a number of factors related to

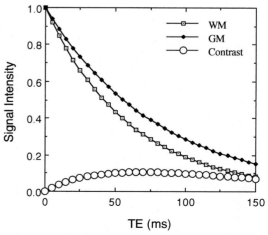

FIGURE 1–51. T2 contrast. Signals and difference (contrast) between two tissues with T2 = 80 ms (GM) and T2 = 60 ms (WM) as a function of TE. Although the peak signal for both tissues occurs at TE = 0, the maximal contrast occurs at TE ~ 70 ms, although it is fairly flat from 50 to 100 ms.

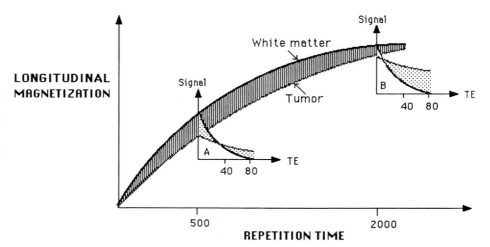

FIGURE 1–52. Crossover. MR images obtained with practical scan parameters always contain some T1 weighting, which is most evident at short TR. Note that the crossover point occurs at relatively long TE in *A* but at shorter TE as the TR is lengthened and T1 weighting diminishes *(B)*.

MAGNETS

The magnets used for clinical MRI range in strength from 0.06 to 2.0 T, where 1 T = 10,000 G. A few whole-body systems have been installed for research into spectroscopy and functional brain imaging with field strengths exceeding 4 T. By comparison, the small magnets used to hold notes on refrigerator doors produce a field of approximately 400 G, and the earth's magnetic field is about 0.5 G. Several types of magnets

are in commercial use. Permanent magnets (Fig. 1–55*A*), which produce field strengths of approximately 0.2 to 0.3 T, are made of special rare earth alloys that can retain strong magnetic fields. Although such magnets were formerly quite massive, newer models are considerably lighter. Permanent magnets are susceptible to ambient temperature changes, so great care must be taken to maintain a constant room temperature.

Electromagnets, on the other hand, require a con-

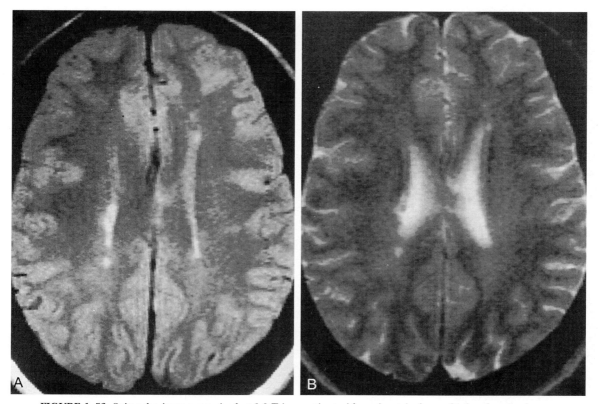

FIGURE 1–53. Spin-echo images acquired at 1.0 T in a patient with periventricular multiple sclerosis plaques. *A*, TR/TE = 2500/30. *B*, TR/TE = 2500/80. Note that the plaques appear brighter than cerebrospinal fluid on the proton density–weighted image but are seen less clearly on the T2-weighted image because of isointensity with cerebrospinal fluid.

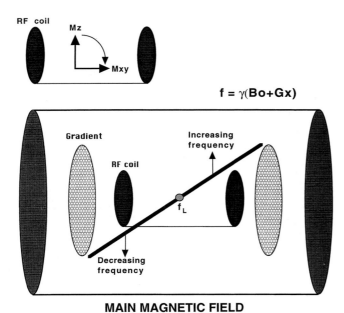

$$f = \gamma(Bo+Gx)$$

MAIN MAGNETIC FIELD
(0.2-1.5 T)

GRADIENT MAGNETIC FIELD
(0-15 mT/m)

FIGURE 1–54. Schematic sketch of the interlocking hardware. The RF coil excites and detects the spins that are imaged; the gradient coil is used to image the spins that are polarized in the MR magnet.

stant input of electrical current. The amount of current increases rapidly with magnetic field strength. Generally, such magnets are limited to less than 0.4 T owing to high power consumption. Permanent magnets and some electromagnets produce fields that are vertical. The stray fields from these magnets are contained within a few feet, simplifying siting requirements.

The more powerful magnets (>0.5 T) use superconducting wire to provide magnetic fields that are usually oriented along the long axis of a cylindric bore. When cooled below their so-called critical temperature (a few degrees above absolute zero), certain alloys, such as niobium-titanium, lose all resistance to the flow of electrical current. Once current is set to flowing, if the magnet is kept cold, the current flows almost indefinitely. Superconducting magnets (Fig. 1–55B) consist of miles of this wire wrapped around a cylinder. To maintain superconductivity, the magnet core is encased in an insulating drum (Dewar) containing liquid helium (at 4 K). Because thermal conductive and convective losses occur, the liquid helium must be regularly replenished. Failure to do so may cause a sudden loss of superconductivity, called a *quench*, which, although not a significant hazard to the patient, may result in costly boil-off of cryogens.[17] Current magnets generally use a chiller pump to keep the inner and outer cryostats (the insulating shields around the Dewar) cold. By keeping the cryostat cold, one can increase the time between expensive helium refills to 1 year or longer.

Each type of magnet has certain advantages. Because the S/N ratio improves approximately linearly with

magnetic field strength (Fig. 1–56), the higher field strengths produced by superconducting magnets yield improved S/N ratios, benefiting both imaging and spectroscopy. Additional considerations, however, make the advantages of high field somewhat less clear. For instance, T1 relaxation times lengthen as the field strength increases, which tends to reduce the S/N ratio if TR is kept fixed. Also, readout bandwidths are usually increased as the field strength increases to compensate for greater chemical-shift and susceptibility artifacts, again tending to reduce the S/N ratio. Thus, the C/N ratio may be less than linearly proportional to field strength. Moreover, devices with high field strength create greater siting problems. The stray fields from superconducting magnets extend for dozens of feet in all directions, posing potential risks to electronic equipment and patients with cardiac pacemakers. Large metal objects in the vicinity of the magnet can distort field homogeneity, and smaller metal objects can be attracted into the magnet bore at dangerously high velocities. Solutions for this problem include passive and active magnetic shielding (see Chapter 14). Although there is a consensus that high-field magnets produce images that are subjectively bet-

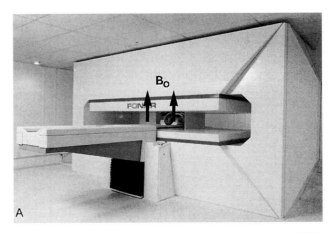

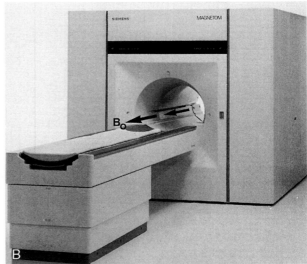

FIGURE 1–55. Main magnetic field (B_0) direction is different for (A) a permanent magnet and (B) a superconducting magnet.

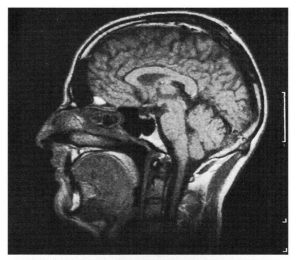

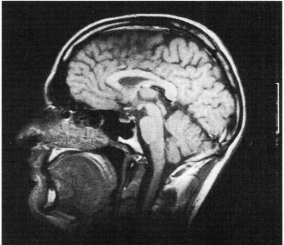

FIGURE 1–56. Comparison of image quality at different field strengths using same pulse sequence and scan parameters: top, 0.5 T; middle, 1.0 T; bottom, 1.5 T.

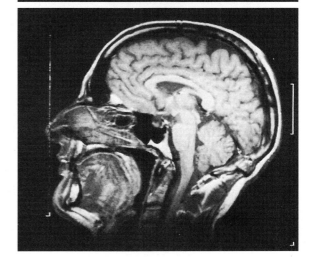

ter (because of higher S/N ratios) than lower field systems, this has not been proved to result in improved accuracy in lesion detection.[64–66] On the other hand, certain specific techniques such as susceptibility-based perfusion imaging and spectroscopy are better done at high field, and very high resolution imaging, includ-

ing MR angiography, clearly benefits from the additional S/N ratio. Newer superconducting magnets are considerably shorter (hence less claustrophobic) and lighter than older ones. Some 1.5-T magnets now weigh as little as 8000 lb, and still lighter models are in development.

Some newer magnet designs have an open architecture, with a reduced risk of claustrophobia compared with standard superconducting magnets. Open magnet architecture permits easy access to the patient with potential uses for interventional MRI (see Chapter 12). Tradeoffs of these newer magnet designs may include a more limited usable FOV and the need for novel hardware such as flat gradient coils.

A homogeneous magnetic field is essential for both MRI and MR spectroscopy. Magnets used for MRI must be carefully "shimmed" to maximize homogeneity. This shimming is accomplished physically by strategic placement of steel plates around the magnet (*passive shimming*), as well as by varying currents into electromagnetic coils (*active shimming*). Homogeneity is especially critical for spectroscopy and chemically specific imaging (i.e., fat suppression), in which field uniformity must be an order of magnitude better than that required for MRI. In general, this homogeneity appears most easily achieved with superconducting magnets.

RADIOFREQUENCY COILS

Transmitter Coils

To excite the protons, an RF magnetic field perpendicular to the main field must be used. The assembly of wires used to deliver the RF pulses is called the transmitter coil. The goal of this coil is usually to deliver a uniform magnetic field over a desired region of interest. As a rule, most scanners use both a large body coil and a second, smaller head coil. As we will see, sometimes the same coil can be used to detect the MR signal as well, although in general different coils are used.

Receiver Coils

The receiver coil, which detects the MR signal, must be designed to have high sensitivity for the body part being imaged. As a rule, because both the signal and the noise come from the body, it is usually desirable to match the size of the receiver coil, and therefore the sensitive volume of the coil, to the region of interest. Such coils are said to have a high *filling factor*. For instance, the smaller head coil has a higher filling factor and provides a better S/N ratio for brain imaging compared with the larger body coil, because 1) it is less sensitive to thermal noise arising from tissues outside the brain and 2) it can be placed closer to the protons of the brain and thus detect their signal more sensitively.

An application of this principle is the use of *surface* or *local* coils (Fig. 1–57). A surface coil is a type of receiver that can be placed close to the region of interest, maximizing the signal it detects from that region and minimizing the noise from outside. There are many types of surface coils. Surface coils may be linear or quadrature coils, as discussed next, with the latter design giving up to a 40% improvement in S/N

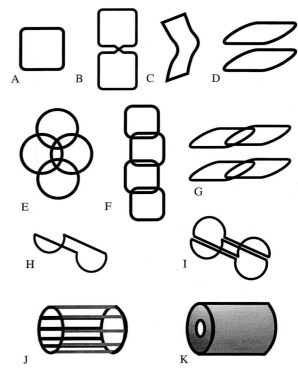

FIGURE 1–57. Schematic drawings of various receiver coils. *A*, Flat loop. *B*, Butterfly coil. *C*, Flexible coil. *D*, Helmholtz coil; the top element is passively coupled to the bottom element. *E*, Four-element array for functional brain imaging. *F*, Four-element array for spine imaging. *G*, Four-element array for body imaging. For coils E to G (also called multicoil, phased-array, or synergy coils), each coil element has its own preamplifier and amplifier. *H*, Half-saddle coil for neck imaging. *I*, Saddle coil for head and extremity imaging at low-to middle-field strengths. *J*, Birdcage coil for head and body imaging. *K*, Cavity resonator for imaging at extremely high field strengths (e.g., 4 T).

ratio over a linear configuration. Flat surface coils are best for imaging of the spine. Helmholtz arrays, consisting of an anterior and a posterior portion, are used for neck imaging. Flexible coils can be wrapped around the body part to give an optimal filling factor and are ideal for shoulder, elbow, or wrist imaging.

Quadrature (Circularly Polarized) Coils

There is one particularly good trick for improving the S/N ratio of the detected protons. The MR phenomenon has a preferred rotation direction. That is, at 1.5 T, the protons precess at 64 MHz in one direction (i.e., clockwise or counterclockwise) and not the other. A simple loop of wire (the simplest MR receiver coil) is equally sensitive to signals that come from either rotation direction. Such a coil is called a linear RF coil and would detect a signal coming from either rotation direction, or *polarization* in MR parlance. In practice, then, a linear coil picks up signal from one polarization but picks up the random thermal noise from both polarizations. However, it is possible to make a coil that is sensitive to signals from only one polarization. If it is assumed that the coil is set up to detect the correct polarization, such a coil picks up

$\sqrt{2}$ less noise for the same amount of signal by ignoring the wrong polarization. Such coils are called *circularly polarized* or *quadrature* coils.

In addition, by not transmitting the ineffective polarization, quadrature coils can, in theory, produce a 90° RF pulse with 50% less RF power deposition. More important, when receiving, they can provide a 40% improvement in S/N ratio over the linear mode. In practice, the gain from quadrature operation is less dramatic, in part because the body is not an ideal spherical, homogeneous object. However, for body and head coils, the near-theoretic advantage is often obtained. In addition, not all coil designs are suitable for quadrature operation, although there have been a number of improvements even to flat coils to allow some quadrature gains. For example, flat quadrature coils for spine imaging can be made using a figure eight configuration.

Phased-Array Coils

Even though they provide a high S/N ratio, one problem with small surface coils is that they cover a limited FOV. However, a series of small surface coils can be combined to form a coil array and thus provide sensitivity for imaging over a large volume. In such coil sets, called *phased-array coils* or *multicoil arrays,* the individual coils (which may be linear or quadrature) are slightly overlapped to decouple them magnetically.[67] Each coil is connected to its own receiver channel. Because each coil in the array is magnetically isolated from the other elements, large phased-array coils provide the same S/N ratio over a large FOV as would be provided by one of the elements over its much smaller FOV. With phased-array coils, high-resolution images of the spine, abdomen, pelvis,[68] and other organs can be acquired in just a few minutes. Drawbacks of phased-array coils are their greater expense and severalfold longer reconstruction times because of the need to combine data from several receiver channels (typically from four to six).

GRADIENTS

As described earlier, MRI systems have three pairs of orthogonal gradient coils, oriented respectively along the x, y, and z axes of the magnet. Activation of an individual gradient coil produces a linear variation of the z magnetic field along one of the orthogonal axes. Simultaneous activation of two or three gradient coils produces a linear gradient along a nonorthogonal direction, which is applied for oblique imaging (Fig. 1–58).

Maximal gradient amplitudes, which limit the available slice thickness and FOV, range from 10 to 15 mT/m, although systems used for echo-planar imaging (see Chapter 10) produce peak gradient amplitudes up to twice as strong. Gradient ramp times—that is, the time required to switch from no gradient to a stable plateau value (rise time) and vice versa (fall time)—ranges from a few hundred microseconds to 1.5 ms. Gradient performance is often characterized by the *slew rate*, which is the gradient change per unit time measured in tesla per meter per second. Fast rise times are critical for minimizing the TE in a variety of sequences.

Several problems result from operation of the gradient coils at their maximal capacity:

1. A large amount of audible noise can be generated by the electromechanical forces on the gradient coils as the magnetic field flux changes rapidly, which can be quite disturbing to the patient lying in the magnet bore.

2. It may be necessary to allow some dead time for the gradients during the pulse sequence (duty cycle < 100% of the TR).

3. With echo-planar imaging–capable systems, the dB/dt (change in magnetic field per unit time) may be sufficient to cause peripheral nerve stimulation.

4. Eddy currents may produce image artifacts (see Chapter 3).

Eddy currents represent undesirable magnetic fields that are induced each time the gradient is pulsed. These magnetic fields, which vary over time and space, occur in conducting structures in proximity to the gradient coil, such as the cryoshield (see Chapter 14). The major effect of eddy currents is to distort the gradient profile and thus reduce the fidelity of the resulting encoded image. As a result, the dephasing and rephasing lobes of a gradient reversal, used in all gradient-echo and spin-echo pulse sequences, may be unequal, so that the echo is not properly refocused. In addition, the frequency-encoding gradient may be unstable during the readout period, resulting in image artifacts. The long time constant (up to tens of milliseconds) of some eddy currents is a particular problem

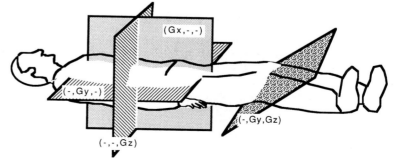

FIGURE 1–58. Oblique imaging uses multiple gradients simultaneously.

for certain spectroscopic experiments. In most imaging systems, the effects of these eddy currents are reduced by electronic preadjustment of the gradient waveforms so that the net (i.e., gradient coil plus eddy currents) field produced more closely resembles the pure gradient. In addition, some gradient coil designs dramatically reduce the eddy currents by using an additional coil set whose purpose is to minimize the field produced outside the gradient coils and thus reduce the source of the eddy current. These *actively shielded gradients* trade some coil efficiency (i.e., field produced per ampere of current) for useful field purity.

EXTREMELY HIGH FIELD MAGNET SYSTEMS

Extremely high field magnets (e.g., ≥ 2 T) are becoming more common for research purposes. Such magnets have been used for decades for high-resolution analytic spectroscopy as well as for in vivo research using small animals. However, the construction of these systems for human use has only more recently been possible. There is particular interest in using these systems for functional brain imaging, brain imaging with high anatomic resolution, and spectroscopy.[69] Potential advantages of such high-field systems include increased magnetic susceptibility effects (giving improved contrast with task activation using the blood oxygen level–dependent [BOLD] functional magnetic resonance imaging [FMRI] technique), better S/N ratio, and larger chemical shifts for better separation of different chemical species. There are many drawbacks to these systems as well. Their cost is high because of the extra expense for the magnet, as well as the fact that such systems are nonstandard and few in number. The weight of the magnet and associated shielding can exceed 50 tons and, along with fringe field considerations, can necessitate stringent siting requirements. Flexibility in pulse sequence design is restricted by several factors. Readout bandwidths tend to be kept high to minimize artifacts resulting from magnetic susceptibility. The RF transmitter, operating at frequencies on the order of 128 to 170 MHz, has high power requirements. Moreover, RF power deposition is a major concern, because it increases with the square of the operating frequency. Echo-planar imaging is commonly used for FMRI studies of the brain. Susceptibility artifacts with echo-planar imaging are problematic even at 1.5 T, particularly near the paranasal sinuses and skull base. These artifacts are much worse at higher field strengths. T2 relaxation times shorten substantially. Torque on the gradient coils as they are pulsed with current, already high with echo-planar imaging, is proportionally worsened as the field strength is increased, so that requirements for mechanical stability are more stringent.

The design of RF coils that operate in extremely high magnetic fields is also different from that of coils for use at field strengths of 1.5 T or lower. Below 2 T, the wave nature of the RF energy used in MRI can generally be neglected. However, at very high field strengths, the operating frequency increases and the wavelength decreases to the point that it approaches the dimensions of the RF coil and the body. Standard "lumped element" designs that are suitable for lower field work suffer from several problems at extremely high field strengths. These include 1) nonuniform current distribution, resulting in worsened homogeneity and fill factor and increased electric field losses; 2) decreased conductor skin depths; 3) self-resonance below the desired frequency; and 4) electromagnetic radiative losses.[70] Vaughan and colleagues[70] have designed RF coils using transmission line theory that may offer at least partial solutions to these problems, and promising results have been obtained. With this coil design, the S/N ratio of head images may approach the linear relationship to field strength that would be expected in the absence of worsened coil performance.

CONCLUSIONS

The goal of this chapter was to introduce the basic concepts and technologies of MRI, as well as point to the larger discussions of issues that form entire chapters in this book. We have described the physical basis of the nuclear magnetic resonance phenomenon and how it can be exploited to make an MR tomogram. We have described the underlying relaxation processes (T1 and T2) that provide most of the useful contrast in current clinical practice, as well as pointed to several of the more complex phenomena that also provide useful contrast. We have introduced the language of MR pulse sequences, by which the user manipulates this contrast, as well as the language of MR image quality, by which we assess this contrast. Finally, we have given a cursory introduction to the actual hardware that is used to make the MR image.

MRI, we believe, differs from the other medical imaging modalities in many fundamental ways. Ultimately, one of the most important differences is its wide flexibility. However, that flexibility implies some fundamental complexities in terms of an initial understanding of the tool and a need for attention to its continually broadening applications. This chapter seeks to serve as a unifying introduction to help the user understand not only the underlying technology but also the current and future innovations.

REFERENCES

1. Abragam A: The Principles of Nuclear Magnetism. London: Oxford University Press, 1961.
2. Slichter CP: Principles of Magnetic Resonance: With Examples from Solid State Physics. 2nd ed. Berlin: Springer-Verlag, 1978.
3. Hinshaw WS, Lent AH: An introduction to NMR imaging: from the Bloch equation to the imaging equation. Proc IEEE 71:338, 1983.
4. Mansfield P, Morris PG: NMR Imaging in Biomedicine. New York: Academic Press, 1982, pp 29–30.
5. Kaufman L, Crooks LE, Margulis AR: Nuclear Magnetic Resonance Imaging in Medicine. New York: Igaku-Shoin, 1981.
6. Rabi II, Millman S, Kusch P, et al: The molecular beam resonance method for measuring nuclear magnetic moments. Phys Rev 55:526, 1939.
7. Bloch F, Hansen WW, Packard M: Nuclear induction. Phys Rev 69:127, 1946.

8. Purcell EM, Torrey HC, Pound RV: Resonance absorption by nuclear magnetic moments in a solid. Phys Rev 69:37, 1946.
9. Lauterbur PC: Image formation by induced local interactions. Nature 242:190, 1973.
10. Damadian R, Goldsmith M, Minkoff L: NMR in cancer. XVI. FONAR image of the live human body. Physiol Chem Phys 9:97–100, 1977.
11. Mansfield P, Maudsley AA: Planar spin imaging by NMR. J Magn Reson 27:101, 1977.
12. Hinshaw WS, Bottomley PA, Holland GN: Radiographic thin section image of the human wrist by NMR. Nature 270:722, 1977.
13. Glover GH, Pauly JM: Projection reconstruction techniques for reduction of motion effects in MRI. Magn Reson Med 28:275–289, 1992.
14. Mugler JP 3d, Brookeman JR: Rapid three-dimensional T1-weighted MR imaging with the MP-RAGE sequence. J Magn Reson Imaging 1:561–567, 1991.
15. Oshio K, Jolesz FA, Melki PS, Mulkern RV: T2-weighted thin-section imaging with the multislab three-dimensional RARE technique. J Magn Reson Imaging 1:695–700, 1991.
16. Cameron IL, Ord WVA, Fullerton GD: Characterization of proton NMR relaxation times in normal and pathological tissues by correlation with other tissue parameters. Magn Reson Imaging 2:97–106, 1984.
17. Mitchell DG, Burk DL, Vinitski S, et al: The biophysical basis of tissue contrast in extracranial MR imaging. AJR 149:831–837, 1987.
18. Bottomley PA, Hardy CJ, Argersinger RE, Allen-Moore G: A review of ¹H NMR relaxation in pathology: are T1 and T2 diagnostic? Med Phys 14:1–37, 1987.
19. Mann J: Stability of gadolinium complexes in vitro and in vivo. J Comput Assist Tomogr 17(suppl 1):S19–S23, 1993.
20. Weinmann HJ, Laniado M, Mützel W: Pharmacokinetics of Gd-DTPA/dimeglumine after intravenous injection into healthy volunteers. Physiol Chem Phys Med NMR 16:167–172, 1984.
21. Russell E, Schaible T, Dillon W, et al: Multicenter double-blind placebo-controlled study of gadopentetate dimeglumine as an MR contrast agent: evaluation in patients with cerebral lesions. AJR 152:813–823, 1989.
22. Yuh W, Engelken J, Muhonen M, et al: Experience with high-dose gadolinium MR imaging in the evaluation of brain metastases. AJNR 13:335–345, 1992.
23. Ross JS, Masaryk TJ, Schrader M, et al: MR imaging of the postoperative lumbar spine: assessment with gadopentetate dimeglumine. AJR 155:867–872, 1990.
24. Niendorf HP, Haustein J, Cornelius I, et al: Safety of gadolinium-DTPA: extended clinical experience. Magn Reson Med 2:222–228, 1991.
25. Young I, Clark G, Bailes D, et al: Enhancement of relaxation rate with paramagnetic contrast agents in NMR imaging. J Comput Assist Tomogr 5:543–547, 1981.
26. Tien RD: Fat-suppression MR imaging in neuroradiology: techniques and clinical application. AJR 158:369–379, 1992.
27. Elster AD, Mathews VP, King JC, Hamilton CA: Improved detection of gadolinium enhancement using magnetization transfer imaging. Neuroimaging Clin North Am 4:185–192, 1994.
28. Hiraishi K, Narabayashi I, Fujita O, et al: Blueberry juice: preliminary evaluation as an oral contrast agent in gastrointestinal MR imaging. Radiology 194:119–123, 1995.
29. Wesbey GE, Brasch RC, Goldberg HI, et al: Dilute oral iron solutions as gastrointestinal contrast agents for magnetic resonance imaging: initial clinical experience. Magn Reson Imaging 3:57–64, 1985.
29a. Albert MS, Cates GD, Driehuys B, et al: Biological magnetic resonance imaging using laser-polarized ¹²⁹Xe. Nature 370:199–201, 1994.
30. Hamm B, Vogl TJ, Branding G, et al: Focal liver lesions: MR imaging with Mn-DPDP—initial clinical results in 40 patients. Radiology 182:167–174, 1992.
31. Weissleder R, Stark DD, Engelstad B, et al: Superparamagnetic iron oxide: pharmacokinetics and toxicity. AJR 152:167–173, 1989.
32. Weissleder R, Papisov M: Pharmaceutical iron oxides for MR imaging. Rev Magn Reson 4:1–20, 1992.
33. Janick PA, Hackney DB, Grossman RI, Asakura T: MR imaging of various oxidation states of intracellular and extracellular hemoglobin. AJNR 12:891–897, 1991.
34. Bryant RG, Marill K, Blackmore C, Francis C: Magnetic relaxation in blood and blood clots. Magn Reson Med 13:133–144, 1990.
35. Wright GA, Hu BS, Macovski A: Estimating oxygen saturation of blood in vivo with MR imaging at 1.5 T. J Magn Reson Imaging 1:275–283, 1991.
36. Ogawa S, Lee TM, Kay AR, Tank DW: Brain magnetic resonance imaging with contrast dependent on blood oxygenation. Proc Natl Acad Sci USA 87:9868–9872, 1990.
37. Haase A, Frahm J, Matthaei D, et al: FLASH imaging: rapid NMR imaging using low flip-angle pulses. J Magn Reson 67:256–266, 1986.
38. Laub G: Displays for MR angiography. Magn Reson Med 14:222–229, 1990.
39. Anderson CM, Saloner D, Lee RE, et al: Assessment of carotid artery stenosis by MR angiography: comparison with x-ray angiography and color-coded Doppler ultrasound. AJNR 13:989–1003, 1992.
40. Ruggieri PM, Masaryk TJ, Ross JS, Modic MT: Magnetic resonance angiography of the intracranial vasculature. Top Magn Reson Imaging 3:23–33, 1991.
41. Finn JP, Goldmann A, Edelman RR: Magnetic resonance angiography in the body. Magn Reson Q 8:1–22, 1992.
42. Wolff SD, Balaban RS: Magnetization transfer contrast (MTC) and tissue water proton relaxation in vivo. Magn Reson Med 10:135–144, 1989.
43. Balaban RS, Ceckler TL: Magnetization transfer contrast in magnetic resonance imaging. Magn Reson Q 8:116–137, 1992.
44. Edelman RR, Ahn SS, Chien D, et al: Improved time-of-flight MR angiography of the brain using magnetization transfer contrast. Radiology 184:359–399, 1992.
45. Tan Hu JI, Sepponen RE, Lipton MJ, Kuusela T: Synergistic enhancement of MRI with Gd-DTPA and magnetization transfer. J Comput Assist Tomogr 16:19–24, 1992.
46. Dousset V, Grossman RI, Ramer KN, et al: Experimental allergic encephalomyelitis and multiple sclerosis: lesion characterization with magnetization transfer imaging. Radiology 182:483–491, 1991.
47. Dixon WT, Engels H, Castillo M, Sardashti M: Incidental magnetization transfer contrast in standard multislice imaging. Magn Reson Imaging 8:417–422, 1990.
48. Erickson SJ, Prost RW, Timins ME: The "magic angle" effect: background physics and clinical relevance. Radiology 188:23–25, 1993.
49. Fullerton GD, Cameron IL, Ord VA: Orientation of tendons in the magnetic field and its effect on T2-relaxation times. Radiology 155:433–435, 1985.
50. Hennig J, Nauerth A, Friedburg H: RARE imaging: a fast imaging method for clinical MR. Magn Reson Med 3:823–833, 1986.
51. Melki PS, Jolesz FA, Mulkern RV: Partial RF echo planar imaging with the FAISE method. I. Magn Reson Med 26:328–341, 1992.
52. Melki PS, Jolesz FA, Mulkern RV: Partial RF echo-planar imaging with the FAISE method. II. Magn Reson Med 26:342–354, 1992.
53. Norbash AM, Glover GH, Enzmann DR: Intracerebral lesion contrast with spin-echo and fast spin-echo. Radiology 185:661–665, 1992.
54. Gronemeyer SA, Langston JW, Hanna SL, Langston JW Jr: MR imaging detection of calcified intracranial lesions and differentiation from iron-laden lesions. J Magn Reson Imaging 2:271–276, 1992.
55. Brateman L: Chemical shift imaging: a review. AJR 146:971–980, 1986.
56. Brix G, Heiland S, Bellemann SE, et al: MR imaging of fat-containing tissues: valuation of two quantitative imaging techniques in comparison with localized proton spectroscopy. Magn Reson Imaging 11:977–991, 1993.
57. Pfleiderer B, Ackerman JL, Garrido L: In vivo ¹H chemical shift imaging of silicone implants. Magn Reson Med 29:656–659, 1993.
58. Anzai Y, Lufkin RB, Jabour BA, Hanafee WN: Fat-suppression failure artifacts simulating pathology on frequency-selective fat-suppression MR images of the head and neck. AJNR 13:879–884, 1992.
59. Spielman D, Meyer C, Macovski A, Enzmann D: ¹H spectroscopic imaging using a spectral-spatial excitation pulse. Magn Reson Med 18:269–279, 1991.
60. Dixon WT: Simple proton spectroscopic imaging. Radiology 153:189–194, 1984.
61. Schneider E, Chan TW: Selective MR imaging of silicone with the three-point Dixon technique. Radiology 187:89–93, 1993.
62. Rose A: The sensitivity performance of the human eye on an absolute scale. J Opt Soc [A] 38:196–208, 1948.
63. Owen RS, Wehrli FW: Predictability of SNR and reader preference in clinical MR imaging. Magn Reson Imaging 8:737–745, 1990.
64. Lee DH, Vellet AD, Eliasziw M, et al: MR imaging field strength: prospective evaluation of the diagnostic accuracy of MR for diagnosis of multiple sclerosis at 0.5 and 1.5 T. Radiology 194:257–262, 1995.
65. Jack CR, Berquist TH, Miller GM, et al: Field strength in neuro-MR imaging: a comparison of 0.5T and 1.5T. J Comput Assist Tomogr 14:505–513, 1990.
66. Steinberg HV, Alarcon JJ, Bernadino ME: Focal hepatic lesions: comparative MR imaging at 0.5 and 1.5 T. Radiology 174:153–156, 1990.
67. Roemer PB, Edelstein WA, Hayes CE, et al: The NMR phased array. Magn Reson Med 16:192–225, 1990.
68. McCauley TR, McCarthy S, Lange R: Pelvic phases array coil: image quality assessment for spin-echo MR imaging. Magn Reson Imaging 10:513–522, 1992.
69. Ugurbil K, Garwood M, Ellerman J, et al: Imaging at high magnetic fields: initial experiences at 4 T. Magn Reson Q 9:259–278, 1993.
70. Vaughan JT, Hetherington HP, Otu JO, et al: High frequency volume coils for clinical NMR imaging and spectroscopy. Magn Reson Med 32:206–218, 1994.

Practical MRI for the Technologist and Imaging Specialist

KATHLEEN DUPUIS ■ VENKATESAN THANGARAJ
ROBERT R. EDELMAN

Magnetic resonance imaging (MRI) is a dynamic field of study, continually evolving with increasing clinical applications. Improvements in both software and hardware have resulted in enhanced image quality and shorter scanning times, providing health care professionals with information not previously available with this modality. Developments such as phased-array coils, fast spin-echo, multislice breath-hold imaging, noninvasive MR angiography, and echo-planar imaging give the technologist and imaging specialist a number of new and exciting approaches that place MRI at the forefront of medical imaging. It is imperative, in these rapidly changing times, that the imaging technologist keep informed of new developments in design and technology and successfully apply these skills to provide both quality care of patients and diagnostic imaging. This chapter serves as an overview of performing an examination in the MRI environment (Fig. 2–1). The reader will find some helpful imaging tips throughout the course of this chapter, which are designated by *italics*.

THE FACILITY

DESIGN AND FUNCTION

The needs for equipment and facility organization will differ somewhat, depending on an MRI facility's affiliation with a clinic, a hospital environment, or a freestanding imaging center. Facility location not withstanding, most MRI centers have a mix of patients consisting of a larger percentage of outpatients than inpatients. Decisions on size and scope of resources should be made with an understanding of market demand for the MRI facility location and population served.

A floor plan common to all facility types has several basic features (Fig. 2–2). The first is a reception area,

where patients register for an appointment and non-MRI health care providers may make inquiries, receive information, and ask for assistance and direction from reception staff. The reception area must be located outside the 5-G field line. Warning signs should be posted at or before the entrance to the MRI suite notifying all persons entering the area of the potentially hazardous magnetic field. These signs should clearly state that no ferromagnetic objects should be brought into the area and that all patients, personnel, and visitors are required to stop at the reception area and check with department personnel before proceeding. A waiting area should be located adjacent to the reception desk. This area should be large enough to serve as a place for patients to complete questionnaires and for their companions to wait comfortably while a patient undergoes the procedure. Rest rooms are necessary outside the suite for visitors or patients not yet cleared by MRI staff for entrance into the MRI suite. Additional facilities should be located within the suite to provide convenience and privacy for gowned patients.

Receptionists need to monitor pedestrian traffic continually. Communication and team support with other team members such as technologists and radiologists are essential. Therefore, it is important to make this area easily accessible to MRI health care workers as well. A technologist should be available to reception staff to assist with scheduling and patient-related questions.

Dressing rooms and lockers are needed, because a patient undergoing MRI will need to remove personal belongings such as credit cards with a magnetic strip; clothing with zippers, snaps, or hooks; jewelry; hairpins; and any other metallic objects. A room designated for preparation of patients should be provided for the following instances: preparation for intravenous (IV) access for examinations that require IV administration of contrast medium; administration and

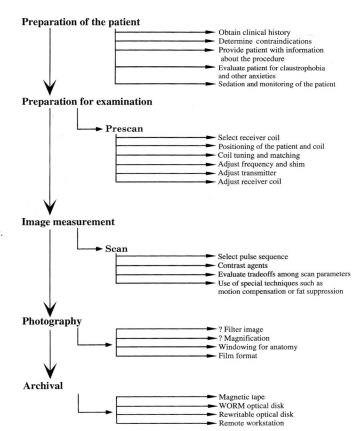

Preparation of the patient
- Obtain clinical history
- Determine contraindications
- Provide patient with information about the procedure
- Evaluate patient for claustrophobia and other anxieties
- Sedation and monitoring of the patient

Preparation for examination

Prescan
- Select receiver coil
- Positioning of the patient and coil
- Coil tuning and matching
- Adjust frequency and shim
- Adjust transmitter
- Adjust receiver coil

Image measurement

Scan
- Select pulse sequence
- Contrast agents
- Evaluate tradeoffs among scan parameters
- Use of special techniques such as motion compensation or fat suppression

Photography
- ? Filter image
- ? Magnification
- Windowing for anatomy
- Film format

Archival
- Magnetic tape
- WORM optical disk
- Rewritable optical disk
- Remote workstation

FIGURE 2–1. Flow chart for patient imaging.

pre- and postexamination monitoring of conscious sedation; and a preprocedure interview and physical examination of the patient by the radiologist. Ideally, the preparation room is located close to the MRI examination room, to reduce movement of patients between the two areas.

The MRI examination room should be as aesthetically pleasing to patients as possible. It must be functional for the technologist's use, as well. Certain stringent technical requirements must be met so the system may perform reliably and produce artifact-free images. Equipment and supplies specifically designed for the MRI environment should be stored within the MRI examination room, including all radiofrequency (RF) coils, MR-compatible vital sign monitoring equipment, earplugs, prism glasses, and blindfolds. Other items that are not unique to the MRI examination requirements but are universal to the hospital or clinic setting should also be stocked in this room. Examples include clean and dirty linen stores, antibacterial cleaning fluids, emesis basins, glucagon, IV supplies, contrast agent reaction kits, and denture cups. A technologist should need to exert minimal effort in gaining access to these items to perform an examination adequately in a comfortable, clean, and safe environment without delay. A well-organized examination room is more reassuring to a patient because it is less technically foreboding. Another advantage is that a technologist familiar with the location of equipment can more easily provide timely, competent, and professional care.

Some surface coils are awkward and heavy. Therefore, proper storage location is an important consideration. If coils are stored in an inconvenient location, they may be subject to damage, or worse, the technologist may suffer injury. *Heavy coils should be stored as nearby as possible and at waist height.* There should be no hindrance between the coil storage area and the examination table. Adequate shelving for coil storage is also important in preventing coil damage. Coils should not be stacked on top of each other in any way, nor should other equipment be stored on top of the coils, or vice versa. When planning for shelf space, it is wise to allow for more than what seems needed in the immediate future to allow for growth of services and changes in technology.

Room decor also plays a role in reducing a patient's level of anxiety. Indirect room lighting has a softer, less abrasive tone. Plants, skylight windows, or wall hangings depicting relaxing scenery may assist to focus and calm the anxious patient. Assisting a patient to perceive the environment as spacious and nonconfining enhances the patient's overall MRI examination experience.

An MR-compatible stereo system provides the patient with relaxing music and better communication capabilities. Patients reported lower levels of anxiety after the MRI scan when able to listen to music of choice during the procedure compared with patients who had no music during MRI.[1] In addition, stereo systems that provide ear protection are an important

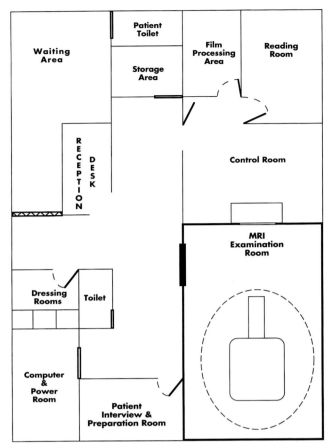

FIGURE 2–2. Typical MRI unit floor plan.

consideration, because some scanning techniques are loud enough to cause temporary hearing loss.[2]

Room ventilation is an important factor to consider for comfort of patients.[3] Adequate air exchange is impeded by the room's copper shielding, which prevents RF interference from the outside environment. It is helpful to have a separate dedicated temperature control for the examination room. In addition, most manufacturers' equipment specifications call for cooler temperatures and higher humidity than in other areas of the hospital. Collaborating with architects and engineers about such requirements during the facility planning stages will prevent future problems in meeting the demands on the heat, ventilation, and air conditioning system, which also controls humidification, required in the MRI environment. The humidity required is higher than most other environments. *A scan room with humidity below 50% will likely produce unpredictable image artifacts.* This point should be stressed with planning engineers, because correcting an inadequate system after it is implemented is costly and disruptive to this environment.

SAFETY

There are many potential risks in the MRI environment. The first concern is related to the high magnetic field strengths used in the clinical and research settings. Strong magnetic fields are measured in tesla (T), whereas the unit of measure for a small field is gauss (G). One tesla is equal to 10,000 G. Field strengths of magnets used for clinical purposes vary from 0.2 to 1.5 T. Magnets stronger than 1.5 T are not approved by the U.S. Food and Drug Administration (FDA) for use with patients but are used in research and development.

A 1-T magnet has more than 30,000 times the earth's magnetic pull. Attention must be given to the avoidance of ferromagnetic objects nearing the vicinity. The magnetic attraction on a ferromagnetic object may not be noticeable until it is brought relatively close to the MRI system, especially for passively and actively shielded magnets. The risk of attracting a projectile increases with the field strength of the magnet. One may have a false sense of security because the attraction is not felt until quite near the bore of the magnet. Personnel should be educated on the types of objects that are potential threats to patients, visitors, or health care workers in the examination room, not to mention potential damage to the system. Unfortunately, there is no finite list of such articles. All metallic objects should be scrutinized carefully regardless of size or location.

An object outside the body, carried or worn by a person, may be screened for potential hazards relatively easily by placing a small bar magnet adjacent to it. It is safest to eliminate all metallic objects. Determining the safety of metallic objects within a person's body from surgery or injury is not as obvious. Innumerable types of surgical clips, sutures, implants, and prostheses exist in medicine today and still more are being developed. Therefore, all MRI technologists have a professional responsibility to question the unknown. Chapter 13 of this text provides a comprehensive listing of the more commonly found metallic implants with information on their compatibility in the MRI environment. Cardiac pacemakers have been considered a contraindication to a patient's undergoing MRI. However, some testing has been done with cardiac pacemakers in place while the pacemaker is inactive, but this procedure must be considered experimental and hazardous. If a patient has an implant and the hazard potential in the MRI environment is unknown, the technologist should postpone the examination until safety can be confirmed. To determine the safety of a metallic implant, it is best to try to obtain that implant from the manufacturer or, if possible, the operating room. *A technologist may tie a string to a small implant and suspend it while slowly bringing it toward the bore of the magnet as another method for testing magnetic attraction.* If the implant in question is pulled or torqued to align with the magnetic field, the implant should be considered a contraindication. An implant or other device with wires may also be considered a contraindication, because of the possibility of inducing a current in a wire and causing a burn on a patient. The risk of burns is highest when imaging sequences are used that are RF intensive, such as fast spin echo.

Medical devices that have moving parts, such as a pump, may malfunction when in the MRI environment, causing potentially serious complications for a patient. Therefore, these devices should be tested for magnetic attraction as well as device malfunction in the MRI examination room. One example of a contraindicated medical device is an IV infusion control pump, commonly used for heparin or other medications that require regulated continual infusion rates. The referring physician may opt to disconnect the device for the duration of the MRI examination and arrange for another method of administering the medication to a patient in the interim.

If it is not considered medically safe to remove the infusion pump and MRI is the first diagnostic method of choice, the medical team can prepare the pump with a sufficiently long piece of extension tubing between the patient and the pump so that the pump remains outside the examination room. Under these circumstances, the IV tubing is unusually long and the flow rate may decrease. This would also require that the examination room door remain open during image acquisition, thus risking image artifact from outside RF sources. Clearly this is not an ideal approach in producing high-quality images, yet it may suffice in obtaining a diagnosis. MRI-compatible IV infusion pumps may be available in the near future.

Every MRI department should provide a physical barrier between the reception area and the clinical MRI environment. Entry doors should be installed with an electronic, manual, or combination lock controlled by appropriate department personnel. An informed staff member, such as a receptionist, should be located near this physical barrier. The reception staff monitors the passage of patients and personnel beyond the barrier. In addition, the boundary may aid in preventing unauthorized patients and personnel from straying into the magnet's fringe field. The reception area should be located at a safe distance from the 5-G line, the defining line for safety purposes.[4] The major concern of entering a fringe field beyond the 5-G line is specific to individuals with a pacemaker, because its function may be altered. This line may be defined by measuring the magnetic force with a magnetometer.

The location of the defining line depends on the magnet strength and the type of shielding employed. Manufacturers offer actively shielded magnets, which consist of additional superconducting loops of wire around the magnet. These coils partially negate the magnetic fringe field, bringing the 5-G line closer to the magnet. Passive shielding is another way to bring the 5-G line closer to the magnet. This method utilizes large pieces of iron placed in strategic locations around the magnet. A major drawback with this system is that the quantity of iron needed greatly increases the overall weight of the system. The excess weight limits its placement in certain locations because it is more challenging and costly to install such heavy equipment several floors above ground level. Permanent magnets tend to have much smaller fringe fields than superconductive ones.

Some patients are nonambulatory and require assis-tance with transportation. It is necessary to purchase an MRI-compatible wheelchair and stretcher so patients can enter the magnetic field without risk of injury. In addition, the facility should be equipped with nonferromagnetic IV poles for patients requiring IV fluids. Many equipment suppliers now provide medical equipment specifically designed for the MRI environment.

Attention should also be given to the arrangement of the MRI scanner in relationship to the scan console. It is best for a technologist to have visual contact with a patient in the bore of the magnet to detect more easily if a patient is in distress or in need of assistance. One scenario for seeing into the bore is by direct viewing through a window between the control room and the examination room. Another way to see a patient in the bore is through a video camera at one end of the magnet bore with an image display located at the scan console. Also, *a patient should be given a call button device, to contact a health care worker at any time during the scan.* This provides a method of communication for a patient who is not able to communicate verbally. All patients may use this as an emergency call button, if claustrophobic, anxious, or in pain.

Another concern arises with regard to the cryogens used to cool the superconducting magnets. These systems use liquid hydrogen and possibly liquid nitrogen. It is possible for rapid burnoff of the liquids into odorless and colorless gases. This is known as a quench. When a quench occurs, it is usually unmistakable. The cryogen burnoff rate is so rapid that a loud rumbling sound is heard, similar to thunder. The room air pressure increases rapidly as well, especially if the quench vent is not sufficiently designed to handle a large output of gases. Therefore, it could be difficult to open the examination room door. Technologists should be aware of potential hazards of both a magnet quench or when Dewars around the magnet are being refilled during routine maintenance. In both situations, these gases replace oxygen and cause a brisk decline of oxygen levels in the room. Patients, health care workers, or service personnel in the room may lose consciousness rapidly and unexpectedly.[5] Therefore, the scan room should be equipped with sensors to measure oxygen levels in the room, with an alarm display panel outside of the scan room accessible to maintenance staff. Because helium rises when released into room air, one sensor should be placed high on a wall. If the superconducting magnet also uses nitrogen, a second sensor should be placed lower on a wall, because the cooled nitrogen is heavier than room air and will fall.

In the event of a quench, the MRI examination room should be vacated of all patients and employees as quickly as possible, and the room should be securely closed until sufficient time has passed to allow the oxygen levels to return to normal. Room air usually contains approximately 20% oxygen. Refer to Chapter 13 for further reading on safety and contraindications.

MRI facilities should have protocols established as a frame-work for the MRI team to use to respond quickly and skill-fully in emergency situations such as a quench. Other crisis situations include patients' medical emergencies. These situations present additional challenges to staff because most equipment used elsewhere in the hospital for emergency medical care, such as stethoscopes, Kelly clamps, and laryngoscopes, become harmful projectiles when introduced into high magnetic fields. Other equipment, such as defibrillators and non–MRI-compatible electrocardiogram (ECG) recorders, may malfunction in a magnetic field. In the event of a medical emergency, the safest environment for implementation of resuscitation or treatment of unexpected medical complications is outside the 5-G line. The MRI receptionist should place a call to a code team or emergency medical technician for assistance. Each health care team member in MRI should be trained in basic cardiac life support or advanced cardiac life support so that resuscitation may begin while a patient is being transported away from the potentially harmful fringe field of the magnet. The patient should be transported immediately from the MRI examination room to an area furnished with all necessary emergency supplies and equipment. This may be in the preparation room or immediately outside the MRI examination room. Cardiopulmonary resuscitation should continue until the specially trained team summoned for this event responds.

Another potential emergency situation may occur if a large ferromagnetic object is brought into an MRI examination room. If the object is brought close to the magnetic field, it would quite likely become a projectile mass and move rapidly toward the magnet, striking any person or object in its path. It may also become bound to the magnet with a person or object pinned between the two. If an object is pinned to the magnet and cannot safely be removed while the main magnetic field is active, a technologist may need to call a service technician to ramp down the magnetic field. This can be performed safely under controlled supervision. However, if a person is constrained by the object to the magnet, there is a need for rapid response on the part of the MRI team to free the individual and call for emergency medical care due to the trauma likely incurred by the victim. *The fastest action would be to quench the magnet, although this may cost tens of thousands of dollars worth of cryogens (all MRI systems have an emergency quench button, and all MRI personnel should know its location), and remove the victim immediately.* This is an extremely dangerous circumstance. Precautions should be strictly enforced and measures taken seriously by all MRI staff to avoid accidents.

ORGANIZATION OF STAFF

Each MRI department member plays an integral role in ensuring competent, reputable service. The MRI team consists of schedulers, receptionists, technologists, and radiologists. Once the examination is requested, the MRI team works to provide expert diagnostic information in a timely manner. The scheduler and receptionist begin the process by obtaining and validating a significant amount of information from the clinician's office, such as clinical history and reason for examination. The demographic and insurance information may be completely or partially procured from the referring clinician's office or from the patient.

After the examination is scheduled, the radiologist reviews the indications for the request and decides on a scanning protocol. The team determines if the examination is scheduled appropriately based on such factors as the time of day, available staff, and the length of the examination. Most scheduled examinations will require few alterations when handled by experienced personnel. Applications for MRI are becoming more complex, and certain examinations require detailed clinical information for the MRI team to plan properly for the scanning protocol. *An integral part of the process of preparing for the study requires continuous flow of communication among all team members.* An adequately prepared team reduces the chance of unanticipated problems, allowing for smooth execution of the examination.

Technical staffing needs vary from site to site. Factors such as hospital-based versus outpatient center and the type and volume of referrals received help to determine the number of imaging technologists required for various shifts. A hospital-based facility will refer more inpatients, thereby increasing the nonambulatory population and patients requiring more medical attention. In a busy hospital setting it is beneficial to have dedicated nursing assistance. Some of the advantages include improved care of patients by having a nurse monitor vital signs as needed; ability to administer sedation to a claustrophobic or physically distressed patient; and ability to start an IV line when technologists are not trained to do so. It is a facility's obligation to provide an inpatient with the same level of care that would normally be received in the inpatient unit. A patient's needs should be met not only during the MRI examination but also before and after the examination while in the department. With these responsibilities removed, the technologist is able to focus on performing the examination in an organized fashion, quickly, and precisely. This is helpful not only for throughput but also for comfort and safety of patients, particularly when a patient's condition is unstable.

Regardless of the facility siting, most MRI centers perform more technically challenging examinations during the weekday, while a radiologist is available to monitor the examination. These examinations usually require more involved protocols for preparation of patients. For example, to perform a study of the pelvis, a radiologist may request that glucagon be prepared for an intramuscular injection. Many examinations require contrast medium administration; therefore, it may be beneficial to have an IV line in place before the examination commences. Abdominal and thoracic cavity imaging usually requires breath-holding by patients. The radiologist may also wish to examine the patient and possibly place a marker over an area of point tenderness or palpable mass. Other examinations may require the use of ECG leads for gated acquisitions, and still other examinations may require unusual positioning of the patient and coil. Each of these steps takes time to execute properly. The MRI examination and all of the previously mentioned steps must be explained to the patient.

Monitored examinations range in duration from 30 to 90 minutes. When scanning has concluded, the technologist will have postprocessing and filming yet to complete. Some of this may begin while the scan is active, but for many monitored examinations a second technologist is required to accomplish this task. During a typical weekday shift at a busy MRI center, many other responsibilities and duties arise, as this is the time of day when referring physicians' offices and other services are open and fully staffed. This time may become easily filled with a wide variety of tasks, such as refilming lost films; postprocessing images of previously scanned unmonitored examinations with a different method than is the usual protocol; testing new scanning techniques, filming, or postprocessing protocols; assisting in scheduling of future or emergent examinations; and speaking to patients or referring physicians about examination-related questions. Therefore, two or three technologists should be available to manage a fully scheduled MRI system on a weekday shift. Facilities that have two MRI systems within proximity to each other may require five technologists between the two systems.

Technical staffing for evening, night, and weekend shifts will vary. The majority of the examinations performed on these shifts are unmonitored, resulting in more straightforward examination protocols. Because examination length is more predictable during these time periods, appointment times may be scheduled with more regularity and closer together, thereby increasing examination throughput. However, because the technical staff is always responsible for final screening of the patient for contraindications and for explaining the procedure as well as for filming, postprocessing, and image archival, if increased examination throughput is expected, then technical staffing should be maintained at a level of two technologists per shift. One technologist working alone will not likely be able to perform more than one routine outpatient examination per hour.

Provisions should be made on all shifts for the likely possibility of urgent or emergent add-on examinations to the daily schedule of patients. Openings throughout the day may also be used as a buffer for times when the actual schedule is delayed compared with the planned schedule. This may happen for a variety of reasons, such as when a patient arrives late for an appointment; a patient unexpectedly experiences a claustrophobic or anxiety attack; or a monitored examination requires additional series of images for diagnosis.

PREPARING A PATIENT FOR MRI

SCHEDULING AN EXAMINATION

When a call is received from the referring physician to perform an examination, the scheduler should be prepared to process the request in as short a time as possible, yet a significant amount of information needs to be obtained to schedule an appointment appropriately. In addition to demographic data and type of insurance, related medical history needs to be obtained. A skilled scheduler will be able to probe for further information as needed. This allows scheduling of a suitable appointment for time of day and week as well as the correct duration of a given appointment. A radiologist should review all requests and determine a scanning protocol before the appointment time.

It is quite costly to a facility to have an open time slot of 45 minutes to 1 hour if a patient does not arrive for an appointment. Because there is no notice, it is nearly impossible to arrange for another patient to come in for the opening. For busy MRI centers, it can be especially frustrating because there are often patients who would have come in for the open appointment. Therefore, a receptionist or scheduler should call all patients scheduled for the MRI examination approximately 2 days in advance to confirm the appointment date and time. Speaking to a patient directly helps to reduce any potential "no-shows." When confirming an appointment time with a patient, a receptionist may also interview patients briefly for a prescreening of metallic implants, claustrophobia, and whether a patient needs special assistance. A receptionist may also give some information to a patient about the length of the visit, how a patient should dress (e.g., no jewelry or eye make-up), bringing family members, or directions to the facility. This is a good opportunity for a patient to ask questions on topics that may have been causing some anxiety. A knowledgeable and skilled receptionist will be able to relieve some fears a patient may have or to decide if it is necessary for a nurse to contact a patient requiring oral or IV sedation. Also, if a patient requires special assistance in ambulating, the appointment time should coincide with adequate staffing.

SCREENING A PATIENT

A referring clinician may or may not be fully aware of the potential hazards inherent in the MRI environment. In providing a service to the referring clinician and the patient, *the MRI department is responsible for ensuring the safety of those entering the MRI environment.* This can begin at the time an appointment is made for an MRI examination by well-informed schedulers. They may begin a preliminary screening of some of the more commonly found contraindicated metallic objects. Examples include a pacemaker or ferromagnetic material embedded in a susceptible anatomic structure such as an aneurysm clip in the brain or metal in the eye.

A scheduler and receptionist should have guidelines to follow for a verbal screening. The guidelines should include steps to take if the presence of a potentially contraindicated object is discovered. Also, a technologist or a radiologist may assist in clarifying any questionable circumstances. This can be a good prescreening tool to avoid having a patient come to the facility unnecessarily. However, a receptionist may not be able to reach every patient scheduled for an examination. Also, a patient may not wish to remain on the telephone to thoroughly review all contraindications. Therefore, this in itself is not adequate. This information should be repeated in written form when the patient checks in for the appointment.

When a patient arrives for the scheduled MRI examination, a receptionist should instruct the patient to complete a detailed screening checklist (see the Appendix in this chapter). The checklist is designed specifically for detecting potentially dangerous ferromagnetic implants or objects outside the body that could also be considered potentially harmful to the patient or anyone else in the area. This checklist should also screen for metallic objects that may degrade image quality, such as dentures or braces. Women of childbearing age should be asked if they are pregnant. It is necessary to document the screening process to ensure consistency in quality of care. Before bringing the patient into the fringe field, a technologist should carefully review the completed checklist and obtain verbal confirmation directly from the patient as well. Repetition in questioning the patient is often necessary, because a patient may have either skimmed through the forms or misunderstood a specific question. Literature has shown that incomplete or incorrect information has resulted in serious consequences for the patient and staff.[6, 7] Reception staff also need to receive visitors and non-MRI health care workers and possibly direct them into areas near the magnetic field. For this reason reception staff need to be well versed on the MRI environment and areas to avoid physical harm or equipment damage.

The screening should also ask for a patient's weight. This is needed for three reasons: all MRI systems have a weight limit defined by the manufacturer for each model to avoid damage to the mechanics that move the patient table; second, when a patient is exposed to RF, the body tissue is prone to warming. The FDA has determined that this warming is not to exceed a rise in core body temperature of 1°C.[4] Third, contrast material dosage is based on body weight, as recommended by the manufacturer.[5]

EDUCATION OF PATIENTS

As with any medical procedure, providing the patient with information about the examination is essential. In doing so, the health care provider must address the patient's needs and anxieties. According to Devine and Cook,[8, 9] three psychoeducational interventional domains should be addressed: procedural, sensory, and psychosocial. The health care provider must be knowledgeable in the subject matter to inform the patient with clear and concise communication.

Addressing the procedural aspect of education of patients entails informing a patient what the procedure is and why it is being performed and that the examination is not painful. Technical staff should educate a patient about what is required of the patient such as the specific positioning required for an examination. In some examinations, as in abdominal imaging, a patient may also need to follow breath-hold instructions, preferably explained before the patient is placed into the bore. A patient should also know that the technologist will be in constant communication, giving information on scan lengths and periodic verification of the patient's comfort.

The sensory aspect of educating the patient includes information on the physical environment of the machine and the bore size. Some patients consider it confining. Additional sensory information should include the noise associated with the scanning and that it may be considered annoying. Also, a patient should be aware of the expected duration of the procedure.

Studies have shown that patients may experience high levels of anxiety while undergoing MRI.[10] The imaging technologist should ascertain specific concerns, using open-ended questions to address the sensory and psychosocial aspects. It may be necessary to use prompts when trying to determine the source of the anxiety. Adverse psychologic reactions to MRI are often referred to as claustrophobia. However, research has shown that anxiety may also result from other factors.[11] A patient may be concerned about the pending diagnosis and the availability of the results. In addition to physical discomfort, noise from the scanner may induce emotional distress. Another common factor may be that a patient feels a lack of control. A patient may have already experienced significant testing or other medical procedures and may be overwhelmed by yet another test about which he or she knows little. The MRI environment may be even more distressing owing to a feeling of confinement and restrictiveness. Once the patient's concerns are discovered, they must be addressed before the patient can reliably comply with the requirements of the procedure.

The technologist should direct efforts to a patient's physical and emotional comfort by asking for suggestions from the patient. The technologist may further assist the patient in alleviating anxieties by using methods described in the section on claustrophobia. Employing psychologic methods in addition to education has shown a reduction in anxiety levels, compared with giving procedural information only.[12] Once a patient's physical and psychologic needs are satisfied, the health care provider may focus on performing the MRI.

After the patient is in the examination room, certain important information and instructions should be reviewed with the patient for reinforcement. Examples include the importance of remaining motionless during image acquisition; methods of communication available to the patient to reach the technologist; reassurance of the technologist's immediate availability; expected examination duration; and, when applicable, a review of breath-hold instructions with a practice session. In short, both the technologist and patient benefit when the health care worker enlists proactive methods in preparation for the MRI examination.

PHYSICAL PREPARATION OF A PATIENT

Patients should be asked to change from their personal clothing into a gown and robe. Patients who are allowed to wear personal clothing during a scan have been known to harbor ferromagnetic objects in the examination room. Attempts to remove the object frees it from restraint, and it then becomes a projectile mass. This is not only a threat to the physical safety of patients and staff but also a means of potential damage to the MRI scanner. A ferromagnetic object could hide in the magnet and may go undetected for a time, resulting in image degradation.

If a protocol includes IV contrast medium administration, a technologist, nurse, or physician should consider establishing IV access before the examination while the patient is in a preparation room. By starting the IV line in advance, some potential problems may be avoided. For instance, starting an IV line can be time-consuming, depending on the condition of a patient's peripheral veins. It places additional emotional and physical stress on a patient who may already be experiencing some duress. Another potential problem occurs when a patient is taken out of the bore to obtain IV access, potentially decreasing the likelihood of obtaining images at the same anatomic location before and after contrast medium administration. Last, if a health care provider, such as an IV nurse, attempting to gain IV access is not familiar with the MRI environment, additional delays and potential safety issues may arise.

Before starting the scan, several details should be considered. A marker may be used to aid in definition of a mass or as a reference point in relation to anatomic structures.[13, 14] The best materials to use for a marker in MRI are those that have a bright signal on a T1-weighted sequence. Because fat appears bright on a T1-weighted scan, many markers are made of a substance that contains animal or vegetable oil. Some examples are cod liver oil, soybean oil, and various nonroasted nuts (e.g., almonds). Vitamin E capsules are also used. It is helpful to use more than one marker. Placing two or three markers side by side may save scanning time because acquired images often have an interslice gap and may not well visualize a single marker.

When the structures in the abdomen and pelvis are imaged, motion of the small intestine can be a significant detractor in image quality. It may be reasonable for the radiologist to give a patient an intramuscular injection of glucagon (1 mg) to slow the peristalsis, thereby reducing motion artifact. Alternatively, glucagon may be given IV shortly before the most critical images are acquired, because the effects of an intramuscular injection given before initial positioning of the patient might not last for a sufficiently long time. Contraindications include patients with a known hypersensitivity to glucagon or history of pheochromocytoma or insulinoma.[15] Health care workers should exercise caution if a patient has a medical history of diabetes. Some patients have experienced a short duration of slight nausea up to 6 hours after completion of the examination. The patient should be informed of this so as not to be alarmed. If the nausea continues, the patient should contact his or her referring physician or the radiologist supervising the MRI examination. *A wide strap may be wrapped snugly around the abdomen to prevent excessive ghost artifact from respiratory motion during long image acquisitions.*

SPECIAL CONSIDERATIONS

Pregnancy

MRI is believed to be a safe imaging modality because there is no ionizing radiation as is used in general radiology or computed tomography (CT). However, it is a relatively new method, which means that long-term effects are yet to be determined. There are two populations to consider: the pregnant patient and the pregnant health care provider.

A patient and a health care worker have different exposures to different factors in the MRI environment. The patient is placed in the center of the bore of the magnet for approximately 45 minutes. She may also be given IV contrast medium. The potential risks a patient faces are from the static magnetic field, changing electromagnetic fields, RF, and contrast agents. The patient's exposure is usually a one time occurrence during a pregnancy, whereas a health care worker is constantly exposed to the static magnetic field.

It is difficult to determine what effects MRI may have on a pregnant woman and her fetus for several reasons. First, the spontaneous abortion rate in the normal pregnant population is 30% during the first trimester.[5] The population of pregnant patients and health care providers exposed to MRI is small. A survey of women of childbearing years working in the MRI environment was conducted in 1990.[16] The results show no statistically significant variations in reproductive health or menstrual cycles of the respondents compared with the general population. Facilities differ on a policy of restriction of work responsibilities for the pregnant health care provider. It has been suggested by Kanal and colleagues[16] in the aforementioned study, that activities should be the same for all employees. The pregnant health care workers may perform examinations, which include entering the MRI examination room in the absence of scanning and attending to the patient's needs, without concern of harmful effects.

Because there is no conclusive evidence that undergoing MRI is completely safe, *it is wise to act conservatively in scanning a pregnant patient.* Before performing an examination on a pregnant patient, a discussion should take place between a referring physician and a diagnosing radiologist to determine the effect the results would have on treatment of the patient and if MRI is the best modality for the clinical indications. Also, as recommended by the Safety Committee of the Society of Magnetic Resonance Imaging, the patient should be made aware "that, to date, there has been no indication that the use of clinical MR imaging during pregnancy has produced deleterious effects. However, as noted by the FDA, the safety of MR imaging during pregnancy has not been proved."[17] See Chapter 13 for further information on this topic.

Claustrophobia and Other Anxieties

Due to the structure of the MRI machine, claustrophobic reactions severe enough to cancel or postpone the study occur in 4% to 5% of the population of patients.[18] Of the patients attempting to undergo a scan, as many as 65% experience some level of anxiety or discomfort.[18] Some manufacturers have designed systems that have a wider or shorter bore size. These systems are less threatening for those affected with mild claustrophobia. Unfortunately, there may be a tradeoff when scanning with these types of systems, because they are typically low-field magnets and imaging times are generally longer. Also, for advanced imaging techniques, such as MR angiography, the image quality is inferior to that of high-field systems.

Some suggestions for the MRI technologist to assist claustrophobic or anxious patients through an MRI examination are listed here:

1. Reassure patients that they will not be kept in the machine against their will. The greatest fear patients may have is a feeling of loss of control.[20]

2. Maintain close, two-way verbal contact with patients throughout the examination, so they do not feel abandoned.

3. Give patients a device that allows them to establish contact at any time, such as a panic button.

4. Whenever possible, try to have patients enter the bore of the magnet feet first, thus giving them the sensation of being farther out of the magnet.

5. Offer the patients a pair of prism glasses, which may be used to look out of the machine through a reflection in the prism.

6. Give patients a blindfold to cover the eyes so they are less aware of the environment.

7. Guide patients through relaxation techniques such as deep breathing exercises immediately before the scan or guided imagery[21] before and during the scan.

8. Give patients either headphones designed specifically for use in the MRI system to play relaxing music or earplugs to reduce the noise level they encounter during imaging.

9. Ask a family member to accompany the patient through the examination, touching and talking to the patient as permitted through the constraints of examination execution. Patients usually find it reassuring to have physical contact with the environment outside of the "tube" of the magnet.

10. Provide good ventilation to patients while in the bore of the magnet.

11. Advise patients to try to "condition" themselves to the MRI environment by resting in a quiet environment at home and practice lying down with a large box over their head for a few minutes at a time.

If these techniques fail, the patient may need oral or IV sedation.

SEDATING A PATIENT

A patient could receive sedation for five possible reasons: 1) prior history of uncompensated claustrophobia when undergoing MRI; 2) previous reaction of claustrophobia in nonrelated situations (e.g., cannot enter an elevator); 3) acute or chronic pain rendering proper positioning intolerable for the duration of the procedure; 4) infant and pediatric patients; and 5) mental incapacitation.

Oral sedation is usually given for mild claustrophobia. The referring physician usually prescribes oral medication for a claustrophobic patient. Instructions may be given to the patient about when to take a prescribed oral sedative by either the prescribing physician or a pharmacist. Arrival time of the patient and the actual examination time do not necessarily coincide, owing to examination-related paperwork, removal of worn metallic objects, obtaining IV access for contrast medium administration, or a preprocedure interview with the radiologist for examination-related medical history. Therefore, *the MRI staff may wish to advise the patient on the timing of ingestion of the prescribed oral medication.*

IV sedation may be arranged for a severely claustrophobic or anxious patient. If IV sedation is planned, it is necessary to obtain a more extensive medical history for a history of respiratory problems. It is also necessary to monitor a patient's vital signs during the MRI examination. Due to the strong magnetic field, MRI-compatible equipment is needed to carry out the monitoring. When IV sedation is needed, the examination should be scheduled with a nurse or physician who can administer IV sedation and monitor a patient's response. A patient's vital signs should be recorded before the administration of IV sedatives for a baseline comparison. Vital signs should be continually monitored throughout the procedure and for a period after the examination is completed, ensuring vital signs have returned to baseline. This may take 2 to 3 hours. A patient scheduled for IV sedation should be instructed not to eat for 8 hours before the examination, and a responsible adult should accompany a patient to the procedure and drive the patient home after being released. The effects of the medication may inhibit motor skills for several hours after the sedation has been given. *Therefore, a health care worker should advise the patient that it is unsafe for the patient to drive or go home alone.*

MONITORING OF PATIENTS

As mentioned earlier, a sedated patient's vital signs should be monitored by reliable equipment. Another population of patients who may require vital sign monitoring is that of critical care/intensive care patients. The nature of the MRI environment makes it difficult, if not impossible, to have proximity to a patient to check for level of responsiveness. Also, some of the imaging times last up to 10 minutes or more, with complete examination times lasting up to 90 minutes. This is too long to wait to monitor a patient's level of consciousness. The Joint Commission on Accreditation of Healthcare Organizations[22] has recommended a protocol for conscious sedation for all procedures. To keep within compliance of these guidelines, *the MRI facility must have the capability to monitor pulse rate, oxygen saturation, respiration, blood pressure, and ECG.* MR-compatible monitoring devices come equipped with fiberoptic cables from the equipment to the patient's contact areas, thus preventing skin burns that might result from monitoring equipment used in other areas of the hospital. In addition, the use of monitoring equipment not specifically designed for the MRI environment during image acquisition may result in gross image artifact. Display screens for the measured vital signs must also be designed for this environment so as to avoid a distorted ECG and other displayed information.

MR-compatible anesthesia machines and ventilators are safer and more reliable than noncompatible equipment.[23] Equipment that has ferromagnetic properties may be affected by the magnetic field. Some equipment with metallic parts without ferromagnetic properties may still be affected by the eddy currents in the fringe field of the magnet and cause equipment malfunction, especially if these have moving parts. It is best to test equipment for safety first and then for function. Unfortunately, this equipment is costly, and only a handful of manufacturers have the necessary FDA approval for use with patients. Those products that do have FDA approval have a limited history for use in the clinical MRI setting. An increasing number of vendors are manufacturing MR-compatible equipment, which may result in a more competitive market. To safely sedate and monitor patients in the MRI environment, it is necessary to have these provisions available and technologists, nurses, and clinicians properly trained in equipment use.

POSITIONING OF PATIENTS

Factors to consider are the anatomic location of the area in question and signal-to-noise (S/N) ratio for the coils available. Manufacturers often design imaging coils shaped to fit specific anatomy. Surface coils, or more accurately named local coils, include spine, neck, knee, wrist, temporomandibular joint (TMJ), shoulder, breast, pelvis, and prostate coils. The head or body coil may also be used and is known as a volume coil. The body coil is typically located within the magnet as a permanent structure and is used for scanning larger areas of anatomy such as the abdomen, chest, or an entire extremity. *The patient should be made as comfortable as possible to achieve cooperation in maintaining the desired position.* For most MRI examinations, the patient lies supine and is centered relative to the coil's center. Additional information on use of surface coils is detailed later in this chapter.

IMAGE OPTIMIZATION

Many factors are involved in producing high-quality images, most of which are discussed in detail in other chapters. The following is a brief overview of the general principles and what an imaging specialist should consider in making decisions when choosing image parameters.

SIGNAL-TO-NOISE RATIO

The sharpness of an image is partly determined by the S/N ratio. A higher S/N ratio means the image will appear to be less grainy, or sharper. Conversely, a low S/N ratio results in a grainy image. Although a high S/N ratio is desirable, increasing the S/N ratio requires more imaging time. The human eye is able to detect differences only up to a certain point. Therefore, it is best to *maximize the S/N ratio to an acceptable level for making a diagnosis without increasing imaging time to a length that is unacceptable to a patient.*

Many factors may have an effect on the S/N ratio. A higher magnet field strength will produce a higher S/N ratio when motion artifacts are suppressed. Low bandwidth pulse sequences produce images with a higher S/N ratio than high bandwidth sequences. Coherent (e.g., respiratory and pulsatile motion causing ghost artifact) noise and incoherent (e.g., RF leak) noise reduce the S/N ratio. Both receiver coil sensitivity, determined by its design, and the distance from the tissue producing a signal to the coil will alter the S/N ratio. As spatial resolution (which is determined by field of view [FOV], matrix, and slice thickness) is increased, the S/N ratio decreases in direct proportion to the volume of the voxel.

IMAGE CONTRAST

Image contrast in MRI refers to differences in signal intensity from different tissue structures. Greater differences in signal intensities account for better contrast. Tissue contrast may be manipulated through selection of scan parameters and pulse sequences. Some factors are repetition time (TR), echo time (TE), matrix, number of signal averages, slice thickness, orientation and location, and bandwidth. A technologist and radiologist may maximize either the T1 or T2 contrast of different tissues through appropriate choices of scan parameters in the area of interest. Because the magnetic field strength and coil selection are also factors that affect image contrast, *selection of the scan parameters should be made specific to the field strength and the receiver coil utilized for each examination.*

SPATIAL RESOLUTION

Spatial resolution of an image determines the viewer's ability to discern two points as separate and distinct. Two factors determining spatial resolution are voxel size and S/N ratio. A voxel can be thought of as a cube, although it may have unequal sides. Voxel size is dependent on slice thickness, which is represented by the depth of the cube; FOV, or the area being imaged; and image matrix, which determines the number of pixels for the given area. A larger slice thickness will increase the voxel size and lower spatial resolution. Increasing the FOV increases the pixel size, which decreases the spatial resolution. Increasing the matrix increases the number of pixels for a given area, thereby increasing the spatial resolution.

PRESCANNING ADJUSTMENTS

Before the scan begins, a technologist must perform prescan adjustments in a specific order. Without the proper implementation, a variety of problems may occur, such as unusable image data or equipment malfunction or breakdown. The following is an overview of the steps required, in the proper order.

RECEIVER COIL

Coil Selection

The first step to consider is receiver coil selection. A receiver coil acts like an antenna for a radio signal tuned to a specific frequency. There are several receiver coils available, each having a different function determined by both shape and design. The technologist and radiologist should choose the coil that best suits the area to be scanned. The general types of coils available are local coils, partial-volume coils, intracavity coils, and whole-volume coils. Solenoid coils are sometimes used in permanent magnet systems, owing to a different orientation of the main magnetic field. These coils are more commonly used in lower field strength magnets. See Figure 2–3 for examples of various coil designs.

Surface coils, also known as local coils, aid in improved image quality but are limited to a smaller FOV. The higher image quality is a result of a better S/N ratio. Surface coils tend to be sensitive to signal close to the receiver coil and relatively insensitive to signal away from the coil. The range of the coil sensitivity directly relates to the size of the surface coil. The boundaries of signal detection are approximately the length of the coil and up to a depth equal to three to four times the coil's radius. *S/N ratio typically remains superior to the body coil up to a depth of one coil diameter.* Local coils are typically used to image areas such as the spine or TMJ. Flex coils are designed to be flexible, as the name would suggest. The flexible material that encases the receiver coil protects the coil from damage yet allows the coil to be wrapped around such anatomic structures as the upper and lower extremities. These coils provide much more uniform signal than other flat surface coils because of their capability of conforming to the shape of the structure.

Partial-volume coils consist of two receiver coils, one

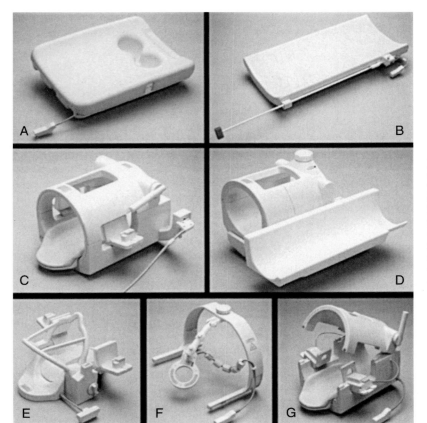

FIGURE 2–3. Examples of surface coils. *A,* Breast coil. *B,* Circularly polarized spine coil. *C,* Circularly polarized head coil. *D,* Circularly polarized extremity coil for knee and lower extremity imaging. *E,* Curved Helmholtz coil designed specifically for neck imaging. *F,* Small-field FOV coil, which may be used for temporomandibular joint (TMJ), orbit, or extremity imaging. *G,* TMJ coil; note the two small surface coils, one on each side, which may be used independently of each other or together. (*A* to *G* courtesy of Siemens Medical Systems, Iselin, NJ.)

on each side of a structure. These are usually receive-only coils and produce images with a more uniform signal than a single receiver coil. The uniformity of the image from these coils, in the area between the coils, approaches that seen with the whole-volume coils, as long as the distance between the two coils is not greater than the radius of the coil. The most common partial-volume coils are the Helmholtz coils, which are used for imaging the neck and shoulder.

Intracavity coils are similar in design to local coils in that they are used for imaging a small area. When these coils are used the signal intensity is much stronger close to the coil and significantly drops off at points away from the coil. Coils of this type are used for clinical purposes and are designed to be inserted into the rectum. These coils receive signal from anatomic structures located quite close to the coil with a high S/N ratio, with less sensitivity to motion from vascular flow or breathing. The coils may be designed to pick up signal from a specific direction. Examples from current clinical work include imaging the prostate gland and the rectum. Also, some experimental intravascular coils are being developed and may prove to have some clinical relevancy.

A whole-volume coil is used to acquire a uniform signal from a large volume. The body, head, body-phased array, and some knee coils are examples of whole-volume coils. These are often both transmit and receive coils, but some are receive-only coils.

Coils are designed as linear or quadrature, also known as circularly polarized coils, the latter consisting of two sets of magnetically decoupled coils. Advantages of a quadrature coil over a linear coil design include 1) a more spatially uniform flip angle from the RF pulse; 2) a reduction in power deposition of up to 50%; 3) increased S/N ratio; and 4) increased homogeneity of the signal. Most head and body coils manufactured today are quadrature coils.

When choosing a surface coil, one should keep in mind that a smaller coil yields a better S/N ratio. Therefore, it is advantageous to select a coil that will cover the area of interest and can be placed at a distance away from the area of interest that is less than the diameter of the receiver coil. For larger areas or deeper anatomic structures, volume coils will give better signal uniformity, but they are also more sensitive to noise produced from the patient's motion. Another variable to consider is the filling factor, which refers to the ratio of the volume of the area being sampled to the volume of the coil. *It is most desirable to have as high a filling factor as possible to maximize the S/N ratio from a given coil.* Therefore, one should not choose a large coil, such as a body coil, for imaging a small structure, such as a pediatric or infant spine.

Phased-array coils consist of a series of small coil elements that are magnetically decoupled from one another and have separate receivers. They offer a much larger FOV than provided by small surface coils. Phased-array coils allow imaging over a large FOV, as seen by its combined coil elements, with a similar S/N ratio to that which would be obtained over a smaller FOV with just one of its coil elements. Depending on hardware configuration, one may be able to select which of several (typically four to six) coil elements are activated. For instance, all elements of a body phased-array coil might be activated for liver or pelvic imaging but only the posterior coil elements might be used for renal imaging because of the dorsal location of the kidneys. *By not utilizing the anterior elements, artifacts from respiratory motion of the anterior abdominal wall are reduced.* Use of the posterior elements only is recommended for kidney imaging, except when the liver must also be evaluated. Some kind of respiratory compensation or fat suppression can be essential for optimal chest or abdominal imaging with phased-array coils. In using a spine phased-array coil, some designs offer more coil elements than receivers, so it may not be possible to image with all elements activated simultaneously. A limitation of phased-array coils is that several times more data must be processed (depending on the number of receivers) than for imaging with standard surface or whole-volume coils. This will increase image reconstruction time and may limit the use of sequences that acquire data rapidly, such as echo-planar imaging, or acquire large amounts of data, such as phase-contrast angiography.

There are times when a coil designed for a specific anatomic structure may not be used. For instance, a patient with severe scoliosis or with a halo for a cervical fracture or stereotactic frame may not be positioned easily in a head or neck coil. In such instances, the body coil may be used to obtain adequate images by using a large FOV, increasing the number of excitations, and using thicker slices to reduce graininess.

Restrictions in Receiver Coil Design and Positioning

Coil design depends on the magnetic field strength. Low- to middle-field magnets may employ saddle-shaped and spherical coils. These coils are incompatible with high-field systems because of self-resonance, which is a physical limitation, preventing the coil from tuning and matching at higher frequencies. The receiver coil is also restricted by design with regard to the orientation of the main magnetic field. The coil will have highest sensitivity to the signal when its magnetic axis (B_1) is positioned perpendicular to the main magnetic field. Therefore, different RF coils must be used with different types of magnets.

In systems with the main magnetic field, B_0, oriented horizontally, the magnetic axis of a coil is oriented vertically. For example, a surface coil, such as a spine coil, is positioned horizontally in the center of the main magnetic field, which results in B_1 being positioned perpendicularly to B_0 (Fig. 2–4). This is the most desirable position, because tilting the coil away from the perpendicular reduces its sensitivity and effectiveness, thereby reducing the S/N ratio.

When the main magnetic field is oriented vertically, such as a permanent magnet, solenoid coils may need to be used (Fig. 2–5). The magnetic field of these coils is oriented horizontally, which is perpendicular to the main magnetic field and therefore most desirable.

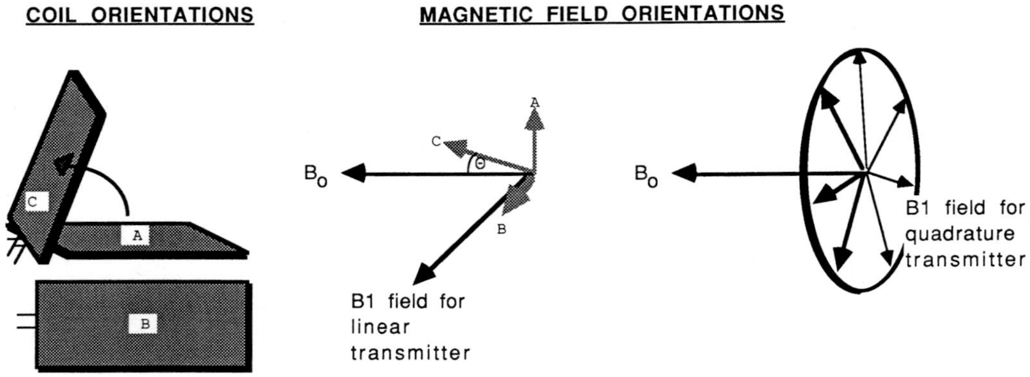

COIL ORIENTATIONS   MAGNETIC FIELD ORIENTATIONS

FIGURE 2–4. Positioning of a flat "license plate" receiver coil in a superconducting magnet. *A,* With horizontal positioning of a receiver coil, its B_1 RF field is perpendicular to the main magnetic field (B_0), resulting in optimal sensitivity for the tissue MR signal. In addition, its B_1 field is perpendicular to that of a linear transmitter coil (i.e., physically decoupled), which is required for safety reasons if the receiver and transmitter coils are not electronically decoupled. Note that the B_1 field of a quadrature (circular polarized) transmitter coil continually changes (i.e., rotates within the x-y plane). Therefore, it is not possible to decouple the receiver coil physically from the transmitter coil, and electronic decoupling is required. *B,* The receiver coil can be rotated to a sagittal orientation with no loss of sensitivity. Electronic decoupling of the coils in now required because the B_1 field of the receiver coil is aligned with that of the transmitter coil. *C,* Tilting a receiver coil toward a coronal orientation results in a loss of sensitivity owing to partial alignment of the B_1 field of the coil with the B_0 field. Optimal sensitivity is attained when the two are perpendicular ($\theta = 90°$), as in *A* or *B.*

There is another factor possibly restricting coil position. If the system does not have electronic decoupling, and if the transmitter and receiver coils are not placed in proper orientation to each other, a number of potential problems could result. The receiver coil position for these older systems is fixed and usually in the horizontal position. Variation from this predetermined location may result in reduced image quality, coil damage, and possibly even burning of the patient. The latter complication occurs when the RF energy from the transmitter goes directly to the receiver coil, which produces arcing to a patient. This is a serious complication, due to a high risk of burning a patient positioned in the bore of the magnet. Most systems now have electronic decoupling, which detunes the receiver coil during RF transmission, thereby avoiding adverse complications. These newer coils allow more freedom in positioning, as long as the magnetic axis is placed perpendicular to the main magnetic field, as previously discussed.

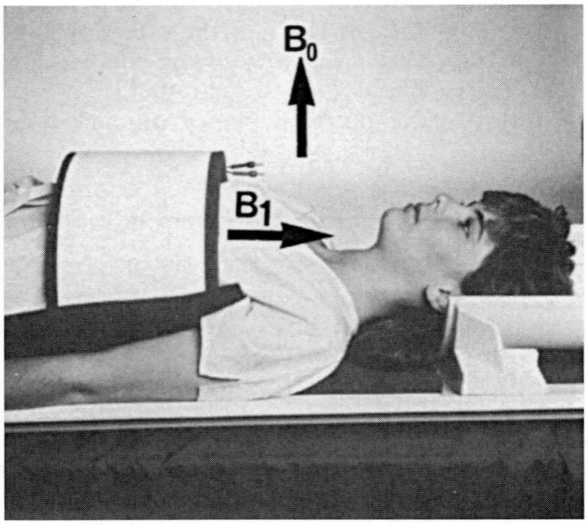

Coil Centering

The magnetic field is most uniform at the magnet isocenter. The magnetic field uniformity and integrity of the gradients decline as one moves from isocenter. Therefore, surface coils should be placed in the center of the magnet to obtain the best image quality possible. When a surface coil is placed in the periphery of the main magnet, the S/N ratio drops and the image may be distorted. However, it may be necessary to place a coil off-center when imaging a shoulder or wrist, owing to the physical limitations in positioning the patient. Imaging techniques that require a high degree of field homogeneity, such as fat suppression, may be problematic far from the isocenter.

COIL TUNING AND MATCHING

Surface coils work best when positioned as close as possible to the signal source. When using volume coils, one should center the area of interest in the center of the volume coil. An incorrectly positioned coil may not tune and match. The coil impedance must also match with the preamplifier used to magnify the signal. When a receiver coil is properly positioned, it is influenced by the electrical properties of the tissues in that area of the patient and is "loaded" by the patient. This change in impedance decreases the quality factor

FIGURE 2–5. Flexible solenoid coil used for spine imaging in a permanent magnet system with a vertical main field (B_0) perpendicular to B_1. (Courtesy of Fonar Medical Systems, Melville, NY.)

(Q factor) of the coil and changes its resonant frequency and matching. This necessitates that the coil be retuned and rematched to the resonant frequency of the local tissue. Coils with a high Q factor are more difficult to tune and match because the acceptable range of frequencies is smaller. Conversely, a coil with a low Q factor tunes more easily because it has a wider range of acceptance. This is not noticeable in most systems today because they are equipped with autotuning.

An incorrectly tuned and matched coil will reflect power that is delivered to it through its connecting cables. Most systems measure the RF power reflected from the coil to observe coil tuning and matching. The coil is optimally tuned and matched when the reflected power is zero at the frequency of operation. Some coils may autotune and match using this reflected power with a simple command by the operator. Yet others require manual tuning, in which the operator makes adjustments while the reflected power is used for tuning and matching. The circuits are either motor driven, as in head and body coils, or electronically driven, as in some surface coils, such as the spine coil. These adjustments continue until an acceptable signal is reached to obtain the highest quality signal possible.

Some manufacturers design the surface coils so that they do not require tuning for each individual patient. Instead, they are pretuned and have a wide range of acceptable frequencies. The advantage in this design is that there are fewer difficulties in scanning a patient because the tuning and matching steps are eliminated. The disadvantage is a reduced S/N ratio because the coils in these systems have a low Q factor.

Occasionally, a coil will not tune to a patient. This may be due to the patient's size being either too small or too large. If the patient is small (e.g., infant or child), the coil may have difficulty tuning because there is not enough signal returning to the receiver coil. *Placing bags of saline within the surface coil area will help load the coil so that it may tune.* Patients who are too large may need to be slightly adjusted in position to have the coil tune successfully. Another scenario that may create difficulty for coil tuning is a patient with a significantly large metallic implant, such as a hip replacement. Slightly adjusting the patient's position in this situation may be all that is required. Another possible remedy is changing coils, when that option is feasible for the type of study being performed.

FREQUENCY ADJUSTMENT

The scanning RF is proportional to the magnetic field strength, as determined by the Larmor equation. However, introducing an object, such as a patient, into the magnetic field alters its homogeneity. A patient's body acts like an antenna, slightly distorting the magnetic field. Because each patient is unique in size and shape, it is necessary to make an adjustment of the transmitted frequency. This is accomplished by emitting a wide range of frequencies, and the result is

Fourier transformed. The transformed information is displayed as a spectrum on a graph, with peaks representing various signal intensities. Ideally, two peaks are displayed, with the higher frequency peak representing water, and the lower frequency peak representing fat. The adjustment process takes this information and adapts the frequency to match that of the water or as close to the water peak as possible, depending on which type of system is employed. For most imaging techniques, it is desirable to match the center frequency on the water peak. Occasionally, the fat peak is larger, and depending on the software, the center frequency is incorrectly set at this value. This is noticeable only in fat or silicone saturation images. In this case, *one can add a value of 220 Hz at 1.5 T, or proportionally less at lower field strengths, to center correctly at the water peak.*

Obtaining fat saturation images may be problematic if there is a poor shim. This will be especially noticeable when imaging the neck and breast, owing to the anatomic contours, or when imaging far off the isocenter, as for the shoulder. An apparatus is available that fits the contours of the neck to reduce the problems associated with a poor shim. It acts as an interface between a curved structure and the coil.

The frequency adjustment process is especially important on mobile systems, as the environment from site to site varies. The shim of the magnet is usually different in different locations owing to adjacent structures of the site location. Hindrances in the adjustment process may be encountered when there is a large metallic object in the imaging area, when a patient is improperly positioned with respect to the receiver coil, or when the main magnetic field is inhomogeneous. These problems result in a reduced S/N ratio. Therefore, *it is important to eliminate all metallic objects, ferrous or nonferrous, whenever possible.* A service engineer is able to check the magnetic field homogeneity when it is suspected to be a problem.

TRANSMITTER ADJUSTMENT

Adjustment of the transmitter is performed to ascertain the correct level of power given to the RF pulse to produce the desired flip angle of the nuclei. It is necessary to readjust the transmitter each time a patient is repositioned or when scanning a new patient, inasmuch as the shape of the body will be different, resulting in a different amount of required power.

The system calculates the power required to produce the desired flip angle, depending on which pulse sequence is chosen by the operator, and other flip angles, as well. The computer generates a string of numbers. These numbers are a representation of the given pulse sequence. The numbers are converted by a digital-to-analog converter, thereby translating the numbers to an analog waveform that produces the voltage in the RF. To accomplish adjustment, most systems start the adjustment process with a low voltage, with successive steps of increased RF voltage to the patient, until a minimal signal is detected by the receiver. The transmitted RF may either cover the entire imaging area, known as a nonselective pulse, or measure the signal from a single slice. This is a selective RF pulse. The latter is more accurate than the nonselective pulse.

Some difficulties may arise when adjusting the transmitter. For instance, larger patients require a higher voltage. The transmitter tube may not be capable of emitting enough power to reach the required minimal signal output. Also, the transmitter tube may not be able to emit enough power on average-sized patients when the tube is old. A service engineer can determine the number of hours the tube has been used and can recommend when it needs replacing. Another potential problem *occurs when the transmitter coil sends enough power to produce a 360° flip angle instead of a 180° flip angle. The resultant images will have a very low S/N ratio.* The user should check the transmitter values when this error is suspected and look for unusually high voltages for the size of the given patient. If the system allows it, the user should reduce the transmitter values and attempt the scan again. Last, if a surface coil has been improperly positioned, or if there is an electronic malfunction, the receiver coil may not decouple from the transmitter coil during the adjustment process. This will result in improper transmitter adjustment.

RECEIVER ADJUSTMENT

The receiver coil detects the MR signal produced by the patient's body after the tissue is excited by the transmitted RF. Different parts of the body emit different frequencies. This is partially due to the gradients used in the MR system and partially due to the changes in the patient's body contour. The receiver is adjusted to listen for the emitted signal at different frequencies.

Also during the receiver adjustment, the signal is amplified and translated back from an analog signal to a digital output, by the analog-to-digital converter. This makes it possible for the MR computer to take the information from the various signal intensities and send it to the Fourier transform to then produce an image. However, the converter has a limited capacity in digitizing the signal. Receiver gain adjustment will keep the range of numbers manageable for the converter.

Systems without automatic receiver adjustment may have problems with this step, and poor images are usually a result of an incorrectly set receiver gain. Most systems today have an automatic receiver gain adjustment. Yet, improper receiver adjustment may still occur. One example is when the patient moves during the scan acquisition, but not during the receiver adjustment, because motion changes signal intensity. The receiver is set at a particular level, but the scan produces more signal. Images appear with altered tissue contrast and a bright background. *One may reduce the receiver gain by about 3 dB from the automatic receiver gain value and rescan a patient.* Another example is when performing an examination of an area using the same pulse sequence before and after IV contrast

medium administration. If the receiver is not adjusted after the contrast agent is injected, the receiver gain may have an improper setting (Fig. 2–6). This is due to the increased signal detected from the contrast material. *A technologist, when anticipating such a situation, may reduce the receiver gain by about 6 dB from the receiver gain value from the automatic adjustment.*

IMAGE MEASUREMENT

Preparation Scans

After all prescan adjustments have been made, the measurement process may commence. However, data

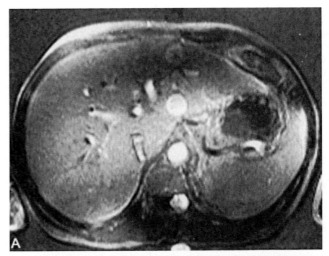
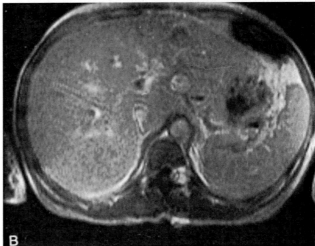

FIGURE 2–6. Bolus administration of gadolinium diethylenetri-aminepentaacetic acid (Gd-DTPA) breath-hold scanning in a patient with suspected liver metastasis. *A,* Immediate postcontrast scan of the upper abdomen. Note the peculiar image contrast and bright background, representing ''clipping'' of an MR signal that exceeds the dynamic range of the analog-to-digital converter. The receiver gain for this scan was adjusted before administration of contrast agent to avoid any delay before initiating dynamic scanning of the liver. However, there was an overall increase in signal intensity after contrast agent administration because of the marked enhancement of the liver, spleen, and blood vessels, so that the previously determined receiver gain was too high. *B,* After manual reduction of the receiver gain by 3 dB, image contrast becomes normal.

are not actually acquired for several seconds after the nominal start of the measurement. The reason for this relates to the need to establish an equilibrium or steady-state magnetization (see Chapter 1). Before any RF pulses are applied, the spins are fully magnetized. Therefore, the first RF pulse produces a strong signal. However, each of the next few RF pulses produces less signal, owing to incomplete T1 relaxation between excitations. Only after several excitations is a balance (i.e., equilibrium) reached between the TR and T1.

To avoid an anomalous change in signal intensity over the first few repetitions, a number of preparation scans are applied for the first few seconds of the scan (Fig. 2–7). Different sequence types have different preparation scans. For instance, with a spin-echo sequence equilibrium is achieved after the first 90° excitation pulse. The first data set is not collected in this case, but all subsequent data are used in image reconstruction. In gradient-echo (GRE) imaging, the number of preparation pulses needed to have the tissue reach a steady-state varies. A lower flip angle sequence means a longer preparation time due to a weaker RF excitation pulse. Conversely, a higher flip angle requires less preparation time because the RF pulse is stronger. When using a fast spin-echo sequence, the tissue will reach equilibrium with a second 90° pulse. Most systems today can automatically calculate the time needed for preparation based on the type of sequence selected, known as "auto prep time."

SPECIFIC ABSORPTION RATE

The specific absorption rate (SAR) refers to the amount of RF power deposition to biologic tissue during image acquisition measured in watts per kilogram. The FDA has set specific limitations on the amount of RF power a patient may receive during each series of images. The upper limits are 0.4 W/kg for the whole-body average and 8.0 W/kg for any 1 g of tissue. The purpose of setting limitations is so that a patient's core body temperature will increase no more than 1°C.

Factors influencing the amount of RF power to the patient are the magnetic field strength, the type of pulse sequence, and the choice of receiver coil used for imaging. Stronger magnets require higher frequency RF and therefore deposit more energy in tissues, whereas lower field systems will use less power and are less likely to reach the SAR limitations. Certain pulse sequences will emit more power than others. For instance, fast spin echo, also known as turbo spin echo, utilizes rapid RF pulses of a high power, thus increasing the RF deposition. This problem can be minimized by reducing the flip angle of the refocusing pulses from 180° to about 130°, without loss of image quality in most cases. Magnetization transfer sequences also increase the power deposition to the patient. Spin-echo imaging and GRE imaging do not usually require as much energy. However, the power emitted also depends on the coil selected. Small coils (e.g., head coil) require less energy for imaging than larger coils (e.g., body coil). The coil design also plays a role in the amount of RF power emitted. Circularly polarized transmitter coils require less power than linearly polarized coils.

Studies have shown that patients with normal heat loss capacity are able to safely undergo MRI with an SAR as much as 4 W/kg averaged over the whole body. The FDA limitations may be overridden at hospital-based facilities if approval is obtained from the institutional review board, the hospital's governing board of clinical research trials. Outpatient centers without hospital affiliation must be designated by an MRI equipment manufacturer as a research site to obtain permission to exceed the SAR limitations. Patients with heat regulation deficiencies may experience discomfort or medical complications. Those potentially at risk include obese or geriatric patients or patients with cardiovascular disease or a disease or medication causing high temperature. Therefore, caution should be taken not to expose these patients to more than 2 W/kg.

Other alternatives exist if SAR limitations are a factor in imaging. For instance, choosing pulse sequences that have fewer RF pulses or longer RF pulses will aid in obtaining images without reaching SAR limitations. Unfortunately, there are drawbacks to implementing these techniques. Longer RF pulses mean a longer minimal TE and therefore less signal or more artifact. Chemical-shift artifacts may also be more prominent

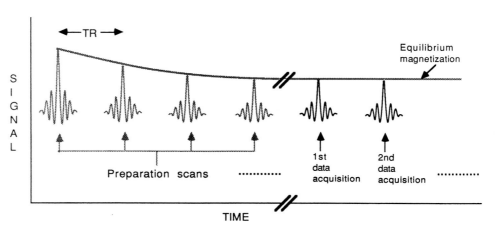

FIGURE 2–7. At the start of the measurement process, a number of preparation scans may be applied to establish an equilibrium magnetization, or steady state. The data acquisition is started only after the preparation scans are finished.

in the slice-select direction on middle- to high-field systems.

CHOOSING A PULSE SEQUENCE

A multitude of types of sequences are available in MRI through conventional imaging (spin echo and GRE), fast imaging (turbo or fast spin echo), and ultrafast imaging (echo planar). The technologist and radiologist need to consider the anatomic structure that is being imaged and decide on the appropriate use of the options available.

SPIN ECHO

Spin-echo imaging is the "bread and butter" of MRI, although it is increasingly being supplanted by faster GRE and fast spin-echo sequences. Adjustments in the TR and TE determine tissue contrast. A combination of short TR and short TE produces a T1-weighted image, a long TR and long TE produce a T2-weighted image, and a long TR and short TE yield a proton or spin density image. There is always some amount of T1, T2, and proton density weighting in images from any of these parameters. However, by maximizing one over the other, or minimizing the effects of two of these, the resultant image is more strongly weighted with the desired tissue contrast.

To produce a T1-weighted image with a spin-echo sequence, the TR ranges between 300 and 800 ms and the TE ranges between 6 and 25 ms. Because the TR is one of the factors determining scan time and the number of slices allowed, the technologist should try to minimize the TR as much as possible. The technologist may increase the number of slices by choosing a high-bandwidth sequence and using a shorter TE. Another method of obtaining coverage over a larger area is to increase the slice thickness or the interslice gap. This may be done without increasing the imaging time. There is less flexibility in choosing the TE of a sequence as it is restricted by the TR, bandwidth, and pulse sequence design. For T1 weighting, the TE should be kept to a minimum to reduce any T2 weighting in the image.

A sequence with a TR greater than 2000 ms and a long TE (greater than 60 ms) will yield T2-weighted images. The long TR provides ample time to sample data at two different TEs without increasing the imaging time. Therefore, two images are usually acquired, one with a short TE and one with a long TE. The first echo image is a proton density–weighted image, and the second is the T2-weighted image. Because the TR is long, adequate coverage of the area of interest is not usually a problem; however, the imaging time can be quite long. The S/N ratio of the second echo is diminished because the sampling takes place after much of the signal has decayed. T2-weighted images are also more susceptible to motion artifacts, causing further image degradation.

GRADIENT ECHO

GRE imaging may be used in place of spin-echo sequences for certain anatomic structures and certain indications. The parameters may be manipulated to obtain either more T1-weighted or more T2-weighted images, although the former is usually more useful. It is not appropriate to use in all cases because of the artifacts experienced by use of this technique. GRE sequences are more sensitive to magnetic field inhomogeneity, which can be caused by metal in or on a patient (e.g., metallic implants, jewelry, braces). Advantages to GRE scanning are that it is faster and it provides better evaluation of vascular structures over spin echo. Faster scanning is achieved by using a partial flip angle instead of the full 90° and 180° induced in a spin-echo sequence.

To obtain a T1-weighted scan with a GRE sequence, the user should choose a larger flip angle (70° to 90°). A higher flip angle results in more T1-weighted contrast in the image. A lower flip angle produces a more strongly T2-weighted image. The resultant images do not, however, produce enough true T2 signal to actually replace a conventional spin-echo T2 sequence. Therefore, the user should consider a patient's clinical history and the pathologic process in question when determining the appropriateness of choice of a GRE sequence. *The signal from a T2-weighted GRE may not be adequate to detect plaques of multiple sclerosis or a faint spinal tumor. Instead, one should select a FLAIR (fluid-attenuated inversion recovery) fast spin-echo sequence.*

The TE should be kept as short as possible to minimize artifacts. An exception to this rule may be when looking for brain hemorrhage. In this case, a long TE is desirable for looking at blood products. A long TE and reduced flip angle produce good contrast between blood and brain tissue. *To accentuate signal intensity from moving blood, one should use flow compensation.*

One can use multislice or sequential two-dimensional (2D) GRE sequences. The former, which uses a moderate TR generally greater than 100 ms, can be used for rapid anatomic imaging (e.g., for breath-hold T1-weighted liver or kidney imaging). The latter is used predominantly for MR angiography because the short TR gives good background suppression.

OTHER IMAGING PARAMETERS

NUMBER OF EXCITATIONS

The number of excitations (NEX), or equivalently the number of acquisitions (ACQ), refers to the number of times the data are acquired for each phase encode. The duration of a sequence is determined by TR × matrix (in the phase encoding direction) × NEX (except in fast spin-echo imaging in which TR is not as much a factor as echo train length). It is desirable to keep imaging times as short as possible. However, image quality may be improved by increasing the NEX, which increases image signal and reduces ghosting artifacts from blood or cerebrospinal fluid

(CSF) flow and respiratory motion. The reduction of signal from ghost artifact is approximately equal to the square root of the NEX. The user must balance the cost of increased time against improved image quality and determine its usefulness for any given anatomic area. Imaging techniques also play a role in determining the cost of imaging times. Increasing from 1 to 2 NEX doubles the imaging time. Doubling the imaging time of a T1-weighted spin-echo or T2-weighted fast spin-echo sequence may be acceptable. However, doubling the number of excitations of a T2-weighted spin-echo sequence is impractical owing to the increase in the acquisition time.

SLICE THICKNESS

Choosing a slice thickness depends on many factors, such as anatomic area to be covered, size of a given structure being imaged, number of slices allowed by the type of scanning sequence, desired S/N ratio, magnetic field strength, and gradient strength. *Thinner (3 mm) slices should be used when scanning smaller structures such as a pituitary gland, metatarsal or metacarpal bones, or seventh and eighth cranial nerves of the internal auditory canal.* However, thinner slices yield less signal. To compensate, the user may increase the NEX. Thicker slices (5 mm) may be used for areas such as a routine screening brain study. Even thicker slices (up to 10 mm) may be used for abdominal or thoracic cavity surveys. Because of the short TR, a T1-weighted sequence may limit the number of slices allowed. The TR may be increased, but only a small amount before the tissue characteristics from T2 effects result in contrast changes. To cover the area of interest, the user may instead increase slice thickness or keep the same slice thickness and run the T1-weighted sequence twice to cover the area. This may be done by selecting contiguous slices and run one set over one half of the area and the remainder for the second half or by interleaving the slice locations from one acquisition to the next. The latter is preferable, as this technique will less likely produce images with cross-talk. A T2-weighted sequence will yield more slices, allowing more flexibility in slice thickness. A low-field magnet may require the use of thicker slices for an adequate S/N ratio. Gradient strength and the RF pulse duration and shape will determine the minimal slice thickness for a particular MR system, which is usually between 2 and 3 mm. Three-dimensional (3D) scanning techniques allow acquisition of slice thicknesses of 1 mm or less.

INTERSLICE GAP AND SLICE PROFILE

It would be ideal to obtain contiguous images in MRI. In practice, it is necessary to insert an interslice gap. The reason for this practice relates to imperfections in slice profiles. A mathematic function known as *sinc* [sin (x)/x] is commonly used to modulate the waveform of the RF pulse. The Fourier transform of this function is a rectangle. However, a perfectly rect-

angular slice profile is produced only by a sinc pulse of infinite duration, which is impractical. RF pulses of shorter duration always produce imperfect slice profiles, so that the flip angle varies across the thickness of the slice. If narrow gaps between the slices are used, then each slice is contaminated by RF excitations from the edges of the adjacent slices (cross-talk) (Fig. 2–8). The result of these extra excitations is that a slice will have an effective TR less than the nominal TR. Cross-talk may be eliminated by using sinc pulses of long (e.g., >5 ms) duration. On T2-weighted images, cross-talk is manifested as a reduction in the signal from structures with long T1 relaxation times, such as CSF and neoplasms (Fig. 2–9). As a result, longer TR and TE are needed to recover the expected T2 contrast. A gap of 20% to 50% will eliminate cross-talk in these images. T1-weighted images are less degraded by cross-talk than are T2-weighted images, so that slice gaps of 10% to 30% may be adequate.

However, use of small gaps may make it difficult to obtain adequate coverage of the region of interest.

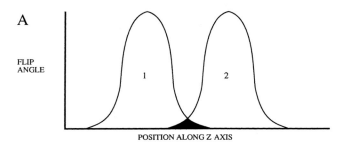

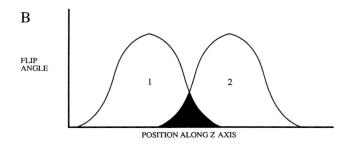

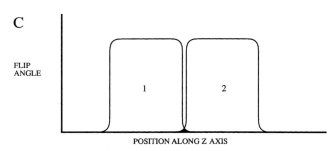

FIGURE 2–8. Slice profiles. *A,* Sinc pulse of moderate duration. *B,* Sinc pulse of shorter duration. Cross-talk *(shaded area)* 1 and 2 is worse in *B* than *A,* owing to the worsened slice profile in the latter case. This necessitates increasing the interslice gap. *C,* Long sinc pulses or computer-optimized RF pulses of shorter duration produce nearly rectangular slice profiles, permitting interslice gaps less than or equal to 10% of the normal slice thickness.

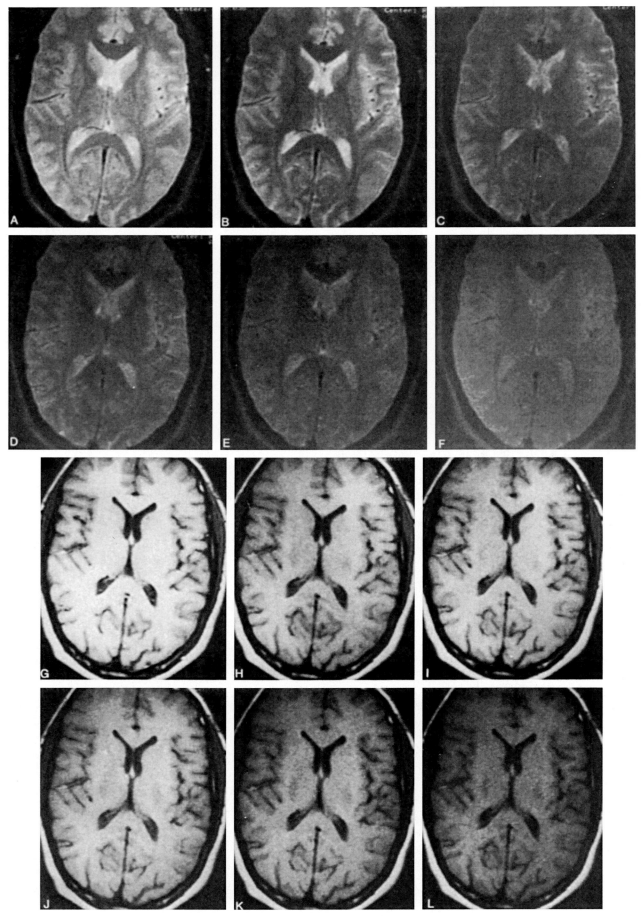

FIGURE 2–9 *See legend on opposite page*

Total coverage, defined as the space between the centers of the outer slices, may be expressed as

$$\text{Coverage} = (\text{number of slices} - 1)$$
$$\times (\text{slice thickness} + \text{gap})$$

For instance, a 20-slice axial acquisition using 5-mm-thick slices and no gap would produce coverage of 95 mm, which is less than the vertical extent of the average adult brain. Older MR systems may be further restricted by the amount of computer memory available for the storage of raw data. To compensate for these limitations, changing the interslice gap to 40% of the slice thickness, or 2 mm, will cover the average adult brain. Unlike 2D acquisitions, 3D acquisitions have no cross-talk between adjacent slices, although cross-talk may occur between adjacent slabs of a multislab (e.g., 3D fast spin-echo) acquisition.

FIELD OF VIEW

The FOV is defined as the horizontal or vertical distance across an image. The minimal FOV is primarily determined by the peak gradient amplitude and gradient duration. Decreases in the FOV are brought about by increasing the strength of the frequency-encoding and phase-encoding gradients. Spatial resolution improves as the FOV is decreased, within the constraints of the S/N ratio limitations. Reductions in FOV produce a rapid decline in the S/N ratio in proportion to the square of the FOV. Reducing slice thickness also reduces the S/N ratio, but on a one-to-one proportion. Therefore, adjusting slice thickness may be a more practical method for reducing partial volume averaging instead of adjusting the FOV.

An FOV is chosen based on the anatomic structure of interest and the chosen imaging coil. Small FOVs (e.g., 8 to 12 cm) are used for detailed anatomic evaluation, as needed in the TMJ or the wrist. *Small FOVs may produce wraparound artifacts unless oversampling methods are used* (Fig. 2–10). Low-bandwidth sequences, because of the weaker readout gradient, typically permit smaller FOVs than do higher bandwidth sequences, but chemical-shift artifact is worse. Larger FOVs (e.g., 32 to 38 cm) are used when more spatial coverage is required, such as in chest, abdominal, pelvic, and spine imaging. Good spatial resolution can be maintained despite the large FOV by using a 512 acquisition matrix.

MATRIX

The image matrix represents the number of pixels along the frequency-encoding and phase-encoding axes. Imaging time is proportional to the number of

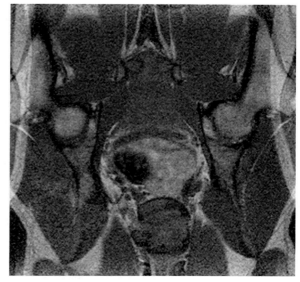

FIGURE 2–10. Pelvic image acquired with 28-cm FOV in the coronal plane. Oversampling was applied in the frequency-encoding (vertical) direction only. The image is degraded by a wraparound artifact in the phase-encoding (horizontal) direction.

phase-encoding steps. (An exception is the class of single-shot imaging techniques, such as echo planar, turboFLASH, or HASTE [half-Fourier single-shot turbo spin echo].) Most systems allow the user to select from several matrix sizes. Typically, 256 pixels are selected along the frequency-encoding axis and from 128 to 256 pixels are selected along the phase-encoding axis. Images acquired with a symmetric FOV and 256 × 256 matrix have equal resolution along both axes.

Images can be acquired using a 256 × 128 (frequency × phase) matrix in half the time of a 256 × 256 matrix, at the expense of a 50% reduction in spatial resolution. Because of the lower spatial resolution, the S/N ratio improves with a reduction in matrix size (Table 2–1). However, objectionable ringing artifacts may result from small matrix sizes so that a compromise may be made between spatial resolution and imaging time by using a 256 × 192 (frequency × phase) matrix.

Ringing artifacts and spatial resolution can also be improved, despite a reduced matrix, by using an asymmetric (rectangular) FOV. As mentioned in Chapter 1, this technique improves resolution along the phase-encoding axis by increasing the amplitude of the phase-encoding gradient, while keeping constant the number of pixels in the matrix. For instance, one can consider an image acquired with a 256 × 128 matrix and a 30 × 30-cm FOV. In the same amount of time, an image can be acquired with 33% more resolution

FIGURE 2–9. Effects of cross-talk on image contrast and S/N ratio. T2-weighted spin-echo images *(A to F)* and T1-weighted images *(G to L)* with decrease in interslice gap from 100% *(A and G)* to 0% *(F and L)*. Note marked worsening in T2 contrast and S/N ratio, even with moderate gaps (e.g., 20% in *D*), whereas T1-weighted images are less severely degraded at the same gap *(J)*. (*A to L* from Kucharczyk W, Crawley AP, Kelly WM, Henkelman RM: Effect of multislice interference on image contrast in T2- and T1-weighted MR images. AJNR 9:443–451, 1988, © by American Roentgen Ray Society.)

TABLE 2–1. SOME EXAMPLES OF THE EFFECTS OF CHANGES IN SCAN PARAMETERS ON ACQUISITION TIME, S/N RATIO, AND SPATIAL RESOLUTION

MATRIX	SLT* (mm)	FOV (cm)	NEX	ACQ TIME† (s)	S/N RATIO‡	RESOLUTION (mm)	VOXEL (mm³)
256 × 256	5	24	1	128	100	0.9 × 0.9	4.4
256 × 256	5	24	1	64	71	0.9 × 0.9	4.4
Half-Fourier							
256 × 192	5	24	1	96	115	0.9 × 1.3	5.9
256 × 256	5	24 × 30	1	128	125	0.9 × 1.2	5.5
Asymmetric FOV							
256 × 128	5	24	1	64	141	0.9 × 1.8	8.8
256 × 128	5	24	2	128	200	0.9 × 1.8	8.8
256 × 256	5	17	1	128	50	0.7 × 0.7	2.2
256 × 256	5	17	4	512	100	0.7 × 0.7	2.2
256 × 128	5	17	2	128	100	0.7 × 1.3	4.4
256 × 128	7	17	1	64	100	0.7 × 1.3	6.2
256 × 256	3	10	1	128	10	0.4 × 0.4	0.5
256 × 128	3	10	8	512	40	0.4 × 0.8	0.9

*SLT = slice thickness.
†Acquisition time for TR = 500 ms.
‡S/N ratio normalized to 100 for 5-mm slice, 256 × 256 matrix, and 1 NEX.

along the y axis by using a 30 × 20-cm (frequency × phase) FOV. However, compared with the image acquired using the symmetric FOV, this image will have 33% less S/N ratio. In addition, wraparound artifact may limit the application of this method with small FOVs, depending on the dimensions of the body part being imaged.

TRADEOFFS AMONG IMAGING PARAMETERS

It is generally desirable to maximize spatial resolution while minimizing imaging time. However, it is also necessary to maintain an adequate level of S/N ratio. For instance, a reduction in slice thickness produces a decrease in S/N ratio that may be compensated for by using a slightly larger FOV or smaller matrix. Some examples of interdependent effects that result from changes in various scan parameters are provided in Table 2–1.

SPECIAL TECHNIQUES

Some of the most recent developments in imaging techniques have specific applications. For instance, FLAIR sequences are most commonly used for detecting the presence of plaques of multiple sclerosis that are not otherwise seen by conventional imaging. The tissue signal to be nulled is the CSF, and the inversion time should be approximately 2200 ms. Alternatively, an inversion time on the order of 150 ms will null the signal from fat (STIR [short-tau inversion recovery] imaging), a technique that has wide applications for detection of tumors, inflammation, and edema.

Magnetization transfer contrast (MTC or MT) is used when it is desirable to or suppress stationary tissue compared with blood. This imaging technique is useful in imaging vessel anatomy in the brain with MR angiographic techniques. *It is also beneficial to use MTC for T1-weighted images immediately after IV contrast medium administration when looking for metastatic disease in the brain.* This technique is much more sensitive to enhancing lesions than the conventional spin-echo method.

HALF-FOURIER

The half-Fourier method reconstructs an image from only half the available data in the matrix and mirroring the other half to fill in the full matrix. This technique provides a reduction of nearly 50% in imaging time. *However, with the faster acquisition, S/N ratio is reduced by 40%, so the method should be employed only when the S/N ratio is not a limiting factor.* Moreover, the half-Fourier images are prone to artifacts produced by magnetic field inhomogeneity or motion of the patient. This technique should be avoided with GRE sequences, as the problem would be compounded when both techniques are applied. In addition, the extra data manipulations required with half-Fourier imaging may increase reconstruction times as much as twofold.

FLOW COMPENSATION (BRIGHT BLOOD SEQUENCE)

Flow compensation, also known as "flow comp," gradient motion rephasing (GMR), gradient moment nulling (GMN), or motion artifact suppression technique (MAST), is a method for reducing flow and motion artifacts (see Chapter 3). The method incorporates into the pulse sequence additional gradient pulses that reduce motion-related phase shifts. In multiechof pulse sequences used for obtaining T2-weighted images, the first or second echoes, or both, may be flow compensated, depending on the pulse sequence and the MR system.

The effect of flow compensation is to increase signal intensity from flowing blood and CSF. Flow compensation should be used in nearly all clinical applications of T2-weighted images when motion is an issue. *This method is particularly useful for suppressing ghost artifacts arising from CSF pulsation in the brain and spine.* When flow compensation is used for abdominal imaging, signal intensity from moving organs, such as the liver, is increased and ghost artifacts are reduced.

The major limitation of flow compensation is that the minimal TE, slice thickness, and FOV may be increased compared with standard pulse sequences. As a result, it may not be possible to use flow compensation in applications that require extremely high spatial resolution, such as imaging the TMJ. In addition, in some patients, flow compensation may not provide adequate suppression of ghost artifacts from CSF pulsation. In these instances, the combination of flow compensation and ECG gating (see later in this chapter) may provide better artifact suppression.

Flow compensation should not be used when it is important that flowing blood or CSF appears dark. For instance, flow compensation will eliminate the CSF flow void sign in the aqueduct of Sylvius. This sign is occasionally used to characterize hydrocephalus. Similarly, flow compensation may not be desirable on T1-weighted images of the spine, because it increases the signal intensity of CSF and may reduce contrast between CSF and spinal cord or cauda equina.

Presaturation (Dark Blood Sequence)

Presaturation is a method that eliminates ghost artifacts resulting from blood flow or respiratory motion (see Chapter 3). The method incorporates into the pulse sequence additional RF pulses that saturate tissue magnetization over user-defined regions. *Presaturation applied along the slice-select direction eliminates flow artifacts and should routinely be used for imaging the brain, neck, chest, abdomen, and extremities, wherever flow artifact may limit image quality.* The use of presaturation aids in image quality by reducing ghost artifact from pulsatile blood flow in vessels such as intracerebral and carotid arteries, aorta, and inferior vena cava, as well as the popliteal artery. It is usually affordable, with regard to imaging time, on a T2 sequence and also quite beneficial for this technique.

The effectiveness of flow presaturation depends on the velocity and direction of flow. Therefore, one should not be surprised if the technique fails to eliminate signal completely from CSF within the thecal sac, where the flow is to and fro rather than unidirectional, or in certain patterns of blood flow. For instance, presaturation does not typically affect artifacts caused by vascular pulsation in the cerebral venous sinuses, because the effects of the presaturation pulses on arteries do not carry through the capillary system into the veins. It may also fail to suppress intravascular signal adequately within large aortic aneurysms, which have slow flow.

Additional limitations of the method include reduced multislice capability and increased RF power deposition.

Presaturation becomes ineffective after IV administration of gadolinium chelates, because the T1 of blood becomes too short. *Direct saturation along the long axis of the aorta can be helpful to reduce ghost artifacts, particularly for coronal imaging of the abdomen.*

Some systems offer the capability of applying presaturation along directions other than slice selection. For instance, presaturation applied along the phase-encoding direction may be useful for spine imaging to suppress ghost artifacts arising from vascular pulsation and respiratory motion, particularly if gradient rotation is not available. Presaturation may also be used to suppress the high signal pattern from subcutaneous fat in the near field of a surface coil, which reduces motion artifacts.

Gradient Rotation (Phase Frequency Swap)

The orientation of the phase-encoding axis is determined by the user. *By reorienting the phase-encoding axis by 90°, it may be possible to keep ghost artifacts off the region of interest.* For axial brain imaging, the phase-encoding axis is typically oriented horizontally (swapped) to direct artifacts from eye motion away from the brain. For spine imaging, the phase-encoding axis may be oriented parallel to the long axis of the spine to prevent ghost artifacts from respiratory motion and vascular pulsation. Axial images of the upper abdomen usually have the phase-encoding axis oriented from anterior to posterior of the patient so that blood flow artifacts from the inferior vena cava and aorta are away from the liver and kidneys. However, if the left lobe of the liver is the area of interest, the user may wish to swap the phase-encoding direction so that it is oriented from left to right, thus moving aortic ghost artifact off the left lobe of the liver.

A major limitation of gradient rotation (also known as swapping phase and frequency-encoding gradients) is wraparound artifact when the phase-encoding axis is oriented along the long axis of the body. Suppression of wraparound requires concomitant use of oversampling methods. If these are not available, presaturation should be used for artifact suppression, rather than gradient rotation. Wraparound artifact may result when a relatively small FOV is used with gradient rotation in an area such as the pelvis. The wraparound artifact may reduce the overall attractiveness of the image. However, this may not be a problem for making a diagnosis because the wraparound may occur in areas outside the region of interest. This is especially true when it is more important to have a smaller FOV of the area of interest for more detailed anatomic evaluation. For instance, the uterus is usually found in the center of the pelvis, so wraparound artifacts extending into the outer hip muscles will not interfere with the region of interest.

RESPIRATION MOTION COMPENSATION

The order of phase-encoding steps may be varied according to the respiratory phase, as monitored by a bellows device around the chest or abdomen. This device should be wrapped snugly around a patient's abdomen, but not so tight so as to be uncomfortable. This method provides a substantial reduction in ghost artifact from respiratory motion. Limitations of this method include difficulty in obtaining adequate sensitivity with the bellows device and increased reconstruction time, because additional data processing is required.

A simpler way of reducing respiratory artifact when imaging in the abdominal area is to use a piece of fabric, available through vendors selling positioning devices, with Velcro for keeping a snug fit around a patient's abdomen. *This limits the up-and-down motion of a patient's abdomen without increasing image acquisition time and therefore reduces ghost artifact from that type of motion.*

Eventually, respiratory gating methods using a mechanical bellows or, better still, navigator echoes will come into routine use for motion suppression. Extra time is required to position the bellows optimally and to choose the thresholds for accepting the data, or in the case of navigator echoes, to position the beam over the region of interest (e.g., lung-diaphragm interface). Moreover, with respiratory gating methods, some data must be rejected so that scan times are increased typically by a factor of 2 to 4. Fast imaging sequences such as fast spin echo are needed to make the increased scan time acceptable.

OVERSAMPLING TO ELIMINATE WRAPAROUND

Oversampling methods acquire an expanded matrix (typically up to 512 pixels) along either or both the frequency and the phase directions to eliminate wraparound artifact (see Chapter 3). The extra pixels that contain the wrapped portion of the image are discarded, so that only the central 256 pixels are displayed. In the frequency direction, there is no time penalty for using oversampling. The only problem that may occur is that the data sampling rate increases, which may prove excessive in some situations when a phased-array coil is used. In the phase direction, the scan time increases in direct proportion to the percentage of oversampling, because additional phase encodes must be acquired. For abdominal and chest imaging, phase oversampling is particularly important for acquisitions in the coronal plane, because the body is typically wider than it is broad. The wraparound artifact on coronal acquisitions is exacerbated when the arms are at the sides of the patient rather than resting on the abdomen or over the head. For similar reasons, use of a rectangular FOV should be avoided on coronal acquisitions.

ELECTROCARDIOGRAPHIC GATING

ECG gating involves synchronization of data acquisition to a patient's ECG tracing to suppress flow arti-

facts, to define cardiac and vessel anatomy more precisely, or to permit dynamic display of cardiac function using cine techniques.

There is some confusion of terminology with respect to the terms *triggering* and *gating*. Although these terms are often used synonymously, some manufacturers use the term triggering specifically to refer to prospective methods of cardiac gating.

Prospective Cardiac Gating

For prospective cardiac gating, data acquisition is initiated after a user-determined time interval following the R wave of the cardiac cycle (Fig. 2–11). This "trigger delay" can be varied so that images are obtained in a particular phase of the cardiac cycle. For instance, triggering with no delay initiates data acquisition at end-diastole, when flow is slow and vascular signal intensity is high on a T1-weighted sequence (Fig. 2–12*A*). Conversely, a trigger delay on the order of 200 to 300 ms initiates data acquisition during systole, when flow is rapid and vascular signal intensity is low for the area imaged (Fig. 2–12*B*). In a multislice acquisition, the images are acquired over a finite period, corresponding to the user-selected TR. As a result, the images usually span a substantial portion of the cardiac cycle.

ECG gating should be used for cardiac imaging and for imaging of structures directly adjacent to the heart, such as the aortic root and main pulmonary arteries. Imaging of other vascular structures, such as renal arteries and inferior vena cava, may benefit from ECG gating as well. However, for several reasons, difficulties may be encountered in obtaining a satisfactory ECG tracing:

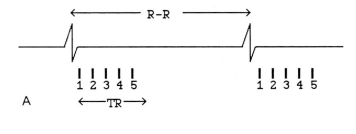

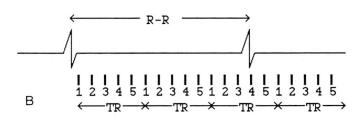

FIGURE 2–11. Comparison of prospective cardiac gating *(A)* and retrospective cardiac gating *(B)* for five-slice acquisition. In prospective gating, the time interval between sequence repetitions is determined by the RR interval, not the TR. The TR determines the duration of the cardiac cycle during which slices are acquired. In retrospective gating, the time interval between sequence repetitions is determined by the TR, as it would be for an ungated acquisition. Retrospective gating provides more consistent image quality for cine imaging than does prospective gating.

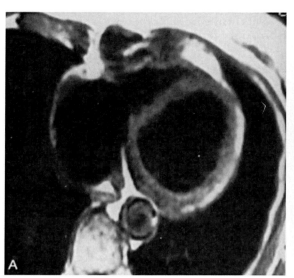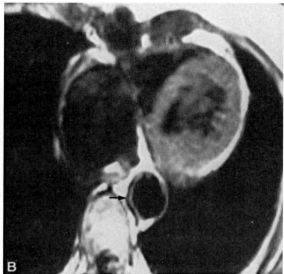

FIGURE 2–12. Axial spin-echo images of a heart at the level of the ventricles. Diastolic spin-echo image *(A)* shows brighter signal in descending aorta, because of slower flow velocity; note the low signal intensity in the aorta (*arrow* in *B*) because the image was acquired during systole when flow is rapid.

1. Poor lead contact may result from inadequate skin preparation. The skin should always be cleansed of oil and debris, by using an alcohol swab or by gently scraping the skin with a piece of thin plastic (the cover from some ECG electrodes will suffice) before applying the electrodes. In some instances, the hair should be shaved where lead contact is to be made. In addition, ECG electrodes should contain a minimal amount of metal to reduce local artifact and to prevent warming or burning of a patient's skin.

2. Respiratory motion causes a variation in the ECG baseline, making it difficult for the system to find and follow the R wave of the cardiac cycle. This problem may be prevented by attaching ECG leads to the back of a patient and using special positioning schemes (Fig. 2–13).

3. Gradient pulsing during imaging induces electrical currents in ECG leads, which may completely obscure the ECG tracing unless electronic filtering is adequate. Positioning the ECG lead wires straight along the magnet axis and twisting the leads around one another can help prevent artifacts. If the leads are placed in so that there are loops, arcing may occur. This could be dangerous to the patient being imaged because this may cause burning, which in some cases can be quite severe. Both conscious and sedated patients may not realize that this is happening at the time. Therefore, a technologist should take precautions when placing ECG leads on a patient. Placing a towel or pillowcase between the lead wires and the patient's skin helps prevent skin warming or burning of a patient. Optimal lead placement is shown in Figure 2–13.

4. Another problem is that intense static magnetic fields may alter the ECG by producing an augmented T wave or other nonspecific ECG changes. These alterations are directly related to the magnetic field strength. The mechanism responsible for increased size of the T wave is postulated to be a superimposition of a low potential on the normally occurring biopotential produced by a magnetohydrodynamic effect, as blood (i.e., a conductive fluid) flows in the presence of a static magnetic field. The computer may confuse the large T wave with an R wave, resulting in gating twice during each RR interval. In general, before using ECG gating methods it is wise to consult applications personnel for the manufacturer of the system being used, because gating methods vary widely among different systems. In difficult cases, peripheral gating using finger plethysmography may be preferred to ECG gating, although problems may then be encountered from finger motion or in patients with severe peripheral artery disease and weak pulses.

As previously mentioned, the user-selected TR has a function different from that in ungated acquisitions. *In ECG-gated acquisitions, the RR interval, rather than the TR, determines the time between successive excitations of a given slice* (see Fig. 2–11*B*). The RR interval may be calculated from the heart rate as follows:

$$\text{RR interval} = 60 \text{ seconds/number of heartbeats per minute}$$

Because each R wave triggers the pulse sequence, tissue contrast is determined by the patient-dependent RR interval rather than the operator-determined TR. When T2-weighted images are desired, data acquisition may be triggered off every third or fourth R wave. However, this practice may produce some inconsistency in data acquisition and worsened image quality, compared with results obtained with triggering off every R wave.

If data acquisition extends into the subsequent R wave, the system will fail to gate off that R wave. *To avoid this problem, the TR should be kept at least 15% shorter than the RR interval,* to account for expected

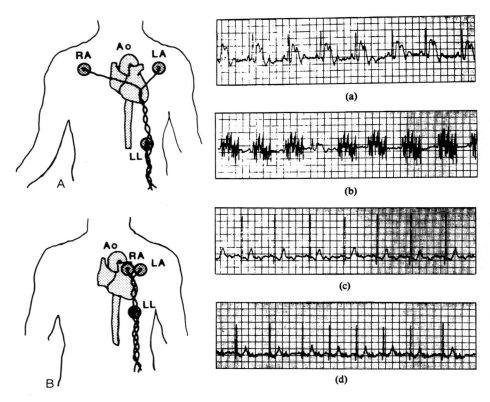

FIGURE 2–13. Examples of cardiac lead placement. *Left*, For optimal results, leads should be twisted, with close placement of limb electrodes *(B)*, rather than placed far apart *(A)*. Corresponding ECG tracings at right show optimal lead placement *(c and d)* and with limb leads placed apart *(a and b)*. Loops in the ECG leads should be avoided to prevent burns. High-impedance (e.g., carbon fiber) electrodes are preferred also to prevent burns. (*Left* and *Right* from Wendt RE, Rokey R, Vick GW, Johnson DL: Electrocardiographic gating and monitoring in NMR imaging. Magn Reson Imaging 6:89–95, 1988, with permission, Pergamon Press, plc.)

physiologic variations in the heart rate. A patient may have such a rapid heart rate that an extremely short TR must be selected, reducing the number of slices that can be obtained. If the heart rate is quite fast, the user may also set the pulse sequence to trigger off every other R wave for T1-weighted images, as long as the effective TR is still within an acceptable range. Otherwise, the user may run contiguous slice sets to cover the area of interest.

Scan parameters for cardiac studies depend on the particular system. Use of the following parameters with prospective ECG gating should provide good diagnostic images: FOV = 32 to 36 cm; acquisition matrix = 256 × 128; slice thickness = 5 to 10 mm; NEX = 2 to 4; and the application of flow presaturation. Although standard orthogonal planes of section may be adequate in many applications, it may be preferable to obtain images oriented along the true short and long axis of the heart.

Retrospective Cardiac Gating

In some patients, conventional ECG triggering fails to produce satisfactory image quality because of physiologic variation of the heart rate or because of arrhythmias. In these patients, retrospective cardiac gating is essential. In retrospective gating methods, data are acquired continuously, independent of the R wave (see Fig. 2–11). The user-selected TR represents the time between excitations, as it would in an ungated acquisition. To permit subsequent data reconstruction, the patient's ECG is continuously stored in memory. At the end of the acquisition, each line of the data is resorted according to the ECG phase in which it was acquired. Errors in the data due to variations in heart rate or, to some extent, respiration can be suppressed during postprocessing of the data. Ultrafast imaging methods such as echo-planar imaging (see Chapter 10) may also prove useful for overcoming artifacts resulting from arrhythmias and respiratory motion.

SEQUENCE BANDWIDTH

Low-bandwidth, or narrow-bandwidth, pulse sequences use a weak frequency-encoding gradient and a prolonged readout period to improve S/N ratio (see Chapter 4). Matched-bandwidth sequences represent a variation on this technique. The method uses an asymmetric readout of the echo to shorten the TE in conjunction with a long readout period. Low-bandwidth methods are particularly useful on low-field systems, in which the intrinsic S/N ratio is worse than on high-field systems.

Low-bandwidth sequences should not be used when a short TE is desired, for example, when obtaining T1-weighted spin-echo images of the liver. The prolonged readout period of these sequences necessitates an increase in the minimal TE. Images obtained with low-bandwidth methods may also be more susceptible to image artifact from the patient's motion, magnetic susceptibility artifacts, and any instrument instabilities such as eddy current effects. Additional drawbacks of low-bandwidth methods include reduced multislice capability and greater chemical-shift artifact, which may be troublesome on high-field systems. If objectionable chemical-shift artifact is present when using a low-bandwidth sequence on a high-field system, the matrix can be increased to 512 pixels in the frequency direction to reduce the artifact, at the expense of decreased S/N ratio.

High-bandwidth sequences allow for a shorter TE and therefore more slices per acquisition. Unfortunately, the use of a broader bandwidth also allows more background noise to be included as part of the image signal, and hence worse S/N ratio.

THREE-DIMENSIONAL GRADIENT-ECHO METHODS

3D GRE methods permit acquisition of thin, essentially contiguous slices (<1 mm) in reasonable amounts of time. It is important to understand that although the data are acquired from a 3D volume, the final result is a set of 2D images. Furthermore, as with 2D methods, one must select an orientation for the acquisition (e.g., axial, sagittal, coronal, or oblique). These images are reconstructed in the same plane as the acquisition plane.

Profiles of the slices acquired by 3D methods are not actually perfectly rectangular because the data are phase encoded along the slice select direction. Ringing (Gibbs or truncation) artifacts occur along this direction (particularly for small numbers of partitions), as they occur along the phase- and frequency-encoding directions in 2D images. Despite this, the slices are truly contiguous.

Two types of 3D acquisitions are possible: isotropic (i.e., the voxel is a cube) and anisotropic (i.e., the voxel is elongated in one dimension, usually the slice-selection axis). In addition, nonselective (i.e., the entire volume of tissue is excited by a nonselective RF pulse) or limited-volume (i.e., a thick slab is excited) 3D acquisitions may be performed. The 3D data differ from 2D data in that, if thin slices are acquired, one can perform high-quality multiplanar reconstructions along orientations different from the one in which the data were acquired, particularly if the acquisition is isotropic. The quality of multiplanar reconstructions of anisotropic 3D and 2D images suffers in comparison with isotropic acquisitions, because of the larger slice thickness.

SLICE THICKNESS

The 3D acquisitions are performed much like 2D acquisitions; considerations of matrix size and FOV are identical. However, 3D methods are unique in other respects. First, only a single excitation is usually selected. Second, *one must define two different slice thicknesses.* These are the *slab thickness,* representing the thickness of tissue that will be excited by the RF pulse, and the *partition thickness,* representing the thickness of the final images. The partition thickness decreases in proportion to the number of partitions:

Partition thickness = slab thickness/number of partitions

For instance, four partitions from a slab that is 2 cm thick produces images with a thickness of 5 mm. Although increasing the number of partitions reduces the partition thickness, it also produces a proportional increase in imaging time. For reasons relating to the imperfect slab profile produced by the RF pulse, as well as the resulting wraparound across the z-phase–encoding direction, the number of useful images may be at least one fewer than the number of partitions (Fig. 2–14).

SCAN PARAMETERS OF THREE-DIMENSIONAL METHODS

The choice of TR, TE, and matrix relates to the application. *Either GRE pulse sequences, which permit a shorter TR than do spin-echo sequences, or fast spin-echo sequences are used.* In general, the TR should be kept as short as possible (e.g., as short as 20 to 40 ms) to minimize imaging time. The effects of the flip angle are similar to those with 2D GRE methods; that is, large flip angles of 50° or more produce T1-weighted images, whereas small flip angles of 10° to 20° produce proton density–weighted or T2*-weighted images, or both, depending on the TE. Flow compensation is useful for evaluating blood vessels and for reducing motion artifact.

With 3D methods, one has several options available, which primarily represent tradeoffs between faster imaging and higher spatial resolution. For instance, the imaging time for an isotropic 3D data set with a slab thickness of 128 mm, a partition thickness of 1 mm, a TR of 100 ms, a matrix of 128 × 128 × 128, and 1 NEX is 27 minutes. If the number of partitions is

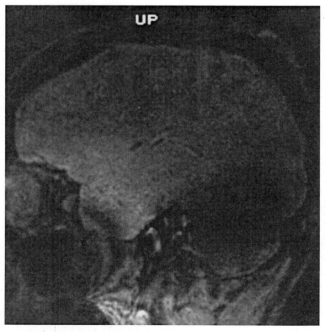

FIGURE 2–14. End slice from 3D acquisition, showing image degradation due to imperfect slab profile and wraparound along the slice-selection axis.

reduced to 32, the partition thickness increases to 4 mm, resulting in an anisotropic acquisition. However, the advantage is that the imaging time is reduced to 6 minutes. What happens if now, in addition to reducing the number of partitions from 128 to 32, one also reduces the slab thickness from 128 mm to 32 mm? The partition thickness once more becomes 1 mm (resolution is again isotropic), but the imaging time is still only 6 minutes instead of 27 minutes. The S/N ratio is proportional to the square root of the number of partitions. Therefore, the penalty for maintaining a high level of spatial resolution while reducing the number of partitions to image faster is a lower S/N ratio. In terms of motion artifact, a large number of partitions have a similar effect to a large number of excitations, that is, it reduces the severity of ghost artifacts.

Clinical applications for 3D methods include evaluation of the cervical spine; evaluation of cruciate ligaments and menisci of the knee, wrist, and other joints for which thin slices are required for optimal assessment; MR angiography (see Chapter 9); *and surface modeling* (Fig. 2–15) for radiation therapy, reconstructive surgery, and, most recently, research developments in MR-guided therapy and surgery. 3D fast spin-echo imaging can be extremely sensitive to motion artifacts in the abdomen unless respiratory gating is used.

MULTISLAB THREE-DIMENSIONAL ACQUISITION

Just as it is possible to perform multislice 2D acquisitions, one can perform multislab 3D acquisitions. Here, "multislab" means that two or more separate tissue volumes are excited. Each of these volumes is then subdivided into thin partitions, as is the case for single-slab 3D acquisitions.

Multislab 3D methods have applications similar to those of single-slab 3D methods but are especially useful for imaging two or more regions that are widely separated. For instance, both carotid bifurcations or TMJs can be imaged simultaneously in a two-slab 3D acquisition. If one attempted to encompass these structures using a single-slab approach, one would need to excite a much larger volume, which consists predominantly of regions that are of no clinical interest. To obtain a reasonably thin partition thickness from such a wide slab, a large number of z-phase–encoding steps would be required, with a proportional increase in imaging time.

Using multislab 3D methods does not, per se, increase the imaging time compared with that in single-slice 3D. However, the minimal TR must be increased to accommodate a larger number of slabs. For instance, if the minimal TR for a single-slab 3D acquisition is 30 ms, the minimal TR for a two-slab 3D acquisi-

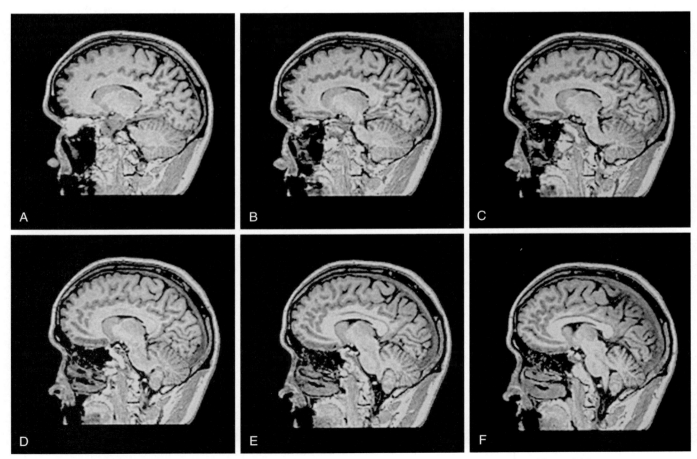

FIGURE 2–15. Series of six sagittal 1.56-mm slices acquired with magnetization-prepared rapid acquisition GRE (MP-RAGE) sequence, a T1-weighted volume acquisition.

tion is 60 ms, thereby doubling the imaging time. In addition, the slab profiles may be nonrectangular, so that a gap should be left between the slabs.

One major problem with 3D methods, from a practical standpoint, is the large number of images that is generated and that must be filmed by a technologist and viewed by a physician. This problem is compounded when multiplanar reconstructions are performed. Total reconstruction time typically increases in proportion to the increase in the number of partitions. Reconstruction time is lengthened severalfold when phased-array coils are used, further worsening the problem. *Efficient use of 3D methods necessitates having a 3D workstation or a satellite console available for off-line data processing.* These workstations generally have their own array processor to permit fast multiplanar and surface reconstruction. Alternatively, the 3D slabs can be acquired sequentially, a method used for MR angiography in multiple overlapping thin-slab acquisition (MOTSA). In this case, the acquisition time is increased compared with a single large slab, because of the nonrectangular slab profile and need to overlap sequential slabs.

The 3D data sets, when acquired to look at blood vessel flow, may also be postprocessed with maximal intensity projection (MIP) manipulations (see Chapter 9), which takes the strongest signal from each row of pixels and makes a composite image. *The user may also choose to reconstruct these images in various planes and degrees of rotation so as to lay out overlapping vessel anatomy.*

USE OF CONTRAST AGENTS

Timing of postcontrast imaging varies, depending on the area being scanned and how rapidly the contrast material is injected. Generally, MR contrast agents are given in a bolus injection over 1 to 2 minutes. To ensure that all contrast material is administered evenly and quickly, the technologist, nurse, or physician may wish to *prepare a second syringe of normal saline as a bolus to follow the contrast agent, using a three-way stopcock on the line, and completely flush the long tubing.* Another technique is to draw up some saline, approximately 40 mL, into a 60-mL syringe, and then carefully draw up the needed contrast agent (up to 20 mL of contrast agent) so that the two substances are layered one over the other (the contrast agent is heavier than the saline, so it will stay closer to the end of the tip of the syringe as long as the syringe is kept in a vertical position with the tip down). This method works best with gadolinium diethylenetriaminepentaacetic acid and not nonionic contrast material, because other FDA-approved IV contrast agents are less dense and mix with saline.

In brain or spine scanning, scanning should begin soon after (usually within 1 minute) the IV contrast agent has been administered, with a follow-up of the drip infusion saline. When imaging liver or kidneys, a technologist or radiologist may wish to begin breath-hold imaging within 20 seconds of the bolus of contrast medium (given over approximately 5 seconds). Delayed (10 minutes) postcontrast imaging may be helpful in characterizing hemangioma versus tumor of the liver.

A note of caution should be made that a rapid bolus injection sometimes causes a patient to feel nauseated (a nonspecific effect resulting from administering a hypertonic solution). The consequences of nausea developing into vomiting are hazardous, as the patient's position in the magnet is supine in most cases and the bore of the magnet is limiting, thus putting a patient at higher risk of aspiration.

Double-dose contrast medium may be helpful for improved detection of brain metastases. Also, double-dose contrast medium administration can be used for *3D MR angiography of the aorta (e.g., in cases of suspected aneurysm or dissection).* Nearly the whole length of the aorta can be covered in an oblique sagittal acquisition using a 45-cm FOV, 256 × 512 matrix, with a flip angle on the order of 40°, TR on the order of 20 ms or less, and 32 partitions. The imaging time is approximately 3 minutes, sufficiently short that enhancement of the inferior vena cava is minimal. The contrast agent is administered over a 3-minute period by hand injection, and the 3D MR angiographic acquisition is initiated after approximately 1 minute into the infusion. Breath-hold 3D MR angiograms may be acquired on systems with enhanced gradient capabilities, using a TR on the order of 5 ms and a flip angle on the order of 40°. In this case, the contrast medium is given over a duration of approximately 30 seconds. Care must be taken to start the acquisition after an appropriate delay, to avoid missing the arrival of the contrast bolus. In some cases, for example, patients with low cardiac output, a small test injection of a few milliliters of contrast medium may be given, followed by a series of fast turbo-FLASH scans to estimate the circulation time (as used in spiral CT angiography).

MEASUREMENT PERIOD

The onset of image measurement period is indicated by a jackhammer-like knocking sound. This sound represents the mechanical vibrations of the gradient coils produced by changing magnetic fluxes during gradient pulsing. Gradient-produced noise is most severe in pulse sequences that use rapid switching of high-amplitude gradients (e.g., GRE scans with thin slices, small FOV, flow compensation, and short TE and TR). *At the start of each measurement, a technologist should forewarn a patient of this noise to prepare a patient psychologically and to prevent motion due to involuntary reaction from a startling noise.* As mentioned earlier, it is advisable to give all patients some protection for the ear from the noise created by the scanning.

Some patients may become agitated after the measurement is under way. Several options are then available:

1. On some systems, selection of a "pause" option temporarily aborts the current acquisition. This allows the technologist to speak with the patient to determine

if the request for a pause is of an urgent nature or if the patient needs a moment to cough, for instance. This option is of value only if the patient is able to continue with the procedure without having moved from the original position. Otherwise, the acquisition will need to be restarted from the beginning.

2. Some systems can reconstruct images from incomplete data sets if more than 50% of the information has been collected. The quality of these images improves as the percentage of data acquired approaches 100%. If the patient starts to move toward the end of the measurement period, it may be prudent to abort the acquisition prematurely and use these images reconstructed from the incomplete data set.

3. If the patient moves transiently during the acquisition, the resultant image degradation may be minimal, particularly if the movement occurs near the beginning or end of the acquisition (i.e., strongest phase-encoding steps). In this case, it may not be necessary to abort the acquisition.

4. The acquisition may be repeated using a smaller matrix, fewer excitations, and shorter TR for faster imaging to improve the likelihood of obtaining a motion-free image. Echo-planar imaging has proved to be somewhat useful for this application, as well, although this technique has yet to come to the point of completely replacing conventional MRI.

BREATH-HOLD IMAGING

Respiration may be voluntarily suspended for a limited time in certain clinical applications. In particular, breath-holding markedly improves the quality of GRE and fast spin-echo images in the abdomen. These techniques can be used to evaluate vessel patency or to detect a lesion in the liver, kidneys, adrenal glands, and pancreas.

Fairly consistent results can be obtained when the data acquisition time is kept to a minimum, perhaps 10 to 20 seconds. Images are acquired at end-expiration so that the diaphragm is as close as possible to the same location for each acquisition. *A technologist should review the breath-hold instructions with a patient before the start of the examination.* If the patient is prepared for the breath-hold instructions, there will be less chance of confusion, especially with systems that may have an inferior quality intercom to the patient or if a patient has hearing loss. A technologist should also review the instructions to obtain consistency in breath-holding (e.g., inhale and exhale the same amount each time the patient is directed to do so). The patient is instructed to breathe in (wait approximately 3 seconds), breathe out (again wait approximately 3 seconds), and stop breathing. Hyperventilation, commonly used before breath-hold spiral CT acquisitions, is equally helpful for MRI. In difficult cases, breath-hold capability can be improved by administration of 100% oxygen. Most systems have a slight computational delay between when the user activates the measurement process and when the measurement actually begins. In addition, preparation scans may add several seconds to the imaging time predicted from the product of TR, matrix, and NEX. This may prolong the required breath-hold period, which a patient may not be able to sustain. *Technologists should be aware of these factors when giving breath-hold instructions to a patient, so that a patient does not begin the suspension of respiration too early and risk not being able to maintain the breath-hold for the duration of the acquisition.* The command to stop breathing should be given at the last possible moment, taking into account the intrinsic delays that occur before the start of data acquisition.

New respiratory compensation techniques such as the use of navigator echoes may obviate the need for breath-holding in many cases.

DATA ACQUISITION

Reconstruction times depend on matrix size, as well as on the capabilities of the computer and array processor. A 256×128 data matrix reconstructs in approximately half the time of a 256×256 matrix. Reconstruction times for images obtained with oversampling, which use even larger matrices, as mentioned earlier, are longer than those for standard 256×256 matrix images. Most systems also have available 512×512 image matrices. Often it is not necessary to use as many pixels in both directions. Instead, it is more reasonable to use a 512×384 matrix. Of course, images acquired with the larger matrix will also increase the reconstruction time.

A variety of filters are available for image smoothing, signal intensity normalization, and reduction of artifacts. The availability of various image filters is system dependent. Some of these filters are applied to the data during reconstruction, whereas others are applied directly to the reconstructed image. Noise reduction filters (e.g., sigma) reduce the background noise in the image by determining if the intensity of a pixel exceeds a certain threshold; pixels with lower intensity are assumed to represent background noise and are assigned a zero intensity. Edge enhancement and edge detection algorithms consider the difference between the signal intensities of adjacent pixels. See Figure 2–16 for examples.

Renormalization filters correct for the signal nonuniformity produced by surface coils, either by using an approximate 3D exponential or polynomial correction or by modeling the falloff in signal from the coil surface based on measurement in phantoms.[24] Smoothing filters (e.g., gaussian or Hanning) smooth the appearance of the image by averaging nearby pixels, at the expense of spatial resolution. A contrast-limited adaptive histogram equalization (CLAHE)[25] filter breaks the image up into smaller regions, which are independently optimized by relative equalization of the histogram, thus enhancing image contrast over the S/N ratio (Fig. 2–17).

PHOTOGRAPHY AND ARCHIVAL

MR images are notoriously difficult to photograph, owing to the wide ranges of tissue contrast as well as

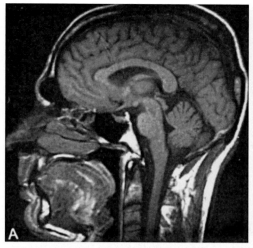
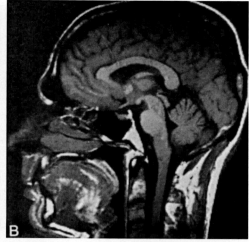

FIGURE 2–16. Effects of various image filters. *A*, Unfiltered sagittal T1-weighted spin-echo image of a brain. *B*, Same as in *A* but with noise reduction by a sigma filter. *C* to *E*, Sagittal images of a cervical spine with smoothing *(C)*, contour enhancement *(D)*, and edge detection *(E)* filters.

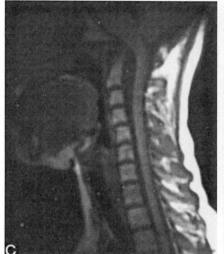
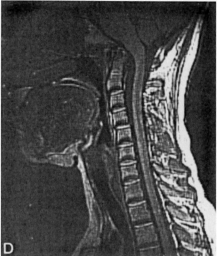
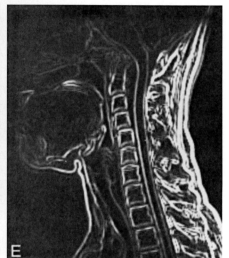

signal inhomogeneity produced by surface coils. One should set two general goals for photography of MR images:

1. Emphasize the region of interest and minimize the conspicuity of background noise, so that an aesthetically pleasing image will be produced.
2. Maximize tissue contrast over the region of interest by using a sufficiently narrow window width, without giving the image a harsh appearance.

With surface coil studies, care must be taken not to choose such a narrow window width that fatty tissues, such as bone marrow, cannot be evaluated (see Fig. 2–16).

Occasionally, two sets of images with different window settings must be photographed for adequate image evaluation. This practice is particularly useful for knee studies, in which one window setting may be used to evaluate menisci and another may be used for bone detail (Fig. 2–18).

To improve the visual presentation, images may be magnified before being photographed. Two-on-one vertical magnifications are particularly useful for sagittal spine images. This filming method also helps to reduce the amount of film needed. Magnification is also helpful for evaluating fine meniscal detail in knee studies. However, one must keep in mind that making the image larger does not improve the in-plane resolution. This can be done only by acquiring the image with a small FOV, acquiring thinner slices or a higher matrix or both (Fig. 2–19).

Because of the large number of images generated by 3D acquisition methods (as many as 256 images from one acquisition), it may be desirable to preselect images for photography. Also, formatting the images to four-on-one will help reduce the number of overall films. However, these images will be small in comparison to a normally displayed image on a sheet of film. It may be difficult to interpret images of this size unless the radiologists are looking in a specific area. On occasion, one may forego photographing these images and instead photograph the postprocessed images only, and the radiologist may choose to view the raw data images on a workstation. For instance, filming of MIP images of the circle of Willis may be adequate for patients with a nonspecific history. However, if a patient presents with headaches and has a family history of intracerebral aneurysm, both

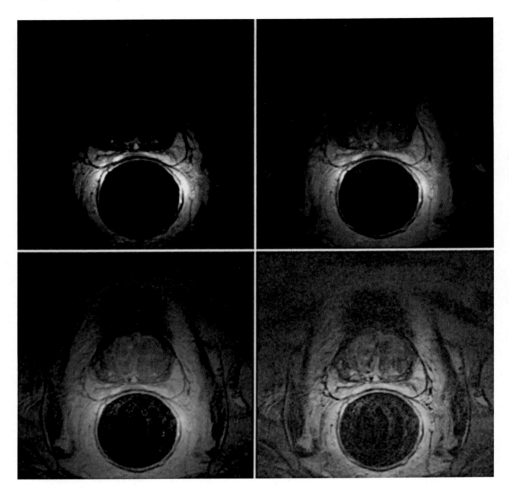

FIGURE 2–17. Filters for images acquired with a surface coil. *A,* Unfiltered axial image of a prostate gland acquired with an endorectal coil windowed with an automatic windowing function (choosing a contrast and brightness at midpoint for the overall image). *B,* Manual windowing of same image demonstrating more image detail. *C,* An exponential, or homomorphic, filtered image demonstrating a less severe signal dropoff. *D,* The same image filtered with the CLAHE algorithm. This method allows for better image contrast. Note that the two filtered images offer better demonstration of overall anatomy.

MIP and raw data images should be filmed for review and diagnosis.

A technologist may set image windows and contrast levels at a desirable level as viewed on an image display monitor or workstation. Yet when the same images are viewed on the resultant film, the images may appear gray or flat (i.e., minimal contrast between tissue types). This appearance could be caused by one or more possible problems: 1) the temperature of the film processor is too low due to a malfunctioning thermostat; 2) developer chemicals are contaminated; 3) the film laser printer contrast or density settings are incorrect; or 4) the image display monitor contrast or brightness has changed due to normal wear over time, thus making the image appear brighter on the monitor. To compensate, the user will attempt to properly set the image contrast and unwittingly bring the window level too high.

Most MR systems use laser printers for producing films. It is preferable to connect the MR system to the camera with a digital interface to a laser camera. A digital interface allows greater flexibility in film formats and a laser camera is able to produce films with a darker background than standard cameras. Other advantages to laser cameras are 1) film contrast reproducibility is easy; 2) error corrections are possible before a film is printed; 3) duplicate copies of films are easily done; 4) most laser printers today are equipped with daylight-loading supply magazines; 5) most laser cameras are docked to a film processor so that films are automatically sent through to a camera, thus freeing up technical staff to carry out other functions more directly related to care of patients and system operation; and 6) laser cameras, because of the digital interface, may also be part of a local computer network with other imaging systems. Compatible systems may be networked to a printer to process requests for film production from an additional system or from a different modality. This is advantageous because it may be adequate to have one laser printer serving two or more systems, thus decreasing the overall cost for every system that is added to it. A disadvantage is the initial cost of a laser camera. Also, laser or helium-neon film is about as costly as copy film.

Even though hard copy films are still produced in most facilities and made a part of the patient's permanent record, it is also necessary to archive image data onto optical disk or, on older systems, magnetic tape. Unfortunately, magnetic tape can store only approximately 200 images of 256×256 matrix or 50 images of 512×512 matrix, which in turn means that only a few examinations will archive onto one tape. Archiving to tape is time-consuming because of the number of images in a typical MRI examination. Images may be

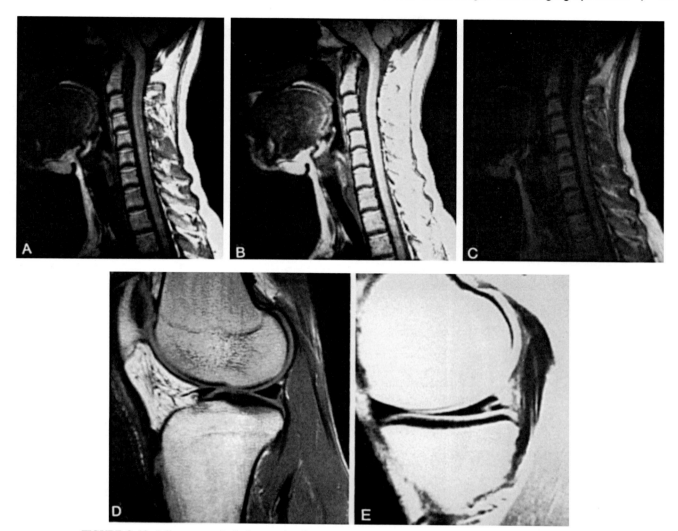

FIGURE 2–18. Adjustment of window setting for photography. *A,* Sagittal T1-weighted spin-echo image of a cervical spine with optimal window settings for spinal cord and vertebra. *B,* Image photographed at narrower window width might be useful for anterior neck structures but is worthless for spinal cord. *C,* Wider window width might be useful for posterior soft tissues, but evaluation of spinal cord is suboptimal. *D,* Sagittal T1-weighted image of a knee, bone windows. Note the good delineation of cartilage, bone marrow, and soft tissues. *E,* Different slice position. With narrower meniscal window and image magnification there is good delineation of tear of posterior horn of medial meniscus but poor representation of other structures.

compressed to allow for more images to be archived onto tape, but compressing the images is also time-consuming. Magnetic tapes can be reused for writing new data over old data, but more errors are encountered the more this is employed. Archival onto optical disk is faster and more convenient because this storage method holds much more data (over 10,000 images of 256×256 matrix). A disadvantage again is the initial cost of an optical disk drive and the optical disks. Some optical disks are WORM (write once, read many) disks, whereas others are rewritable disks. However, even though the optical disks are rewritable, one should check with a product specialist to determine if a particular MR system will actually write new image data over old image data on a rewritable disk, because the cost of a WORM disk is much more economical than a rewritable disk.

Temporary storage of images may be made on a workstation. This is usually used for short-term storage for physicians to review image data on a daily basis. Some larger clinics and hospitals with smaller affiliate sites in remote, rural, or suburban locales are also networking images between satellite facilities and main departments, usually to a workstation. In larger hospitals, remote workstations may be provided to areas of high volume of referrals such as a clinic or an intensive care unit. This is being used for all imaging modalities, not just MRI.

TROUBLESHOOTING

Quality control is a more complex process for MRI systems than for other imaging modalities such as CT. Numerous artifacts may occur in MR images from a variety of causes. MR image artifacts are reviewed in

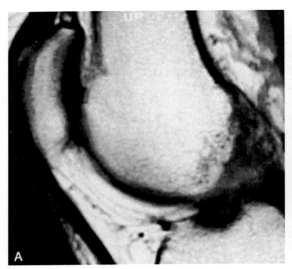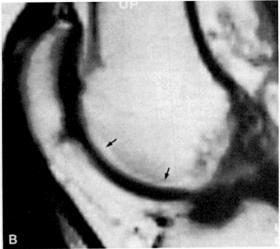

FIGURE 2–19. Sagittal T1-weighted spin-echo image of knee: comparison between image magnification and gradient zoom. *A,* Gradient zoom shows fine detail. *B,* Magnification of larger FOV image to same size shows less detail and greater chemical-shift artifact *(arrows)*.

detail in Chapter 3. Although many of these artifacts require the attention of service personnel, it is helpful to know when image quality problems are related to hardware rather than to inappropriate selection of pulse sequence or scan parameters or to the patient. Therefore, the technologist and physician should be aware of basic troubleshooting procedures.

The most important aspect of quality control is to maintain a daily log of S/N ratio measurements performed on phantoms. Ideally, these measurements should be performed with all receiver coils. However, this practice may be extremely time-consuming, so it is reasonable to perform measurements with various receiver coils on alternate days. S/N ratio measurements with surface coils may be difficult to standardize, owing to depth dependence of coil sensitivity, so service personnel should be consulted with regard to proper procedures. In addition, it is recommended that at least a weekly log of transmitter voltages for various types of patient's studies be recorded. Significant changes in average transmitter voltages may herald impending failure of the RF tube, excessive magnetic coupling of the RF coils, or other hardware problems.

A consistent downward trend in S/N ratio measurements warrants a call for service. *One should note whether the noise has any "structure" to it.* For instance, discrete vertical lines oriented to the frequency-encoding axis represent RF noise. RF noise may be caused by a defective RF enclosure for the magnet room, and one should check to make sure that the door is tightly closed and that the copper tabs surrounding the door are intact. One should also check for flickering within the magnet room. One or more discrete lines oriented perpendicular to the phase-encoding axis may represent ghost artifact from respiration from pulsatile flow. If this cause is excluded, the artifacts likely relate to hardware problems, such as RF or gradient instability or inadequate eddy current compensation. Intermit-

tent diagonal lines or "snowstorm" artifacts (Fig. 2–20*A*) may relate to hardware problems or to static discharges, which tend to occur during conditions of low humidity. One should check the humidity levels in both the magnet room and the room containing the gradient subsystems and should consult service personnel. This type of problem may occur more frequently in colder seasons or when quite cold for even a short period. Heating systems are running for long periods, causing a decrease in humidity. Artifacts that occur only intermittently may also be caused by temperature instability in the magnet room or the room housing the computer and other hardware. Ambient temperature greater than 72°F is not usually well tolerated and may result in damage to electronic components. Also, intermittent artifacts can be encountered from a loose screw or other hardware adjoining the body coil or a gradient coil, which results in abnormal mechanical vibration and arcing. These artifacts may be intermittent because the vibrations are problematic only with particular pulse sequences. Direct inspection by service personnel may be required to troubleshoot this problem.

Unstructured noise may be due to a variety of causes. Although service is probably required, one can check the integrity of the connectors and cables for the receiver coils, because these, on occasion, are mangled during positioning of the patient. Metallic implants such as Harrington rods or dental plates produce localized regions of geometric distortion and may also cause poor S/N ratio, owing to improper coil tuning. More generalized evidence of geometric distortion suggests problems with magnet shimming or gradient linearity. If intermittent, this artifact might be caused by the movement of large metal objects, such as cars or elevators, in the vicinity of the magnet. Mobile MR sites may be more affected by this type of incident, as the siting of the magnet is usually in a parking lot adjacent to a building.

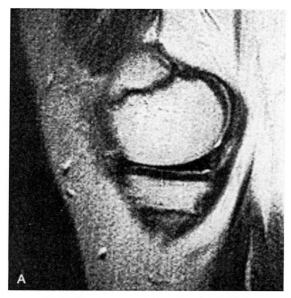

FIGURE 2–20. Diagonal snowstorm artifacts usually suggest a hardware problem or static discharges. In this case, the problem was a loose screw in the body coil, resulting in abnormal vibrations and arcing. *A,* Sagittal knee imaging is degraded by these artifacts. *B,* Raw data set corresponding to *A.* Each column corresponds to a specific time interval or frequency sample; each row or "line" corresponds to data acquired from one phase-encoding step. The semiperiodic nature of the artifacts, suggesting the presence of abnormal vibrations, is evident in the raw data but not the image.

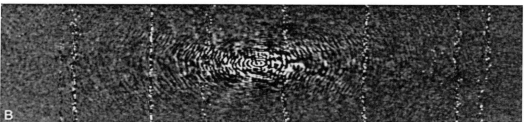

For any of these artifacts, it is important to save raw data (Fig. 2–20*B*), which often provide additional information about the source of the artifacts. However, in most commercial systems, the raw data must be saved immediately after the scans, because the data may be deleted when the next prescan is initiated.

Finally, whether because the service personnel are temporarily unavailable or because the schedule of patients cannot be interrupted, it may be necessary to continue scanning despite problems with image quality. In this case, thicker slices, larger FOVs, or more excitations may be used to improve image quality. If artifacts are particularly severe with certain pulse sequences or planes of section, these should obviously be avoided.

In conclusion, we see that there are numerous practical considerations involved in the production of high-quality MR images. Although this chapter offers recommendations for optimizing MRI examinations, there are no panaceas. One must experiment with different imaging parameters and decide for oneself what best suits the needs of a particular MRI site and the physicians involved there.

Appendix

SAMPLE CHECKLIST FOR SCREENING PATIENTS

Date: _____

Patient Name: _____   Weight: _____

An MRI examination involves the use of an extremely strong magnet. For safety purposes, the presence of certain metallic objects must be determined *before* you enter the examination room. Place a mark in the appropriate column for each listing as it applies to you. If you answer "yes" to any item, please describe in detail below.

	YES	NO
Pacemaker/wires/implantable defibrillator	_____	_____
Metallic heart valve prosthesis	_____	_____
Implanted pump (insulin, breast)	_____	_____
Coronary artery bypass clips (CABG)	_____	_____
Limb or joint replacement or pinning	_____	_____
Biostimulator, neurostimulator, or TENS device	_____	_____
Aneurysm clips (e.g., brain, aorta)	_____	_____
Other vascular clips	_____	_____
Intracranial clips (brain surgery)	_____	_____
Middle ear prosthesis (surgery on bones in ear)	_____	_____
Cochlear implant	_____	_____
Filter in a blood vessel (e.g., IVC, Gianturco coil)	_____	_____
Tattooed eyeliner	_____	_____
Penile implant/prosthesis	_____	_____
Surgical clips or wires	_____	_____
Dental implant (held in place by a magnet)	_____	_____
Shrapnel or bullet fragments (anywhere in the body)	_____	_____
Have you had an injury of metal to the eye?	_____	_____
Have you ever been a metal worker?	_____	_____
Have you had any previous surgery?	_____	_____
Have you had an MRI scan before?	_____	_____
Have you ever experienced claustrophobia?	_____	_____

If yes, please describe in detail any item above that you answered with "yes." Also, list all surgical procedures:

_____
_____
_____

Female Patients:

IUD (intrauterine device)	_____	_____
Are you pregnant?	_____	_____

If yes, how many weeks? _____

Before you enter the examination room, please remove any of the following:

Eye make-up	Retainers (a cup will be provided)	
Wigs or hair pieces	Watches	Bobby pins
Wallets	Jewelry	Bra

You will be asked to remove your clothing. We will provide a robe, johnny, and pajama pants.

Please circle if any of the following apply to you:

Dentures	Hearing aids	Eyeglasses	Braces

Signed: _____

Relationship (if not the patient): _____

REFERENCES

1. Slifer KJ, Penn-Jones K, Cataldo MF, et al: Music enhances patients' comfort during MR imaging. AJR 156:403, 1991. Letter.
2. Brummett RE, Talbot JM, Charuhas P: Potential hearing loss resulting from MR imaging. Radiology 169:539–540, 1988.
3. Freinhar JP, Alvarez WA: Organic claustrophobia: an association between panic and carbon dioxide? Int J Psychosom 34(2):18–19, 1987.
4. Saunders RD, Smith H: Safety aspects of NMR clinical imaging. Br Med Bull 40:148–154, 1984.
5. Shellock FG, Kanal E: Policies, guidelines, and recommendations for MR imaging safety and patient management. J Magn Reson Imaging 1:97–101, 1991.
6. Stephenson GM, Freiherr G: Indifference to safety heightens MRI risks. Diagn Imag June:79–83, 1990.
7. Kanal E, Shellock FG, Talagala L: Safety considerations in MR imaging. Radiology 176:593–606, 1990.
8. Devine EC, Cook TD: Clinical and cost-saving effects of psychoeducational interventions with surgical patients: a meta-analysis. Res Nurs Health 9:89–105, 1986.
9. Devine EC, Cook TD: A meta-analytic analysis of effects of psychoeducational interventions on length of postsurgical hospital stay. Nurs Res 32:267–273, 1983.
10. Flaherty JA, Hoskinson K: Emotional distress during magnetic resonance imaging. N Engl J Med 320:467–468, 1989.
11. Melendez JC, McCrank E: Anxiety related reactions associated with magnetic resonance imaging examination. JAMA 270:745–747, 1993.
12. Quirk ME, Letendre AJ, Coittone RA, Lingley JF: Evaluation of three psychologic interventions to reduce anxiety during MR imaging. Radiology 173:759–762, 1989.
13. Abrahams JJ, Lange RC: Coil holder and marker system for MR imaging of the total spine. Radiology 172:869–871, 1989.
14. Henck ME, Simpson EL: Superiority of cod liver oil as a marker for lesions in MR imaging of the extremities. AJR 161:904–905, 1993.
15. Chernish SM, Maglinte DD: Glucagon: common untoward reactions—review and recommendations. Radiology 177:145–146, 1990.
16. Kanal E, Gillen J, Evans J, et al: Survey of reproductive health among female MR workers. Radiology 187:395–399, 1993.
17. U.S. Food and Drug Administration: Magnetic resonance diagnostic device: panel recommendation and report on petitions for MR reclassification. Final rule. Fed Regist 54(20):5077–5078, 1988.
18. Quirk ME, Letendre AJ, Coittone RA, Lingley JF: Anxiety in patients undergoing MR imaging. Radiology 170:463–466, 1989.
19. Brennan S, Redd W, Jacobsen P, et al: Anxiety and panic during magnetic resonance scans. Lancet 2:512, 1988.
20. Beck A, Emery G: Anxiety Disorders and Phobias. New York: Basic Books, 1985.
21. Thompson MB, Coppens NM: The effects of guided imagery on anxiety levels and movement of clients undergoing magnetic resonance imaging. Holistic Nurse Pract 8(2):59–69, 1994.
22. Accreditation Manual for Hospitals, Volume I—Standards. Oakbrook Terrace, IL: Joint Commission on Accreditation of Healthcare Organizations, 1994.
23. Holshouser BA, Hinshaw DB, Shellock F: Sedation, anesthesia, and physiologic monitoring during MR imaging: evaluation of procedures and equipment. J Magn Reson Imaging 3:553–558, 1993.
24. Lufkin RB, Sharpless T, Flannigan B, Hanafee W: Dynamic range compression in surface-coil MRI. AJR 147:379–382, 1986.
25. Heckbert PS: Graphics Gems IV. New York: Academic Press, 1994, pp 474–485.

Artifacts in MRI: Description, Causes, and Solutions

GEORGE WESBEY ▪ MARY K. ADAMIS
ROBERT R. EDELMAN

Since the first edition of this book was published, considerably more than 100 original scientific manuscripts have been published on the subject of magnetic resonance imaging (MRI) artifacts. This chapter reviews the various artifacts encountered in MRI today and considers their causes and solutions. Although certain artifacts related to older software and hardware configurations are seldom encountered, there is no shortage of other kinds of artifacts, including those related to the use of MR angiography (MRA) and fast imaging techniques.

The radiologist relies on visual impressions to make a diagnosis. But in the case of MRI, what one sees can sometimes be a far cry from reality. Images stretch, wrinkle, or distort in ways that are alien to other less complex imaging modalities (radiography, computed tomography [CT], nuclear medicine, ultrasonography). Some of these artifacts are due to equipment malfunctions, whereas others are due to improper technique selection or are simply inherent to the MRI process. One needs to understand the sources and appearances of these artifacts, not only to interpret the images properly but also to be able to eliminate these artifacts to obtain the highest quality images. Prerequisite to an understanding of artifacts is a knowledge of the physical principles and instrumentation that form the basis for the infinite variety of signal intensity patterns obtainable in the MR image. We consider artifacts under several distinct categories, although in reality artifacts arise from an interplay of these factors (Fig. 3–1).

An MRI artifact is defined as any signal intensity, or void, that does not have an anatomic basis in the image. The classification of artifacts is complicated by the multifactorial basis of production: the interrelationship among software, hardware, and radiofrequency (RF) or static magnetic field components; the pulse sequence parameters; and the system-dependent nature of artifacts related to static magnetic field

strength, magnetic gradient strengths, RF coil type, and body part examined. Bellon and colleagues[1] have categorized artifacts by cause as sequence, reconstruction algorithm, patient, and system related. In their thorough and comprehensive review article, Henkelman and Bronskill[2] classified artifacts based on both their appearance and cause. This chapter is intended to serve as a relatively complete "atlas" of MRI artifacts, with an effort to provide explanations geared to physicians involved in clinical imaging.

Realizing that any classification of MRI artifacts is arbitrary and incomplete, we propose the following general outline based on the predominant causative agent or affected system component: static magnetic field (B_0), RF magnetic field (RF or B_1), gradient magnetic field (G_x, G_y, G_z), motion, sequence parameters, MRA, and miscellaneous. A brief description of the classic appearance of the artifact, a concise explanation of its origin, and various solutions accompany examples of more frequently seen MRI artifacts. In light of the variability of MRI systems from various manufacturers, we have tried to include artifacts common to all MRI systems, including examples from several different vendors.

STATIC MAGNETIC FIELD ARTIFACTS

A fundamental prerequisite for MRI is a homogeneous static magnetic field, B_0. Imperfections in magnet construction or, more commonly, in shimming (the process of compensating for B_0 inhomogeneities) may disrupt the B_0 homogeneity. Areas of image distortion or focal signal loss along the readout axis are the result (Fig. 3–2). Rarely, B_0 inhomogeneity may present as propagation of signal loss or noise in the phase-encoding direction across the entire image.[3]

Other causes of B_0 inhomogeneity are temporal fluctuations in the power supply and thermal instabil-

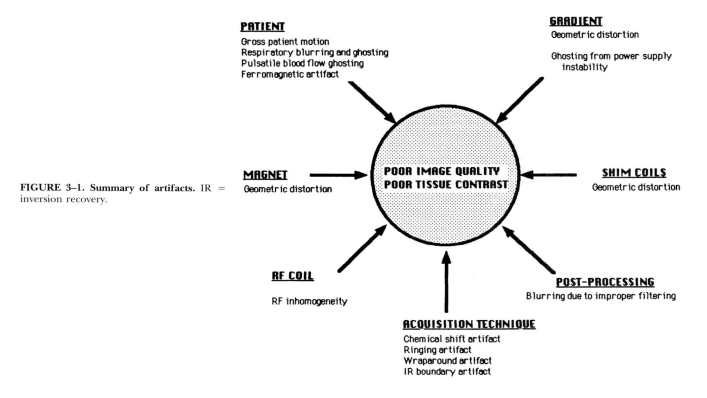

PATIENT
Gross patient motion
Respiratory blurring and ghosting
Pulsatile blood flow ghosting
Ferromagnetic artifact

GRADIENT
Geometric distortion

Ghosting from power supply instability

POOR IMAGE QUALITY POOR TISSUE CONTRAST

MAGNET
Geometric distortion

SHIM COILS
Geometric distortion

RF COIL
RF inhomogeneity

POST-PROCESSING
Blurring due to improper filtering

ACQUISITION TECHNIQUE
Chemical shift artifact
Ringing artifact
Wraparound artifact
IR boundary artifact

FIGURE 3–1. Summary of artifacts. IR = inversion recovery.

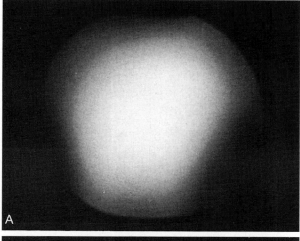

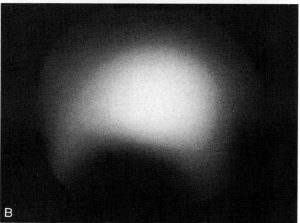

FIGURE 3–2. Transaxial MR image of a homogeneous 28-cm-diameter by 40-cm-long cylindrical phantom taken at *(A)* 15 cm superior to the z axis isocenter and *(B)* 15 cm inferior to the z axis isocenter reveals focal signal inhomogeneity in the periphery caused by imperfect shimming of the static field in this region. Such inhomogeneity was readily evident in clinical off-isocenter images.

ity. Foo and Hayes[4] addressed the correction of view-to-view phase shifts caused by B_0 instability by applying a phase correction to the low-spatial-frequency views. Their algorithm assumes that the signal intensity in the space outside an object represents only noise. A set of phases for the low-spatial-frequency views are calculated by minimizing, in the image, the intensity of the induced artifacts in the space outside the object. Resistive magnets are susceptible to accidental power interruption, and images may demonstrate severe artifacts resulting from B_0 inhomogeneity many hours after restoration of power. State-of-the-art superconducting magnets operate with temporal stabilities of 0.1 to 1 ppm over days to weeks.[5]

However, without routine active shimming, the thermal fluctuation of the system results in accumulated B_0 inhomogeneity that can degrade image quality rapidly. Proper magnet design and production and regular shimming by service personnel maintain B_0 inhomogeneity at a minimum.

Objects both external and internal to the imaging volume of the MRI system may interfere with static magnetic field linearity. Sizable ferromagnetic structures in motion near the magnet, such as a truck or elevator, generate magnetic forces of their own. If static field shielding fails to compensate for these forces, these external fields may create B_0 inhomogeneity artifacts.

FERROMAGNETIC MATERIALS

Magnetic susceptibility is the tendency of a substance to attract magnetic lines of force. Most materials may be classified as ferromagnetic (strongly attracting lines of force), paramagnetic (weakly attracting lines of force), or diamagnetic (weakly repelling lines of force). These three classes of magnetic properties are thus all related by the relative magnetic susceptibilities. Magnetic susceptibility simply represents the ratio of induced magnetization to applied magnetization and is therefore a dimensionless quantity. Diamagnetic substances (e.g., water) have an induced magnetization that is a millionfold less than the applied field, with opposite polarity (repelling). For example, in a 1.5-T (15,000-G) clinical MRI system, water has an induced magnetization of roughly -0.015 G (flux lines opposite the direction of the magnet). Paramagnetic compounds (e.g., elemental gadolinium) have an induced magnetization four orders of magnitude greater than that of diamagnetic compounds and are attracted to the applied field (induced magnetization of approximately $+150$ G in the preceding example). Ferromagnetic substances (e.g., iron-containing alloys) have a magnetic susceptibility four orders of magnitude greater than that of paramagnetic compounds (roughly $+1.5$ million G of induced magnetization in a 1.5-T imager).

Titanium, tantalum, and aluminum are nonferromagnetic.[6] Stainless steel alloys that have a high content of nickel, such as 304 and 316L, are nonferromagnetic. However, cold working of these materials (as when they are bent to form surgical clips) can impart

a mild degree of ferromagnetism[7] (Fig. 3–3). Ferromagnetic artifacts may also result from minute metallic particles that wear off surgical instruments, particularly metal suction tips, which occasionally come in contact with diamond surgical drills.[8–10] These artifacts simulate hypertrophic bone formation with cord compression and are particularly prominent on gradient-echo images (Fig. 3–4), because these images are acquired without a refocusing 180° RF pulse.

BASIS OF FERROMAGNETISM

Ferromagnetic materials contain macroscopic magnetic "domains" in which the molecules align with the main magnetic field. These materials have high magnetic susceptibilities; that is, they strongly attract magnetic lines of force and distort magnetic field homogeneity in their vicinity. Because magnetic susceptibility is proportional to magnetic field strength, ferromagnetic artifacts worsen at high fields.[11] A ferromagnetic artifact has a specific appearance, consisting

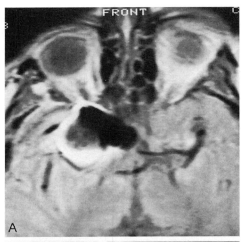

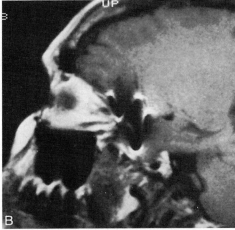

FIGURE 3–3. Cold working of nonferromagnetic materials can impart a degree of ferromagnetism. A titanium intracerebral aneurysm clip, which is supposed to be nonferromagnetic, causes a strong ferromagnetic artifact, a result of bending of the clip. *A,* Axial proton density–weighted spin-echo image. *B,* Sagittal T1-weighted spin-echo image.

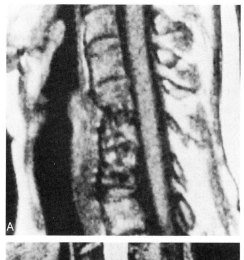

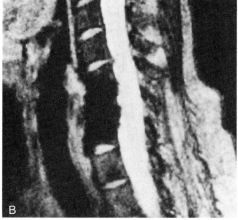

FIGURE 3–4. A ferromagnetic artifact can be caused by metallic particles that wear off surgical devices. A, T1-weighted image of cervical spine status post anterior interbody fusion demonstrates signal inhomogeneity caused by metallic particles worn off surgical drill. B, Gradient-echo image (fast low-angle shot, repetition time [TR]/echo time [TE]/flip angle [FA] = 200/13/20°) shows increased artifact, greatly exaggerating the extent of central canal compromise. (A and B courtesy of M. Modic, MD, Cleveland Clinic, Cleveland, OH.)

of signal abnormality and geometric distortion: a region of decreased signal intensity abutted on one side by a curvilinear region of marked hyperintensity[12, 13] (Figs. 3–5 to 3–8; see Fig. 3–3).

The explanation for this artifact is illustrated in Figure 3–9. Spatial localization for two-dimensional Fourier transform (2DFT) image formation depends on the presence of a highly linear magnetic field gradient. Ferromagnetic objects distort the magnetic field in their vicinity. On one side, the field generated by the ferromagnetic object augments the applied magnetic field gradient, stretching the image as well as causing signal loss. On the other side, the increased field from the ferromagnetic object opposes the applied gradient; the MR signals from the tissue protons, over the region where the gradient is attenuated, collapse to a high-intensity line. In addition to generating artifacts, larger ferromagnetic objects (such as dental plates) can worsen RF coil performance because they alter the

coil tuning; in bad cases, imaging may be impossible, particularly on systems with high-quality coils.

Small ferromagnetic objects in the volume imaged cause characteristic focal MRI aberrations. Artifact-generating ferromagnetic objects include some types of surgical clips (see Fig. 3–6B), interventional radiologic coils (see Fig. 3–5), steel implants such as ventriculoperitoneal shunts (see Fig. 3–6A), dental steel in orthodontic braces and dentures, hair and safety pins, mascara (see Fig. 3–7), and zippers.[7, 14, 15] These artifacts classically consist of a central signal void and asymmetric margins of higher signal intensity in bizarre, nonanatomic configurations (see Fig. 3–8). Ventriculoperitoneal shunts (Fig. 3–10) and various clips, such as internal mammary coronary artery bypass clips (Fig. 3–11) and carotid endarterectomy metal clips, can all produce artifactual stenosis or occlusion of vessels on maximal intensity projections (MIPs) in MRA studies[16, 17] (see later section on artifacts in MRA).

Nonferromagnetic metallic implants, such as some small surgical clips, may be invisible but can generate artifacts in the form of localized signal voids. Nonetheless, because of the different acquisition and reconstruction method employed, MR images are usually

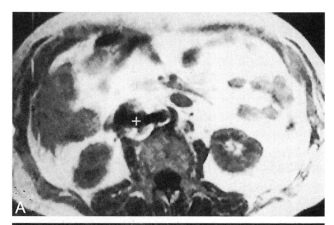

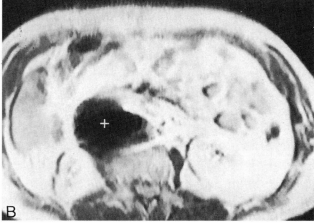

FIGURE 3–5. Ferromagnetic artifact from a Gianturco coil. A, T1-weighted image demonstrates central signal void (cross) and high-intensity curvilinear rim along left. B, T2 weighted image demonstrates a larger artifact because the frequency-encoding gradient is reduced (to improve S/N ratio; sampling time increased, same field of view [FOV] as in A).

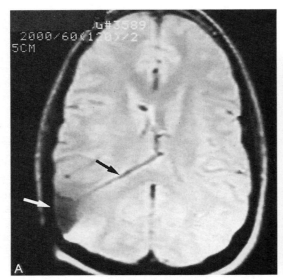
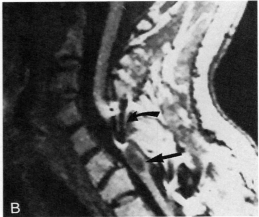

FIGURE 3–6. Shunt artifact. *A,* Shunt tube produces a minimal artifact *(black arrow)*, whereas ferromagnetic connectors produce a larger artifact *(white arrow). B,* Patient with post-traumatic syrinx *(straight arrow).* Apparent cord deformity *(curved arrow)* above syrinx cavity is caused by ferromagnetic artifact resulting from surgical clips.

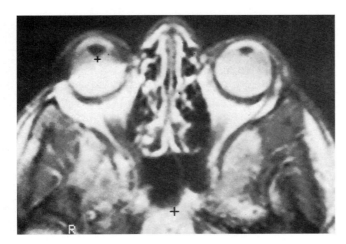

FIGURE 3–7. Mascara artifact *(cross)* caused by ferromagnetic iron ores.

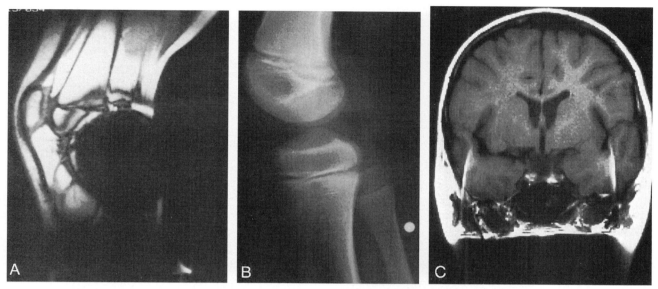

FIGURE 3–8. Ferromagnetic foreign object. *A,* Sagittal image of the knee of a 10-year-old boy with a BB pellet in the soft tissues posteroinferior to the joint line. Note the bizarre shape and disproportionate size of the signal void caused by the 5-mm metallic object. *B,* Radiograph. *C,* MR image of patient with ferromagnetic dental hardware. An artifactual bright signal overlapping temporal lobes bilaterally represents frequency-shifted signals from the mouth.

FIGURE 3–9. Explanation of geometric distortion and signal changes caused by a ferromagnetic object. Ferromagnetic object produces a localized increase in the magnetic field (1). Normally, there is a linear increase in magnetic field strength along the direction of the frequency-encoding gradient (2). In conjunction with the magnetic field gradient, the field distortions by the ferromagnetic object cause either stretching and signal loss as a result of an increased gradient (region B) or increased signal collapsed to a line because of a decreased gradient (region C).

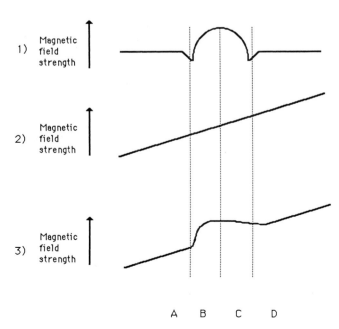

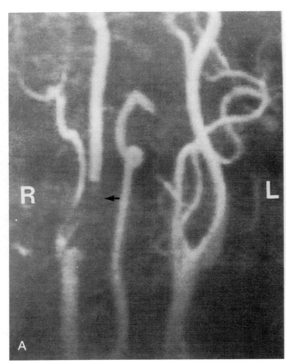

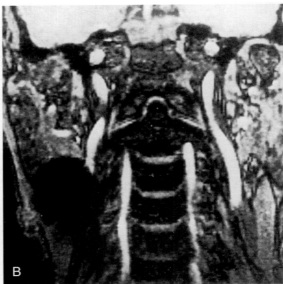

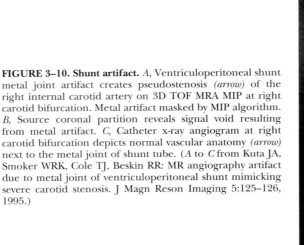

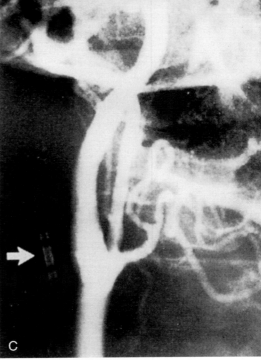

FIGURE 3–10. Shunt artifact. *A,* Ventriculoperitoneal shunt metal joint artifact creates pseudostenosis *(arrow)* of the right internal carotid artery on 3D TOF MRA MIP at right carotid bifurcation. Metal artifact masked by MIP algorithm. *B,* Source coronal partition reveals signal void resulting from metal artifact. *C,* Catheter x-ray angiogram at right carotid bifurcation depicts normal vascular anatomy *(arrow)* next to the metal joint of shunt tube. *(A* to *C* from Kuta JA, Smoker WRK, Cole TJ, Beskin RR: MR angiography artifact due to metal joint of ventriculoperitoneal shunt mimicking severe carotid stenosis. J Magn Reson Imaging 5:125–126, 1995.)

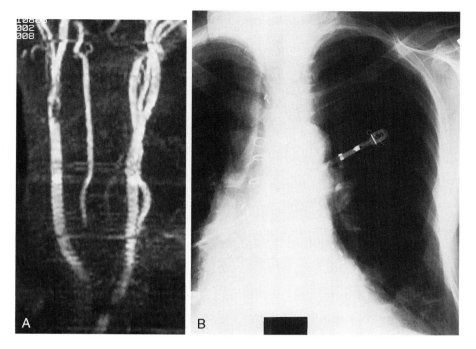

FIGURE 3–11. Bypass clip artifact. *A,* High left internal mammary coronary artery bypass graft clip creates pseudo-occlusion of the left common carotid artery 2 cm from its origin on 2D TOF MRA MIP. *B,* Radiograph of region of interest demonstrating the metal clip.

more interpretable in the presence of metal than are the radially streaked x-ray CT images (Fig. 3–12). The severity of the artifact depends on the shape of the object, because this determines whether closed conducting pathways exist; for instance, a U-shaped clip may generate less artifact than a closed loop. The orientation of the long axis of a surgical nail relative to the readout gradient axis also influences the degree of artifact present.

Rarely, nonferromagnetic metallic objects may cause focal signal loss, with the mechanism involving RF field–induced eddy currents within the diamagnetic object as discussed by Camacho and colleagues.[18] They found that this artifact was due to the perturbations of the transmit and receive sensitivities of the RF coil. They proposed correction schemes based on a multiexcitation postprocessing method, use of sequences that are less sensitive to B_1 amplitude (gradient-echo, adiabatic pulses), or breaking the conduction pathway when feasible. RF eddy currents caused by nonferromagnetic metallic objects result in negligible local heating, despite often substantial local signal artifacts.[19]

SUSCEPTIBILITY ARTIFACT

At the boundary between two tissues with different magnetic susceptibilities, there is local distortion of the magnetic field. Spin dephasing across the slice as well as within the slice results in miscentering of the echo; when severe, this produces signal loss. Geometric distortion is also produced. The geometric distortion can be manifested by a change in shape of the object, as well as by slight mispositioning of the slice. The variation in susceptibility can occur between voxels, resulting in loss of signal at the boundary between

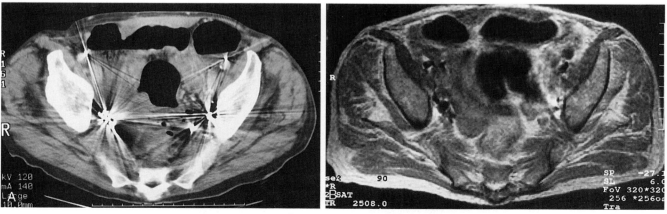

FIGURE 3–12. Metal clip artifact. *A,* Axial CT image of the pelvis shows severe artifact caused by surgical clips. *B,* Axial proton density–weighted MR image of the same patient shows minimal artifact.

tissues, or, if susceptibilities vary within the voxel, loss of signal from that voxel. In contrast, Kim and coworkers[20] found that hemosiderin deposits within intracerebral cavernous hemangiomas behave like a point magnetic dipole, causing intravoxel signal interference patterns that appear as a ring of enhanced signal intensity within the expected signal void around many of the individual lesions on axial gradient-echo sequences (Fig. 3–13). Knowledge of this artifact should allow radiologists to avoid misinterpreting a single lesion as multiple contiguous lesions.

Although a ferromagnetic artifact is the extreme example, susceptibility artifacts are also commonly seen at the boundary between materials with different magnetic susceptibilities, such as air, bone, brain, nonferrous metal implants,[21] and hemorrhage. Although susceptibility artifacts are less extreme than ferromagnetic artifacts, signal loss and geometric distortion are present and may mimic partial-volume averaging or calcification (Fig. 3–14). These artifacts are most prominent with high-field systems and on images acquired with gradient-echo, rather than spin-echo, techniques.[22] The artifacts can be seen above the petrous bones and around the paranasal sinuses, as well as around bowel loops on gradient-echo abdominal images.

Magnetic susceptibility artifacts in the sella turcica on spin-echo MR images have been studied by Sakurai and colleagues.[23] They showed a high-signal-intensity "spot" (Fig. 3–15) or distortion of the contour of the floor of the sella turcica on coronal T1-weighted spin-echo MR images of the sella at the junction of the sellar floor with the sphenoid septum. When no sphenoid septum was present, they found distortion of the inferior surface of the pituitary gland. They attributed these phenomena to magnetic susceptibility effects. Elster[24] found that a focal artifact larger than 1 mm² was observed in MR studies of 7 (14%) of 50 subjects and was sufficiently large to mask or mimic disease in all cases. The location of this artifact was always within the pituitary gland but closely related to the junction of the sphenoid septum and sellar floor. Its magnitude was shown to be linearly related to the strength and direction of the readout gradient. This focal susceptibility artifact may mimic or obscure a microadenoma.

Tien and coworkers[25] quantified the susceptibility artifact–induced pseudonarrowing of the cervical neural foramina. The gradient-echo images showed more apparent narrowing than did the spin-echo images. The absolute distortion of the neural foramina was rather constant (less than two pixels) on the gradient-echo images. The absolute and relative distortion increased as the echo time (TE) increased. At a constant TE, the structural distortion did not change with different repetition time (TR) values or flip angles. They recommended the shortest possible TE for evaluation of the cervical spine. Similar observations on gradient-echo MRI cervical neural foraminal pseudostenoses were reported by Tsuruda and Remley.[26] Compared with CT, MRI consistently underestimated the diameters of the neural foramina, leading to overestimation of neural foraminal stenosis. The degree of overestimation varied directly with increasing TE values, from 8% (TE = 11 ms) to 27% (TE = 22 ms). Motion artifacts also increased foraminal overestimation and mimicked osseous hypertrophy. The effect of image degradation caused by motion was noted to increase with longer TE values. They also suggested minimizing image degradation resulting from magnetic susceptibility and motion artifacts by using the shortest TE possible. In another paper on cervical spine three-dimensional Fourier transform (3DFT) MRI, Tsuruda and associates[27] also noted wraparound artifact in the slice-selection direction with this pulse sequence. In comparison with 4-mm-thick axial T1-weighted spin-echo 2DFT or gradient-echo 2DFT studies, diagnostic confidence was improved with 3DFT as a result of the reduction of partial-volume artifact with the thinner slices (1.5- to 2.0-mm-thick axial sections).

Gradient-echo images obtained at a location remote

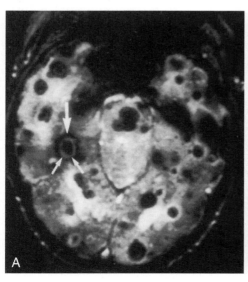
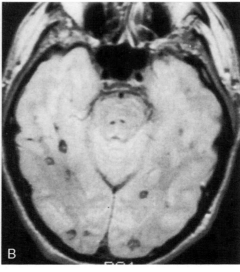

FIGURE 3–13. *A*, Gradient-echo image (60/44/24°) of multiple intracerebral hemangiomas. High-intensity ring *(small arrows)* inside low-intensity periphery *(large arrow)* from susceptibility-induced intravoxel phase interference induced by magnetic point dipole–like field perturbation. *B*, Spin-echo image at same slice location with far less susceptibility-induced signal loss shows central nidus. (*A* and *B* from Kim JK, Kucharczyk W, Henkelman RM: Cavernous hemangiomas: dipolar susceptibility artifacts at MR imaging. Radiology 187:735–741, 1993.)

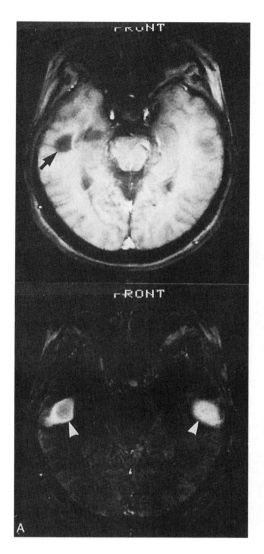

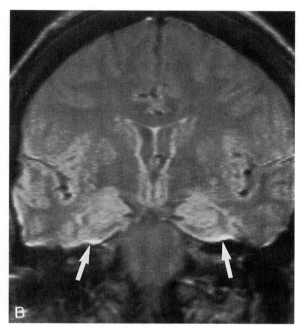

FIGURE 3–14. Magnetic susceptibility artifacts on fast low-angle gradient-echo images caused by boundary between petrous ridges and brain. *A, top,* With echo time TE = 13 ms, localized area of decreased signal intensity is seen in right temporal lobe *(arrow).* This does not represent partial-volume averaging. Also note decreased signal intensity surrounding maxillary antra. *Bottom,* With longer TE (40 ms), susceptibility artifacts *(arrowheads)* are much worse. *B,* Coronal proton density image of brain, obtained with low-bandwidth spin-echo pulse sequence, demonstrates artifactual high signal intensity under temporal lobes *(arrows),* representing susceptibility artifact.

from the magnet isocenter also suffer from susceptibility artifacts (Fig. 3–16). On gradient-echo images, bone marrow has a lower signal intensity than expected for the TE. This is due to spin dephasing produced by the presence of substances with different susceptibilities (calcium, water, and fat) within the same voxel.

The characteristic appearance of a susceptibility artifact is geometric distortion of a structure's shape; that is, round objects are depicted as spear or flower shaped (susceptibility "flowering"),[28] with alterations in pixel signal intensity caused by the overlapping of displaced images.

MOVING SUSCEPTIBILITY ARTIFACT: GASTROINTESTINAL CONTRAST AGENTS

A bowel-labeling agent may be useful in some cases for abdominal MRI. Besides providing contrast between the bowel and other organs, the contrast agent itself can be a potential source of artifacts.[29] Apart from the expected static effects of the superparamagnetic particle gastrointestinal contrast agent, movement-induced artifacts were seen as signal displacements in the phase-encoding direction. The artifacts were obvious at an iron concentration of 1 mg/mL, barely visible at 0.2 mg/mL, and completely absent at 0.1 mg/mL. Artifacts were also evident with the superparamagnetic particle outside the imaging slice. The authors further emphasized the importance of choosing the lowest effective dose when using superparamagnetic particle contrast agents. For the paramagnetic agent, motion-propagated artifacts consisted of regions of high and low signal intensity in a mosaic pattern. The gastrointestinal contrast agent perfluorocarbon emulsion (perfluorooctylbromide) does not produce an MR signal. It is not associated with a statistically significant increase in image artifacts before versus after contrast agent administration.[30]

REDUCE ARTIFACTS BY USING AN APPROPRIATE PULSE SEQUENCE

Many practical solutions to correcting susceptibility artifacts have appeared in the past 6 years. A significant

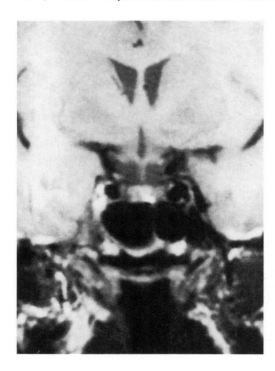

FIGURE 3–15. Focal high-signal-intensity "spot" at junction of sphenoid septum with the floor of the sella from magnetic susceptibility effect. (From Sakurai K, Fujita N, Harada K, et al: Magnetic susceptibility artifact in spin-echo MR imaging of the pituitary gland. AJNR 13[5]:1301–1308, 1992, © by American Society of Neuroradiology.)

advance has been the fast spin-echo (also called turbo spin-echo or rapid acquisition with relaxation enhancement, RARE) pulse sequence.[31] Sagittal T2-weighted conventional spin-echo and fast spin-echo paired images with metallic artifacts from various sources, including fixation rods or plates, posterior fixation wires, drill particles from anterior cervical diskectomy, and an inferior vena cava filter, were compared, and the metal artifact signal void was found to be less apparent with fast spin-echo sequences in 39 of 45 cases. In 8 of 45 evaluations, the reading of the region of interest was feasible only on the fast spin-echo images (Fig. 3–17). Fast spin-echo imaging, particularly when accomplished with shorter echo spacing, reduces magnetic susceptibility effects.

Spurious signal intensities may be decreased with stronger readout gradients at any given field of view

(FOV). Ludeke and colleagues[28] demonstrated that with constant FOVs, a 0.2 G/cm readout gradient (shorter sampling window, higher receiver bandwidth) reduced the magnetic susceptibility artifact at air-water interfaces compared with that at a 0.08 G/cm readout gradient (longer sampling window, narrower receiver bandwidth). Young and colleagues[32] noted the advantage of heightening spatial resolution as a method of diminishing artifacts caused by field inhomogeneities.

Short TE values (see Fig. 3–5A) allow less time for spin dephasing than long TE values (see Fig. 3–5B), so susceptibility artifacts are reduced. Susceptibility artifacts can also be minimized by the use of thin slices, which reduces dephasing across the slice. For gradient-echo images, three-dimensional (3D) volume methods are particularly effective for reducing dephasing across the slice. If enough phase-encoding steps are acquired

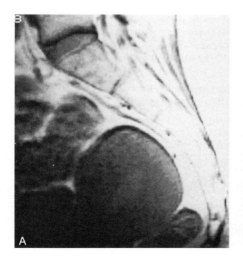

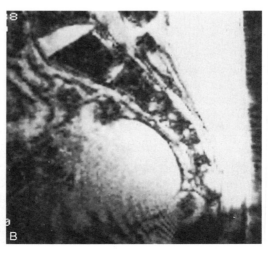

FIGURE 3–16. Gradient-echo images are particularly sensitive to magnetic field inhomogeneity, which worsens with distance from the isocenter of the magnet. A, T1-weighted spin-echo image of the lower lumbar spine and pelvis demonstrates normal uterine anatomy. Magnetic field inhomogeneity is not apparent. B, Gradient-echo (fast imaging with steady-state precession) image acquired with TE = 11 ms demonstrates multiple ring-like artifacts along the inferior edge of the image, which is distant from the magnet center.

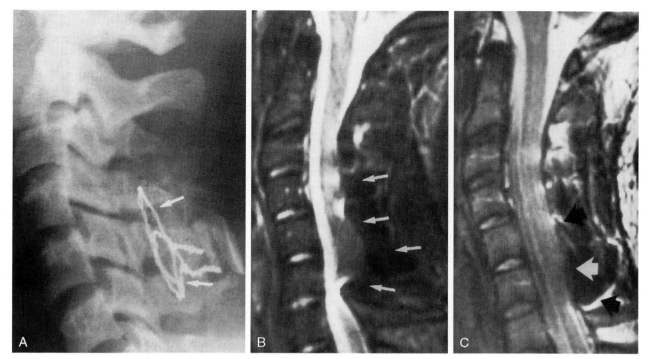

FIGURE 3–17. *A,* Radiograph of posterior fusion wires C-4 to C-6. *B,* Conventional T2-weighted spin-echo MR image (2000/80) shows posterior spinal canal and cord distorted by metal artifact *(arrows). C,* Fast spin-echo T2-weighted MR image (2000/102), obtained in one fourth the acquisition time of the image in *B,* illustrates far less distortion *(arrows). (A* to *C* from Tartaglino LM, Flanders AE, Vinitski S, Friedman DP: Metallic artifacts on MR images of the postoperative spine: reduction with fast spin-echo techniques. Radiology 190:565–569, 1994.)

along the selection axis, then for some values of the selection gradient the effects of local magnetic field inhomogeneities are compensated. As the severity of the susceptibility artifact worsens, more phase-encoding steps are needed to correct for the local field inhomogeneity. Compared with two-dimensional (2D) gradient-echo images, 3D gradient-echo images of the head show improved definition of the pituitary gland because susceptibility effects resulting from the interface between brain and air-containing sphenoid sinus are reduced; 3D gradient-echo images of the spine show increased signal intensity from bone marrow.

Another B_0 artifact was described by Erickson and coworkers.[33] Orientation in the static field is responsible for the frequent occurrence of increased signal intensity from normal tendons on MR images. Increased signal intensity from the wrist, ankle, and shoulder caused by the "magic angle" effect may be misdiagnosed as tendinous degeneration (tendinosis, tendinopathy), tendinitis, or frank tear (Fig. 3–18). Markedly increased intratendinous signal intensity was observed at the magic angle of 55° in relation to the constant magnetic induction field (B_0). Intermediate signal intensity was observed at 45° and 65°, and no signal intensity was observed at 0° and 90°. Peterfy and colleagues[34] noted that augmented signal intensity is often visible in the upsloping, medial division of the posterior horn of the normal lateral meniscus on standard short-TE MR images of the knee (Fig. 3–19). This characteristic can imitate or conceal irregularities in this section of the meniscus. A magic angle phenome-

non results from the angular orientation of this meniscal section and its concentrically arranged collagen fibers relative to the B_0 field. Increased signal intensity was present in the medial segment of the posterior horn of the lateral meniscus in 74% of images. In 81% of these, this meniscal segment was oriented at 55° to 60°. Increased signal intensity was also displayed in this meniscal segment in three (60%) of five asymptomatic knees imaged in the neutral position. In each of these, abduction of the leg decreased the meniscal signal

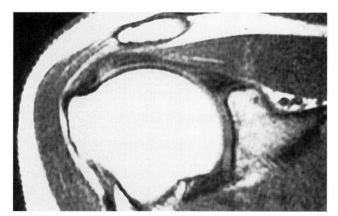

FIGURE 3–18. Magic angle. T1-weighted (500/25) oblique coronal spin-echo image of the shoulder in an asymptomatic 14-year-old patient, depicting increased signal intensity in the rotator cuff just proximal to the insertion site on the greater tuberosity. This segment approximates the magic angle (55°).

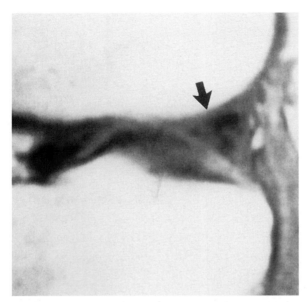

FIGURE 3–19. T1-weighted (400/20) sagittal MR image of the knee, with increased intrameniscal signal intensity in the upsloping medial division of the posterior horn of the lateral meniscus in an asymptomatic volunteer *(arrow)*. This segment approximates the magic angle (55°). (From Peterfy CG, Janzen DL, Tirman PF, et al: "Magic-angle" phenomenon: a cause of increased signal in the normal lateral meniscus on short-TE MR images of the knee. AJR 163:149–154, 1994.)

intensity by 52% to 80%. Increased signal intensity in the upsloping segment of the posterior horn of the lateral meniscus on short-TE images is commonly due to the magic angle phenomenon rather than to meniscal tear or degeneration.

RADIOFREQUENCY FIELD ARTIFACTS

The RF pulses utilized to excite protons in MRI share frequency ranges with many extraneous RF sources, including fluorescent lights; television and radio broadcasts; distant shortwave broadcasts appearing in the evening; electric motors (particularly direct current) such as in CT scanners, pumps, and floor-cleaning equipment; electric trains; forklift trucks; elevator switching gear; defective diodes; bad connections; a leaky magnet room RF-shielding enclosure; devices for monitoring patients; typewriters; and computers.[1, 3] Penetration of these extrinsic RF energies into an MRI system results in image noise, with the degree of image degradation dependent on the frequency range of the noise source and the MRI system resonance frequency and bandwidth. Broad-band noise may degrade an entire image, whereas an extrinsic narrow-frequency signal commonly causes linear bands of interference perpendicular to the frequency-encoding axis (Fig. 3–20). The exact location of the artifactual band is related to the difference between the center frequency of the scanner and the frequency of the extraneous signal.

Specifically, amateur radio operators operate within the frequency range of 21.0 to 21.5 MHz. The Larmor frequency for a 0.5-T MRI system of 21.3 MHz falls within this range. A 1.5-T MRI system has a proton resonance frequency of 64.0 MHz, which lies within the frequency domain of 60 to 66 MHz assigned to television channel 3.[1]

Obviously, shielding from extrinsic RF sources is necessary for MR image preservation from external noise. The magnet room enclosure should attenuate extrinsic noise by a factor on the order of 80 to 100 dB, depending on the installation. RF leaks can occur through pipes and electrical lines; this can be avoided by enclosing the lines in wave-guides. RF noise enters if the door is left open or if the flexible copper tabs along the sides, top, and bottom of the door break off. Of course, poor image quality is not always due to excessive noise; poor quality also results from low signal intensity caused by a bad choice of imaging technique, RF coil, or improper prescan adjustments. Optimization of image quality requires proper maintenance procedures, including keeping a log of ambient noise levels and signal-to-noise (S/N) ratio in a standard phantom. In analogous fashion, an object on the surface of a patient may act as a shield from the system RF pulses, generating local B_1 defects and signal loss or distortion.[3] Potential internal (to the system) RF shields are metal-containing dressings, electrode disks, or RF-impermeable objects in the patient's clothing.

Removal of the shielding objects restores RF homogeneity. Prevention of extraneous RF noise in images is achieved through proper planning of MRI system location and effective shielding. If discrete RF noise lines perpendicular to the readout axis persist in the image despite all shielding efforts, field service can always change the magnetic field and RF synthesizer frequency up or down within 200,000 Hz to find a

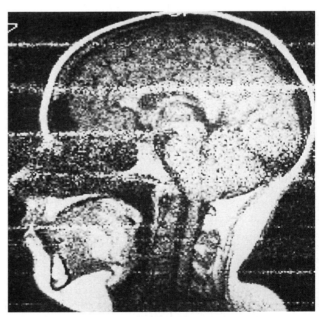

FIGURE 3–20. RF interference resulting from defective magnet room enclosure. Note multiple vertical lines, oriented perpendicular to the frequency-encoding axis, representing RF interference at multiple frequencies.

"clean" imaging bandwidth. Discrete RF noise lines oriented along both the readout and phase-encoding axes arise from the imaging system itself (synchronous RF noise),[2] most often from bad electrical or RF grounding, and are the responsibility of field service.

Artifactual loss of signal is an inherent problem in surface coil imaging because of loss of RF intensity away from the center of the coil (Fig. 3–21). The peripheral drop-off of signal intensity occurs in all possible modes of operation with RF surface coils: transmit-only, receive-only, and transmit-receive. Optimal positioning of the coil minimizes the loss of diagnostically useful information. Signal inhomogeneity across the image can be improved by appropriate rescaling of the image.[35]

The phased-array coil provides an improved S/N ratio over that available with the body coil, especially in pelvic MRI with a small FOV.[36] Two factors that can limit image quality in phased-array MRI are increased motion artifact, largely caused by the high signal intensity from moving subcutaneous fat in the anterior near field of the coil, and nonuniformity of signal with distance from the coils. Significant improvements in image quality may occur with improved techniques for decreasing motion artifact, particularly breath-hold imaging.

RF flip angle inhomogeneity may cause asymmetric brightness in an image (Fig. 3–22). This problem may originate in the RF transmitter attenuation setting or RF coil geometry. In the former instance, the RF 90° or 180° pulse is calibrated to obtain the optimal amount of nuclear MR signal in the center slice of the multislice imaging volume. Selected slices of interest away from the center slice may experience more or less RF attenuation than the center slice, resulting in

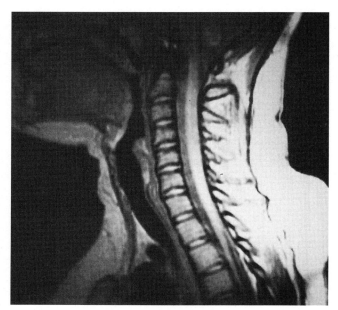

FIGURE 3–21. Surface coil signal loss. Sagittal image of the neck obtained with a planar surface coil (body coil transmit, surface coil receive). The cervical spinal cord is well visualized but signal drops off rapidly in adjacent deeper areas.

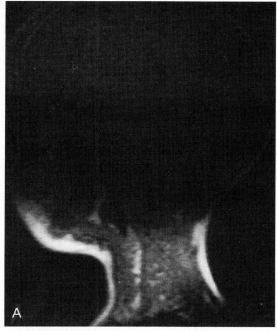

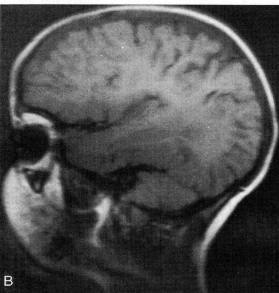

FIGURE 3–22. Incorrect RF attenuation of setting. A, Sagittal T1-weighted study of the head with RF pulse attenuation erroneously peaked over the neck. As a result, the intended 90° to 180° RF pulses produced actual tip angles of 180° to 360° in the head, with a loss of signal in the region of interest. B, Correct RF attenuation peaking at the same level yields satisfactory head study.

RF flip angles greater or less than 90° or 180°. Signal intensity of spins in that slice diminishes corresponding to the decrease in transverse magnetization. Similarly, inhomogeneous energy deposition across the volume of tissue may occur as a result of asymmetric RF coil geometry or off-center positioning of the patient. The artifactual variation in signal intensity over the image is identical to that caused by RF flip angle inhomogeneity but is correctable by proper positioning of the patient. Adiabatic pulses are useful for in-

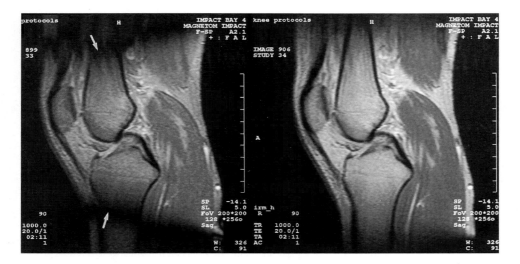

FIGURE 3–23. Adiabatic inversion. Sagittal inversion recovery fast spin-echo images of the knee, using transmit-receive knee coil. *Left,* Standard sinc pulse used for inversion shows banding *(arrows)* due to drop-off in RF at the edges of the knee coil, so that the inversion pulse has a flip angle less than 180°. *Right,* Same, using a hyperbolic secant adiabatic pulse for inversion. The adiabatic pulse ensures a uniform inversion even in the presence of B_1 field inhomogeneity and eliminates the banding artifact.

verting spins for inversion recovery pulse sequences, because they provide a uniform inversion even in the presence of B_1 field inhomogeneity (Fig. 3–23). Unfortunately, adiabatic pulses cannot be used as refocusing pulses for spin-echo pulse sequences. RF eddy currents occur in biologic tissues even without metal implants and result in a B_1 nonuniformity known as the quadrupole artifact with linearly polarized RF coils.[37]

RF pulses may be selective, exciting spins in a discrete volume of finite thickness, or nonselective, exciting spins in the entire tissue volume. The assumption that a selective RF pulse excites protons in a well-defined geometric slab of tissue is often incorrect, especially with nominal 180° RF pulses. Some MR image slice profiles are gaussian or even M shaped. Artifactual loss of signal intensity in a stack of multislice images acquired contiguously may occur because of saturation of spins by overlapping, nonsquare slice profiles in contiguous slice imaging. Interleaving slices in data acquisition, lengthening the TR, or increasing the interslice gap alleviates this "cross-talk" problem. Sophisticated tailored RF excitation pulses resulting in negligible cross-talk with gapless multislice spin-echo imaging are commercially available.[38] Unlike spin-echo sequences, which require the use of 180° pulses, low-flip-angle gradient-echo pulse sequences can routinely provide gapless contiguous multislice sections without significant cross-talk.

Random thermal or incoherent noise degrades spatial resolution and contrast over the entire object imaged. Thermal noise can be reduced by increasing the number of signal averages (excitations) or using surface coils, thereby limiting detection of thermal noise in more distant tissues not containing the region of interest and increasing the S/N ratio.[39]

Physical contact between the patient and the RF coil produces signal loss and image distortion similar to those that occur with ferromagnetic artifacts. A contact artifact is distinguished by its peripheral location on the image and the bizarre configuration of the anatomic part involved, usually the upper extremity, abdomen, or pelvis. Remedies include repositioning the

patient or utilizing a smaller FOV. Alternatively, the technique of inner volume imaging of Feinberg and coworkers[40] is able to "focus in" on a central region of interest not affected by peripheral body coil contact artifact.

CENTRAL POINT ARTIFACT

The central point artifact is a central bright or dark area of signal intensity (occasionally with a column of truncation ringing bordering it) and occurs generally in the exact center of the image[3] (Fig. 3–24). It results from a constant direct current offset in the level of the

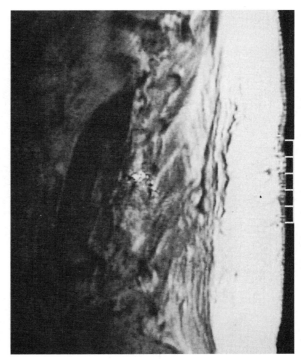

FIGURE 3–24. Central field artifact. Proton density–weighted sagittal images of the lumbar spine demonstrate a classic central field artifact of bright signal intensity covering several pixels.

receiver voltage of each phase-encoding step. If the direct-current level of each phase-encoding step is variable, a line parallel to the phase-encoding axis can result (similar to RF feedthrough; see the next section). This artifact can be reduced by phase alternation of two RF excitation pulses at each phase-encoding step, resulting in cancellation of the two averaged extraneous signals.

CENTRAL LINES

Central line artifacts can be divided into those parallel to the phase-encoding axis and those parallel to the frequency-encoding axis. Figure 3–25 demonstrates an example of the central line artifact in the phase-encoding direction. This artifact results from RF feedthrough[2] detected by the sensitive RF receiver, which by necessity must reside close to the strong RF transmitter. In addition to phase alternation of paired excitation pulses, one-excitation acquisitions can be obtained free of central lines parallel to the phase-encoding axis by substitution of the spurious central data point in each phase-encoding step with a point interpolated from adjacent points.[2] This interpolation would take place between the first and second Fourier transformations, so this technique would be ineffective if digital smoothing filters were applied along the readout axis before the first Fourier transformation (because the filter distributes the RF feedthrough over many frequencies, rendering single-point interpolation impossible).[2]

Central line artifact parallel to the readout axis can be caused by residual transverse magnetization (in the form of a free induction decay or stimulated echo signals), primarily resulting from imperfections of the 180° pulses directly preceding the corresponding spin echoes. The imperfections are unavoidable in any practical instrument, especially for multiple slice sequences requiring selective 180° RF pulses. A selective pulse must have some finite transition region between its center (where it does its main function) and its exterior (where it is supposed to do nothing). In this transition, a 180° pulse passes through lesser values that generate a free induction decay. In multiecho pulse sequences, additional echoes can be generated because of imperfections in the 90° and 180° RF pulses. If these stimulated echoes happen to fall within the readout period, a central line (''zipper'') can be produced. Stimulated echoes can also produce an inverted image ghost (as opposed to a 180° rotated image from quadrature-phase error), because the phase of the stimulated echo is opposite in polarity to the Carr-Purcell nth echo (n > 1)[2] (Fig. 3–26).

In Figure 3–27, we see a basic imaging pulse sequence. There are 90° and 180° RF pulses and three gradient waveforms. Note two things in addition. There is a free induction decay following the 180° RF pulse much like the one from the 90° RF pulse. (It has been exaggerated in Fig. 3–27.) Also, the spatial information in the phase-encoded direction is imposed before this free induction decay associated with the 180° pulse exists.

The reconstructed image from this sequence has a thin line of hash through the center of the phase-encoded direction, parallel to the readout axis (see Fig. 3–27A). The hash piles up there because it missed being phase encoded, and it is treated as a direct-current component and dumped in the central row along the phase-encoding axis.

A solution to a wholly analogous problem in a different nuclear MR application was given in 1977 by Bodenhausen and coworkers.[41] The suggestion was to alternate the phase of the 180° RF pulse across phase-encoding steps. Again, the spin echoes are unchanged but the hash from the free induction decay changes sign, apparently at the Nyquist frequency. The reconstructed image still contains the hash but it is no longer in the center of the image but rather at one edge (see Fig. 3–27B). Other phase-cycling techniques can be employed as well.[42, 43]

Residual transverse magnetization can also be limited by using short readout periods and by adjusting timing parameters within the pulse sequence. In addition, improvement of the slice excitation profile by better RF pulse tailoring should reduce this artifact, but little agreement on the ''ideal'' selective pulse has been achieved.[38, 44–49] A commonly employed technique is to insert paired pulsed gradients (''crushers'')[50, 51] to spoil the residual transverse magnetization. Increasing the interslice gap can also reduce the formation of the readout zipper. The stimulated echo ghost problem can be eliminated by display strategies or by inversion of the polarity of the second spin-echo signal (relative to the first echo) by use of an additional phase-encoding gradient between the first echo and the second 180° RF pulse.[2]

Artifacts caused by residual transverse magnetization in 3DFT MRI were described by Wood and Runge.[52] One artifact is caused by differential spoiling of trans-

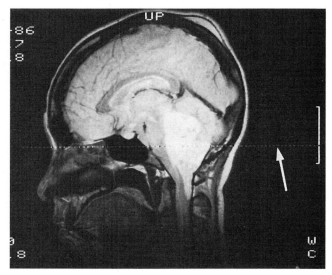

FIGURE 3–25. Center line artifact, parallel to phase-encoding axis, in a proton density–weighted image of a patient with an ependymoma.

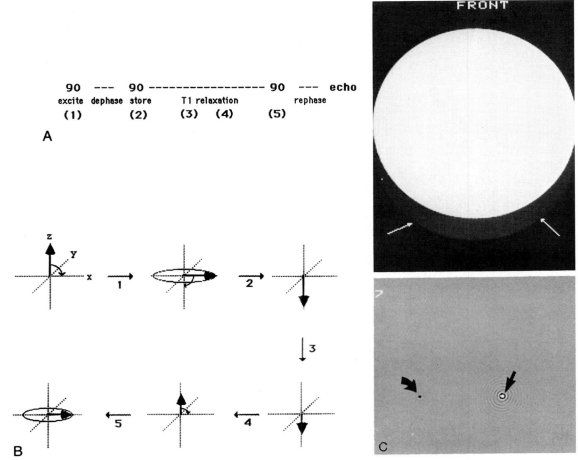

FIGURE 3–26. Stimulated echo artifacts. *A,* Three RF pulses can produce a stimulated echo. *B,* Illustration of magnetization is stored and then read out to produce a stimulated echo. *C,* Effect of a stimulated echo seen in an image of a water bottle. *Top,* In addition to normal image, there is a striated inverted ghost image that is displaced inferiorly along the phase-encoding axis. *Bottom,* Raw data demonstrate a normal echo *(straight arrow)* as well as a lower intensity stimulated echo *(curved arrow).*

verse magnetization by the two separate phase-encoding gradients in a 3DFT sequence (slice selection, phase encoding, and in-plane phase encoding). The image intensity in different slices becomes artifactually altered, especially for a short TR and a large flip angle, which are conditions for achieving strong T1-weighted contrast. The further addition of constant spoiler gradients reduces this intensity increase by one half.

PARTIAL-VOLUME AVERAGING

Partial-volume averaging occurs when the voxel dimensions are comparable to the dimensions of the object being imaged. Because most MRI is performed by using anisotropic techniques (i.e., lower resolution in one dimension than in the other two), partial-volume averaging is most severe in the direction of slice selection (Figs. 3–28 and 3–29). Curtin and associates[53] found that transverse scans of the cervical spinal cord ordinarily show signal changes associated with the inner structure of the cord that do not correctly correspond to histologic cross sections. The appearance of

the central sections of the gray and white matter was influenced variably by partial-volume averaging, depending on the matrix size. High-contrast structures (e.g., lipid-containing iophendylate [Pantopaque] droplets on a T1-weighted image) can be visualized even when they are smaller than the voxel (Fig. 3–30); however, low-contrast structures (e.g., small meningiomas) may not be detected. Retained intraspinal iophendylate may mimic the appearance of intra- or extradural lesions, magnetic susceptibility artifact, and flow on gradient-echo MR images of the spine.[54]

Partial-volume averaging is minimized by improving spatial resolution. This can be accomplished by reducing the section thickness or by reducing the FOV. However, either maneuver results in a reduction in the S/N ratio, which may necessitate increased signal averaging and proportionately increased acquisition time. Because the voxel is usually much larger in the direction of slice selection, a reduction in section thickness generally provides a greater reduction in partial-volume averaging than a reduced FOV. Reductions in the FOV may result in wraparound artifacts (discussed later).

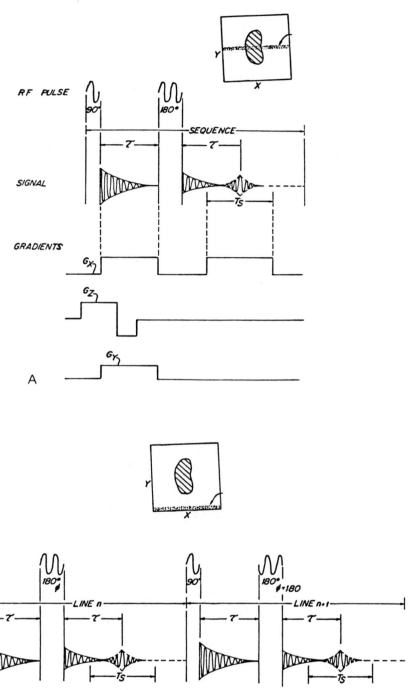

FIGURE 3–27. Explanation of center line artifact. *A,* Without alternating phase of 180° RF pulse, residual transverse magnetization in the form of a free induction decay from the imperfect 180° RF pulse spills over into the spin-echo sampling window (T_s). Because this spurious signal was created after phase encoding, its multiple frequencies are all dumped into the zeroth phase-encoding column in the image, creating the center line parallel to the phase-encoding axis. *B,* With phase alternation of successive 180° pulses, this residual transverse magnetization is shifted to the edge of the image.

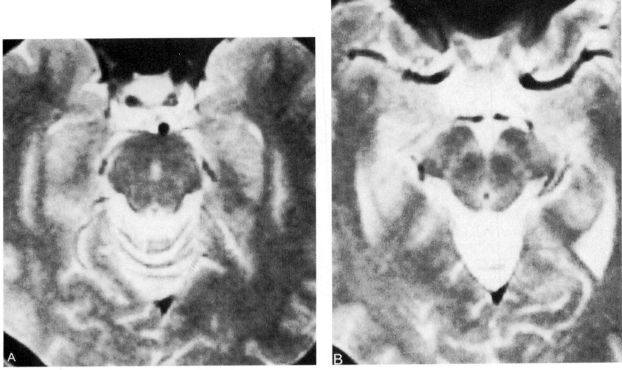

FIGURE 3–28. *A,* T2-weighted image with horizontal phase encoding demonstrates inferior midbrain central high signal intensity (5-mm-thick section). *B,* Adjacent slice centered 7.5 mm superior shows the high-signal-intensity interpeduncular cistern as the source of this partial-volume averaging artifact.

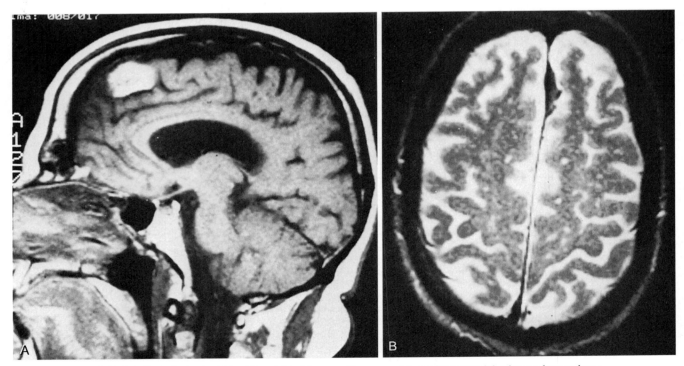

FIGURE 3–29. *A,* Sagittal midline T1-weighted image with apparent frontal intracranial subacute hemorrhage. *B,* Axial T2-weighted section shows the short T2 nature and falx cerebri location, diagnostic of normal bone marrow lipid in an ossified falx.

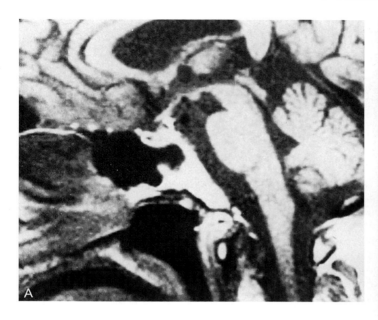

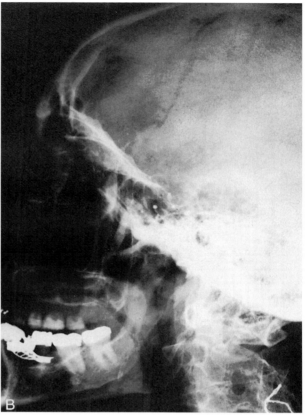

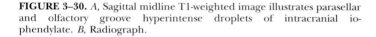

FIGURE 3–30. *A,* Sagittal midline T1-weighted image illustrates parasellar and olfactory groove hyperintense droplets of intracranial io-phendylate. *B,* Radiograph.

DATA-CLIPPING ARTIFACT

On occasion one may encounter an image with a peculiar ghost-like quality, with a "snowstorm" background and loss of contrast between soft tissues (Fig. 3–31). This is a data-clipping artifact, resulting from having signal intensity that is outside the digitization range (saturation) of the analog-to-digital converter. The artifact may be encountered on some sections and not others in a multisection acquisition. The problem is most severe on surface coil images, where subcutaneous fat contributes a high signal intensity; in obese patients; and in techniques that use large numbers of slices or thick sections. Normally, the receiver adjustment is performed using the zero-phase line (i.e., no phase-encoding gradient), because this data line produces the highest signal intensity. However, interactions between the magnetic field of a surface coil and the main field can change the line that produces the maximal signal. As a result, the maximal signal occurs a few lines away from zero rather than at the zero line. If the automatic receiver adjustment results in clipping, the receiver gain can be manually reduced, typically by a few decibels. Operator misadjustment of the receiver attenuation has diminished in frequency with the advent of automatic adjustment procedures on most commercial systems.

Several sources of artifacts do not clearly fit into the categories already mentioned. Asymmetric brightness, described previously as a result of nonuniform slice thickness secondary to slice-selection gradient inhomo-

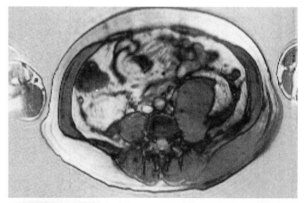

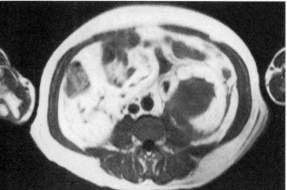

FIGURE 3–31. Data-clipping artifact. *Top,* T1-weighted image of the abdomen demonstrates ghost-like appearance caused by an incorrect setting of receiver gain. *Bottom,* Lower receiver gain produces a normal-appearing image.

geneity, can be due to low-pass filters that are too narrow about the signal band. This leads to inappropriate rejection of a portion of the signal emitted by the protons in the section of interest. The characteristic appearance is a uniform decrease in signal intensity on one side of an image. The problem may be corrected by widening the bandpass of the frequency filter.

LOSS OF DATA

Loss of one or more lines of data causes a variable degree of artifact; loss of the central data lines (weakest phase-encoding steps) results in the largest artifacts. Loss of data can result from communication problems, gradient instability, or excessive receiver noise (Fig. 3–32). Analog-to-digital converter errors are unavoidable on any MRI system, because more than 10 million analog-to-digital conversions take place in a study of a single patient.[2] An error in the digitization of a single data point can result in a uniform background of vertical, horizontal, or obliquely oriented stripes (Fig. 3–33). The intensity of the stripes can be severe or barely noticeable, depending on where the bad data point falls in the raw data. Spontaneous occurrence of single data point digitization errors cannot be prevented but can be eliminated by postacquisition processing of the raw image data. It has been suggested that spontaneous discharge of static electricity from patients' blankets can result in these single data point errors.[2] We have observed this artifact to result from corroded scan room light bulbs, noisy cryogen scavenger systems, and defectively arcing RF body coil inductive drive bars (Fig. 3–34). The last cause is important to consider, as we had a patient experience a second-degree forearm skin burn despite no physical contact with the sidewalls of the magnet. With a fast spin-echo

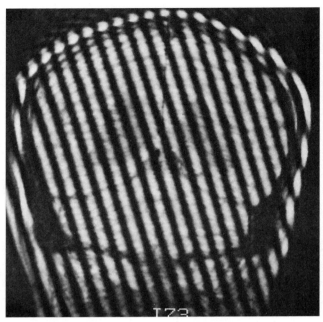

FIGURE 3–33. Digitization error in a single data point results in an annoying blanket of diagonal stripes in the conventional magnitude reconstruction.

sequence, this artifact was observed in the presence of a body coil inductive drive bar meltdown.

QUADRATURE PHASE-SENSITIVE DETECTOR ERRORS

Improper tuning of the real and imaginary channels of the quadrature phase-sensitive detector in the RF receiver can result in a ghost image rotated 180° relative to the center of the image. Tuning the phase angle between the two channels to 90° corrects this problem.

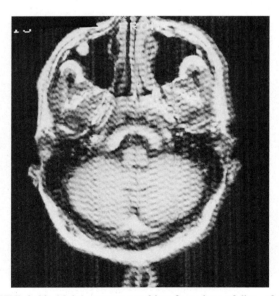

FIGURE 3–32. Moiré pattern resulting from loss of line of data during acquisition. In this case, loss of the data line was produced by excessive receiver noise, secondary to a defective service light bulb.

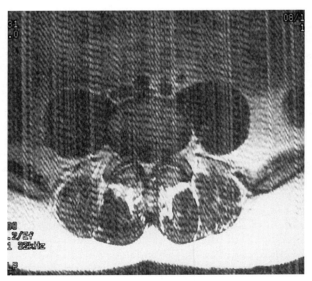

FIGURE 3–34. "Herringbone" background artifact resulting from arcing of a defectively melted inductive drive bar in an RF coil subsystem.

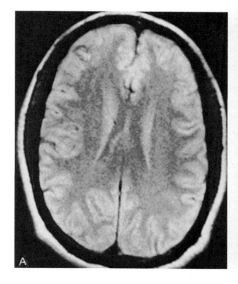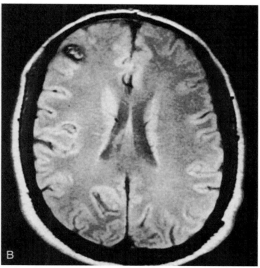

FIGURE 3–35. Gradient power drop-off. *A*, Axial (2000/30) image of the head of a patient with an intracerebral hemorrhage from an arteriovenous malformation. The dolichocephalic appearance of the head is due to gradient power drop-off. *B*, Evaluation of the same patient 7 weeks later with a different MRI system shows a normal head configuration and lesion with a peripheral rim of low-intensity signal secondary to a paramagnetic effect of hemosiderin-laden macrophages.

GRADIENT ARTIFACTS

Magnetic field gradients transform an MR experiment into the MR image, as they provide the information necessary for slice selection and spatial encoding. As a result, even minor gradient problems may render clinical images inaccurate (Fig. 3–35) or uninterpretable. The gradient fields must be designed to switch on and off rapidly, usually within 1 ms. This demand exacts strict requirements on gradient coil power supplies and generates mechanical stress on the coil itself that may lead to malfunction. In addition to gradient coil mechanical problems causing artifacts, the 2DFT reconstruction of gradient-generated spatial-encoding data produces inherent MR artifacts, which are discussed later.

The frequency-encoding gradient is the gradient most sensitive to inherent B_0 static field inhomogeneities.[3] An image obtained with the frequency-encoding gradient selected along the axis of greatest B_0 inhomogeneity, conventionally the z axis in most systems, may show bands or areas of signal loss corresponding to the areas of B_0 nonuniformity. By exchanging the orientations of the frequency- and phase-encoding axes (phase-encoding axis in the z direction), the S/N ratio over the entire image can be increased.

RINGING ARTIFACT

Ringing artifacts (also called Gibbs, edge ringing, spectral leakage, or truncation artifacts) appear as concentric curvilinear low-intensity lines that cross through the entire image.[55] These artifacts arise primarily in two circumstances: 1) because of data interpolation (zero filling), when a smaller acquisition matrix (e.g., 256 × 128) is interpolated into a larger display matrix (e.g., 256 × 256), and 2) near edges where there are abrupt transitions in signal intensity along relatively linear portions of tissue interfaces (e.g., between bright scalp fat and dark cortex of the calvaria) (Fig. 3–36). On occasion, ringing may mimic a motion artifact or a fine structure such as a small syrinx in the spinal cord,[56, 57] intervertebral disk,[58, 59] muscle bundles, or nerve fibers.[2]

Unlike the other kinds of artifacts we have described, ringing artifacts occur in both the frequency-encoding and phase-encoding directions and are always present to some degree in MR images. On images obtained with short TR and TE, a ring of high signal intensity at the periphery of the cervical spinal cord can be found because of truncation artifact.[53] Ringing artifacts are clinically most likely to be present along the phase-encoding axis, because throughput and economic pressures often constrain imaging time to the least number of phase-encoding steps possible (e.g., 128). It must be emphasized that with greater sampling of the higher frequencies in k-space (e.g., 256 phase-encoding steps), the spacing of the ringing lines is cut

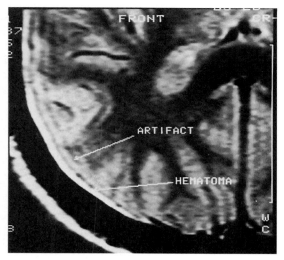

FIGURE 3–36. Patient with a small subdural hematoma; 256 × 128 acquisition matrix; no filtering. Note curvilinear lines (ringing artifacts) that parallel the high-signal-intensity hematoma along the horizontal phase-encoding axis.

in half but their amplitude is not diminished.[2] Despite this theoretic limitation of this solution to truncation ringing, it remains the most practical and effective remedy because the closer spacing of the ringing lines vastly reduces their conspicuity.

An artifact that is similar in appearance to ringing artifacts but different in etiology and orientation can be seen on images acquired with marked bandwidth reduction (used to improve the S/N ratio). Bandwidth reduction techniques use a weak readout gradient; ringing artifacts along the readout axis arise when the gradient is so small that the ratio (duration of readout period/T2) approaches unity.[1] So-called matched bandwidth techniques that employ a long narrow-band sampling window that is asymmetrically displaced earlier in time than the center of the echo (to achieve earlier minimal TE values for a given bandwidth) also suffer from ringing artifacts along the frequency-encoding axis.

Filter to Reduce Ringing Artifact

During the calculation of an image from the raw data, one has the opportunity to introduce some filter functions into the process to improve the image quality with little or no increase in the time required for reconstruction. This is accomplished by a general technique known as digital filtering. A review of the basic applications of digital filters[60] reveals that they are particularly applicable in Fourier transform (FT) signal processing.

The edge ringing artifact is caused by sudden truncation of the raw data at the high-frequency ends of the spectrum. Another way to reduce this common artifact is to apply a filter that reduces the contribution of the extremely high frequency components. This has the side effects of reducing the noise content without removing much anatomic information and of enhancing edges.[61] The result, if this is done properly, is generally desirable, although there is necessarily a small loss of edge definition (spatial blurring)[62] or spurious thickening of structures that do not match assumed step edge models using a modified iterative method.[63] Constable and Henkelman[64] described a data extrapolation approach to the reduction of ringing artifacts in MRI.

In general, filters are used to modify the frequency content of a signal, such as the filter in an audio receiver that removes static and hissing. When one has a set of digitally recorded data, one can see its frequency content by submitting it to FT analysis. If one could tell by inspection that some of the frequencies in the raw data could not be part of the desired information, then those frequencies could be suppressed. After a second FT, which takes one back to the original format of the data, the quality of the desired information has been improved. If it were an audio recording that contained hiss, one would observe a high intensity in the high frequencies that is rather constant, even when the character of the music changes dramatically. One can then test whether the suspect frequencies are hissing by performing the FT back into the normal sound data and listening again. We are not usually able to eliminate any of our data as noise by any simple means. We are, however, able to nip some well-known artifacts in the bud, including edge ringing artifacts and central point artifacts. An artifact similar in appearance to the Gibbs phenomenon can result from inadequate peak power output from the gradient power supply during the strongest phase-encoding steps. This can be corrected by purposely overpowering the gradient during these steps.[2]

Gradient amplifiers can also fail to meet power requirements during the weaker steps of phase encoding, because of dynamic range problems in the digitization of the gradient, especially for wide-FOV acquisitions.[2] *Translated* ghosts (as opposed to 180°-*rotated* or *inverted* ghosts) result from this error in software pulse sequence design. This error can be avoided by ensuring that all phase-encoding steps for all possible FOVs have a whole integer value assigned to them by the digital-to-analog converter, avoiding digital roundoff problems for the lower order phase-encoding steps. This approach may not be feasible for oblique sections, requiring interpolation schemes in the reconstruction of the second dimension of the 2DFT.

Sixty-hertz electrical noise (from imager or environmental hardware) can result in translated ghosts, as persistent view-to-view errors in the gradient amplifier are introduced. As opposed to translated ghosts associated with gradient digital-to-analog converter error, these ghosts are reduced by signal averaging[2] or gating the excitation sequence to 60 Hz (TR = a whole integer multiple of $\frac{1}{60}$ second, or 16.67 ms). This approach is entirely analogous to averaging and gating with biologic respiratory or cardiac motion (see Motion-Related Artifacts). Room lights can be a cause of 60-cycle noise–induced translated ghosts.

CHEMICAL-SHIFT ARTIFACT

Chemical-shift artifact can occur along either the readout or slice-selection axis. Along the readout axis, it is seen at the border between fat-containing tissue (e.g., retroperitoneal fat, bone marrow) and water-containing tissue (e.g., renal cortex, intervertebral disk). Fat protons resonate at a frequency approximately 3.5 ppm lower than that of water protons. However, MR images are usually obtained using the water peak as the central reference frequency. Because frequency is equivalent to position in 2DFT imaging and fat protons resonate at a lower frequency, they appear shifted in position along the frequency-encoding axis to the lower frequency side of the image (Fig. 3–37). As shown in Figure 3–38 for the kidney (which is embedded in fat), when the chemical shift is comparable to or greater than the pixel size, it results in a dark line on the low-frequency border of the kidney and a bright line on the high-frequency border.[65] Areas in which a chemical-shift artifact may cause diagnostic problems include the optic nerves, kidneys, pericardium, and vertebral end plates. Note that chemical-shift artifact does not occur in brain, despite the fat content of myelin, because these fat protons have short

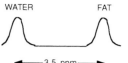

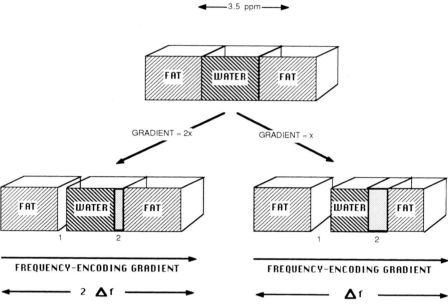

FIGURE 3–37. Chemical-shift artifact. Fat and water protons resonate at slightly different frequencies, so water protons appear to be displaced relative to fat protons. In region 1, fat protons appear shifted to the left, leaving a pixel with no signal. In region 2, fat and water signals overlap, resulting in high signal intensity on T2-weighted images. For frequency-encoding gradient = 2x, artifact is half as wide as for gradient = x.

T2 values and are MR invisible. The chemical-shift artifact is diminished when curvilinear or planar lipid-water interfaces are not oriented along the axis of slice selection.[66]

Chemical-shift artifact can also occur along the slice-selection axis (Fig. 3–39). In the head, lipid protons from an axial section from skull bone marrow can be misregistered (with reference to the same section's water protons) along the z axis, resulting in bilaterally symmetric "pseudo–subdural hematomas."[2] In the kidney, a chemical-shift artifact along the section-selection axis can mimic a renal mass and was observed adjacent to 39% of all renal poles imaged in abdominal MRI.[67] This artifact can be corrected by reversal of the polarity of the slice-selection gradient between the 90° pulse and the 180° pulse.

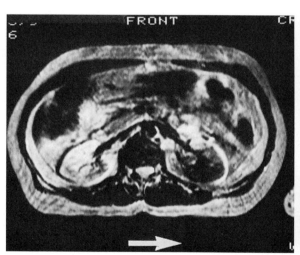

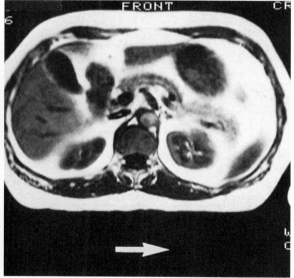

FIGURE 3–38. Chemical-shift artifact. White arrow = direction of readout gradient. *Left,* Note bright curvilinear line along the right (high-frequency) side and the dark line along the left (low-frequency) side of each kidney, representing a chemical-shift artifact on this T2-weighted image (spin echo, 2000/60). *Right,* T1-weighted acquisition, which uses a stronger readout gradient because of the shorter TE, demonstrates only a minimal chemical-shift artifact.

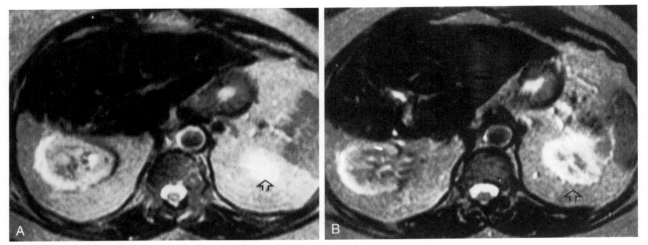

FIGURE 3–39. Chemical-shift artifact. Spin-echo (2500/100) axial MR image at the top of the kidney *(A)* showing hyperintense left-sided pseudomass *(arrow)* caused by a chemical-shift artifact along the slice-selection axis. *B,* The top of the kidney *(arrow)* is seen in the next slice. *A* and *B* from Wachsberg RH, Mitchell DG, Rifkin MD, et al: Chemical shift artifact along the section-select axis. J Magn Reson Imaging 2:589–591, 1992.)

Solutions for Chemical-Shift Artifact

Like ferromagnetic artifacts, chemical-shift artifacts worsen in proportion to the magnetic field strength and improve in proportion to the frequency-encoding gradient.[68] Doubling the frequency-encoding gradient (e.g., using a higher bandwidth pulse sequence) reduces the chemical-shift artifact by a factor of 2 but at the expense of a 1.4-fold worsening in S/N ratio caused by the bandwidth increase. Chemical-shift artifacts can be minimized for certain structures (e.g., optic nerve) by reorienting the frequency-encoding gradient so that it parallels the tissue's long axis. More complex methods are also under development.[69] For instance, chemical-shift–selective imaging can be used to eliminate selectively signals from fat or water protons. Although various methods are available for reducing the chemical-shift artifact, we have found that it seldom presents significant diagnostic problems even at high fields.

WRAPAROUND ARTIFACT AND ALIASING

Have you ever watched an old Western on television and noticed that wagon wheels appear to rotate slowly backward when in actuality the wagon is moving rapidly forward? This is an example of aliasing, which arises from insufficiently rapid sampling of a periodic function and causes a high frequency to appear artifactually as a lower frequency. Examples of sampling functions include digital recording of sound, shooting a movie (each frame is one sample), and measuring the MR signal. The Nyquist theorem states that, when sampling a periodic function, one must sample at least as frequently as

$$f_N > 2 \times f_{max}$$

where f_N is the Nyquist frequency and f_{max} is the highest frequency in the periodic function (Fig. 3–40). In our

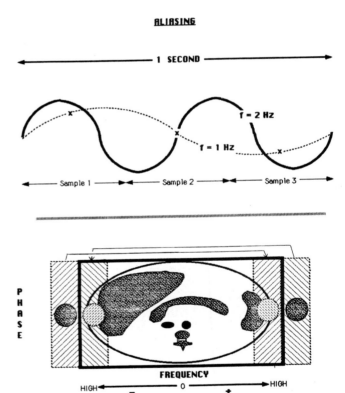

FIGURE 3–40. Aliasing. *Top,* Solid line represents a periodic wave with the frequency = 2 Hz. If the wave is sampled at less than the Nyquist frequency (4 Hz), an artifactually low-frequency wave is represented *(dotted line)*. *Bottom,* Wraparound artifact, an expression of aliasing, causes structures, such as the arms, at the outer edges of the FOV to be folded into the middle of the image (right arm to left side, left arm to right side).

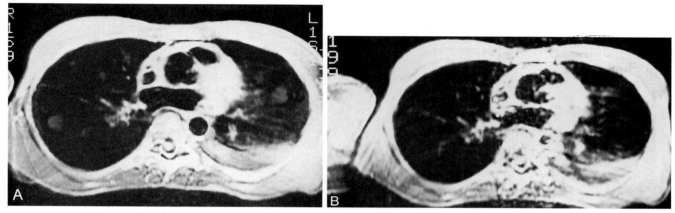

FIGURE 3–41. Aliasing mimicking pulmonary nodules. Transverse images from a respiratory and cardiac gated chest study with an FOV of 32 cm demonstrate aliasing of humeral marrow fat bilaterally into the lung parenchyma *(A)*, which disappears on wider FOV acquisition *(B)*.

movie example, a wagon wheel appears to turn the way it does because the movie frames are acquired at less than twice the rotational frequency of the wheel, resulting in aliasing to a lower rate of rotation. In this phenomenon, known as foldover, frequencies exceeding the Nyquist frequency are assigned a frequency below the Nyquist frequency.

Appearance of Wraparound

One manifestation of aliasing, not encountered in CT, is wraparound.[70] Wraparound can occur on MR images as one reduces the FOV. Objects near the sides of the image (e.g., the arms on chest images) overlap structures in the middle of the image, creating "pseudolesions" (Fig. 3–41). The appearance is similar to that of a piece of paper that has been folded to fit into an envelope. Wraparound occurs because, in reducing the FOV, one increases the precessional frequencies in the object but does not correspondingly increase the number of phase-encoding steps or frequency samples. Wraparound is simply a variation of the foldover concept, because the phase-sensitive method of signal reception in MRI results in assignment of the aliased signal to a corresponding negative frequency (rather than a lower positive frequency in foldover). Mild wraparound is seldom of significance, but severe wraparound renders images uninterpretable (Fig. 3–42).

Solutions to Wraparound

Wraparound along the frequency-encoding axis can be prevented by matching the receiver bandpass filter to the reciprocal of the sampling time and by oversampling along the frequency-encoding axis (e.g., acquiring 512 rather than the usual 256 samples). Wraparound along the phase-encoding axis is a more intractable problem. Reducing the strength of the phase-encoding gradient reduces wraparound but also reduces spatial resolution. Wraparound along the phase-encoding axis can also be reduced by oversampling along the phase-encoding axis (e.g., "high sort"

no phase wrap method).[71, 72] This technique is effective but minimal acquisition time is increased. The inner volume method can eliminate wraparound by limiting the RF excitation to a restricted volume of tissue.[40] With this method, slice selection is performed sequentially along two intersecting planes to define a limited central volume. However, inner volume imaging is essentially a single-slice technique, which reduces its efficiency for 2DFT imaging. Presaturation of signals from tissues outside the region of interest is a more practical method and does not have any significant drawbacks other than a slight increase in the minimal TR per slice, typically a few milliseconds[73] (Fig. 3–43).

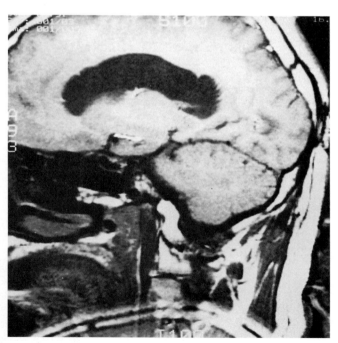

FIGURE 3–42. Aliasing in both phase- and frequency-encoding directions. Sagittal head image (spin echo, 600/25) with FOV of 20 cm demonstrates wraparound posterior and inferior to skull. The region of interest in the pituitary is unaffected by peripheral aliasing. (Frequency gradient is vertical.)

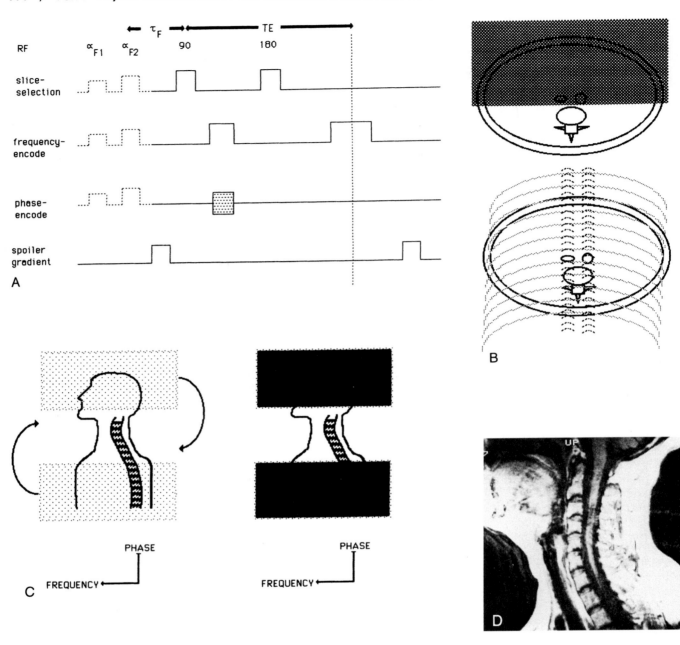

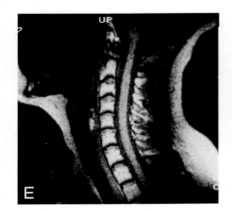
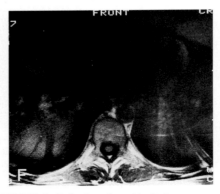
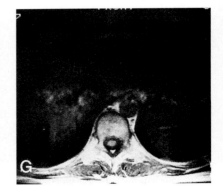

FIGURE 3–43 *See legend on opposite page*

Aliasing can also occur along the slice-selection axis in 3D volume MRI acquisitions, because of incorrectly tailored selective excitation RF pulses.[2] This artifact resembles a bizarre variation of the partial-volume averaging phenomenon (ear projecting into upper spinal canal of midsagittal cervical spine section).

EDDY CURRENTS

Eddy currents are residual, undesirable magnetic gradients that persist for a variable time after the pulse of electrical current from the gradient power supply is terminated. Eddy currents can be induced in shim coils, other gradient coils, magnet windings, cryostat shields, or RF resonant structures.[2] They can result in more rapid dephasing of the transverse magnetization, resulting in reduced spin-echo or gradient-echo amplitude (shortening the observed T2 decay).

Eddy current problems are much more noticeable in images obtained off the magnet z axis isocenter, because of generally longer time constants of the z axis gradients than the x or y axis gradients.[2] Longer TE values also bring out these effects on reducing the observed T2 decay. Residual magnetic gradients can also shift the temporal position of the spin echo from the standard TE (by introducing a spatially varying phase shift). This phase shift can become manifest in image artifact ghosts identical to motion-induced phase shift artifacts (discussed in the next section). Gradient power supply temporal instability also causes translated phase axis ghosts, similar in appearance to 60-cycle noise ghosts as well as eddy current ghosting. The key to eliminating motion as the cause of "ghosting" is to image a stationary phantom. A pattern of dark bands superimposed on the image can also result from eddy currents.[2] The spin-echo signal can be adversely affected by a stimulated echo signal that has experienced an entirely different gradient pattern. This is most noticeable in later echoes of a multiecho train and in oblique slices.

With short TE values in spin-echo studies, eddy currents from the dephasing lobe of the readout gradient can interfere with the 180° slice-selection gradient, resulting in an oblique plane of 180° nutation (despite an orthogonal plane of 90° excitation). This results in a major loss of signal from the outer edges of the image along the readout axis, similar to the intentional in-plane saturation obtained with presaturation techniques (see Motion-Related Artifacts).

Eddy Currents: Solutions

Most manufacturers commonly use eddy current compensation circuits in the gradient power supply. This approach does not work for all pulse sequences and all spatial locations within the magnet, because the spatial and temporal characteristics of the eddy currents vary from sequence to sequence.[2] Other approaches include meticulous physical adjustment of the gradient coils during initial installation. The ultimate approach is to eliminate the production of the eddy currents with the use of "mirror" gradient coils.[74] These coils have been installed on most commercial imagers and have vastly improved image quality in cinecardiac angiographic MRI.

An MRI artifact that has not been reported in the literature, to our knowledge, is one we call *telescoping*. The image of the structure under examination, generally the abdomen in a multislice stack of transaxial sections, is reduced in apparent size in all dimensions while anatomic proportion is maintained, with gradual tapering of the dimensions from the isocenter to the most peripheral section (Fig. 3–44). Gradient nonlinearity off the z axis isocenter is the cause of this artifact. Software correction algorithms (e.g., GRADWARP; General Electric Medical Systems, Milwaukee, WI) eliminate this artifact.

THIRD ARM ARTIFACT

Gradient nonlinearity at the edges of the gradient coil can cause a bright artifact to appear in images acquired at slice positions far from the isocenter (Fig. 3–45). The artifact shifts slightly in position in successive slices, unlike a standard wraparound artifact.

FIGURE 3–43. Application of presaturation techniques for reduction of motion artifact. *A,* Presaturation pulses can be introduced into any pulse sequence. In this example of a spin-echo sequence, two presaturation RF pulses (α_{F1} and α_{F2}), in conjunction with extra gradient pulses, define two thick slabs in which protons are presaturated. No signal is generated within these regions, and therefore there are no artifacts. *B,* Ghost artifacts caused by swallowing, respiration, and vascular pulsations *(top)* are reduced by applying a presaturation slab over the offending regions, using the phase-encoding gradient for slab selection *(bottom)*. *C,* With small FOVs, extraneous tissue signal can fold into the region of interest *(left)*. Two presaturation slabs, displaced along the phase-encoding axis, can be used to eliminate signal from outside the FOV and thereby eliminate the wraparound artifact *(right)*. *D,* Surface coil image of the cervical spine in a patient with multiple sclerosis. Ghost artifacts produce a low-intensity area in the spinal cord, simulating a syrinx cavity. *E,* With double presaturation slabs applied over the anterior and posterior soft tissues, ghost artifacts from swallowing and respiration are eliminated. The apparent syrinx has disappeared. *F,* Axial surface coil image of the cervical spine, obtained with swapping of the frequency- and phase-encoding gradients. Note artifactual variation in signal intensity caused by wraparound along the phase-encoding axis. *G,* Double presaturation slabs, displaced just outside the FOV, reduce wraparound and result in an improved image. (*A to G* from Edelman RR, Atkinson DJ, Silver MS: FRODO pulses: a new method for elimination of motion, flow, and wraparound artifact. Radiology 166:231–236, 1988.)

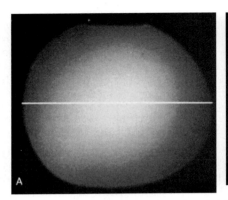
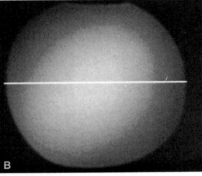
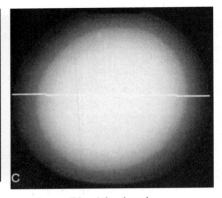

FIGURE 3–44. Telescoping. Axial scans of a 28-cm-diameter by 40-cm-long phantom from a T2-weighted study. Images *A* (150 mm inferior to the magnet's z isocenter) and *B* (150 mm superior to the magnet's isocenter) demonstrate an artifactual decrease in diameter in all dimensions caused by gradient power drop-off in the periphery. Image *C* is 10 mm superior to the isocenter of the study and shows less phantom geometric distortion.

MOTION-RELATED ARTIFACTS

MOTION ARTIFACT

Motion artifact is a common problem in MRI, particularly when the head, spine, chest, abdomen, or pelvis is imaged. Two types of artifact are encountered. Motion causes the signal from an object to spread out spatially, producing blurring. Blurring can occur along any axis. In addition to blurring, motion causes ghost artifacts (Fig. 3–46). Unlike blurring, these artifacts, which appear as alternating high- and low-intensity ghost-like images of a moving object, occur only along the phase-encoding axis. Before we discuss biologic ghosting, let us briefly review the various causes and signatures of "imager" ghosting. Before accepting the technologist's plea that motion of the patient resulted in ghost artifact, the radiologist should check the daily morning quality assurance phantom for the following:

GHOST ORIENTATION	CAUSE	EFFECT OF AVERAGING
Inverted	Stimulated echo	None
180° rotation	Quadrature phase-sensitive detector	None
Translated	Gradient digital-to-analog converter	None
Translated	60-Hz noise	Reduced
Translated	Eddy currents	Reduced
Translated	Gradient amplifier instability	Reduced

Ghost artifacts result from temporal variations in signal intensity; the usual culprits are cardiac motion, pulsatile flow of blood or cerebrospinal fluid (CSF), and respiration. The intensity of the ghost artifact increases with the amplitude of the periodic motion, because the greater the amplitude of motion, the greater the variation in signal intensity. The intensity of the ghost also increases in proportion to the signal intensity of the moving tissue. For instance, ghost artifacts resulting from pulsatile flow are worse on en-

trance sections because of the high signal intensity from unsaturated blood protons. Ghost artifacts in the abdomen arise predominantly from motion of high-intensity structures, such as subcutaneous fat on T1-weighted images or fluid-filled bowel loops and spleen on T2-weighted images. Note that nonperiodic motion, such as bowel peristalsis, generates diffuse image noise along the phase-encoding axis rather than periodic ghosts. Ghost artifact conspicuity can also be a function of the temporal relationship of the motion (e.g., a cough or sneeze or deep sigh) to the phase-encoding cycle (Fig. 3–47).

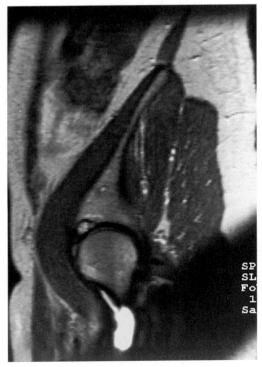

FIGURE 3–45. Third arm artifact. Sagittal turbo spin-echo T2-weighted image of the hip shows a bright artifact just inferior to the femoral head.

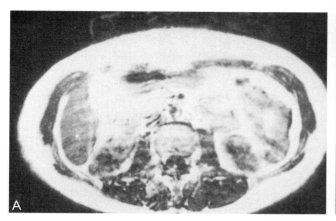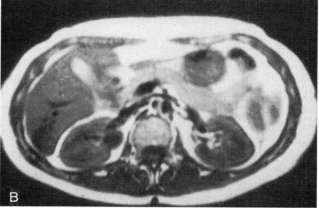

FIGURE 3–46. **Reordering of phase-encoding steps to reduce respiratory artifact.** *A,* T1-weighted axial image of the abdomen obtained with two excitations. Note respiratory ghost artifacts, arising primarily from motion of the subcutaneous fat, which cause severe image degradation. *B,* By reordering the phase-encoding steps according to the phase of the respiratory cycle (EXORCIST method), most of the artifacts can be eliminated. (Courtesy of General Electric Medical Systems, Milwaukee, WI.)

Reducing Motion Artifact

A multitude of proposed solutions and effective techniques have become available for reducing motion artifact in all facets of MRI. A number of papers have reviewed this subject.[75–79] The traditional approaches include gating, dynamic reordering of the phase-encoding gradient steps (e.g., respiratory-ordered phase encoding [ROPE], centrally ordered phase encoding [COPE], EXORCIST) (see Fig. 3–46B), varying the repetition time and number of excitations (NEX), reducing the intrinsic signal of moving tissue, physically restraining body motion, swapping phase-encoding and frequency-encoding axes, gradient refocusing, and presaturation. Techniques also exist that permit images to be acquired within a breath-holding interval[80, 81] or so rapidly that motion is essentially frozen (e.g., echo planar on a standard MR imager)[82]; these rapid

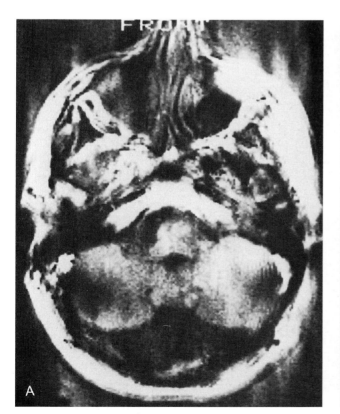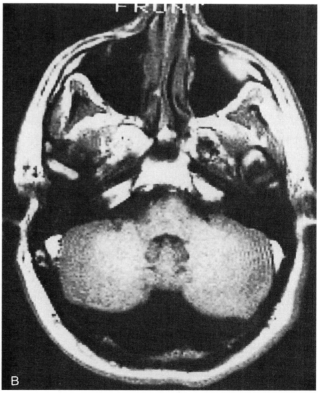

FIGURE 3–47. Images from a volunteer whose head motion was limited to the lower and zeroth order phase-encoding steps in the middle of the scan *(A)* versus motion limited to the higher order phase-encoding steps at the end of the scan *(B)*. Notice the profoundly greater motion artifacts in *A*.

imaging techniques are covered elsewhere in this book. Major advances in the reduction of motion artifact in MRI include the fast spin-echo pulse sequence, short-TE sequences (both breath-hold and breathing approaches), and postprocessing advances.

1. *Gating.* Ghost artifacts can be eliminated by ensuring that an object is in the same position and has the same signal intensity during the acquisition of each view. This can be accomplished by using physiologic gating techniques, which limit data acquisition to a specific phase of the cardiac or respiratory cycle. Respiratory gating requires measurement of chest wall expansion (e.g., with a mechanical bellows) or airflow (e.g., nasal thermistor); cardiac triggering requires electrocardiographic monitoring or measurement of the peripheral pulse (plethysmography).

An advance in the reduction of motion artifact associated with gated MRI was described by Rogers and Shapiro.[83] In conventional spin-echo imaging, impaired longitudinal recovery connected with physiologic respiration-induced heart rate alterations causes signal intensity to fluctuate and results in image replicates and spattering along the phase direction. In volunteers, respiration-induced heart rate changes created a mean 17.2% ± 4.9% fluctuation in the raw data signal, with an average frequency of 0.36 ± 0.06 Hz. Image artifacts created by heart rate changes within the imaging period are expected and may be diminished by adjusting signal intensity for each phase view before 2DFT.

Respiratory gating effectively eliminates both ghosting and blurring[84, 85] (Fig. 3–48). However, respiratory gating is inefficient. Data collected during phases of the respiratory cycle other than end-expiration must be discarded. This inefficiency typically leads to a two- to fourfold increase in acquisition time. Technical difficulties may also be encountered in obtaining consistent gating. Cardiac triggering is also inefficient, because the TR is locked to the RR interval.[86] Furthermore, cardiac triggering does not completely eliminate ghosting, because variations in signal intensity occur with beat-to-beat variations in the RR interval.

2. *Phase-reordering methods.* If the patient's respiration is monitored, the periodicity of motion responsible for ghosting can be destroyed by matching the order in which the views are acquired to the appropriate phase of the respiratory cycle.[87] These techniques are referred to as ROPE, COPE, and EXORCIST (see Fig. 3–46B). For instance, the COPE method relies on the fact that motion during phase-encoding steps of high amplitude results in lower amplitude ghosts than motion during the weaker (central) phase-encoding steps (see Fig. 3–47). In the COPE method, the phase-encoding gradient is maximized during end-inspiration (maximal displacement of diaphragm) and minimized during end-expiration (minimal displacement of diaphragm) (Fig. 3–49). Unlike respiratory gating, phase-reordering methods are efficient because data from the entire respiratory cycle are used; these techniques typically prolong acquisitions by less than 15%.

3. *Varying TR and NEX.* The distance separating ghost artifacts along the phase-encoding axis is a function of the period of the respiratory motion (TB) relative to the time between acquisition of views, given by TR × NEX. For fixed NEX, the spacing of the ghost artifacts increases with TR until

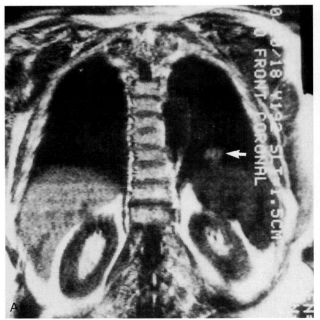
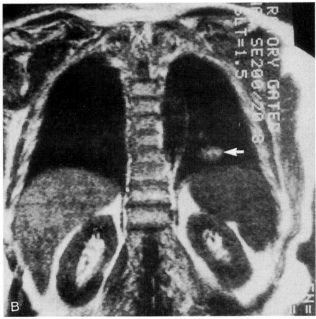

FIGURE 3–48. T1-weighted coronal images of the chest of a patient with a pulmonary hamartoma *(arrow)*. *A,* Ungated image obtained with 18 excitations demonstrates blurring of the fat-kidney boundary. Hamartoma appears contiguous with the left diaphragm. *B,* With respiratory gating and only eight excitations, kidneys and diaphragms are more sharply delineated. Mass is clearly separated from left diaphragm.

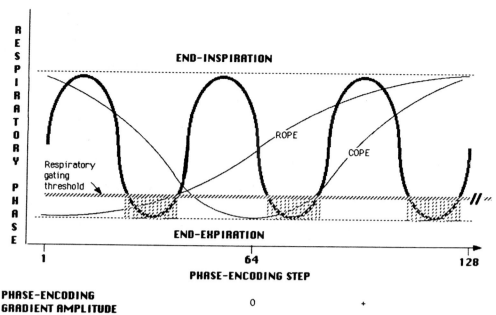

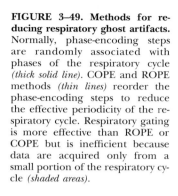

FIGURE 3–49. Methods for reducing respiratory ghost artifacts. Normally, phase-encoding steps are randomly associated with phases of the respiratory cycle *(thick solid line)*. COPE and ROPE methods *(thin lines)* reorder the phase-encoding steps to reduce the effective periodicity of the respiratory cycle. Respiratory gating is more effective than ROPE or COPE but is inefficient because data are acquired only from a small portion of the respiratory cycle *(shaded areas)*.

$$TB = 2(TR \times NEX)$$

at which point the ghost artifacts are completely displaced off the body.[88] If TB is further increased to equal TR × NEX, one is effectively gating to respiration and the ghosts disappear completely (pseudogating). However, these techniques do not permit the free selection of TR, which is needed to optimize the S/N ratio and tissue contrast.

4. *Signal averaging*. Rather than displace the ghosts, one can reduce their intensity by signal averaging. Unlike respiratory gating and phase-reordering techniques, signal averaging reduces the intensity of ghost artifacts arising from both respiration and pulsatile flow. Signal averaging does not improve motion-induced blurring. The signal intensity of ghost artifacts, like background noise, is reduced by the square root of NEX. This technique has proved particularly effective in imaging of the chest and abdomen.[89, 90] However, signal averaging causes a proportionate increase in acquisition time, rendering it impractical for T2-weighted acquisitions because of the long TR. The technique of signal averaging can be made more effective by increasing the time interval between averages.[91] This technique of so-called serial averaging (as opposed to customary parallel averaging) reduces the likelihood of acquiring multiple averages at the same point in the respiratory cycle; put another way, spreading out the averages improves the sampling of the respiratory cycle (Fig. 3–50).

5. *Reducing the signal intensity of the moving tissue that is the source of the ghost artifacts*. Still another approach to reducing the intensity of the ghosts is to reduce the intensity of the source tissue. For instance, T2-weighted images of the spine demonstrate negligible CSF pulsation artifact because of the low intensity of CSF. For imaging of the abdomen, fat signal can be selectively eliminated by the application of lipid frequency–selective RF saturation pulses or by short-tau (inversion time) inversion recovery (STIR)[92] sequences. STIR sequences have been suggested to be useful for detecting liver masses at both low fields (0.15 T) and high fields (1.5 T). STIR sequences have the drawback of a relatively low S/N ratio, but good results are now obtained with short scan times by using a STIR fast spin-echo sequence. Another drawback for abdominal imaging is that, although ghost artifacts from subcutaneous fat are suppressed, ghost artifacts from liver masses and

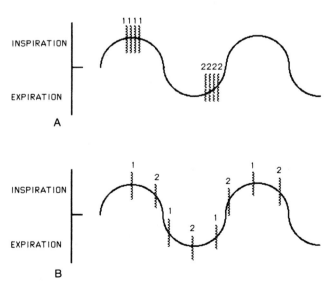

FIGURE 3–50. *A,* Signal averaging with short TR but without regard for the order of acquisitions is relatively inefficient, because the averaged measurements tend to be obtained in the same part of the respiratory cycle (parallel averaging). *B,* By increasing the interval between averaged measurements (serial averaging), a better sampling distribution of the respiratory cycle is obtained with concomitant reduction in ghost artifacts. However, the latter approach requires more data processing.

bowel loops are enhanced, because these tissues demonstrate high intensity on STIR images.

6. *Restraining body motion.* One can also reduce ghosting by splinting the motion of subcutaneous fat. Compression devices are moderately effective but are uncomfortable. In conjunction with surface coil imaging, it can be useful to position the patient so that moving tissue is dependent and restrained by the patient's weight. To restrain motion of subcutaneous fat in the near field of a surface coil, supine positioning would be preferred for imaging of the spine, whereas prone positioning would be preferred for the pancreas.

7. *Gradient reorientation.* Ghost artifacts are detrimental only if they cross a region of interest. Because ghost artifacts propagate along the direction of phase encoding, they can be reoriented away from the region of interest by rotating the phase-encoding axis (Fig. 3–51). However, new pitfalls may compound gradient swapping, as noted by Mirowitz.[93] Popliteal artery pulsatile anterior-posterior phase axis ghosts on sagittal MR images can be removed from the cruciate ligaments and their depiction improved by swapping the phase axis to superior-inferior. The new problem that Mirowitz noted is knee motion ghosting along the superior-inferior axis from the bone marrow traversing the menisci, which mimics a tear. Meniscal pseudotears associated with superior-inferior phase encoding can also be caused by truncation artifact; Turner and colleagues[94] recommended 192×256 or 256×256 acquisition matrices or an anterior-posterior phase-encoded 128×256 matrix.

Swapping the phase-encoding and frequency-encoding axes can also be useful for obtaining a better myelogram effect in the cervical and thoracic spine on T2-weighted images. Normally, the frequency-encoding gradient is oriented along the long axis of the spine, which is also the direction of CSF flow. This results in large phase shifts, associated signal loss, and ghost artifacts that obscure the spinal cord, spondylitic changes, and disk herniations. By orienting the frequency-encoding gradient perpendicular to the direction of flow, signal loss is minimized. An additional benefit of this method is that artifacts arising from motion of subcutaneous fat in the anterior neck, which is prominent with Helmholtz and solenoidal surface coils, are directed off the spine. However, rotating the motion artifacts also rotates the chemical-shift artifact, which is now parallel to the axis of the intervertebral disks. Small disk protrusions can be obscured by the chemical-shift artifact.[95]

8. *Motion compensation using gradient rephasing.* Ghost artifacts are a reflection of phase shifts resulting from motion. This motion may occur between phase-encoding views, as well as during the acquisition of each view. Gating techniques are directed toward elimination of artifacts resulting from motion between views, whereas motion compensation techniques using refocusing gradients are directed toward reducing phase shifts resulting from within-view motion.

Within-view motion results in imperfect rephasing of spins at TE, causing signal loss and ghosting artifact.

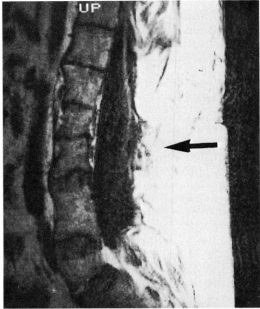

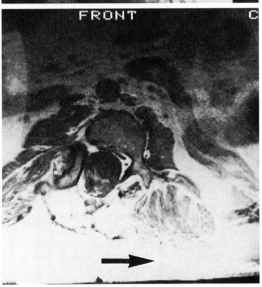

FIGURE 3–51. Reduction of motion artifact by gradient rotation (swapping). Black arrow shows the direction of the phase-encoding gradient. *Top,* Claustrophobic patient hyperventilated during study despite sedation, resulting in image degradation by ghost artifacts originating in the anterior abdomen and posterior subcutaneous fat. *Bottom,* Axial image. Frequency- and phase-encoding axes have been swapped compared with normal orientation so that motion artifacts are kept off the spine. Note the absence of artifact over the spine. With a smaller FOV, wraparound would degrade image.

Additional gradient pulses within either a spin-echo or a gradient-echo pulse sequence can be used to correct for phase shifts resulting from within-view motion, resulting in higher, more uniform signal intensity and reduced ghost artifacts.[96–102] This effect is similar to that achieved by even-echo rephasing in a multiecho sequence, except that, compared with even-echo rephasing, gradient-rephasing techniques are more consistently effective (Fig. 3–52). Gradient moment nulling is particularly important with the steady-state free

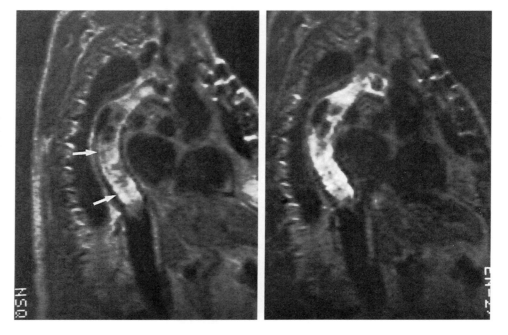

FIGURE 3–52. Even-echo rephasing in aortic dissection. Gated T2-weighted sagittal images. *Left,* First echo image. Signal intensity in the aortic lumen *(arrows)* measures 110. *Right,* Second echo image. Signal intensity measures 130, an absolute increase from the first echo. This must represent flow rather than thrombus. (Courtesy of R. Felder, MD, Desert MRI, Phoenix, AZ.)

precession pulse sequences such as PSIF, which are perhaps the most motion sensitive of all MRI sequences.[103]

Three gradient pulses can correct for constant-velocity motion, regardless of velocity. Four gradient pulses are needed to correct for acceleration, and still more are needed to correct for higher order effects such as jerk. Compensation is usually performed along all three gradient axes. However, some manufacturers have given their users the option to choose the axis of motion compensation, to keep TE at a minimum. This has proved useful in reducing motion artifact where

flow is relatively unidirectional, as in the CSF. Fast spin-echo sagittal spinal T2-weighted sequences (superior-inferior [frequency axis] motion compensation) and axial fast spin-echo spinal T2-weighted sequences (superior-inferior [slice-selection axis] motion compensation) are two common examples of use of this feature in daily scanning protocols (Fig. 3–53).

The major clinical application of motion compensation using gradient rephasing is in the elimination of signal loss and ghost artifacts caused by CSF pulsation in the spine (Fig. 3–54) and brain. It is also useful for abdominal imaging, particularly on T2-weighted

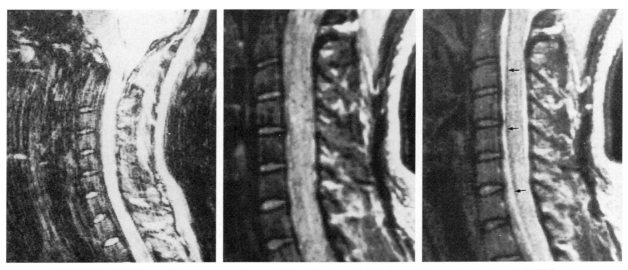

FIGURE 3–53. Effect of flow compensation on T2-weighted sagittal images of the cervical spine. *Left,* Without flow compensation, there are extensive ghost artifacts caused by CSF pulsation. *Middle,* With improperly calibrated flow compensation, the interface between CSF and spinal cord is obscured. *Right,* With properly calibrated flow compensation, CSF interfaces are sharp and ghost artifacts are mostly eliminated. The dark band along anterior surface of cord represents residual boundary layer phase dispersion. (Courtesy of M. Modic, MD, Cleveland Clinic, Cleveland, OH.)

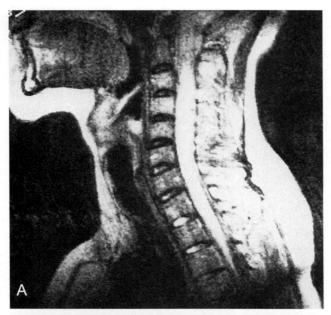

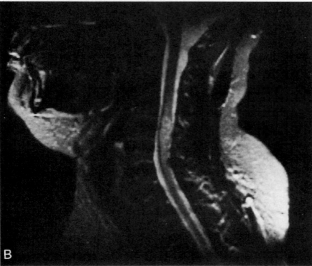

FIGURE 3–54. Sagittal T2-weighted image without ECG gating *(A)* fails to demonstrate intramedullary mass, which is well seen with ECG gating *(B)*.

images, because the latter use long TE values. Long TE values allow more within-view motion, making T2-weighted images particularly susceptible to motion artifacts. The use of gradient rephasing for motion compensation is not without drawbacks, however. Because of the stringent timing requirements for the gradient pulses, choice of TE, FOV, slice thickness, and multi-echo capability may be restricted. In addition, because the extra gradient pulses require extra time within the pulse sequence, the time available for readout of the MR signal may be reduced, necessitating the use of a stronger readout gradient. Because of the stronger readout gradient, the bandwidth is increased and the S/N ratio reduced. However, this reduction in S/N ratio may be more than adequately compensated by the reduction in motion artifact. Also, gradient rephas-

ing does not eliminate ghost artifacts produced by variable flow-related enhancement associated with saturation effects. These are more effectively suppressed by presaturation methods.

9. *Presaturation.* It is obvious that artifacts cannot arise from tissues unless they produce a signal. Methods have been developed that use presaturation to eliminate the signal over a selected region without affecting other areas (Fig. 3–55). Artifacts arising from tissues in the selected area can thereby be eliminated, without affecting tissues in the region of interest.[73, 104]

Presaturation is accomplished by use of special RF pulses inserted before the conventional pulse sequence. An example of such a pulse sequence is shown in Figure 3–43. A crafted RF pulse provides a highly rectangular slice profile even when thick slices are used. Any gradient can be used for definition of the presaturation volume in conjunction with the presaturation pulse, independent of the gradients used for the rest of the pulse sequence. As illustrated by Figure 3–43*B* and *C*, presaturation pulses can be used to eliminate two types of artifact: ghost artifact and wraparound artifact.

As demonstrated in Figure 3–43*D* and *E*, presaturation pulses can be applied along the phase-encoding axis to eliminate ghost artifacts caused by swallowing, respiration, and vascular pulsation. This is routinely useful for spine imaging. In addition, two presaturation pulses or a single cosine-modulated pulse can be used to eliminate signal from tissues outside the FOV, thus eliminating wraparound artifact along the phase-encoding axis (see Fig. 3–43*F* and *G*). In addition to these two applications, presaturation along the slice-selection direction can be used to selectively eliminate signal from inflowing spins[105] (Fig. 3–56). With this method, intraluminal flow signal and associated ghost artifacts are vastly reduced. By eliminating intraluminal flow signal, flow presaturation can help avoid confusion between flow-related enhancement and thrombus.

A tradeoff one encounters with spatial presaturation sequences is lengthening of TR and thus prolonging the scan time. Ro and Cho[106] described a new flow suppression technique, based on spin dephasing, using a set of tailored RF pulses. Their proposed method does not require additional saturation RF pulses or spoiling gradient pulses, making it advantageous over most presaturation methods that lengthen TR. In addition, the method is relatively robust to flow velocity. Their proposed technique is equivalent to the existing flow saturation technique except that the elimination of the flow component is achieved by a pair of tailored 90° and 180° RF pulses in the spin-echo sequence. The principle of the proposed method is the creation of a linear phase gradient within the slice along the slice-selection direction for the moving material by use of two opposing quadratic-phase RF pulses, that is, 90° and 180° RF pulses with opposing quadratic-phase distributions. All the spins of the moving materials along the slice-selection direction become dephased. Therefore, no observable signal is generated.

10. *Short-TE, fast sequences.* Several newer pulse sequences have been developed that reduce both ghost-

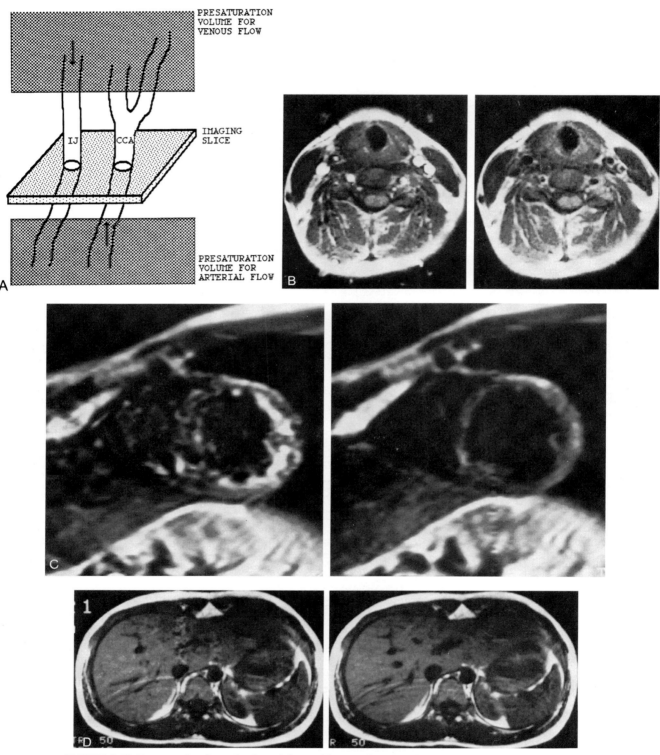

FIGURE 3–55. Presaturation for reduction of flow artifacts. *A,* Presaturation *(dark stippling)* above and below the plane of section can be used to eliminate signal from inflowing spins, illustrated for the carotid artery and jugular veins. *B,* Axial T1-weighted spin-echo image of neck. *Left,* Without presaturation, there are ghost artifacts, as well as a prominent vascular signal, which could mimic thrombus. *Right,* Presaturation eliminates the artifacts. *C,* Short-axis T2-weighted spin-echo images of heart. *Left,* Without presaturation, there is increased signal intensity adjoining the endocardium of the left ventricle, representing flow-related enhancement. This signal intensity may be mistaken for a subendocardial infarction. *Right,* Presaturation eliminates the pseudoinfarct. *D,* Axial T1-weighted images of abdomen. Ghost artifacts resulting from pulsatile flow in the inferior vena cava and aorta obscure left lobe of liver *(left).* With presaturation *(right),* ghost artifacts are eliminated.

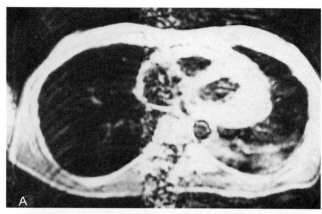
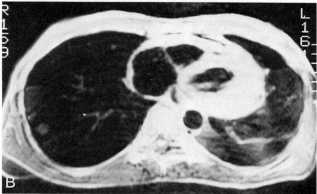

FIGURE 3–56. ECG-gated images with respiration-ordered phase encoding *(A)* without z axis RF spatial presaturation and *(B)* with z axis RF spatial presaturation. The image obtained with presaturation demonstrates a marked reduction in cardiac blood pool ghost artifact.

ing and blurring caused by motion. They all feature as a common denominator either a short TE or a short echo space time between the phase-encoding 180° RF pulses in fast spin-echo MRI. Because dephasing and therefore motion-related artifacts worsen with lengthened TE, a significant incentive is present to reduce TE, especially for MRA. Many of these allow breath-holding during "fast" (less than 25 seconds) acquisitions, without resorting to additional hardware upgrades (e.g., special gradient amplifiers).[107, 108] Snapshot MRI can produce abdominal images with 192 (or 256) × 256 resolution, negligible motion artifact, and contrast-to-noise ratios 1.29 (± 0.48) times higher than that in T1-weighted spin-echo imaging.[107]

Echo-planar MRI can be implemented on a standard MR scanner without resorting to special gradient hardware.[82] Butts and colleagues developed a multisection whole-body echo-planar imaging system. This capability was achieved by dividing the data acquisition period into eight interleaved segments rather than one or two as implemented previously with echo-planar imaging systems having high-power gradient subsystems. The interleaved echo-planar images had excellent depiction of anatomy and no identifiable respiratory artifact.

Another pulse sequence, rapid acquisition spin-echo (RASE) MRI, allows coverage of the entire liver with spin-echo images during a single 23-second breath-

holding period.[109] Images obtained with this pulse sequence were devoid of respiration-related ghost artifacts or edge blurring.

Segmented k-space acquisitions for breath-hold cine MRI have also proved extremely effective in reducing artifacts in cardiovascular studies.[110] The breath-hold studies show no ghost artifact, and cardiac edges are clearly identified because of the reduced blurring.

The rapid acquisition with relaxation enhancement imaging sequence, now more commonly known as fast spin echo, was first described by Hennig and colleagues[111] and was refined by Mulkern and coworkers.[112] Usually used for T2-weighted imaging, it has had a substantial benefit in clinical practice for motion artifact reduction in the abdomen,[113] pelvis,[114] and spine.[115] Improvements include axis-specific motion compensation gradient-rephasing options. In fast spin-echo imaging, T2 decay in short-T2 tissues (liver, muscle, lung, cartilage, tendon, atherosclerotic plaque) and motion between echoes can result in image blurring and ghost artifacts. Vinitski and colleagues[116] decreased TE in conventional spin-echo imaging to 5 ms (compared with a usual value of 12 ms) and echo spacing in fast spin-echo imaging to 6 ms (compared with a typical value of 17 ms). Short TE significantly improved the liver-spleen contrast-to-noise ratio on T1 weighted spin-echo images, reduced the intensity of ghost artifacts, increased the number of available imaging planes by 30%, improved delineation of cranial nerves, and reduced susceptibility artifacts. On short echo space, fast spin-echo images, spine, lung, upper abdomen, and musculoskeletal tissues appeared more sharply defined, and the measured spleen-liver contrast-to-noise ratio increased significantly. The depiction of tissues with short T2 (e.g., cartilage) and motion artifact suppression were also improved.

Zhou and associates[117] described a simple method for reducing ringing and blurring artifacts caused by discontinuous T2 weighting of k-space data in fast spin-echo MRI. The method demodulates the weighting function along the phase-encoding direction by using multiple T2 values derived from a set of non–phase-encoded echoes obtained with an extra excitation. Although the authors designed this sequence for MR microscopy, its use in clinical whole-body imagers should be equally efficacious.

11. Postprocessing advances. A general overview of postprocessing techniques for inter-view motion artifact correction can be found in Hedley and Yan.[118] These authors described an iterative technique for reducing artifacts resulting from motion along the slice-selection axis[119] and translational motion.[120] A contribution by Wood and coworkers[121] demonstrated a correction scheme for irregular body movements such as head nodding or body shifting. They manually measured rotational and translational displacements of each Fourier-transformed image of each k-space segment without the use of navigator echoes or external markers. Translational corrections were applied to both k-space and the spatial domain; rotational corrections were applied only to the spatial domain. This method reduced ghosts and blurring substantially in sagittal T1-weighted images of the brain of a subject who was head nodding.

Xiang and Henkelman[122] described a novel method for ghost artifact suppression in any direction, as well as other types of quasi-periodic signal modulation. The method is based on the concept of decomposition of a ghosted complex image into a ghost mask and an ideal image. The ideal image obtained (representing the time-averaged spin-density distribution) is shown to be a truer representation of physical reality than the ghost-free image obtained with ordered phase encoding. The technique is also useful in simultaneously suppressing ghosts from multifrequency signal modulations such as respiratory and cardiac motions. As reported by Hinks and coworkers,[123] "a set of . . . ghosted images . . . may be acquired in which the ghost mask is intentionally phase shifted by varying amounts relative to [the spin-density distribution] with interleaved acquisitions that have shifted phase-encoding orders or by acquiring multiple images during a single readout period in the presence of an oscillating phase-encoding gradient. . . . Simulations and experiments with the phase-encoding gradient modulation method show good general ghost suppression for a variety of quasi-periodic motion sources including both respiratory-type artifacts and flow artifacts. The primary limitation of the method is the need for rapid gradient switching."

Navigator echoes are interleaved with the imaging sequence to provide an accurate and highly detailed record of the displacements and phase shifts that are due to tissue motion during imaging. Navigator echoes are collected without phase encoding, so they represent data along a projection of the body. The area excited for the navigator echo can be restricted to a cylindrical volume using a 2D RF excitation. Navigator echoes can be used to determine the motion of the diaphragm. Depending on the phase of the respiratory cycle, data are accepted or rejected in a hurry. As with respiratory gating, the method increases scan time but eliminates ghost artifacts and blurring. Navigator echoes are often more accurate than mechanical bellows for assessing respiratory phase.

In another approach that does not increase scan time, Ehman and Felmlee[124] used navigator echoes along with a set of algorithms that can reverse the effects of object displacements and phase shifts. These algorithms essentially transfer the frame of reference of the image reconstruction from the static frame of the imager couch to the moving "visceral" frame. The technique can directly correct image degradation caused by motion. In contrast to conventional artifact reduction techniques, such as ordered phase encoding and gradient moment nulling, this newer method has a unique capacity to reduce motion unsharpness, particularly that associated with respiratory motion in thoracoabdominal imaging.

Doyle and coworkers[125] introduced an image processing method that reduces random artifacts and white noise in sets of high-resolution, time-resolved images. At each pixel, the processing consists of the isolation of a time-intensity curve, Fourier transformation of each time-intensity curve, application of a threshold to remove low-intensity coefficients, and inverse transformation to generate noise-reduced time-intensity curves. These are recombined to form images with an improved S/N ratio.

FLOW ARTIFACT

In analyzing MRA or MRI, two main flow effects are observed: phase phenomena and time-of-flight (TOF) effects. The interested reader is referred to in-depth reviews by Axel,[126] Bradley and Waluch,[127] Moran and colleagues,[128] and von Schulthess and Higgins.[129] TOF effects are due to wash-in of spins that have not undergone prior RF excitation at the Larmor resonance frequency. With flowing fully magnetized blood, hydrogen nuclei enter the imaging section and are excited by the RF pulse; they are able to produce a brighter signal than either blood that is stagnant or stationary tissue. As flowing blood within a vascular lumen may cross a succession of imaging planes in a multislice sequence, the flow-related enhancement is maximal at the initial slice proximal in the vessel, the so-called entrance slice phenomenon (Figs. 3–57 and 3–58). A saturation result occurs with increasing distance into the stack of sections, which is commensurate with flow velocity, slice thickness, and the excitation wave (con-

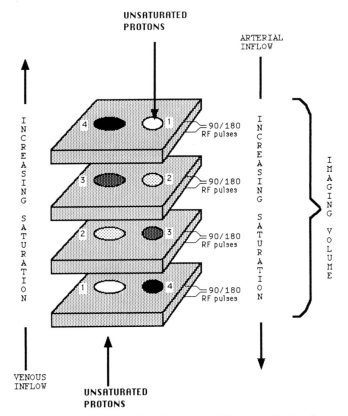

FIGURE 3–57. Entrance slice phenomenon. Unsaturated spins flowing into the entrance slice appear bright. As blood flows through the imaging volume, the likelihood increases that the spins were previously saturated by an RF pulse. As a result, vascular signal decreases within the inner slices.

current or countercurrent to flow). Flow-related enhancement is most conspicuous in short-TR single-slice gradient-echo MRI with flow perpendicular to the plane of section and when circumstances exist so that all protons in flowing blood within the plane of section are replaced between pulse repetitions. Another TOF effect is seen with washout of spins between a selective 90° RF pulse and a selective 180° RF pulse in a multislice spin-echo study. This ''high-velocity'' signal loss is nonexistent in gradient-echo imaging.

The major contribution of flow effects in standard spin-echo MRI sequences is that of spin-phase phenomena. Unlike incoherent x-ray photons or γ-emitting photons, the MR signal is basically a coherent vectorial entity, possessing both magnitude and phase properties. The phase angle is simply the arctangent I/R, where I and R represent the imaginary (y axis) and real (x axis) transverse magnetization signals received by the quadrature phase-sensitive detector. Magnitude or ''modulus'' phase-insensitive images are routinely reconstructed after the 2DFT of the raw time domain MR image data and are equal to the square root of the sum of the squares of the real and imaginary components of transverse magnetization.

Blood flowing along a magnetic gradient induces a differential phase change depending on the velocity distribution; direction of flow; presence or absence of flow compensation gradients; echo delay time, TE; gradient strength, duration, and lobe-to-lobe time separation; and character of flow (linear [constant flow], quadratic [acceleration], cubic [jerk], turbulence). Of these diverse details influencing the phase shift, the echo delay time, TE, is the most important, because the phase shift is proportional to the square of the echo delay time. Laminar flow, with its parabolic profile, produces greater flow at the median of the vessel than at the border, which creates a variance of phase angles across the lumen (Fig. 3–59). A voxel that comprises all of these protons across the lumen of the vessel contains a phase incoherence among the hydrogen protons, resulting in the flow void seen routinely in patent vessels in normal spin-echo MRI studies. Electrocardiographic (ECG) gating can reduce the intravoxel velocity distribution in arterial vessels by synchronizing acquisition with a unique temporal phase of the cardiac cycle. Thus, despite the seeming absence of direct phase information in modulus reconstruction MR images, destructive cancellation within the MR voxel of the randomly distributed transverse magnetization signal vectors from flowing blood produces the ''black blood'' spin-phase phenomenon.

In theory, if the MR voxel were infinitely small and one could image an individual nuclear spin within a single MR voxel, no intravoxel phase incoherence and

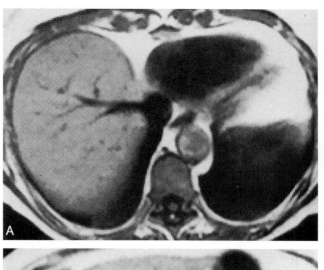

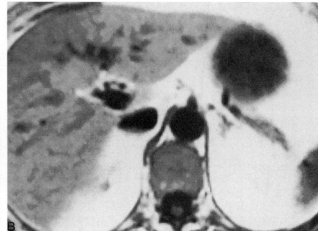

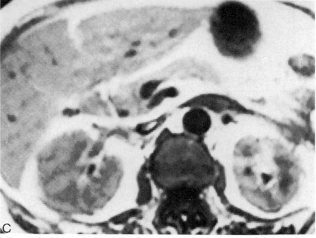

FIGURE 3–58. Axial sections from a multislice study of the abdomen. Location of the entrance slice effect depends on the direction of flow. *A,* Most cephalad sections show high signal intensity in the aorta and low signal intensity in the inferior vena cava. *B,* Center section shows low signal intensity in both aorta and inferior vena cava. *C,* Most caudal sections show high signal intensity in the inferior vena cava and low signal intensity in the aorta.

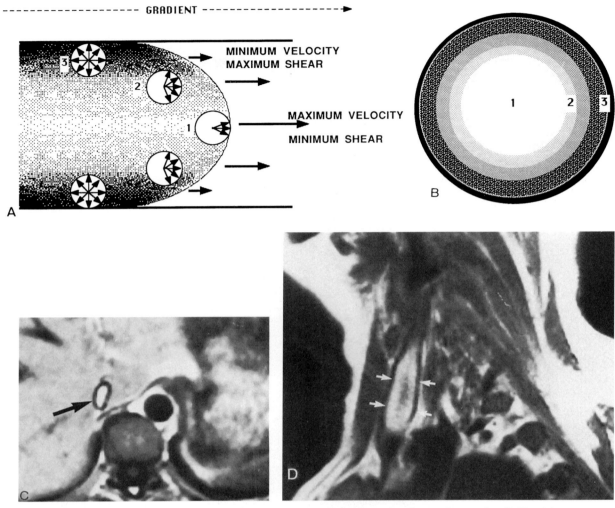

FIGURE 3–59. "Donut" sign. *A,* Shear flow is most pronounced in region 3 near the vessel wall. Signal loss caused by phase dispersion is most pronounced in this region despite slower flow. Signal intensity is greater in region 1 despite faster flow because shear is minimal. *B,* Vessel shown in cross section shows marked signal loss peripherally in region 3, with higher signal intensity centrally in regions 1 and 2. *C,* Axial image of abdomen shows central high signal intensity in the inferior vena cava with a peripheral low-intensity donut sign, representing slow flow rather than vessel wall. *D,* Thrombosis of the internal jugular vein caused by an indwelling catheter. Peripheral low intensity *(arrows),* which could mimic the donut sign in patent vessel, represents residual flow around the thrombus.

resultant signal darkening would exist in spin-echo MR images. The spin-phase phenomenon is contingent on the spatial resolution of the MR voxel and the layout of spin velocities across the voxels. Smaller voxels result in smaller phase shifts not only because of a small distribution of velocities but also because of a diminished distribution of the magnetic field values across the voxel (from stronger gradients). Oblique flow misregistration artifact[129] and flow ghosts along the phase-encoding dimension are two other important effects of flow-induced phase shifts.

Direct insight into phase information is lost with the modulus reconstruction techniques employed in more than 99% of clinical MR images generated today. Direct display of phase angle on a pixel-by-pixel basis can be performed and the arctangent I/R calculated.[130] Perturbations of the MR signal's phase angle can be produced by flowing blood, bulk tissue motion, alter-ations of magnetic susceptibility, Hahn echo–gradient echo mismatch, RF inhomogeneity, static field inhomogeneity, or residual magnetic gradients (eddy currents).

The flow of blood and CSF can generate a variety of artifacts: 1) flow can be high or low in signal intensity, depending on the balance of TOF and phase shift effects (Fig. 3–60); 2) pulsatile flow generates ghost artifacts that propagate along the phase-encoding axis; and 3) the flow signal can be displaced outside the vessel lumen along the direction of the frequency-encoding axis (Fig. 3–61). The flow signal and associated motion artifact are most prominent on images acquired with short-TE and gradient-echo images. Cardiac triggering and gradient rephasing both help to reduce flow-related ghost artifacts. Three examples of flow artifacts mimicking anatomic lesions are shown in Figures 3–62, 3–63, and 3–64.

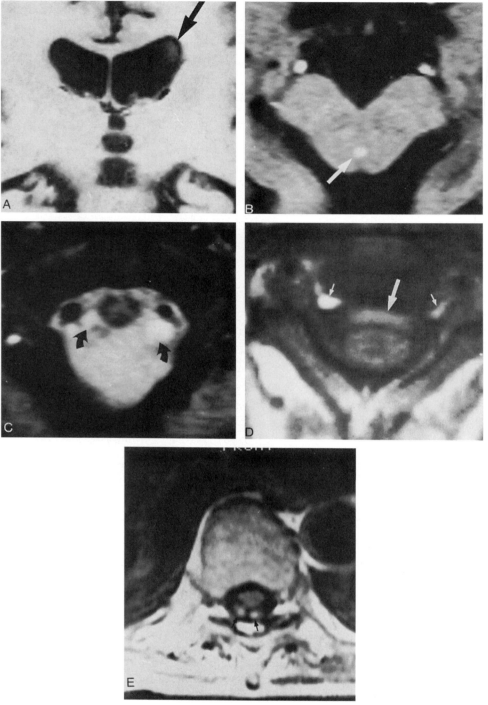

FIGURE 3–60. Flow-related enhancement caused by CSF flow is usually seen in the first and last slices from a multisection acquisition. These flow artifacts may simulate disease. *A,* Most anterior slice from coronal T1-weighted spin-echo acquisition shows bright signal *(arrow)* caused by flow, simulating mass in the anterior horn of the left lateral ventricle. *B,* Top slice from axial T1-weighted spin-echo acquisition shows bright signal *(arrow)* in the aqueduct of Sylvius. *C,* Bottom slice from axial T2-weighted head acquisition demonstrates flow-related enhancement *(arrows)* adjacent to vertebral arteries. *D,* Top slice from axial T1-weighted spin-echo acquisition shows bright signal in the anterior subarachnoid space *(large arrow),* caused by inflow of unsaturated spins. This signal could be confused with disk protrusion. Epidural veins *(small arrows)* within neural foramina also appear bright. *E,* On the bottom slice, an axial T1-weighted image of thoracic spine demonstrates paired pseudolesions posterior to the spinal cord, again representing inflow of unsaturated CSF into the slice.

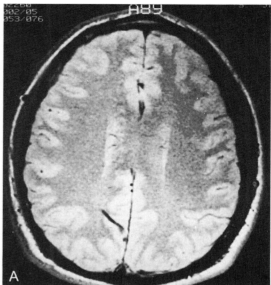

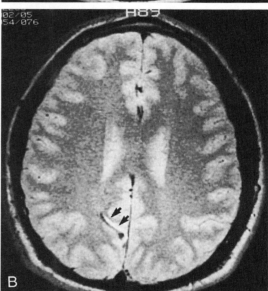

FIGURE 3–61. Flow artifacts. T2-weighted multiecho study. Image *A* (TE = 20 ms) shows a signal void in a large feeding vessel to an arteriovenous malformation. Image *B* (second echo, TE = 40 ms) demonstrates both even-echo flow rephasing high signal intensity and artifactual signal shift of obliquely flowing spins caused by phase-encoding gradient spatial misregistration.

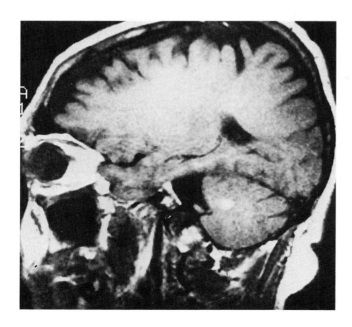

FIGURE 3–62. Left cerebellar pseudohemorrhage. Mismapping of flow signal from the lateral dural sinus along the phase-encoding axis creates a focus of spurious intracerebellar high signal intensity.

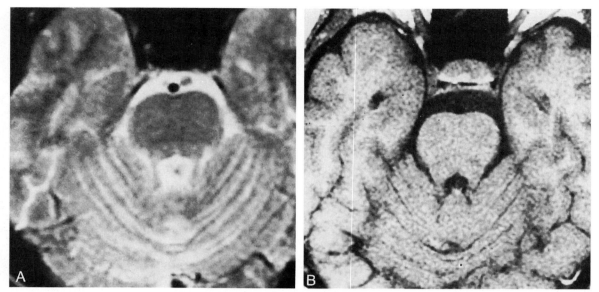

FIGURE 3–63. CSF flow artifact. T2 weighted image through the basilar cisterns with an apparent mass adjacent to the basilar artery *(A)*; the "mass" disappears on the T1-weighted image *(B)*.

OBLIQUE FLOW MISREGISTRATION

Spatial misregistration of the signal recovered from obliquely flowing spins within vascular structures is a common phenomenon in MRI, particularly of the central nervous system[131] (Figs. 3–65 and 3–66). The condition is displayed as a bright line or dot offset from the true anatomic location of the lumen of the imaged vessel. Its origin is the time delay between applications of the phase- and frequency-encoding gradients used to locate spins within the plane of section. The principal condition necessary for the production of spatial misregistration is flow oblique to the axis of the phase-encoding gradient. Flow-related enhancement (entry

slice phenomenon), even-echo rephasing, and gradient-moment nulling contribute to the production of the bright signal of spatial misregistration. Familiarity with the typical appearance of flow-dependent spatial misregistration permits confirmation of a vessel's patency; identification of the direction of flow; estimation of the velocity of flow; and differentiation of this flow artifact from atheromas, dissection, intraluminal clot, and artifacts such as chemical shift. Frank and coworkers[132] showed that for flow that has constant velocity between the start of the phase encoding and the center of the echo it is possible to eliminate these artifacts by gradient moment nulling in the phase-encoding direction (Fig. 3–67). Correction for oblique flow dis-

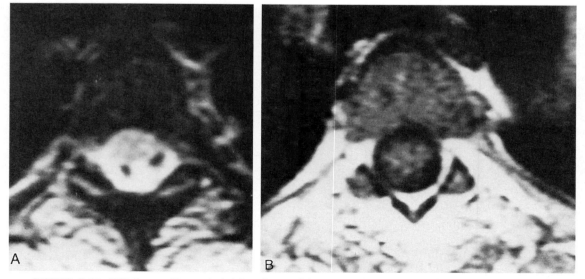

FIGURE 3–64. CSF flow artifacts. *A,* Axial surface coil image of the thoracic spine employing multislice interleaved gradient echoes (300/15/15°) shows twin filling defects initially confused with extramedullary intradural anatomic lesions. *B,* Axial T1-weighted image fails to confirm these findings; normal CT myelogram.

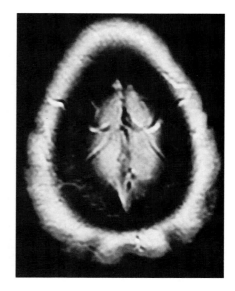

FIGURE 3–65. Flow misregistration artifact. First echo (TE = 40 ms) T2-weighted axial spin-echo brain MR image using flow compensation gradients demonstrates misregistered hyperintense signal adjacent to obliquely coursing superficial cortical draining veins.

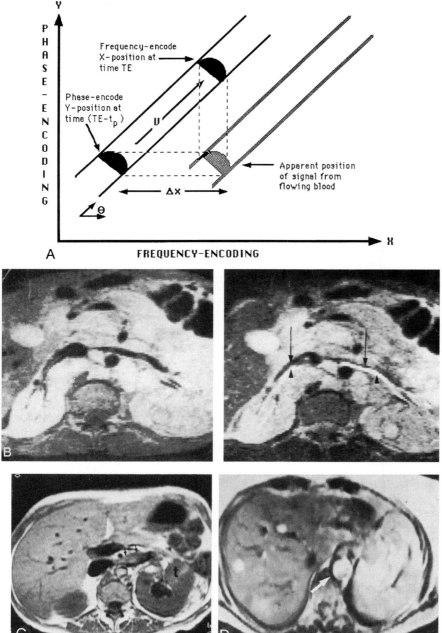

FIGURE 3–66. Flow displacement artifact. *A,* Time delay between excitation and position encoding causes signal from flowing blood to be displaced from its actual position. Because phase encoding occurs first, the apparent position of the intravascular signal *(shaded semicircle)* appears to be displaced farther along the frequency- than the phase-encoding axis. *B,* First *(left)* and second *(right)* echo images of renal veins demonstrate even-echo rephasing on the second image. Intravascular signal *(arrowheads)* appears displaced out of the vessel lumen *(arrows)* on the second image. *C,* Patient with left hypernephroma. Pattern of increased signal intensity *(arrows)* in the left renal vein mimics a flow displacement artifact but actually represents eccentric tumor thrombus with residual flow seen posteriorly in the vein. T = tumor. *D,* Axial T2-weighted image in patient with liver metastases. Chemical-shift artifact *(arrow)* may be difficult to distinguish from flow displacement artifact. (*A* to *D* from von Schulthess GK, Higgins CB: Blood flow imaging with MR: spin-phase phenomena. Radiology 57:687–695, 1985.)

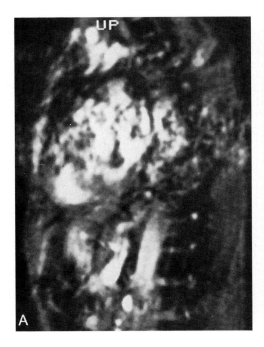
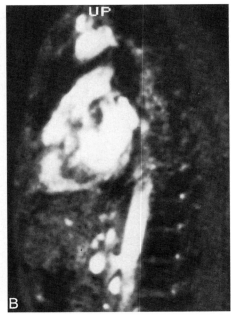

FIGURE 3–67. Sagittal gradient-echo images of chest obtained without *(A)* and with *(B)* flow compensation. Note that flow compensation increases intravascular signal intensity and reduces ghost artifact.

placement artifacts may be particularly useful in quantitative flow and angiographic applications.

ARTIFACTUAL ASYMMETRY OF INTRACRANIAL VASCULAR SIGNAL

Fujita and coworkers[133] analyzed right-to-left signal intensity differences arising from intracranial vessels during routine spin-echo axial MRI of the head. By using a normal imaging sequence in which the default directions of the frequency and phase axes were horizontal and vertical, respectively, differences in signal intensity arising from the vertebral arteries were observed in a healthy subject. With the exchange of the frequency and phase axes relative to the normal sequence, no signal intensity differences between the vertebral arteries were recognized. Other pulse sequence modifications—that is, the use of motion-compensating gradients and the reversed polarity of the frequency-encoding gradient—also resulted in variable appearances of the vertebral arteries, indicating that the right-to-left signal asymmetry of the vertebral arteries observed on the normal spin-echo image resulted from a pulse sequence–dependent phenomenon. Frequency-encoding and slice-selection gradients both produce motion-induced phase shifts. These phase shifts depend on the angle between the direction of flow and that of the effective vector sum of these gradients. The asymmetric appearance of the vertebral arteries during normal spin-echo imaging was found to result from the angle dependence of motion-induced phase shifts. Awareness of this artifactual phenomenon is important to avoid confusing it with conditions such as stenosis or occlusion, dissection, or slow flow.

FLOW ARTIFACTS IN FAST IMAGING

Phasic flow artifacts, particularly in the inferior vena cava and aorta, can degrade image quality, even with a breath-hold acquisition.[134] Fast magnetization–prepared MRI sequences allow clinical acquisitions in about 1 second but still can suffer from flow phase ghosting.[135] Recording all encodings within one cardiac cycle reduced pulsatile flow artifacts in nonsegmented acquisitions with sequential phase-encoding order, regardless of the location of magnetization preparation within the cardiac cycle. In segmented acquisitions, however, the sequential order always increased flow artifacts. To reduce the artifacts in short–inversion time acquisitions, the magnetization should be prepared during diastole.

AORTIC PSEUDODISSECTION

The clinical question of acute aortic dissection is a common and high-stakes problem faced all over the world by diagnostic imagers. Mortality related to acute ascending aortic dissection is 1% per hour in the first 48 hours, making early diagnosis essential. Detection of the intraluminal intimal flap is the sine qua non for this diagnosis. Adding to the challenge is the threat of acute cardiopulmonary arrest in this setting. There is no room for the luxury of a leisurely review of the images; the clinical setting demands a quick "yes" or "no" answer, with no time for waffling about possible intimal flap artifacts.

In a landmark German study of 110 patients comparing CT, catheter aortography, transesophageal and transthoracic echocardiography, and ECG-gated MRI, MRI proved to be the most accurate technique,

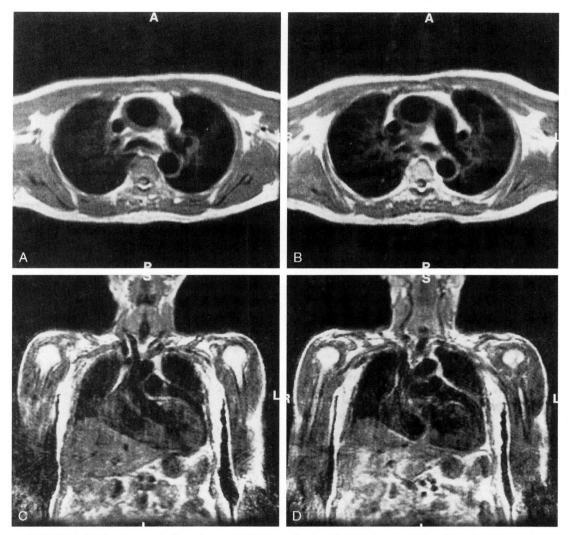

FIGURE 3–68. Aortic pseudodissection. Axial ECG-gated spin-echo MR images (TE = 20 ms) with superior-inferior spatial presaturation pulses and respiration-ordered phase encoding. *A* and *B,* Apparent ascending aortic dissection with crescentic thrombosed posterior false lumen. *C* and *D,* Coronal images with the same pulse sequence show a large pericardial effusion as the cause of this artifactual pseudodissection.

with the highest sensitivity (98.3%) and specificity (97.8%).[136] The authors' conclusion recommended transesophageal echocardiography for hemodynamically unstable patients and MRI for stable patients. Pitfalls and artifacts that mimic the intimal flap of aortic dissection occur in 64% of thoracic MRI examinations.[137] These authors classified grade 1 artifacts and pitfalls as mimics of aortic dissection on individual images, but they could be demonstrated not to represent a dissection when other images from the same sequence were evaluated. Of the 53 cases examined, 34 (64%) had artifacts or pitfalls of grade 1 or higher. An example of this pitfall is a pseudoflap appearance created by the walls of the adjacent left brachiocephalic vein and aortic arch on axial planes of section, origins of arch arteries, superior pericardial recess, motion ghost artifact in the phase-encoding direction, and aortic plaque. Grade 2 artifacts and pitfalls (19%) required the use of images from other planes or se-

quences to distinguish them from a dissection (Fig. 3–68). Motion ghosts, arch vessel origins, and superior pericardial recess all produced grade 2 artifacts. Grade 3 artifacts and pitfalls could not be distinguished from a dissection without the use of other imaging modalities (2%). Mediastinal fibrosis mimicked aortic dissection on multiple pulse sequences in the authors' study. We have been fooled by the converse as well: an acute dissection with thrombosis of the false lumen can mimic mediastinal fibrosis.

PULSE SEQUENCE–RELATED ARTIFACTS

A fourth category of MRI artifacts consists of those that are pulse sequence related; that is, they are observed only in studies utilizing specific techniques and timing of RF pulses and data acquisition. In general, these artifacts appear as nonanatomic signal voids, of-

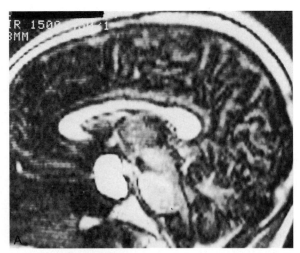

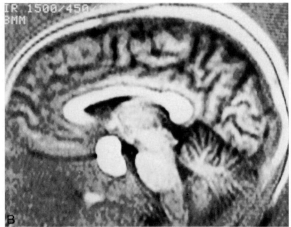

FIGURE 3–69. Inversion recovery bounce point artifact. *A,* Conventional magnitude reconstruction demonstrates an artifactual dark line highlighting gray matter–white matter boundary. *B,* Corresponding phase reconstruction demonstrates no artifact.

ten at the interface between dissimilar tissues or structures. We call this phenomenon *spurious etching* and review its various forms, causes, and solutions. The common denominator for all causes of this artifact is its presence in magnitude-reconstructed images and elimination by phase-sensitive reconstruction.

INVERSION RECOVERY BOUNCE POINT

Let us briefly review what happens in an inversion recovery sequence. The first pulse inverts all of the signals in the slice and the recovery period inversion time begins. The faster relaxing spins lead the pack and at some point pass through zero on their way to regaining the full "positive" alignment. The slowest relaxing signals are still pointing in a "negative" direction. Any two tissues with different spin-lattice relaxation times, T1, are in such a state for a period between their respective zero crossings. The readout part of the sequence is now applied.

What happens to the image? If full attention is paid to the sign of the signals, the reconstruction shows the longer T1 tissue as negative image intensity (Fig. 3–69). If, as is usually the case, the magnitude FT is displayed, then the signs are dropped and all image intensities are taken to be positive. This changes the appearance of the would-be negative tissue dramatically and always reduces the original contrast. If one were extraordinarily unlucky, the tissue contrast would vanish because the signals from two tissues of interest were of opposite sign but equal strength. In the interface between two signals that would have been opposite in sign the image intensity abruptly shoots through zero, hence the dark rim.

The inversion recovery bounce point artifact refers to an apparent loss of contrast on inversion recovery scans.[138] There is also a thin dark rim, one picture element in width, around some of the features (Fig. 3–69A). This is an artifact that can best be described as a display error. It is a result of using the magnitude of the FT output as the final image. Preserving the full phase information is often not practical. In addition, most imaging pulse sequences produce data for which the magnitude FT is always sufficient.

This artifact may simulate the lack of signal seen in calcification, air, or rapidly flowing blood. In the STIR sequence, the inversion time is chosen at the null point (inversion time = 0.63 × T1 of fat), taking advantage of the signal void for subcutaneous fat, which reduces ghost artifact from body wall motion. The bounce point artifact may be eliminated through phase-sensitive reconstruction in which image intensities constitute the entire dynamic range from negative to positive values.

FREQUENCY-SELECTIVE SUPPRESSION FAILURE ARTIFACTS

Fat suppression failure artifacts (high-signal-intensity lipid) can occur at magnetic susceptibility interfaces on frequency-selective fat suppression MRI of the head and neck[139] and abdomen (bowel air–bowel wall interface) and at the periphery of the FOV and imaging volumes. Water suppression failure artifacts are a common problem in MRI of silicone breast implants.[140]

FUNCTIONAL IMAGING

An application of the previously described navigator echo technique to correct for motion artifact was described by Hu and Kim[141] for functional MRI. Stimulus-correlated motion is a common artifact in functional MRI described by Hajnal and coworkers.[142] Motion causes subtraction artifacts that simulate brain activity; sophisticated statistical methods are required to eliminate these artifacts. Artifacts in functional MRI are considered elsewhere in greater depth (see Chapters 8 and 26).

ARTIFACTS IN MR ANGIOGRAPHY

Although the first MR angiogram was published before the gradient-echo era by Wedeen and associates,[143] the seminal development was the use of the maximal intensity projection (MIP) combined with a gradient-echo TOF flow-sensitive acquisition.[144] To provide functional information, novel MRA techniques of acquisition, information processing, and display are used, generating an entire new category of artifacts.[145] It must be emphasized that MRA acquisition techniques are inherently physiologic, and anatomic structure is indirectly presumed. Fundamentally, the two major sources of flawed flow information are the acquisition sequence and the reconstruction algorithm (typically the MIP). Tsuruda and colleagues[145] proposed that MRA artifacts can be categorized into six prevalent types: overestimation of stenosis, view-to-view variations, poor visualization of small vessels, vessel overlap, false-positives, and false-negatives. They proposed four generalized solutions for MRA artifacts: edit volume boundaries before performing MIP reconstructions, optimize acquisition parameters, refer to the individual source images, and use alternative image processing.

CAUSE AND SOLUTION FOR MR ANGIOGRAPHY STENOSIS OVERESTIMATION ARTIFACT

Despite the good correlation of MRA with intra-arterial angiography and carotid duplex ultrasonography in depicting carotid bifurcation disease,[17] a consistent overestimation of stenosis by MIP images has plagued this modality.[146, 147] Lin and coworkers[148] were the first to show the advantages of multiplanar reformations in MRA. Flow and background anatomy are depicted at oblique planes of section in an image that looks similar to the source partition. Multiplanar reformatting (MPR) of images of 3D TOF MR angiograms was done at the obliquity that shows the greatest stenosis on the MIP images, and the resulting images depicted the low-contrast flow-related enhancement seen at the margins of the carotid arteries better than standard MIP images.[149] The vessel margins are better defined with MPR images, improving the measurement of carotid stenosis. MPR of the 3D TOF MR angiograms does not lead to overestimation of carotid stenosis in the way that 2D and 3D TOF MIPs do. MPR of the 3D TOF data decreases the mean overestimation to nearly zero. The patent but highly stenotic vessel lumens that result in flow gaps on the MIP images of the 3D and 2D TOF MR angiograms are seen on the MPR images (Fig. 3–70).

The MIP algorithm results in reduced noise by decreasing the projected variance of the background compared with that in the source axial images. For the MIP to be accurate, the vessel signal intensity must be at least two standard deviations above the mean of the background signal intensity.[150] This generally leads to an increased contrast-to-noise ratio in the MIP images.[151] However, in the case of a projection through an area with minimal flow-related enhancement (as commonly occurs in the vicinity of a stenosis), the MIP algorithm can actually decrease the contrast-to-noise ratio so that the vessel is less apparent in the final MIP image than in the source axial images. This occurs because the projected mean intensity of the background increases more than that of the vessel. In regions in which flow-related enhancement is good, this difference in mean intensities is insignificant and the contrast-to-noise ratio is improved. The weighted sum average used with MPR to reformat the data leads to an improvement in contrast-to-noise ratio as a result of the averaging effect. The improvement in contrast-to-noise ratio is not dependent on background suppression by decreased variance. No change in the relative mean intensities of the vessel and background signals occurs with MPR as with the MIP algorithm. Therefore, the vessel contrast is maintained even in areas of minimal flow-related enhancement. The margins of the vessel are better preserved against the background.

MPR of the 3D TOF MR angiogram reliably shows the percentage of carotid stenosis with no statistically significant difference compared with intra-arterial angiography. MPR is a powerful and readily available solution to the problem of overestimation of extracranial carotid stenosis in MRA, especially in the display of oblique coronal or oblique sagittal views provided by transaxial source image data from body coil transmit and volume neck receive coils. Few clinical MRI sites have "neurovascular" transmit-receive head-neck coils to perform sagittal 3D TOF MRA of the carotid bifurcations and avoid inflow saturation from the aortic arch and great vessels. If sagittal acquisitions can be ob-

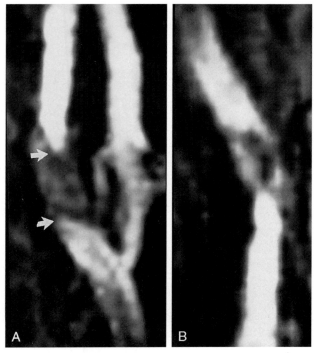

FIGURE 3–70. *A*, MIP of 3D TOF MRA shows a flow gap of 8 mm *(arrows)* in internal carotid artery. *B*, MPR MR angiogram successfully recovers signal in the highly stenotic vessel.

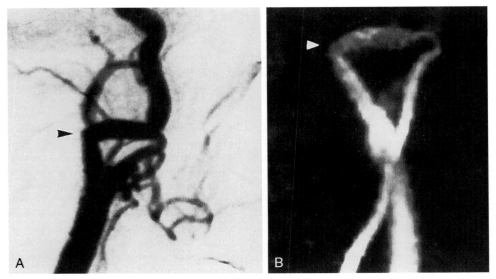

FIGURE 3–71. *A,* Lateral carotid digital subtraction angiogram shows a kink within the proximal internal carotid artery *(arrowhead). B,* 3D TOF MIP from MRA with pseudostenosis at the kink *(arrowhead).*

tained, then editing the volume boundaries by limiting the number of input sagittal partitions to those at the carotid bifurcation improves lumen definition.

As illustrated by Patel and colleagues,[152] kinks and tortuosity in the carotids can lead to overestimation of stenosis on the MIPs (Fig. 3–71) or even false-positive occlusion (Fig. 3–72). Ulcers can be missed, and "string" signs can also be hard to see even on 2D TOF sequences. We have found that the use of MPR image synthesis often overcomes these problems. It is well accepted that sole reliance on conventional 3D TOF MRA for the carotid bifurcation eventually leads to a mistaken diagnosis of internal carotid artery occlusion, when in fact a string sign is found on 2D TOF and x-ray angiography (Fig. 3–73). Disordered flow can also simulate stenotic disease (Fig. 3–74).

VIEW-TO-VIEW VARIATIONS IN MR ANGIOGRAPHY: CAUSE AND SOLUTION

Sometimes a set of MIPs from an MRA data set shows discrepant depiction of a vessel in different projections (e.g., visible vessel on anterior-posterior projection, invisible on lateral projection). The cause of this artifact is the variation of the background signal intensity in the source images. Solutions are directed at homogenizing the background signal intensity with appro-

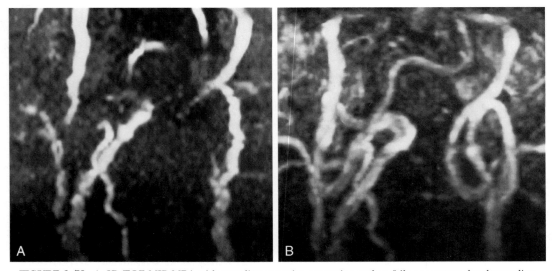

FIGURE 3–72. *A,* 2D TOF MIP MRA with traveling superior saturation pulses fails to portray the descending course of the looping cervical internal carotid artery on the right and left sides. *B,* 3D TOF MIP MRA with a superior saturation pulse above the slab faithfully depicts the normal luminal caliber of the descending course of cervical internal carotid artery on both the left and right sides.

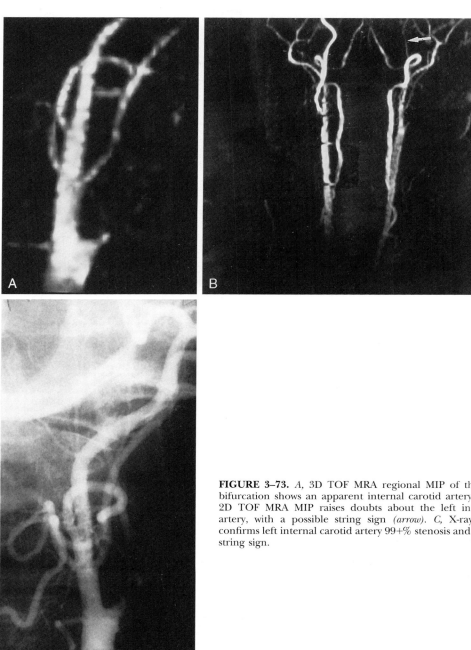

FIGURE 3–73. *A*, 3D TOF MRA regional MIP of the left carotid bifurcation shows an apparent internal carotid artery occlusion. *B*, 2D TOF MRA MIP raises doubts about the left internal carotid artery, with a possible string sign *(arrow)*. *C*, X-ray angiography confirms left internal carotid artery 99+% stenosis and a poststenotic string sign.

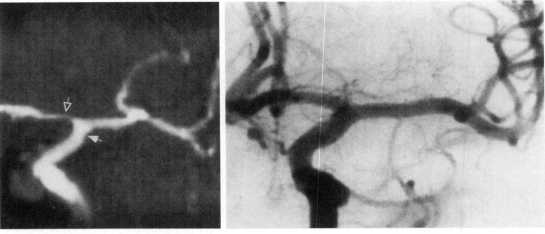

FIGURE 3–74. *A,* 3D TOF MRA MIP shows apparent stenosis of the supraclinoid internal carotid artery and proximal anterior cerebral artery caused by disordered flow *(arrows). B,* X-ray angiogram shows a normal appearance. (*A* and *B* from Tsuruda J, Saloner D, Norman D: Artifacts associated with MR neuroangiography. AJNR 13[5]:1411–1422, 1992, © by American Society of Neuroradiology.)

priate pulse sequences (e.g., avoiding rectangular FOV cutoff of background signal).

POOR VISUALIZATION OF SMALL VESSELS IN MR ANGIOGRAPHY: CAUSE AND SOLUTION

Because the vessel signal intensity must be at least two standard deviations above the background signal intensity for reliable visualization of vessels,[150] factors that reduce small vessel signal intensity, such as slow flow saturation, poor background suppression, large background volume, and partial-volume averaging, result in small vessel MIP nonvisualization. Inspection of the original slice-partition data is essential (Fig. 3–75). For slow-flow states such as cardiomyopathy, dolichoec-

tasia, giant aneurysms, or arteriovenous malformations, or downstream from a stenosis, TOF MRA acquisitions should be focused on 2D TOF sequences, which are less sensitive to slow flow saturation than their 3D TOF counterparts. Phase-contrast sequences[153] may not suffer as much from saturation effects as TOF sequences but probably do not match the sensitivity of 2D TOF for the depiction of slow-flow states (<5 cm/ s) when standard gradient power supplies are employed.

Poor background suppression in TOF MRA can be improved by using magnetization transfer pulses or volume editing before the MIP, editing out high-signal-intensity areas such as those representing fat, methemoglobin, inspissated paranasal sinus mucus, posterior pituitary bright spot, or gadolinium. Because of the

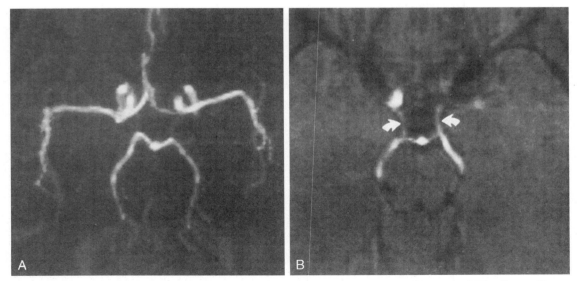

FIGURE 3–75. Small vessels such as the posterior communicators, often not visible on the MIP collapse *(A),* are seen easily in the source axial partition *(arrows) (B).* Notice the higher background signal intensity in the MIP compared with the source axial partition.

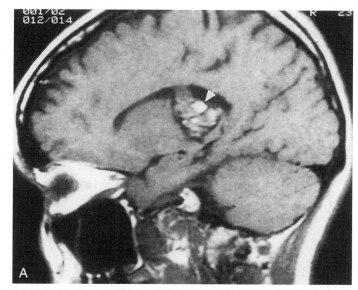

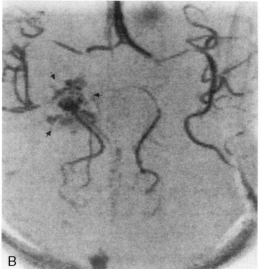

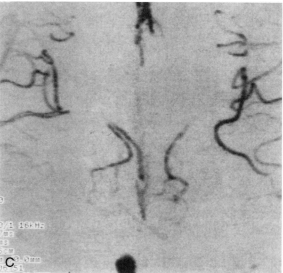

FIGURE 3–76. *A,* T1-weighted image shows hyperintense extravascular methemoglobin *(arrow). B,* False-positive MIP depiction of flow on 3D TOF MRA caused by extravascular methemoglobin *(arrows). C,* 3D phase-contrast MIP showing no flow because of lack of phase shift in the region of methemoglobin.

paramagnetic effect of methemoglobin, blood within a stationary hematoma may appear as an area of active flow with these postprocessing techniques. The methemoglobin problem is not an issue with phase-contrast techniques (Fig. 3–76). Background suppression and depiction of small vessels can also be improved in TOF MRA by the use of off-resonance magnetization transfer RF preparation pulses.[154] Spin saturation effects in 3D TOF MRA can be reduced by using RF pulses with linearly increasing flip angles (ramp pulses) in the main direction of flow.[155]

Large background volumes increase the statistical likelihood that a background voxel will have a higher signal intensity than a vessel voxel. If the ray-tracing algorithm passes through both voxels, the vessel is lost in the MIP ("MIPped out"). One solution to this problem is to use volume editing not only in the in-plane dimensions but also along the slice-selection axis before performing the MIP. Partial-volume averaging effects in reducing small vessel conspicuity can be ad-

dressed only by reducing voxel size. This carries with it the associated tradeoff of loss of contrast-to-noise ratio for a given scan time.

VESSEL OVERLAP: CAUSE AND SOLUTION

The MIP does not portray vessel overlap in the traditional "summation density" fashion of projective contrast x-ray angiography. The intensity of a projected voxel in an MIP intersected by two overlapping vessels is not different from the voxel intensity in either vessel proximal or distal to the intersection. This is in contradistinction to the summation density phenomena of projective x-ray angiography, in which overlapping vessels project a higher density than the voxel intensity in either vessel proximal or distal to the intersection.[156]

Pulsatile flow generates artifacts in 2D and 3D MRA acquisitions. Time variations in the MR signal during the heart cycle lead to more complex patterns of artifacts in 3D imaging than in 2D imaging.[157] The appearance and location of these artifacts within the image volume are describable as displacements along a line in a plane parallel to that defined by the phase- and volume-encoding directions. The angle of the line in the plane depends solely on the imaging parameters, whereas the ghost displacement along the line is proportional to the signal modulation frequency. Aliasing of these ghosts leads to a variety of artifact patterns that are sensitive to the pulsation period and TR of the pulse sequence.

Korin and coworkers[158] proposed a centric method of reordering phase and slab encoding that can be used to address some of the inherent problems related to motion in 3D imaging. The method was shown to be more robust than conventional 3D slab and phase encoding with respect to reducing artifacts resulting from several fundamental types of motion. It can be readily implemented on a standard MR scanner with essentially no increase in total imaging time.

MULTIPLE OVERLAPPING THIN-SLAB ACQUISITION: VENETIAN BLIND ARTIFACT

Multiple overlapping 3D TOF carotid MRA potentially combines many of the desirable features of 2D and single-volume 3D MRA techniques. Blatter and colleagues[159] described a modified multiple overlapping thin-slab acquisition (MOTSA) technique that did not lead to overestimation of carotid bifurcation stenosis. However, the MIP images from such acquisitions are often degraded by artifacts caused by nonuniform signal intensity of contiguous imaging volumes. This has been termed the venetian blind artifact.[160] The severity of the artifact has been minimized by the use of thin slabs with a large percentage of overlap. The combined use of spatially variable excitation pulses and an automatic postprocessing technique can improve the uniformity of the signal from blood across the slab and allow thicker slabs to be acquired with less overlap. However, with a different commercial implementation of multiple overlapping thin-slab acquisition and ramped pulses, we see the venetian blind artifact actually increase (Fig. 3–77) with the use of ramped pulses.

MOTION ARTIFACT REDUCTION IN CINE PHASE-CONTRAST IMAGING

2D cine phase-contrast MRA acquires projections through the entire thickness of the subject, permitting excitation geometries to be independent of image orientation. Early experience with cine phase-contrast MRA with the bipolar flow-encoding gradient pulse application split in two successive cardiac cycles found chest and abdominal breathing and gastrointestinal peristalsis motion artifacts particularly problems. Dumoulin and associates[161] described a new technique in which they employed minimal delays within the same

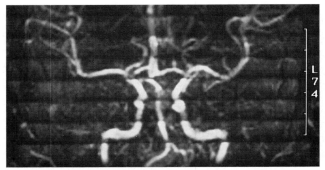

FIGURE 3–77. Conspicuous venetian blind artifact in 3D TOF MIP, obtained with multiple overlapping thin-slice requisition and a 1995 commercial imager, despite use of ramped inferior-to-superior RF tip angles and magnetization transfer. Eight 16-partition (1-mm-thick) slabs with 2-mm interslab overlap (56/6.9/20°).

cardiac cycle between the acquisition of oppositely flow-encoded data, resulting in fewer artifacts caused by movement of nominally stationary tissue for aortic arch and iliac MRA.

METAL CLIPS, MR ANGIOGRAPHY, AND THE MAXIMAL INTENSITY PROJECTION: A GIANT POTENTIAL PITFALL

Although metallic clips from prior surgery are generally recognized with ease on the individual source images from any MRA data set and any MRA pulse sequence, total reliance on the MIPs and collapse for a diagnosis could prove disastrous, leading to a carotid endarterectomy for a normal internal carotid artery, for instance. The bizarre signal voids resulting from metal clips are lost in the MIP process, with the clip looking like an ordinary stenosis or occlusion.[162] Metal clip recognition is less of a problem if MPR is performed.[163] Of course, metal clips often render an MRA interpretation regionally nondiagnostic; it is much better to say "I don't know" than to "drop the blade" on a noncritical or nonexistent lesion. We have taken great precautions to guard against this potential catastrophe at the extracranial carotid bifurcation, including careful screening of patients, liberal use of correlative radiographs, filming of all source images, and insistence on a corroborative duplex examination if endarterectomy is to be performed without catheter angiography.

MAXIMAL INTENSITY PROJECTION SATURATION BANDING

The impact of the normal triphasic arterial waveform of the peripheral arterial circulation on 2D TOF MRA MIP images of the lower extremity was first discovered by Caputo and coworkers.[164] In MIP images of normal volunteers, they noticed an artifact of horizontal "banding" throughout the course of a lower extremity artery, whose existence was dependent on the traveling RF presaturation gap distance along the z axis. With a large gap (20 mm), spins would return relatively "fresh" through the "back door" of the slice during the early diastolic flow reversal phase of the arterial waveform, without banding. With a presaturation gap distance of 5 mm, the returning spins would be hit hard by the traveling spatial presaturation RF pulse, bringing "dark" blood back into the slice and resulting in low-intensity horizontal stripes in the MIP projection. A drawback of a large presaturation gap distance in lower extremity 2D TOF MR arteriograms is the appearance of venous structures.

CHEMICAL-SHIFT ETCHING

Work in proton spectroscopic imaging by Dixon[165] has led to clinically useful MR images of separate water- and fat-containing tissues. The opposed, or out-of-phase, images are obtained with the magnetization vectors of fat and water, which precess at different frequencies because of chemical-shift differences of 3 to 4 ppm, pointing in opposite directions. The net transverse magnetization in such an experiment therefore represents water minus fat magnetization, resulting in a minimal signal intensity. If a given voxel contains similar proportions of fat and water protons, the out-of-phase image registers a signal void in the corresponding pixel. This technique contrasts with the standard Hahn spin-echo experiment, in which the echo is obtained at the point at which water and fat spins are aligned to produce maximal signal intensity. Clinically, the opposed-phase artifact may be seen at any boundary where the voxels at the interface contain both fat and water. This artifact differs from readout axis chemical-shift artifact by the absence of any orientation along the readout axis. Swapping the phase and frequency axes has no effect on chemical-shift–induced spurious etching.

A similar out-of-phase image may be obtained with gradient echoes. The timing of the TE determines whether the fat and water protons in a voxel of interest are in or out of phase, yielding maximal or minimal spurious etching.[166]

MOTION INTERFACE ETCHING

Spurious etching can also occur at the interface between moving and nonmoving tissues. At the boundary, a spectrum of velocities (and phase angles) can be produced in a single voxel. The distribution of phase angles leads to signal loss in magnitude-reconstructed images. This produces an artifactually "thicker" pericardium in gated cardiac images, as first pointed out by Moran and Moran.[167] This artifact can be reduced by using higher in-plane spatial resolution (e.g., 256 phase-encoding steps instead of 128). The presence or absence of the pericardial etching artifact can be used to clinical advantage in assessing the degree of malignant invasion of the pericardium by adjacent cancers.

CONCLUSION

The most important new artifacts to be recognized, in terms of potential grave consequences to the patient (unnecessary surgical or medical treatment for normal anatomy), are metal clip signal void MIP MRA simulation of vascular stenosis or occlusion and magic angle effects on tendinous and meniscal structures, simulating degeneration or tear. MRI artifacts are commonly seen at all clinical imaging sites, and the more frequently encountered ones should be recognized by practitioners so as to avoid diagnostic errors and to maintain image quality. Some artifacts, such as aliasing and motion artifacts, are predictable and can be manipulated to reduce their degradation of the image in the anatomic region of interest. Others, such as RF pulse inhomogeneity and gradient-induced eddy current artifacts, are more sporadic and difficult to diagnose, and correcting them requires field service engineers. The clinical impact of MRI artifacts is minimized by routine preventive maintenance, daily quality control checks, and heightened awareness on the part of the radiologist.

REFERENCES

1. Bellon EM, Haacke EM, Coleman PE, et al: MR artifacts: a review. AJR 147:1271–1281, 1986.
2. Henkelman RM, Bronskill MJ: Artifacts in magnetic resonance imaging. Rev Magn Reson 2:1–126, 1987.
3. Porter BA, Hastrup W, Richardson ML, et al: Classification and investigation of artifacts in magnetic resonance imaging. Radiographics 7:271–287, 1987.
4. Foo TK, Hayes CE: Phase-correction method for reduction of B_0 instability artifacts. J Magn Reson Imaging 3:676–681, 1993.
5. Partain L, James EE, Rollo P: Nuclear Magnetic Resonance Imaging. Philadelphia: WB Saunders, 1983.
6. Mirvis SE, Geisler F, Joslyn JN, Zrebeet H: Use of titanium wire in cervical spine fixation as a means to reduce MR artifacts. AJNR 9:1229–1231, 1988.
7. New PFJ, Rosen BR, Brady TJ, et al: Potential hazards and artifacts of ferromagnetic and non-ferromagnetic surgical and dental materials and devices in nuclear magnetic resonance imaging. Radiology 147:139–148, 1983.
8. Heindel W, Friedmann G, Bunke J, et al: Artifacts in MRI after surgical intervention. J Comput Assist Tomogr 10:596–599, 1986.
9. Peterman SB, Hoffman JC Jr, Malko JA: Magnetic resonance artifact in the postoperative cervical spine. A potential pitfall. Spine 16:721–725, 1991.
10. Levitt M, Benjamin V, Kricheff II: Potential misinterpretation of cervical spondylosis with cord compression caused by metallic artifacts in magnetic resonance imaging of the postoperative spine. Neurosurgery 27:126–129, 1990.
11. Farahani K, Sinha U, Sinha S, et al: Effect of field strength on susceptibility artifacts in magnetic resonance imaging. Comput Med Imaging Graph 14:409–413, 1990.
12. Vaccaro AR, Chesnut RM, Scuderi G, et al: Metallic spinal artifacts in magnetic resonance imaging. Spine 19:1237–1242, 1994.
13. Haramati N, Penrod B, Staron RB, Barax CN: Surgical sutures: MR artifacts and sequence dependence. J Magn Reson Imaging 4:209–211, 1994.
14. Teitelbaum GP, Bradley WG, Klein BD: MR imaging artifacts, ferromagnetism, and magnetic torque of intravascular filters, stents, and coils. Radiology 166:657–664, 1988.
15. Hinshaw DB, Holshouser BA, Engstrom HIM, et al: Dental material artifacts on MR images. Radiology 166:777–779, 1988.
16. Kuta JA, Smoker WRK, Cole TJ, Beskin RR: MR angiography artifact due to metal joint of ventriculoperitoneal shunt mimicking severe carotid stenosis. J Magn Reson Imaging 5:125–126, 1995.
17. Wesbey GE, Bergan JJ, Moreland SI, et al: Cerebrovascular magnetic resonance angiography: a critical verification. J Vasc Surg 16:619–628, 1992.
18. Camacho CR, Plewes DB, Henkelman RM: Nonsusceptibility artifacts due to metallic objects in MR imaging. J Magn Reson Imaging 5:75–78, 1995.

19. Buchli R, Boesiger P, Meier D: Heating effects of metallic implants by MRI examination. Magn Reson Med 7:255–261, 1988.

20. Kim JK, Kucharczyk W, Henkelman RM: Cavernous hemangiomas: dipolar susceptibility artifacts at MR imaging. Radiology 187:735–741, 1993.

21. Girard MJ, Hahn PF, Saini S, et al: Wallstent metallic biliary endoprosthesis: MR imaging characteristics. Radiology 184:874–876, 1992.

22. Czervionke LF, Daniels DL, Wehrli FW, et al: Magnetic susceptibility artifacts in gradient-recalled echo MR imaging. AJNR 9:1149–1155, 1988.

23. Sakurai K, Fujita N, Harada K, et al: Magnetic susceptibility artifact in spin-echo MR imaging of the pituitary gland. AJNR 13:1301–1308, 1992.

24. Elster AD: Sellar susceptibility artifacts: theory and implications. AJNR 14:129–136, 1993.

25. Tien RD, Buxton RB, Schwaighofer BW, Chu PK: Quantitation of structural distortion of the cervical neural foramina in gradient-echo MR imaging. J Magn Reson Imaging 1:683–687, 1991.

26. Tsuruda JS, Remley K: Effects of magnetic susceptibility artifacts and motion in evaluating the cervical neural foramina on 3DFT gradient echo MR imaging. AJNR 12:237–241, 1991.

27. Tsuruda JS, Norman D, Dillon W, et al: Three-dimensional gradient-recalled MR imaging as a screening tool for the diagnosis of cervical radiculopathy. AJR 154:375–383, 1990.

28. Ludeke KM, Roschmann A, Tischler R: Susceptibility artifacts in NMR imaging. Magn Reson Imaging 3:329–343, 1985.

29. Bach-Gansmo T, Ericsson A, Leander P, et al: Motion associated susceptibility artifacts. Acta Radiol 33:606–610, 1992.

30. Mattrey RF, Trambert MA, Brown JJ, et al: Perflubron as an oral contrast agent for MR imaging: results of a phase III clinical trial. Radiology 191:841–848, 1994.

31. Tartaglino LM, Flanders AE, Vinitski S, Friedman DP: Metallic artifacts on MR images of the postoperative spine: reduction with fast spin-echo techniques. Radiology 190:565–569, 1994.

32. Young IR, Cox IJ, Bryant DJ, Bydder GM: The benefits of increasing spatial resolution as a means of reducing artifacts due to field inhomogeneities. Magn Reson Imaging 6:585–590, 1988.

33. Erickson SJ, Cox IH, Hyde JS, et al: Effect of tendon orientation on MR imaging signal intensity: a manifestation of the ''magic angle'' phenomenon. Radiology 181:389–392, 1991.

34. Peterfy CG, Janzen DL, Tirman PF, et al: ''Magic-angle'' phenomenon: a cause of increased signal in the normal lateral meniscus on short-TE MR images of the knee. AJR 163:149–154, 1994.

35. Axel L, Costantini J, Listerud J: Intensity correction in surface-coil MR imaging. AJR 148:418–420, 1987.

36. McCauley TR, McCarthy S, Lange R: Pelvic phased array coil: image quality assessment for spin-echo MR imaging. Magn Reson Imaging 10:513–522, 1992.

37. Glover GH, Hayes CE, Pelc NJ, et al: Comparison of linear and circular polarization for magnetic resonance imaging. J Magn Reson 64:255–270, 1985.

38. Conolly S, Nishimura D, Macovski A: Optimal control solutions to the magnetic resonance selective excitation problem. IEEE Trans Med Imaging 5:106–115, 1986.

39. White EM, Edelman RR, Stark DD, et al: Surface coil MR imaging of abdominal viscera: Part II. The adrenal glands. Radiology 157:431–436, 1985.

40. Feinberg DA, Hoenninger JC, Crooks LE, et al: Inner volume MR imaging: technical concepts and their application. Radiology 156:743–747, 1985.

41. Bodenhausen G, Freeman R, Turner D: Suppression of artifacts in 2D J-spectroscopy. J Magn Reson 27:511–514, 1977.

42. Kramer DM, Murdoch JB: Artifact minimization in multislice multiecho MR imaging. In: Society of Magnetic Resonance in Medicine, Fifth Annual Meeting, 1986, pp 1436–1437. Abstract.

43. Graumann R, Oppelt A, Stetter E: Multiple spin-echo imaging with a 2-D method. Magn Reson Med 3:707–721, 1986.

44. Tycko R, Cho HM, Schneider E, Pines A: Composite pulses without phase distortion. J Magn Reson 6:90–101, 1985.

45. Yan H, Gore JC: Improved selective 180 degree radiofrequency pulses for magnetization inversion and phase reversal. J Magn Reson 71:116–131, 1987.

46. Murdoch JB, Lent AH, Kritzer MR: Computer-optimized narrowband pulses for multislice imaging: asymmetric amplitude-modulated 180 degree pulses. In: Society of Magnetic Resonance in Medicine, Fifth Annual Meeting, 1986, pp 1432–1433. Abstract.

47. O'Donnell M, Adams WJ: Selective time-reversal pulses for MR imaging. Magn Reson Imaging 3:377–382, 1985.

48. Lurie DJ: A systematic design procedure for selective pulses in NMR imaging. Magn Reson Imaging 3:235–243, 1985.

49. Silver MS, Joseph RI, Hoult DI: Highly selective 90 and 180 degree pulse generation. J Magn Reson 59:347–351, 1984.

50. Duijn JH, Creyghton JHN, Smidt J: Suppression of artifacts due to imperfect pi pulses in multiple echo Fourier imaging. In: Society of Magnetic Resonance in Medicine, Third Annual Meeting, 1984, pp 197–198. Abstract.

51. Crawley AP, Henkelman RM: A stimulated echo artifact from slice interference in magnetic resonance imaging. Med Phys 14:842–848, 1987.

52. Wood ML, Runge VM: Artifacts due to residual magnetization in three-dimensional magnetic resonance imaging. Med Phys 15:825–831, 1988.

53. Curtin AJ, Chakeres DW, Bulas R, et al: MR imaging artifacts of the axial internal anatomy of the cervical spinal cord. AJR 152:835–842, 1989.

54. Jack CR Jr, Gehring DG, Ehman RL, Felmlee JP: Cerebrospinal fluid-iophendylate contrast on gradient-echo MR images. Radiology 169:561–563, 1988.

55. Czervionke LF, Czervionke JM, Daniels DL, Haughton VM: Characteristic features of MR truncation artifacts. AJR 151:1219–1228, 1988.

56. Bronskill MJ, McVeigh ER, Kucharczyk W, Henkelman RM: Syrinx-like artifacts on MR images of the spinal cord. Radiology 166:485–488, 1988.

57. Hashimoto M, Shingyouchi H, Seino Y, et al: Syrinx-like artifact on MR images of the spinal cord. Rinsho Hoshasen 34:697–701, 1989.

58. Levy LM, Di Chiro G, Brooks RA, et al: Spinal cord artifacts from truncation errors during MR imaging. Radiology 166:479–483, 1988.

59. Breger RK, Czervionke LF, Kass EG, et al: Truncation artifact in MR images of the intervertebral disk. AJNR 9:825–828, 1988.

60. Haacke EM: The effects of finite sampling in magnetic resonance imaging. Magn Reson Med 4:407–421, 1987.

61. Hu XP, Johnson V, Wong WH, Chen CT: Bayesian image processing in magnetic resonance imaging. Magn Reson Imaging 9:611–620, 1991.

62. Harris FJ: On the use of windows for harmonic analysis with the discrete Fourier transform. Proc IEEE 66:51–83, 1978.

63. Amartur S, Haacke EM: Modified iterative model based on data extrapolation method to reduce Gibbs ringing. J Magn Reson Imaging 1:307–317, 1991.

64. Constable RT, Henkelman RM: Data extrapolation for truncation artifact removal. Magn Reson Med 17:108–118, 1991.

65. Soila KP, Viamonte M, Starewicz PM: Chemical shift misregistration effect in MRI. Radiology 153:819–820, 1984.

66. Smith RC, Lange RC, McCarthy SM: Chemical shift artifact: dependence on shape and orientation of the lipid-water interface. Radiology 181:225–229, 1991.

67. Wachsberg RH, Mitchell DG, Rifkin MD, et al: Chemical shift artifact along the section-select axis. J Magn Reson Imaging 2:589–591, 1992.

68. Lufkin R, Anselmo M, Crues J, et al: Magnetic field strength dependence of chemical shift artifacts. Comput Med Imaging Graph 12:89–96, 1988.

69. Vinitski S, Mitchell DG, Rifkin MD, Burk DL Jr: Improvement in signal-to-noise ratio and reduction of chemical shift and motion-induced artifacts by summation of gradient and spin echo data acquisition. J Comput Assist Tomogr 13:1041–1047, 1989.

70. Pusey E, Yoon C, Anselmo ML, Lufkin RB: Aliasing artifacts in MR imaging. Comput Med Imaging Graph 12:219–224, 1988.

71. Kurihara N, Kamo O, Umeda M, et al: Applications in one dimensional and two dimensional NMR of a pseudofilter by jittered time averaging. J Magn Reson 65:405–416, 1985.

72. Axel L, Dougherty L: Reduction of aliasing in 2-D FT MRI by pseudofiltering. Magn Reson Imaging 5:63, 1987. Abstract.

73. Felmlee JP, Ehman RL: Spatial presaturation: a method for suppressing flow artifacts and improving depiction of vascular anatomy in MR imaging. Radiology 164:559–564, 1987.

74. Roemer PB, Edelstein WA, Hickey JS: Self shielded gradient coils. In: Society of Magnetic Resonance in Medicine, Fifth Annual Meeting, 1986, pp 1067–1068. Abstract.

75. Mitchell DG: Abdominal magnetic resonance imaging: optimization and artifact suppression. Top Magn Reson Imaging 4:18–34, 1992.

76. Chezmar JL: Magnetic resonance imaging of the liver. Technique. Radiol Clin North Am 29:1251–1258, 1991.

77. Powers T, Lum A, Patton JA: Abdominal MRI artifacts. Semin Ultrasound CT MR 10:2–10, 1989.

78. Mitchell DG, Vinitski S, Burk DL Jr, et al: Multiple spin-echo MR imaging of the body: image contrast and motion-induced artifact. Magn Reson Imaging 6:535–546, 1988.

79. Wedeen VJ, Wendt RE 3d, Jerosch-Herold M: Motional phase artifacts in Fourier transform MRI. Magn Reson Med 11:114–120, 1989.

80. Edelman RR, Hahn P, Buxton R, et al: Rapid magnetic resonance imaging with suspended respiration: clinical application in the liver. Radiology 161:125–131, 1986.

81. Atkinson DJ, Edelman RR: Cineangiography of the heart in a single breath hold with a segmented turboFLASH sequence. Radiology 178:357–360, 1991.

82. Butts K, Riederer SJ, Ehman RL, et al: Echo-planar imaging of the liver with a standard MR imaging system. Radiology 189:259–264, 1993.

83. Rogers WJ Jr, Shapiro EP: Effect of RR interval variation on image quality in gated, two-dimensional, Fourier MR imaging. Radiology 186:883–887, 1993.

84. Runge VM, Clanton JA, Partain CL, James AE: Respiratory gating in magnetic resonance imaging at 0.5 tesla. Radiology 151:521–523, 1984.

85. Ehman RL, McNamara MT, Pallack M, et al: Magnetic resonance imaging with respiratory gating: techniques and applications. AJR 143:1175–1182, 1984.

86. Lanzer P, Botvinick EH, Shiller NB, et al: Cardiac imaging using gated magnetic resonance. Radiology 150:121–127, 1984.

87. Bailes DR, Gildendale DJ, Bydder GM, et al: Respiratory ordered phase

encoding (ROPE): a method for reducing respiratory motion artifacts in MR imaging. J Comput Assist Tomogr 9:835–838, 1985.

88. Axel L, Summers RM, Kressel HY, Charles C: Respiratory effects in two-dimensional Fourier transform imaging. Radiology 160:795–801, 1986.

89. Stark DD, Wittenberg J, Edelman RR, et al: Detection of hepatic metastases by MRI: analysis of pulse sequence performance. Radiology 159:365–370, 1986.

90. Gazelle GS, Saini S, Hahn PF, et al: MR imaging of the liver at 1.5 T: value of signal averaging in suppressing motion artifacts. AJR 163:335–337, 1994.

91. Dixon WT, Brummer ME, Malko JA: Acquisition order and motional artifact reduction in spin warp images. Magn Reson Med 6:74–83, 1988.

92. Bydder GM, Steiner E, Blumgart LH, et al: MR Imaging of the liver using short T1 inversion recovery sequences. J Comput Assist Tomogr 9:1084–1089, 1985.

93. Mirowitz SA: Motion artifact as a pitfall in diagnosis of meniscal tear on gradient reoriented MRI of the knee. J Comput Assist Tomogr 18:279–282, 1994.

94. Turner DA, Rapoport MI, Erwin WD, et al: Truncation artifact: a potential pitfall in MR imaging of the menisci of the knee. Radiology 179:629–633, 1991.

95. Enzmann DR, Griffin C, Rubin JB: Potential false-negative MR images of the thoracic spine in disk disease with switching of phase- and frequency-encoding gradients. Radiology 165:635–637, 1987.

96. Haacke EM, Lenz GW: Improving MR image quality in the presence of motion by using rephasing gradients. AJR 148:1251–1258, 1987.

97. Quencer RM, Hinks RS, Pattany PH, et al: Improved MR imaging of the brain by using compensating gradients to suppress motion-induced artifacts. AJR 151:163–170, 1988.

98. Mitchell DG, Vinitski S, Burk DL Jr, et al: Motion artifact reduction in MR imaging of the abdomen: gradient moment nulling versus respiratory-sorted phase encoding. Radiology 169:155–160, 1988.

99. Lipcamon JD, Chiu LC, Phillips JJ, Pattany PM: MRI of the upper abdomen using motion artifact suppression technique (MAST). Radiol Technol 59:415–418, 1988.

100. Elster AD: Motion artifact suppression technique (MAST) for cranial MR imaging: superiority over cardiac gating for reducing phase-shift artifacts. AJNR 9:671–674, 1988.

101. Zee CS, Boswell WD Jr, Norris SL, et al: The motion artifact suppression technique (MAST) in magnetic resonance imaging: clinical results. Magn Reson Imaging 6:293–299, 1988.

102. Hirohashi S, Otsuji H, Uchida H, et al: The usefulness of motion artifact suppression technic (MAST) in the MRI diagnosis of liver tumors. Rinsho Hoshasen 34:591–597, 1989.

103. Wood ML, Zur Y, Neuringer LJ: Gradient moment nulling for steady-state free precession MR imaging of cerebrospinal fluid. Med Phys 18:1038–1044, 1991.

104. Mugler JP 3d, Brookeman JR: The design of pulse sequences employing spatial presaturation for the suppression of flow artifacts. Magn Reson Med 23:201–214, 1992.

105. Felmlee JP, Ehman RL: Spatial presaturation: a method for suppressing flow artifacts and improving depiction of vascular anatomy in MR imaging. Radiology 164:559–564, 1987.

106. Ro YM, Cho ZH: A novel flow-suppression technique using tailored RF pulses. Magn Reson Med 29:660–666, 1983.

107. Holsinger-Bampton AE, Riederer SJ, Campeau NG, et al: T1-weighted snapshot gradient-echo MR imaging of the abdomen. Radiology 181:25–32, 1991.

108. de Lange EE, Mugler JP 3rd, Bosworth JE, et al: MR imaging of the liver: breath-hold T1-weighted MP-GRE compared with conventional T2-weighted SE imaging—lesion detection, localization, and characterization. Radiology 190:727–736, 1994.

109. Mirowitz SA, Lee JK, Gutierrez E, et al: Dynamic gadolinium-enhanced rapid acquisition spin-echo MR imaging of the liver. Radiology 179:371–376, 1991.

110. Sakuma H, Fujita N, Foo TK, et al: Evaluation of left ventricular volume and mass with breath-hold cine MR imaging. Radiology 188:377–380, 1993.

111. Hennig J, Naureth A, Friedburg H: RARE imaging: a fast imaging method for clinical MR. Magn Reson Med 3:823–833, 1986.

112. Mulkern RV, Wong STS, Winalski C, Jolesz FA: Contrast manipulation and artifact assessment of 2D and 3D RARE sequences. Magn Reson Imaging 8:557–566, 1990.

113. Low RN, Francis IR, Sigeti JS, Foo TK: Abdominal MR imaging: comparison of T2-weighted fast and conventional spin-echo, and contrast-enhanced fast multiplanar spoiled gradient-recalled imaging. Radiology 186:803–811, 1993.

114. Smith RC, Reinhold C, Lange RC, et al: Fast spin-echo MR imaging of the female pelvis. Part I. Use of a whole-volume coil. Radiology 184:665–669, 1992.

115. Ross JS, Ruggieri PM, Tkach JA, et al: Lumbar degenerative disk disease: prospective comparison of conventional T2-weighted spin-echo imaging and T2-weighted rapid acquisition relaxation-enhanced imaging. AJNR 14:1215–1223, 1993.

116. Vinitski S, Mitchell DG, Einstein SG, et al: Conventional and fast spin-echo MR imaging: minimizing echo time. J Magn Reson Imaging 3:501–507, 1993.

117. Zhou X, Liang ZP, Cofer GP, et al: Reduction of ringing and blurring artifacts in fast spin-echo imaging. J Magn Reson Imaging 3:803–807, 1993.

118. Hedley M, Yan H: Motion artifact suppression: a review of post-processing techniques to correct for motion. Magn Reson Imaging 10:627–635, 1992.

119. Hedley M, Yan H: Slice selection axis motion artifact correction in MRI. Australas Phys Eng Sci Med 14:234–239, 1991.

120. Hedley M, Yan H: An algorithm for the suppression of translational motion artifacts in MRI. Australas Phys Eng Sci Med 13:177–184, 1990.

121. Wood ML, Shivji MJ, Stanchev PL: Planar-motion correction with use of K-space data acquired in Fourier MR imaging. J Magn Reson Imaging 5:57–64, 1995.

122. Xiang QS, Henkelman RM: Motion artifact reduction with three-point ghost phase cancellation. J Magn Reson Imaging 1:633–642, 1991.

123. Hinks RS, Xiang QS, Henkelman RM: Ghost phase cancellation with phase-encoding gradient modulation. J Magn Reson Imaging 3:777–785, 1993.

124. Ehman RL, Felmlee JP: Adaptive technique for high-definition MR imaging of moving structures. Radiology 173:255–263, 1989.

125. Doyle M, Chapman BL, Blackwell G, et al: Adaptive Fourier threshold filtering: a method to reduce noise and incoherent artifacts in high resolution cardiac images. Magn Reson Med 31:546–550, 1994.

126. Axel L: Blood flow effects in magnetic resonance imaging. AJR 143:1159–1166, 1984.

127. Bradley W, Waluch V: Blood flow: magnetic resonance imaging. Radiology 154:443–450, 1985.

128. Moran PR, Moran RA, Karstaedt N: Verification and evaluation of internal flow and motion. True magnetic resonance imaging by the phase gradient modulation method. Radiology 154:433–441, 1985.

129. von Schulthess GK, Higgins CB: Blood flow imaging with MR: spin-phase phenomena. Radiology 57:687–695, 1985.

130. Wesbey GE, Higgins CB, Amparo EG, et al: Peripheral vascular disease: correlation of MR imaging and angiography. Radiology 156:733–739, 1985.

131. Larson TC 3d, Kelly WM, Ehman RL, et al: Spatial misregistration of vascular flow during MR imaging of the CNS: cause and clinical significance. AJR 155:1117–1124, 1990.

132. Frank LR, Crawley AP, Buxton RB: Elimination of oblique flow artifacts in magnetic resonance imaging. Magn Reson Med 25:299–307, 1992.

133. Fujita N, Harada K, Hirabuki N, et al: Asymmetric appearance of intracranial vessels on routine spin-echo MR images: a pulse sequence-dependent phenomenon. AJNR 13:1153–1159, 1992.

134. Silverman PM, Patt RH, Baum PA, Teitelbaum GP: Ghost artifact on gradient-echo imaging: a potential pitfall in hepatic imaging. AJR 154:633–634, 1990.

135. Tasciyan TA, Mitchell DG: Pulsatile flow artifacts in fast magnetization-prepared sequences. J Magn Reson Imaging 4:217–222, 1994.

136. Nienaber C, Kodolitsch Y, Nicolas V, et al: The diagnosis of thoracic aortic dissection by noninvasive imaging procedures. N Engl J Med 328:1–9, 1993.

137. Solomon SL, Brown JJ, Glazer HS, et al: Thoracic aortic dissection: pitfalls and artifacts in MR imaging. Radiology 177:223–238, 1990.

138. Hearshen DO, Ellis JH, Carson PL, et al: Boundary effects from opposed magnetization artifacts in IR images. Radiology 160:543–547, 1986.

139. Anzai Y, Lufkin RB, Minoshima S, et al: Fat suppression failure artifacts at the susceptibility interface on frequency selective fat suppression MR imaging in the head and neck. Nippon Igaku Hoshasen Gakkai Zasshi 54:1–7, 1994.

140. Gorczyca DP, Schneider E, DeBruhl ND, et al: Silicone breast implant rupture: comparison between three-point Dixon and fast spin-echo MR imaging. AJR 162:305–310, 1994.

141. Hu X, Kim SG: Reduction of signal fluctuation in functional MRI using navigator echoes. Magn Reson Med 31:495–503, 1994.

142. Hajnal JV, Myers R, Oatridge A, et al: Artifacts due to stimulus correlated motion in functional imaging of the brain. Magn Reson Med 31:283–291, 1994.

143. Wedeen VJ, Meuli RA, Edelman RR, et al: Projective imaging of pulsatile flow with magnetic resonance. Science 230:946–948, 1985.

144. Rossnick S, Laub G, Braeckle R, et al: Three dimensional display of blood vessels in MRI. In: Proceedings of the IEEE Computers in Cardiology Conference. New York: Institute of Electrical and Electronic Engineers, 1986, pp 193–196.

145. Tsuruda J, Saloner D, Norman D: Artifacts associated with MR neuroangiography. AJNR 13:1411–1422, 1992.

146. Riles TS, Eidelman EM, Litt AW, et al: Comparison of magnetic resonance angiography, conventional angiography, and duplex scanning. Stroke 23:341–346, 1992.

147. Buijs PC, Klop RB, Eikelboom BC, et al: Carotid bifurcation imaging: magnetic resonance angiography compared to conventional angiography and Doppler ultrasound. Eur J Vasc Surg 7:245–251, 1993.

148. Lin W, Haacke EM, Smith AS: Lumen definition in MR angiography. J Magn Reson Imaging 1:327–336, 1991.

149. De Marco JK, Nesbit GM, Wesbey GE, Richardson D: Prospective comparison of extracranial carotid stenosis with intraarterial angiography versus MR angiography using maximum-intensity projections and multiplanar reformations. AJR 163:1205–1212, 1994.

150. Anderson CM, Saloner D, Tsuruda JS, et al: Artifacts in maximum-intensity-projection display of MR angiograms. AJR 154:623–629, 1990.

151. Brown DG, Riederer SJ: Contrast-to-noise ratios in maximum intensity projection images. Magn Reson Med 23:130–137, 1992.

152. Patel MR, Klufas RA, Kim D, et al: MR angiography of the carotid bifurcation: artifacts and limitations. AJR 162:1431–1437, 1994.

153. Dumoulin CL, Souza SP, Walker MF, Wagle W: Three-dimensional phase contrast angiography. Magn Reson Med 9:139–149, 1989.

154. Edelman RR, Ahn SS, Chien D, et al: Improved time-of-flight MR angiography of the brain with magnetization transfer contrast. Radiology 184:395–399, 1992.

155. Nagele T, Klose U, Grodd W, et al: The effects of linearly increasing flip angles on 3D inflow MR angiography. Magn Reson Med 31:561–566, 1994.

156. Huston J 3d, Rufenacht DA, Ehman RL, Wiebers DO: Intracranial aneurysms and vascular malformations: comparison of time-of-flight and phase-contrast MR angiography. Radiology 181:721–730, 1991.

157. Frank LR, Buxton RB, Kerber CW: Pulsatile flow artifacts in 3D magnetic resonance imaging. Magn Reson Med 30:296–304, 1993.

158. Korin HW, Riederer SJ, Bampton AE, Ehman RL: Altered phase-encoding order for reduced sensitivity to motion in three-dimensional MR imaging. J Magn Reson Imaging 2:687–693, 1992.

159. Blatter DD, Bahr AL, Parker DL, et al: Cervical carotid MR angiography with multiple overlapping thin-slab acquisition: comparison with conventional angiography. AJR 161:1269–1277, 1993.

160. Ding X, Tkach JA, Ruggieri PR, Masaryk TJ: Sequential three-dimensional time-of-flight MR angiography of the carotid arteries: value of variable excitation and postprocessing in reducing venetian blind artifact. AJR 163:683–688, 1994.

161. Dumoulin CL, Steinberg FL, Yucel EK, Darrow RD: Reduction of artifacts from breathing and peristalsis in phase-contrast MRA of the chest and abdomen. J Comput Assist Tomogr 17:328–332, 1993.

162. McCarty M, Gedroyc WMW: Surgical clip artifact mimicking arterial stenosis: problem with magnetic resonance angiography. Clin Radiol 48:232–235, 1993.

163. De Marco JK, Nesbit GM, Wesbey GE, Richardson D: Prospective comparison of extracranial carotid stenosis with intraarterial angiography versus MR angiography using maximum-intensity projections and multiplanar reformations. AJR 163:1205–1212, 1994.

164. Caputo GR, Masui T, Gooding GA, et al: Popliteal and tibioperoneal arteries: feasibility of two-dimensional time-of-flight MR angiography and phase velocity mapping. Radiology 182:387–392, 1992.

165. Dixon WT: Simple proton spectroscopic imaging. Radiology 153:189–194, 1984.

166. Wehrli FW, Perkins TG, Shimakawa A, Roberts F: Chemical shift–induced amplitude modulations in images obtained with gradient refocusing. Magn Reson Imaging 5:157–158, 1987.

167. Moran PR, Moran RA: Imaging true motion velocity and higher order motion quantities by phase gradient modulation techniques in NMR scanners. In: Esser PD, Johnston RE, eds: Technology of Nuclear Magnetic Resonance. New York: Society of Nuclear Medicine, 1984, pp 149–163.

Pulse Sequence Design in MRI

J. PAUL FINN ■ ORLANDO P. SIMONETTI

The magnetic resonance imaging (MRI) community has witnessed a rapid proliferation of new pulse sequences and techniques. With advances in hardware and computer technology, there has been explosive development in fast and ultrafast imaging methods. At the same time, the range of clinical applications for MRI has widened, so that virtually every organ system is now a focus for MRI developers and clinical scientists alike. For the MRI developer, these are exciting times; the pace of development has never been faster. For the MRI user, these are confusing times; the diversity of new techniques is perceived to have added layers of complexity to what was never considered a simple modality. However, ideas are rarely original, and much of what is hailed as new today is as much a consequence of improvements in implementation as in design. MRI scientists have quite correctly built on the wealth of ideas generated over the years in pulse nuclear magnetic resonance (NMR) spectroscopy, and concepts of single-shot MRI were expounded several years before the hardware was available for their practical implementation (just as the mathematic basis for cross-sectional image reconstruction was worked out before the development of computed tomography). We mention these facts not to detract from the creativity of pulse sequence developers but rather to emphasize that the basic concepts of a wide range of pulse sequences have been around for some time. Moreover, these can be built on and understood with some basic tools that include a clear grasp of the underlying MR physics and relevant aspects of signal processing theory. Although one's ability to implement new concepts or extend current ones may be limited by hardware and software constraints, these limitations are being increasingly eroded by advances in digital technology, electronics, and materials science.

MRI is a multiparametric technique, and many parameters can be associated in a more or less arbitrary manner. A confounding array of different pulse sequences is therefore possible. However, relatively few techniques have found their way into routine clinical practice. There are several reasons for this; in some cases there is no clear clinical application for a pulse sequence; in some cases there is a substantial time lag between initial concept and dissemination as a commercial product; and in some cases a technique proves unwieldy or unreliable in a clinical context. An important point to emphasize at this stage is that an MRI pulse sequence is more likely to find a place in clinical practice if it is *designed* to tackle a clinical problem than if it serendipitously finds a niche. To some extent, then, a grasp of the clinical focus is the first step in designing a pulse sequence to solve a problem.

Pulse sequence design is a huge topic, comprising elements from many disciplines in the physical and clinical sciences, and a comprehensive treatment of the subject is beyond the scope of any book chapter. However, it is our hope that once the reader has grasped the relevant basic principles, the leap from 10-minute spin-echo imaging of the brain to subsecond imaging of the heart will be greater in time scale than in concept. In this chapter, we confine the scope of the discussion to a description of the relevant physics, data acquisition, signal processing, and image reconstruction as they relate to conventional and ultrafast MRI techniques. We do not deal with hardware issues. For an in-depth treatment of this subject, the reader is referred to Chapter 14. We also do not deal with clinical applications, which are dealt with in several other chapters (see, for example, Chapter 10).

We take as our working definition of an *MRI pulse sequence* a series of radiofrequency (RF) pulses and magnetic field gradient pulses generating NMR signals that, when appropriately processed, result in the formation of an image. The details of how the RF and gradient pulses are played out determine the form, speed, and information content of the image. We concern ourselves with these processes.

SUMMARY OF BACKGROUND PHYSICS

MAGNETIZATION

Of central importance to a consideration of pulse sequence design is the behavior of the net magnetization vector, **M.** This is the vector sum of all the individual spin moments, $\Sigma\ \mathbf{\mu}_i$, aligned parallel to the main magnetic field $\mathbf{B}_0$ (Fig. 4–1). The magnitude and direction of **M** are determined by the Boltzmann distribution,[1] which favors alignment of a small majority of spins parallel to $\mathbf{B}_0$. At equilibrium, **M** is invariant along $\mathbf{B}_0$ and experiences no torque. However, the individual spin moments $\mathbf{\mu}_i$ contributing to **M** are each aligned at an angle to $\mathbf{B}_0$ and do experience a torque $\mathbf{\tau}$ described by[2]

$$\mathbf{\tau} = \frac{d\mathbf{p}_i}{dt} = \mathbf{\mu}_i \times \mathbf{B}_0 \qquad (1)$$

where $\mathbf{p}_i$ is the angular momentum vector of the spinning nucleus. Equation 1 states that the torque is equal to the rate of change of the angular momentum vector and that this in turn is the cross-product of the magnetic moment and main field vectors. As shown graphically in Figure 4–1, the torque in such an arrangement causes the spin to precess about the main field axis. An ensemble of identical spins each with a random starting phase therefore describes a cone-shaped precession about $\mathbf{B}_0$ at a frequency $\omega_0 = \gamma\mathbf{B}_0$ (see Fig. 4–1*B*). Here, γ is the gyromagnetic ratio, defined as the ratio of the spin magnetic moment to the angular moment:

$$\mathbf{\mu} = \gamma\mathbf{p} \qquad (2)$$

γ is also the proportionality constant relating the Larmor precessional frequency ω_0 to the applied field strength. The Larmor frequency for protons is 42.577 $\times\ 10^6$ Hz/T.

Equations 1 and 2 can be combined to give

$$\frac{d\mathbf{\mu}_i}{dt} = \gamma\frac{d\mathbf{p}_i}{dt} = \gamma\mathbf{\mu}_i \times \mathbf{B}_0 \qquad (3)$$

The phases of the individual spins are uncorrelated, so the components of the spin vectors lying in the plane perpendicular to $\mathbf{B}_0$ sum to zero. In what follows, we consider only the classic (as opposed to quantum mechanical) treatment of the behavior of the net magnetization **M.**

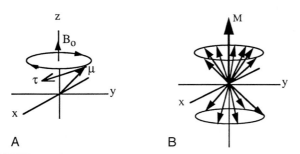

FIGURE 4–1. Spin precession around $\mathbf{B}_0$. As shown in *A*, the torque $\mathbf{\tau}$ acting on a typical spin is always perpendicular both to $\mathbf{\mu}$ and to the main field. This results in a circular motion of the tip of the $\mathbf{\mu}$ vector around the axis of the main field. As shown in *B*, there is a slight excess of vectors pointing with the field in accordance with the Boltzmann distribution. Because the spins are randomly orientated in the x-y plane, there is no net x-y magnetization.

THE BLOCH EQUATIONS

Because the nuclear spin moments $\mathbf{\mu}_i$ add vectorially to give **M,** the torque on **M** is given by

$$\frac{d\mathbf{M}}{dt} = \gamma(\mathbf{M} \times \mathbf{B}) \qquad (4)$$

where **B** is the effective field experienced by **M;**[3] this may or may not be equal to $\mathbf{B}_0$. Equation 4 states that the net magnetization **M** experiences a torque only if it has a component perpendicular to the effective magnetic field **B.** By convention, magnetic fields and magnetic moments are referenced to a right-handed cartesian frame in which the main magnetic field $\mathbf{B}_0$ is taken to lie parallel to the z axis. The unit vectors along the x, y, z directions are denoted by **i, j, k,** respectively.

$$\mathbf{M} \times \mathbf{B} = \begin{bmatrix} \mathbf{i} & \mathbf{j} & \mathbf{k} \\ M_x & M_y & M_z \\ B_x & B_y & B_z \end{bmatrix} \qquad (5)$$

Equation 5 implies that changes in **M** along each of the axes are caused only by components of **M** and **B** lying in the plane orthogonal to that axis.[3] In other words,

$$\frac{dM_x}{dt} = \gamma(M_yB_z - M_zB_y),$$

$$\frac{dM_y}{dt} = \gamma(M_zB_x - M_xB_z), \qquad (6)$$

$$\frac{dM_z}{dt} = \gamma(M_xB_y - M_yB_x)$$

THE ROTATING FRAME

When aligned along z, the magnetization is essentially static and does not generate a detectable signal. When rotated away from z, the magnetization precesses coherently about $\mathbf{B}_0$ at the Larmor frequency and is detectable in the x-y plane by a suitable probe. The rotation is accomplished by the magnetic field of an RF pulse, generally designated the $\mathbf{B}_1$ field. From the arguments presented so far, we can see that to rotate **M** away from the z direction:

- A magnetic field must lie somewhere in the x-y plane.
- The $\mathbf{B}_1$ field must be synchronous with the magnetization by rotating at the same (Larmor) frequency as **M** (Fig. 4–2*A*).[2]

In this case, as $\mathbf{B}_1$ tips **M** off axis, the motion of **M** relative to $\mathbf{B}_1$ is characterized by a simple rotation around the $\mathbf{B}_1$ axis (Fig. 4–2*B*).

With the components of the rotating $\mathbf{B}_1$ field, the total field along the three axes can be expressed by $B_x = B_1\cos(2\pi f_0 t)$, $B_y = -B_1\sin(2\pi f_0 t)$, $B_z = B_0$, and these values can be substituted into Equations 6. For completeness, relaxation effects must be taken into account. Equations 6 then become the *Bloch equations,*[4]

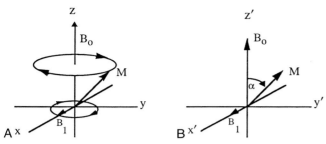

FIGURE 4–2. Rotating frame. *A,* In the laboratory frame xyz, B_1 rotates with **M** in the x-y plane. *B,* In the frame rotating with B_1 (x'y'z'), B_1 is static and the only motion of **M** is due to the torque **M** × B_1, which nutates **M** through α toward y' at a rate γB_1.

defining the motion of **M** in the presence of static field B_0 and rotating field B_1:

$$\frac{dM_x}{dt} = \gamma(M_y B_0 + M_z B_1 \sin 2\pi f_0 t) - \frac{M_x}{T2} \tag{7}$$

$$\frac{dM_y}{dt} = \gamma(M_z B_1 \cos 2\pi f_0 t - M_x B_0) - \frac{M_y}{T2} \tag{8}$$

$$\frac{dM_z}{dt} = -\gamma(M_x B_1 \sin 2\pi f_0 t + M_y B_1 \cos 2\pi f_0 t) - \frac{M_z - M_0}{T1} \tag{9}$$

where M_0 is the equilibrium magnetization along z and T1 and T2 are the longitudinal and transverse relaxation times, respectively.

Consideration of the response of **M** to an RF field can be simplified by referring the motion of **M** to a frame rotating at the B_1 frequency. The time derivative of a vector in a frame rotating at angular velocity $\mathbf{\Omega}$ is given by[4]

$$\left(\frac{d\mathbf{M}}{dt}\right)_{lab} = \left(\frac{\partial\mathbf{M}}{\partial t}\right)_{rot} + \mathbf{\Omega} \times \mathbf{M} \tag{10}$$

where the subscripts lab and rot refer to the laboratory (fixed) and rotating frames, respectively. By combining Equations 4 and 10 we obtain

$$\left(\frac{\partial\mathbf{M}}{\partial t}\right)_{rot} = \gamma\mathbf{M} \times \left(\mathbf{B}_0 + \frac{\mathbf{\Omega}}{\gamma}\right) = \gamma(\mathbf{M} \times \mathbf{B}_{eff}) \tag{11}$$

Equation 11 states that the motion of **M** in the rotating frame is a precession about an "effective" field $\mathbf{B}_{eff} = \mathbf{B}_0 + \mathbf{\Omega}/\gamma$. $\mathbf{\Omega}/\gamma$ is often referred to as a "fictitious" field consequent on the rotation. If $\mathbf{\Omega}$ is at the Larmor angular frequency $-\gamma\mathbf{B}_0$, $\mathbf{B}_{eff}$ is zero and **M** does not move in the rotating frame. When B_1 is now applied in the x-y plane, it rotates at the Larmor frequency in the laboratory frame but is fixed in the rotating frame. We define a new set of coordinate axes for the rotating frame labeled x'y'z'. z' is identical to z, and x' and y' rotate at $\mathbf{\Omega}$ relative to x and y. One can now define an arbitrary orientation in the rotating frame for the B_1 field; this is usually taken along the x' axis. Equation 11 suggests that, at the Larmor frequency, the motion of **M** describes a precession around B_1 so that **M** lies within the y'-z' plane. The precessional frequency of **M** around B_1 is γB_1 and the angle α that **M** rotates through is given by

$$\alpha = \gamma B_1 t \tag{12}$$

where t is the duration for which B_1 is applied (see Fig. 4–2*B*).

RADIOFREQUENCY EVENTS

In MRI, RF energy is typically applied as a pulse lasting from tens of microseconds to tens of milliseconds, depending on the application. When the RF is applied on resonance, that is, at the Larmor frequency, the magnetization is rotated α° about B_1 according to Equation 12. When α is 90°, all magnetization is nutated into the x-y plane, and the potential signal is maximal. As discussed later, however, for many applications flip angles other than 90° are used. For example, 180° pulses are used for inversion and refocusing, and pulses substantially less than 90° may be appropriate for short repetition time (TR) imaging.

Spin Echoes

When the magnetization is nutated into the x-y plane, initially all of it is available for detection and the MR signal is maximal. However, through relaxation processes, the signal begins to decay exponentially. The falling signal profile over time is known as a free induction decay, and the rapidity with which the signal falls off is determined by how efficient transverse relaxation processes are.[1] Spins dephase through a combination of T2 decay, main field nonuniformity, and local field distortions caused by susceptibility gradients. The inhomogeneity in the main field ΔB_0 causes spins to dephase at a rate γΔB_0 in addition to the intrinsic spin-spin interaction 1/T2. The net rate of decay is therefore the sum (1/T2 + γΔB_0). In the presence of main field nonuniformity, the effective decay time is expressed by T2* = 1/(1/T2 + γΔB_0). The rate of decay of the transverse magnetization is therefore greater in the presence of significant ΔB_0.

Hahn[5] described a technique of RF refocusing to neutralize the effects of B_0 inhomogeneity and local susceptibility effects, which is termed *spin echo*. After the 90° excitation, a 180° pulse is applied, and an echo is formed at a time determined by twice the interval between the two pulses. As outlined in Figure 4–3, the 180° pulse has the effect of refocusing spins that fanned out before its application. The spin echo refocuses dephasing caused by fixed differences such as ΔB_0, chemical-shift effects (see later discussion of fat suppression), and local susceptibility gradients. It does not refocus dephasing caused by random processes such as spin-spin interaction[1] ("true T2") and diffusion.[6] The refocusing pulse can be reapplied multiple times to generate a train of spin echoes as described by Carr and Purcell.[7] The T2 decay envelope can then be measured and values of T2 computed.

In the modification of the Carr-Purcell spin-echo experiment described by Meiboom and Gill,[8] the phase of the refocusing 180° pulses is offset by 90° relative to the excitatory 90° pulse (see Fig. 4–3*C'* and *D'*). Thus, if a π/2 pulse is applied along x, the refocusing π pulses are applied along y. The effect of the π pulse is

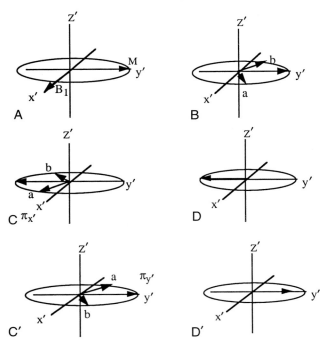

FIGURE 4–3. Spin echo. In *A*, a 90° pulse has been applied along x′ and the magnetization lies along y′. *B,* At time t = TE/2 later, the spins have dephased in the x-y plane through T2* decay. In *C*, a 180° refocusing pulse applied along x′ reflects the spin vectors through the x′ axis. The spins continue to precess as before the refocusing pulse, and in *D*, at time t = TE, a spin echo occurs. With multiple refocusing pulses, imperfections in the RF are propagated. When the refocusing pulse is applied along y′ as in *C′*, the spin echo occurs along y′ without phase inversion as in *D′*. Flip angle errors are corrected on alternate echoes and are not propagated. This is the Meiboom-Gill modification of the Carr-Purcell multiecho pulse. It is standard in long spin-echo train sequences.

to form the complex conjugate **M*** of **M** by rotation about y. This serves to prevent propagation of imperfections in the π pulses as follows. Consider a situation in which instead of π refocusing pulses, 150° pulses are applied along x, the same axis as the excitatory 90° pulse. At the first spin echo, the magnetization **M** lies 30° below the x-y plane, at the second spin echo **M** lies 60° above the x-y plane, and so on for subsequent spin echoes. If the refocusing RF pulses are applied along y, then the undershoot on the first echo is corrected on the second, the undershoot on the third is corrected on the fourth, and so on. Every second spin echo now has the correct amplitude, and the initial error is not propagated. Formerly, generation of multiple spin echoes had as its main application the measurement of T2 values. With the development of rapid acquisition with relaxation enhancement (RARE)[9] and related rapid spin-echo imaging techniques,[10–12] the use of multiecho sequences has increased significantly. This buffering effect of offsetting the phase of the π pulses may be useful clinically when the application of multiple refocusing pulses results in RF energy deposition outside recommended limits. The flip angle of the π pulses can be scaled back as described earlier with little perceptible change in image quality but substantial reduction in specific absorption rate. This

is particularly relevant in the design of hybrid fast RF refocused sequences such as turbo (fast) spin echo.

Stimulated Echoes

Stimulated echoes occur when a train of three or more RF pulses is applied sequentially.[13] Each stimulated echo is formed by three (nominal) 90° pulses. The first pulse nutates the magnetization into the x-y plane so that it initially lies, for example, along y′ (Fig. 4–4). Subsequently, over an interval TE/2, where TE is the echo time, the spins fan out in the x-y plane as a result of T2* decay. The second pulse now rotates the plane of magnetization so that it has one axis parallel to z. The components lying along z no longer precess, and those lying along y′ undergo irreversible T2 decay. The third pulse recalls the magnetization stored along ±z to ±x′. After another interval TE/2, the magnetization has a component along +y′; this is the stimulated echo. As illustrated in Figure 4–4, the delay between the first two pulses is the same as the delay between the last pulse and the stimulated echo.

The following are noteworthy about stimulated echoes:

- The amplitude of the echo is smaller than that of a spin echo of comparable TE. This is because only half the available magnetization is used in the stimulated echo.
- For the same reason, not all spins are exactly in phase along y′ at the echo (only spins 3 and 7 in Fig. 4–4 are), as would occur with a spin echo. Rather, there is a distribution of spin vectors oriented in the positive y′ direction; the largest are refocused along y′ and others also have a component along ±x′.
- The interval between the second and third pulses can be substantially larger than TE. This long interval can be exploited to heighten sensitivity to diffusion and flow effects.
- T1 relaxation occurs between the second and third pulses. If this is significant, the amplitude of the stimulated echo is decreased still further.
- Stimulated echoes occur in a variety of circumstances in which one might not expect them. For example, in multiecho spin-echo imaging, three sequential RF pulses produce a stimulated echo that may be superimposed on a spin echo. It is important in fast or turbo spin-echo (TSE) imaging to be aware of the effects stimulated echoes can have on image contrast[14, 15] and to engineer them appropriately. In certain forms of fast gradient-echo imaging, stimulated echoes modulate the amplitude of subsequent gradient and RF echoes and can alter image contrast and signal-to-noise (S/N) ratio.
- Stimulated-echo imaging[16, 17] has found applications in several areas, including ultrafast imaging,[18] motion tracking,[19] and black blood cardiac imaging.[20]

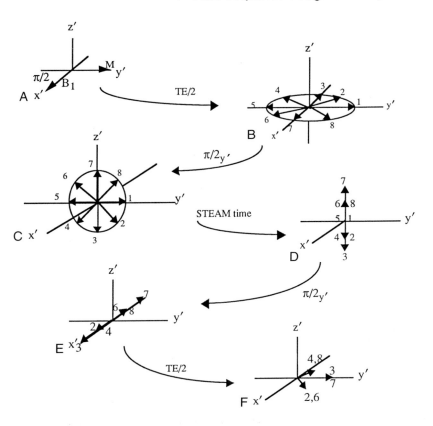

FIGURE 4–4. Stimulated-echo acquisition mode (STEAM). A stimulated echo is formed by a train of three 90° pulses. In *A*, $\mathbf{B}_1$ is applied along x′ and the magnetization is laid down along y′. *B*, After a suitable time TE/2, the spins have dephased in the x-y plane as a result of T2* processes or applied gradients. A 90° pulse is now applied along y′, rotating the plane of magnetization to the y′-z′ plane *(C)*. Spins aligned along z′ undergo no further phase changes, whereas those along y′ dephase completely *(D)*. We refer to this interval as the STEAM time. Another 90° pulse is now applied along y′, rotating the z magnetization along x′ *(E)*. After TE/2, these spins all have components along positive y′ *(F)*, forming a stimulated echo. Note that only half the magnetization is recoverable in this way.

Adiabatic Pulses and Off-Resonance Effects

The discussion so far has assumed that the RF is applied uniformly throughout the relevant field of view (FOV), in other words, that α is invariant over space. In practice, this is not the case, and the spatial variation in the $\mathbf{B}_1$ field is strongly influenced by the design of the transmitter and how the subject loads the coil. Generally, large transmitter coils have spatial $\mathbf{B}_1$ profiles that vary only slowly, whereas the RF field of small transmitter coils may fall off dramatically toward the periphery. It may be important in the design of a pulse sequence to take these effects into account and in the case of a surface receiver coil to determine whether it also serves as transmitter.

When the $\mathbf{B}_1$ profile of a coil is known, it is possible to generate a correction algorithm for postprocessing and normalization in the same way as for a surface receiver coil. Although useful for display purposes, such a scheme does not address S/N ratio or contrast deficiencies that arise as a consequence of the RF field. $\mathbf{B}_1$ nonuniformity is most apparent and most damaging when large flip angles are used, as in inversion recovery (IR) imaging. Because the contrast in IR images is largely determined by the inversion pulse, IR images are sensitive to the $\mathbf{B}_1$ profile during inversion.

Although the motion of $\mathbf{M}$ is significantly simplified when the $\mathbf{B}_1$ field rotates at the Larmor frequency, we often encounter situations in which the $\mathbf{B}_1$ frequency differs from f_0. In such cases, $\mathbf{B}_0$ is not cancelled, and the effective field is the vector sum of $\mathbf{B}_1$ and the residuum of the $\mathbf{B}_z$ field. This is illustrated in Figure 4–5.

As can be seen from Figure 4–5, the magnitude of $\mathbf{B}_{\text{eff}}$ is given by

$$| \mathbf{B}_{\text{eff}}| = \left[\left(B_0 + \frac{\Omega}{\gamma}\right)^2 + B_1^2 \right]^{1/2}$$

$$= \frac{1}{\gamma}\left[(\omega_0 - \Omega)^2 + (\gamma B_1)^2\right]^{1/2} \quad (13)$$

$\mathbf{M}$ therefore precesses about $\mathbf{B}_{\text{eff}}$ at an angular velocity

$$\omega = \left[(\omega_0 - \Omega)^2 + (\gamma B_1)^2\right]^{1/2} \quad (14)$$

Off-resonance effects may arise from main field nonuniformities, chemical shift, or susceptibility effects. Obviously, when $\Omega = \omega_0$, Equation 14 reduces to the first derivative of Equation 12.

Adiabatic Passage

MRI evolved from pulse NMR, which in turn evolved from continuous wave NMR.[1] In continuous wave

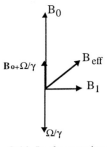

FIGURE 4–5. Effective field. In the rotating frame, when $\mathbf{B}_1$ is not at the Larmor frequency, there is a residual $\mathbf{B}_z$ field given by $B_0 + \Omega/\gamma$ that sums vectorially with $\mathbf{B}_1$ to give $\mathbf{B}_{\text{eff}}$.

NMR, a spectrum is acquired by slowly sweeping the magnetic field while irradiating a sample continuously with pure tone RF (recall that for a waveform to have a single frequency it must be continuous over time). As the field passes through resonance for a given species, the RF is absorbed at that frequency and a spectrum is recorded. An equivalent experiment can be performed by sweeping the RF frequency while the magnetic field is kept constant. The frequency of the B_1 field is offset well to one side of the Larmor frequency and is slowly brought through resonance. This process has several consequences that we now consider, some of which are highly desirable from an imaging standpoint.

Consider the motion of $\mathbf{M}$ in the rotating frame as the RF field is swept through resonance. When the frequency offset $\Delta\omega = (\omega_0 - \Omega)$ is large, there is a large residual B_z field $B_0 + \Omega/\gamma$ (Fig. 4–6). $\mathbf{B}_{eff}$ is therefore coincident with $\mathbf{B}_0$ and $\mathbf{M}$ precesses about the main field. As the frequency offset is *slowly* decreased, $\mathbf{B}_{eff}$ approaches $\mathbf{B}_1$ but at all times remains the precession axis for $\mathbf{M}$. In other words, $\mathbf{M}$ follows $\mathbf{B}_{eff}$ as it changes its orientation from along z through $\mathbf{B}_1$ to $-z$. The magnitude of $\mathbf{B}_{eff}$ decreases to a minimum when aligned along $\mathbf{B}_1$ and then grows again. The fact that $\mathbf{B}_{eff}$ rotates at a velocity $\delta\theta/\delta t$, determined by the sweep rate, means that in the rotating frame another field $-(\delta\theta/\delta t)/\gamma$ exists along y'.[21] A new effective field can be described by $\mathbf{B}'_{eff}$, with magnitude given by

$$|\mathbf{B}'_{eff}| = \left[\left(B_0 + \frac{\Omega}{\gamma} \right)^2 + B_1^2 + \frac{(\partial\theta/\partial t)^2}{\gamma^2} \right]^{1/2} \quad (15)$$

Equation 15 states that with a changing offset frequency, there are now three orthogonal contributions to the effective field around which $\mathbf{M}$ precesses. The orientation of $\mathbf{M}$ therefore depends on the relative magnitude of these components (see Fig. 4–6). The rate of precession of $\mathbf{M}$ around $\mathbf{B}_{eff}$ must be large compared with $(\delta\theta/\delta t)/\gamma$ for $\mathbf{M}$ to follow $\mathbf{B}_{eff}$. This is the *adiabatic* condition. Also, the sweep must be fast enough that no significant relaxation occurs during the RF irradiation. These boundary conditions can be summarized as

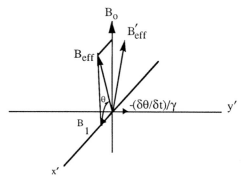

FIGURE 4–6. Changing effective field. As $\mathbf{B}_{eff}$ changes its magnitude and rotates around y', the new effective field is $\mathbf{B}'_{eff} = \mathbf{B}_{eff} - (\delta\theta/\delta\tau)/\gamma$. When the frequency sweep is slow, such that $\delta\theta/\delta t$ is small, $\mathbf{M}$ follows $\mathbf{B}_{eff}$ in the $\mathbf{B}_{eff}$-$\mathbf{B}_1$ plane.

$$\frac{B_1}{T2} << \frac{\partial\theta}{\partial t} << \gamma B_1^2 \quad (16)$$

When the offset frequency is incremented linearly over time, the RF power requirements can be significant. Noting that $\mathbf{B}_{eff}$ is much larger at the beginning and end of the passage than at the center (when $\mathbf{B}_{eff} = \mathbf{B}_1$), Hardy and colleagues[22] suggested a tangential frequency sweep of the form $\omega_t - \omega_0 = \omega_1 \tan(\alpha\omega_1 t)$, where $\omega_t - \omega_0$ is the frequency offset at time t during the sweep, ω_1 is the $\mathbf{B}_1$ frequency, and α is a scaling factor given by $\alpha = (2/\omega_1 T_0) \arctan(\theta/\omega_1)$, where T_0 is the sweep time, 2θ is the range of the angular frequency sweep, and $0 < \alpha < 1$. This scheme provides an order of magnitude increased efficiency compared with a linear sweep and has good inversion properties.

Because the $\mathbf{B}_1$ frequency is offset from the spin (Larmor) frequency, the $\mathbf{B}_1$ field is said to be frequency modulated. In the scheme outlined by Hardy and coworkers,[22] the amplitude of the $\mathbf{B}_1$ field is constant. Other workers have described adiabatic pulses that are amplitude and frequency modulated.[23, 24] These pulses provide insensitivity to inhomogeneity in the $\mathbf{B}_1$ spatial profile and can therefore be of value when the RF transmitter field is nonuniform. $\mathbf{B}_1$ insensitivity is especially important for inversion pulses as described in the following.

For spins lying at arbitrary orientations (not along z) at the start of the pulse, the trajectory in the spatially varying $\mathbf{B}_1$ field is not defined. Classic adiabatic pulses can therefore be used for inversion and excitation, but because they cannot induce plane rotations about an axis of the rotating frame, they are inappropriate for refocusing. For a detailed analysis of the behavior of several classes of adiabatic pulses, the interested reader is referred to the work of Ugurbil and colleagues.[25] Following their notation, the functions for amplitude and frequency modulation, respectively, of adiabatic pulses have the form

$$B_1(t) = 2\pi A v f_B(t) \quad (17)$$

$$\Delta\omega(t) = 2\pi A f_\omega(t) \quad (18)$$

where v is the ratio of the peak RF amplitude to the frequency modulation amplitude A, and f_B and f_ω are time waveforms. Function pairs for f_B/f_ω include constant/tan,[22] sech/tanh,[23] and sin/cos.[24]

By reversing the polarity of the $\mathbf{B}_1$ field at the half-passage point, Ugurbil and colleagues[26] produced refocusing adiabatic pulses of the form

$$B_1(t) = 2\pi A v \sin 2\pi v t (x''), \quad 0 < 2\pi v t < \frac{\pi}{2} \quad (19)$$

$$B_1(t) = 2\pi A v \sin 2\pi v t (-x''), \quad \frac{\pi}{2} < 2\pi v t < \pi \quad (20)$$

$$\Delta\omega(t) = 2\pi A (|\cos 2\pi v t| + s)(z''), \quad 0 < 2\pi v t < \pi \quad (21)$$

The effect of this pulse scheme is to invert magnetization oriented along z' at the beginning of the pulse as for standard adiabatic passage. Spin vectors orthogonal to $\mathbf{B}_{eff}$ at the beginning of the pulse remain orthogonal to $\mathbf{B}_{eff}$ throughout, but the phase "scrambling" that occurs during the first half of the rotation is reversed during the second half by reversing the polarity of $\mathbf{B}_{eff}$. Spins within the entire plane are therefore refocused (or inverted). The pulse described by Equations 19 to 21 breaks down for spins far off-resonance. The hyperbolic secant pulse described by Silver and coworkers,[23] in addition to being insensitive to RF non-uniformity, has excellent slice profile properties for inversion. Above a threshold $\mathbf{B}_1$ intensity, the magnetization remains inverted, and outside the slice the spins are returned to their equilibrium position along the z axis. Connolly and colleagues[27] described a slice-selective, self-refocusing pulse that leaves no phase variation across the slice and maintains insensitivity to $\mathbf{B}_1$ non-uniformity. Their pulse is a composite one of 2π and π pulses; the 2π pulse performs no rotation, just compensates for the phase scrambling caused by the π pulse.

Adiabatic pulses have many advantages for certain imaging applications (such as IR sequences and blood-tagging studies[28]) but they are relatively long, and significant relaxation can take place in some tissues during irradiation. Tissue components with short relaxation times can lose signal during the pulse, insensitivity to $\mathbf{B}_1$ variations may be compromised, and spurious high signal intensity may originate from outside the slice.[29]

Chemical-Shift–Selective Radiofrequency Pulses

Hydrogen nuclei in different molecules are surrounded by varying electron clouds. These orbital electrons are constantly in motion within the cloud and, when subjected to an external magnetic field, according to Lenz's law adjust their trajectories so as to induce an opposing field. The induced fields shield the nuclei from the applied field $\mathbf{B}_0$ to different degrees, expressed by the shielding constant σ, such that the net field seen by the nuclei is $\mathbf{B}_0 (1 - \sigma)$. This phenomenon forms the basis for NMR spectroscopy.[2] Protons in lipid molecules are associated with denser electron cloud cover than those in water molecules, and so, when placed in a magnetic field, lipid protons precess at a lower frequency. The difference in precessional frequencies between nuclei in various chemical environments is expressed by the chemical shift. The units used to quantify chemical shift are either hertz or parts per million, depending on whether normalization for field strength has been performed. For example, at 1.5 T, hydrogen nuclei in fat molecules precess at about 210 Hz below hydrogen nuclei in water. The Larmor frequency for water protons at 1.5 T is 63.75 MHz, and the chemical shift for fat protons is $(-210$ $Hz/63.75 \times 10^6$ $Hz) \times 10^6 = -3.3$ ppm. Conversion from parts per million to shift in hertz is performed simply by multiplying by the frequency of RF irradiation in megahertz.

For many clinical applications, it is desirable to eliminate the signal from protons in one or other chemical environment. This most commonly involves suppression of the fat signal either by exciting and then crushing the fat[30–32] or by exciting the water selectively.[33, 34] Chemical-shift–selective fat saturation is accomplished

by applying a frequency-selective, spatially nonselective excitation pulse to the fat protons and then spoiling the transverse magnetization with a strong gradient pulse. The water spins are unaffected and can then be excited and imaged without interference from the fat. The technical challenge in chemical-shift–selective saturation is selecting only the fat or the water without selecting the other species. This is not a problem when there is no overlap between fat and water resonances. For example, at 1.5 T an RF pulse could be centered on the fat frequency with a bandwidth of, say, ± 100 Hz. Such a pulse would leave water spins relatively untouched. However, in practice there are nonuniformities $\Delta\mathbf{B}_0$ in the main field, caused mainly by patient-induced susceptibility gradients that may exceed the fat-water chemical-shift separation. Water protons precessing at $(\gamma/2\pi)(\mathbf{B}_0 + \Delta\mathbf{B}_0)$ may well lie within the bandwidth of the fat saturation pulse. The result is that in some portions of the image fat is suppressed, whereas in other portions water is suppressed. To minimize this effect, $\mathbf{B}_0$ homogeneity must be optimized by shimming before all spectral selective measurements.

Fat suppression is most often carried out by using either a gaussian pulse centered on the fat frequency or a binomial excitation scheme with short, wide-bandwidth ("hard") pulses. Because the frequency separation of fat and water is small, the RF saturation bandwidth must be narrow (typically less than 200 Hz) to avoid cross-talk.

Binomial excitation is performed by applying a series of hard RF pulses.[32] The series describes a binomial distribution when the amplitude of the pulses is plotted over time, and the time between pulses corresponds to a chosen phase evolution between the fat and water spins. For example, if the interpulse interval is 2.38 ms, the fat-water phase evolution between pulses is 180° at 1.5 T. The pulses may be designed to excite water or fat selectively by appropriate choice of the RF phase.[33, 34] If the phase is kept constant, the sense of nutation for fat resonances is reversed with alternate pulses, and because the binomial distribution is symmetric, the net flip angle is zero. For the water resonances, the pulses are additive, such that the net flip angle is the sum of the individual pulses. For example, with a 1:2:1 excitation scheme, if each unit contains enough energy for a flip of α, the maximal achievable flip angle is 4α for spins on resonance (Fig. 4–7). To excite and then spoil the fat resonances, the RF phase would be alternated (e.g., from x to $-$x) so that the phase of the RF always coincides with the phase of the fat spins and the net flip angle for water is zero.

Better spectral selectivity is achieved with higher order binomial schemes such as 1:3:3:1 or higher. However, the time penalty can be costly, and in some cases the minimal TR of a gradient-echo sequence may be more than doubled. This may have undesirable effects not only on acquisition time but also on image contrast in sequences that depend on steady-state effects. The simplest binomial series is a 1:1 "jump return," where one species sees $\theta/2:\theta/2 = \theta$ and the other sees $\theta/2: -\theta/2 = 0$. This approach has been extended by Thomasson and coworkers,[34] who offset

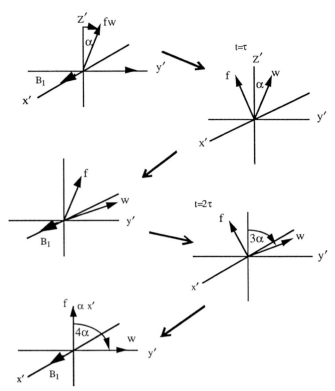

FIGURE 4–7. A 1:2:1 binomial water-selective pulse sequence. Fat spins (**f**) and water spins (**w**) evolve a π phase shift in a time τ. When a series of pulses are applied at intervals of τ, the effects on fat and water spins are opposite, so the flip angle for water sums to 90° whereas that for fat is zero.

the phase of the second RF pulse by $\pi/2$ or less, shortening the interpulse delay by a factor of 2 or more. They achieved a substantial time saving in short-TR three-dimensional (3D) gradient-echo sequences and extended the concept to spatial-spectral excitation.[35]

Practical Considerations in Radiofrequency Pulse Design

As summarized in Equation 12, the integral of the $\mathbf{B}_1$ field over time determines the flip angle, and that required for a π pulse is twice that needed for a $\pi/2$ pulse. In practice, one typically fixes the duration of the RF pulse and calibrates the $\mathbf{B}_1$ intensity. The RF transmitter voltage may be adjusted so that the output that causes the first signal maximum is defined as a $\pi/2$ pulse. A more widely used algorithm finds the first signal minimum and defines this as a π pulse; a $\pi/2$ pulse is half this value. It follows that a flip α can be reached with a short pulse of intense $\mathbf{B}_1$ or a longer pulse of less intense $\mathbf{B}_1$. In most situations, it is desirable to achieve α as quickly as possible. However, a number of factors considered later may limit how quickly this can be achieved:

- The peak voltage of the RF transmitter sets a limit on the $\mathbf{B}_1$ field intensity, such that the flip angle required may not be reached in the allotted time.

- For spatially selective pulses, the slice profile becomes degraded with truncation. The availability of strong slice-selection gradients helps to offset this limitation, but it must still be considered.
- For clinical imaging, the specific absorption rate for RF energy must remain within allowed limits. Shorter RF pulses require higher power, and therefore higher specific absorption rate values, to attain the same flip angle as longer pulses.

It is clear from Equation 12 that if the $\mathbf{B}_1$ field is not homogeneous in the volume of interest, α is not a single flip angle but is a distribution of flip angles. This may have unwanted effects on image contrast.

GRADIENT EVENTS

Magnetic field gradients are used in MRI to encode spatial information. The Larmor equation states that the precessional frequency (ω) of a spin is directly proportional to the magnetic field strength (**B**):

$$\omega = \gamma \mathbf{B} \qquad (22)$$

The mapping of position to frequency by a magnetic field gradient follows directly from the Larmor equation. A spatial variation in the magnetic field causes a corresponding spatial variation in precessional frequency. The gradient field (**G**) is produced by pulsing current through some combination of coils to generate three spatially orthogonal, linear variations in the main field (G_x, G_y, and G_z). Whereas the main magnetic field, $\mathbf{B}_0$, is generally fixed in direction and magnitude, the gradient field **G** can assume a range of values.

It should be emphasized at this point that the field generated by the gradient coils is in the direction of the main field (z), so that the magnitude of the $\mathbf{B}_z$ field is made to be a function of position along the direction of the gradient. For example, if the slice-selection direction is the sagittal plane, the slice-selection gradient $\mathbf{G}_s$ is along the x direction and is defined by

$$\mathbf{G}_s = \frac{\partial \mathbf{B}_z}{\partial s} = \frac{\partial \mathbf{B}_z}{\partial x} = \mathbf{G}_x \qquad (23)$$

Thus, "gradient" refers to the rate of change of the $\mathbf{B}_z$ field in the specified direction. Following Equation 23, when the x gradient $\mathbf{G}_x$ is active, the net field $\mathbf{B}_{net}$ has components from the main field, $\mathbf{B}_0$, and $\mathbf{G}_x$ such that

$$\mathbf{B}_{net} = \mathbf{B}_0 + x\mathbf{G}_x \qquad (24)$$

and combining with Equation 22 yields

$$\omega_x = \gamma(\mathbf{B}_0 + x\mathbf{G}_x) \qquad (25)$$

Equation 25 expresses resonance frequency as a linear function of position along the gradient direction, where x is the offset from the magnet isocenter. At the isocenter, the net field is $\mathbf{B}_0$ at all times, because x (and therefore $x\mathbf{G}_x$) is zero. The actual field at any position within the magnet bore is the sum of contributions from all sources including the main field, applied gradients, and intrinsic susceptibility gradients.

In the preceding example, $\mathbf{G}_s$ happens to coincide with the x gradient direction. It may, however, assume any orientation, and the physical meaning of $\mathbf{G}_s$ is defined by the slice plane chosen at the time of the measurement. For an arbitrary orientation (e.g., double oblique plane), $\mathbf{G}_s$ may have contributions from all three orthogonal gradient sets, as represented by

$$\mathbf{G}_s = G_x\mathbf{i} + G_y\mathbf{j} + G_z\mathbf{k} \qquad (26)$$

Similar considerations apply to the "read" and "phase-encode" gradients.

For clinical machines, the maximal gradient strength typically lies in the range 10 to 25 mT/m. In typical imaging systems, the gradient field is about two orders of magnitude smaller than the main field. For example, if $\mathbf{B}_0$ is 1.5 T, the maximal field caused by the gradients is about ± 2.5 to ± 6.5 mT, assuming maximal gradient amplitudes in the range 10 to 25 mT/m over a linear range of ± 25 cm (Fig. 4–8). The gradient in frequency corresponding to the field gradient is given by $\gamma/2\pi G$, where γ is the gyromagnetic ratio. For G = 10 mT/m = 10^{-5} T/mm, the frequency gradient is therefore 426 Hz/mm.

SLICE SELECTION

One of the primary advantages of MRI over other imaging modalities is the ability to image planes or slices of tissue with effectively any arbitrary orientation, thickness, and position. The process of slice selection is carried out by applying band-limited RF energy simultaneously with a magnetic field gradient. A slice is defined by its

- Orientation, determined by the gradient direction
- Thickness, determined by the interplay between gradient amplitude and RF bandwidth
- Offset (position along the slice-selection direction), determined by the modulation of the RF

To excite a slice plane, the resonance frequency of the spin system along the slice-selection direction (ω_s) is made to vary linearly with position by a slice-selection field gradient $\mathbf{G}_s$ superimposed on the main field $\mathbf{B}_0$:

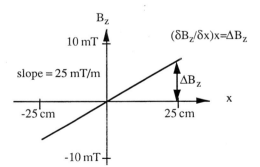

FIGURE 4–8. Gradient field. Magnetic field gradient causes the frequency at position x to change by x(δG/δx). The field experienced by spins far off center in the positive direction is therefore greater than that seen by spins close to the magnet isocenter. As illustrated, the gradient strength is 25 mT/m.

$$\omega_s = \gamma\mathbf{B}_0 + \mathbf{G}_s \qquad (27)$$

A slice of a given thickness therefore contains spins precessing over a range of frequencies—the *bandwidth*, Δf. By pulsing RF only in this frequency range, the slice of interest can be selectively excited. The slice thickness (d) is related to the RF bandwidth by

$$d = \frac{\Delta\omega}{\gamma G_s} = \frac{2\pi\Delta f}{\gamma G_s} \qquad (28)$$

Inspection of Equation 28 reveals that for a given bandwidth,

- Stronger gradients produce thinner slices

and for a given gradient amplitude,

- Narrower bandwidths (longer pulses) produce thinner slices

The task is now reduced to limiting the excitation to a frequency band covering no more than the desired slice thickness.

SLICE PROFILE

Ideally, one would fully excite all magnetization, **M**, within the slice of interest and leave everything outside the slice unaffected. The formal representation of this arrangement is a square wave, where **M** has its full value for all frequencies within the specified bandwidth, $\pm f_0$, and is zero for f greater than $|f_0|$. We must now prescribe an RF pulse waveform, played out over time, having this well-defined frequency bandwidth. The frequency content of any time waveform is described by its Fourier transform, such that

$$P(f) = \int_{-\infty}^{\infty} p(t)e^{-j2\pi ft}\, dt \qquad (29)$$

where $P(f)$ is the amplitude of the sinusoid whose frequency is f and $P(t)$ is the amplitude of the time waveform at time t. $P(f)$ and $p(t)$ define a Fourier transform pair $p(t) \Leftrightarrow P(f)$. For in-depth background on Fourier transforms and their applications, the interested reader is referred to two excellent texts.[36, 37] It must be noted that the Fourier transform relationship between the RF pulse envelope and the resultant magnetization holds only for flip angles less than approximately 30°. The nonlinearity of the Bloch equations must be accounted for at higher flip angles.[38] Nevertheless, the Fourier transform offers a good first approximation to the response of the spin system to RF excitation in the presence of a linear field gradient.

Equation 29 tells us that if we require a specific frequency domain waveform P(f) (defined for present purposes as a square wave), we need to apply a time domain RF pulse given by the integral on the right-hand side of Equation 29. This is evaluated as a sinc function of infinite duration, defined by sinc(t) = $\sin(\pi t)/\pi t$, and illustrated in Figure 4–9. Nodes or zero crossings occur when the argument of the sinc function is an integral multiple of π, and the function is even with a maximum at t = 0. The bandwidth of

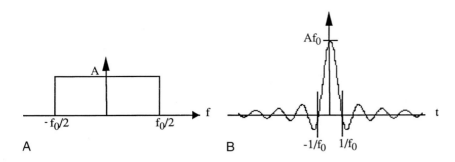

FIGURE 4–9. Slice selection. Rectangular frequency band *(A)* and its Fourier transform *(B)*. A sinc RF profile over time produces a well-defined spectrum in the frequency domain. The vertical lines in *B* denote the times of the first zero crossings, which determine the bandwidth, $\pm (f_0/2)$. The nodes of the sinc function in this example occur at integer multiples of $1/f_0$. The example illustrated assumes the sinc function is infinite, not truncated.

the RF pulse is $\Delta f = \pm f_0$, and this in turn is defined by the (reciprocal) time to the first zero crossing in the sinc function.

- The broader the sinc function, the narrower the bandwidth, and vice versa.

If we fix the gradient at 10 mT/m (426 Hz/mm), a 5-mm slice spans a 2.1-kHz range of resonance frequencies. The sinc function that produces a 5-mm-thick slice has a bandwidth of 2.1 kHz and has its first zero crossing 470 μs after maximal amplitude. If the gradient is increased to 25 mT/m (1064.5 Hz/mm), a 2.1-kHz band covers only 2 mm, and the same pulse and bandwidth now excite a slice only 2.0 mm thick. To excite a 2.0-mm slice using a 10 mT/m gradient, the RF pulse must have a bandwidth of 852 Hz and its first zero crossing 1175 μs after maximal amplitude.

The definition of the Fourier transform considered here assumes that the RF pulse is played out over infinite time! This is, of course, impractical, and for many applications severe constraints are placed on the time available for RF excitation. A typical pulse lasts several milliseconds and may last as little as a few hundred microseconds. The result of truncating the RF pulse is a distortion or "rippling" of the slice

profile. Truncation can be described mathematically as the multiplication of an infinite-duration pulse (p(t)) with a square wave of unit amplitude (a(t)). Equation 30,

$$F(p(t)a(t)) = P(f) \otimes A(f) \qquad (30)$$

where F represents the Fourier transform and $\otimes$ is the convolution operator, is the frequency-convolution theorem. It tells us that for two functions p(t) and a(t), the Fourier transform of the product p(t)a(t) is the convolution of the individual transforms, P(f) and A(f). That is, multiplication in one domain corresponds to convolution in the other domain.

From inspection of Figure 4–10, we can see that

- The slice profile is expressed by the convolution of the square wave P(f) and the sinc function A(f).
- Convolution with the sinc causes blunting and rippling of the slice profile, and the amount of deviation from ideal square wave behavior is inversely related to the width of the truncation function.
- In the limit as the truncation function gets wider (approaching infinite time), its transform (sinc) gets narrower and approaches an impulse; convolution of any function with the unit impulse yields

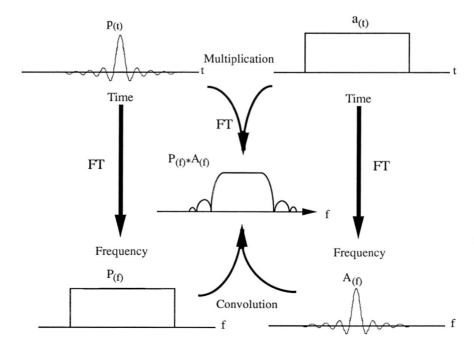

FIGURE 4–10. Slice profile. Slice profile resulting from truncated RF pulse. Because the RF pulse is truncated in time, the frequency convolution theorem implies that the attenuated sinc RF pulse transforms not to the square wave P(f) but to the convolution of P(f) with the transform A(f) of the sampling envelope a(t). This effect introduces ripples into the edges of the slice, most pronounced for extremely short pulses.

the original function. So, the longer the duration of a sinc RF pulse (or the more zero crossings), the better the slice profile.

In practice, one cannot spend too long playing out the RF, and the slice profile may be improved by filtering in the time domain. Most commonly, the amplitude of the RF time envelope is weighted with a gaussian or Hanning filter function, smoothing out the ripples at the expense of widening the main central lobe of the profile. One can use a gaussian RF envelope directly in the time domain, and this produces a gaussian slice profile, formally described by

$$p(t) = e^{-(t^2/2\sigma^2)} \Leftrightarrow P(f) = \sqrt{2\pi}\sigma e^{(-2\pi^2 f^2 \sigma^2)} \quad (31)$$

where σ is the standard deviation of the distribution. Again,

- A broad function in the time domain is a narrow function in the frequency domain and vice versa.

Recall that another factor of practical importance in improving the slice profile is the strength of the slice-selection gradient. Because of the Larmor relationship between magnetic field strength and precessional frequency, a field gradient can be expressed in terms of hertz per millimeter. Thus, if the gradient is stronger, for a given slice thickness the bandwidth in the RF pulse is greater. This means more zero crossings can be used for the same pulse duration, decreasing truncation effects. So stronger gradients can be used to get either thinner slices for a given pulse duration and bandwidth, better slice profiles for a given pulse duration and slice thickness, or shorter RF pulses for a given slice profile and thickness.

As the bandwidth of the pulse increases, the peak transmitter power must increase to achieve the same flip angle. For a given flip angle α,

$$\alpha \propto A \int_{-\infty}^{\infty} p^2(t) \, dt = A \int_{-\infty}^{\infty} (P(f))^2 \, df \quad (32)$$

so that as the integral decreases, the amplitude A of the RF envelope must increase. The equivalence of the RF energy in the time domain and the frequency domain (Parseval's theorem) is expressed in Equation 32.

Digitization Constraints

The arguments put forward so far are valid for a pulse envelope with a continuous range of values over the truncation interval. However, pulse envelopes are specified digitally by a finite number of support points as digital-to-analog converter values over the duration of the RF pulse. As a result, synthesized pulse waveforms are subject to the limitations of discrete sampling—specifically, aliasing—and they must be designed with this in mind.

- According to the Nyquist theorem, frequency ambiguity occurs for frequencies greater than half the sampling rate.

The waveform is reproduced periodically in the positive and negative frequency domain. The high-frequency copies of the pulse waveform are filtered out by low-pass filters—hardware crystals with a well-defined frequency response. For example, if the pulse duration is 5120 μs and there are 512 sample points, the sampling frequency is 10^{-5} s^{-1} = 100 kHz, and no aliasing occurs below 50 kHz. The low-pass filter cutoff frequency is therefore set at 50 kHz.

As pointed out earlier, for larger flip angles (>30°), the response of the spin system deviates from linearity and the slice profile can no longer be predicted simply by Fourier transformation of the RF envelope. This is particularly true for 180° pulses. In practice, optimization by numerical methods is often utilized in RF pulse design.

Modulation

In addition to defining the thickness of the slice, its offset or displacement along the gradient axis needs to be specified. This is done by modulating the RF waveform with a sinusoid of the appropriate carrier frequency f_m:

$$p(t)e^{j2\pi f_m t} \Leftrightarrow P(f - f_m) \quad (33)$$

Equation 33 shows that multiplication by a sinusoid in the time domain shifts the frequency envelope of the pulse without distorting its shape. The bandwidth (and slice thickness) is the same, but it is now centered at $f = f_m$, not $f = 0$. By making f_m continuously variable, any slice shift can be defined. The frequency offset, f_m, that corresponds to a slice position x is given by

$$f_m = \frac{xG(x)\gamma}{2\pi} \quad (34)$$

As an example, if G(x) is 10 mT/m and x is 20 cm, f_m is 85.2 kHz. Because it is necessary to be able to shift the slice several times its thickness, the modulation frequency (slice shift in hertz) is usually significantly greater than the bandwidth (slice thickness in hertz). In practice, modulation may be performed by applying an incremented phase change over time to the RF pulse envelope. For example, assume that we have a 5.12-ms sinc pulse defined by 512 discrete points at 10-μs intervals. The phase at each point is incremented by

$$\varphi = \frac{2\pi\tau f_m}{\text{number of points}} \quad (35)$$

where φ is in radians, τ is the duration of the RF pulse in seconds, and f_m is the modulation frequency in hertz.

Gradient Refocusing

When an RF pulse is applied in the presence of a field gradient, the spins within the slice have a distribution of frequencies determined by their position along the gradient axis. The phases therefore fan out across the slice, but they can be brought back into alignment by a reverse gradient.

- When the RF pulse is complete and the gradient is turned off, a representative spin at position **r** has accumulated a phase, ϕ_r, according to

$$\phi_r = \gamma \int_0^t \mathbf{G}_s \cdot \mathbf{r} \, dt \qquad (36)$$

Equation 36 refers only to magnetization lying in the x-y plane, and before excitation all magnetization is assumed to lie along z. The flip angle within the slice ranges from 0 at the start of the RF pulse to some angle $\alpha \le \pi/2$ at the end. An approximation used in slice-selection gradient waveform design is that the transverse magnetization is generated instantaneously halfway through the RF pulse. To determine the phase accumulated by stationary spins during slice selection, the limits of integration in Equation 36 are set from the center of the RF pulse to the end of the slice-selection gradient. This phase can be "unwound" by a gradient of equal and opposite area as shown in Figure 4–11.

IN-PLANE SPATIAL ENCODING

An MR image is a map of the spatial distribution of spins. Conventionally, the imaging volume is mapped onto a 3D cartesian grid, the axes of which are labeled generically read, phase encode, and slice selection. The basis of spatial encoding with MRI is that the Larmor frequency depends on the magnetic field experienced by the spins. When this field is made to vary

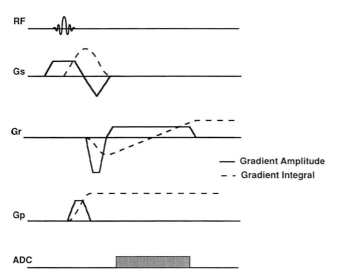

FIGURE 4–11. Gradient refocusing. During slice selection, the phases of the spins are dispersed over the width of the slice. For stationary spins, these phases are unwound by a rephrasing lobe equal to half the area of the primary lobe and of opposite sign. In the read direction, the phase dispersion caused by the first lobe is reversed by the rephasing lobe at the gradient echo. As long as the integral of the second lobe exactly counterbalances the first lobe, the relative durations of the gradient lobes may be different. The duration of the readout lobe can therefore be expanded or contracted and its amplitude changed accordingly. In this way the bandwidth of the detected signal may be modified. In the phase-encode direction, a unipolar pulse imparts a constant phase to spins, proportional to position along the gradient axis.

with position by a gradient, the local frequency is also made to vary in a known way. By means of the Fourier transform, it is possible to unravel the spectrum of frequencies generated by the encoding gradient and derive from them a map of signal amplitude versus position.

We assume for the moment that the process of slice selection has reduced the task to encoding the remaining two dimensions of the slice plane. In this case, the resolution in the slice direction is reflected directly by the slice thickness in millimeters.

FREQUENCY ENCODING AND K-SPACE

As discussed earlier, the application of a field gradient makes the precessional frequency a function of position along the gradient axis. Analogous to slice selection, when a linear gradient $\mathbf{G}(r)$ is applied in the read direction, the precessional frequency $\omega(r)$ of a spin at position r along this direction is in the rotating frame

$$\omega(r) = \gamma \mathbf{G}(r)r = 2\pi \mathbf{f}(r) \qquad (37)$$

where $\omega(r)$ is in radians per second and $\mathbf{f}(r)$ is in hertz. For a read gradient $\mathbf{G}(r)$,

- The precessional frequency in a plane perpendicular to $\mathbf{G}(r)$ at a displacement r from the isocenter is uniquely defined. The signal amplitude at a given frequency is proportional to the number of spins at that frequency, as determined by the Fourier transform of the time domain signal.

Immediately after a 90° excitation pulse and ignoring relaxation and flow effects, the signal S sampled at time t after the application of a linear gradient G(r) is given by

$$S(t) = C \int \rho(r) \exp\left[j\gamma r \left(\int_0^t G(r) \, dt \right) \right] dr \qquad (38)$$

where C is a proportionality constant that includes such factors as coil sensitivity and receiver bandwidth and p(r) is the spin density as a function of position. By reference to Equation 29, it can be seen that S(t) and p(r) are a Fourier transform pair, so that Fourier transformation of the time domain signal gives the spin distribution p(r).

Here we introduce the concept of *k-space*[39] or *frequency space* as the representation of the gradient-encoded image before Fourier transformation. The raw time signal contains all the information about the frequency distribution of the spins in the direction of the read gradient, but it must be transformed from a map of signal versus spatial frequency into a readable image as signal versus position. Each value of k is proportional to the zeroth time moment (or area), which is determined by the strength and duration of the gradient waveform (Equation 39). A list of such values (spatial frequencies) is collected in the gradient direction to be input to the Fourier transform.

Defining

$$k(r) = \gamma \int_0^t G(r) \, dt \qquad (39)$$

and substituting into Equation 38 gives

$$S(t) = C \int \rho(r) e^{jk(r)r} \, dr \qquad (40)$$

With reference to Equation 40,

- k(r) has the dimension of inverse distance or spatial frequency.
- When k(r) is multiplied by a position coordinate r, the result is a phase determined by the magnitudes of k(r) and r (analogous to the product of temporal frequency and time).
- The temporal sequence in which values for k(r) are encoded is termed the k-space trajectory (Fig. 4–12). However, the same value of k(r) can be arrived at in a variety of ways, with the trajectory controlled by gradient waveforms. This may have an indirect effect on the image in several ways (e.g., contrast and motion sensitivity).
- The FOV is the longest finite spatial wavelength (reciprocal of spatial frequency) that can be encoded with discrete sampling. This corresponds to the minimal nonzero value of k. If N discretely sampled data points are acquired equally spaced at intervals Δt during a constant-amplitude read gradient, FOV in the frequency encoded direction can be defined as

$$FOV = 1/(\Delta k) = 1/(\gamma G \Delta t) \qquad (41)$$

- In the spatial frequency domain, small values of k (low spatial frequencies) are linked to large objects in the image space. For a gradient to rotate the phase through 2π across an object, the object must have a linear dimension $\lambda = 2\pi/k$ along the direction of the gradient. The maximal value of k defines the smallest dimension encoded; therefore, k_{max} defines the spatial resolution (Δx). Again, assuming equidistant discrete sampling and equal coverage of negative and positive spatial frequencies, the resolution in the read direction can be defined as

$$\Delta x = 2/(N\Delta k) = 2/(\gamma G N \Delta t) \qquad (42)$$

- Equations 41 and 42 define the basic relationships between FOV and resolution, as well as the read gradient strength (G), duration ($N\Delta t$), and sampling bandwidth ($1/\Delta t$).

Sampling the Signal

If the read gradient is turned on and the signal is sampled immediately after excitation, a free induction decay is acquired. Usually, a dephasing read gradient is applied before the rephasing read gradient, and an echo rather than a free induction decay is acquired. A gradient echo is said to occur when the dephasing effect of one gradient lobe is exactly balanced by the rephasing effect of another. For this to occur, the two counterbalancing gradient pulses must subtend equal

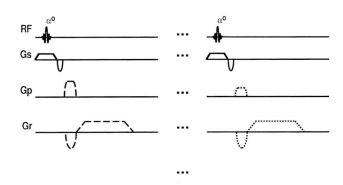

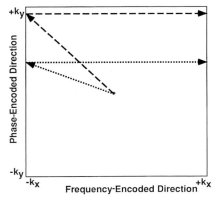

FIGURE 4–12. 2D FLASH k-space trajectory. Prephasing lobes in the phase-encode (k_y) and read (k_x) directions assign the spins to the top left corner of the 2D k-space matrix. The read component is unwound by the rephasing read gradient during signal sampling, causing the k trajectory to run from left to right across the matrix. For the next phase-encode step, the amplitude of the phase-encoding gradient is decreased, so that the k_y offset is diminished at the start of the readout period. A table of such incremental offsets spans the k_y axis from maximal negative through zero to maximal positive values. At each value of k_y, an otherwise identical set of points is acquired along k_x. The trajectory is therefore a horizontal raster in the read direction, incremented in the vertical direction by each phase-encoding iteration, analogous to scanning lines of print. The gradient echo occurs halfway along k_x, and the maximal signal is generated when k_y is zero, corresponding to zero amplitude of the phase-encoding gradient. The k_y values close to zero are low spatial frequencies, generally regarded as the primary determinants of image contrast.

areas of opposite sign. In the simplest gradient-echo measurement, a read gradient preparatory lobe is applied immediately after RF excitation, as shown in Figure 4–11. This causes the spins to evolve a phase given by Equation 36, proportional to the gradient area or k-space value as described earlier. If a gradient of opposite polarity is now applied, the spins rephase when the area under the second lobe is the same size as that of the first. As the area of the second lobe exceeds that of the first, the process of spin dephasing recurs, as shown in Figure 4–11. By acquiring data from the start of the rephasing gradient lobe, the buildup and decay of the magnetization can be sampled. During the first half of the rephasing lobe, the free induction decay is rebuilt to (potentially) its original amplitude, and during the second half it becomes dephased again.[1]

In the laboratory frame, the raw time signal is in megahertz. This is down modulated to frequencies in the audio range by a sinusoid at the Larmor frequency. The bandwidth in the signal is then determined by the frequency distribution around the Larmor frequency associated with the read gradient. Although a continuous range of frequencies is contained in the analog signal, the signal is sampled discretely and is digitized by an analog-to-digital converter at a rate determined by the signal bandwidth.

To prevent aliasing, the sampling rate must be at least twice the bandwidth. For example, 256 complex points are typically sampled during the readout period (analog-to-digital converter ON time) by a quadrature detector (see Chapter 14). If the readout time is 5.12 ms and 256 complex points are sampled (256 real and 256 imaginary), the sampling rate is 100 kHz and the resolvable bandwidth is 50 kHz (± 25 kHz). Low-pass filters are set to exclude signal (and noise) outside the sampled frequency bandwidth.

Occasionally, the sampling rate is inadequate to prevent aliasing of parts outside the region of interest. The low-pass filters are not effective, because the signal is wrapped around into the low-frequency range and appears as a phantom limb or other body part. The only way to prevent this phenomenon is to sample rapidly enough that the unwanted signal is correctly localized outside the imaging bandwidth. If the sampling frequency is doubled, an FOV twice as large can be correctly localized. Overfolding is therefore prevented by oversampling the signal, which effectively increases the FOV but does not change the resolution, S/N ratio, or gradient strength. Resolution is determined only by the k value as described earlier. Oversampling increases both the number of pixels and FOV proportionately.

It is convenient to normalize the sampling bandwidth to the number of pixels in the read direction, so that a 50-kHz bandwidth corresponds to 50,000/256 = 195 Hz/pixel in a 5.12-ms readout time. If the readout time is 10.24 ms, the bandwidth is 97.5 Hz/pixel and so on. This nomenclature is desirable because

- The bandwidth in hertz per pixel is not influenced by oversampling or variations in matrix size.
- The fat-water displacement caused by chemical shift can be conveniently expressed in pixels.

For extremely high bandwidth sequences, digitization of the signal must be fast. In echo-planar imaging (EPI), for example, with a typical sampling bandwidth of 1667 Hz/pixel (corresponding to a 600-μs readout window) and a 16-bit analog-to-digital converter, the digitizer must be able to handle at least 4 megabytes per second. If multiple channels are used simultaneously in a phased-array coil, this number goes up proportionately. The rates are correspondingly increased if oversampling is used.

Chemical-Shift Artifact

Protons in fat precess about 3.3 ppm more slowly than those in water (see the section on chemical-shift–

selective RF pulses). Therefore, at any given position in the read direction, fat spins have a frequency offset from water of 3.3 times the main field in megahertz, or 210 Hz at 1.5 T. This offset is fixed and is independent of readout bandwidth. Therefore, if the bandwidth is 210 Hz/pixel or greater, the fat image is shifted one pixel or less downfield of the water, and this is generally acceptable. If, however, much narrower bandwidths are used, the fat-water shift can be several pixels, and this may result in an unacceptable artifact. At the extreme, with single-shot EPI, a severe chemical shift artifact occurs in the phase-encode direction, where the bandwidth may be as low as 10 Hz/pixel. This would result in a fat-water displacement of more than 20 pixels! Fat suppression is therefore mandatory in EPI.

Signal-to-Noise Ratio Considerations

The S/N ratio increases in proportion to the square root of the time spent sampling the signal. More time is spent sampling when the bandwidth is narrow and when more acquisitions are averaged. For a voxel of dimensions dx dy dz, the S/N ratio is

$$\frac{S}{N} = k\, dx\, dy\, dz\, \sqrt{\frac{N_x N_y N_{acq}}{\Delta f}} \qquad (43)$$

where N_x and N_y are the numbers of samples in dimensions x and y, N_{acq} is the number of acquisitions, Δf is the bandwidth, and k is a constant that includes all other factors such as coil sensitivity, subject loading, field strength, and relaxation effects. It can be seen from Equation 43 that the S/N ratio scales as the size of the voxels and as the square root of the sampling time.

PHASE ENCODING

Phase encoding is a process whereby a spatially dependent phase shift in a direction orthogonal to the read gradient is introduced by an additional gradient pulse. A series of such phase-modulated echoes generated by a table of sequential pulses, as shown in Figures 4–13 and 4–14, forms the basis for spatial encoding in this second dimension. Each phase-modulated echo translates to one spatial frequency in the phase-encoding direction, so the process must be repeated N times to encode N spatial frequencies. This differs from the read direction, where N values of k are encoded during a single pulse of the read gradient (a single readout period). We now consider this in more detail.

We have seen that a given value of k for a spin at position r results in a predictable phase shift. However, as pointed out earlier, the definition of k as used in Equation 39 makes no assumptions about how k was generated. Moreover, the expression is a generic one, equally applicable to any spatial orientation. Recall that k is proportional to the gradient-time integral, so

- k may be made a function of time if the gradient

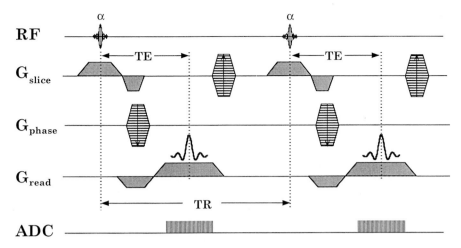

FIGURE 4–13. 2D FLASH sequence structure. After slice selection, the rephasing slice-selection, dephasing read, and phase-encoding gradients are applied simultaneously. This is followed by the rephasing read gradient and signal sample window (ADC on time). To destroy coherent magnetization between excitations, a gradient spoiling table is applied after data acquisition. RF spoiling is typically also employed with this structure.

is constant and time is incremented, as is the case during readout, or

- k may be made a function of gradient strength, G, if the time is constant and the gradient amplitude is incremented

Now suppose that $k(p)$ defines a gradient event in the phase-encoding direction y orthogonal to read; then the phase of the echo is modulated as

$$\phi(p) = \gamma \int_0^t G(p) y \, dt = k_{py} \qquad (44)$$

Application of one such gradient event simply shifts the phase of the echo from each pixel in the read direction by an amount determined by the mean contribution from all y offsets, and this provides no useful information. However, if $k(p)$ is successively incremented in value by $\Delta k(p)$ during a series of measurements, the phase at position y undergoes periodic change as a function of $k(p)$. This is analogous to the periodic phase change at position r in the read direction as a function of $k(r)$. Therefore, when $k(p)$ steps through a table of 256 values from $-k(p)_{max}$ to $+k(p)_{max}$ in 256 equal increments $\Delta k(p)$ and $k(r)$ steps through the same set of values under the read gradient, then successive two-dimensional (2D) Fou-

rier transformation along the read and phase-encoding directions yields an image with isotropic spatial resolution.

Although the processes of spatial encoding in the read and phase-encoding directions are mathematically similar, physically they are different and prone to different artifacts. In conventional spin-warp imaging, adjacent values of k along the read direction are typically separated in time by about 20 μs, and this is not long enough for significant changes to occur in the status of the magnetization. In the phase-encoding direction, however, the interval between successive k values is typically the TR of the sequence. Depending on the sequence structure, TR ranges from tens of milliseconds to several seconds, and during this interval substantial changes may occur to the amplitude and phase of the MR signal. The sampled function may therefore be modulated by a variety of mechanisms, and the function modulating the signal is convolved in the reconstructed image. Depending on the nature of the changes (e.g., motion, flow, nonuniform relaxation effects), they may be manifest in the image as a loss of resolution, altered contrast, or, in the case of periodic fluctuations, ghost artifact projected along the phase-encoding direction. In practice, phase en-

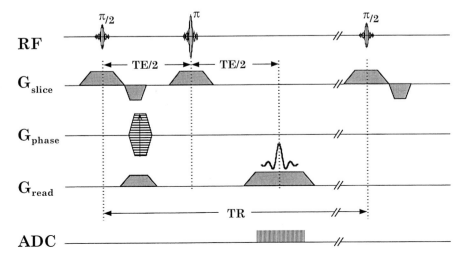

FIGURE 4–14. Spin-echo pulse sequence diagram. After a $\pi/2$ excitation pulse, a π refocusing pulse is applied at TE/2. A spin echo occurs at TE as outlined in Figure 4–3. By comparison with Figure 4–13, note that the polarity of the dephasing read gradient is the same as that of the rephasing read gradient. This is a consequence of the π pulse, which inverts the phase of the echo.

coding is carried out by applying a gradient pulse for a time t_p after excitation and before readout. If t_p is constant and G_p is varied, the process is termed *spin-warp imaging*.[40] A 2D image is calculated by carrying out a 2D Fourier transform on the time domain data—first line by line, then column by column.

Speeding Up the Phase-Encoding Process

A practical point to note about phase encoding is that it is time-consuming. Whereas in the read direction all spatial frequencies are encoded in a matter of milliseconds, in the phase-encoding direction the process may take several minutes. It is the iterative nature of phase encoding and the influence of longitudinal relaxation that necessitate the use of a TR in pulse sequences. Total acquisition time is determined by TR × N × Acq, where N is the number of phase-encode iterations and Acq is the number of acquisitions or averages (Acq is more than 1 if the S/N ratio needs to be boosted or motion artifacts need to be averaged out). Depending on the required contrast in the image, spins may need to relax for a longer or shorter time between phase-encode steps. For pure T2-weighted images, the TR should be several times the longest T1 in the region of interest. This typically includes water, so TR should be several seconds. Conventional T2-weighted images are therefore time intensive. In the case of IR imaging, the requirements for a long TR are even more stringent. T1-weighted spin-echo measurements are designed to suppress partially the signal from long-T1 tissues, so these are done with a relatively short TR—usually 300 to 600 ms.

RECTANGULAR FIELD OF VIEW. Because the high-cost item in terms of acquisition time is the number of iterations of the excitation process (the number of repetitions of TR), time can be saved by decreasing this number. Reducing the FOV in the phase-encoding direction by phase encoding along the short axis of the subject (rectangular FOV) yields equivalent spatial resolution in a shorter imaging time. For example, if the FOV in the read direction is 350 mm with 256 points in read and the FOV in the PE direction is 175 mm, then 128 PE steps yield an image with square

pixels; the imaging time is halved. Because the S/N ratio is proportional to the square root of the number of phase-encode steps, there is a penalty in the S/N ratio with this method, depending on the aspect ratio. Where the S/N ratio is not limiting, the technique is successful.

ACQUIRING MULTIPLE LINES PER EXCITATION. In conventional gradient-echo and spin-echo imaging (see Figs. 4–13 and 4–14), one line of k-space is acquired per α or 90° pulse, and the number of iterations required is equal to the number of phase-encoding steps. If transverse magnetization persists after the signal is read, in principle this can be used to encode further echoes. By reapplying the read gradients, interleaved with additional PE gradients, several Fourier lines can be acquired in much less time than with conventional encoding. Two extreme forms of this process include the single-shot techniques of EPI[41, 42] and RARE. Intermediate between conventional and single-shot techniques are the hybrid fast imaging methods of turbo or fast spin-echo and segmented EPI. All of these methods are considered in more detail later.

Three-Dimensional Encoding

Phase encoding can also be applied to the slice-selection direction to add a third dimension of spatial encoding. If a thick slab rather than a thin slice is selected, the slab can be resolved into thin slices (partitions) by incrementing a phase-encoding table in this direction, analogous to the 2D case. The number of iterations (excitations) required to encode a 3D image is N_yN_z, where N_y and N_z refer to the numbers of iterations in the phase-encoding and slice-selection directions, respectively. A 3D gradient-echo pulse sequence is diagrammed in Figure 4–15. With conventional acquisition, the minimal time required for this process is TR × N_y × N_z. Because acquisition times with long TR sequences would be prohibitively long, the applications of 3D imaging techniques were formerly limited to fast gradient-echo techniques.

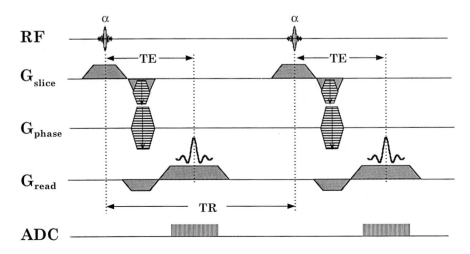

FIGURE 4–15. 3D gradient-echo pulse sequence. The basic structure differs from the 2D case in the addition of a phase-encoding table in the slice-selection direction. The amplitude of the slice-selection gradient is generally smaller and slice thickness correspondingly greater than in the 2D case. Slice selection is therefore quicker, and the minimal TE is shorter than with 2D imaging. The 3D gradient table may be applied as a list of offsets to the rephasing lobe of the slice-selection gradient, simultaneously with the dephasing read and in-plane phase-encoding gradients.

Phase-Encode Ordering

In conventional gradient-echo and spin-echo imaging, the magnetization is sampled in a steady state and no significant variations in the magnetization occur from one phase-encoded readout to the next. In this case, the order in which the phase-encoding table is stepped through is unimportant. However, in many fast imaging techniques, such as turbo fast low-angle shot (turboFLASH), segmented RARE, and EPI, the magnetization is not in a steady state during acquisition and relaxation causes a modulation of signal amplitude in the phase-encoded direction.[43-45] Image contrast is determined mainly by the low spatial frequencies (low phase-encode pulse amplitudes) and resolution by high spatial frequencies (high phase-encode pulse amplitudes). Thus, signal modulation can have a profound effect on the image contrast and effective resolution and can be manipulated by reordering the phase-encoding table.

In turboFLASH imaging (Fig. 4–16), an inversion preparation is typically applied, followed by a rapid gradient-echo acquisition of all of the image data during the IR of the longitudinal magnetization. The longitudinal magnetization may be negative for the initial phase-encoded steps, pass through a null point, and become positive for the remaining phase-encoded steps. Reordering the phase-encoding table so that the central lines are acquired at the zero point of magnetization recovery of specific tissues is a strategy used to "null" the signal from blood or specific organs. The "effective" inversion time (TI) is determined by the time between the inversion pulse and the acquisition of the central lines of k-space.

In multishot RARE (fast or turbo spin echo), a 90° excitation is followed by multiple 180° refocusing pulses and readouts (Fig. 4–17). T2 relaxation progressively attenuates the signal available with each readout. The "effective" TE of a segmented RARE sequence is determined by the echo that is encoded to provide the lowest spatial frequency information and, thus, the dominant image contrast characteristics.

Phase Accumulation

In most imaging pulse sequences, phase encoding of each echo is accomplished with a single discrete gradient pulse. The amplitude of the pulse is varied from echo to echo to encode a unique line of k-space

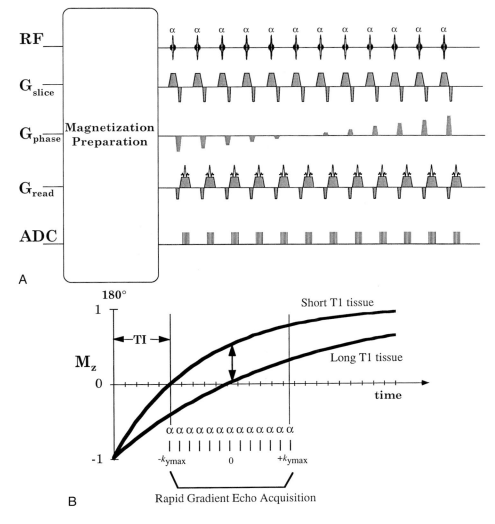

FIGURE 4–16. TurboFLASH pulse sequence diagram. After a single magnetization preparation phase (A), a fast FLASH sequence is played out. The time between the preparation event and the zero phase-encoding step (here illustrated halfway through the FLASH sequence) determines the image contrast. For example, in the case of inversion (B), the effective inversion time is the interval from the inversion pulse to the central phase-encode step (arrow). With centric phase-encode reordering, this step occurs at the beginning of the FLASH sequence, and the effective TI is the nominal TI.

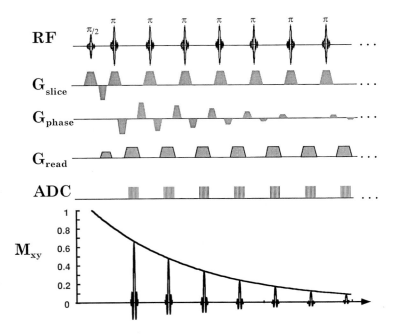

FIGURE 4–17. Turbo spin echo. TSE sequence diagram showing T2 decay that occurs from one echo to the next. The exact modulation function that this decay imposes on the image data is determined by the phase-encode ordering.

in each readout. The phase generated with each pulse is typically "rewound" with a pulse of equal and opposite area, or the phase-encoded transverse magnetization is dephased or "spoiled" after each readout. In this manner, no phase is accumulated from one echo to the next.

However, phase accumulation is an alternative means of phase encoding. This strategy is used in EPI in two modes: "blipped" phase encoding, in which a series of constant-amplitude gradient pulses are used for phase encoding, and constant phase encoding, in which a constant-amplitude gradient is applied throughout the entire acquisition. In both cases, phase accumulates from one echo to the next as the total area of the phase-encoding gradient increases. In EPI, the T2* relaxation modulates the MR signal from line to line (Figs. 4–18 and 4–19).

In EPI with constant phase encoding, it becomes difficult to distinguish the readout gradient from the phase-encoding gradient in the traditional sense. Both gradient axes are active during data acquisition. In fact, in examining the EPI sequence diagram in Figure 4–19, the similarity between the phase-encoding gradient and the readout gradient of a conventional gradient-echo sequence is apparent. Spiral scanning takes this blending of frequency and phase encoding one step further[46]; identical gradient waveforms (with a phase shift between the two) are applied to the two in-plane gradient axes, as shown in Figure 4–20. Data are sampled throughout as the gradient waveforms generate a spiral trajectory through k-space.

RADIOFREQUENCY PREPULSES

RF prepulses may be applied to spins inside or outside the FOV in a variety of forms and for a variety of reasons.

PREINVERSION

Conventional Inversion Recovery

Preinversion may be used to generate T1-based contrast, as in IR imaging. As originally implemented in spectroscopy, IR preparation was used to eliminate spectra from unwanted chemical species, based on their T1.

Immediately after inversion, all magnetization lies along the $-z$ axis and spins begin to relax exponentially toward $+z$. At the halfway stage, the z magnetization is zero, and no longitudinal magnetization is available to tip into the transverse plane (Fig. 4–21). The time between inversion and excitation pulse or TI appropriate to null a species is related to its T1 as TI $= 0.693$T1, for TR much greater than T1. A long TI is required to null long-T1 components, whereas short-T1 components are nulled in a short TI.

Spins with long T1 (e.g., in fluids such as cerebrospinal fluid) may still be aligned along $-z$ and have negative phase at the time of readout. With phase-sensitive reconstruction (as opposed to magnitude reconstruction), the phase as well as the amplitude of the signal is represented in the image. To spins with negative phase, a pixel intensity less than background is ascribed. Spins with positive phase have relaxed past zero (have short T1), and to these a pixel intensity greater than background is ascribed. So the order of pixel intensity for a long-TI, IR brain image (assuming phase-sensitive reconstruction) is white matter greater than gray matter greater than background greater than cerebrospinal fluid.

Because long-TI, IR imaging has poor slice efficiency and requires long acquisition times, it has come into clinical use only with the advent of segmented RARE techniques. However, short-TI (tau) IR (STIR) imaging has found many applications.[47, 48] In vivo, because spins with large T1 values also tend to have large T2

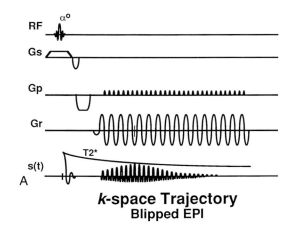

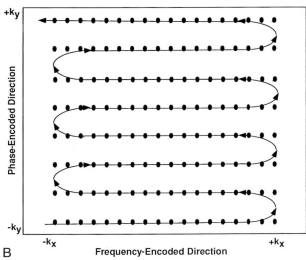

FIGURE 4–18. Blipped phase-encoding EPI pulse sequence *(A)*. The k-space is traversed by monotonic progression of phase from a series of small, discrete gradient pulses *(B)*. Of particular importance in EPI is the time reversal of the echoes from line to line. The k trajectory in read therefore alternates between left-right and right-left, and the blipped phase-encoding gradient increments the offset in k_y between lines. Without proper correction for phase drift between odd and even lines, N/2 ghosts may be severe.

values, contrast between long-T1, long-T2 and short-T1, short-T2 tissues is increased by superimposing T2 effects on a short-TI preparation. In practice, this is done by using a moderately long TE so that long-T2 components retain signal and short-T2 components do not. STIR imaging is generally done with magnitude reconstruction, because the shortest T1 tissues are near the null point and all other tissues have negative phase; the range in signal is therefore $-M_z$ to zero. Long-T1 and long-T2 tissues appear hyperintense compared with tissues with short T1 and short T2.

STIR is typically implemented with a TI value appropriate to null fat, so a narrow-bandwidth readout can be used to boost the S/N ratio without producing a chemical-shift artifact. The longer TE that accompanies long readout times has a beneficial rather than a deleterious effect on contrast with STIR, because the T1 and T2 effects are additive.

STIR has been shown to be an effective and sensitive

technique for detection of a variety of disorders in the liver,[48] brain,[48] and musculoskeletal system.[49] As a fat suppression technique, STIR is generally more robust than chemical-shift methods because it does not have stringent requirements for B_0 homogeneity and is not vulnerable to susceptibility gradients. It can, however, fail with poor B_1 homogeneity, and one must be careful in the design of inversion pulses. In general, one should use pulses that are B_1 insensitive, particularly with local transmit-receive coils.

Black Blood Preparation

As discussed earlier, blood can be nulled effectively with a nonselective inversion pulse, based on its T1 and independent of flow. A limitation of this process is that all spins in the slice plane are also inverted and have their contrast behavior so determined. Magnetization within the slice plane can be "reset" after inversion by a selective 180° pulse, as described by Edelman and colleagues[50] and shown in Figure 4–22. The effect

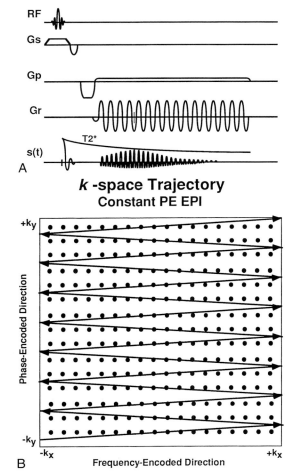

FIGURE 4–19. Constant phase-encoding EPI pulse sequence *(A)*. The k-space is traversed by accumulation of phase throughout a constant, low-amplitude gradient *(B)*. Because k_y is incremented continuously and not as a series of discrete steps as with blipped EPI, the k trajectory now oscillates obliquely rather than horizontally. This must be interpolated onto a cartesian k-space grid before Fourier transformation.

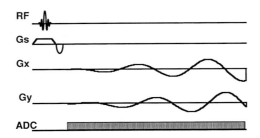

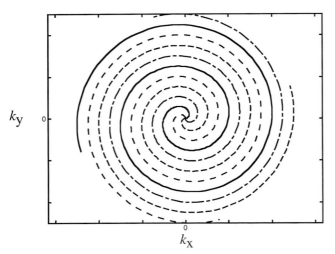

FIGURE 4–20. Spiral scanning. Readout occurs continuously during simultaneous application of sinusoidal read and phase-encoding gradients. A phase offset of $\pi/2$ between the gradients causes the k trajectory to describe a spiral, starting at $k_x = k_y = 0$. As illustrated, the data are acquired in an interleaved mode of four shots (analogous to turbo spin echo or segmented turboFLASH). Because the spins pass repeatedly through zero along k_x and k_y, phase accumulation caused by flow is reversed, and the resulting images are intrinsically flow compensated. Also, the low spatial frequencies are acquired early, so the minimal TE is small.

and then spoiling coherent magnetization with a crusher gradient. The effect persists until longitudinal magnetization is restored and so is T1 limited. The most common application for spatial presaturation is to eliminate artifact from flowing blood or to perform selective MR angiography (see Chapter 9). It can also be used to decrease signals from organs or soft tissues that are the source of motion artifact, such as the larynx or anterior abdominal fat.

MAGNETIZATION TRANSFER

Spins in the body result in a narrow or broad spectral peak depending on whether they have a long or short T2, respectively. Spins that are bound to macromolecules have a short T2 and a broad spectral peak. This pool can therefore be excited by RF irradiation centered anywhere in the spectrum. By the process of magnetization transfer, the energy is exchanged between the bound and unbound pools. Unbound spins, on the other hand, have a narrow-frequency bandwidth and must be excited at or near the Larmor frequency. By applying a long RF pulse, typically centered 1.5 kHz off-resonance, the pool of bound spins can be saturated before exciting the unbound pool by a pulse at the Larmor frequency. The effect of magnetization transfer preparation is to suppress partially the signal from certain "solid" tissues such as muscle and brain, depending on the relative populations of bound and unbound spins.[53] Applications of magnetization transfer preparation include background suppression in MR angiography,[54] T2-type contrast in the heart at shorter TE values,[55] and gadolinium-enhanced T1-weighted imaging of the brain.

of the combined pulses on spins within the slice is as if they had seen no RF, while all spins outside the slice (most relevantly in blood) are inverted. As originally described, a fast gradient-echo readout of the slice is timed to coincide with the null point of blood, so that blood that has entered (and exited) the slice during TI gives no signal but the image is otherwise proton density weighted. Excellent contrast between stationary tissue and the blood pool has been shown with this technique, and it has been used to distinguish between blood and thrombus in abdominal aneurysms.

In studies of the heart, blood nulling has been used as a preparatory event in breath-hold T1- and T2-weighted TSE imaging and breath-hold STIR imaging by Simonetti and coworkers[51] with promising results.

SPATIAL PRESATURATION

Unwanted signal from within or outside the slice plane may be suppressed by means of spatial presaturation pulses.[52] This is typically implemented by selectively exciting the region of interest with a $\pi/2$ pulse

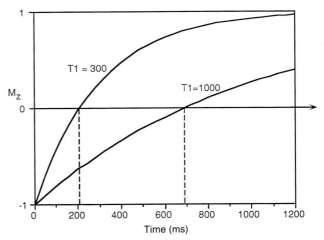

FIGURE 4–21. T1 recovery curves. After inversion, spins recover longitudinal magnetization at a rate dependent on their T1. Short-T1 components (such as fat) reach the null point quickly, whereas long-T1 components (such as water) recover slowly. The TI appropriate to null a given component then varies with its T1 and with the TR of the sequence. Assuming TR is much greater than T1, spins with T1 = 300 ms are nulled when TI = 200 ms and spins with T1 = 1000 ms are nulled when TI = 700 ms, as illustrated.

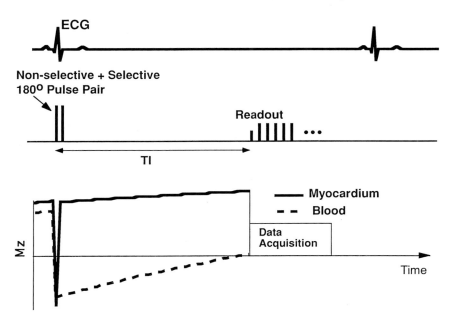

FIGURE 4–22. Double-inversion black blood RF preparation. After non–spatially selective inversion, a spatially selective "reversion" pulse is immediately applied to spins within the slice plane. In-plane spins (in this case in myocardium) effectively see no inversion pulse. Spins outside the slice plane (of relevance to flowing blood) remain inverted and begin to relax. If the acquisition is timed so that the low spatial frequencies are acquired during the null point of blood relaxation, no signal is seen from blood that enters the slice between inversion and readout. ECG = electrocardiography. (From Simonetti OP, Finn JP, White RD, et al: Black-blood T2-weighted IR imaging of the heart. Radiology, in press.)

IMAGE RECONSTRUCTION

FOURIER TRANSFORM MRI

One beauty of MRI is the simplicity of image reconstruction. The raw data are the complex 2D Fourier transform of the final image. Therefore, with most MRI techniques, a 2D (inverse) Fourier transform is all that is required to reconstruct an image from the acquired data. The magnitude result is typically utilized, although phase information is useful in flow quantification. The fast Fourier transform[56] can be applied to data sets that consist of a power of two data points and significantly increases the speed of reconstruction. Thus, many MR images are matrices of 128×128 or 256×256 pixels. To reduce acquisition time, the number of phase-encoded lines is often reduced, with or without a corresponding reduction in the FOV in the phase-encoded direction. In either case, the raw data matrix is typically "zero padded" out to a full power of 2 square matrix before reconstruction to allow the use of the fast Fourier transform. In any case, the resolution in the phase-encoded direction is determined by the extent of k-space that is sampled. This is what defines the spatial frequency content of the image. Zero padding of data generates additional pixels by sinc interpolation and does not increase the true image resolution.[37]

ASYMMETRIC AND PARTIAL DATA SAMPLING

Raw data space can be asymmetrically sampled[57] in either the frequency- or phase-encoded direction. In the frequency-encoded direction, an asymmetric echo is often utilized to keep TE to a minimum either to obtain a desired image contrast or to avoid the effects of motion and magnetic susceptibility (T2*). In the phase-encoded direction, asymmetric sampling is used to reduce acquisition time without fully sacrificing image resolution. Recall that the raw data cover both positive and negative spatial frequencies, and without system and sample imperfections (e.g., random noise, eddy currents, motion, susceptibility differences) a complex conjugate symmetry would exist in the raw data. This is exploited in some reconstruction schemes (partial or half-Fourier imaging) to synthesize a symmetric data set.[58, 59] Simple zero filling of the data is also often utilized with reasonable results.

SOME SPECIFIC PULSE SEQUENCE TYPES

The building blocks of all sequences in common use have now been described, and several features specific to certain classes of pulse sequences have also been outlined. We now review the major categories of pulse sequences in use or in development for clinical imaging, highlight similarities and differences among them, and allude to their major applications. For detailed treatment of clinical applications of these and other techniques, the reader is referred to the relevant chapters in this edition (see, for example, Chapter 10).

SPIN ECHO VERSUS GRADIENT ECHO

A spin echo occurs by the refocusing effect of a 180° RF pulse as outlined in Figure 4–3. The timing of the spin echo is determined by the time interval between the 90° and 180° pulses, independent of gradient events. A gradient echo occurs when the area subtended by a gradient pulse is exactly neutralized by an equal and opposite area. The parameter that determines when the gradient echo occurs is the rate at which these areas are traced out, and this is proportional to the gradient amplitude. In general, sequences are designed so that the gradient echo is made to coincide with a spin echo (if one exists), but it should be noted that these are independent processes. For example, it may be desirable to offset the spin echo and gradient echo for opposed-phase fat-water imaging. The steps outlined earlier for spatial encoding can be applied to data acquired under either a spin-echo or gradient-echo envelope. With spin-echo refocusing, dephasing effects caused by magnetic field nonuniformities and chemical shift are reversed. Irreversible dephasing persists because of T2 decay and diffusion, providing mechanisms for tissue contrast. Gradient reversal does not undo dephasing effects resulting from chemical shift or magnetic field inhomogeneity, whether caused by nonuniformity of the B_0 field or magnetic susceptibility gradients. The choice of TE in a gradient-echo sequence may profoundly influence image contrast, depending on whether fat and water are in phase or opposed in phase.

GRADIENT-ECHO PULSE SEQUENCES

FLASH or Spoiled GRASS

Gradient-echo techniques have proved useful for fast MRI in a variety of circumstances. Yet another contrast parameter is available with gradient echoes: the flip angle. The simplest of all gradient-echo imaging techniques is the FLASH[60] or spoiled GRASS (gradient-recalled acquisition in the steady state) sequence (see Fig. 4–13), widely used for fast T1-weighted imaging.

In short-TR gradient-echo imaging, phase coherences may build up in the transverse magnetization.[61] Depending on the desired contrast in the image, these coherences may be detrimental or beneficial. To generate T1 contrast in a short-TR gradient-echo sequence, it is desirable to eliminate all transverse coherence between phase-encoding steps, because such coherences accentuate signal from long-T2* (and therefore long-T1) components. These coherences can be suppressed by applying a crusher gradient[62] after sampling the echo and before the next excitation; this process is termed *gradient spoiling*. The aim is to cause dephasing of all coherent x-y magnetization. Another technique, called *RF spoiling*,[62] uses a table of pseudorandom values for the phase of the B_1 field on successive iterations, so preventing the buildup of transverse coherences. The phase of the echo is varied between phase-encoding steps; this phase is also locked into the receiver reference signal so that image calculation is not affected. Unlike gradient spoiling, RF spoiling is effective even in the center of the magnetic field. Attention must be paid to the details of the B_1 phase series over time, to avoid unexpected coherences.

The spin-warp sequence structure for gradient-spoiled 2D FLASH as outlined in Figure 4–13 provides a good template for illustration of conventional spatial encoding and signal sampling. After slice selection, gradients in slice, phase encode, and read are applied simultaneously to maximize time efficiency. The rephasing lobe in slice selection is to undo the dephasing effects of the first lobe. Simultaneous application of the dephasing read gradient and maximal-amplitude phase-encoding gradient sets the magnetization to one corner of k-space in a diagonal trajectory, as shown in Figure 4–12. The rephasing read gradient then unwinds the phase of the dephasing lobe and causes maximal rephasing in read at the time of the echo. The k-space trajectory of this last step is linear in the read direction, at an offset in the phase-encoding direction determined by the strength of the phase-encoding gradient pulse (see Fig. 4–12). Because the phase-encoding gradient steps through a table of values from $-G(p)_{max}$ to $G(p)_{max}$, the k-space trajectory is a linear raster of values. Discrete signal sampling occurs via the analog-to-digital converter during the buildup and decay of the gradient echo. In Figure 4–13, a gradient spoiling table is shown. When present, this increases the minimal TR of the sequence and slightly decreases slice efficiency. The same basic FLASH structure (typically with a wide bandwidth) is used as the readout module after the preparatory period in turboFLASH.

TurboFLASH

TurboFLASH is a gradient-echo sequence that uses an RF preparation followed by multiple, short TE and TR FLASH acquisitions, as diagrammed in Figure 4–16. The Ernst angle is small because of the short TR, and, without preparation of the magnetization, the images would be basically proton density weighted and appear "flat." To introduce T1 contrast, a single inversion pulse is applied before acquiring all of the image data (k-space lines). This differs substantially from the classic method of IR imaging in which an inversion pulse precedes every line of data (every phase-encoding step). Nonetheless, turboFLASH images have IR-type contrast that is typically greater than can be achieved with non-IR spin-echo or gradient-echo methods. T1 relaxation is changing throughout the acquisition period, and the data are modulated in the phase-encoded direction by the T1 recovery curve. Despite this, image quality with turboFLASH is typically limited more by S/N ratio than by image blurring.

The type of T1 contrast generated with turboFLASH depends on how much relaxation has progressed by the time the central lines of k-space are collected. This in turn is influenced by the order in which the phase-encoding steps are acquired. To clarify this point, consider that a nominal delay time T1 follows the inversion pulse and that the FLASH readout is acquired with centric phase encoding. The center of k-space that dominates image contrast is therefore acquired at the nominal TI, and the contrast is comparable to that of an IR image at that TI. If, however, the FLASH readout is acquired with linear phase encoding, then the central lines of k-space are acquired not at the nominal TI but at an effective TI of TI + (TR × N/2), where N is the number of phase-encoding steps. Thus, if TI = 500 ms, TR = 12 ms, and N = 128, then TI_{eff} = 500 + (12 × 64) = 1268 ms! Therefore, with linear phase encoding, TI_{eff} scales with the number of phase-encoding steps. If TI = 0, then TI_{eff} =

768 ms, a typical value for T1-weighted abdominal imaging at 1.0 or 1.5 T. It should be noted, however, that with linear ordering TI_{eff} is related to the number of phase-encoding steps and that with reasonable spatial resolution the minimal TI_{eff} is large. TurboFLASH has been extended to a 3D acquisition by Mugler[63] for rapid T1-weighted imaging of the brain.

The inversion prepulse for turboFLASH may be spatially selective or nonselective. A spatially nonselective RF pulse is typically applied over a wide bandwidth in the absence of a field gradient. To excite spins evenly over a wide range of frequencies, the envelope of the RF pulse approaches a spike function in the time domain; its Fourier transform approaches a constant value in the frequency domain. Such a pulse is often referred to as a "hard" pulse, and in practice it is applied as a short rectangular pulse that excites a broad frequency envelope. Because hard pulses are short, they require relatively high peak transmitter voltage.

In turboFLASH, a hard inversion pulse is combined with spatially selective α pulses for slice selectivity. For single-slice imaging, the main difference between using selective and nonselective inversion pulses is the effect on spins outside the slice. There are two major consequences of using a nonselective inversion pulse:

- Because the entire FOV of the transmitter is inverted, the blood signal may be uniformly nulled without interference from flow-related effects and independent of the blood flow velocity. Flow artifacts may therefore be completely eliminated by choice of the appropriate TI_{eff}, for example, in coronal imaging of the abdomen.
- Because the entire FOV of the transmitter is inverted, sufficient time must be allowed for relaxation before the next slice is acquired. This decreases time efficiency in multislice applications.

If selective inversion pulses are used, sequential slice acquisition may proceed without waiting for adjacent slice positions to relax. The blood signal is less predictable with selective pulses and is often bright because of inflow effects. Selective inversion pulses are best implemented with the hyperbolic secant (sech) or other optimized pulses discussed in the section on adiabatic pulses in this chapter.

Segmented TurboFLASH

By shortening the acquisition window of the FLASH readout, both the T1 filtering effect and the minimal TI limitation can be addressed. This has been accomplished by segmenting[64] the acquisition into several sequential windows, each containing a fraction of the data, as shown in Figure 4–23. For example, 128 phase-encoding steps can be acquired as four segments, each containing 32 lines. An inversion pulse precedes each segment and a delay time separates the segments from each other to allow relaxation to occur. The intersegment delay should be several seconds, and one dummy segment should precede the first segment acquisition to establish a steady state for the remaining ones. The concept of segmentation of k-space in the phase-encoding direction has been applied to several other techniques for fast imaging, including breath-hold cine[65] MRI of the heart, breath-hold–triggered MR angiography, TSE, and segmented EPI.

TurboSTEAM

Stimulated-echo acquisition mode (STEAM) imaging can be carried out, like turboFLASH, as a single-shot technique.[20] In the method described by Frahm and colleagues,[20] two 90° pulses are applied TE/2 apart. A series of fast, low-flip-angle readouts is used to capture the magnetization stored along z, each separately phase encoded as a stimulated echo (Fig. 4–24). The method can be used for fast diffusion imaging or black blood imaging of the heart.

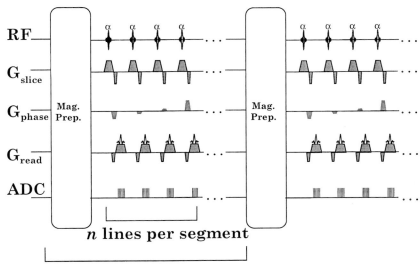

FIGURE 4–23. Segmented turboFLASH. The basic structure is similar to that of turboFLASH, but the acquisition is broken into a number of segments, each preceded by magnetization preparation. The k-space is traversed in a number of interleaved shots, and the acquisition window of the FLASH sequence is correspondingly narrowed compared with the single-shot case. Less relaxation time filtering of the data occurs, and image contrast can be more finely controlled.

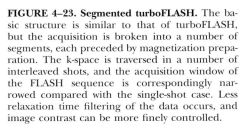

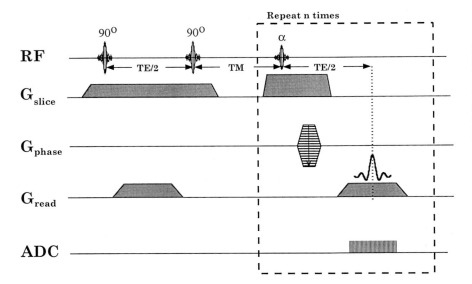

FIGURE 4–24. TurboSTEAM sequence. Slice-selective $\pi/2$ pulses are separated in time by TE/2. Slice-selection and read gradient lobes ensure full dephasing of transverse magnetization, which is aligned along the z axis by the second $\pi/2$ pulse. A series of fast, low-flip-angle gradient-echo readouts follows, each separately phase encoded. Within STEAM time (TM), the slice-selection lobe balances the initial dephasing lobe and the read gradient balances the earlier dephasing read gradient lobe. The gradient echo occurs at TE/2 after the α pulse, coinciding with the stimulated echo (see Fig. 4–4). Because α is small, only a portion of the stored z magnetization is read with each phase-encode step, so the process can be repeated many times.

FISP

Fast imaging with steady-state precession (FISP)[66] is a fast gradient-echo technique used to enhance the signal from long-T2* components (such as fluid). When TR is short compared with the rate of decay of transverse magnetization, it is possible to recycle a large part of the magnetization by alternating the phase of the RF pulse on successive excitations; that is, the direction of the $\mathbf{B}_1$ field is alternated. The effect is to realign along z the component of magnetization that lies along y at a time TR after the previous excitation, while at the same time tilting longitudinal magnetization from z to $-y$. It follows that the phase of $\mathbf{M}_{xy}$ is alternated from positive to negative with successive phase-encoding steps; this is accounted for by matching the transmitter and receiver phase. Also, for this scheme to be effective in restoring $\mathbf{M}_{xy}$ along z, $\mathbf{M}_{xy}$ must be made to lie coherently along y, because B_{1x} has no effect on spins aligned along $\pm x$. In general, at the end of a readout period, the spins are dephased in x-y because of a combination of gradient moments from the readout and phase-encoding directions. To rephase $\mathbf{M}_{xy}$ along y, these gradient moments must be reversed before the next excitation (Fig. 4–25). Balancing the gradients rephases spins that have not moved over the duration of the interval. However, flowing spins have acquired a velocity-dependent phase shift that is not unwound with zero-order gradient balancing.

As illustrated in Figure 4–25, the gradients in FISP are not fully balanced in the slice-selection and read directions. In true FISP, the gradient structure is symmetrically balanced in slice, phase-encoding, and read directions (Fig. 4–26). The structure generates motion insensitivity because of first-order gradient moment nulling, and the RF echoes generated by the train of α pulses in the steady state are superimposed on the gradient echo (assuming a uniform main field). Signal is therefore highlighted from long-T2* and long-T2 components.

PSIF

Unlike FLASH and FISP, which both acquire the primary gradient echo, the time-reversed FISP (PSIF)

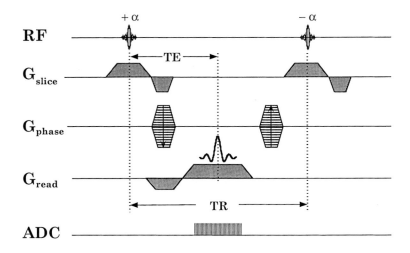

FIGURE 4–25. 2D FISP sequence structure. Compared with the structure in FLASH, the phase of the RF is alternated from one line to the next, and the gradient spoiling table in the FLASH sequence is replaced by a phase-encoding rewinding table. Coherent magnetization that persists after signal sampling (for example, for fluid) is realigned along z and is made available for re-excitation with the subsequent α pulse. Long-T2* components are therefore accentuated.

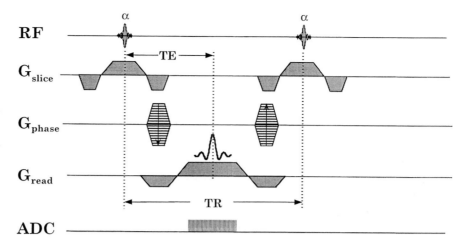

FIGURE 4–26. True FISP. The gradients are balanced along all three axes so that steady-state effects related to long-T2* species are emphasized. The gradient echo and the RF echo are superimposed at TE, and the gradient structure is motion insensitive.

or contrast-enhanced Fourier-acquired steady-state (CE-FAST)[67, 68] acquisition utilizes the RF echo formed by the repeated α pulses. The signal intensity of the RF-refocused echo is weighted by T2 over the interval from one α pulse to the readout after the next α pulse, as diagrammed in Figure 4–27. Stimulated echoes as well as spin echoes contribute to the PSIF signal, making the contrast highly dependent on flip angle. PSIF is useful in rapid acquisition of fluid-sensitive images.

DESS

The double echo in the steady state (DESS)[69] or fast acquisition double echo (FADE)[70] sequence (Fig. 4–28) utilizes both the free induction decay gradient echo used in in the FISP sequence, and the RF echo of PSIF. The gradient echo is offset from the RF echo, and they may be used to generate separate images that can be combined or displayed separately. The RF echo tends to accentuate long-T2 components such as fluid. This may be superimposed on a more T1-weighted anatomic image related to the FISP echo.

SPIN-ECHO PULSE SEQUENCES

Conventional spin-echo pulse sequences have formed the basis for clinical MRI since the modality was introduced. Various derivative techniques have been proposed that dramatically speed up image acquisition and make possible applications that would otherwise not be feasible. Strictly speaking, any technique that uses a 180° refocusing RF pulse and acquires data under the RF echo is a spin-echo pulse sequence. With the explosive pace of development in fast imaging, a rapidly increasing number of techniques now fall within the scope of this definition.

Conventional Spin-Echo Sequences

The design of a conventional spin-echo pulse sequence is straightforward and is illustrated in Figure 4–14. The initial gradient and RF events are similar to the 2D FLASH structure of Figure 4–13, but a refocusing π pulse is applied at time TE/2, immediately after the phase-encoding, slice-rephasing, and read-dephas-

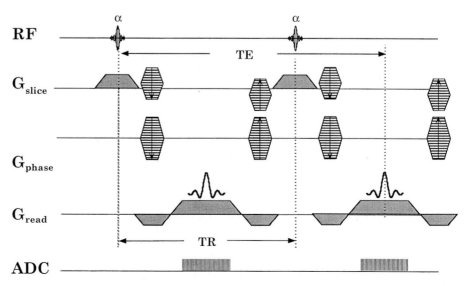

FIGURE 4–27. PSIF pulse sequence diagram. In this technique, the RF echo is of prime importance in generating image contrast. It is mainly the RF portion of the steady-state signal that is acquired. The gradient structure is balanced within the TR scope, and the RF echo occurs during readout in the following cycle.

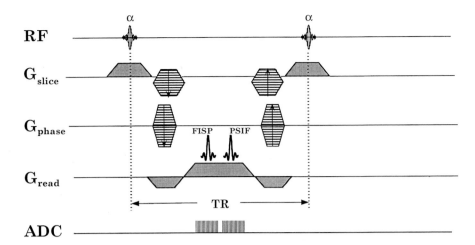

FIGURE 4–28. DESS pulse sequence diagram. The basic structure is similar to that of true FISP, but the gradient and RF echoes are offset. They may be used to generate separate images, which can be combined or displayed separately.

ing lobes. Note that the polarity of the dephasing and rephasing read gradients is the same, because the π pulse has inverted all phase accumulations. Note also that the π pulse is slice selective but does not have a rephasing lobe; π pulses are self-refocusing (for stationary spins). The spin echo occurs at TE, and the gradient echo is made to coincide with this. In the sequence diagram in Figure 4–14, the shortest possible TE is used, so this corresponds to the structure for a T1-weighted, short-TR, short-TE sequence. For a T2-weighted spin-echo sequence, a delay time is added on either side of the π pulse. In Figure 4–14, the area of the gradient pulses from the 90° pulse to the center of the echo is zero when the phase-reversal effect of the 180° pulse is taken into account. First-order or higher order gradient moment nulling may be employed to diminish sensitivity to flow and motion artifact on spin-echo as well as gradient-echo sequences.

Turbo (Fast) Spin-Echo Sequences

The concept of independently phase encoding sequential spin echoes of a multiecho train and using all the echoes to generate one image was first expounded by Hennig and colleagues.[9] Their original implementation of a single-shot technique, which they called RARE, acquired all the data for an image with just one 90° pulse and multiple 180° pulses. The phase-encoding gradient was incremented with each spin echo, such that all of k-space was traversed in a single excitation. This was an extension of an earlier concept of Mansfield for single-shot imaging, which he called EPI, using a rapidly oscillating read gradient and a constant, low-amplitude phase-encoding gradient. Whereas EPI requires fast gradients and associated hardware, RARE techniques are feasible on conventional MRI machines. Both RARE and EPI are subject to significant artifacts. With RARE, T2 decay progresses between points in k-space, whereas with EPI T2* decay progresses between points in k-space. The net effect of these dependences is that RARE images are highly T2 filtered, causing severe blurring of all but long T2 components, and EPI images are highly susceptibility weighted. Both of these effects are minimized by the

use of shorter acquisition windows, either by enhanced gradient performance or by segmenting the acquisition into several narrower windows. This latter technique is employed in TSE and segmented EPI. Whatever technique is used, relaxation time filtering is diminished when the interval between successive echoes is minimized. This requires short gradient rise times and relatively short readout periods (wide bandwidths).

The method of TSE or segmented RARE employs a variable number of separately phase-encoded echoes per 90° excitation pulse, as shown in Figure 4–17. The number of spin echoes per excitation is called the echo train length or turbo factor. If, for example, the turbo factor is 15, then for each pass of the TR, 15 phase-encoding steps rather than 1 are acquired, speeding acquisition of a single slice by a factor of 15. It should be noted, however, that with multislice acquisition, the minimal TR per slice is increased, so that overall multislice acquisition time is decreased by a factor less than the turbo factor.

The T2 contrast in TSE is determined by the TE of the echoes used to encode the center of k-space.[44] If, for example, the low spatial frequencies correspond to TE values of about 100 ms, the T2 weighting is similar to that for a conventional spin-echo image with TE = 100 ms. The order in which the echoes are phase encoded is important in TSE and variants. Sharp discontinuities and periodicities in k-space must be avoided to minimize ring and ghost artifacts, and this generally implies that the acquisition order must be interleaved from segment to segment. Blurring is more of a problem with short TE values because short-T2 components contribute more to the signal, and these are the source of the worst T2 filtering. One feature that distinguishes TSE T2-weighted images from conventional T2-weighted images is the intensity of the fat signal. With conventional T2, fat is subdued, whereas with TSE, fat is intense[71]; this can be a source of confusion. For this reason, TSE images may sometimes give the false impression of being T1 weighted. Another feature of TSE that has caused some concern in brain imaging is its relative insensitivity to the susceptibility effects of blood products. Repeated and rapid application of refocusing RF pulses prevents the dephasing by diffusion through local fixed field nonuniformities that is responsible for the signal loss in hematomas and hemosiderin.

A half-Fourier version of single-shot RARE, termed half-Fourier single-shot TSE (HASTE),[72] can be used to acquire a single image with standard spatial resolution in a few hundred milliseconds. An inversion prepulse can be appended to any of the TSE group of sequences to give IR-type contrast. Also, because of the increased time efficiency of TSE, it is feasible to run a 3D version for isotropic coverage of the brain or spine in less than 10 minutes.

Turbo Inversion Recovery

Conventional STIR imaging is time inefficient, and this has limited its widespread clinical use. With the advent of TSE techniques, turboSTIR imaging (Fig. 4–29) became an obvious and immediate extension.[73] In fact, some of the less desirable features of TSE imaging may be offset by using a STIR preparation. The bright fat signal, distracting on many TSE images, is nulled on turboSTIR, and the T2 filtering effect, caused largely by short-T2 components, is less of a problem. For these reasons, turboSTIR may have higher contrast and less blurring than its TSE counterpart, and turboSTIR is the only TSE technique in widespread clinical use for musculoskeletal imaging.

When used in imaging of the brain, STIR produces bright cerebrospinal fluid, which may render periventricular white matter lesions difficult to see. It has been shown that by using a long TI to null the cerebrospinal fluid, together with a long TE for T2 weighting, periventricular white matter lesions are made conspicuous in the brain. This technique, called fluid-attenuated IR (FLAIR),[74] is time-consuming but is much more efficient when used as a turboIR implementation. Slice looping structures for IR imaging can be optimized at the extremes of TI:

- For short TI, the most efficient loop structure has the inversion and readout completed on one slice before inverting the next.
- For long TI, an interleaved structure is used,

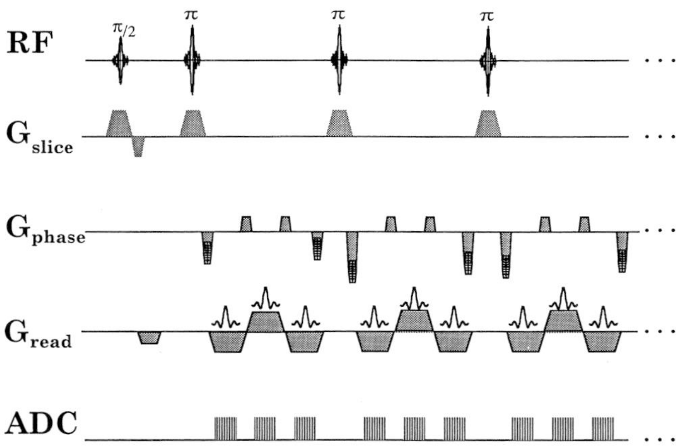

FIGURE 4–30. GRASE pulse sequence diagram. The structure differs from that of TSE in that additional gradient refocusings surround the spin echoes. These additional gradient echoes are separately phase encoded, increasing time efficiency and lowering RF power deposition. Note that the polarity of the additional read gradient refocusings is opposite to that of the central lobe. Time reversal of alternate echoes can give rise to artifacts analogous to those in segmented EPI. Because of the frequent spin echoes, however, sensitivity to susceptibility gradients is less than with EPI. In general, the low spatial frequencies coincide with the spin echoes. The k-space offset between adjacent gradient-echo and spin-echo refocusings is constant, and the gradient tables are incremented between adjacent gradient-echo refocusings.

whereby slices 1 to N are first inverted and then slices 1 to N are excited and read.

With intermediate values of TI, either limitations are imposed on the number of slices available or acquisition time is prolonged.

GRASE

One of the limitations of TSE is its high specific absorption rate in multislice applications with large turbo factors. A solution to this problem has been suggested by Feinberg and Oshio[75] in a technique that they called gradient and spin echo (GRASE). By combining data from spin-echo refocusings with gradient-echo refocusings, images can be acquired with fewer RF pulses and more quickly than with TSE (Fig. 4–30).

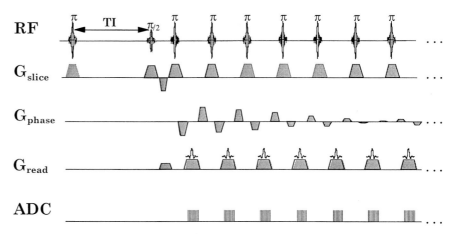

FIGURE 4–29. TurboIR pulse sequence diagram. The structure is that of a TSE sequence after an inversion pulse. After a suitable TI, a 90° excitation pulse is followed by a train of refocusing RF pulses, each giving rise to a spin echo. Each echo is separately phase encoded, and the effective TE is determined by the low-spatial-frequency echoes.

In principle, sensitivity to blood products, which is diminished in TSE, can be recovered in GRASE through the gradient-echo refocusings. Because the polarity of the read gradient in GRASE is alternated, additional steps must be taken to prevent N/2 ghosting. GRASE can also be used as a single-shot technique.

ECHO-PLANAR IMAGING

EPI is the fastest MRI method to have found potential clinical applications.[41, 42, 76] All of the spatial encoding is carried out after a single excitation under a spin-echo or gradient-echo envelope. The read gradient is oscillated, generating a series of rapid gradient-echo refocusings, during each of which one Fourier line is read. Phase encoding is carried out with either a constant, low-amplitude pulse or a series of blipped pulses between readouts, which progressively increase the gradient moment in discrete steps (see Figs. 4–18 and 4–19). The polarity of the read gradient is alternated plus and minus, resulting in a rectilinear zigzag raster in k-space. With blipped phase encoding, the k-space trajectory is mapped directly to a cartesian grid, so no interpolation is necessary before image reconstruction. With constant phase encoding, the k-space trajectory is an oblique zigzag, so the k values do not fit exactly on a cartesian grid and must be interpolated before Fourier transformation.

Signal sampling with EPI depends on the read gradient waveform. When ''resonant'' gradients are used, the fastest waveform is a sinusoidal pattern at the resonant frequency of the gradient coil (see Chapter 10). This generates a smooth transition without sharp discontinuities at plateaus. It also means that the signal can be sampled through the sinusoidal half-period, including the ramps. In this case, correction must be made for the unequal rate of k-space encoding with linear sampling, again with interpolation. An alternative scheme samples nonlinearly in time but linearly in k-space, and this requires matching the sampling window to the gradient waveform with high precision.[77]

With EPI, a variety of contrast-altering preparatory schemes may be used. These include preinversion and diffusion encoding with either a spin-echo or a stimulated-echo readout.

MOTION AND FLOW

Because conventional MR image acquisition typically takes several minutes, significant motion and flow can take place within the body, giving rise to a variety of effects and artifacts.[78, 79] These can be separated into two classes: time-of-flight effects, which are based on the macroscopic motion of fluid and tissue both through and within the image plane, and phase effects, which are due to the motion of spins along the applied imaging field gradients. Both classes of motion effects have been exploited in MR angiographic techniques[80, 81] and quantitative flow measurement.[82, 83]

TIME-OF-FLIGHT EFFECTS

In conventional spin-echo imaging, washout and signal loss occur when spins initially excited in the slice plane move out of the slice in the time interval between the 90° and 180° pulses. This effect can be useful in generating black blood contrast and eliminating motion artifact by suppressing the signal from flowing blood. Washout of flowing blood occurs by the same mechanism in TSE, in which each 90° excitation is followed by a train of 180° refocusing pulses, and in spin-echo EPI, in which the 90° to 180° pulse pair is followed by the readout of multiple echoes.

Black blood contrast is deliberately enhanced through the use of spatial presaturation pulses and out-of-slice inversion pulses to reduce selectively the signal from blood flowing into the image plane from either or both sides (see Fig. 4–22). Ordering the slice acquisition in the direction of flow also serves to saturate the signal from blood before it enters the slice plane. Alternatively, ordering the slice acquisition opposite to the flow direction emphasizes in-flow enhancement.

When TR is short, the signal from stationary tissue saturates, while the blood signal is constantly refreshed by inflow. Inflow enhancement occurs when the TR between RF excitations is sufficient to allow partially saturated spins to be replaced by fully magnetized spins from outside the imaged slice. Inflow enhancement is the mechanism of contrast in time-of-flight angiography techniques. This is described in detail in Chapter 9.

For the case of constant flow velocity, bulk motion generates the signal suppression or enhancement patterns just described but no discernible image artifacts. On the other hand, if flow or motion is time varying throughout the image acquisition, the washout and inflow effects are time varying as well and cause a modulation of the amplitude of the MR image data. Any modulation of the signal amplitude not generated intentionally by spatial encoding gives rise to image artifacts. Most physiologic motion is approximately periodic with cardiac and respiratory cycles and generates discrete ''ghost'' artifacts in the image. Cardiac and respiratory triggering or gating is commonly employed to eliminate this signal modulation by acquiring data at the same point in the cardiac or respiratory cycles. Fast image acquisition techniques can be used to reduce the data acquisition to a reasonable breath-hold period (<20 seconds); this is an effective means of eliminating respiratory motion artifact. A similar approach of avoiding motion can be used in cardiac imaging by gating image acquisition to diastole, when the heart is relatively stationary.

Another time-of-flight effect is the misregistration artifact, which is due to motion with components along at least two of the imaging axes. This is often referred to as the oblique flow artifact.[84] This artifact occurs because in conventional 2D Fourier transform imaging, the spatial positions along the imaging axes are encoded at different distinct points in time: at the center of the RF pulse on the slice-select axis, at the center of a unipolar phase-encoding pulse on the phase-encoded axis, and at the echo on the read axis. Motion with directional components along two or three axes causes a misregistration of spins to appear in the image at a location they never actually occupy. This effect is most obvious when blood vessels are lying in the image plane and oriented oblique to the read-out and phase-encoded axes. It is possible to design the phase-encoding waveform to encode position at an arbitrary point in time, eliminating misregistration between two of the three axes. By extending this to a 3D Fourier transform pulse sequence, where two of the three axes are phase encoded, oblique flow misregistration can be eliminated entirely.

PHASE EFFECTS

In addition to time-of-flight effects, motion in the presence of magnetic field gradients contributes to the phase of the MR signal. The phase of the magnetization at a specific point in space and time is defined in terms of the gradient waveform, $\mathbf{G}(t)$, and the position, $\mathbf{r}$, of a spin by the equation

$$\phi(r, T) = \gamma \int_0^T \mathbf{G}(t) \cdot \mathbf{r} \, dt \qquad (45)$$

This equation is central to the design of gradient waveforms for imaging but is valid only under the assumption that the positions of spins remain unchanged over the interval of integration, that is, during the application of the gradient. When human subjects are imaged, this assumption is frequently violated. If a spin is moving along the direction of a time-varying magnetic field gradient $\mathbf{G}(\tau)$, Equation 45 becomes

$$\phi(t) = \int_0^t \gamma \, \mathbf{G}(\tau) \cdot \mathbf{r}(\tau) \, d\tau \qquad (46)$$

where τ is the variable of integration and $\mathbf{r}(\tau)$ is the time-varying position of a moving spin in the direction defined by the gradient. Thus, the phase is a function of not only the applied gradient but also the motion itself. It is important to understand the effects that motion may have on the phase of the MR signal when designing a pulse sequence for clinical application. At times it may be desirable to quantify physiologic motion, to utilize motion as a contrast mechanism, or to minimize the effects of motion in the final image. Gradient waveforms can be defined that exploit the motion dependence of the phase of the NMR signal to achieve these goals.

To facilitate an understanding of the effects of motion on the MR signal phase, it is helpful to expand the instantaneous position as a Taylor series, which expresses a function in terms of its value and its instantaneous derivatives. For example, substituting

$$r(t) = x_0 + x_0't + \frac{1}{2}(x_0''t^2) + \cdots \qquad (47)$$

where x_0 = position at time t_0
  $x_0' = v_0$ = velocity at time t_0
  $x_0'' = a_0$ = acceleration at time t_0

back into Equation 46 and rearranging terms yield

$$\phi(t) = \gamma x_0 \int_{t_0}^t G(\tau) \, dt + \gamma v_0 \int_{t_0}^t G(\tau) t \, dt$$
$$+ \gamma a_0 \int_{t_0}^t G(\tau) t^2 \, dt + \cdots \qquad (48)$$

Thus, the phase can be separated into terms proportional to specific instantaneous derivatives of position. The gradient waveform moment integrals define the sensitivity of a gradient waveform to each order of motion. This forms the basis for motion artifact suppression by gradient moment nulling, phase-contrast angiography, and flow velocity quantification.

Gradient Moment Nulling

The relationship between data space (k-space) and image space can be corrupted by motion-induced phase, resulting in image artifacts by several mechanisms. Dispersion of phase by spatial variation of motion within a voxel causes a loss of signal intensity. If this phase dispersion is time varying as well, it may cause ghosting and blurring. If all of the spins within a voxel are moving in the same manner, they all acquire the same phase shift as a result of motion. This can result in a misregistration artifact if there is a motion component in more than one imaging axis and in ghosting and blurring if it varies from view to view. All of these deleterious effects of motion can be suppressed by the technique of gradient moment nulling.[85, 86]

Examining Equation 48, one can see that phase related to velocity and higher derivatives of position can be nullified by designing the gradient waveform $G(t)$ so that its first-order moment is zero. This can be extended to higher order derivatives as well, although for the relatively short time intervals defined by the typical TE values used in MRI, most physiologic motion may be represented by a finite Taylor series expansion of two or three terms. A gradient waveform consisting of $n + 1$ pulses is required to null n moments. For example, a three-lobe gradient waveform is required to achieve zero phase related to position and velocity, as shown in Figure 4–31. Gradient waveforms with any order of motion compensation are easily designed by using linear algebra techniques.[85]

Equation 46 is usually evaluated at the echo (t = TE), where the result indicates the phase shift of the dominant $k_x = 0$ spatial frequency component of the image. Phase at other spatial frequencies is measured relative to the linear phase generated by the spatial encoding of stationary spins and cannot be fully compensated by standard moment-nulling techniques. Spins moving along a constant linear field gradient exhibit a nonlinearly varying phase as a function of time, and this causes a blurring in the image.

Gradient moment nulling can also be used to compensate for the oblique flow misregistration artifact described in the previous section. Defining the TE as the time origin, or center of the moment expansion, and designing the phase-encoding waveform with the first moment nulled effectively encode the position at

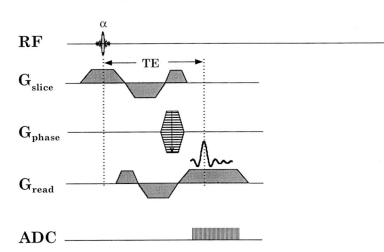

FIGURE 4–31. FLASH gradient waveforms with first-order moment nulling (velocity compensation). The waveform is designed so that the zeroth- and first-order gradient moments are nulled. Position-dependent phase shifts and velocity-dependent phase shifts (independent of position) are nulled. Note that the echo occurs asymmetrically during the readout window. This is designed to shorten the TE and minimize sensitivity to higher order motion.

TE of spins with a constant velocity component along the phase-encoded axis. Thus, the phase-encoded and readout coordinates of a spin are defined simultaneously, eliminating misregistration. This can be extended to the slice-select direction in a 3D sequence as well.

TSE pulse sequences differ from conventional spin-echo imaging in that stimulated echo components are included in the MR signal. Moment nulling for the stimulated echoes must consider only the time that the signal spends in the transverse plane, as this is the only time that phase caused by motion can accumulate. Hinks and Constable[87] described a technique for moment nulling the spin echo and stimulated echoes in TSE; resultant waveforms are shown in Figure 4–32.

Despite its speed, EPI can be highly sensitive to flow and motion effects,[88, 89] particularly when in-plane velocities are high. The time-of-flight and phase effects found in conventional MRI have analogues in EPI. The washout effect described for spin-echo imaging occurs in spin-echo EPI and can be used to suppress the signal from blood. Inflow enhancement does not normally occur in single-shot EPI because the TR is effectively infinite. However, intentional presaturation of stationary spins can be used to generate inflow

enhancement if desired. Misregistration artifacts caused by directional components of motion along multiple axes can occur in EPI, particularly in single-shot techniques, in which the TE values are typically long and the time difference between encodings along the slice-select and phase-encoding axes is significant.

Phase effects of motion in EPI are somewhat different from those in conventional MRI. Whereas the phase-encoded axis in EPI is directly analogous to the conventional readout axis in terms of motion sensitivity, significant differences exist in the EPI slice-selection and readout axes. Single-shot EPI is insensitive to motion along the slice direction for two reasons: the high-powered gradient system required for EPI can be used to keep the duration (and motional dephasing) along the slice-select axis to a minimum, and there is no line-to-line variation in effects caused by through-plane motion. Slice selection occurs only once per image, effectively freezing motion and eliminating any signal modulation. The EPI phase-encoded axis, either blipped or constant, can be treated exactly like a conventional readout axis in terms of moment nulling. It should be noted that the duration of the EPI readout is typically on the order of 20 to 100 ms, and significant dephasing can occur. The oscillating EPI readout gra-

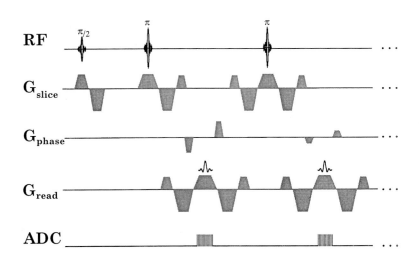

FIGURE 4–32. Velocity-compensated TSE pulse sequence. First-order moment nulling is applied in slice-selection and read directions. Both the primary spin echoes and stimulated echoes are flow compensated.

dient has no analogue in conventional MRI. The first moment of this waveform oscillates between two values and causes a modulation of signal phase even with constant-velocity motion. Fortunately, these oscillating moments are typically quite small, and high velocities along the read direction are required for this effect to be significant. The line-to-line oscillation results in N/2 ghosts. In practice, the same strategies of keeping TE short, gradient moment nulling, and blood signal suppression are effective in suppressing motion artifacts in EPI.

CONCLUSION

We have seen that, although the details of how a specific pulse sequence is designed may vary greatly from one technique to another, all pulse sequences share a set of common elements. Spins must be excited and the resulting signal spatially encoded, detected, and digitally processed to produce an image. Within this general framework, a variety of RF prepulses and gradient pulse modifications may be used for specific purposes, as described. The resulting images may contain information that focuses on detailed anatomic structure or on correlates of organ function such as flow, perfusion, diffusion, oxygenation, muscle mechanics, or kinematics. The power of MRI lies in its flexibility, and its clinical potential will continue to grow with developments in its underlying technology. Pulse sequence design will remain a cornerstone for future development.

REFERENCES

1. Fukushima E, Roeder SB: Experimental Pulse NMR: A Nuts and Bolts Approach. Reading, MA: Addison-Wesley Publishing, 1981, pp 270–275.
2. Emsley J, Feeney J, Sutcliffe LH: High Resolution NMR Spectroscopy. Oxford: Pergamon Press, 1965.
3. Farrar TC, Becker ED: Pulse and Fourier Transform NMR. New York: Academic Press, 1971.
4. Bloch F: Nuclear induction. Phys Rev 70:460, 1946.
5. Hahn EL: Spin echoes. Phys Rev 80:580–594, 1950.
6. Stejskal EO, Tanner JE: Spin diffusion measurements: spin-echoes in the presence of a time-dependent field gradient. J Chem Physiol 42:288–292, 1965.
7. Carr HY, Purcell EM: Effects of diffusion on free precession in nuclear magnetic resonance experiments. Phys Rev 94:630–638, 1954.
8. Meiboom S, Gill D: Modified spin echo method for measuring nuclear relaxation rates. Rev Sci Instrum 29:688, 1958.
9. Hennig J, Nauerth A, Friedburg H: RARE imaging: a fast imaging method for clinical MR. Magn Reson Med 3:823–833, 1986.
10. Melki PS, Jolesz FA, Mulkern RV: Partial RF echo-planar imaging with the FAISE method. I. Experimental and theoretical assessment of artifact. Magn Reson Med 26:328–341, 1992.
11. Melki PS, Jolesz FA, Mulkern RV: Partial RF echo-planar imaging with the FAISE method. II. Contrast equivalence with spin echo sequences. Magn Reson Med 26:342–354, 1992.
12. Oshio K, Feinberg DA: GRASE (gradient- and spin-echo) imaging: a novel fast MRI technique. Magn Reson Med 20:344–349, 1991.
13. Hennig J: Echoes—how to generate, recognize, use or avoid them in MR imaging sequences. I. Fundamental and not so fundamental properties of spin echoes. Concepts Magn Reson 3:125–143, 1991.
14. Constable RT, Smith RC, Gore JC: Signal to noise and contrast in fast-spin-echo (FSE) and inversion recovery FSE imaging. J Comput Assist Tomogr 16:41–47, 1992.
15. Constable RT, Anderson AW, Zhong J, Gore JC: Factors influencing contrast in fast-spin-echo MR imaging. Magn Reson Imaging 10:497–511, 1992.
16. Frahm J, Merboldy KD, Hanicke W, et al: Stimulated echo imaging. J Magn Reson 64:81–93, 1985.
17. Sattin W, Mareci T, Scott K: Exploiting the stimulated echo in nuclear magnetic resonance imaging. I. Method. J Magn Reson 64:177–182, 1985.
18. Hennig J, Hoddap M: Burst imaging. MAGMA 1:39–48, 1993.
19. Wedeen VJ, Weisskoff RM, Reese TG, et al: Motionless movies of myocardial strain-rates using stimulated echoes. Magn Reson Med 33:401–408, 1995.
20. Frahm J, Hanicke W, Bruhn H, et al: High-speed STEAM MRI of the human heart. Magn Reson Med 22:133–142, 1991.
21. Ugurbil K, Garwood M, Rath AR, Bendall MR: Amplitude- and frequency/phase-modulated refocusing pulses that induce plane rotations even in the presence of inhomogeneous B₁ fields. J Magn Reson 78:472–497, 1988.
22. Hardy CJ, Edelstein WA, Vatis D: Efficient adiabatic fast passage for NMR population inversion in the presence of radiofrequency field inhomogeneity and frequency offsets. J Magn Reson 66:470–482, 1986.
23. Silver MS, Joseph RI, Hoult DI: Highly selective π/2 and π pulse generation. J Magn Reson 59:347–351, 1984.
24. Bendall MR, Garwood M, Ugurbil K, Pegg DT: Adiabatic refocusing pulse which compensates for variable RF power and off-resonance effects. Magn Reson Med 4:493–499, 1987.
25. Ugurbil K, Garwood M, Rath AR: Optimization of modulation functions to improve insensitivity of adiabatic pulses to variations in B₁ magnitude. J Magn Reson 80:448–469, 1988.
26. Ugurbil K, Garwood M, Bendall MR: Amplitude- and frequency-modulated pulses to achieve 90° plane rotations with inhomogeneous B₁ fields. J Magn Reson 72:177–185, 1987.
27. Connolly S, Nishimura D, Macovski A: A selective adiabatic spin-echo pulse. J Magn Reson 83:324–344, 1989.
28. Edelman RR, Siewert B, Darby DG, et al: Qualitative mapping of cerebral blood flow and functional localization with echo-planar MR imaging and signal targeting with alternating radiofrequency. Radiology 192:513–520, 1994.
29. Norris DG, Ludemann H, Leibfritz D: An analysis of the effects of short T₂ values on the hyperbolic-secant pulse. J Magn Reson 92:94–101, 1991.
30. Frahm J, Haase A, Hanicke W, et al: Chemical shift selective MR imaging using a whole-body magnet. Radiology 156:441–444, 1985.
31. Rosen BR, Wedeen VJ, Brady TJ: Selective saturation NMR imaging. J Comput Assist Tomogr 8:813–818, 1984.
32. Hore PJ: Solvent suppression in Fourier transform nuclear magnetic resonance. J Magn Reson 55:283–300, 1983.
33. Flamig DP, Pierce WB, Harms SE, Griffey RH: Magnetization transfer contrast in fat-suppressed steady-state three dimensional MR images. Magn Reson Med 26:122–131, 1992.
34. Thomasson DM, Purdy DE, Finn JP: Fast spectrally selective excitation in 3D gradient echo imaging. J Magn Reson Imaging 4(P):56, 1994. Abstract.
35. Thomasson DM, Moore JR, Purdy DE, Finn JP: Minimum-time spatial-spectral pulses using a phase modulated 1-1 binomial pulse design. In: Proceedings of the Second Annual Meeting of the Society of Magnetic Resonance, San Francisco, 1994, p 120.
36. Bracewell R: The Fourier Transform and Its Applications. 2nd ed. New York: McGraw-Hill, 1986.
37. Brigham EO: The Fast Fourier Transform and Its Applications. Englewood Cliffs, NJ: Prentice-Hall, 1988.
38. Hoult D: The solution of the Bloch equations in the presence of a varying B₁ field: an approach to selective pulse analysis. J Magn Reson 35:69–86, 1979.
39. Tweig DB: The k trajectory formulation of the NMR imaging process with applications in analysis and synthesis of imaging methods. Med Phys 10:610–621, 1983.
40. Edelstein WA, Hutchison JMS, Johnson G, Redpath TW: Spin-warp NMR imaging and application to whole-body imaging. Phys Med Biol 25:751–756, 1980.
41. Mansfield P, Pykett IL: Biological and medical imaging by NMR. J Magn Reson 29:355–373, 1978.
42. Stehling MK, Turner R, Mansfield P: Echo-planar imaging: magnetic resonance imaging in a fraction of a second. Science 254:43–50, 1991.
43. Chien D, Atkinson DJ, Edelman RR: Strategies to improve contrast in k-space coverage: reordered phase encoding and k-space segmentation. J Magn Reson Imaging 1:63–70, 1991.
44. Mulkern RV, Melki PS, Jakab P, et al: Phase-encode order and its effect on contrast and artifact in single-shot RARE sequences. Med Phys 18:1032–1037, 1991.
45. Mulkern RV, Wong STS, Winalski C, Jolesz FA: Contrast manipulation and artifact assessment of 2D and 3D RARE sequences. Magn Reson Med 8:557–566, 1990.
46. Meyer CH, Hu BS, Nishimura DG, Macovski A: Fast spiral coronary artery imaging. Magn Reson Med 28:202–213, 1992.
47. Bydder GM, Young IR: MR imaging: clinical use of the inversion recovery sequence. J Comput Assist Tomogr 9:659–675, 1985.
48. Bydder GM, Steiner RE, Blumgart LH, et al: MR imaging of the liver using short TI inversion recovery sequences. J Comput Assist Tomogr 9:1084–1089, 1985.
49. Dewyer AJ, Frank JA, Sank VJ, et al: Short TI inversion recovery pulse sequence: analysis and initial experience in cancer imaging. Radiology 168:827–836, 1988.
50. Edelman RR, Chien D, Kim D: Fast selective black blood imaging. Radiology 181:655–660, 1991.

51. Simonetti OP, Finn JP, White RD, et al: Black-blood T2-weighted IR imaging of the heart. Radiology, in press.
52. Felmlee JP, Ehman RL: Spatial presaturation: a method for suppressing flow artifacts and improving depiction of vascular anatomy in MR imaging. Radiology 164:559–564, 1987.
53. Wolff SD, Balaban RS: Magnetization transfer contrast (MTC) and tissue water proton relaxation in vivo. Magn Reson Med 10:135–144, 1989.
54. Edelman RR, Ahn SS, Chien D, et al: Improved time-of-flight MR angiography of the brain with magnetization transfer contrast. Radiology 184:395–399, 1992.
55. Balaban RS, Chesnick S, Hedges K, et al: Magnetization transfer contrast in MR imaging of the heart. Radiology 180:671–675, 1991.
56. Cooley JW, Tukey JW: An algorithm for the machine calculation of complex Fourier series. Math Comput 19:297–301, 1965.
57. Margosian PM: Faster MR imaging: imaging with half the data. Health Care Instrum 161:527–531, 1986.
58. Haacke EM, Lindskog ED, Lin W: Partial Fourier imaging: a fast, iterative POCS technique capable of local phase recovery. J Magn Reson 92:126–145, 1991.
59. Hurst GC, Hua J, Simonetti OP, Duerk JL: Signal-to-noise, resolution, and bias function analysis of asymmetric sampling with zero-padded magnitude FT reconstruction. Magn Reson Med 27:247–269, 1992.
60. Haase A, Frahm J, Matthaei D, et al: FLASH imaging: rapid NMR imaging using low flip-angle pulses. J Magn Reson 67:256–266, 1986.
61. Frahm J, Merboldt KD, Hanicke W: Transverse coherence in rapid FLASH NMR imaging. J Magn Reson 277:304–314, 1987.
62. Crawley AP, Wood ML, Henkelman RM: Elimination of transverse coherences in FLASH MRI. Magn Reson Med 8:248–260, 1988.
63. Mugler JP: Three-dimensional magnetization-prepared rapid gradient-echo imaging (3D MP-RAGE). Magn Reson Med 15:152–157, 1990.
64. Edelman RR, Wallner B, Singer A, et al: Segmented turboFLASH: method for breath-hold MR imaging of the liver with flexible contrast. Radiology 177:515–521, 1990.
65. Atkinson DJ, Edelman RR: Cine-angiography of the heart in a single breath-hold with a segmented turboFLASH sequence. Radiology 178:357–361, 1991.
66. Oppelt A, Graumann R, Barfuss H, et al: FISP: a new fast MRI sequence. Electromedica (English ED) 3:15–18, 1986.
67. Gyngell ML: The steady-state signals in short repetition-time sequences. J Magn Reson 81:474–483, 1989.
68. Gyngell ML: The application of steady-state free precession in rapid 2DFT NMR imaging: FAST and CE-FAST sequences. Magn Reson Imaging 6:415–419, 1988.
69. Bruder H, Fischer H, Graumann R, Deimling M: A new steady-state imaging sequence for simultaneous acquisition of two MR images with clearly different contrasts. Magn Reson Med 7:35–42, 1988.
70. Redpath TW, Jones RA: FADE: a new fast imaging sequence. Magn Reson Med 6:224–234, 1988.
71. Listerud J, Einstein S, Outwater E, Kressel HY: First principles of fast spin echo. Magn Reson Q 8:199–244, 1992.
72. Kiefer B, Grassner J, Hausmann R: Image acquisition in a second with half-Fourier acquisition single shot turbo spin echo. J Magn Reson Imaging 4(P):86–87, 1994.
73. Smith RC, Constable RT, Reinhold C, et al: Inversion recovery fast spin echo imaging. Radiology 181:202, 1991. Abstract.
74. White SJ, Hajnal JV, Young IR, Bydder GM: Use of fluid-attenuated inversion-recovery pulse sequences for imaging the spinal cord. Magn Reson Med 28:153–162, 1992.
75. Feinberg DA, Oshio K: Gradient-echo shifting in fast MRI techniques (GRASE imaging) for correction of field inhomogeneity errors and chemical shift. J Magn Reson 97:177–183, 1992.
76. Cohen MS, Weisskoff RM: Ultra-fast imaging. Magn Reson Imaging 9:1–37, 1991.
77. Bruder H, Fischer H, Reinfelder HE, Schmitt F: Image reconstruction for echo planar imaging with nonequidistant k-space sampling. Magn Reson Med 23:311–323, 1992.
78. Axel L: Blood flow effects in magnetic resonance imaging. AJR 148:1157–1166, 1984.
79. Mills CM, Brant-Zawadzki M, Crooks LE, et al: Nuclear magnetic resonance: principles of blood flow imaging. AJR 142:165–170, 1984.
80. Laub GA, Kaiser WA: MR angiography with gradient motion refocusing. J Comput Assist Tomogr 12:377–382, 1988.
81. Dumoulin CL, Hart HR: Magnetic resonance angiography. Radiology 161:717–720, 1986.
82. Moran PR: A flow velocity zeugmatographic interlace for NMR imaging in humans. Magn Reson Imaging 1:197–203, 1982.
83. Edelman RR, Mattle HP, Kleefield J, et al: Quantification of blood flow with dynamic MR imaging and presaturation bolus tracking. Radiology 171:551–556, 1989.
84. Nishimura DG, Jackson JI, Pauly JM: On the nature and reduction of the displacement artifact in flow images. Magn Reson Med 22:481–492, 1991.
85. Pattany PM, Duerk JL, McNally JM: Motion artifact suppression technique in multislice MR imaging. Magn Reson Imaging 5(suppl 1):107–108, 1987.
86. Haacke EM, Lenz GW: Improving image quality in the presence of motion by using rephasing gradients. AJR 148:1251–1258, 1987.
87. Hinks RS, Constable RT: Gradient moment nulling in fast spin echo. Magn Reson Med 32:698–706, 1994.
88. Butts K, Riederer ST: Analysis of flow effects in echo-planar imaging. J Magn Reson Imaging 2:288–293, 1992.
89. Duerk JL, Simonetti OP: Theoretical aspects of motion sensitivity and compensation in echo-planar imaging. J Magn Reson Imaging 1:643–650, 1991.

MRI Contrast Agents: Basic Principles

RANDALL B. LAUFFER

As magnetic resonance imaging (MRI) became a routine clinical tool during the past 15 years, contrast agents played an increasingly important role. It is estimated that roughly 30% of MRI examinations today include the use of an intravenously administered contrast agent. The convergence of new contrast agent approaches and new imaging technology is likely to increase their use considerably.

As with imaging agents used in x-ray and scintigraphic imaging, MRI contrast agents are a unique class of pharmaceuticals. The combined goals of image enhancement and safety place severe demands on agent developers. The challenges of therapeutic agent design are equal or greater, but the breadth of disciplines involved in developing MRI contrast agents is enormous, spanning the whole of the chemical, physical, and biologic sciences.

This chapter serves to introduce the most important background information and current topics related to MRI contrast media. These tools should allow one to understand the chemical and physical basis of MRI enhancement and critically evaluate new agents as they are introduced into the clinical arena. More detailed accounts of the chemistry, biophysics, and pharmacology of MRI agents have been published.[1–4]

HISTORICAL BACKGROUND

Fundamental investigations leading to the new area of MRI contrast agents are briefly discussed here. Bloch[5] first described the use of a paramagnetic salt, ferric nitrate, to enhance the relaxation rates of water protons. The standard theory relating solvent nuclear relaxation rates in the presence of dissolved paramagnetic substances was developed by Bloembergen, Solomon, and others.[6–9] Eisinger and colleagues[10] demonstrated that binding of a paramagnetic metal ion to a macromolecule—in their case, DNA—enhances the water proton relaxation efficiency via lengthening of the rotational correlation time. This phenomenon, which came to be known as proton relaxation enhancement, has been utilized extensively to study hydration and structure of metalloenzymes.[11–13]

The pioneering 1973 work of Lauterbur[14] in imaging with MR was extended to human imaging in 1977.[15–17] Lauterbur and colleagues[18] were first to show the feasibility of paramagnetic agents for tissue discrimination on the basis of differential water proton relaxation times. In their experiments, a salt of manganese(II), a cation known to localize in normal myocardial tissue in preference to infarcted regions, was injected into dogs with an occluded coronary artery. The longitudinal proton relaxation rates ($1/T1$) of tissue samples correlated with Mn^{II} concentration, and thus normal myocardium could be distinguished from the infarcted zone by relaxation behavior alone. Brady, Goldman, and colleagues[19, 20] subsequently confirmed the feasibility of paramagnetic agents in imaging studies of excised dog hearts treated in a similar fashion. Normal myocardium, containing Mn^{II}, exhibited greater signal intensity than did infarcted regions on MR images; no contrast was present without Mn^{II}.

The first human MRI study involving a paramagnetic agent was performed by Young and associates[21]; orally administered ferric chloride was used to enhance the gastrointestinal tract. The diagnostic potential of paramagnetic agents was first demonstrated in patients by Carr and coworkers.[22] Gadolinium(III) diethylenetriaminepentaacetic acid ($[Gd-DTPA]^{2-}$) was administered intravenously to patients with cerebral tumors and provided enhancement of the lesion in the region of cerebral capillary breakdown.

MAGNETIC PROPERTIES AND NUCLEAR RELAXATION

Substances used as MRI contrast agents affect nuclear relaxation rates because they possess electrons whose spins are unpaired. Electron spin is analogous to the quantum mechanical property of spin possessed by nuclei. For most molecules, electrons are distributed in pairs into various *orbitals* (an orbital defines a region in space where an electron has some probability

TABLE 5–1. MAGNETIC MOMENTS OF SELECTED PARAMAGNETIC METAL IONS

ION	NUMBER OF UNPAIRED ELECTRONS	MAGNETIC MOMENT (BOHR MAGNETONS)
Transition Metal Ions		
Copper(II)	1	1.7–2.2
Nickel(II) (high spin)*	2	2.8–4.0
Chromium(III)	3	3.8
Iron(II) (high spin)	4	5.1–5.5
Manganese(II), iron(III)	5	5.9
Lanthanide Metal Ions		
Praseodymium(III)	2	3.5
Gadolinium(III)	7	8.0
Dysprosium(III)	5	10.6
Holmium(III)	4	10.6

*The number of unpaired electrons depends on the chemical environment around the metal ion. The table shows the maximal number of unpaired electrons, that is, the high-spin state. Under some conditions, electrons can pair, giving a low-spin state; for instance, Fe^{II} in the low-spin state has no unpaired electrons.

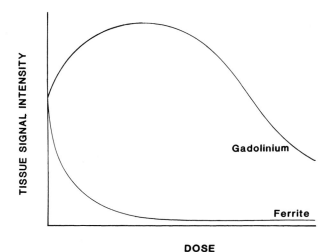

FIGURE 5–1. Dose- or concentration-dependent effect of typical MRI contrast agents on tissue signal intensity. Gadolinium agents generally increase signal intensity except where present in high concentrations. Larger iron particles (e.g., AMI-225) usually lead to signal loss. Small iron particles (e.g., nanopolymers such as AMI-227) have higher T1 relaxivity and can cause a signal intensity increase on T1-weighted images or decrease on T2-weighted images.

of residing). The two electrons in a given orbital must have opposite spins (one up and one down), as described by the Pauli exclusion principle. Because these two spins cancel, there is no net electron spin associated with the molecule, and it is said to be *diamagnetic*.

Some substances, however, have several orbitals at identical (or similar) energy levels. In this case, only one electron may be placed into each orbital, and the electrons all have parallel spins. A net electron spin results, and the substance is said to be *paramagnetic*. The unpaired electrons of paramagnetic substances generate strong, fluctuating magnetic fields at nearby nuclei, thus stimulating nuclear relaxation.

The most common paramagnetic species in nature are metal ions, which usually possess incompletely filled d or f orbitals. These ions possess between one and seven unpaired electrons, as shown in Table 5–1. For the transition metal ions and Gd^{III}, the strength of the magnetic moment of the ion (which is one factor that determines the efficiency of nuclear relaxation enhancement) is roughly proportional to the number of unpaired electrons. For the lanthanide ions other than Gd^{III}, the orbital motion of the unpaired electrons adds to the angular momentum from their respective spins to create magnetic moments larger than that predicted by the number of unpaired electrons.

Other paramagnetic substances include organic free radicals (e.g., nitroxides) and molecular oxygen. These have rather low magnetic moments and thus have received less attention as MRI contrast agents.

Paramagnetism generally involves the magnetism of small, isolated ions, but the collection of paramagnetic ions into crystalline arrays creates stronger forms of magnetism. In relation to MRI contrast agents, the most important forms of magnetism are ferromagnetism and superparamagnetism, which exist in iron particles (Table 5–2). In ferromagnetism, the individual magnetic dipoles align cooperatively in a magnetic field, creating a much stronger form of magnetism that persists even when the substance is removed from the magnetic field. A weaker form of this is superparamagnetism, wherein the crystalline arrays are imperfect or small, resulting in reduced magnetism. Superparamagnets thus behave like strong paramagnets.

Table 5–3 lists the effects that different forms of contrast agents have on MR image intensity. At equilibrium concentrations in tissues, gadolinium- and iron particle–based agents lead to drastically different effects on image intensity (Fig. 5–1). The T1-lowering effect of the small-molecule gadolinium chelates dominates at low concentrations, leading to increases in signal intensity. At higher concentrations, the T2-lowering effect becomes significant and the signal intensity decreases. Iron particles, on the other hand, generally lead to signal loss. However, smaller iron particles with more balanced T1 and T2 effects can increase image intensity on heavily T1-weighted sequences.

TABLE 5–2. PROPERTIES OF DIFFERENT FORMS OF MAGNETISM

TYPE OF MAGNETISM	NET ALIGNMENT TO EXTERNAL FIELD	RELATIVE MAGNETIC SUSCEPTIBILITY	EXAMPLE OF SUBSTANCE
Diamagnetism	Antiparallel	−1	Most organic materials
Paramagnetism	Parallel	+10	Metal chelates
Superparamagnetism	Parallel	+5,000	Small iron particles
Ferromagnetism	Parallel	+25,000	Large iron particles

TABLE 5–3. EFFECT OF CONTRAST AGENTS ON MRI SIGNAL INTENSITY*

CONTRAST AGENT	T1-WEIGHTED IMAGE	T2-WEIGHTED IMAGE
Gadolinium chelate: equilibrium tissue concentration	+ + +	+
Gadolinium chelate: first pass or high concentration	+	− −
Iron particle	+ / −	− − −
Nonproton (oral use, e.g., perfluorocarbons)	−	−
Diamagnetic (oral use)	−	−

*+ = increase in signal intensity; − = decrease in signal intensity.

DISTINCTION BETWEEN T1 AND T2 AGENTS

For the purposes of this discussion, it is useful to classify MRI contrast agents into two broad groups based on whether the substance increases the 1/T2 of water protons by roughly the same amount that it increases 1/T1 or whether the transverse relaxation rate (1/T2) is altered to a much greater extent. (Relaxation rates, the reciprocals of relaxation times, are additive and thus much more useful in quantitative discussions.) We can refer to the first category as T1 agents, because, on a percentage basis, these generally alter 1/T1 of tissue more than 1/T2 owing to the fast endogenous transverse relaxation in tissue. With most conventional pulse sequences, this dominant T1-lowering effect gives rise to increases in signal intensity; thus, these are positive contrast agents. On the other hand, T2 agents largely increase the 1/T2 of tissue rather selectively; this leads to decreases in signal intensity, and thus these represent negative contrast agents. Contrast agents constituting a third class—nonproton agents, such as certain perfluorocarbons—do not affect relaxation rates but produce low signal intensity by virtue of the absence of hydrogen; these agents are not considered in this chapter.

GENERAL REQUIREMENTS FOR MRI CONTRAST AGENTS

MRI contrast agents must be biocompatible pharmaceuticals in addition to nuclear relaxation probes. Aside from standard pharmaceutical features, such as water solubility and shelf stability, the requirements relevant for metal ion–based agents can be classified into three general categories.

RELAXIVITY

The efficiency by which the agent enhances the proton relaxation rates of water, referred to as *relaxivity*, must be sufficient to increase significantly the relaxation rates of the target tissue. The dose of the agent at which such alteration of tissue relaxation rates occurs must, of course, be nontoxic. Increases in 1/T1 as small as 10% to 20% could be detected by MRI.

SPECIFIC IN VIVO DISTRIBUTION

Ideally, to be of diagnostic value, the agent should localize for a period in a target tissue or tissue compartment in preference to nontarget regions. This is a basic tenet in any agent-based imaging procedure, in which detection of the agent is usually a simple function of its tissue concentration. For MRI relaxation agents, however, this requirement should be qualified: It is sufficient that the relaxation rates of the target tissue be enhanced in preference to the rates of other tissues. This goal might be accomplished by means other than concentration differences if the agent has a higher relaxivity in the environment of one tissue.

IN VIVO STABILITY, EXCRETABILITY, AND LACK OF TOXICITY

The acute and chronic toxicity of an intravenously administered metal complex is related in part to its stability in vivo and its tissue clearance behavior. The transition metal and lanthanide ions are relatively toxic at doses required for MRI relaxation rate changes, and thus dissociation of the complex cannot occur to any significant degree. (The toxicity of the free ligand also becomes a factor in the event of dissociation.) In addition, a diagnostic agent should be excreted within hours of administration.

T1 AGENTS

GADOLINIUM CHELATES APPROVED FOR HUMAN USE

Since the introduction of Gd-DTPA (gadopentetate dimeglumine, Magnevist) in 1988, three other similar gadolinium chelates have been approved for clinical use in different countries. The chemical structures of these agents are shown in Figure 5–2. The similarities among the agents include 1) rather strong chelation of the relatively toxic but highly magnetic gadolinium ion using a multiarmed organic ligand, 2) nearly identical effects on signal intensity of tissue, 3) substantially equivalent biodistribution and plasma half-life, and 4) good to excellent safety and tolerance record in millions of applications. The main differences among the agents are 1) the electrical charge of the gadolinium chelate and 2) whether or not the chelating ligand

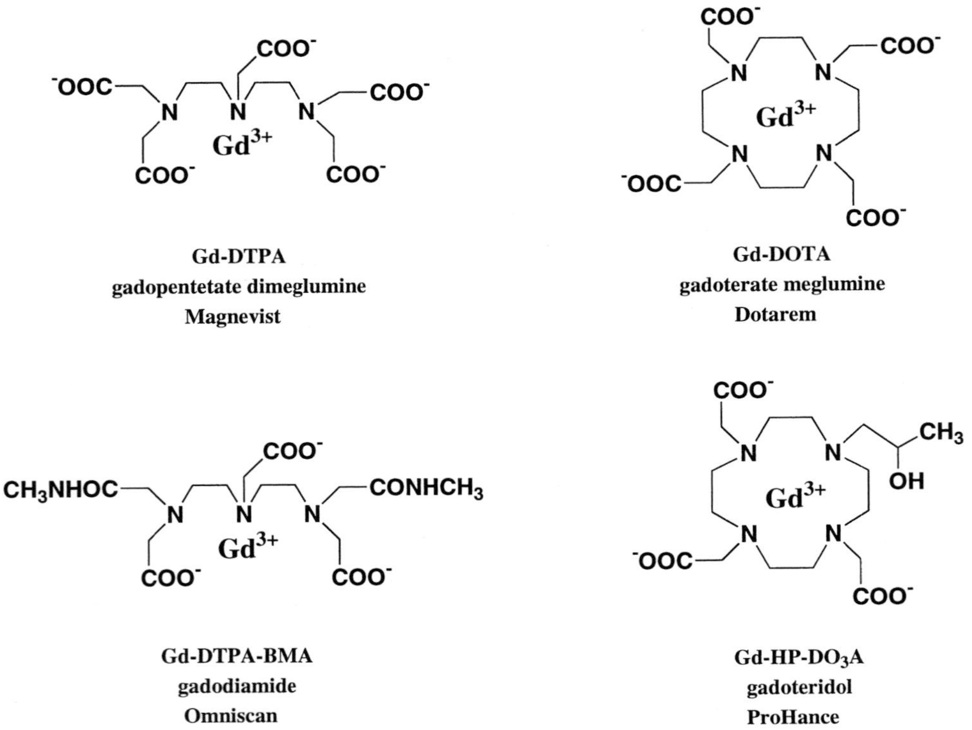

Gd-DTPA
gadopentetate dimeglumine
Magnevist

Gd-DOTA
gadoterate meglumine
Dotarem

FIGURE 5–2. Chemical structures of currently approved MRI contrast agents.

Gd-DTPA-BMA
gadodiamide
Omniscan

Gd-HP-DO₃A
gadoteridol
ProHance

is cyclic in nature. The relative importance of these properties is discussed in the appropriate following sections.

RELAXIVITY

Theory

The addition of a paramagnetic solute causes an increase in the 1/T1 and 1/T2 of solvent nuclei. The diamagnetic and paramagnetic contributions to the relaxation rates of such solutions are additive and given by

$$(1/Ti)_{obs} = (1/Ti)_d + (1/Ti)_p \quad i = 1, 2 \quad (1)$$

where $(1/Ti)_{obs}$ is the observed solvent relaxation rate in the presence of a paramagnetic species, $(1/Ti)_d$ is the (diamagnetic) solvent relaxation rate in the absence of a paramagnetic species, and $(1/Ti)_p$ represents the additional paramagnetic contribution. In the absence of solute-solute interactions, the solvent relaxation rates are linearly dependent on the concentration of the paramagnetic species ([M]); relaxivity, R_i, is defined as the slope of this dependence in units of $M^{-1} s^{-1}$ or, more commonly, $mM^{-1} s^{-1}$:

$$(1/Ti)_{obs} = (1/Ti)_d + R_i[M] \quad i = 1, 2 \quad (2)$$

The large and fluctuating local magnetic field in the vicinity of a paramagnetic center provides this additional relaxation pathway for solvent nuclei. Because these fields fall off rapidly with distance, random translational diffusion of solvent molecules and the complex and specific chemical interactions that bring

the solvent molecules near the metal ion (e.g., within 5 Å) are important in transmitting the paramagnetic effect. Different types of chemical interaction can yield different relaxation efficiencies, as governed by the distance and time scale of the interaction; the sum of these contributions and that related to translational diffusion gives the total relaxivity of the paramagnetic species.

For the discussion that follows, it is useful to classify the relevant contributions to water proton relaxivity with respect to three distinct types of interactions, as shown in Figure 5–3. In case A, a water molecule binds in the primary coordination sphere of the metal ion and exchanges with the bulk solvent. The term *inner sphere relaxation* is often applied loosely to this type of relaxation mechanism. Case B represents hydrogen-bonded waters in the second coordination sphere. Because of the lack of understanding of second coordination sphere interactions, investigators often do not distinguish between this relaxation mechanism (case B) and that involving translational diffusion of the water molecule past the chelate (case C), referring simply to *outer sphere relaxation*. The total relaxivity of a paramagnetic agent is therefore generally given by

$$(1/Ti)_p = (1/Ti)_{inner\ sphere} + (1/Ti)_{outer\ sphere} \quad i = 1, 2 \quad (3)$$

The longitudinal relaxation contribution from the inner sphere mechanism results from a chemical exchange of the water molecule between the primary coordination sphere of the paramagnetic metal ion (or any hydration site near the metal) and the bulk solvent, as shown in Figure 5–4, yielding the following expression:

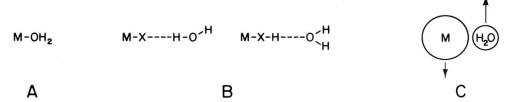

A   **B**   **C**

FIGURE 5–3. Interactions between water and metal complexes (M). *A*, Inner sphere relaxation resulting from binding of water molecules to primary coordination sphere of metal ion. *B* and *C*, Outer sphere relaxation resulting from hydrogen-bonded water in outer coordination sphere *(B)* and motion of water past the metal ion *(C)*.

$$\left(\frac{1}{T1}\right)_{\substack{inner \\ sphere}} = \frac{P_M q}{T1_M + \tau_M} \qquad (4)$$

Here, P_M is the mole fraction of metal ion, q is the number of water molecules bound per metal ion, $T1_M$ is the relaxation time of the bound water protons, and τ_M is the residence lifetime of the bound water. The value of $T1_M$ is in turn given by the Solomon-Bloembergen equation[7, 9]:

$$\frac{1}{T1_M} = \frac{2}{15} \frac{\gamma_I^2 g^2 S(S+1)\beta^2}{r^6} \left(\frac{7\tau_c}{1 + \omega_S^2 \tau_c^2} + \frac{3\tau_c}{1 + \omega_I^2 \tau_c^2}\right) \qquad (5)$$

where γ_I is the proton gyromagnetic ratio, g is the electronic g-factor, S is the total electron spin of the metal ion, β is the Bohr magneton, r is the proton–metal ion distance, and ω_S and ω_I are the electronic and proton Larmor precession frequencies, respectively. The dependence on the last two quantities makes relaxivity a function of magnetic field as well as other physical and chemical properties. (Equation 5 includes only the dipolar ["through space"] contribution to relaxivity; the scalar, or contact ["through bonds"] contribution is rarely significant for metal ion species used as contrast agents.)

The key feature of paramagnetically induced nuclear relaxation is that the local magnetic field from the electron spin must fluctuate at proper frequencies to stimulate nuclear relaxation. The time scale of these fluctuations is characterized by the overall correlation time τ_c; the characteristic rate of these fluctuations, $1/\tau_c$, is dominated by the fastest of three processes:

$$\frac{1}{\tau_c} = \frac{1}{T1_e} + \frac{1}{\tau_M} + \frac{1}{\tau_R} \qquad (6)$$

where $T1_e$ (also called τ_S) is the longitudinal electron spin relaxation time; τ_M is the water residence time, as already mentioned; and τ_R is the rotational tumbling time of the entire metal-water unit. These processes, all of which alter the magnetic field at the nucleus, are shown in Figure 5–4.

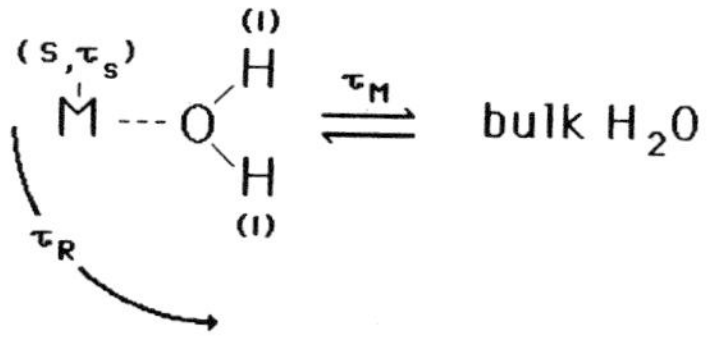

Similar theories exist for outer sphere relaxation. It should be pointed out, however, that the quantitative understanding of both inner and outer sphere relaxivities of metal complexes is still at an early stage.[1]

Relaxivity in Solution

Table 5–4 lists the 20-MHz longitudinal relaxivities for various simple metal complexes; structures of selected ligands are shown in Figure 5–5. Relaxivity is proportional to the number of inner sphere water molecules (q), which decreases when large ligands (e.g., DTPA) are bound to the metal ion to ensure stability of the complex. For example, chelation of Gd^{III} with DTPA decreases q from 8 or 9 to 1; the structure of the resulting complex is shown in Figure 5–6. All four gadolinium chelates approved for human use have q = 1 and thus comparable relaxivities. When q = 0, relaxation is limited to outer sphere mechanisms; from Table 5–4 one can see that outer sphere relaxivities are quite sizable. In the design of MRI contrast agents, the use of multidentate ligands to ensure in vivo stability of the complexes reduces the number of coordinated water molecules; the outer sphere contribution to these low-molecular-weight

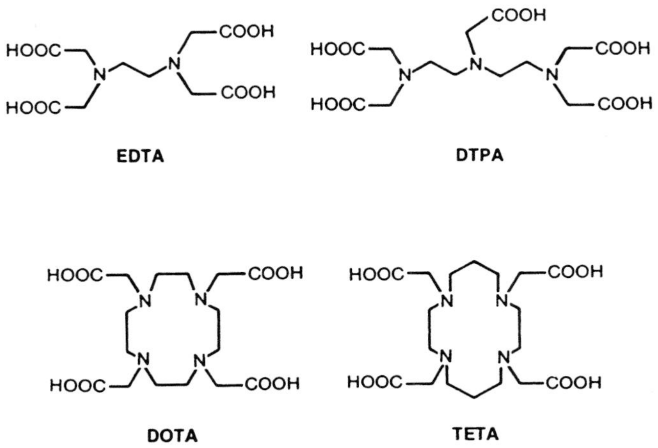

FIGURE 5–4. Proton relaxation by paramagnetic metal ions. The proton spin I on a metal-bound water molecule experiences the fluctuating magnetic field of the electron spin S; this water exchanges with the bulk solvent. The rates of water exchange (τ_M^{-1}), rotation of the paramagnetic complex (τ_R^{-1}), and electron spin relaxation (τ_S^{-1}) determine the relaxation rate (1/T1) of the bound water, as expressed by the Solomon-Bloembergen equations.

EDTA

DTPA

DOTA

TETA

FIGURE 5–5. Structures of selected chelating agents.

TABLE 5–4. LONGITUDINAL RELAXIVITIES (R_1) AT 20 MHz AND THE NUMBER OF COORDINATED WATER MOLECULES (q) FOR SELECTED METAL COMPLEXES*

COMPLEX†	q	R_1 (mM^{-1} s^{-1})
Gd^{III}		
Aquo ion	8,9	9.1
EDTA	2,3	6.6
DOTA	1	3.4
DTPA	1	3.7
DTPA-BMA	1	4.6‡
HP-DO3A	1	3.7
TTHA	0	2.0
Mn^{II}		
Aquo ion	6	8.0
EDTA	1	2.0
DTPA	0	1.1
Fe^{III}		
Aquo ion	6	8.0
EDTA	1	1.8
EHPG	0	0.95
DTPA	0	0.73
Cr^{III}		
Aquo ion	6	5.8
EDTA	1	0.2
Cu^{II}		
Aquo ion	6	0.84
Dy^{III}		
Aquo ion	8,9	0.56
EDTA	2,3	0.17
DTPA	1 (?)	0.096

*Relaxivity values given for the temperature range of 35°C to 39°C.
†BMA = bismethylamide; TTHA = triethylenetetraaminehexaacetic acid.
‡10 MHz.

Reprinted with permission from Lauffer RB: Paramagnetic metal complexes as water proton relaxation agents for NMR imaging: theory and design. Chem Rev 87:901–927, 1987. Copyright 1987 American Chemical Society.

complexes thus becomes a significant fraction (if not all) of the total relaxivity.

In general, relaxivities are also proportional to the magnetic moment of the metal ion. However, we can see from Table 5–4 that dysprosium(III) with DTPA

Coordination of Gd^{3+} with DTPA · H$_2$O

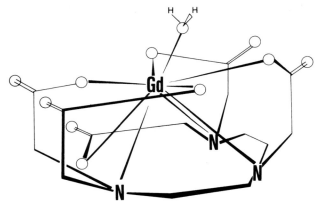

FIGURE 5–6. Structure of Gd-DTPA. (Courtesy of Schering AG, Berlin, Germany.)

has a much lower relaxivity than the analogous Gd^{III} complex despite the larger magnetic moment of Dy^{III}. As it turns out, for all of the lanthanide(III) ions except Gd^{III} and for certain transition metal ions, electron spin relaxation occurs so rapidly (T1$_e$ ~ 1 ps) that fluctuations at the proper frequencies for nuclear relaxation are less probable and thus relaxivities are low. (This is equivalent to saying that a short T1$_e$ leads to a small value of τ_c [τ_c = T1$_e$ in this case], which, in turn, leads to low relaxivity, as shown in Equation 5.)

For metal ions with relatively long T1$_e$ values—Gd^{III}, Mn^{II}, and iron(III) are good examples—alteration of the rotational tumbling time τ_R is the single most important source of relaxivity enhancement. The degree of enhancement possible, which is limited by the values of T1$_e$ and τ_M according to Equation 6, exceeds that which is realistically available from optimizing any of the other relevant parameters. Figure 5–7 shows the magnetic field dependence of relaxivity (also known as nuclear magnetic relaxation dispersion profile, or NMRD) as a function of τ_R calculated from the Solomon-Bloembergen equation. Parameters typical of Gd^{III} complexes are utilized. The enhancement in R$_1$ predicted at longer τ_R values (the proton relaxation enhancement effect) has been experimentally observed for metal ions bound to DNA or proteins. One can see from Figure 5–7 that both the magnitude of relaxivity and the functional form of its field dependence are altered when the rotation rate is decreased. The prominent peak that forms is noteworthy, because

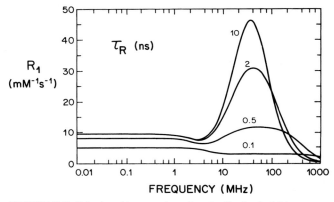

FIGURE 5–7. Calculated inner sphere longitudinal relaxivities versus Larmor frequency, or NMRD profiles, as a function of different values of the rotational correlation time, τ_R, of a metal complex. Values chosen are typical of a Gd^{III} complex with q = 1. The lowest value of τ_R chosen, 0.1 ns, is roughly that of low-molecular-weight complexes such as (Gd-DTPA)$^{2-}$; the single dispersion at approximately 5 MHz is that of the 7τ_c term in Equation 5 (the 3τ_c term does not disperse under these conditions until ~1000 MHz). Increasing τ_R (e.g., by increasing size of complex) allows the frequency dependence of T1$_e$ to be expressed; T1$_e$ is thought to rise dramatically with increasing frequency beginning at 10 MHz, creating the peak characteristic of slowly rotating paramagnetic ions. The increase in τ_c pushes the 7τ_c dispersion to lower frequency (~2 MHz) and brings the 3τ_c dispersion down to about 100 MHz. With the parameters used here, raising τ_R above 10 ns does not increase relaxivity further, as T1$_e$ or τ_M or both become the dominant correlation times. (Reprinted with permission from Lauffer RB: Paramagnetic metal complexes as water proton relaxation agents for NMR imaging: theory and design. Chem Rev 87:901–927, 1987. Copyright 1987 American Chemical Society.)

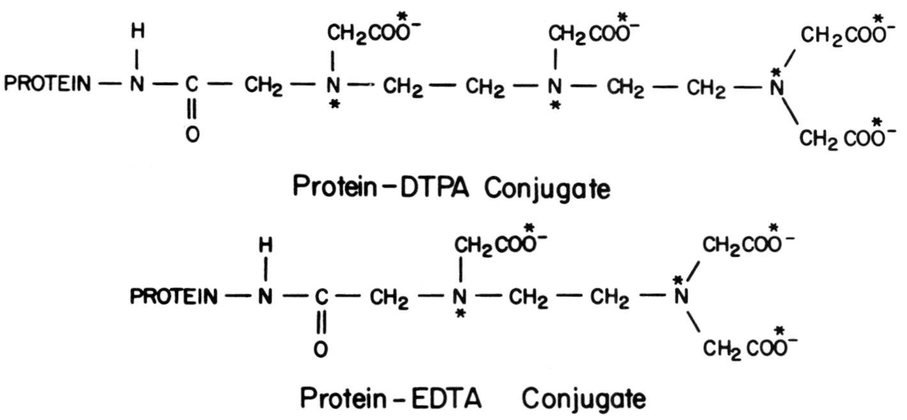

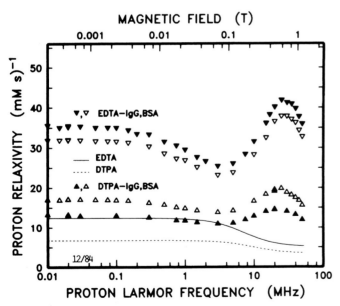

FIGURE 5–8. Anticipated structure of the DTPA and EDTA ligands when covalently attached to protein amino groups. Heteroatoms most likely involved in Mn^{II} or Gd^{III} binding are denoted with asterisks. These protein-bound complexes can be used to slow molecular rotation and thereby enhance relaxivity. (From Lauffer RB, Brady TJ, Brown RD, et al: 1/T1 NMRD profiles of solutions of Mn^{2+} and Gd^{3+} protein-chelate complexes. Magn Reson Med 3:541–548, 1986.)

it is predicted to occur over the clinically relevant field range.

The proton relaxation enhancement effect has been shown to be operative when intact chelates are covalently attached to protein amino acid residues. The ligands ethylenediaminetetraacetic acid (EDTA) and DTPA were attached to amino groups on bovine serum albumin and bovine immunoglobulins using cyclic anhydride forms of the ligands.[23, 24] The structure of the bound ligands, shown in Figure 5–8, most likely involves an amide linkage between a ligand carboxylate and the lysine or terminal amino group. Metal ions can be titrated selectively into the chelating sites on the proteins. Figure 5–9 displays the complete NMRD profiles of the free and bound Gd^{III} chelates. Binding

is generally accompanied by an increase in the amplitudes of the curves and a change in their functional form, resembling that calculated from theory and observed in slowly rotating metalloenzyme systems. This finding implies that despite the potentially flexible linkage to the protein the chelates appear to be fairly immobilized. The magnitudes of the relaxivities are most likely related to the average number of coordinated waters in each case, which is greater for the EDTA conjugates than for the DTPA conjugates.

Relaxivity in Tissue

The efficiency by which a metal complex influences tissue relaxation rates is dependent on two factors:

1. The chemical environment (or environments) encountered by the complex in vivo. By far the greatest effect is exerted by binding of the agent to macromolecular structures, which can potentially cause significant relaxivity enhancement.

2. Compartmentalization of the complex in tissue. Generally, tissue water is compartmentalized into intravascular, interstitial (fluid space between cells and capillaries), and intracellular space constituting roughly 5%, 15%, and 80% of the total water, respectively. Cellular organelles further subdivide the intracellular component. If water exchange between any of these compartments is slow relative to the relaxation rate in the compartment with the longest T1, multiexponential longitudinal relaxation may result. This can decrease the effective tissue relaxivity of an agent because not all of the tissue water is encountering the paramagnetic center.

Estimates of tissue relaxivities of metal complexes require the measurement of T1 values of excised tissue from two groups of animals: those receiving the agent and a control group. The tissue concentration of the complex should be determined by analysis of the tissue for metal content or by use of a suitable radioactive tracer. The largest source of error in these determinations is the animal-to-animal variation in baseline relaxation rates.

For low-molecular-weight, hydrophilic metal complexes, the available data show clearly that the relaxi-

FIGURE 5–9. NMRD profiles of Gd^{III} chelates covalently attached to protein amino groups. Data are shown for Gd-EDTA attached to bovine immunoglobulins (IgG,▼) and bovine serum albumin (BSA,▽) and the corresponding Gd-DTPA conjugates (▲, △). The solid and dashed curves in the lower portion of the figure indicate data for the free chelates (Gd-EDTA)$^{-}$ and (Gd-DTPA)$^{2-}$, respectively. (From Lauffer RB, Brady TJ, Brown RD, et al: 1/T1 NMRD profiles of solutions of Mn^{2+} and Gd^{3+} protein-chelate complexes. Magn Reson Med 3:541–548, 1986.)

vity in blood and soft tissue is within experimental error of that in aqueous solution; this has been shown, for example, for $(Gd-DTPA)^{2-}$ and $(Gd-DOTA)^{-}$ (DOTA = 1,4,7,10-tetraazacyclododecane-N,N',N'',N'''-tetraacetate) by Tweedle and colleagues.[25, 26] This observation suggests that no binding interactions between the chelate and proteins or membrane structures are taking place. The early use of cobalt(II) EDTA as an extracellular marker suggests that the distribution of these Gd^{III} complexes is the same.[27] The hydrophilic nature of the complexes, as well as their extracellular localization (where protein concentrations are lower relative to intracellular environments), apparently results in unhindered rotational mobility.

Koenig and associates[28] have measured NMRD profiles for blood containing $(Gd-DTPA)^{2-}$. The single exponential decay of the longitudinal relaxation in these samples indicates that water exchange between erythrocytes and plasma must be fast relative to the relaxation rates. It is interesting that the NMRD difference curves obtained after subtracting out the diamagnetic contribution to the observed rates were identical in amplitude and functional form to that of the complex in aqueous solution.

Compartmentalization effects have been noted for the kidney by Koenig and coworkers[29] in another study of $(Gd-DTPA)^{2-}$. Longitudinal relaxation in the renal medulla was found to be biexponential in the presence of the paramagnetic agent, resulting from concentration of the agent in the collecting tubules.

The most prominent evidence for a paramagnetic agent binding in vivo and generating greater relaxivity is that of the Mn^{II} ion. Although not relevant as a contrast agent because of its toxicity, Mn^{II} has both a historical and an instructive importance. Lauterbur and colleagues,[18] in their landmark 1978 contribution, noted an approximately 50% increase in relaxivity for Mn^{II} in heart tissue at 4 MHz. Kang and Gore[30] measured enhancement factors (relative to the aquo ion in aqueous solution) of 4 to 6 at 20 MHz for Mn^{II} in heart, liver, spleen, and kidney. Kang and colleagues[31] found that Mn^{II} binding to serum albumin in blood induces a 10-fold enhancement in relaxivity. Koenig and colleagues[32] measured NMRD profiles of liver and kidney tissue after injection of Mn^{II} (or weakly chelated complexes) and found peaks in relaxation rate centered at approximately 10 to 20 MHz, indicative of Mn^{II} in slowly tumbling environments, possibly bound to proteins or membrane surfaces. The field dependence of relaxation is thus valuable in that it can qualitatively indicate binding interactions in tissue without independent determinations of agent concentration.

TOXICITY

It is important to understand the acute and chronic toxic effects of paramagnetic metal complexes in view of the likely possibility of routine intravenous administration of such compounds for MRI examinations in the future. The required doses of such compounds

(roughly 0.5 to 5.0 g per patient) greatly exceed those of metal ions or complexes used in radioscintigraphy. However, iodine-containing contrast agents are used in computed tomography and other radiologic procedures at much higher doses than are MRI agents (~50 to 200 g per patient). With the development of relatively nontoxic chelates, the contrast-enhanced MRI examination is likely to be safer than similar computed tomography procedures.

Toxicity and stability are discussed together here to emphasize the historical importance of metal complex stability in determining toxicity in early evaluations of MRI agents. The dissociation of a complex generally leads to a higher degree of toxicity stemming from the free metal ion or free chelating ligand.

Toxic effects from a metal complex can arise from 1) free metal ion, released by dissociation; 2) free ligand, which also arises from dissociation; and 3) the intact metal complex. In the last two cases, one may also have to consider metabolites, which may be more toxic than the parent compound.

The available toxicologic data point to the importance of metal complex dissociation as an important source of toxicity. Table 5–5 lists acute LD_{50} values (interpolated doses at which 50% of the animals would die) determined for metal ions, complexes, and ligands. Both metal ions and free ligands tend to be more toxic than metal chelates. This finding is reasonable if one considers that complexation itself "neutralizes" the coordinating properties of both the ligand and the metal ion to some degree, decreasing their avidity for binding to proteins, enzymes, or membranes via electrostatic or hydrogen-bonding interactions or covalent bonds.

In the simplest view, the degree of toxicity of a metal chelate is related to its degree of dissociation in vivo before excretion. A good example of the dependence of toxicity and in vivo stability on the chelating ligand is the comparison between $(Gd-EDTA)^{-}$ and $(Gd-DTPA)^{2-}$. The latter is a stable complex (metal-ligand formation constant, $\log K_{ML} = 22.5$) that is excreted intact readily by the kidneys, exhibiting a low degree of toxicity ($LD_{50} \sim 10$ to 20 mmol/kg).[33] $(Gd-EDTA)^{-}$, on the other hand, has a toxicity comparable to that of $GdCl_3$ ($LD_{50} \sim 0.5$ mmol/kg), despite its apparently high thermodynamic stability ($\log K_{ML} = 17.4$). The straightforward interpretation is that the latter complex quantitatively dissociates in vivo, yielding the toxicity of the free ion.

The toxicity of metal ions has been extensively reviewed.[34] The coordination of ions to oxygen, nitrogen, or sulfur heteroatoms in macromolecules and membranes alters the dynamic equilibria necessary to sustain life. Gd^{III}, for example, can bind to calcium(II) binding sites, often with higher affinity owing to its greater charge/radius ratio.

The toxicity of free ligands, which is less understood, can stem from the sequestration of essential metal ions, such as Ca^{II}, in addition to "organic" toxicity.

The toxicity of intact metal complexes can stem from a wide variety of specific and nonspecific effects. At the high doses required in LD_{50} determinations

TABLE 5–5. ACUTE LD_{50} VALUES FOR METAL SALTS, METAL COMPLEXES, AND FREE LIGANDS

COMPOUND*	LD_{50} (mmol/kg)	ANIMAL	ADMINI-STRATION†
$GdCl_3$	0.5	Rat	IV
	0.4	Mouse	IV
	0.26	Rat	IV
	1.4	Mouse	IP
$Gd(OH)_3$	0.1	Mouse	IV
$(MEG)[Gd(EDTA)(H_2O)_n]$	0.3	Rat	IV
	0.62	Mouse	IP
$MEG[Gd(CDTA)(H_2O)_n]$	<2.5	Rat	IV
$MEG[Gd(EGTA)(H_2O)_n]$	<2.5	Rat	IV
$(MEG)^2[Gd(DTPA)(H_2O)]$	10	Rat	IV
	>10	Mouse	IV
$Na^2[Gd(DTPA)(H_2O)]$	>10	Mouse	IV
	20	Rat	IV
$(MEG)[Gd(DOTA)(H_2O)]$	>10	Mouse	IV
$Na[Gd(DOTA)(H_2O)]$	>10	Mouse	IV
Gd(DTPA-BMA)	34‡	Mouse	IV
Gd(HP-DO3A)	12‡	Mouse	IV
$(MEG)_3[Gd(TTHA)]$	6	Rat	IV
$MnCl_2$	0.22	Rat	IV
	1.5	Mouse	IP
$Na_2[Mn(EDTA)(H_2O)]$	7.0	Rat	IV
	5.9	Mouse	IP
$Na_3[Mn(DTPA)]$	1.9	Rat	IV
$FeCl_3$	1.6	Mouse	IP
$Na[Fe(EDTA)(H_2O)]$	3.4	Mouse	IV
	1.7	Mouse	IP
$Na_3[Ca(DTPA)]$	5.0	Rat	IV
	3.5	Mouse	IV
$(MEG)_3H_2DTPA$	0.15	Mouse	IV
Na_3H_3DTPA	0.1	Mouse	IV
$Na_2[Ca(DOTA)]$	>7.0	Mouse	IV
$(MEG)_2H_2DOTA$	0.18	Mouse	IV

*MEG = N-methylglucamine; CDTA = trans-1,2-cyclohexylenedinitrilo-tetraacetic acid; EGTA = ethylene glycol(2-aminoethylether)tetraacetic acid; TTHA = triethylenetetraaminehexaacetic acid.

†IV = intravenous; IP = intraperitoneal.

‡Data from Watson AD, Rocklage SM, Corrlin MJ: Contrast agents. In: Stark DD, Bradley WG, eds. Magnetic Resonance Imaging. St. Louis: Mosby–Year Book, 1992, pp 372–437.

Reprinted with permission from Lauffer RB: Paramagnetic metal complexes as water proton relaxation agents for NMR imaging: theory and design. Chem Rev 87:901–927, 1987. Copyright 1987 American Chemical Society.

of relatively nontoxic hydrophilic chelates like (Gd-DTPA)$^{2-}$, the nonspecific hypertonic effect is thought to be important. A difference in osmolality between intracellular and extracellular compartments is established after injection of large quantities of the ionic complexes and appropriate counter-ions. Water is drawn out of cells as a result of the osmotic gradient, causing cellular and circulatory damage. The two non-ionic gadolinium agents, Gd-DTPA-BMA (gadodiamide, Omniscan) and Gd-HP-DO3A (gadoteridol, Pro-Hance), were developed to reduce the osmolality of the injected formulations.[2-4] Judging from the excellent safety record of the ionic Gd-DTPA[35] (even at doses > 0.3 mmol/kg), it is not clear whether the nonionic concept is medically relevant or just a convenient marketing tool. Low osmolality may reduce the apparent acute toxicity in animals of large doses (100 times the clinical dose) (see Table 5–5), but the relevance of these findings to the clinical setting is uncertain.

Other possible mechanisms of chelate toxicity in-clude enzyme inhibition, nonspecific protein conformational effects, and alteration of membrane potentials. The interactions between metal chelates and biologic macromolecular structures, which are not well understood, represent an important area of investigation relevant to understanding toxicity on a molecular basis.

BIODISTRIBUTION

Targeting a paramagnetic agent to a particular site within the body is one of the most challenging aspects of MRI contrast agent design. The diagnostic utility of a contrast-enhanced MRI examination depends on the absolute concentration of the agent in the desired tissue and the selectivity of the distribution relative to other tissues. True targeting is rarely achieved. After administration, the agent equilibrates in several body compartments before excretion; preferential distribution of the agent to the desired site is all that can be expected in most circumstances. MRI agents are similar to radiopharmaceuticals or iodinated computed tomography agents in that the MR image enhancement depends on the concentration of a paramagnetic metal complex. The principles of distribution governing these other agents are directly applicable to MRI agents. New approaches to targeting magnetopharmaceuticals in this fashion are discussed in the Chapter 6.

However, the dependence of relaxivity on the chemical environment of a paramagnetic complex alters this simple view. What is directly relevant to MRI is not the actual distribution of the agent but the distribution of the relaxation rate changes induced by the agent. The enhancement in relaxivity induced by binding the agent to a macromolecule (the proton relaxation enhancement effect) is of central importance. By targeting a complex to desired sites where such binding interactions occur, the target/nontarget ratio in terms of relaxation rate changes may be increased above that in terms of concentration. This "binding enhancement" concept has been put into practice in the design of a high-relaxivity liver agent (discussed later).

Figure 5–10 illustrates potential distribution sites and excretion pathways relevant for soluble metal complexes. An intravenously administered chelate rapidly

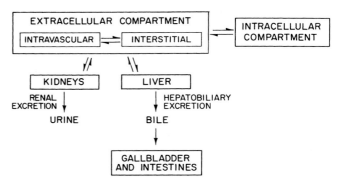

FIGURE 5–10. Principal distribution sites and excretion pathways for intravenously administered soluble metal complexes.

equilibrates in the intravascular and interstitial (space between cells) fluid compartments; these are referred to collectively as the extracellular compartment. Depending on its structure, the complex may also be distributed into various intracellular environments (including that of liver and kidney) by passive diffusion or specific uptake processes.

The structure of the complex determines its excretion pathway. Most commonly, low-molecular-weight hydrophilic chelates that do not bind to plasma proteins are nonspecifically filtered out in the kidneys (glomerular filtration).[36] If the molecule possesses a balance between hydrophobic and hydrophilic character, particularly if it contains aromatic rings, some fraction of the complex is taken up by liver cells and excreted into the bile (hepatobiliary excretion).[37] Such molecules often exhibit some degree of plasma protein binding, particularly to albumin, which reduces the free fraction available for glomerular filtration. The hepatobiliary and renal pathways can thus be competitive. Generally, the greater the lipophilicity of a molecule, the greater the hepatobiliary excretion. The complete clearance of the agent from the body by either route is, of course, desirable to minimize toxicity. If, however, the complex is quite lipophilic, it can 1) distribute into fat storage sites or membranes or 2) precipitate in blood and be taken up by reticuloendothelial cells in the liver and spleen. Both possibilities lead to long-term retention of the agent, which may be associated with chronic toxicity.

The following is a discussion of the various classes of metal complexes under investigation as MRI agents. Owing to the relatively high concentration of a paramagnetic agent required for image enhancement, the targeting of low-concentration receptor sites (<1 μM), as in traditional radioscintigraphy or positron emission tomography,[38] is not feasible for MRI. Therefore, the diagnostic utility of most of the complexes under examination is linked to their general distribution or excretion pathway or both, and this fact is reflected in the classifications that follow.

Extracellular Distribution: Renal Excretion

$(Gd-DTPA)^{2-}$ and the other approved agents are members of this class of agents. Compared with other substances discussed later, these agents are nonspecific in reference to their nonselective extracellular distribution. Their localization in tissues does not usually reflect specific cellular processes. They nevertheless form an important class of potential MRI agents that resemble iodinated computed tomography contrast media as well as more analogous radiopharmaceuticals, such as the DTPA complexes of technetium 99m (^{99m}Tc) or indium 113 (^{113}In).[38]

The structural requirements for these agents are satisfied by simple metal complexes. The presence of charged or hydrogen-bonding groups such as carboxylates and the lack of large hydrophobic groups ensure minimal interaction with plasma proteins, other macromolecules, and membranes. This situation allows equilibration of the complex in the extracellular space

and efficient renal excretion. The stereochemistry of the complex or other subtle structural features are not likely to be important. Most members of this class are anionic.

The renal excretion of these agents yields the obvious application of imaging the kidneys, both for structural and for functional information.[39, 40] The status of blood flow to a tissue (perfusion) may be another application of these agents[1–4, 41]; this requires the use of fast imaging techniques to follow the rapid passage through the tissue.

The major use of these nonspecific agents is in the detection of cerebral capillary breakdown or the enhancement of tissues with an increased extracellular volume. Both applications stem from the dependence of the bulk tissue $1/T1$ on the volume of distribution of the paramagnetic agent. If we assume that water exchange between the extracellular and intracellular compartments is fast relative to their T1 values, then the bulk tissue $1/T1$ before injection of the agent is given by

$$(1/T1)_{preinj} = f_{ex}(1/T1)_{ex, pre} + f_{in}(1/T1)_{in} \quad (7)$$

where f_{ex} is the fraction of water protons in the extracellular space, $(1/T1)_{ex, pre}$ is the extracellular relaxation rate in the absence of the paramagnetic species, and f_{in} is the intracellular fraction characterized by $(1/T1)_{in}$. The extracellularly localized agent increases $(1/T1)_{ex}$ directly, and the net change in the overall tissue $1/T1$ is given by

$$\begin{aligned}
\Delta(1/T1) &= (1/T1)_{postinj} - (1/T1)_{preinj} \\
&= [f_{ex}(1/T1)_{ex, post} + f_{in}(1/T1)_{in}] \\
&\quad - [f_{ex}(1/T1)_{ex, pre} - f_{in}(1/T1)_{in}] \\
&= [f_{ex}[(1/T1)_{ex, post} - (1/T1)_{ex, pre}] \quad (8)
\end{aligned}$$

If an agent equilibrates to roughly the same concentration in the extracellular space, and therefore $(1/T1)_{ex, post}$ is relatively constant in different tissues, then the tissues with the greatest fraction of extracellular space yield the greatest signal intensity changes. This finding has been observed for tumors and abscesses, which often exhibit increased interstitial volume.[25, 40]

The most dramatic enhancement of lesions with these agents is seen in the brain (Fig. 5–11), where normal tissue exhibits little enhancement because of the impermeable nature of brain capillaries (the blood-brain barrier) and the small intravascular volume of distribution (5%) of the agent. The capillaries of tumors, however, do allow the passage of the complex into the interstitial space, allowing selective enhancement.

Extracellular Distribution: Hepatobiliary Excretion

Hepatobiliary agents are another important class of potential MRI contrast agents. By virtue of their efficient excretion from the body, the development of safe derivatives of this class seems likely. In addition, in contrast to the nonspecific renal agents, hepatobiliary

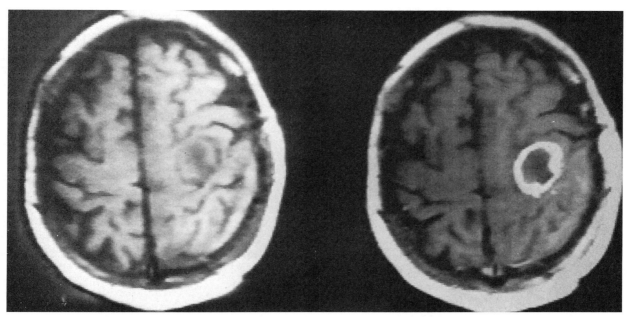

FIGURE 5–11. Transverse MR images (0.6 T, 24 MHz) through the brain of a patient before *(left)* and 3 minutes after *(right)* intravenous injection of $(Gd-DTPA)^{2-}$ (dimeglumine salt) at a dose of 0.1 mmol/kg. Characteristic ring enhancement of a tumor (high-grade astrocytoma) is seen in the postinjection image. Pulse sequence: spin echo, repetition time (TR) = 500 ms, and echo time (TE) = 20 ms. (Courtesy of T. Brady, MD, Massachusetts General Hospital, Boston, MA.)

agents may give an indication of the status of specific cellular function: that of the hepatocytes of the liver.

The potential diagnostic utility of this class of MRI agents includes the following:

1. Selective enhancement of normal, functioning liver tissue to aid in the detection of small lesions, such as metastatic tumors (focal liver disease).

2. Indication of the status of liver function to detect diffuse liver disease such as cirrhosis.

3. High-resolution visualization of bile ducts and the gallbladder.

Other forms of diagnostic hepatobiliary agents are radioactive ^{99m}Tc complexes[38, 42] and iodinated computed tomography agents.[43, 44] Currently, various substituted ^{99m}Tc–acetanilidoiminodiacetic acid (^{99m}Tc-IDA) complexes are used in scintigraphic imaging to detect obstruction of bile ducts. However, the image resolution is low compared with that in MRI, limiting biliary visualization. Furthermore, detection of small lesions in the liver by these complexes or other radiopharmaceuticals is not possible. The hepatobiliary agents for computed tomography that have been evaluated are not used clinically owing to their toxicity and high dose requirements.[44]

The mechanisms by which the hepatocytes of the liver extract certain molecules from the blood and secrete them into bile have not been refined.[37, 45] Diagnostic hepatobiliary agents are generally anionic and are therefore thought to be taken up by the carrier system that transports bilirubin, the dicarboxylic acid breakdown product of heme, and various anionic dyes, such as sulfobromophthalein sodium (bromosulfophthalein). Membrane proteins that are thought to play a crucial role in the uptake of these compounds have been identified, and it is likely that some type of carrier-mediated transport is at work, at least for some types of molecules. Separate anionic transport systems for fatty acids and bile acids apparently exist in addition to that for bilirubin. However, Okuda and coworkers[46] have suggested that anionic compounds such as the ^{99m}Tc-IDA chelates may actually be taken up by more than one of the three carriers. In addition, simple diffusion through the hepatocyte membrane may account for a large part of the uptake, especially for lipophilic molecules.

The structural and physicochemical properties required for hepatocellular uptake are poorly defined.[37] It is generally believed that high molecular weight (>300 for rats and >500 for humans) and the presence of both hydrophilic and lipophilic moieties direct a compound to the bile in preference to the urine. The molecular weight requirement probably reflects the need for large lipophilic groups, especially aromatic rings, which may interact favorably with membranes or the hydrophobic regions of transport proteins. The ^{99m}Tc-IDA complexes, bilirubin, and various cholephilic dyes (such as bromosulfophthalein) possess at least two delocalized ring systems. The more polar moieties, especially ionized groups, are probably required for water solubility; molecules lacking these might precipitate in blood or become deposited in fat tissue or membranes. It is also likely that these groups, especially anionic residues, are important for electrostatic or hydrogen-bonding interactions at macromolecular binding sites.

Early work with a prototype iron agent, iron(III) ethylenebis-(2-hydrophenylglycine) (Fe-EHPG), established that functional hepatobiliary MRI was possible.[1, 47–50] This agent and various chemical derivatives showed strong enhancement of the liver and gallbladder in animals and excellent contrast enhancement of small metastatic tumors in mice (Figs. 5–12 and 5–13). Nonetheless, the relatively low relaxivity of these agents prompted a search for gadolinium-based analogues.

Three gadolinium chelates, gadobenate dimeglumine (Gd-BOPTA), gadolinium ethoxybenzyl DTPA (Gd-EOB-DTPA), and MS-264, are under investigation as hepatobiliary MRI contrast agents.[51–53] The structures of the ligands for these complexes are shown in Figure 5–14. All three chelates have a net charge of -2 and a benzene ring; the anionic charge and aromatic character of these chelates are similar to those of the ^{99m}Tc-IDA complexes. The gadolinium chelates thus have some affinity for the liver, although to varying degrees. Figure 5–15 shows the percentage of the injected dose of the three chelates that is excreted into the feces of various animal species (the remainder is renally excreted). For Gd-BOPTA and Gd-EOB-DTPA, the percentage of biliary excretion is strongly species dependent, showing a marked decrease in humans or in animals whose hepatobiliary physiology more closely resembles that of humans (rabbit and monkey). MS-264, on the other hand, was selected in part on the basis of strong biliary excretion in all species.[53] The greater liver uptake of MS-264 than of Gd-EOB-DTPA was demonstrated directly in whole-body ^{153}Gd scintig-

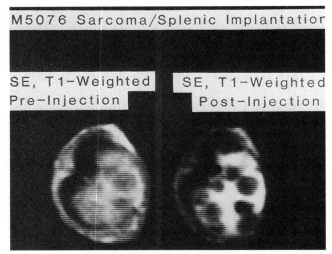

FIGURE 5–13. MR images (spin echo, 200/15) of a mouse exhibiting multiple liver metastases. M5076 sarcoma cells were implanted in the spleen and allowed to metastasize to the liver. Figure shows enhancement of normal liver parenchyma with 0.1 mmol/kg Fe-EHPG, facilitating the detection of the lesions (image at right was obtained 15 minutes after injection). (Courtesy of F. Shtern, MD, and T. Brady, MD, Massachusetts General Hospital, Boston, MA.)

raphy studies. The higher hepatobiliary specificity of MS-264 is expected to permit greater and more persistent liver MRI enhancement and robust performance even in the presence of liver disease.

As noted for other cholephilic anions, these hepatobiliary MRI agents bind with varying degrees of affinity to proteins inside the hepatocyte. Because macromolecular binding alters the molecular tumbling rate of a chelate, considerable enhancement in relaxivity can occur. Figure 5–16 shows the relaxivities of the three chelates in buffer and rat hepatocyte cytosol.[52] MS-264 shows the greatest enhancement in relaxivity, followed by Gd-EOB-DTPA and Gd-BOPTA. The higher relaxivity of MS-264 than of Gd-EOB-DTPA correlated with the percentage of the chelate (at 0.1 mM) that is protein bound as measured by ultrafiltration: 47% versus 15%. MS-264 is therefore a good example of exploiting the unique biophysics of MRI contrast media for signal enhancement.

Intravascular Distribution

A paramagnetic agent that would be confined in the intravascular space by molecular size or by binding to plasma proteins may have potential for the enhancement of normal, perfused tissues in preference to tissue with decreased blood supply. In addition, these agents may be useful for MR angiography.

An intravascular agent could be composed of a paramagnetically labeled protein or polymer. Alternatively, a low-molecular-weight chelate could be designed to bind strongly to human serum albumin. Both the noncovalent and covalent attachments would yield relaxivity enhancement.

The labeled macromolecule approach has yielded a wealth of animal data on the potential diagnostic uses

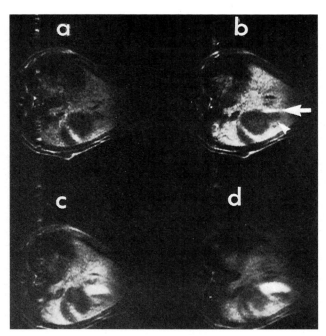

FIGURE 5–12. Transverse MR images (0.6 T, 24 MHz) of the dog abdomen before (a) and 14, 50, and 60 minutes after (b to d, respectively) intravenous injection of Fe-EHPG (0.2 mmol/kg). Enhancement of the liver and gallbladder is evident. Bile in the gallbladder before injection of the agent appears dark (arrowhead), whereas newly formed bile containing the paramagnetic agent appears bright (arrow) and layers on top. (a to d from Lauffer RB, Greif WL, Stark DD, et al: Iron-EHPG as an hepatobiliary MR contrast agent: initial imaging and biodistribution studies. J Comput Assist Tomogr 9:431–438, 1985.)

OCH₂CH₃

EOB

BOPTA

(CH₂)₃CH₃

MS-264

FIGURE 5–14. Structures of the ligands for three gadolinium-based hepatobiliary agents in development.

for a blood pool agent.[2–4, 54] Human serum albumin, dextran, polylysine, and polyethylene glycol have all been labeled with gadolinium groups and shown to have long half-life in blood and good enhancement of blood in arteries, veins, and tissues. However, the immunogenic potential, long-term retention, and other problems with these agents have prevented them from entering clinical trials to date.

The noncovalent human serum albumin–targeting approach gets around these problems by employing reversible binding to the macromolecule.[55, 56] This prevents rapid extravasation and clearance of the chelate but allows complete excretion after the MRI examination. A number of gadolinium chelates have been reported for this application.[56, 57] Clinical trials are expected soon.

Tumor-Localizing Agents

Two groups have described the use of synthetic paramagnetic metalloporphyrins to decrease the proton relaxation times of tumors.[58, 59] The properties of these complexes are somewhat different from those of the free porphyrin ligand mixture, known as hematoporphyrin derivative, which localizes in tumors and is used in phototherapy.[60] Nevertheless, some degree of retention of synthetic complexes, such as Mn[III] tetrakis(4-sulfonatophenyl)porphyrin, in tumors has been observed. The mechanism for this retention is not known, and this prevents a rational approach to the design of these agents. However, the stability and high relaxivity of these complexes, in addition to their unexplained tumor localization, make them attractive prototype contrast agents.

An alternative approach to tumor imaging involves the use of labeled monoclonal antibodies specific to a particular tumor line. Although greeted initially with enthusiasm, this method is likely to be useful only in radioimaging, in which only minuscule concentrations of the label are needed. For MRI, the required concentration of paramagnetic species is roughly 10 to 100 μM, whereas the concentration of antigenic sites in

FIGURE 5–15. Biliary excretion of gadolinium chelates in multiple species. Higher mammals generally excrete a smaller fraction of an administered chelate into feces than do rodents. MS-264, on the other hand, shows high hepatobiliary specificity in all species. The values shown in parentheses are the injected dose in millimoles per kilogram. The rabbit value for MS-264 is a lower estimate determined by [153]Gd scintigraphy.

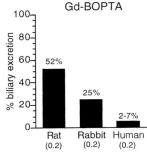

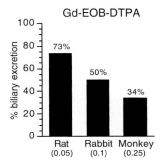

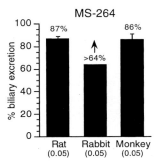

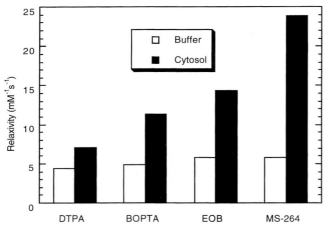

FIGURE 5–16. Relaxivity in buffer and rat hepatocyte cytosol for three gadolinium chelates (20 MHz, 37°C, pH 7.4). The enhancement in relaxivity in cytosol stems from protein binding, which is greatest for MS-264.

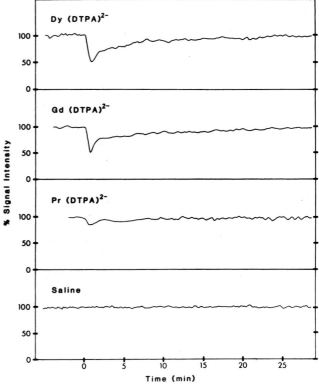

FIGURE 5–17. Effect of different lanthanide chelates on rat brain signal intensity using a one-dimensional rapid imaging technique designed to isolate the brain intensity with 8-second temporal resolution (spin echo, 1000/120). In each case, 1 mmol/kg of the agent was injected intravenously. The selected complexes exhibit varying magnetic moments: dysprosium (Dy) (III), 10.6 Bohr magnetons; gadolinium (Gd) (III), 8.0; and praseodymium (Pr) (III), 3.5. The percent decrease in signal intensity was found to correlate with the magnetic moment of the ion. (From Villringer A, Rosen BR, Belliveau JW, et al: Dynamic imaging with lanthanide chelates in normal brain: contrast due to magnetic susceptibility effects. Magn Reson Med 6:164–174, 1988.)

tumors is 0.1 μM or less.[61] Even if these sites could be saturated with paramagnetically labeled antibody molecules, such conjugates would require 100 to 1000 chelates per molecule for significant relaxation time differences. Because of this factor, coupled with the obvious problems of the potential toxicity and lower antigenic affinity of these conjugates, this approach is not likely to be clinically feasible. Perhaps other diagnostically useful target sites of higher concentration exist for magnetoimmunoimaging.

T2 AGENTS

T2 agents are also referred to as *homogeneity spoilers*. An early example of this class of agents is ferromagnetic (or superparamagnetic) particles, such as ferrite (Fe_3O_4). When water molecules diffuse through the microscopic magnetic field gradients around such particles, the protons experience efficient spin dephasing and transverse relaxation, leading to *decreases in signal intensity*. Because particulates are efficiently scavenged by reticuloendothelial cells, various compositions incorporating such particles are being evaluated as "negative" contrast agents for the liver, spleen, lymph nodes, and bowel (oral use). These and other applications are discussed in Chapter 6.

It has also been shown that soluble metal chelates such as Gd-DTPA can be used as T2 contrast agents. If present in sufficient concentration in the blood or extracellular space (such as immediately after injection), paramagnetic substances increase the bulk magnetic susceptibility of a given tissue compartment, leading (apparently) to field gradients at compartment interfaces and enhanced transverse relaxation. Early studies showed that injection of Dy-DTPA causes a transient decrease in rat liver image intensity using conventional spin-echo pulse sequences (Lauffer RB, Saini S, Brady TJ, unpublished results). Further work using different lanthanide DTPA chelates confirmed the effect on rat brain signal intensity and showed that

the degree of signal loss correlated with the magnetic moment of the metal ion[62] (Fig. 5–17). It is thought that this type of contrast agent will be especially useful in examining cardiac, brain, and tumor perfusion, particularly when combined with fast imaging techniques (echo planar or gradient echo).[63] Indeed, it has been shown that this technique can be used to examine subtle blood volume changes in the human brain during thought.[64]

REFERENCES

1. Lauffer RB: Paramagnetic metal complexes as water proton relaxation agents for NMR imaging: theory and design. Chem Rev 87:901–927, 1987.
2. Watson AD, Rocklage SM, Carvlin MJ: Contrast agents. In: Stark DD, Bradley WG, eds. Magnetic Resonance Imaging. 2nd ed. St. Louis: Mosby–Year Book, 1992, pp 372–437.
3. Tweedle M: Physicochemical properties of gadoteridol and other MR contrast agents. Invest Radiol 27(suppl 1):S2–S6, 1992.
4. Oksendal AN, Hals PA: Biodistribution and toxicity of MR imaging contrast media. J Magn Reson Imaging 3:157–165, 1993.
5. Bloch F, Hansen WW, Packard M: The nuclear induction experiment. Phys Rev 70:474, 1948.
6. Bloembergen N, Purcell EM, Pound RV: Relaxation effects in nuclear magnetic resonance absorption. Phys Rev 73:679, 1948.

7. Bloembergen N: Proton relaxation times in paramagnetic solutions. J Chem Phys 27:572, 1957.
8. Kubo R, Tomita K: Paramagnetic relaxation. J Phys Soc Jpn 9:888, 1954.
9. Solomon I: Relaxation processes in a system of two spins. Phys Rev 99:559, 1955.
10. Eisinger J, Shulman RG, Blumberg WE: Relaxation enhancement by paramagnetic iron binding in deoxyribonucleic acid solutions. Nature 192:963, 1961.
11. Dwek RA: Nuclear Magnetic Resonance in Biochemistry: Applications to Enzyme Systems. Oxford: Clarendon Press, 1973.
12. Mildvan AS: Proton relaxation enhancement. Annu Rev Biochem 43:357, 1974.
13. Burton DR, Forsen S, Karlstrom G, Dwek RA: Proton relaxation enhancement (PRE) in biochemistry: a critical survey. Prog NMR Spectrosc 13:1, 1979.
14. Lauterbur PC: Image formation by induced local interactions: examples employing nuclear magnetic resonance. Nature 242:190, 1973.
15. Hinshaw WS, Bottomley PA, Holland GN: Radiographic thin-section image of the human wrist by nuclear magnetic resonance. Nature 270:722, 1977.
16. Andrew ER, Bottomley PA, Hinshaw WS, et al: NMR images by the multiple sensitive point method: application to larger biological systems. Phys Med Biol 22:971, 1977.
17. Damadian R, Goldsmith M, Minkoff L: NMR in cancer. XVI. Fonar image of the live human body. Physiol Chem Phys 9:97, 1977.
18. Lauterbur PC, Mendonca-Dias MH, Rudin AM: Augmentation of tissue water proton spin-lattice relaxation rates by in vivo addition of paramagnetic ions. In: Dutton PL, Leigh LS, Scarpaa A, eds. Frontier of Biological Energetics. New York: Academic Press, 1978, p 752.
19. Brady TJ, Goldman MR, Pykett IL, et al: Proton nuclear magnetic resonance imaging of regionally ischemic canine hearts: effect of paramagnetic proton signal enhancement. Radiology 144:343, 1982.
20. Goldman MR, Brady TJ, Pykett IL, et al: Quantification of experimental myocardial infarction using nuclear magnetic resonance imaging and paramagnetic ion contrast enhancement in excised canine hearts. Circulation 66:1012, 1982.
21. Young IR, Clarke GJ, Gailes DR, et al: Enhancement of relaxation rate with paramagnetic contrast agents in NMR imaging. Comput Tomogr 5:534, 1981.
22. Carr DH, Brown J, Bydder GM, et al: Intravenous chelated gadolinium as a contrast agent in NMR imaging of cerebral tumors. Lancet 1:484, 1984.
23. Lauffer RB, Brady TJ: Preparation and water relaxation properties of proteins labeled with paramagnetic metal chelates. Magn Reson Imaging 3:11, 1985.
24. Lauffer RB, Brady TJ, Brown RD, et al: 1/T1 NMRD profiles of solutions of Mn^{2+} and Gd^{3+} protein-chelate complexes. Magn Reson Med 3:541–548, 1986.
25. Tweedle MF, Brittain HG, Eckelman WC, et al: Principles of contrast-enhanced MRI. In: Partain CL, Price RR, Patton JA, et al, eds. Magnetic Resonance Imaging. 2nd ed. Philadelphia: WB Saunders, 1988, pp 793–809.
26. Tweedle MF, Gaughan GT, Hagan J, et al: Considerations involving paramagnetic coordination compounds as useful NMR contrast agents. Nucl Med Biol 15:31, 1988.
27. Brading AF, Jones AW: Distribution and kinetics of CoEDTA in smooth muscle and its use as an extracellular marker. J Physiol (Lond) 200:387, 1969.
28. Koenig SH, Spiller M, Brown RD III, Wolf GL: Relaxation of water protons in the intra- and extracellular regions of blood containing Gd(DTPA). Magn Reson Med 3:791, 1986.
29. Spiller M, Koenig SH, Wolf GL, Brown RD III: Presented at the 4th Annual Meeting of the Society of Magnetic Resonance in Medicine, London, 1985.
30. Kang YS, Gore JC: Studies of tissue NMR relaxation enhancement by manganese. Dose and time dependences. Invest Radiol 19:399, 1984.
31. Kang YS, Gore JC, Armitage IM: Studies of factors affecting the design of NMR contrast agents: manganese in blood as a model system. Magn Reson Med 1:396, 1984.
32. Koenig SH, Brown RD III, Goldstein EJ, et al: Magnetic field dependence of tissue proton relaxation rates with added Mn^{2+}: rabbit liver and kidney. Magn Reson Med 2:159, 1985.
33. Weinmann H-J, Brasch RC, Press RC, Wesbey GE: Characteristics of gadolinium-DTPA complex: a potential NMR contrast agent. AJR 142:619, 1984.
34. Luckey TD, Venugopal B: Metal Toxicity in Mammals, Volume 1. New York: Plenum Publishing, 1977.
35. Niendorf HP, Alhassan A, Haustein J, Claus W: Safety review of Gd-DTPA: extended clinical experience after more than 5,000,000 applications. Presented at the Contrast Media Research Conference, San Antonio, TX, October 1993.
36. Venkatachalam MA, Rennke HG: The structural and molecular basis of glomerular filtration. Circ Res 43:337, 1978.
37. Klaassen CD, Watkins JB III: Mechanisms of bile formation, hepatic uptake, and biliary formation. Pharmacol Rev 36:1, 1984.
38. Heindel ND, Burns HD, Honda T, Brady LW: The Chemistry of Radiopharmaceuticals. New York: Masson, 1978.
39. Wolf GL, Fobben ES: The tissue proton T1 response to gadolinium DTPA injection in rabbits: a potential renal contrast agent for NMR imaging. Invest Radiol 19:324, 1984.
40. Brasch RC, Weinmann H-J, Wesbey GE: Contrast-enhanced NMR imaging: animal studies using gadolinium-DTPA complex. AJR 142:625, 1984.
41. McNamara MT, Tscholakoff D, Revel D, et al: Use of gadolinium DTPA in assessing myocardial perfusion. Radiology 158:765, 1986.
42. Chervu LR, Nunn AD, Loberg MD: Radiopharmaceuticals for hepatobiliary imaging. Semin Nucl Med 12:5, 1984.
43. Koehler RE, Stanley RJ, Evans RG: Isofemate meglumine: an iodinated contrast agent for hepatic computed tomography scanning. Radiology 132:115, 1979.
44. Moss AA: Computed tomography of the hepatobiliary system. In: Moss AA, Gamsu G, Genant HK, eds. Computed Tomography of the Body. Philadelphia: WB Saunders, 1983, p 615.
45. Berk PD, Stremmel W: Hepatocellular uptake of organic anions. Prog Liver Dis 8:125–144, 1986.
46. Okuda H, Nunes R, Vallabhajosula S, et al: Studies of the hepatocellular uptake of the hepatobiliary scintiscanning agent ^{99m}Tc-DISIDA. J Hepatol 3:251–259, 1986.
47. Lauffer RB, Greif WL, Stark DD, et al: Iron-EHPG as an hepatobiliary MR contrast agent: initial imaging and biodistribution studies. J Comput Assist Tomogr 9:431, 1985.
48. Greif WL, Buxton RB, Lauffer RB, et al: Pulse sequence optimization for MR imaging using a paramagnetic hepatobiliary contrast agent. Radiology 157:461, 1985.
49. Lauffer RB, Vincent AC, Padmanabhan S, et al: New hepatobiliary MR contrast agents: 5-substituted iron-EHPG derivatives. Magn Reson Med 4:582–590, 1987.
50. Shtern F, Garrido L, Compton C, et al: MR imaging of blood-borne liver metastases in mice: contrast enhancement with Fe-EHPG. Radiology 178:83–89, 1991.
51. Schuhmann-Giampieri G: Liver contrast media for magnetic resonance imaging: interrelations between pharmacokinetics and imaging. Invest Radiol 28:753–761, 1993.
52. Lauffer RB, Parmalee DJ, Jenkins BJ, et al: Liver enhancement in normal and tumor-bearing rats with MS-264, a new high-relaxivity hepatobiliary agent. In: Proceedings of the Second Annual Meeting of the Society of Magnetic Resonance, San Francisco, August 1994, p 1513.
53. Walovitch RC, McMurry TJ, Tyeklar Z, et al: Biodistribution and safety studies of MS-264, a new liver agent with high hepatobiliary specificity. In: Proceedings of the Second Annual Meeting of the Society of Magnetic Resonance, San Francisco, August 1994, p 387.
54. Brasch RC: New directions in the development of MR imaging contrast media. Radiology 183:1–11, 1992.
55. Lauffer RB: Targeted relaxation enhancement agents for MRI. Magn Reson Med 22:339–342, 1991.
56. Lauffer RB, Parmelee DJ, Ouellet HS, et al: MS-325, the first small-molecule blood pool agent for MRI. Presented at the Contrast Media Research Conference, Naantali, Finland, June 1995, p 58.
57. Lauffer RB, U.S. Patent 4,880,008, 1989.
58. Lyon RC, Faustino PJ, Cohen JS, et al: Tissue distribution and stability of metalloporphyrin MRI contrast agents. Magn Reson Med 4:24, 1987.
59. Fiel RJ, Button TM, Gilani S, et al: Proton relaxation enhancement by manganese (III) TPPS4 in a model tumor system. Magn Reson Imaging 5:149, 1987.
60. Doiron DR, Gomer CJ (eds): Porphyrin Localization and Treatment of Tumors. New York: Alan R. Liss, 1984.
61. Unger EC, Totty WG, Neufeld DM, et al: Magnetic resonance imaging using gadolinium labeled monoclonal antibody. Invest Radiol 20:693, 1985.
62. Villringer A, Rosen BR, Belliveau JW, et al: Dynamic imaging with lanthanide chelates in normal brain: contrast due to magnetic susceptibility effects. Magn Reson Med 6:164–174, 1988.
63. Rosen BR, Belliveau JW, Chien D: Perfusion imaging by nuclear magnetic resonance. Magn Reson Q 5:263–281, 1989.
64. Belliveau JW, Kennedy DN, McKinstry RC, et al: Functional mapping of the human visual cortex by magnetic resonance imaging. Science 254:716–719, 1991.

Organ- and Tissue-Directed MRI Contrast Agents

W. SCOTT ENOCHS ▪ RALPH WEISSLEDER

The use of nonspecific extravascular, extracellular contrast agents in magnetic resonance imaging (MRI) is well established. Approximately 30% of all MRI examinations in the United States are performed with the use of a gadolinium chelate (e.g., Gd-DTPA [gadolinium(II) diethylenetriaminepentaacetic acid], Gd-HP-DO3A [gadolinium(II) 10-(2′-hydroxypropyl)-1,4,7,10-tetraazacyclododecane-$N,N′,N″$-triacetic acid], and Gd-DTPA-BMA [gadolinium(II) diethylenetriaminepentaacetic acid-bis(methylamide)]). These were the first contrast agents to be developed, and their pharmacologic profiles, indications for use, and mechanisms of action are detailed in Chapter 5.

A recognized need exists for contrast agents having a limited biodistribution (Fig. 6–1). Such agents are intended to improve the diagnosis of disease by selectively changing the signal intensity of normal or abnormal tissues, but preferably not both. Changes in signal intensity can be used to improve the detection of lesions (increased contrast-to-noise ratio) and their characterization. The more specific the accumulation of a contrast agent within the target tissue without distribution to surrounding tissue, the better is the resulting lesion-tissue contrast. The characterization of lesions also depends critically on the specificity of the contrast agent for a certain tissue type.

Our intent in this chapter is to critically review MRI contrast agents with tissue or organ specificity. Because of the large number of agents reported, this review is restricted largely to the clinically most relevant agents in each class and to those agents that have been described in peer-reviewed journals. The first two sections on gastrointestinal and blood pool agents cover agents that rely on a restricted biodistribution for their efficacy, that is, to the gut and vascular lumen, respectively. The next four sections discuss metabolic agents (metalloporphyrins and hepatobiliary agents) and particulate agents (magnetic liposomes and superparamagnetic iron oxides) that show characteristic specificities for various organs and tissues. Finally, the last section on target-specific agents summarizes and describes results with a variety of sophisticated agents that bind to particular cells and cellular receptors.

GASTROINTESTINAL AGENTS

Applications of MRI to the abdomen and upper pelvis (excluding the liver) have been lagging because of motion artifacts associated with respiration and

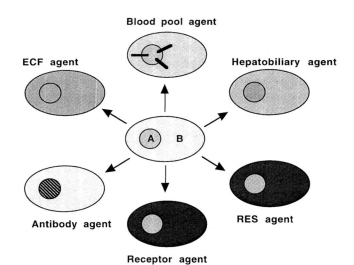

FIGURE 6–1. Types of parenteral MRI contrast agents. Diagnostic MRI pharmaceuticals for detecting tumor (A, e.g., tissue) in a parenchymal organ (B, e.g., liver). Extracellular fluid (ECF) agents (e.g., Gd-DTPA) are usually not tissue specific and are therefore distributed to both liver and tumor; the change in observable tumor-liver contrast is therefore low. Blood-pool agents primarily enhance the intravascular signal intensity and are thus used primarily for MR angiography. Hepatobiliary agents (e.g., Gd-EOB-DTPA and Mn-DPDP) are characterized by high hepatobiliary, rather than renal, excretion. Reticuloendothelial system (RES) agents (e.g., iron oxides and liposomes) accumulate primarily in Kupffer cells of the liver and phagocytes of the spleen. Receptor agents show the greatest promise for improving the detection of hepatic tumors. Tumor-directed antibody agents can be selective in organs devoid of phagocytically active cells or that metabolize immunoglobulin G.

bowel peristalsis and also because of the lack of a single accepted gastrointestinal contrast agent. As in computed tomography (CT), such an agent would be helpful for distinguishing bowel from adjacent normal or pathologic structures and thus for delineation of the bowel wall. All of the primary determinants of MRI contrast have been exploited in the search for an efficacious agent[1, 2] (Table 6–1). Candidates are typically classified by their miscibility with bowel contents and their effect on the signal intensity, but they have a biodistribution that is restricted to the gut lumen with no or only limited absorption. The ideal contrast agent should be well tolerated, safe, and inexpensive; become uniformly distributed throughout the entire gastrointestinal tract; be efficacious over wide ranges of intraluminal concentrations, pulse sequences, and timing parameters; and not exacerbate image artifacts.

None of the agents described in this chapter satisfy all of the preceding requirements, but some are remarkably efficacious in most respects. If delineation of the upper gastrointestinal tract is desired (e.g., in the setting of pancreatic cancer or lymphoma), water or feeding formulas are inexpensive and approved agents that show reasonable efficacy. Water is technically not a contrast agent but can be used effectively to distend the stomach and duodenum; it is not useful in the imaging of the small bowel and colon, however, because of rapid absorption.[3] If delineation of the small bowel is desired, an osmotically active agent must be used. In this regard, controversy exists over whether contrast agents having T1 (paramagnetic) or T2 (superparamagnetic) effects are preferable. Reliable delineation of the colon is even more challenging because water absorption often leads to artifacts from hyperconcentrations of the agents, particularly in the case of iron oxides. Fortunately, few indications exist in which opacification of the small bowel or colon is required that cannot be achieved with other imaging techniques such as CT. However, the advent of lymphotropic contrast agents for the staging of lymph node metastases may boost the use of oral MRI contrast agents.

HYDROGEN REPLACEMENT AGENTS

Two hydrogen replacement agents are gas, either carbon dioxide from ingested effervescent crystals (EZ gas, E-Z-EM, Westbury, NY)[4, 5] or air introduced by a rectal tube,[6] and liquid perfluorooctylbromide (PFOB) (Imagent GI, Alliance Pharmaceuticals, San Diego, CA).[7–12] Both agents cause a complete lack of intraluminal signal with all pulse sequences by replacing bowel contents and distending bowel with a medium lacking hydrogen altogether[4–6] (Figs. 6–2 and 6–3). Gas has been effectively applied in the stomach, duodenum, and rectum but can cause susceptibility artifacts at

TABLE 6–1. OVERVIEW OF GASTROINTESTINAL CONTRAST AGENTS*

CLASS	ACTIVE INGREDIENT	OTHER INGREDIENTS	STATUS	CONCENTRATION OF INGESTED METAL (mM)	ORAL DOSE (mL)	DISADVANTAGES	REFERENCES
Diamagnetic	Water or modified water (Readi-cat 2)	Suspending agents	Human	NA	500	Small bowel absorption; ultrafast imaging required	3, 26
	Gas	None	Human	NA	400–800†	Susceptibility artifacts	4–6
	PFOB	None	Human	NA	300–1000†	Expensive	7–12
	Oil emulsions		Human	NA	500	Absorbed in small bowel; weak T1 effect	5, 13–17
	Sucrose polyester		Animal	NA		Not tested in humans	14
	Clay minerals	Yes	Human	NA	450–900†	Unpalatable, biphasic dose response	5, 18, 19
	Barium sulfate	Suspending agents	Human	20–85 (% w/w)	400–900†	Inconsistent bowel distribution	5, 19–25
Paramagnetic	Ferric ammonium citrate	Alcohol in Geritol, flavoring in OMR	Human	1	500–600	Biphasic dose response; phase artifacts	3, 5, 27–30
	Iron phytate	Viscosity enhancer, volume expander, buffer	Human	3.6	900	Biphasic dose response; phase artifacts	34
	Manganese chloride (LumenHance)	Proprietry polymer	Human	1	NR	Biphasic dose response; phase artifacts	2, 35, 36
	Mn-DPDP	Commercial barium sulfate preparation	Animal	2		Biphasic dose response; phase artifacts; not tested in humans	37
	Gd-DTPA	Mannitol	Human	0.5–1	400–700†	Phase artifacts	40–43
Superparamagnetic	OMP	Viscosity enhancer	Human	2	800	Susceptibility artifacts	42, 48–62
	AMI-121	Suspending agent	Human	2–4	600–900	Susceptibility artifacts	43, 63, 64
	AMI-227	Suspending agent	Animal	NA		Biphasic dose response; phase artifacts	43

*PFOB = perfluorooctylbromide; OMR = proprietary ferric ammonium citrate; NA = not applicable; NR = not reported.
†Typically given with glucagon.

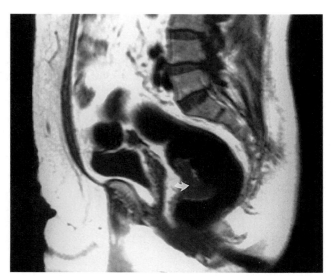

FIGURE 6–2. Air as MRI contrast agent. Rectal air insufflation is used to evaluate rectal carcinoma. Mildly T1-weighted sagittal image (spin echo, repetition time/echo time = 500/30) shows a large polypoid tumor (*arrow*) arising from the anterior rectal wall. Linear strands extending into perirectal fat from the base of the tumor indicate transmural invasion. After bowel preparation, air is instilled through a rectal catheter until the patient feels full. Between pulse sequences, the patient is encouraged to squeeze the air bulb insufflator on the end of the tube to maintain distention. (From Hahn PF: Oral contrast agents for abdominal MRI. In: Thrall JH, ed: Current Practice of Radiology. Philadelphia: BC Decker, 1993, pp 172–174. By permission of Mosby–Year Book, Inc.)

the air–bowel wall interface. By comparison, PFOB undergoes rapid transit and has been especially useful in studying the bowel wall.[7–12] Although the latter agent is relatively expensive, it has become the first oral agent for MRI to be approved by the U.S. Food and Drug Administration.[2] Minor side effects include an oily taste, rectal leakage, nausea, and vomiting; the last two may be associated with the concomitant administration of glucagon.

LIPIDS

The reported lipid agents have been prepared as emulsions of vegetable oils and thus behave as miscible substances.[5, 13–15] These agents increase the intraluminal signal intensity on T1- and, to a lesser extent, T2-weighted images owing to the faster relaxation of lipid protons compared with water protons. With appropriate flavorings, these agents can be tolerated but have a relatively weak T1 effect compared with paramagnetic agents. Extensive absorption in the small bowel limits their utility to the upper gastrointestinal tract. Sucrose polyester, a dietary fat substitute that is nondigestible and thus circumvents this problem, has been tested in animals.[14] The efficacy of a variety of infant and adult feeding formulas in the upper gastrointestinal tract is attributable to their contents of both lipid emulsions and paramagnetic metal ions.[16, 17]

MINERALS

The clay minerals tested as oral contrast agents include kaolin and attapulgite, which are the major ingredients of Kaopectate and New-Formula Kaopectate, respectively (Upjohn, Kalamazoo, MI)[5, 18, 19]; these substances form miscible suspensions in water. Barium sulfate as a standard commercial preparation has been used for applications in both the upper (E-Z-Pake) and lower (Sol-O-Pake, E-Z-EM) gastrointestinal tract[5, 19–25]; although insoluble in aqueous solution, barium sulfate is made miscible by the presence of suspending agents. Both the clay minerals and barium sulfate cause reductions in the intraluminal signal on T1- and T2-weighted images through diamagnetic interactions between the suspended particles and solvent water protons. Although these agents have the advantages of established safety, wide availability, and relative low cost, the clay minerals are unpalatable and are required in large doses that may cause constipation. Readi-cat 2 (E-Z-EM) has also been used as a gastrointestinal contrast agent for MRI,[26] but its efficacy is probably related to its content of an undisclosed paramagnetic agent rather than the barium (only 2%).

PARAMAGNETIC AGENTS

Paramagnetic agents consist of paramagnetic metals in ionic form or as soluble chelate complexes that primarily increase the intraluminal signal intensity on T1-weighted images. Because of its established safety, one of the first such agents to be investigated was ferric

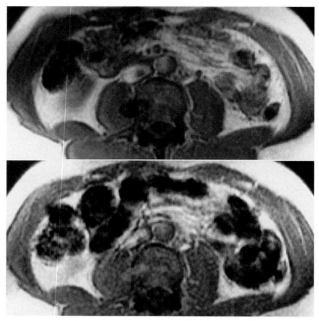

FIGURE 6–3. Perfluorooctylbromide. Gradient-echo (GRE) image of the abdomen after ingestion of perfluorooctylbromide (PFOB). Note the low signal intensity of bowel due to the absence of water protons, which are replaced by PFOB. (Courtesy of Peter F. Hahn, MD, PhD, Massachusetts General Hospital, Boston, MA.)

ammonium citrate, which is contained in the dietary iron supplement Geritol (Beecham Products, Bristol, TN)[3, 5, 27, 28] (Fig. 6–4). Geritol contains alcohol as an additive, and this restricts ingestion of the large quantities required for MRI. The efficacy of ferric ammonium citrate has led to its incorporation into a granular powder (OMR, Oncomembrane, Seattle, WA), which forms a flavored, effervescent drink when added to water and has passed phase III clinical trials.[29, 30] One potential disadvantage of such preparations of ferric ammonium citrate is their lack of volume expanders, which generally limits their use to the upper gastrointestinal tract. Compared with other paramagnetic metal ions used in oral contrast agents (i.e., manganese and gadolinium), the relaxivity of the ferric aquoion, and hence its molar efficiency as a contrast agent, is relatively low; incorporating the ion into a large molecular complex, however, increases its rotational correlation time and thus its relaxivity.[31–33] This strategy has been applied in the development of iron phytate, an oligomeric complex formed between ferric ion and phytate (inositol hexaphosphate) that has been tested as an oral agent in a pilot study.[34]

Manganese has been attractive as the paramagnetic component of MRI contrast agents because 1) it has a large magnetic moment and 2) it is a natural trace metal. Although initial enthusiasm has been tempered by observed cardiac and central nervous system (CNS) toxicities of ionic manganese, it has been investigated as an oral contrast agent.[2, 35–37] Early studies showing substantial systemic absorption of manganese when ingested as manganese chloride have resulted in formulations of relatively stable chelate complexes.[36] One example is manganese dipyridoxal diphosphate (Mn-DPDP, Salutar, Sunnyvale, CA), which has been used successfully in animals as a mixture with commercial barium preparations (E-Z-Paque, E-Z-EM) to allow radiographic assessment of the intraluminal distribution of the agent before imaging.[37] Another preparation is manganese combined with a proprietary polymer (LumenHance, Bristol-Myers Squibb, Princeton, NJ), which is undergoing phase III clinical trials.[2] All of these preparations have a biphasic effect on signal intensity, increasing the signal intensity in bowel on T1-weighted images and decreasing it on T2-weighted images. Although some investigators have thought this to be a disadvantage, it may prove to be useful for abdominal imaging.

Gadolinium has also been a desirable component of MRI contrast agents because it has one of the largest magnetic moments in the periodic table. This metal was first used as an oral contrast agent in the form of gadolinium oxalate, an insoluble compound that was prepared as a suspension of paramagnetic particles in analogy to commercial barium sulfate.[38, 39] A more recent formulation of Gd-DTPA combined with mannitol as a volume expander has been shown to be effective and safe in humans.[40–43] Gd-DTPA mixed with barium paste has also been used successfully to delineate the esophageal lumen on MR images.[44]

One considerable design issue in the development of oral MRI contrast agents has been the need to maintain the concentrations of paramagnetic ions at relatively constant levels throughout the gastrointestinal tract. Changes in local concentration (dilutional mixing with secretions in the upper gastrointestinal tract or hyperconcentration in the colon) can be minimized by the presence of a volume expander such as mannitol, although this increases the incidence of diarrhea.[40, 41] A frequently cited disadvantage of the T1 agents is that increased luminal signal intensities may cause image degradation through phase artifacts associated with peristaltic motion. This problem can be addressed by pretreatment with glucagon (0.5 mg given intravenously or 1 to 2 mg given subcutaneously or intramuscularly) to reduce bowel peristalsis, but the incidence of nausea and vomiting is reportedly increased.[40, 41] Alternatively, fast imaging can be performed, and this frontier will be advanced by developments in hardware and software.

IRON OXIDES

This class of gastrointestinal contrast agents uses the T2 and susceptibility effects of superparamagnetic iron oxides to markedly reduce the intraluminal signal intensity on T2- and especially gradient-echo (GRE) T2*-weighted MR images. After the demonstration of efficacy in early feasibility studies[15, 45–47] (Fig. 6–5), two commercial formulations of large, miscible particulates of iron oxide have been developed and tested clinically. The most extensively documented of the two

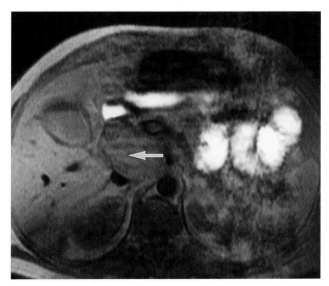

FIGURE 6–4. Ferric ammonium citrate. Ferric ammonium citrate is used to evaluate a peripancreatic lymph node metastasis. Fat-saturated T1-weighted spin-echo image after ingestion of 12 oz of 1:10 aqueous dilution of Geritol shows high signal intensity contrast material in the stomach, proximal jejunum, and duodenal bulb, which is displaced anteriorly by the mass (arrow). Note the phase artifacts arising from jejunal loops moving during the 3.5-minute acquisition. (From Hahn PF: Oral contrast agents for abdominal MRI. In: Thrall JH, ed: Current Practice of Radiology. Philadelphia: BC Decker, 1993, pp 172–174. By permission of Mosby–Year Book, Inc.)

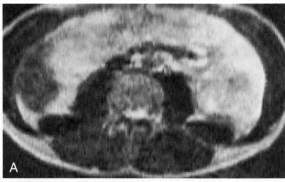
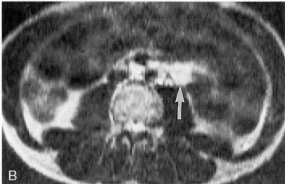

FIGURE 6–5. Iron oxide (AMI-121). *A*, Precontrast spin-echo image (2350/60) shows the small bowel to be of high signal intensity. *B*, After ingestion of 900 mL of 175 mg Fe/L of AMI-121, the signal intensity of the small bowel is diminished and a structure *(arrow)* next to the aorta is demonstrated. (*A* and *B* from Hahn PF, Stark DD, Lewis JM, et al: First clinical trial of a new superparamagnetic iron oxide for use as an oral gastrointestinal MR contrast agent. Radiology 175:695–700, 1990.)

consists of monodisperse 300- to 400-nm particles of sulfonated styrene-divinylbenzene copolymer coated with small crystals (<50 nm) of iron oxide (OMP, Nycomed, Oslo, Norway; WIN 39996, Winthrop-Sterling); this preparation has passed phase III clinical trials.[42, 48–62] The second formulation consists of 200-nm particles of crystalline iron oxide coated with silicone (Ferumoxsil or AMI-121, Advanced Magnetics, Cambridge, MA) and is being evaluated in phase II and III trials.[43, 63, 64] Both formulations are stable and effective throughout the entire gastrointestinal tract. Early problems with susceptibility artifacts caused by intraluminal aggregation of particles have been solved by the addition of viscosity enhancers, suspending agents, volume expanders, or a combination of these. Reported side effects of nausea, vomiting, bloating, diarrhea, and flatulence are typically mild and are believed to be due to large administered volumes rather than to the active ingredient.

AMI-227, an ultrasmall iron oxide (see section on reticuloendothelial system agents), also has considerable R1 relaxivity so that it can be used to increase the intraluminal signal intensity on T1-weighted images and to decrease it on T2-weighted images.[43] This flexibility may prove to be clinically desirable, and results from further clinical trials should be available soon.

BLOOD-POOL AGENTS

The use of intravenous Gd-DTPA to study organ and tissue perfusion (except in the brain) has been restricted to fast imaging techniques because of rapid equilibration of this agent between the intravascular and extravascular, extracellular compartments. An MRI contrast agent having a biodistribution restricted to the intravascular space (blood-pool agent), as well as a prolonged plasma half-life, would have myriad applications in imaging, and one of the most useful applications would be in MR angiography. Because in-phase spin saturation is common in nonenhanced three-dimensional (3D) sequences, contrast agents that reduce the T1 of blood efficiently increase the signal-to-noise ratio of vessels. Blood-pool agents are particularly promising in detecting small vessels with abnormalities (e.g., arteriovenous malformations, CNS vasculature, and coronary arteries), vessels with slow flow (e.g., pulmonary embolism and tumor invasion of the portal vein), and vessels with complex flow (e.g., stenoses and aneurysms). Other exciting applications for blood-pool agents include perfusion imaging, functional imaging, equilibrium imaging of hepatic tumors, imaging of tumor neovascularity, and serving as the basis for developing tissue-specific MRI contrast agents. Two classes of potential blood-pool and perfusion agents that meet the previous criteria are under development: paramagnetic macromolecules tagged with Gd-DTPA and certain preparations of iron oxide (Table 6–2). Iron oxides have the advantage of being more advanced in clinical trials, but timing and dosing constraints may make gadolinium-based agents ultimately the more desirable.

PARAMAGNETIC MACROMOLECULES

At least four prototypic agents have been described that contain numerous groups (tens to hundreds) of Gd-DTPA covalently linked to a macromolecular backbone such as a protein, a polysaccharide, or a synthetic polymer[65] (see Table 6–2). The high molar relaxivity (twofold to fivefold higher per gadolinium when compared with Gd-DTPA) of these complexes is attributable to slow rotation of the macromolecules in solution.[31–33] All four reported agents have molecular masses equal to or greater than 50 kd, which prolongs their plasma half-life by slowing renal excretion.

Albumin tagged with up to 35 groups of Gd-DTPA was the first such agent developed and has been used in animals with conventional spin-echo sequences to image 1) patterns of perfusion in normal and abnormal tissues[66–74]; 2) abnormal perfusion in normal tissues (myocardial ischemia/reperfusion and zonal renal ischemia)[67, 75–78]; and 3) flowing blood in large blood vessels to form MR angiograms.[68, 79, 80] Concerns about the potential immunogenicity of albumin have led to the subsequent development of dextran tagged with 15 groups of Gd-DTPA[81–87] and polylysine (PL) tagged with up to 60 groups,[74, 88–98] both of which are efficacious in imaging normal perfusion and flowing

TABLE 6–2. PROTOTYPIC BLOOD-POOL AGENTS

CLASS	COMPOUND	n	kd	AQUEOUS R1 (PER MOLECULE OR PARTICLE) AT 0.47 T/37°C–39°C (mM^{-1}/s^{-1})	AQUEOUS R1 (PER Gd) AT 0.47 T/37°C (mM^{-1}/s^{-1})	PLASMA HALF-LIFE—RAT (min)	LD_{50}—MICE (mmol/kg)	IMAGING DOSE (μmol/kg)	REFERENCES
Extracellular agents	Gd-DTPA	1	0.5	4.5	4.5	20	10	100	340, 341
Macromolecules	Albumin-(Gd-DTPA)$_n$	35	92	420*	14*	250	NR†	30–100	66–71, 73–80, 87, 342
	Dextran-(Gd-DTPA)$_n$	15	75	160*	10*	43	NR	10–50	81–84
	PL-(Gd-DTPA)$_n$	60	50	790	13	150	17	20–100	74, 88–98
	MPEG-PL-(Gd-DTPA)$_n$	110	430	2000–2500	18	840	NR	20–30	105, 108
Iron oxides	AMI-227	NA†	NR	24	NA	120	>10	10–30	109, 110
	MION-46	NA	NR	16	NA	180	NR	15–50	111, 343

*0.25 T, 37°C.

†NR = not reported; NA = not applicable.

blood in animals.[74, 82, 87, 89–91, 93, 95–97] The latter agent also has been used in animals to enhance time-of-flight (TOF) MR angiograms[89, 98] and as the perfusion component of a preliminary ventilation-perfusion technique that relies solely on MRI[95–97]; ventilation is assessed by using aerosolized gadolinium.[96, 99, 100] Three proprietary synthetic polymers (Starburst dendrimer, Michigan Molecular Institute, Midland, MI; Gd-DTPA–polyethylene glycol (PEG), Sterling Winthrop, Collegeville, PA; and 24-cascade-polymer, Schering, Berlin, Germany) have appeared as blood-pool agents,[101–103] but their characterization is preliminary.

Concerns linger about the potential immunogenicity of the previously mentioned agents, stimulated by the demonstration that Gd-DTPA bound to macromolecules may act as a hapten in the formation of antibodies against these agents,[104] particularly after repeated administrations. This problem has been addressed in the development of a unique copolymer of monomethoxypolyethylene glycol (MPEG) and PL, which contains up to 110 groups of Gd-DTPA (Gd-DTPA-PL-MPEG).[105] This agent is novel in three aspects: 1) it is the first graft copolymer for MRI, 2) it utilizes nonimmunogenic polyethylene glycol to decrease toxicity, and 3) it is one of the most effective enhancers of proton relaxation times in this class because it is extremely hydrophilic. Because surface-bound Gd-DTPA may be recognized as a hapten, Gd-DTPA-PL-MPEG contains the paramagnetic chelates "in its interior" where they are masked with surface-bound MPEG (steric protection). Polyethylene glycols have long been known to reduce the immunogenicity of a large number of proteins and antibodies.[106, 107] Because of the repeating oxygen group in the glycol unit, each repeating segment in this macromolecule attracts water through vander Waals forces, further increasing the relaxivity and hydrodynamic diameters of the proteins to which it is fixed.

Preclinical trials with Gd-DTPA-PL-MPEG have corroborated that the MRI appearance of peripheral vascular anatomy is significantly improved and that vessels with slow and nonorthogonal flow are better visualized.[105, 108] In one study, vessels less than 1 mm in size could be resolved because of the high signal-to-noise ratio between the vessels and the background (Fig. 6–6). Gd-DTPA-PL-MPEG seems to be particularly useful for assessing vessels showing slow flow (pulmonary vasculature and peripheral arterial disease) or small vessels such as the coronary arteries. Animal studies in our laboratory indicate that this agent improves the detection of pulmonary emboli in MR angiography of the pulmonary vessels, even the presence of small peripheral emboli in fourth-order branches (Fig. 6–7). Other experiments in animals have shown the superiority of this agent over Gd-DTPA-PL and Gd-DTPA-albumin, and initial data indicate that it has a high safety profile.

IRON OXIDES WITH LONG BLOOD HALF-LIVES

In addition to their susceptibility effect on the T2 relaxation of solvent water protons, small superparamagnetic iron oxides can have a substantial effect on T1 relaxation. When used at concentrations low enough that their relaxation behavior is not dominated by the susceptibility effect (1 to 2 mg Fe/kg), these agents can increase the signal intensity on heavily T1-weighted images.[109–111] Certain preparations of these compounds show sufficiently long half-lives (hours) in plasma[109–111] that their use as blood-pool agents is feasible. Advantages of the iron oxides over gadolinium-tagged macromolecules include their known favorable safety profile in animals and their advanced development as clinical agents.

The first iron oxide to be used for MR angiography was a monocrystalline iron oxide nanocompound (MION-46).[111] Using 3D TOF sequences, this agent caused a threefold to fourfold increase in the signal intensity of the aorta compared with muscle at ideal peak imaging doses (1.7 mg/kg). Phantom studies indicated that heavily T1-weighted spoiled gradient-recalled sequences (SPGR) with flip angles of 50° to 70° result in maximal vascular enhancement. In an animal model, this agent led to superb delineation of small abdominal vessels[111] (Fig. 6–8). Another iron oxide with a long blood half-life and significant R1 relaxivity is AMI-227, which is undergoing phase II and

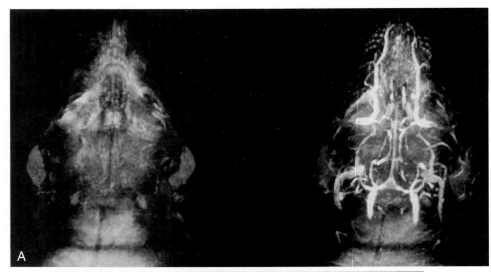

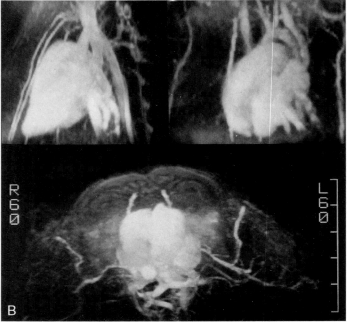

FIGURE 6–6. Gd-DTPA-PL-MPEG. *A,* Maximal intensity projection spoiled gradient-recalled acquisition in the steady state (GRASS) (SPGR) images of a rat head, obtained before and after intravenous administration of Gd-DTPA-PL-MPEG. The precontrast image was obtained at 60/8 (repetition and echo times in milliseconds) with a flip angle of 20°. The postcontrast image was obtained at 60/8 with a flip angle of 60°. Arteries and veins are much better visualized after administration of the contrast agent, and vessels less than 1 mm in diameter are seen because of the high vessel-to-muscle ratio. Note the areas of high vascularity in the whisker region. *B,* Lateral, oblique, and craniocaudal maximal intensity projection images of a rabbit thorax after intravenous administration of Gd-DTPA-PL-MPEG (25 μmol Gd/kg). Note the excellent delineation of the cardiac atria and ventricles as well as the large vessels and internal mammary vessels. (*A* from Bogdanov AA Jr, Weissleder R, Frank HW, et al: A new macromolecule as a contrast agent for MR angiography: preparation, properties, and animal studies. Radiology 187:701–706, 1993.)

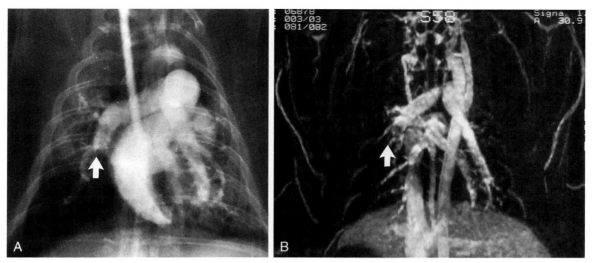

FIGURE 6–7. Pulmonary embolism. *A,* Conventional pulmonary angiography after right ventricular injection of 7 mL of Hypaque. The embolus in the right pulmonary artery is seen as a cutoff *(arrow). B,* Corresponding coronal maximal intensity projection (see Fig. 6–6 for imaging parameters) after administration of Gd-DTPA-PL-MPEG (35 μmol Gd/kg) demonstrates central embolus *(arrow).* (*A* and *B* from Frank H, Weissleder R, Bogdanov AA, Brady TJ: Detection of pulmonary emboli by using MR angiography with MPEG-PL-Gd-DTPA: an experimental study in rabbits. AJR 162:1041–1046, 1994.)

III clinical trials. This agent similarly increases the signal-to-noise ratio of vessels, but little information is available on optimal sequences, timing parameters, or dosages.

METABOLIC AGENTS WITH SOME TISSUE SPECIFICITY

The search for molecular compounds that, when injected intravenously, display preferential biodistribu-tion to specific organs and tissues has a long history in radiology, nuclear imaging, and pharmacology. One active and fruitful area of research in developing novel MRI contrast agents has been the identification of molecules having known organ or tissue specificity and their modification to carry paramagnetic groups while maintaining their original specificity. Two major classes of such compounds are the metalloporphyrins, which are known to accumulate to some extent in tumors, and a group of agents that show selective hepatobiliary uptake and excretion.

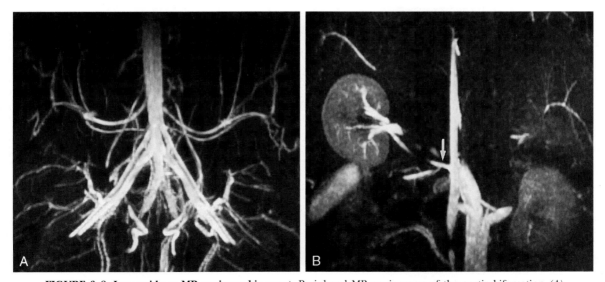

FIGURE 6–8. Iron oxide as MR angiographic agent. Peripheral MR angiograms of the aortic bifurcation *(A)* and origins of the renal arteries *(B)* (SPGR 50/5/60°) after intravenous administration of MION-46. A series of five collapsed images shows the origin of the left renal artery *(arrow).* (*A* and *B* from Frank H, Weissleder R, Brady TJ: Enhancement of MR angiography with iron oxide: preliminary studies in whole-blood phantom and in animals. AJR 162:209–213, 1994.)

METALLOPORPHYRINS

Distinguishing tumors from normal soft tissues non-invasively is a fundamental goal of diagnostic imaging, and the relatively high intrinsic contrast between soft tissues on early unenhanced MR images raised the possibility that this goal had been achieved. Although tumors in the absence of a contrast agent are often relatively hypointense on T1-weighted images and hyperintense on T2-weighted images, these findings are not completely reliable or specific. Therefore, a tumor-specific MRI contrast agent remains desirable for improved detection of tumors, staging, and the characterization ("typing") of tumors.

Porphyrins were the first potential "tissue-specific" MRI contrast agents to be evaluated because of their ability to form stable chelate complexes with paramagnetic metal ions and their well-known selective retention by tumors[112] (Table 6–3). Furthermore, complexes containing manganese were identified as potentially the most useful ones because of the high relaxivity of this metal when so coordinated.[113] Manganese (II) tetrakis-(4-sulfonatophenyl) porphyrin (Mn-TPPS$_4$) is the best characterized of these compounds and has shown uptake by a variety of tumors in mice sufficient to increase their signal intensities on T1-weighted MR images; furthermore, uptake is prompt (minutes) and retention is prolonged (days).[113–128] This compound is water soluble and excreted by the kidneys. Disadvantages of Mn-TPPS$_4$ that have prevented testing in humans are a low ratio between the useful imaging dose and the median lethal dose (LD$_{50}$), as well as the undesirable side effect of greenish discoloration of the skin.

Alternative porphyrins have been investigated to circumvent the disadvantages of Mn-TPPS$_4$. Manganese mesoporphyrin does not cause cutaneous discoloration but has a toxicity similar to that of Mn-TPPS$_4$.[124, 129] Substituted porphyrins containing gadolinium have been prepared to achieve comparable efficacy at lower doses by exploiting the higher relaxivity of gadolinium; however, these compounds are usually unstable because of the large size of the gadolinium atom relative to the dimensions of the binding core of conventional porphyrins.[130–132] This problem has been addressed by the synthesis of novel expanded porphyrins that have an enlarged binding core.[133–135] The prototypic agent gadolinium texaphyrin has been shown to be effective and safe in a preliminary study with rats and rabbits.[136]

The uptake of porphyrins by tumors is not well understood but is thought to be due to binding to benzodiazepine receptors on the outer membrane of mitochondria.[136] Pharmacologically, Mn-mesoporphyrin and Gd-texaphyrin show predominant hepatobiliary excretion, whereas Mn-TPPS$_4$ is excreted mainly by the kidneys. Given the multitude of other attractive MRI contrast agents and significant disadvantages of currently available porphyrins, it appears unlikely that these agents will be developed for clinical use.

HEPATOBILIARY AGENTS

The hepatobiliary agents (Table 6–4) share the property of substantial hepatic uptake and biliary excretion, and all but one appear to do so through an affinity for the organic anion transport system.[137, 138] The compound that does not show a specificity for this transport system (Mn-DPDP) is an analogue of vitamin B$_6$, which may be extracted by the hepatocyte by means of the transport system for this vitamin. All of these agents show a higher relaxivity in liver than in aqueous solution, which probably is due to binding to a slowly rotating intracellular protein that carries the agent from the basal pole of the hepatocyte to the apical pole for excretion into the bile. On T1-weighted MR images, these agents cause a preferential enhancement of the liver and biliary tree, beginning within minutes and lasting up to 2 hours. One of the first compounds to be investigated as a hepatobiliary agent was Fe-EHPG (iron(III) ethylenebis-(2-hydroxyphenylglycine)) followed by subsequent derivatives.[139–144] These compounds are structurally related to the ^{99m}Tc-iminodiacetate (Tc-IDA) complexes used in nuclear imaging of the hepatobiliary system. One derivative of Fe-EHPG, Fe-HBED (iron(III)-bis(2-hydroxybenzyl) ethylenediaminediacetic acid), shows more than three times greater hepatobiliary excretion in rats than the parent compound. The efficacy of both compounds in enhancing the liver and biliary tree on T1-weighted MR images has been demonstrated in animals, and proof of the concept of improved detection of hepatic tumors has been shown with Fe-EHPG.

Another iron-containing complex examined as a hepatobiliary agent in preliminary studies was Fe-PGDF (iron(III)-N-(3-phenylglutaryl)desferrioxamine).[145, 146] Desferrioxamine B is a siderophore that shows prompt renal excretion and is used as a drug in chelation

TABLE 6–3. METALLOPORPHYRINS

COMPOUND	AQUEOUS R1/R2 (mM^{-1} s^{-1})	ACCUMULATION—MICE	ELIMINATION—MICE	LD$_{50}$—MICE (μmol/kg)	CUTANEOUS DISCOLORATION	IMAGING DOSE—MICE (μmol/kg)	REFERENCES
Mn-TPPS$_4$	10/13*	Kidney > tumor > liver	Renal	500	Yes	20–150	113–128, 344
Mn-mesoporphyrin		Liver > tumor	Hepatobiliary	300–500	No	10–100	124, 129
Gd-texaphyrin	19/22†	Liver > tumor	Hepatobiliary	NR‡	NR	2.5–17	133, 135, 136

*0.47 T.
†1.5 T.
‡NR = not reported.

TABLE 6–4. HEPATOBILIARY CONTRAST AGENTS*

COMPOUND	MANUFACTURER	AQUEOUS R1/R2 AT 0.47 T/ 37°C–39°C (mM^{-1}/s^{-1})	EX VIVO (RAT LIVER) R1 AT 0.47 T/37°C–39°C (mM^{-1}/s^{-1})	HEPATIC ELIMINATION —RAT (%)	PLASMA HALF-LIFE —RAT (min)	LD$_{50}$—MICE (mmol/kg)	STATUS	IMAGING DOSE (µmol/kg)	SIDE EFFECTS	REFERENCES
Fe-EHPG	NA	0.9/1.1	NR	26 (mice)	80	NR	Animal	50–200	NA	31, 139, 141–143
Fe-PGDF	NA	2.0†/NR	NR	32	NR	NR	Animal	100	NA	144–146
Gd-BOPTA (gadobenate dimeglumine)	Bracco	4.6/5.6	15	39‡	15	5.8	Human	50–100	Nausea, vomiting, pruritus, muscle cramps	141, 150–154
Gd-EOB-DTPA	Schering	5.3/6.1	17	63§	10	7.5	Human	30–100		155–165
MS264	Metasyn	5.8/NR	24	87‖	NR	NR	Animal	NR		167
Mn-DPDP	Salutar	2.8/3.7	22	47	120	5.4	Human	3–10	Facial flushing, nausea, vomiting, tightness in throat, transient hypertension and tachycardia; lightheadedness and/or dizziness; increased α-antitrypsin	147, 154, 168–184

*NA = not applicable; NR = not reported.
†0.25 T/37°C.
‡/Decreases to 25% in rabbits.
§Decreases to 34% in monkeys.
‖Species independent.

therapy. However, phenylglutaryl and phenylsuccinyl derivatives of desferrioxamine B show substantial and rapid excretion by the biliary route. Contrary to Fe-EHPG and its derivatives, Fe-PGDF after intravenous administration to rats caused dramatic enhancement of the small bowel on MR images but relatively little hepatic enhancement, which was attributed to markedly faster transport of Fe-PGDF within the hepatocyte. Because of this observation and the comparatively low relaxivity of iron-containing complexes in general, none of the compounds just mentioned have been further investigated in clinical trials.

Other compounds have been examined as potential hepatobiliary agents in preliminary studies but have not been pursued further. One such compound is Cr-HIDA (chromium(III)-bis(N-2,6-diethylphenylcarbamoylmethyl)iminodiacetic acid), which, like Fe-EHPG, is an analogue of ^{99m}Tc-IDA and undergoes sufficient hepatobiliary uptake in rats to alter MR signal intensity.[147, 148] Another class of compounds is the nitroxyl lipids, which are members of the heterogeneous group of paramagnetic nitroxides.* The nitroxyl lipids demonstrate selective hepatic uptake and also increase the signal intensity of the liver, but apparently not that of the biliary tree, on MR images.

The three potential clinical hepatobiliary contrast agents that contain gadolinium are Gd-BOPTA or gadobenate (gadolinium(III)-3,6,9-triaza-12-oxa-3,6,9-tricarboxylmethylene-10-carboxy-13-phenyltridecanoic acid), Gd-EOB-DTPA (gadolinium(III)-3,6,9-triaza-3,6,9-tris-(carboxymethyl)-4-(4-ethoxybenzyl)-undecandicarboxylic acid), and MS264 (see Table 6–4). All three complexes consist essentially of a hydrophilic Gd-DTPA moiety covalently coupled to a lipophilic benzene ring that may show further substitution; these complexes are thus amphiphilic and undergo both hepatobiliary and renal excretion. Gd-BOPTA was the first such compound to be described and has shown efficacy both in animals and in phase I and II clinical trials.[141, 150–154] Gd-EOB-DTPA has been studied extensively in animals and also in clinical trials.[155–165] Fifteen percent of volunteers had mild side effects with the latter agent, but no serious adverse events were observed. At an imaging dose of approximately 50 μmol Gd/kg, the plasma half-life of Gd-EOB-DTPA in humans was 1.5 hours with a biliary excretion of 40% to 50%,[166] considerably higher than that of Gd-BOPTA. This agent has been efficacious in animal models of transplanted and acutely rejecting livers[161] and has shown complete excretion by the hepatobiliary or renal routes when the other pathway was severely obstructed.[157, 163] Preliminary studies in animals with MS264, the newest compound in this group, do not appear to show this behavior.[167]

Mn-DPDP (manganese(II)-N,N'-dipyridoxylethylene-

diamine-N,N'-diacetate-5,5'-bis(phosphate)) is the best studied of the hepatobiliary contrast agents in both animals and humans.[147, 154, 168–184] This compound has an efficacy comparable to those of the agents described earlier, despite its distinguishing feature of bypassing the organic anion transporter during uptake into the hepatocyte. An additional characteristic unique to Mn-DPDP is that its uptake by the liver does not appear to be affected by the presence of biliary obstruction.[147, 179] Mn-DPDP has also been shown to have an unexpected affinity for the pancreas in humans,[174] which has unexplored potential applications.

Mn-DPDP shows an unusually high affinity for primary hepatic neoplasms, such as well-differentiated hepatocellular carcinoma, focal nodular hyperplasia, and regenerating nodules.[175, 180, 182–184] Although this finding could mean a reduced sensitivity in detecting these lesions on MR images, it suggests a means of distinguishing them from secondary hepatic neoplasms. Another phenomenon unique to Mn-DPDP is peritumoral rim enhancement seen on delayed images in highly malignant primary and secondary hepatic tumors, which is associated with proliferation of bile ducts and bile stasis at the periphery of these lesions.[183] Such observations may further the use of MRI in the noninvasive diagnosis of focal hepatic lesions. Disadvantages of Mn-DPDP over the other hepatobiliary agents are the susceptibility of manganese(II) to oxidation to the less paramagnetic form manganese(III) and a higher toxicity, which is probably due to the relative instability of the complex and the potential for release of free manganese. In clinical trials, mild side effects (flushing and metallic taste) were common (>50%) but usually resolved within minutes after administration[176]; dose-dependent increases in blood pressure and heart rate were also observed.

CALCIUM-AVID AGENTS

Two related paramagnetic phosphates have been synthesized that, like their analogues in nuclear imaging, display affinities for soft tissues undergoing calcification.[185–188] These agents, Gd-DTPA-HPDP (1-hydroxy-3-aminopropane-1,1-diphosphonate–modified Gd-DTPA) and Gd-DTPA-BDP (4-aminobutane-1,1-diphosphonate–modified Gd-DTPA), have been evaluated in preliminary studies and show preferential biodistribution to bone and infarcted myocardium at concentrations sufficient to alter the signal intensity on MR images. At least one MR image has been published showing enhancement of a myocardial infarct in a rat.[186]

RETICULOENDOTHELIAL SYSTEM AGENTS

Particulate agents (liposomes and iron oxides) preferentially distribute to the reticuloendothelial system (RES), that is, to Kupffer cells in the liver and macrophages in spleen, bone marrow, and lymph nodes. The biodistribution of these agents and their plasma half-

---

*Nitroxides were one of the first chemical species to be evaluated as potential extracellular contrast agents for MRI, due to their well-known characteristics and versatility.[149] They are relatively stable free radicals that are paramagnetic because of a single unpaired, nitrogen-centered electron. However, the nitroxides have since been overshadowed by the more potent paramagnetic metal ions.

lives are determined by their size, charge, and surface coating. Thus, large particles (over 100 nm) rapidly undergo phagocytosis by hepatic Kupffer cells and splenic macrophages, whereas small particles bypass these cells and become more slowly distributed to macrophages in the bone marrow and lymph nodes.

MAGNETIC LIPOSOMES

Liposomes are artificial lipid vesicles of microscopic size, composed of either a single (unilamellar) or multiple concentric (multilamellar) spherical lipid bilayers, that can be prepared to encapsulate or surface bind specific magnetic labels.[189, 190] Liposomes were originally developed as a target vehicle for delivering toxic chemicals such as chemotherapeutic agents to specific tissues in vivo, but their rapid uptake and degradation by the RES, primarily in the liver and spleen, have been a major impediment to further development of this concept. However, this problem was recognized as an advantage in the early search for MRI contrast agents showing specificity for these particular organs.

One approach to the development of magnetic liposomes has been the encapsulation of soluble metal ions,[191–196] chelate complexes,[197–209] or nitroxides[194, 210–212]; the entrapped compound carries a charge that prevents its escape from the interior of the vesicle. The most extensively studied of this type of liposome consists of a mixture of phosphatidylcholine and cholesterol that contains a solution of Gd-DTPA (Table 6–5). The relaxivity of a paramagnetic agent thus entrapped is limited by the diffusion of water across the lipid bilayer,[207] which in turn is inversely proportional to the size of the liposome and its content of cholesterol.[200, 203, 204] The stability of a liposome in vivo also has an inverse dependence on size and the content of cholesterol.[202–205] Therefore, preparations having the most favorable relaxation characteristics in vitro are often the most unstable in vivo. A satisfactory formulation for MRI appears to be liposomes composed of phosphatidylcholine and cholesterol in an 8:2 molar ratio and filtered to an average size of 50 nm (see Table 6–5).

A second approach in developing magnetic liposomes has been to incorporate a lipid that is first modified with a paramagnetic chelate complex[213–220] or nitroxide[194, 221] so that the paramagnetic group becomes an intrinsic component of the lipid bilayer. The paramagnetic moiety in this class of liposome gains in relaxivity by rotating at the much slower rate of the liposome.[209] A typical formulation of such liposomes is phosphatidylcholine, cholesterol, and stearylamide at a molar ratio of 1:1:1, the last of which is coupled to Gd-DTPA (Gd-DTPA-SA) (see Table 6–5).

During the vascular distribution phase, magnetic liposomes of both classes act as blood-pool agents[199]; they subsequently function as preferential contrast agents for the liver and spleen as they become trapped by Kupffer cells and macrophages, respectively.* Differential enhancement between liver and secondary hepatic tumors on MR images of animals has been demonstrated after intravenous administration of such liposomes.[196, 201, 202] During the process of phagocytosis, liposomes of both classes disassemble, their contents (Gd-DTPA or water) are released in situ, and the lipid bilayer undergoes subsequent degradation within lysosomes. The half-life for hepatic clearance of Gd-DTPA entrapped within liposomes is several days, consistent with gradual release of Gd-DTPA from Kupffer cells and hepatocytes.[204, 206] By comparison, a half-life for clearance of incorporated Gd-DTPA-SA of several weeks indicates slow intralysosomal degradation; indeed, analogous but more labile lipids coupled to Gd-DTPA are cleared much more rapidly.[216]

Other liposomes have been synthesized that contain certain superparamagnetic iron oxides[223–227] ("ferrosomes"), and one has been used as an intermediate in the preparation of magnetically labeled human leukocytes.[226, 228] However, applications of these interesting preparations to MRI have not yet been described and, judging from the decline in publications, the use of liposomes in general as specific MRI contrast agents for the liver and spleen has been overshadowed by the other agents.

IRON OXIDES

Although still in the early stages of clinical development, an already extensive literature indicates that superparamagnetic iron oxides are poised to become one of the most important and versatile category of MRI contrast agents (e.g., RES, blood-pool, and gastrointestinal agents).[229–232] Once these agents are in a magnetic field, the magnetic moments of individual iron atoms in these particles become aligned to produce a net magnetic moment that is several times larger than those of typical paramagnetic molecules. This net magnetic moment in turn causes a substantial disturbance in the magnetic field around the particle (susceptibility effect) that leads to increased dephasing of the water protons diffusing nearby (T2 effect). The result is a large increase in R2 relaxivity that causes a loss of signal intensity on T2- and especially GRE T2*-weighted images. By this mechanism, superparamagnetic iron oxides can be detected on MR images at low concentrations, and this feature is the basis of cellular and subcellular applications.[233, 234]

STRUCTURE

The literature shows an often confusing plethora of different types of superparamagnetic iron oxides and proprietary formulations. The best-characterized agents are summarized in Table 6–6, and other agents are reviewed in more detail elsewhere.[229, 230] Some

---

*References 191, 192, 195, 196, 199, 201, 202, 213, 214, 216, 218–222.

TABLE 6–5. REPRESENTATIVE MAGNETIC LIPOSOMES

CLASS	ACTIVE INGREDIENT	COMPONENT LIPIDS*	MOLAR PROPORTION	MEAN SIZE (nm)	AQUEOUS R1/R2 AT 0.47 T/37°C (mM^{-1}/s^{-1})	PLASMA HALF-LIFE—RAT (h)	HEPATIC CLEARANCE OF Gd-DTPA	IMAGING DOSE (μmol Gd/kg)	REFERENCES
Paramagnetic	Entrapped Gd-DTPA	PC:Ch	1:0–1	70–400	0.4–2.9/1.2–2.8	4	Days	25–100	199–206
	Surface-bound Gd-DTPA	PC:Ch:Gd-DTPA-SA	1:1:1	30–50	NR†	2	Weeks	15	213, 214, 216–219
Superparamagnetic	MION-46	PC/SM:DOPE:Ch	9:2:9	170–360	14.8/130.3	NR	NR	NR	227
	Magnetite–carboxydextran	PC:PS:Ch	5:2:1	200–280	5.8/247.7	NR	NR	NR	226

*PC = phosphatidylcholine; Ch = cholesterol; SA = stearylamide; NR = not reported; SM = sphingomyelin; DOPE = dioleoylphosphatidylethanolamine; PS = phosphatidylserine.
†R1/R2 = ~ 15/13 for similar liposomes.[215]

TABLE 6-6. SUPERPARAMAGNETIC IRON OXIDES

CLASS	COMPOUND	MANUFACTURER	COATING	MEAN SIZE—CORE (nm)	MEAN SIZE—PARTICLE (nm)	AQUEOUS R2/R1 AT 0.47 T/37°C (mM⁻¹/s⁻¹)	PLASMA HALF LIFE—RAT (min)	LD₅₀—MICE (mmol/kg)	STATUS	IMAGING DOSE (µmol/kg)	SIDE EFFECTS	REFERENCES
SPIO	MSM	Nycomed	Starch	10	300–400	180/28*	~2	~3	Animal	3–20	NA†	252–256, 258, 259
	AMI-25	AMI	Dextran		50–100	160/40	10/90‡	>3	Human	10–50	Mild: 10%–15%; rarely: back pain, hypotension	109, 241, 266, 268, 269–284, 286–289, 291, 301–306, 345–352
USPIO	AMI-227	AMI	Dextran	4–6	17–20	53/24*	120	>10	Human	5–30	<10%	109, 110, 293–297
	SHU 555	Meito Sangyo	Carboxy-dextran	3–5	30–50	190/24	<10		Human	5–40	NR†	352
MION	MION-37	MGH	Dextrans	4–6	16–28	35/16	90	NR	Animal	20–200	NA	329, 353
	MION-46	MGH	Dextran, strain B512F	3.5–5.7	18–24	35/16	180	NR	Animal	20–200	NA	111, 343, 351, 353

*39°C–40°C.

†Biphasic elimination.

‡NA = not applicable; NR = not reported.

pharmaceutical iron oxides have been referred to as ferrites and magnetites. Both ferrite ($Fe_2M_xO_4$, where M is a metal cation) and magnetite (Fe_3O_4) are water-insoluble crystals that are not suitable for clinical use. To be used pharmaceutically, iron oxides must be chemically modified while their magnetic properties remain unchanged. The model structure of a pharmaceutically acceptable compound contains a magnetically responsive core, which may be made up of one or many aggregates of individual iron oxide crystals. Surface molecules are then attached to this magnetic core to stabilize the colloidal solution, and target specificity is conferred by attaching an inert, target-specific molecule to this construct.

The most commonly used synthesis for obtaining superparamagnetic iron oxides involves the alkaline precipitation of a magnetite-like compound from aqueous salt solutions of Fe^{2+} and Fe^{3+} in the presence of a colloidal stabilizing agent. During the increase in pH, hydrolysis of iron(III) occurs, which forms different intermediary iron complexes. The chemical structures of these complexes may be given by $(Fe^{II}_1Fe^{III}_1)$, $(Fe^{III}_2Fe^{III}_1)$, $[(Fe^{II}_1Fe^{III}_2)O_x(OH)_{2(3-x)}]_n^{2n+}$, $(Fe^{II}_1O_xFe^{III}_2)^{(11-2x)+}$.[235] Further synthesis encompasses dehydration (and sometimes oxidation) of the intermediary complexes to form Fe_3O_4 (magnetite), α-Fe_2O_3, γ-Fe_2O_3, or FeOOH (iron oxyhydroxide). The reaction conditions and the ratio of Fe^{2+} to Fe^{3+} are crucial for the formation of different types of iron oxides.[235]

Anchored surface molecules grafted onto the core during synthesis are necessary to stabilize the iron oxide in aqueous colloidal solution. This surface molecule usually consists of a biocompatible polymer such as a polysaccharide. The molecular arrangement of the surface molecule in solution depends on its molecular structure, charge, and flexibility and determines the overall size, biokinetics, and biodistribution of the superparamagnetic construct.

Biologic Properties

The pharmacokinetic behavior of iron oxide preparations has been assessed scintigraphically with ^{99m}Tc-labeled iron oxides[236, 237] and echo-planar MR techniques.[238] If a decrease in the MR signal intensity of an organ is assumed to be proportional to the concentration of iron oxide in the tissue, plots of signal intensity versus time have been generated by fast MRI techniques. During the first minute after intravenous administration of an iron oxide, a steep decrease in MR signal intensity occurs in all well-perfused tissues, including liver, kidney, and heart[238]; this initial decrease corresponds to the vascular phase of the contrast agent. Organs that accumulate iron oxides after initial perfusion show a further decrease in signal intensity with time. These organs belong either to the RES and contain phagocytic activity or contain specific receptor systems (e.g., asialoglycoprotein) or antigenic sites to which certain iron oxides bind. The kinetics of this attachment and the cellular internalization process

vary between agents and depend on blood flow, receptor affinity constants, and the recycling of receptors. Mathematic models of particle pharmacokinetics have been derived[236, 237] and can be used to calculate organ-specific capture coefficients.

The biodistribution of conventional dextran-stabilized preparations of iron oxide has been investigated extensively.[239–243] One study found the following biodistribution of ^{59}Fe-AMI-25 in rats: 83% ± 0.3% of the injected dose to liver and 6.2% ± 7.3% to spleen.[241] When the biodistribution is expressed as a percentage of the injected dose per gram of tissue, liver and spleen show the highest concentrations (6.31% ± 0.52%/g and 11% ± 7.6%/g, respectively). Only minimal amounts of ^{59}Fe are detectable in other tissues, such as kidney, lung, and brain.[241]

Iron oxide particles are internalized by phagocytic cells (presumably by the scavenger receptors) or hepatocytes (e.g., through the asialoglycoprotein receptor). Once inside the cells, the particles are channeled into lysosomes. As observed by means of electron microscopy, this process has been shown not to affect the magnetic properties of iron oxides in tissues.[238] Observed organ half-lives of ^{59}Fe-AMI-25 are 3 days for liver and 4 days for spleen. Interestingly, spleen displays a second peak of radioactivity after 60 days that is most likely due to secondary ^{59}Fe uptake from senescent erythrocytes. Degradation of iron oxides into iron and oxygen is presumed to occur within intracellular lysosomes of macrophages under the influence of a variety of hydrolytic enzymes and low pH. Twenty percent of molecular ^{59}Fe is found in hemoglobin 14 days after intravenous administration.[241] Similar rates of incorporation into erythrocytes have been reported for radiolabeled ferritin (21%).[244]

The chemical toxicity of iron and its derivatives has been studied in detail.[245, 246] Human tissues may contain iron or iron oxides in the form of hemosiderin, ferritin, and transferrin. Normal liver contains approximately 0.2 mg of iron per gram wet weight of tissue,[247] and total human iron stores amount to 3500 mg. The quantity of iron oxide proposed for diagnostic imaging (50 to 100 mg Fe/kg body weight) thus is small compared with the normal iron store. Chronic iron toxicity (cirrhosis and hepatocellular carcinoma) develops only after the liver iron concentration exceeds more than 4 mg/g wet weight of tissue.

Individual Iron Oxide Agents

Paramagnetic metallic particulates (i.e., iodinated manganese sulfide[248] and gadolinium oxide[249]) were used to alter the relaxivity of liver in animals as early as 1984. The first demonstrations that iron oxide particles decrease the signal intensity of liver on T2-weighted images of animals were published in 1986.[250, 251] Within 6 months, superparamagnetic particles embedded in a matrix of denatured albumin were used to show differential changes in contrast between liver and implanted hepatic tumors in rabbits.[45] During the next several years, superparamagnetic particles consisting of

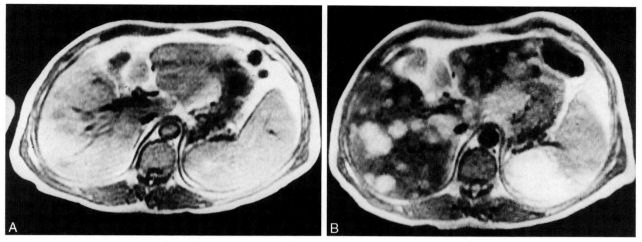

FIGURE 6–9. Detection of hepatic and splenic metastases with AMI-25. *A,* Nonenhanced spin-echo image (500/28). *B,* After intravenous administration of AMI-25, both hepatic and splenic metastases become easily detectable. (*A* and *B* from Weissleder R, Hahn PF, Stark DD, et al: Superparamagnetic iron oxide: enhanced detection of focal splenic tumors with MR imaging. Radiology 169:399–403, 1988.)

iron oxide crystals either embedded in a starch matrix (magnetic starch microspheres, Nycomed)[252–259] or surrounded by a coat of dextran (M4125 or Biomag, AMI, Cambridge, MA)[240, 260–267] were investigated in preliminary studies as MRI contrast agents for the liver and spleen.

AMI-25 has since been used extensively in numerous studies of malignant and benign diseases of the liver, spleen, and lymph nodes of animals[241, 268–278] (Figs. 6–9 and 6–10), culminating in the first clinical studies of iron oxides in humans[279–282] and more recent phase II and III trials.[283–289] Clinical trials of this agent are reviewed in detail elsewhere.[232] At the time of this writing, more than 1500 patients have received intravenous injections of AMI-25. Results from these clinical trials show an unequivocal increase in contrast-to-noise ratio between tumor and liver, significantly more detectable lesions on postcontrast images, and occasionally the ability to differentiate between malignant and nonmalignant tumors. Results of these clinical trials also demonstrate that side effects occur in 10% to 15% of patients, with most side effects being mild and not requiring treatment. Overall, the most common side effect is back pain (3% to 4%). Hypotension initially reported to be common with the first formulation of AMI-25 has subsequently been shown to occur infrequently; in phase III clinical trials, hypotension has been observed in 1% to 2% of the 1500 patients.

The next agent to receive widespread attention was an ultrasmall superparamagnetic iron oxide (USPIO),

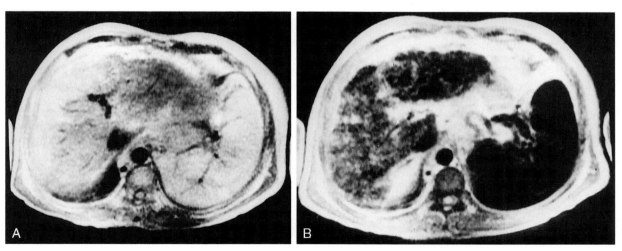

FIGURE 6–10. Use of AMI-25 for evaluation of splenomegaly. Spin-echo images (1500/42) of benign splenomegaly due to congestion caused by hepatic cirrhosis. *A,* Before administration of AMI-25, spleen size is increased and the signal intensity is slightly higher than that of liver. *B,* After administration of AMI-25 (40 μmol Fe/kg), the signal intensity of liver and spleen is decreased, indicating phagocytosis and benign splenomegaly. Malignant splenomegaly such as in lymphoma is not expected to decrease in SI to a degree that allows differentiation. (*A* and *B* from Bohdiewicz PJ, Lavallee DK, Fawwaz RA, et al: Mn[III] hematoporphyrin, a potential MR contrast agent. Invest Radiol 25:765–770, 1990.)

which originally consisted of the smallest 10% to 15% of the particles of AMI-25. This agent was initially obtained by ultrafiltration[233, 278, 290–292] but was later synthesized directly as AMI-227 (Advanced Magnetics).[109, 110, 293–297] The particles have been found to have a much longer plasma half-life and different biodistribution than the original AMI-25, showing preferential accumulation in the lymph nodes (Fig. 6–11) and bone marrow[278, 290–293, 295, 296] (Fig. 6–12). The prolonged plasma half-life (approximately 120 minutes in rats) has also allowed their use as a blood-pool agent on T1-weighted images.[109, 110] The pharmacologic properties of AMI-227 have been reported in detail elsewhere. This agent has also been shown to be a safe MRI contrast agent in initial clinical trials.[297]

TARGET-SPECIFIC CONTRAST AGENTS

In general, target-specific MRI contrast agents consist of two components: a magnetic label capable of altering the signal intensity on MR images and a target-specific carrier molecule having a characteristic affinity for a specific type of cell, a specific receptor, or both. After intravenous administration, such agents show preferential accumulation with time in the organ or tissue containing the target cell or receptor. For the agent to cause a macroscopic alteration in the MR signal intensity of the organ or tissue, however, it must have a large enough relaxivity and the density of target cells or receptors must be sufficiently high. This was recognized in early attempts at labeling antibodies with insufficient numbers of paramagnetic chelates[298–300] and is the basis for the versatility of the iron oxides. The large variety of target-specific agents that have

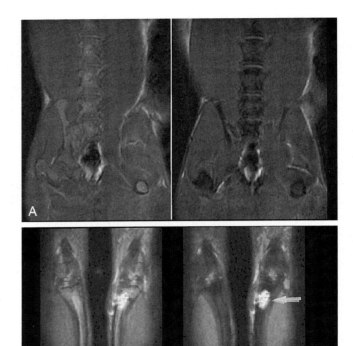

FIGURE 6–12. Use of USPIO as a bone marrow imaging agent. USPIO can be used to decrease the signal intensity of red bone marrow. A, After intravenous administration of USPIO (160 μmol Fe/kg) in a rabbit, there is a significant decrease of bone marrow signal intensity in the spine, iliac bone, and femurs (spin echo, 1500/40). B, In a rat tumor model, intravenous administration of USPIO (160 μmol Fe/kg) results in enhanced detection of a tibial metastasis (arrow).

been synthesized and successfully tested in vitro or in vivo are summarized in Table 6–7. In the present section, these agents are classified according to their surface-bound carrier molecules.

POLYSACCHARIDES

Many polysaccharides are recognized by mammalian endogenous glycoprotein receptors, and some have been used as carrier molecules in model target-specific contrast agents. The most widely tested compound is probably arabinogalactan, a polysaccharide obtained from larchwood. This naturally occurring polysaccharide has multiple terminal galactose and arabinose groups, which confer an affinity for asialoglycoprotein (ASG) receptors on hepatocytes and possibly other galactose receptors. Ultrasmall iron oxides synthesized with an arabinogalactan coating have been used extensively in experiments for ASG receptor MRI.[278, 301–307] The large number of ASG binding sites per hepatocyte[308] and the rapid internalization and reutilization of the receptor[309] make this receptor system convenient for targeted drug delivery. Hepatocyte-directed magnetopharmaceuticals have three potential advantages over iron oxides directed at Kupffer cells: 1) improved contrast-to-noise ratio of tumor to liver at equimolar

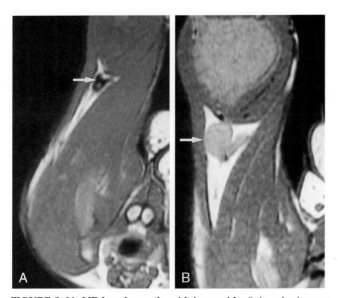

FIGURE 6–11. MR lymphography with iron oxide. Spin-echo images (1500/40) after intravenous administration of MION-46 (100 μmol Fe/kg) to rabbits. A, In normal lymph nodes, there is a homogeneous decrease in the signal intensity of a popliteal lymph node (arrow). B, Metastatic lymph nodes are enlarged (arrow) and do not take up iron oxides; hence, their signal intensity is unchanged on contrast-enhanced images.

TABLE 6–7. TARGET-SPECIFIC AGENTS*

ORGAN OR TISSUE	TARGET	AGENT	STATUS	REFERENCES
Liver	Kupffer cells	All liposomes	In vivo	192, 195–197, 199, 201, 202, 204, 206, 212–216, 218–220, 222, 224
		All iron oxides	In vivo	45, 109, 110, 239, 240, 242, 243, 250–256, 259–262, 264–267, 269, 270, 272, 273, 275–277, 279, 280, 285, 287, 290, 296, 297, 353, 354
	Hepatocytes (ASG receptors)	AG-USPIO-(BMS-180550)	In vivo	278, 301–307
		MION-AG	In vivo	306
		MION-ASF	In vivo	314
		AG-PCA	In vivo	311
Spleen	Macrophages	All liposomes	In vivo	197, 204, 206, 212, 214–216, 218, 219, 220, 222, 224
		All iron oxides	In vivo	45, 110, 240, 241, 243, 250, 251, 253, 254, 255, 258–260, 262, 263, 266, 268, 280, 281, 290, 296, 297, 353, 354
Lymph nodes	Macrophages	AMI-25, SC	In vivo	271
		Dextran magnetite, SC	In vivo	355
		AMI-227, IV (BMS-180549)	In vivo	290, 291, 293, 295, 296, 356
		MION-46, IV	In vivo	351
		Gd-DTPA-PGM, IV, SC	In vivo	313a
Bone marrow	Macrophages	Liposomes	In vivo	204, 212
		MION-46	In vivo	292
Adrenal	Amine receptors	PL-(Gd-DTPA)$_{30\%}$	In vivo	313b
Pancreas	CCK receptors	MION-CCK	In vitro	326
Nervous system	Neurons	MION-PL-WGA	In vivo	318
		MION-46	In vivo	357
	Axons	MION-PL	In vivo	319
		MION-PL-WGA	In vivo	318
Heart	Myosin	MION-Fab	In vitro	329
Tumor	Human gastrointestinal adenocarcinoma	MAb-(Gd-DTPA)$_{16–25}$	In vivo	331, 332
	Human T cells	MAb-(Gd-DTPA)$_{10}$	In vivo	333
	Neuroblastoma	SPIO-albumin/ polymer MAb	In vivo	327
	Human colon cancer	SPIO-MAb	In vivo	328
	Human squamous cell carcinoma	MION-L6	In vitro	Weissleder, unpublished data
Inflammation	Phagocytes	MION-IgG	In vivo	358
	Leukocyte common antigen	SPIO-biotin-streptavidin-biotin-MAb	In vitro	359
	Phagocytes	SPIO-lipid	In vivo	225, 360
	Leukocytes	Liposome	In vitro	361

*AG = arabinogalactan; ASF = asialofetuin; SC = subcutaneous; IgG = immunoglobulin G; IV = intravenous; MAb = monoclonal antibody; CCK = cholecystokinin; WGA = wheat germ agglutinin; PGM = polyglucose-associated macrocomplex; PCA = pyrrolidinoxylcarboxylic acid.

doses (i.e., lower dose requirements, 2) the ability to assess organ function, and 3) the potential for differential diagnoses of tumors.[302, 303] ASG-directed agents have been used not only to detect both primary and secondary hepatic tumors in animals[301–303, 305, 307] (Fig. 6–13) but also to evaluate benign diffuse liver diseases such as hepatitis.[304] The usefulness of ASG-targeted agents for the differentiation of liver tumors has also been demonstrated in an ex vivo human specimen.[310] Surgical human specimens demonstrated high ASG activity and binding of receptor agents to normal liver, focal nodular hyperplasia, adenoma, hepatitic liver, and cirrhotic liver. In contrast, neither primary hepatic tumors (hepatocellular carcinoma or hemangioma)

nor metastatic tumors (colon or renal cell carcinoma) showed significant accumulation of receptor agents. A nitroxide spin label covalently linked to arabinogalactan has similarly been used to increase the signal intensity of liver on T1-weighted images.[311]

Other polysaccharides that have been attached to iron oxides during synthesis include fucoidan (terminal fucose residues), mannan (terminal mannose residues), mannose 6-phosphate–containing polysaccharides, and chitosan (terminal N-acetylglucosamine residues).[312] Most of these compounds show predominant biodistribution to liver, spleen, kidneys, and lungs. This biodistribution is similar to that of glycosylated neoglycoproteins.[313]

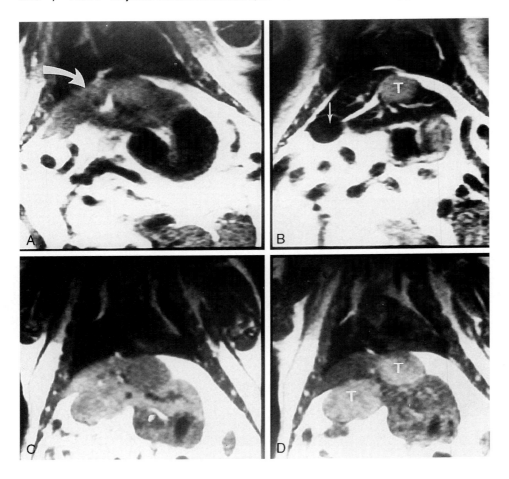

FIGURE 6–13. Receptor versus RES imaging. Woodchuck hepatoma (T = tumor) imaged (spin echo, 500/30) before *(A and C)* and after *(B and D)* intravenous administration of 10 μmol Fe/kg of arabinogalactan-USPIO (AG-USPIO) *(A and B)* or AMI-25 *(C and D)*. Note that AG-USPIO decreases liver signal intensity to a greater degree than does AMI-25. As a result, liver–hepatocellular carcinoma contrast is higher in *B*. A hyperintense area *(curved arrow)* in *A* was found to correspond to a regenerating nodule. Note that the signal intensity of this area decreases homogeneously after intravenous administration of AG-USPIO *(B)*. The straight arrow in *B* denotes the gallbladder. *(A to D* from Reimer P, Weissleder R, Brady TJ, et al: Experimental hepatocellular carcinoma: MR receptor imaging. Radiology 180:641–645, 1991.)

POLYMERS

Two target-specific paramagnetic polymers containing Gd-DTPA have been tested in animals. One is Gd-DTPA–polyglucose–associated macrocomplex (Gd-DTPA-PGM), which shows characteristic uptake by lymph nodes[313a] (Fig. 6–14). Another is PL-(Gd-DTPA)$_{30\%}$, an incompletely substituted polylysine that has a large number of amino groups. This agent displays a unique specificity for the adrenal gland (Fig. 6–15), possibly due to binding to amine uptake receptors.[313b]

PROTEINS

Many proteins are readily available for use as carrier molecules in potential target-specific contrast agents. One group of macromolecular carriers is the ASGs, which have a high affinity for the ASG receptor that is unique to hepatic parenchymal cells. Using asialofetuin as the carrier molecule, monodisperse, monocrystalline iron oxide nanoparticles (MION) have been targeted to the ASG receptor for MR receptor imaging.[314] The blood clearance of MION is changed dramatically when asialofetuin is covalently linked to the iron oxide. Specifically, the blood half-life of the superparamagnetic label decreases from more than 3 hours to less than 3 minutes after coupling to asialofetuin, with a virtually exclusive biodistribution to the liver.

Lectins are glycoproteins that bind with some selectivity to various sugar receptors on cells and may have considerable potential as carrier molecules. The best example is wheat germ agglutinin (WGA), which has been used as a carrier to study axonal transport. The property of axonal uptake and subsequent transport of lectins is exploited by neuroscientists to determine the connectivity of specific brain regions. Lectins have been attached to different iron oxides,[315–319] and MION-PL-WGA has exhibited axonal transport in a sciatic nerve model that could be visualized by MRI in vivo[318, 319] (Fig. 6–16). This method holds largely unexplored potential for clinical applications.

Polyclonal, nonspecific human immunoglobulin G (IgG) has been used as a carrier molecule in clinical trials to detect areas of inflammation[320] (Fig. 6–17). Although the exact mechanism of IgG localization in areas of inflammation is not known, several explanations have been offered. An initial proposal that expression of the Fc receptor on macrophages, polymorphonuclear leukocytes, and lymphocytes is enhanced in the presence of focal inflammation[321] has been refuted.[322] Rather than specific binding to the Fc receptor, accumulation of nonspecific IgG may occur through nonspecific extravasation of plasma proteins due to enhanced vascular permeability.[323, 324] Although controversy about the exact mechanism exists, human

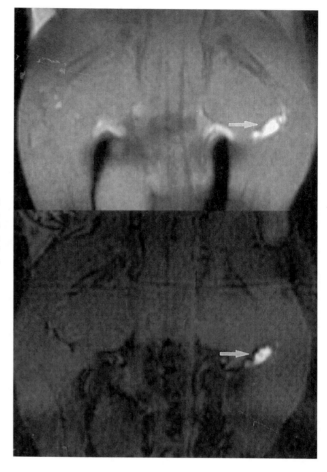

FIGURE 6–14. MR lymphography. MR lymphography (fat-suppressed spin-echo, 300/17 top row, SPGR 50/7/60° bottom row) of a normal rat. Popliteal lymph nodes are markedly enhanced *(arrow)* after subcutaneous administration of Gd-DTPA-PGM (6 μmol Gd/kg). (From Harika L, Weissleder R, Poss K, et al: MR lymphography with a lymphotrophic T1-type MR contrast agent: Gd-DTPA-PGM. Magn Reson Med 33:88–92, 1995.)

polyclonal IgG attached to MION has been used for MRI of inflammation.[325]

PEPTIDES

Several peptides have been used as carrier molecules for scintigraphy and MRI. Cholecystokinin (CCK) has been attached to an iron oxide label and the complex (MION-CCK) used for MRI of the pancreas. CCK binds to pancreatic acinar cells at their basolateral surface and is subsequently internalized and transported to the endoplasmatic reticulum. Uptake of MION-CCK by receptors in the exocrine pancreas can be blocked with a CCK receptor antagonist such as proglumide. After intravenous administration of this compound to rats, the MR signal intensity of pancreas decreased as expected, but that of a pancreatic tumor remained

FIGURE 6–15. Adrenal imaging. Coronal spin-echo images (300/20) before *(A)* and immediately after *(B)* intravenous administration of PL-(Gd-DTPA)$_{30\%}$ (80 μmol Gd/kg). Note the immediate increase in signal intensity in the kidney and adrenal gland *(arrows)*. Two hours after administration of the agent, the signal intensity of the adrenal gland was still substantially increased. (*A* and *B* from Weissleder R, Wang YM, Papisov M, et al: Polymeric contrast agent for MR imaging of adrenal glands. J Magn Reson Imaging 3:93–97, 1993.)

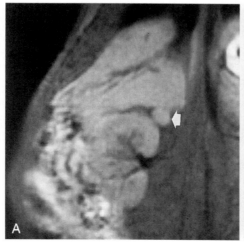
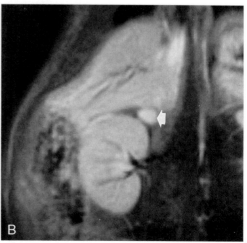

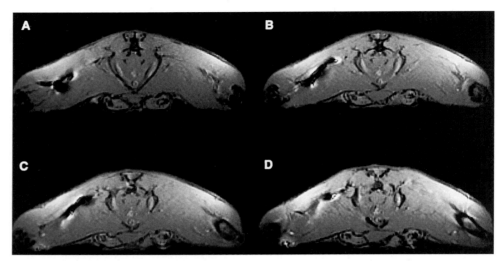

FIGURE 6–16. Axonal transport imaging. Serial axial 3D GRE images *(A and D)* through the hindquarters of a prone rat obtained 2 days after injection of MION-PL-WGA into the site of focal crush injury to the left sciatic nerve. The nerve is identified on the left as a thick, hypointense structure surrounded by thigh muscles; the other hypointense structures seen bilaterally are cortical bone of the femurs and pelvis. The approximate location of the injection site at the popliteal fossa is shown after injection in *A.* The contrast agent has undergone bidirectional transport within axons of the nerve and has reached the greater sciatic foramen proximally. *(A to D* from Enochs WS, Schaefer B, Bhide P, et al: MR imaging of slow axonal transport in vivo. Exp Neurol 123:235–242, 1993.)

unchanged.[326] These initial feasibility studies indicate the possibility of extrahepatic receptor–targeted MRI.

ANTIBODIES

Antibodies appear to be a logical choice as carrier molecules in target-specific contrast agents because of their high specificity in vitro. Preparations of antibody linked to iron oxide both noncovalently and covalently have been made and tested in vivo or in vitro using monoclonal antibodies against neuroblastoma,[327] human colon cancer,[328] human squamous cell carcinoma (Weissleder R, unpublished observations), antimyosin,[329] and leukocyte common antigen.[330] Monoclonal antibodies against human gastrointestinal adenocarci-

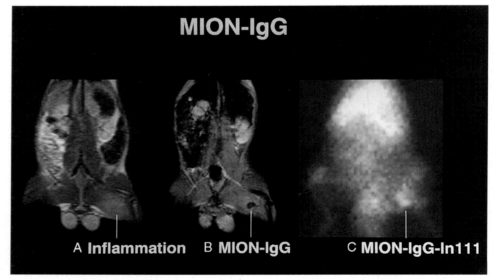

FIGURE 6–17. Inflammation imaging with MION-IgG-[111]In. Coronal spin-echo images (1500/40) before *(A)* and 1 hour after *(B)* the administration of MION-IgG. On the precontrast image, an area of inflammation in the left hindleg has a slightly increased signal intensity due to edema. After administration of MION-IgG, there is a focal decrease in signal intensity in the center of inflammation, indicating specific uptake of MION-IgG. Decreases in signal intensity are also seen in liver and bone marrow. *C,* Corresponding scintigraphic image demonstrates increased radiotracer activity in the left hindleg. *(A to C* from Weissleder R, Lee A, Fischman A, et al: Polyclonal human immunoglobulin G labeled with polymeric iron oxide: antibody MR imaging. Radiology 181:245–249, 1991.)

noma[331, 332] and human T cells tagged with multiple groups of Gd-DTPA[333] have also been prepared and tested in vivo. Attachment of a sufficiently large number of metallic chelates directly to an antibody usually is not feasible, so lanthanide chelates are often assembled on linking molecules (PL,[90, 92] dextran,[82] or albumin[334]) before the latter are attached to the antibody. Such antitumor antibody complexes labeled with PL-$(Gd-DTPA)_n$ have been used to detect tumors by MRI.[334, 335]

Clinical studies have shown that certain antibody-drug complexes can be used successfully in vivo. In spite of its appeal, the antibody carrier approach is associated with a number of problems. Of these, specificity in vivo and scarcity of target antigen remain the most important concerns. This is exemplified in a report that an antitumor antibody labeled with iron oxide showed good tumor binding in vitro but that results were not as convincing in an in vivo situation,[328] presumably because of the rapid extraction of the complex by phagocytic cells. Nonspecific phagocytosis of antibody-label complexes by phagocytic cells in liver, spleen, and lymph nodes will render the tumor antibody approach diagnostically useless in these organs unless carrier systems are developed that can evade phagocytosis. However, if the tumor is located outside of organs with phagocytic activity (e.g., soft tissues and the peritoneal cavity), this approach may ultimately be successful for improving tumor diagnosis.

Another application involves antibodies that recognize components of normal tissues. An example is the use of antimyosin antibody or its Fab fragment to detect myocardial infarction.[336, 337] Antimyosin Fab is a murine monoclonal antibody that binds human myosin and V_3 isomyosin in rodents.[338] In infarcted myocardial cells, exposed myosin is recognized by the antibody, whereas normal myocardial cells with intact cell membranes do not react with the antibody. This difference permits the assessment of myocardial viability (Fig. 6–18). Antimyosin Fab has been labeled with MION in several studies by both noncovalent[336] and covalent[337] means.

CELLS

In a different approach to achieving target selectivity, advantage has been taken of the ability of certain cells to phagocytose or bind a magnetic label and thus transport it to their destination. A notable example is neutrophils that localize in inflammatory lesions after incubation with various types of iron oxides.[330, 339] These studies generally showed good intracellular uptake of the label, particularly if an iron oxide tagged with the Fc fragment of IgG or bovine serum albumin was used rather than one containing a simple coat of dextran.[339]

Lymphocytes have also been marked with magnetic labels for in vitro[226] and in vivo (Bogdanov A., unpublished observations) applications. In one study,[226] lymphocytes were labeled with antilymphocyte-biotinylated dextran magnetite particles, a compound similar to those used for magnetic cell separation. These dextran magnetite particles were shown to bind to the surface of lymphocytes, and the labeled lymphocytes decreased the MR signal intensity of gel phantoms. In another

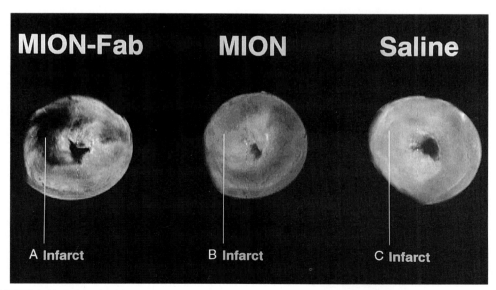

FIGURE 6–18. Infarct imaging with MION-Fab. After injection of contrast agents into rats with infarcts, hearts were excised and spin-echo images were obtained. *A*, T2-weighted (6000/20) image of infarcted heart from rat injected with MION-tagged with antimyosin Fab shows loss of signal intensity in the myocardium supplied by the anterior coronary artery. Although this T2-shortening effect is visible on the T1-weighted image (not shown), its effect is less pronounced. *B* and *C*, Rats that received injections of a control solution containing free MION not tagged with Fab *(B)* failed to show uptake in the area of the infarct. Similarly, the infarct showed no loss of signal intensity when saline was injected *(C)*. *(A to C* from Weissleder R, Lee A, Khaw B, et al: Antimyosin labeled monocrystalline iron oxide allows detection of myocardial infarct: MR antibody imaging. Radiology 182:381–385, 1992.)

study (Bogdanov A, personal communication, 1994) lymphocytes were labeled with MION to be used for in vivo MRI. Results of these studies should be available in the near future.

Acknowledgment

We would like to thank Dr. Peter Hahn and Dr. Alexei Bogdanov for fruitful discussions and helpful comments. A special thanks goes to Ms. Dianne Moschella, who assisted in the collection of data, typing, editing, and proofreading.

REFERENCES

1. Hahn PF: Gastrointestinal contrast agents. AJR 156:252–254, 1991.
2. Pels Rijcken TH, Davis MA, Ros PR: Intraluminal contrast agents for MR imaging of the abdomen and pelvis. J Magn Reson Imaging 4:291–300, 1994.
3. Wesbey GE, Brasch RC, Goldberg HI, et al: Dilute oral iron solutions as gastrointestinal contrast agents for magnetic resonance imaging: initial clinical experience. Magn Reson Imaging 3:57–64, 1985.
4. Weinreb JC, Maravilla KR, Redman HC, Nunnally R: Improved MR imaging of the upper abdomen with glucagon and gas. J Comput Assist Tomogr 8:835–838, 1984.
5. Tart RP, Li KCP, Storm BL, et al: Enteric MRI contrast agents: comparative study of five potential agents in humans. Magn Reson Imaging 9:559–568, 1991.
6. Butch R, Stark D, Wittenberg J, et al: Staging rectal cancer by MR and CT. AJR 146:1155–1160, 1986.
7. Mattrey RF, Hajek PC, Gylys-Morin VM, et al: Perfluorochemicals as gastrointestinal contrast agents for MR imaging: preliminary studies in rats and humans. AJR 148:1259–1263, 1987.
8. Rubin DL, Muller HH, Nino-Murcia M, et al: Intraluminal contrast enhancement and MR visualization of the bowel wall: efficacy of PFOB. J Magn Reson Imaging 1:371–380, 1991.
9. Brown JJ, Duncan JR, Heiken JP, et al: Perfluorooctylbromide as a gastrointestinal contrast agent for MR imaging: use with and without glucagon. Radiology 181:455–460, 1991.
10. Mattrey RF, Trambert MA, Brown JJ, et al: Results of the phase III trials with Imagent GI as an oral magnetic resonance contrast agent. Invest Radiol 26:S65–S66, 1991.
11. Anderson CM, Brown JJ, Balfe DM, et al: MR imaging of Crohn disease: use of perflubron as a gastrointestinal contrast agent. J Magn Reson Imaging 4:491–496, 1994.
12. Mattrey RF, Trambert MA, Brown JJ, et al: Perflubron as an oral contrast agent for MR imaging: results of a phase III clinical trial. Radiology 191:841–848, 1994.
13. Li KCP, Ang PGP, Tart RP, et al: Paramagnetic oil emulsions as oral magnetic resonance imaging contrast agents. Magn Reson Imaging 8:589–598, 1990.
14. Ballinger R, Magin RL, Webb AG: Sucrose polyester: a new oral contrast agent for MRI. Magn Reson Med 19:199–202, 1991.
15. Rubin DL, Muller HH, Young SW: Formulation of radiographically detectable gastrointestinal contrast agents for magnetic resonance imaging: effects of a barium sulfate additive on MR contrast agent effectiveness. Magn Reson Med 23:154–165, 1992.
16. Gerscovich EO, McGahan JP, Buonocore MH, et al: The rediscovery of infant feeding formula with magnetic resonance imaging. Pediatr Radiol 20:147–151, 1990.
17. Mirowitz SA, Susman N: Use of nutritional support formula as a gastrointestinal contrast agent for MRI. J Comput Assist Tomogr 16:908–915, 1992.
18. Listinsky JJ, Bryant RG: Gastrointestinal contrast agents: a diamagnetic approach. Magn Reson Med 8:285–292, 1988.
19. Mitchell DG, Vinitski S, Mohamed FB, et al: Comparison of Kaopectate with barium for negative and positive enteric contrast at MR imaging. Radiology 181:475–480, 1991.
20. Marti-Bonmati L, Vilar J, Paniagua JC, Talens A: High density barium sulphate as an MRI oral contrast. Magn Reson Imaging 9:259–261, 1991.
21. Li KCP, Tart RP, Fitzsimmons JR, et al: Barium sulfate suspension as a negative oral MRI contrast agent: in vitro and human optimization studies. Magn Reson Imaging 9:141–150, 1991.
22. Ros PR, Steinman RM, Torres GM, et al: The value of barium as a gastrointestinal contrast agent in MR imaging: a comparison study in normal volunteers. AJR 157:761–767, 1991.
23. Panaccione JL, Ros PR, Torres GM, Burton SS: Rectal barium in pelvic MR imaging: initial results. J Magn Reson Imaging 1:605–607, 1991.
24. Langmo L, Ros PR, Torres GM, Erquiaga E: Comparison of MR imaging after barium administration with CT in pelvic disease. J Magn Reson Imaging 2:89–91, 1992.
25. Liebig T, Stoupis C, Ros PR, et al: A potentially artifact-free oral contrast agent for gastrointestinal MRI. Magn Reson Med 30:646–649, 1993.
26. Hahn PF, Saini S, Cohen MS, et al: An aqueous gastrointestinal contrast agent for use in echo-planar MR imaging. Magn Reson Med 25:380–383, 1992.
27. Wesbey GE, Brasch RC, Engelstad BL, et al: Nuclear magnetic resonance contrast enhancement study of the gastrointestinal tract of rats and a human volunteer using nontoxic oral iron solutions. Radiology 149:175–180, 1983.
28. Jenkins JPR, Braganza JM, Hickey DS, et al: Quantitative tissue characterisation in pancreatic disease using magnetic resonance imaging. Br J Radiol 60:333–341, 1987.
29. Patten RM, Moss AA, Fenton TA, Elliott S: OMR, a positive bowel contrast agent for abdominal and pelvic MR imaging: safety and imaging characteristics. J Magn Reson Imaging 2:25–34, 1992.
30. Patten RM, Lo SK, Phillips JJ, et al: Positive bowel contrast agent for MR imaging of the abdomen: phase II and III clinical trials. Radiology 189:277–283, 1993.
31. Lauffer R, Brady T: Preparation and water relaxation properties of proteins labeled with paramagnetic metal chelates. Magn Reson Imaging 3:11–16, 1985.
32. Koenig SH, Baglin C, Brown RD III: Magnetic field dependence of solvent proton relaxation induced by Gd^{3+} and Mn^{2+} complexes. Magn Reson Med 1:496–501, 1984.
33. Lauffer R, Brady T, Brown R, et al: $1/T_1$ NMRD profiles of solutions of Mn^{2+} and Gd^{3+} protein-chelate conjugates. Magn Reson Med 3:541–548, 1986.
34. Unger EC, Fritz TA, Palestrant D, et al: Preliminary evaluation of iron phytate (inositol hexaphosphate) as a gastrointestinal MR contrast agent. J Magn Reson Imaging 3:119–124, 1993.
35. Mamourian AC, Burnett KR, Goldstein EJ, et al: Proton relaxation enhancement in tissue due to ingested manganese chloride: time course and dose response in the rat. Physiol Chem Phys Med NMR 16:123–128, 1984.
36. Cory DA, Schwartzentruber DJ, Mock BH: Ingested manganese chloride as a contrast agent for magnetic resonance imaging. Magn Reson Imaging 5:65–70, 1987.
37. Rubin DL, Muller HH, Young SW: Methods for the systemic investigation of gastrointestinal contrast media for MRI: evaluation of intestinal distribution by radiographic monitoring. Magn Reson Imaging 9:285–293, 1991.
38. Runge VM, Stewart RG, Clanton JA, et al: Work in progress: potential oral and intravenous paramagnetic NMR contrast agents. Radiology 147:789–791, 1983.
39. Runge WM, Foster MA, Clanton JA, et al: Particulate oral NMR contrast agents. Int J Nucl Med Biol 12:37–42, 1985.
40. Laniado M, Kornmesser W, Hamm B, et al: MR imaging of the gastrointestinal tract: value of Gd-DTPA. AJR 150:817–821, 1988.
41. Kaminsky S, Laniado M, Gogoll M, et al: Gadopentetate dimeglumine as a bowel contrast agent: safety and efficacy. Radiology 178:503–508, 1991.
42. Vlahos L, Gouliamos A, Athanasopoulou A, et al: A comparative study between Gd-DTPA and oral magnetic particles (OMP) as gastrointestinal (GI) contrast agents for MRI of the abdomen. Magn Reson Imaging 12:719–726, 1994.
43. Rogers J, Lewis J, Josephson L: Use of AMI-227 as an oral MR contrast agent. Magn Reson Imaging 12:631–639, 1994.
44. Pavone P, Cardone GP, Cisternino S, et al: Gadopentetate dimeglumine-barium paste for opacification of the esophageal lumen on MR images. AJR 159:762–764, 1992.
45. Widder DJ, Greif WL, Widder KJ, et al: Magnetite albumin microspheres: a new MR contrast material. AJR 148:399–404, 1987.
46. Hahn P, Stark D, Saini S, et al: Ferrite particles for bowel contrast in MR imaging: design issues and feasibility studies. Radiology 164:37–41, 1987.
47. Tilcock C, Unger EC, Ahkong QF, et al: Polymeric gastrointestinal MR contrast agents. J Magn Reson Imaging 1:463–467, 1991.
48. Lönnemark M, Hemmingsson A, Carlsten J, et al: Superparamagnetic particles as an MRI contrast agent for the gastrointestinal tract. Acta Radiol 29:599–602, 1988.
49. Lönnemark M, Hemmingsson A, Bach-Gansmo T, et al: Effect of superparamagnetic particles as oral contrast medium at magnetic resonance imaging: a phase I clinical study. Acta Radiol 30:193–196, 1989.
50. Bach-Gansmo T, Hemmingson A, Lönnemark M, et al: Safety and tolerance of oral magnetic particles for abdominal magnetic resonance imaging. Clin Trials J 26:216–225, 1989.
51. Lönnemark M, Hemmingsson A, Ericsson A, et al: Oral superparamagnetic particles for magnetic resonance imaging: effect in plain and viscous aqueous suspensions. Acta Radiol 31:303–307, 1990.
52. Niemi P, Katevuo K, Kormano M, et al: Superparamagnetic particles as gastrointestinal contrast agent in magnetic resonance imaging of lower abdomen. Acta Radiol 31:409–411, 1990.
53. Rinck P: Oral magnetic properties in MR imaging of the abdomen and pelvis. Radiology 178:775–779, 1991.

54. Lönnemark M, Hemmingsson A, Bach-Gansmo T, et al: Superparamagnetic particles as oral contrast medium in MR imaging of malignant lymphoma. Acta Radiol 32:232–238, 1991.

55. van Beers B, Grandin C, Jamart J, et al: Magnetic resonance imaging of lower abdominal and pelvic lesions: assessment of oral magnetic particles as an intestinal contrast agent. Eur J Radiol 14:252–257, 1992.

56. Øksendal AN, Jacobsen RF, Gundersen HG, et al: Superparamagnetic particles as an oral contrast agent in abdominal magnetic resonance imaging. Invest Radiol 26:S67–S70, 1991.

57. Boudghène FP, Bach-Gansmo T, Grange JD, et al: Contribution of oral magnetic particles in MR imaging of the abdomen with spin-echo and gradient-echo sequences. J Magn Reson Imaging 3:107–112, 1993.

58. Prayer L, Stiglbauer R, Kramer J, et al: Superparamagnetic particles as oral contrast medium in magnetic resonance imaging of patients with treated ovarian cancer—comparison with plain MRI. Br J Radiol 66:415–419, 1993.

59. Bach-Gansmo T, Dupas B, Gayet-Delacroix M, Lambrechts M: Abdominal MRI using a negative contrast agent. Br J Radiol 66:420–425, 1993.

60. MacVicar D, Jacobsen TF, Guy R, Husband JE: Phase III trial of oral magnetic particles in MRI of abdomen and pelvis. Clin Radiol 47:183–188, 1993.

61. Rubin DL, Muller HH, Sidhu MK, et al: Liquid oral magnetic particles as a gastrointestinal contrast agent for MR imaging: efficacy in vivo. J Magn Reson Imaging 3:113–118, 1993.

62. Rubin DL, Muller HH, Young SW, et al: Optimization of an oral magnetic particle formulation as a gastrointestinal contrast agent for magnetic resonance imaging. Invest Radiol 29:81–86, 1994.

63. Hahn PF, Stark DD, Lewis JM, et al: First clinical trial of a new superparamagnetic iron oxide for use as an oral gastrointestinal MR contrast agent. Radiology 175:695–700, 1990.

64. Torres GM, Erquiaga E, Ros PR, et al: Preliminary results of MR imaging with superparamagnetic iron oxide in pancreatic and retroperitoneal disorders. Radiographics 11:785–791, 1991.

65. Brasch RC: Rationale and applications for macromolecular Gd-based contrast agents. Magn Reson Med 22:282–287, 1991.

66. Schmiedl U, Ogan MD, Moseley ME, Brasch RC: Comparison of the contrast-enhancing properties of albumin-(Gd-DTPA) and Gd-DTPA at 2.0 T: an experimental study in rats. AJR 147:1263–1270, 1986.

67. Schmiedl U, Ogan M, Paajanen H, et al: Albumin labeled with Gd-DTPA as an intravascular, blood pool-enhancing agent for MR imaging: biodistribution and imaging studies. Radiology 162:205–210, 1987.

68. Schmiedl U, Moseley M, Ogan M, et al: Comparison of initial biodistribution patterns of Gd-DTPA and albumin-(Gd-DTPA) using rapid spin echo MR imaging. J Comput Assist Tomogr 11:306–313, 1987.

69. Wikström MG, Moseley ME, Shite DL, et al: Contrast-enhanced MRI of tumors: comparison of Gd-DTPA and a macromolecular agent. Invest Radiol 24:609–615, 1989.

70. Aicher KP, Dupon JW, White DL, et al: Contrast-enhanced magnetic resonance imaging of tumor-bearing mice treated with human recombinant tumor necrosis factor α. Cancer Res 50:7376–7381, 1990.

71. Niemi P, Reisto T, Hemmilä I, Kormano M: Magnetic field dependence of longitudinal relaxation rates of solutions of various protein-gadolinium^{3+} chelate conjugates. Invest Radiol 26:820–824, 1991.

72. Niemi P, Koskinen S, Reisto T: Tissue relaxation enhancement after intravenous administration of (ITCB-DTPA)-gadolinium conjugated albumin and intravascular magnetic resonance imaging contrast agent. Invest Radiol 26:674–680, 1991.

73. Vexler VS, Berthezéne Y, Wolfe CL, et al: Magnetic resonance imaging demonstration of pharmacologic-induced myocardial vasodilatation using a macromolecular gadolinium contrast agent. Invest Radiol 27:935–941, 1992.

74. Vexler VS, Clément O, Schmitt-Willich H, Brasch RC: Effect of varying the molecular weight of the MR contrast agent Gd-DTPA-polylysine on blood pharmacokinetics and enhancement patterns. J Magn Reson Imaging 4:381–388, 1994.

75. Schmiedl U, Sievers RE, Brasch RC, et al: Acute myocardial ischemia and reperfusion: MR imaging with albumin-Gd-DTPA. Radiology 170:351–356, 1989.

76. Wolfe CL, Moseley ME, Wikstrom MG, et al: Assessment of myocardial salvage after ischemia and reperfusion using magnetic resonance imaging and spectroscopy. Circulation 80:969–982, 1989.

77. Vexler VS, Berthezene Y, Moseley ME, Brasch RC: Magnetic resonance imaging enhanced with a macromolecular contrast agent: detection of the zonal renal ischemia. Invest Radiol 26:S131–S133, 1991.

78. Vexler VS, Berthèzene Y, Clément O, et al: Detection of zonal renal ischemia with contrast-enhanced MR imaging with a macromolecular blood pool contrast agent. J Magn Reson Imaging 2:311–319, 1992.

79. Ogan MD, Schmiedl U, Moseley ME, et al: Albumin labeled with Gd-DTPA, an intravascular contrast-enhancing agent for magnetic resonance blood pool imaging: preparation and characterization. Invest Radiol 22:665–671, 1987.

80. Moseley ME, White DL, Wang SC, et al: Vascular mapping using albumin-(Gd-DTPA), an intravascular contrast agent, and projection MR imaging. J Comput Assist Tomogr 13:215–221, 1989.

81. Gibby WA, Bogdan A, Ovitt TW: Cross-linked DTPA polysacharides for magnetic resonance imaging. Invest Radiol 24:302–309, 1989.

82. Wang S, Wikstrom M, White D, et al: Evaluation of Gd-DTPA-labeled dextran as an intravascular MR contrast agent: imaging characteristics in normal rat tissues. Radiology 175:483–488, 1990.

83. Armitage FE, Richardson DE, Li KCP: Polymeric contrast agents for magnetic resonance imaging: synthesis and characterization of gadolinium diethylenetriaminepentaacetic acid conjugated to polysaccharides. Bioconjug Chem 1:365–374, 1990.

84. Meyer D, Schaffer M, Bouillot A, et al: Paramagnetic dextrans as magnetic resonance contrast agents. Invest Radiol 26:S50–S52, 1991.

85. Niemi P, Reisto T, Kormano M: Relaxometry of dextran and albumin labeled with Gd-chelates. Invest Radiol 26:S48–S49, 1991.

86. Bligh S, Harding C, Sadler P, et al: Use of paramagnetic chelated metal derivatives of polysaccharides and spin-labeled polysaccharides as contrast agents in magnetic resonance imaging. Magn Reson Med 17:516–532, 1991.

87. Li KCP, Quisling RG, Armitage FE, et al: In vivo MR evaluation of Gd-DTPA conjugated to dextran in normal rabbits. Magn Reson Imag 10:439–444, 1992.

88. Sieving PF, Watson AD, Rocklage SM: Preparation and characterization of paramagnetic polychelates and their protein conjugates. Bioconjug Chem 1:65–71, 1990.

89. Marchal G, Bosmans H, Van Hecke P, et al: MR angiography with gadopentetate dimeglumine-polylysine: evaluation in rabbits. AJR 155:407–411, 1990.

90. Van Hecke PV, Marchal G, Bosmans H, et al: NMR imaging study of the pharmacodynamics of polylysine-gadolinium-DTPA in the rabbit and the rat. Magn Reson Imaging 9:313–321, 1991.

91. Berthezène Y, Vexler V, Jerome H, et al: Differentiation of capillary leak and hydrostatic pulmonary edema with a macromolecular MR imaging contrast agent. Radiology 181:773–777, 1991.

92. Schuhmann-Giampieri G, Schmitt-Willich H, Frenzel T, et al: In vivo and in vitro evaluation of Gd-DTPA-polylysine as a macromolecular contrast agent for magnetic resonance imaging. Invest Radiol 26:969–974, 1991.

93. Brasch RC, Berthezene Y, Vexler V, et al: Facilitated magnetic resonance imaging diagnosis of pulmonary disease using a macromolecular blood-pool contrast agent, polylysine-(Gd-DTPA). Invest Radiol 26:S42–S45, 1991.

94. Marchal G, Bosmans H, van Hecke P, et al: Experimental Gd-DTPA polylysine enhanced MR angiography: sequence optimization. J Comput Assist Tomogr 15:711–715, 1991.

95. Berthezène Y, Vexler V, Price D, et al: Magnetic resonance imaging of an experimental pulmonary perfusion deficit using a macromolecular contrast agent. Invest Radiol 27:346–351, 1992.

96. Berthezène Y, Vexler V, Clément O, et al: Contrast-enhanced MR imaging of the lung: assessments of ventilation and perfusion. Radiology 183:667–672, 1992.

97. Berthezène Y, Vexler V, Kuwatsuru R, et al: Differentiation of alveolitis and pulmonary fibrosis with a macromolecular MR imaging contrast agent. Radiology 185:97–103, 1992.

98. Böck JC, Pison U, Kaufmann F, Felix R: Gd-DTPA-polylysine-enhanced pulmonary time-of-flight MR angiography. J Magn Reson Imaging 4:473–476, 1994.

99. Montgomery AB, Paajanen H, Brasch RC, Murray JF: Aerosolized gadolinium-DTPA enhances the magnetic resonance signal of extravascular lung water. Invest Radiol 22:377–381, 1987.

100. Berthezène Y, Mühler A, Lang P, et al: Safety aspects and pharmacokinetics of inhaled aerosolized gadolinium. J Magn Reson Imaging 3:125–130, 1993.

101. Wiener EC, Brechbiel MW, Brothers H, et al: Dendrimer-based metal chelates: a new class of magnetic resonance imaging contrast agents. Magn Reson Med 31:1–8, 1994.

102. Desser TS, Rubin DL, Muller HH, et al: Dynamics of tumor imaging with Gd-DTPA-polyethylene glycol polymers: dependence on molecular weight. J Magn Reson Imaging 4:467–472, 1994.

103. Adam G, Neuerburg J, Spüntrup E, et al: Gd-DTPA-cascade-polymer: potential blood pool contrast agent for MR imaging. J Magn Reson Imaging 4:462–466, 1994.

104. Baxter AB, Melnikoff S, Stites DP, Brasch RC: Imunogenicity of gadolinium-based contrast agents for magnetic resonance imaging. Invest Radiol 26:1035–1040, 1991.

105. Bogdanov AA Jr, Weissleder R, Frank HW, et al: A new macromolecule as a contrast agent for MR angiography: preparation, properties, and animal studies. Radiology 187:701–706, 1993.

106. Abuchowski A, McCoy J, Palczuk N, et al: Effect of covalent attachment of polyethylene glycol on immunogenicity and circulating life of bovine liver catalase. J Biol Chem 252:3582–3586, 1977.

107. Abuchowski A, Es T, Palczuk N, Davis F: Alteration of immunological properties of bovine serum albumin by covalent attachment of polyethylene glycol. J Biol Chem 252:3578–3581, 1977.

108. Frank H, Weissleder R, Bogdanov AA, Brady TJ: Detection of pulmonary emboli by using MR angiography with MPEG-PL-GdDTPA: an experimental study in rabbits. AJR 162:1041–1046, 1994.

109. Chambon C, Clement O, Le Blanche A, et al: Superparamagnetic iron oxides as positive MR contrast agents: in vitro and in vivo evidence. Magn Reson Imaging 11:509–519, 1993.

110. Small WC, Nelson RC, Bernardino ME: Dual contrast enhancement of both T_1 and T_2-weighted sequences using ultrasmall superparamagnetic iron oxide. Magn Reson Imaging 11:645–654, 1993.

111. Frank H, Weissleder R, Brady TJ: Enhancement of MR angiography with iron oxide: preliminary studies in whole-blood phantom and in animals. AJR 162:209–213, 1994.

112. Nelson JA, Schmiedl U: Porphyrins as contrast media. Magn Reson Med 22:366–371, 1991.

113. Koenig SH, Brown RD III, Spiller M: The anomalous relaxivity of Mn^{3+} (TPPS$_4$). Magn Reson Med 4:252–260, 1987.

114. Chen C, Cohen JS, Myers CE, Sohn M: Paramagnetic metalloporphyrins as potential contrast agents in NMR imaging. FEBS Lett 168:70–74, 1984.

115. Patronas NJ, Cohen JS, Knop RH, et al: Metalloporphyrin contrast agents for magnetic resonance imaging of human tumors in mice. Cancer Treat Rep 70:391–395, 1986.

116. Lyon RC, Faustino PJ, Cohen JS, et al: Tissue distribution and stability of metalloporphyrin MRI contrast agents. Magn Reson Med 4:24–33, 1987.

117. Fiel RJ, Button RM, Gilani S, et al: Proton relaxation enhancement by manganese(III)TPPS$_4$ in a model tumor system. Magn Reson Imaging 5:149–156, 1987.

118. Ogan MD, Revel D, Brasch RC: Metalloporphyrin contrast enhancement of tumors in magnetic resonance imaging: a study of human carcinoma, lymphoma and fibrosarcoma in mice. Invest Radiol 22:822–828, 1987.

119. Furmanski P, Longley C: Metalloporphyrin enhancement of magnetic resonance imaging of human tumor xenografts in nude mice. Cancer Res 48:4604–4610, 1988.

120. Fiel RJ, Musser DA, Mark EH, et al: A comparative study of manganese meso-sulfonatopenyl porphyrins: contrast-enhancing agents for tumors. Magn Reson Imaging 8:255–259, 1990.

121. Bockhorst K, Höhn-Berlage M, Kocher M, Hossmann K-A: Proton relaxation enhancement in experimental brain tumors—in vivo NMR study of manganese(III)TPPS in rat brain gliomas. Magn Reson Imaging 8:499–504, 1990.

122. Place DA, Faustino PJ, van Jijl PCM, et al: Metalloporphyrins as contrast agents for tumors in magnetic resonance imaging. Invest Radiol 25:S69–S70, 1990.

123. Hoehn-Berlage M, Norris D, Bockhorst K, et al: T1, snapshot FLASH measurement of rat brain glioma: kinetics of the tumor-enhancing contrast agent manganese (III) tetraphenylporphine sulfonate. Magn Reson Med 27:201–213, 1992.

124. Schmiedl UP, Nelson JA, Starr FL, Schmidt R: Hepatic contrast-enhancing properties of manganese-mesoporphyrin and manganese-TPPS$_4$: a comparative magnetic resonance imaging study in rats. Invest Radiol 27:536–542, 1992.

125. Place DA, Faustino PJ, Berghamns KK, et al: MRI contrast-dose relationship of manganese(III)tetra(4-sulfonatophenyl) porphyrin with human xenograft tumors in nude mice at 2.0 T. Magn Reson Imaging 10:919–928, 1992.

126. Bockhorst K, Hoehn-Berlage M, Ernestus RI, et al: NMR-contrast enhancement of experimental brain tumors with MnTPPS: qualitative evaluation by in vivo relaxometry. Magn Reson Imaging 11:655–663, 1993.

127. Wilmes LJ, Hoehn Berlage M, Els T, et al: In vivo relaxometry of three brain tumors in the rat: effect of Mn-TPPS, a tumor-selective contrast agent. J Magn Reson Imaging 3:5–12, 1993.

128. Huang LR, Straubinger TM, Kahl SB, et al: Boronated metalloporphyrins: a novel approach to the diagnosis and treatment of cancer using contrast-enhanced MR imaging and neutron capture therapy. J Magn Reson Imaging 3:351–356, 1993.

129. Nelson JA, Schmiedl U, Shankland EG: Metalloporphyrins as tumor-seeking MRI contrast media and as potential selective treatment sensitizers. Invest Radiol 25:S71–S73, 1990.

130. Marzola P, Cannistraro S: Gd^{3+}-TPPS: a potential paramagnetic contrast agent in NMR imaging. Physiol Chem Phys Med NMR 19:279–282, 1987.

131. Hindré F, Le Plouzennec M, de Certaines JD, et al: Tetra-p-aminophenylporphyrin conjugated with Gd-DTPA: tumor-specific contrast agent for MR imaging. J Magn Reson Imaging 3:59–65, 1993.

132. Bockhorst K, Els T, Hoehn-Berlage M: Selective enhancement of experimental rat brain tumors with Gd-TPPS. J Magn Reson Imaging 4:451–456, 1994.

133. Sessler JL, Murai T, Hemmi G: A water-stable gadolinium(III) complex derived from a new pentadentate "expanded porphyrin" ligand. Inorg Chem 28:3390–3393, 1988.

134. Sessler JL, Murai T, Lynch V, Cyr M: An "expanded porphyrin": the synthesis and structure of a new aromatic pentadentate ligand. J Am Chem Soc 110:5586–5588, 1988.

135. Sessler JL, Mody TD, Hemmi GW, et al: Gadolinium(III) texaphyrin: a novel MRI contrast agent. J Am Chem Soc 115:10368–10369, 1993.

136. Young SW, Sidhu MK, Qing F, et al: Preclinical evaluation of gadolinium(III) texaphyrin complex: a new paramagnetic contrast agent for magnetic resonance imaging. Invest Radiol 29:330–338, 1994.

137. Schuhmann-Giampieri G: Liver contrast media for magnetic resonance imaging: interrelations between pharmacokinetics and imaging. Invest Radiol 28:753–761, 1993.

138. de Haën C, Gozzini L: Soluble-type hepatobiliary contrast agents for MR imaging. J Magn Reson Imaging 3:179–186, 1993.

139. Lauffer R, Greif WL, Stark DD, et al: Iron-EHPG as an hepatobiliary MR contrast agent: initial imaging and biodistribution studies. J Comput Assist Tomogr 9:431–438, 1985.

140. Lauffer RB, Vincent AC, Padmanabhan S, et al: Hepatobiliary MR contrast agents: 5-substituted iron-EHPG derivatives. Magn Reson Med 4:582–590, 1987.

141. Vittadini G, Felder E, Musu C, Tirone P: Preclinical profile of Gd-BOPTA. A liver-specific MRI contrast agent. Invest Radiol 25:S59–S60, 1990.

142. Shtern F, Garrido L, Compton CC, et al: MR imaging of blood-borne liver metastasis in mice: contrast enhancement with Fe-EHPG. Radiology 178:83–89, 1991.

143. Hoener BA, Engelstad BL, Ramos EC, et al: Comparison of Fe-HBED and Fe-EHPG as hepatobiliary MR contrast agents. J Magn Reson Imaging 1:357–362, 1991.

144. Hoener BA, Tzika AA, Englestad BL. White DL: Hepatic transport of the magnetic resonance imaging contrast agent Fe(III)-N-(3-phenylglutaryl)desferrioxamine B. Magn Reson Med 17:509–515, 1991.

145. Muetterties K, Hoerner B, Englestad B, et al: Ferrioxamine B derivatives as hepatobilary contrast agents for magnetic resonance imaging. Magn Reson Med 22:88–100, 1991.

146. White DL, Eason RG, Alkire AL, et al: Hepatic transport of magnetic resonance imaging contrast agents: ferrioxamine B derivatives. Invest Radiol 26:S146–S147, 1991.

147. Leander P, Golman K, Klaveness J, et al: MRI contrast media for the liver: efficacy in conditions of acute biliary obstruction. Invest Radiol 25:1130–1134, 1990.

148. Golman K, Klaveness J, Holtz E, et al: A magnetic resonance imaging contrast medium for the liver and bile. Invest Radiol 23:S243–S245, 1988.

149. Brasch RC, London DA, Wesbey GE, et al: Nuclear magnetic resonance study of a paramagnetic nitroxide contrast agent for enhancement of renal structures in experimental animals. Radiology 147:773–779, 1983.

150. Vittadini G, Felder E, Tirone P, Lorusso V: B-19036, a potential new hepatobiliary contrast agent for MR proton imaging. Invest Radiol 23(suppl):S246–S248, 1988.

151. Pavone P, Patrizio G, Buoni C, et al: Comparison of Gd-BOPTA with Gd-DTPA in MR imaging of rat liver. Radiology 176:61–64, 1990.

152. Cavagna F, Depra M, Maggioni F, et al: Gd-BOPTA/Dimeg: experimental disease imaging. Magn Reson Med 22:329–333, 1991.

153. Vogl TJ, Pegios W, McMahon C, et al: Gadobenate dimeglumine—a new contrast agent for MR imaging: preliminary evaluation in healthy volunteers. AJR 158:887–892, 1992.

154. Kreft BP, Tanimoto A, Baba Y, et al: Enhanced tumor detection in the presence of fatty liver disease: cell-specific contrast agents. J Magn Reson Imaging 4:337–342, 1994.

155. Weinmann HJ, Schuhmann-Giampieri G, Schmitt-Willich H, et al: A new lipophilic gadolinium chelate as a tissue-specific contrast medium for MRI. Magn Reson Med 22:233–237, 1991.

156. Schuhmann-Giampieri G, Schmitt-Willich H, Press WR, et al: Preclinical evaluation of Gd-EOB-DTPA as a contrast agent in MR imaging of the hepatobiliary system. Radiology 183:59–64, 1992.

157. Clément O, Mügler A, Vexler V, et al: Gadolinium-ethoxybenzyl-DTPA, a new liver-specific magnetic resonance contrast agent: kinetic and enhancement patterns in normal and cholestatic rats. Invest Radiol 27:612–619, 1992.

158. Mühler A, Clément O, Vexler V, et al: Hepatobiliary enhancement with Gd-EOB-DTPA: comparison of spin-echo and STIR imaging for detection of experimental liver metastases. Radiology 184:207–213, 1992.

159. Clément O, Mühler A, Vexler V, et al: Comparison of Gd-EOB-DTPA and Gd-DTPA for contrast-enhanced MR imaging of liver tumors. J Magn Reson Imaging 3:71–77, 1993.

160. Clément O, Mühler A, Vexler V, et al: Evaluation of radiation-induced liver injury with MR imaging: comparison of hepatocellular and reticuloendothelial contrast agents. Radiology 185:163–168, 1992.

161. Mühler A, Freise CE, Kuwatsuru R, et al: Acute liver rejection: evaluation with cell-directed MR contrast agents in a rat transplantation model. Radiology 186:139–146, 1993.

162. Mühler A, Clément O, Saeed M, et al: Gadolinium-ethoxybenzyl-DTPA, a new liver-directed magnetic resonance contrast agent. Invest Radiol 28:26–32, 1993.

163. Mühler A, Heinzelmann I, Weinmann HJ: Elimination of gadolinium-ethoxybenzyl-DTPA in a rat model of severely impaired liver and kidney excretory function: an experimental study in rats. Invest Radiol 29:213–216, 1994.

164. Ni Y, Marchal G, Lukito G, et al: MR imaging evaluation of liver enhancement by Gd-EOB-DTPA in selective and total bile duct obstruction in rats: correlation with serologic microcholangiographic, and histologic findings. Radiology 190:753–758, 1994.

165. van Beers BE, Grandin C, Pauwels S, et al: Gd-EOB-DTPA enhancement pattern of hepatocellular carcinomas in rats: comparison with Tc-99m-IDA uptake. J Magn Reson Imaging 4:351–354, 1994.

166. Mühler A, Staks T, Frenzel T, et al: First use of hepatobiliary MR contrast agent Gd-EOB-DTPA in man: pharmacokinetics and tolerability in phase I clinical trials. In: Proceedings of the Second Annual Meeting of the Society of Magnetic Resonance, San Francisco, 1994, p 894.

167. Walovitch RC, McMurry TJ, Tyeklar Z, et al: Biodistribution and safety studies of MS-264, a new liver agent with high hepatobiliary specificity. In: Proceedings of the Second Annual Meeting of the Society of Magnetic Resonance, San Francisco, 1994, p 387.

168. Young SW, Simpson BB, Ratner AV, et al: MRI measurement of hepatocyte toxicity using the new MRI contrast agent manganese dipyridoxal diphosphate, a manganese/pyridoxal 5-phosphate chelate. Magn Reson Med 10:1–13, 1989.

169. Rocklage SM, Cacheris WP, Quay SC, et al: Manganese(II) N,N'-dipyridoxylethylenediamine-N,N'-diacetate5,5′-bis(phosphate). Synthesis and characterization of a paramagnetic chelate for magnetic resonance imaging enhancement. Inorg Chem 28:477–485, 1989.

170. Young SW, Bradley B, Muller HH, Rubin DL: Detection of hepatic malignancies using Mn-DPDP (manganese dipyridoxal diphosphate) hepatobiliary MRI contrast agent. Magn Reson Imaging 8:267–276, 1990.

171. Lim KO, Stark DD, Leese PT, et al: Hepatobiliary MR imaging: first human experience with MnDPDP. Radiology 178:79–82, 1991.

172. Elizondo G, Fretz CJ, Stark DD, et al: Preclinical evaluation of MnDPDP: new paramagnetic hepatobiliary contrast agent for MR imaging. Radiology 178:73–78, 1991.

173. Nelson RC, Chezmar JL, Newberry LB, et al: Manganese dipyridoxyl diphosphate: effect of dose, time, and pulse sequence on hepatic enhancement in rats. Invest Radiol 26:569–573, 1991.

174. Gehl H, Vorwerk D, Klose K, Günther R: Pancreatic enhancement after low-dose infusion of Mn-DPDP. Radiology 180:337–339, 1991.

175. Hamm B, Vogl TJ, Branding G, et al: Focal liver lesions: MR imaging with Mn-DPDP—initial clinical results in 40 patients. Radiology 182:167–174, 1992.

176. Bernardino ME, Young SW, Lee JKT, Weinreb JC: Hepatic MR imaging with Mn-DPDP: safety, image quality, and sensitivity. Radiology 183:53–58, 1992.

177. Bernardino ME, Young SW, Lee JKT, Weinreb J: Contrast-enhanced magnetic resonance imaging of the liver with Mn-DPDP for known or suspected focal hepatic disease. Invest Radiol 26:S148–S149, 1991.

178. Rummeny E, Ehrenheim CH, Gehl HB, et al: Manganese-DPDP as a hepatobiliary contrast agent in the magnetic resonance imaging of liver tumors. Invest Radiol 26:S142–S145, 1991.

179. Marchal G, Ni Y, Zhang X, et al: Mn-DPDP enhanced MRI in experimental bile duct obstruction. J Comput Assist Tomogr 17:290–296, 1993.

180. Ni Y, Marchal G, Zhang X, et al: The uptake of manganese dipyridoxaldiphosphate by chemically induced hepatocellular carcinoma in rats. Invest Radiol 28:520–528, 1993.

181. Nelson RC, Chezmar JL, Thompson EH, et al: Preliminary reports: magnetic resonance imaging after arterial portography with manganese dipyridoxal diphosphate. Invest Radiol 28:335–340, 1993.

182. Rofsky NM, Weinreb JC, Bernardino ME, et al: Hepatocellular tumors: characterization with Mn-DPDP enhanced MR imaging. Radiology 188:53–59, 1993.

183. Ni Y, Marchal G, Yu J, et al: Experimental liver cancers: Mn-DPDP enhanced rims in MR-microangiographic-histologic correlation study. Radiology 188:45–51, 1993.

184. Liou J, Lee JKT, Borrello JA, Brown JJ: Differentiation of hepatomas from nonhepatomatous masses: use of MnDPDP-enhanced MR imaging. Magn Reson Imaging 12:71–79, 1994.

185. Adzamli IK, Gries H, Johnson D, Blau M: Development of phosphonate derivatives of gadolinium chelates for NMR imaging of calcified soft tissues. J Med Chem 32:139–144, 1989.

186. Adzamli IK, Blau M, Pfeffer MA, Davis MA: New magnetic resonance imaging contrast agents for infarct imaging based on phosphonate derivatives of Gd-DTPA. Invest Radiol 26:S242–S244, 1991.

187. Adzamli IK, Blau M: Phosphonate-modified GdDTPA complexes. I. NMRD study of the solution behavior of new tissue-specific contrast agents. Magn Reson Med 17:141–148, 1991.

188. Adzamli IK, Johnson D, Blau M: Phosphonate-modified Gd-DTPA complexes. II. Evaluation in a rat myocardial infarct model. Invest Radiol 26:143–148, 1991.

189. Seltzer SE: The role of liposomes in diagnostic imaging. Radiology 171:19–21, 1989.

190. Unger EC, Shen D, Fritz TA: Status of liposomes as MR contrast agents. J Magn Reson Imaging 3:195–198, 1993.

191. Parasassi T, Bombieri G, Conti F, Croatto U: Paramagnetic ions trapped in phospholipid vesicles as contrast agents in NMR imaging. Inorg Chim Acta 106:135–139, 1985.

192. Magin R, Wright S, Niesman M, et al: Liposome delivery of NMR contrast agents for improved tissue imaging. Magn Reson Med 3:440–447, 1986.

193. Navon G, Panigel R, Valensin G: Liposomes containing paramagnetic macromolecules as MRI contrast agents. Magn Reson Med 3:876–880, 1986.

194. Bacic G, Niesman MR, Bennett HF, et al: Modulation of water proton relaxation rates by liposomes containing paramagnetic materials. Magn Reson Med 6:445–458, 1988.

195. Bacic G, Niesman MR, Magin RL, Swartz HM: NMR and ESR study of liposome delivery of Mn^{2+} to murine liver. Magn Reson Med 13:44–61, 1990.

196. Niesman M, Bacic G, Wright S, et al: Liposome encapsulated $MnCl_2$ as a liver specific contrast agent for magnetic resonance imaging. Invest Radiol 25:545–551, 1990.

197. Caride VJ, Sostman HD, Winchell RJ, Gore JC: Relaxation enhancement using liposomes carrying paramagnetic species. Magn Reson Imaging 2:107–112, 1984.

198. Turski P, Kalinke T, Strother L, et al: Magnetic resonance imaging of rabbit brain after intracarotid injection of large multivesicular liposomes containing paramagnetic metals and DTPA. Magn Reson Med 7:184–196, 1988.

199. Unger E, Needleman P, Cullis P, Tilcock C: Gadolinium-DTPA liposomes as a potential MRI contrast agent: work in progress. Invest Radiol 23:928–932, 1988.

200. Tilcock C, Unger E, Cullis P, MacDougall P: Liposomal Gd-DTPA: preparation and characterization of relaxivity. Radiology 171:77–80, 1989.

201. Unger EC, Winokur T, MacDougall P, et al: Hepatic metastases: liposomal Gd-DTPA-enhanced MR imaging. Radiology 171:81–85, 1989.

202. Unger EC, MacDougall P, Cullis P, Tilcock C: Liposomal Gd-DTPA: effect of encapsulation on enhancement of hepatoma model by MRI. Magn Reson Imaging 7:417–423, 1989.

203. Tilcock C, MacDougall P, Unger E, et al: The effect of lipid composition on the relaxivity of Gd-DTPA entrapped in lipid vesicles of defined size. Biochim Biophys Acta 1022:181–186, 1990.

204. Unger E, Cardenas D, Zerella A, et al: Biodistribution and clearance of liposomal gadolinium-DTPA. Invest Radiol 25:638–644, 1990.

205. Unger E, Tilcock C, Ahkong QF, Fritz T: Paramagnetic liposomes as magnetic resonance contrast agents. Invest Radiol 25:S65–S66, 1990.

206. Unger E, Fritz T, Tilcock C, New T: Clearance of liposomal gadolinium: in vivo decomplexation. J Magn Reson Imaging 1:689–693, 1991.

207. Koenig SH, Ahkong QF, Brown RD III, et al: Permeability of liposomal membranes to water: results from the magnetic field dependence of T_1 of solvent protons in suspensions of vesicles with entrapped paramagnetic ions. Magn Reson Med 23:275–286, 1992.

208. Koenig SH: Relaxometry of paramagnetic liposomes. Invest Radiol 26:S260–S262, 1991.

209. Tilcock C, Ahkong QF, Koenig SH, et al: The design of liposomal paramagnetic MR agents: effect of vesicle size upon the relaxivity of surface-incorporated lipophilic chelates. Magn Reson Med 27:44–51, 1992.

210. Chan HC, Magin RL, Swartz HM: Delivery of nitroxide spin label to cultured cells by liposomes. Magn Reson Med 8:160–170, 1988.

211. Chan HC, Magin RL, Swartz HM: Rapid assessment of liposomal stability in blood by an aqueous nitroxide spin label. J Biochem Biophys Methods 18:271–276, 1989.

212. Federico M, Iannone A, Chan HC, Magin RL: Bone marrow uptake of liposome-entrapped spin label after liver blockade with empty liposomes. Magn Reson Med 10:418–425, 1989.

213. Kabalka G, Buonocore E, Hubner K, et al: Gadolinium-labeled liposomes: targeted MR contrast agents for the liver and spleen. Radiology 163:255–258, 1987.

214. Kabalka GW, Buonocore E, Hubner K, et al: Gadolinium-labeled liposomes containing paramagnetic amphipathic agents: targeted MR contrast agents for the liver. Magn Reson Med 8:89–95, 1988.

215. Grant CWM, Karlik S, Florio E: A liposomal MRI contrast agent: phosphatidylethanolamine-DTPA. Magn Reson Med 11:236–243, 1989.

216. Kabalka GW, Davis MA, Moss TH, et al: Gadolinium-labeled liposomes containing various amphiphilic Gd-DTPA derivatives: targeted MRI contrast enhancement agents for the liver. Magn Reson Med 19:406–415, 1991.

217. Kabalka GW, Davis MA, Duonocore E, et al: Gd-labeled liposomes containing amphipathic agents for magnetic resonance imaging. Invest Radiol 25:S63–S64, 1990.

218. Schwendener RA, Wüthrich R, Duewell S, et al: Small unilamellar liposomes as magnetic resonance contrast agents loaded with paramagnetic Mn-, Gd- and Fe-DTPA-stearate complexes. Int J Pharm 49:249–259, 1989.

219. Schwendener RA, Wüthrich R, Duewell S, et al: A pharmacokinetic and MRI study of unilamellar gadolinium-, manganese-, and iron-DTPA-stearate liposomes as organ-specific contrast agents. Invest Radiol 25:922–932, 1990.

220. Unger E, Shen D, Wu G, Fritz T: Liposomes as MR contrast agents: pros and cons. Magn Reson Med 22:304–308, 1991.

221. Grant CW, Barber KR, Florio E, Karlik S: A phospholipid spin label used as a liposome-associated MRI contrast agent. Magn Reson Med 5:371–376, 1987.

222. Karlik S, Florio E, Grant CWM: Comparative evaluation of two membrane-based liposomal MRI contrast agents. Magn Reson Med 19:56–66, 1991.

223. Margolis LB, Namiot VA, Kljukin LM: Magnetoliposomes: another principle of cell sorting. Biochim Biophys Acta 735:193–195, 1983.

224. Kiwada H, Sato J, Yamada S, Kato Y: Feasibility of magnetic liposomes as a targeting device for drugs. Chem Pharm Bull 34:4253–4258, 1986.

225. De Cuyper M, Joniau M: Magnetoliposomes: formation and structural characterization. Eur Biophys J 15:311–319, 1988.

226. Bulte JWM, Ma LD, Magin RL, et al: Selective MR imaging of labeled human peripheral blood mononuclear cells by liposome mediated incor-

poration of dextran-magnetite particles. Magn Reson Med 29:32–37, 1993.

227. Bodganov AA Jr, Martin C, Weissleder R, Brady TJ: Trapping of dextran-coated colloids in liposomes by transient binding to aminophospholipid: preparation of ferrosomes. Biochim Biophys Acta 1193:212–218, 1994.

228. Go KG, Bulte JWM, de Ley L, et al: Our approach towards developing a specific tumor-targeted MRI contrast agent for the brain. Eur J Radiol 16:171–175, 1993.

229. Weissleder R, Papisov MI: Pharmaceutical iron oxides for MR imaging. Rev Magn Reson Med 4:1–20, 1992.

230. Fahlvik AK, Klaveness J, Stark DD: Iron oxides as MR imaging contrast agents. J Magn Reson Imaging 3:187–194, 1993.

231. Weissleder R, Reimer P: Superparamagnetic iron oxides for MRI. Eur J Radiol 3:198–212, 1993.

232. Weissleder R: Liver MR imaging with iron oxides: towards consensus and clinical practice. Radiology 193:593–595, 1994.

233. Weissleder R: Target-specific superparamagnetic MR contrast agents. Magn Reson Med 22:209–212, 1991.

234. Weissleder R, Bogdanov A, Papisov M: Drug targeting in magnetic resonance imaging. Magn Reson Q 8:55–63, 1992.

235. Misawa T, Hashimoto K, Shimodaira S: Formation of Fe(II), -Fe(III) intermediary green complex on oxidation of ferrous iron in neutral and slightly alkaline sulphate solutions. J Inorg Nucl Chem 35:4107–4174, 1973.

236. Papisov M, Savelyev V, Sergienko V, et al: Magnetic drug targeting. I. In vivo kinetics of radiolabeled magnetic drug carriers. Int J Pharm 40:201–206, 1987.

237. Papisov M, Torchilin V: Magnetic drug targeting. II. Targeted drug transport by magnetic microparticles: factors influencing therapeutic effect. Int J Pharm 40:207–214, 1987.

238. Reimer P, Kwong K, Brady TJ, et al: Single shot echo planar imaging allows assessment of pharmacokinetics of MR contrast agents. In: Proceedings of the 10th Annual Meeting of the Society of Magnetic Resonance in Medicine, San Francisco, 1991, p 839.

239. Kawamura Y, Endo K, Watanabe Y, et al: Use of magnetite particles as a contrast agent for MR imaging of the liver. Radiology 174:357–360, 1990.

240. Majumdar S, Zoghbi S, Pope CF, Gore JC: Quantitation of MR relaxation effects of iron oxide particles in liver and spleen. Radiology 169:653–655, 1988.

241. Weissleder R, Stark DD, Engelstad B, et al: Superparamagnetic iron oxide: pharmacokinetics and toxicity. AJR 152:167–173, 1989.

242. Magin RL, Bacic G, Niesman MR, et al: Dextran magnetite as a liver contrast agent. Magn Reson Med 20:1–16, 1991.

243. Pouliquen D, Le Jeune JJ, Perdrisot R, et al: Iron oxide nanoparticles for use as an MRI contrast agent: pharmacokinetics and metabolism. Magn Reson Imaging 9:275–283, 1991.

244. Hershko C, Cook J, Finch C: Storage iron kinetics. II. Study of desferrioxamine action by selective radioiron labels of RE and parenchymal cells. J Lab Clin Med 81:876–886, 1973.

245. Weir M, Gibson J, Peter T: Haemosiderosis and tissue damage. Cell Biochem Funct 2:186–194, 1984.

246. Tavill A, Bacon B: Hemochromatosis: how much is too much? Hepatology 6:142–145, 1986.

247. Bassett M, Halliday J, Powell L: Value of hepatic iron measurements in early hemochromatosis and determination of the critical iron level associated with fibrosis. Hepatology 6:24–29, 1986.

248. Chilton HM, Jackels SC, Hinson WH, Ekstrand KE: Use of a paramagnetic substance, colloidal manganese sulfide, as an NMR contrast material in rats. J Nucl Med 25:604–607, 1984.

249. Burnett KR, Wolf GL, Shumacher HR, Goldstein EJ: Gadolinium oxide: a prototype agent for contrast enhanced imaging of the liver and spleen with magnetic resonance. Magn Reson Imaging 3:66–71, 1985.

250. Renshaw PF, Owen CS, McLaughlin AC, et al: Ferromagnetic contrast agents: a new approach. Magn Reson Med 3:217–225, 1986.

251. Mendonca-Dias MH, Lauterbur PC: Ferromagnetic particles as contrast agents for magnetic resonance imaging of liver and spleen. Magn Reson Med 3:328–330, 1986.

252. Olsson MBE, Persson BRB, Salford LG, Schröder U: Ferromagnetic particles as contrast agent in T2 NMR-imaging. Magn Reson Imaging 4:437–440, 1986.

253. Hemmingsson A, Carlsten J, Ericsson A, et al: Relaxation enhancement of the dog liver and spleen by biodegradable superparamagnetic particles in proton magnetic resonance imaging. Acta Radiol 28:703–705, 1987.

254. Fahlvik AK, Holtz E, Leander P, et al: Magnetic starch microspheres, efficacy and elimination: a new organ-specific contrast agent for magnetic resonance imaging. Invest Radiol 25:113–120, 1990.

255. Fahlvik AK, Holtz E, Schroder U, Klaveness J: Magnetic starch microspheres, biodistribution and biotransformation: a new organ-specific contrast agent for magnetic resonance imaging. Invest Radiol 25:793–797, 1990.

256. Fahlvik AK, Holtz E, Klaveness J: Relaxation efficacy of paramagnetic and superparamagnetic microspheres in liver and spleen. Magn Reson Imaging 8:363–369, 1990.

257. Fahlvik AK, Artursson P, Edman P: Magnetic starch microspheres: interactions of a microsphere MR contrast medium with macrophages in vitro. Int J Pharm 65:249–259, 1990.

258. Kreft B, Tanimoto A, Leffler S, et al: Contrast-enhanced MR imaging of diffuse and focal splenic disease with use of magnetic starch microspheres. J Magn Reson Imaging 4:373–379, 1994.

259. Bach-Gansmo T, Fahlvik AK, Ericsson A, Hemmingsson A: Superparamagnetic iron oxide for liver imaging: comparison among three different preparations. Invest Radiol 29:339–344, 1994.

260. Saini S, Stark DD, Hahn PF, et al: Ferrite particles: a superparamagnetic MR contrast agent for the reticuloendothelial system. Radiology 162:211–216, 1987.

261. Saini S, Stark D, Hahn P, et al: Ferrite particles: A superparamagnetic MR contrast agent for enhanced detection of liver carcinoma. Radiology 162:217–222, 1987.

262. Bacon BR, Stark DD, Park SH, et al: Ferrite particles: a new magnetic resonance imaging contrast agent: lack of acute or chronic hepatotoxicity after intravenous administration. J Lab Clin Med 110:164–171, 1987.

263. Weissleder R, Hahn PF, Stark DD, et al: MR imaging of splenic metastases: ferrite-enhanced detection in rats. AJR 149:723–726, 1987.

264. Weissleder R, Stark DD, Compton CC, et al: Ferrite-enhanced MR imaging of hepatic lymphoma: an experimental study in rats. AJR 149:1161–1165, 1987.

265. Weissleder R, Saini S, Stark DD, et al: Dual-contrast MR imaging of liver cancer in rats. AJR 150:561–566, 1988.

266. Majumdar S, Zoghbi S, Pope CF, Gore JC: A quantitative study of relaxation rate enhancement produced by iron oxide particles in polyacrylamide gels and tissue. Magn Reson Med 9:185–202, 1989.

267. Kawamori Y, Matsui O, Kadoya M, et al: Differentiation of hepatocellular carcinomas from hyperplastic nodules induced in rat liver with ferrite-enhanced MR imaging. Radiology 183:65–72, 1992.

268. Weissleder R, Stark DD, Rummeny EJ, et al: Splenic lymphoma: ferrite-enhanced MR imaging in rats. Radiology 166:423–430, 1988.

269. Tsang YM, Stark DD, Chen MCM, et al: Hepatic micrometastases in the rat: ferrite-enhanced MR imaging. Radiology 167:21–24, 1988.

270. Majumdar S, Zoghbi SS, Gore JC: The influence of pulse sequence on the relaxation effects of superparamagnetic iron oxide contrast agents. Magn Reson Med 10:289–301, 1989.

271. Weissleder R, Elizondo G, Josephson L, et al: Experimental lymph node metastases: enhanced detection with MR lymphography. Radiology 171:835–839, 1989.

272. Marchal G, Van Hecke P, Demaerel P, et al: Detection of liver metastases with superparamagnetic iron oxide in 15 patients: results of MR imaging at 1.5 T. AJR 152:771–775, 1989.

273. Fretz CJ, Elizondo G, Weissleder R, et al: Superparamagnetic iron oxide-enhanced MR imaging: pulse sequence optimization for detection of liver cancer. Radiology 172:393–397, 1989.

274. Majumdar S, Zoghbi SS, Gore JC: Pharmacokinetics of superparamagnetic iron-oxide MR contrast agents in the rat. Invest Radiol 25:771–777, 1990.

275. Fretz CJ, Stark DD, Metz CE, et al: Detection of hepatic metastases: comparison of contrast-enhanced CT, unenhanced MR imaging, and iron oxide-enhanced MR imaging. AJR 155:763–770, 1990.

276. Clement O, Frija G, Chambon C, et al: Liver tumors in cirrhosis: experimental study with SPIO-enhanced MR imaging. Radiology 180:31–36, 1991.

277. Clement O, Frija G, Chambon C, Schouman-Clayes E: Superparamagnetic iron oxide-enhanced magnetic resonance imaging of experimental liver tumors after mitomycin C administration. Invest Radiol 27:230–235, 1992.

278. Reimer P, Kwong K, Weisskoff R, et al: Dynamic signal intensity changes in liver with superparamagnetic MR contrast agents. J Magn Reson Imaging 2:177–181, 1992.

279. Stark DD, Weissleder R, Elizondo G, et al: Superparamagnetic iron oxide: clinical application as a contrast agent for MR imaging of the liver. Radiology 168:297–301, 1988.

280. Weissleder R, Hahn PF, Stark DD, et al: Superparamagnetic iron oxide: enhanced detection of focal splenic tumors with MR imaging. Radiology 169:399–403, 1988.

281. Weissleder R, Elizondo G, Stark DD, et al: The diagnosis of splenic lymphoma by MR imaging: value of superparamagnetic iron oxide. AJR 152:175–180, 1989.

282. Elizondo G, Weissleder R, Stark DD, et al: Hepatic cirrhosis and hepatitis: MR imaging enhanced with superparamagnetic iron oxide. Radiology 174:797–801, 1990.

283. Hagspiel KD, Eichenberger AC, Neidl KFW, et al: The role of AMI-25 in the assessment of liver metastases: a comparative study between pre- and post-contrast MRI, CT, delayed CT, ultrasound (US) and intraoperative ultrasound (IOUS). In: Proceedings of the 11th Annual Meeting of the Society of Magnetic Resonance in Medicine, Berlin, 1992, p 3222.

284. Ros PR, Freeny PC, Harms SE, Seltzer SE, Davis PL, Green AM: Efficacy of superparamagnetic iron oxide as an adjunct to MR imaging of the liver: results of a multicenter trial. Presented at the Annual Meeting of the Radiological Society of North America, Chicago, 1992, p 202.

285. Winter TC III, Freeny PC, Nghiem HV, et al: MR imaging with IV superparamagnetic iron oxide: efficacy in the detection of focal hepatic lesions. AJR 161:1191–1198, 1993.

286. Bruel JM, Group European SPIO Collaborative Study: Superparamag-

netic iron oxide for the detection of hepatic lesions with MR imaging: results of phase III trial. Presented at the Annual Meeting of the Radiological Society of North America, Chicago, 1993, p 273.

287. Duda SH, Laniado M, Kopp AF, et al: Superparamagnetic iron oxide: detection of focal liver lesions at high-field-strength MR imaging. J Magn Reson Imaging 4:309–314, 1994.

288. Denys A, Arrive L, Servois V, et al: Detection and characterization of hepatic tumors by MR imaging at one tesla with AMI-25: analysis by means of receiver operating characteristic curve. Radiology 193:665–669, 1994.

289. Bellin MF, Zaim S, Auberton E, et al: Safety and efficacy of superparamagnetic iron oxide in the detection of liver metastases. Radiology 193:657–663, 1994.

290. Weissleder R, Elizondo G, Wittenberg J, et al: Ultrasmall superparamagnetic iron oxide: characterization of a new class of contrast agents for MR imaging. Radiology 175:489–493, 1990.

291. Weissleder R, Elizondo G, Wittenberg J, et al: Ultrasmall superparamagnetic iron oxide: an intravenous contrast agent for assessing lymph nodes with MR imaging. Radiology 175:494–498, 1990.

292. Seneterre E, Weissleder R, Jaramillo D, et al: Bone marrow: ultrasmall superparamagnetic iron oxide for MR imaging. Radiology 179:529–533, 1991.

293. Tanoura T, Bernas M, Barkazanli A, et al: MR lymphography with iron oxide compound AMI-227: studies in ferrets with filariasis. AJR 159:875–881, 1992.

294. Trillaud H, Degrèze P, Combe C, et al: Evaluation of intrarenal distribution of ultrasmall superparamagnetic iron oxide particles by magnetic resonance imaging and modification by furosemide and water restriction. Invest Radiol 29:540–546, 1994.

295. Guimaraer R, Clément O, Bittoun J, et al: MR lymphography with superparamagnetic iron nanoparticles in rats: pathologic basis for contrast enhancement. AJR 162:201–207, 1994.

296. Bengele HH, Palmacci S, Rogers J, et al: Biodistribution of an ultrasmall superparamagnetic iron oxide colloid, BMS 180549, by different routes of administration. Magn Reson Imaging 12:433–442, 1994.

297. McLachlan SJ, Morris MR, Lucas MA, et al: Phase I clinical evaluation of a new iron oxide MR contrast agent. J Magn Reson Imaging 4:301–307, 1994.

298. Unger EC, Totty WG, Neufeld DM, et al: Magnetic resonance imaging using gadolinium labeled monoclonal antibody. Invest Radiol 20:693–700, 1985.

299. Shreve P, Aisen AM: Monoclonal antibodies labeled with polymeric paramagnetic ion chelates. Magn Reson Med 3:336–340, 1986.

300. Macri MA, DeLuca F, Maraviglia B, et al: Study of proton spin-lattice relaxation variations induced by paramagnetic antibodies. Magn Reson Med 11:283–287, 1989.

301. Josephson L, Groman EV, Menz E, et al: A functionalized superparamagnetic iron oxide colloid as a receptor directed MR contrast agent. Magn Reson Imaging 8:637–646, 1990.

302. Weissleder R, Reimer P, Lee AS, et al: MR receptor imaging: ultrasmall iron oxide particles targeted to asialoglycoprotein receptors. AJR 155:1161–1167, 1990.

303. Reimer P, Weissleder R, Lee A, et al: Receptor imaging: Application to MR imaging of liver cancer. Radiology 177:729–734, 1990.

304. Reimer P, Weissleder R, Lee A, et al: Asialoglycoprotein receptor function in benign liver disease: evaluation with MR imaging. Radiology 178:769–774, 1991.

305. Reimer P, Weissleder R, Brady TJ, et al: Experimental hepatocellular carcinoma: MR receptor imaging. Radiology 180:641–645, 1991.

306. Reimer P, Weissleder R, Wittenberg J, Brady T: Receptor-directed contrast agents for MR imaging: preclinical evaluation with affinity assays. Radiology 182:565–569, 1992.

307. Small WC, Nelson RC, Sherbourne GM, Bernardino ME: Enhancement effects of a hepatocyte receptor-specific MR contrast agent in an animal model. J Magn Reson Imaging 4:325–330, 1994.

308. Schwartz AL, Rup D, Lodish HF: Difficulties in the quantification of asialoglycoprotein receptors on the rat hepatocyte. J Biol Chem 255:9033–9036, 1980.

309. Tolleshaug H: Binding and internalization of asialoglycoproteins by isolated rat hepatocytes. Int J Biochem 13:45–51, 1981.

310. Reimer P, Weissleder W, Wittenberg JW, Brady TJ: Affinity assays allow preclinical evaluation of receptor directed MR contrast agents. Radiology 182:565–569, 1992.

311. Gallez B, Lacour V, Demeure R, et al: Spin labeled arabinogalactan as MRI contrast agent. Magn Reson Imaging 12:61–69, 1994.

312. Shen T, Weissleder R, Papisov M, Brady T: Polymeric iron oxide compounds for MR imaging. Presented at 10th Annual Meeting of the Society of Magnetic Resonance in Medicine, San Francisco, 1991, p 870.

313. Kojima S, Ishido M, Kubota K, et al: Tissue distribution of radioiodinated neoglycoproteins and mammalian lectins. Biol Chem Hoppe Seyler 371:331–338, 1990.

313a. Harika L, Weissleder R, Poss K, et al: MR lymphography with a lymphotrophic T1-type MR contrast agent: Gd-DTPA-PGM. Magn Reson Med 33:88–92, 1995.

313b. Weissleder R, Wang YM, Papisov M, et al: Polymeric contrast agent for MR imaging of adrenal glands. J Magn Reson Imaging 3:93–97, 1993.

314. Schaffer BK, Linker C, Papisov M, et al: MION-ASF: biokinetics of an MR receptor agent. Magn Reson Imaging 11:411–417, 1993.

315. Gosh P, Hawrylak N, Broadus J, et al: NMR imaging of transplanted iron-oxide labeled cells in rat brain. In: Proceedings of the 9th Annual Meeting of the Society of Magnetic Resonance in Medicine, New York, 1990, p 749.

316. Gosh P, Zhou X, Lin W, et al: Neuronal tracing with magnetite labels. In: Proceedings of the 9th Annual Meeting of the Society of Magnetic Resonance in Medicine, New York, 1990, p 1042.

317. Filler AG, Winn HR, Howe FA, et al: Axonal transport of superparamagnetic metal oxide particles: potential for magnetic resonance assessment of axoplasmatic flow in clinical neuroscience. In: Proceedings of the 10th Annual Meeting of the Society of Magnetic Resonance in Medicine, San Francisco, 1991, p 985.

318. Enochs WS, Schaefer B, Bhide P, et al: MR imaging of slow axonal transport in vivo. Exp Neurol 123:235–242, 1993.

319. van Everdingen K, Enochs WS, Bhide PG, et al: Determinants of in vivo MR imaging of slow axonal transport. Radiology 193:485–491, 1994.

320. Rubin RH, Fischman AJ, Callahan RJ, et al: ^{111}In-labeled nonspecific immunoglobulin scanning in the detection of focal infection. N Engl J Med 321:935–940, 1989.

321. Fischman AJ, Rubin RH, White JA, et al: Localization of Fc and Fab fragments of nonspecific polyclonal IgG at focal sites of inflammation. J Nucl Med 31:1199–1205, 1990.

322. Eckle I, Reifer R, Hoferichter A, et al: High affinity binding of immunoglobulin G fragments to human polymorphonuclear leukocytes. Biol Chem Hoppe Seyler 371:1107–1111, 1990.

323. Juweid M, Strauss HW, Yaoita H, et al: Accumulation of IgG at focal sites of inflammation. Eur J Nucl Med 19:159–165, 1992.

324. Morrel E, Tompkins RG, Fischman AJ, et al: Autoradiographic method for quantitation of radiolabeled proteins in tissues using In-111. J Nucl Med 30:1538–1545, 1989.

325. Weissleder R, Lee AS, Fischman AJ, et al: MR antibody imaging: polyclonal human IgG labelled with polymeric iron oxide. Radiology 181:245–249, 1991.

326. Reimer P, Weissleder R, Knoefel WT, et al: Pancreatic receptors: initial feasibility studies with a targeted contrast agent. Radiology 193:527–531, 1994.

327. Renshaw PF, Owen CS, Evans AE, Leigh JS Jr: Immunospecific NMR contrast agents. Magn Reson Imaging 4:351–357, 1986.

328. Cerdan S, Lötscher HR, Künnecke B, Seelig J: Monoclonal antibody–coated magnetite particles as contrast agents in magnetic resonance imaging of tumors. Magn Reson Med 12:151–163, 1989.

329. Weissleder R, Lee A, Khaw B, et al: Antimyosin labeled monocrystalline iron oxide allows detection of myocardial infarct: MR antibody imaging. Radiology 182:381–385, 1992.

330. Bulte JWM, Hoekstra Y, Kamman RL, et al: Specific MR imaging of human lymphocytes by monoclonal antibody-guided dextran-magnetite particles. Magn Reson Med 25:148–157, 1992.

331. Curtet C, Tellier C, Bohy J, et al: Selective modification of NMR relaxation time in human colorectal carcinoma by using gadolinium-diethylenetriaminepentaacetic acid conjugated with monoclonal antibody 19-9. Proc Natl Acad Sci USA 83:4277–4281, 1986.

332. Curtet C, Bourgoin C, Bohy J, et al: Gd-25 DTPA-MAb, a potential NMR contrast agent for MRI in the xenografted nude mouse: preliminary studies. Int J Cancer 2(suppl):126–132, 1988.

333. Kornguth SE, Turski PA, Perman WH, et al: Magnetic resonance imaging of gadolinium-labeled monoclonal antibody polymers directed at human T lymphocytes implanted in canine brain. J Neurosurg 66:898–906, 1987.

334. Brasch R: New directions in the development of MR imaging contrast media. Radiology 183:1–11, 1992.

335. Göhr-Rosenthal S, Schmitt-Willich H, Ebert W, et al: An immunoselective contrast medium for MRI: detection of colorectal tumor transplants in mice with a Gd-labeled monoclonal antibody. Presented at the 10th Annual Meeting of the Society of Magnetic Resonance in Medicine, San Francisco, 1991, p 356.

336. Weissleder R, Lee AS, Khaw BA, et al: MR antibody imaging: antimyosin labelled with monocrystalline iron oxide allows detection of myocardial infarct. Invest Radiol 26:1125, 1991. Abstract.

337. Papisov M, Weissleder R, O'Donnell S, et al: Target-specific nuclear magnetic resonance imaging with antibody-iron-oxide particles. In: Book of Abstracts: Society of Nuclear Medicine 1991. New York: Society of Nuclear Medicine, 1991. Abstract.

338. Khaw BA, Torchilin VP, Klibanov AL, et al: Modification of monoclonal antimyosin antibody: enhanced specificity of localization and scintigraphic visualization in acute experimental myocardial infarction. J Mol Cell Cardiol 21:31–35, 1989.

339. Chan TW, So A, Kressel HY: In vitro incorporation of iron oxide particles into peripheral phagocytic cells. Presented at the 9th Annual Meeting of the Society of Magnetic Resonance in Medicine, New York, 1990, p 749.

340. Weinmann HJ, Brasch RC, Press WR, Wesbey GE: Characteristics of gadolinium-DTPA complex: a potential NMR contrast agent. AJR 142:619–624, 1984.

341. Brasch RC, Weinmann HJ, Wesbey GE: Contrast-enhanced NMR imaging: animal studies using gadolinium-DTPA complex. AJR 142:625–630, 1984.

342. Schmiedl U, Moseley ME, Sievers R, et al: Magnetic resonance imaging of myocardial infarction using albumin-(Gd-DTPA), a macromolecular blood-volume contrast agent in a rat model. Invest Radiol 22:713–721, 1987.

343. Shen T, Weissleder R, Papisov M, et al: Monocrystalline iron oxide nanocompounds (MION): physicochemical properties. Magn Reson Med 29:599–604, 1993.

344. Helpern JA, Curtis JC, Hearshen D, et al: The development of a pH-sensitive contrast agent for NMR ^{1}H imaging. Magn Reson Med 5:302–305, 1987.

345. Josephson L, Lewis J, Jacobs P, et al: The effects of iron oxides on proton relaxivity. Magn Reson Imag 6:647–653, 1988.

346. Kent TA, Quast MJ, Kaplan BJ, et al: Assessment of a superparamagnetic iron oxide (AMI-25) as a brain contrast agent. Magn Reson Med 13:434–443, 1990.

347. Hahn PF, Stark DD, Weissleder R, et al: Clinical application of superparamagnetic iron oxide to MR imaging of tissue perfusion of vascular liver tumors. Radiology 174:361–366, 1990.

348. Rozenman Y, Zou X, Kantor HL: Signal loss induced by superparamagnetic iron oxide particles in NMR spin-echo images: the role of diffusion. Magn Reson Med 14:31–39, 1990.

349. Rozenman Y, Zou XM, Kantor HL: Cardiovascular MR imaging with iron oxide particles: utility of a superparamagnetic contrast agent and the role of diffusion in signal loss. Radiology 175:655–659, 1990.

350. Rozenman Y, Zou X, Kantor H: Magnetic resonance imaging with superparamagnetic iron oxide particles for the detection of myocardial reperfusion. Magn Reson Imaging 9:933–939, 1991.

351. Weissleder R, Heautot JF, Schaffer BK, et al: MR lymphography: study of a high-efficiency lymphotrophic agent. Radiology 191:225–230, 1994.

352. Hamm B, Staks T, Taupitz M, et al: Contrast enhanced MR imaging of liver and spleen: first experience in humans with a new superparamagnetic iron oxide. J Magn Reson Imaging 4:659–668, 1994.

353. Papisov MI, Bogdanov AA Jr, Schaffer B, et al: Colloidal magnetic resonance contrast agents: effect of particle surface on biodistribution. J Magnetism Magn Methods 122:383–386, 1993.

354. Summers RM, Joseph PM, Renshaw PF, Kundel HL: Dextran-magnetite: a contrast agent for sodium-23 MRI. Magn Reson Med 8:427–439, 1988.

355. Hamm B, Taupitz M, Hussmann P, et al: MR lymphography with iron oxide particles: dose-response studies and pulse sequence optimization in rabbits. AJR 158:183–190, 1992.

356. Lee AS, Weissleder R, Brady TJ, Wittenberg J: Lymph nodes: microstructural anatomy at MR imaging. Radiology 178:519–522, 1991.

357. Neuwelt EA, Weissleder R, Nilaver G, et al: Delivery of virus-sized iron oxide particles to rodent CNS neurons. Neurosurgery 34:777–784, 1994.

358. Weissleder R, Lee A, Fischman A, et al: Polyclonal human immunoglobulin G labeled with polymeric iron oxide: antibody MR imaging. Radiology 181:245–249, 1991.

359. Bulte JWM, Hoekstra Y, Kamman RL, et al: Specific MR imaging of human lymphocytes by monoclonal antibody-guided dextran-magnetite particles. Magn Reson Med 25:148–157, 1992.

360. Chan TW, Eley C, Liberti P, et al: Magnetic resonance imaging of abscess using lipid-coated iron oxide particles. Invest Radiol 27:443–449, 1992.

361. Bulte JWM, Ma LD, Magin RL, et al: Selective MR imaging of labeled human peripheral blood mononuclear cells by liposome mediated incorporation of dextran-magnetite particles. Magn Reson Med 29:32–37, 1993.

Biochemical Basis of the MRI Appearance of Cerebral Hemorrhage

KEITH R. THULBORN ■ THOMAS J. BRADY

The highly variable appearance of cerebral hemorrhage by magnetic resonance imaging (MRI) holds a wealth of information about the underlying biochemical processes. This information is often neglected in the MRI evaluation of hemorrhagic pathologic processes. A complete analysis using the full information content of MR images requires an understanding of the biochemical processes influencing the relaxation mechanisms controlling signal intensity.

Extrapolating from in vitro studies and clinical observations, researchers have proposed hypotheses to explain the evolution of the features of cerebral hematomas on MR images.[1-6] The explanations have emphasized the role of iron from hemoglobin in determining relaxation mechanisms of these variable patterns. This is based on the high concentration and changing magnetic properties of iron as the biochemical form, oxidation state, and spatial distribution change with time. Other pathophysiologic processes such as changes in integrity of the blood-brain barrier with alteration of the degree of edema and protein concentration have explained other features of these images. In this chapter, the physiochemical principles of the magnetic properties of biologic systems are reviewed, the biochemical pathways of iron metabolism in resolving hematoma are discussed, and a nonmathematic scheme is presented for relating these biochemical aspects to the relaxation phenomena that produce the variable signal contrast observed in MR images of hemorrhage. Clinical aspects involved in using MRI to evaluate hemorrhage are considered in Chapter 21.

BIOCHEMICAL EVOLUTION OF IRON IN CEREBRAL HEMATOMA

Hemorrhage is a complex process, biochemically and pathologically, evolving over many months. The pattern of evolution of hemorrhage described by computed tomography is relatively simple, reflecting the protein content of the tissues at the site of the lesion,[7, 8] as compared with the richness of information content reflected in the variability reported for MR images of the same process.[3-6] The rate of the many biochemical changes depends on the location and size of the lesion and on the physiologic status of the patient.[9] Better vascularized areas would be expected to show more rapid repair. The integrity of the blood-brain barrier makes intraparenchymal repair and clearance processes different from subarachnoid and subdural hemorrhages. Such variability in hematoma-induced repair response has been reported also from biochemical studies of hemorrhage at different sites outside the central nervous system.[10]

IRON METABOLISM IN HEMORRHAGE

Iron is a transition metal with an atomic number of 26 and an electronic configuration described as

$$1s^2 2s^2 2p^6 3s^2 3p^6 3d^6 4s^2$$

The distribution of electrons in the outer 3d electronic orbital is dependent on the number of electrons. As the oxidation state increases, outer electrons are lost, leaving the ferrous ion (Fe^{2+}) with six 3d electrons and the ferric ion (Fe^{3+}) with five 3d electrons. Unpaired electrons within the outer 3d orbitals of iron are of critical importance in determining the magnetic properties of this atom.

As the most abundant transition metal in the human body, iron is vital for oxygen transport by hemoglobin in the erythrocyte of blood, oxygen storage by myoglobin in the tissues, and multiple catalytic functions in enzyme systems throughout the body. In contrast to its functional chelated form, free iron is toxic, as is evident from toxic ingestions and iron overload states.[11-13] Toxicity is believed to be due to enhanced catalysis of free radical production by unchelated iron.[14] Hemorrhage can be thought of as having a tightly controlled iron salvage pathway, in which iron from the extravasated erythrocytes is mobilized from hemoglobin, detoxified by chelation to short-term iron transport proteins for transfer back to the reticuloendothelial system, or converted to long-term storage proteins for local deposition.[12, 15, 16] The different forms of iron in this still incompletely understood pathway have different magnetic properties that can influence the magnetic relaxation properties of the proton spin system used to form the MR image.

The iron salvage pathway of arterial hemorrhage is now examined stepwise in terms of the magnetic properties of the iron (Fig. 7–1). No time scale is given because this can only be misleading, given the multiple factors that determine rate of repair as described previously.

Arterial Blood

In arterial hemorrhage, the freshly extravasated erythrocytes contain fully oxygenated hemoglobin. Hemoglobin is a tetramer of polypeptide chains, with each polypeptide chain having considerable ordered secondary and tertiary structure.[11] Each chain has a prosthetic heme group bound within a hydrophobic cleft. The heme group is protoporphyrin IX with a centrally chelated ferrous ion. Initially, in arterial blood, iron is bound in octahedral geometry with six ligands. The tetrapyrrole nitrogens of the protoporphyrin constitute four ligands in a plane around the iron. The imidazole group of a histidine from the polypeptide chain is the axial ligand below the protoporphyrin plane, whereas molecular oxygen is the

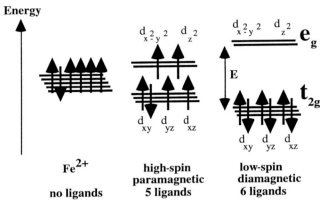

FIGURE 7–2. Energy diagram of the 3d electronic orbitals of the ferrous form of iron with different ligands. In the absence of ligands, all 3d orbitals have the same energy. In deoxyhemoglobin, the five ligands produce little energy separation between the e_g and t_{2g} groups of 3d orbitals, allowing the six electrons to distribute such that four electrons are unpaired (i.e., paramagnetic). In oxyhemoglobin, the six ligands produce marked energy difference E between the e_g and t_{2g} groups of 3d orbitals, causing electron pairing in the lowest energy state of the t_{2g} orbitals (i.e., diamagnetic).

sixth exchangeable ligand above the plane. The interaction of the six ligands with the metal center in oxyhemoglobin causes the six outer electrons of the ferrous ion to pair in the t_{2g} group of 3d orbitals of the lowest energy (Fig. 7–2). Because all the electrons of the iron and other atoms that constitute hemoglobin are paired, oxygenated blood is diamagnetic ($\chi < 0$).

Deoxygenation

In tissues undergoing aerobic respiration, the partial pressure of dissolved oxygen is lower than that required to fully saturate the oxygen binding sites of hemoglobin. The binding equilibrium is reversed, and molecular oxygen is delivered to the tissues. A cerebral hematoma has a mass effect compressing surrounding tissue, thereby reducing perfusion to these regions. A gradient in the partial pressure of oxygen from the hematoma to the compromised surrounding tissue results in hemoglobin desaturation. In addition, there is reduced washout of byproducts, such as carbon dioxide from remaining aerobic respiration and lactate from anaerobic glycolysis, which results in a decline in pH as the buffering capacity of the tissue is exceeded. This leads to further deoxygenation of the hemoglobin by displacement of the hemoglobin oxygen-binding equilibrium toward dissociation (the Bohr effect). The removal of molecular oxygen changes the coordinate geometry of the heme ferrous ion to a five-ligand system of deoxyhemoglobin, which decreases the energy separation between the e_g and t_{2g} groups of electronic orbitals. The six 3d electrons redistribute among the five 3d orbitals, leaving four unpaired electrons of parallel spin (see Fig. 7–2). These unpaired electrons confer deoxyhemoglobin with its paramagnetic properties ($\chi > 0$). Because the paramagnetic ferrous ion is bound to the heme group in the hydrophobic cleft

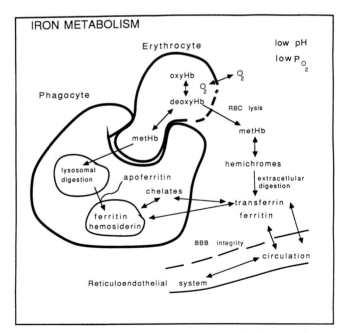

FIGURE 7–1. Schematic depiction of iron metabolism in a hematoma showing simplified iron salvage pathways in the red blood cell, phagocyte, and extracellular space. oxyHb = oxyhemoglobin; deoxyHb = deoxyhemoglobin; metHb = methemoglobin; BBB = blood-brain barrier; P_{O_2} = partial pressure of oxygen.

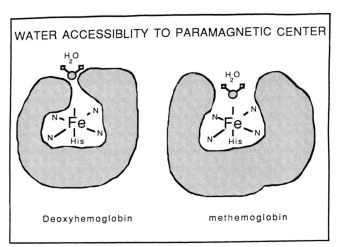

WATER ACCESSIBLITY TO PARAMAGNETIC CENTER

Deoxyhemoglobin   methemoglobin

FIGURE 7–3. Schematic representation of the exclusion of water from the paramagnetic iron of deoxyhemoglobin by the surrounding globin protein until the protein undergoes conformational changes that lead to access of water to the heme cleft and oxidation of the ferrous iron to ferric iron in methemoglobin. Water access explains relaxivity effects of methemoglobin and the absence of such effects for deoxyhemoglobin, although both are paramagnetic.

of the globin protein, water molecules are unable to approach the iron center. This restricts relaxivity effects (Fig. 7–3). As the deoxyhemoglobin is packaged in red blood cells, the magnetic susceptibility of the interior of the cell is different from that of the suspending fluid, resulting in susceptibility variations within the hematoma (Fig. 7–4). The importance of the integrity of the red blood cell membrane has been demonstrated in vitro.[18, 19]

The time course and distribution of deoxygenation

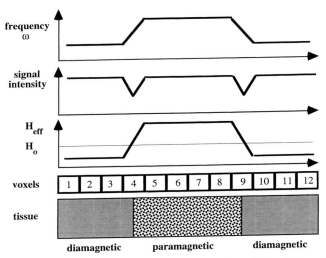

FIGURE 7–4. Simplified schematic representation of the different effective magnetic fields H_{eff} produced by tissues of diamagnetic ($\chi_1 < 0$) and paramagnetic ($\chi_2 > 0$) magnetic susceptibilities in the applied field H_0. The signal frequency ω is shifted by H_{eff} according to the Larmor equation ($\omega = \gamma H_{eff}$). The signal intensity of the voxels (4 and 9 of voxels 1 through 12) at the boundaries are reduced owing to diffusion in the field gradients on spin-echo images and, in addition, due to intravoxel dephasing on gradient-echo images.

can be used to explain some features of hyperacute hemorrhage (Atlas S, personal communication, 1992) in which a peripheral rim of reduced signal intensity is observed around parenchymal hematomas of less than 24 hours on T2-weighted images. The hematoma-tissue interface is not smooth but rather shows interdigitation of strands of blood clot containing intact red blood cells with tissue. This geometry results in proximity of aerobic tissue that has compromised perfusion and on clot that causes rapid deoxygenation in this peripheral location of the lesion. This configuration causes rapid deoxygenation and hence produces the magnetic susceptibility effects underlying the signal loss.

Red Blood Cell Lysis

The tissue damage elicits an inflammatory repair response within the surrounding tissue, with phagocytes, such as macrophages, infiltrating the boundaries of the hematoma to clear extravasated materials and damaged tissues. Glial cells also show phagocytic activity. Red blood cells may be phagocytosed entirely or partially or lysed by enzymes released into the region by the inflammatory cells.[8, 9] Loss of red blood cell membrane integrity releases hemoglobin. In the absence of the functional reductase enzymes of the red blood cell (NADH–cytochrome b_5 reductase, NADPH–flavin reductase),[17] hemoglobin is rapidly converted to methemoglobin, in which the iron, still bound to the heme moiety within the globin protein, is oxidized to the ferric state with five 3d electrons. Once in the ferric oxidation state, the iron is paramagnetic ($\chi > 0$). The protein undergoes a number of changes, ultimately irreversible, in secondary, tertiary, and quaternary structures in which the ferric iron is no longer protected from the surrounding solvent.[20] The electronic configuration of the iron changes from initially five unpaired electrons, one in each of the five 3d suborbitals, to one unpaired electron as the weak sixth ligand of water is exchanged for a hydroxide and then another imidazole nitrogen of a histidyl residue of the protein. These changes define the hemichromes as described by electron paramagnetic resonance spectroscopy.[21] The time course of these processes in vivo remains unknown.

Extracellular Iron-Binding Proteins

Extracellular protein is further degraded with release of the iron to localized extracellular binding proteins such as lactoferrin and transferrin. Some extracellular ferritin is also present. These binding proteins detoxify free iron for recycling to the reticuloendothelial system through the circulation and for local storage by glial cells and macrophages. The chelated iron remains paramagnetic.[22–24]

Intracellular Iron Processing

Red blood cells and hemoglobin, phagocytosed by macrophages and glial elements of the central nervous system, are digested by the lysosomal system, with the iron being stored as ferric oxyhydroxide in the hydrophobic center of the major iron storage protein called *ferritin*.[15, 25] Ferritin is a water-soluble protein of about 450 kd with 24 polypeptide subunits surrounding a core of as many as 4500 ferric ions. If the quantity of available iron exceeds the capacity of the cell to synthesize apoferritin, excess iron is stored as hemosiderin.[16] Hemosiderin is an insoluble larger aggregation of ferric oxyhydroxide with less protein than ferritin and, as yet, a poorly characterized biochemical structure. These storage forms with large aggregates of iron behave antiferromagnetically and ferromagnetically, sometimes with superparamagnetic properties ($\chi > 0$).[26–28] These aggregates of iron have reduced accessibility to surrounding water, thereby minimizing relaxivity effects. However, magnetic susceptibility variations can be expected in tissues containing such materials. The iron storage processes occur throughout resolution of hemorrhage but become significant later, presumably reflecting concentration changes and the cessation of other relaxation processes. Much of the ferritin is intracellular within both macrophages and astrocytes, whereas the hemosiderin is in macrophages.[29]

INTEGRITY OF THE BLOOD-BRAIN BARRIER

EDEMA

The loss of the blood-brain barrier around the site of hemorrhage causes vasogenic edema. The damage to the tissue in and around the site from mass effect, reduced perfusion, and inflammation worsen the edema. Although such changes do not affect the magnetic properties of the tissues that remain diamagnetic ($\chi < 0$), other magnetic relaxation phenomena occur to alter the MR image.

COAGULATION

The extravasated blood initiates the coagulation cascade, leading to clot formation that limits further bleeding. The protein network of the clot with trapped red blood cells is expected to undergo a number of changes, including clot contraction with changes in the concentration and distribution of blood products, which can change magnetic properties of the tissue and thus the MRI characteristics. This has not been systematically studied in vivo.[30, 31]

RELAXATION MECHANISMS

For totally diamagnetic tissues, the most important relaxation mechanism for both longitudinal and transverse relaxation is attributed to dipole-dipole interactions.[32, 33] Other mechanisms of scalar-spin coupling, chemical shift anisotropy, and quadripolar and spin-

rotational effects are usually less important in p MRI and are described elsewhere.[32–37] Paramagnet substances have several effects of much greater magnitude than diamagnetic substances, as discussed in the Appendix at the end of this chapter and in Chapters 5 and 6. These effects include 1) relaxivity effects due to dipole-dipole interactions, which produce T1 and T2 relaxation, generally with T1 effects dominating to produce increased signal intensity; and 2) susceptibility effects, which produce only T2 relaxation and signal loss on MR images.

The dipole-dipole effects of paramagnetic substances are discussed in the Appendix, but consideration must be given to other exchange processes not involving paramagnetic species.

Changes in the protein content within the hematoma are also seen as clot formation, clot contraction, and necrosis occur. From in vitro studies,[37] increasing protein concentration would be expected to promote T1 and T2 relaxation rates, although rigorous in vivo studies have not been reported. It is possible that the exchange of water between bulk and protein-bound phases may be a significant relaxation process in some situations. Increasing edema has been suggested to allow increased diffusion by removing diffusional barriers such as macromolecules and cell membranes, thereby promoting T2 relaxation. In areas of necrosis, diffusional barriers may not be removed to the same degree as in vasogenic edema in intact, albeit damaged, tissue. The relative influences of diffusion and protein exchange on in vivo relaxation processes cannot be predicted as yet.

SENSITIVITIES OF MRI PULSE SEQUENCES

The basic principles of imaging pulse sequences have been presented in numerous excellent texts,[38–42] and only features pertaining to hemorrhage are elaborated on here.

SPIN-ECHO PULSE SEQUENCE

The spin-echo (SE) sequence, shown in Figure 7–5, uses a 180° radiofrequency (RF) pulse centered between the initial 90° RF pulse and the center of the acquisition time period to refocus nuclear spins of variable Larmor frequencies into an echo, producing the MR signal. This minimizes the effect of static H_0 inhomogeneities on transverse relaxation that would otherwise reduce the signal intensity. By selecting appropriate timing parameters for the pulse sequence, the MR image can be made selectively sensitive to relaxivity and magnetic susceptibility effects. If significant diffusion through field inhomogeneities occurs during the echo time (TE), signal loss occurs, as discussed in the Appendix. As TE is made longer relative to the diffusional correlation time, the pulse sequence becomes more sensitive to these inhomogeneities. Because susceptibility differences are a source of field

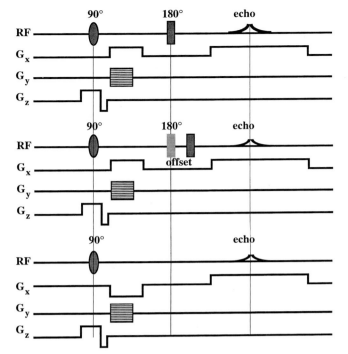

FIGURE 7–5. Simplified schematic of timing diagrams of the spin-echo (SE) *(top)*, asymmetric-echo (ASE) *(middle)*, and gradient-echo (GRE) *(bottom)* pulse sequences with slice selection by gradient G_z shown only on the 90° RF pulse, frequency encoding using G_x, and phase encoding using G_y. The echoes are labeled. The pre-encode G_x gradient is positive for the SE sequence as it is before the 180° RF pulse but negative for the GRE sequence because there is no 180° RF pulse.

nonuniformity, increasing TE increases sensitivity of SE images to processes such as hemorrhage that generate such susceptibility variation. The effect is readily recognized as signal loss on T2-weighted images, which is not present on T1-weighted images.

Two other imaging sequences can be used to enhance detection of the susceptibility effects on T2 relaxation. These are the gradient- or field-echo (GRE) and the asymmetric spin-echo (ASE) sequences that have been described in detail elsewhere[43, 44] (see Fig. 7–5).

ASYMMETRIC SPIN-ECHO PULSE SEQUENCE

The ASE sequence offsets the 180° refocusing pulse by a time interval that can be varied to alter the amount of signal refocusing. This sequence is sensitive not only to the effects of diffusion through magnetic field gradients as used by the SE sequence but also to variations of Larmor frequencies within a single voxel due to nonuniform magnetic susceptibility (Fig. 7–6). This results in rapid loss of phase coherence among the nuclear spins within the voxel and hence rapid signal loss. The amount of signal loss, and thus the sensitivity to intravoxel susceptibility heterogeneity, can be altered by varying the size of the offset. Comparison with ASE and SE images of the same TE allows

calculation of T2* and has been suggested as a means of quantifying the iron content of tissue.[44]

This sequence has been adapted to an echo-planar sequence for detection of magnetic susceptibility effects arising from tissue oxygenation changes during neuronal activation in functional MRI.[45]

GRADIENT-ECHO PULSE SEQUENCE

The GRE sequence does not use a 180° refocusing pulse and is thus sensitive to both static magnetic field inhomogeneities (magnet imperfections and tissue susceptibility heterogeneity) and the effects of diffusion.[43] Magnet imperfections over the volume of the imaging voxel have become less important with improved magnet technology, allowing detection of tissue susceptibility variations by means of the diffusional effects. Even without diffusion, signal cancellation occurs owing to the range of Larmor frequencies caused by susceptibility variations within a voxel, as is also the case for the ASE sequence. This makes the GRE sequence useful for enhancing detection of susceptibility effects that may be less clearly identified on SE images. The artifacts from unwanted susceptibility effects, such as from the paranasal sinuses on intracranial lesions close to the base of the skull,[46] make the GRE sequence less useful for initial clinical screening examinations.

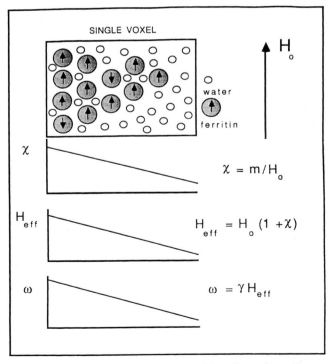

FIGURE 7–6. Schematic representation of the effects of nondiamagnetic substances on the intravoxel distribution of susceptibility χ, H_{eff}, and resonance frequency ω. Variation of resonance frequencies within the voxel produces signal loss on GRE images.

FIELD STRENGTH DEPENDENCE

The variation of $1/T1$ and $1/T2$ with magnetic field strength is termed *nuclear magnetic relaxation dispersion*. Because the mathematic treatment of nuclear magnetic relaxation dispersion is beyond the scope of this chapter, the interested reader is referred elsewhere for a more formal introduction.[26] Only the observations relevant to hemorrhage are discussed here. At the limit of zero field, $1/T1 = 1/T2$. As field strength changes, the efficiency of relaxation is dependent on matching correlation times of local fluctuating magnetic fields generated by diffusional processes to the Larmor frequency. This occurs over a wide range (10^{-10} to 10^{-11} second) corresponding to low imaging field strengths, and the effects on T1 and T2 relaxation rates are comparable. In contrast, at higher fields, $1/T1$ tends toward zero and $1/T2$ tends to a nonzero value termed the *secular* contribution to T2 relaxation. Therefore, higher magnetic field strengths emphasize susceptibility effects. In vitro studies of deoxygenated red blood cells indicate a quadratic dependence of $1/T2$ on magnetic field strength over a range of 2 to 5 T.[18] The susceptibility effects of ferritin as a function of field strength in vivo have been measured, and less than a quadratic dependence was found.[47] The distribution of the iron aggregates in vivo is not known, and modeling is difficult. Although the theoretic treatment is incomplete for susceptibility effects induced by ferritin and hemosiderin (speculated to be due to antiferromagnetic and ferromagnetic properties of these iron aggregates), it is clear that higher imaging magnetic field strengths increase sensitivity of MR images to susceptibility-induced relaxation mechanisms, regardless of the source of the susceptibility variation.[26, 27]

EVALUATION OF HEMORRHAGE WITH MRI

ROLE OF IRON PRODUCTS

The magnetic properties of the iron products of resolving hematoma have been discussed earlier. Although deoxygenated hemoglobin and all the products containing iron in the ferric oxidation state are paramagnetic (methemoglobin, hemichromes, transferrin, lactoferrin, low-molecular-weight iron chelates) or antiferromagnetic (ferritin, hemosiderin), the production of relaxivity effects is dependent on the close approach of water protons to the iron and the production of the susceptibility effects is dependent on the distribution of the iron. The relaxation properties and the imaging characteristics are discussed and summarized in Table 7–1.

Oxyhemoglobin

The MR image of the center of an acute hematoma is essentially a collection of protein-rich diamagnetic fluid. Relaxivity and susceptibility effects are not observed for the diamagnetic iron of oxygenated hemoglobin. Image intensity is determined by other dipole-dipole mechanisms as operating in normal surrounding tissue. This means a variably long T1 (isointense to dark on T1-weighted images) and relatively long T2 (bright on T2-weighted images). The change in water content and distribution is clearly evident as areas of long T1 (dark on T1-weighted SE images) and long T2 (bright on T2-weighted SE images) in the areas bordering the hematoma.[48] Changes in the protein content within the hematoma also occur as clot formation, clot contraction, and necrosis occur. From in vitro studies,[49] increasing protein concentration would be expected to promote T1 and T2 relaxation rates, although rigorous in vivo studies have not been reported. Exchange of water between bulk phase and protein-bound phases may provide an explanation for small modulations in image intensity.

Deoxygenated Hemoglobin

The paramagnetic iron of deoxygenated hemoglobin is held within a hydrophobic cleft. The exclusion of water from close approach to the paramagnetic center prevents relaxivity effects. T1 relaxation is not affected so that the hematoma remains dark on T1-weighted images. The packaging of the paramagnetic centers within the red blood cells produces susceptibility variations that produce transverse relaxation. This explains the loss of signal on T2-weighted SE and GRE

TABLE 7–1. THE INFLUENCE OF IRON METABOLISM ON THE MRI APPEARANCE OF HEMORRHAGE*

STAGE	BIOCHEMICAL FORM	LOCATION	MAGNETIC PROPERTY	RELAXATION MECHANISM		MR SIGNAL INTENSITY†	
				R	χ	T1	T2
Oxyhemoglobin	Fe^{II} oxyHb	RBC	Diamag	−	−	Dark	Bright
Deoxygenation	Fe^{II} deoxyHb	RBC	Paramag	−	+	Dark	Dark
RBC lysis + oxidation	Fe^{III} metHb, hemichromes	Extracellular	Paramag	+	−	Bright	Bright
Extracellular iron processing	Fe^{III} transferrin, lactoferrin	Extracellular	Paramag	+	−	Bright	Bright
Intracellular iron storage	Fe^{III} ferritin, hemosiderin	Phagocytes	Superpar	−	+	Iso	Dark

*Paramag = paramagnetic; Diamag = diamagnetic; Superpar = superparamagnetic; oxyHb = oxyhemoglobin; deoxyHb = deoxyhemoglobin; metHb = methemoglobin; RBC = red blood cell; R = relaxivity; χ = susceptibility; T1 = T1 weighted; T2 = T2 weighted; iso = isointense.
†Signal intensities are estimated relative to cerebral cortex.

images (dark on T2-weighted images). The deoxygenation extends inwardly over time from the periphery of the hematoma where there is close interdigitation of clot and tissue.

Red Blood Cell Lysis

Loss of integrity of the red blood cells homogenizes the distribution of paramagnetic iron to minimize the susceptibility variations and reduces transverse relaxation. As the enzyme systems employed within the red blood cell to maintain the ferrous oxidation state of the iron become nonfunctional, methemoglobin and other hemichromes are formed. These proteins allow water access to the paramagnetic iron to induce the relaxivity effects that shorten T1 and to a lesser degree T2. Thus, a hematoma at this stage shows increasing brightness on T1-weighted SE images. Although the concomitant shortening of T2 from relaxivity effects may suggest further loss of brightness on T2-weighted SE and GRE images, the loss of red blood cell integrity removes the paramagnetic aggregation responsible for susceptibility-induced relaxation effects. Because this is the dominant T2 relaxation process, loss of this mechanism means that the effective T2 is still longer than with intact red blood cells. Hence T2-weighted SE and GRE images appear brighter after cell lysis has occurred. This effect extends from the periphery inwardly to the center of the hematoma.

Extracellular Iron-Binding Proteins

The specific relaxivity and susceptibility effects of ferric ions chelated to these proteins described in vitro[22–24] remain unknown for resolving in vivo hemorrhage. The concentration of these substances may be too low to have a significant role in determining signal intensity within an MR image.

Intracellular Iron Storage

The structure of iron storage proteins such as ferritin excludes water from close approach to most of the paramagnetic ferric ions, minimizing relaxivity effects. The antiferromagnetic properties of these crystalline aggregates of ferric oxyhydroxide induce susceptibility variations from surrounding tissue. The implications for imaging of old resolving hematomas are that T1-weighted MR images are isointense with surrounding tissue owing to the absence of relaxivity effects and that T2-weighted and GRE images show signal loss owing to susceptibility effects. If the T2 is significantly shortened below the TE used for T1-weighted images, then the susceptibility effect is observed on these images. This is not a relaxivity effect. Rather, the term T1 weighted is inappropriate under these conditions. This assumes that cavitation has not occurred. If a cavity develops in the region of tissue loss, then the signal characteristics of cerebrospinal fluid that fills the cavity dominate the image.

IMAGES OF EVOLVING CEREBRAL HEMATOMA

The best controlled longitudinal study of resolving intraparenchymal hematoma was reported for an experimental model of hemorrhage in the monkey in which venous blood was injected into the right cerebral hemisphere and followed by MRI for several months.[48] Selected images from this study are reproduced with permission for discussion.

At 2 hours after injection of blood (Fig. 7–7A and B), the acute hematoma has low signal intensity on the T1-weighted and high signal intensity on the T2-weighted images relative to normal cortex. This is consistent with the absence of significant relaxivity and susceptibility relaxation mechanisms in the acute setting. Although the injection used venous blood, marked susceptibility effects are not observed, suggesting that greater deoxygenation is required. The T1-weighted image shows greater signal loss in the periphery consistent with edema in surrounding tissue having slightly different relaxation phenomena from the center of the hematoma. During the next 2 days (Fig. 7–7C and D), the signal intensity of the center of the hematoma on the T1-weighted image increases, presumably from the relaxivity mechanism of methemoglobin, hemichromes, and other paramagnetic centers, allowing close approach of water protons. The signal intensity from the surrounding edematous zone shows little change. In contrast, the same area of hematoma on the T2-weighted image displays decreased signal intensity, presumably from susceptibility-induced relaxation mechanisms as the intact red blood cells become increasingly deoxygenated and from any intracellular methemoglobin that may form as the energy status of the cells declines. It is not clear whether the methemoglobin and hemichromes form intracellularly or that the hematoma is a mixture of intact deoxygenated cells suspended within a solution of hemoglobin degradation products. Over 6 to 10 days (Fig. 7–7E to H), the T1-weighted images show increasing signal intensity due to relaxivity effects from increasing concentrations of hemoglobin degradation products. The T2-weighted images show increasing signal intensity when susceptibility effects diminish as red blood cell integrity is lost within the hematoma. The edematous periphery of the lesion shows minimal changes during this time interval. After 2 months (Fig. 7–7I and J), the T1-weighted image shows little evidence of the lesion, whereas an area of decreased signal intensity remains on the T2-weighted image. This can be attributed to the susceptibility-induced relaxation mechanism of the iron storage products.

CONCLUSION

The basis of the highly variable MRI appearance of resolving intraparenchymal cerebral hematoma reported clinically can be rationalized largely in terms of a model encompassing current concepts of iron

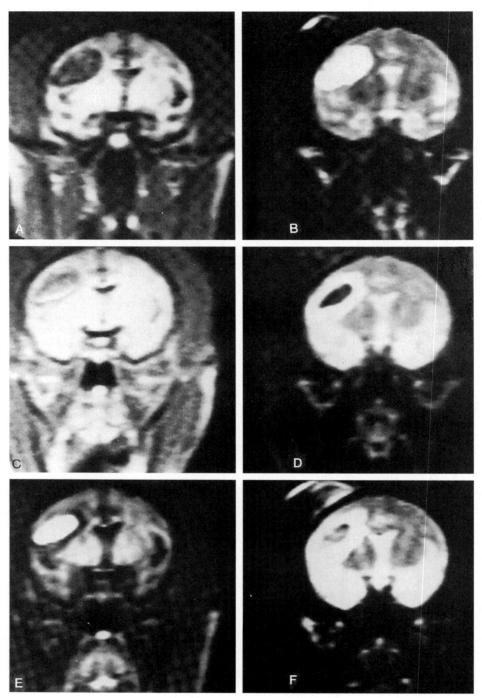

FIGURE 7–7. Longitudinal study, using inversion recovery (T1-weighted) SE *(A, C, E,* and *I)* and T2-weighted SE coronal images *(B, D, F,* and *J)* of a monkey after injection of 3 mL of venous blood into the right cerebral hemisphere. Images were selected at 2 hours *(A* and *B),* 2 days *(C* and *D),* 6 days *(E* and *F).*

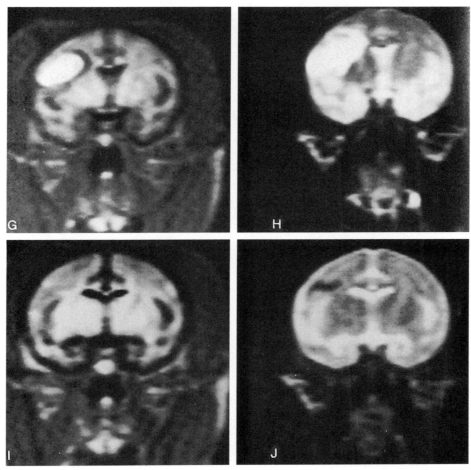

FIGURE 7–7 *Continued* 10 days *(G* and *H)*, and 2 months *(I)* and *(J)* from a more complete study *(A* to *J* from Di Chiro G, Brooks RA, Girton ME, et al: Sequential MR studies of intracerebral hematomas in monkeys. AJNR 7:193–199, 1986 © by American Society of Neuroradiology 1986.)

metabolism and integrity of the blood-brain barrier. The time scale is dependent on the size of the lesion, its location with respect to both vascular supply and white and gray matter, and the physiologic status of the patient. The model should be regarded as a working hypothesis. The delineation of the in vivo biochemistry of iron metabolism and water balance remains to be performed. It is unlikely that descriptive analysis of the MRI appearance of cerebral hemorrhage can be verified with biochemical studies in patients, making animal models a necessary vehicle for further detailed studies.

Appendix
MAGNETIC PROPERTIES OF BIOLOGIC TISSUES

ORIGIN OF MAGNETIC PROPERTIES

A magnetic field is generated by a moving electric charge, that is, an electric charge with momentum.[50]

The strength of the magnetic field is determined by the magnitude of both the charge and momentum. Such a charge with a magnetic field is termed a *magnetic dipole.* Electrons moving in orbitals about a nucleus represent moving charges with both orbital angular momentum and spin angular momentum and generate a magnetic field. The nucleus also has momentum and charge. However, because the magnetic moment of the charged particle is inversely proportional to its mass, and the mass of the nucleus is three orders of magnitude greater than that of the electron, the contribution of the nucleus to the magnetic properties of the atom is much less than that of the electrons. Hence, although nuclear magnetic interactions occur and nuclear magnetization is the source of the signal in the MR image, the magnetic properties of tissue are determined predominantly by the electronic configuration of the atoms and molecules. The dominant effects encountered on MR images are discussed in the following.

DIAMAGNETISM

Most biologic materials consist of low-atomic-weight elements such as carbon and hydrogen in which the electrons are paired in atomic and molecular suborbitals. When the electrons are paired, the spin angular momentum is canceled and no magnetic dipole is observed. However, the paired electrons still have orbital angular momentum that produces a magnetic field (termed a *Lenz field*) opposing the applied magnetic field. The resultant field within such a material is less than that of the original applied magnetic field. Such materials are termed *diamagnetic*.

PARAMAGNETISM

Some biologic substances have atomic or molecular structures in which some of the electrons are unpaired. Transition metal ions, such as iron with the ferrous and ferric oxidation states, are important examples in which the number of unpaired electrons varies with the biochemical state of the metal ion. An unpaired electron has a spin angular momentum and therefore a magnetic moment that is not canceled as in the paired state. At physiologic temperatures, more electrons align parallel to the applied field, resulting in an enhancement of that applied field. Materials that have no magnetic field in the absence of an applied magnetic field but that respond to enhance an applied magnetic field are termed *paramagnetic*. Examples of paramagnetic substances include gadolinium, used as an MRI contrast agent, and ferrous and ferric iron. On T1-weighted images, uniform distributions of such species produce increased signal intensity. However, nonuniform distributions of such species alter the MR image by producing a range of effective magnetic fields within the sample and therefore a range of resonance frequencies of the MR signal. Depending on the type of imaging pulse sequence used, the frequency dispersion can be manipulated to decrease signal in the area of the paramagnetic species (see earlier section on sensitivities of MRI pulse sequences).

OTHER FORMS OF MAGNETISM

There are other biologically important closely packed ensembles of atoms, such as crystalline structures, in which unpaired electrons of neighboring atoms interact to minimize the magnetic forces outside the material in the absence of an applied magnetic field. The magnetic forces producing preferred patterns of spin alignments to reach magnetic equilibrium are termed *exchange forces*.

Antiferromagnetism (Individual Opposition). If unpaired electrons of neighboring atoms interact to align with opposing spins, the magnetic forces are minimized. In an applied magnetic field, spin pairing must be disrupted for realignment. Thus, the response to the applied field is less than that of a paramagnetic substance, but the effective field is still enhanced. Such materials are termed *antiferromagnetic*. The alignment pattern can be disrupted if the thermal energy is increased, and initially the response to an applied field

is enhanced as the temperature is increased. Above a critical temperature, known as the Neel temperature, adjacent spin pairing is disrupted and the substance becomes paramagnetic. The effects of antiferromagnetic substances on MR images are similar to those of paramagnetic substances although reduced in magnitude and with a different temperature dependence.

Ferromagnetism (Group Opposition). If the unpaired electrons of a group of atoms can align in domains, each domain has a net magnetic field. Adjacent domains can then interact by means of these magnetic fields to minimize, although not completely cancel, the field outside the material. If that material is immersed in a high magnetic field, domains respond to both the applied field and neighboring domain fields to markedly enhance the field. Such materials show a magnetic field in the absence of an applied magnetic field and are termed *ferromagnetic*. The effect of such substances on the MR image is of greater magnitude than for paramagnetic substances.

If a ferromagnetic crystal is reduced in size to that of a single domain, this single-domain particle has a net magnetic dipole equivalent to that of a domain. If a collection of such particles is free to rotate in an applied magnetic field on a time scale that is shorter than the observation time, the magnetic dipoles behave as expected for paramagnetism discussed previously. However, the larger magnetic moments of the particles produce a greater enhancement of the applied magnetic field. Such particles are termed *superparamagnetic*.[51, 52]

If the size of the particles, usually containing many domains, is reduced *below* the size of a single domain, the aligning exchange forces and disaligning thermal forces become comparable. If the time scale of the observation is longer than the switching rate of the equilibrium between the aligned and disordered states, then the magnetic properties of the particles are dependent on the temperature-volume relationships that determine the switching frequency. An aggregate of such particles behaves paramagnetically but with a greater magnetic dipole than if no domain formed at all and thus is termed *supermagnetic*.[50] Thus, the effects of superparamagnetic and supermagnetic substances on the MR image are similar to those of paramagnetic substances but of a magnitude between that of paramagnetic and ferromagnetic species.

MAGNETIC SUSCEPTIBILITY

Because all biologic materials have at least one of the previously discussed magnetic properties, they interact with a static magnetic field, H_0, to produce a magnetization, m, that reduces (diamagnetism) or enhances (paramagnetism, antiferromagnetism, ferromagnetism) the effective magnetic field, H_{eff}, established within the material. Note that m in this sense is usually referring to the effects of electronic configurations, not nuclear magnetization M. This effect can be expressed in terms of the magnetic susceptibility χ of the material in which

$$H_{eff} = H_0 + m = H_0(1 + \chi) \qquad (1)$$

where $\chi = m/H_0$. Thus, $\chi < 0$ for diamagnetic materials, $\chi > 0$ for paramagnetic materials, and $\chi = 0$ for a vacuum.

When placed in a static magnetic field of the imaging magnet, tissues of different magnetic susceptibilities establish different effective magnetic fields experienced by the nucleus under observation. Thus, the response of the nuclear magnetization generated in the MRI study is altered with resultant changes in the image. Susceptibility-induced field variations within a voxel broaden the Larmor frequency range (see Fig. 7–6). SE imaging minimizes this effect by using a 180° RF pulse to refocus the dispersion that occurs in the transverse magnetization M_{xy}, during the pulse sequence. If significant molecular diffusion occurs during TE (time from initial 90° RF pulse to formation of the echo) through regions of variable H_{eff}, due to either magnet imperfections or susceptibility variations in the tissue, incomplete refocusing results in loss of transverse magnetization and thus signal loss in the MR image. The effect becomes more apparent as the TE exceeds the diffusional correlation time (time taken for a proton to move from one position to the next position). Spins diffusing in the x-y plane experience these variations in H_{eff} as a fluctuating magnetic field h_z, with resultant transverse but not longitudinal relaxation. This effect is well known in MR spectroscopy, [33-35] in which a known magnetic field gradient (G) can be applied to a sample to measure the diffusion coefficient (D) of protons through a solvent. The signal intensity (S) for a Hahn spin echo at TE is given as

$$S = S_0 \exp([TE/T_2 + 1/12\gamma^2 G^2 D TE^3]) \qquad (2)$$

Hence, differences in susceptibilities at the boundary of a hematoma containing paramagnetic blood products and surrounding normal diamagnetic tissue produce T2 relaxation if sufficient diffusion is permitted to occur during the imaging sequence. Such effects cause signal loss at these boundaries on T2-weighted MR images of sufficiently long TE without corresponding signal loss on T1-weighted images.

RELAXIVITY

The relative rotational and translational motions of water molecules and paramagnetic entities in biologic systems occur on a time scale that produces an apparent isotropically fluctuating magnetic field in the range of the Larmor frequencies for protons at current imaging field strengths. If the water molecules are able to approach the paramagnetic center, then magnetic interactions allow efficient energy exchange to occur and the magnetically perturbed water proton spin system can relax to its equilibrium state.[53] The phenomenologic equation for intermolecular relaxation

interactions of a paramagnetic agent (P) in bulk solution is

$$(1/Ti)_{obs} = (1/Ti)_d + (1/Ti)_p \qquad (3)$$

$$(1/Ti)_p = R[P] \qquad (4)$$

where $i = 1, 2$; R is the relaxivity constant ($mM^{-1} s^{-1}$); and [P] is the concentration (mM) of the paramagnetic substance P. $(1/T)_d$ is the rate attributable to diamagnetic relaxation processes and $(1/T)_p$ is the relaxation rate in the presence of P. In the presence of a suitable paramagnetic substance, the paramagnetic term dominates over the diamagnetic term of Equation 3. The same equation applies for both longitudinal and transverse relaxation. Because T1 is generally longer than T2, 1/T1 is smaller than 1/T2, and so the constant term R[P] contributes a greater proportion to the longitudinal relaxation rate (1/T1) than transverse relaxation rate (1/T2). The implication to MRI is that the relaxivity effects of paramagnetic substances are detected with greater sensitivity on T1-weighted images than on T2-weighted images. The paramagnetic relaxation rate can be further analyzed mechanistically as inner sphere (ligand exchange in which water molecules are in the first coordination sphere of P) and outer sphere (diffusion with close approach of water near to but without coordination to P) contributions, but it is not the purpose of this review to describe the more mechanistic Solomon-Bloembergen equations that are presented in detail elsewhere.[53] Application of Equation 3 in biologic systems as complex as cerebral hematomas can only be approximate because of the heterogeneity in type and distribution of the various paramagnetic substances involved. When water is unable to approach the paramagnetic center, no magnetic interaction and therefore no relaxation occurs by relaxivity mechanisms (see Fig. 7–3). However, susceptibility effects can still be manifested so that, whereas T1 is unaffected, T2 is shortened and the MR signal is decreased.

REFERENCES

1. Sipponen JT, Sepponen RE, Sivula A: Nuclear magnetic resonance (NMR) imaging of intracranial hemorrhage in the acute and resolving phases. J Comput Assist Tomogr 7:954–959, 1983.
2. DeLaPaz RL, New PFJ, Buonanno FS, et al: NMR imaging of intracranial hemorrhage. J Comput Assist Tomogr 8:599–607, 1984.
3. Gomori JM, Grossman RI, Goldberg HI, et al: Intracranial hematomas: imaging by high-field MR. Radiology 157:87–93, 1985.
4. Gomori JM, Grossman RI: Head and neck hemorrhage. In: Kressel HY, ed. Magnetic Resonance Annual 1987. New York: Raven Press, 1987, pp 71–112.
5. Gomori JM, Grossman RI, Hackney DB, et al: Variable appearances of subacute intracranial hematomas on high-field spin-echo MR. AJNR 8:1019–1026, 1987.
6. Zimmerman RD, Heier LA, Snow RB, et al: Acute intracranial hemorrhage: intensity changes on sequential MR scans at 0.5 T. AJNR 9:47–57, 1988.
7. New PFJ, Scott WR: Blood. In: New PFJ, Scott WR, eds. Computed Tomography of the Brain and Orbit (EMI Scanning). Baltimore: Williams & Wilkins, 1975, pp 263–267.
8. Enzmann DR, Britt RH, Lyons BE, et al: Natural history of experimental intracerebral hemorrhage: sonography, computed tomography and neuropathology. AJNR 2:517–526, 1981.
9. Kreindler A, Marcovici G, Florescu I: Histoenzymologic and biochemical investigations into the nervous tissue round an experimentally-induced cerebral hemorrhagic focus. Rev Roum Neurol 9:313–319, 1972.

10. Lalonde JMA, Ghadially FN, Massey KL: Ultrastructure of intramuscular haematomas and electron-probe X-ray analysis of extracellular and intracellular iron deposits. J Pathol 125:17–23, 1978.
11. Finch CA, Huebers HA: Iron metabolism. Clin Physiol Biochem 4:5–10, 1986.
12. Trump BF, Valigorsky JM, Arstila AU, et al: The relationship of intracellular pathways of iron metabolism to cellular iron overload and the iron storage diseases. Am J Pathol 72:295–324, 1973.
13. Weinberg ED: Iron, infection and neoplasia. Clin Physiol Biochem 4:50–60, 1986.
14. Southern PA, Powis G: Free radicals in medicine. I. Chemical nature and biologic reactions. II. Involvement in human disease. Mayo Clin Proc 63:390–408, 1988.
15. Munro HN, Linder MC: Ferritin: structure, biosynthesis and role in iron metabolism. Physiol Rev 58:317–396, 1978.
16. Wixon RL, Prutkin L, Munro HN: Hemosiderin: nature, formation and significance. Int Rev Exp Pathol 22:193–225, 1980.
17. Bunn HF, Forget BG, eds. Hemoglobin: Molecular, Genetic and Clinical Aspects. Philadelphia: WB Saunders, 1986, pp 13–35, 634–662.
18. Thulborn KR, Wateron JC, Matthews PM, Radda GK: Oxygenation dependence of the transverse relaxation time of water protons in whole blood at high field. Biochim Biophys Acta 714:265–270, 1982.
19. Brindle KM, Brown FF, Campbell ID, et al: Application of spin-echo nuclear magnetic resonance to whole cell systems: membrane transport. Biochem J 180:37–44, 1979.
20. Koenig SH, Brown RD, Lindstrom TR: Interactions of solvent with the heme region of methemoglobin and fluoro-methemoglobin. Biophys J 34:397–408, 1981.
21. Blumberg WE: The study of hemoglobin by electron paramagnetic resonance spectroscopy. Methods Enzymol 76:312–329, 1981.
22. Windle JJ, Weirsema AK, Clarke JR, Feeney RE: Investigation of the iron and copper complexes of avian conalbumins and human transferrins by electron paramagnetic resonance. Biochemistry 2:1341–1345, 1963.
23. Aasa R, Aisen P: An electron paramagnetic resonance study of the iron and copper complexes of transferrin. J Biol Chem 243:2399–2404, 1968.
24. Koenig SH, Schillinger WE: Nuclear magnetic relaxation dispersion in protein solutions. II. Transferrin. J Biol Chem 244:6520–6526, 1969.
25. Harrison PM, Fischbach FA, Hoy TG, Haggis GH: Ferric oxyhydroxide core of ferritin. Nature 216:1188–1190, 1967.
26. Koenig SH, Brown RD: Relaxometry of magnetic resonance imaging contrast agents. In: Kressel HY, ed. Magnetic Resonance Annual 1987. New York: Raven Press, 1987, pp 263–286.
27. Gillis P, Koenig SH: Transverse relaxation of solvent protons induced by magnetized spheres: application to ferritin, erythrocytes and magnetite. Magn Reson Med 5:323–345, 1987.
28. Weir MP, Peters TJ, Gibson JF: Electron spin resonance studies of splenic ferritin and haemosiderin. Biochim Biophys Acta 828:298–305, 1985.
29. Boas JF, Troup GJ: Electron spin resonance and Mossbauer effect studies of ferritin. Biochim Biophys Acta 229:68–74, 1971.
30. Darrow YC, Alvord EC, Hodson WA: Histological evolution of the reactions to hemorrhage in the premature human infant's brain: a combined autopsy study and a comparison with the reaction in adults. Am J Pathol 130:44–58, 1988.
31. Cohen MD, McGuire W, Cory DA, Smith JA: MR appearance of blood and blood products: an in vitro study. AJR 146:1293–1297, 1986.
32. Hayman LA, Ford JJ, Taber KH, et al: T2 effect of hemoglobin concentration: assessment with in vitro spectroscopy. Radiology 168:489–491, 1988.
33. Abragam A: Principles of Nuclear Magnetism. Oxford: Clarendon Press, 1985.
34. Becker ED: High Resolution NMR. Theory and Chemical Applications. New York: Academic Press, 1980.
35. Farrar TC, Becker ED: Pulse and Fourier Transform NMR. New York: Academic Press, 1971, pp 2–15.
36. Fukushima E, Roeder SBW: Experimental Pulse NMR. A Nuts and Bolts Approach. London: Addison-Wesley Publishing, 1981, pp 1–125.
37. Yoder CH, Schaeffer CD Jr: Introduction to Multinuclear NMR. Menlo Park, CA: Benjamin/Cummings Publishing, 1987.
38. Fullerton GD: Basic concepts for nuclear magnetic resonance imaging. Magn Reson Imaging 1:39–53, 1982.
39. Bottomley PA: NMR imaging techniques and applications. Rev Sci Instrum 53:1319–1337, 1982.
40. Brant-Zawadzki M, Norman D: Magnetic Resonance Imaging of the Central Nervous System. New York: Raven Press, 1987.
41. Pykett IL, Newhouse JH, Buonanno FS, et al: Principles of nuclear magnetic resonance imaging. Radiology 143:157–168, 1982.
42. Wehrli FW: Principles of magnetic resonance. In: Stark DD, Bradley WG, eds. Magnetic Resonance Imaging. St. Louis: CV Mosby, 1988, pp 1–23.
43. Edelman RR, Buxton RB, Brady TJ: Rapid MR imaging. In: Kressel HY, ed. Magnetic Resonance Annual 1988. New York: Raven Press, 1988, pp 189–216.
44. Wismer GL, Buxton RB, Rosen BR, et al: Susceptibility induced magnetic resonance line broadening: applications to brain iron mapping. J Comput Assist Tomogr 12:259–265, 1988.
45. Hoppel BE, Weisskoff RM, Thulborn KR, et al: Measurement of regional blood oxygenation and cerebral hemodynamics. Magn Reson Med 30:715–723, 1993.
46. Ludeke KM, Roschmann P, Tischler R: Susceptibility artefacts in NMR imaging. Magn Reson Imaging 3:329–343, 1985.
47. Schenck JF, Mueller OM, Souza SP, Dumoulin CL: Magnetic resonance imaging of brain iron using a 4 Tesla whole-body scanner. In: Frankel RB, Blakemore RP, eds. Iron Biominerals. New York: Plenum Publishing, 1990, pp 373–385.
48. Di Chiro G, Brooks RA, Girton ME, et al: Sequential MR studies of intracerebral hematomas in monkeys. AJNR 7:193–199, 1986.
49. Kamman RL, Go KG, Brouwer W, Berendsen HJC: Nuclear magnetic resonance relaxation in experimental brain edema: effects of water concentration, protein concentration and temperature. Magn Reson Med 6:265–274, 1988.
50. Burke HE: Handbook of Magnetic Phenomena. New York: Van Nostrand Reinhold, 1986, pp 9–57.
51. Bean CP, Livingston JD: Superparamagnetism. J Appl Phys 30:120S–129S, 1959.
52. Bean CP: Hysteresis loops of mixtures of ferromagnetic micropowders. J Appl Phys 26:1381–1383, 1955.
53. Lauffer RB: Paramagnetic metal complexes as water proton relaxation agents for NMR imaging: theory and design. Chem Rev 87:901–927, 1987.

Principles of Diffusion and Perfusion MRI

RICHARD B. BUXTON ■ LAWRENCE R. FRANK
POTTUMARTHI V. PRASAD

Diffusion is a basic physical process important in a number of physiologic functions. Transport of metabolic substrates such as glucose and oxygen into the cells ultimately depends on the diffusion of molecules from the capillaries to the cells through a liquid medium. These diffusional motions arise because the molecules of the liquid possess an intrinsic kinetic energy, leading to random molecular motions. The effect of diffusion is that labeled molecules initially present in a high local concentration spread out over time, like a drop of ink in a glass of water. Diffusion is often thought of in this way, as a net motion of solute molecules down a concentration gradient. However, even with no concentration gradients the water molecules are still in random motion. The effect of this is that a particular molecule wanders over time from its starting point, a process described as the *self-diffusion* of water. Nuclear magnetic resonance (NMR) is an ideal method for investigating the self-diffusion of water because it is possible to label the molecules by manipulating the magnetization of the hydrogen nuclei without interfering with the process of diffusion.

The discovery that diffusion affects the NMR signal was made by Hahn[1] and reported in the paper in which he described spin echoes (SEs) for the first time. Studies of these diffusion effects have continued over the years and form the basis for using NMR as a tool to measure diffusion.[2–6] These spectrometer-based methods have been extended to magnetic resonance imaging (MRI),[7] and the diagnostic utility of diffusion-weighted imaging is now being tested in a range of pathologic states. Diffusion imaging has been used in tumor studies to distinguish cystic or edematous tumor from solid tumor.[8, 9] Changes in the apparent diffusion coefficient after stroke show considerable promise as a sensitive early indication of ischemia.[10–13] In white matter, diffusion has been found to be anisotropic, with greater water mobility along the myelinated fiber tracts than perpendicular to them.[14, 15] By measuring this asymmetry, diffusion imaging provides a way to map these tracts and also a way to investigate myelination.[16, 17] Diffusion in the heart[18, 19] and abdomen[20] has also

been investigated. Because diffusion is a temperature-dependent process, measurement of changes in the local rate of diffusion can be used as an indicator of changes in tissue temperature.[21]

Perfusion is related to the blood supply of an element of tissue and at first glance would seem to have little to do with the process of diffusion. However, one of the early approaches to developing perfusion-sensitive MRI was to consider the motion of blood in randomly oriented capillaries as akin to the random motions of diffusion, so that diffusion-weighted methods could potentially reveal useful information about perfusion.[22] Today, this approach has been largely eclipsed by newer methods based on magnetic susceptibility effects and inflow effects. When certain MR contrast agents (such as gadolinium diethylenetri-aminepentaacetic acid [Gd-DTPA]) pass through a capillary bed, they produce a transient signal loss caused by these susceptibility effects, and this provides a way to measure the first-pass kinetics of the agent.[23] Local blood volume can be calculated from a kinetic analysis of the dynamic signal changes. The magnitude of these signal changes on SE images depends on the local water diffusion. Alternative methods for directly assessing perfusion based on inflow effects have also been developed.[24] Also, there has been a flurry of work on functional MRI (FMRI) techniques for measuring changes in the perfusion state of the tissue based on changes in the oxygenation of blood.[25, 26] These methods are now being used extensively to map activated regions of the brain during sensory, motor, and cognitive tasks. The physical basis of these methods is again related to diffusion and magnetic susceptibility effects, in this case associated with the intrinsic paramagnetism of deoxyhemoglobin.

These new methods for diffusion and perfusion imaging have considerably broadened the field of MRI. In addition to providing high-resolution anatomic images, MRI can now be used to probe physiologic function. In this chapter we focus on the principles underlying diffusion and perfusion MRI to lay the groundwork for understanding and interpreting the growing body of applications reported in the literature and discussed in Chapter 26.

DIFFUSION IMAGING

The effects of random thermal motions on the NMR signal can be somewhat subtle and nonintuitive. In the next section, the basic physical principles of diffusion are developed. We present a physical picture of diffusion in terms of a random walk of individual molecules and show how this model is related to the more common understanding of diffusion in terms of Fick's law. The effect of randomly varying magnetic fields on the decay of the NMR signal is described to show that the key parameter for understanding signal decay is the spread of precessional phases. These physical arguments are combined to show that signal decays caused by relaxation and motion in a field gradient have quite different characteristics, even though both are due to random molecular motions. In the next section, the important case of diffusion in a linear field gradient, which forms the basis for in vivo diffusion imaging, is considered in more detail. The effects of restricted and anisotropic diffusion, which are often encountered in biologic tissues, are discussed. Different pulse sequences for measuring diffusion and the data analysis methods used are described. Finally, the more complex problem of diffusion around local field perturbations is discussed to provide the groundwork for understanding the perfusion methods discussed later.

PHYSICS OF DIFFUSION AND ITS EFFECT ON THE NUCLEAR MAGNETIC RESONANCE SIGNAL

The Random Walk

At the heart of diffusional motions is the concept of the random walk.[27] Because of random thermal motions, the water molecules in a liquid are constantly colliding with one another. With each collision a molecule is deflected and rotated, so that both the orientation and the position of the molecule tend to change in a random way. The interaction and scattering of densely packed water molecules are, of course, complicated processes, but we can model the displacements over time of a particular molecule in a simple way as a series of random steps (a *random walk*), which yields quantitatively accurate results. We assume that a molecule stays in one position for a time Δt and then through interaction with the other molecules moves a distance d in a random direction. After another interval Δt, it makes another random step, and so on.

This view of diffusion as a random walk may seem at odds with the classic concept of diffusion as a flux of particles down a concentration gradient as described by Fick's law:

$$\mathbf{J} = -D\nabla C \qquad (1)$$

where $\mathbf{J}$ is the particle flux (number of particles passing through a unit area per second), ∇C is the gradi-

ent of the particle concentration, and D is the diffusion coefficient. On the basis of this equation, it is sometimes said that diffusion is "driven" by a concentration gradient. This seems inconsistent with the random walk model, in which each step is random regardless of the concentration. However, Equation 1 is the natural result of random motions: there is a net flux from high to low concentrations simply because more particles start out from the region of high concentration.

To relate the parameters of a random walk (d and Δt) to D, consider a one-dimensional random walk and the net flux past a particular point x. The local density of particles along the line is C(x), and for one time step we need only look at the particles within a distance d of x to calculate the flux, because these are the only particles that can cross x in one step. Let $C_1 = C(x - d/2)$ be the mean concentration on the left and $C_2 = C_1 + d\,(dC/dx)$ the mean concentration on the right of x. In a time interval Δt (one step), on average half of the particles within a distance d to the left of x move to the right past x, giving a positive flux $J^+ = dC_1/2\Delta t$. Similarly, half of the particles within a distance d to the right move left to form a negative flux $J^- = dC_2/2\Delta t$. The net flux $J = J^+ - J^-$ is then

$$J = -\frac{d^2}{2\Delta t}\,\frac{dC}{dx} \qquad (2)$$

The classic diffusion coefficient D can thus be related to the parameters of a random walk as

$$D = \frac{d^2}{2\Delta t} \qquad (3)$$

In understanding the effects of diffusion on the MR signal, however, Fick's law is no help, because it deals only with a net flux and the random motions of water molecules happen in the absence of any concentration gradient. But in terms of a random walk we can ask the key question: How far will a water molecule have moved after N steps? For one molecule this is impossible to predict, but if many molecules are undergoing their own separate random walks, we can predict the *distribution p(x)* of the distances moved. That is, p(x) is the probability of finding a molecule at a distance x from its starting point after N steps. For example, consider a one-dimensional random walk, in which each step is equally likely to be to the left or the right (Fig. 8–1). Because there is no preference for left or right, we expect the mean displacement after many steps to be zero. But as the number of steps increases we would also expect to find some molecules farther from their starting point, so that the width (or standard deviation) of the distribution should increase.

For a random walk of N steps there are a final position Δx and an average position x_{av}, and for any particular walk they are likely to be different from zero (see Fig. 8–1). If we now imagine following many particles, each undergoing its own individual random walk, we can ask about the average values (denoted by $<\ >$) of these two quantities. Because there is no preference for left or right steps, we clearly must have $<\Delta x> = <x_{av}> = 0$. But each of these quantities has

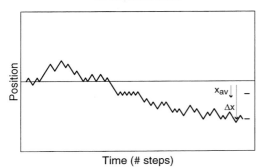

1D Random Walk

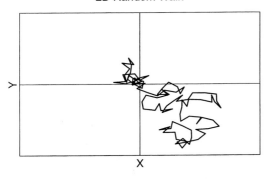

2D Random Walk

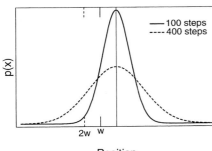

Distribution of Final Positions

$$\Delta x^2 = 2DT \qquad (4a)$$

$$x_{av}^2 = \frac{2DT}{3} \qquad (4b)$$

The key relationship in Equations 3 and 4 is that the mean square displacement is proportional to a constant characteristic of the medium (D) and the elapsed time (T). These arguments were developed for a one-dimensional random walk, but they can easily be extended to two- and three-dimensional random walks. Figure 8–1 shows an example of a two-dimensional random walk in which the steps are of the same size but the direction is random. Equations 3 and 4 also hold true if the step size is not always the same, with d^2 then being replaced by the mean square step size.

Equations 3 and 4 are the basic equations of diffusion, showing that displacement grows only as the square root of time. This is fundamentally different from motion at a constant velocity, for which displacement is proportional to time. For example, compare the average displacement of a water molecule diffusing with a diffusion coefficient $D = 10^{-5}$ cm^2/s (a typical number for brain) and a water molecule being carried along in the blood of a capillary with a speed of 1 mm/s. In 2 ms each moves about 2 μm, but whereas the time for the flowing molecule to move 20 μm is only 20 ms, the time for the diffusing molecule to move the same distance is 200 ms. Diffusion is thus reasonably efficient for moving molecules short distances but highly inefficient for transport over large distances. It is a remarkable fact that such small displacements as these (tens of micrometers) can have a measurable effect on the MR signal.

Effect of Time-Varying Magnetic Fields on the Nuclear Magnetic Resonance Signal

When a radiofrequency (RF) pulse is applied to a collection of spins, the longitudinal magnetization is tipped over to create a local transverse magnetization, which then precesses with a frequency proportional to the local magnetic field strength. We can picture this as each spin precessing around its local field and creating a small signal. The net signal is the sum of all of these individual signals. If the magnetic field is not uniform, some spins precess faster than others and there are phase differences between the individual signals. The net signal is reduced, and the signal decreases further as time progresses and the phase differences grow. We can describe this signal reduction by writing $S(t) = A(t)S_0$, where $A(t)$ is the signal attenuation factor and varies from 1 (no attenuation) down to 0 (complete signal loss) and S_0 is the unattenuated net signal.

It is a common practice to write $A(t)$ in the form $A(t) = \exp(-R_2t)$, where R_2 is the transverse relaxivity (1/T2). We can extend this and use the symbol ΔR_2 as the additional transverse relaxation resulting from diffusion in a linear field gradient. It is important to bear in mind, however, that writing $A(t)$ as a simple decaying exponential is a convenience motivated by T2 decay, for which the mathematic form is correct

FIGURE 8–1. The random walk. *Top,* A one-dimensional random walk in which a particle moves randomly left or right with each step (step size d = 1, time between steps $\Delta t = 1$). After N steps the final position is Δx and the average position occupied by the particle during the walk is x_{av}. *Middle,* A two-dimensional random walk in which each step is equally likely to be in any direction. *Bottom,* The distribution of final positions, showing that the width increases in proportion to $\sqrt{N}$. The full width at half-maximum of each distribution is indicated on the horizontal axis.

some scatter about the mean, and it is a somewhat more difficult problem to calculate the standard deviations. One can show that for a large number of steps N, both distributions are gaussian, the variance of the final position is $\sigma^2 = \langle \Delta x^2 \rangle = Nd^2$ and the variance of the average position $\sigma_{av}^2 = \langle x_{av}^2 \rangle$ is one third of the variance of the final position. But the number of steps N is simply an indication of how much time has elapsed (total time $T = N\Delta t$). In terms of the diffusion coefficient D, the mean square displacement after a time T and the mean square average displacement during T can be expressed as

and R_2 is thus a constant. More generally, transverse relaxivity is not always a simple exponential, and then ΔR_2 must be considered a function of time. For example, in the following sections we show that for diffusion in a linear field gradient, $\Delta R_2 \propto t^2$, a much stronger time dependence than that for T2 decay.

To develop a more quantitative understanding of the attenuation A(t), consider a collection of spins diffusing through a nonuniform magnetic field as their magnetization precesses. The net magnetization after a time t depends on the distribution of the final phases of the individual signals, and each final phase depends on the history of magnetic fields felt by the individual spin. The field at the spin could vary for two reasons: 1) as the water molecule tumbles, the orientation of the spin relative to another nearby magnetic moment (e.g., the other hydrogen nucleus in the molecule) changes, creating a change in the magnetic field, or 2) the spin diffuses into another region where the field is different. The first effect is the basis for T2 relaxation, and the second is more directly related to displacements caused by diffusion. Both of these effects follow from the random thermal motions of the molecules.

To calculate this dephasing more precisely, we can imagine following an individual spin and plotting the variation with time of the magnetic field at the spin. We can approximate this process by imagining that the molecular motions (tumbling and displacement) take place in small jumps. We picture the spin as "sitting" in a constant field B_1 for a short time Δt and then jumping to a new field B_2 and remaining in that field for the same time Δt. In each instant Δt the spin precesses at a rate set by the current value of B and acquires a phase increment $\Delta \phi = \gamma B \, \Delta t$, where γ is the gyromagnetic ratio for the proton. The final phase value after a time T is the sum of these phase increments. But because each phase increment is proportional to the current value of B, the final phase ϕ is the same as it would have been if the spin felt only the average field B_{av} for the total time T: $\phi = \gamma T B_{av}$. At the end of the elapsed time T, there is a distribution of phase values for the signals from different spins because each spin has experienced a different B_{av}. The standard deviation σ_ϕ of the final phase values is thus proportional to the standard deviation σ_B of the average field felt by a nucleus:

$$\sigma_\phi{}^2 = (\gamma T)^2 \, \sigma_B{}^2 \qquad (5)$$

The standard deviation σ_ϕ of the phase distribution $p(\phi)$ can be thought of as a measure of the width of the distribution. When the individual signals are added (e.g., all spins within an imaging voxel), the net signal is strongly attenuated if σ_ϕ is large. However, the exact form of the attenuation factor A(T) depends on the shape of $p(\phi)$ as well as the width σ_ϕ at time T. For any phase distribution, A(T) is calculated by integrating $p(\phi) \cos \phi$ over all phase angles. To illustrate how the shape of $p(\phi)$ affects the net attenuation, we can compare two distributions that arise in NMR: the gaussian and the lorentzian (or Cauchy) distributions (Fig. 8–2). The width of the gaussian is characterized

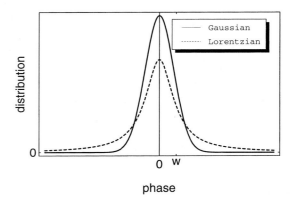

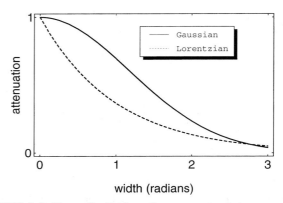

FIGURE 8–2. Phase distributions. Because each of the spins that contribute to the net signal feels a different pattern of fluctuating magnetic fields, there is a spread in the final phases of the signals from each. The effect of this phase spread on the signal attenuation A(t) depends on the shape of the phase distribution as well as its width. Two distributions are illustrated: the gaussian $p(\phi) \propto \exp(-\phi^2/2\sigma_\phi{}^2)$ and the lorentzian (or Cauchy distribution) $p(\phi) \propto 1/[1 + (\phi/w)^2]$, where w is half of the full width at half of the maximal peak value. The width of the gaussian is characterized by the standard deviation σ_ϕ, but for the lorentzian we must use w to characterize the width, rather than the standard deviation, because σ is infinite for this distribution. The equivalent half-width for the gaussian is w = $1.17\sigma_\phi$. *Top*, Examples of the two distributions with equal half-widths. *Bottom*, The resulting attenuation curves plotted as a function of the width of the distribution. Both curves are exponential but depend on different powers of the width: ln A is proportional to w for the lorentzian but w^2 for the gaussian.

by σ_ϕ, and the width of the lorentzian is characterized by the half-width w at half of the maximal value. The attenuation factors resulting from these two distributions are

$$A(T) = \exp[-\sigma_\phi{}^2(T)/2] \qquad \text{(gaussian)} \qquad (6a)$$

$$A(T) = \exp[-w(T)] \qquad \text{(lorentzian)} \qquad (6b)$$

Equations 5 and 6 provide a general method for understanding the attenuation of the MR signal in a variety of circumstances. We simply determine the width of the phase distribution for a collection of spins at time T and apply Equations 6a and 6b. (Of course, if the phase distribution is neither gaussian nor lorentzian, a different form of Equations 6a and 6b must be developed.) The time dependence of the attenuation factor A(T) thus depends on how the width of the phase distribution changes with time and on the shape of that distribution. For example, a monoexponential form for A(T) can arise in two ways: from a lorentzian phase distribution with a width that is proportional to T or from a gaussian phase distribution with a width proportional to $\sqrt{T}$.

We can now apply these ideas to two important examples: 1) relaxation resulting from fields varying randomly in time (R_2) and 2) diffusion through a linear field gradient (ΔR_2). These two examples are in many respects limiting cases and essentially bracket the range of diffusion effects encountered in both diffusion-sensitive imaging and perfusion-sensitive imaging based on magnetic susceptibility effects.

Comparison of Relaxation and Diffusion in a Field Gradient

Although T2 relaxation and attenuation resulting from diffusion in a field gradient both have their origins in random thermal motions, their dependence on those motions is decidedly different. To focus the arguments of the next sections, consider a simple idealized experiment. The SE signal is measured from a sample of pure water, and the echo time (TE) is varied to measure R_2. Then a magnetic field gradient is added and ΔR_2 is measured. The temperature of the water sample is raised (thus increasing the thermal motions) and R_2 and ΔR_2 are measured again. The somewhat surprising result is that R_2 decreases but ΔR_2 increases with increasing temperature. In this section the reason for this important difference is discussed. In both cases, random motions lead to each spin feeling a variable magnetic field so that the signals gradually become out of phase. But it is how the phase distribution evolves in time that determines the form of A(t).

To illustrate how random motions lead to these two different phenomena, we can apply a simplified random walk model to describe both the changing magnetic field associated with other nuclei as the water molecule tumbles and the changing field as the molecule diffuses to a different location. We assume that a molecule remains stationary for a time τ_c (the correlation time) and then randomly moves a distance d and also tumbles to a new random orientation. In a water molecule, a proton feels a small field caused by the other hydrogen nucleus (as well as other nearby nuclear dipoles on other molecules) in addition to the main magnetic field. As the molecule tumbles, the orientation of the nuclear dipoles changes, and each nucleus thus feels a fluctuating field B caused by the other. We can further simplify the model by assuming that the magnitude of the field variation associated with reorientation is always the same (B) but the sign ($\pm$) fluctuates randomly. With this simple model, R_2 depends only on τ_c and B and ΔR_2 depends on τ_c and d. Both the tumbling and the displacement lead to fluctuating magnetic fields; the important difference is in the character of those fluctuations (Fig. 8–3).

Consider first the form of R_2 in a uniform field. The key physical parameter that determines A(t) is the standard deviation of the distribution of average fields

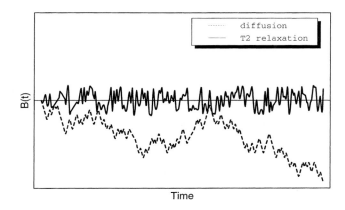

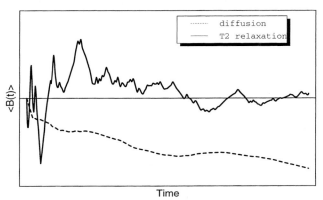

FIGURE 8–3. Fluctuating magnetic fields. Because of random thermal motions a water molecule tumbles and moves in position, both of which can lead to fluctuating fields at a particular nucleus. The tumbling leads to a reorientation of the magnetic moment with respect to other magnetic moments and is characterized by each new value of the field B being independent of the previous one. Random diffusional motions through a field gradient also lead to field fluctuations but differ in that each new field B is still close to the previous B. The different effects of these two processes on signal attenuation are due primarily to the different character of the curves B(t). *Top*, Plot of B(t) for both processes. *Bottom*, Plot of the average field experienced by a nucleus up to a time t. Note that the random field related to tumbling (labeled T2 relaxation) leads to an average field offset magnitude that tends to decrease with time, whereas the average field offset related to diffusion increases with time.

felt by the spins. As we average more values of $\pm$B, we would expect the average field for each spin to move closer to zero. To calculate the average field we can use the mathematics developed earlier for a random walk. If we add up the individual B values for N time steps, the sum is the end result of a random walk with step size B and the standard deviation of the sum is $\sigma = B\sqrt{N}$. But to calculate the average field we must divide this by N. Because $N = T/\tau_c$, the result is that $\sigma^2(B_{av}) = B^2\tau_c/T$. Furthermore, the distribution is gaussian in shape. When this result is combined with Equations 5 and 6a, A(t) becomes a simple decaying exponential. The transverse decay rate R_2 is thus proportional to $B^2\tau_c$.

Suppose now that a linear magnetic field gradient G exists in the sample, so that as spins diffuse to different positions, they feel different fields. After a time T, how is the net signal from a small region (e.g., near position x_0) attenuated? To answer this question we must determine the width of the phase distribution for all possible random walk paths that start at any point in the sample but end on x_0 at time T. However, a simpler way to think about this task is to realize that the net phase acquired in a random walk from point x_1 to point x_0 is the same as that for the same random walk done in reverse (from x_0 to x_1). So the problem of determining the phase distribution at a point after time T can be restated: If many spins start at $x = x_0$ at $t = 0$ and then diffuse for a time T, what is the distribution of phases for the signals from these spins? This can be calculated directly from the earlier random walk results. Because the field varies linearly with position (B = Gx), the variance of the average field felt by a diffusing molecule is simply G^2 times the variance of the position: $\sigma^2(B_{av}) = G^2d^2N = G^2d^2T/\tau_c$. Combining this with Equations 5 and 6a, we have that ΔR_2 is proportional to d^2T^2/τ_c.

Thus, the effects of random motions are different for T2 relaxation and diffusion in a field gradient in two important ways. 1) The relaxivities depend in an inverse way on the correlation time τ_c: R_2 is proportional to τ_c and ΔR_2 is proportional to $1/\tau_c$. This explains the opposite behavior described for the temperature experiment: If the temperature increases τ_c decreases, and R_2 then decreases while ΔR_2 increases. 2) The time dependence of ΔR_2 is much stronger than that for relaxation. The essential reason for these differences is that the variance of the average field felt by a spin decreases with time for the case of T2 relaxation but increases with time for diffusion in a linear field gradient. The source of this difference is that for diffusion through a field gradient each new value of the field offset is *not* independent of the values before. Although each diffusion step is random (i.e., equally likely to be toward higher or lower fields), the new field the spin finds itself in is still close to the old field because the distance moved is small. That is, even though the spin is undergoing a random walk, so that each step in position is independent of the previous one, the phase acquired in each step depends on the current position (the sum of all of the previous steps). As time increases, the spins spread into a broader range of fields, and the width of the phase dispersion increases more rapidly than it would if each new field value was independent.

SIGNAL ATTENUATION CAUSED BY DIFFUSION IN A LINEAR MAGNETIC FIELD GRADIENT

The preceding arguments were cast in terms of the parameters of a random walk to clarify the relationship between relaxation and diffusional signal losses. However, for practical applications it is more convenient to express the diffusion attenuation in terms of the diffusion coefficient D. The attenuation caused by diffusion in a linear field gradient is then[1]

$$A(T) = \exp[-(\gamma G)^2DT^3/3] \qquad (7)$$

Effect of Spin Echoes

If field gradients are present in a sample, diffusion can lead to strong attenuation of the signal because of the strong time dependence in Equation 7. However, Carr and Purcell[2] showed that multiple SEs substantially reduce the effects of diffusion. To see why this is so, consider again the variations in B plotted in Figure 8–3. If a 180° RF pulse is applied at TE/2, all of the previously acquired phase values are reversed in sign. This is effectively equivalent to reversing all of the B values up to TE/2. Figure 8–4 shows the effects of one 180° pulse and of eight pulses. The folding of the phase by multiple 180° pulses effectively reduces the average field felt by each spin. Because the net phase acquired on a particular random walk path is simply proportional to the average B value, the net phase of each path is reduced and thus the phase dispersion is reduced. Mathematically, the SE attenuation caused by diffusion through a linear field gradient for a total time T with n 180° pulses is[2]

$$A(T) = \exp[-(\gamma G)^2DT^3/12n^2] \qquad (8)$$

Multiple 180° pulses thus substantially reduce the signal attenuation caused by diffusion. Note that if the 180° pulses are applied with only a small gap between them, so that the number of pulses n is proportional to T, the decay becomes a single exponential. That is, for many pulses the additional decay caused by diffusion appears simply as a small change in the T2 relaxation. Physically, this occurs because the folding effect of the 180° pulses makes the pattern of fields felt by a spin look more like a randomly varying field.

Restricted Diffusion

The foregoing arguments are based on free diffusion in an infinite medium. That is, there are no barriers to prevent a molecule from drifting farther and farther from its starting point as time increases. But in biologic structures diffusion is restricted by natural barriers such as cell membranes and large protein molecules.[28] As a result, the MR signal attenuation is different from the free diffusion case. A simple example based on the random walk illustrates the nature of restricted diffusion effects.

Consider a molecule diffusing through a linear field gradient with step size d but confined within a box of size 10d. If a step would carry it out of the box, it is reflected off the wall. Figure 8–5 shows typical random walks for the restricted case and for free diffusion. For short time intervals there is not much difference between the two cases. But as time increases and the restricted molecule encounters the wall more frequently, the paths diverge and the restricted molecule is prevented from straying very far from its starting point. As a result, the mean field felt by the restricted molecule is less than that felt by the free molecule, so the signal attenuation is not as severe with restricted diffusion. That is, the variance of the mean position is smaller for restricted diffusion than for free diffusion.

As time increases further, the restricted molecule encounters the barriers many times, and the plot of B versus t begins to look more like the plot for random variations in the relaxation example. That is, the curve tends to cross and recross zero many times. As in the

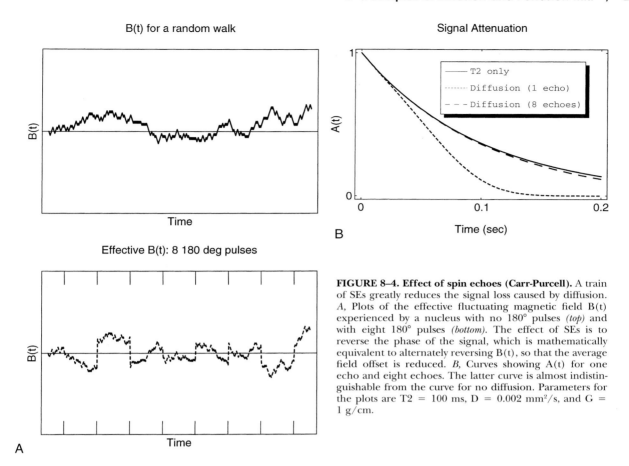

FIGURE 8–4. Effect of spin echoes (Carr-Purcell). A train of SEs greatly reduces the signal loss caused by diffusion. *A,* Plots of the effective fluctuating magnetic field B(t) experienced by a nucleus with no 180° pulses *(top)* and with eight 180° pulses *(bottom).* The effect of SEs is to reverse the phase of the signal, which is mathematically equivalent to alternately reversing B(t), so that the average field offset is reduced. *B,* Curves showing A(t) for one echo and eight echoes. The latter curve is almost indistinguishable from the curve for no diffusion. Parameters for the plots are T2 = 100 ms, D = 0.002 mm²/s, and G = 1 g/cm.

relaxation example, in this situation the variance of the average field felt by a molecule tends to decrease with time.

The attenuation curve A(t) for restricted diffusion is thus not a simple curve. For short times $\Delta R_2 \propto T^2$, for long times ΔR_2 is constant, and for intermediate times the dependence varies between these extremes. In the first regime a typical molecule has not yet encountered the barrier, whereas in the final regime it has encountered the barrier many times. The crossover between these regimes occurs when the molecule has diffused a distance comparable to the size of the restricted region. Thus, measurements of A(t) may provide information on the size of the restricted region.

Anisotropic Diffusion

At this point we have considered diffusion that occurs with equal probability in any direction and that is characterized by a single diffusion constant D. Such diffusion is said to be *isotropic.* In general, however, diffusion can be influenced by the structure of the local environment. For example, in white matter of the brain, water readily diffuses along the fiber tracts but diffusion perpendicular to the fiber is restricted by the myelin sheath.[7, 14, 15, 29–31] This is called *anisotropic* diffusion. This more general description of diffusion requires a more generalized form of D, and it must now be considered to be a tensor rather than a scalar.

Figure 8–6 illustrates the more complicated behavior of anisotropic diffusion for a two-dimensional example. Consider a set of parallel fiber tracts with diffusion coefficients D_1 along the tracts and D_2 perpendicular to the tracts and with D_1 greater than D_2. The tracts are oriented at an angle to the x and y axes of a reference frame. If the water molecules at a small point in this anisotropic medium could be labeled, it would be seen that over time they spread out by diffusion. However, the pattern of dispersion is an asymmetric ellipse with the long axis aligned with the fibers. That is, the mean square displacement is proportional to D_1 along the fibers and proportional to D_2 perpendicular to the fibers. A somewhat surprising result of the anisotropy is that a concentration gradient in one direction can create a flux in a perpendicular direction. For example, a concentration gradient in x creates a flux along the fibers, but because they are angled this flux has a y component as well. This effect also leads to the result that the particle flux **J** and the concentration gradient are no longer parallel. These effects are described mathematically by treating D as a tensor.

As described at the beginning of the chapter, the diffusive flux **J** in a medium is proportional to the concentration gradient ∇C through Fick's law (Equation 1) and D is the proportionality constant. For this isotropic diffusion the flux vector is in the same direction as the concentration gradient. When we replace the scalar D with the tensor **D** in Fick's law, the

Free Diffusion

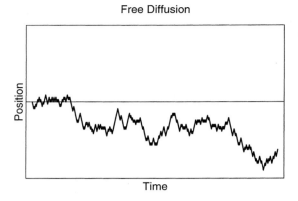

Restricted Diffusion

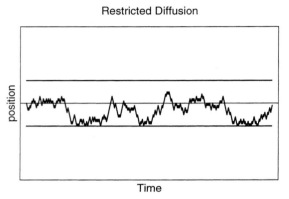

FIGURE 8–5. Restricted diffusion. Typical one-dimensional numeric random walk paths (d = 1 and Δt = 1) for free diffusion and diffusion restricted by an impenetrable barrier at position ± 10. At early times the two paths are the same, but for later times they are quite different because the restricted particle has enountered the barrier many times. The average displacement is less for the restricted particle, so the average field offset when a linear field gradient is present is also less.

flux is not necessarily parallel to the concentration gradient vector. In other words, the flux in each of the three spatial dimensions {x, y, z} is affected by the concentration gradient in all three directions. The diffusion tensor has nine components and can be written in the form of a matrix D_{ij}, where i refers to the ith component of the flux and j to the jth component of the concentration gradient. An important property of D is that it is symmetric (i.e., $D_{ij} = D_{ji}$), so that there are only six different components. This fact reduces the experimental time necessary to determine the tensor D.

The mathematic formalism of the diffusion tensor can also be applied to signal attenuation in NMR. The Bloch equation[32] can be modified to include both isotropic[33] and anisotropic[4, 34] diffusion. From this it is possible to derive analytic expressions relating the measured echo intensity to the applied pulsed gradient sequence in an SE. Considerable simplification is achieved by defining an *effective* diffusion tensor as the diffusion tensor averaged over TE.[9, 35] The signal intensity as a function of TE is then related to the effective diffusion tensor by the expression

$$\ln \frac{A(b)}{A(0)} = - \sum_{i=1}^{3} \sum_{j=1}^{3} b_{ij} D_{ij} \qquad (9)$$

where A(0) is the signal intensity with no gradients applied and b_{ij} incorporates the effects of the prescribed magnetic field gradients,[35, 36] including effects of interactions between the imaging and diffusion-sensitizing gradients.

MEASUREMENT OF THE DIFFUSION COEFFICIENT WITH NUCLEAR MAGNETIC RESONANCE

Water Self-Diffusion Measurements with Pulsed Field Gradients

The measurement of the self-diffusion coefficient D of water in its simplest form consists of carrying out an SE experiment while a linear field gradient is applied continuously to the sample. Both the free induction decay signal (the signal immediately following the application of an excitation pulse) and the SE signal at time TE are measured. The ratio of the SE signal to the free induction decay signal is A(TE), and D is then calculated from Equation 8. (A correction must also be made for natural T2 decay during the interval TE.)

However, this simple approach has some technical difficulties. From Equation 8 it is apparent that larger G values provide more sensitive measurements of D. However, the measured signals (both free induction decay and SE) become narrow as the gradient increases. A compression in the time domain corresponds to expanded width in the frequency domain, so the signal receiving system must have a wider bandwidth. With wider bandwidth, the noise level also increases. This problem was solved by Stejskal and Tan-

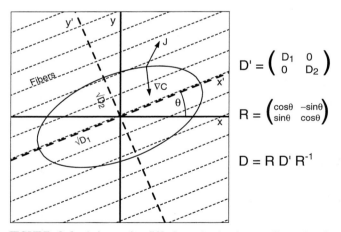

FIGURE 8–6. Anisotropic diffusion. A simple two-dimensional model for diffusion in white matter, in which the diffusion coefficient along the fiber tracts is D_1 and that perpendicular to the tracts is D_2, with D_2 less than D_1 because of the restriction imposed by the myelin sheath. The diffusion properties of this system are defined by three parameters: D_1, D_2, and the orientation angle θ. An initial localized concentration of particles spreads out over time in an elliptic pattern with major and minor axes proportional to $\sqrt{D_1}$ and $\sqrt{D_2}$, respectively. Because of the anisotropy, the flux vector J is no longer parallel to the concentration gradient (∇C). Fick's law still applies, but D must be taken to be a two-by-two tensor rather than a scalar. In the principal axis coordinate system *(dashed lines)*, the form of the diffusion tensor simplifies so that all the off-diagonal components are zero.

ner[4] and Tanner,[5, 37] who introduced the use of pulsed gradients for the measurement of diffusion coefficients. Because the gradients are turned off during data collection, the gradient strength can be increased without increasing the signal bandwidth. A typical pulsed gradient SE (PGSE) sequence is shown in Figure 8–7.

For a PGSE experiment the attenuation caused by diffusion is[2]

$$A(\Delta,\delta,G) = \exp[-\gamma^2 G^2 \delta^2 (\Delta - \frac{\delta}{3})D]$$

$$= \exp(-bD) \qquad (10a)$$

where

$$b = \gamma^2 G^2 \delta^2 (\Delta - \frac{\delta}{3}) \qquad (10b)$$

The attenuation factor $A(\Delta,\delta,G)$ depends on the gradient strength and two time parameters (the width and separation of the gradient pulses) but not on TE itself. The resulting signal attenuation can be characterized by the single operator-controlled parameter b, which depends on the timing parameters and the amplitude of the gradient pulses and has dimensions (seconds per square centimeter) that are the inverse of the dimensions of D. For diffusion to create an appreciable (and thus measurable) attenuation of the signal, the product bD must be on the order of 1. A typical value of D is 10^{-5} cm^2/s (= 0.001 mm^2/s), so b must be on the order of 1000 s/mm^2. For example, if the maximal gradient strength is G = 10 mT/m (a typical value for conventional MR scanners), one set of pulses that produce a b value of about 1000 s/mm^2 is δ = 40 ms and Δ = 100 ms.

A typical diffusion measurement requires repeating the PGSE pulse sequence with different gradient strengths or delays and fitting the curve ln A versus b to a straight line; the slope of this curve is D (Fig. 8–8). Because all measurements are made with the same TE, there is no need to correct for intrinsic T2 decay.

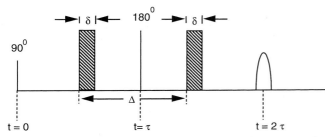

FIGURE 8–7. PGSE pulse sequence. The basic pulse sequence for measuring diffusion is an SE with identical gradient pulses added before and after the 180° RF pulse. The attenuation related to diffusion depends on the gradient amplitude G, duration δ, and separation of the pulses Δ. The form of this dependence can be expressed by a single parameter b such that the attenuation is e^{-bD}. The diffusion coefficient D can be measured by repeating the pulse sequence with different values of b.

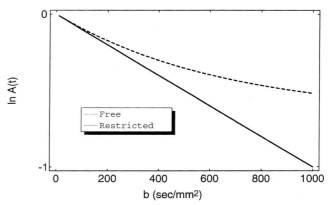

FIGURE 8–8. Measuring the diffusion coefficient. The PGSE pulse sequence is repeated a number of times with different values of b. A plot of ln A versus b is a straight line for free diffusion with a slope of D (in this example D = 0.001 mm^2/s). The parameter b can be varied by changing either G or Δ in the PGSE pulse sequence, and for free diffusion the curves are the same. For restricted diffusion, however, the curves are different, depending on whether G or Δ is varied. The curve labeled Restricted results if b is varied by changing Δ. Another way to describe this phenomenon is that the value of D measured by varying G for a fixed Δ is different for different Δ values.

Analysis of Diffusion Attenuation Curves

The simplest measurement of D requires measurement of attenuation for two different b values. However, it is often desirable to have more data points to increase the precision and allow investigation of more complex systems in which the signal decay may not be a single exponential. The latter could result from restricted diffusion or the presence of several components with significantly different diffusion coefficients in a sampled voxel (e.g., brain tissue and cerebrospinal fluid). One could then use multiexponential fits to estimate the individual diffusion coefficients.

The PGSE sequence offers other advantages because it provides additional parameters that influence the diffusion sensitivity. The possibility of measuring the diffusion coefficient by varying Δ offers a means of studying time-dependent diffusion. Tanner and Stejskal[38] showed that by repeating the diffusion measurement (by varying G) for different values of Δ one can investigate restricted diffusion. (Figure 8–8 shows schematically how the measured D varies with Δ.) In their original experiments with yeast cells, which are nearly spherical and have an average diameter of 6 µm, they were able to estimate accurately the size of the restricted region (the cell size) from diffusion measurements.[38]

The acquisition of diffusion-weighted images is discussed in the following, but the analysis of imaging data is similar to that for spectrometric data. The same kind of analysis as described earlier can be applied pixel by pixel to form a diffusion coefficient map. Alternatively, one could measure regions of interest in each diffusion-weighted image and apply the preceding analysis to the measurements. Both methods are used commonly in practice. When performing pixel-by-pixel analysis, it is important that there are no misregistration artifacts. These could result from motion between image acquisitions or from eddy current generation. Proper corrections should be performed before the calculation of diffusion maps.

In analyzing diffusion imaging data, it is important to realize that other gradient pulses are applied for spatial encoding and may lead to additional diffusion weighting. Thus, calculations of b values in principle have to take into account all of the imaging gradients as well as the gradients added for diffusion sensitivity.[36, 39] On whole-body scanners, the effects of imaging gradients are usually a minor correction, but they become crucial when microscopy or imaging is done with small-bore animal scanners, where the imaging gradient strengths can be considerably larger. Another potential source of error in calculating b is background gradients inherent in the sample or the imaging hardware because of field inhomogeneity or magnetic susceptibility variations in the sample. More complicated pulse sequences have been proposed to eliminate the effect of these undesired gradient fields.[40] On the other hand, the effect could be exploited to estimate the strength of the internal gradient,[41] which may be useful in both medical applications (estimation of brain iron content) and nonmedical applications (study of fluid flow in porous media).

Measuring Anisotropic Diffusion

As discussed earlier, the general description of three-dimensional diffusion depends on the diffusion tensor D, which contains six distinct components. The components of D can be estimated experimentally using linear regression analysis of Equation 9 with seven measurements: six for each of the unique components of D_{ij} and one for A(0).[35] For example, consider again the simple two-dimensional example of Figure 8–6, in which D_{ij} is a two-by-two matrix with three distinct components. Separate measurements of attenuation associated with gradients along the x axis, y axis, and an axis at 45° provide enough information to calculate the components of D.

The values of the components of D_{ij} depend on the reference coordinate system used. If we had used a coordinate system in which one of the axes was aligned with the fibers, the matrix D_{ij} would have been diagonal (all off-diagonal components zero). This is the *principal axis* coordinate system, and the diagonal components are the *principal diffusivities* (D_1 and D_2 in the example of Fig. 8–6). If D is measured in an arbitrary coordinate system, the principal axes and diffusivities can be calculated by computing the eigenvectors and eigenvalues of D.

The principal axes of D accurately reflect the directional diffusion characteristics of the tissue. In particular, the principal axis associated with the largest diffusivity represents the primary diffusion orientation of the tissue. For a white matter voxel containing parallel fibers, for instance, this would define the fiber orientation. This property has been exploited to map the fiber orientations in brain noninvasively, which may prove to be useful in studying myelination in the brain,

especially in neonates.[16] Hajnal and colleagues[17] have provided a comprehensive compilation of anisotropic diffusion measurements in different white matter tracts in human brain in both normal and pathologic states.

One point should be kept in mind about the interpretation of the principal axes of the diffusion tensor in terms of fiber orientation. If the voxel contains a mixture of anisotropic components, such as two collections of fibers with different orientations, the interpretation of the principal axes is not as clear. The principal axes then reflect the composite nature of the voxel and generally do not lie on either of the fiber directions unless they are perpendicular to each other.

It is also useful to find properties of the diffusion tensor that are independent of the reference frame in which D is measured. This has the obvious practical significance that such a quantity would be characteristic of the medium yet not be influenced by its orientation within the magnet. One of these invariant properties is the trace of D, denoted $Tr(D)$, which is just the sum of the diagonal components of D. Pulse sequences have been developed that can measure this quantity.[42, 43] These sequences have the added advantage of being much faster, requiring only the orthogonality of the diffusion-sensitizing gradients and thereby allowing single-shot imaging of $Tr(D)$. In contrast, manipulation of a standard diffusion-weighted sequence to measure the components of D separately can take an exceedingly long time, which reduces its clinical utility.[35]

Measuring Temperature

The diffusion coefficient is temperature dependent,[44] with an estimated 2.4% change in D for a 1°C change in temperature.[21] Thus, by means of proper calibration, it should be possible to measure temperature distributions with good accuracy using diffusion MRI. This may have important consequences for hyperthermia and laser therapy by providing a means of monitoring temperature in real time.[45, 46] Other NMR parameters such as T1 are also temperature dependent and have been proposed as a basis for temperature measurement,[47] but these approaches rely on extensive modeling and trials in the exact site of interest.[48] Basing temperature measurements on changes in the diffusion coefficient appears less problematic, although there can be significant errors in temperature calibrations, mainly because of anisotropy in tissue.[48]

METHODS FOR IN VIVO DIFFUSION IMAGING

With the evolution of MRI systems, the PGSE technique was extended to the imaging domain, opening up the possibility of obtaining spatially resolved diffusion measurements in vivo. Numerous imaging techniques have been proposed for in vivo diffusion imaging, and the following is a brief summary of some of the major methods used. The basic diffusion-sensitive NMR pulse sequences are illustrated in Figure 8–9.

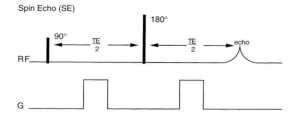

Spin Echo (SE)

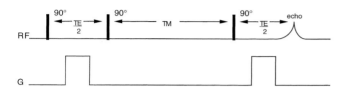

Stimulated Echo (STE)

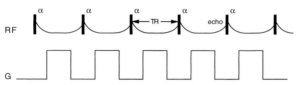

Steady-State Free Precession (SSFP)

FIGURE 8–9. Basic diffusion-sensitive pulse sequences. Three pulse sequences sensitive to diffusion are spin echo (SE), stimulated echo (STE), and steady-state free precession (SSFP). Diffusion sensitivity increases with greater separation between the gradient pulses. For the SE sequence this requires increasing TE and thus a greater signal loss related to T2 decay. With the STE sequence the echo is only half as strong as with SE, but the magnetization decays by T1 rather than T2 during the interval TM. This interval can be extended to increase the diffusion sensitivity without increasing T2 signal loss. The SSFP sequence with a low flip angle α is the most sensitive to diffusion because the signal consists primarily of STEs from previous RF pulses. However, quantitation of D is more difficult because the degree of attenuation depends on the relaxation times as well as D.

Spin-Echo Methods

SE pulse sequences are most commonly used for diffusion measurements. A pair of strong gradient pulses is added to a conventional imaging sequence before and after the 180° RF pulse. Early attempts to perform diffusion imaging were based on conventional SE sequences with readout gradients played for longer durations[49] or additional gradients used along the slice-selection direction.[50] The diffusion pulse sequence proposed by Ahn and coworkers[49] involved obtaining a set of diffusion-encoded images by varying the duration of the readout gradient and the associated compensation gradient. This simple technique had practical advantages (employment of low-amplitude gradient fields and elimination of residual gradient fields arising from eddy current effects) and was used for early clinical studies.[51–53] However, this sequence is limited by a low signal-to-noise (S/N) ratio and sensitivity to motion artifacts. With the development of stronger gradient coils, SE pulse sequences became more flexible and are now widely used.

Stimulated-Echo Methods

One important limitation of SE sequences is that long TE values are required to accommodate the long durations of the diffusion-sensitizing gradient pulses, and the resulting T2 decay compromises the S/N ratio in the diffusion-weighted image. This has serious consequences when studying objects with short T2 and small D values, which is often the case of interest. The use of stimulated echoes (STEs) for diffusion studies was proposed as a way to solve this problem.[54, 55] STE methods have advantages when one works with systems in which T1 is much greater than T2, which is virtually always the case for in vivo imaging.

Three RF pulses are required to form an STE, and for a typical implementation they are all 90° pulses (see Fig. 8–9). The initial 90° pulse tips the longitudinal magnetization into the transverse plane, the second pulse tips a portion of the transverse magnetization back onto the longitudinal axis, and the final 90° pulse again tips the magnetization back to the transverse plane. One can think of the magnetization as evolving through three periods: for a time TE/2 after the first pulse it is transverse, for a time TM between the second and third pulses it is longitudinal, and for another period TE/2 after the third pulse it is again transverse. At the end of this time the STE occurs.

The key effect of this pulse sequence is that any phase changes acquired by the local transverse magnetization during the first transverse period are partially preserved during the longitudinal period. The magnetization is then returned to the transverse plane flipped by 180° (the combined effect of the two 90° pulses), and after evolution for another TE/2 period an echo forms. Furthermore, during the longitudinal period the magnetization decays with time constant T1 rather than T2, so this period can be made quite long. The effect is as if we froze the precessing magnetization during the time TM, applied a 180° RF pulse, and then let the transverse magnetization continue to evolve to create an echo. However, the STE amplitude is only half of a conventional SE amplitude for the same TE, because only one component of the transverse magnetization can be stored along the longitudinal axis; the other component continues to decay by T2 during TM and so does not contribute to the STE. STEs are the basis for the stimulated-echo acquisition mode (STEAM) imaging pulse sequence.

STE pulse sequences are useful for extending the diffusion time Δ. By placing diffusion-sensitizing gradient pulses during the two transverse periods, the diffusion time Δ can be made much longer than T2 by increasing TM without suffering a severe signal loss. For imaging applications, diffusion sensitivity can be combined with STEAM imaging. This implementation is desirable especially when time-dependent diffusion (i.e., restricted diffusion) is of interest. Also, as shown later, the STEAM implementation combined with a single-shot technique such as echo-planar imaging (EPI) can be utilized for diffusion imaging even for rapidly moving organs like the heart.

Steady-State Free Precession Methods

Fast imaging using steady-state techniques has also been used to perform diffusion imaging.[56, 57] When RF pulses are applied with repetition time (TR) less than T2, the magnetization reaches a condition called steady-state free precession (SSFP). In SSFP the magnitude of the magnetization depends on both T1 and T2 and on the flip angle α. This pulse sequence is much more sensitive to diffusion than either SE or STE pulse sequences, and the sensitivity depends strongly on the flip angle.[58, 59] The SSFP signal can be viewed as the sum of many echoes: each RF pulse creates an echo of previous transverse magnetization. These echoes can be either direct SEs or STEs, but the STEs are strongly attenuated by diffusion because of the long diffusion times. With small flip angles, the SSFP signal is mostly composed of STEs, so diffusion sensitivity is enhanced.[59] Although these techniques have short acquisition times and high diffusion sensitivity, they are also highly susceptible to motion artifacts. But owing to the short acquisition times, it is possible to perform several averages to reduce these effects.[60] Quantitation of diffusion coefficients is not straightforward with these steady-state techniques because of complex signal dependence on the relaxation times in addition to diffusion.[58, 59, 61]

Motion Artifact Reduction

Because diffusion imaging pulse sequences are made sensitive to microscopic motions, they are also highly sensitive to any other undesired motions that may be present in the object.[62] This high sensitivity to motion has serious consequences when performing in vivo studies. Tissue pulsations, microcirculation, motion of the patient, and so forth lead to artifacts (increased signal attenuation and ghosting) in the diffusion-sensitive image.[63] Studies of brain parenchymal motions using phase-contrast MRI have shown that brain tissues are displaced up to 0.5 mm during the cardiac cycle.[64, 65] Even though these are small displacements for conventional imaging, they can produce a significant effect in diffusion-weighted imaging. Several approaches to minimizing motion artifacts in diffusion imaging have been proposed, including projection reconstruction in place of Fourier encoding, motion compensation or correction techniques, and fast or ultrafast imaging techniques.

The most prominent motion artifact is the ghosting caused by phase contamination resulting from the motion between phase-encoding steps. One way to avoid these artifacts is to use projection reconstruction in place of phase encoding.[66] With projection reconstruction methods, motion artifacts tend to average out, but these methods are more sensitive to resonance frequency offsets caused by field inhomogeneity, magnetic susceptibility variations, and chemical shift. A modified version of projection reconstruction imaging was proposed to minimize these artifacts[67]; however, this technique has not come into general use.

Motion compensation techniques using bipolar diffusion gradients to minimize the effect of bulk motion[62] have also been proposed. Each of the gradient pulses of a standard PGSE sequence is replaced by a pair of pulses with opposite sign (a bipolar pulse). The cost of motion compensation is that the sensitivity to diffusion is significantly reduced as well (i.e., the maximal b is reduced). For equal TE values, the gradient pulse duration for the unipolar implementation could be twice that of the bipolar version, making the difference in b values about a factor of 5 with the value for unipolar implementation being higher.

Navigator echoes have been used to correct for motion artifacts[68, 69] in diffusion-weighted images. In this technique, additional echoes with no phase encoding are acquired to estimate the phase errors caused by motion during application of diffusion gradients and used to correct the phase-encoded image data. Although the technique has been shown to provide diffusion-weighted images free of ghost artifacts, there are certain restrictions on the diffusion gradient orientation. The correction is found to be most effective only when the diffusion gradients are applied along the phase-encode direction.

Fast Diffusion Imaging Methods

Fast imaging techniques collect all of the phase-encode steps required for imaging in a short period. Ultrafast gradient echo (GE) techniques (turbo fast low-angle shot [turboFLASH]) use short TR values (typically 4 to 6 ms) with low flip angles to provide a proton density–weighted image in less than 1 second. Contrast can be augmented by applying suitable preparation modules. One such technique applied to diffusion imaging was high-speed STEAM[70] (Fig. 8–10). Two 90° RF pulses prepare the longitudinal magnetization, which is then read out by the application of n low-flip-angle pulses. The technique has several advantages. Unlike GE techniques, high-speed STEAM acquires RF-refocused STE signals and thus the images resemble conventional SE images. They are also free from flow, chemical shift, and susceptibility-related artifacts. One disadvantage is that the low S/N ratio available necessitates multiple averages. Also, the diffusion weighting varies with each phase-encode step, leading to blurring.

EPI, proposed first by Mansfield,[71] is the fastest clinically useful imaging technique and allows collection of data required for image reconstruction in 30 to 100 ms. The entire image data set is acquired after a single excitation pulse with rapid gradient switching to generate GEs (see Fig. 8–10). Because a single shot is used, the magnetization is not saturated by previous RF pulses, so the S/N ratio is high. EPI is ideally suited for diffusion imaging, because ghost artifacts due to motion are virtually eliminated. Owing to short image acquisition times, diffusion-weighted images with several gradient values can be obtained, making quantitation more robust. Volume coverage can also be improved.[72]

With the evolution of enhanced gradient systems,

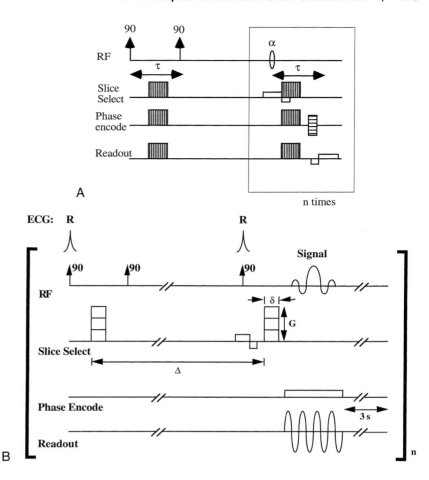

FIGURE 8–10. Fast imaging diffusion-weighted pulse sequences. *A,* Diagram of the high-speed STEAM imaging pulse sequence. The first two RF pulses prepare the magnetization, which is then read out with a series of closely spaced low-flip-angle pulses. Total data collection for an image can be done in less than 1 second. *B,* Diagram of an STE sequence combined with an EPI pulse sequence. The data are read out as a series of rapidly switched gradient echoes after a single excitation pulse. Total data collection time is 30 to 100 ms. ECG = electrocardiogram.

it is now possible to perform EPI with commercially available whole-body imagers. This has opened up new areas of interest for diffusion imaging, for example, in the heart[18] and in the abdomen.[20, 73] Application to the heart requires the diffusion imaging sequence to have minimal bulk motion sensitivity. For this purpose an STE EPI sequence has been used that combines STEAM excitation and EPI readout to obtain diffusion-weighted images during a breath-hold.[18] The use of STEAM for the heart is particularly suitable because the myocardium has a short T2. Also, it is possible to gate the sequence in such a way that the first and third 90° RF pulses are synchronized to identical phases of two sequential cardiac cycles via the electrocardiogram. By applying diffusion gradient pulses after the first and third RF pulses, the gradient pulses are applied at identical phases of the cardiac cycle. To further avoid any misregistration artifacts, the first two RF pulses are made nonselective.

Hardware Considerations

There are several stringent hardware requirements for diffusion imaging. Because images obtained with different b values are used to calculate the diffusion coefficient, stability of the equipment is important. Because the b factor depends primarily on the strength and duration of the gradient pulse, it is important that the exact gradient waveform applied be known. This requires exact gradient amplifier calibration and good eddy current compensation. Eddy currents become more important when strong gradient pulses are applied. This not only affects the diffusion coefficient quantification but also can introduce image artifacts because of interactions with the imaging gradients. Several approaches have been proposed for reducing the effects of eddy currents. These include use of passive shielding[74] or self-shielded gradient coils.[75] Shielded gradient coils are designed to generate no magnetic field external to the gradient coil set, thus removing the source of eddy currents.

The standard gradient systems on commerical scanners are limited to a gradient strength of 10 mT/m, and thus the b values are usually limited to a few hundred seconds per millimeter squared for reasonable TE values. For the brain, b values up to 1000 s/mm² are usually desired. Also, EPI requires stronger and faster gradient systems than are needed for conventional imaging, and eddy currents caused by the imaging gradients as well as the diffusion-sensitizing gradients need to be considered. In addition, the production of currents in the body by the rapidly switched gradients is of concern for safety reasons. The U.S. Food and Drug Administration has imposed a limit on the rate of magnetic field change of 20 T/s along the long axis of the magnet. This safety limitation sets the ultimate limit on the speed of EPI.

DIFFUSION AROUND LOCAL FIELD PERTURBATIONS

Effect of Local Field Perturbations

The preceding arguments dealt with the effects of diffusion in a linear gradient on the resulting MR signal. For most applications, the field gradient is applied by the experimenter and so is controllable in magnitude and orientation. But in a number of important situations there are local field variations caused by the intrinsic heterogeneity of the tissue or the presence of exogenous contrast agents. The most common example is the field distortion caused by variations in magnetic susceptibility. The effects of susceptibility variations are often seen at the boundaries of different types of tissue (e.g., bone and brain). In the past few years, techniques for measuring the local perfusion state of the tissue have been developed that are based on microscopic susceptibility differences between blood vessels (particularly capillaries and other small vessels) and the surrounding fluid. In one class of techniques, a contrast agent with a high magnetic moment, such as a gadolinium or dysprosium compound, is injected and causes a transient change in the blood susceptibility.[23, 76, 77] It was realized that intrinsic changes in blood susceptibility caused by changes in the oxygenation of hemoglobin can also have a measurable effect on the MR signal.[78–82] To understand these susceptibility-based methods, we must consider the effects of diffusion through local field perturbations.

Early studies in the imaging literature focused on understanding the effects of contrast agents such as microscopic magnetized particles that primarily affect T2.[83–86] The physical picture of this process is that the particles are scattered randomly throughout the medium with each particle creating a local distortion (or perturbation) in the magnetic field (Fig. 8–11). If there was no diffusion, spins near a particle would precess at a different rate than spins far from a particle. For a simple GE pulse sequence, which has only the initial excitation RF pulse, the phase difference between the signals from the near and far spins continues to grow and the net signal from a macrosopic voxel decays away more rapidly than it would if the particles were not present. This is usually characterized by a relaxation time T2* that is less than T2, and this effect for GE pulse sequences is described as a T2* effect. But for an SE pulse sequence the 180° RF pulse refocuses the effects of field offsets so that the signals from the near and far spins come back into phase and create the SE. If there is no diffusion, the SE signal at the echo peak should be unaffected by the presence of field perturbations.

With diffusion, however, the SE signal is also affected. The nature of the diffusion effect is quite different from that of the effects in a linear gradient. We can imagine a hypothetic experiment in which we begin with no diffusion (D = 0) and then slowly increase D, repeating our SE and GE experiments as we go. As we start with D = 0, we see a substantial signal loss in the GE experiment and no signal loss in

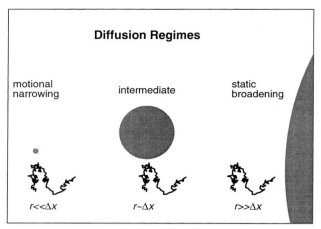

FIGURE 8–11. Diffusion through field perturbations. Microscopic magnetized bodies create local field distortions, and diffusion through these inhomogeneous fields leads to a relaxivity change ΔR_2. The form of ΔR_2 depends on how the typical distance moved by diffusion Δx compares with the size of the field perturber r (e.g., for spherical perturbers r is the sphere radius). Three regimes are illustrated by showing the same random walk path next to spheres of different sizes. These regimes can be described as motional narrowing (r $<<$ Δx), intermediate (r $\sim$ Δx), and static broadening (r $>>$ Δx). The effects are similar for magnetized cylinders (capillaries), with r the radius of the cylinder.

the SE experiment. From the preceding discussion of diffusion in linear field gradients, we might naively expect more signal loss as D increases, and initially we do see the SE signal decrease. However, the GE signal increases with increasing D (i.e., there is less signal loss). As we continue to increase D, the GE signal continues to increase but the SE signal exhibits more complex behavior. As D increases the SE signal first decreases but then begins to level off and finally, when D is large enough, the SE signal begins to increase. In this regime the SE and GE signals are nearly the same. The effect that leads to this odd behavior is called *motional narrowing*, and it occurs when the typical distance moved by a spin as a result of diffusion during the experiment is much larger than the size of the local field perturbation. In the following sections we try to explain how this odd behavior comes about and consider some of the quantitative details of these magnetic susceptibility effects.

Effects of Nonuniform Magnetic Susceptibility

The magnetic susceptibility (χ) is a measure of the degree to which a material becomes magnetized when placed in a magnetic field.[87] In a strong magnetic field B_0, the intrinsic magnetic moments within a material tend to align with the field, creating a magnetization $M = \chi B_0$. The magnetization M has the same physical dimensions as magnetic field, so χ is dimensionless. For nonferromagnetic materials, χ is on the order of 10^{-6} and is usually expressed in parts per million. The susceptibility χ arises mainly from internal dipole moments resulting from 1) nuclei with an odd number of neutrons or protons, 2) unpaired electrons, and 3) the molecular orbital motions of electrons. The first effect, that of nuclear dipole moments, is, of course, the basis of NMR. However, the contribution of the nuclei to χ is negligible compared with the contributions from the other two sources. The magnetic moment of an electron is larger by three orders of magnitude than the moment of the proton, so the alignment of unpaired electrons with B_0 creates a large contribution to χ (paramagnetism). The orbital motions of electrons also create a magnetic dipole moment, but the nature of these orbital moments is that they align opposite to the field (diamagnetism). For this reason χ may be positive or negative, depending on the balance of the diamagnetic and paramagnetic components. Exogenous contrast agents are primarily paramagnetic.

The effects of nonuniform magnetic susceptibility can be seen in conventional MRI. When χ varies from one tissue to another (e.g., at tissue-bone or tissue-air interfaces), the local magnetic field varies and there are intrinsic field gradients near tissue interfaces. Because the precession frequency of nuclei is proportional to the local magnetic field, the local signal phase acquired after a time TE is also proportional to the field offset. For this reason the phase of GE images is essentially a map of the field offsets. Figure 8–12 shows typical large-scale field gradients through the brain associated with the sinus cavities. In addition to this bulk phase effect, field variations within a voxel lead to phase variations in the signal of the precessing spins and a loss of net signal from the voxel (T2* effect). For GE pulse sequences these effects can be pronounced (e.g., at 1.5 T a field difference of 1 ppm causes the spins to become 180° out of phase after only about 8 ms of precession). GE imaging with long TE is thus quite sensitive to susceptibility variations. On the other hand, the 180° RF pulse in an SE pulse sequence is designed to refocus inhomogeneity effects such as this, and to a large degree it does. However, as described earlier, diffusion of water molecules through nonuniform fields leads to imperfect refocusing and

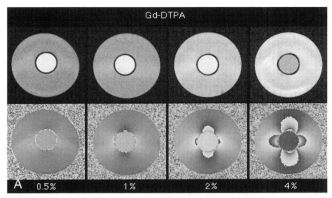

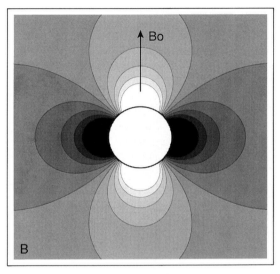

FIGURE 8–13. Field distortions around a magnetized cylinder. *A,* Magnitude and phase images of concentric cylinders with water in the outer cylinder and different concentrations of Gd-DTPA in the inner cylinder. The phase images show a dipolar field distortion outside the inner cylinder caused by the magnetic susceptibility difference $\Delta\chi$ between the two liquids. The concentrations are volume fractions of commercial Gd-DTPA. A bolus injection of Gd-DTPA is probably diluted to about 3% during the first pass through the brain. Fully deoxygenated blood with a hematocrit of 40% produces a $\Delta\chi$ equivalent to about 0.5% Gd-DTPA. For the highest concentration the field distortions are sufficiently large that the magnitude image shows some spatial distortion. *B,* For comparison, a plot of the theoretic field distortion (B_z) outside a magnetized infinite cylinder, in good agreement with the experimental images. A field offset of zero is colored a medium gray, so white and black indicate positive and negative field offsets.

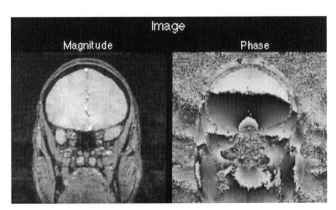

FIGURE 8–12. Field variations caused by magnetic susceptibility variations in the brain. The phase of a GE image primarily reflects local magnetic field offsets and can be taken as a map of the local field. Field distortions caused by the different magnetic susceptibilities of the sinus cavities (air) and the brain (water) are clearly seen. On the phase images the gray scale is mapped over the range 0° to 360°, so larger phase values are wrapped, producing sharp transitions from white to black.

signal loss in SE imaging as well, although SE imaging is still much less sensitive to susceptibility effects than is GE imaging.

When a body is surrounded by a medium with a different susceptibility, the local field distortions depend on both the susceptibility difference $\Delta\chi$ and the geometry of the perturber. For example, Figure 8–13 shows maps of the field distortions around a cylinder with different concentrations of gadolinium. In each image the central cylinder contains a gadolinium solution and the outer cylinder contains pure water. Inside the cylinder the field is uniform (but shifted); outside the field has a dipole pattern.

These images can serve as a model for the effects of microscopic susceptibility variations in tissues. When the susceptibility of the blood is altered (e.g., by injecting Gd-DTPA or by a change in the concentration of deoxyhemoglobin), the magnetic field around the vessels is distorted. For a magnetized cylinder the field offset is largest at the surface and falls off with increasing distance. The magnitude of this maximal field distortion depends on the susceptibility difference between the cylinder and the surrounding medium but is independent of the cylinder radius. However, the field falls off more rapidly with distance for smaller cylinders. Thus, for smaller cylinders the field gradient produced is larger but the extent of the field distortion is smaller. Because of the larger gradients, we expect the smaller vessels (capillaries, arterioles, and venules) to show the strongest diffusion-related effects. But the fact that the field distortions are small suggests that the nature of the diffusion effects may be quite different from that for diffusion in a linear field gradient.

Motional Narrowing

The key physical difference between diffusion through an array of magnetized cylinders and diffusion in a linear field gradient is that in the former the range of fields a spin can experience is limited. In a linear field gradient, the farther a spin moves the larger the field offset, and spins that tend to diffuse in different directions acquire large phase differences. If the cylinders are small enough (or the diffusion coefficient is high enough), it is possible for a spin to diffuse past many cylinders and thus sample the full range of field distortions. If all of the diffusing spins also sample all of the field variations, the spins acquire about the same net phase, corresponding to precession in the average field. With relatively little phase dispersion present, the signal is only slightly decreased. If D increases (or the cylinder diameter decreases), the averaging is even more effective and there is less attenuation. This phenomenon is often described as *motional narrowing*, in reference to the fact that the local spectral line width becomes narrower. (The local signal decay rate R_2 and the spectral line width are proportional to one another; if there is less signal loss, R_2 is smaller and so the line is narrower.)

Motional narrowing affects both the GE and SE signals, and indeed the two signals are nearly the same in this regime. The reason is that when spins are moving through variable fields the pattern of field fluctuations felt before the 180° pulse has no relation to the fields felt after the 180° pulse, so the SE process is ineffective. Motional narrowing is similar to T2 decay, discussed at the beginning of this chapter. In this regime ΔR_2 decreases when D increases, the opposite of the dependence on D in a linear gradient.

Modeling Diffusion Around Field Perturbations

We can develop a more quantitative understanding of diffusion effects by introducing a few physical pa-

rameters that characterize the system. Let $\tau_R = R^2/D$ be the typical time required for a spin to diffuse past the region of field distortion of size R produced by a local perturbing body. For example, for a magnetized capillary bed τ_R is the time required to diffuse a distance equal to the capillary radius. The magnitude of the field perturbation can be characterized by the maximal field offset at the surface of the cylinder (or for a sphere the equatorial field offset at the surface). Different authors have expressed this field offset in different ways (e.g., in milligauss or angular frequency), but for this discussion it is convenient to express it as a resonance frequency offset ν in hertz, following Ogawa and coworkers.[88] Finally, the observation time of an experiment, TE, is also an important factor.

The physical system can thus be characterized by three time-related parameters: τ_R, ν, and TE. For the case of diffusion around magnetized capillaries, it is a remarkable fact that these time constants have similar magnitudes. For a capillary radius of 4 μm and a typical value of D = 0.001 mm²/s for brain, τ_R is about 16 ms. For fully deoxygenated blood with a hematocrit of 40%, the susceptibility difference between the capillary and the surrounding fluid is about 0.07 ppm, and for a main magnetic field strength of 1.5 T this gives a ν of about 28 Hz, so $1/\nu$ is about 36 ms. A typical TE value for imaging studies is 40 ms.

That these three time constants are similar is a source of difficulty in developing a quantitative understanding of diffusion-related signal loss. If instead τ_R was much smaller than $1/\nu$ or TE, as it would be with particles smaller than 1 μm, we could assume that a diffusing spin sampled the fields around a number of cylinders. Analytic solutions based on motional narrowing could then be applied.[83] On the other hand, if τ_R was much larger than $1/\nu$ or TE, we could assume that each spin does not stray far from where it starts. Then the problem could be treated as an extension of the linear gradient theory by assuming that each spin is diffusing in a local linear gradient but there is a distribution of gradient values.[85] For the case of diffusion around capillaries, neither of these approximations applies, and investigators have been forced to use numeric simulations to probe this regime.

With a Monte Carlo numeric simulation, the geometry of the perturbing field (usually assumed to be due to either magnetized spheres or cylinders) is first established. Then many random walks are explicitly calculated for spins diffusing through the perturbed fields, and the results are appropriately averaged to determine signal attenuation for either GE or SE experiments.[84, 86, 89–91] The calculated attenuation is taken to be of the form $\exp(-\Delta R_2 t)$, and the observed change in relaxation rate ΔR_2 for SE experiments or ΔR_2^* for GE experiments is then plotted as a function of different parameters of the problem (e.g., perturber size, density, or $\Delta \chi$).

Weisskoff and colleagues[91] compared Monte Carlo calculations with direct experiments for spheres with diameters ranging from 1 to 20 μm suspended in solutions of Dys-DTPA to alter the susceptibility difference and found excellent agreement. In Figure 8–14, their plots of ΔR_2 and ΔR_2^* versus sphere diameter have been redrawn as a plot of relaxivity versus τ_R. These curves illustrate the important features of relaxation resulting from diffusion through field perturbations. Consider the GE curve first, and bear in mind that an increase in relaxivity corresponds to a decrease in signal. When τ_R is large (large sphere diameter), the GE relaxivity is large and independent of the exact value of τ_R. This is the static broadening regime, where diffusion is not important and there is substantial GE signal loss simply because there is a range of fields within the voxel. As τ_R is decreased, spins begin to feel more of the range of field variations and motional narrowing begins to be effective, so ΔR_2^* decreases and the GE signal increases. For short τ_R there is little signal loss in the GE experiment. For SE the relaxivity is similar to that for GE when τ_R is small, again because of motional narrowing. When τ_R is large, the SE effectively refocuses the field offsets, so there is little loss of the SE signal (unlike the GE signal). The maximal SE relaxivity occurs at an intermediate regime, where τ_R is not small enough for motional narrowing to work and not large enough for the SE process to work. For these data the peak of the SE curve occurs at about $\tau_R = 7$ ms for $1/\nu = 35$ ms and TE = 40 ms.

The MR effects of diffusion through nonlinear gradients are thus somewhat complex and depend on several properties of the tissue. In the following sections we consider two methods for assessing the perfusion state of tissue that are based on creating a susceptibility difference between blood and the surrounding extravascular space. The first is based on injection of an appropriate contrast agent, and the second is based on intrinsic susceptibility changes in the blood itself.

PERFUSION IMAGING

In the previous sections we have described in some detail the effects of diffusion on the MR signal. Diffusion in a linear field gradient is the prototypic example

of these effects and forms the basis for measuring diffusion by applying carefully controlled and geometrically simple gradient fields. Diffusion through field perturbations introduces qualitatively different features and a more complex behavior. Diffusion around magnetized blood vessels is the primary example we have considered, and this biophysical system is central to understanding methods for assessing the perfusion state of a tissue based on changes in blood susceptibility. Before applying the diffusion ideas developed earlier to these applications, we must broaden the scope of the discussion to define precisely what we mean by perfusion. Several distinct physiologic parameters are related to the perfusion state of a tissue, and each may produce measurable effects on the MR signal. Exactly how each of these parameters changes in different physiologic states is not well known, so it is important to try to clarify exactly what each of the MR methods measures. In the following we also review some of the principles of kinetic modeling, which originated in tracer studies but are now finding increasing application in MR studies. In this discussion we focus on the brain, but the principles apply to other organs as well.

PERFUSION STATE OF TISSUE

Perfusion-Related Physiologic Parameters

Perfusion describes the nutritive blood supply to an element of tissue.[92] For this discussion we take a specific quantitative definition of perfusion to distinguish it from other physiologic parameters that may also affect the MR signal, such as blood volume, blood velocity, and blood oxygenation (Fig. 8–15 and Table 8–1).

PERFUSION. Consider a volume of tissue (V). The capillary beds within V are supplied with arterial blood at a rate F (milliliters per minute). The perfusion (f) is then f = F/V, the milliliters of arterial blood delivered per minute per milliliter of tissue. With this definition of perfusion, f has dimensions of 1/minute and

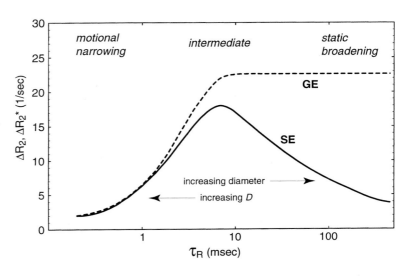

FIGURE 8–14. Relaxivity changes related to diffusion through field perturbations. Transverse relaxivity changes observed for SE (ΔR_2) and GE (ΔR_2^*) pulse sequences plotted as a function of τ_R, the typical time required to diffuse past the local field perturbation (specifically, $\tau_R = r^2/D$, where r is the radius of a magnetized sphere). Curves were calculated from experimental data and numeric Monte Carlo simulations reported by Weisskoff and colleagues[91] for magnetized spheres 1 to 20 μm in diameter suspended in a 11.2 mM solution of Dys-DTPA ($\Delta\chi \sim 0.6$ ppm). Two other time parameters in addition to τ_R are needed to describe these effects fully: the reciprocal of the resonant frequency offset ν at the surface of the sphere and TE. For these data typical values are $1/\nu \sim 35$ ms and TE ~ 40 ms, and the peak SE relaxivity occurs at $\tau_R \sim 7$ ms. For small τ_R, diffusing spins sample all of the field variations so that the relaxivity changes with motional narrowing are small. For large τ_R, diffusion is a small effect, so the GE signal is strongly reduced (large ΔR_2^*) as a result of static field broadening. In this regime the SE process is effective, so the SE relaxivity change is reduced.

Perfusion

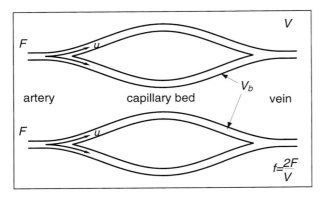

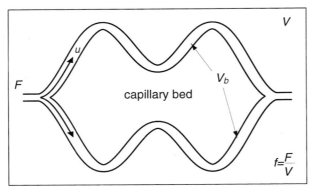

FIGURE 8–15. The meaning of perfusion. Two idealized capillary beds illustrating the distinction between blood volume (V_b), blood velocity (u), and perfusion (f). In each bed V_b and u are the same, but f is twice as large in the top configuration. In the top panel a tissue volume V is fed by two arteries each with flow F (milliliters per minute), so the perfusion is f = 2F/V. In the bottom panel the capillaries are twice as long (so the blood volume is the same) but fed by only one artery, so f = F/V. Thus, blood volume and velocity do not uniquely define perfusion unless capillary length is uniform for all capillary beds. (In practice, the interpretation of measurements of V_b and u is further complicated by the fact that most of the tissue blood volume is venous rather than capillary.)

is thus a rate constant. In fact, f is the fundamental rate constant that governs the delivery of metabolic substrates (e.g., glucose and oxygen) and the clearance of products of metabolism (e.g., CO_2 and lactate). This definition differs slightly from the standard definition of perfusion as milliliters of blood per minute per 100 g of tissue (the standard definition of cerebral blood flow [CBF]).[93] The latter definition is more practical for experimental studies in which tissue samples are measured for concentrations of radioactive tracers, but the definition we use is convenient for imaging studies that sample a known volume of tissue.

BLOOD VOLUME. The fraction of the total tissue volume within a voxel occupied by blood (arteries, capillaries, and veins) is V_b, a dimensionless quantity. The blood volume V_b and the perfusion f are distinct quantities, and in principle there need not be any consistent relation between them. Experimentally, however, f and V_b are often strongly correlated in the normally functioning brain.[94]

BLOOD VELOCITY. The velocity (u) of flowing blood is, of course, quite different in arteries, capillaries, and veins. Nevertheless, because the MR signal can be quite sensitive to motion, it is useful to consider the mean blood velocity u as another parameter describing the perfusion state of the tissue. If changes in the perfusion f are accompanied by changes in velocity at all levels of the vascular tree, u may correlate with f. However, it should be noted that f, V_b, and u are in general distinct and independent physiologic quantities. Figure 8–15 illustrates in a schematic way that determination of V_b and u is not sufficient to determine f. In practice, these three quantities (f, V_b, and u) are usually strongly correlated, but this correlation may not hold in pathologic states. Often the term perfusion is used loosely to describe measurements that are sensitive to V_b or u as well as f.

OXYGEN EXTRACTION FRACTION. As already noted, f is the fundamental rate constant for delivery of metabolic substrates to the tissue. However, we must introduce another parameter, the extraction fraction E, to describe the fraction of delivered substrate that is taken up (extracted) by the tissue. For example, only 30% to 50% of the O_2 delivered to brain tissue is metabolized[95]; the rest is cleared by venous flow. The local cerebral metabolic rate of O_2 (CMRO$_2$) can be written as $CMRO_2 = EfC_a(O_2)$, where E is the net extraction fraction and $C_a(O_2)$ is the arterial O_2 concentration. In this expression all of the complexities of O_2 transport are lumped into the parameter E, and it is important to remember that E is also likely to vary as f changes. The extraction fraction is also simply related to the arterial and venous concentrations ($C_a(O_2)$ and $C_v(O_2)$, respectively) as $E = (C_a(O_2) - C_v(O_2))/C_a(O_2)$. Changes in venous blood oxygenation resulting from changes in E are the basis for the blood oxygenation level–dependent (BOLD) contrast brain activation studies described later.

TABLE 8–1. PERFUSION-RELATED PHYSIOLOGIC PARAMETERS

PARAMETER	DESCRIPTION	UNITS	EXAMPLE
f	Perfusion	mL blood/min/mL tissue (1/min)	Cerebral blood flow
V_b	Blood volume	mL blood/mL tissue (dimensionless)	Cerebral blood volume
u	Blood velocity	cm/s	
E	Extraction fraction	Dimensionless	Oxygen extraction fraction
C_a	Arterial concentration of substrate	mmol/mL	
C_v	Venous concentration of substrate	mmol/mL	
p	Partition coefficient	Dimensionless	
τ	Mean transit time	Seconds	

TISSUE-BLOOD PARTITION COEFFICIENT. A key parameter for describing the kinetics of an agent as it passes through a tissue is the partition coefficient p. The partition coefficient measures the equilibrium distribution of the agent between blood and tissue. If C_a is held constant for a long time, the tissue concentration C_T approaches an asymptotic value pC_a. When C_a and C_T are expressed in the same units (e.g., moles per milliliter), p is dimensionless. If the agent is simply diffusing between tissue volumes (i.e., it is never bound in a particular space), p is simply the volume of distribution of the agent. For example, for an agent that remains in the blood (such as Gd-DTPA in the normal brain) p is the local blood volume (V_b); for an agent that freely diffuses into the tissue (such as labeled H_2O) p is about 1.0.

MEAN TRANSIT TIME THROUGH THE TISSUE. Another important parameter for describing the transport kinetics of an agent is the mean transit time τ through the tissue. For agents that remain in the blood (such as Gd-DTPA), τ is only a few seconds, whereas for agents that diffuse out of the blood and into the larger tissue space (such as labeled H_2O) τ is much longer.

Physiologic Changes in the Brain Perfusion State

More than 100 years ago, Roy and Sherrington[96] proposed the theory that blood flow adjusts to meet the changing metabolic demands of the brain. Confidence in this idea has waxed and waned,[97] but on the whole it is still the dominant principle for understanding changes in normal brain perfusion. Several techniques have been developed for assessing brain blood flow in humans, beginning with the Kety-Schmidt technique in 1948[98] and continuing with radioactive ^{133}Xe methods and positron emission tomography (PET) methods using water labeled with ^{15}O.[93] With these techniques, reproducible local changes in blood flow have been found to occur during performance of a variety of motor, sensory, and cognitive tasks.[99] In addition, changes in the CO_2 content or pH of the blood strongly affect CBF, with increased CO_2 or decreased pH stimulating CBF.[95] This sensitivity to one of the products of oxidative metabolism certainly suggests the basis for a coupling of blood flow to metabolic needs. But other factors also affect blood flow (such as NO, K^+, and adenosine), and the nature of the coupling between flow and metabolism is still not well understood.[100]

Fox and coworkers[101, 102] reported some surprising results that make the nature of the relationship between flow and metabolism more puzzling and even cast doubt on the Roy and Sherrington hypothesis itself. In PET studies of somatosensory and visual stimulation in humans, they found a large imbalance in the local changes in CBF, O_2 metabolism, and glucose metabolism. During these tasks, the CBF and glucose metabolic rate increased by 30% to 50% focally in the appropriate regions of the brain, but O_2 metabolism increased only about 5%. These data have been interpreted in a number of ways, ranging from viewing them as evidence for an uncoupling of flow and oxidative metabolism[102] to viewing them as evidence for tight coupling in the presence of limited O_2 extraction from the capillaries.[103]

MRI has provided an unexpected confirmation of this imbalance in flow and metabolic changes.[80–82] If flow increases more than O_2 metabolism, less O_2 is removed from the blood and the venous blood oxygenation must increase. The MR signal is sensitive to this change because deoxyhemoglobin is paramagnetic.[104] As the concentration of deoxyhemoglobin increases, the susceptibility difference between the blood and the surrounding space also increases, and the resulting microscopic field variations lead to a decrease in the MR signal. In the resting state the normal brain extracts about 40% of the O_2 delivered to it, and this level of venous and capillary deoxyhemoglobin attenuates the signal by a few percent with T2*-weighted pulse sequences in a 1.5-T field. If the flow then increases by 50% while the O_2 metabolism increases by only 5%,[102] the O_2 extraction fraction must drop to about 28%. The deoxyhemoglobin concentration is then reduced and the MR signal increases slightly. This MR signal increase during brain activation has now been measured during a wide range of sensory, motor, and cognitive tasks.[26] Although the underlying reasons are still unknown, it appears that a strong imbalance in blood flow and O_2 metabolism is a common occurrence during brain activation. In the last section of this chapter the applications of this effect in FMRI are discussed in more detail.

MR is also potentially sensitive to the other perfusion-related physiologic parameters defined earlier. Animal and human studies using radioactive tracers and altered partial pressure of carbon dioxide (PCO_2) as a means of changing global brain perfusion have consistently shown an increase in cerebral blood volume (CBV) accompanying increased flow.[94, 105–107] Most of these studies used labeled red blood cells as the blood volume marker, but Sakai and colleagues[107] also used a plasma marker. They found that inhalation of 5% CO_2 produced a larger change in the plasma volume than in the red blood cell volume, a finding that may bear on MR perfusion studies. In Gd-DTPA studies the plasma susceptibility is altered, but with BOLD studies the red blood cell susceptibility is altered. We may thus expect these different methods to have different sensitivities to blood volume changes.

The physiologic mechanism by which perfusion increases is still unclear. We can imagine two distinct scenarios that bracket a range of possibilities, and evidence has been presented for both views. The first is capillary recruitment, in which the flow characteristics within a capillary (e.g., velocity and size) remain constant but more capillaries open up. The second is increased velocity through a fixed capillary bed. Whereas some studies have indicated that at rest as few as 60% of available capillaries are perfused and that this fraction increases when perfusion increases,[108–110] a number of other studies have found that at least 90% of capillaries are open at rest so that perfusion must increase through increased capillary velocity.[111–115] Note that the observation of increased total blood volume is consistent with either mechanism because the methods used cannot distinguish among capillary, venule, and arteriole volume changes. Even with a completely fixed capillary bed the venules may swell as a passive response to a local pressure increase, which would be expected after the arterioles dilate to reduce the local vascular resistance. In addition to the possibility of recruitment, capillary volume may increase by dilatation.[116]

The physiologic picture of what happens during brain activation is thus still incomplete. But the evidence to date suggests the following scenario: perfusion f and total blood volume V_b increase substantially; the O_2 extraction fraction E drops substantially; the local blood velocity u in the arterioles, capillaries, and venules probably increases with an accompanying drop in the transit time τ; and the capillary density probably stays about the same (but may increase).

PRINCIPLES OF KINETIC MODELING

Tissue Concentration-Time Curve

In nuclear medicine studies, the concentration of a radioactive tracer in a tissue is measured over time, and a kinetic model is used to interpret the measured concentration curve in terms of physiologic parameters such as those in Table 8–1.[117–120] With the development of MR perfusion imaging methods the same kinetic modeling ideas can be applied to measurements of the MR signal. With MR the "tracer" could be an injected contrast agent or, as discussed later, a volume of blood labeled with a tagging RF pulse. In this section we summarize some basic kinetic modeling results needed for the interpretation of MR data. The important question is: How is the measured tissue concentration of an agent related to local physiologic parameters such as perfusion and blood volume?

After injection of an agent (such as Gd-DTPA), the local tissue concentration as a function of time $C_T(t)$ can be written in terms of the arterial concentration $C_a(t)$ as

$$C_T(t) = \int_0^t fC_a(t')R(t-t')\,dt' = fC_a(t)*R(t) \quad (11)$$

where f is the local perfusion, R(t) is the local residue function (or impulse response of the system), and * indicates convolution. Specifically, R(t) is the probability that a molecule of the agent that entered the voxel at time t = 0 is still there at time t. Equation 11 can be interpreted as simply adding up the amount of the agent that entered the voxel at all times in the past weighted with the probability that the agent is still in the voxel at time t. The condition required for the validity of Equation 11 is that when each molecule of the agent enters the capillary bed it has the same possible fates as every other molecule of the agent. This condition could break down if the underlying physiology is not in a steady state (e.g., if f is changing

during the experiment) or if the agent is present in such a high concentration that there is competition for a saturable transport system (e.g., glucose extraction from the capillary bed in the brain has a limited capacity and can be saturated). In the latter case a molecule that enters when the agent concentration is low would have a higher probability of being extracted than one that entered when the concentration is high. But for tracer studies Equation 11 is an accurate general expression for the tissue concentration as a function of time.

The form of R(t) depends on the details of the transport of the agent between blood and tissue and the clearance of the agent from the voxel volume. For example, in MR studies the contrast agent Gd-DTPA remains confined to the vascular space (in normal brain) but labeled water freely diffuses into the tissue space. Regardless of the form of R(t), there is always a simple mathematic relationship between R(t) and the mean transit time:

$$\tau = \int_0^\infty R(t)\,dt \quad (12)$$

Central Volume Principle

The central volume principle (CVP) is an important and useful relationship between key physiologic parameters that has been recognized for the past hundred years.[119–121] The CVP states that the perfusion f, partition coefficient p, and mean transit time τ are always related by

$$f = \frac{p}{\tau} \quad (13)$$

The CVP can be derived by combining Equation 11 with the definition of p. If C_a is held constant for a long time compared with the time required for R(t) to become small, then from Equation 11 C_T approaches $f\tau C_a$. But by the definition of p, this equilibrium value of C_T is pC_a and Equation 13 then follows directly.

The CVP is a remarkably general relationship. It applies to any agent, whether or not it is extracted from the capillary bed, and we can use Equation 13 to estimate the lifetime of different agents in the brain. For a typical human CBF of 60 mL/min per 100 g, f in our units is 0.01 s^{-1}. For an agent confined to the vascular space ($p = V_b = 0.04$), the mean tissue transit time is 4 seconds, but for a freely diffusible agent ($p = 1.0$) τ is about 100 seconds.

Equations 11 and 13 provide a useful and robust interpretation of a measured local tissue concentration curve:

$$\int_0^\infty C_T\,dt = p\int_0^\infty C_a\,dt \quad (14)$$

where we have made use of the fact that the integral of a convolution is the product of the separate integrals. Because C_a is the same for all tissue elements, the integral of the local tissue curve is simply proportional to the local value of p. For an agent that remains in the blood $p = V_b$, and a measured tissue concentration curve then provides a direct measure of local blood volume. Note that we can apply this result to obtain relative values of V_b without knowing $C_a(t)$ or the form of $R(t)$.

Measuring Perfusion

Equation 11 applies to a wide range of agents, but we have achieved this generality by lumping all of the details of transport and uptake of the agent into the single function $R(t)$. In particular, Equation 11 hides the full dependence of the tissue curve on perfusion because $R(t)$ usually depends on f as well. A more detailed consideration of the form of $R(t)$ for different agents is therefore necessary to clarify how the measured kinetics of an agent can be used to measure the local perfusion. By definition, $R(t)$ is the probability that a molecule of the agent that entered the capillary bed at $t = 0$ is still there at time t, so $R(0) = 1$ because there has been no time for it to leave. Furthermore, $R(t)$ must decrease monotonically with increasing time and must be of a form that satisfies the CVP (Equation 13): $\int R(t)\, dt = \tau = p/f$.

Consider first how Equation 11 can be applied to microsphere studies in which injected labeled spheres are too large to fit through the capillaries and so remain lodged in the tissue. For this agent, $R(t) = 1$ for all time (because the microspheres never leave the tissue), and so by Equation 11 the measured tissue concentration is simply the perfusion f times the integral of the arterial concentration. This is a robust method for measuring f and is usually considered the "gold standard" for perfusion measurements. The integrated arterial curve can be measured from any convenient artery and need not be measured locally. (The form $R(t) = 1$ does mathematically satisfy the CVP because both the integral of $R(t)$ and the partition coefficient p are infinite.)

A diffusible tracer is one that freely crosses the blood-brain barrier and enters the extravascular space, such as an inert gas (e.g., ^{133}Xe) or labeled water (e.g., $H_2^{15}O$). A simple form for $R(t)$ that satisfies the CVP and is commonly used to model the kinetics of these agents is $R(t) = e^{-ft/p}$. This exponential form naturally arises in compartmental models in which the rate of transport out of a compartment is taken to be a rate constant times the concentration in the compartment. Indeed, this form of $R(t)$ is equivalent to modeling the tissue as a single well-mixed compartment. We can now consider an ideal prototypic experiment. The agent is quickly introduced into the tissue so that the arterial concentration curve is a narrow function of time (a sharp bolus). In the limit of a perfect bolus, by Equation 11 the tissue curve is proportional to $R(t)$, and the initial value is $f \int C_a\, dt$. In practice, a perfectly sharp bolus cannot be achieved, but this idealization is a fruitful thought experiment for understanding the basic approaches for measuring perfusion.

The local flow thus affects the tissue curve in two distinct ways: the amount of agent delivered to the tissue is directly proportional to f, and the clearance of the agent depends on f through the form of $R(t)$. So either delivery or clearance of the agent can be used as the basis for a measurement of f. With the $H_2^{15}O$ method the tracer is administered rapidly and the initial concentration in the tissue (averaged over the first 40 seconds) is measured locally with PET, directly yielding a measurement proportional to f based on the delivery of the agent.[93] The concentration maps can be calibrated by also measuring the arterial curve. In the ^{133}Xe method the agent is administered by inhalation and the clearance curve is measured with an external detector.[93] The measured tissue curve can then be fit to a decaying exponential and the time constant for clearance is p/f. Provided that p is known (and for diffusible tracers it is near 1), f can be measured directly from the clearance curve. An advantage of this approach is that it is necessary to measure not the *absolute* tissue concentration but just a signal that is proportional to it in order to measure the decay constant. For example, calibration of an external detector for absolute measurements can be difficult because of unknown attenuation in the skull and scalp, but as long as the detector is in a fixed position with respect to the head a clearance curve can be measured.

Although perfusion can be measured with a diffusible tracer either from delivery or from clearance of the agent, measurements based on delivery are more robust. Delivery is always proportional to flow, as with microspheres, and is independent of $R(t)$. But to model clearance a form of $R(t)$ must be assumed, and calculated perfusion is always somewhat model dependent. For example, consider measuring f in a voxel that contains two types of tissue with different perfusion (e.g., gray matter and white matter). Delivery of the tracer is then governed simply by the average value of f in the voxel, but clearance is now more complicated than the simple exponential form; $R(t)$ should be modeled as a biexponential.

From the foregoing arguments we see that the local kinetics of an agent depend on both the local perfusion and the local volume of distribution. Curves of $C_T(t)$ obtained by using Equations 11 and 14 are illustrated in Figure 8–16 to show the sensitivity of the measured curve to these two physiologic parameters. Note that for a vascular agent the curves are strongly sensitive to CBV but only weakly sensitive to CBF. In principle, it is also possible to interpret measured tissue curves in terms of Equation 11 and arrive at an estimate of f. However, measurement of f requires[122] 1) a separate measurement of $C_a(t)$ and 2) knowledge of the form of $R(t)$.

On the basis of the principles that have been outlined, we can broadly characterize different agents in the following way. Agents that remain in the blood can be used for a robust measurement of blood volume, but measurement of perfusion is much more difficult.[122] Diffusible tracers that readily leave the capillary and diffuse through the entire tissue space can be used for a measurement of perfusion, based either on how much of the agent is delivered to the local tissue or on how quickly the agent is cleared from the tissue (washout). The latter effect requires more specific

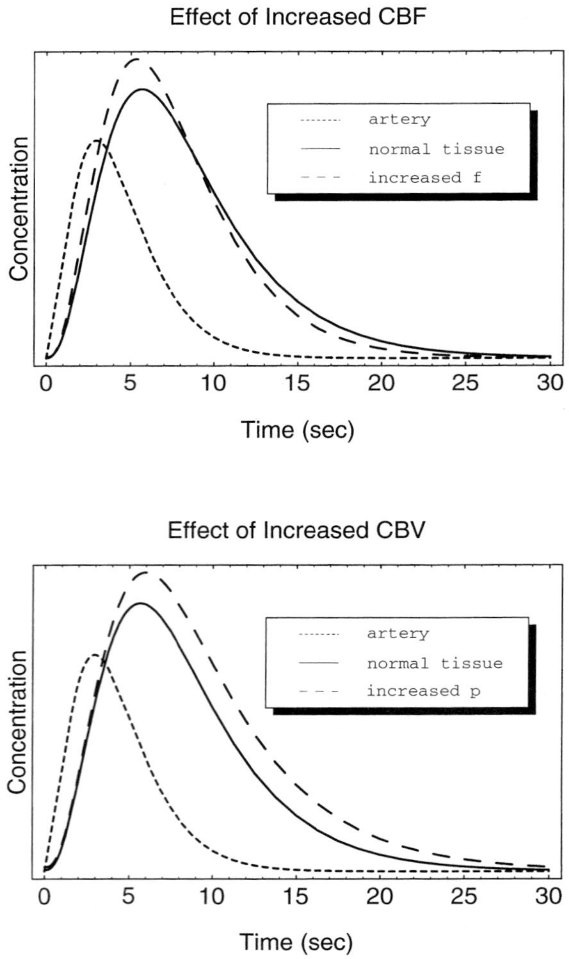

Effect of Increased CBF

Effect of Increased CBV

FIGURE 8–16. Tissue concentration-time curve. Theoretic concentration curves illustrating the sensitivity of the tissue curve to changes in perfusion and blood volume for an ideal vascular agent that remains in the blood. *Top,* Effect of a 30% increase in perfusion. *Bottom,* Effect of a 30% increase in blood volume. Note that a blood volume change simply scales up the tissue curve, so changes are readily measured from the integrated tissue curve. However, a change in perfusion has a more subtle effect on the tissue curve, which depends on the arterial curve (shown as small dashes) and the details of clearance from the tissue.

modeling, so the measured perfusion is potentially more model dependent.

INTRAVOXEL INCOHERENT MOTIONS

An early attempt to develop perfusion-sensitive MR methods was the intravoxel incoherent motion (IVIM) method,[123, 124] an outgrowth of the development of earlier diffusion-weighted imaging. The basic motivation for this approach is that motion of blood in a randomly oriented capillary network should have an effect on the MR signal similar to that of random diffusional motions: when bipolar gradient pulses are applied, the signal should decrease. Because typical blood velocities (>1 mm/s) lead to larger displacements than do diffusional motions, the blood signal

should decrease more rapidly than the extravascular signal. The expected diffusion curve, with signal intensity plotted as a function of b, should have two components, with an initial steep drop reflecting the blood component followed by the normal slow decrease related to diffusion in the rest of the tissue. Careful analysis of the early part of the curve may then allow estimates of the blood volume, based on the size of the initial drop, and the blood velocity, based on the magnitude of b required to reduce the initial signal.

However, the interpretation of IVIM data has proved to be more difficult. One problem is that other factors may also lead to a biphasic signal curve.[125] Cerebrospinal fluid has an intrinsically large diffusion coefficient, and the normal convective motions of cerebrospinal fluid lead to an apparent diffusion coefficient that can be much larger. As a result, partial-volume averaging of gray matter with cerebrospinal fluid can naturally lead to a biphasic signal curve. This problem is compounded by the fact that the signal of interest (that from the blood) is only a small fraction of the total signal. Neil and colleagues[126] proposed a novel pulse sequence using two inversion pulses for suppressing extravascular signal based on the T1 of tissue water and cerebrospinal fluid. By adding Gd-DTPA to reduce the T1 of blood, the contribution of blood to the total signal is substantially increased. Using this method, they demonstrated in a rat model that the flowing volume estimated from the early part of the diffusion curve correlated with increasing P_{CO_2}.[127]

The interpretation of IVIM data is still far from clear. Even in principle, IVIM is not a direct measure of perfusion.[128] As noted before, blood volume and blood velocity are not sufficient to measure perfusion. Although these three quantities (f, u, V_b) may be physiologically correlated in the normal brain, this correlation may well break down in pathologic states. Furthermore, the basic model of the diffusion curve as two components is probably too simple.[129] Studies using ^{19}F imaging of perfluorocarbons that remain in the blood (so that there is no extravascular signal) still show a multiexponential diffusion curve.[130, 131] Henkelman and coworkers[131] argued that such data can be interpreted as a result of the geometry of the vasculature. They showed that a fractal model of the vascular bed naturally leads to a nonmonoexponential diffusion curve. Nevertheless, the IVIM methods are in some way sensitive to changes in the tissue perfusion state. Although interpretation in terms of classic perfusion as we define it here may not be possible, the IVIM methods may provide information on the manner in which flow increases to address the question of capillary recruitment versus increased velocity.[132]

DYNAMIC GD-DTPA STUDIES

Transient Kinetics

One fruitful approach to assessing the perfusion state of tissue with MRI began with the observation that a bolus of Gd-DTPA creates a transient MR signal drop as it passes through the brain.[133, 134] This clearly suggested that dynamic measurement of the kinetics of Gd-DTPA could provide measurements of the perfusion state of the tissue. However, the observed effect was rather surprising, given that Gd-DTPA is commonly used to enhance the MR signal by reducing the T1. This well-understood relaxivity effect is exploited when Gd-DTPA is used routinely as a contrast agent to enhance tumors with a leaky blood-brain barrier. The gadolinium enters the tumor, T1 is reduced, and the tumor is brighter on a T1-weighted image. But in normal brain with an intact blood-brain barrier the gadolinium remains confined to the vascular space, so there should be no relaxivity effects. This suggests that the observed signal drop is due to an effect of gadolinium different from its relaxivity effect.

The source of the new effect is that gadolinium possesses a large magnetic dipole moment. When present in sufficient concentration, gadolinium appreciably alters the local magnetic susceptibility. Because the gadolinium is confined to the vascular space, there are variations in magnetic susceptibility on a microscopic scale (i.e., on the scale of a capillary diameter, about 8 μm). These variations in magnetic susceptibility lead to magnetic field variations and a drop in the MR signal. To make use of this effect to assess the perfusion state of the tissue we must 1) quantitatively relate the signal change to the local concentration of gadolinium and 2) apply tracer kinetic principles to relate the gadolinium concentration-time curve to the physiologic parameters described earlier that characterize the perfusion state of the tissue.

Field Perturbations and Signal Loss Caused by Gadolinium

Because of the large magnetic dipole moment of gadolinium, a solution of Gd-DTPA has a susceptibility different from that of pure water. Commercially available gadolinium contrast agents have a gadolinium concentration of 0.5 mol/L, so a 0.2% solution is about 1 mM gadolinium. The magnetic susceptibility difference $\Delta\chi$ between pure water and a dilute solution of gadolinium is proportional to the gadolinium concentration, and for 1 mM gadolinium, $\Delta\chi = 0.026$ ppm.[90, 91, 135] When Gd-DTPA is injected reasonably rapidly (over a few seconds) into a human subject, the peak concentration of the bolus reaching the brain is probably about 15 mM because of mixing with the blood.[136] The susceptibility difference between capillaries containing gadolinium and the surrounding extravascular space is then about $\Delta\chi = 0.4$ ppm.

To make use of this transient effect of gadolinium to measure some aspect of the perfusion state of the tissue, we must know how the magnitude of the signal loss depends on the local physiologic parameters. In particular, if we can relate the signal loss to the local tissue concentration of gadolinium, we can apply the tracer kinetic methods outlined earlier. The signal attenuation caused by the gadolinium is taken to be of the form $A(t) = \exp(-\Delta R_2 \, TE)$, and the key assumption is that ΔR_2 (or ΔR_2^* for a GE signal) is simply proportional to the gadolinium concentration[23, 76, 77]:

$$\Delta R_2 = KC_{Gd} \qquad (15)$$

where C_{Gd} is the local tissue concentration of gadolinium and K is a proportionality constant. If this relation holds, it is a simple matter to take a curve of signal versus time and convert it to a curve of concentration versus time. Then the kinetic analysis principles described earlier can be applied to determine local physiologic parameters. In particular, because the volume of distribution of Gd-DTPA in the brain is the vascular space ($p = V_b$), the integrated ΔR_2 curve is proportional to the local blood volume V_b by Equation 14.

However, Equation 15 is a simple model for a complex process of signal loss, and it is an important question whether K is indeed constant and uniform in the normal brain and in pathologic conditions (e.g., tumors). In general, we might expect K to depend on the concentration of gadolinium in the vasculature, the local blood volume, and perhaps the exact geometry of the capillary bed. To focus this question more sharply, we can break it into two questions: 1) For a given vascular geometry, is ΔR_2 (or ΔR_2^*) proportional to the local tissue gadolinium concentration as the concentration varies? 2) If so, is K uniform throughout the brain?

To date, the validity of Equation 8 has not been systematically established. However, Weisskoff and coworkers[77] have reported experimental data from several animal studies supporting a linear relationship. In rat brain at 4.7 T, both ΔR_2 and ΔR_2^* were found to vary linearly with the blood concentration of a superparamagnetic blood pool agent. Experiments in canine myocardium at 1.5 T also showed a linear relationship. Earlier hypercapnia studies in a canine model by Belliveau and colleagues[76] provide some evidence for the uniformity of K in the brain. Dynamic gadolinium studies were performed at several values of P_{CO_2}, which is known to alter blood volume, and maps proportional to CBV were calculated by integrating ΔR_2. The MR-measured CBV for both white matter and gray matter increased with increasing P_{CO_2}, as expected for CBV changes. In addition, the ratio of the blood volumes (gray/white) was about 2, also in good agreement with other studies, suggesting that K is similar for white matter and gray matter.

Theoretic analyses of diffusion and signal loss in nonlinear field gradients give a somewhat mixed level of support for the validity of Equation 15. In terms of modeling the signal loss process, the validity of Equation 15 has two requirements: 1) that ΔR_2 for a fixed capillary geometry is proportional to $\Delta\chi$ (and thus to the vascular concentration of gadolinium and 2) that as the capillary geometry changes (e.g., increased CBV accompanying increased CBF) ΔR_2 depends only on the tissue concentration of gadolinium and not on the vessel geometry. Weisskoff and coworkers[91] found in studies of spherical field perturbers that there are limited regimes in which ΔR_2 and ΔR_2^* are proportional to $\Delta\chi$. For GE methods $\Delta R_2^* \propto \Delta\chi$ in the static broadening regime (the plateau in Fig. 8–14), but for shorter τ_R

the dependence is more like $\Delta\chi^2$, in agreement with earlier calculations for cylinders by Ogawa and coworkers.[88] For SE methods the proportional regime corresponds to the peak relaxivity, suggesting that in practice we should expect $\Delta R_2 \propto \Delta\chi$ when there is a substantial signal change. Kennan and associates[90] reported numeric simulations for cylinders addressing the second question. They examined whether ΔR_2^* varies linearly with changes in the vessel volume fraction for two scenarios: volume increase by dilatation and volume increase by recruitment (increasing the density of capillaries without changing their size). For both cases they found an approximately linear relation between ΔR_2^* and volume fraction for V_b = 2% to 6%. However, for volume increase by dilatation they found that the regression line did not pass through zero, so that ΔR_2^* is not proportional to V_b in this case. Ogawa and coworkers,[88] however, found that their numeric simulation results (also for cylinders) were consistent with $\Delta R_2^* \propto V_b$ for either scenario of volume increase. If indeed the calculated signal changes are not strongly dependent on the exact vessel geometry, that would provide support for the uniformity of K in different tissues.

There is thus some experimental and theoretic support for Equation 15, but more work is needed to establish its validity, particularly experimental studies of the uniformity of K in different tissues.

Measurement and Analysis of Dynamic Gd-DTPA Curves

The intrinsic transit time of gadolinium through the normal brain is only a few seconds. Because the gadolinium is administered in a venous injection, even an initially narrow bolus is broadened to a width of 5 to 10 seconds by the time it reaches the brain (Fig. 8–17). To resolve a transient signal drop of such a short duration it is necessary to have rapid imaging (approximately one image per second). Initial studies and many current studies use EPI image acquisitions,[77] but Edelman and coworkers[137] showed that it is also possible to perform dynamic gadolinium studies with turboFLASH techniques.

Typical analysis of the data consists of the following procedure.[77] From a dynamic data set the signal versus time curve S(t) is measured for each pixel. The curve S(t) is then normalized to the initial signal value (before gadolinium administration) to create a curve of the attenuation factor A(t). (Note that A(t) is used in a slightly different way here than in the earlier discussions of diffusion effects. Previously, when we referred to A(t) the t indicated the evolution time TE. For each image in the dynamic data set TE is the same. Time t now refers to the change in A with successive images.) The apparent change in relaxation rate (either ΔR_2 or ΔR_2^*) is then calculated as $-TE(\ln A)$, where ln signifies natural logarithm. Equation 15 is then used to convert relaxation rate changes into local concentration. In practice, the proportionality constant K is usually not known, and calculations are based on ΔR_2 itself with the understanding that it is proportional to

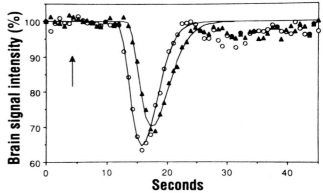

FIGURE 8–17. Dynamic MR signal curves after Gd-DTPA administration. Original data of Belliveau and coworkers[184] demonstrating brain activation with MRI. The two curves were measured in the visual cortex of a human volunteer with eyes closed and while watching a flashing checkerboard pattern. For each pixel the measured attenuation curve was assumed to be of the form $A(t) = \exp[-\Delta R_2(t)TE]$ and converted to a relaxivity curve. The integral of $\Delta R_2(t)$ was then assumed to be proportional to the local blood volume based on the assumed proportionality of relaxivity changes to gadolinium concentration (Equation 15) and on principles of tracer kinetics (Equation 14). In this way the blood volume change accompanying visual stimulation was found to be 32% ± 10% (for seven subjects). (To simplify the integration, each curve was fit to a γ variate function.) (Reprinted with permission from Belliveau JW, Kennedy DN, McKinstry RC, et al: Functional mapping of the human visual cortex by magnetic resonance imaging. Science 254:716–719, 1991. Copyright 1991 American Association for the Advancement of Science.)

the concentration. The curve $\Delta R_2(t)$ is then integrated for each pixel, and an image of this integral is interpreted as being proportional to a map of CBV.

In principle, one can also try to determine f from the measured kinetics of Gd-DTPA using Equation 11. However, this requires knowledge of $C_a(t)$ and $R(t)$. The first requirement can be satisfied by a dual acquisition scheme in which the plane of interest in the brain and a slice through the major arteries feeding the brain are imaged in an interleaved fashion.[77, 138, 139] However, there is no clear way to satisfy the second requirement, so we must rely on an assumed form for $R(t)$. The simplest form for $R(t)$ is a rectangle: $R(t) = 1$ for t less than τ and 0 for larger t. This assumes that all paths through the tissue have the same transit time. Alternatively, one could assume a single compartment form $R(t) = e^{-ft/p}$. Weisskoff and coworkers[140] have discussed some of the complexities involved in trying to measure perfusion with gadolinium.

INFLOW METHODS OF PERFUSION IMAGING

Inflow Effects on the Longitudinal Magnetization

In the perfusion imaging methods described earlier, the presence of gadolinium in the vessels changes the MR signal by affecting the net transverse magnetization. But perfusion can also have a direct effect on the MR signal by altering the local longitudinal magnetization. Fresh spins are delivered to a voxel by flow, so if the arterial magnetization of the water in arterial blood is different from that of the water in the tissue, the longitudinal magnetization is changed and the resulting signal after an RF excitation pulse is also changed. A simple example of this effect was demonstrated by Kwong and colleagues,[141] who compared two inversion recovery experiments, one with a slice-selective 180° pulse and one with a nonselective pulse. After the inversion pulse the magnetization in the slice begins to relax back toward equilibrium with a time constant T1. In the nonselective pulse experiment the magnetization of the arterial blood is also inverted. As a result, the magnetization delivered by the arterial flow is the same as that cleared by the venous flow, so perfusion makes no difference to the net magnetization in the voxel. But with a selective inversion pulse fully relaxed magnetization is delivered by arterial flow, while the venous flow carries away inverted magnetization. The effect thus appears as an apparent increase in the relaxation rate (i.e., the magnetization approaches equilibrium more rapidly because of refreshment and thus appears to have a slightly shorter T1). Several methods designed to exploit this inflow effect have been developed and are described in the following.

Arterial Tagging Methods

A promising approach to measuring perfusion is to use arterial presaturation pulses to invert or saturate the magnetization of the arterial blood[24, 142, 143] (Fig. 8–18). Early demonstrations of arterial tagging in rats combined adiabatic continuous inversion[142] (or saturation pulses[24]) in the neck with imaging in a slice through the brain. In this way the magnetization of the arterial blood leaving the saturation region is inverted, and as long as the transit delay from the saturation region to the brain slice is not too long, the magnetization of the arterial blood entering the brain is still inverted. The water molecules carrying the inverted magnetization are extracted from the capillary bed and join the larger pool of brain water. Over time, the inverted magnetization disappears primarily by relaxation back to equilibrium but also by clearance of the water molecules by flow. If the adiabatic inversion is applied continuously for a long time, the magnetization in the brain approaches a steady-state value such that the delivery of inverted magnetization by flow is balanced by the clearance by relaxation. The result is that the apparent equilibrium magnetization of the tissue is reduced in proportion to the local perfusion f. This method is thus similar to the equilibrium ^{15}O method[144] for measuring perfusion with PET. In the NMR methods, relaxation plays the same role as radioactive decay.

Potential problems with this method are unwanted magnetization transfer effects in the slice of interest caused by the off-resonance inversion pulse, incomplete inversion of the arterial blood, and relaxation during the transit from the inversion region to the slice. In a series of papers, Koretsky and coworkers[24, 142, 145, 146] have modeled and analyzed these effects and

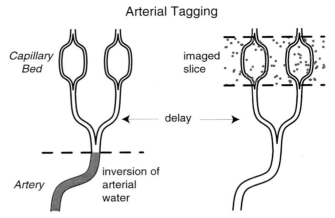

FIGURE 8–18. Arterial tagging for measurement of perfusion. The basic scheme for three similar approaches to measuring perfusion directly with MR is illustrated. Each method is a subtraction technique designed to isolate the signal of entering arterial blood in a slice of interest. For the first image the magnetization of the water protons in the arterial blood is inverted in the large vessels, and after a delay the inverted spins reach the capillary and diffuse out into the tissue water space of the imaged slice. The experiment is then repeated without inverting the arterial blood, and the two images are subtracted. Ideally, the only spins in the imaged slice that have different magnetizations in the two images are those that entered from the arterial blood during the time delay, so the difference signal is proportional to the amount of blood delivered and thus to local perfusion. In the Kwong method,[141] inversion recovery images with a slice-selective 180° pulse and a nonselective 180° pulse are subtracted. In the Edelman method,[143] images with and without an initial inversion pulse below the slice of interest are subtracted. In the original Williams method,[142] images with and without a continuous adiabatic inversion in the neck are subtracted. For all of these methods the measured signal changes are small because the fraction of tissue water replaced by perfusion during the experiment is small (on the order of fT1), but the quantitative changes can be interpreted directly in terms of perfusion.

have developed correction algorithms so that quantitative perfusion measurements can be made. Initial animal studies involving CBF alterations by altering P_{CO_2} showed excellent agreement with microsphere measurements of CBF.[147]

Edelman and colleagues[143] introduced a similar method that grew out of MR angiography techniques.[148] The EPI signal targeting with alternating radiofrequency (EPISTAR) method is an EPI version of an earlier MR angiography approach[149] and is essentially a non–steady-state form of the method of Williams and coworkers[142] that does not require adiabatic RF pulses. In EPISTAR imaging, a selective 180° inversion pulse is applied to a thick slab just below the slice of interest to invert the magnetization of the arterial blood. A 90° saturation pulse is then applied to the slice of interest to suppress the static tissue signal. After a delay inflow time, a 90° pulse is applied with an EPI readout to form an image. This procedure is repeated a second time without the arterial inversion pulse and the two images are subtracted. (In practice, for the second image an inversion pulse is applied above the slice of interest so that magnetization transfer and off-resonance excitation effects of the inversion pulse are the same but the arterial blood is not tagged.) Essentially, the EPISTAR method is designed to image only blood that has entered the slice during the time interval inflow time. The static tissue signal is largely suppressed with the saturation pulse, and any remaining signal should be subtracted out by taking the image difference. However, the magnetization carried by the incoming arterial blood is inverted in the first image but completely relaxed in the second, and the amount of blood that has entered the voxel is proportional to the perfusion. So the difference signal ΔS in EPISTAR is proportional to f. For both the EPISTAR method and the steady-state method a detailed model of the process combining kinetics and relaxation is needed to extract a quantitative measurement of f.

Modeling Inflow Effects

There are thus three experimental approaches for measuring perfusion from inflow effects:

1. Method of Kwong and colleagues[141]: difference of inversion recovery images with selective and nonselective 180° pulses.
2. Method of Williams and coworkers[142]: difference of images with and without continuous inversion of arterial blood. (The equilibrium MR method can be performed with arterial saturation instead of inversion but with a loss of a factor of 2 in the magnitude of the MR signals produced.[24])
3. Method of Edelman and coworkers[143]: difference of images with and without preinversion of arterial blood with a 180° RF pulse.

Each of these is a difference technique requiring two images, and ideally the only difference in the signal is due to the different ways in which the arterial blood is treated. However, it should be kept in mind that each of these methods may suffer from nonideal conditions (e.g., imperfect RF pulses, magnetization transfer effects). Detailed quantitative models for the interpretation of inflow effects have been developed by combining single-compartment kinetics with the Bloch equations for relaxation.[24, 142] However, the general quantitative features of inflow effects in these methods can be understood by simply considering the amount of blood entering the voxel and the magnetization carried by that blood.

For each method the measured signal difference ΔS is proportional to the difference in longitudinal magnetization ΔM for the voxel. And ΔM is simply the difference in magnetization of the arterial blood delivered to the voxel. Specifically, let

m_0 = equilibrium magnetization of 1 mol of water molecules
C_a = concentration of water in arterial blood (mol/mL)
C_t = concentration of water in tissue (mol/mL)
V = volume of the voxel (mL)
f = perfusion (s^{-1})

Then the equilibrium magnetization in the voxel (in the absence of flow effects) is $M_0 = m_0VC_t$, and the partition coefficient of water is $p = C_t/C_a$. For each method we can view the magnetization in the voxel as

the result of two conflicting processes: magnetization is delivered to the voxel by arterial flow and then lost from the voxel by relaxation and by venous flow. Because water is nearly 100% extracted from the blood as it passes through the capillary bed, the rate of loss of magnetization by venous flow is much less than that by relaxation, and we neglect it in the following arguments. To simplify the analysis further, we assume that the T1 values of blood and tissue are the same. With these definitions we can derive approximate expressions for ΔM for each of the methods.

The Kwong method and the Edelman method are identical as far as the mathematics is concerned. For each method the arterial magnetization per mole at time t after the inversion pulse is m_0 for one image (with the selective pulse in the Kwong method and without a preinversion pulse in the Edelman method) and $m_0(1 - 2e^{-t/T1})$ for the other image, so $\Delta m = 2e^{-t/T1}$ in both cases. Furthermore, the number of spins that entered the voxel up to time t after the inversion pulse is $N = fVC_at$. Then the total magnetization difference is $\Delta M = N\Delta m$ or with the relations defined earlier:

$$\Delta M = 2M_0 \frac{f}{p} te^{-t/T1} \qquad (16)$$

The Williams method is conceptually different. We assume that the adiabatic inversion has been applied continuously for a long time, so that inverted magnetization has been entering the voxel for all times in the past but has relaxed since it entered. We assume that our measurement is made at time t, so we have to consider the contributions of all spins that entered at time t' in the past. Without the inversion, the magnetization of the blood entering at t' was m_0 and it would still be m_0 at time t. But with the inversion the blood entered with magnetization $-m_0$ at time t' but has relaxed to $m_0(1 - 2e^{-(t-t')/T1})$ by time t. The magnetization difference is then $2e^{-(t-t')/T1}$. The number of spins that entered between t' and $t' + dt'$ is $dN = fVC_a dt'$, so adding up the contributions from all times in the past, ΔM is the integral of $\Delta m dN$, or

$$\Delta M = 2M_0 \frac{f}{p} T1 \qquad (17)$$

The form of ΔM is similar for the different methods. For each we can write $\Delta M \propto fT$, where $T = T1$ for the Williams method and $T = te^{-t/T1}$ for the Kwong and Edelman methods. Physically, fT is simply the milliliters of blood entering 1 mL of tissue in the time T, and for fT much less than 1 we can interpret it as the fraction of the tissue water that has been replaced by fresh arterial water during T. For typical values of $f = 0.01$ s^{-1} and $T = 1$ second, fT is about 1%. Note also that T for the Kwong and Edelman methods is maximized when $t = T1$, and then $T = T1/e$, about 37% of the T value for the Williams experiment.

We thus see that inflow perfusion imaging methods are limited by T1, and the fact that $fT1$ is small means that the magnitude of the signal changes observed is also small. Nevertheless, with state-of-the-art MRI systems, sufficiently high S/N ratios can be achieved that these small changes can readily be measured. In addition, the observed signal changes can be modeled directly in terms of f, thus providing the potential for obtaining quantitative measurements of perfusion.

In analogy with classic tracer kinetic studies, we can think of these inflow methods as effectively creating labeled water in the arteries and observing how it distributes in the tissues. Furthermore, because clearance of the tracer is dominated by relaxation rather than venous flow, we would expect the measured flow to be fairly independent of the details of the assumed model for clearance (R(t)). Instead, the kinetics should be dominated by delivery of the labeled blood, so the measurement of f is more robust. However, the ideal experiments considered here may not be realizable in practice, and some of the limitations have already been discussed. An additional potential problem is related to the definition of perfusion as the amount of arterial blood delivered to the capillary bed of a tissue voxel. With arterial tagging methods larger arteries that simply pass through a tissue voxel (and thus do not end on a capillary bed) nevertheless carry labeled blood into the voxel and so are counted as part of the local perfusion. Gradient spoiling techniques that reduce the signal of moving blood may help to reduce the contribution of magnetization that has not been extracted from the capillaries. A second potential problem is that the arterial blood is labeled based on its position below the slice of interest. In regions where the vasculature has a more complex geometry, the labeling pulse may miss some arteries feeding the slice and hit some veins that pass through the slice. Both effects lead to errors in the measurement of f. Although more work is needed to sort out these issues of quantitation, inflow methods nevertheless show great promise for providing a measurement of local perfusion.

OTHER METHODS OF PERFUSION IMAGING WITH NUCLEAR MAGNETIC RESONANCE

The methods described so far have all been used in human subjects. A number of other methods have been proposed and used in animal studies. The following is a brief survey of these methods; a more extensive review can be found elsewhere.[150]

Labeled Water

The use of labeled water as a diffusible tracer for measuring perfusion is the basis of the PET $H_2^{15}O$ method. Ackerman and coworkers[151] showed that water with deuterium substituted for hydrogen can also be used as a diffusible tracer with deuterium-sensitive NMR serving as the means for following the kinetics of the tracer. In this way all of the machinery of tracer kinetic analysis discussed earlier can be applied to the NMR-derived concentration curves. The advantage of deuterium labeling is that D_2O (or HDO) behaves much like native water, and the partition coefficient is thus reasonably well known in different tissues. This

method has been applied successfully to a number of organ systems.[152–154] Limitations of this method are low NMR sensitivity and a short T2 that limit the S/N ratio. Also, the labeled water takes several days to clear from the system, which limits the number of sequential measurements that can be made.

Another way to label water for NMR detection is to use $H_2^{17}O$.[155] The ^{17}O nuclide is intrinsically more sensitive for NMR detection than deuterium, but the T2 is much shorter.[150] However, $H_2^{17}O$ is also an effective contrast agent, altering the proton relaxation time through the coupling with ^{17}O. This provides an alternative approach for assessing the concentration of ^{17}O from relaxation measurements with proton NMR that overcomes the short-T2 limitation of direct ^{17}O measurement.[156, 157] These methods are promising but are currently limited by the high cost of the agent.

^{19}F Compounds

The ^{19}F nuclide is readily observable with NMR with high sensitivity (its resonance frequency is relatively close to that of protons). Furthermore, ^{19}F is the most abundant naturally occurring isotope of fluorine. Methods involving detection of the ^{19}F NMR signal have been developed to investigate several aspects of perfusion. Fluorinated gases, such as trifluoromethane (CHF_3), chlorodifluoromethane ($CHClF_2$), and halothane, readily diffuse through the tissues and are cleared through the lungs and can be used as diffusible agents for perfusion measurement.[158–162] Other fluorine compounds, particularly perfluorocarbon emulsions used as blood substitutes, can be used as blood markers for blood volume studies.[163] As noted in the discussion of IVIM methods, use of a fluorinated blood substitute overcomes the dynamic range problem encountered in proton imaging of the vascular system.[130] The proton signal from blood is only a small fraction of the total signal, whereas with fluorine the signal is still small but all of it comes from the blood. Finally, these compounds have another feature that shows considerable promise for assessing the metabolic state of the tissue. The relaxation times of the ^{19}F are sensitive to the local oxygenation, so that measurement of T1 provides a way of estimating the local Po_2.[164–167] The many applications of ^{19}F NMR in perfusion studies have been reviewed elsewhere.[168]

Superparamagnetic Iron Oxide Crystals

One of the advantages of the Gd-DTPA (or Dys-DTPA) methods for assessing local blood volume is that even though the agent is confined to the blood, its effects are much more widespread and thus more readily detectable. The changes in susceptibility of the vascular compartment create field gradients in the surrounding space and a resulting measurable signal loss. Other contrast agents that can produce a similar effect are superparamagnetic iron oxide crystals.[169] These particles are small (4 to 25 nm) and structurally similar to magnetite.[170]

The term superparamagnetic describes the fact that

the magnetic properties of these crystals lie in between paramagnetism and ferromagnetism.[170] In paramagnetism individual magnetic moments align randomly because of thermal motions but tend to align with an externally applied magnetic field. However, this alignment is due to the independent interaction of each magnetic moment with the field; there is little interaction between the magnetic moments. In ferromagnetism, however, there is a strong interaction among the individual magnetic moments, so that neighboring particles align together. This ordering extends over a certain range of distance and defines a domain of magnetization. A large crystal contains a number of domains, each with a different local orientation of the magnetization. At the domain boundaries there is a sharp change in the magnetization orientation. This leads to magnetic properties different from those of paramagnetic materials, including the familiar example of a ferromagnetic material remaining magnetized after the magnetic field is removed. Superparamagnetic crystals are sufficiently small that they contain only one domain and so do not display all of the ferromagnetic (or ferrimagnetic) properties of a larger crystal. Because of the iron spins, they become strongly magnetized in a magnetic field but do not retain the magnetization when the field is removed.

Superparamagnetic iron crystals are finding widespread application as general contrast agents.[170] The use of these agents for specific perfusion-related studies has been demonstrated in the brain,[169, 171, 172] heart,[173] and kidney.[174]

BRAIN ACTIVATION STUDIES BASED ON DEOXYHEMOGLOBIN CHANGES

One of the remarkable developments in MRI is the recognition that changes in the metabolic state of the brain affect the signal in a detectable fashion and therefore provide an intrinsic mechanism of contrast for brain activation studies. The effect is the result of the fact that the magnetic state of hemoglobin depends on its oxygenation: it is diamagnetic when oxygenated and paramagnetic when deoxygenated. As discussed earlier, during neural stimulation the local flow increase in the brain is much larger than the oxygen metabolism increase. As a result the venous blood becomes more oxygenated and thus the local magnetic susceptibility of the blood changes during activation. Diffusion through the local field perturbations around the vessels then leads to a change in the local MR signal on both GE and SE images. Brain activation studies based on this BOLD contrast typically employ an experimental paradigm in which a subject alternates between periods of stimulation and rest while a series of MR images is rapidly collected.

The fact that the magnetic state of hemoglobin changes with its state of oxygenation was discovered in 1936 by Pauling and Coryell,[175] before the discovery of NMR itself. In 1982, Thulborn and colleagues[104] demonstrated T2 changes in blood samples resulting from the susceptibility changes caused by the presence

of the paramagnetic deoxyhemoglobin. In 1990, Ogawa and colleagues[78] showed that controlled O_2-dependent susceptibility changes in rats caused visible changes in brain images obtained with GE acquisition schemes that are particularly sensitive to susceptibility effects. Then in 1992, Kwong,[80] Ogawa,[81] Bandettini,[82] and their coworkers showed that similar changes evoked by changes in brain oxygenation during human visual or motor stimulation were detectable on a clinical scanner and thus provided a method for mapping regions of activation.

BLOOD OXYGENATION LEVEL–DEPENDENT CONTRAST STUDIES

Pre–Functional MRI Oxygen Contrast Studies

The initial studies concerning BOLD contrast were not activation studies but animal studies in which the metabolic conditions were controlled as closely as possible. Ogawa and colleagues[78] regulated the O_2 intake of mice while imaging their brains in high-field (7- and 8.4-T) systems with GE images. The signal intensity was found to be significantly larger when the mice breathed 100% O_2 than when they breathed 20% O_2 (Fig. 8–19). Furthermore, the effect was greatly reduced in SE images. Both observations were consistent with the source of the effect being related to the susceptibility changes (to which GE images are highly sensitive) brought on by the presence of the deoxygenated hemoglobin. Ogawa and associates[78] suggested that this phenomenon could form the basis for monitoring regional O_2 use in the brain and speculated that during activation more O_2 would be removed from the blood and the deoxyhemoglobin concentration would increase. Turner and coworkers[79] imaged cat brains under the controlled conditions of anoxia, apnea, and euthanasia with an EPI sequence on a 2-T system. They also found MR signal changes that were dependent on the oxygenation of the blood. These early studies suggested that the distribution of the cerebral perfusion might be visualized.

Functional MRI Activation Studies

The detectability of blood oxygenation effects in these well-controlled animal experiments at high fields at least suggested that such effects might be seen in humans during tasks that altered the O_2 utilization in the brain. Kwong and coworkers[80] acquired images of a normal human subject during visual stimulation with a GE EPI sequence using a long TE (40 ms) to enhance the susceptibility effects. Temporally resolved images acquired during and in the absence of stimulation showed clear differences in signal intensity (Fig. 8–20). However, the signal increased during stimulation, rather than decreased, suggesting that the deoxyhemoglobin concentration decreased with activation. This surprising result was just the opposite of what had been predicted based on the earlier MR studies[78] but is consistent with the earlier PET results. The unex-

functional activation and its relation to handedness.[179] Schneider and colleagues[180] used FMRI to investigate activation of the visual cortex along the cortical ribbon and were able to identify four topographically distinct areas of activation. Engel and associates[181] used an ingenious method for measuring visual cortex properties based on temporal correlations of the FMRI activation with a periodic stimulus and were able to demonstrate that the movement of a stimulus from the fovea to the periphery generates stimulation from the posterior to the anterior portions of the calcarine sulcus.

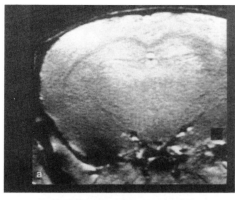

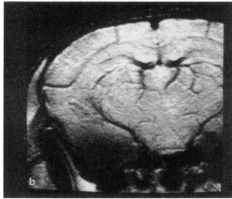

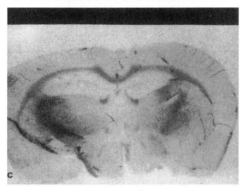

FIGURE 8–19. Effect of deoxyhemoglobin on the MR signal. Original images of Ogawa and coworkers[78] demonstrating that increased deoxyhemoglobin produces measurable signal loss in the brain. GE images of a mouse brain at 7 T. *a,* Breathing 100% oxygen; *b,* breathing air; *c,* a fixed slice of an excised mouse brain. Most of the observed dark lines correspond to blood vessels. (*a* to *c* from Ogawa S, Lee T-M, Nayak AS, Glynn P: Oxygenation-sensitive contrast in magnetic resonance image of rodent brain at high magnetic fields. Magn Reson Med 14:68–78, 1990.)

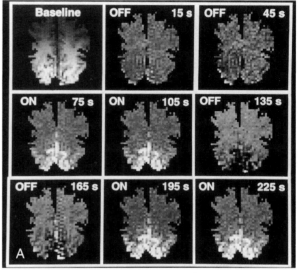

Gradient Echo Images

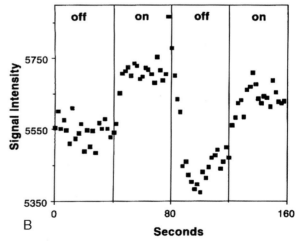

FIGURE 8–20. FMRI demonstration of brain activation in the human visual cortex. Original data of Kwong and coworkers[80] showing brain activation caused by intrinsic MR signal changes in the visual cortex of a human subject. The subject was exposed to a flashing checkerboard pattern alternated with darkness while EPI GE images were collected. *A,* A series of images over time, with the baseline image subtracted to show dynamic signal changes. *B,* Time course of intensity changes for a pixel in the visual cortex. The signal changes are small but readily detectable. Subtraction images clearly show the pattern of activation. (*A* and *B* from Kwong KK, Belliveau JW, Chesler DA, et al: Dynamic magnetic resonance imaging of human brain activity during primary sensory stimulation. Proc Natl Acad Sci USA 89:5675–5679, 1992.)

pected nature of the metabolic response to brain activation is that less O_2 is removed from the blood. Other FMRI studies of the visual cortex with a high-field (4-T) scanner[81] and the motor cortex with an echoplanar system with specially designed gradient coils[82] also demonstrated signal increases with activation. Similar results were soon obtained on a conventional clinical scanner as well.[176–178]

The FMRI technique has been utilized for a variety of applications. FMRI of the motor cortex has been used to study the possible hemispheric asymmetry of

Another group used FMRI to study the cognitive task of internal speech word generation on a high-field (4-T) system.[182] Using a conventional T2*-weighted FMRI sequence, activation in Broca's area was demonstrated. Although much of the interest in FMRI application has focused on its use in cognitive neuroscience, it is also of great potential clinical significance in surgical planning when tumor resection endangers nearby functioning areas of the brain. Tumor growth can displace brain regions, making recognition of healthy regions difficult. FMRI provides a means of identifying functional areas preoperatively.[183]

NATURE OF BLOOD OXYGENATION LEVEL–DEPENDENT CONTRAST

Modeling BOLD Contrast

The basic model for understanding this blood oxygenation effect is a cylindrical vessel with a magnetic susceptibility different from that of the surrounding fluid. This is the model used for interpreting gadolinium effects, but there are two important differences. First, the susceptibility difference for BOLD effects is about an order of magnitude smaller than for gadolinium studies. For fully deoxygenated blood with a hematocrit of 40%, the susceptibility difference between blood and water is about 0.07 ppm.[136] This corresponds to a gadolinium concentration of about 3 mmol/L (i.e., about a 0.5% solution of commercially available Gd-DTPA). As a result the signal changes with BOLD contrast are small, typically a few percent at 1.5 T. Second, the basic effect with gadolinium is a drop in the local MR signal intensity and during activation the drop is more severe, but with BOLD contrast the signal intensity increases during activation. Both of these effects are consistent with the model of the susceptibility effect, but the immediate causes of the changes are different. The greater signal loss with gadolinium is interpreted as a result of the increased blood volume during activation, with a constant susceptibility difference.[184] The increased blood volume would also be expected to decrease the BOLD signal, but the accompanying decrease in the susceptibility difference resulting from the drop in deoxyhemoglobin concentration more than compensates for the volume change, so the BOLD signal increases.

The actual fields within a voxel depend on the field strength, the vessel geometry, the strength of the inhomogeneity $\Delta\chi$, and the distribution of vessels within the voxel, as well as the local diffusion characteristics. Because of the intrinsic complexity of the brain anatomy, it is not possible to create a simple analytic model that captures the essential features of the system. Rather, extensive work has been done on creating computer models that simulate both the geometry and the intrinsic physiologic effects appropriate to particular imaging sequences.[88–91] These models focus on the role of diffusion around field perturbations, as discussed earlier, and have clarified the subtle role that diffusion plays in affecting the SE and GE signals.

The results of the modeling studies can be broadly characterized in the following way. For GE pulse sequences the effect on the signal is greatest for the larger vessels (for the same susceptibility difference) and increases as the blood volume fraction increases. The effect also increases as the magnitude of the field offset at the surface of the vessel increases. Because the field offset is on the order of $\Delta\chi B_0$, either an increase in the main magnetic field B_0 or an increase in the susceptibility difference increases the effect. With SE pulse sequences the magnitude of the signal change is less, and the effect is greatest for a particular size of vessel. For the susceptibility changes expected for deoxyhemoglobin the effect is strongest for the smallest vessels (capillaries) and reduced for the larger vessels. That is, in Figure 8–14 the peak SE relaxivity occurs approximately at the τ_R corresponding to capillary sizes.

Physiologic Changes During Brain Activation

A full understanding of the signal changes in an FMRI activation study also requires modeling of several physiologic changes that occur during stimulation and their effects on the MR signal. In experiments at high field (e.g., 4 T), the signal changes accompanying activation are as large as 20%, and the dominant source of this change is likely to be the BOLD effect.[181, 185] BOLD contrast is due to the imbalance in the changes of flow and O_2 metabolism during stimulation. A large change in flow accompanied by a much smaller change in the O_2 metabolic rate requires that the O_2 extraction fraction drop, and the venous blood is then more oxygenated. But at moderate fields (1.5 T) the BOLD effect is expected to be only 1% to 5%,[88] and other physiologic changes may make comparable contributions to the signal change. Changes in blood volume and flow can also affect the signal, and the quantitative nature of these changes in the brain during stimulation is still not well understood. A blood volume increase (at a constant level of blood oxygenation) should lead to a reduction of the signal, the opposite of the effect associated with the oxygenation change. An increase in flow could lead to a signal increase (the basis of the inflow perfusion imaging methods discussed earlier). But increased velocity in the vessels might lead to a decrease in the net signal of the blood (the basis of the IVIM method). In addition, susceptibility effects related to the shape of the erythrocytes may substantially alter the signal from the blood itself, and these changes may be a significant portion of the total observed signal change.[186] Each of these effects may be small, but the signal changes found at 1.5 T are also small. More sophisticated models incorporating physiologic changes along with the susceptibility effects are being investigated[187] and offer hope for understanding the magnitude and time course of FMRI activation studies in terms of basic physiologic processes.

FUNCTIONAL MRI TECHNIQUES

Specificity of Localized Activation Measured with Different Pulse Sequences

One of the primary difficulties in localizing brain activity with FMRI is that the brain's response is really a chain of events that occur on many spatial and temporal levels, many of which potentially have some effect on the MR signal. Arteriolar dilatation initiates changes in blood volume, velocity, and oxygenation in the downstream capillaries, venules, and draining veins. It is generally accepted that detection of signal changes on the capillary level is desired for studies of localized brain activation, because both feeding arteries and draining veins may be located some distance from the site of activation. But the MR signal is potentially sensitive to changes at all levels of the vascular tree, and it is thus important to consider the sensitivity of different pulse sequences to these effects.

For the susceptibility effect, the modeling studies suggest that a GE pulse sequence should be the most sensitive for detecting activation. However, because the GE signal is more sensitive to larger vessels, the strongest activations are likely to be near draining veins.[188, 189] With the use of conventional GE pulse sequences, activations as large as 30% or more have been found, far larger than the expected 1% to 5% resulting from the capillary BOLD effect.[188, 190] Furthermore, the magnitude of the signal change was found to increase when the voxel size was reduced. Lai and colleagues[188] compared the regions of strong activation with high-resolution MR angiography and found a close association between the location of small vessels and areas of activation. Menon and coworkers[189] also found large signal changes at 4 T in the vicinity of vessels. This evidence supports the view that the largest signal changes measured with a GE pulse sequence are due to draining veins. The increased effect with smaller voxels is consistent with the vessel occupying a larger volume fraction and so having a larger effect on the net signal. The signal from such voxels may be affected by flow-induced phase variations as well as susceptibility effects.[188]

An SE pulse sequence is less sensitive to the BOLD effect but may be more specific to smaller vessels.[77] That is, the SE signal change may more accurately reflect changes at the capillary level. Larger vessels such as draining veins are expected to have a much smaller effect on the SE signal because of the size dependence of the relaxation curve (see Fig. 8–14), so the SE signal change may more accurately reflect changes at the capillary level.

A third type of pulse sequence that involves features of both SE and GE pulse sequences is the asymmetric spin-echo (ASE) sequence[191] (Fig. 8–21). In a standard SE pulse sequence there are actually two echoing processes at work. The 180° RF pulse creates an RF echo, and the frequency-encoding gradients (the compensation gradient and the readout gradient) create a GE. Normally the pulse sequence is tuned so that both the

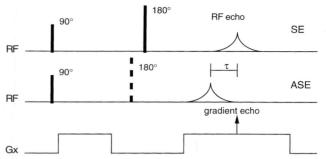

FIGURE 8–21. ASE pulse sequence. In a conventional SE pulse sequence for imaging there are two echoing processes at work: an RF echo related to the 180° pulse and a GE related to the imaging gradients. The GE determines the center of k-space sampling, and normally the RF echo is tuned to occur at the same time. In the ASE pulse sequence *(dashed line)*, the 180° pulse is shifted by a time $\tau/2$ so that the RF and gradient echoes are shifted by τ. This increases the sensitivity to field variations by allowing phase evolution for a time τ, similar (although not identical) to the phase evolution in a GE image with $\tau = TE$. The ASE sequence thus provides a bridge between conventional SE and GE sequences, allowing finer control over the sensitivity to local field distortions.

RF echo and the GE occur at the center of the data collection window. In this way phase changes resulting from resonant frequency offsets are refocused in the image. An ASE pulse sequence is created by separating the times of the two echoes by a time τ (e.g., by shifting the time of the 180° pulse by $\tau/2$). Then the signals from spins sitting in different fields acquire phase differences equivalent to evolution for a time τ. That is, with an ASE pulse sequence with an offset τ the phase evolution is similar to that of a GE sequence with TE = τ. The two are not precisely alike because T2 decay affects the two signals differently. With GE imaging, the T2 effects and the field nonuniformity effects are combined in T2*. But with an ASE pulse sequence it is possible to examine the field nonuniformity separately by using different τ offsets with the same TE, so that T2 effects are unchanged. (The signal decay with increasing τ is sometimes described by a time constant T2′.[191]) The ASE pulse sequence thus offers a bridge between SE and GE that allows finer control over the tradeoff between sensitivity and specificity.[77] With larger τ the sensitivity to the BOLD effect is increased, but with smaller τ the signal is more specifically sensitive to changes at the capillary level.

Inflow effects after changes in perfusion can also affect the signal, as discussed earlier. The source of this effect is that the signal of the static spins is partly saturated, so that fresh unsaturated blood entering the voxel increases the signal intensity. When flow is increased, more unsaturated blood enters. These effects are likely to be largest in voxels with a large blood volume fraction. If there is a general increase in blood velocity at all levels during activation, we can expect voxels containing either feeding arteries or draining veins near the activated area to show the largest signal changes related to inflow refreshment. Because these regions may not be well localized to the site of activation, it is often desirable to try to eliminate inflow effects in BOLD studies.

The inflow effect can be reduced by preventing saturation of the stationary spins. This can be done either by using a long TR (several times T1) or by using a low flip angle (e.g., 10°) with a GE pulse sequence. The first approach is practical only for an EPI acquisition, but the second can be used with a more conventional acquisition. An alternative approach for reducing inflow effects is to try to eliminate the signal from blood in large vessels by adding spoiler gradients (effectively adding diffusion-weighting pulses). Inflow effects with SE and ASE pulse sequences are probably less of a problem because of the flow void phenomenon. For the signal to appear in the image a flowing spin must be hit by both the 90° and 180° pulses. If the TE is long, the fastest flows do not generate a signal.

High Fields

The effects of functional susceptibility changes are more pronounced on systems of higher field strength. Comparative studies of the BOLD effect at different fields indicated that the increase in the magnitude of the signal change was larger than the field increase.[185] Standard MR imagers have a 1.5-T field strength, but advances in FMRI have prompted several manufacturers to build 3- and 4-T imaging systems, which have been used to investigate the possible advantages of high-field systems for FMRI. Imaging at high fields is complicated because susceptibility-induced artifacts can be exacerbated, there is diminished T1 contrast, and there are dielectric and penetration effects with RF at high frequencies that are pronounced in SE images.[192] However, the increased susceptibility effects are potentially advantageous in FMRI, and the intrinsic MR S/N ratio increases with higher field as well. To overcome RF penetration effects, Ugurbil and colleagues[192] used a driven equilibrium sequence that has decreased sensitivity to B_1 deviations and regains the T1 contrast lost with conventional sequences at high fields. The functional images obtained with high-field systems have been quite promising.[81, 179, 189, 192]

Fast Image Acquisition

One of the difficulties in functional imaging is that the signal changes are often small compared with the resting signal, particularly at low fields. With conventional imaging the magnitude of the signal change caused by activation is often comparable to the magnitude of artifacts produced by physiologic motions, such as bulk motion artifacts and flow artifacts, which are often lumped together under the category of *physiologic pulsations*. Any signal that changes during the image acquisition causes confusion in the phase-encoding process. Although the region of signal change may be localized within the subject, because the data are collected in k-space the resulting images can have intensity artifacts spread throughout the image. In many clinical applications of conventional imaging, when the detection of small signal changes is not as critical, such effects can be reduced to a sufficient degree by various means such as partial echoes and cardiac gating. But for the detection of small signal changes, a more efficient method of artifact suppression is often desirable. One way to accomplish this is simply to collect entire images on a time scale that is short compared with physiologic motion. This may be accomplished by scanning all of k-space after a single excitation pulse with EPI.[193] Images can be acquired in 30 to 100 ms and physiologic motions are thus frozen within any particular image.

In addition to motion insensitivity, EPI acquisitions generally have a high S/N ratio, primarily because the signal is relatively unsaturated.[194] To achieve short imaging times with a conventional pulse sequence requires short TR values and usually reduced flip angles, so the measured signal is much less than the fully relaxed signal. Disadvantages of EPI are that the spatial resolution is typically coarser than with conventional MRI, and the EPI images are more sensitive to susceptibility artifacts. This sensitivity is a result of the fact that the data acquisition window is much longer with EPI (30 to 100 ms) than with conventional MRI (8 ms). As a result, unwanted phase changes caused by field inhomogeneities accrue during the entire acquisition period and lead to distortion in the images. For example, the chemical-shift artifact leads to a shift in the apparent position of fat by a couple of pixels in a conventional image but by many pixels in an EPI image. For this reason, fat suppression and careful shimming of the magnet are required.

Fast scanning methods are also possible on conventional scanners using low-flip-angle GE methods, but these offer less S/N ratio than EPI. EPI can also be used for either GE, SE, or ASE acquisitions. However, to have EPI capabilities, imagers must have specialized gradient hardware. Sites without such a capability can still efficiently employ functional imaging methods with conventional fast scan methods.[176–178]

Spiral k-space imaging methods have shown great promise as fast acquisition schemes well suited to functional imaging and employable on a conventional scanner.[181, 195] With spiral imaging, k-space is sampled by a small set of interleaved spiral trajectories. Each trajectory starts at the center of k-space, making the images relatively insensitive to in-plane motion.[195, 196] These methods make efficient use of the available gradient power and available imaging time, and motion artifacts have a different character, similar to those in projection reconstruction imaging.[197]

DATA PROCESSING STRATEGIES

The Problem of Detecting Small MR Signal Changes

The data in a functional imaging experiment are typically collected as a set of temporally resolved images obtained during alternating periods of stimulation and rest. Ideally, comparison of the images collected during periods of stimulation with those collected during rest (by subtraction, for example) reveals locations that experienced changes during those periods. However, FMRI data suffer from several problems that complicate this analysis. The BOLD signal changes are typically small, at most a few percent of the resting signal at 1.5 T, so the intrinsic S/N ratio of the individual images limits the sensitivity of the method. The S/N ratio can be improved by appropriate averaging of the images, but this brings in two other problems. First, over the several minutes required for a study the MR imager may drift, introducing a slowly varying trend into the time course for each pixel. Second, the response of the brain to stimulation is not immediate, nor is its "shutting off" after a stimulation has been completed. Therefore, the periods in which the images show activation and those in which they do not are not precisely the same as the periods of stimulation and rest themselves. Typically, the MR signal change is delayed 6 to 10 seconds from the initiation of the stimulus, and the characteristics of the brain's response may be different in different regions of the brain.[80, 82, 176]

In addition to being sensitive to random thermal noise, MR images are sensitive to more structured, systematic noise related to physiologic motions. Cardiac pulsations, brain pulsations, or bulk body motions can result in signal intensity changes as a function of time.[198] The most insidious of these changes are due to bulk body motions that result from activities performed as a part of the activation portion of the FMRI protocol and thus result in intensity changes strongly correlated with the activation periods but unrelated to brain activation.[199] Pixels near a high-contrast tissue boundary (e.g., at the edge of the brain) are particularly sensitive to small head motions that alter the partial-volume averaging within the pixel. For example, if a visual stimulus causes the subject to tip his or her head slightly each time the stimulus is turned on, pixels near an edge may appear to be activated. It is critical for the experimenter to eliminate such motion with the use of a head restraining device or a bite bar. If such motions cannot be eliminated, image coregistration software may be required.

Physiologic pulsations cannot be eliminated in this way but can be removed to some degree in postprocessing by recognition of the frequency components of the signal related to such pulsations.[200] It is therefore important that the frequency of stimulation is chosen to be well separated from the physiologic frequencies related to cardiac and brain pulsations. It is also important that the images be collected with a TR short enough to sample these pulsations critically so that they are not aliased (i.e., TR should be less than one half the pulsation period). If the TR is too long, the aliased pulsation frequencies may appear to be at much lower frequencies, similar to those related to activation. This may pose a problem for multislice FMRI, which is limited by short TR values.

The data analysis methods described next are all motivated by a consideration of ideal data that are not contaminated by drifts of the imaging system or systematic motion effects. That is, we assume that baseline trends in the time course of each pixel have been removed, so that what remains is a simple response curve with added random noise.

Statistical Significance Tests

Several questions might be asked of FMRI data, but the most obvious is whether or not there is an activation in any particular pixel. The simplest approach is to calculate the mean value at each pixel of the images collected during the stimulated or "on" periods and subtract them from the mean value at each pixel of the images collected during the control or "off" periods. Regions with different mean values during the two periods would show up as activated regions.[189] Because the data are contaminated by noise, however, one might ask just how significant a measured difference in the mean really is, particularly for the small changes found at 1.5 T. This may be formulated by constructing a statistic that measures the confidence with which one may say two means are significantly different. If one assumes that the data from the stimulated periods and the data from the control periods come from two independent sets of observations, each with a gaussian distribution and with potentially different means but the same variance, then this statistic takes the form of a t-test to test the hypothesis that these sample populations have the same mean (the null hypothesis).

For each pixel a value of the t-statistic can be calculated, and a threshold chosen to distinguish activated pixels.[177] The logic of this approach is that the threshold value of the t-statistic can be chosen large enough so that it is highly unlikely that a pixel for which the means are actually the same would reach the threshold. Then the pixels above the threshold can with reasonable confidence be interpreted as activated. The criterion for identifying an activated pixel can, of course, be adjusted by changing the threshold value.

The t-test is one of the most commonly used, but caution should be exercised when interpreting FMRI data based on a t-test. Any time a threshold is applied, an artificial boundary (activated or not activated) is placed between pixels whose signal characteristics may be only slightly different. Furthermore, an image of the t-statistic for each pixel is really a map of significance, not a map of change. Two pixels with the same magnitude of signal change (e.g., 1%) may nevertheless have different values of the t-statistic if the signal variance is different between the two regions. The interpretation of t-statistic maps is therefore somewhat subtle. We can with some confidence conclude that a pixel above the threshold was activated, but we are not justified in concluding that a pixel below the threshold was not activated.

Finally, if the data are not ideal, the statistical foundation for using the t-test may be invalidated. Any trend in the data biases the results because it affects the mean values of the two populations and makes them nongaussian. If the delay in the onset of the MR signal change after stimulation is not taken into account, the sensitivity of the t-test is compromised by the mixing of rest and stimulation samples. The proper choice of a statistical test for FMRI data is a matter of ongoing debate in the literature.[201]

Correlation Methods

An alternative method is a correlation technique[200] in which the data from each pixel are correlated with a model function that describes the expected activation response time profile (e.g., a square wave). For each pixel the time course of signal values is treated as a vector S_i ($i = 1$ to N, the number of images). The expected response (the model) is another vector M_i. From each of these vectors the mean is subtracted to form s_i and m_i. Then if σ_s and σ_m are the standard deviations of the data and the model, respectively, the correlation coefficient cc is

$$cc = \frac{<sm>}{\sigma_s \sigma_m} \qquad (18)$$

where $<sm>$ is the average value of $s_i m_i$. The correlation coefficient reflects the degree to which the shapes of m and s are similar but does not reflect their relative amplitudes. For relative amplitude information to be included, the correlation coefficient must be multiplied by σ_s/σ_m. Bandettini and colleagues[200] concluded that such an image, which they termed a cross-correlation image, is the preferred way to present FMRI data.

As with the t-test, the correlation methods are designed for the analysis of ideal data. Any trends in the time course must be identified and removed before processing.[200] An advantage of these methods is that the model function adds flexibility to the analysis. If the signal response is expected to be delayed and possibly to ramp up at the beginning of the stimulation and ramp down at the end, these features can easily be incorporated in the model function. In fact, one could even use the measured response of a highly activated pixel (or group of pixels) as the model function for analyzing the other pixels.[200]

Fourier Methods

Another related processing method utilizes the presumed periodicity of the activation.[200] Periodicities in the data may be identified by Fourier transformation, which reflects both the frequency and amplitude of the response, as well as the phase information, which reflects delays in the response. These Fourier methods are relatively fast and efficient because of the fast Fourier transform routines that are readily available. For each pixel the time course data is Fourier transformed and the spectral intensity at the fundamental frequency of stimulation is displayed. In fact, this method is closely related to the correlation method; the Fourier transform is essentially a correlation with a sine wave model function.

COMPARISON OF FUNCTIONAL MRI AND POSITRON EMISSION TOMOGRAPHY

PET methods have been used for the past two decades for investigating brain activity.[93, 99] FMRI, with its

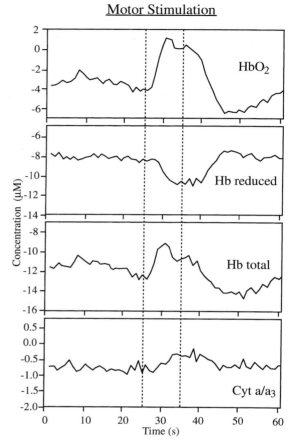

FIGURE 8–22. Influence of brain activation on near-infrared spectroscopy parameters. Brain activation was achieved by performing a finger opposition task. The spectroscopic parameters, HbO_2 (oxygenated hemoglobin), Hb reduced (deoxygenated hemoglobin), and Hb total (reflecting blood volume) are given in concentration changes. Cyt = cytochrome. (From Kwong KK: Functional MRI with echo planar imaging. Magn Reson Q 11:1–20, 1995. By permission of Raven Press, New York.)

better spatial and temporal resolution, is now a strong competitor with PET for performing these studies. A typical $H_2{}^{15}O$ PET perfusion study requires 40 seconds and the spatial resolution is limited to 5 to 10 mm. With FMRI, subsecond imaging allows the possibility of directly measuring local hemodynamic response times, and with spatial resolution of 1 to 3 mm partial-volume averaging problems are much reduced. FMRI does not require radioactive tracers, so the number of studies that can be performed on one subject is limited only by the subject's cooperativity. Furthermore, FMRI appears to be a sensitive indicator of perfusion changes, so that statistically meaningful activations can be recorded for a single subject. With PET it is often necessary to pool the results of a number of studies and draw conclusions from the pooled data, and normal variability in human anatomy complicates this type of data analysis. Because PET does not provide any anatomic reference image, localization must also include registration of the PET images with a high-resolution image (usually MR), which can introduce more computational complexity as well as misregistration errors.

With FMRI, high-resolution reference images are easily obtained as part of the FMRI protocol. Finally, MR imagers are much more widely available than PET imagers.

However, an advantage of PET is that the measured signal changes are well understood. With PET the tissue concentration of the tracer is directly measured, and the tracer kinetic models that relate this measurement to perfusion are well defined and have been tested in a number of ways. With FMRI the quantitative relationship between the measured signal changes and physiologic parameters is still an area of intense research and debate. If the signal changes in FMRI are due primarily to the BOLD effect, then FMRI is really a measure of the imbalance in the changes in flow and O_2 metabolism. It cannot be used to measure resting perfusion, whereas PET can. Furthermore, our understanding of the physiologic changes that accompany activation is incomplete. Because we do not know why the flow change is so much larger than the O_2 metabolism change, we cannot be sure that this imbalance is uniform throughout the brain or even if it always happens. A promising approach for clarifying the dynamics of brain metabolism is the combination of FMRI with other techniques that allow direct measurement of cerebral blood oxygenation, such as near-infrared spectroscopy, as illustrated in Figure 8–22. Although much work still needs to be done to address these issues, FMRI promises to be an essential tool for studying the working brain.

REFERENCES

1. Hahn EL: Spin echoes. Phys Rev 80:580–593, 1950.
2. Carr HY, Purcell EM: Effects of diffusion on free precession in nuclear magnetic resonance experiments. Phys Rev 94:630–639, 1954.
3. Woessner DE: Effects of diffusion in nuclear magnetic resonance spin-echo experiments. J Chem Phys 34:2057–2061, 1961.
4. Stejskal EO, Tanner JE: Spin diffusion measurements: spin echoes in the presence of a time-dependent field gradient. J Chem Phys 242:288–292, 1965.
5. Tanner JE: Pulsed field gradients for NMR spin-echo diffusion measurements. Rev Sci Instrum 36:1086–1087, 1965.
6. Kaiser R, Bartholdi E, Ernst RR: Diffusion and field-gradient effects in NMR Fourier spectroscopy. J Chem Phys 60:2966–2979, 1974.
7. LeBihan D: Molecular diffusion nuclear magnetic resonance imaging. Magn Reson Q 7:1–30, 1991.
8. Patronas N, Turner R, Chiro GD, Le Bihan D: Intravoxel incoherent motion (IVIM) imaging of intra-axial brain tumors. Presented at the Society of Magnetic Resonance in Medicine Workshop on Future Direction in MRI of Diffusion and Microcirculation, Bethesda, MD, 1990, p 230.
9. Tsuruda JS, Chew WM, Moseley ME, Norman D: Diffusion-weighted MR imaging of extra-axial tumors. Magn Reson Med 19:316–320, 1991.
10. Moseley ME, Cohen Y, Mintorovitch J, et al: Early detection of regional cerebral ischemia in cats: comparison of diffusion- and T2-weighted MRI and spectroscopy. Magn Reson Med 14:330–346, 1990.
11. Moseley ME, Kucharczyk J, Mintorovitch J, et al: Diffusion-weighted MR imaging of acute stroke: correlation with T2 weighted and magnetic susceptibility–enhanced MR imaging in cats. AJNR 11:423–429, 1990.
12. Warach S, Chien D, Li W, et al: Fast magnetic resonance diffusion-weighted imaging of acute human stroke. Neurology 42:1717–1723, 1992.
13. van Gelderen P, de Vleeschouwer MHM, DesPres D, et al: Water diffusion and acute stroke. Magn Reson Med 31:154–163, 1994.
14. Moseley ME, Cohen T, Kucharczyk J: Diffusion weighted MR imaging of anisotropic water diffusion in cat central nervous system. Radiology 176:439–446, 1990.
15. Doran M, Hajnal JV, Van Bruggen N, et al: Normal and abnormal white matter tracts shown by MR imaging using directional diffusion weighted sequences. J Comput Assist Tomogr 14:865–873, 1990.
16. Rutherford MA, Cowan FM, Manzur AY, et al: MR imaging of anisotropically restricted diffusion in the brain of neonates and infants. J Comput Assist Tomogr 15:188–198, 1991.
17. Hajnal JV, Doran M, Hall AS, et al: MR imaging of anisotropically restricted diffusion of water in the nervous system: technical, anatomic and pathologic considerations. J Comput Assist Tomogr 15:1–18, 1991.
18. Edelman RR, Gaa J, Wedeen VJ, et al: In vivo measurement of water diffusion in the human heart. Magn Reson Med 32:423–428, 1994.
19. Garrido L, Wedeen VJ, Spencer U, Kantor H: Anisotropy of water diffusion in the myocardium of the rat. Circ Res 74:789–793, 1994.
20. Müller MF, Prasad PV, Siewert B, et al: Abdominal diffusion-mapping using a whole body echo planar system. Radiology 190:475–478, 1994.
21. Le Bihan D, Delannoy J, Levin RL: Temperature mapping with MR imaging of molecular diffusion: application to hyperthermia. Radiology 171:853–857, 1989.
22. Le Bihan D, Breton E, Lallemand D, et al: MR imaging of intravoxel incoherent motions: application to diffusion and perfusion in neurologic disorders. Radiology 161:401–407, 1986.
23. Rosen BR, Belliveau JW, Chien D: Perfusion imaging by nuclear magnetic resonance. Magn Reson Q 5:263–281, 1989.
24. Detre JA, Leigh JS, Williams DS, Koretsky AP: Perfusion imaging. Magn Reson Med 23:37–45, 1992.
25. Shulman RG, Blamire AM, Rothman DL, McCarthy G: Nuclear magnetic resonance imaging and spectroscopy of human brain function. Proc Natl Acad Sci USA 90:3127–3133, 1993.
26. Prichard JW, Rosen BR: State-of-the-art review: functional study of the brain by NMR. J Cereb Blood Flow Metab 14:365–372, 1994.
27. Berg HC: Random Walks in Biology. Princeton, NJ: Princeton University Press, 1983.
28. Cooper RL, Chang DB, Young AC, et al: Restricted diffusion in biophysical systems. Biophys J 14:161–177, 1974.
29. Chenevert TL, Brunberg JA, Pipe JG: Anisotropic diffusion in human white matter: demonstration with MR techniques in vivo. Radiology 177:401–405, 1990.
30. Douek P, Turner R, Pekar J, et al: MR color mapping of myelin fiber orientation. J Comput Assist Tomogr 15:923–929, 1991.
31. Le Bihan D, Turner R, Douek P: Is water diffusion restricted in human brain white matter? An echo-planar NMR imaging study. Neuroreport 4:887–890, 1993.
32. Bloch F: Nuclear induction. Phys Rev 70:460–474, 1946.
33. Torrey HC: Bloch equations with diffusion terms. Phys Rev 104:563–565, 1956.
34. Stejskal EO: Use of spin echoes in a pulsed magnetic field gradient to study anisotropic, restricted diffusion and flow. J Chem Phys 43:3597–3603, 1965.
35. Basser PJ, Mattiello J, Le Bihan D: MR diffusion tensor spectroscopy and imaging. Biophys J 66:259–267, 1994.
36. Mattiello J, Basser PJ, Le Bihan D: Analytical expressions for the b matrix in NMR diffusion imaging and spectroscopy. J Magn Reson Ser A 108:131–141, 1994.
37. Tanner JE: Magnetic resonance in colloid and interface science. ACS (Am Chem Soc) Symp Ser 34:16, 1976.
38. Tanner JE, Stejskal EO: Restricted self-diffusion of protons in colloidal systems by the pulsed-gradient, spin echo method. J Chem Phys 49:1768–1777, 1968.
39. Neeman M, Freyer JP, Sillerud LO: Pulsed gradient spin echo diffusion studies in NMR imaging: effects of the imaging gradients on the determination of diffusion coefficients. J Magn Reson 90:303–312, 1990.
40. Karlicek RF Jr, Lowe IJ: A modified pulsed gradient technique for measuring diffusion in the presence of large background gradients. J Magn Reson 37:75–91, 1980.
41. Zhong J, Keenan RP, Gore JC: Effects of susceptibility variations on NMR measurements of diffusion. J Magn Reson 95:267–280, 1991.
42. Mori S, van Zijl PCM: Single scan magnetic resonance imaging of the trace of the diffusion tensor. In: Proceedings of the Second Annual Meeting of the Society of Magnetic Resonance, San Francisco, August 1994, p 135.
43. Wong EC, Cox RC: Single shot imaging with isotropic diffusion weighting. In: Proceedings of the Second Annual Meeting of the Society of Magnetic Resonance, San Francisco, August 1994, p 136.
44. Simpson JH, Carr HY: Diffusion and nuclear spin relaxation in water. Phys Rev 111:1201–1202, 1958.
45. Delannoy J, Chen C, Turner R, et al: Noninvasive temperature imaging using diffusion MRI. Magn Reson Med 19:333–339, 1991.
46. Bleier AR, Jolesz GA, Cohen MS, et al: Real-time magnetic resonance imaging of laser heat deposition in tissue. Magn Reson Med 21:132–137, 1991.
47. Parker DL, Smith V, Sheldon P, et al: Temperature distribution measurements in two-dimensional NMR imaging. Med Phys 10:321–325, 1983.
48. Young IR, Hand JW, Oatridge A, Prior MV: Modeling and observation of temperature changes in vivo using MRI. Magn Reson Med 32:358–369, 1994.
49. Ahn CB, Lee SY, Nalcioglu O, Cho ZH: An improved nuclear magnetic resonance diffusion coefficient imaging method using an optimized pulse sequence. Med Phys 13:789–793, 1986.
50. Taylor DG, Bushell MC: The spatial mapping of translational diffusion

coefficients by the NMR imaging technique. Phys Med Biol 30:345–349, 1985.

51. Chien D, Buxton RB, Kwong KK: Quantitative diffusion imaging in the human brain. In: Proceedings of the Seventh Annual Meeting of the Society of Magnetic Resonance in Medicine, San Francisco, 1988, p 218.
52. Chien D, Kwong KK, Buonanno RS, et al: MR Diffusion imaging of cerebral infarction. In: Proceedings of the Seventh Annual Meeting of the Society of Magnetic Resonance in Medicine, San Francisco, 1988, p 889.
53. Mikulis D, Chien D, Kwong K, et al: Diffusion magnetic resonance imaging in multiple sclerosis. In: Proceedings of the Seventh Annual Meeting of the Society of Magnetic Resonance in Medicine, San Francisco, 1988, p 762.
54. Tanner JE: Use of stimulated echo in NMR diffusion studies. J Chem Phys 52:2523–2526, 1970.
55. Merboldt KD, Hanicke W, Frahm J: Self-diffusion NMR imaging using stimulated echoes. J Magn Reson 64:479–486, 1985.
56. Le Bihan D: Intravoxel incoherent motion imaging using steady-state free precession. Magn Reson Med 7:346–351, 1988.
57. Merboldt KD, Hanicke W, Gyngell ML, et al: Rapid NMR imaging of molecular self-diffusion using a modified CE-FAST sequence. J Magn Reson 82:115–121, 1989.
58. Wu EX, Buxton RB: Effect of diffusion on the steady-state magnetization with pulsed field gradients. J Magn Reson 90:243–253, 1990.
59. Buxton RB: The diffusion sensitivity of fast steady-state free precession imaging. Magn Reson Med 29:235–243, 1993.
60. Merboldt KD, Hanicke W, Gyngell ML, et al: The influence of flow and motion in MRI of diffusion using a modified CE-FAST sequence. Magn Reson Med 12:198–208, 1989.
61. Le Bihan D, Turner R, Macfall JR: Effects of intravoxel incoherent motions (IVIM) in steady-state free precession (SSFP) imaging: application to molecular diffusion imaging. Magn Reson Med 10:324–337, 1989.
62. Prasad PV, Nalcioglu O: A modified pulse sequence of in vivo diffusion imaging with reduced motion artifacts. Magn Reson Med 18:116–131, 1991.
63. Merboldt KD, Bruhn H, Frahm J, et al: MRI of "diffusion" in the human brain: new results using a modified CE-FAST sequence. Magn Reson Med 9:423–429, 1989.
64. Poncelet BP, Wedeen VJ, Weisskoff RM, Cohen MS: Brain parenchyma motion: measurement with cine echo-planar MR imaging. Radiology 185:645–651, 1992.
65. Enzmann DR, Pelc NJ: Brain motion: measurement with phase-contrast MR imaging. Radiology 185:653–660, 1992.
66. Mulkern RV, Spencer RGS: Diffusion imaging with paired CPMG sequences. Magn Reson Imaging 6:623–631, 1988.
67. Jung KJ, Cho ZH: Reduction of flow artifacts in NMR diffusion imaging using view-angle tilted line-integral projection reconstruction. Magn Reson Med 19:349–360, 1991.
68. Ordidge RJ, Helpern JA, Qing Z, et al: Correction of motional artifacts in diffusion-weighted MR images using navigator echoes. Magn Reson Imaging 12:455–460, 1994.
69. Anderson AW, Gore JC: Analysis and correction of motion artifacts in diffusion weighted imaging. Magn Reson Med 32:379–387, 1994.
70. Merboldt KD, Hanicke W, Bruhn H, et al: Diffusion imaging of the human brain in vivo using high-speed STEAM MRI. Magn Reson Med 23:179–192, 1992.
71. Mansfield P: Multi-planar image formation using NMR spin echoes. J Phys C 10:L55, 349–352, 1977.
72. Warach S, Wielopolski P, Edelman RR: Identification and characterization of the ischemic penumbra of acute human stroke using echo planar diffusion and perfusion imaging. In: Proceedings of the 12th Annual Meeting of the Society of Magnetic Resonance in Medicine, New York, 1993, p 249.
73. Müller MF, Prasad PV, Bimmler D, et al: Functional imaging of the kidney by measurement of the apparent diffusion coefficient. Radiology 193:711–715, 1994.
74. Turner R, Bowley RM: Passive screening of switched magnetic field gradients. J Phys E Sci Instrum 19:876, 1986.
75. Mansfield P, Chapman B: Active magnetic screening of gradient coils in NMR imaging. J Magn Reson 66:573–576, 1986.
76. Belliveau JW, Rosen BR, Kantor HL, et al: Functional cerebral imaging by susceptibility-contrast NMR. Magn Reson Med 14:538–546, 1990.
77. Weisskoff RM, Belliveau JW, Kwong KK, Rosen BR: Functional imaging of capillary hemodynamics. In: Potchen EJ, Haacke EM, Siebert JE, Gottschalk A, eds. Magnetic Resonance Angiography Concepts and Applications. St. Louis: CV Mosby, 1993, pp 473–484.
78. Ogawa S, Lee T-M, Nayak AS, Glynn P: Oxygenation-sensitive contrast in magnetic resonance image of rodent brain at high magnetic fields. Magn Reson Med 14:68–78, 1990.
79. Turner R, Le Bihan D, Moonen CTW, et al: Echo-planar time course MRI of cat brain oxygenation changes. Magn Reson Med 22:159–166, 1991.
80. Kwong KK, Belliveau JW, Chesler DA, et al: Dynamic magnetic resonance imaging of human brain activity during primary sensory stimulation. Proc Natl Acad Sci USA 89:5675–5679, 1992.
81. Ogawa S, Tank DW, Menon R, et al: Intrinsic signal changes accompa-

nying sensory stimulation: functional brain mapping with magnetic resonance imaging. Proc Natl Acad Sci USA 89:5951–5955, 1992.
82. Bandettini PA, Wong EC, Hinks RS, et al: Time course EPI of human brain function during task activation. Magn Reson Med 25:390–397, 1992.
83. Gillis P, Koenig SH: Transverse relaxation of solvent protons induced by magnetized spheres: application to ferritin, erythrocytes, and magnetite. Magn Reson Med 5:323–345, 1987.
84. Muller RN, Gillis P, Moiny F, Roch A: Transverse relaxivity of particulate MRI contrast media: from theories to experiments. Magn Reson Med 22:178–182, 1991.
85. Majumdar S, Gore JC: Studies of diffusion in random fields produced by variations in susceptibility. Magn Reson Med 78:41–55, 1988.
86. Hardy P, Henkelman RM: On the transverse relaxation rate enhancement induced by diffusion of spins through inhomogeneous fields. Magn Reson Med 17:348–356, 1991.
87. Purcell E: Electricity and Magnetism. Berkeley Physics Series. New York: McGraw-Hill, 1965.
88. Ogawa S, Menon RS, Tank DW, et al: Functional brain mapping by blood oxygenation level–dependent contrast magnetic resonance imaging: a comparison of signal characteristics with a biophysical model. Biophys J 64:803–812, 1993.
89. Fisel CR, Ackerman JL, Buxton RB, et al: MR contrast due to microscopically heterogeneous magnetic susceptibility: numerical simulations and applications to cerebral physiology. Magn Reson Med 17:336–347, 1991.
90. Kennan RP, Zhong J, Gore JC: Intravascular susceptibility contrast mechanisms in tissues. Magn Reson Med 31:9–21, 1994.
91. Weisskoff RM, Zuo CS, Boxerman JL, Rosen BR: Microscopic susceptibility variation and transverse relaxation: theory and experiment. Magn Reson Med 31:1–10, 1994.
92. Edvinsson L, MacKenzie ET, McCulloch J: Cerebral Blood Flow and Metabolism. New York: Raven Press, 1993.
93. Raichle ME: Brain blood flow and metabolism. In: Plum F, ed. Handbook of Physiology, Section 1, The Nervous System, Volume V, Part 2, Higher Functions of the Brain. New York: Oxford University Press, 1987, pp 643–674.
94. Grubb RL, Raichle ME, Eichling JO, Ter-Pogossian MM: The effects of changes in P_{CO_2} on cerebral blood volume, blood flow, and vascular mean transit time. Stroke 5:630–639, 1974.
95. Siesjo BK: Brain Energy Metabolism. New York: John Wiley & Sons, 1978.
96. Roy CS, Sherrington CS: On the regulation of the blood supply of the brain. J Physiol (Lond) 11:85–108, 1890.
97. Kety SS: The early history of the coupling between cerebral blood flow, metabolism and function. In: Lassen NA, Ingvar DH, Raichle ME, Friberg L, eds. Brain Work and Mental Activity: Quantitative Studies with Radioactive Tracers. Copenhagen: Munksgaard, 1991, pp 19–28.
98. Kety SS, Schmidt CF: Nitrous oxide method for the quantitative determination of cerebral blood flow in man: theory, procedure and normal values. J Clin Invest 27:475–483, 1948.
99. Roland PE: Brain Activation. New York: Wiley-Liss, 1993.
100. Lassen NA, Ingvar DH, Raichle ME, Friberg L, eds: Brain Work and Mental Activity: Quantitative Studies with Radioactive Tracers. Copenhagen: Munksgaard, 1991.
101. Fox PT, Raichle ME: Focal physiological uncoupling of cerebral blood flow and oxidative metabolism during somatosensory stimulation in human subjects. Proc Natl Acad Sci USA 83:1140–1144, 1986.
102. Fox PT, Raichle ME, Mintun MA, Dence C: Nonoxidative glucose consumption during focal physiologic neural activity. Science 241:462–464, 1988.
103. Buxton RB, Frank LR: A physiological model for the interpretation of functional MR brain activation studies. In: Proceedings of the 12th Annual Meeting of the Society of Magnetic Resonance in Medicine, New York, 1993, p 4.
104. Thulborn KR, Waterton JC, Matthews PM, Radda GK: Oxygenation dependence of the transverse relaxation time of water protons in whole blood at high field. Biochim Biophys Acta 714:265–270, 1982.
105. Smith AL, Neufeld GR, Ominsky AJ, Wollman H: Effect of arterial CO_2 tension on cerebral blood flow, mean transit time, and vascular volume. J Appl Physiol 31:701–707, 1971.
106. Greenberg JH, Alavi A, Reivich M, et al: Local cerebral blood volume response to carbon dioxide in man. Circ Res 43:324–331, 1978.
107. Sakai F, Nakazawa K, Tazaki Y, et al: Regional cerebral blood volume and hematocrit measured in normal human volunteers by single-photon emission computed tomography. J Cereb Blood Flow Metab 5:207–213, 1985.
108. Weiss HR: Measurement of cerebral capillary perfusion with a fluorescent label. Microvasc Res 36:172–180, 1988.
109. Shockley RP, LaManna JC: Determination of rat cerebral cortical blood volume changes by capillary mean transit time analysis during hypoxia, hypercapnia and hyperventilation. Brain Res 454:170–178, 1988.
110. Frankel HM, Garcia E, Malik F, et al: Effect of acetazolamide on cerebral blood flow and capillary patency. J Appl Physiol 73:1756–1761, 1992.
111. Pawlik G, Rackl A, Bing RJ: Quantitative capillary topography and blood flow in the cerebral cortex of cats: an in vivo microscopic study. Brain Res 208:35–58, 1981.

112. Gobel U, Klein B, Schrock H, Kuschinsky W: Lack of capillary recruitment in the brains of awake rats during hypercapnia. J Cereb Blood Flow Metab 9:491–499, 1989.

113. Gobel U, Theilen H, Kuschinsky W: Congruence of total and perfused capillary network in rat brains. Circ Res 66:271–281, 1990.

114. Bereczki D, Wei L, Otsuka T, et al: Hypoxia increases velocity of blood flow through parenchymal microvascular systems in rat brain. J Cereb Blood Flow Metab 13:475–486, 1993.

115. Wei L, Otsuka T, Acuff V, et al: The velocities of red cell and plasma flows through parenchymal microvessels of rat brain are decreased by pentobarbital. J Cereb Blood Flow Metab 13:487–497, 1993.

116. Duelli R, Kuschinsky W: Changes in brain capillary diameter during hypocapnia and hypercapnia. J Cereb Blood Flow Metab 13:1025–1028, 1993.

117. Lassen NA, Perl W: Tracer Kinetic Methods in Medical Physiology. New York: Raven Press, 1979.

118. Meier P, Zierler KL: On the theory of the indicator-dilution method for measurement of blood flow and volume. J Appl Physiol 6:731–744, 1954.

119. Zierler KL: Theoretical basis of indicator-dilution methods for measuring flow and volume. Circ Res 10:393–407, 1962.

120. Axel L: Cerebral blood flow determination by rapid-sequence computed tomography: a theoretical analysis. Radiology 137:679–686, 1980.

121. Stewart GN: Researches on the circulation time in organs and on the influences which affect it. Parts I–III. J Physiol (Lond) 15:1–89, 1894.

122. Lassen N: Cerebral transit of an intravascular tracer may allow measurement of regional blood volume but not regional blood flow. J Cereb Blood Flow Metab 4:633–634, 1984.

123. Le Bihan D, Breton E, Lallemand D, et al: MR imaging of intravoxel incoherent motions: application to diffusion and perfusion in neurologic disorders. Radiology 168:497–505, 1988.

124. Le Bihan D, Turner R, Moonen CTW, Pekar J: Imaging of diffusion and microcirculation with gradient sensitization: design, strategy and significance. J Magn Reson Imaging 1:7–28, 1991.

125. Kwong KK, McKinstry RC, Chien D, et al: CSF suppressed quantitative single-shot diffusion imaging. In: Proceedings of the 10th Annual Meeting of the Society of Magnetic Resonance in Medicine, San Francisco, 1991, p 215.

126. Neil JJ, Scherrer L, Ackerman JJH: An approach to solving the dynamic range problem in measurement of the pseudodiffusion coefficient in vivo with spin echoes. J Magn Reson 95:607–614, 1991.

127. Neil JJ, Bosch CS, Ackerman JJH: An evaluation of the sensitivity of the intravoxel incoherent motion (IVIM) method of blood flow measurement to changes in cerebral blood flow. Magn Reson Med 32:60–65, 1994.

128. Henkelman RM: Does IVIM measure classical perfusion? Magn Reson Med 16:470–475, 1990.

129. Kennan RP, Gao JH, Zhong J, Gore JC: A general model of microcirculatory blood flow effects in gradient sensitized MRI. Med Phys 21:539–545, 1994.

130. Neil JJ, Ackerman JJH: Detection of pseudodiffusion in rat brain following blood substitution with perfluorocarbon. J Magn Reson 97:194–201, 1992.

131. Henkelman RM, Neil JJ, Xiang QS: A quantitative interpretation of IVIM measurements of vascular perfusion in the rat brain. Magn Reson Med 32:464–469, 1994.

132. Le Bihan D, Turner R: The capillary network: a link between IVIM and classical perfusion. Magn Reson Med 27:171–178, 1992.

133. Villringer A, Rosen BR, Belliveau JW, et al: Dynamic imaging with lanthanide chelates in normal brain: contrast due to magnetic susceptibility effects. Magn Reson Med 6:164–174, 1988.

134. Belliveau JW, Rosen BR, Buxton RB, et al: Dynamic imaging with gadolinium of magnetic susceptibility effects in experimental brain ischemia. In: Proceedings of the Sixth Annual Meeting of the Society of Magnetic Resonance in Medicine, New York, 1987, p 7.

135. Josephson L, Bigler J, White D: The magnetic properties of some materials affecting MR images. Magn Reson Med 22:204–208, 1991.

136. Weisskoff RM, Kiihne S: MRI susceptometry: image-based measurement of absolute susceptibility of MR contrast agents and human blood. Magn Reson Med 24:375–383, 1992.

137. Edelman RR, Mattle HP, Atkinson DJ, et al: Cerebral blood flow: assessment with dynamic contrast-enhanced T2*-weighted MR imaging at 1.5 T. Radiology 176:211–220, 1990.

138. Perman WH, Gado MH, Larson KB, Perlmutter JS: Simultaneous MR acquisition of arterial and brain signal-time curves. Magn Reson Med 28:74–83, 1992.

139. Taylor NJ, Rowland IJ, Tanner SF, Leach MO: A rapid interleaved method for measuring signal intensity curves in both blood and tissue during contrast agent administration. Magn Reson Med 30:744–749, 1993.

140. Weisskoff RM, Chesler D, Boxerman JL, Rosen BR: Pitfalls in MR measurement of tissue blood flow with intravascular tracers: which mean transit time? Magn Reson Med 29:553–558, 1993.

141. Kwong KK, Chesler DA, Weisskoff RM, Rosen BR: Perfusion MR imaging. In: Proceedings of the Second Annual Meeting of the Society of Magnetic Resonance, San Francisco, August 1994, p 1005.

142. Williams DS, Detre JA, Leigh JS, Koretsky AP: Magnetic resonance imaging of perfusion using spin inversion of arterial water. Proc Natl Acad Sci USA 89:212–216, 1992.

143. Edelman RR, Siewert B, Darby DG, et al: Qualitative mapping of cerebral blood flow and functional localization with echo-plan or MR imaging and signal targeting with alternating radiofrequency. Radiology 192:513–520, 1994.

144. Lammertsma AA, Jones T: Correction for the presence of intravascular oxygen-15 in the steady-state technique for measuring regional oxygen extraction ratio in the brain: 1. Description of the method. J Cereb Blood Flow Metab 3:416–424, 1983.

145. Zhang W, Williams DS, Detre JA, Koretsky AP: Measurement of brain perfusion by volume-localized NMR spectroscopy using inversion of arterial water spins: accounting for transit time and cross-relaxation. Magn Reson Med 25:362–371, 1992.

146. Zhang W, Williams DS, Koretsky AP: Measurement of rat brain perfusion by NMR using spin labeling of arterial water: in vivo determination of the degree of spin labeling. Magn Reson Med 29:416–421, 1993.

147. Walsh EG, Minematsu K, Leppo J, Moore SC: Radioactive microsphere validation of a volume localized continuous saturation perfusion measurement. Magn Reson Med 31:147–153, 1994.

148. Nishimura DG, Macovski A, Pauly JM: Magnetic resonance angiography. IEEE Trans Med Imaging MI-5(3):140–151, 1986.

149. Edelman RR, Siewert B, Adamis M, et al: Signal targeting with alternating radiofrequency (STAR) sequences: application to MR angiography. Magn Reson Med 31:233–238, 1994.

150. Evelhoch JL: Tracer measurements of blood flow. In: Gillies RJ, ed. NMR in Physiology and Biomedicine. San Diego: Academic Press, 1994, pp 209–220.

151. Ackerman JJH, Ewy CS, Becker NN, Shalwitz RA: Deuterium nuclear magnetic resonance measurements of blood flow and tissue perfusion employing ^2H_2O as a freely diffusible tracer. Proc Natl Acad Sci USA 84:4099–4102, 1987.

152. Kim SG, Ackerman JJH: Quantification of regional blood flow by monitoring of exogenous tracer via nuclear magnetic resonance spectroscopy. Magn Reson Med 14:266–282, 1990.

153. Evelhoch JL, McDouall JB, Mattiello J, Simpson NE: Measurement of relative regional tumor blood flow in mice by deuterium NMR imaging. Magn Reson Med 24:42–52, 1992.

154. Neil JJ, Song S-K, Ackerman JJH: Concurrent quantification of tissue metabolism and blood flow via $^2H/^{31}P$ NMR in vivo. II. Validation of the deuterium NMR washout method for measuring organ perfusion. Magn Reson Med 25:56–66, 1992.

155. Pekar J, Ligeti L, Ruttner Z, et al: In vivo measurement of cerebral oxygen consumption and blood flow using ^{17}O magnetic resonance imaging. Magn Reson Med 21:313–319, 1991.

156. Hopkins AL, Haacke EM, Tkach J, et al: Improved sensitivity of proton MR to oxygen-17 as a contrast agent using fast imaging: detection in brain. Magn Reson Med 7:222–229, 1988.

157. Kwong KK, Hopkins AL, Belliveau JW, et al: Proton NMR imaging of cerebral blood flow using $H_2^{17}O$. Magn Reson Med 22:154–158, 1991.

158. Eleff SM, Schnall MD, Ligetti L, et al: Concurrent measurements of cerebral blood flow, sodium, lactate, and high-energy phosphate metabolism using ^{19}F, ^{23}Na, ^1H, and ^{31}P nuclear magnetic resonance spectroscopy. Magn Reson Med 7:412–424, 1988.

159. Ewing JR, Branch CA, Helpern JA, et al: Cerebral blood flow measured by NMR indicator dilution in cats. Stroke 20:259–267, 1989.

160. Rudin M, Sauter A: Non-invasive determination of cerebral blood flow changes by ^{19}F NMR spectroscopy. NMR Biomed 2:98–103, 1989.

161. Barranco D, Sutton LN, Florin S, et al: Use of ^{19}F spectroscopy for measurement of cerebral blood flow: a comparative study using microspheres. J Cereb Blood Flow Metab 9:886–891, 1989.

162. Pekar J, Ligeti L, Sinnwell T, et al: ^{19}F magnetic resonance imaging of cerebral blood flow with 0.4-cc resolution. J Cereb Blood Flow Metab 14:656–663, 1994.

163. Thomas C, Counsell C, Wood P, Adams GE: Use of fluorine-19 nuclear magnetic resonance spectroscopy and hydralazine for measuring dynamic changes in blood perfusion volume in tumors in mice. J Natl Cancer Inst 84:174–180, 1992.

164. Parhami P, Fung BM: Fluorine-19 relaxation study of perfluorocarbons as oxygen carriers. J Phys Chem 87:1928–1931, 1983.

165. Fishman JE, Joseph PM, Carvlin MJ, et al: In vivo measurements of vascular oxygen tension in tumors using MRI of a fluorinated blood substitute. Invest Radiol 24:65–71, 1989.

166. Thomas SR, Clark LC Jr, Ackerman JL, et al: MR imaging of the lung using liquid perfluorocarbons. J Comput Assist Tomogr 10:1–9, 1986.

167. Hees PS, Sotak CH: Assessment of changes in murine tumor oxygenation in response to nicotinamide using ^{19}F NMR relaxometry of a perfluorocarbon emulsion. Magn Reson Med 29:303–310, 1993.

168. London RE: In vivo NMR studies utilizing fluorinated probes. In: Gillies RJ, ed. NMR in Physiology and Biomedicine. San Diego: Academic Press, 1994, pp 263–277.

169. Majumdar S, Zoghbi SS, Gore JC: Regional differences in rat brain displayed by fast MRI with superparamagnetic contrast agents. Magn Reson Imaging 6:611–615, 1988.

170. Fahlvik AK, Klaveness J, Stark DD: Iron oxides as MR imaging contrast agents. J Magn Reson Imaging 3:187–194, 1993.

171. Kent T, Quast M, Kaplan B, et al: Assessment of a superparamagnetic iron oxide (AMI-25) as a brain contrast agent. Magn Reson Med 13:434–443, 1990.

172. Forsting M, Reith W, Dorfler A, et al: MRI in acute cerebral ischaemia: perfusion imaging with superparamagnetic iron oxide in a rat model. Neuroradiology 36:23–26, 1994.

173. Rozenman Y, Zou X, Kantor HL: Magnetic resonance imaging with superparamagnetic iron oxide particles for the detection of myocardial reperfusion. Magn Reson Imaging 9:933–939, 1991.

174. Trillaud H, Grenier N, Degreze P, et al: First-pass evaluation of renal perfusion with turboFLASH MR imaging and superparamagnetic iron oxide particles. J Magn Reson Imaging 3:83–91, 1993.

175. Pauling L, Coryell CD: The magnetic properties and structure of hemoglobin and carbonmonoxyhemoglobin. Proc Natl Acad Sci USA 22:210–216, 1936.

176. Frahm J, Bruhn H, Merboldt K-D, Hanicke W: Dynamic MR imaging of human brain oxygenation during rest and photic stimulation. J Magn Reson Imaging 2:501–505, 1992.

177. Constable RT, McCarthy G, Allison T, et al: Functional brain imaging at 1.5 T using conventional gradient echo MR imaging techniques. Magn Reson Imaging 11:451–459, 1993.

178. Cao Y, Towle VL, Levin DN, Balter JM: Functional mapping of human motor cortical activation with conventional MR imaging at 1.5 T. J Magn Reson Imaging 3:869–875, 1993.

179. Kim S-G, Ashe J, Hendrich K, et al: Functional magnetic resonance imaging of motor cortex: hemispheric asymmetry and handedness. Science 261:615–617, 1993.

180. Schneider W, Noll DC, Cohen JD: Functional topographic mapping of the cortical ribbon in human vision with conventional MRI scanners. Nature 365:150–153, 1993.

181. Engel SA, Rumelhart DE, Wandell BA, et al: fMRI of human visual cortex. Nature 369:525, 1994. Letter.

182. Hinke RM, Hu X, Stillman AE, et al: Functional magnetic resonance imaging of Broca's area during internal speech. Neuroreport 4:675–678, 1993.

183. Connelly A, Jackson GD, Frackowiak RS, et al: Functional mapping of activated human primary cortex with a clinical MR imaging system. Radiology 188:125–130, 1993.

184. Belliveau JW, Kennedy DN, McKinstry RC, et al: Functional mapping of the human visual cortex by magnetic resonance imaging. Science 254:716–719, 1991.

185. Turner R, Jezzard P, Wen H, et al: Functional mapping of the human visual cortex at 4 and 1.5 tesla using deoxygenation contrast EPI. Magn Reson Med 29:277–279, 1993.

186. Boxerman JL, Weisskoff RM, Kwong KK, et al: The intravascular contribution to fMRI signal change: modeling and diffusion-weighted in vivo studies. In: Proceedings of the Second Annual Meeting of the Society of Magnetic Resonance, San Francisco, August 1994, p 619.

187. Davis TL, Weisskoff RM, Kwong KK, et al: Temporal aspects of fMRI task activation: dynamic modeling of oxygen delivery. In: Proceedings of the Second Annual Meeting of the Society of Magnetic Resonance, San Francisco, August 1994, p 69.

188. Lai S, Hopkins AL, Haacke EM, et al: Identification of vascular structures as a major source of signal contrast in high resolution 2D and 3D functional activation imaging of the motor cortex at 1.5T: preliminary results. Magn Reson Med 30:387–392, 1993.

189. Menon RS, Ogawa S, Tank DW, Ugurbil K: 4 tesla gradient recalled echo characteristics of photic stimulation–induced signal changes in the human primary visual cortex. Magn Reson Med 30:380–386, 1993.

190. Frahm J, Merboldt K-D, Hanicke W: Functional MRI of human brain activation at high spatial resolution. Magn Reson Med 29:139–144, 1993.

191. Hoppel BE, Weisskoff RM, Thulborn KR, et al: Measurement of regional blood oxygenation and cerebral hemodynamics. Magn Reson Med 30:715–723, 1993.

192. Ugurbil K, Garwood M, Ellermann JM, et al: Imaging at high magnetic fields: initial experiences at 4T. Magn Reson Q 9:259–277, 1993.

193. Edelman RR, Wielopolski P, Schmitt F: Echo-planar MR imaging. Radiology 192:600–612, 1994.

194. Cohen MS, Weisskoff RM: Ultra-fast imaging. Magn Reson Imaging 9:1–37, 1991.

195. Noll DC, Cohen JD, Meyer CH, Schneider W: Spiral k-space MR imaging of cortical activation. J Magn Reson Imaging 5:49–56, 1995.

196. Meyer CH, Hu BS, Nishimura DG, Macovski A: Fast spiral coronary artery imaging. Magn Reson Med 28:202–213, 1992.

197. Glover GH, Pauly JM: Projection reconstruction techniques for reduction of motion effects in MRI. Magn Reson Med 28:275–289, 1992.

198. Weisskoff RM, Baker J, Belliveau J, et al: Power spectrum analysis of functionally-weighted MR data: What's in noise? In: Proceedings of the 12th Annual Meeting of the Society of Magnetic Resonance in Medicine, New York, 1993, p 7.

199. Hajnal JV, Myers R, Oatridge A, et al: Artifacts due to stimulus correlated motion in functional imaging of the brain. Magn Reson Med 31:283–291, 1994.

200. Bandettini PA, Jesmanowicz A, Wong EC, Hyde JS: Processing strategies for time-course data sets in function MRI of the human brain. Magn Reson Med 30:161–173, 1993.

201. Biswal B, DeYoe EA, Cox RW, Hyde JS: FMRI analysis for aperiodic task activation using nonparametric statistics. In: Proceedings of the Second Annual Meeting of the Society of Magnetic Resonance, San Francisco, August 1994, p 624.

MR Angiography: Basic Principles

DAISY CHIEN ▪ CHARLES M. ANDERSON ▪ RALPH E. LEE

Magnetic resonance angiography (MRA) has attained an important position in the evaluation of vascular diseases. Through technical advances, substantial improvements in image quality and vessel depiction have been made in a relatively short time (Fig. 9–1). In intracranial examinations, vascular resolution of MRA begins to approach that of conventional x-ray angiography. MRA has a number of potential advantages over conventional angiography. First, it is noninvasive. Second, it uses the intrinsic mechanisms of blood flow instead of the exogenous introduction of a contrast material to depict flow. Third, MRA offers a range of information not available with conventional angiography. MRA goes beyond the mere depiction of vascular anatomy; it provides insight into underlying functions.

BEHAVIOR OF BLOOD FLOW

Flow contrast in MRA is a result of blood motion. Hemodynamics of blood flow has profound effects on vessel appearance in MRA. Therefore, a good understanding of the fundamental properties of flow is useful for selecting the best protocol for MRA.

STREAMLINES AND FLOW PROFILES

Blood flow is complex and highly variable in vivo. It can, however, be described by simple flow models. In fluid dynamics, streamlines and flow profiles are often used to provide a graphic description of flow in vessels. Common examples of streamline flow include plug flow and laminar flow (Fig. 9–2). In plug flow, all fluid particles move forward in parallel lines with the same speed. Plug flow has a characteristic blunt profile and is often observed in the descending thoracic aorta. Laminar flow, on the other hand, has a parabolic flow profile with the fastest moving fluid particles at the center of the lumen. It is called laminar because the particles move along in concentric sheets or laminae.[1] The flow velocity at any radial location in steady laminar flow is precisely described by the following equation:

$$V(r) = V_{max}[1 - (r/R)^2] \qquad (1)$$

where $V(r)$ is the velocity at distance r from the center of the lumen, R is the radius of the vessel, and V_{max} is the maximal flow velocity. Note that the velocity is maximum (V_{max}) for particles at the center of the lumen (r = 0), whereas the velocity is zero for fluid particles at the vessel wall (r = R). Friction and the resulting drag at the vessel wall are responsible for this zero velocity.

Flow profiles have a significant impact on the flow contrast obtained in MRA. In addition, they can affect the interpretation of measured flow velocity in different blood vessels. For example, the average velocity in laminar flow is exactly 50% of the peak velocity at the center of the lumen, whereas the average velocity in plug flow is equal to the peak velocity.

VESSEL GEOMETRY AND ENTRANCE EFFECT

Geometry plays an important role in fluid dynamics. Variations in vessel geometry, such as vessel tortuosity, stenosis, and bifurcations, can alter the appearance of flow in MRA. For example, signal heterogeneity in MRA of the carotid artery siphons is due to local vessel curvature that causes the fastest moving fluid particles to swing toward the outer curve of the vessel (as a result of inertia).[2]

The local flow profile often changes when the geometry of a blood vessel deviates from a long cylinder. For example, the U shape of the aortic arch results in blood traveling with a helical flow pattern. In the vicinity of a bifurcation, flow separation occurs. Flow separation is the formation of a local fluid recirculation zone that does not move with the main streamlines. This can be observed in the carotid bulb. It can also occur adjacent to a stenosis (Fig. 9–3). The separation zone often appears dark in MRA and is due to saturation, which is described in greater detail in this chapter.

271

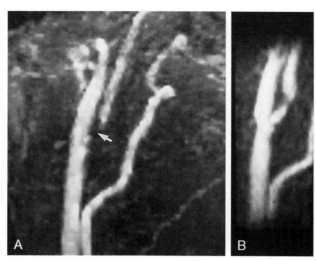

FIGURE 9–1. *A,* A three-dimensional (3D) time-of-flight (TOF) image of the carotid bifurcation of a patient with proximal internal carotid stenosis *(arrow)* acquired in 1989 (TR/TE = 40/9). *B,* Acquisition repeated 3 years later showing less signal loss related to turbulence at the stenosis with the use of a shorter TE (7 ms) and increased image resolution.

Another important flow phenomenon occurs when laminar flow proceeds from a larger vessel or fluid cavity into a smaller vessel. It is known as the entrance effect. Immediately at the entrance of the smaller vessel, the flow profile is blunt and it takes a certain distance for flow to develop fully to the parabolic flow profile[3] (Fig. 9–4). As a result of the entrance effect, the measured flow profile and velocity distribution can vary depending on the location of the measurement.

FLOW BEHAVIOR IN THE HUMAN VASCULATURE

Blood flow in the major arteries is highly pulsatile, with flow velocity varying from greater than 100 cm/s during systole to almost no flow during diastole. Flow quantification by MR has shown that blood flows in the ascending aorta with a skewed velocity profile during systole (with an axis of skew symmetric about the plane of the aortic arch) and flows in the descending aorta with a plug profile with minimal skew.[4] During diastole, blood flow actually reverses for a short time in medium to large arteries, such as the aorta. This flow reversal typically occurs during early diastole. One of its causes is reflection of the pulse pressure wave at the distal vessels. Wave reflection at the peripheral vessels also results in the distinctive triphasic (forward-backward-forward) waveform in the popliteal artery observed by MR flow quantification. This triphasic

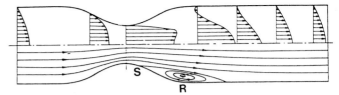

FIGURE 9–3. Schematic diagram of the change in streamline and flow profile caused by a vessel stenosis. Immediately distal to the stenosis is a flow separation (S) and recirculation (R) zone. (From Milnor WR: Hemodynamics. Baltimore: Williams & Wilkins, 1989, p 35.)

waveform may be lost when significant atherosclerotic disease is present.

There is always resistance to blood flow in a vessel. Flow resistance depends on the fluid viscosity as well as the shape of the vessel. It has a strong dependence on the vessel diameter (it decreases with the fourth power of the radius). This is because most of the resistance occurs at the vessel wall. As a result, flow encounters increasing resistance as it goes from larger vessels to smaller ones. Because of vessel tapering and higher and higher resistance to flow at the distal vessels, the arterial tree has considerable damping of cardiac pulsations as blood travels from the arteries to the veins.

VISCOSITY AND NON-NEWTONIAN PROPERTIES OF BLOOD

Viscosity is the internal friction of a fluid. Unlike flow resistance, it depends only on the nature of the fluid and is totally independent of the vessel geometry. Viscosity of blood is approximately three times higher than that of water as a result of the red blood cells exerting frictional drag on neighboring cells and against the wall of the vessel. A newtonian fluid has, by definition, a viscosity that is constant regardless of the shear rate (steepness of the velocity profile). At low shear rates, blood becomes viscous as the red blood cells adhere to each other and its viscosity is no longer constant. At high shear rates, on the other hand, there is much less tendency for the cells to aggregate and blood behaves more like a newtonian fluid. This is true for swift blood flow in large arteries.

TURBULENCE AND THE REYNOLDS NUMBER

Within the radiology community, the term *turbulence* is used loosely to refer to chaotic flow patterns, which are often associated with unwanted signal loss in MRA.

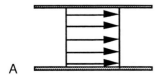
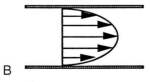

FIGURE 9–2. Schematic diagrams of streamline flow showing *(A)* plug flow and *(B)* laminar flow.

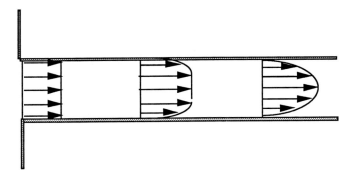

FIGURE 9–4. Schematic diagram of the flow entrance effect.

In fluid mechanics, turbulence has a more precise definition. It refers to shuddering disturbances throughout a fluid and is associated with the formation of eddies and vortices. The onset of turbulence is determined by the Reynolds number, which is given by

$$Re = \rho vD/\mu \qquad (2)$$

where ρ is the density of the fluid, v is the average velocity, D is the diameter of the vessel, and μ is the viscosity. Flow becomes turbulent when the Reynolds number is 2000 and above. As shown in Equation 2, the Reynolds number increases with the diameter of the tube and the average velocity and decreases with the viscosity. In the human aorta, the Reynolds number is about 1500. True turbulence is seldom encountered in vivo. Even before reaching turbulence, nonstreamline flow can lead to phase incoherence and loss of signal in MRA.

As can be seen from this brief discussion of flow dynamics, different flow conditions can have a significant impact on the results of MRA. With this in mind, optimal flow contrast can be achieved with an understanding of both the flow behavior and the principles of MRA.

MR ANGIOGRAPHY

Myriad MRA techniques have been proposed and evaluated over the years.[5, 6] It would be beyond the scope of this chapter to describe all the methods that can be used to depict flow. Rather, this chapter focuses on the techniques that have established applicability and are used routinely in a clinical setting for diagnosis of vascular abnormalities.

There are two major mechanisms by which moving blood affects the MR signal. They are the time-of-flight (TOF) effect, first observed more than four decades ago, and the phase effect, also discovered in the early days of MR.[7–9] These two principles form the basis of MRA. Both can be used to generate MR angiograms, evaluate vessel stenosis, detect flow direction, and quantify blood flow.

TIME OF FLIGHT

TOF is the most commonly chosen angiographic technique. This technique has been successful in ad-

dressing a wide range of clinical questions. TOF imaging has been used to depict the intracranial, extracranial, thoracic, abdominal, and peripheral arteries and veins.[10–12] Clinical studies of TOF are numerous[13–20] and are testimony to the flexibility of this approach. For many practitioners, TOF is the first and often the only MRA method they employ.[21]

BASIC MECHANISM

TOF imaging typically consists of 1) suppression of background tissue signal and 2) generation of a bright flow signal.

Background Tissue Suppression

Signal from background tissue is suppressed by saturating the spins with a rapid succession of radiofrequency (RF) pulses (using a repetition time, TR, that is short compared with the T1 of the stationary tissue) so that the spins do not have enough time to regain their longitudinal magnetization. Saturation refers to the reduction in longitudinal magnetization as a result of repeated RF excitations. Saturated spins produce a dim signal, whereas unsaturated spins produce a bright signal. Intentional saturation of stationary tissues makes them appear dark (Figs. 9–5 and 9–6).

Bright Inflow Signal

Blood outside the imaging slice is not affected by the slice-selective RF pulses. It is unsaturated, and as it flows into the volume with full magnetization, it produces a bright signal and gives rise to the inflow enhancement (also known as flow-related enhancement). The vascular signal in TOF increases with the velocity of blood flow. The increase in signal with flow is linear until the blood is completely replaced with each TR, that is, all the spins in the imaging volume are entirely replenished after each pulse.[22] For flow orthogonal to the imaging slice, complete inflow occurs when

$$TR = th/v \qquad (3)$$

where TR is the repetition time, th is the slice thickness, and v is the blood velocity. For a given TR, total replenishment of spins occurs at lower velocities for a thin slice than a thick one. The actual amount of

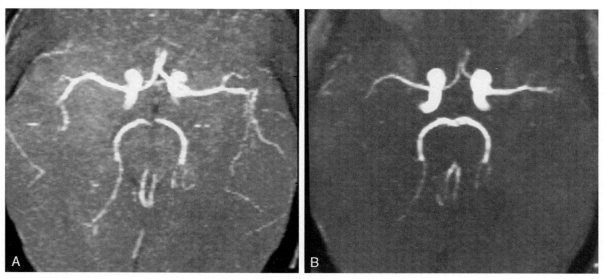

FIGURE 9–5. *A,* 3D TOF image of the circle of Willis (TR/TE/FA = 60/6/15°). *B,* Acquisition repeated with a shorter TR and a larger FA (TR/TE/FA = 18/6/30°) demonstrates background suppression. Some saturation of slow flow can also be seen.

flow enhancement depends on the number of spins entering the slice with full magnetization. For TOF imaging, the flow signal increases linearly until it reaches a plateau at which all the spins within the slice are replaced with fully magnetized ones (Fig. 9–7).

EFFECTS OF TIME-OF-FLIGHT ACQUISITION PARAMETERS ON VASCULAR CONTRAST

MRA offers much flexibility in the depiction of flow. Flow typically appears bright, but it can also be made

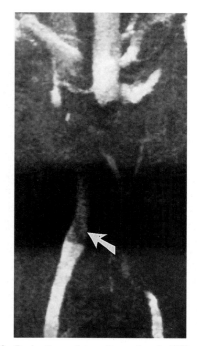

FIGURE 9–6. Projection of two-dimensional (2D) coronal TOF breath-hold images of the abdominal vasculature (TR/TE/FA = 50/10/30°). The application of an axial saturation band demonstrates the suppression of background tissue. Inflow of the iliac vein can be seen *(arrow)*. The patient had an occluded aorta below the renal arteries.

to appear dark. Flow contrast in TOF varies with the choice of a number of image parameters, including the TR, echo time (TE), flip angle (FA), size of the imaging volume, pixel size, and slice orientation. Angiographic contrast also depends on flow conditions such as velocity, pulsatility, and vessel tortuosity. A good understanding of how the sequence parameters affect vascular contrast enables one to tailor sequences for specific applications.

Repetition Time, Flip Angle, and Inflow

To suppress background signal, RF pulses are delivered at a TR much shorter than the T1 of tissue to cause effective spin saturation. Typical TR values range between 25 and 70 ms. A shorter TR also results in a shorter acquisition time. Therefore, there is further incentive to select short TR values. However, TR values must not be so short that there is insufficient time for the inflow of fresh spins.

Effective saturation is also achieved by using large FA values. The same RF pulses that reduce the tissue signal, however, can also affect the blood signal. This is particularly true for slow-moving blood that spends a relatively long time within the imaging volume, which results in a diminished signal (see Fig. 9–5*B*). To maximize the blood signal, a long TR and a small FA should be used to minimize spin saturation of blood. Unfortunately, the background signal is then relatively high and flow contrast (the difference in signal between flowing blood and stationary tissue) is low. Therefore, the selection of TR and FA is a compromise between saturating background tissue and not saturating blood. The optimal values of TR and FA depend on the velocity of blood and the anatomic distances to be covered. Typical FA values range between 20° and 35° for three-dimensional (3D) TOF and 30° and 90° for two-dimensional (2D) TOF.

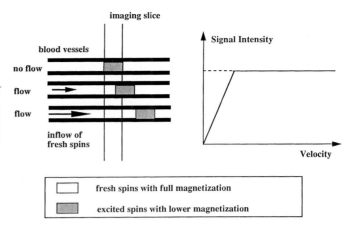

FIGURE 9–7. *Left*, Schematic diagram showing increased inflow of fresh spins into the imaging slice with increasing flow velocity. *Right*, Plot of the flow signal intensity versus velocity for gradient-echo imaging. The flow signal increases linearly with velocity until all the spins within the slice are replaced by fresh spins entering with full magnetization.

Slice Orientation

When performing 2D acquisition, inflow can be maximized by positioning the imaging slice perpendicular to the direction of flow. This provides effective replenishment of fresh spins into the slice and allows the use of a large FA excitation for maximal flow contrast. A drawback of a large FA excitation is an increase in ghost artifacts resulting from pulsatile flow. Placing the imaging slice in the plane of the vessel is undesirable because slow-moving spins become progressively saturated; this effect worsens as the FA is increased. This is known as in-plane saturation. When performing 3D TOF, the vessel segment of interest should be near the entry point for flowing blood and not at the far end of a large slab, by which point the flowing blood is saturated.

Voxel Size

Incoherent flow leads to phase cancellation and therefore loss of signal. This signal loss can be reduced by using smaller voxels (i.e., higher spatial resolution) to diminish the amount of intravoxel dephasing. Therefore, a small voxel is often used to better visualize small vessels, given a sufficient signal-to-noise ratio. 3D sequences usually give a better signal-to-noise ratio for small voxels than do 2D sequences.

Echo Time and Flow Compensation

Unwanted loss of flow signal occurs when there is phase dispersion caused by turbulent flow. This is discussed in greater detail later in this chapter. The amount of phase dispersion can be reduced by using flow compensation with the shortest TE.[23] Flow compensation works by achieving phase coherence of both the stationary and moving spins at the time of the echo.[24] At least three gradient lobes are needed to have velocity compensation (also known as first-order flow compensation) (Fig. 9–8A). Higher order motions, such as acceleration, are not refocused by first-order flow compensation and are best dealt with by using a short TE. The TOF method typically uses a gradient-echo sequence with a short TE and velocity compensation.[25–27] Figure 9–8B shows a pulse sequence

diagram of a 2D TOF sequence that is flow compensated along the read and slice-select directions. A short TE minimizes phase dispersion related to higher order motions (Fig. 9–8C). Furthermore, one can sample the echo earlier in time by using an asymmetric echo. This shortens the time the spins are allowed to dephase in the presence of the readout gradient, at the expense of slight blurring in the read direction.

Another important impact of the TE in MRA is its effect on the signal intensity of fat. An unwanted bright fat signal can be a problem for MRA of the thoracic, abdominal, and peripheral vasculature. The presence of fat is troublesome for MRA particularly when projections of the vasculature are generated from a stack of 2D or 3D slices (Fig. 9–9A). The bright fat signal can mask the region of interest and confound the results. To minimize the fat signal, MRA is performed with a TE such that protons in fat and water are out of phase. On a 1.5-T machine, this occurs at approximately 7, 12, or 17 ms. The out-of-phase time is inversely proportional to the field strength of the instrument. For example, the TE for fat and water out of phase is 11 ms at 1 T. An alternative way to minimize the fat signal is to use fat suppression RF pulses, as described next.

Fat Suppression

Protons in fat have a different frequency from protons in blood (the frequency offset is about 220 Hz at 1.5 T). The fat suppression pulses are applied at this frequency offset to saturate selectively the signal from fat. Removal of the competing background fat signal is particularly useful for MRA of the lower extremities (Fig. 9–9B). Effective fat suppression requires a homogeneous magnetic field, so shimming may be required. Otherwise, the region of fat saturation may not extend across the entire imaging volume if the field has spatial variations. As an alternative to fat suppression, selective water excitation using spectral-spatial pulses has been proposed as a more robust technique that is less sensitive to field inhomogeneities and produces less inadvertent saturation of arterial signal.

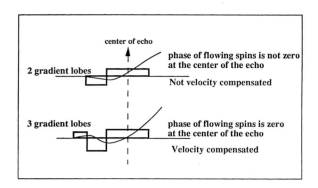

A

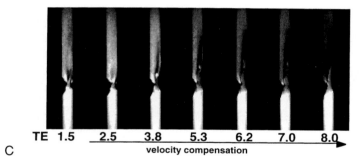

B

FIGURE 9–8. *A,* Gradient lobes in velocity compensation. *B,* Pulse sequence diagram of a 2D TOF gradient-echo sequence with flow compensation along the read and the slice-select directions. *C,* Pulsatile flow phantom showing influence of TE on signal loss resulting from flow-related dephasing. A 70% stenosis was incorporated into the phantom with a maximal flow velocity of 95 cm/s proximal to the stenosis. Signal loss resulting from flow-related dephasing is minimized as the TE is shortened. Signal loss is negligible with a TE of 2.5 ms and flow compensation or a TE of 1.5 ms without flow compensation. Strong gradients, such as those provided by echo-planar imaging systems, are required to obtain such short TEs if small fields of view (e.g., 20 cm) are needed.

C

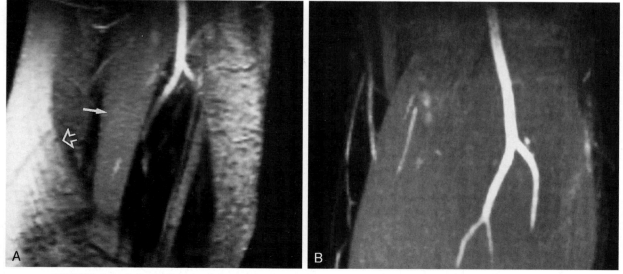

FIGURE 9–9. *A,* Projection of 2D coronal TOF images of the popliteal artery (TR/TE/FA = 40/10/40°). Note the high signal intensity from subcutaneous fat *(open arrow)* and fat within the bone marrow *(solid arrow). B,* Projection of 2D coronal TOF images acquired with fat suppression showing clear depiction of the vessels without overlapping fat signal. (*A* and *B* courtesy of David Saloner, PhD, University of California, San Francisco, CA.)

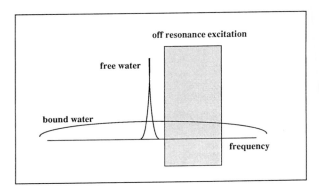

FIGURE 9–10. Diagram showing an MT pulse that is applied off-resonance to the free water peak.

Background Tissue Suppression

Stationary tissue can be selectively suppressed by using magnetization transfer (MT) pulses. An MT pulse is an off-resonance RF pulse that saturates the protons in bound water, which have a broad resonance peak compared with the sharp, narrow peak of protons in free water (Fig. 9–10). These pulses selectively remove signal from stationary tissue while causing only slight attenuation of the blood signal[28] (Fig. 9–11). Because of the diffusion of water, saturated bound protons exchange with free water protons. This causes some of the free water to become saturated as well. MT tissue suppression is most effective when the ratio of bound to free water in a tissue is large. MT has been particularly effective in intracranial angiography, in which the large number of bound protons in brain parenchyma contrasts with the mostly free water in blood serum.

A second technique for background suppression combines TOF with a slice-selective inversion recovery pulse.[29] This pulse is delivered to the imaging slice, and then data are acquired while the magnetization of fat or some other background tissue is crossing zero[30] (Fig. 9–12). More complete elimination of background tissue signal can be achieved by the signal targeting with alternating RF (STAR) technique, which involves subtracting two sets of TOF acquisitions in which the longitudinal magnetization of the flowing spins is inverted in alternate acquisitions (Fig. 9–13), giving excellent flow contrast with nearly perfect background suppression.[31] The STAR technique has evolved from previously described subtraction methods such as selective inversion recovery that rely on preinversion of inflowing spins.[32–35] The basic idea is to tag blood in a feeding vessel and then image it after it has flowed into a target vessel. For instance, to image the renal arteries, blood in the suprarenal abdominal and thoracic aorta is tagged by using an adiabatic inversion pulse, concomitant with presaturation of the imaging volume encompassing the renal arteries. A segmented turbo fast low-angle shot (turboFLASH) sequence is used to acquire the data, gated to the electrocardiogram. The tagging pulse is applied on alternate acquisitions, and the images are then subtracted. The image subtraction eliminates background tissue while maintaining a large intravascular signal. Thick sections (10 to 40 mm) are used, so that even tortuous vessels are encompassed in the section. The entire renal artery is usually depicted in a single image acquired in one breath-hold. First- and second-order branches of the renal arteries are routinely shown in normal subjects. Even small accessory renal arteries are shown. Because the technique is so simple and efficient, it should be ideal for depiction of normal vascular anatomy (e.g., for presurgical work-up of renal transplant donors) and for detection of renal artery stenosis.

STAR sequences offer certain advantages over other TOF methods:

1. Background suppression is complete, unlike that with standard 2D and 3D TOF sequences. With the STAR method, the even- and odd-numbered acquisitions are identical except for the FA of the tagging RF pulse, so that gradient-induced eddy currents and their effects are identical on the alternate acquisitions. MT

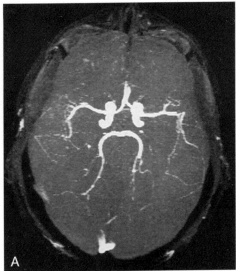
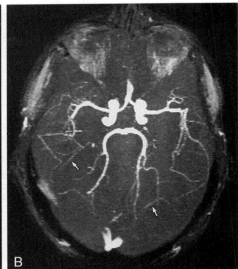

FIGURE 9–11. 3D TOF images of the circle of Willis (TR/TE/FA = 35/7/20°) *(A)* without and *(B)* with MT (frequency offset = 1500 Hz). Note that MT increases background suppression and improves depiction of smaller vessels *(arrows).*

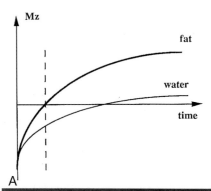

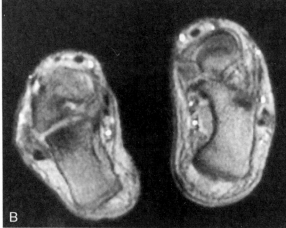

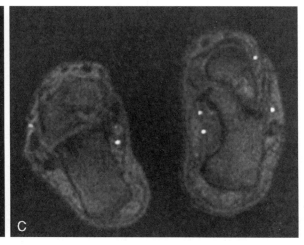

FIGURE 9–12. *A,* Diagram showing the longitudinal magnetization of fat and water after the application of an inversion pulse. To null out the signal from adipose tissue, data are acquired when the magnetization of fat crosses zero. *B* and *C,* Axial 2D TOF images of the feet (TR/TE/FA = 30/9/60°) without *(B)* and with *(C)* in-plane inversion to reduce the background tissue signal.

effects can be made similar by applying 180° RF tagging pulses that are positioned equidistant from the slice during both odd and even acquisitions. However, we found that the MT effects are small when a segmented turboFLASH acquisition is used, because the 180° pulse is applied infrequently (only once every two RR intervals).

2. Maximal intensity projections (MIPs) from standard 2D or 3D MRA acquisitions may show artifactual narrowing of the vessels, because of poor flow contrast along the vessel edges.[36] This is less of a problem with STAR angiography because of the extreme degree of background suppression.

3. A cine implementation of the technique permits visualization of vessels that have significant flow only during limited portions of the cardiac cycle.

4. The application of a presaturation pulse to the plane of section suppresses signal from in-plane moving structures such as bowel loops that could otherwise cause ghost artifacts.

Clinical experience with this technique is limited at present, but potential applications include imaging of the circle of Willis, extracranial carotid bifurcation, and renal arteries.

PRESATURATION

Arteries and veins are often companion structures. An unobscured view of the arteries therefore requires removal of venous signal and vice versa. This may be readily achieved by saturating the unwanted vessel upstream from the region of interest, using a presaturation band (Fig. 9–14). For most applications, the presaturation band should be close to the acquired slice and may partially overlap it. A presaturation band that moves in tandem with the acquired slice in sequential 2D TOF is termed a *walking* or *traveling* saturation band.

Saturation bands may also be used to reduce flow artifacts or artifacts resulting from respiratory and/or cardiac motion.[37] For example, a saturation band can be applied to the anterior chest wall to minimize ghost artifacts related to breathing.[38, 39] A clever use of saturation bands is to determine the feeding vessels of an arteriovenous malformation, the cervical vessels supplying a middle cerebral artery, or the direction of flow[40] (Fig. 9–15). When a saturation band is placed over the vessel, all branches downstream from it disappear from the angiogram.

BOLUS TAGGING

In addition to determining direction of flow and source of perfusion, saturation bands may be used to quantify blood velocity. This technique, known as bolus tagging, uses an RF pulse to generate a saturation band across the image. The saturation band, placed orthogonal to flow, serves as a flow tag (Fig. 9–16).

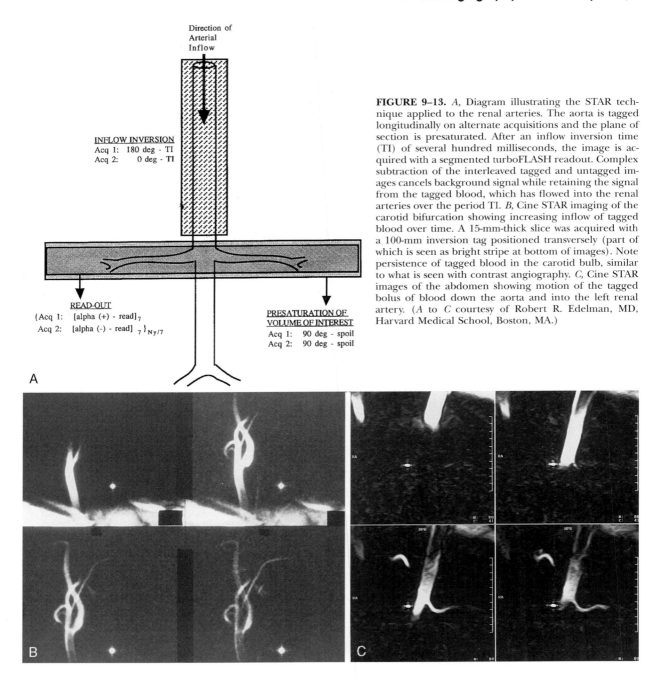

Direction of
Arterial
Inflow

INFLOW INVERSION
Acq 1: 180 deg - TI
Acq 2: 0 deg - TI

READ-OUT
{Acq 1: [alpha (+) - read]$_7$
Acq 2: [alpha (-) - read] $_7$ }$_{Ny/7}$

PRESATURATION OF
VOLUME OF INTEREST
Acq 1: 90 deg - spoil
Acq 2: 90 deg - spoil

A

B

C

FIGURE 9–13. *A,* Diagram illustrating the STAR technique applied to the renal arteries. The aorta is tagged longitudinally on alternate acquisitions and the plane of section is presaturated. After an inflow inversion time (TI) of several hundred milliseconds, the image is acquired with a segmented turboFLASH readout. Complex subtraction of the interleaved tagged and untagged images cancels background signal while retaining the signal from the tagged blood, which has flowed into the renal arteries over the period TI. *B,* Cine STAR imaging of the carotid bifurcation showing increasing inflow of tagged blood over time. A 15-mm-thick slice was acquired with a 100-mm inversion tag positioned transversely (part of which is seen as bright stripe at bottom of images). Note persistence of tagged blood in the carotid bulb, similar to what is seen with contrast angiography. *C,* Cine STAR images of the abdomen showing motion of the tagged bolus of blood down the aorta and into the left renal artery. (*A* to *C* courtesy of Robert R. Edelman, MD, Harvard Medical School, Boston, MA.)

There is an adjustable time delay in the sequence between the saturation pulse and the echo readout. In the stationary tissue the tag remains where it is applied, but in the blood vessel the tag moves along with flow. To determine velocity, one simply divides the bolus displacement by the delay time. Bolus tagging has been used to quantify flow velocity in the portal vein and in the intracranial vessels.[41, 42]

Compared with phase contrast (PC), bolus tagging has advantages and disadvantages. With bolus tagging, the results are directly available without further processing, no special software is required, and it is not necessary to set a velocity-encoding sensitivity as required with PC. On the other hand, it may be difficult to image small vessels in long axis over a substantial length, which is required with bolus tagging; the vessel can be more easily viewed in cross section for PC imaging. Also, the edges of the tagged bolus may become indistinct with rapid flow or over long distances, making precise measurements a problem.

TWO- AND THREE-DIMENSIONAL TIME OF FLIGHT

TOF may be implemented as either a 2D or a 3D sequence. 2D TOF consists of individual, thin sections usually acquired in a sequential fashion.[43] As pointed out earlier, these sections are often positioned perpen-

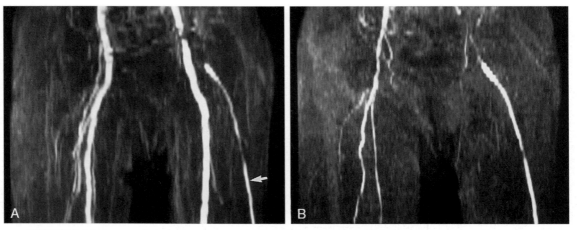

FIGURE 9–14. A coronal projection from axial 2D TOF through the pelvic region in a patient with an arterial bypass graft *(arrow)* (TR/TE = 35/10) acquired *(A)* without and *(B)* with venous saturation to demonstrate the use of spatial presaturation to eliminate venous signal. Without venous saturation, the femoral vein was obscuring the patient's native arteries.

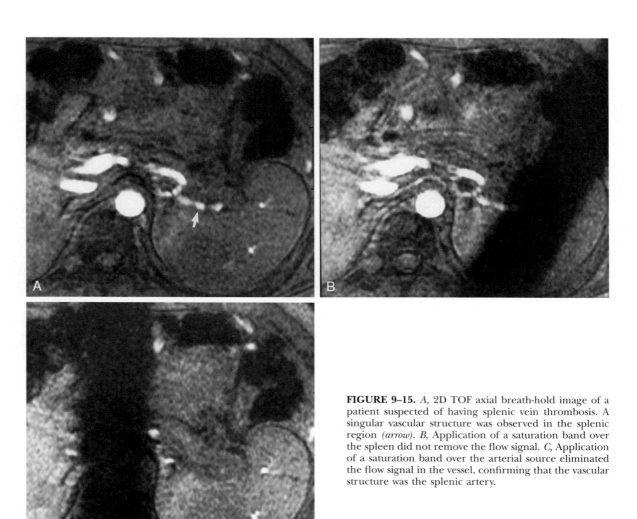

FIGURE 9–15. *A,* 2D TOF axial breath-hold image of a patient suspected of having splenic vein thrombosis. A singular vascular structure was observed in the splenic region *(arrow). B,* Application of a saturation band over the spleen did not remove the flow signal. *C,* Application of a saturation band over the arterial source eliminated the flow signal in the vessel, confirming that the vascular structure was the splenic artery.

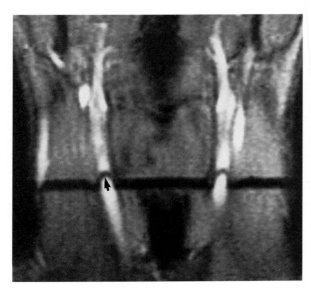

FIGURE 9–16. Coronal 2D bolus tag image of the carotid arteries acquired with the use of a presaturation band to generate a flow tag (*arrow*). Flow direction and profile are depicted by the bolus tag and flow velocity can be calculated from the tag displacement.

dicular to the direction of the blood flow to maximize inflow effects. After the first section is acquired, a second acquisition is made adjacent to the first, followed by a third, and so on. Note that this method of acquisition, in which slices are acquired sequentially, is different from the familiar multislice 2D acquisition used in spin-echo imaging, in which the slices are all acquired at the same time. Sequential 2D acquisition maximizes the inflow effect. Multisection 2D acquisitions may also have applications in MRA, particularly in conjunction with the administration of paramagnetic contrast agents, as discussed later.

3D TOF has substantially better spatial resolution than 2D TOF and has many useful clinical applications.[44–46] As with any 3D sequence, the volume is subdivided into smaller sections called partitions. Also as with any 3D sequence, the partitions are typically quite thin (<1 mm) and are contiguous with no interslice gap. The increase in resolution, however, comes at a price. Blood must enter a larger volume and travel a longer distance within the imaging volume. The inflow effect persists for only a short distance into the volume before the signal from blood is lost and the vessel intensity fades. The challenge is therefore to provide RF pulses that adequately suppress the background tissue without noticeably diminishing the blood signal. The selection of an optimal RF pulse is especially difficult for imaging vessels with slow flow. Use of 3D TOF is therefore limited to vessels with moderately high rates of flow.

The progressive saturation of blood as it flows across a thick 3D TOF slab often results in high blood signal intensity at the entry side of the slab and lower signal intensity at the exit side. This gradient in blood intensity may be partly corrected by gradually increasing the FA across the slab, a technique called tilted optimized nonselective excitation (TONE).[47] Lower FA values are

applied at the entry side of the imaging volume to minimize saturation effects, and higher FA values are applied at the exit side to maximize blood signal more distally (Fig. 9–17). In a TONE 3D TOF axial acquisition of the circle of Willis, for instance, vascular structures at the inflow end of the slab (e.g., carotid siphons) can be made as bright as structures at the outflow end (e.g., small distal vessels). Although this technique is effective at evening out the angiographic intensity across a 3D volume, it does not eliminate the tendency for vessels with unusually slow flow to become saturated. It also presumes that flow crosses the slab in one direction, which may not be the case for tortuous vessels such as renal arteries.

COMPARISON OF TWO-DIMENSIONAL AND THREE-DIMENSIONAL TIME OF FLIGHT

Some applications are best performed with 2D TOF, others with 3D TOF. Seldom are these sequences interchangeable. The choice of 2D or 3D techniques is made on the basis of several factors.

2D TOF is sensitive to slow blood flow, whereas 3D TOF often cannot detect vessels with slowly flowing blood such as veins and peripheral arteries (Fig. 9–18). This results from the difference in thickness between the volumes into which blood must enter: a thin slice in the case of 2D, a thick slab in 3D.

2D TOF can be acquired with breath-holding to minimize respiratory motion artifacts. This makes 2D a favorite sequence for abdominal venous studies, because the anatomy may be covered by a series of breath-holds. 3D TOF requires a longer scan time and is typically not compatible with breath-holding. However, with the advent of enhanced gradient systems, breath-hold 3D TOF imaging has become feasible with TR values as short as 5 ms.

3D TOF provides higher spatial resolution than 2D TOF.[48] The partitions of 3D acquisition are usually less than 1 mm thick, which compares favorably with the 2-mm or thicker slices of 2D acquisition.[23]

3D TOF is less susceptible to turbulent signal loss (e.g., within a stenotic segment) than 2D TOF (Fig. 9–19). This results from a smaller voxel size. Thus, one can select a 3D TOF acquisition to grade the percent stenosis within an internal carotid artery lesion but use a 2D TOF sequence to reliably visualize slow flow beyond a stenosis.

A technique that seeks to combine the advantages of 2D and 3D acquisition is the 3D multislab approach, also known as multiple overlapping thin-slab acquisition (MOTSA).[49] As the name indicates, this consists of a series of thin-slab 3D acquisitions (Fig. 9–20). Thin slabs are chosen to reduce blood saturation and improve sensitivity to slow flow. The slabs are acquired with overlap because the slices at the end of a 3D slab often have low signal intensity. The redundant slices are discarded. Otherwise, they would result in a "venetian blind" appearance in the projected image. MOTSA is often used when high-resolution images are

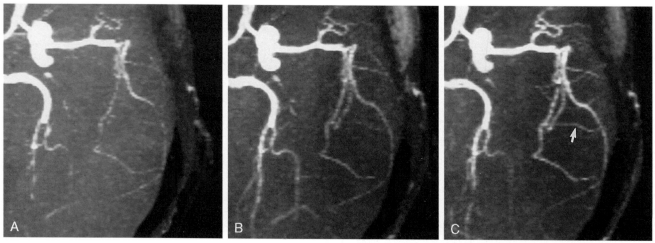

FIGURE 9–17. *A*, Standard 3D TOF acquisition of the circle of Willis (TR/TE/FA = 35/7/20°, 55-mm slab with 64 partitions). *B* and *C*, Same acquisition but with *(B)* MT and *(C)* MT and TONE. Note the appearance of small vessels not previously seen *(arrow)*. The TONE ratio was 1:2 (15° to 30°) in the cranial direction.

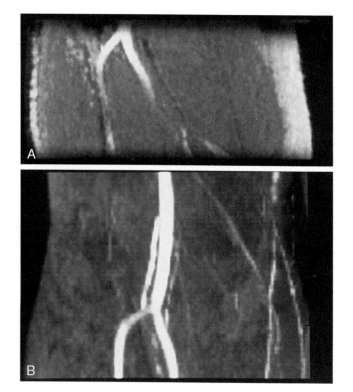

FIGURE 9–18. A pair of images comparing the degree of spin saturation in 2D versus 3D MRA. *A*, Coronal projection from an axial 3D acquisition in the area of the popliteal artery. Note the rapid loss of vascular signal. The 3D acquisition was acquired with TR/TE/FA = 40/7/20°, effective slice thickness = 1 mm, and 64 partitions. *B*, Coronal projection of 2D axial acquisitions (TR/TE/FA = 44/10/40°, and slice thickness = 3 mm). The degree of spin saturation is reduced in the 2D compared with the 3D acquisition.

FIGURE 9–19. A pair of images comparing the extent of intra-voxel dephasing in 2D versus 3D MRA of a patient with proximal internal carotid artery stenosis. *A*, Sagittal projection from 2D axial acquisitions (TR/TE/FA = 35/9/35°, slice thickness = 3 mm). Note the complete loss of vascular signal in the area of the stenosis *(arrow)*. *B*, Sagittal projection from a 3D axial acquisition from the same patient (TR/TE/FA = 35/7/25°, effective slice thickness = 1 mm). Reduction of signal loss caused by turbulence in the 3D acquisition resulted in a more accurate depiction of the true vessel lumen *(open arrow)*.

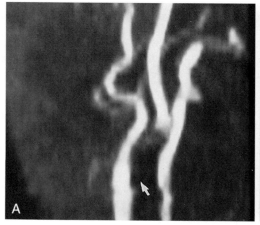
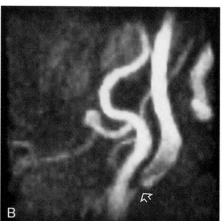

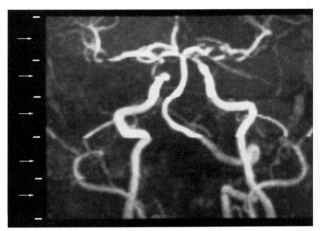

FIGURE 9–20. MOTSA acquisition: a coronal projection of five overlapping axial 3D thin slabs *(arrows)* of the intracranial circulation. This multislab sequential 3D technique offers coverage of an extended volume of interest.

required over a large anatomic area, for instance, the aortic arch, carotid, and intracranial arteries.

GADOLINIUM

The vascular signal can be further increased by using a small amount of contrast agent. Gadolinium chelates such as gadolinium diethylenetriaminepentaacetic acid (Gd-DTPA), a paramagnetic contrast agent, increase the blood signal by shortening its T1 relaxation time.[50, 51] After intravenous injection of gadolinium chelates, blood regains its longitudinal magnetization more rapidly and gives a stronger signal. Although it is not in widespread use for MRA, contrast enhancement has many advantages. The FA used for excitation can be increased for greater vascular signal and reduced background signal without risk of saturating slowly flowing blood. The conspicuity of small peripheral vessels is improved. The nidus of an arteriovenous malformation is better seen. With dynamic first-pass imaging, the arteries but not veins are enhanced. In the abdomen and pelvis, selective water excitation (which eliminates the signal from fat) is helpful for improved background suppression, particularly for contrast-enhanced multisection 2D acquisitions. Subtraction of pre- from postcontrast images in the absence of motion of the patient gives excellent background suppression and better vessel conspicuity than are possible using standard MRA techniques. Contrast-enhanced vessels appear bright regardless of the presence of slow flow.

One can use 3D, sequential 2D, or multisection 2D MRA for contrast-enhanced studies. An advantage of multisection 2D MRA is that a series of contiguous or slightly overlapping sections can be obtained in a single breath-hold. Because the TR (e.g., 100 to 300 ms) is of the same order as the T1 of contrast-enhanced blood, an FA of 90° can be used for maximal signal-to-noise ratio (Fig. 9–21). This is advantageous compared

with contrast-enhanced 3D MRA, in which a much shorter TR and therefore a higher dose of contrast medium are needed.[52] Breath-hold double-dose contrast-enhanced 3D imaging may be particularly useful for MRA of renal artery stenosis and peripheral artery disease.[52a] Interestingly, our experience has shown that ghost artifacts resulting from pulsatile flow are negligible with contrast-enhanced MRA.

The use of contrast enhancement, however, has some important limitations. First, venous structures may be difficult to eliminate because the use of presaturation regions is less effective. Second, background tissues such as the cavernous sinus and nasal mucosa are enhanced and can appear in the MIP images. Third, one must acquire all the data quickly while the agent is still predominantly intravascular. Repeated acquisitions are not always possible because gadolinium chelates are interstitial agents that are rapidly distributed into the extravascular spaces. The use of double or triple doses of gadolinium chelates has been proposed for 3D acquisitions that use short TRs, but the cost of the contrast agent is substantial.

SEGMENTED K-SPACE ACQUISITIONS

MRA of the thorax poses a greater challenge than intracranial MRA. This is due to motion artifacts caused by cardiac pulsation and respiration. Removal of such ghost artifacts requires fast acquisitions, for instance, high-speed cardiac-triggered MRA with a segmented k-space data acquisition scheme. With segmented k-space, the entire cardiac-triggered acquisition can be completed within a single breath-hold, and such a technique is especially effective for thoracic studies.[53, 54]

The substantial reduction in scan time is achieved by acquiring N phase-encode lines per segment (i.e., multiple phase-encode lines are acquired in each heartbeat) (Fig. 9–22). The saving in scan time is determined by N. For example, for N = 16, the scan time for a triggered acquisition is decreased by a factor of 16. Faster acquisition is achieved at the expense of precise electrocardiographic triggering to a single time point within the cardiac cycle. When performing segmented acquisitions, the time interval over which the N echoes are acquired spans a portion of the cardiac cycle. Typically, for TR = 10 ms, the acquisition window spans 160 ms for N = 6. This time interval increases with increasing N. When imaging moving objects, care should be taken to find the optimal N because there is more time for blurring to occur as N is increased. An acquisition window of 300 ms is acceptable for renal artery imaging but not for coronary artery imaging, where cardiac motion is a problem.

By using segmented acquisitions, cardiac-triggered acquisitions that previously took 3 to 5 minutes can now be completed within 20 seconds. When segmented acquisition is combined with breath-holding, both cardiac pulsations and respiratory motion are eliminated (Fig. 9–23). This has revolutionized tho-

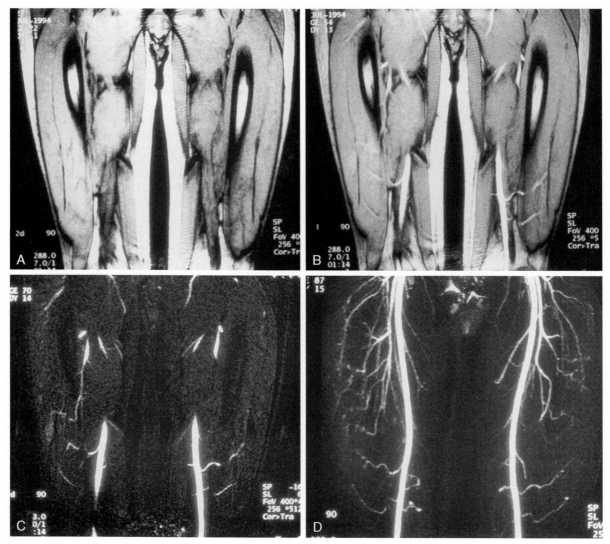

FIGURE 9–21. Typical coronal-oblique MRA images of the lower extremities of a healthy volunteer. A multisection 2D fast imaging with steady-state precession (FISP) MRA sequence was performed in the coronal-oblique plane. Image parameters were 40 cm field of view, TR/TE/FA = 291/7/90°, 256 × 512 matrix, one acquisition, 5-mm section thickness, and 16 sections with 0.5-mm overlap. The imaging protocol was completed with three measurements; the first measurement was used as the mask. The second was a transition measurement, with manual injection of 20 mL of gadoteridol beginning with 35 seconds remaining in the sequence and continuing over a 1-minute interval. The sole purpose of this measurement was to avoid interrupting the steady noise level associated with the measurement process, as our experience has shown that interruption or initiation of the noise from a measurement may cause the patient to move. The data from this measurement were discarded. The third measurement was performed during and after contrast agent injection. The total examination time was less than 4 minutes. The magnitude data of the first measurement were then subtracted on a section-by-section basis from the magnitude data of the third measurement. *A,* Precontrast 2D FISP image; *B,* postcontrast 2D FISP image; *C,* subtracted image *(B − A); D,* MIP of the subtracted images for all 16 slices. (*A* to *D* courtesy of Robert R. Edelman, MD, Harvard Medical School, Boston, MA.)

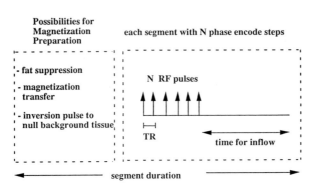

FIGURE 9–22. Schematic diagram of segmented k-space acquisition with magnetization preparation pulses to obtain flexible image contrast.

ward flow approaching −80 cm/s is assigned the darkest signal intensity. The V_{enc} of the pulse sequence can be adjusted by varying the gradient strength and duration. The sequence can be tailored to image fast flow or slow flow. The V_{enc} is particularly important when imaging slow flow (Fig. 9–27). When the vessel of interest is anticipated to have a peak velocity of 15 cm/s, reducing the V_{enc} from 100 to 20 cm/s improves the dynamic range of the study. This is true for both MRA and flow quantification. Choosing the proper V_{enc} results in better visibility of vessels in PC MRA.

One should always choose a V_{enc} that is slightly higher than the maximal anticipated velocity in the vessel of interest. When the peak velocity exceeds the V_{enc}, velocity aliasing results and artifacts are produced within the vessel of interest. For example, when the chosen V_{enc} is 20 cm/s and the blood is traveling at 21 cm/s, the image of blood is not assigned to the brightest signal plus one. Rather, the signal is wrapped around and has a low intensity in the image (Fig. 9–28). This gives a misleading impression that flow is going in the opposite direction. Velocity aliasing, when present, can be readily detected in the image (Fig. 9–29). Normal phase images show a gradual transition of phase within the vessel lumen. Velocity aliasing, on the other hand, shows abrupt transition of phase from positive to negative within a vessel. When that occurs, the study should be repeated with the correct V_{enc}.

CORRECTION OF PHASE ERRORS

Magnetic field inhomogeneities and eddy currents can induce local phase shifts. When these are present, stationary spins no longer have zero phase. To achieve background suppression, a subtraction of two phase images is performed: two phase images are acquired, one with flow encoding and one with flow compensation. Stationary spins have the same phase in both images. A subtraction of the two phase images produces zero phase shift for the stationary material.[63, 64] Flowing spins, on the other hand, have a phase shift in the flow-encoded image but not in the flow-compensated image. As a result, a subtraction of the two images gives a net phase shift for the flowing spins and each pixel is then assigned a signal intensity that increases with the phase shift. An alternative way is to subtract two images, one acquired with a pair of bipolar gradient lobes and the second acquired with the polarity of the gradient lobes reversed. This also produces a net phase shift for flow while subtracting out the background (Fig. 9–30).

Based on the linear relationship between phase shift and flow, fast-flowing spins are depicted with a brighter signal than are slower moving spins. The advantage of the first technique is that the same acquisition without encoding may be subtracted from each of the three encoded acquisitions, assuming three-directional sensitivity, thereby reducing the total acquisitions from six to four.

Yet another technique is the Hadamard algorithm, in which four different acquisitions are made, each with a different combination of bipolar gradients, applying the gradients simultaneously in two directions for each acquisition.[65] These are then added or subtracted to extract the flow encoding for each axis separately. The purpose of this algorithm is again to reduce the total number of acquisitions necessary to encode in all three directions from six to four.

SPEED, COMPLEX DIFFERENCE, AND PHASE DIFFERENCE DISPLAY

Once the phase shifts resulting from flow encoding have been acquired, they may be displayed in several ways.

Net phase shift (phase difference) is used for flow quantification. The phase difference image is computed from the difference in phase between the positive-encoded and negative-encoded acquisitions. The value of the phase difference is proportional to velocity; therefore, this image is also called a velocity map and is used for velocity and flow volume calculations (Figs. 9–31 and 9–32). Flow encoding is performed in one direction only.

Complex difference is used mainly for 2D scout imaging. The complex difference image is the magnitude of the vector difference (rather than the phase difference) between the positive-encoded and negative-encoded acquisitions (Fig. 9–33). Rather than being simply a reflection of velocity, it is also proportional to the magnitude of the magnetization. As with speed images, there is no indication of whether flow is along the positive or negative direction of the flow-encoding gradient. When the peak velocity exceeds the V_{enc}, the flow signal remains bright. As with phase difference images, flow encoding is performed in one direction only. Complex difference is used in 2D PC acquisition (when special background spoiler gradients are employed) because it is less susceptible to phase artifacts than are phase difference images. The complex difference obtained in these images, however, no longer follows a simple linear relationship with velocity. As a result, velocity quantification is not so straightforward in the complex difference image.

Speed information is often used to generate an angiogram. The speed image shows simply the speed of flow. Speed is calculated at each pixel based on the following:

$$\sqrt{v_x^2 + v_y^2 + v_z^2} \tag{5}$$

where v_x, v_y, and v_z are velocities along the x, y, and z directions. In the speed image, there is no information about the direction of flow. Aliasing is less of a problem with speed display, because the peak positive-encoded flow is identical in intensity to the peak negative-encoded flow. There is no sudden change from bright to dark as the V_{enc} is exceeded. Speed images are ideal for anatomic depictions of vascular anatomy.

Magnetization vectors within pixels that have little or no signal, such as those representing air and bone cortex, have random and meaningless phases. Air might therefore contribute a speckled appearance on

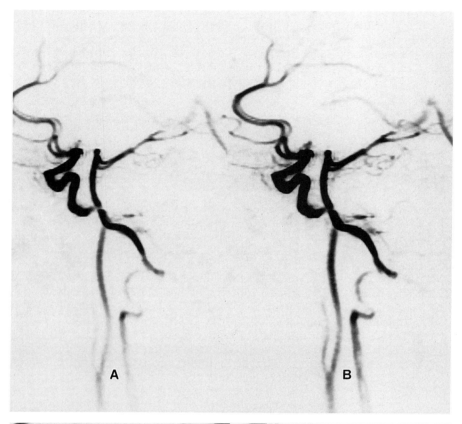

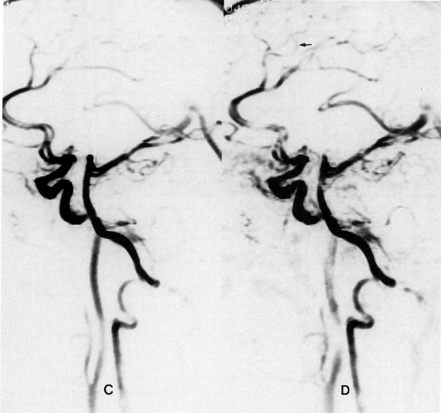

FIGURE 9–27. Sagittal 2D thick slab of the head and neck with *(A)* $V_{enc} = 80$ cm/s, *(B)* $V_{enc} = 60$ cm/s, *(C)* $V_{enc} = 40$ cm/s, and *(D)* $V_{enc} = 20$ cm/s. The use of a reduced V_{enc} improved depiction of smaller vessels *(arrow)*. (*A* to *D* courtesy of Patrick Turski, MD, University of Wisconsin, Madison, WI.)

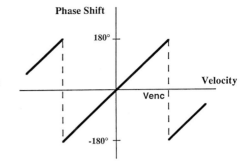

FIGURE 9–28. Graph showing the linear relationship between phase and velocity. When the velocity surpasses V_{enc}, velocity wraparound (aliasing) occurs.

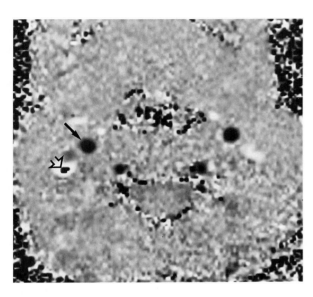

FIGURE 9–29. Axial subtracted phase image of the carotid arteries and jugular veins showing aliasing in the right jugular vein *(open arrow)*. Flow in the caudal direction appears bright and flow in the cranial direction (in the carotid artery) appears dark *(solid arrow)*.

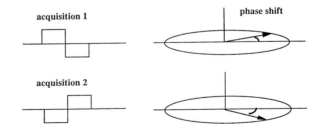

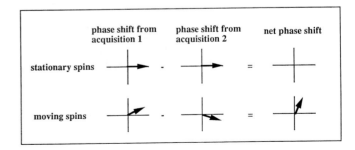

FIGURE 9–30. Diagram showing the use of bipolar gradient lobes in PC flow quantification to obtain zero phase shift for the stationary tissue and a net phase shift for flow.

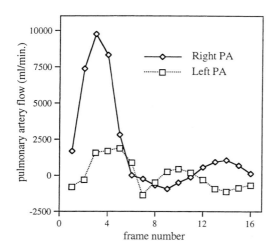

FIGURE 9–31. Flow measured by cine PC of a patient who was treated for primary pulmonary hypertension with a single lung transplant. The flow was measured in the left and right pulmonary arteries. Note the normal flow to the transplanted right lung but bidirectional flow with little net flow to the diseased left lung. (From Pelc NJ, Sommer FG, Li KCP, et al: Quantitative magnetic resonance flow imaging. Magn Reson Q 10:125–147, 1994.)

FIGURE 9–32. *(A)* Preprandial and *(B)* postprandial blood flow as a function of time in the cardiac cycle in the superior mesenteric artery of a normal volunteer. (*A* and *B* from Applegate GR, Talagala SL, Applegate LJ: MR angiography of the head and neck: value of two-dimensional phase-contrast projection technique. AJR 159: 369–374, 1992.)

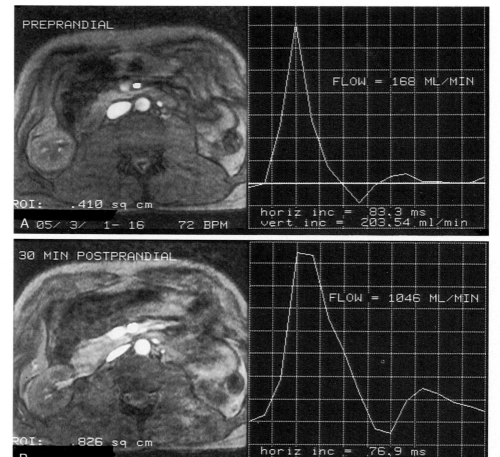

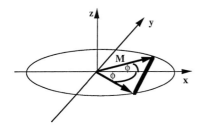

FIGURE 9–33. The complex difference process involves determining the absolute value of 2M sin φ, where M is the magnitude of the magnetization and φ is the phase shift. Complex difference is used mainly for thick-slab acquisitions.

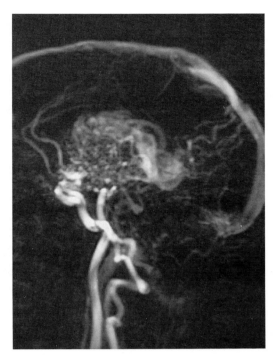

FIGURE 9–34. 2D thick-slab PC acquisition (TR/TE = 33/8, slice thickness = 60 mm, matrix = 256 × 192, number of excitations = 8, with V_{enc} = 60 cm/s). Note the excellent depiction of the vascular structures in the arteriovenous malformation. (Courtesy of Patrick Turski, MD, University of Wisconsin, Madison, WI.)

the angiogram, obscuring the true vascular signal. This can be removed by setting pixels corresponding to small magnetic vectors to the value of the background signal. This is called applying a mask.

THICK-SLAB TWO-DIMENSIONAL PHASE CONTRAST

Thick-slab 2D PC offers a quick assessment of flow and is often used to obtain a projective view of the vasculature[66, 67] (Fig. 9–34). This can be performed rapidly, unlike 3D PC. The slab thickness ranges from 2 to 10 cm. Because of the thicker slice, partial voluming does occur and the spatial resolution may sometimes be suboptimal. Most important, when two vessels cross within the slice, the acquired phase is the sum of the two, so various phase artifacts may be present that are worse with increasing slice thickness. When pulsatile flow is present, multiple acquisitions are acquired to reduce respiratory and pulsatility artifacts. Alternatively, one may use electrocardiographic triggering.

DIRECTIONAL FLOW IMAGING

A simple and rapid application of 2D PCA is to determine direction of flow (Fig. 9–35). An image is acquired with flow encoding in one direction. Based on image intensity, one can readily determine whether flow is in the positive or negative direction along the

flow-encoding axis.[68] For example, if the V_{enc} is 100 cm/s, the normal convention is to assign white to blood that is flowing at 100 cm/s in the positive direction, black to flow at −100 cm/s, and shades of gray to velocities in between. Stationary tissue is midgray. Note that if flow in a vessel is perpendicular to the encoding axis, there is no evidence of motion as long as there is no motion component in the encoded direction.

FLOW VELOCITY QUANTIFICATION AND CINE PHASE CONTRAST

Flow quantification is a major application for PC acquisitions.[69] Typically, a pair of phase images are acquired (with and without flow-encoding gradients) as described earlier. To remove inhomogeneities of the static field, the net phase shift is obtained by subtracting the flow-sensitive phase image from the flow-compensated phase image.[64] By using the linear relationship between flow velocity and the net phase shift (Equation 4), the velocity can be calculated.

Cine PC allows the measurement of pulsatile flow velocity[70–72] (see Figs. 9–31 and 9–32). This is done by acquiring data at multiple time points throughout the cardiac cycle (known as a cine measurement) using electrocardiographic triggering. The time resolution of the series is given by TR, which is typically 30 to 40 ms. Multiple pairs of flow-sensitive and flow-compensated images are acquired in a triggered study. A time-velocity curve can be obtained by subtraction of the images and determination of the net phase shift at each time point.[73] In addition, volumetric flow rates can be calculated.[74–76] The volumetric flow rate is given by the product of the measured velocity and the cross-sectional area of the vessel lumen, which can be determined.

Rapid flow quantification has been achieved that enables measurements to be completed within a single breath-hold. High-speed acquisitions are particularly important for flow quantification in the thorax, for example, measurements in the coronary arteries.[77]

V_{enc} is an important parameter in phase acquisitions and particularly for flow quantification. It must be chosen with care. Otherwise, aliasing can occur, which produces misleading results. For example, consider an acquisition in which the V_{enc} is 20 cm/s. For symmetric velocity encoding, a forward flow of 20 cm/s would accumulate a +180° phase shift whereas a backward flow of −20 cm/s would accumulate a −180° phase shift. Flow that exceeds this V_{enc} would have a phase shift larger than 180°. For example, flow at 60 cm/s would accrue a 540° phase shift, which is equivalent to a net phase shift of 180°, and this would erroneously suggest a flow velocity of 20 cm/s. As another example, flow at 30 cm/s would have a phase shift of 270° (which is equivalent to −90°) and the velocity measurement would incorrectly indicate a flow velocity of −10 cm/s (i.e., 10 cm/s in the opposite direction). The problem of aliasing can be readily corrected by

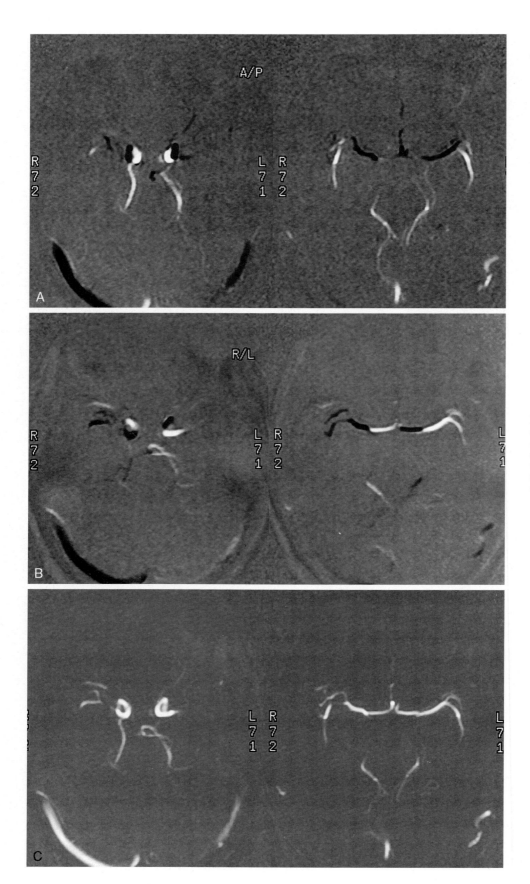

FIGURE 9–35. 2D adjacent axial slab PC acquisitions. *A,* Flow encoding along the anteroposterior direction. *B,* Flow encoding along the left-right direction. *C,* Speed images obtained from the same data set.

choosing a V_{enc} that is larger than the maximal flow velocity.

Because the measured velocity varies substantially over the pulsatile cycle, one may wish to use a smaller V_{enc} during diastole and a larger V_{enc} during systole.[78] This ensures increased dynamic range for all the cardiac phases.[79] Care must be taken to avoid velocity aliasing at any time over the pulsatile cycle. It is therefore helpful to have an estimate of the anticipated time-velocity waveform when specifying the variable V_{enc}.

The following are the causes and remedies for the more common artifacts that can occur with MR PC velocity quantification:

1. Velocity aliasing (phase wrapping). The peak velocity exceeds the V_{enc}. Remedy: increase the V_{enc} to have it larger than the maximal velocity.

2. Local signal loss. Phase incoherence is due to higher order motions or turbulent flow. Remedy: use a short TE and a small voxel to minimize the amount of intravoxel dephasing.

3. Background phase inhomogeneity. Local variations of phase shift are caused by magnetic field inhomogeneity. Remedy: do careful shimming and phase map correction using a static reference.

THREE-DIMENSIONAL PHASE CONTRAST

3D PC MRA, like 3D TOF, generates a volumetric data set that can be reformatted and displayed in any chosen orientation by using the MIP algorithm. In addition to MR angiograms, flow directional images can be generated to show flow along different axes. Repeated acquisitions are needed to encode flow along all three orthogonal directions. 3D streamline profiles of flow have been generated from 3D PC data[80] (Fig. 9–36). Cardiac triggering is not used with 3D PC because of prohibitive acquisition times. As a result, the flow velocity obtained is averaged over the cardiac cycle. Common applications of 3D PC are in cerebral angiography, renal and other visceral angiography, and studies of distal extremities.

EFFECTS OF PULSE SEQUENCE PARAMETERS

Typically, both 2D PC and 3D PC use a short TR (approximately 30 to 40 ms), a short TE (8 ms or less), and a small FA of 20° to 30°. Saturation of blood occurs with PCA, just as it does with TOF. However, because the image intensity is related to the phase rather than the magnitude of the magnetization, the vessel remains bright until the magnetization is quite small or falls below the level of the mask.

Phase incoherence related to turbulent or disorderly flow patterns can lead to signal loss, just as in TOF. In TOF, such phase incoherence is minimized by using flow-compensated gradients. In PCA, however, the flow-encoding portion of the acquisition does not have flow compensation. To minimize phase incoherence in

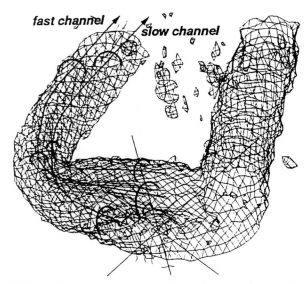

FIGURE 9–36. Streamlines showing fast and slow channels of blood flow through the carotid bulb determined from 3D PC data. (From Buonocore MH: Algorithms for improving calculated streamlines in 3-D phase contrast angiography. Magn Reson Med 31:22–30, 1994.)

the flow-sensitive image, a small voxel size is used, which also reduces the effects of partial voluming.

ADVANTAGES AND LIMITATIONS OF PHASE-CONTRAST ANGIOGRAPHY

PCA has several qualities that distinguish it from TOF. First, the values portrayed in an image are phase shifts rather than magnitudes. Second, PCA is a reflection of blood motion along a gradient rather than inflow into a slice. Third, nearly complete background elimination is achieved, whereas in TOF the vessel wall and other structures are faintly visible.

PCA enjoys the following strengths. First, it improves the detection of small vessels by virtue of its excellent background elimination. All stationary materials, even those with a short T1 (such as fat and methemoglobin), are eliminated. As a result, hematomas are not mistaken for vascular structures, as may happen with TOF (Fig. 9–37). PCA can often provide an MIP of larger volumes than TOF because of its superior background suppression.[81] Second, PCA is well suited for imaging of slow flow, as in vein structures or large aneurysms. By adjusting the gradient strength and duration, one can make a pulse sequence that is sensitive even to velocities as slow as that of cerebrospinal fluid motion. Third, cine PC can be used to perform flow quantification and to obtain the velocity-time curve in pulsatile flow.

PCA also has limitations. First, PC acquisitions, particularly in 3D PCA, take approximately two to three times longer than TOF acquisitions of comparable resolution. This is because flow-encoded data along each of the three axes are separately acquired. Second, PC MRA is sensitive to instrument imperfections. The presence of eddy currents or field instabilities degrades

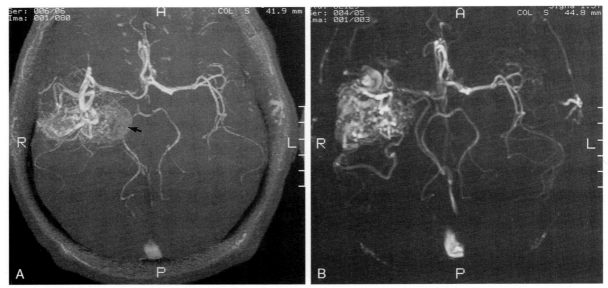

FIGURE 9–37. *A,* 3D TOF image showing an arteriovenous malformation with hematoma *(arrow)*. *B,* The hematoma is subtracted from the 3D PC flow image. (*A* and *B* courtesy of Patrick Turski, MD, University of Wisconsin, Madison, WI.)

the background suppression. The use of self-shielded gradient coils and careful eddy current compensation alleviate these problems. Having to partially dephase flowing spins to obtain flow sensitivity makes PC images more sensitive than TOF images to artifacts resulting from complex flow, which may occur distal to a stenosis or in some aneurysms.

DISPLAY AND INTERPRETATION

The introduction of the MIP algorithm first allowed realistic angiograms to be calculated and displayed.[82] It allowed individual slices of blood vessels, acquired over a 3D volume, to be combined and rendered in a 2D projection[83] (Fig. 9–38). Projection angiograms can be generated from either a series of 2D images or a 3D data set.[84, 85] The method has become so universal that it is nearly synonymous with MRA. Yet MIP is not always the best technique for vascular display. Here the most important features of these methods are summarized.

MAXIMAL INTENSITY PROJECTION

Blood vessels course across many slices in a typical angiographic acquisition. To display the entire vessel, one must combine the slices. If one simply sums the intensities on the slices, an immediate problem presents itself—the background signal added from the many slices exceeds that of the vessels, with the result that vessels are no longer visible. The MIP algorithm was designed to overcome this problem. Rather than adding intensities, it uses only the largest single intensity at each position in the projection in the combined image.

First, the direction of projection is chosen; the com-

puter algorithm then goes through the 3D data along that direction and automatically picks out and displays the highest signal intensity from the slices. Because the program does not differentiate between blood and background tissue, the selection is based on signal intensity alone.

Although MIP is much better than simple pixel addition, weak vascular features can be lost in the projection because the vessel signal intensity is exceeded by the background signal intensity. Vessels may appear narrowed or absent on an MIP. Therefore, when interpreting a study, the original images should be consulted to determine the true vessel width.

Vessel depiction can be improved by targeted MIP, in which a selected volume of the 3D data is projected (Fig. 9–39). By limiting the projection volume, signals from other vessels or bright structures are removed, and the chance that vessel intensity is exceeded by background intensity is reduced. Another approach that can be helpful is to first perform multiplanar reconstructions of the 3D data and then obtain an MIP of these reconstructions.

VESSEL TRACKING

In vessel tracking one tries to identify the signal corresponding to blood vessels and then remove all nonvascular voxels (Fig. 9–40). This is done by picking out an object with contiguous voxels that have signal intensity over a chosen threshold. With the program, a volume is separated into different contiguous objects, many of which are vessels.[86] The nonvascular objects are then edited out by the operator.

The algorithm may be assisted by "seeding," in which a point in the vessel is selected by the operator. The computer then looks for bright voxels contiguous

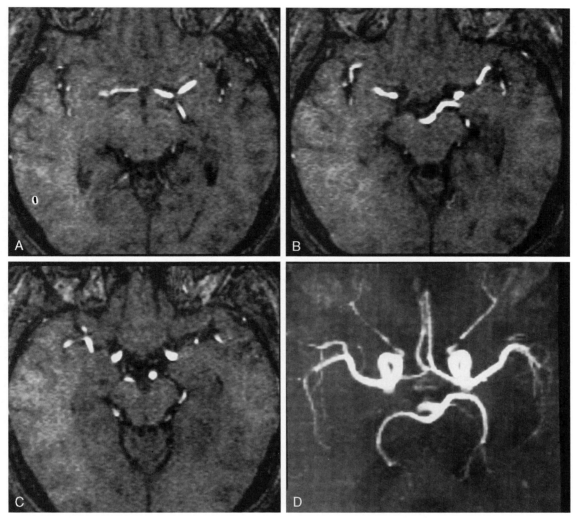

FIGURE 9–38. A set of four images showing three source images of the intracranial vessels *(A to C)* and *(D)* the MIP.

with that seed. These voxels in turn are used as seeds for the next iteration. The object grows outward until it reaches the vessel wall. The progression of the seed is based on signal comparison between neighboring voxels and is governed by criteria set by the user.

SURFACE RENDERING

Once the voxels corresponding to a vessel are identified, and assuming the angiogram is of adequate resolution, one may calculate the position of the outer margin of the lumen. This can be rendered into a realistic surface with shading and perspective, as if a model had been made of the vessel.[87] Although still uncommon, this method of presentation is effective for displaying complex anatomy.

SOURCE DISPLAY

The original source images are important for determination of vessel widths and the degree of stenosis. The true lumen size is better evaluated in the cross-sectional views than in the projections[36] (Fig. 9–41). Furthermore, vessels with slow flow are always better visualized on the original images. It is prudent to photograph both MIP and selected source images when interpreting a study.

PATTERNS OF BLOOD FLOW AND THEIR APPEARANCE ON MR ANGIOGRAMS

Blood flow can sometimes be disorderly, turbulent, or highly pulsatile. Furthermore, blood can follow a tortuous course. In some instances, the depiction of the vessel lumen in MRA may not resemble the true shape or size of the lumen. The image may suggest disease when none is present or lead to an overestimation of disease. These abnormal patterns are predictable and can be recognized when they are present.

TURBULENCE AND PHASE DISPERSION

The term turbulent flow in the context of MR means chaotic or incoherent flow in which there is consider-

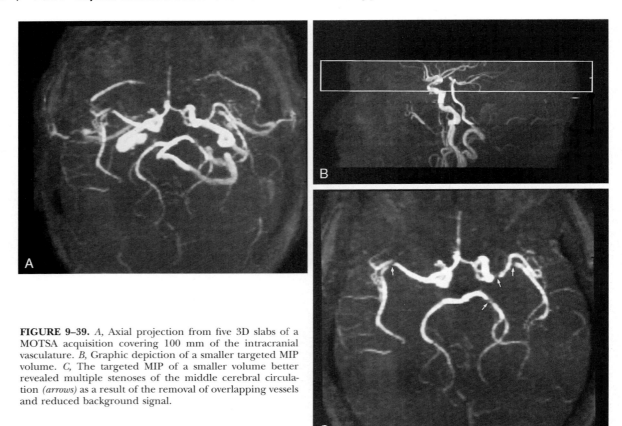

FIGURE 9–39. *A,* Axial projection from five 3D slabs of a MOTSA acquisition covering 100 mm of the intracranial vasculature. *B,* Graphic depiction of a smaller targeted MIP volume. *C,* The targeted MIP of a smaller volume better revealed multiple stenoses of the middle cerebral circulation *(arrows)* as a result of the removal of overlapping vessels and reduced background signal.

able mixing of spins, which no longer travel along straight streamlines. Such a flow pattern often occurs just beyond a tight vascular stenosis, where blood is decelerating and mixing with much lower velocity blood. Turbulent flow, or more precisely incoherent flow, often results in an unwanted loss of signal caused by phase incoherence.

Within regions of turbulent flow, acceleration and higher order motions introduce variations in phase within each voxel that cannot be corrected by flow

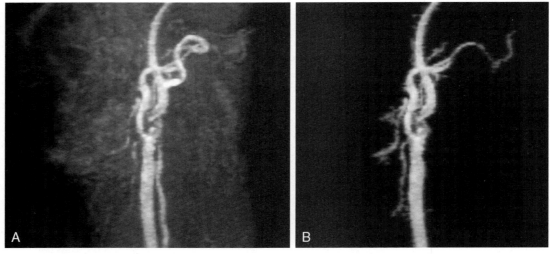

FIGURE 9–40. *A,* MIP projection of the carotid bifurcation acquired with a 3D sagittal TOF acquisition. The severity of stenosis at the bifurcation is obscured by the overlapping vertebral artery. *B,* MIP calculated after performing a connected voxel algorithm search to identify the carotid artery alone. Overlapping vessels and stationary signal not connected to the carotid artery are eliminated. (*A* and *B* from Saloner D, Hanson WA, Tsuruda JS, et al: Application of a connected-voxel algorithm to MR angiographic data. J Magn Reson Imaging 1:423–430, 1991.)

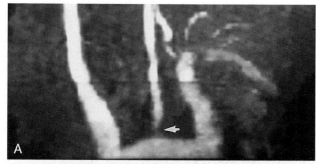

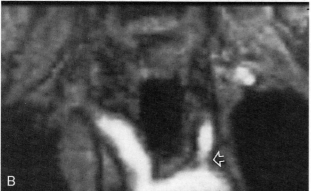

FIGURE 9–41. Comparison of stenosis depiction by MIP versus source images. *A,* Paracoronal MIP projection (from a four-slab axial MOTSA acquisition) of the great vessels of the aortic arch showing a stenosis at the origin of the left common carotid artery *(arrow)*. *B,* Reconstructed 3D source image shows a more accurate depiction of the vessel stenosis *(arrow)*.

compensation. As a result, the magnetization vectors of spins in the voxel point in different directions and cancel each other. The intensity of the voxel becomes reduced. This phenomenon can be readily observed at a vascular stenosis or near cardiac valves as a focal dropout in signal. The degree of signal loss depends on the amount of turbulence. Sometimes this phenomenon is seen as a flame-shaped dark jet beyond the lesion orifice, sometimes as an exaggeration of the degree of stenosis, and sometimes as an apparent complete interruption in the vessel. Note that only transverse magnetization is affected by this phenomenon—beyond the turbulence the blood again appears bright because longitudinal magnetization is still available to be excited.

Several measures can be taken to mitigate this loss of signal. One can acquire small voxels so that fewer spins are placed together in a voxel, as described earlier in this chapter. One can select a short TE with an asymmetric echo so that the duration of the frequency-encoding gradient is minimized. This gradient is thought to be the greatest contributor to phase dispersion. One can employ 3D rather than thin-slice 2D acquisition, which reduces the size of the slice-select gradient. Most important, one can inspect the individual, unprojected sections when assessing the degree of stenosis. Often, residual, uncanceled signal within the stenosis may be faintly visible.

PULSATILE FLOW

Arterial flow is periodic in nature. The variation in the wash-in rate of spins between systole and diastole creates alterations in the amplitude of echoes acquired during the course of the acquisition. This "view-to-view" variation results in ghost artifacts along the phase-encoding direction of TOF images. The amount of ghosting is made worse by using large FA values (Fig. 9–42). These ghost artifacts can be selectively removed by using presaturation bands to eliminate the arterial signal when performing MR venography.[37]

The variation in velocity over the cardiac cycle also causes modulations of phase in both TOF and PCA acquisition, which cannot be eliminated by first-order flow compensation. Cardiac triggering can be used to synchronize data collection to the cardiac cycle to address this problem. When triggering is not used, the blood signal can be variable and ghost artifacts can be seen. Pulsatile artifacts can be quite complex in 3D imaging.[88] With 3D there are two phase-encoding directions (in plane and slice select), and ghost artifacts resulting from respiration and pulsatile flow can propagate in both directions. Artifacts in the slice-select direction may cause slice-to-slice variations in signal intensity.

FLOW SEPARATION AND RECIRCULATION

Flow saturation can be pronounced at regions of a vessel where blood flow circles in one place (*recirculation*) or is stagnant (Fig. 9–43). The most common example of this is the carotid bulb, where blood moves forward in the anterior portion of the proximal internal carotid artery and in the reverse direction in the posterior portion. The laminar streamlines of flow separate from the vessel wall at that point, a phenomenon called *flow separation*. Blood in the posterior bulb spends a long time in the acquired volume and appears dark, which might simulate the appearance of a plaque. Flow separation may also occur beyond a stenosis or with an ulcer or aneurysm, again with the result that those areas appear more dark.

FLOW MISREGISTRATION

A blood signal often seems to arise from a point outside the vessel, as if the image of the blood and the image of the background were misregistered. This artifact occurs as a result of flow during the time delay between the phase-encoding and the frequency-encoding portions of the sequence.[89] In other words, the position on the phase-encoding axis is determined at one point in time and the position along the frequency-encoding axis is determined at a slightly later point in time. Blood flowing at an angle to the phase-encoding axis appears displaced along the frequency-encoding axis (Fig. 9–44). Displacement artifacts and signal "pileup" are often seen in tortuous vessels such as the carotid siphon.[90] The presence of misregistra-

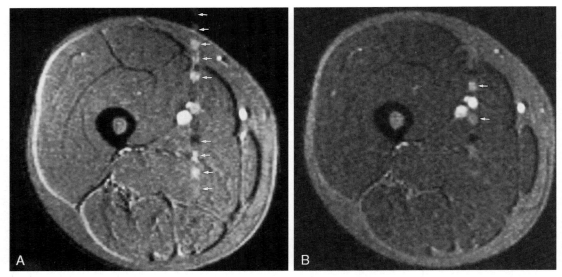

FIGURE 9–42. A pair of 2D TOF images of the popliteal artery showing a decrease in pulsatile artifacts *(arrows)* when a smaller FA is used. The images were acquired with FA values of *(A)* 90° and *(B)* 60° (both with TR/TE = 25/10).

tion can be discovered by repeating the MRA sequence with the frequency and phase axes swapped. If the vessel takes on a new shape or position, a displacement artifact is present.

The degree of misregistration depends on the blood velocity, the angle of the vessel with respect to the phase-encoding direction, and the time delay between phase encoding and frequency encoding. The displacement is in the same direction as the flow. This artifact differs from a chemical-shift artifact, which also occurs along the frequency-encoding direction. Reduction of this artifact requires changes in pulse sequence design so that the time between phase encoding and frequency encoding is minimized.

ECHO-PLANAR ANGIOGRAPHY

Relatively little flow-related dephasing occurs with single-shot echo-planar imaging (EPI), even without flow compensation. Dephasing is minimal because of the ultrashort interval between sequential echoes and the fact that even-echo rephasing occurs on alternate echoes. Ghost artifacts are absent, because all data for a section are acquired within a small portion of a single cardiac cycle. Although ghost artifacts do not occur, flow displacement artifacts can be large if data are acquired during rapid systolic flow, because of the long readout period.[91] Nonetheless, EPI has potential value as an ultrafast method for MRA[92] and flow quan-

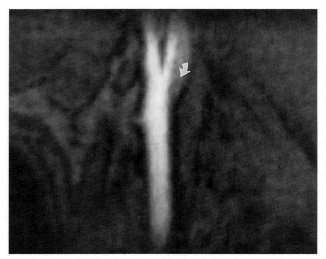

FIGURE 9–43. Sagittal projection from a 3D axial TOF image of the carotid bifurcation showing spin saturation caused by recirculation in the carotid bulb *(arrow)*. The image was acquired with TR/TE/FA = 35/7/20° and 64 partitions.

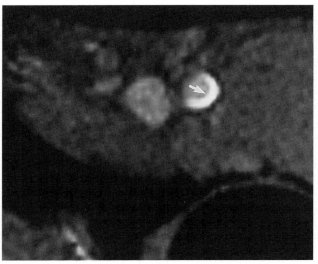

FIGURE 9–44. Example of signal pileup in a gradient-echo image (TE = 25 ms) related to flow displacement artifact *(arrow)* in the femoral artery, which was at an angle to the imaging slice.

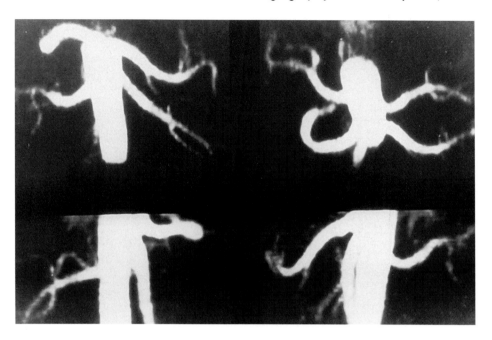

FIGURE 9–45. MIPs from a breath-hold STAR acquisition using a segmented 3D echo-planar pulse sequence. The renal arteries and other aortic branches are well shown in multiple projections. (Courtesy of P. Wielopolski, PhD, Harvard Medical School, Boston, MA.)

tification.[93] Angiographic results are best if the data are acquired during diastole, when acceleration and associated displacement artifacts resulting from oblique flow are minimal.[94] The readout period should be kept to a minimum.

The EPISTAR sequence, a tagging and subtraction technique similar to the STAR technique described earlier but using an echo-planar readout, can also be used for MRA.[95] The long inflow times afforded by EPISTAR permit extensive lengths of the vessels to be filled by tagged protons, and the excellent background suppression and use of thick slabs for imaging make it possible to encompass the entire vessel in one section, without the need for subsequent image processing. The single-shot readout renders the images relatively insensitive to peristaltic motion for abdominal MRA. A 3D segmented EPI sequence has been developed that permits imaging of an entire volume within a single breath-hold.[96] Multiplanar reconstructions and MIPs can then be performed on the volumetric data (Fig. 9–45). With this technique, unlike standard 3D acquisitions, there is no degradation from respiratory artifacts. Present drawbacks include limited signal-to-noise ratio and the need for stronger, faster gradients than are generally available.

Another approach under investigation is spiral scan imaging,[97] which involves oscillating the readout and frequency-encoding gradients in tandem. The method is intrinsically flow compensated, as the center of k-space is acquired early on. Thus, it suffers from fewer flow artifacts than does EPI.

SUMMARY

In the past decade, MRA has become widely accepted as a noninvasive method for vascular imaging. TOF has been extensively applied to nearly every part of the body and is effective in addressing numerous clinical questions. PC MRA is also useful in many clinical applications. Although PC MRA is slightly more complex to use than TOF, it provides excellent tissue background suppression and flexibility in flow sensitivity. As a result, PC MRA provides better depiction of small vessels and slow flow. Moreover, it enables flow quantification and the generation of directional flow maps.

In the future, we will see techniques that allow higher image resolution and depict even finer vascular details. Specialized coils will be available for higher signal-to-noise ratio for specific applications. Furthermore, faster image acquisitions will enable the complete elimination of physiologic motions in both 2D and 3D acquisitions. Further work is needed to determine the potential clinical role of flow quantification. As the technology advances and clinical validation is done, MRA will probably replace diagnostic contrast angiography in an increasing variety of clinical applications.

REFERENCES

1. Caro CG, Pedley JG, Schroter RC, Seed WA: The Mechanics of Circulation. Oxford: Oxford University Press, 1978.
2. McDonald DA: Blood Flow in Arteries. London: Edward Arnold, 1974.
3. Milnor WR: Hemodynamics. Baltimore: Williams & Wilkins, 1989.
4. Kilner PJ, Yang GZ, Mohiaddin RH, et al: Helical and retrograde secondary flow patterns in the aortic arch studies by three-directional magnetic resonance velocity mapping. Circulation 88:2235–2247, 1993.
5. Edelman RR: Magnetic resonance angiography. An overview. Invest Radiol 28(suppl 4):S43–S46, 1993.
6. Saloner D, Chien D: Historical development of MRA. In: Anderson CM, Edelman RR, Turski PA, eds. Clinical Magnetic Resonance Angiography. New York: Raven Press, 1993, pp 161–180.
7. Hahn E: Spin echoes. Phys Rev 80:580–594, 1950.
8. Suryan G: Nuclear resonance in flowing liquids. Proc Indian Acad Sci A33:107–113, 1951.
9. Hahn E: Detection of sea water motion by nuclear precession. J Geophys Res 65:776–777, 1960.

10. Masaryk TJ, Laub GA, Modic MT, et al: Carotid-CNS MR flow imaging. Magn Reson Med 14:308–314, 1990.
11. Edelman RR, Manning WJ, Burstein D, Paulin S: Coronary arteries: breath-hold MR angiography. Radiology 181:641–643, 1991.
12. Manning WJ, Li W, Boyle NG, Edelman RR: Fat-suppressed breath-hold magnetic resonance coronary angiography. Circulation 87:94–104, 1993.
13. Rother J, Wentz KU, Rautenberg W, et al: Magnetic resonance angiography in vertebrobasilar ischemia. Stroke 24:1310–1315, 1993.
14. Durham JR, Hackworth CA, Tober JC, et al: Magnetic resonance angiography in the preoperative evaluation of abdominal aortic aneurysms. Am J Surg 166:173–177 (discussion 177–178), 1993.
15. Anderson CM, Saloner D, Lee RE, et al: Assessment of carotid artery stenosis by MR angiography: comparison with x-ray angiography and color-coded Doppler ultrasound. AJNR 13:989–1008, 1992.
16. Lewis WD, Finn JP, Jenkins RL, et al: Use of magnetic resonance angiography in the pretransplant evaluation of portal vein pathology. Transplantation 56:64–68, 1993.
17. Turnipseed WD, Kennell TW, Turski PA, et al: Combined use of duplex imaging and magnetic resonance angiography for evaluation of patients with symptomatic ipsilateral high-grade carotid stenosis. J Vasc Surg 17:832–839 (discussion 839–840), 1993.
18. Anson JA, Heiserman JE, Drayer BP, Spetzler RF: Surgical decisions on the basis of magnetic resonance angiography of the carotid arteries. Neurosurgery 32:335–343 (discussion 343), 1993.
19. Finn JP, Kane RA, Edelman RR, et al: Imaging of the portal venous system in patients with cirrhosis: MR angiography vs duplex Doppler sonography. AJR 161:989–994, 1993.
20. Mohiaddin RH, Paz R, Theodoropoulos S, et al: Magnetic resonance characterization of pulmonary arterial blood flow after single lung transplantation. J Thorac Cardiovasc Surg 101:1016–1023, 1991.
21. Anderson CM, Lee RE: Time-of-flight angiography. In: Anderson CM, Edelman RR, Turski PA, eds. Clinical Magnetic Resonance Angiography. New York: Raven Press, 1993, pp 11–42.
22. Wehrli FW: Time-of-flight effects in MR imaging of flow. Magn Reson Med 14:187–193, 1990.
23. Schmalbrock P, Yuan C, Chakeres DW, et al: Volume MR angiography: methods to achieve very short echo times. Radiology 175:861–865, 1990.
24. Laub GA, Kaiser WA: MR angiography with gradient motion refocusing. J Comput Assist Tomogr 12:377–382, 1988.
25. Wehrli FW, Shimakawa A, Gullberg GT, MacFall JR: Time-of-flight MR flow imaging: selective saturation recovery with gradient refocusing. Radiology 160:781–785, 1986.
26. Axel L: Blood flow effects in magnetic resonance imaging. Magn Reson Annu :237–244, 1986.
27. Nishimura DG: Time-of-flight angiography. Magn Reson Med 14:194–201, 1990.
28. Edelman RR, Ahn SS, Chien D, et al: Improved time-of-flight MR angiography of the brain with magnetization transfer contrast. Radiology 184:395–399, 1992.
29. Dixon WT, Sardashti M, Castillo M, Stomp GP: Multiple inversion recovery reduces static tissue signal in angiograms. Magn Reson Med 18:257–268, 1991.
30. Edelman RR, Chien D, Atkinson DJ, Sandstrom J: Fast time-of-flight magnetic resonance angiography with improved background suppression. Radiology 179:867–870, 1991.
31. Edelman RR, Siewert B, Adamis M, et al: Signal targeting with alternating radiofrequency (STAR) sequences: application to MR angiography. Magn Reson Med 31:233–238, 1994.
32. Nishimura DG, Macovski A, Pauly JM: Considerations of magnetic resonance angiography by selective inversion recovery. Magn Reson Med 7:472–484, 1988.
33. Sardashti M, Schwartzberg DG, Stomp GP, Dixon WT: Spin-labeling angiography of the carotids by presaturation and simplified adiabatic inversion. Magn Reson Med 15:192–200, 1990.
34. Dixon WT, Du LN, Faul DD, et al: Projection angiograms of blood labeled by adiabatic fast passage. Magn Reson Med 3:454–462, 1986.
35. Wang SJ, Nishimura DG, Macovski A: Fast angiography using selective inversion recovery. Magn Reson Med 23:109–121, 1992.
36. Anderson CM, Saloner D, Tsuruda JS, et al: Artifacts in maximum-intensity-projection display of MR angiograms. AJR 154:623–629, 1990.
37. Ehman RL, Felmlee JP: Flow artifact reduction in MRI: a review of the roles of gradient moment nulling and spatial presaturation. Magn Reson Med 14:293–307, 1990.
38. Felmlee JP, Ehman RL: Spatial presaturation: a method for suppressing flow artifacts and improving depiction of vascular anatomy in MR imaging. Radiology 164:559–564, 1987.
39. Edelman RR, Atkinson DJ, Silver MS, et al: FRODO pulse sequences: a new means of eliminating motion, flow, and wraparound artifacts. Radiology 166:231–236, 1988.
40. Edelman RR, Mattle HP, O'Reilly GV, et al: Magnetic resonance imaging of flow dynamics in the circle of Willis. Stroke 21:56–65, 1990.
41. Edelman RR, Zhao B, Liu C, et al: MR angiography and dynamic flow evaluation of the portal venous system. AJR 153:755–760, 1989.
42. Mattle H, Edelman RR, Wentz KU, et al: Middle cerebral artery: determination of flow velocities with MR angiography. Radiology 181:527–530, 1991.
43. Gullberg GT, Wehrli FW, Shimakawa A, Simons MA: MR vascular imaging with a fast gradient refocusing pulse sequence and reformatted images from transaxial sections. Radiology 165:241–246, 1987.
44. Masaryk TJ, Modic MT, Ross JS, et al: Intracranial circulation: preliminary clinical results with three-dimensional (volume) MR angiography. Radiology 171:793–799, 1989.
45. Ruggieri PM, Laub GA, Masaryk TJ, Modic MT: Intracranial circulation: pulse-sequence considerations in three-dimensional (volume) MR angiography. Radiology 171:785–791, 1989.
46. Lewin JS, Laub G, Hausmann R: Three-dimensional time-of-flight MR angiography: applications in the abdomen and thorax. Radiology 179:261–264, 1991.
47. Purdy D, Cadena G, Laub G: The design of a variable tip angle slab selection (TONE) pulse for improved 3D MRA. In: Proceedings of the 11th Annual Meeting of the Society of Magnetic Resonance in Medicine, Berlin, 1992, p 882.
48. Haacke EM, Masaryk TJ, Wielopolski PA, et al: Optimizing blood vessel contrast in fast three-dimensional MRI. Magn Reson Med 14:202–221, 1990.
49. Parker DL, Yuan C, Blatter DD: MR angiography by multiple thin slab 3D acquisition. Magn Reson Med 17:434–451, 1991.
50. Creasy JL, Price RR, Presbrey T, et al: Gadolinium-enhanced MR angiography. Radiology 175:280–283, 1990.
51. Lin W, Haacke EM, Smith AS, Clampitt ME: Gadolinium-enhanced high-resolution MR angiography with adaptive vessel tracking: preliminary results in the intracranial circulation. J Magn Reson Imaging 2:277–284, 1992.
52. Prince MR, Yucel EK, Kaufman JA, et al: Dynamic gadolinium enhanced three-dimensional abdominal MR angiography. J Magn Reson Imaging 3:877–882, 1993.
52a. Holland GA, Slossman F, Baum RA, et al: Fast 3D time-of-flight (3D-TOF) MR angiography (MRA) of the aortoiliac arteries using gadolinium: optimization and preliminary experience. In: Proceedings of the Society of Magnetic Resonance, Third Scientific Meeting, Nice, France, August 19–25, Volume 3. Berkeley, CA: Society of Magnetic Resonance, 1995, p 1577.
53. Atkinson DJ, Edelman RR: Cine-angiography of the heart in a single breath-hold with a segmented turboFLASH sequence. Radiology 178:357–360, 1991.
54. Chien D, Edelman RR: Ultra-fast imaging using gradient echoes. Magn Reson Q 7:31–56, 1991.
55. Wielopolski PA, Haacke EM, Adler LP: Three-dimensional imaging of the pulmonary vasculature: preliminary experience. Radiology 183:465–472, 1992.
56. Edelman RR, Chien D, Kim D: Fast selective black blood MR imaging. Radiology 181:655–660, 1991.
57. Chien D, Goldmann A, Edelman RR: High-speed black blood imaging of vessel stenosis in the presence of pulsatile flow. J Magn Reson Imaging 2:437–441, 1992.
58. Edelman RR, Mattle HP, Wallner B, et al: Extracranial carotid arteries: evaluation with "black blood" MR angiography. Radiology 177:45–50, 1990.
59. Wedeen V, Rosen B, Chesler D, Brady T: MR velocity imaging by phase display. J Comput Assist Tomogr 9:530–536, 1985.
60. Moran P: A flow velocity zeugmatographic interlace for NMR imaging in humans. Magn Reson Imaging 1:197–203, 1982.
61. von Schulthess G, Higgins C: Blood flow imaging with MR: spin-phase phenomena. Radiology 157:687–695, 1985.
62. Firmin DN, Nayler GL, Kilner PJ, Longmore DB: The application of phase shifts in NMR for flow measurement. Magn Reson Med 14:230–241, 1990.
63. Dumoulin CL, Souza SP, Walker MF, et al: Three-dimensional phase-contrast angiography. Magn Reson Med 9:139–149, 1989.
64. Pelc NJ, Bernstein MA, Shimakawa A, Glover GH: Encoding strategies for three-direction phase-contrast MR imaging of flow. J Magn Reson Imaging 1:405–413, 1991.
65. Dumoulin C, Souza S, Darrow R, et al: Simultaneous acquisition of phase-contrast angiograms and stationary tissue images with Hadamard encoding of flow-induced phase shifts. J Magn Reson Imaging 1:399–404, 1991.
66. Turski PA, Korosec F: Technical features and emerging clinical applications of phase contrast MRA. Neuroimaging Clin North Am 2:785–800, 1992.
67. Applegate GR, Talagala SL, Applegate LJ: MR angiography of the head and neck: value of two-dimensional phase-contrast projection technique. AJR 159:369–374, 1992.
68. Pernicone JR, Siebert JE, Laird TA, et al: Determination of blood flow direction using velocity-phase image display with 3-D phase-contrast MR angiography. AJNR 13:1435–1438, 1992.
69. Underwood SR: Cine magnetic resonance imaging and flow measurements in the cardiovascular system. Br Med Bull 45:948–967, 1989.
70. Enzmann DR, Ross MR, Marks MP, Pelc NJ: Blood flow in major cerebral arteries measured by phase-contrast cine MR. AJNR 15:123–129, 1994.
71. Debatin JF, Ting RH, Wegmuller H, et al: Renal artery blood flow: quantitation with phase-contrast MR imaging with and without breath holding. Radiology 190:371–378, 1994.
72. Applegate GR, Thaete FL, Meyers SP, et al: Blood flow in the portal

vein: velocity quantitation with phase-contrast MR angiography. Radiology 187:253–256, 1993.

73. Meier D, Maier S, Bosiger P: Quantitative flow measurements on phantoms and on blood vessels with MR. Magn Reson Med 8:25–34, 1988.

74. Glover GH, Pelc NJ: A rapid gated cine MR technique. Magn Reson Annu 299–333, 1988.

75. Bogren HG, Klipstein RH, Firmin DN, et al: Quantitation of antegrade and retrograde blood flow in the human aorta by magnetic resonance velocity mapping. Am Heart J 117:1214–1222, 1989.

76. Li KCP, Whitney WS, McDonnell CH, et al: Chronic mesenteric ischemia: evaluation with phase-contrast cine MR imaging. Radiology 190:175–179, 1994.

77. Edelman RR, Manning WJ, Gervino E, Li W: Flow velocity quantification in human coronary arteries with fast breath-hold MR angiography. J Magn Reson Imaging 3:699–703, 1993.

78. Korosec FR, Mistretta CA, Turski PA: ECG-optimized phase contrast line scanned MR angiography. Magn Reson Med 24:221–235, 1992.

79. Swan S, Weber D, Grist T, et al: Peripheral MR angiography with variable velocity encoding. Radiology 184:831–817, 1992.

80. Buonocore MH: Algorithms for improving calculated streamlines in 3-D phase contrast angiography. Magn Reson Med 31:22–30, 1994.

81. Steinberg FL, Yucel EK, Dumoulin CL, Souza SP: Peripheral vascular and abdominal applications of MR flow imaging techniques. Magn Reson Med 14:315–320, 1990.

82. Rossnick S, Laub G, Braeckle R: Three dimensional display of blood vessels in MRI. In: Proceedings of the IEEE Computers in Cardiology. New York: Institute of Electrical and Electronic Engineers, 1986, pp 193–195.

83. Keller PJ, Drayer BP, Fram EK, et al: MR angiography with two-dimensional acquisition and three-dimensional display. Work in progress. Radiology 173:527–532, 1989.

84. Dixon W, Du L, Faul D, et al: Projection angiograms of blood labeled by adiabatic fast passage. Magn Reson Med 3:454–462, 1986.

85. Laub G: Displays for MR angiography. Magn Reson Med 14:222–229, 1990.

86. Saloner D, Hanson WA, Tsuruda JS, et al: Application of a connected-voxel algorithm to MR angiographic data. J Magn Reson Imaging 1:423–430, 1991.

87. Hu X, Alperin N, Levin D, et al: Visualization of MR angiographic data with segmentation and volume-rendering techniques. J Magn Reson Imaging 1:539–546, 1991.

88. Frank LR, Buxton RB, Kerber CW: Pulsatile flow artifacts in 3D magnetic resonance imaging. Magn Reson Med 30:296–304, 1993.

89. Nishimura DG, Jackson JI, Pauly JM: On the nature and reduction of the displacement artifact in flow images. Magn Reson Med 22:481–492, 1991.

90. van Tyen R, Saloner D, Jou LD, Berger S: MR imaging of flow through tortuous vessels: a numerical simulation. Magn Reson Med 31:184–195, 1994.

91. Butts K, Riederer SJ: Analysis of flow effects in echo-planar imaging. J Magn Reson Imaging 2:285–293, 1992.

92. Goldberg MA, Yucel EK, Saini S, et al: MR angiography of the portal and hepatic venous systems: preliminary experience with echo planar imaging. AJR 160:35–40, 1993.

93. Firmin DN, Klipstein RH, Hounsfield GL, et al: Echo-planar high-resolution flow velocity mapping. Magn Reson Med 12:316–327, 1989.

94. Simonetti OP, Wielopolski P, Duerk JL: Experimental evaluation of flow effects in echo planar imaging. In: Proceedings of the Society of Magnetic Resonance, San Francisco, August 6–12, Volume 1. Berkeley, CA: Society of Magnetic Resonance, 1994, p. 460.

95. Adamis MK, Gaa J, Edelman RR: STAR (signal targeting with alternating radio-frequency) renal artery imaging. J Magn Reson Imaging 4:S22, 1994.

96. Wielopolski PA, Edelman RR: Ultrafast, high resolution 3D STAR MR angiography using interleaved segmented echo planar readouts. In: Proceedings of the Society of Magnetic Resonance, San Francisco, August 6–12, Volume 2. Berkeley, CA: Society of Magnetic Resonance, 1994, p. 948.

97. Meyer C, Mu B, Nishimura D, Macouski A: Fast spiral coronary artery imaging. Magn Reson Med 28:202–213, 1992.

10

Fast MRI

ROBERT R. EDELMAN ■ PIOTR A. WIELOPOLSKI

Magnetic resonance imaging (MRI) has progressed at a spectacular rate in the past few years. Technical innovations and clinical needs have prompted an expansion of its uses from a few initial applications in the central nervous system to a host of applications throughout the body, including the liver, pelvis, musculoskeletal system, and heart. Moreover, there is increasing interest in using MRI to study organ function rather than simply to depict anatomy.

Along with this expansion of applications has come a heightened appreciation of the problems posed by respiratory and cardiac motion and the need for fast imaging to overcome these artifacts and to provide the speed needed for functional imaging studies (Fig. 10–1). Although standard spin-echo (SE) pulse sequences are well validated and in general use, they lack the flexibility to address these problems. Fortunately, solutions now exist in the area of fast MRI techniques. It is now possible, for instance, to eliminate artifacts from respiratory motion by use of subsecond imaging methods such as turbo fast low-angle shot (turboFLASH); cardiac motion can be tamed by use of electrocardiogram-gated cine gradient echo (GRE), segmented turboFLASH, or ultimately the speediest approach, echo-planar imaging (EPI) (Fig. 10–2). In addition, fast MRI methods can produce images with enhanced tissue contrast and improved spatial resolution, completely aside from the ability to reduce scan times.

The technical aspects of pulse sequences have been reviewed in Chapter 4. In this chapter, the basic concepts of fast MRI are reviewed along with examples of useful clinical applications. Although the field is progressing rapidly and new pulse sequences are being created all the time, these sequences have common underlying principles. These methods, summarized in Table 10–1, can greatly improve the image quality and breadth of applications of MRI.

TYPES OF PULSE SEQUENCES

A pulse sequence is a collection of events designed to create an MR image with particular characteristics. Radiofrequency (RF) pulses are applied to excite the protons and, for SE sequences, to refocus the MR signal. For standard pulse sequences, the protons are excited once, one amplitude of the phase-encoding gradient is applied, and a single *line* of data is acquired for each repetition time (TR) interval. A complete image typically requires 128 to 512 lines and, for sequences that acquire only one phase-encoding line per excitation such as conventional SE or GRE, 128 to 512 repetitions of the pulse sequence. Gradient magnetic fields are applied to localize the MR signal spatially. The signal is read out during a time that may range from a few milliseconds to tens of milliseconds.

The signal-to-noise (S/N) ratio is inversely proportional to the square root of the readout period; this readout period determines the *bandwidth* of the MR signal. For instance, a readout period of 10 ms (with a bandwidth of 1/10 ms = 10 kHz) gives half the bandwidth and a 41% higher S/N ratio than a readout period of 5 ms. The flip side is that a long readout period necessitates a lengthened minimal echo time (TE) and TR; low-bandwidth sequences also have a weak readout gradient that exacerbates chemical-shift and magnetic susceptibility artifacts. At 1.5 T a readout bandwidth per pixel of 110 Hz gives a chemical shift of two pixels, compared with a shift of one pixel for a higher bandwidth per pixel of 220 Hz. These issues figure prominently in the design of fast imaging sequences, and the optimal design depends on magnetic field strength, hardware configuration, part of the body being imaged, and other factors.

SPIN ECHO

In spite of continuing sequence developments, variants of SE remain the most commonly used sequences

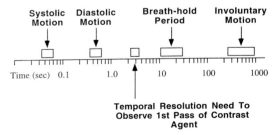

FIGURE 10–1. Time line showing the different time frames of certain body functions.

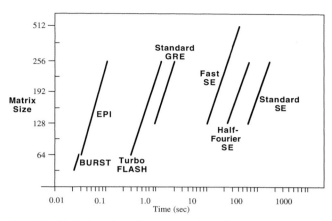

FIGURE 10–2. Imaging time comparison for various pulse sequences.

for MRI. The single-echo SE sequence consists of a pair of RF pulses and can be represented as

90°-(wait TE/2)-180°-(wait TE/2)-(signal readout)

where TE defines the center of the SE signal. The pulse sequence is repeated at time intervals equal to TR. For each excitation, the number of times the sequence is repeated is determined by the spatial resolution (specifically the number of pixels) along the phase-encoding axis and is equal to the number of phase-encoding steps. A large number of phase-encoding steps is needed for high spatial resolution.

The first pulse in the SE sequence, used to excite the spins, is set to 90° to tip the existing longitudinal magnetization completely into the transverse plane. This maximizes the amount of signal that can be obtained per measurement. However, immediately after the 90° pulse, the remaining longitudinal magnetization is zero. If the spins were again excited at this time, no signal would be produced. The next 90° pulse produces a signal proportional to the accumulated magnetization, as expressed by

$$S = S_0[1 - \exp(-TR/T1)]$$

where S_0 is the signal that would be produced by a 90° pulse when the spins are fully aligned with the magnetic field. The signal (S) depends on the amount of T1 relaxation that occurs during the interval TR. To maintain a sufficient degree of tissue contrast and S/N ratio, the TR cannot be made much shorter than approximately 300 to 400 ms. This limitation essentially precludes a conventional SE sequence from being used for fast imaging, the reason being that scan time is proportional to TR, as given by the following equality:

$$\text{Scan time} = TR \times N_y \times NEX$$

where N_y is the number of phase-encoded lines and NEX is the number of excitations (also called Naq, for number of acquisitions).

TABLE 10–1. SUMMARY OF RAPID IMAGING METHODS*

HOW SCAN TIME IS REDUCED	TYPICAL SCAN TIMES	SPECIAL FEATURES
Shorten TR		
GRE	3 s–3 min	Contrast depends on flip angle; sensitive to B_0 inhomogeneities
Spoiled GRE		T1, proton density contrast; breath-hold T1-weighted image of abdomen
Steady-state GRE		Bright fluids if TR < T2*, motion sensitive
Contrast-enhanced GRE		T2 contrast, motion sensitive, TE ~ 2TR
Single-shot turboFLASH	0.5–2 s	Motion insensitive; good T1 contrast; some blurring; dynamic contrast-enhanced perfusion imaging, e.g., kidneys, heart
Segmented turboFLASH	10–20 s	Breath-hold cineangiography
Fast STEAM	0.5–2 s	Dark blood images; some blurring
SE with optimized flip angle: FLAME	4–8 min	SE contrast
Decrease number of views		
Reduced acquisition matrix	—	Reduced spatial resolution unless rectangular field of view used
Half-Fourier	—	Scan time reduced by nearly half if applied along phase-encoding axis; worsened signal-to-noise ratio; some artifacts
Acquire multiple views per excitation		
Fast SE	30 s–6 min	Excellent for T2, inversion recovery contrast; wide range of applications; slight blurring compared with SE
HASTE	1 s	Motion-insensitive single-shot fast SE with half-Fourier; T2 contrast for long-T2 tissues; some blurring; used for MR cholangiography, MR urography
GRASE	10 s–2 min	Like fast SE but with reduced scan time and radiofrequency power deposition, more blurring than fast SE
Single-shot GRASE	0.5 s	Motion insensitive; T2 contrast for long-T2 tissues; much blurring
Single-shot echo planar	0.05–0.1 s	Motion insensitive; good T2, inversion recovery contrast; usually low resolution; sensitive to B_0 inhomogeneities, ideal for functional studies, unstable patients
Segmented echo planar	10–30 s	Breath-hold T2-weighted images
Decrease number of excitations		
Single excitation	—	Motion artifacts more noticeable than with number of excitations >1

*FLAME = fast low-angle multiecho; FLASH = fast low-angle shot; GRASE = gradient and spin echo; GRE = gradient echo; HASTE = half-Fourier single-shot turbo spin echo; STEAM = stimulated-echo acquisition mode.

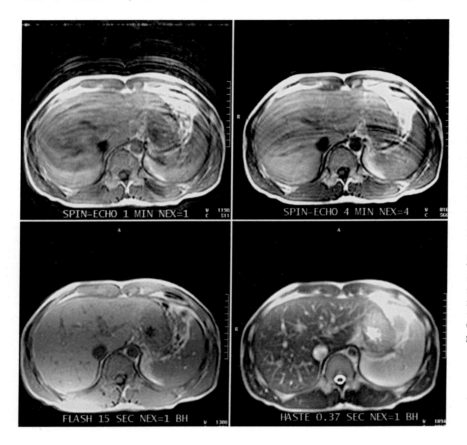

FIGURE 10–3. Signal averaging: issues for abdominal imaging. Abdominal images of a normal subject acquired in a multicoil array. *Upper left,* SE image (TR/TE/NEX = 500/12/1) obtained in 1 minute during breathing shows blurring and ghost artifacts from respiratory motion. *Upper right,* Same with 4 NEX obtained in 4 minutes shows improved S/N ratio and a reduction in ghost artifacts, but the image remains blurred. *Lower left,* Breath-hold FLASH image (TR/TE/flip angle/NEX = 120/4.8/80°/1) obtained in 15 seconds shows no ghost artifacts and greatly improved detail. The S/N ratio is better for the FLASH than the SE images despite the much shorter scan time, because of the reduction of coherent noise from respiratory ghost artifacts. *Lower right,* Breath-hold HASTE image (TE/NEX = 60/1) acquired in only 370 ms also shows good S/N ratio and good detail.

Each 180° pulse in a conventional SE sequence refocuses the MR signal at a time interval TE/2 after the center of the pulse. At the center of the SE, the effects of static magnetic field inhomogeneities (like those occurring at air–soft tissue interfaces) are eliminated.[1] Additional 180° pulses may be applied to generate additional SEs; each echo is used to create a single image. An alternative SE method is to phase encode each echo individually; this method is called rapid acquisition with relaxation enhancement (RARE). An optimized version of RARE has evolved into a clinically valuable fast imaging technique, called *fast spin echo,* that is considered later.

COLLECTING FEWER DATA

The fact that TR is constrained to fairly long values in SE imaging leaves open the possibility of speeding up the imaging process by decreasing the NEX or the matrix size of the image. There are several ways to take advantage of decreases in these parameters, but there may also be undesirable side effects that need to be understood.

REDUCED NUMBER OF EXCITATIONS

The parameter NEX refers to the number of times the pulse sequence is repeated *in each projection* during the process of acquiring an image. The reason for using more than one excitation is to eliminate certain undesirable features in the image. The features include artifacts resulting from thermal noise and artifacts resulting from repetitive motion (e.g., ghost artifacts from respiration).

By adding together the signals acquired from multiple excitations, undesirable features tend to be averaged out. This is represented in an improved S/N ratio, where

$$S/N \sim \sqrt{NEX}$$

Scan time is proportional to the NEX, so that using a single excitation cuts the scan time in half compared with that for two excitations. However, the penalty is a 41% reduction (i.e., $\sqrt{2}$) in S/N ratio, manifested as increased graininess in the image.

Single-excitation imaging is routinely used with high-field MRI systems. Even with lower field systems, which have an intrinsically lower S/N ratio, the loss in S/N ratio resulting from using fewer acquisitions can be compensated by slight increases in TR. For instance, an image produced with TR = 3000 ms and one acquisition may be similar in quality to one acquired with TR = 2000 ms and two acquisitions, although the scan time is less (13 minutes versus 17 minutes for a 256×256 matrix). As discussed later, one advantage of fast SE sequences is that one can benefit from the improved tissue contrast at long TR (e.g., >4 to 5 seconds), yet keep scan times less than for conventional SE sequences using a much shorter TR.

Loss of S/N ratio is not the only problem with single-excitation imaging. Ghost artifacts resulting from respiration and pulsatile flow are decreased by imaging with multiple excitations. The details of this process are quite complex, but if the motion is not correlated with TR, motion artifacts average out in much the same fashion as thermal noise. Therefore, motion artifacts decrease roughly as $\sqrt{NEX}$.

Ghost artifacts may be objectionable on images acquired with a single excitation. In the abdomen, where motion artifacts are most pronounced, it is usually better to use multiple-NEX scans unless a breath-holding study is possible (Fig. 10–3). One can avoid increasing the scan time despite the increased NEX by reducing the number of phase encodes and using a rectangular field of view (FOV) to maintain the level of spatial resolution.

REDUCED MATRIX SIZE

Scan time is proportional to the number of phase-encoding steps, so scan time can be decreased by using a smaller matrix size along the phase-encoding direction (changing the matrix size along the frequency-encoding direction has no effect on scan time). Decreasing the matrix size blurs the image and exacerbates the truncation or the Gibbs ringing artifact, which appears as multiple ghost images of certain features. Truncation artifacts are difficult to discern in images acquired with 256 phase encodes but are more apparent in images made with 128 phase encodes. Truncation artifacts can be reduced by utilizing a different reconstruc-

tion algorithm, for example, constrained reconstruction methods[2] (see Chapter 3).

For a given FOV, a 256 × 256 matrix has twice the spatial resolution of a 128 × 256 matrix. However, 128 phase encodes can be acquired in half as much time as 256 phase encodes. In many applications, a 128 × 256 matrix provides adequate spatial resolution. Furthermore, despite the shorter scan time, an image acquired with a 128 × 256 matrix has a 41% higher S/N ratio than one acquired with a 256 × 256 matrix. The reason is that the S/N ratio of the 128 × 256 image is decreased by a factor of $\sqrt{2}$ because of the twofold reduction in the amount of data that is collected but the pixel is twice as large (net change in S/N ratio is $2/\sqrt{2} = \sqrt{2}$ or 41%). An intermediate matrix (e.g., 192 × 256) is more time-consuming but produces fewer truncation artifacts and is therefore commonly used. Truncation artifacts are also made less apparent by using an asymmetric FOV.

RECTANGULAR FIELD OF VIEW

There is one situation in which the matrix size can be reduced with minimal or no loss in spatial resolution. If the anatomy being imaged is elliptic (e.g., head or abdomen), a rectangular or asymmetric FOV can be used to recover some or all of the resolution lost by using an asymmetric matrix (Fig. 10–4). For instance, consider 1) a 256 × 256 image with a symmetric 24

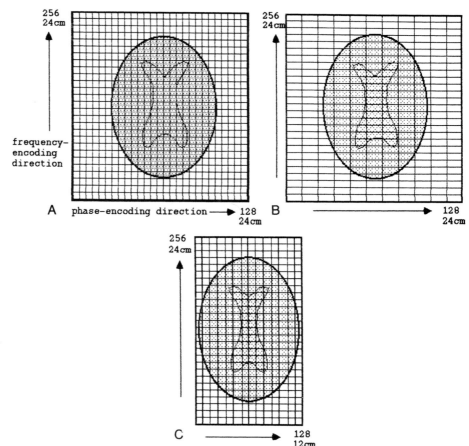

FIGURE 10–4. Schematic comparison of the effects of acquisition with different matrices on pixel size and image appearance. Note that subtle differences, such as truncation artifacts, are not shown here. *A*, A 256 × 256 (frequency × phase) image has square pixels (0.9 × 0.9 mm). *B*, A 256 × 128 image has rectangular pixels (0.9 × 1.8 mm) with half the spatial resolution of *A*, but the image is acquired in half as much time. Area under the phase-encoding gradient is half of that in *A*. *C*, A 256 × 128 image acquired using asymmetric FOV along the phase-encoding direction with one half the FOV in the frequency-encoding direction (24 × 12 cm). The resolution is the same as that in *A*, but the image is acquired in half as much time. It may not always be possible to reduce the FOV by such a large amount in the phase-encoding direction because of wraparound.

× 24-cm FOV versus 2) an image with 128 phase-encoding steps and a rectangular FOV of 12 cm (phase-encoding direction) × 24 cm (frequency-encoding direction). These images have equal pixel resolutions of 0.9 × 0.9 mm, but the image with the smaller matrix is acquired in half the time.

By permitting smaller acquisition matrices to be used without unacceptable compromises of spatial resolution, rectangular FOVs are routinely useful for reducing scan time, provided that the FOV accommodates the anatomy. If the anatomy does not fit in the rectangular FOV, substantial wraparound artifacts may occur along the phase-encoding direction. Wraparound is not a problem along the frequency-encoding direction because oversampling in this direction does not require extra time and, in conjunction with the application of a bandpass filter, cuts off signals arising from outside the prescribed FOV.

The S/N ratio is a consideration in the use of rectangular FOVs but is not a limiting factor as long as the FOV is not too asymmetric. Consider 1) an image acquired with a 256 × 256 matrix and a symmetric 24 × 24-cm FOV and 2) an image acquired in half the time with a 128 × 256 matrix and a 17 × 24-cm (41% smaller) FOV along the phase-encoding direction. Surprisingly, these two images have the same S/N ratio. The loss of S/N ratio resulting from the reduced FOV in the second image is precisely compensated by the gain in S/N ratio from the larger pixel size.

GRADIENT-ECHO SEQUENCES

A GRE sequence generates a *gradient echo* (also called a *gradient-recalled echo* or *field echo*) simply by applying a pair of balanced gradients of opposite sign along the frequency-encoding direction (see Chapter 4). The first gradient, called a dephasing or compensatory gradient, spreads out the transverse magnetization over 180° (π) or more and thereby dephases the spins. The readout gradient exactly undoes the dephasing at the TE so that there is no residual gradient dephasing effect. Unlike an SE sequence, which uses at least two RF pulses to generate an SE, a GRE sequence uses a single RF pulse to generate the GRE, usually with a flip angle less than 90°. A major advantage of GRE sequences is that good image quality can be maintained even with quite short TR (e.g., 30 ms).

The amount of signal generated by an RF pulse is proportional to the longitudinal magnetization existing at the moment before the pulse is applied. Now consider the effect of a 90° RF pulse. After applying this pulse, one must wait a considerable time, on the order of the tissue T1 relaxation time, before repeating the excitation. Otherwise, as mentioned before, the tissue magnetization becomes saturated (i.e., approaches a value of zero) and insufficient signal is produced. On the other hand, if a reduced flip angle (e.g., 30°) is used with a GRE sequence, saturation effects are much less and the TR can be substantially shortened (Fig. 10–5). The flip angle that produces

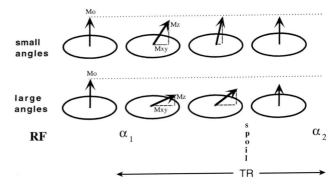

FIGURE 10–5. Relationship of flip angle to signal for a spoiled GRE sequence. The time between α_1 and α_2 is TR. *Top,* Signal is directly proportional to spin density if α^2 is much less than 2TR/T1. Only a small amount of transverse magnetization (M_{xy}) and signal is generated from the first small flip angle RF pulse (α_1), but the protons are almost fully magnetized by the time of the second RF pulse (α_2) and produce nearly the same amount of signal as from the first excitation. *Bottom,* More transverse magnetization is initially generated with a large flip angle excitation, but the protons have recovered only a portion of the magnetization by the time of the next RF pulse and produce substantially less signal intensity from this excitation.

the most signal for a given TR and T1 is known as the Ernst angle (α_E), as given by

$$\cos(\alpha_E) = \exp(-TR/T1)$$

However, the Ernst angle is not necessarily the best choice for flip angle. More critical for lesion detection than the S/N ratio is the signal difference to noise or contrast to noise ratio (i.e., the difference in signal between two tissues, such as a metastasis and the liver, divided by the standard deviation of the background noise). The flip angle is a key determinant of GRE image contrast[6, 7] (Figs. 10–6 and 10–7). For T1-weighted GRE images, a flip angle larger than the Ernst angle produces better T1 contrast; for proton density–weighted images, a smaller flip angle is desirable.

Because short TR values are permissible with GRE sequences, three-dimensional (3D) acquisitions can be completed in a reasonable time (e.g., 5 to 10 minutes).[8] With 3D acquisitions, a thick volume of tissue rather than a thin two-dimensional (2D) section is excited by the RF pulse. 3D GRE imaging has the advantage of allowing quite thin (e.g., 1 mm or less) contiguous sections with good S/N ratio, because acquisition of multiple 3D partitions is comparable to using multiple excitations in terms of boosting the S/N ratio (S/N ratio $\alpha \sqrt{\text{3D partitions}}$).

Several variants of GRE sequences have been developed[9-11] (Table 10–2).

SPOILED GRADIENT ECHO

In spoiled GRE sequences such as FLASH or spoiled gradient recalled (SPGR), a spoiler gradient (i.e., a strong gradient that is either constant or stepped through a different value after each excitation) is ap-

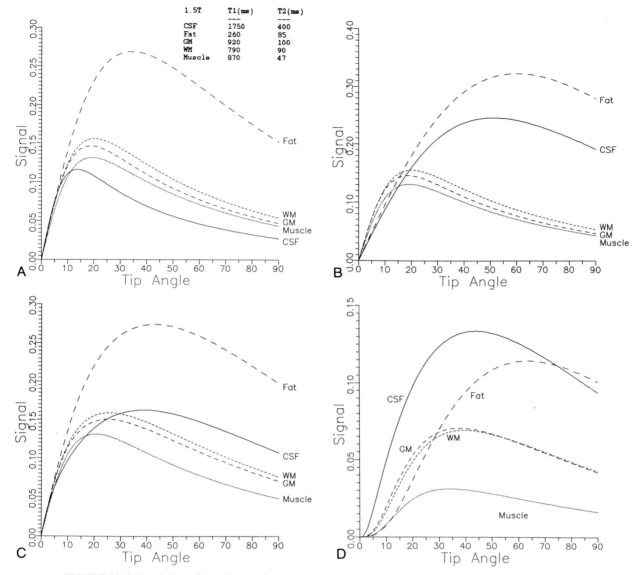

1.5T	T1(ms)	T2(ms)
CSF	1750	400
Fat	260	85
GM	920	100
WM	790	90
Muscle	870	47

FIGURE 10–6. Simulation of signal strengths from various tissues using different GRE methods. All calculations obtained with TR/TE = 50/12. Vertical axis represents signal strength as a fraction of maximal signal intensity (unweighted image). *A,* Spoiled GRE. T1 contrast is highest with large flip angles. However, signal is maximal at smaller flip angles (Ernst angle), here shown to be approximately 15° to 30°. Note that signal curve in region of Ernst angle is relatively flat, suggesting that there is considerable leeway in the choice of flip angles. *B,* Steady-state coherent GRE obtained with phase alternation of RF pulses. Note marked enhancement of CSF because of its small T1/T2 ratio. *C,* Contrast-enhanced steady-state GRE sequence, first echo. Contrast is similar to that in *B. D,* Contrast-enhanced steady-state GRE sequence (CE-FAST, PSIF). Note the increased T2 contrast compared with *A* and *B.*

plied at the end of the readout. The spoiler gradient disperses any residual transverse magnetization that remains after the signal has been read and the analog-to-digital converter is turned off.[12] If a spoiler is not applied, buildup of transverse coherences over multiple RF excitations leads to horizontal striping in the image, particularly if short TR and large flip angles are used[13] (see Chapter 3). Spoiling is most effective if, in addition to the use of a spoiler gradient, the residual magnetization is dispersed by randomizing the phases of the RF pulses, a method called *RF spoiling.* Contrast for spoiled GRE sequences is summarized in

Figure 10–8. In a spoiled GRE sequence, the transverse magnetization decays in much the same fashion as in an SE sequence. The signal intensity in spoiled GRE images is given by

$$S = S_0[(1 - E_1) \sin \alpha / (1 - E_1 \cos \alpha)]E_2^*$$

where $E_1 = \exp(-TR/T1)$, $E_2^* = \exp(-TE/T2^*)$, and α is the flip angle. S_0 is the maximal obtainable signal, that is, using a long TR, a short TE, and a 90° flip angle. The third term, E_2^*, contributes the T2* weighting. The T2* weighting is somewhat different from the T2 weighting in an SE because, as denoted

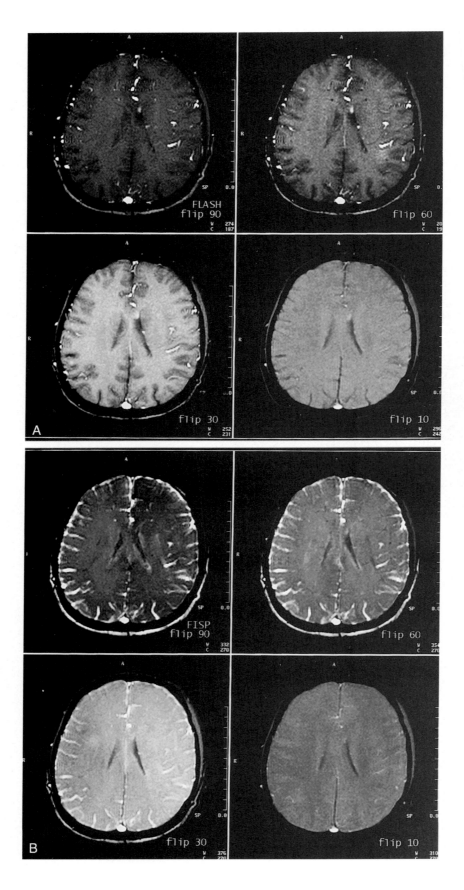

FIGURE 10–7. Axial brain images showing comparisons of spoiled GRE and steady-state GRE sequences. *A*, Spoiled GRE (FLASH). TR was 15 ms and the flip angle varied from 90° *(upper left)* to 10° *(lower right)*. *B*, Steady-state coherent GRE (FISP). TR was 15 ms and the flip angle varied from 90° *(upper left)* to 10° *(lower right)*. T1 contrast is inferior to that in *A* and the CSF signal intensity over the cerebral convexities is high. Note that the lateral ventricles do not appear bright because CSF pulsation destroys the steady-state signal.

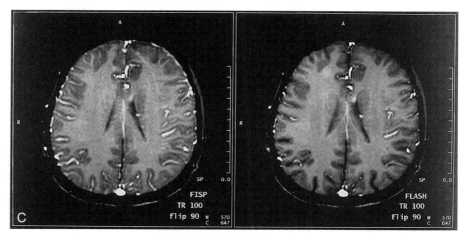

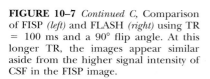

FIGURE 10–7 *Continued C,* Comparison of FISP *(left)* and FLASH *(right)* using TR = 100 ms and a 90° flip angle. At this longer TR, the images appear similar aside from the higher signal intensity of CSF in the FISP image.

by the asterisk, magnetic field inhomogeneity contributes to the loss of signal. The rate of signal loss is given by

$$1/T2* = 1/T2 + \gamma\pi\Delta B_0$$

where ΔB_0 is the magnetic field variation across a pixel and γ is the gyromagnetic ratio for hydrogen (approximately 42 MHz/T). Because artifacts resulting from magnetic field inhomogeneity worsen with long TE, strong T2* weighting is problematic with spoiled GRE sequences. Susceptibility effects are minimized by the use of a short TE, high readout bandwidth, and thin slice.[14] Although susceptibility artifacts are often the cause of low signal intensity in GRE images, other causes must be considered as well:

1. Hemorrhage: intracellular deoxyhemoglobin and methemoglobin in acute hemorrhage; hemosiderin and ferritin in chronic hemorrhage
2. Dense calcifications
3. Air
4. Disordered flow
5. Fat-water signal cancellation on out-of-phase images
6. Gadolinium during first pass through brain or on delayed image as a result of hyperconcentration in the renal collecting system (Fig. 10–9)

STEADY-STATE COHERENT GRADIENT ECHO

Rather than discard the transverse magnetization that persists after readout, *steady-state coherent* (SSC) GRE sequences recycle this magnetization to increase the signal intensity of certain tissues.[15, 16] One example of an SSC GRE sequence is fast imaging with steady-state precession (FISP),[17] or gradient-recalled acquisition in the steady state (GRASS). This sequence is similar to a spoiled GRE sequence except that there is no spoiler gradient; instead, an extra phase-encoding gradient, of opposite sign to the regular phase-encoding gradient, is appended after the readout gradient. The purpose of this extra gradient is to eliminate spoiling by the phase-encoding gradient of the transverse component of the steady-state magnetization. The difference in contrast behavior between spoiled and SSC GRE is manifested only at short TR, when TR is less than T2, and with large flip angle excitations (Fig. 10–10). When TR is less than T2, the transverse magnetization persists long enough after the readout that a portion of it can be tipped back onto the longitudinal axis by the next RF excitation; it adds to the magnetization recovered by T1 relaxation over the TR interval. Subsequent RF pulses then tip this enhanced magnetization back into the transverse plane, so that the signal intensity is greater than that produced by spoiled GRE sequences. Some tissues (particularly fluids) appear bright in SSC GRE images, but the images are not T2 weighted in the usual sense of T2-weighted SE images. The contrast depends on the ratio of T2 and T1; only tissues with a small T1/T2 ratio show high signal intensity. With longer TR (e.g., >100 ms), spoiled and SSC GRE sequences produce images that are more or less identical. Moreover, motion destroys the residual transverse magnetization so that moving fluids do not appear uniformly bright in SSC GRE images.[18] From a practical standpoint, it usually matters

TABLE 10–2. TYPES OF GRADIENT-ECHO SEQUENCES*

SEQUENCE TYPE	ACRONYMS	M_z COMPONENT	M_{xy} COMPONENT	CONTRAST DEPENDENCE
Spoiled GRE	FLASH, SPGR	Yes	No	T1, proton density, T2*
Steady-state coherent GRE	FISP, GRASS	Yes	Yes	T2*, T1/T2
Contrast-enhanced GRE	CE-FAST, PSIF	No	Yes	T2, T2*, T1/T2

*FISP = fast imaging with steady-state precession; GRASS = gradient-recalled acquisition in the steady-state; CE-FAST = contrast-enhanced Fourier-acquired steady-state technique; PSIF = time-reversed FISP.

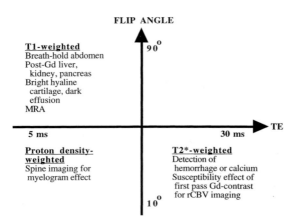

FLIP ANGLE

90°

T1-weighted
Breath-hold abdomen
Post-Gd liver,
  kidney, pancreas
Bright hyaline
  cartilage, dark
  effusion
MRA

5 ms   30 ms   TE

**Proton density-
weighted**
Spine imaging for
  myelogram effect

T2*-weighted
Detection of
  hemorrhage or calcium
Susceptibility effect of
  first pass Gd-contrast
  for rCBV imaging

10°

FIGURE 10–8. Effect of flip angle and TE on tissue contrast for spoiled GRE sequences. MRA = MR angiography; rCBV = regional cerebral blood volume.

little for clinical imaging whether one chooses a spoiled or SSC GRE sequence, as long as TR is much greater than T2.

A modification of FISP and GRASS called *true FISP* has a balanced structure that eliminates phase shifts caused by motion. Fluids such as cerebrospinal fluid (CSF) or blood appear bright with this sequence even when moving. MR angiographic images can be acquired with subsecond scan times with this sequence (Fig. 10–11). Using a 3D true FISP sequence, one can produce 3D MR myelograms that appear similar to conventional myelograms using intrathecal contrast.[19] A drawback of true FISP is that off-resonance effects (i.e., effects due to frequency shifts) produce dark stripes in the image, particularly in regions where the magnetic field is inhomogeneous. The striping can be reduced by the use of short TR and TE (e.g., 5 and 2 ms). Power deposition can be quite high with the large excitation flip angles and ultrashort TR needed for optimal true FISP imaging. Alternatively, a maximal intensity projection of two true FISP acquisitions (one

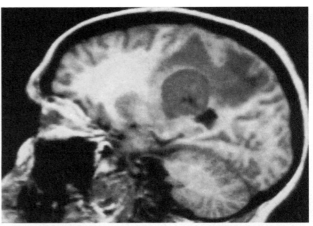

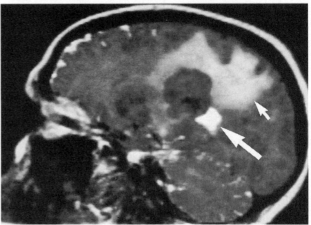

FIGURE 10–10. Spoiled GRE *(top)* and steady-state coherent GRE *(bottom)* images show divergent contrast behavior with short TR. Parasagittal images of a patient with a brain metastasis. TR/TE/FA = 30/14/90°. Note that the spoiled GRE image appears T1 weighted, but with same scan parameters the steady-state coherent GRE image shows marked enhancement of CSF *(large arrow)* and edema *(small arrow)* (small T1/T2 ratio).

with alternating RF phase, one with constant RF phase) is done to eliminate the striping.[19]

REACHING THE STEADY STATE

Depending on the imaging parameters, the application of multiple RF pulses leads to the establishment of a steady-state or equilibrium condition. With both spoiled and SSC GRE sequences using small flip angle excitations and short TR, many (typically dozens of) preparatory RF excitations must be applied before starting the acquisition of data for the spins to reach a steady-state magnetization; otherwise, there are initial fluctuations in the tissue magnetization that produce variations in the signal intensity and hence artifacts.[20] When spoiling is effective with short TR values, the approach to steady state is smooth for any RF excitation flip angle and involves only longitudinal magnetization components. Nonetheless, for SSC GRE sequences and repetition times much shorter than T2, the approach to equilibrium is rather complex and

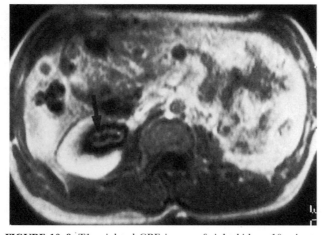

FIGURE 10–9. T1-weighted GRE image of right kidney 10 minutes after administration of gadolinium diethylenetriaminepentaacetic acid (Gd-DTPA) demonstrates loss of signal intensity in and around renal pelvis *(arrow)* as a result of susceptibility effects (T2* shortening) caused by concentrated paramagnetic agent.

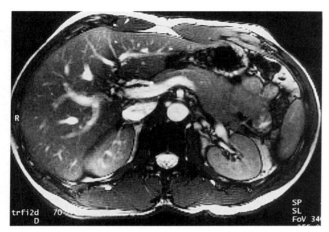

FIGURE 10–11. Axial true FISP image acquired with TR/TE/FA = 5/2.5/70°. Tissues with a small T1/T2 ratio, including CSF, blood, and fat, all appear bright. The blood vessels and CSF would not appear as bright with standard steady-state GRE sequences like FISP or GRASS because of motion effects.

involves a mixture of transverse and longitudinal magnetization components that regain coherence at every RF excitation, making the approach highly oscillatory with large flip angles (Fig. 10–12). This situation differs from SE imaging, in which the steady state is essentially reached after the first 90° excitation. Imaging during the transient behavior before the establishment of an equilibrium condition has been exploited extensively with many ultrafast GRE techniques to improve S/N ratio and to obtain different tissue contrasts with short imaging times.[21]

CONTRAST-ENHANCED STEADY-STATE GRADIENT ECHO

The time-reversed FISP (PSIF), or contrast-enhanced Fourier-acquired steady-state technique (CE-FAST), sequence has a structure that is reversed from a standard SSC GRE sequence.[22, 23] The result is that a heavily T2-weighted RF echo, rather than a GRE, is generated. The degree of T2 weighting is exponentially dependent on twice the TR; thus, the effective TE is actually longer than the TR. Contrast-enhanced steady-state GRE sequences render fluids and tumors bright but have the drawback of being sensitive to motion (Fig. 10–13). The technique has been used for MR cholangiography: the stationary bile in dilated bile ducts appears bright, whereas flowing blood appears dark because motion destroys the steady-state magnetization. It is also possible to generate two echoes with different degrees of T2 weighting in the same acquisition. The first echo has FISP-like contrast, the second is PSIF-like. These two echoes can be added together (double echo in the steady state [DESS]) to produce an image with a good S/N ratio but the high signal intensity of fluid, which may be helpful for the evaluation of hyaline cartilage in the knee when an effusion is present. Interest in T2-weighted GRE sequences has waned considerably with the advent of fast SE imaging, because more reliable T2 weighting and less motion sensitivity are found with the latter method.

SLICE PROFILE EFFECTS IN GRADIENT-ECHO IMAGING

With short TR values as used in GRE imaging, the slice profile may be different from that obtained with longer TR. The problem is compounded by the fact that short RF pulses are often used for GRE imaging to minimize TE. These RF pulses have poor slice profiles compared with longer pulses, so that the flip angle varies across the slice thickness. The degradation in the slice profile is most severe when the TR is short and the flip angle is large. Near the center of the slice, the flip angle is correct, but the edges of the slice experience smaller flip angles. Using a spoiled GRE sequence, one finds that the portions of the slice that experience large flip angles show T1 contrast, whereas portions that experience smaller flip angles show proton density contrast. The combination of these signals results in overall reduced tissue contrast. A dynamic transformation of the slice profile also occurs for ultrafast GRE acquiring data during the approach to steady state.[24] As just noted, distortions in the slice profile are worst with short TR values and high flip angles. In the center of the profile, tissues saturate faster than in the outer portions of the profile, shifting the maximal signal received on early excitations from tissues in the center of the profile to tissues at the edges of the profile. The tissues at the edge of the slice have higher signal intensity because they are closer to the steady-state condition and the Ernst flip angle (optimal signal for spoiled GRE). This effect is more complicated in steady-state GRE than in spoiled GRE, because the transient to the steady state is oscillatory at larger flip angles.

CLINICAL USES OF GRADIENT-ECHO SEQUENCES

GRE sequences are used in several clinical applications. Some examples are given in the following subsections.

BRAIN

MR ANGIOGRAPHY. 2D and 3D GRE sequences are essential for time-of-flight MR angiography (see Chapter 9). With short TR, the signal intensities of stationary tissues are suppressed. Inflowing blood appears bright, a phenomenon known as flow-related enhancement. This effect is improved by the use of *flow compensation*.[25, 26] With flow compensation, an extra gradient pulse is incorporated in the sequence to eliminate phase shifts caused by motion. Bright blood GRE images allow the differentiation of blood flow from calcium or old blood. Sequential 2D or 3D GRE images can be processed by a maximal intensity projection

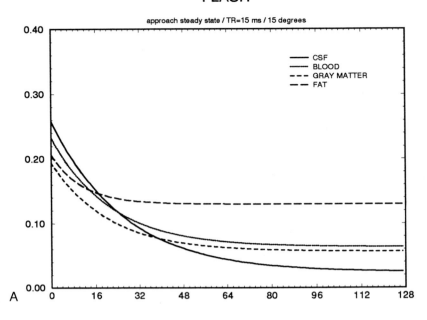

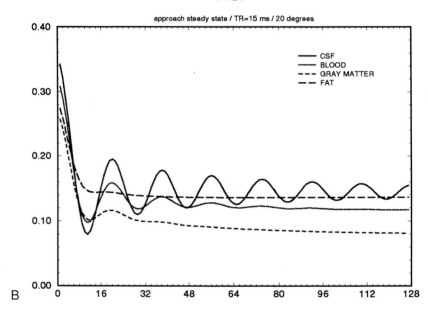

FIGURE 10–12. Approach to the steady state for spoiled and steady-state coherent GRE sequences. Calculated signal intensity as a function of excitation number for TR/FA = 15/20°. *A,* Spoiled GRE sequence. Note the smooth approach to the steady state. *B,* Steady-state coherent GRE sequence. Note the marked oscillation in signal intensity as a function of excitation number, particularly for long-T2 tissues such as blood and CSF.

algorithm, which displays the brightest pixels along a user-selected orientation. The resultant projection images show blood vessels much like a digital subtraction angiogram.

MULTIPLANAR RECONSTRUCTION. 3D GRE and its variant, 3D magnetization-prepared rapid gradient echo (MP-RAGE), permit whole-brain screening with high-quality reformatting in arbitrary plane orientations (Fig. 10–14).

SUSCEPTIBILITY CONTRAST. Because GRE sequences lack a 180° pulse, they are sensitive to mag-

netic field distortions (*susceptibility* effects) caused by the presence of iron or air–soft tissue or bone–soft tissue interfaces. This results in image degradation (signal loss and geometric distortion) around the paranasal sinuses, bowel, or ferromagnetic implants. It is also the source of "zebra stripe" artifacts, particularly seen on coronal GRE images (Fig. 10–15). Zebra stripe artifacts are produced by severe spatially dependent phase variations caused by magnetic field inhomogeneity near the sides of the magnet. On the other hand, GRE sequences permit more sensitive detection than

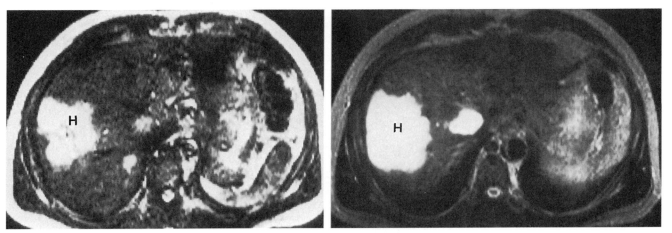

FIGURE 10–13. Patient with three cavernous hemangiomas (H) in the liver. PSIF image *(left)* obtained with TR = 30 ms in less than 10 seconds provides similar contrast to that obtained in 10 minutes using a T2-weighted SE image *(right,* slightly different slice position). However, sensitivity to motion (e.g., from pulsatile flow, cardiac pulsations transmitted to left lobe of liver) is much worse with PSIF.

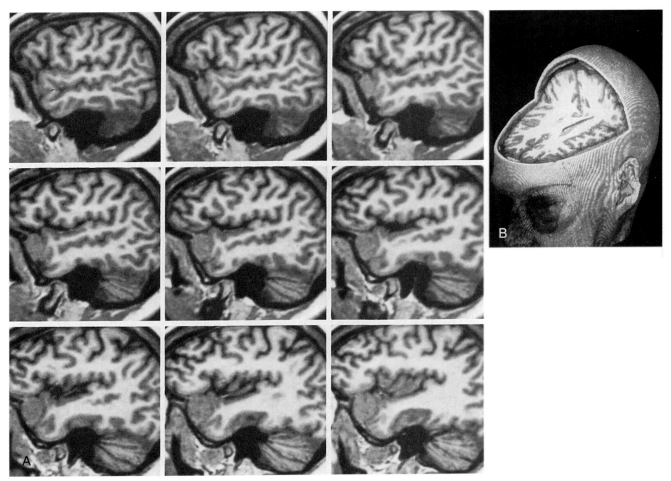

FIGURE 10–14. 3D spoiled GRE acquisitions permit thin, contiguous slices to be obtained in a reasonable amount of time. *A,* Patient with meningioma: 9 of 126 contiguous images acquired in 20 minutes using 3D spoiled GRE (40/15/40°) with a slice thickness of 1.5 mm, FOV = 28 cm. (Courtesy of P. Ruggieri, MD, The Cleveland Clinic Foundation, Cleveland, OH.) *B,* Segmentation (separation of different tissue types) of 3D images is possible if tissue contrast is adequate. A surface-rendered image of the scalp and brain has been created from a 3D MP-RAGE acquisition with a section of brain removed to depict the internal brain structures. Such displays can be particularly helpful to the neurosurgeon in planning approaches for tumor resection.

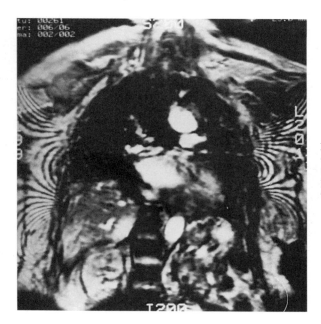

FIGURE 10–15. Coronal GRE image obtained with TR/TE = 21/12 and a 40-cm FOV. Note the zebra-striped patterns of signal loss at the periphery of the FOV caused by the arms and shoulders lying in an inhomogeneous portion of the static magnetic field. This artifact would not usually be encountered in an SE image or in a sagittal or axial GRE image.

SE sequences of hemorrhagic brain lesions such as occult vascular malformations or those that occur in shear injuries or amyloid (Fig. 10–16). They are useful as well for evaluation of brain perfusion (see Chapter 8). Rapid administration of a bolus of a gadolinium chelate causes an alteration in the magnetic susceptibility of intracerebral blood vessels and nearby tissues, thereby causing a drop in tissue signal intensity as a function of regional blood volume. The sensitivity to this effect increases as the TE is lengthened.

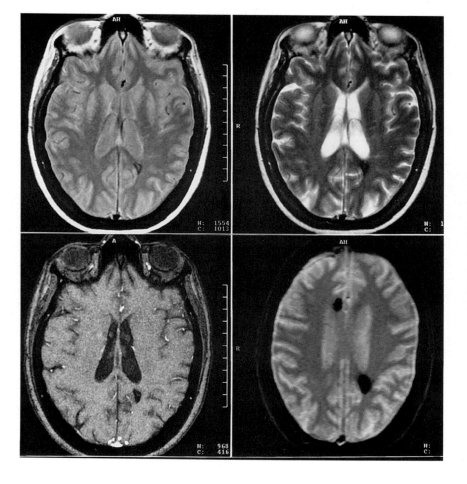

FIGURE 10–16. Comparison of sequences for sensitivity to hemorrhage. Patient with presumed amyloid angiopathy. *Upper left,* Proton density–weighted fast SE, 5-mm slice thickness, TR/TE = 4500/22; *upper right,* T2-weighted fast SE, 5-mm slice thickness, TR/TE = 4500/85; *lower left,* 3D GRE with 0.8-mm slice thickness, TE = 10 ms; *lower right,* 2D GRE with 5-mm slice thickness, TE = 28 ms. The GRE sequences are most sensitive to hemorrhage, with 2D more sensitive than 3D because of the longer TE and thicker slice.

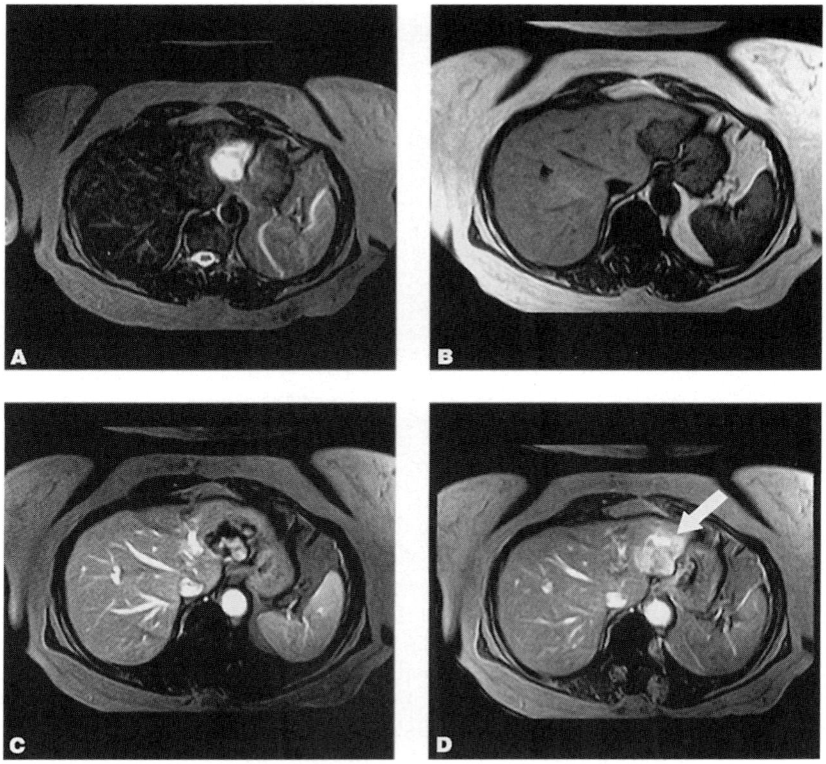

FIGURE 10–17. Cavernous hemangioma of left lobe of liver. *A,* Axial 13-minute, T2-weighted SE study of the liver. *B,* Breath-hold T1-weighted spoiled GRE image (TR/TE/FA = 122/6/80°) acquired in 16 seconds. *C,* Same immediately after bolus infusion of 0.1 mmol/kg Gd-DTPA shows typical nodular and blotchy rim enhancement. *D,* Same 10 minutes delayed shows filling in of the lesion *(arrow).*

ABDOMEN

EVALUATION OF LIVER MASSES. Multisection T1-weighted GRE images can be acquired within a breath-hold, thereby eliminating respiratory artifacts. The TR must be reasonably short for breath-holding; a single-acquisition study with a 128 × 256 matrix and a TR of 110 ms takes 14 seconds. Multiple slices can be acquired, the exact number depending on pulse sequence design. With much shorter TR, T1 contrast in GRE images may be deficient for standard clinical work but is adequate for dynamic contrast-enhanced studies to characterize cavernous hemangiomas and other hepatic masses[27] (Fig. 10–17).

Unlike the situation with SE sequences, with GRE sequences the choice of TE is critical. A short TE is desirable to minimize image distortions caused by air-containing bowel loops. A longer TE may be helpful for detecting iron-containing regenerating nodules in a cirrhotic liver. However, a complicating factor is that fat-water phase-contrast effects occur with GRE, but not SE, sequences (see Chapter 1). Depending on the field strength and TE, fat and water signals arising from the same voxel can either add or subtract.[28] At 1.5 T, an oscillation in the signal intensity of a fat-water mixture occurs approximately every 2.3 ms; for instance, a TE of 2.3 ms gives an *opposed-phase* image with signal cancellation in tissues containing fat-water mixtures such as fatty liver or red bone marrow, but a TE of 4.6 ms gives an *in-phase* image in which fat and water signals add. A TE-dependent oscillation in signal intensities also occurs to a minor degree in subcutaneous and deep fat because of the presence of fatty acid

and triglyceride components having different proton chemical shifts but to a much lesser degree than in fatty liver.

Opposed-phase images permit detection of fatty infiltration (which appears dark) within the liver. They also permit accurate characterization of adrenal adenomas, which contain fat, unlike most metastases.[29] However, when searching for liver masses one should choose an in-phase TE for T1-weighted images, because fatty infiltration would reduce the parenchymal signal and therefore contrast with metastases in an opposed image. With opposed images, care must also be taken not to misinterpret the artifactual dark line that occurs at fat-water interfaces surrounding viscera.

SPINE

MR MYELOGRAM. Because of its elevated proton density, CSF appears brighter than disk material and the spinal cord on proton density–weighted GRE images. This creates a myelogram-like effect that is particularly helpful for sagittal and axial imaging of the cervical spine. T1-weighted GRE images are helpful for showing the cord-CSF interface and nerve roots (Fig. 10–18). Fast SE sequences have largely replaced GRE for sagittal spine imaging because of better T2 contrast for cord lesions, but we still prefer GRE sequences for axial myelographic images because there are fewer artifacts from CSF pulsation.

MUSCULOSKELETAL SYSTEM

Hyaline cartilage appears bright on T1-weighted GRE images acquired with long TR (e.g., TR/TE/FA

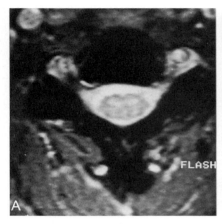
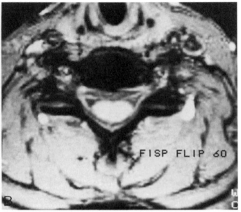

FIGURE 10–18. Comparison of T1-weighted and proton density–weighted axial GRE images of the cervical spine. *A,* Proton density–weighted GRE image (300/18/15°) demonstrates excellent gray-white matter differentiation and the neural foramina. *B,* T1-weighted GRE image (300/18/60°) demonstrates dorsal and ventral nerve rootlets entering the neural foramina.

= 300/10/80°), whereas effusions appear dark (Fig. 10–19). Alternatively, steady-state GRE sequences with large flip angles render effusions bright. Either technique can be helpful for detection of cartilage defects. GRE images are highly sensitive to degeneration of the fibrocartilages of the knee and shoulder (menisci and glenoid labrum). In fact, this sensitivity can be excessive, making it difficult to distinguish a torn from a degenerated meniscus (Fig. 10–20). Fast 2D GRE sequences permit kinematic imaging of joints. 3D GRE sequences routinely permit the acquisition of submillimeter slices, which may increase sensitivity for cartilage defects (Fig. 10–21).

HEART

Data acquisition can be synchronized to a constant phase of the cardiac cycle by using electrocardio-graphic or peripheral pulse gating. More commonly, GRE sequences are used for cine imaging of the heart, which involves acquiring data over multiple phases of the cardiac cycle (see Chapters 54 and 55). With cine GRE imaging, the signal intensities of myocardium and stationary tissues are suppressed by the short TR (e.g., 30 ms), but fresh blood flowing into the plane of section appears bright.[30] Cine GRE imaging is used to evaluate functional parameters such as ejection fraction and wall motion. In conjunction with phase-contrast imaging, cine permits flow quantification over the cardiac cycle.[31]

K-SPACE

A useful concept for understanding the differences among fast imaging sequences is k-space.[32] The raw data (i.e., the data as collected before the 2D Fourier transform) can be depicted as a 2D matrix of spatial frequencies (k_x, k_y) (Fig. 10–22). In generic form, k = $\gamma \int G(t)\, dt$, where γ is the gyromagnetic ratio and G(t) is the time-dependent gradient amplitude. Various parts of k-space influence the appearance of the image in different ways. Because magnetic field gradients cause dephasing, the MR signal is strongest when the weakest phase-encoding gradients are applied. The center of k-space consists of data acquired during the weakest phase-encoding gradients. Because the signals are so large in this part of k-space, these data control image contrast. The weaker signals in the outer part of k-space (strongest phase-encoding gradients) contain the high spatial frequencies that determine image detail (Fig. 10–23). The manner in which the various spatial frequencies are collected determines the k-space *trajectory.* The MR data are collected to encode both low and high spatial frequencies (i.e., the image should have good tissue contrast as well as high spatial resolution). Independent of the acquisition matrix size selected, the relative speed at which k-space is covered determines the time savings possible with a particular MRI technique.

The k-space trajectory for any pulse sequence must span all the (k_x, k_y) points to generate a complete image. For instance, with standard GRE or SE se-

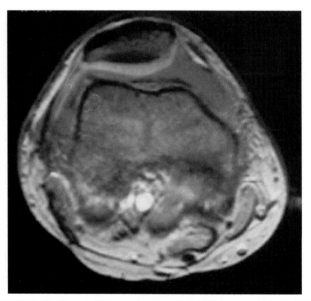

FIGURE 10–19. Axial T1-weighted spoiled GRE image (300/10/80°) of a patient with a knee effusion. The effusion, which appears dark, contrasts well with the moderate signal intensity of the hyaline articular cartilage of the patella.

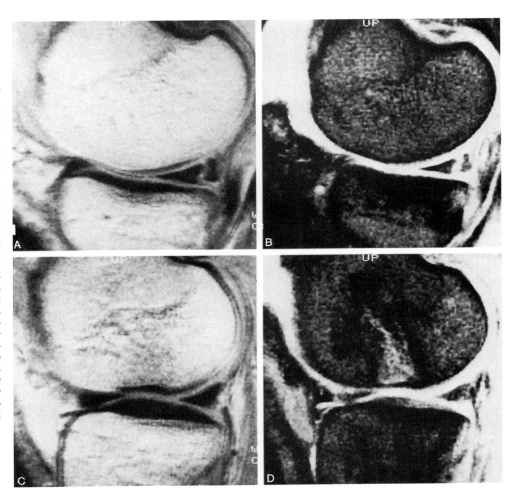

FIGURE 10–20. Comparison of SE (TR/TE = 1200/16) and GRE (600/18/15°) images of patient with torn posterior horn of medial meniscus and osteochondral fracture. *A*, SE image shows meniscal tear and articular cartilage as moderate signal intensity. *B*, GRE image shows meniscal tear and articular cartilage as high intensity. Excessive sensitivity of GRE sequences to meniscal degeneration can make it difficult to distinguish degeneration from tear. Note decreased signal intensity of bone marrow relative to SE image, in part related to phase-contrast effects between fat and water signals and in part to T2* dephasing caused by the inhomogeneous honeycomb structure of cancellous bone. *C*, SE image poorly demonstrates subchondral fracture. *D*, On the GRE image the subchondral fracture appears bright because of bone marrow edema and is better seen. Marrow edema would be even better detected by inversion recovery fast SE.

quences, one phase-encoding step is applied and one line of data is collected (i.e., all k_x points for one value of k_y) after each RF excitation. The k-space trajectory thus consists of a series of horizontal lines as shown in Figure 10–24. This is repeated as many times as necessary to complete the full raw data. All frequency samples in k-space are acquired in each readout period, corresponding to one pulse of the readout gradient. On the other extreme, advanced sequences using the EPI encoding, for example, use a strong bipolar oscillating gradient field to generate a train of GREs that are phase encoded independently after the application of a single RF excitation, thus collecting the full k-space matrix in a single shot.

FASTER SPIN-ECHO IMAGING: HALF-FOURIER, REDUCED FLIP ANGLE, AND FAST SPIN ECHO

HALF-FOURIER

Normally, the phase-encoding gradient is gradually increased from a large negative amplitude, to zero, to a large positive amplitude (or vice versa) over the course of an acquisition. In the *half-Fourier* method, only the positive phase-encoding steps are acquired, along with the zero step and a few negative ones.[33–35] A mirror image copy of the positive data is created, and a complete image is reconstructed from the acquired and synthetic data (Fig. 10–25). As only a little more than half the data is acquired, scan time is reduced nearly twofold. In practice, half-Fourier techniques reduce scan time by slightly less than 50%, because the mirror image symmetry of the data is only true for a hypothetic "ideal" acquisition. The actual MR data have phase offsets that distort the symmetry of the matrix. Most half-Fourier techniques require the acquisition of some extra negative phase-encoding steps to calculate phase corrections for the data (Fig. 10–26).

The first step in the process of half-Fourier image reconstruction is to reflect the positive data to generate an entire raw data matrix. The data are then phase corrected based on a low-resolution phase shift map generated from the positive and extra negative projections. Finally, the data are processed using ordinary Fourier reconstruction algorithms to produce an image.

There are several drawbacks to the half-Fourier method. The extra steps required for image processing significantly increase image reconstruction time. Other drawbacks include a 41% reduction in S/N ratio, which may or may not be acceptable depending on

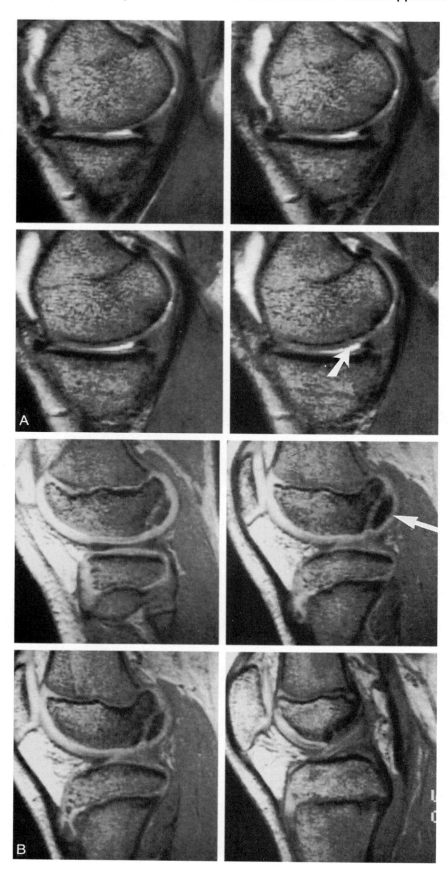

FIGURE 10–21. Examples of contiguous 1.7-mm knee images from 3D GRE acquisitions for two different patients (TR/TE/FA = 30/14/40°). Imaging time less than 10 minutes for 64 slices. *A,* Truncated posterior horn of medial meniscus *(arrow). B,* Osteochondral fragment *(arrow).* Note high signal intensity of hyaline cartilage. (*A* and *B* courtesy of R. Tyrell, MD, University Hospitals of Cleveland, Cleveland, OH.)

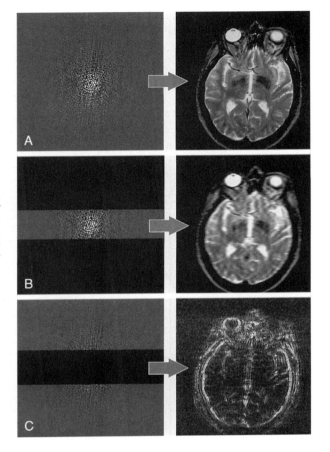

FIGURE 10–22. Raw data. *A,* The amount and manner in which data are acquired can dramatically alter the appearance of the MR image. The raw data *(left)* are converted into an image *(right)* by the Fourier transform. *B,* With removal of the outer lines of the raw data (high spatial frequencies), details are lost but contrast is preserved. *C,* With removal of the central lines of the data (low spatial frequencies), image contrast is lost, leaving a ghostly image showing tissue boundaries only.

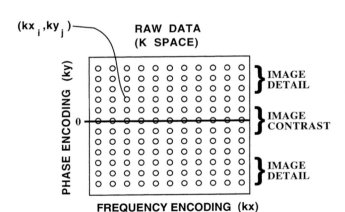

FIGURE 10–23. Illustration of raw data (k-space) showing the relationship of the central lines (weakest phase-encoding gradient amplitudes and strongest signal) to image contrast and of the outer lines to image detail. For a complete image, all (k_x, k_y) points must be covered by the acquisition.

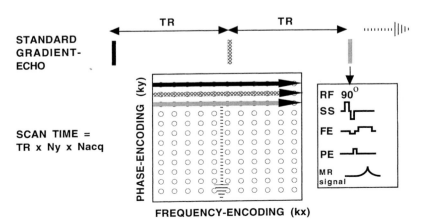

FIGURE 10–24. The k-space trajectory for standard GRE sequence. Data are acquired one line at a time for each TR interval.

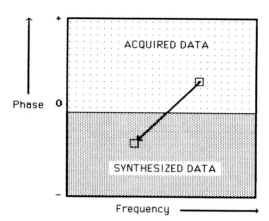

FIGURE 10–25. The k-space representation of conjugate synthesis in half-Fourier imaging. Compared with a conventional image, only slightly more than half of the data are acquired. The rest are synthesized from the acquired data, reducing imaging time almost by a factor of 2.

the application, increased sensitivity to motion artifacts, and image distortions caused by RF or magnetic field inhomogeneities. Half-Fourier works less well with GRE than SE sequences because of the greater sensitivity of GRE sequences to magnetic field inhomogeneities, but it can be used if the TE is sufficiently short. More robust half-Fourier methods that are less sensitive to rapid local phase changes have been developed, using an iterative approach to reconstruct the missing portion of k-space.[36] The steps involved in the calculation require the acquisition of a sufficient number of extra points before the echo to permit the calculation of a low-frequency phase map. The phase map is then applied to the magnitude reconstruction of a Hanning filtered version of the truncated data set, and the resulting image is transformed back to obtain the "synthetic" raw data. The composite raw data, formed by combining the synthetic data and the originally measured data, are transformed back again to obtain an improved magnitude reconstruction that is multiplied once again by the low-frequency phase estimate originally calculated. This loop is repeated until convergence is achieved, but generally three iterations in the loop are sufficient to obtain the desired image. The S/N ratio is generally better for the iterative approach because the contribution to the signal from the extra points sampled before the echo is not eliminated as in the conjugate synthesis methods. Half-Fourier reconstructions can also be applied along the frequency-encoding direction in conjunction with asymmetric sampling of the echo. Asymmetric sampling allows a reduced readout period and thus a shorter TE, at the expense of increased blurring. By synthesizing the missing portion of the data, half-Fourier eliminates this blurring. Further reductions in imaging time may be possible using constrained reconstruction techniques.[37, 38] These techniques can be applied perpendicularly to the axis on which half-Fourier was first applied. However, the slowness of these methods makes them impractical for general use.

REDUCED FLIP ANGLE SPIN ECHO

A second approach to reducing scan time with SE sequences is to decrease the excitation flip angle from 90°, a method known as the fast low-angle multiecho (FLAME) technique.[39, 40] As with low-flip-angle GRE sequences, the reduced flip angle decreases saturation effects with short TR. For this approach to work, an even number of 180° RF pulses (e.g., two) must be used. The reduced flip angle excitation tilts the longitudinal magnetization partway into the transverse plane, so there are a transverse component and a longitudinal component (along the +z direction). The first 180° pulse refocuses the transverse component of the magnetization as an SE, which is read out. This 180° pulse also flips the longitudinal component of the magnetization into the −z direction. The second 180° pulse flips the longitudinal magnetization back along the +z direction (Fig. 10–27). Using the FLAME technique, an SE sequence with a TR of 1500 ms and a flip angle of 60° might generate T2 contrast similar to that obtained with a TR of 2500 ms and a 90° flip angle. The advantage of the shorter TR is a reduced scan time; the drawback is a decreased multislice capability because of the shorter TR. Although of potential value, the FLAME technique has mostly been superseded by fast SE.

FAST SPIN ECHO

The most robust approach for speeding up SE imaging is to use the fast SE technique.[41, 42] Fast SE (also called turbo SE) is an optimized version of RARE.[43, 44] It is a multiecho SE sequence in which each SE signal is separately phase encoded, rather than being used to produce a separate image. Like SE, fast SE has the advantage over GRE that it uses 180° pulses to eliminate susceptibility artifacts. Heavily T2-weighted images can be acquired; this is not easily done with GRE. Thin-section T2-weighted 3D scans, not practical with conventional SE, can be acquired using fast SE in 10 minutes or less. Drawbacks of fast SE include increased RF deposition and magnetization transfer effects arising from the application of multiple 180° pulses, increased signal intensity of fat, and blurring artifacts particularly at short TE. Depending on the sequence implementation and choice of imaging parameters, some lesions may not be seen as well with fast SE as with conventional SE images. In spite of these limitations, fast SE has largely replaced conventional SE imaging for the brain, spine, and pelvis and will soon do so in the abdomen as well.

The scan time for a fast SE sequence is given by

$$\text{Scan time} = \text{TR} \times N_y \times \text{NEX/ETL}$$

The *echo train length* (ETL) or *turbo factor* is the number of echoes that are phase encoded after each 90° pulse. For instance, if eight echoes are acquired, the scan time is reduced by a factor of 8. The duration of the echo train can be called the *echo train time* (ETT). A large ETL provides the greatest reduction in scan time,

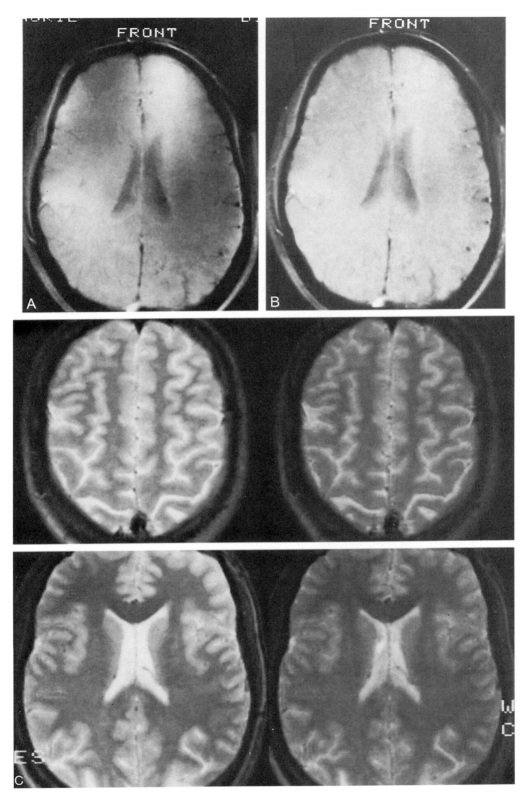

FIGURE 10–26. Half-Fourier GRE images acquired with 2 extra negative projections *(A)* and 16 extra projections *(B)*. Note signal inhomogeneity in *A*, caused by spurious phase shifts. This inhomogeneity is reduced by acquiring extra projections *(B)*. Successful use of half-Fourier for GRE sequences requires a short TE to minimize sensitivity to susceptibility-induced phase shifts. *C*, Comparison of standard SE images *(left)* and half-Fourier images *(right)* acquired in almost half the time (eight extra projections). TR/TE = 3500/60. Image contrast and resolution are identical. Despite lower S/N ratio of half-Fourier images, images have comparable diagnostic utility.

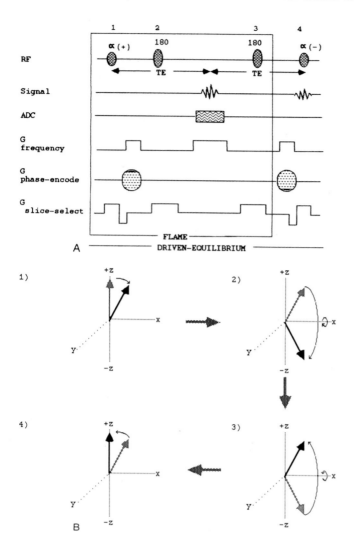

FIGURE 10–27. Driven-equilibrium methods use modified SE sequences that realign the magnetization along the magnetic field after signal readout. *A,* Pulse sequence diagram for driven equilibrium–type sequences. Sequences 1 through 3 correspond to methods of the FLAME type; sequences 1 through 4 correspond to classic DEFT (driven-equilibrium Fourier transform) method. In theory, these sequences exhibit behavior similar to that of reduced flip angle GRE methods, except that the effects of magnetic field inhomogeneities have been eliminated by the addition of an RF refocusing pulse. Driven-equilibrium methods produce maximal signal enhancement for tissues with a small T1/T2 ratio, such as CSF. *B,* Path of magnetization vector with these methods. 1) Reduced flip angle excitation tips part of longitudinal magnetization (+z direction) into transverse (x-y) plane. 2) First 180° RF pulse tips transverse magnetization around x axis to −z direction. 3) Second 180° RF tips magnetization back to +z direction. 4) Additional RF pulse, used in classic DEFT method, tips magnetization into alignment with main magnetic field.

but beyond a factor of 8 or so blurring artifacts may become objectionable for some tissues with current sequence implementations because of signal loss from T2 relaxation over the long ETT. It is possible to acquire as many as 128 echoes in less than 1 second. In conjunction with half-Fourier, one can use this technique (called HASTE [half-Fourier single-shot turbo spin echo]) for subsecond imaging. HASTE images

provide good depiction of fluids, but other tissues with shorter T2 values tend to show some blurring artifacts.

EFFECTIVE ECHO TIME

As mentioned earlier, image contrast depends on the characteristics of the MR signals acquired with the central phase-encoding lines. The central lines are selected simply by setting the amplitude of the phase-encoding gradient to low values; this can be done for any of the echoes in the fast SE echo train, although the order must be appropriate to avoid artifacts. The timing of the central phase-encoding lines determines the *effective TE*. If the central lines are timed to occur late, allowing T2 decay of the echo, the image appears T2 weighted; if it is timed to occur early, the image appears proton density weighted (or T1 weighted if the TR is short). One can split the echo train, for instance, to acquire proton density– and T2-weighted images simultaneously. Then four echoes are used for each image, and the ETL and scan time reduction is only a factor of 4. To save scan time, an echo-sharing technique can be used.[45] Two images with different effective TE values are acquired using the same high-frequency data. The central (low-frequency) lines are acquired twice at different TE values, as part of the same echo train.

PHASE-ENCODING ORDER

Because the MR signal strength decreases with each successive echo as a result of T2 decay, the image appearance is dramatically altered with changes in the phase-encoding order. The T2-modulated time-dependent decrease in signal intensity acts as a filter of high spatial frequencies, causing blurring. Phase-encoding order is a critical determinant of image quality with fast SE sequences.[46–48] The phase-encoding order must be such that abrupt discontinuities in the signal intensity from line to line as well as gradient-induced eddy current effects are minimized. Discontinuities can cause blurring and ghost artifacts. Although fast SE imaging can be done on systems without active gradient shielding, our experience has been that results are better with active shielding because of reduced eddy currents. Reordered phase encoding is an essential ingredient for optimizing tissue contrast and eliminating artifacts not only for fast SE but also for turboFLASH, EPI, and still newer approaches such as spiral scanning.

The amount of blurring with fast SE imaging depends on the T2 of the tissue, because signal loss occurs over the ETT as a result of T2 relaxation. For instance, T2 decay over the ETT is worse for white matter than for CSF. Thus, one could use a much longer echo train (e.g., 64 to 128 echoes) in conjunction with a single-shot fast SE acquisition if a fluid is the tissue of interest (e.g., MR myelography, MR cholangiography) than for imaging of white matter lesions (e.g., 4 to 16 echoes). Paradoxically, in addition

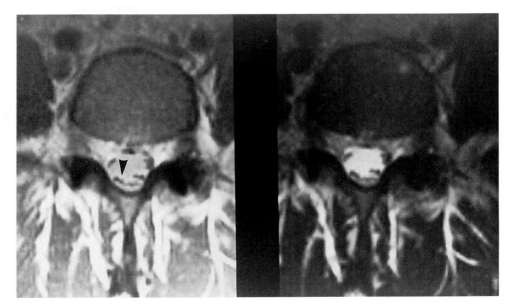

FIGURE 10–28. Edge enhancement on fast SE images. *Left,* Axial proton density–weighted fast SE image (4500/22) shows artifactual bright line *(arrowhead)* around the dark nerve roots. *Right,* Artifact is less obvious on T2-weighted fast SE image (4500/85). The edge enhancement effect improves the conspicuity of the nerve roots.

to blurring, there can be an edge enhancement effect that in some circumstances improves depiction of normal anatomy or lesion detection.[49] For instance, blurring is minimal for CSF because of its long T2. On the other hand, nerve roots are blurred because of their shorter T2. The net effect is that the interface between nerve root and CSF is enhanced, thereby increasing the conspicuity of the root, while there is artifactually low signal intensity within the root (Fig. 10–28). Another consideration is motion artifact. The blurring caused by long echo trains may in some cases be more than compensated by the reduction in motional blurring resulting from the shorter scan time with fast SE. Interecho spacing is also important. The ETT is minimized by keeping the time between echoes to a minimum, thereby reducing signal modulation resulting from T2 decay. Thus, for a given ETL, blurring is less for a short interecho spacing than for a long one; alternatively, for a given duration of the echo train, the ETL can be longer.[50] The drawbacks of short interecho spacing are a reduced S/N ratio because the readout bandwidth must be increased (assuming that gradient ramp times are already minimized), brighter fat signal, lower conspicuity of hemorrhagic lesions, and higher power deposition if the RF pulse duration is shortened.

THREE-DIMENSIONAL FAST SPIN ECHO

Although 3D imaging with conventional SE sequences is impractical because of the long scan times, 3D fast SE is feasible with scan times less than 10 minutes.[51] The sequence is similar to 2D fast SE but incorporates an extra phase-encoding step in the slice-select direction. Multiple 3D volumes spanning the region of interest are acquired within each TR interval. The volumes must be slightly overlapped because of the nonrectangular slab profile of each 3D volume. Compared with 2D fast SE imaging, thinner sections

can be obtained and multiplanar reformations can be done.

MAGNETIZATION TRANSFER EFFECTS

A slice-selective RF pulse excites protons over a range of hundreds to thousands of hertz. Although the frequency of the pulse is selected to be on-resonance (at the Larmor frequency) for the particular slice being excited, it is off-resonance for the other slices of a multislice acquisition. The result is that each slice in a multislice volume experiences some degree of magnetization transfer effect from the RF excitations of each of the other slices, particularly from the 180° pulses, which deposit more power than the 90° pulses[52] (see Chapter 1). Magnetization transfer effects, which are relatively minor with conventional multislice SE sequences, become much more significant with fast SE sequences because of the larger number of 180° pulses.[53] The result is a change in tissue contrast that may or may not be desirable. Magnetization transfer effects are more pronounced with long ETLs and in tissues that contain both mobile and restricted pools of protons. Thus, the signal intensity of brain, liver, or muscle is reduced by magnetization transfer effects, but the signal intensity of tissues that contain only a small pool of restricted protons, such as CSF, blood, or cavernous hemangiomas,[54] is affected less. The net result is that CSF appears brighter than expected compared with brain, and a hemangioma appears relatively enhanced compared with liver parenchyma.

STIMULATED ECHOES

Any combination of three RF pulses has the potential to generate a stimulated echo. With all the RF pulses applied in a fast SE sequence, stimulated echoes are unavoidable. In fact, the stimulated echoes are deliberately added to the SE signals to increase signal intensity, although some alteration in tissue contrast occurs as a result.[55]

To control stimulated-echo artifacts and reduce power deposition, it is helpful to reduce the flip angle of the fast SE refocusing pulses from 180° to about 130° to 150°. Despite the lower flip angle, image quality and tissue contrast are as good or better than with a 180° refocusing pulse and power deposition is reduced.

FLOW EFFECTS WITH FAST SPIN ECHO

Outflow of blood from the slice during the interval TE/2 between the 90° and 180° RF pulses (washout) tends to make flowing blood appear dark in conventional SE images. Washout effects are still greater with fast SE sequences, which use longer echo trains than conventional SE. Thus, fast SE imaging could be a useful way to create "dark blood" angiograms.

APPEARANCE OF HEMORRHAGE ON FAST SPIN-ECHO IMAGES

Intracellular deoxyhemoglobin and methemoglobin are largely responsible for the signal loss in acute hemorrhage seen on T2-weighted SE images.[56] Iron storage products (ferritin and hemosiderin) cause the signal loss in chronic bleeding. The paramagnetic iron in hemorrhage causes local magnetic field distortions[57] (see Chapters 7 and 21). Although static field effects are canceled by the refocusing pulse in SE sequences, diffusion of spins through these regions of inhomogeneous magnetic susceptibility causes dephasing that is not completely refocused by the SE. This dephasing results in signal loss within the hemorrhage.[58] Signal loss resulting from diffusion can be minimized by using a train of closely spaced SEs, originally described in the Carr-Purcell sequence[59] and modified by Meiboom and Gill.[60] Fast SE is basically a Carr-Purcell-Meiboom-Gill (CPMG) sequence, so it also minimizes signal loss resulting from diffusion. The greatest reduction in signal loss from diffusion occurs with fast SE sequences that have a short interecho spacing. The bottom line is that fast SE sequences are less sensitive to T2-dependent signal loss in hemorrhage than are conventional T2-weighted SE sequences. This insensitivity to susceptibility effects may also prove useful for lung imaging. We have obtained good images of lung parenchyma using a HASTE sequence with a short interecho spacing.

APPEARANCE OF FAT ON FAST SPIN-ECHO IMAGES

The most obvious difference in the appearance of fast SE images compared with conventional SE images is the higher signal intensity of fat. Several factors may contribute to this difference, the most important of which are diffusion effects and J coupling.[61, 62] Other factors, such as stimulated echoes and steady-state effects, are considered to be less important.

Diffusion of fat molecules normally causes some degree of signal loss in conventional SE images. Because the sensitivity to diffusional effects is less with fast SE imaging, fat should appear brighter, although the scale of this loss in vivo is uncertain. J coupling represents the *intramolecular* interactions of spins with different chemical shifts through their electron bonds. It is responsible for splitting the spectrum of a molecule. Acquisition of a train of SEs with a short interecho spacing minimizes J-coupling effects and thereby increases the signal intensity of fat. Again, the relative importance of this effect in vivo is uncertain.

Fat suppression can be achieved in fast SE imaging by application of a chemical-shift–selective saturation pulse before each repetition of the sequence. Alternatively, the fat signal can be reduced by varying the timing of odd and even echoes so that there is a 90° phase shift between fat and water resonances. This gives a Carr-Purcell, rather than CPMG, condition for fat that increases dephasing.[63]

CLINICAL APPLICATIONS OF FAST SPIN-ECHO IMAGING

There are numerous clinical applications of fast SE imaging. These applications include ones that were previously accomplished by conventional SE sequences and new ones enabled by the shorter scan times or longer TR values possible with fast SE.

BRAIN

At many institutions, fast SE has replaced conventional SE for T2-weighted scans.[64, 65] Lesion detection is generally comparable for both sequences, although fast SE may be slightly less sensitive for small, low-contrast lesions. One implementation of fast SE, called fluid-attenuated inversion recovery (FLAIR) fast SE, uses an inversion prepulse and a long inversion time (TI) (on the order of 2.2 seconds) to null the CSF signal. With this sequence, periventricular multiple sclerosis plaques appear bright compared with dark CSF in the adjoining ventricles and thus are more conspicuous than in standard SE or fast SE sequences (Fig. 10–29). This sequence has also proved highly sensitive for subarachnoid blood and may overcome previous limitations of MRI in this regard. Fast SE sequences acquired with long TE for greater T2 weighting can improve differentiation of fluid from tumor (Fig. 10–30).

The bright fat signal seen with some fast SE implementations can be reduced by chemical-shift–selective saturation pulses or by shifting the timing of the 180° pulses, as mentioned earlier; however, field inhomogeneity can cause inadvertent saturation of nonfatty tissues, particularly near the orbits or skull base. Short-tau inversion recovery (STIR) fast SE uses a short TI (on the order of 150 ms) to null the fat signal and improves the conspicuity of orbital lesions as well as other lesions embedded in fat. 3D fast SE produces exquisite images of the brain stem and cranial nerves.

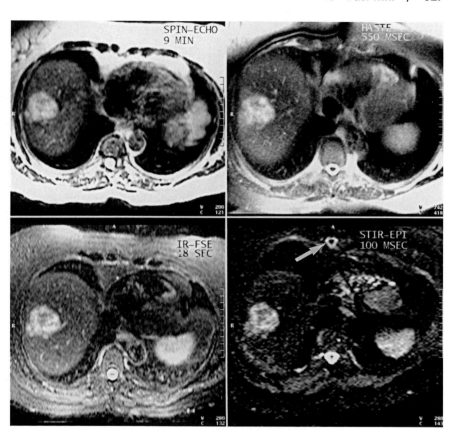

FIGURE 10–33. Sequence comparison in a patient with liver metastasis from colon adenocarcinoma. *Upper left,* SE (TR/TE = 2500/90, 9-minute scan time); *upper right,* breath-hold fat-suppressed HASTE (TE = 60 ms, 550-ms scan time); *lower left,* breath-hold inversion recovery (IR) fast SE (TR/TE/TI 4500/60/150, 18-second scan time); *lower right,* breath-hold fat-suppressed IR EPI (TE/TI = 60/150, scan time 100 ms excluding the TI interval). Arrow = N/2 ghost from spinal canal, present only with EPI. The IR fast SE sequence provides the best lesion-liver contrast-to-noise ratio and sharpest image, but all three breath-hold sequences show the lesion well in a fraction of the time for the standard SE sequence. Note that the IR fast SE and EPI sequences show more uniform fat suppression than the HASTE sequence, which uses a chemical-shift–selective saturation pulse, which is sensitive to B_0 inhomogeneities. Also note the greater signal from lung parenchyma in the fast SE and HASTE images compared with the SE image.

lesions may be less well shown than with conventional SE sequences.[70, 71]

We have found that a STIR fast SE sequence (ETL = 33) using an extremely short interecho spacing (4 ms) allows multislice breath-hold imaging with better image contrast and quality than provided by much lengthier SE or fast SE acquisitions. The uniformity of fat suppression is better with the STIR preparation than with chemical-shift–dependent fat suppression. The STIR fast SE sequence has the potential to replace slower, non–breath-hold sequences for abdominal imaging. Alternatively, promising results have been obtained with the HASTE sequence, although blurring may obscure small lesions. Breath-holding is not a requirement with HASTE because of the short period of data acquisition, although sequentially acquired slices may not be properly registered if the patient breathes.

There is general agreement that fast SE is useful for pelvic imaging.[72–74] The 512 × 512 acquisitions show the detailed architecture of the uterus and prostate and in the latter case may be particularly useful in conjunction with intrarectal surface coils. Fast SE sequences with long echo trains (e.g., 25 to 30 echoes) allow a multislice acquisition within a single breath-hold of 20 seconds or less. If a long TE (e.g., >200 ms) and long TR (e.g., >3500 ms) are used, fluids appear bright. This is the basis for the techniques of MR cholangiography[75] and MR urography.[76, 77] Steady-state GRE sequences can also be used to render fluids bright[78] but suffer signal loss when there is motion, such as transmitted cardiac pulsations affecting the left lobe of the liver. The STIR fast SE sequence gives

improved detection of lymphadenopathy (see Fig. 10–32*B*) in the abdomen, pelvis, and elsewhere.

MUSCULOSKELETAL SYSTEM

There is no consensus about the role of fast SE imaging for the musculoskeletal system. Fast SE may be less sensitive for subtle meniscal tears, and the blurring on proton density–weighted fast SE images may create pseudotears. The high fat signal intensity with fast SE can be difficult to distinguish from the bright T2 signal of effusions. The STIR fast SE sequence has proved particularly useful, as it is highly sensitive for bone marrow edema resulting from bone bruises, fractures, and other marrow abnormalities (Fig. 10–34). For shoulder imaging, it is used to distinguish fat from fluid in the subacromial bursa.

MR CHOLANGIOGRAPHY AND UROGRAPHY USING FAST SPIN ECHO

Steady-state GRE sequences render fluids bright. Breath-hold images collected by 2D or 3D steady-state GRE techniques can be used to create projection images of the biliary tree or urinary tract. However, steady-state GRE images are sensitive to motion, which can cause undesirable artifacts. A heavily T2-weighted multislice fast SE acquisition using a long TE (e.g., >200 ms) can be completed in a single breath-hold by using a long ETL (e.g., >20) and is less prone to motion artifact. Our best results to date have used

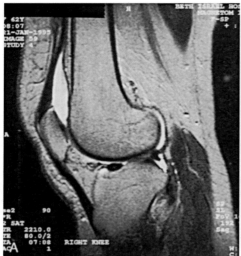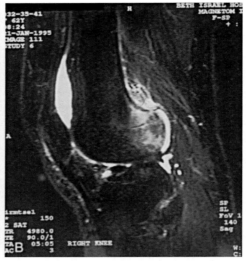

FIGURE 10–34. Images of a patient with a bone bruise of posterior femoral condyle. *A,* Sagittal T2-weighted SE (TR/TE = 2210/80, 7-minute acquisition) image shows knee effusion and faintly elevated bone marrow signal intensity in the posterior femoral condyle. *B,* The elevated marrow signal is much better shown on a STIR fast SE image (TR/TE/TI = 4980/90/150, 5-minute acquisition).

single-shot fast SE imaging with an ETL of 128 to 192 and very short interecho spacing (4 ms). Instead of breath-holding, motion compensation techniques such as respiratory gating or navigator echoes can greatly improve image quality.[78a] A maximal intensity projection of multiple slices yields the desired cholangiogram or urogram (Fig. 10–35). We generally use relatively thick slices, on the order of 5 mm or greater, acquired in an appropriate plane to span the region of interest. However, with such thick slices the projection cannot be rotated from the orientation in which the images were acquired without losing resolution; this would not be the case for a 3D fast SE sequence, which allows thinner slices to be acquired. Also, it must be recognized that any tissue with a long T2 appears bright, including ascites and other fluid collections. Small nondistended structures such as a normal-sized ureter may not be well shown. MR cholangiography is proving of great clinical value for noninvasive detection of stones and strictures of the biliary and pancreatic ducts and detection of ductal anomalies such as pancreas divisum.

GRASE

Fast SE offers a major improvement in acquisition speed over conventional SE, but still faster imaging is possible using the gradient- and spin-echo (GRASE) sequence.[79] With fast SE, the application of multiple 180° RF pulses is time-consuming. Each 180° pulse has a finite duration, typically from 3 to 5 ms; moreover, these pulses are specific absorption rate-intensive. If the interecho interval is shortened too much, the specific absorption rate limits may be exceeded, especially when the body coil is used as the transmitter.

GRASE solves this problem by acquiring several gradient echoes (e.g., three) in place of the single SE of fast SE. Each of these gradient echoes is separately phase encoded. Because multiple phase-encoding steps are acquired after each 180° pulse instead of just one, scan times are shorter than with fast SE. For instance,

an entire brain study can be completed in as little as 20 seconds, compared with 1 minute or longer with fast SE. There is a price to be paid, however. Unlike SEs, GREs decay according to T2* and are more sensitive to variations in magnetic susceptibility as well as chemical shift. In principle, GRASE sequences are more sensitive to the susceptibility effects of hemorrhage than fast SE, but the sensitivity depends on the particular sequence implementation. In our experience to date there has been little difference in the sensitivity to hemorrhage of GRASE and fast SE (Fig. 10–36). Phase or amplitude corrections must be made to the data to eliminate abrupt jumps in phase or signal intensity from one line of data to the next (these procedures are less crucial with fast SE). With GRASE, it is difficult to achieve a smooth transition between the signal intensities of lines containing SE and GRE signals. These signal discontinuities cause ringing artifacts that are more apparent than with fast SE. At present, we find GRASE of limited value because of artifacts that occur if B_0 homogeneity is suboptimal (e.g., for imaging near the dome of the liver). Single-shot GRASE using a long ETL allows subsecond imaging, although with considerable blurring except for tissues with long T2 values (i.e., fluids).

TURBOFLASH AND MP-RAGE

With short TR values (e.g., <10 ms), scan times less than 1 second are feasible with GRE sequences. However, these images show poor contrast and are best used as localizer scans. The addition of an RF preparatory pulse substantially alters tissue contrast, so that the images can be clinically useful. This approach is called snapshot FLASH,[80] turboFLASH, or MP-RAGE. The most commonly used turboFLASH sequence has a 180° prepulse followed by a waiting period TI before data acquisition. This sequence gives inversion recovery (IR)–like contrast.

In using IR turboFLASH clinically, one aims to make one tissue appear bright (e.g., liver parenchyma) and

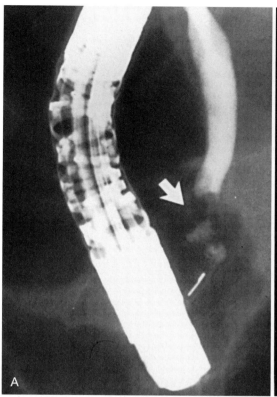

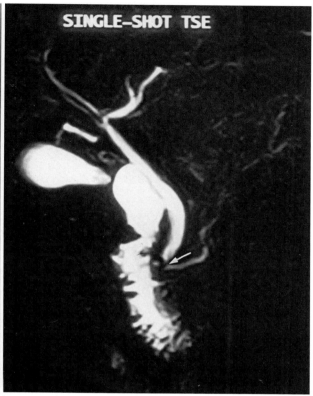

SINGLE-SHOT TSE

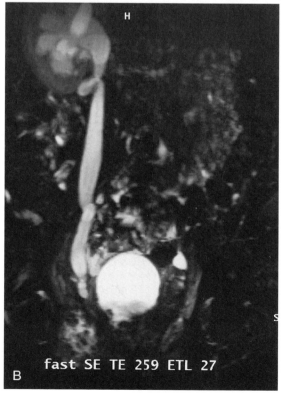

fast SE TE 259 ETL 27

FIGURE 10–35. *A,* Endoscopic retrograde cholangiogram *(left)* of patient with a filling defect *(arrow)* in the distal common bile duct. The MR cholangiogram *(right)* is a maximal intensity projection of a breath-hold series of coronal fat-suppressed single-shot fast SE images using an ETL of 128, a TE of 400 ms, and 13 slices. The arrow indicates the filling defect. *B,* MR urogram of a patient with obstruction of right ureter by tumor at the ureterovesical junction. Maximal intensity projection of coronally acquired fast SE images, TR/TE = 3500/259, ETL = 27, 6-mm-thick slices. The distended right ureter and collecting system are well shown, but the normal-sized left ureter is not apparent.

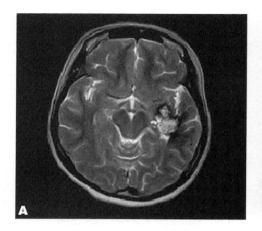
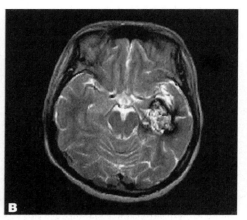

FIGURE 10–36. Comparison of fast SE *(A)* with GRASE *(B)* in a case of a left temporal cavernous hemangioma. *A,* TR/TE = 3500/119, 23-cm FOV, 250 × 256 matrix, 3 minutes, 3 seconds acquisition. *B,* TR/TE = 3500/110, 24-cm FOV, 420 × 512 matrix, 2 minutes, 23 seconds acquisition. The GRASE image appears slightly more sensitive to blood products. (*A* and *B* courtesy of NYU Faculty Practice.)

another appear dark (e.g., metastasis). As with a conventional IR sequence, at a certain time after the 180° pulse, the longitudinal magnetization of the metastasis recovers from a negative value to a positive one and in so doing transiently crosses through a value of zero. Because the data are obtained over a period of up to a second for 64 to 128 phase-encoding steps, it is impossible to acquire the entire image at this zero crossing. Instead, the essential trick is to acquire the central lines near this time period.

For instance, consider an IR turboFLASH sequence with a TR of 7 ms and 128 phase-encoding steps. At 1.5 T, a typical metastasis might be nulled with a nominal TI of 700 ms. Using a standard phase-encode order, the effective TI (i.e., the time from the 180° pulse to the central phase-encoding step) of this sequence is equal to the nominal TI of 700 ms + (7 ms × 64 steps) = 1148 ms. On the other hand, it would not be possible to null tissues having a short T1, such as fat or liver, with this sequence. Even with a nominal TI of 0 (effective TI of 448 ms), the longitudinal magnetization of these tissues would already have recovered well past zero by the time the central lines were acquired. This problem can be overcome by reordering the phase-encoding steps to acquire the central lines first.[81] For instance, the so-called centric approach acquires the steps as follows: 0, 1, −2, 2, −2, 3, −3, ...

There are several clinical applications of IR turboFLASH.

BRAIN

3D IR turboFLASH gives strongly T1-weighted brain images with nearly isotropic spatial resolution.[82] The resulting 1-mm or thinner sections can be reformatted for multiplanar imaging and may improve detection of small lesions. However, contrast enhancement of lesions after gadolinium administration may be less apparent than with T1-weighted SE or 3D spoiled GRE sequences.

SPINE

3D IR turboFLASH with multiplanar reformatting can provide detailed views of the obliquely oriented cervical neural foramina.

CHEST

Single-shot turboFLASH is too slow for detailed evaluation of the heart. Nonetheless, one can use it in conjunction with contrast agent administration to evaluate qualitatively myocardial perfusion in patients with suspected myocardial ischemia. First-pass turboFLASH scanning can also be used as a substitute for radionuclide scanning to detect and quantify intracardiac shunts and with ultrashort TE (1 ms) can be used to evaluate lung perfusion (Hatabu H, unpublished).[83]

ABDOMEN

Subsecond IR turboFLASH minimizes respiratory motion and provides good-quality T1-weighted images of the liver in patients who are unable to breathhold (Fig. 10–37). It is especially helpful for dynamic perfusion imaging of the liver and kidneys after bolus administration of a paramagnetic contrast agent like gadolinium diethylenetriaminepentaacetic acid.

Care must be taken in the interpretation of images acquired with turboFLASH, as well as other fast imaging methods. For instance, turboFLASH images may suffer from substantial blurring along the phase-encoding direction, related to T1 relaxation that occurs during the acquisition. IR turboFLASH can show an artifactual ring around a lesion, called a *bounce point artifact* (also seen with conventional IR sequences). Also, turboFLASH images are less sensitive to breathing artifacts than standard sequences, but some blurring occurs particularly with high respiratory rates.

SEGMENTED TURBOFLASH

In this modification of turboFLASH, the acquisition is divided into groups or *segments* of phase-encoding

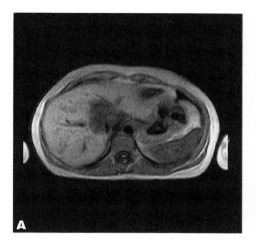 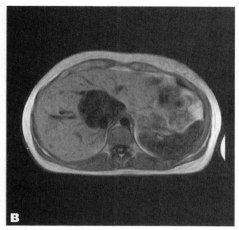

FIGURE 10–37. Single-shot turboFLASH *(A)* versus segmented turboFLASH *(B)*. The segmented turboFLASH image has much higher resolution with stronger liver-spleen contrast. However, the single-shot turboFLASH image (acquired in <2 seconds) is less motion sensitive; the segmented image was acquired in approximately 13 seconds.

steps. The advantage of segmented turboFLASH (also called phase-encoded groups [PEG] or fastCARD) over single-shot turboFLASH is that the data acquisition period is greatly shortened, so that better T1 or T2 contrast is obtained or, in the case of the heart, there is less blurring from cardiac motion. Typically, 8 to 32 steps are acquired in each segment followed by a recovery period before the next segment. Thus, for a four-segment acquisition with 128 phase-encoding lines, one might acquire lines 1 to 32 in the first segment, followed by a 2-second recovery period, then lines 33 to 64, then another 2-second wait, then lines 65 to 96, and after a final 2-second wait lines 97 to 128. In practice, this approach creates artifacts caused by jumps in signal intensity from the last step in one segment (e.g., line 32) to the first step in another segment (e.g., line 33). Therefore, one usually interleaves the steps so that segment 1 contains lines 1, 5, 9, . . . , segment 2 contains lines 2, 6, 10, . . . , and so forth until all the data are acquired. For small numbers of lines per segment (e.g., six), the time period for data acquisition can be as short as 50 ms. This is sufficiently brief to freeze cardiac motion. Thus, by acquiring electrocardiogram-gated segmented turboFLASH images, high-quality breath-hold cine imaging of the heart, including the coronary arteries, is feasible[84] (Fig. 10–38). A low-flip-angle excitation (e.g., 10° to 30°) is generally used. To improve the S/N ratio, a series of incremented flip angles increasing from a small value (e.g., 10°) for the first RF excitation in the segment to a peak value on the order of 40° to 50° for the central phase-encoding step can be used. The use of an incremented flip angle may cause some blurring in the phase-encoding direction.

BURST

A newly described fast imaging technique, called BURST, is so named because it applies a burst of brief RF pulses.[85–87] Multiple echoes are generated, separated by the interval that separates the RF pulses; each echo can be individually phase encoded. The data acquisition speed is nearly as fast as for EPI but without the need for high-speed gradients. Much work remains to be done to eliminate artifacts and motion sensitivity and to define the contrast behavior of this technique. The method appears particularly promising for perfusion imaging and other kinds of functional brain imaging, because the whole brain can be imaged using a 3D BURST sequence in just a few seconds.

URGE

Ultrarapid gradient echo (URGE) is a novel ultrafast technique that utilizes a string of short, low-flip-angle nonselective RF pulses during the application of a constant, negative gradient and generates a train of GREs that are equal in number to the RF pulses applied using a constant, positive readout gradient, as in conventional GRE imaging. URGE departs from other concepts such as utilized in BURST, SUNBURST,[88] optimized ultrafast imaging sequence (OUFIS),[89] DANTE ultrafast imaging sequence (DUFIS),[90] or quick-echo split imaging technique (QUEST),[91] in which SEs rather than GREs are acquired, so that one obtains maximal spin utilization and consequently better S/N ratios. Images can be generated as quickly as in EPI but do not require the stringent gradient hardware necessary to achieve the performance of the latter, because the data are acquired during a constant gradient readout. Using an interleaved trajectory, such as that explored in segmented turboFLASH or segmented EPI sequences,[92] produces URGE images of good quality with small effects of field inhomogeneities, T2* decay, or diffusion and flow. Only a 3D version of URGE has been implemented because of the nonselective nature of the RF excitation process. Magnetization-prepared URGE has also been demonstrated with strong T1 weighting.

FAST STEAM

A stimulated-echo acquisition mode (STEAM)[93–95] can be used for fast imaging.[96] The magnetization is stored along the −z axis using two 90° RF pulses and

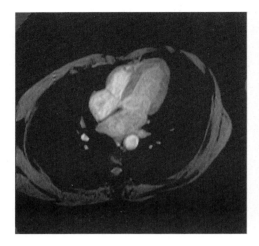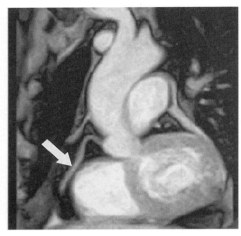

FIGURE 10–38. *Left,* Segmented turboFLASH long-axis heart image acquired with seven lines per segment, a segment duration of 104 ms, 17-second acquisition, 133 × 256 matrix. *Right,* Fat-suppressed segmented turboFLASH image of the right coronary artery *(arrow).*

is then read out using a series of independently phase-encoded low-flip-angle excitations. Subsecond acquisition times are possible with this approach. The images are T1 weighted according to the length of the interval between the second RF pulse and the central phase-encoding step. Flowing blood is effectively dephased with STEAM imaging, so that it appears uniformly dark. Rapid STEAM imaging has been proposed for cardiac and perfusion imaging.[97] However, image quality is less than can be obtained by other fast imaging methods, so the method has not come into widespread use.

MR FLUOROSCOPY

X-ray fluoroscopy or ultrasonography permits the visualization of dynamic processes with image acquisition times of several milliseconds, making it feasible to maintain a high image refreshment rate with good spatial resolution. MRI is a much slower imaging modality, but the implementation of an MR fluoroscopic system has been attempted.[98, 99] Special considerations related to the image reconstruction hardware are necessary to permit the real-time reconstruction of raw data generated continuously. Interactive color flow MRI[100] permits the superimposition of flow information over the images in real time, as in color duplex Doppler ultrasound imaging.[101] Although the initial implementation used a short TR GRE sequence, the clinical availability of EPI in the near future should make it possible to obtain images with much higher time resolution and S/N ratio. Future applications of MR fluoroscopic systems will be in the field of interventional MRI.

Other approaches to real-time data collection with MRI have been attempted using a line scan technique.[102, 103] RF pulses that are spatially selective in two dimensions (using time-varying gradients applied during the excitation) can be used to excite a beam of tissue selectively. This technique permits the encoding of spatial information along the beam with each RF excitation, making it possible to obtain data in several milliseconds. The technique is similar to that used in M-mode ultrasonography and permits the real-time quantification of processes occurring along the excited beam. With the addition of velocity-encoding gradients (V mode), velocity information can be obtained along any voxel along the beam.

KEYHOLE IMAGING

In many cases, the observation of contrast agent uptake in several organs is required after a rapid bolus injection to observe deficits in tissue perfusion. Trading off coverage and resolution against time resolution is sometimes not a desirable choice, depending on the time scale of the dynamic process that is to be observed. Based on the fact that the center of k-space is responsible for the contrast in the final image (the outer portion of k-space determines the finer detail), the keyhole technique acquires only the low-spatial-frequency information during the dynamic process, thus reducing the imaging time, and forms a composite data set that uses the high-spatial-frequency information acquired from a base image before the dynamic acquisition to permit the reconstruction of a high-resolution dynamic data set.[104, 105] The keyhole concept can be applied with any imaging sequence, although it is commonly used with fast GRE sequences because the low-spatial-frequency information can be obtained quickly.

A drawback of the keyhole technique is that the objects within the FOV of interest must remain stationary during the experiment; otherwise, the high-spatial-frequency k-space data collected in the high-resolution image do not match the corresponding low-spatial-frequency information and cause blurring and spatial misregistration of the fine detail. The number of phase-encoding lines replaced determines the size of the features that exhibit the changes. In general, a loss in contrast-to-noise ratio is apparent in small enhanced structures and the quantification of the effects may be erroneous (small structures have energy across the entire k-space data).[106] Furthermore, dramatic changes in the signal intensity between the full k-space data and the segment of data replaced can create significant signal discontinuities that can lead to increased blurring and ghost artifacts along the phase-encoding direction (as in cases in which a susceptibility-weighted sequence is used to obtain brain perfusion maps).

Other methods have been explored that do not employ data replacement strategies to maintain the high spatial resolution with the reduced raw data collected dynamically. Instead, the higher resolution image is utilized to impose constraints on the reconstruction of the high-spatial-frequency features of the dynamic image. One of these methods, reduced encoding by generalized series reconstruction (RIGR), uses a generalized series model to maintain data consistency when combining the dynamic and the high-resolution reference data sets.[107] RIGR has an advantage over keyhole imaging in that the edge information and contrast in small features are retained at the resolution of the reference image.

WAVELET-ENCODED MRI

Wavelet-encoded MRI is a new encoding modality that departs radically from the traditional Fourier-based method.[108, 109] The Fourier transform is a global transform and the entire k-space must be acquired to resolve images with a particular pixel resolution across the entire FOV. By using wavelets, the resolution in a particular portion of the FOV can be selectively enhanced.[110] This is possible because wavelets are spatially localized and the spatial information is contained within each wavelet coefficient, which encodes a specific portion of the FOV. A wavelet-based encoding technique has been implemented in the form of a line-scanning sequence using an SE technique in which the frequency encoding is acquired as in conventional imaging but the second dimension is wavelet encoded instead, using a wavelet-shaped RF profile that changes from one excitation to the next based on the Battle-Lemarie wavelet basis.[111] Although the NEX required to reconstruct the same resolution across the entire FOV is the same as in the Fourier transform case, wavelet encoding has a worse S/N ratio. Nonetheless, the use of wavelet encoding can be advantageous in some cases, as it has better immunity to motion degradation and, because of the spatial selectivity within the FOV, the NEX necessary to resolve a particular region of the FOV decreases. This feature allows one to update only information that significantly changes over time within the FOV. Wavelet encoding can be used to speed up the acquisition process for dynamically changing features without a loss in resolution or to track the motion of edge information without having to search over the entire image.[112]

ECHO-PLANAR AND SPIRAL SCAN IMAGING

EPI, proposed by Mansfield and Pykett in 1977,[113] is a fast imaging technique that allows one to collect all the data required to reconstruct an image in a brief interval, as short as the duration of a single readout period (~32 to 100 ms).[114–116] With image acquisition times on the order of a 10th of a second, EPI represents the fastest clinically useful imaging technique. The BURST technique is faster in principle, but image quality has not yet been sufficient for routine clinical use. A number of new clinical applications have become feasible with the introduction of EPI, including real-time imaging of cardiac motion, multisection imaging of the brain or upper abdomen in a few seconds, and functional brain imaging (including imaging of perfusion, diffusion, and cortical activation) (Table 10–3). Moreover, the stronger and faster gradients of EPI-capable MRI systems can be used advantageously to collect images with short TE values that minimize dephasing from flow or magnetic susceptibility variations, for example, for applications such as MR angiography or lung imaging.

BASIC PRINCIPLES OF ECHO-PLANAR IMAGING

Single-Shot Echo-Planar Imaging

An EPI image can be acquired in a single measurement or *shot*, with all the data collected after one RF excitation, or as multiple shots using repeated RF excitations, as discussed later. The single-shot approach differs from standard SE and GRE sequences, with which only a portion of the data is collected after each RF excitation. Echo-planar data are collected during the application of a rapidly oscillating gradient along the readout (frequency-encoding) direction. With each reversal of the gradient polarity from positive to negative and vice versa, a GRE is produced that is independently phase encoded, resulting in the generation of a train of echoes. One can use a terminology for EPI similar to that used in fast SE imaging

TABLE 10–3. POTENTIAL CLINICAL APPLICATIONS OF ECHO-PLANAR IMAGING–CAPABLE MRI SYSTEMS

Brain
  Replace T2 SE or fast SE with segmented EPI
  Single-shot EPI (2-s whole-brain study) for uncooperative subjects
  Perfusion imaging with contrast agents (e.g., for detection of ischemia, differentiation of recurrent tumor from radiation necrosis)
  Perfusion imaging without contrast agents (e.g., EPISTAR)
  Diffusion imaging (e.g., for early detection of ischemia)
  Cortical activation
Neck
  Ultrashort-TE MR angiography to reduce flow-related dephasing
Abdomen
  Replace T2 SE with segmented EPI
  Single-shot EPI (2-s upper abdominal study) for uncooperative subjects, lesion characterization
  Ultrashort TE breath-hold
    3D MR angiography with double-dose contrast enhancement
  MR angiography with EPISTAR
  Renal perfusion imaging with EPISTAR
  Abdominal diffusion imaging
Heart
  Rapid functional or anatomic evaluation

TABLE 10–4. COMPARISON OF FEATURES OF STANDARD AND ECHO-PLANAR IMAGING–CAPABLE MRI SYSTEMS

STANDARD MRI SYSTEMS	EPI-CAPABLE MRI SYSTEMS
Image acquisition time $\geq$ 1 s	Single-shot acquisition time 30–150 ms
Gradient rise times of 0.5–1 ms for amplitudes of 10–15 mT/m	Gradient rise times of 0.1–0.3 ms for amplitudes of 15–25 mT/m
Gradient coil nonresonant	Gradient coil nonresonant or resonant
Standard RF coils	Special RF coils to minimize gradient-induced eddy currents on metallic components
256 readout samples in $\geq$2.5 ms	128 readout samples in ~0.5 ms; requires special analog-to-digital converter for high digitization rate
Linear sampling for constant readout gradient	Linear sampling for constant readout gradient
	Nonlinear sampling or interpolation for sinusoidal readout gradient
Modest chemical-shift artifact	Severe chemical-shift artifact
	Requires good fat suppression
Modest magnetic susceptibility artifact	Severe susceptibility artifact; improved by use of thin sections, minimal TE, SE EPI, segmented EPI
Arbitrary spatial resolution	Limited in-plane spatial resolution (FOV $\geq$ 25 cm for 128 × 128 matrix) with single-shot EPI; depends on T2*, readout duration, and so on
	Arbitrary spatial resolution with segmented EPI, but longer image acquisition time (15–60 s)
No hazard from gradients	Potential neuromuscular stimulation hazard from gradients

with respect to the echo train. Thus, the ETL represents the number of echoes collected and the ETT represents the duration of the echo train. A single-shot sequence has a long ETL and a long ETT, whereas a multishot or segmented EPI sequence has a shorter ETL and a shorter ETT, depending on the number of segments. The image acquisition time is simply the ETT, typically from 30 to 150 ms. To accumulate the data sufficiently rapidly, EPI-capable MRI systems must have special features, as summarized in Table 10–4.

EPI collects data in a markedly different way from standard pulse sequences, but differences exist even among various EPI implementations (e.g., blipped versus constant phase encoding; single shot versus multishot). Figure 10–39 shows k-space trajectories for single-shot EPI. With single-shot EPI, the need for a TR interval between data collections is eliminated. The TR is essentially infinite, eliminating any degree of T1 weighting. T2 contrast is thereby improved, which is helpful for characterization of long-T1, long-T2 lesions such as cysts and hemangiomas.

Radiofrequency Excitation for Echo-Planar Imaging

Virtually any combination of RF pulses used in conventional pulse sequences can be used in EPI (Figs.

10–40 and 10–41). For instance, a 90° pulse and a 180° RF pulse can be applied so that the EPI data are collected under the T2-dependent decay envelope of an SE signal (SE EPI). Alternatively, a single RF pulse can be applied with a flip angle of 90° or less so that the EPI data are collected under the T2*-dependent decay envelope of a GRE signal (GRE EPI). GRE EPI makes the blood pool appear bright. The bright blood pool is useful for real-time cine imaging and MR angiography. GRE EPI is also used for imaging of susceptibility-dependent contrast enhancement. SE EPI is best for anatomic imaging because it is less sensitive to magnetic susceptibility variations and because flowing blood can be rendered dark, thus avoiding flow artifacts.

Echo-Planar Imaging Gradient Systems

To keep the ETT brief (necessary because of signal loss resulting from T2* decay), the rise and fall times

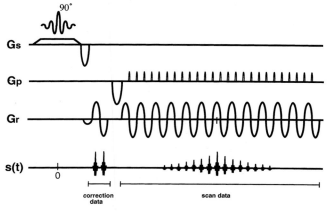

FIGURE 10–40. Pulse sequence diagram for single-shot GRE EPI using a two-echo phase correction to suppress n/2 artifacts. The correction data are acquired without phase encoding immediately after the 90° RF excitation. A blipped phase-encoding approach is illustrated, but a constant phase-encoding gradient could also be used. Gs = slice-selection gradient; Gp = phase-encoding gradient; Gr = readout gradient; s(t) = MR signal.

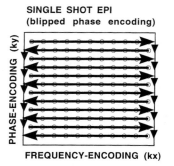
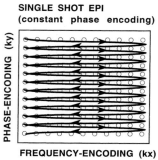

FIGURE 10–39. The k-space trajectories for single-shot EPI. Comparison of blipped *(left)* and constant *(right)* phase encoding.

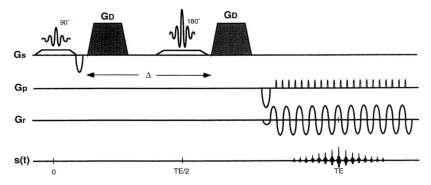

FIGURE 10–41. Diffusion-weighted SE EPI sequence. A pair of diffusion gradients (G_D) of equal area and separated in time by Δ are applied around the 180° RF pulse to dephase and cause signal loss from diffusing protons but not from stationary spins.

for the readout gradient must be short. For instance, if the gradient rise and fall times are each 0.25 ms, one readout gradient pulse can be applied in as little as 0.5 ms, and 128 echoes could be collected in 128 × 0.5 ms or 64 ms. Not only must the gradient rise times be several times shorter than for standard gradient systems, the gradients must also be capable of reaching higher peak amplitudes. This is because the spatial resolution is determined by the integral of the gradient waveform. Because the duration of each readout gradient pulse is so short, its amplitude must be correspondingly high. The gradient performance may be characterized in terms of *slew rate* (Fig. 10–42),

which is the gradient magnetic field change per unit time, given in tesla per meter per second. For instance, for trapezoidal gradients, a slew rate of 200 T/m/s could mean that the gradient rise time is 0.1 ms for a peak gradient amplitude of 20 mT/m or 0.05 ms for a peak gradient amplitude of 10 mT/m. The definition of slew rate is trickier for sinusoidal gradients, as the slew rate varies over the duration of the sinusoid. Potential advantages of high slew rates include 1) shorter TE for non-EPI applications; 2) reduction in the ETT, so that susceptibility and T2* filtering effects are reduced; and 3) higher spatial resolution, because the gradient can be ramped more rapidly. This allows more time at the plateau of peak gradient amplitude and a larger area under the gradient. Drawbacks of high slew rates include greater risk of neuromuscular stimulation and more stringent hardware requirements. With the use of high-slew-rate gradient pulses, good eddy current compensation is essential to avoid image artifacts. This is accomplished by active gradient shielding or, in the case of small insert gradient coils, by physical separation of the gradient coils from the cryoshield of the magnet. Special low-inductance gradient coils are required for EPI to avoid energy dissipation in the coil.

Two kinds of gradient systems have been used for the readout gradient: resonant[117] and nonresonant.[118] A resonant gradient system stores a large voltage in a bank of capacitors, which discharges into the gradient coil. The energy is then returned to the capacitor, and the process is repeated. The energy rapidly oscillates back and forth between the capacitors and gradient coil, like the to-and-fro motion of a pendulum. The system is designed to resonate at a specific frequency, determined by the capacitance (C) and inductance (L) of the system, according to $1/(LC)^{1/2}$. This frequency can be changed by adding or subtracting capacitors. With a simple resonant system, the gradient amplitude cannot be sustained at a fixed nonzero value. Therefore, a "catch and hold" circuit is incorporated that permits the gradient amplitude to be maintained at a plateau for an extended period after a quarter–sine wave ramp of the gradient. This modification is needed for ultrashort TE MR angiography or diffusion imaging.

Alternatively, the gradients can be nonresonant, as in conventional gradient systems but faster and with higher peak amplitudes. Powerful amplifiers are used

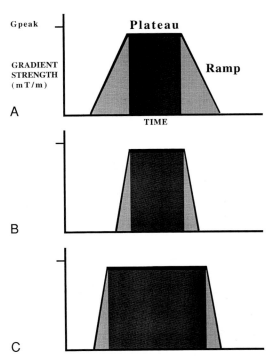

FIGURE 10–42. Uses of high slew rates. *A*, Standard gradient systems typically have gradient ramp times on the order of 1 ms from zero to peak amplitude. *B*, EPI-capable systems have much higher slew rates, so that the duration of the gradient ramps can be shortened. This technique can be used to reduce TE without increasing the signal bandwidth compared with that in *A*. *C*, Alternatively, the use of faster ramps allows the plateau sampling period to be extended, thereby lowering the signal bandwidth and improving the S/N ratio without increasing the total duration of the frequency-encoding gradient waveform compared with that in *A*.

that can quickly drive the gradients to the required amplitude. Nonresonant systems permit arbitrary gradient waveforms to be designed. The main drawback compared with resonant systems is the higher cost of the more powerful gradient amplifier, at least in the case of large gradient coils, because the power requirements increase with the square of the gradient amplitude and with the fifth power of coil diameter.

Data Sampling

For both conventional MRI and nonresonant EPI, trapezoidal gradient waveforms are typically applied. Data are collected during a constant-amplitude readout gradient and the sampling rate is fixed for the entire readout period. In contrast, resonant EPI typically uses a sinusoidal readout gradient. In this case, the gradient amplitude changes during readout, so a different approach for sampling is required (see Fig. 10–39). Either the data can be sinc interpolated onto a rectilinear k-space grid or nonlinear sampling of the data can be performed (Fig. 10–43).

Phase Encoding in Echo-Planar Imaging

Because the data for EPI are collected as a series of ultrafast GREs, the techniques for phase encoding are different from those used for standard imaging. One of two methods for phase encoding is generally used: 1) a constant phase-encoding gradient is applied over the entire duration of the EPI readout or 2) a phase-encoding "blip" of short duration is applied at the end of each readout gradient pulse. The trajectory along the phase-encoding direction is slightly different for each approach and is treated differently during the image reconstruction.[119] Echo-planar images can also be acquired in a 3D mode by applying a standard phase-encoding gradient along the section-select direction, with much shorter image acquisition times (as little as 10 seconds for 128 partitions) than for standard 3D GRE sequences.

Artifacts in Echo-Planar Imaging

N/2 GHOSTS. Ghost artifacts are typically caused by periodic fluctuations in image signal intensity. Because single-shot EPI data are accumulated within an interval that is short compared with periods of physiologic motion, the images do not suffer from ghost artifacts caused by breathing or cardiac pulsation. However, they can suffer from ghost artifacts of a different kind. Odd and even EPI echoes are collected with readout gradients of alternating polarity. Imperfections in the gradients, gradient-induced eddy currents, flow, or field inhomogeneities may cause slight mismatches in the timings of the odd and even echoes, which translate into phase errors after the Fourier transform. These phase errors are manifested in EPI as duplicate images of the object, called N/2 ghosts, that propagate along the phase-encoding direction (see Fig. 10–33). If N/2 ghosts are severe, they can degrade image quality. To suppress N/2 ghosts, care must be taken to ensure gradient stability and minimize eddy currents. The N/2 ghosts can also be suppressed by a phase correction determined from two echoes collected during a single bipolar readout gradient (see Fig. 10–40).

SUSCEPTIBILITY AND CHEMICAL-SHIFT ARTIFACTS. The amplitude of the phase-encoding gradient for EPI is much weaker than for standard pulse sequences. As a result, EPI is sensitive to the effects of static magnetic field inhomogeneities (susceptibility and chemical shift artifacts); however, the sensitivity is directed along the phase-encoding rather than the frequency-encoding direction, as is typical of standard pulse sequences. Susceptibility artifacts may be severe at the skull base, near the paranasal sinuses, at the anterior orbits, at the lung-heart interface, and near air-containing bowel loops. Because chemical-shift artifacts with single-shot EPI are many times larger than with standard sequences, efficient fat suppression is essential (Fig. 10–44). This can be problematic in certain areas, such as the dome of the liver, where field inhomogeneities are unavoidable. The problem is worsened when a body multicoil is used, because of the high signal intensity of subcutaneous fat. More uniform fat suppression is obtained by the use of an inversion (STIR) preparation. Susceptibility artifacts are reduced by shimming, that is, adjusting the currents in the shim coils of the magnet to maximize static field homogeneity. Susceptibility artifacts are further reduced by using thin sections, using a shorter TE (which can be achieved by reducing the ETL or by asymmetric k-space sampling along the phase-encoding direction), or augmenting the amplitude of the phase-encoding gradient (e.g., using a rectangular FOV). The TE also can be shortened by increasing the readout bandwidth (i.e., reducing the duration of echo sampling), but this approach is ultimately limited by the gradient capabilities of the system.

T2* FILTERING. Data collection with EPI is fast

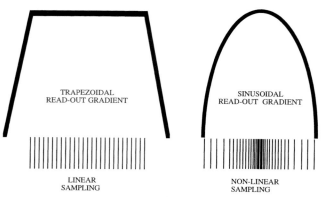

TRAPEZOIDAL READ-OUT GRADIENT

SINUSOIDAL READ-OUT GRADIENT

LINEAR SAMPLING

NON-LINEAR SAMPLING

FIGURE 10–43. Data-sampling schemes. *Left,* Linear sampling with a trapezoidal readout gradient. The data are collected with a constant sampling rate. Under a sinusoidal gradient, constant sampling translates into nonequidistant coverage of k-space and interpolation must be performed to remap k-space. *Right,* Nonlinear sampling with a sinusoidal readout gradient. Samples are collected at different points in time so that the resulting sampling maps directly into the k-space grid. The timing for data sampling is dependent on equal area increments (nonlinear sampling), compared with equal time increments (linear sampling) during the readout.

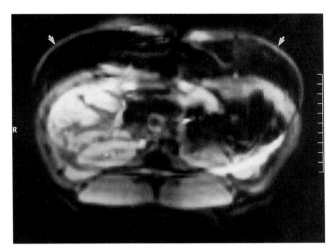

FIGURE 10–44. Abdominal echo-planar image acquired without fat suppression. Note the enormous chemical-shift displacement of the subcutaneous fat *(arrows)*.

relative to conventional MRI techniques and to periods of physiologic motion; it is not fast with respect to T2* decay. T2* decay during the ETT causes blurring (filtering of high spatial frequencies) along the phase-encoding direction because the signal intensity changes substantially over this period.[120] The shorter the T2*, the worse the blurring. This filtering effect can be minimized by shortening the ETT and the TE.

IN-PLANE SPATIAL RESOLUTION. In-plane spatial resolution along the x and y directions is determined, respectively, by the integrals of the readout and phase-encoding gradient waveforms. Because the ETT must be kept short to minimize T2* decay and resultant blurring, the FOV of single-shot EPI is ultimately limited by the peak gradient amplitude. As a result, the minimal FOV of current whole-body EPI systems is on the order of 25 cm or greater for a 128 × 128 acquisition matrix, giving a typical pixel size of 2 to 3 mm.

Multishot or Segmented Echo-Planar Imaging

One can substantially overcome the FOV limits and susceptibility artifacts that occur with single-shot EPI by accumulating the data over multiple excitations. This procedure decreases the ETL and ETT per segment (one excitation per segment) in proportion to the number of segments collected. Multishot EPI greatly reduces the demands on gradient performance and allows in-plane spatial resolution to be improved to a level comparable to that with standard pulse sequences. There are several possibilities for multishot imaging. For instance, one could simply acquire half of k-space in the first shot and concatenate the other half acquired in the second shot. When done along the frequency-encoding direction, this is called *mosaic imaging*.[121] Half-Fourier imaging can also be used to improve spatial resolution, at the expense of a loss in S/N ratio and some increase in artifacts. A more flexi-

ble alternative is segmented EPI; with this method, a limited portion or segment of data (e.g., 8 to 32 lines) is collected within each TR interval. The data from all the segments are interleaved before image reconstruction[122] (Fig. 10–45A), in a manner similar to that used for segmented turboFLASH.[123] Interleaving minimizes signal intensity fluctuations that occur from the end of one segment to the beginning of another. To smooth out phase and amplitude modulations in the raw data, which otherwise introduce artifacts into the image, the technique of *echo shifting* is used. With this technique, the timing of the echoes is varied slightly from segment to segment.[124, 125] Segmented EPI images of diagnostic quality can be acquired in a single breath-hold period even using a conventional MRI system.[126, 127]

Spiral Scanning

Spiral scanning is another fast imaging method that can be implemented, like segmented EPI, on a conventional MRI system.[128] With spiral scanning, two gradients are oscillated in tandem to describe a spiral k-space trajectory (Fig. 10–45B). Because the central part of k-space (which determines image contrast) is covered early in the spiral and because the gradient moments pass through zero repeatedly as a result of the spiral trajectory, little flow-related dephasing occurs. As a result, spiral scanning is intrinsically flow compensated, a property that is advantageous for MR angiography. However, it is quite sensitive to static magnetic field inhomogeneities, and off-resonance effects can cause marked blurring. Motion artifacts appear as rings instead of ghosts. The advantages and disadvantages of spiral scanning versus EPI require further study.

Signal-to-Noise Ratio in Echo-Planar Imaging

The S/N ratio is proportional to 1/(readout bandwidth)$^{1/2}$. The duration of each GRE readout in the EPI echo train is many times shorter than that of the readout of a conventional pulse sequence; therefore, the readout bandwidth is correspondingly higher and the S/N ratio lower. Despite this limitation, the S/N ratio of single-shot EPI images can be surprisingly good. One reason is the limited in-plane spatial resolution, as the S/N ratio scales with the pixel area. For instance, a 128 × 128 or 64 × 128 acquisition matrix is commonly used for EPI with pixel dimensions on the order of 2 to 4 mm, versus 1 to 2 mm with standard sequences. Furthermore, all the echoes are collected after a single RF excitation, so that one does not have the inefficiency of data collection encountered with standard pulse sequences, with which one must wait a TR interval between successive readouts. Although the S/N ratio of EPI images is lower than that of images acquired using standard pulse sequences, the S/N ratio per unit acquisition time is higher. An interesting feature of EPI is that image quality may improve (up to a point), rather than worsen, as the section thickness is reduced. This is because T2* decay caused by intravoxel variations in magnetic susceptibility is reduced

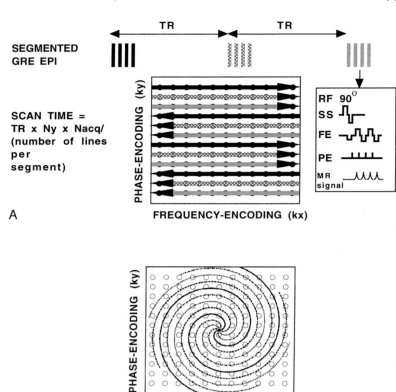

SEGMENTED GRE EPI

SCAN TIME = TR x Ny x Nacq/ (number of lines per segment)

A

FIGURE 10–45. The k-space trajectories for multishot imaging techniques. *A,* Trajectory for segmented EPI. The data from multiple segments are interleaved, rather than simply concatenated, to minimize jumps in signal intensity from one line to the next. The technique of echo shifting also helps to reduce these jumps. *B,* Trajectory for spiral scan. Two magnetic field gradients are oscillated in tandem to trace a spiral k-space trajectory.

as the section thickness is decreased. Although the best EPI images to date have been acquired at 1.5 T, one can obtain EPI images of good quality with lower field systems by increasing the ETT. The ETT can be lengthened either by increasing the ETL or by reducing the readout bandwidth (i.e., increasing the duration of echo sampling). This is possible because T2* is longer at lower field strengths. However, if the ETT is too long, filtering effects resulting from T2* decay and motion artifacts become a problem.

Safety

The RF power deposition with EPI is low, because few RF pulses are applied. The gradients are another issue entirely. A change in the magnetic field (B field) can create an electric field (E field) directly proportional to the rate of change of the B field, thus giving rise to electric currents when the changes occur in a conductive surrounding. The fast-changing magnetic field gradients needed for EPI can induce rapidly changing electric currents in the body that are potentially hazardous. These currents can cause neuromuscular stimulation and have raised concerns about the safety of EPI for human studies. Because of the different geometries of the three gradient coils, the stimulation hazard is worst when the z gradient is used for readout (i.e., for sagittal or coronal EPI imaging). Swapping the phase- and frequency-encoding gradients for an EPI axial acquisition increases the risk of neuromuscular stimulation compared with an unswapped axial acquisition because of greater stimulation when the y gradient is used for readout compared

with the x gradient. Sinusoidal gradients may have a lower threshold for stimulation than trapezoidal ones.[129, 130] Currently, the dB/dt (rate of change of the magnetic field with time) limits imposed by the U.S. Food and Drug Administration[131] are 60 T/s for the transverse (x and y) gradients for a pulse width (duration of a rectangular pulse or sinusoidal half period) greater than 120 μs and 20 T/s for the z gradient (these regulations are currently being modified, so these particular values may soon be out of date). By comparison, the peak dB/dt of standard gradient systems is typically less than 20 T/s.

Two studies have reported sensations ranging from mild twitching to pain, depending on the maximal change in B over time when the magnetic field gradients oscillate during EPI data collection.[132, 133] The sensation is felt near the physical extremes of the gradient coil, where the gradient field change (and therefore dB/dt) is largest. For instance, the trunk muscles or buttocks are typically affected when the head is positioned at the center of the magnet for brain imaging, because they lie near the edge of the magnet bore and thus the ends of the gradient coils. Similarly, the bridge of the nose may be affected during abdominal imaging. Fortunately, the cardiac stimulation threshold is at least 10-fold higher than for skeletal muscle. Nonetheless, further study is warranted to determine the safety of EPI for patients who are prone to arrhythmias or suffer from metabolic abnormalities, such as hypocalcemia, that can predispose to tetany.

The risk of stimulation can be reduced by shortening the gradient coil, which reduces the peak dB/dt at the ends of the coil. Figure 10–46 shows field plots for

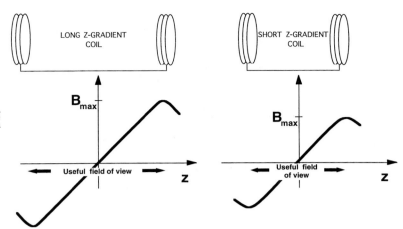

FIGURE 10–46. Field plot of a z gradient coil. A long gradient coil has a higher dB/dt at its ends than does a shorter gradient coil.

long and short z gradient coils. A disadvantage of a short gradient coil is that spatial distortions are seen for positions far off center. These distortions can be corrected at least in part if the gradient field distribution is known.[134]

CLINICAL ASPECTS OF ECHO-PLANAR IMAGING

Some potential clinical applications of EPI are summarized in Table 10–3. Before now, EPI has been available at only a few sites. As a result, large-scale validation studies have not been done and these applications must still be considered investigational.

BRAIN

Echo-Planar Imaging as a Substitute for Spin-Echo Imaging

Currently, image acquisition times for T2-weighted brain studies using standard MRI equipment are on the order of 5 to 15 minutes for SE and 1 to 5 minutes for fast SE sequences. With single-shot EPI, a 20-section study of the entire brain can be acquired in as little as 2 seconds (Fig. 10–47). This fast imaging capability is particularly helpful for uncooperative patients and pediatric subjects. In a preliminary study of patients with multiple sclerosis,[135] we found that lesions larger than a few millimeters in diameter were detected as well by single-shot EPI as by T2-weighted SE sequences. That single-shot EPI was insensitive for small brain lesions is related in part to the minimal pixel size, on the order of 2×2 mm, which is twice that of standard T2-weighted SE sequences. T2* filtering effects may make actual spatial resolution even worse than expected from the pixel size. Moreover, lesion conspicuity around the base of the brain may be degraded by magnetic susceptibility artifacts and poor fat suppression. As a result, single-shot EPI is not a substitute for high-resolution SE imaging. On the other hand, segmented EPI can provide images of comparable quality to SE images in as little as 30 seconds to 1 minute.[136] The sensitivity to B_0 field inhomogeneity is less than that with single-shot EPI but still more than that with SE or fast SE imaging.

Functional Brain Imaging

With the advent of EPI and other subsecond imaging techniques, the field of functional brain imaging has rapidly progressed. Functional imaging encompasses diffusion, perfusion, and cortical activation studies.

Diffusion Imaging

Although MR was proposed to measure molecular diffusion in the early 1950s, only in the past few years have in vivo measurements been practical.[137] Diffusion is the process of random thermal motion of molecules, also called brownian motion. It occurs at a microscopic scale. Whereas water molecules in blood vessels move as much as a meter or more per second, water molecules diffuse on the order of only hundredths or tenths of a millimeter per second.

Diffusion through a magnetic field gradient causes intravoxel dephasing and a loss of signal intensity as expressed by

$$S/S_0 = \exp(-bD)$$

where S/S_0 is the signal intensity ratio between two images acquired with and without diffusion-sensitizing gradients and D is the diffusion coefficient (given in millimeters squared per second or centimeters squared per second), which characterizes the rate of diffusional motion.[138] The diffusion coefficient depends on the temperature and physical characteristics of the molecules. For instance, small molecules such as water diffuse rapidly and have a high D, whereas large molecules such as proteins diffuse more slowly and have a lower D. In biologic systems, factors other than diffusion (e.g., perfusion, water transport, or bulk motion) might contribute to the signal loss, so that the term apparent diffusion coefficient (ADC) is used instead of D. The b value (given in seconds per millimeters squared or seconds per centimeter squared) is related to the strength, duration, and separation of the diffu-

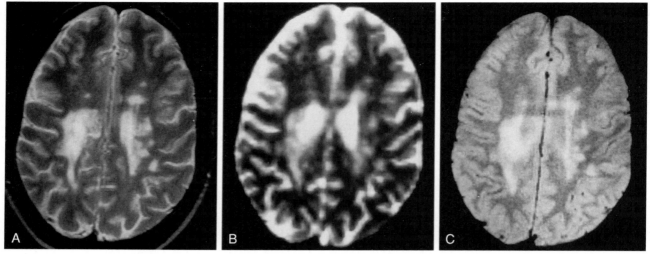

FIGURE 10–47. Sequence comparison for a patient with multiple sclerosis. *A,* T2-weighted SE image with TR/TE 2400/80, scan time 7 minutes, 44 seconds. *B,* Single-shot SE EPI with 128 × 128 matrix, FOV = 25 cm, TE = 80 ms, scan time = 120 ms. Spatial resolution is lower than in *A. C,* Segmented SE EPI, 252 × 256 matrix (28 lines per segment × 9 segments), FOV = 27 cm, TR/TE = 3500/21, two acquisitions, scan time 1 minute, 6 seconds. Image quality is comparable to that in *A.* All EPI images shown were obtained with spectral fat suppression.

sion-sensitizing gradients. We typically use b values in the range of several hundred to more than 1000 s/mm^2 for diffusion-weighted imaging. High b values improve diffusion sensitivity at the expense of S/N ratio.

Because the molecular displacements are so small, a large gradient amplitude or duration is required to produce observable signal loss from diffusion. However, the scale of molecular displacements related to physiologic motion, such as breathing or brain pulsation, is much larger than for diffusional displacements. Therefore, diffusion-weighted images acquired with conventional pulse sequences suffer from severe motion artifacts. These artifacts are minimal in single-shot EPI images. Approaches for diffusion-weighted imaging include SE EPI and stimulated-echo EPI. Stimulated-echo EPI allows shorter TE values and longer diffusion-sensitizing intervals than SE EPI, so that there is less T2* decay and higher b values can be obtained; drawbacks are T1 decay over the diffusion-sensitizing interval and loss of half the signal by virtue of the stimulate-echo readout. Alternatively, diffusion-weighted images can be acquired with a fast stimulated-echo acquisition method on a conventional MRI system[139]; however, image quality and multisection imaging capability are worse than with EPI.

At present, the most important clinical applications of diffusion imaging involve the detection and characterization of cerebral ischemia. Within a few minutes of the onset of ischemia, there is a marked decrease in the ADC of brain tissue, causing the ischemic zone to appear brighter than healthy tissue on a diffusion-weighted image. This effect is most likely related to energetic failure, with impairment of membrane ion pumps and the consequent onset of intracellular edema. However, the precise manner in which intracellular edema lowers the ADC is not known.

Ischemia is detected much earlier by diffusion-

weighted imaging than by conventional MRI, which depends on the presence of vasogenic edema and may miss infarcts earlier than 6 hours after onset of ischemia.[140, 141] Early stroke detection will become increasingly important as clinical trials of potentially effective stroke therapies are initiated. Diffusion changes in early ischemia are reversible, so that the efficacy of therapy can be monitored on a real-time basis. As stroke patients may have difficulty cooperating for the examination, EPI is especially useful for completing the study quickly.

Another potential application of diffusion EPI is for mapping of white matter development and anatomy. Unlike diffusion in gray matter, diffusion in white matter is *anisotropic,* that is, dependent on the direction of the diffusion-sensitizing gradient.[142] The myelin sheath acts as a barrier to water motion, so that diffusion along axons is faster than across them. Myelination in infants can be monitored by measuring the amount of diffusional anisotropy in white matter. Aside from white matter, diffusion is markedly anisotropic in other organs, such as muscle and renal medulla. Diffusion imaging also distinguishes solid neoplasms such as epidermoids, which despite their cystic appearance on T1- and T2-weighted images have a low ADC, from subarachnoid cysts that have a high ADC.[143]

Perfusion Imaging

FIRST-PASS CONTRAST-ENHANCED IMAGING. Relative cerebral blood volume maps can be created by first-pass EPI imaging after a bolus intravenous injection of a paramagnetic contrast agent.[144-146] With a T1-weighted pulse sequence such as IR SE EPI, the contrast agent produces an increase in the signal intensity of the perfused regions of the brain. More clinical experience has been accumulated with the use of susceptibility (T2*)–weighted contrast-enhanced studies.

With a T2*-weighted pulse sequence such as GRE EPI, the contrast agent bolus produces a decrease in the signal intensity of perfused brain tissue. Alternatively, one can use a T2-weighted SE EPI sequence. The susceptibility effect resulting from the contrast agent bolus is reduced compared with T2*-weighted EPI. However, the effect is better localized to brain tissue, with fewer artifacts resulting from long-range susceptibility effects related to the presence of contrast agent within large vessels. A series of multisection brain perfusion images spanning the entire brain can be acquired as often as every 2 seconds. These methods have been successfully applied for studies of human brain perfusion using fast non-EPI and EPI sequences in patients with various neurologic lesions.[147, 148] The method is especially useful for detecting hypoperfused regions in patients with cerebral ischemia[149] and is complementary to diffusion imaging in the information it provides about them. It can be used to assess tumor vascularity,[150] distinguish recurrent tumor from radiation necrosis, and depict hypervascularity associated with an epileptic focus during a seizure.[151]

EPISTAR. We have described a noninvasive, EPI-based approach for qualitative mapping of cerebral blood flow, called EPI with signal targeting with alternating RF (EPISTAR).[152] The basic idea is to acquire alternately two sets of data that are identical except for the longitudinal magnetization of inflowing arterial spins.[153, 153a] During alternate acquisitions, a single 180° adiabatic RF pulse is applied to invert the inflowing arterial spins. Magnitude subtraction of the images yields a qualitative map of cerebral blood flow. The TI between the inversion that tags the arterial spins and readout can be varied from a few milliseconds to several seconds. The portion of the vasculature shown is dependent on the TI. With a short TI (e.g., 400 ms), flow in major arteries is seen. With delays on the order of 800 ms, distal branch arteries are shown. With delays greater than 1 second, the arteries tend to disappear and cortical enhancement is seen as the tagged blood protons enter the capillaries and exchange with cortical tissue protons. The method can be applied as often as desired, without the problem of accumulated contrast agent load that can limit the repeated use of first-pass contrast-enhanced imaging. Potential clinical applications include detection of abnormal tumor vascularity[154] and ischemic regions in stroke. The method could also be useful for evaluation of renal perfusion (Fig. 10–48).

Cortical Activation Studies

One of the most active fields of study in neuroscience is the localization of brain activity. Previously, this was mostly the domain of positron emission tomography, which has limited availability and requires administration of a radioactive isotope. MRI provides better spatial resolution than positron emission tomography and, because MRI is noninvasive, activation studies can be repeated at will. The MRI techniques used to date have been based on the susceptibility effects of either paramagnetic contrast agents[155] or deoxyhemoglobin (blood oxygen level–dependent [BOLD] contrast imaging).[156–158] With the BOLD method, activated cortical areas show an increase of signal intensity in T2*-weighted images (see Chapters 8 and 26). It is believed

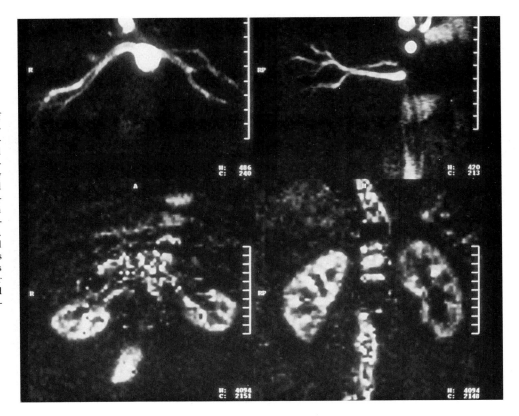

FIGURE 10–48. Applications of EPISTAR sequence for renal angiography *(top)* and perfusion imaging *(bottom)*. *Top,* Axial *(left)* and coronal *(right)* EPISTAR angiograms acquired in approximately 10 seconds. The aorta was labeled longitudinally on alternate acquisitions by an adiabatic inversion pulse. The time delay between labeling and readout was 250 ms. *Bottom,* Axial *(left)* and coronal *(right)* EPISTAR perfusion images acquired in the same manner as the angiograms but with a longer time delay between labeling and readout of 950 ms. Note the presence of cortical enhancement.

that activation increases cerebral blood flow without a proportionate increase in tissue oxygen extraction. Therefore, an excess of oxyhemoglobin-containing arterial blood, which has a longer T2* than venous blood, flows into the venous bed with activation. This causes a lengthening of the T2* of the venous blood and an increase in signal intensity on T2*-weighted images. BOLD images can be acquired with a GRE or asymmetric SE EPI sequence; the latter is a modified SE EPI sequence in which the 180° pulse is deliberately miscentered to introduce some T2* weighting. Alternatively, standard GRE sequences can be used with conventional MR hardware, although EPI has the advantages of less motion sensitivity and greater multisection capability. Promising results have also been obtained with the EPISTAR technique.

ABDOMEN

Although high-quality T1-weighted images of the upper abdomen can be acquired during a breath-hold by using spoiled GRE sequences,[159] GRE sequences are less useful for T2-weighted acquisitions. However, with single-shot T2-weighted SE EPI, a multisection study of the upper abdomen can be completed in as little as 2 seconds (Fig. 10–49). One can also use long-TE EPI for rapid lesion characterization[160] (Fig. 10–50). With single-shot EPI, artifacts may be encountered as a result of magnetic field distortions caused by air-containing bowel loops or imperfect fat suppression. Butts and colleagues[122] showed that breath-hold T2-weighted images can be acquired on a conventional MRI system by using segmented EPI, with lesion-liver contrast comparable to that of standard SE images. Segmented EPI has the potential to replace standard SE for liver imaging, but potential limitations include its sensitivity to motion artifacts resulting from cardiac pulsation and bowel peristalsis and magnetic susceptibility artifacts. Because they are less artifact prone, fast SE sequences will likely prove more useful than EPI for abdominal imaging.

Diffusion-weighted EPI images of the abdomen can be acquired.[161] Cardiac triggering is occasionally necessary for accurate diffusion measurements, especially for the left lobe of the liver. The abdominal viscera have distinctive ADCs; for instance, the spleen has a low ADC despite the high vascularity of this organ, for reasons as yet undetermined. By contrast, the kidney has a higher ADC than water at body temperature, indicating contributions from water transport processes and blood flow. Thus, diffusion measurements have the potential to provide functional information about the kidneys. For instance, preliminary animal studies in our laboratory indicate that renal ischemia produced by arterial occlusion causes an immediate and marked decrease in the ADC of the kidney.[162]

HEART

MRI has had a limited impact to date on the field of cardiac imaging. Currently, the only common applications are for the diagnosis of aortic dissection and pericardial disease. This could change with the advent of EPI,[163] which greatly extends the robustness and functional capabilities of MRI. Other fast imaging techniques, such as single-shot and segmented[164] turboFLASH, should also benefit from the faster gradients (and therefore shorter TR and TE) of EPI-capable systems. EPI may be helpful for pediatric subjects to avoid motion artifacts in the evaluation of congenital heart disease.[165, 166]

Several EPI sequences have been tested for cardiac imaging[167, 168] (Fig. 10–51). One must contend with the fact that the heart is surrounded by air-containing lung, causing susceptibility artifacts that may be pronounced in GRE EPI images but are minimal in SE EPI images. Given the long interval over which the MR signal is read out and phase encoding is performed, accelerating or turbulent blood flow may cause severe flow displacement artifacts in GRE EPI images. These artifacts are reduced with SE EPI because of washout

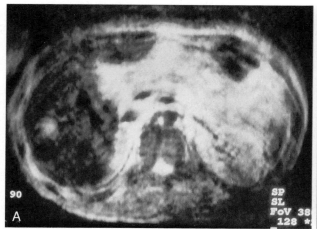
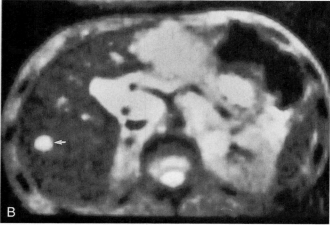

FIGURE 10–49. Images of a patient with liver metastasis from lymphoma. *A*, Thirteen-minute T2-weighted SE image with TR/TE = 3000/90, 128 × 256 matrix, two acquisitions. *B*, Single-shot SE EPI image with TE-100 ms, 128 × 128 matrix, 1 of 20 sections acquired in approximately 3 seconds. The lesion *(arrow)* is better shown by EPI, even though the spatial resolution of the EPI image is lower because of the smaller acquisition matrix. Blurring related to respiration has been eliminated by the short acquisition time.

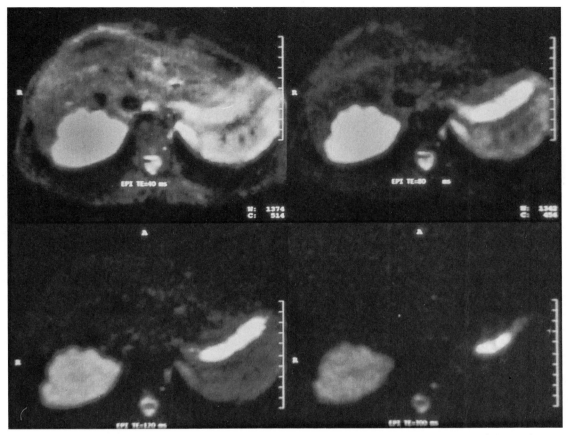

FIGURE 10–50. Liver lesion characterization using SE EPI. Cavernous hemangioma. Progressively increasing TE values were used during separate breath-holds from 40 ms *(upper left)* to 300 ms *(lower right)*. There was no T1 contamination of the single-shot EPI image contrast because of the long interval between acquisition of successive images.

from the plane of section between the 90° and 180° RF pulses and still more so if the blood-pool signal is suppressed by the application of balanced dephasing gradients placed around the 180° pulse. GRE EPI is best used for T2*-weighted perfusion studies and for real-time cine imaging. For cine imaging, one can acquire the GRE EPI images in rapid sequence and create a series of images over multiple cardiac cycles, without the need for electrocardiographic gating. Thus, the method would be particularly helpful for patients with arrhythmias who are not otherwise amenable to cardiac MRI. One can also observe beat-to-beat variability, which is not possible with pulse sequences such as SE, conventional cine, or segmented turboFLASH that create a composite image from data acquired over multiple heart cycles.

Cardiac perfusion can be evaluated by first-pass imaging after bolus administration of a paramagnetic contrast agent.[169, 170] In a first-pass study, the signal intensity of normally perfused myocardium decreases on T2*-weighted GRE images with less change in ischemic myocardium.[171] Alternatively, a T1-weighted IR SE EPI sequence can be used, in which case the signal intensity of perfused myocardium is higher after administration of a contrast agent than that of the ischemic region. The spatial resolution and temporal reso-

lution are sufficient to permit one to distinguish perfusion patterns in the subendocardial, middle, and subepicardial zones of the left ventricular myocardium. Cardiac diffusion imaging has also been attempted, although it is obviously a major technical challenge to measure diffusion in the beating heart. Some progress has been made by using a stimulated-echo EPI sequence with cardiac triggering and breath-holding. With this method, there is an indication of diffusional anisotropy within the myocardium, perhaps related to muscle fiber orientation.[172] Cardiac diffusion measurements are sensitive to myocardial strain as well as diffusion.

With the introduction of EPI into commercial MRI systems, the combination of breath-hold fast imaging of cardiac anatomy, coronary artery MR angiography, wall motion evaluation using cine and myocardial tagging,[173] first-pass imaging of contrast enhancement patterns, and possibly diffusion imaging could provide a cost-effective alternative to current strategies for workup in ischemic heart disease. However, clinical validation and availability of the necessary hardware and software are prerequisites.

ECHO-PLANAR MR ANGIOGRAPHY

Relatively little flow-related dephasing occurs with single-shot EPI scans, even without flow compensation.

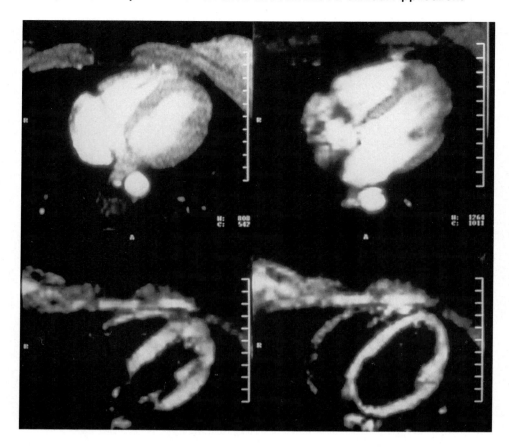

FIGURE 10–51. Comparison of fast techniques for imaging of the heart. *Upper left,* Segmented turboFLASH image acquired in 14 seconds. *Upper right,* GRE EPI image with TE of 18 ms. Magnetic susceptibility artifact partially obscures the apex. *Lower left,* SE EPI image with TE of 53 ms and paired dephasing gradients acquired during systole. *Lower right,* Same acquired during diastole. The SE EPI images are not particularly degraded by magnetic susceptibility artifact.

Dephasing is minimal because of the ultrashort interval between sequential echoes and the fact that even-echo rephasing occurs on alternate echoes. Ghost artifacts are absent, because all data for a section are acquired within a small portion of a single cardiac cycle. Although flow artifacts do occur,[174] EPI has potential value as an ultrafast method for MR angiography[175] and flow quantification.[176, 177] Angiographic results are best if the data are acquired during diastole, when acceleration and associated displacement artifacts resulting from oblique flow are minimal. The EPISTAR sequence, similar to the technique described earlier but using complex subtraction, can also be used for MR angiography.[178] The long inflow times afforded by EPISTAR permit extensive lengths of the vessels to be filled by tagged protons, and the excellent background suppression and use of thick slabs for imaging make it possible to encompass the entire vessel in one section, without the need for subsequent image processing.

MISCELLANEOUS APPLICATIONS OF ECHO-PLANAR IMAGING

Rapid fetal movement, especially during the first two trimesters, makes it difficult to image the fetus with MRI. EPI freezes fetal motion and has been used to identify anomalies,[179] although its role compared with that of ultrasonography is not yet defined. Bowel peristalsis can be observed in real time.[180] Diffusion imaging allows real-time temperature monitoring,[181] at least until a tissue undergoes a phase transition (e.g., coagulation or freezing). Echo-planar MRI can be used to guide minimally invasive surgery using focused ultrasound or thermal lasers.[182] Kinematic studies of joint motion are also possible, although with lower spatial resolution than with conventional sequences.

NON–ECHO-PLANAR IMAGING USES OF ECHO-PLANAR IMAGING–CAPABLE SYSTEMS

The enhanced gradient capabilities provided by EPI-capable MRI systems can be used to improve the performance of non-EPI sequences. Interecho spacing can be reduced for fast SE sequences. One can implement TE values as short as 1 to 2 ms even with a small FOV (e.g., 20 cm). With such short TE values, GRE images show minimal or no evidence of flow-related dephasing[183] (Fig. 10–52). Ultrashort TE values may prove useful for lung parenchymal imaging by minimizing magnetic susceptibility artifacts. However, there is a reduction in S/N ratio because the readout duration must be decreased (and signal bandwidth increased) to accommodate the short TE. There is a benefit from using EPI-capable systems even for MR angiograms acquired with standard TE values, because the duration of the flow-compensating gradients can be reduced, allowing a longer readout, lower bandwidth, and therefore improved S/N ratio.

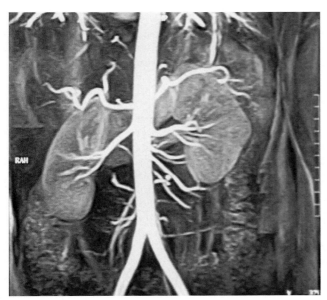

FIGURE 10–52. Maximal intensity projection from a breath-hold coronal 3D acquisition using an ultrashort TR/TE = 5/2, 32 partitions, 128 lines, 20-second breath-hold. A double dose of gadolinium chelate was given over a 30-second period. An enhanced gradient system was required to obtain such short TR/TE values.

SUMMARY OF ECHO-PLANAR IMAGING

EPI-compatible MRI equipment is gradually being introduced by commercial vendors. Considering the paucity of clinical data for such systems, choosing a system can be difficult, and, with the pace of technical development, the risk of obsolescence is substantial. Important considerations include gradient rise time and peak gradient amplitude, gradient duty cycle, multiplanar and oblique imaging capabilities, bore size (which may be reduced with gradient insert coils and certain volume gradient coil designs), availability of EPI-compatible receiver coils, pulse programming flexibility, and hardware upgradability to accommodate rapid changes in the technology. A short gradient rise time and high peak gradient amplitude are irrelevant considerations if the neuromuscular stimulation threshold precludes their use, so the latter must be carefully weighed for the particular gradient design. Also, the sensitivity of the system to gradient-induced eddy currents should be evaluated, as these can introduce artifacts especially if high dB/dt is used. If one wishes to use EPI mainly for functional brain imaging, a small gradient insert coil might suffice. Stimulation is avoided because of the small dimensions of the coil. On the other hand, one must weigh the inconvenience and time required to install and remove the coil and the inability to perform EPI of the heart, abdomen, and other areas of the body. Service issues may be particularly important in the context of EPI, as there is little long-term experience with EPI-capable systems, especially considering the severe mechanical stresses on the gradient coil and associated components.

Single-shot EPI is not a technique that is likely to replace conventional scanning protocols in the near future. The impact of single-shot EPI will be dictated by its temporal resolution and immunity to physiologic motion rather than by its spatial resolution. It will serve as an adjunct to current imaging protocols to help increase diagnostic accuracy and will be essential for optimal functional studies of the brain, heart, and abdomen. Segmented EPI techniques substantially reduce scan time and provide image quality that is competitive with that of conventional sequences but without the extreme demands on the gradients of single-shot EPI. However, segmented EPI is less versatile than single-shot EPI for functional studies. Further study is needed to determine the eventual clinical roles and cost-efficacy of EPI.

Appendix

STEADY-STATE IMAGING

Fast imaging, as described several years ago, referred mostly to a group of GRE imaging techniques that used shorter TR values than were previously possible with conventional SE techniques to obtain images in a much shorter time. Conventional fast imaging offers a variety of different tissue contrast possibilities, including proton density weighting, T1 weighting, T2 weighting, and T1/T2 weighting, depending on the state of transverse and longitudinal magnetization components with respect to T1, T2, TR, and the RF excitation angle. The term steady state refers to the presence of a constant signal for the longitudinal magnetization only or both the longitudinal and transverse magnetization components together during the application of all the RF pulses during imaging. The term steady state also provides a way to differentiate conventional fast imaging from many techniques that employ the basic sequence structures from conventional steady-state sequences to collect the data while the magnetization signal is still evolving to a steady-state condition. Here, a steady-state incoherent (SSI) technique is a technique in which only the longitudinal magnetization is maintained constant during the acquisition. Techniques that combine both longitudinal and transverse magnetization components to generate the signal are referred to as steady-state coherent (SSC) techniques. SSI and SSC form the basics of many new imaging techniques and a complete understanding is necessary to apply them successfully in new applications.

STEADY-STATE INCOHERENT TECHNIQUES

An SSI technique is an imaging modality in which the signal contribution to the image formation comes only from longitudinal magnetization that has recovered between two successive RF excitations. FLASH is an SSI technique (other acronyms are spoiled GRASS and SPGR). The signal that each SSI imaging technique provides is found by solving the Bloch equations considering that the transverse magnetization before each RF excitation does not contribute to building up the signal. The transverse magnetization can be eliminated by using gradient spoilers or by imparting a controlled phase increment to each spin isochromat through changes in the RF phase or frequency of the transmitter. Likewise, motion can destroy transverse coherences. The signal for FLASH is then given by

$$M_y^+ = \frac{M_0 \sin \alpha (1 - E_1) E_2^*}{1 - \cos \alpha E_1} \quad (A1)$$

where α is the RF flip angle, $E_1 = \exp(-TR/T1)$, and $E_2^* = \exp(-TE/T2^*)$. For sufficiently small flip angles and short TR, the image contrast is predominantly proton density weighted; otherwise, T1 contrast is possible by choosing larger flip angles. T2* weighting can be generated only by lengthening TE, making the image more sensitive to signal loss resulting from susceptibility changes between air-tissue interfaces (e.g., near the sinuses, bone, and lungs). For an SE sequence, a 90° angle is always chosen, making the signal increase in proportion to TR/T1. For FLASH, the maximal signal can be obtained by choosing the RF excitation at the optimal angle, usually referred to as the Ernst angle or α_E, for a particular TR. The Ernst angle is given by

$$\alpha_E = \cos^{-1}(E_1) \quad (A2)$$

At α_E, the signal is

$$M_y^+ = \sqrt{\frac{1 - E_1}{1 + E_1}} \quad (A3)$$

which is roughly proportional to $\sqrt{TR/2T1}$. For a fixed TR, the Ernst angle decreases as T1 increases.

STEADY-STATE COHERENT TECHNIQUES

An SSC technique uses both longitudinal and transverse magnetization components to form the image. The signal equations for SSC sequences are considerably more complex than the corresponding equation for FLASH. This additional complexity results from the persistence of transverse magnetization from one TR interval to the next. Because signal buildup relies on transverse coherences that accumulate on successive excitations, appreciable motion of any kind creates signal fluctuations in an otherwise homogeneous tissue. For moving blood and some regions where the CSF is pulsatile, the same signal that FLASH generates for the particular TR and flip angle is used during imaging.

In all the SSC techniques, the signal arises from contributions from the steady-state transverse and longitudinal components of the magnetization. The mixing of the transverse and longitudinal magnetization components is better understood if each RF excitation is considered to separate the magnetization into three components, one proportional to the longitudinal magnetization that has recovered during the interpulse interval and the other two proportional to the transverse magnetization and its complex conjugate before the RF excitation. At the RF excitation, a portion of M_{xy}^-, weighted by $\cos^2(\alpha/2)$, does not change its phase and continues dephasing until it experiences the next RF excitation; the remaining portion of M_{xy}^-, weighted by $\sin^2(\alpha/2)$, reverses its phase (similarly to the effect of a pure 180° refocusing pulse) and after being rotated by the next RF excitation is refocused by the subsequent RF pulse, producing a primary echo. The longitudinal magnetization also has components proportional to M_{xy}^- and its conjugate. The RF pulse stores these components along the z axis, and after the next RF excitation the stored M_{xy}^{-*} experiences a phase reversal to form a stimulated echo. The term M_{xy}^- after a subsequent RF pulse behaves as if its previous in-phase condition were moved forward in time by a reversal equal to the repeat time, and after being excited again by another RF pulse it generates a virtual stimulated echo. The process is repeated for all the RF pulses exciting the system until an equilibrium condition is reached. Interestingly, this simple transformation that a single RF pulse can produce can be considered one of the main building blocks of several ultrafast imaging techniques such as BURST, OUFIS, DUFIS, and QUEST. These techniques are basically the imaging extension of the stopped pulsed RF experiment that can use a conventional imaging system to generate an image by sampling the train of SEs generated during constant readout and phase-encoding gradients as opposed to those considering the acquisition of several gradient echoes to sweep k-space after a single RF excitation, as in EPI techniques.

The condition for the generation of such a delicate equilibrium is that the phases accumulated by spins within every interpulse interval must be always maintained the same. This is reflected in the construction of the different SSC sequences, in which all the phase-encoding tables applied before the acquisition window are rewound before the application of the next RF excitation while keeping the frequency-encoding and slice-selection gradient waveforms constant in every interpulse interval. Whether gradients are left balanced or unbalanced, meaning that the area integral of the gradient waveform is zero or not over a repetition interval (between the centers of two adjacent RF excitations), determines the type of contrast behavior and sensitivity to field inhomogeneities and motion, as outlined later.

As already mentioned, the SSC techniques rely on the contributions of longitudinal and transverse magnetization components to form the signal. In the design of an SSC imaging sequence, specific components of the dynamic longitudinal-transverse magnetization equilibrium can be enhanced. Two distinct signals occur: 1) the free induction decay (FID) is produced by tipping the steady-state longitudinal magnetization and the signal is read using a typical GRE structure along the frequency-encoding direction, and 2) an RF echo can be generated by refocusing the steady-state transverse magnetization with a time-reversed gradient waveform instead (often called time-reversed FID). Sequences that use the FID portion, or M_y^+, are known by several acronyms, such as FISP (fast imaging with steady-state precession), GRASS, ROAST (resonant offset averaging in the steady state), and FAST (Fourier acquired steady-state technique). On the other hand, sequences that collect the RF echo component, or M_y^-, are known as PSIF (time-reversed FISP), CE-FAST (contrast-enhanced FAST), and CE-ROAST (contrast-enhanced ROAST). Assuming for the moment that the integral of the gradient area is not zero between two RF excitations, the FID portion of the signal is given by

$$M_y^+ = \frac{M_0 \sin \alpha}{1 + \cos \alpha} \left(1 + \frac{1 + \cos \alpha - a}{\sqrt{a^2 - b^2}} \right) E_2^* \quad (A4)$$

and the time-reversed portion is given by

$$M_y^- = \frac{M_0 \sin \alpha}{1 + \cos \alpha} \left[1 + \frac{(1 + \cos \alpha) E_2^2 - a}{\sqrt{a^2 - b^2}} \right] E_2^* \quad (A5)$$

with a and b defined by

$$a = \frac{1 - E_1 E_2^2 + \cos \alpha (E_2^2 - E_1)}{1 - E_1}$$

$$b = (1 + \cos \alpha) E_2$$

The signal and contrast with M_y^- are similar to those with M_y^+ except that there is additional T2 weighting with an effective TE that is defined as the time between the echo formation and the preceding RF pulse (introduced by the term E_2^2 appearing in the numerator of Equation A5). The decay is a true T2 decay although the signal is weighted by T2*, which is computed from the time of the echo and the subsequent RF excitation.

To yield the maximal signal for a specific T1/T2 combination, it is assumed that TR is much less than T2, in which case the optimal flip angle is given by

$$\cos \alpha_{opt} = \frac{(T1/T2) - 1}{(T1/T2) + 1} \quad (A6)$$

This relation demonstrates that for tissues that have a T1/T2 ratio closer to 1, the optimal flip angle approaches 90°. Unfortunately, these techniques provide poor contrast between gray and white matter, because the T1/T2 ratio is similar for both tissues (about 10 at 1.5 T).

Alternating and nonalternating RF excitations provide the same signal for M_y^+ and M_y^- because there is a 2π integration over the resonant offset β, which is present because a nonzero gradient area is present between two adjacent RF excitations. The resonant offset for one TR is defined by

$$\beta(TR) = \gamma[\Theta_{RF} + \Delta B_f TR + x \int_0^{TR} G_x(t) \, dt$$
$$+ y \int_0^{TR} G_y(t) \, dt + z \int_0^{TR} G_z(t) \, dt] \quad (A7)$$

which is made equal to 2π to provide a homogeneous signal in an inhomogeneous main magnetic field, given by ΔB_f, and where the integrals represent the effective gradient area within TR and Θ_{RF}, the phase difference between two consecutive RF excitations. The signal is different only if a true FISP acquisition is used in which both the FID echo and the RF echo

are combined under the same acquisition window by making sure that the gradient area between RF pulses is zero. In this case, the only contributors to β are $\Theta_{RF} + \Delta B_f TR$. Thus, to obtain good results with true FISP, completely balanced gradients and perfect field homogeneity are necessary. The signal for a true FISP acquisition is given by

$$M_{xy}(TE) = \\ \frac{M_0 (1 - E_1) \sin \alpha E_2(TE) \sqrt{1 + E_2(TR)^2 - 2E_2(TR) \cos \beta}}{(1 - E_1 \cos \alpha)[1 - E_2(TR) \cos \beta] - (E_1 - \cos \beta)[E_2(TR) - \cos \beta] E_2(TR)} \quad (A8)$$

which exhibits the complicated behavior of the signal with respect to the resonant offset β. Here $E_2(TE) = \exp(-TE/T2)$ and $E_2(TR) = \exp(-TR/T2)$. Assuming a completely homogeneous field, an alternating RF excitation ($\beta = \pi$) provides a signal proportional to $\sqrt{1 + E_2(TR)}$. Otherwise, with nonalternating RF ($\beta = 0$), the signal is proportional to $\sqrt{1 - E_2(TR)}$, which provides little signal when imaging is performed at the optimal flip angle.

The optimal flip angle has an intricate dependence on β as well and it is given by

$$\cos \alpha_{opt} = \frac{E_1 + E_2(\cos \beta - E_2)/(1 - E_2 \cos \beta)}{1 + E_1 E_2(\cos \beta - E_2)/(1 - E_2 \cos \beta)} \quad (A9)$$

By varying α it is possible to obtain the optimal signal for each value of β. For β close to zero, the optimal angle is low, whereas for β close to π, the optimum occurs at higher flip angles. In any case, the signal generated for any value of β is always the same. Nevertheless, small variations in β around zero produce rapid signal fluctuations, whereas values close to $\beta = \pi$ have broader maxima and hence less variation with small variations in β around $\beta = \pi$.

The signal is roughly independent of TR as long as TR is kept much shorter than T2 for all the SSC techniques. If we forget for a moment readout bandwidth arguments, the optimal TR is always the shortest possible with the system hardware. Unless a technique collecting M_y^- is used, in which T2 weighting is introduced by lengthening TR, TR should be always the shortest possible to obtain the best S/N ratio (additional averaging can be performed by keeping a short TR). Also, by keeping a low flip angle (which reduces the weighting of transverse coherences generated several TRs before the current acquisition window), better T2 weighting is possible for M_y^-, although an S/N penalty is paid because of the lower flip angles used. Among all the techniques, true FISP provides the best S/N ratio because it combines both FID and RF echo components. True FISP is also less susceptible to the motion that may destroy the delicate transverse coherence because it is intrinsically velocity compensated and variations in β are small between adjacent intervals even when motion is present.

IMAGING DURING NON–STEADY-STATE CONDITIONS

Many of the current fast imaging techniques do not refer as much to imaging under steady-state conditions but take advantage of short TR and a magnetization preparation period to create a specific contrast or to choose specific k-space trajectories to collect data in a more efficient fashion. In the magnetization-prepared techniques, the signal development during the approach to equilibrium can better determine the contrast in the final image by managing appropriately the evolution of the transient behavior between thermal equilibrium and steady state as it relates to the trajectory chosen to cover k-space.

In general, images collected with FLASH during the approach to equilibrium lack tissue contrast. The magnetization preparation period permits modification of the initial longitudinal magnetization and increases the tissue contrast. Thus, to increase T1 weighting, an inversion pulse can be introduced to affect the initial longitudinal magnetization before data collection. The treatment used to calculate the signal is analogous to the one described for the approach to equilibrium without the magnetization preparation structure.

The magnetization of a spin system experiences a dynamic evolution when driven by a string of RF pulses. Depending on the imaging parameters, the application of multiple RF pulses leads to the establishment of a steady-state or equilibrium condition. Imaging during the transient behavior, before the establishment of an equilibrium condition, has been exploited extensively with many GRE techniques to improve the S/N ratio and obtain different tissue contrasts with short imaging times.

The characteristics of the magnetization signal during this approach to equilibrium are dependent on the type of imaging sequence as well as imaging parameters with respect to the T1 and T2 properties of the tissues. For instance, for TR values shorter than T2, the approach to equilibrium is rather complex and involves a mixture of transverse and longitudinal magnetization components that regain coherence at every RF excitation (e.g., when using SSC techniques). Nonetheless, depending on the sequence structure chosen and the state of "motion" in the tissue, the signal received is weighted only by the longitudinal magnetization component or by both the longitudinal and transverse magnetization components. The advantage of the latter is that the utilization of the transverse magnetization can lead to substantial increases in the S/N ratio when tissues are stationary.

FLASH is the most frequently utilized sequence because it permits shorter TR values and hence faster acquisitions. Another reason for using FLASH is its simple structure and smooth approach to equilibrium, which has only a mild filtering effect on the final image. The approach to equilibrium is driven by

$$M_y^+(n) = M_0 \sin \alpha [M_s + (1 - M_s) r^{n-1}] \quad \text{for } n \geq 1 \quad (A10)$$

where $r = E_1 \cos \alpha$, $E_1 = \exp(-TR/T1)$, $M_s = (1 - E_1)/(1 - r)$, and n indicates the number of RF excitations seen by the system from thermal equilibrium conditions. The rate at which equilibrium is reached is dependent only on T1, TR, and the RF excitation angle α. Also, assuming a steady TR much less than T1, the approach for low flip angles (1° to 3°) is long. For example, for TR = 5 ms, a flip angle of 2°, and T1 = 1200 ms, it takes

approximately 400 RF excitations to come within 5% of the steady-state signal. However, the starting value is only 9% away from the equilibrium value. Evaluating the limit as $n \to \infty$, Equation A10 converges to the well-known signal at equilibrium conditions for FLASH imaging, as described by Equation A1.

Note that Equation A9 has been written in a form that permits the visualization of a steady-state component (first term) and a transient component (second term), the latter decreasing in strength with a larger value of n. The introduction of magnetization preparation before data collection modifies only the coefficient that accompanies the term r^{n-1}. This permits a compact expression for the interpretation of the signal dynamics during the approach to steady state in all the fast imaging sequences using a FLASH readout module and a magnetization preparation before data collection. A more general expression is

$$M_0 \sin \alpha [M_s + (M_t - M_s) r^{n-1} cb] \quad \text{for } n \geq 1 \quad (A11)$$

in which the term M_t is directly related to the state of the magnetization after the application of the particular RF scheme that encodes the desired contrast (e.g., T1, T2, diffusion weighting). Equations A12 indicate some useful values for M_t.

$$M_t = 1 \quad (A12a)$$

$$M_t = 1 - 2E_{TI} \quad (A12b)$$

$$M_t = \frac{M_s q(1 - r^{N-1}) + 1 - E_{TW}}{1 - qr^{N-1}} \quad (A12c)$$

$$M_t = \frac{E_{TI}[M_s q(r^{N-1} - 1) + E_{TW} - 2] + 1}{1 - E_{T1} qr^{N-1}} \quad (A12d)$$

where

$$
\begin{aligned}
E_1 &= \exp(-TR/T1) \\
r &= E_1 \cos \alpha \\
M_s &= (1 - E_1)/(1 - r) \\
E_{TI} &= \exp(-TI/T1) \\
E_{TW} &= \exp(-TW/T1) \\
q &= E_{TW} \cos \alpha
\end{aligned}
$$

Equation A12a demonstrates that the longitudinal magnetization starts from M_0 for a simple 2D FLASH experiment that collects data during the approach to steady state. Equation A12b is the typical signal received for a turboFLASH experiment in which an inversion pulse is used and TI is the inversion time to the start of data collection. Equations A12c and A12d are general extensions of Equations A12a and A12b in which the experiment is repeated with an effective pause or recovery interval, TW, between experiments. The latter expressions are useful for scans in which k-space segmentation is used to collect the data, permitting the calculation of the exact timing for a TI and TW that null a particular tissue when TW is not infinity, as in the case of Equation A12a and Equation A12b.

The approach to equilibrium for SSC sequences is not as easily visualized as in the case of SSI sequences, as in FLASH, because, as outlined before, the transverse magnetization plays a major role in the signal formation. This case is not treated here because it involves a direct simulation of the Bloch equations and the analytic solutions are not straightforward.

FILTERING EFFECTS WITH MAGNETIZATION-PREPARED SCANS

Nonuniformity in the signal strength of Fourier lines in k-space introduces a nonideal point spread function that degrades, in general, the resolution of the reconstructed images. The filtering function that arises from the transient behavior of the magnetization for a magnetization-prepared acquisition is not as simple, as tissues with different T1 and T2 values can have radically dissimilar behaviors during the transition to steady state. Similar effects occur as well when collecting data with RARE, fast SE, or EPI (see next section), in which the effective acquisition window with respect to the T2 or T2* decay defines the loss or resolution enhancement associated.

The point spread function that affects the resolution in the reconstructed image depends on the specific pattern utilized to span k-space during the dynamic evolution of the magnetization after the magnetization preparation period. Analytic expressions for the filtering function associated with a specific phase-encoding ordering scheme may be difficult to find and numeric simulations are commonly performed. However, in the simplest case of a sequential phase-encoding data collection order, a filtering function h(k), independent of position, can be characterized by rewriting Equation A11 in terms of k, the current phase-encoding step accessed during the application of the kth RF excitation,

$$h(k) = \begin{cases} M_s + (M_t - M_s)r^{k-1} & \text{for } -\dfrac{N}{2}\Delta k \leq k \leq \left(\dfrac{N}{2} - 1\right)\Delta k \quad \text{(A13)} \\ 0 & \text{elsewhere} \end{cases}$$

where N is the number of phase-encoding steps collected with the other parameters as defined in the previous section. H(y), the filtering function in the data domain, is derived by applying the Fourier transform on h(k):

$$H(y) = M_s \int_{-K}^{K} e^{2\pi k y}\, dk + (M_t - M_s) \int_{-K}^{K} r^{k-1} e^{2\pi k y}\, dk \quad \text{(A14)}$$

where $K = 1/(2\Delta y)$ and the pixel dimension Δy is defined as FOV/N. The solution to Equation A14 becomes

$$H(y) = \frac{M_s}{\Delta y} \sin c\left(\frac{\pi y}{\Delta y}\right)$$
$$+ \frac{M_t - M_s}{r} \frac{r^{1/2\Delta y}e^{i\pi y/\Delta y} - r^{-1/2\Delta y}e^{-i\pi y/\Delta y}}{\ln r + 2\pi y i} \quad \text{(A15)}$$

The first term in Equation A15 is related to the loss of resolution resulting from the finite number of phase-encoding steps used to reconstruct the image; this effect is known as *Gibbs ringing* and it occurs for any acquisition using a finite number of phase-encoding steps. The second term, related to the dynamic of the magnetization signal during the data collection, introduces a complex filtering function with a full width at half-maximum (FWHM) that is wider when larger flip angles and a lim-

ited number of phase-encoding steps are acquired. The effects are better seen as a high-pass filtering function in which the information from edges is enhanced and more prominent when using an inversion pulse for the magnetization preparation, in which the signal for an object with a specific T1 can be well suppressed but its edges might be enhanced depending on the number of phase-encoding steps collected. The edge enhancement effect can be reduced by using a segmented k-space acquisition, which effectively reduces N to N/n_s, where n_s is the number of excitations utilized to collect each portion of k-space.

T2 FILTERING EFFECTS IN ECHO-PLANAR IMAGING

Filtering artifacts, manifested as blurring along the phase-encoding direction, arise from the long readout time needed for single-shot EPI to encode the entire raw data matrix relative to the T2* decay of most tissues. Filtering along the frequency-encoding direction is not problematic as little T2* decay occurs during the collection of each single line (0.5 to 1.2 ms). For a GRE EPI sequence, the train of echoes decays according to T2* over the entire image acquisition time. Assuming an exponential decay $e^{-t/T2*}$ starting at the time of the data collection window, the FWHM is

$$\text{FWHM} = \frac{\sqrt{3}}{\pi}\left(\frac{\text{Ta}}{\text{T2*}}\right)\Delta y \quad \text{(A16)}$$

for GRE EPI, were Ta denotes the image acquisition window. On the other hand, for an SE EPI acquisition, the FWHM is

$$\text{FWHM} = \frac{1}{\pi}\left(\frac{\text{Ta}}{\text{T2*}}\right)\Delta y \quad \text{(A17)}$$

considering an exponential decay that is symmetric about the center of the data collection window, for example, a filtering function defined by $\exp\left(\left|\dfrac{t - \text{Ta}}{2}\right|/\text{T2*}\right)$. This indicates that the filtering effects for an SE EPI scan are smaller by roughly a factor of $\sqrt{3}$ than those for a GRE EPI scan. In the case of GRE EPI, the filtering effects decrease as longer TE values are selected (T2* decay starts from the time the RF excitation is applied), whereas in the case of SE EPI filtering is the same for all TE values (T2* decay always starts at the time of the echo). The filtering function for a fast SE acquisition is similar to that of a GRE EPI scan with T2* replaced by the natural T2 decay. In this case, filtering is worse as the ETL or the echo spacing is increased.

To keep the resolution loss constrained within the pixel size along the phase-encoding direction, the length of the EPI readout should be set such that the FWHM is less than the spatial resolution Δy. Blurring can be reduced by shortening the duration of the readout period, for example, by speeding up the gradients (possible only within the physical limits of the gradient system and stimulation threshold) or by reducing the number of phase-encoding lines acquired and using a rectangular FOV acquisition or a half-Fourier reconstruction but at the expense of some loss in S/N ratio.

REFERENCES

1. Hahn EL: Spin echoes. Phys Rev 80:580–594, 1950.
2. Haacke EM, Liang ZP, Izen SH: Constrained reconstruction: a superresolution, optimal signal-to-noise alternative to the Fourier transform in magnetic resonance imaging. Med Phys 16:388–397, 1989.
3. Haase A, Frahm J, Matthaei D, et al: FLASH imaging: rapid NMR imaging using low flip-angle pulses. J Magn Reson 67:256–266, 1986.
4. Frahm J, Haase A, Matthaei D: Rapid NMR imaging of dynamic processes using the FLASH technique. Magn Reson Med 4:48–60, 1986.
5. van der Meulen P, Groen JP, Cuppen JJ: Very fast MR imaging by field echoes and small angle excitation. Magn Reson Imaging 3:297–299, 1985.
6. Buxton RB, Fisel CR, Chien D, Brady TJ: Signal intensity in fast imaging. J Magn Reson 83:576–585, 1989.
7. Van der Meulen P, Groen JP, Tinus AMC, Bruntink G: Fast field echo imaging: an overview and contrast calculations. Magn Reson Imaging 6:355–368, 1988.
8. Frahm J, Haase A, Matthaei D: Rapid three-dimensional NMR imaging using the FLASH technique. J Comput Assist Tomogr 10:363–368, 1986.
9. Chien D, Edelman RR: Ultrafast imaging using gradient echoes. Magn Reson Q 7:31–56, 1991.
10. Haacke EM, Wieloposki PA, Tkach JA: A comprehensive technical review of short TR, fast, magnetic resonance imaging. Rev Magn Reson Med 3:53–170, 1991.
11. Haacke EM, Tkach J: A review of fast imaging techniques and applications. AJR 155:951–964, 1990.
12. Crawley AP, Wood ML, Henkelman RM: Elimination of transverse coherences in FLASH MRI. Magn Reson Med 8:248–260, 1988.
13. Frahm J, Merboldt KD, Hänicke W: Transverse coherence in rapid FLASH NMR imaging. J Magn Reson 27:307–314, 1987.
14. Haacke EM, Tkach JA, Parrish TB: Reduction of T2* dephasing in gradient field-echo imaging. Radiology 170:457–462, 1989.
15. Patz S: Steady-state free precession: an overview of basic concepts and applications. Adv Magn Reson Imaging 1:73–102, 1989.
16. Gyngell ML: The steady-state signals in short repetition-time sequences. J Magn Reson 81:474–483, 1988.
17. Oppelt A, Graumann R, Barfuss H, et al: FISP. A new fast MRI sequence. Electromedica 3:15–18, 1986.
18. Hawkes RC, Patz S: Some factors that influence the steady state in steady-state free precession. Magn Reson Imaging 5:117–127, 1989.
19. Haacke EM, Wielopolski P, Tkach JA, Modic MT: Steady state free precession imaging in the presence of motion: an application to cerebrospinal fluid. Radiology 175:545–552, 1990.
20. Hänicke W, Merboldt KD, Chien D, et al: Signal-to-noise in subsecond FLASH NMR imaging. Considerations of the dynamic approach to the steady state by successive saturation. Med Phys 17:1004–1010, 1991.
21. Haase A: Snapshot FLASH MRI, applications to T1, T2 and chemical-shift imaging. Magn Reson Med 13:77–89, 1990.
22. Gyngell ML: The application of steady-state free precession in rapid 2DFT NMR imaging: fast and CE-FAST sequences. Magn Reson Imaging 6:415–419, 1988.
23. Bruder H, Fischer H, Graumann R, Deimling M: A new steady-state imaging sequence for simultaneous acquisition of two MR images with clearly different contrasts. Magn Reson Med 7:35–42, 1988.
24. Hänicke W, Merboldt KD, Chien D, et al: Signal strength in subsecond FLASH magnetic resonance imaging: the dynamic approach to steady state. Med Phys 17:1004–1010, 1990.
25. Haacke EM, Lenz GW: Improving image quality in the presence of motion by using rephasing gradients. AJR 148:1251–1258, 1987.
26. Pattany PM, Philips JJ, Lee CC, et al: Motion artifact suppression technique (MAST) for MR imaging. J Comput Assist Tomogr 11:369–377, 1987.
27. Edelman RR, Siegel J, Singer A, et al: Dynamic magnetic resonance imaging of liver cancer using gadolinium-DTPA: initial clinical results. AJR 153:1213–1219, 1989.
28. Wehrli FW, Perkins TG, Shimakawa A, Roberts F: Chemical shift-induced amplitude modulations in images obtained with gradient refocusing. Magn Reson Imaging 5:157–158, 1987.
29. Mitchell DG, Crovello M, Matteucci TM, et al: Benign adrenocortical masses: diagnosis with chemical shift MR imaging. Radiology 185:345–351, 1992.
30. Glover GH, Pelc NJ: A rapid-gated cine MRI technique. Magn Reson Annu:299–333, 1988.
31. Pelc NJ, Herfkens RJ, Shimakawa A, Enzmann DR: Phase contrast cine magnetic resonance imaging. Magn Reson Q 7:229–254, 1991.
32. Twieg DB: The k-trajectory formulation of the NMR imaging process with applications in analysis and synthesis of imaging methods. Med Phys 10:610–621, 1983.
33. Feinberg DA, Hale JD, Watts JC, et al: Halving MR imaging time by conjugation: demonstration at 3.5 kG. Radiology 1:195–197, 1986.
34. Margosian PM: Faster MR imaging: imaging with half the data. Health Care Instrum 161:527–531, 1986.
35. Haacke EM, Mitchell J, Lee D: Improved contrast using half-Fourier imaging: application to spin-echo and angiographic imaging. Magn Reson Imaging 8:79–90, 1990.
36. Haacke EM, Lindskog ED, Lin W: Partial-Fourier imaging. A fast, iterative, POCS technique capable of local phase recovery. J Magn Reson 92:126–145, 1991.
37. Haacke EM, Liang ZP, Boada FE: Image reconstruction using projection reconstruction onto convex sets model constraints, and linear prediction theory for the removal of phase, motion and gibbs artifacts in magnetic resonance and ultrasound imaging. Opt Eng 29:555–566, 1990.
38. Liang ZP, Haacke EM, Thomas CW: High resolution inversion of finite Fourier transform data through localized polynomial approximation. Inverse Problems 5:831–838, 1989.
39. Hackney DB, Lenkinski RE, Grossman RI, et al: Initial experience with fast low angle multiecho (FLAME) imaging of the central nervous system. J Comput Assist Tomogr 12:171–174, 1988.
40. Mitchell DG, Vinitski S, Burk DL, et al: Variable flip angle SE MR imaging of the pelvis: more versatile T2-weighted images. Radiology 171:525–529, 1989.
41. Melki PS, Jolesz FA, Mulkern RV: Partial RF echo-planar imaging with the FAISE method. II. Contrast equivalence with spin echo sequences. Magn Reson Med 26:342–354, 1992.
42. Melki PS, Mulkern RV, Panych LP, Jolesz FA: Comparing the FAISE method with conventional dual-echo sequences. J Magn Reson Imaging 1:319–326, 1991.
43. Hennig J, Nauerth A, Friedburg H: RARE imaging: a fast imaging method for clinical MR. Magn Reson Med 3:823–833, 1986.
44. Hennig J, Friedburg H: Clinical applications and methodological developments of the RARE technique. Magn Reson Imaging 6:391–395, 1988.
45. Johnson BA, Fram EK, Drayer BP, et al: Evaluation of shared-view acquisition using repeated echoes (SHARE): a dual-echo fast spin-echo MR technique. AJNR 15:667–673, 1994.
46. Mulkern RV, Wong STS, Winalski C, Jolesz F: Contrast manipulation and artifact assessment of 2D and 3D RARE sequences. Magn Reson Imaging 8:557–566, 1990.
47. Melki PS, Jolesz FA, Mulkern RV: Partial RF echo planar imaging with the FAISE method. I. Experimental and theoretical assessment of artifact. Magn Reson Med 26:328–341, 1992.
48. Mulkern RV, Melki PS, Jakab P, et al: Phase-encode order and its effect on contrast and artifact in single-shot RARE sequences. Med Phys 18:1032–1037, 1991.
49. Listerud JL, Einstein S, Outwater E, Kressel HY: First principles of fast spin echo. Magn Reson Q 8:199–244, 1992.
50. Vinitski S, Mitchell DG, Einstein SG, et al: Conventional and fast spin-echo MR imaging: minimizing echo time. J Magn Reson Imaging 3:501–507, 1993.
51. Oshio K, Jolesz FA, Melki PS, Mulkern RV: T2-weighted thin-section imaging with the multislab three-dimensional RARE technique. J Magn Reson Imaging 1:695–700, 1991.
52. Dixon WT, Engels H, Castillo M, Sardashti M: Incidental magnetization transfer contrast in standard multislice imaging. Magn Reson Imaging 8:417–422, 1990.
53. Melki PS, Mulkern RV: Magnetization transfer effects in multislice RARE sequences. Magn Reson Med 24:189–195, 1992.
54. Outwater E, Schnall MD, Braitman LE, et al: Magnetization transfer of hepatic lesions: evaluation of a novel contrast technique in the abdomen. Radiology 182:535–540, 1992.
55. Constable RT, Smith RC, Gore JC: Signal-to-noise and contrast in fast spin echo (FSE) and inversion recovery FSE imaging. J Comput Assist Tomogr 16:41–47, 1992.
56. Gomori JM, Grossman RI, Goldberg HI, et al: Intracranial hematomas: imaging by high-field MR. Radiology 157:87–93, 1985.
57. Thulborn KR, Wateron JC, Matthrews PM, Radda GK: Oxygenation dependence of the transverse relaxation time of water protons in whole blood at high field. Biochim Biophys Acta 714:265–270, 1982.
58. Gomori JM, Grossman RI, Yu-Ip C, Asakura T: NMR relaxation times of blood: dependence on field strength, oxidation state, and cell integrity. J Comput Assist Tomogr 11:684–690, 1987.
59. Carr HY, Purcell EM: Effects of diffusion on free precession in nuclear magnetic resonance experiments. Phys Rev 94:630, 1954.
60. Meiboom S, Gill D: Modified spin-echo method for measuring nuclear relaxation times. Rev Sci Instr 29:688, 1958.
61. Henkelman RM, Hardy PA, Bishop JE, et al: Why fat is bright in RARE and fast spin-echo imaging. J Magn Reson Imaging 2:533–540, 1992.
62. Constable RT, Anderson AW, Zhong J, Gore JC: Factors influencing contrast in fast spin-echo MR imaging. Magn Reson Imaging 10:497–511, 1992.
63. Higuchi N, Hiramatsu K, Mulkern RV: A novel method for fat suppression in RARE sequences. Magn Reson Med 27:107–117, 1992.
64. Jones KM, Mulkern RV, Schwartz RB, et al: Fast spin-echo MR imaging of the brain and spine: current concepts. AJR 158:1313–1320, 1992.

65. Norbash AM, Glover GH, Enzmann DR: Intracerebral lesion contrast with spin-echo and fast spin-echo. Radiology 185:661–665, 1992.

66. Atlas SW, Hackney DB, Listerud J: Fast spin-echo imaging of the brain and spine. Magn Reson Q 9:61–83, 1993.

67. Hennig J, Friedburg H, Stroebel B: Rapid non-tomographic approach to MR myelography without contrast agents. J Comput Assist Tomogr 10:375–378, 1986.

68. Hennig J, Friedburg H, Ott D: Fast three dimensional imaging of cerebrospinal fluid. Magn Reson Med 5:380–383, 1987.

69. Siewert B, Muller MF, Foley M, et al: Fast MR imaging of the liver: quantitative comparison of techniques. Radiology 193:37–42, 1994.

70. Outwater EK, Mitchell DG, Vinitski S: Abdominal MR imaging: evaluation of a fast spin-echo sequence. Radiology 190:425–429, 1994.

71. Mitchell DG, Outwater EK, Vinitski S: Hybrid RARE: implementations for abdominal MR imaging. J Magn Reson Imaging 4:109–117, 1994.

72. Smith RC, Reinhold C, Lange RC, et al: Fast spin-echo imaging of the female pelvis. I. Use of a whole-volume coil. Radiology 184:665–669, 1992.

73. Smith RC, Reinhold C, McCauley TR, et al: Multicoil high-resolution fast spin-echo MR imaging of the female pelvis. Radiology 184:671–675, 1992.

74. Nghiem HV, Herfkens RJ, Francis IR, et al: The pelvis: T2-weighted fast spin-echo MR imaging. Radiology 185:213–217, 1992.

75. Guibaud L, Bret PM, Reinhold C, et al: Diagnosis of choledocholithiasis: value of MR cholangiography. AJR 163:847–850, 1994.

76. Sigmund G, Stoever B, Zimmerhackl LB, et al: RARE-MR-urography in the diagnosis of upper urinary tract abnormalities in children. Pediatr Radiol 21:416–420, 1991.

77. Rothpearl A, Frager D, Subramanian A, et al: MR urography: technique and application. Radiology 194:125–130, 1995.

78. Hall-Craggs MA, Allen CM, Owens CM, et al: MR cholangiography: clinical evaluation in 40 cases. Radiology 189:423–427, 1993.

78a. Barish MA, Yucel EK, Soto JA, et al: MR cholangiopancreatography: efficacy of three-dimensional turbo spin-echo technique. AJR 165:295–300, 1995.

79. Oshio K, Feinberg DA: GRASE (gradient- and spin-echo) imaging: a novel fast MRI technique. Magn Reson Med 20:344–349, 1991.

80. Haase A: Snapshot FLASH MRI. Applications to T1, T2 and chemical shift imaging. Magn Reson Med 13:77–89, 1990.

81. Chien D, Atkinson DJ, Edelman RR: Strategies to improve contrast in k-space coverage: reordered phase encoding and k-space segmentation. J Magn Reson Imaging 1:63–70, 1991.

82. Mugler JP, Brookeman JR: Three-dimensional magnetization-prepared rapid gradient-echo imaging (3D MP-RAGE). Magn Reson Med 15:152–157, 1990.

83. Manning WJ, Atkinson DJ, Parker JA, Edelman RR: Assessment of intracardiac shunts using gadolinium-DTPA enhanced ultrafast MR imaging. Radiology 184:357–361, 1992.

84. Atkinson DJ, Edelman RR: Cine-angiography of the heart in a single breath-hold with a segmented turboFLASH sequence. Radiology 178:357–360, 1991.

85. Hennig J: Burst imaging on a clinical whole body system. In: Proceedings of the 11th Annual Meeting of the Society of Magnetic Resonance in Medicine, Berlin, August 8–14, 1992, p 101.

86. Hennig J, Hoddap M: Burst imaging. MAGMA 1:39–48, 1993.

87. Duyn JH, van Gelderen P, Liu G, Moonen CTW: Fast volume scanning with frequency-shifted BURST MRI. Magn Reson Med 32:429–432, 1994.

88. Wong EC: Magnetic Resonance Functional Neuroimaging using interleaved SUNBURST. In: Proceedings of the Second Annual Meeting of the Society of Magnetic Resonance, San Francisco, 1994, p 25.

89. Zha L, Lowe IJ: Optimized ultra-fast imaging sequence (OUFIS). Magn Reson Med 33:377–395, 1995.

90. Lowe IJ, Wysong RE: DANTE ultrafast imaging sequence (DUFIS). J Magn Reson B101:106–109, 1993.

91. Heid O, Deimling M: Quest-a quick echo split imaging technique. In: Proceedings of the 11th Annual Meeting of the Society of Magnetic Resonance in Medicine, Berlin, August 8–14, 1992, p 433.

92. Heid O, Deimling M, Huk WJ: Ultra-rapid gradient echo imaging. Magn Reson Med 33:143–149, 1995.

93. Sattin W, Mareci T, Scott K: Exploiting the stimulated echo in nuclear magnetic resonance imaging. I. Method. J Magn Reson 64:177, 1985.

94. Sattin W, Mareci T, Scott K: Exploiting the stimulated echo in nuclear magnetic resonance imaging. II. Applications. J Magn Reson 65:298, 1985.

95. Frahm J, Merboldy KD, Hanicke W, et al: Stimulated echo imaging. J Magn Reson 64:81–93, 1985.

96. Frahm J, Haase A, Matthaei D, et al: Rapid NMR imaging using stimulated echo imaging. J Magn Reson 64:81–93, 1985.

97. Warach S, Chien D, Li W, et al: Fast magnetic resonance diffusion-weighted imaging of acute human stroke. Neurology 42:1717–1723, 1992.

98. Holsinger AE, Wright RC, Riederer SJ, et al: Real-time interactive magnetic resonance imaging. Magn Reson Med 14:547–553, 1990.

99. Farzaneh F, Riederer SJ, Lee JN, et al: MR fluoroscopy: initial clinical studies. Radiology 71:545–549, 1987.

100. Riederer SJ, Wright RC, Ehman RL, et al: Real-time interactive color flow MRI. Radiology 181:33–39, 1991.

101. Taylor KJW, Holland S: Doppler US: Part I. Basic principles, instrumentation, and pitfalls. Radiology 174:297–307, 1990.

102. Cline HE, Hardy CJ, Pearlman JD: Fast MR cardiac profiling with two-dimensional selective pulses. Magn Reson Med 17:390–401, 1991.

103. Pearlman J, Moore J, Lizak M: Real-time NMR beam-directed velocity mapping: V-mode NMR. Radiology 86:1433–1438, 1992.

104. van Vals JJ, Tuithof HH, Dixon WT: Increased time resolution in dynamic imaging. In: Proceedings of the 10th Annual Meeting of the Society of Magnetic Resonance in Medicine, New York, 1992, p 1108.

105. Chenevert TL, Pipe JG: Dynamic 3D imaging at high temporal resolution via reduced k-space sampling. In: Proceedings of the 12th Annual Meeting of the Society of Magnetic Resonance in Medicine, New York, 1993, p 1262.

106. Spraggins TA: Simulation of spatial and contrast distortions in keyhole imaging. Magn Reson Med 31:320–322, 1994.

107. Liang Z-P, Hanson JM, Potter CS, Lauterbur PC: Efficient high-resolution dynamic imaging with explicit boundary constraints. In: Proceedings of the Second Annual Meeting of the Society of Magnetic Resonance, San Francisco, 1994, p 53.

108. Healy DM, Weaver JB: Two applications of wavelet transforms in magnetic resonance imaging. IEEE Trans Inform Theory 38:840–862, 1992.

109. Weaver JB, Xu Y, Healy DM, Driscoll JR: Wavelet-encoded MR imaging. Magn Reson Med 24:275–287, 1992.

110. Panych LP, Jakab PD, Jolesz FA: An implementation of wavelet encoded MRI. J Magn Reson Imaging 3:649–655, 1993.

111. Battle G: Cardinal spline interpolation and the block spin contruction of wavelets. In: Chui CK, ed. Wavelets: A Tutorial in Theory and Applications, Volume 2. San Diego, CA: Academic Press, 1992, pp 73–90.

112. Panych LP, Jolesz FA: A dynamically adaptive imaging algorithm for wavelet-encoded MRI. Magn Reson Med 32:738–748, 1994.

113. Mansfield P, Pykett IL: Biological and medical imaging by NMR. J Magn Reson 29:355–373, 1978.

114. Stehling MK, Turner R, Mansfield P: Echo-planar imaging: magnetic resonance imaging in a fraction. Science 254:43–50, 1991.

115. Edelman RR, Wielopolski P, Schmitt F: Echo-planar MR imaging. Radiology 192:600–612, 1994.

116. DeLaPaz RL: Echo-planar imaging. Radiographics 14:1045–1058, 1994.

117. Ideler KH, Nowak S, Borth G, et al: A resonant multi purpose gradient power switch for high performance imaging. In: Proceedings of the 11th Annual Meeting of the Society of Magnetic Resonance in Medicine, Berlin, August 8–14, 1992, p 4044.

118. Mueller OM, Roemer PB, Park JN, Souza SP: A general purpose non-resonant gradient power system. In: Proceedings of the 10th Annual Meeting of the Society of Magnetic Resonance in Medicine, San Francisco, August 10–16, 1991, p 130.

119. Bruder H, Fischer H, Reinfelder H-E, Schmitt F: Image reconstruction for echo planar imaging with nonequidistant k-space sampling. Magn Reson Med 23:311–323, 1992.

120. Farzaneh F, Riederer SJ, Pelc NJ: Analysis of T2 limitations and off-resonance effects on spatial resolution and artifacts in echo-planar imaging. Magn Reson Med 14:123–139, 1990.

121. Cohen MS, Weisskoff RM: Ultra-fast imaging. Magn Reson Imaging 9:1–37, 1991.

122. Butts K, Riederer SJ, Ehman RL, et al: Echo-planar imaging of the liver with a standard MR imaging system. Radiology 189:259–264, 1993.

123. Edelman RR, Manning WJ, Burstein D, Paulin S: Coronary arteries: breath-hold MR angiography. Radiology 181:641–643, 1991.

124. Farzaneh F, Riederer SJ: Hybrid imaging with gradient-recalled sliding echoes. In: Proceedings of the Seventh Annual Meeting of the Society of Magnetic Resonance Imaging, 1989, p 70.

125. Feinberg DA, Oshio K: Gradient-echo shifting in fast MRI techniques (GRASE imaging) for correction of field inhomogeneity errors and chemical shift. J Magn Reson 97:177–183, 1992.

126. Butts K, Riederer SJ, Ehman RL, et al: Interleaved echo planar imaging on a standard MR system. Magn Reson Med 31:67–72, 1994.

127. McKinnon GC: Ultrafast interleaved gradient-echo-planar imaging on a standard scanner. Magn Reson Med 30:609–616, 1993.

128. Meyer C, Hu B, Nishimura D, Macovski A: Fast spiral coronary artery imaging. Magn Reson Med 28:202–213, 1992.

129. Mansfield P, Harvey PR: Limits to neural stimulation in echo-planar imaging. Magn Reson Med 1993; 29:746–758.

130. Schmitt F, Wielopolski P, Fischer H, Edelman RR: Peripheral stimulations and their relation to gradient pulse shapes. In: Proceedings of the Second Annual Meeting of the Society of Magnetic Resonance, San Francisco, 1994, p 102.

131. Safety parameter action levels. In: Guidance for Content and Review of 510(k) Applications for Magnetic Resonance Imaging Devices. Attachment I. Rockville, MD: Center for Devices and Radiological Health, U.S. Food and Drug Administration, August 2, 1988, pp 1–2.

132. Cohen MS, Weisskoff RM, Rzedzian RR, Kantor HL: Sensory stimulation by time-varying magnetic fields. Magn Reson Med 14:409–414, 1990.

133. Budinger TF, Fischer H, Hentschel D, et al: Physiological effects of fast oscillating magnetic field gradients. J Comput Assist Tomogr 15:909–914, 1991.

134. Schmitt F: Correction of geometrical distortions in MR-images. In: Pro-

ceedings of the International Symposium on Computer Assisted Radiology, 1985, pp 14–23.

135. Siewert B, Warach S, Patel MR, et al: Value of echo-planar imaging in the detection of brain lesions. J Magn Reson Imaging 4(P):S13, 1994.

136. DeLaPaz RL, Krol G, O'Malley B: Comparisons of EP imaging and FSE for clinical brain MR imaging. J Magn Reson Imaging 4(P):S48, 1994.

137. LeBihan D: Molecular diffusion nuclear magnetic resonance imaging. Magn Reson Q 7:1–30, 1991.

138. Stejskal EO, Tanner JE: Spin diffusion measurements: spin-echoes in the presence of a time-dependent field gradient. J Chem Physiol 42:288–292, 1965.

139. Merboldt KD, Hanicke W, Bruhn H, et al: Diffusion imaging of the human brain in vivo using high-speed STEAM MRI. Magn Reson Med 23:179–192, 1992.

140. Moseley ME, Kucharczyk J, Mintorovitch J, et al: Diffusion-weighted MR imaging of acute stroke: correlation with T2-weighted and magnetic susceptibility-enhanced MR imaging in cats. AJNR 11:423–429, 1990.

141. Mintorovitch J, Moseley ME, Chileuitt l, et al: Comparison of diffusion- and T2-weighted MRI for the early detection of cerebral ischemia and reperfusion in rats. Magn Reson Med 18:39–50, 1991.

142. Moonen CTW, Pekar J, de Vleeschouwer MHM, et al: Restricted and anisotropic displacement of water in healthy cat brain and in stroke studied by NMR diffusion imaging. Magn Reson Med 19:317–332, 1991.

143. Tsuruda J, Chew WM, Moseley ME, Norman D: Diffusion-weighted MR imaging of the brain: value of differentiating between extraaxial cysts and epidermoid tumors. AJR 155:1059–1065, 1990.

144. Belliveau JW, Rosen BR, Kantor HL: Functional cerebral imaging by susceptibility-contrast NMR. Magn Reson Med 14:538–546, 1990.

145. Rosen BR, Belliveau JW, Vevea JM, Brady TJ: Perfusion imaging with NMR contrast agents. Magn Reson Med 14:249–266, 1990.

146. Rosen BR, Belliveau JW, Chien D: Perfusion imaging by nuclear magnetic resonance. Magn Reson Q 5:263–281, 1989.

147. Edelman RR, Mattle HP, Atkinson DJ, et al: Cerebral blood flow: assessment with dynamic contrast-enhanced T2*-weighted MR imaging at 1.5T. Radiology 176:211–220, 1990.

148. Warach S. Wielopolski P, Edelman RR: Identification and characterization of the ischemic penumbra of acute human stroke using echo planar diffusion and perfusion imaging. In: Proceedings of the 12th Annual Meeting of the Society of Magnetic Resonance in Medicine, New York, 1993, p 249.

149. Kucharczyk J, Vexler ZS, Roberts TP, et al: Echo-planar perfusion-sensitive MR imaging of acute cerebral ischemia. Radiology 188:711–717, 1993.

150. Aronen HJ, Pardo FS, Gazit IE, et al: Multisection MR imaging of cerebral blood volume of gliomas: clinical utility. Radiology 189(P):109, 1993.

151. Warach S, Levin JM, Schomer DL, et al: Hyperperfusion of ictal seizure focus demonstrated by magnetic resonance pefusion imaging. AJNR 15:965–968, 1994.

152. Edelman RR, Siewert B, Darby DG, et al: Qualitative mapping of cerebral blood flow and functional localization with echo-planar MR imaging and signal targeting with alternating radio frequency. Radiology 192:513–520, 1994.

153. Wang SJ, Nishimura DG, Macovski A: Fast angiography using selective inversion recovery. Magn Reson Med 23:109–121, 1992.

153a. Edelman RR, Siewert B, Adamis M, et al: Signal targeting with alternating radiofrequency (STAR) sequences: application to MR angiography. Magn Reson Med 31:233–238, 1994.

154. Gaa J, Warach S, Wen P, et al: EPISTAR perfusion echo-planar imaging of human brain tumors. J Magn Reson Imaging 4(P):S8, 1994.

155. Belliveau JW, Kennedy DN, McKinstry RC, et al: Functional mapping of the human visual cortex by magnetic resonance imaging. Science 254:716–719, 1992.

156. Ogawa S, Lee TM, Kay AR, Tank DW: Brain magnetic resonance imaging with contrast dependent on blood oxygenation. Proc Natl Acad Sci USA 87:9868–9872, 1990.

157. Ogawa S, Tank DW, Menon R, et al: Intrinsic signal changes accompanying sensory stimulation: functional brain mapping with magnetic resonance imaging. Proc Natl Acad Sci USA 89:5951–5955, 1992.

158. Kwong KK, Belliveau JW, Chesler DA, et al: Dynamic magnetic resonance imaging of human brain activity during primary sensory stimulation. Proc Natl Acad Sci USA 89:5675–5679, 1992.

159. Semelka RC, Simm FC, Recht M, et al: T1-weighted sequences for MR imaging of the liver-comparison of three techniques for single breath whole volume acquisition at 1.0T and 1.5T. Radiology 180:629–635, 1991.

160. Goldberg MA, Hahn PF, Saini S, et al: Value of T1 and T2 relaxation times from echoplanar MR imaging. AJR 160:1011–1017, 1993.

161. Müller MF, Prasad PV, Siewert B, et al: Abdominal diffusion mapping using a whole body echo planar system. Radiology 190:475–478, 1994.

162. Müller MF, Prasad PV, Bimmler D, et al: Functional imaging of the kidney by means of measurement of the apparent diffusion coefficient. Radiology 193:711–716, 1994.

163. Pykett IL, Rzedzian RR: Instant images of the body by magnetic resonance. Magn Reson Med 5:563–571, 1987.

164. Manning WJ, Li W, Edelman RR: A preliminary report comparing magnetic resonance coronary angiography with conventional angiography. N Engl J Med 328:828–832, 1993.

165. Chrispin A, Small P, Rutter N, et al: Transectional echo planar imaging of the heart in cyanotic congenital heart disease. Pediatr Radiol 16:293–297, 1986.

166. Chrispin A, Small P, Rutter N, et al: Echo planar imaging of normal and abnormal connections of the great vessels. Pediatr Radiol 16:289–292, 1986.

167. Rzedzian RR, Pykett IL: Instant images of the human heart using a new, whole body MR imaging system. AJR 149:245–250, 1987.

168. Edelman RR, Li W: Contrast-enhanced echo-planar MR imaging of myocardial perfusion: preliminary study in humans. Radiology 190:771–777, 1994.

169. Wendland MF, Saeed M, Masui T, et al: Echo-planar MR imaging of normal and ischemic myocardium with gadodiamide injection. Radiology 186:535–542, 1993.

170. Wilke N, Simm C, Machnig T, et al: First pass myocardial perfusion imaging with gadolinium: correlation with myocardial blood flow in dogs. In: Proceedings of the 11th Annual Meeting of the Society of Magnetic Resonance in Medicine, New York, 1992, p 244.

171. Wendland MF, Saeed M, Masui T, et al: Echo-planar MR imaging of normal and ischemic myocardium. Radiology 186:535–542, 1993.

172. Edelman RR, Gaa J, Wedeen VJ, et al: In vivo diffusion measurement in the human heart. Magn Reson Med 32:423–432, 1994.

173. McVeigh ER, Atalar E: Cardiac tagging with breath-hold cine MRI. Magn Reson Med 28:318–327, 1992.

174. Butts K, Riederer SJ: Analysis of flow effects in echo-planar imaging. J Magn Reson Imaging 2:285–293, 1992.

175. Goldberg MA, Yucel EK, Saini S, et al: MR angiography of the portal and hepatic venous systems: preliminary experience with echo planar imaging. AJR 160:35–40, 1993.

176. Firmin DN, Klipstein RH, Hounsfield GL, et al: Echo-planar high-resolution flow velocity mapping. Magn Reson Med 12:316–327, 1989.

177. Poncelet BP, Weisskoff RM, Wedeen VJ, et al: Time of flight quantification of coronary flow with echo-planar MRI. Magn Reson Med 30:447–457, 1993.

178. Adamis MK, Gaa J, Edelman RR: STAR (signal targeting with alternating radio-frequency) renal artery imaging. J Magn Reson Imaging 4(P):S22, 1994.

179. Mansfield P, Stehling MK, Ordidge RJ, et al: Echo planar imaging of the human fetus in utero at 0.5 T. Br J Radiol 63:833–841, 1990.

180. Stehling MK, Evans DF, Lamont G, et al: Gastrointestinal tract: dynamic MR studies with echo-planar. Radiology 171:41–46, 1989.

181. LeBihan D, Dellanoy J, Levin RL: Temperature mapping with MR imaging of molecular diffusion: application to hyperthermia. Radiology 171:853–857, 1989.

182. Cline HE, Schenck JF, Hynynen K, et al: MR-guided focused ultrasound surgery. J Comput Assist Tomogr 16:956–965, 1992.

183. Wielopolski P, Zisk J, Patel M, Edelman RR: Evaluation of ultra-short echo time MR angiography with a whole body echo planar imager. In: Proceedings of the 12th Annual Meeting of the Society of Magnetic Resonance in Medicine, New York, 1993, p 384.

Spectroscopy: Basic Principles and Techniques

LIZANN BOLINGER ■ ERIK K. INSKO

The ability of spectroscopy to monitor noninvasively metabolic processes in living systems provides an attractive complementary method of characterizing tissue for the radiologist. In many pathologic processes, metabolic changes are most likely to precede anatomic changes during disease progression and treatment. Because spectroscopy is potentially sensitive to such metabolic changes, it offers a method for early detection of new disease and can influence the success or failure of therapeutic intervention. Much of the early work in the application of ^{31}P spectroscopy to humans in a clinical setting was done to monitor tumor response to treatment.[1-3] Today, ^{1}H spectroscopy is being applied in the clinical setting to many diseases and conditions that affect the brain. In this chapter, we hope to provide an understanding of how spectroscopic data are both acquired and interpreted.

WHAT IS SPECTROSCOPY?

In general, magnetic resonance spectroscopy (MRS), unlike imaging, utilizes the frequency-encoding direction to encode chemical-shift information. This allows spectra to be obtained that can provide detailed chemical information about tissues. We can also use MRS to obtain tissue concentrations of MR-visible chemicals. Unfortunately, MRS is an inherently weak form of spectroscopy and requires that chemicals or metabolites be present in concentrations greater than 0.1 mM (detecting this low concentration is possible only in special circumstances). Therefore, even though MRS is a powerful means of noninvasively obtaining in vivo chemical information, it is limited in terms of the metabolites it can monitor. This has probably hindered its immediate use in the clinical setting, which was promised many years back. Many of the metabolites that are known a priori to be important to physicians for diagnostic or therapeutic evaluation are not present in high enough concentrations to be observed by MRS. However, with the introduction of localized spectroscopy packages on most commercial spectrometers, much research is now under way to determine the origins of the metabolites that are observable as well as their role in normal function and pathologic processes. Thus, MRS has remained a promising but as yet underutilized tool for both diagnosis and monitoring of therapeutic intervention.

WHAT IMAGING AND SPECTROSCOPY HAVE IN COMMON (THE BLOCH EQUATIONS)

Imaging can be considered the ultimate spectral localization method. It produces a spatial map of the distribution of water and fat. Mostly, this map is utilized to obtain anatomic information. However, diagnostic information has been gained by exploring the relative amounts of fat and water in tissues. This allows improved diagnostic specificity as well as more precise staging of tumors. When used in this way, imaging and spectroscopy have much in common. Likewise, despite the fact that the true description of spin is quantum mechanical, the signal observed in both imaging and spectroscopy experiments can be described by the Bloch equations. The Bloch equations are the appropriate description when discussing the interaction of magnetic fields, either stationary or rotating, with the net spin magnetization. We can ignore the quantum mechanical description of this type of interaction as long as we agree never to discuss the interactions of a single spin with an externally applied magnetic field (either $\mathbf{B}_0$ or $\mathbf{B}_1$). This interaction is appropriately addressed only by the use of quantum electrodynamics and is well beyond the scope of this chapter and most books on MR. Instead, we always utilize a net magnetization vector. Such a vector is the result of summing the magnetizations from a large number of individual spins. The equations that describe the motion of this magnetization vector in a magnetic field are called the Bloch equations.

The Bloch equations were developed by Felix Bloch[4] to describe, in a phenomenologic way, any MR experiment. These equations describe the motion of a magnetization vector in response to its interaction with magnetic fields. The equations are exactly analogous to the equations that describe the motion of a small spinning top in the large gravitational field of the earth.

$$\frac{dM_x}{dt} = \gamma(M_y B_z - M_z B_y) - \frac{M_x}{T2} \tag{1a}$$

$$\frac{dM_y}{dt} = \gamma(M_z B_x - M_x B_z) - \frac{M_y}{T2} \tag{1b}$$

$$\frac{dM_z}{dt} = \gamma(M_x B_y - M_y B_x) - \frac{M_z - M_0}{T1} \tag{1c}$$

where M_0 is the maximal equilibrium magnetization. What do these equations tell us? If a static field is applied along the z direction—that is, B_z has a nonzero value but B_x and B_y are 0—then the magnetization vector precesses around B_z.

$$\frac{dM_x}{dt} = \gamma M_y B_z \tag{2a}$$

$$\frac{dM_y}{dt} = -\gamma M_x B_z \tag{2b}$$

$$\frac{dM_z}{dt} = 0 \tag{2c}$$

Thus, M_y is converted to M_x and M_x to M_y, but M_z remains constant. To change M_z, we must apply a magnetic field that is not aligned along the z axis. Almost universally, the main external magnetic field is taken to point in the z direction. To tip the net magnetization vector, we apply a radiofrequency pulse given through the probe coil. This produces another magnetic field. For the most efficient use of power, it is best if that new magnetic field is perpendicular to the main magnetic field.

In general, the Bloch equations tell us one thing, that the magnetization vector precesses around a magnetic field. This is all it can do. The components of the magnetization, **M,** that are not aligned with the applied field precess around the field at a constant angle with respect to the field. This is the sum of what can happen in the absence of relaxation, which we address in a moment. It tells us that when a sample is placed in a magnetic field, the net magnetization vector precesses around the main magnetic field. Note that we did not describe a cone of spin vectors precessing around the main magnetic field. This does not happen; it is an often used description that is incorrect and unphysical. We would need to resort to quantum electrodynamics to describe what really does happen to each individual spin. However, the precession of the net magnetization vector is described by the classic Larmor equation:

$$\omega = \gamma B_0 \tag{3}$$

The angular frequency ω, expressed in radians per second, is equal to $2\pi f$, where f is the frequency in hertz.) Note that the frequency of precession is dependent on two parameters, the magnetogyric (or gyromagnetic) ratio, γ, which is an intrinsic property of the spin, and the strength of the static magnetic field, B_0.

When a radiofrequency pulse is applied to the sample, only the component of the B_1 field that is perpendicular to B_0 acts on the net magnetization vector. The problem with the B_1 field is that it varies in time. This introduces an extra time-dependent term into the differential equations. If the radiofrequency pulse is applied perpendicular to the static B_z field, the transverse components of the magnetic field vary in time as given by

$$B_x = B_1 \cos \omega_{RF} t \tag{4a}$$

$$B_y = B_1 \sin \omega_{RF} t \tag{4b}$$

where ω_{RF} is the frequency of the radiofrequency pulse applied. To eliminate this additional time dependence, we shift our reference coordinate system into the rotating frame. Instead of watching the B_{xy} vector precess around the main magnetic field at ω_{RF}, our frame of reference rotates at the same angular velocity, causing the vector to appear stationary (Fig. 11–1). This is similar to watching the horses on a carousel while it is rotating; it is much easier to do if we are on the carousel than if we are on the ground. Usually, we choose to have the rotating frame rotate at a frequency equal to the frequency of the radiofrequency pulse applied. This makes the magnetic field created by the radiofrequency pulse appear stationary. In addition, the equations change so that the external magnetic field now appears small. In fact, if the radiofrequency pulse applied is at the Larmor frequency of the spins, the net vector no longer precesses when not aligned with M_z but appears stationary. This is exactly analogous to the horses on the carousel appearing stationary while we are on the carousel. In that rotating frame, it is the rest of the world that is spinning. The magnetization vector now precesses around the magnetic field at a constant angle with respect to this new field produced by the radiofrequency pulse. This is summarized in the Bloch equations, which have been transformed to the rotating frame:

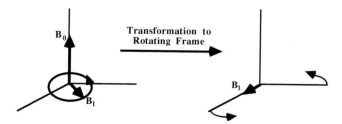

FIGURE 11–1. The rotating frame transformation. The mathematic transformation of the Bloch equations from the laboratory frame to a frame that rotates around the z axis at a rate equal to the frequency of the radiofrequency pulse removes the extra time dependence caused by the radiofrequency pulse. This is similar to viewing the world from the ground or a carousel. This transformation has physical significance because the detector on the spectrometer demodulates the MR signal from megahertz frequencies to kilohertz ranges.

$$\frac{dM_x}{dt} = (\omega_0 - \omega_1)M_y - \frac{M_x}{T2} \quad (5a)$$

$$\frac{dM_y}{dt} = (\omega_0 - \omega_1)M_x + \gamma B_1 M_z - \frac{M_y}{T2} \quad (5b)$$

$$\frac{dM_z}{dt} = \gamma B_1 M_y - \frac{M_z - M_0}{T1} \quad (5c)$$

where it is assumed that the magnetic field associated with the radiofrequency pulse is applied along the x direction and $\omega_0 - \omega_1$ is the difference in frequency between the radiofrequency pulse, ω_1, and the resonance frequency of the magnetization vector, ω_0.

The solution of the Bloch equations in special conditions allows us to explore the motion of the magnetization vector during our MR experiments. For instance, during a radiofrequency pulse applied along the x direction (also stated as a phase shift of 0) and at a frequency equal to the Larmor frequency of the spin, $\omega_0 = \omega_1$ (on-resonance), and ignoring chemical shift and relaxation during the pulse, the results of the preceding differential equations are the following:

$$M_x(+) = M_x(-) \quad (6a)$$

$$M_y(+) = M_y(-)\cos(\gamma B_1 t) + M_z(-)\sin(\gamma B_1 t) \quad (6b)$$

$$M_z(+) = M_z(-)\cos(\gamma B_1 t) - M_y(-)\sin(\gamma B_1 t) \quad (6c)$$

where the + stands for the magnetization just after the pulse and the − for the magnetization just before the pulse. This is exactly what you expect from the foregoing statement; the magnetization vector simply rotates around the $\mathbf{B}_1$ field applied in the x direction (Fig. 11–2). How far it rotates depends on the length of time the $\mathbf{B}_1$ field is applied and the strength of the $\mathbf{B}_1$ field:

$$\Theta = \gamma B_1 \tau \quad (7)$$

where Θ is the flip angle of the pulse, τ is the length of the pulse, and $\gamma B_1 = \omega_1$ is the strength of the $\mathbf{B}_1$ field, typically given in units of hertz.

Often in pulsed MR experiments, the radiofrequency pulse is not applied exactly at the Larmor frequency of the spins. This is appropriately described as applying an off-resonance pulse. When this occurs, the axis around which the magnetization vector rotates is no longer in the x-y plane (Fig. 11–3). It is raised out of the plane by an amount proportional to the off-resonance amount, $\delta\omega = \omega_0 - \omega_1$. This off-resonance $\mathbf{B}_1$ vector is called $\mathbf{B}_{eff}$. The magnetization that is off-resonance effectively feels a stronger $\mathbf{B}_1$ than the mag-

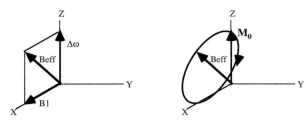

FIGURE 11–3. Off-resonance radiofrequency pulse. Radiofrequency pulses that create a $\mathbf{B}_1$ field along the x axis in the rotating frame cause the magnetization vector of spins at $\Delta\omega$ from the frequency of the radiofrequency pulse to precess not around the x axis but rather around $\mathbf{B}_{eff}$. $\mathbf{B}_{eff}$ is the vector sum of ω_{RF} and $\Delta\omega$. Off-resonance magnetization does not respond in the same way to pulses as on-resonance magnetization. Although this can cause off-resonance magnetization to be inappropriately excited, it also allows frequency-selective radiofrequency pulses to be obtained.

netization that is on-resonance. However, the axis of rotation is no longer in the x-y plane. This means, for example, that we may force the magnetization vector to rotate around the $\mathbf{B}_{eff}$ by 180° but the magnetization does not end up along the −z axis. In fact, if $\mathbf{B}_{eff}$ is 45° out of the x-y plane, a 180° rotation results in what looks like an on-resonance 90° pulse with a phase shift of 90°, in other words, a $\mathbf{B}_y$ pulse (see Fig. 11–3). This occurs when the off-resonance shift is equal to γB_1. When the radiofrequency pulse is applied far off-resonance, the fact that $\mathbf{B}_{eff}$ is stronger than $\mathbf{B}_1$ does not have much of an affect. When $\delta\omega$ is much larger than γB_1, the magnetization vector merely precesses around the main magnetic field, $\mathbf{B}_z$, as if there was no radiofrequency pulse at all.

We have not yet said anything about relaxation. In MR there are two relaxation times, T1 and T2. The two relaxation processes are independent. In general, there should be three relaxation times, one for each component of the magnetization vector. However, the application of the main magnetic field in a single direction makes the physics cylindrically symmetric and hence what would be a T_x and T_y are equivalent and not independent, so we describe them as a single value, T2. The processes in the sample that cause relaxation can all be described as a time-dependent fluctuation in the local magnetic field. Much of this fluctuation arises from the motion of the molecules that contain the spins. Fluctuations at frequencies near zero cause the local magnetic field to appear greater or less than the main magnetic field. This causes spins nearby to change their precession frequency for a short time. These spins now have a phase offset from spins that did not feel the fluctuation. Thus, we see a dephasing of the magnetization vector not dissimilar to that seen with phase encoding. However, it results from random fluctuations of the local field and is not recoverable, because these spins do not easily reverse themselves in a coherent manner. This makes the component of the magnetization vector in the x-y plane grow shorter. For T1, the local magnetic field must fluctuate at a frequency equivalent to the Larmor frequency. This is required because there must be a transfer of energy to cause T1 relaxation. This energy transfer can occur only if we put in energy at the Larmor

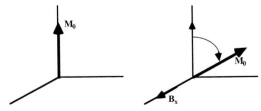

FIGURE 11–2. Effect of the radiofrequency pulse on the magnetization vector. A radiofrequency pulse that creates a $\mathbf{B}_1$ field along the x direction in the rotating frame causes the magnetization vector to precess around the x axis.

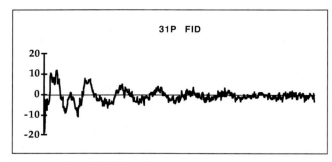

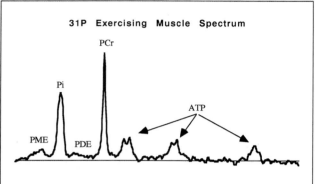

FIGURE 11–4. [31]P spectrum of human muscle. *Top,* An FID obtained after applying a 90° pulse to the exercising muscle of a volunteer. *Bottom,* When a Fourier transform is applied to this FID, the spectrum shown is obtained. Typically, seven signals are observable in ^{31}P spectra: phosphomonoesters (PME) like phosphoethanolamine, phosphocholine, inositol phosphate, and glucose 6-phosphate; inorganic phosphate (Pi); phosphodiesters (PDE); phophocreatine (PCr); and the three phosphates of adenosine triphosphate (ATP).

frequency. This fluctuation is similar to applying a radiofrequency pulse. Once again, however, it is not coherent and does not affect all the spins at once. Describing these processes in more detail is beyond the scope of this chapter and not really necessary for understanding the methods described later. Suffice it to say that T2 relaxation causes an exponential decrease in the transverse magnetization with a rate constant equal to 1/T2, and T1 causes the magnetization to return to equilibrium with a rate constant of 1/T1.

HOW DOES SPECTROSCOPY DIFFER FROM IMAGING?

The major difference between spectroscopy and imaging is the type of information found in the frequency domain. For imaging this is a spatial dimension, but for spectroscopy a chemical shift is encoded in the frequency. This occurs because the data are acquired without the application of a gradient. Thus, the simplest pulse sequence, 90°-acquire, produces a free induction decay (FID) (Fig. 11–4), in which all the spins are merely precessing at frequencies determined by the local magnetic field. A Fourier transform of this FID yields a spectrum as also shown in Figure 11–4. Spectra contain information about the chemical composition of the tissue being probed. For example, the

spectrum in Figure 11–4 is the result of a simple pulse-acquire sequence applied at the ^{31}P nuclear magnetic resonance (NMR) frequency with a surface coil placed under the gastrocnemius muscle of a man. The observable metabolites are phosphocreatine, inorganic phosphate, and adenosine triphosphate (ATP). All of these are found in muscle at concentrations in the range of 1 to 40 mM. In addition, small amounts of phosphodiesters are observed. This signal most likely arises from phospholipid bilayer precursors. This spectrum shows some features of spectroscopy that are not observable in imaging. Each of the chemically distinct phosphorus nuclei has a distinct resonance that results from an interaction with the local electron environment, resulting in a chemical shift. The three chemically distinct phosphorus nuclei on ATP have their own characteristic resonance frequencies. In addition, the phosphorus nucleus at the site of one of the phosphates is influenced by the state of the spin at the neighboring nuclei. This gives rise to scalar coupling, which is observed in these spectra as a splitting of the resonance into multiple peaks. This aids in the identification of resonance peaks. The powers of spectroscopy lie in obtaining chemical information noninvasively and in the ability to study function. Spectra of exercising muscle in real time allow kinetic information to be acquired that can be useful in diagnosing oxygen delivery problems as well as enzyme deficiencies.[5] Both ^{31}P spectroscopy and ^{1}H spectroscopy have been used for this task (Fig. 11–5).

BASIC PRINCIPLES

SPIN, RESONANCE, AND ENERGY LEVELS

The concept of spin was developed in quantum mechanics as a model for experimental observations for

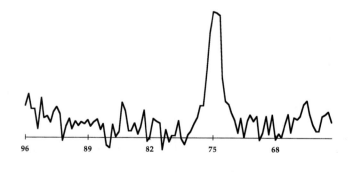

PPM

FIGURE 11–5. Deoxymyoglobin spectrum of human forearm. [31]P spectroscopy has been used as an indicator of the oxygenation state of tissues. However, in muscle a more direct indicator is myoglobin. The deoxymyoglobin signal is observable with ^{1}H spectroscopy and occurs 75 ppm downfield of the water signal. With healthy resting muscles and even healthy working muscles, the deoxymyoglobin signal is not visible. However, under ischemic conditions, such as those found in working muscles of subjects with intermittent claudication of peripheral limbs, this signal can be observed even at low mild exercise levels. The maximal possible concentration of deoxymyoglobin in human muscle is in the range 350 to 500 μM. Thus, this is the weakest signal observable by MRS. (Spectrum provided by Elizabeth A. Noyszewski, PhD, Department of Radiology, University of Pennsylvania, Philadelphia, PA.)

which there was no previous explanation. As spin is a quantum mechanical concept, we often use energy level diagrams to aid in the understanding of experimental observations. For a spin ½ system such as a proton, there are two energy levels. If we were to look at a single spin, we would have no way to know a priori whether the spin would align with the field (lower energy level for a proton spin) or against the field (the higher energy level for a proton spin). The two energy levels are simply representations of the stationary states of the system. If the spin system was not dynamic, a spin would be in one or the other of the states, but in general it is in some linear combination of these two possible states. The spin has a defined state only if we measure it. If we measured the state of a single spin many times, we would find that it was in one energy level or the other in nearly 50% of these measurements. In MR, we deal not with a single spin but with a large number of spins. Therefore, when we place a bulk sample of spins into a magnetic field, we can calculate, using statistical mechanics, the relative difference in population between the two states. Although we often say that this tells us the number of spins that are in each energy level, this is not formally true. It actually tells us only the probability of finding a certain number in that state when we measure the spins. In addition, the population difference is the magnetization that we detect in an MR experiment and it is the vector we manipulate when we utilize the Bloch equations. The polarization or the length of the vector depends directly on the strength of the externally applied static magnetic field. For typical field strengths used in modern clinical imaging systems, the population difference is about 1 part in 10^5. This is an extremely small difference. We shall find, however, that this small difference is also important and relevant.

Let us stop here and consider an important question. What is the meaning of having two preferred orientations with respect to the static magnetic field? This indicates that the nucleus has the spin property of I = ½. Not all nuclei have a spin of ½. Not even all nuclei that may be of clinical importance have I = ½. Thus, the concept of being aligned with or against the magnetic field loses it meaning. Table 11–1 lists nuclei that may have biologic relevance. Also given in Table 11–1 is the spin quantum number, I, for each nucleus. This tells us that the nuclei may be in one of 2I + 1 energy levels. For spin ½ there are two possible energy levels, but for sodium, which has a spin value of ³⁄₂, there are four energy levels (Fig. 11–6).

The difference in energy between two energy levels

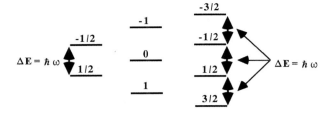

FIGURE 11–6. Energy level diagrams and quantum numbers for nuclei in a magnetic field. Notice that there are 2I + 1 levels for each spin type.

is determined by the strength of the magnetic field. This difference increases linearly with the strength of the magnetic field. We can measure this difference accurately with an MR experiment. As in most spectroscopies, when a nucleus makes a jump from one energy level to another, energy at a certain frequency is either released or absorbed. In our case, the frequency of this energy is directly proportional to the magnetic field strength:

$$E = \hbar\omega = \hbar\gamma B_0 \qquad (8)$$

where γ is the magnetogyric ratio, an intrinsic property of each nucleus with spin; ω is the frequency in radians per second; $\hbar$ is Planck's constant divided by 2π, 1.05459×10^{-34} J s; and B_0 is the strength of the magnetic field in tesla. It is a strength of MRS that we can measure the frequency extremely accurately, usually to better than 1 part in 10^8. The importance of this is discussed in the section on chemical shift.

Just as the resonance frequency increases with the magnetic field strength, so does the inherent sensitivity of the MR experiment. To first order, this increase is strictly due to an increase in the difference in spin population between the two energy levels. The difference can be calculated with the Boltzmann equation:

$$\frac{N_-}{N_+} = e^{-\Delta E/kT} = e^{-\hbar\omega/kT} \qquad (9)$$

where N_- is the population of the higher energy level; N_+ is the population of the lower energy level; k is the Boltzmann constant, 1.38×10^{-23} J/K; and T is the temperature in kelvins. At body temperature, 310.5 K, and a field strength of 1.5 T, the ratio for proton spins is 0.999990129. Unlike the situation in optics, we can observe only a small fraction of the spins when per-

TABLE 11–1. BIOLOGICALLY RELEVANT SPIN NUCLEI

NUCLEI	I	NATURAL ABUNDANCE (%)	FREQUENCY AT 1.5 T	SOME OBSERVABLE METABOLITES
^{1}H	½	100	63.89	Lactate, N-acetylaspartate, taurine, glutamate, glutamine
^{7}L				Lithium-containing drugs
^{13}C	½	1.18	16.06	Glycogen, glucose, lipids
^{19}F	½	100	60.08	Drugs containing fluorine and anesthetics like halothane
^{23}Na	³⁄₂	100	16.89	Intra- versus extracellular sodium
^{31}P	½	100	25.85	Phosphocreatine, ATP, inorganic phosphate

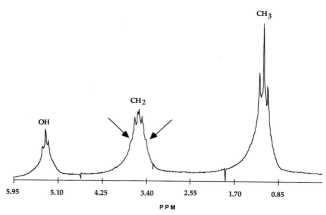

FIGURE 11–7. ¹H spectrum of ethanol at 1.5 T. This spectrum of ethanol illustrates both chemical shift and scalar coupling. Each chemically distinct proton has a specific resonance frequency. This resonance is split by scalar coupling interactions with neighboring spins. The arrows indicate the barely resolvable peaks on the shoulder of the CH₂ resonance, which help make up the doublet of quartets that is the CH₂ resonance. When water is present in the ethanol, the proton of the oxygen chemically exchanges with the protons of water and coupling of CH₂ with these protons no longer occurs. This is called exchange decoupling.

forming MRS. Note that this ratio can be decreased (i.e., we can have a larger proportion of the spins in the lower energy state) by increasing the field strength. Other factors besides the Boltzmann distribution enter into the equation for sensitivity as a function of magnetic field strength.

Chemical Shift

In addition to the main magnetic field and the radiofrequency field, there are internal local magnetic fields that affect the resonance of the spin. One of these internal magnetic fields causes the effect known as chemical shift. The best known example of this is seen in a spectrum of ethanol. Ethanol (CH_3CH_2OH) has three proton resonances because it has three chemically distinct protons (Fig. 11–7). The areas of the three resonances are in a 3:2:1 ratio, corresponding to the relative number of protons of each chemically distinct type. Because we have already learned that the frequency at which a spin resonates is proportional to the total magnetic field, we can assume that the local fields of these three types of protons are different. If we measure the difference in frequency between the three resonances as a function of external field strength, we find that it is linearly proportional to the field strength. Thus, a particular proton species has a resonance frequency that obeys the following equation:

$$\omega = \gamma(\mathbf{B}_0 + \mathbf{\Delta B}) \tag{10}$$

where $\mathbf{\Delta B}$ is proportional to $\mathbf{B}_0$. Therefore, we can define a quantity, σ, the shielding constant, that is independent of the main magnetic field.

$$\mathbf{\Delta B} = \sigma\mathbf{B}_0 \tag{11}$$

$$\omega = \gamma\mathbf{B}_0(1 + \sigma) \tag{12}$$

If σ is positive, there must be a field larger than the externally applied field at the nucleus. This additional field is caused by the local electronic environment of the nucleus. A bare nucleus, with no electrons present, would always resonate at the frequency calculated from Equation 3. Fortunately for the spectroscopist, the electrons have a great influence on the exact resonance frequency of any given nucleus. This fact can be employed to gain a great deal of chemical information about a system. The beauty of this is the potential to obtain chemical and metabolic information about tissues without a biopsy.

We can intuitively understand why the electrons create a local magnetic field that creates the chemical-shift effect. Quantum mechanics tell us that electrons are moving in atomic or molecular orbitals around the nucleus. Our experience with electricity and magnetism tells us that moving electrons create a magnetic field. Thus, we expect the electrons in the atomic or molecular orbitals to produce local magnetic fields (Fig. 11–8). In the presence of an external magnetic field, electrons have a tendency to move in directions that create a magnetic field that opposes the external field. Thus, the external field influences the movement of the electrons in both direction and speed. This in turn affects the direction and strength of the local magnetic field produced by the electrons. This is the origin of the observed behavior of chemical shift with respect to the strength of the externally applied field. We find that the amount of shift, ΔB, and therefore $\Delta\omega$, increases linearly with the applied magnetic field. This has two implications. First, at higher fields our spectral resolution in chemical shift increases. Thus, a higher external magnetic field is advantageous. The second implication is that it is impossible to compare $\Delta\omega$ values, because magnets do not all have the precisely same field strength. Thus, the concept of using a field-independent scale of parts per million (ppm) was developed. The following equation allows you to

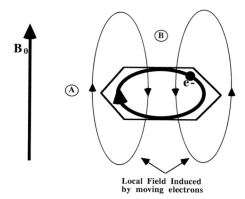

FIGURE 11–8. Local magnetic field produced by a benzene ring. A classic example of the local magnetic field produced by circulating electrons is the benzene ring. The electrons circulate in a direction that produces a magnetic field opposing the externally applied magnetic field. Thus, a nuclear spin at position B feels a net magnetic field that is less than the external magnetic field, whereas a nuclear spin at position A feels a greater magnetic field.

calculate parts per million values as long as you have a point of reference for zero:

$$ppm = \frac{\Delta f}{F_{spec}} + R \qquad (13)$$

where Δf is the difference in hertz of the resonance position from the reference, F_{spec} is the frequency of the spectrometer or carrier frequency, and R is the parts per million value of the reference peak. In all spectra, a resonance, which has been identified and has a known parts per million value, is used as the reference for all other resonances in the spectrum. For in vivo ^1H spectra, water is often used as the chemical-shift reference and is assigned a value of 4.8 ppm. However, the exact resonance frequency of water is known to vary with temperature, although not strongly over physiologic ranges. For ^{31}P spectra, phosphocreatine, which has been observed to have a stable chemical-shift value for a wide variety of physiologic conditions including changes in pH, is usually used for the chemical-shift reference when it is present in the spectrum. Otherwise, the resonance for the α-phosphate group of ATP is used.

We said earlier that the external magnetic field affected both the direction and strength of the ΔB term in the resonance equation. We have discussed the consequences of the strength but not of the direction. In general, chemical shift cannot be thought of as a single value associated with σ, the shielding value. In reality, σ is a tensor, which means that it can have different values in different directions. For most cases, the molecules that we observe tumble freely in space at a rate faster than $1/\delta\omega$, where δω is the largest frequency difference spanned by the spatial dependence of the chemical shift, and thus average out the tensor nature of σ, making it appear to be a single, spatially averaged value. However, the fact that the externally applied magnetic field has a single direction implies that if molecules do not tumble fast, the chemical shift varies if we change the orientation of the sample with respect to the main magnetic field. This is known as chemical-shift anisotropy. Chemical-shift anisotropy is always observed in solids. If molecules do not tumble fast or have restricted tumbling motion, it is possible that the chemical-shift anisotropy is only partially averaged and the lines are broadened beyond their natural T2 line width. Our samples of biologic tissues often contain liquids and solids, making it inevitable that chemical-shift anisotropy is to some extent a factor in the spectra acquired. The speed at which a molecule must tumble to average this anisotropy is field dependent, because the Larmor frequency changes with field strength, requiring that a molecule tumble faster as the field strength increases to average out chemical-shift anisotropy. As high-field magnets become more widely available for in vivo studies, incomplete averaging of chemical-shift anisotropy should become more of a problem. In addition, this incomplete averaging may partially account for the broad lines commonly seen in lipid resonances at current field strengths.

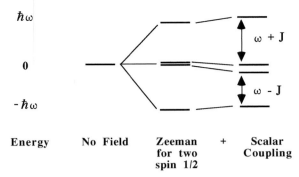

FIGURE 11–9. Energy level diagram associated with scalar coupling. When the scalar coupling interaction between two spins is added to the energy of the system, the middle degenerate energy level splits and the spacing between the energy levels is no longer the same. Thus, the resonance splits into two resonances.

SCALAR COUPLING

Many resonances are split into a pattern of resonant peaks. This is the result of a second internal interaction for nuclei, which is scalar coupling (or J coupling as it is sometimes called) (Fig. 11–9). This coupling arises from an indirect interaction of two nuclear spins via the intervening electronic structure of the molecule. Unlike chemical shift, it is not induced by an external magnetic field and is therefore always present and has no field dependence. It arises from the field produced by one nuclear spin that interacts with the electrons near it. These in turn, through chemical bonds, interact with other electrons, which then influence the field at a neighboring nucleus. The strength of this interaction is measured in hertz and is called the scalar coupling constant, J. The value for J does not change with field strength. This is why we measure its value in hertz instead of parts per million.

The number of peaks arising from the scalar coupling has to do with the number of nuclei nearby. Using ethanol as an example, we find that the CH_3 resonance is split into three resonances through the influence of the two protons on the neighboring carbon (Fig. 11–10). In turn, the CH_2 resonance is split into four peaks because of the CH_3, and this pattern is split again by a factor of 2 by the proton on the oxygen. Thus, the peak pattern for the CH_2 is called a doublet of quartets. The pattern is almost resolvable in the ethanol spectrum in Figure 11–7. When we observe the spectrum of a mixture of ethanol and water, we do not see this pattern. This is due to the chemical exchange of the proton on the OH with the water protons. This effect is discussed more in the section on chemical exchange.

There is no orientation dependence with respect to the external static magnetic field of the scalar coupling constant similar to that of chemical-shift anisotropy. However, the effect of the field strength on the scalar coupling arises in the complexity of the multiplet patterns observed. For high fields, all scalar coupling is assumed to be in the weak coupling regime. This occurs when the field strength is large enough that the chemical-shift difference in hertz between the coupled

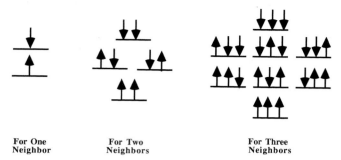

For One Neighbor   **For Two Neighbors**   **For Three Neighbors**

FIGURE 11–10. Spin states available with scalar coupling. The number of peaks that result from the splitting of a resonance by neighboring spins through the scalar coupling interaction is determined by the number of energy configurations possible for the neighboring spins. For spin ½ systems, each of the neighboring spins has two possible orientations. Therefore, for a single neighbor there are two possible energy configurations, which splits the resonance into two peaks of equal intensity. For two neighbors, there are four possible energy configurations but two have equal energy. Therefore, the resonance is split into three peaks with a 1:2:1 ratio. For three neighbors, there are eight possible combinations distributed between four energies. The resulting coupling pattern is 1:3:3:1.

resonances is much larger than the scalar coupling constant.

$$\Delta\omega >> J \qquad (14)$$

When this condition does not hold, the spin system is said to be in the strong coupling regime. At 1.5 T, it is possible for some of the spin systems of the amino acids, for example, glutamate, to be in the strong coupling regime. This means that the simple rules for evolution under the influence of scalar coupling that exist in the weak coupling case no longer apply. Thus, multiple quantum effects are bound to be more prevalent and less straightforward. As discussed later, localization sequences like those in the stimulated-echo acquisition mode (STEAM) are likely to be influenced heavily by coupling effects. Although these effects have been explored for weak coupling cases, the strong coupling cases have not yet been fully explored. This has implications for identification of resonances as well as for quantifying metabolites.

DIPOLE INTERACTION

Chemical shift and scalar coupling are two interactions that produce local magnetic fields at the nucleus through the use of electrons in the molecule. However, a nuclear spin creates a local magnetic field of its own that can be felt by other neighboring spins. This interaction, the dipole-dipole interaction, does not need electrons or chemical bonds to convey the field to the neighboring nucleus. The interaction between the two spins occurs in much the same way as the interaction between two bar magnets, through space. The strength of this interaction is dependent on the relative orientation of the two spins with respect to the external magnetic field direction and the distance between the two spins as given in the equation for the energy of the system related to this dipolar interaction:

$$E_{DD} = -\frac{\mu_1\mu_2}{r^3} + \frac{3(\mu_1 \cdot r)(\mu_2 \cdot r)}{r^5} \qquad (15)$$

where **r** is the vector distance between spin 1 and spin 2 and μ_1 and μ_2 are the spin magnetic moments given by $\gamma\hbar\mathbf{I}$, where **I** is the nuclear spin quantum number. Figure 11–11 illustrates this equation. From this equation it is clear that the distance dependence for the dipole-dipole interation is $1/r^3$. Therefore, the local field created by one spin falls off rather rapidly. For dipolar coupling to occur, the spins must be relatively close, usually within 3 to 6 Å.

In addition to the distance dependence, the strength of the dipolar coupling is determined by the relative angle the vector connecting the two spins makes with the external magnetic field. When this angle is 54.7°, the so-called magic angle, the dipolar interaction is zero and has no affect on the signal. The dipolar interaction acts to couple the two spins together in much the same way as scalar coupling. The energy level diagram in Figure 11–12 illustrates the effect dipolar coupling has on the energy levels. The result of dipolar coupling is a shift in the resonance frequency of the spins. The size of this shift is dependent on the strength of the dipolar coupling constant. The result is an angle-dependent frequency shift much like that discussed for chemical-shift anisotropy. Except in the case of single crystals, whose spectrum is a single narrow line that shifts its resonance position as the crystal orientation in the field is changed, dipolar coupling acts to broaden the resonance lines. In small molecules that can tumble rapidly at rates that are high compared with the dipolar coupling constant, a narrow resonance is still observed, which is the population-weighted average resonance position of all possible angles. Thus, it looks as if the dipolar interaction is zero. However, some biologic molecules tumble slowly enough to allow dipolar broadening to occur. This broadened line can be observed in the ^{31}P MR spectrum of phospholipid vesicles. Signals from these phospholipids can be observed in a ^{31}P spectrum of brain,[6] as shown in Figure 11–13.

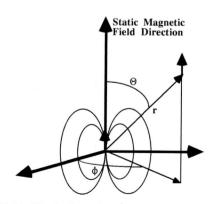

Static Magnetic Field Direction

Θ

r

ϕ

FIGURE 11–11. Dipole-dipole interaction between two spin ½ nuclei. Each spin creates a local magnetic field much like that of a bar magnet. The strength of the field felt by a second spin is dependent on both the distance between the spins, r, and the angle the vector between the two spins makes with the direction of the external magnetic field, Θ.

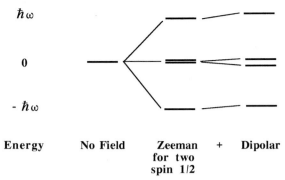

FIGURE 11–12. Energy level diagram resulting from dipolar coupling. Dipolar coupling between two spin ½ systems acts much the same as scalar coupling on the energy levels. The difference is that the exact positions of the energy levels changes with orientation of the two spins relative to the external magnetic field. If the two spins change their relative orientation rapidly with respect to the maximal value of the dipolar coupling, the interaction averages to zero. Therefore, in many liquids this coupling is not observed as a splitting of the resonance but the interaction remains a source of relaxation.

The dipole interaction is also a mechanism by which relaxation can occur. Random motions of molecules in solution cause randomly fluctuating local magnetic fields, which is a requirement for relaxation. An indication that relaxation occurs by dipolar interaction can be obtained by measuring the nuclear Overhauser effect (NOE). This is measured by perturbing one type of spin in the dipolar coupled pair and seeing the effect it has on the signal from the other spin. If one of the spin species is a slow-moving molecule, a reduction of the signal intensity is observed in the signal for the second spin species. This is part of the interaction responsible for the reduction in water signal observed in magnetization transfer contrast imaging. However, if both spin types tumble fast, we get an increase in signal intensity. This is often used to enhance the signal intensity of ^{13}C spectra. Figure

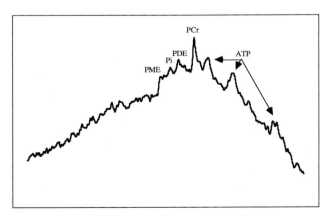

FIGURE 11–13. ^{31}P spectrum of human brain. This spectrum was acquired with a 10-cm surface coil placed on the back of the head of a healthy human volunteer. A pulse optimized to give maximal signal was used. The repetition time TR was 4 seconds and total data acquisition time was 1 minute. The broad resonance below the signals from the phosphorus metabolites is not a baseline problem but a resonance from the dipolar-broadened signal of phospholipids in membrane bilayers.

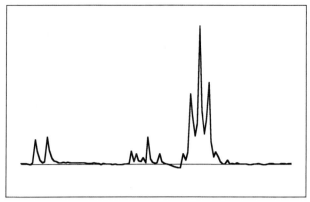

FIGURE 11–14. ^{13}C spectrum of human quadriceps muscle. Natural abundance ^{13}C spectra are difficult to obtain because of the low percentage (1%) of the ^{13}C isotope. However, the lipid and fat resonances are quite prominent in this spectrum, which was obtained in about 5 minutes from a normal volunteer using a surface coil and nuclear Overhauser enhancement via dipole-dipole interactions between the ^1H nuclei and the carbon nuclei to which they are attached. Use of ^{13}C to study lipid storage disorders or glycogen buildup in muscle has often been proposed. Most clinical scanners do not have the second radiofrequency channel necessary to perform the NOE experiment. Thus, widespread use of ^{13}C spectroscopy is not currently possible. (Spectrum provided by Keith Kendrick, PhD, Department of Radiology, University of Pennsylvania, Philadelphia, PA.)

11–14 shows a natural abundance ^{13}C spectrum of muscle lipids that was enhanced via the dipolar interaction between the ^{13}C nuclei and the ^1H nuclei directly attached to them.

QUADRUPOLE INTERACTION

Most biologically interesting nuclei have spin ½. However, several biologically interesting nuclei have spin greater than ½. The implications of having spin greater than ½ are many. There are no longer only two different spin states. In nuclei of spin I = 1, such as deuterium, there are three possible spin states separated by equal energy. In nuclei of spin I = ³⁄₂, there are four possible spin states separated by equal energy. The number of accessible nondegenerate spin states of different energy is computed as 2I + 1 and the energy levels as $I\hbar\omega B_0$, where the spin states, I, are ³⁄₂, ½, −½, and −³⁄₂. Because the spin energy levels are all separated by equal energies, the spectral lines of all possible spin flip ($\Delta m = \pm\frac{1}{2}$) transitions occur at the same frequency. Another difference between spin ½ and spin greater than ½ is that nuclei of spin greater than ½ have nonspherical charge distributions. Any nucleus with a nonspherical charge distribution is said to have a nonzero quadrupole moment, **Q**. Quadrupole moments can be either greater than zero, as in nuclei with prolate charge distributions, or less than zero, as in nuclei with oblate charge distributions.

Such nonspherical charge distributions create the opportunity for a different type of spin interaction. We are already familiar with the dipole-dipole interaction that occurs between spin dipole nuclei that have spher-

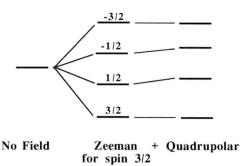

**No Field   Zeeman + Quadrupolar
for spin 3/2**

FIGURE 11–15. Energy level diagram for quadrupole interaction. The quadrupole interaction changes the energy levels of a four-level system in much the same way as scalar and dipolar coupling. The difference is that two spins are not coupling through some interaction; rather, an electric field gradient is perturbing the system. In the absence of the electric field gradient, the energy levels are equally spaced and therefore only one resonance is observed. The presence of an electric field gradient causes an unequal shift of the two outer energy levels compared with the two inner levels. The result is three different spacings between the four levels, and thus three resonance peaks are observed.

ical charge distributions. In nuclei with nonzero quadrupole moments a different type of energetic interaction occurs when the nucleus enters a region of space with an electric field gradient. In such a region, the nonspherical charge distribution has a preferred orientation or lower energy state. Thus, it is clear that the electric field gradient energetically couples to the quadrupole nucleus to a degree that depends on both the strength of the electric field gradient and the quadrupole moment of the nucleus.[7, 8] In doing so, it shifts the energy levels of the spin states such that they are no longer separated by equal amounts (Fig. 11–15). Thus, the spectral lines of all the $\Delta m = \pm \frac{1}{2}$ spin

flip transitions, which were once degenerate, are now spectrally distinct. In addition, spin flip transitions $\Delta m > \pm \frac{1}{2}$, which were previously not allowed by the so-called selection rules, are now possible. Thus, multiple quantum transitions may occur when the quadrupole interactions are strong.

^{23}Na has perhaps the most biologically important quadrupole nucleus. Because of its highly nonspherical nucleus it has a strong quadrupole interaction with electric field gradients that typically occur in association with larger molecules such as proteins. This interaction provides the dominant source of relaxation in ^{23}Na and leads to rather short T1 and T2 relaxation times. In addition, the large quadrupole interaction experienced by sodium ions bound to large protein complexes with associated electric field gradients allows the creation of multiple quantum coherences.[9–11] The multiple quantum coherences created in ^{23}Na may be of particular interest because they occur only when sodium is bound to a large molecule (Fig. 11–16). Sodium certainly binds to proteins, and to a first approximation any sodium that displays quadrupole relaxation–induced multiple quantum coherences is intracellular. Thus, any shifts in the sodium pool from extracellular to intracellular would probably affect both the character and the size of the multiple quantum signal observed. However, sodium also binds to albumin and proteoglycans associated with connective tissues such as cartilage, tendons, or ligaments. Therefore, not all multiple quantum signals from sodium need arise from intracellular sodium.

MAGNETIZATION TRANSFER

In general, the population difference (or magnetization) established when a sample is placed in a mag-

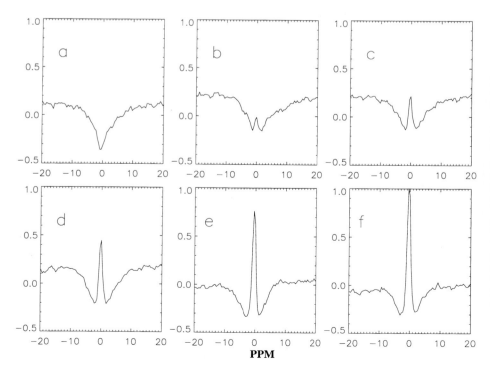

FIGURE 11–16. Double-quantum filtered sodium spectra of human skeletal muscle in vivo. The spectra from *A* through *F* were obtained with increasing time allowed for the relaxation-induced multiple-quantum signal to build up. The negative lobes on the sides of the resonance are part of the normal line shape of a double-quantum sodium signal. Because sodium relaxes rapidly, both TR, 0.3 second, and the buildup times, 0.4, 0.5, 0.6, 1.0, 2.0, and 3.0 ms for *A* through *F*, are short. The double-quantum signal is not visible unless some portion of the sodium in the muscle is bound to proteins or other macromolecules. (Spectra provided by Ravinder Reddy, PhD, Department of Radiology, University of Pennsylvania, Philadelphia, PA.)

PPM

netic field and calculated by using the Boltzmann equation is not a value we can change easily. However, when two spins are coupled through some process such as dipolar coupling, scalar coupling, or chemical exchange processes, we can employ these interactions to transfer magnetization between spins by redistributing the spins in the available energy levels. We can use any or all of these processes to transfer magnetization. This transfer may be obtained in a number of different ways, and the information obtained exposes numerous facts about the interacting spins and their local environment. We begin by exploring chemical exchange processes that allow us to determine tissue pH, to study enzyme kinetics in vivo, and even to play havoc with spectral resolution. Next, we discuss the NOE, which is partially responsible for magnetization transfer contrast imaging but can also be used in some cases to improve the sensitivity of spectra. The final topic is polarization transfer via scalar coupling, which may also be used to improve sensitivity, help identify the chemicals with which resonant peaks are associated, and even edit spectra so that only the spins associated with chemicals of interest are observed.

Chemical Exchange

Chemical exchange effects can be explored by studying two spins jumping between two different chemical environments. When there is no jumping, we observe two distinct resonance peaks as depicted in Figure 11–17. Now let us explore what happens if one of the molecules containing an A spin is converted through a chemical process to the B-type molecule. When the chemical changes from A to B, spin A now feels the local magnetic field of a B spin. Thus, its chemical shift has now changed to the resonance frequency of a B spin. When this happens, the signal intensity of A decreases because the old spin A is now resonating at the frequency of spin B. The signal intensity of the B resonance increases. If spins jumped only from the A environment to the B environment, we would soon see no more A. However, in many chemical exchange events, B is also converted to A. If the exchange rate

in both directions is low compared with the difference in frequency of the two resonances, $1/\Delta\omega$, we would still detect two distinct resonances. Now if the exchange rate between A and B is increased, we observe that the resonant lines for A and B begin to broaden. The spin that was in the A environment at the beginning of data acquisition suddenly jumped to the B environment while the acquisition was in progress. Thus, the spin spent some time at the A frequency and some time at the B frequency. This process acts similarly to a dephasing at the second frequency. Thus, the lines broaden in a T2-like process. In addition, the mean frequency value of each resonance begins to move toward the other resonance. It is as if the resonance frequencies of the two spins are some average of the two frequencies weighted by the length of time the magnetization stays at each frequency.

Now as the exchange rate increases, the two broad lines coalesce into one broad line. At this point the spins are exchanging between two chemical environments at a rate similar to the reciprocal of the difference between the two original resonance frequencies. If the exchange rate increases beyond this point, this single line begins to narrow. The line narrows because at this exchange rate, all spins appear to be in a similar average magnetic field. The exact value of this average field is related to the populations of the two chemical environments and the exchange rates. When the chemical reaction is at equilibrium, the center of this now chemical exchange–narrowed line is determined by a population-weighted average of the original resonant positions of A and B. Thus, the resonance need not be in the center of the two original resonances but appears nearer to the resonant position of the spin environment with the most spins. This phenomenon is critical in measuring cellular pH. It also explains the narrow lines seen in the spectra of liquids compared with those of solids in terms of chemical-shift anisotropy. In fact, we may think of the tumbling of the molecules as an exchange process. The local magnetic environment of the spin in a molecule changes as the molecule tumbles because the external magnetic field that induces chemical shift has a specific, static spatial

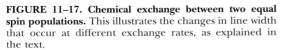

FIGURE 11–17. **Chemical exchange between two equal spin populations.** This illustrates the changes in line width that occur at different exchange rates, as explained in the text.

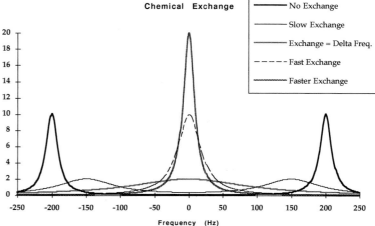

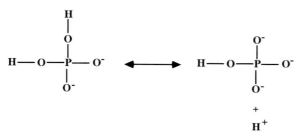

FIGURE 11–18. Inorganic phosphates. The two forms of inorganic phosphate responsible for pH-dependent chemical shift of the inorganic phosphate resonance.

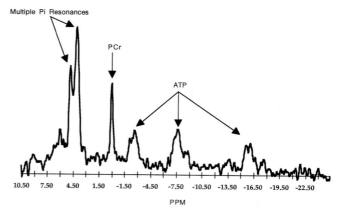

FIGURE 11–19. ^{31}P NMR spectrum of an exercising human gastrocnemius muscle. The two inorganic phosphate resonances indicate that some of the muscle fibers ar at a different pH than others. This may be due to the different metabolic responses of muscle fiber types of exercise[59] or differential activation of fibers. (Data provided by Sarah Englander, PhD, Department of Radiology, University of Pennsylvania, Philadelphia, PA).

direction. As the molecule rotates in the external magnetic field, the electron motion changes with respect to the molecule and thus the local magnetic environment changes as well. This results in a broadened line if the molecule tumbles slowly as compared with the maximal difference in chemical shift caused by chemical-shift anisotropy.

One of the most useful aspects of rapidly chemically exchanging systems in vivo is that they allow noninvasive monitoring of intracellular pH, the result being that the exact chemical shift of a resonance is determined by the pH of the environment in which the molecule exists. Figure 11–18 shows the two protonated forms of inorganic phosphate that are the basis for the ^{31}P MRS determination of intracellular pH. The resonance frequency of A, the diprotonated form, would be 5.7 ppm from phosphocreatine if it was the only form present, and for B it would be 3.3 ppm. At pH values between 5.0 and 8.0, a solution of inorganic phosphate has a mixture of these two forms, which exchange rapidly enough that in the phosphorus spectrum we observe only one resonance. The exact resonance position of this peak changes as a function of pH because the relative concentrations of HPO_4^{2-}, the basic form, and $H_2PO_4^{-}$, the acidic form, change. The ability to determine intracellular pH noninvasively has become one of the most important capabilities of ^{31}P NMR[12] (Fig. 11–19):

$$pH = 6.75 + \log\left(\frac{\delta\omega - 3.3}{5.8 - \delta\omega}\right) \qquad (16)$$

Not only can we use the fast exchange processes seen in vivo to obtain information about the workings of the cell, we can also use the slow exchange times when there are still two distinct peaks. One example of this is the use of the saturation transfer experiment to study enzyme kinetics. For example, creatine kinase catalyzes the reaction

$$PCr + ADP + H^+ \rightleftharpoons Cr + ATP$$

The resonance of the γ-phosphate of ATP is saturated with a long low-power radiofrequency pulse. This phosphate is in chemical exchange with the phosphate on PCr. During the saturation pulse, the two chemical pools mix and the phosphate nuclei that were on the ATP during the saturation pulse but jumped to a PCr molecule remain saturated. When we observe this spectrum we notice first that there is no γ-phosphate peak

because of the direct saturation and the PCr resonance has decreased. The amount of decrease of the PCr resonance depends 1) on the length of the saturation pulse and 2) on the T1 recovery of PCr (Fig. 11–20). There are several ways to perform this experiment, but they all involve perturbing one of the resonances through saturation or inversion and then observing the effect this has on the spectrum.

Nuclear Overhauser Effect

A second form of magnetization transfer occurs via relaxation processes. In general, a transfer of energy is

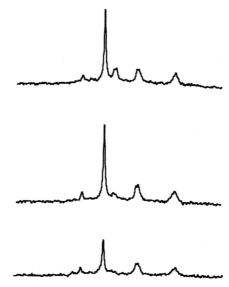

FIGURE 11–20. Saturation transfer data. The three spectra shown are part of a saturation transfer data set for resting human gastrocnemius muscle. The top spectrum is the normal one with no saturating pulse. The middle spectrum was taken after a saturation pulse applied at the resonance of γ-phosphate of ATP for 0.3 second. For the bottom spectrum, the saturation pulse was left on for 4.8 seconds. Note the reduction in the PCr signal caused by a chemical exchange of the γ-phosphate of ATP with the phosphate on PCr.

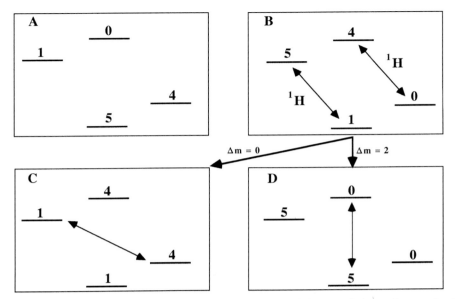

FIGURE 11–21. Population diagram explanation of the NOE. *A,* Relative populations of energy levels for a ^{13}C-^1H spin system. The ratio of the magnetogyric ratios for ^1H and ^{13}C is approximately 4. Therefore, the relative population difference between the ^1H energy levels and the ^{13}C energy levels is also 4 as determined by the Boltzmann distribution. *B,* Population diagram after a 180° pulse has been applied at the ^1H frequency. The 180° pulse acts to invert the population distribution of the ^1H energy levels. The NOE occurs because of dipolar relaxation resulting from a transfer of energy between two spins that are spatially close. This can occur in two ways: by a $\Delta m = 0$ total transition, $|-+>$ to $|+->$, as shown in *C,* or by a $\Delta m = 2$ total transition, $|-->$ to $|++>$, as shown in *D.* The result is quite different in these two cases. The $\Delta m = 0$ process makes the ^{13}C energy levels have a negative enhancement. This happens if the molecules containing the two spins tumble slowly with respect to the difference in resonance frequency between the ^{13}C and ^1H. If the molecule tumbles fast, the $\Delta m = 2$ process dominates and a positive enhancement of the ^{13}C signal occurs. In general, these two mechanisms compete as does the $\Delta m = 1$ relaxation process, so full enhancement is rarely achieved.

needed for T1 relaxation to occur. To transfer energy, there must be some process ready to acquire that energy. Often, this is another spin that is located close to the first spin. We have already discussed a process, dipolar coupling, that could cause such a relaxation process. The beauty of this process is that we can use it to our advantage to increase the sensitivity of some of our weaker spectroscopy experiments. Historically, this has been most important for ^{13}C spectroscopy. The polarization of the protons attached to the ^{13}C nuclei can be used to enhance the ^{13}C signal. Figure 11–21 shows the population diagram that helps explain this process. The pathway of cross-relaxation, $\Delta m = 0$, shown in the figure is partly the source of magnetization transfer that allows magnetization transfer contrast imaging to be performed. This is usually a transfer of magnetization between large bulky molecules and water via an NOE-like process and chemical exchange. It results in a negative enhancement of the signal and thus a decrease in the signal intensity in the images. In addition, the NOE associated with saturating the water proton signal and transferring magnetization to the ^{31}P signal can be observed in the ^{31}P spectra of muscle shown in Figure 11–22. This signal enhancement is surprising, because the water protons cannot get close to the phosphorus nucleus in the middle of a phosphate group. However, this NOE is utilized to increase the sensitivity of ^{31}P spectra to increase the time resolution of many dynamic experiments, such as the study of recovery of PCr in muscle after exercise.

Polarization Transfer

The third form of magnetization transfer is called polarization transfer. It utilizes scalar coupling to couple two spins together in much the same way as the NOE uses dipolar coupling. However, this process is governed not by relaxation processes but rather by scalar coupling evolution. Thus, it can occur on a shorter time scale and does not require random processes in order to occur. The time required for enhancement to occur is determined by the scalar coupling constant between the two spins. This magnetization transfer approach has been utilized to obtain lactate signals in the presence of fat, a technique called spectral editing. Figure 11–23 demonstrates polarization transfer using energy level diagrams and selective pulses. The trick is to redistribute the spin population so that the observed spin has an increased population and is therefore observed with increased signal intensity. This is done at the expense of the population of the second spin, which we can arrange to be uninterested in. Because the efficiency of this method depends on the coupling constant value, the enhancement can be accomplished quite selectively.

MULTIPLE-QUANTUM EFFECTS[13]

For any spin flip transitions to occur, the appropriate type of energetic spin interaction must be present. For

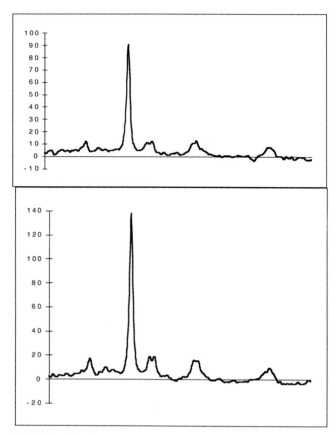

FIGURE 11–22. ³¹P spectra of resting human gastrocnemius muscle without and with NOE. *Top,* Normal ³¹P spectrum of human gastrocnemius muscle at rest. The data were acquired with an 8-cm surface coil placed under the gastrocnemius muscle of a human volunteer. A simple pulse-acquire sequence was used with a TR of 4 seconds. *Bottom,* The same spectrum except that a low-power pulse was applied at the ¹H frequency at all times except during the ³¹P pulse and data acquisition. Note the increase in signal intensity of all the resonances as a result of an NOE between the ¹H and ³¹P nuclei.

example, radiofrequency pulses couple directly into spin systems, resulting in transitions between spin states in which the spin quantum number, m_I, changes by ± 1 ($\Delta m_I = \pm 1$). In simple spin ½ systems such as the proton, we refer to the two spin states as *spin up* and *spin down* and a transition between such states as a *spin flip*. In systems with more than one spin energy state, however, the concepts of spin up, spin down, and spin flip transitions become much less clear and are appropriately abandoned.

The simplest examples of a system with multiple spin energy states are nuclei in which the total nuclear spin quantum number, I, is greater than ½. The most biologically important of these nuclei is probably ²³Na. The total number of accessible spin states for ²³Na is four. When a single radiofrequency pulse is applied to a complex system of spin states such as this, it couples the states separated by a single unit of spin. Thus, although no true spin flip has occurred, it is still true that only the allowed, $\Delta m_I = \pm 1$, transitions are induced. In nuclei with spin greater than ½, such as ²³Na, however, transitions previously regarded as unal-

lowed by the selection rules may be possible. To produce transitions between states separated by more than one unit of spin, or multiple-quantum transitions, a special type of spin interaction must exist. In nuclei of spin greater than ½, the interaction that allows the creation of multiple-quantum coherences is the quadrupole interaction. Simply stated, when nuclei of spin greater than ½ enter a region in which an electric field gradient exists, such as a region near large proteins, the spin energy levels are shifted and transitions may now occur between states separated by more than one unit of spin. For example, a spin in the $+\frac{3}{2}$ state may now make double-quantum transitions to the spin state $-\frac{1}{2}$. A triple-quantum transition would take such a spin all the way to the $-\frac{3}{2}$ spin state.

Multiple-quantum effects are quite common in spin ½ systems as well. However, two requirements must be met before multiple-quantum transitions can occur in spin ½ systems. First, it is necessary that at least two spin ½ nuclei, protons for example, be in close association, or coupled, for a time period, roughly 50 μs at 1.5 T. The second requirement is that there is a spin interaction that allows the coupled spin system to perform previously unallowed spin transitions. Interactions such as the dipole-dipole interaction and spin-spin coupling both make multiple-quantum transitions possible. For example, two coupled spin ½ nuclei may behave somewhat like a spin 1 system. If the spin ½ nuclei make transitions in tandem, then the spin quantum number m_I has changed by more than 1. It is a double-quantum transition. If enough protons are coupled together, as occurs in many metabolites, triple and higher quantum transitions may occur.[14] Also, unlike nuclei with spin greater than ½, coupled spin ½ systems can have zero-quantum coherence, $\Delta m = +1$ for one spin transition and -1 for the other. These can be bothersome in spectroscopy experiments because they cannot be dephased by gradient pulses as are other coherence levels. This type of effect is typically due to the effects of intramolecular spin-spin coupling. Dipole-dipole–induced multiple-quantum effects may be either intra- or intermolecular, however. If, for example, a water proton becomes associated with a proton that is part of a large protein, multiple-quantum effects may be created in this system. This may be related to imaging, because the multiple-quantum effects between the two protons may be partly responsible for the magnetization transfer contrast observed from the free water in systems with large protein moieties.

Interestingly, the multiple-quantum transitions are induced directly by molecular mechanisms and not by externally applied radiofrequency pulses. Radiofrequency pulses do play extremely important roles in multiple-quantum spectroscopy, however. First, radiofrequency pulses prepare the system in such a state that multiple-quantum coherences are more likely to be formed; that is a nonequilibrium state. Second, radiofrequency pulses allow phase cycling. If applied appropriately, such phase-cycling schemes may be employed to eliminate all coherences except for the coherence level desired. Once all undesired coherences

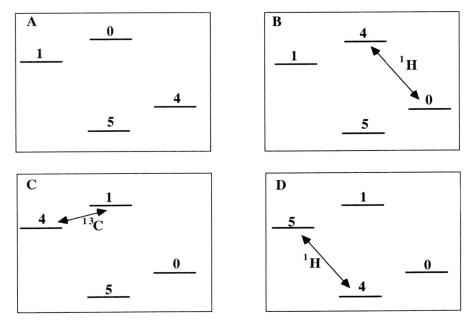

FIGURE 11–23. Polarization transfer. Population distribution of spins in the energy levels for a ^{13}C-^{1}H system similar to the one in Figure 11–18 except that in this case the two spins are scalar coupled. In addition, the enhancement in the population differences of the ^{13}C energy levels is due not to relaxation but to the scalar interaction. To bring about this transfer of polarization, frequency-selective 180° pulses are used. *A,* Starting configuration. *B,* Relative population distribution after a 180° ^{1}H pulse is applied to one of the proton resonances. This is followed by a selective 180° pulse at one of the ^{13}C resonances *(C).* Then a selective 180° pulse at the other ^{1}H resonance is applied *(D).* Finally, an excitation pulse, 90°, is applied at both ^{13}C resonances. The result is an increase in the carbon signal of 4. Because this method does not rely on relaxation, there are no competing mechanisms and the full enhancement can be obtained. However, there is a requirement to wait a length of time, related to the scalar coupling constant between the spins, between the application of the pulses. Although this gives an adequate picture of polarization transfer, the pulse sequence generally used to obtain this enhancement is quite different.

have been eliminated, the final multiple-quantum coherence must be converted, by a final radiofrequency pulse, back to a single-quantum coherence. This must be done because the radiofrequency coils used to detect spin coherences are able to receive a signal only from the single-quantum coherence.

TECHNIQUES: LOCALIZATION METHODS

The need to obtain tissue-specific spectra was recognized early in the field of in vivo NMR spectroscopy. Initially, this condition was met by using local surface coils.[15] Although this is adequate for surface tissue such as muscle and, using a few tricks, liver, most in vivo spectroscopy requires a combination of imaging and spectroscopy concepts to remain noninvasive. In animal experiments, deeper tissues and organs are surgically exposed and sampled by placing a surface coil directly on the organ. In the clinical setting, however, the goal is to be able to obtain a user-selectable region or regions using spatial localization methods rather than surgery.

Every MR signal, S(t), whether it is in an imaging or spectroscopy experiment, has three components:

$$S(t) = \sum_i A_i \cos(\omega_i t + \phi_i) \qquad (17)$$

where A is the amplitude; ω, the frequency; and ϕ, the

phase. In standard clinical imaging, we usually utilize the frequency of the signal to encode spatial information in one direction (frequency encoding) and the phase to encode a second direction (phase encoding), and the amplitude contains the image intensity. The exact value of the image intensity is determined by the spin properties of the water in the tissue, spin density, T1 and T2, and the pulse sequence used to acquire the image. For localized spectroscopy, the intensity is still determined by the spin properties and the pulse sequence. However, the number of spin properties involved is greater because we are no longer observing merely water, a simple spin ½ system. Many of the properties have already been discussed. In addition, the frequency of the signal is used not to encode spatial information but rather to record the natural frequency differences caused by the local magnetic fields responsible for chemical shift. When an FID is acquired with a simple pulse-acquire sequence, two components of the signal already contain information: the frequency, which contains chemical shift, and the amplitude, which gives us the area of the resonance. The phase is utilized only to tell the difference between positive and negative frequencies. Thus, the first localization method, chemical-shift imaging, utilized the phase to perform the spatial encoding. Methods developed later utilized slice selection in multiple directions to obtain a single volume. We describe both multivolume or spectroscopic imaging methods and single-volume localized spectroscopic methods that are currently utilized to perform in vivo spectroscopy. The single-volume methods avoid using any of the components of the signal to encode information, and the multivolume methods utilize either the phase or the amplitude. It seems best to have only chemical-shift information in the frequency of the signal. If one uses the frequency to encode spatial information as well as chemical shift, methods for dissecting the chemical shift from the spatial information must be developed as well. Before describing the most commonly used localization methods, some practical considerations that enter into the choice of a technique are discussed. Some of these considerations are similar to those contemplated for imaging experiments; others are specific to spectroscopy.

PRACTICAL CONSIDERATIONS IN CHOICE OF TECHNIQUE

Radiofrequency Coils

When choosing a radiofrequency coil with which to perform a spectroscopic study, many of the same considerations that are used to select a coil for imaging are employed. Often, for example, there are volume coils that are specifically designed for imaging certain parts of the body, such as the head or the knee. Such coils have uniform B_1 fields over the region of interest and are often well suited to spectroscopic experiments involving the same anatomy. However, there are certain disadvantages to using volume coils in spectroscopic studies. Although volume coils have intrinsically superior B_1 homogeneity, they often have rather poor inherent sensitivity. In certain cases, the limited sensitivity of volume coils is not adequate to observe the signal from metabolites of low in vivo concentration in a reasonable amount of time. If the study time is limited or the metabolite concentration low, modifications must be made to increase the sensitivity level of the study. If a quadrature volume coil can be used instead of a linear radiofrequency coil, the inherent sensitivity of the experiment is increased by up to a factor of $\sqrt{2}$. If additional sensitivity is required, the only remaining option is to make use of a surface coil or some other noncylindrical coil. Surface coils have intrinsically poor B_1 homogeneity but greatly superior sensitivity. The increase in sensitivity of the surface coil may make studies of otherwise undetectable metabolites possible or greatly increase the speed with which spectroscopic studies may be performed. In spectroscopic studies of relatively superficial regions of the anatomy, such as leg muscles or the visual cortex, surface coils are often not the choice of last resort but the clear first choice simply because of superior sensitivity.

Many newer clinical scanners have capabilities that greatly enhance their imaging function but are of limited facility in spectroscopic studies. The use of two separate radiofrequency coils in a study, one volume coil as a radiofrequency transmitter and the other as a local surface coil receiver, limits the effect of B_1 inhomogeneity on images. However, it also distorts the phase characteristics of the signal received by the surface coil so that it is typically more advantageous to employ the surface coil alone when performing spectroscopy. Multiple-coil receivers have also been used to expand the sensitive regions of the imaging experiment. In most spectroscopic experiments this is of limited usefulness because the object is typically to localize the region from which the signal is observed.

Eddy Currents

When the gradients are turned on or off during a pulse sequence, there may be a short time during which they are not at the value expected. Usually, the electronic hardware demands a square pulse for the gradients, but rarely is that achievable. Several physical factors account for the inability to achieve this desired response. The first factor is the finite inductance of the gradient coils. This is not a true eddy current phenomenon but is often described as one. The finite inductance causes a lag in the rise time of the gradient as well as gradient persistence after the demand has been switched off. The effects of this phenomenon may be partially corrected by modifying the demand waveform through pre-emphasis. In essence, the gradient is requested to produce a type of transition that, when combined with the known characteristics of the gradient coil, is closer to square. The application of such a correction has become standard in all commercial whole-body spectrometers.

The second source of gradient waveform distortion is true eddy currents. These are induced by interactions between the gradient coil and conducting elements within the magnet structure. The effect of these eddy currents is a time-dependent variation in the main magnetic field (B_0). Such field variations may persist much longer than the residual gradient field. The effects of eddy currents on MR images have been analyzed by Ahn and Cho.[16] The effects on spectroscopy are much more evident, as shown in Figure 11–24. Note the increase in width of the resonance as well as the distortion of the shape. Thus, more stringent requirements are placed on the performance of the gradient system during spectroscopy than during imaging sequences. Several approaches to eliminating the spectral distortions have been entertained. One is to eliminate the source of the eddy currents by eliminating the interaction of the gradient coils with the conducting elements within the magnet structure. This is accomplished by using shielded gradient coils. The gradient coil shield is, in fact, a second gradient set placed outside the primary set and run in opposition to the inner set. This ensures that there are no magnetic field changes outside the cylinder of the gradient coil set and thus no interaction with the magnet structure. Unfortunately, shielded gradients require much more current than conventional gradients to get the same strength. Most magnet manufacturers now offer shielded gradient coils. In general, this gradient coil

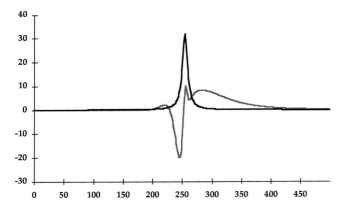

FIGURE 11-24. Effect of eddy currents on resonance line shapes. The result of residual eddy currents during data acquisition of spectra can be quite detrimental to the interpretation of spectra. The original resonance (*dark line*) has a line width of 10 Hz and a resonance frequency of 250 Hz. If an eddy current with a single time constant of 10 Hz and an initial shift of the resonance by 100 Hz occurs during data acquisition, the shaded resonance line is obtained.

set takes up more room inside the bore of the magnet than a conventional gradient coil set. However, by clever design, the body radiofrequency coil has been placed inside the space between the two gradient coils, allowing most clinical magnets to maintain the normal bore size. This eliminates much of the eddy currents, but these designs are not always perfect or available. Thus, methods for correcting the effects of eddy currents on the spectra have also been developed.[17–19] These methods usually involve obtaining a reference spectrum of water with the same pulse sequence and utilizing this simple spectrum to correct the sample spectrum. Many of these algorithms are simple to implement. Thus, any eddy currents that are not fully corrected in the hardware can be removed by post-processing.

Slice Misregistration

Localization methods that rely on slice selection in one or more directions experience slice misregistration of chemically shifted species. This misregistration can complicate the process of obtaining quantitative values from localized spectroscopy, especially because the total signal from each resonance may not arise from the same volume as another resonance in the spectrum. Figure 11–25 illustrates this. The problem arises from the difference in frequencies of the resonances associated with various chemical structures. When a gradient is applied to a sample containing chemically shifted species, there is a displacement of the sensitive volume for each of the different chemical species. This occurs in the frequency-encoding direction in a normal image as well. The bandwidth of the radiofrequency pulse, BW, with respect to the chemical-shift difference, $\delta\omega$, sets the percentage of overlap one can expect from two chemically shifted species in the same volume:

$$\% = \frac{BW - \delta\omega}{BW} \times 100 \qquad (18)$$

The size of the volume is then set by the gradient strengths used. Unfortunately, gradient strengths are limited to about 10 mT/m on most commercial spectrometers operating at 1.5 T. To get small volumes, the bandwidth of the excitation pulse must be made small to accommodate this limitation. Even with stronger gradients, the radiofrequency deposition at larger bandwidths forces a limitation. For instance, if we would like the entire proton spectrum, with a total range of 10 ppm or 640 Hz at 1.5 T, to have an overlap of at least 80%, the radiofrequency pulse must have a bandwidth of 3200 Hz. If we would like this volume to be 1 cm along one side, the gradient strength required is 8 mT/m. If we would like to increase the overlap to 90%, the radiofrequency bandwidth would double to 6400 Hz and the gradient strength would also double to 16 mT/m. Because $\delta\omega$ becomes larger at higher magnetic field strengths, larger gradients and larger radiofrequency bandwidths are necessary to obtain the same amount of overlap for the chemically shifted species.

The second problem with this slice mislocation is where the rest of the signal ends up. The volume adjacent to the one of interest receives this signal contamination. Therefore, signal can be observed in a localized volume even though none of that compound is truly present. Thus, it is important to minimize this slice mislocation even if only qualitative spectra are being obtained.

Water Suppression

The predominant proton signal in most tissues is from water. On average, the tissue in the body is about 80% water. It is this high water content combined with the variation in water percentage that makes proton imaging such a powerful and sensitive tool for gaining anatomic information. The same high water content makes proton spectroscopy of tissues extremely difficult. The water protons produce a signal that results from a concentration of 88 M, whereas most of the metabolites are at the 1 to 20 mM level. Thus, a difference in signal intensity on the order of 10^4 to 10^5 can be expected. Unfortunately, the dynamic range of the instrumentation does not allow the small signals to be observed in the presence of the large one. Therefore, much effort has been given to methods of suppressing the water signal. There are usually two classifications of water suppression methods: selective nonexcitation and saturation of the water signal. One or both of these suppression methods may be used. It is generally believed that combinations of suppression methods provide increased suppression.

One of the first water suppression methods used was a selective nonexcitation scheme in which a frequency-selective pulse was used to excite only the spectral region of interest. The frequency profile of the selective pulse shows no deposition of power at the frequency of water. A sinc pulse of the type commonly

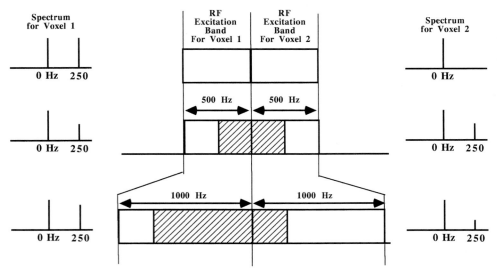

FIGURE 11–25. Slice misregistration. A major source of localization error in slice-selective localization schemes is mislocation of chemically shifted species. This figure illustrated the problem and shows how increasing both the bandwidth of the pulse and the gradients can lead to minimization of the problem. The top row shows the expected spectra from voxels 1 and 2. Note that none of the 250-Hz component exists in voxel 2. If a radiofrequency pulse of bandwidth 500 Hz is used to select voxel 1, the equivalent volume of the 250-Hz species is shifted 250 Hz as well. Thus, only half of the 250-Hz signal is excited by the slice-selection pulse and the spectrum reflects this. The rest of the signal from the 250-Hz component ends up in the next voxel. To minimize this loss of signal from voxel 1 and hence the contamination signal in voxel 2, a radiofrequency pulse of wider bandwidth must be used. To keep the size of the volume the same, the gradient strength must also be increased. The last row of the figure demonstrates the result of increasing both the bandwidth of the pulse and the strength of the gradient by a factor of 2.

used in imaging or a gaussian-shaped pulse performs this function quite well. However, we normally utilize the frequency selectivity of these pulses to provide spatial selectivity. Two-dimensional frequency-selective pulses have been utilized to obtain combined spatial and spectral selectivity. The trouble with the use of simple selective excitation schemes is the limitation of exciting only one band of frequencies either higher or lower than the frequencies of the water. Resonances for metabolites exist on both sides. Thus, a selective pulse with a notch of nonexcitation is more desirable. This is the advantage of binomial pulses,[20] the most commonly used one being the $1\bar{3}3\bar{1}$ sequence. (The bars above the numbers indicate a 180° phase shift of the pulse with respect to the first pulse.) Figure 11–26 demonstrates vectorially the operation of this pulse sequence. Water is placed on-resonance and the delay time between the pulses is set so that spins of one of the metabolites precess 180° during each delay. This pulse sequence has a fairly broad nonexcitation region at 0 Hz, which is where the water resonance is normally placed.

Selective saturation of water is the second scheme for water suppression. The simplest method is to apply a long, low-power pulse at the frequency of the water resonance until the signal is reduced. This is effective if the water resonance is quite narrow. Because the in vivo water resonance can be quite broad, 0.2 to 0.5 ppm, many spectroscopy sequences on clinical machines use chemical-shift–selective (CHESS) pulses to perform water suppression. These pulses selectively excite water and then the water signal is spoiled or dephased using gradient pulses. The frequency-selective pulses just described are good candidates for CHESS pulses. Adequate water suppression is often obtained if three of these pulses are used, one with each gradient direction. In addition, the flip angle of the radiofrequency pulse can be adjusted until the maximal water suppression is obtained.

Out-of-Volume Suppression

One way to minimize contamination from signal outside the volume of interest is to utilize out-of-volume signal suppression. Such methods have been utilized in commercial imaging sequences for many years. Out-of-volume suppression provides a solution to the problem of lipid contamination in proton spectroscopy when the lipid signal arises from regions outside the volume of interest. This situation exists especially in the brain, as most of the lipid signal arises from regions outside the brain. Contamination resulting from this signal can be the result of slice misregistration as described earlier; pixel bleed in Fourier chemical-shift imaging, to be described later; or nonideal radiofrequency pulse excitation profiles that distort the shape of the localized volume. The essence of all the volume localization schemes is to saturate the signal outside the volume of interest with tailored excitation pulses similar to the water suppression pulses described earlier. The saturation can occur via a sequence of low-flip-angle pulses applied in the presence of a gradient[21] or a series of 90° pulses with gradient dephasing.[22, 23] Both of these methods have been applied and give reasonable suppression.[24]

Pulse-Induced Signal Saturation

In imaging, one mechanism for developing contrast is the differential signal saturation that occurs in the tissues as a result of T1 weighting. What is powerful in imaging causes great problems in spectroscopy. Not all metabolites have the same T1 value even within the same tissue. Therefore, pulsing at times shorter than 5 T1 causes different amounts of saturation in the resonance signals from the metabolites. Unfortunately, the T1 values for many small metabolites are quite long, 1 to 2 seconds at 1.5 T for ^{1}H, 4 to 6 seconds for ^{31}P, and even longer for [13]C. Thus, to optimize data

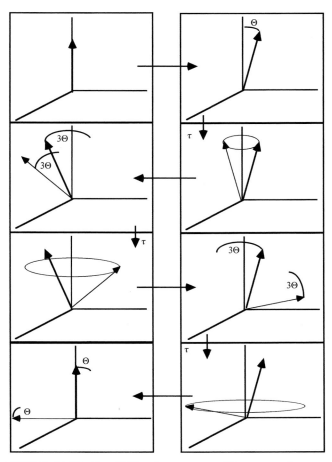

FIGURE 11–26. The 1$\bar{3}$3$\bar{1}$ pulse sequence. The vector diagrams show how the 1$\bar{3}$3$\bar{1}$ pulse sequence excites magnetization at one frequency while leaving the water magnetization along the z axis. The first pulse, Θ, rotates both components around the x axis by one eighth of a 90° pulse. Then a short delay occurs. During this time, τ, the water magnetization does not precess because it has been placed at 0 Hz. However, τ has been chosen so that the magnetization from some metabolite, such as lactate, precesses 180° about the z axis. Now a 3Θ pulse is given along the $-x$ axis, that is, with a 180° phase shift. This rotates the two vectors in the opposite direction from the first pulse. The water magnetization travels back past the z axis and ends up at one fourth of the distance to the $-x$ axis. The lactate magnetization is now 45° from the z axis. Another τ delay, equal to the first, occurs and rotates the lactate 180° around z. Now a zero-phase 3Θ pulse is applied. The water magnetization is back where it was after the first pulse, but the lactate has rotated another 3Θ toward the x-y plane. After another τ delay, the last Θ pulse is given around the $-x$ axis. The water magnetization ends up along the z axis and the lactate magnetization is along the $-y$ axis.

acquisition, spectroscopists rarely wait 5 T1 for TR pulsing, which is usually done at 1 to 1.5 T1. This makes absolute quantification difficult and even the comparison of ratios of peak intensities dependent on TR. If the T1 values are known, the data can be corrected for this saturation effect according to the following equation:

$$M_0 = \frac{M_s}{1 - e^{-TR/T1}} \qquad (19)$$

where M_0 is the equilibrium magnetization that exists before any pulses, M_s is the saturated magnetization obtained using 90° pulses, and TR is the repetition time. This equation does assume 90° pulses and becomes more complicated if any other flip angle is used for the excitation.[25] The equations for the signal expected from the different localization methods have been written out by one of the authors[26] and can be used to correct for saturation and pulse angle effects if all parameters are known.

Scalar Coupling and Echoes

The beauty of the spin echo is its ability to refocus both chemical shift and $\mathbf{B}_0$ inhomogeneities. This allows the data acquisition to be moved away from the radiofrequency pulse and the switching gradients. However, the spin echo does not refocus scalar coupling. The reason for this is depicted in Figure 11–27. For convenience, the figure has been drawn as if 0 Hz is exactly centered between the two resonances of a doublet. Thus, the magnetization precesses with a frequency of $+J/2$ or $-J/2$. For simplicity, component 1 is the $+J/2$ magnetization, which has a neighboring spin aligned against the external magnetic field, and component 2 is the $-J/2$ magnetization, which has a neighboring spin aligned with the external magnetic field. For a simple 90°x-t/2-180°x-t/2 acquisition sequence the following occurs. The 90°x pulse rotates the magnetization vector around the x axis onto the y axis. Now the two components precess with the frequencies $+J/2$ and $-J/2$. The 180° pulse now does two things; it flips both these vectors 180° around the x axis and it flips the neighboring spins. Thus, component 1 now has a neighbor that is aligned with the external magnetic field and precesses at $-J/2$ and component 2 has a neighbor aligned against and precesses at $+J/2$. If we wait another t/2 period so that chemical shift is refocused, we find that the components of the scalar-coupled magnetization have now picked up twice the phase difference. However, if we wait the correct time, these two components come back into alignment on the $-y$ axis. For a doublet this happens when t is a multiple of $1/2J$. However, for a triplet, the spins do not align again until they reach the $+y$ axis, which requires a multiple of $1/J$, and for a quartet, $t = 2n/J$ where n is an integer. Note that even if J is the same for all the scalar coupling constants of interest, t must be chosen so that all multiplet patterns are in phase at the time of the data acquisition.

The consequence of not waiting an appropriate length of time for scalar coupling to come into phase can be devastating for spectra obtained for in vivo samples, where the couplings are almost never resolved. For the doublet, if the data were acquired at $t = 1/4J$, the two components of the multiplet would be exactly out of phase. For unresolved couplings, this can make the resonance peak go to zero. Thus, inadequate information can be obtained even if quantitative data are not required. This creates a problem for T2 measurements as well. Remember, even if the

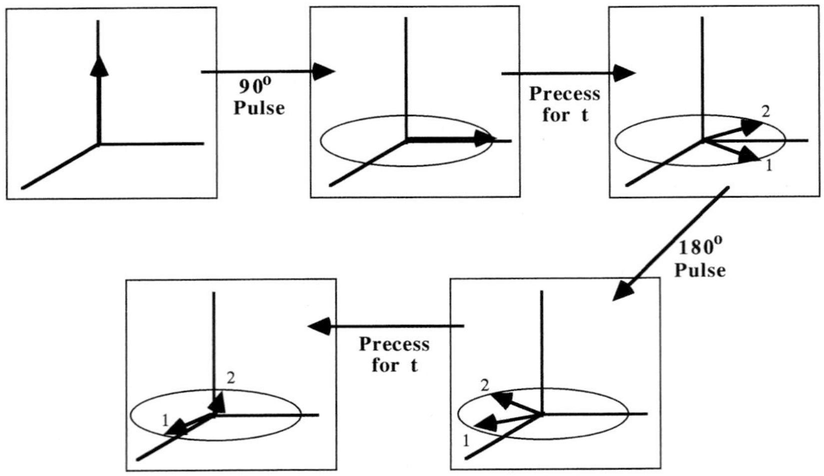

FIGURE 11–27. Effect of spin echoes on scalar-coupled resonances. The spin-echo sequence does not rephase scalar-coupled resonances. After a 90° pulse, the two components of the scalar-coupled resonance precess at a frequency of ± J/2. After a 180° pulse, the magnetization not only flips around the x axis but also changes its sense of rotation. Thus, the two vectors continue to accumulate a phase difference. For unresolved scalar couplings, an echo time of 2t can be chosen so that the two components are exactly out of phase and the resulting signal is zero.

couplings are unresolved, if they exist, they affect the resulting spectrum.

B_1 METHODS

B_1 methods of localization rely in some way on the nonuniform B_1 profile of the radiofrequency coil being used to obtain localization. Most imaging coils are designed to provide spatially uniform excitation of the sample. These designs are usually cylindrical and require that the sample be placed inside the cylinder. Unfortunately, this means that signal is then obtained from all regions of the sample within the coil. One method of localization is to relax the condition of homogeneous excitation and build coils with a limited field of view.

Surface Coils

The first localized spectrum was obtained with a surface coil.[15] Surface coils are typically circular, rectangular, or square loops of wire. The sensitive region of a circular surface coil, for example, arises roughly from a hemisphere with a radius equal to the radius of the coil. Most of the signal observed is from this region. This rule is not completely accurate, however. The field of view of the surface coil may extend beyond this volume, and regions close to the coil can experience a 180° pulse generating no induced signal. In addition, multiple pulse sequences can have drastically different excitation profiles from those of the single pulse-acquire sequence simply because of the inherent inhomogeneity of the B_1 field produced by the surface coil. This apparent disadvantage has been used to give additional localization beyond that of the surface coil alone. The resulting technique is called Fourier series windowing.[27] In spite of these drawbacks, the surface coil does an adequate job of obtaining signals localized to the surface tissues and has been used for many years in both animal and human studies. For studies requiring more precise localization or to quantitate metabolites, a measure of the homogeneity of the coil

or B_1 map is required. As the sample has an effect on the coil performance, the map should be obtained directly with the sample of interest. A few methods for obtaining such a map now exist in the literature.[28–30]

Rotating Frame Imaging

The lack of homogeneity of the surface coil can be used to advantage in localization procedures. The homogeneity of the coil can be designed to be almost linear as a function of spatial coordinates. Thus, an image can be produced using B_1 gradients instead of B_0 gradients. This imaging method was first proposed by Hoult in 1979[31] and was made practical for use with surface coils by Styles and colleagues.[32] Styles and coworkers designed a concentric double surface coil system. The large coil is used to transmit signals and has a nearly linear B_1 gradient over the field of view of the second smaller circular coil. Spectroscopic imaging may be performed in this manner by a modulation of the intensity of the signal received from a point in space by varying the length of the applied radiofrequency pulse linearly. Because $\Theta = \gamma B_1 \tau$, the flip angle of a point in the sample and hence its signal intensity are determined by the duration of the applied pulse and the strength of the B_1 at that point. Thus, the nonuniformity of the B_1 field can be used to advantage to encode one spatial dimension. The other two dimensions are limited by the field of view of the second small coil. A two-dimensional Fourier transform gives spatial information in one direction and chemical shift information in the other. A slight twist on this method that improves the signal-to-noise ratio was introduced by Blackledge and colleagues.[33] This method moves the encoding from the amplitude of the signal to the phase by applying a second pulse of nominal 90° flip angle with a phase shift of 90° with respect to the encoding pulse. Essentially, this takes the signal that was dispersed in the y-z plane and now places it in the x-y plane (Fig. 11–28).

Something akin to slice misregistration occurs in this technique because of off-resonance affects. At places in the sample away from the coil, the B_1 field is quite

FIGURE 11–28. Rotating frame imaging. Four different encoding steps in the rotating frame imaging localization method are shown. The top row demonstrates the motion of the magnetization vector at two spatial locations for the amplitude-encoded version; the bottom row is the equivalent picture for the phase-encoded method. For *A* and *E*, the encoding pulse had zero rotation. The amplitude encoding has no signal and the phase-encoded version has a full unit of signal from both vectors. For *B* and *F*, the encoding pulse was applied for a set length of time and rotated one vector around the x axis 45° and the other 90°. Applying a second 90° pulse along the y axis rotates the y-z plane into the x-y plane to produce the phase-encoded version. Similarly, *C* and *G* demonstrate an en-

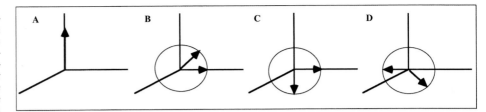

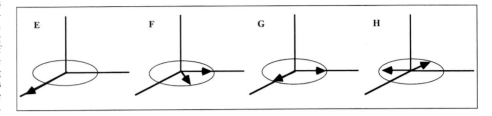

coding in which the encoding pulse was applied twice as long as in *B* and *F*. For *D* and *H*, the pulse was applied for 3t. The signal generated by the amplitude-encoded version comes only from the component of each vector that can be projected onto the x-y plane. For the phase-encoded version, the entire vector is in the x-y plane; therefore, more signal is observed.

weak. Thus, chemical species not on-resonance with the radiofrequency pulse do not rotate around the x axis but rather around $\mathbf{B}_{eff}$. The spins do so faster than if they were on-resonance and therefore appear spatially closer to the coil than they really are. This can be overcome only by increasing the power of the radiofrequency pulse applied. In addition to the off-resonance problem, it is difficult to obtain exact volume sizes with this method. In spite of some of its handicaps, Radda's group[32, 33] has used this method extensively to obtain localized ^{31}P spectra without the use of $\mathbf{B}_0$ gradients.

Depth-Resolved Surface Coil Spectroscopy

Another method for obtaining ^{31}P spectra using a surface coil, depth-resolved surface coil spectroscopy (DRESS), was described by Bottomley and coworkers.[34, 35] This uses the limited field of view of the surface coil in a plane parallel to the plane of the coil but uses a selective pulse in the presence of a $\mathbf{B}_0$ gradient to obtain a localized disk. The method is simple and allows one to adjust the flip angle in the volume of interest to obtain a maximal signal. The use of a $\mathbf{B}_0$ gradient means that eddy currents could affect the spectrum. In addition, there is a delay in the data acquisition while the slice-selection gradient is refocused. This distorts the spectrum, as shown in the later section on data processing. Because this technique utilizes slice selection, there can be slice mislocation artifacts in the direction of the applied gradient.

B_0 Methods

A large number of spatial localization methods utilize switched gradients to obtain localization. Both single-voxel and multivoxel methods are currently employed in the clinical setting. We concentrate on the most commonly used methods and point out some of their strengths and weaknesses. However, to give a historical perspective on this field, we take this opportunity to discuss a few early localization schemes. Initially, localization was achieved mainly by limiting the extent of the $\mathbf{B}_1$ field through the use of surface coils. When this approach was no longer feasible, a modification of the normal imaging scheme was proposed. This technique eliminated the frequency-encoding gradient and utilized phase encoding in multiple spatial dimensions. We discuss this in greater detail later. The first single-volume localization method was proposed by Aue and colleagues[36] and strives to produce localization in a single encoding step. Although this method, volume-selective excitation (VSE), did not become useful because of the radiofrequency power requirements, it did pave the way for many other methods. Modifications of the VSE approach led to the spatially resolved spectroscopy (SPARS) technique.[37, 38] Both VSE and SPARS work on the principle of exciting all the spins in the sample and then placing the spins in the volume of interest back along the z axis while the signal from the rest of the sample is dephased. It is difficult to get reliable localization with such a scheme, because any signal that is not entirely dephased appears in the spectrum of the volume of interest. In addition, stringent timings and good out-of-volume suppression are required. Neither of these approaches has achieved routine use.

Stimulated-Echo Acquisition Mode and Point-Resolved Spectroscopy

Two popular techniques for single-voxel, water-suppressed proton spectroscopy are STEAM[39–43] and point-resolved spectroscopy (PRESS).[44] Both of these methods directly excite the volume of interest with minimal excitation of the rest of the sample. The encoding of a single volume can be obtained in a single pulse sequence, which is why these sequences became known as single-shot localization methods. Both also use three

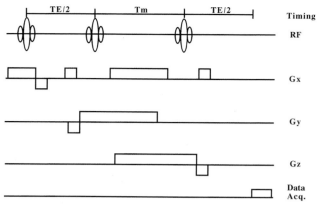

FIGURE 11–29. The STEAM pulse sequence.

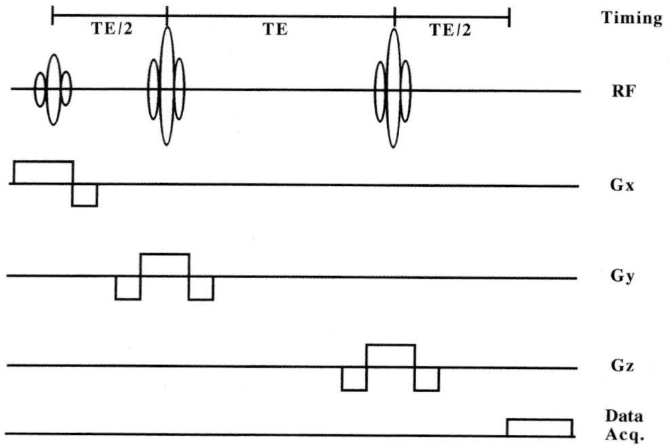

FIGURE 11–30. The PRESS pulse sequence.

slice-selective pulses, one each along the x, y, and z directions, to obtain localization. The difference is that STEAM does the excitation with three 90° pulses and PRESS uses one 90° pulse and two 180° pulses (Figs. 11–29 and 11–30).

PRESS is simple to understand. The first pulse excites all the magnetization in a slice. The second pulse is applied in a direction perpendicular to this slice. Thus, only magnetization in a column or row of intersection between these two slices is refocused. The third slice is perpendicular to the previous two slices. The end result is an echo that consists of only magnetization from the intersection of these three slices. Crusher gradients around the 180° pulses dephase any FID produced from imperfect 180° pulses.

STEAM utilizes 90° excitations only to attain the same localization as the PRESS sequence. However, the stimulated echo produced by the STEAM sequence gives only half the possible signal from the volume. The pulse sequence proceeds in the following manner (Fig. 11–31). The first excitation pulse is the same as in the PRESS sequence. A gradient is applied before the second pulse to dephase the magnetization inside

the slice selected by the first pulse. This helps reduce the frequency-dependent excitation obtained with a normal 90°-t-90° sequence. The second 90° pulse then rotates the plane of magnetization in the spatial column, which is the intersection of the slices from the first and second pulses, into the x-y plane. During the next delay time, spoiler gradients are applied that dephase any FID off the second 90° pulse as well as dephase any portion of the signal left in the x-y plane. This causes the loss of half of the possible signal, because this gradient is not rephased later. Now only the magnetization along the ±z axes is left. The third selective 90° pulse excites magnetization in a third plane that is perpendicular to the other two planes. It also takes the magnetizations left along the ±z axes and places them in the x-y plane. Another gradient both dephases the FID of this 90° pulse and refocuses the magnetization dephased by the gradient before the second pulse. Now, at a time equal to the time between the first and second pulses, the magnetization in the volume defined by the intersection of the planes excited by the three pulses forms an echo. Note that

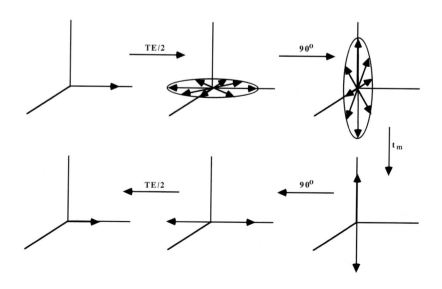

FIGURE 11–31. The STEAM sequence utilizes three 90° slice-selective pulses to provide a spatially localized spectrum. The first pulse rotates the magnetization 90° in a plane. During the time TE/2 (where TE is echo time), a gradient is applied that dephases the magnetization in this plane. The second 90° pulse excites a plane perpendicular to the first. For magnetization in the intersection between these two slices, this 90° pulse rotates the x-y plane of magnetization into the x-z plane. A spoiler gradient applied during t_m dephases any component of the magnetization left in the x-y plane, leaving on the magnetization along the ±z axis. The third 90° pulse rotates the magnetization along the ±z axis resulting from the previous two pulses onto the ±y axis. The gradient applied here serves two purposes. It dephases the FID that occurs from magnetization inside the third slice but outside the volume of interest. It also rephases the magnetization in the volume of interest that was dephased between the first and second pulses. At a time TE/2 after the third pulse, a stimulated echo occurs.

the time between the second and third pulses does not affect the echo time. During this time the magnetization in the volume is along the z axis and does not continue to precess around the z axis.

Both STEAM and PRESS can be preceded by CHESS pulses to obtain water suppression. Out-of-volume suppression can also be done before the sequence. The shape of the volume obtained in these two techniques depends in detail on the radiofrequency pulse profile and the gradients used. It is easy to obtain parallelograms with this method, although most people prefer cube-like voxels.

Because these two methods utilize slice selection to perform the localization, they are both susceptible to slice mislocation. Unless radiofrequency pulses of wide bandwidth are used, the volume for each chemically shifted species is not precisely in the same spatial position of the sample. In addition, the radiofrequency pulses must have fairly precise flip angles and thus require a fairly homogeneous B_1 coil. Current B_1-insensitive excitation pulses and refocusing pulses do not have adequate bandwidth to perform these sequences with surface coils.

One of the advantages of both of these methods is that they are echo techniques. This allows the data acquisition to be moved away from the slice-selection pulses and the switching gradients associated with them. Thus, the influence of eddy currents can be minimized by pushing the data acquisition to long echo times. Unfortunately, this echo also causes problems in the presence of scalar coupling. Unlike chemical shift, scalar coupling does not reverse its direction after a 180° pulse, so it does not refocus. For this reason, only specific echo times can be used. The echo timing is dependent on both the scalar coupling constant and the coupling pattern. Thus, one echo time does not suffice for all resonances. The influence of scalar coupling on the STEAM sequence has been worked out in detail for spin systems similar to the CH_3 resonance of lactate.[45] These results and the effects of scalar coupling on the same spin system have been compared for both STEAM and PRESS.[46] The results of these analyses show that there is a limitation on the echo times that can be used for these two sequences when scalar-coupled spins are being observed. For STEAM, both the echo time and the time between the second and third pulses, t_m, have limitations. All but the zero-quantum signal are dephased by the spoiler gradient used during t_m. However, zero-quantum signals are not affected by this gradient. Therefore, t_m must also be chosen appropriately to ensure that the zero-quantum signal is zero at the time of the third pulse. It is also possible to use a simple two-step phase-cycling scheme to get rid of the zero-quantum signal.[46]

Most of the rest of the difficulties with STEAM and PRESS arise if quantitative information is desired. In both these sequences the signal intensity is affected by T2 and, because most spectra are acquired at short TR values, the T1 as well. In addition, the scalar-coupling constant can affect the signal intensity observed especially for unresolved lines. Thus, all three of these numbers must be obtained to correct the data for

relaxation times or to set up the parameters correctly so that scalar coupling does not interfere.

PRESS and STEAM have been used only for ^{1}H spectroscopy because the T2 values are long and the signal-to-noise ratio is sufficient to take advantage of the single-shot methods. However, versions of these sequences with short echo times should allow ^{31}P spectroscopy to be done with these methods.

Fourier Chemical-Shift Imaging

The first and still commonly used B_0 localization method is a logical extension of multidimensional imaging methods, Fourier chemical-shift imaging (FCSI).[47–49] The technique encodes all spatial dimensions into the phase of the MR signal. Data acquisition is performed in the absence of a frequency-encoding gradient, so chemical-shift information can be retained. Slice selection can also be performed to reduce the number of directions for phase encoding. Both spin-echo and nonecho sequences have been used (Fig. 11–32). The advantage of the echo method is that it moves the data acquisition away from the switching gradients and allows all the resonances to come into phase for acquisition. However, the peak intensity of short-T2 species is greatly affected, as are scalar-coupled resonances. Nonecho versions can acquire data with a shorter delay but chemically shifted species now have different phases.

One of the problems with FCSI is the need for a large number of encodings to obtain a single volume. However, it is excellent at obtaining metabolic maps. To obtain a single volume, a minimum of eight encodings in each direction is required. Thus, for a slice-selected two-dimensional phase-encoded sequence at least 64 encodings are necessary. Even at this large number of encodings, significant pixel bleeding occurs. Pixel bleeding arises from the inability of a sine and cosine encoding scheme to encode a square volume adequately without an infinite number of encodings. Thus, signal from voxels far from the voxel of interest can be found in the spectrum of this voxel. Methods for postprocessing the data to reduce this bleeding have been proposed.[26, 46, 50] In spite of the problems with localization, FCSI has been used extensively for both ^{1}H and ^{31}P NMR imaging. It is a good method for obtaining a large number of voxels or for mapping metabolites. A reduction in pixel bleeding can be obtained by increasing the number of encodings to 16 or 32 in each direction, but this also greatly increases the imaging time.

One great advantage of FCSI is that it has no voxel mislocation caused by chemical shift. The spatial phase difference accumulated by each chemical-shifted species is merely a function of the gradient at that spatial location. Therefore, there is no chemical-shift mislocation in phase-encoding directions. The same is observed in imaging; the chemical-shift artifacts occur only in the frequency-encoding direction in images.

Image-Selected In Vivo Spectroscopy

Image-selected in vivo spectroscopy (ISIS) was proposed as a localization technique by Ordidge and col-

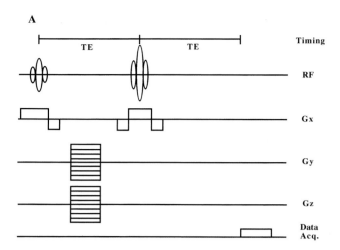

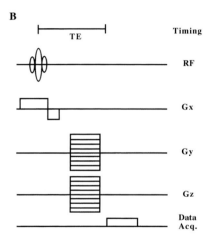

FIGURE 11–32. FCSI pulse sequence. *A*, Echo method. *B*, Non-echo method.

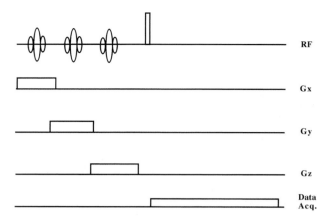

FIGURE 11–33. ISIS pulse sequence. The gradients are turned on and off in eight different combinations to encode the spatial information (see Table 11–2). After appropriately adding and subtracting the eight FIDs, a spectrum from the volume localized by the slice-selection pulses is obtained.

leagues.[51] It performs its localization without placing the magnetization in the x-y plane, where T2, chemical shift, and scalar coupling could affect it before data acquisition. It was one of the first so-called pre-encoding schemes, in which magnetization is encoded along the ±z axes using slice-selective 180° pulses before excitation. Then the excitation pulse converts the encoding into phase information. The sequence is shown in Figure 11–33. A single encoding does not produce a single volume. It requires eight encodings as indicated in Table 11–2. The regions of the sample are encoded using ±1 values indicating placement along the ±z axes during the pre-encoding. The excitation pulse then places this along the ±y axes. The resulting eight FIDs are then added and subtracted to get the single volume.

This technique has several advantages and disadvantages. First, it is a slice-selection method and suffers from slice mislocation caused by chemical shift. Second, eight separate encodings are necessary to obtain the localized volume. Any motion in between these

scans can cause localization errors through incomplete cancellation of the regions of the sample outside the volume. In addition, great machine stability is required. However, the eight encodings are signal averages in the true sense, which makes this localization or stability problem not much worse than problems with signal-averaged single-shot methods. Unlike the situation in the single-shot methods, the magnetization is not in the x-y plane except for data acquisition; therefore, short-T2 species or scalar-coupled resonances are not affected. However, the encoding does require long-T1 relaxation. This makes ISIS a perfect localization method for ^{31}P NMR spectroscopy. Another nicety of this pre-encoding scheme is that localization is separated from excitation, so just about any pulse sequence can be used for excitation, even FCSI.

Multivolume ISIS and Hadamard Spectroscopic Imaging

One problem with ISIS is that a volume is not obtained for every encoding as with FCSI; rather it takes eight encodings to get one volume. Two extensions of the ISIS method allow a more favorable volume-to-encoding ratio: multivolume ISIS[52] and Hadamard

TABLE 11–2. COMBINATION OF RADIOFREQUENCY PULSE APPLICATION IN THE ISIS SEQUENCE AND WHETHER RESULTING FREE INDUCTION DECAY SHOULD BE ADDED OR SUBTRACTED

	INVERSION PULSE			ADD OR SUBTRACT
OPERATION	G_x	G_y	G_z	
1	Off	Off	Off	Add
2	On	Off	Off	Subtract
3	On	On	Off	Add
4	On	On	On	Subtract
5	Off	On	On	Add
6	Off	On	Off	Subtract
7	On	Off	On	Add
8	Off	Off	On	Subtract

spectroscopic imaging (HSI).[26, 53] Developed independently but simultaneously, both methods use multiple magnetization inversion regions to increase the number of volumes to be encoded. Multivolume ISIS uses the sequential application of single-band inversion pulses, and HSI uses specially crafted pulses to produce multiband inversions. HSI looks similar to ISIS in pulse sequence, but the selective inversion pulses are replaced with multiband inversion pulses.

The pulses designed for HSI are fashioned after Walsh functions, square wave equivalents of sine and cosine functions (Fig. 11–34). Up to eighth-order Walsh function pulses have been designed, allowing $8 \times 8 \times 8$ Hadamard encoding. This is a practical limit for both HSI and multivolume ISIS because of radiofrequency power deposition concerns and bandwidth requirements for reduction of slice mislocation. Past this eight-point limit, FCSI is a more practical choice. However, a major advantage of these methods over FCSI is that volumes need not all be the same size. In other words, the space need not be equally sampled. HSI is currently being used for ^{31}P spectroscopy using both volume and surface coils.[54] Also, a hybrid HSI and FCSI method is being used.[55] This hybrid utilizes HSI in the slice direction and FCSI for encoding within the slice.

QUANTIFYING SPECTRA

To obtain numeric results from spectroscopy data, we must be especially careful to note the conditions under which the data were acquired. Often spectroscopists are trying to economize on the time the subject spends in the scanner; however, no amount of data processing can make up for data that are just not there. Sometimes the best that can be done is to spend more time acquiring the data correctly, which in turn makes the data processing itself a bit easier. However, it is not always true that all data-processing troubles can be solved with data acquisition. Therefore, it is important to understand the nature of the data acquisition as well as the data processing before attempting to gather quantitative information from a spectrum. Unfortunately, the data-processing options are numerous and beyond the scope of this chapter. This area is currently active, with both highly interactive or manual processing methods and fully automatic processing methods available.

It is easy to imagine a situation, either clinical or research oriented, in which it would be critical to have the exact concentration of certain in vivo metabolites. It would be even more elegant if the metabolite levels could be obtained noninvasively. The goal, therefore, is to use the noninvasive capability of MRS to obtain a spectrum from which we extract an in vivo metabolite concentration from each signal obtained. To accomplish this, all of the factors that affect the size of the signal from a given metabolite must be accounted for and appropriately corrected. In addition, to obtain the final metabolite concentration, comparison with a normalization standard of well-known NMR characteristics must be performed.

Unfortunately, the metabolite signals obtained from typical spectra are the result of the complex interaction of both internal and external factors. The internal factors that affect the metabolite signal level are many. For example, the signal obtained from a metabolite clearly depends on the level of magnetization present before the application of the acquisition pulse. Indeed, it is this value that we would like to obtain. The observed metabolite magnetization depends not only on the Boltzmann value of the equilibrium magnetization but also on the T1 of the metabolite and the details of the sequence of pulses in terms of both pulse strength and timing. Although this is certainly a complex set of factors to determine only the preacquisition level of magnetization, all of this information is typically well known a priori and requires no additional time to gather. In some cases, however, the T1 of the metabolite may have to be directly determined for each subject. In addition, it is clear that the T2 relaxation time of the metabolite affects the signal level observed.

Characteristics of the hardware and instrumentation used in the study may also affect the level of signal obtained from in vivo metabolites. For example, the radiofrequency pulses transmitted into the subject are often presumed to be perfectly calibrated and applied homogeneously over the region of interest. In practice, this is often untrue, and the error can have a large effect on the amount of signal obtained from any metabolite. In addition, the reception sensitivity of the radiofrequency coil is not as uniform as is presumed. In the case of a surface coil, the fact that the transmission and reception qualities of the coil are often characterized by an effective depth of penetration makes the necessity of knowledge of its $\mathbf{B}_1$ field characteristics obvious. If the $\mathbf{B}_1$ field characteristics of a surface coil are known, it is possible to correct for any inhomogeneities in transmission or reception sensitivity. With volume coils, it is often assumed that the reception and transmission characteristics of the coil are such that all regions of interest within the coil are sampled

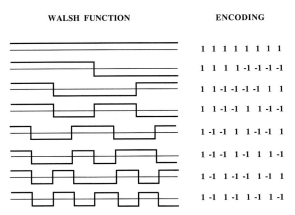

WALSH FUNCTION	ENCODING
	1 1 1 1 1 1 1 1
	1 1 1 1 -1 -1 -1 -1
	1 1 -1 -1 -1 -1 1 1
	1 1 -1 -1 1 1 -1 -1
	1 -1 -1 1 1 -1 -1 1
	1 -1 -1 1 -1 1 1 -1
	1 -1 1 -1 -1 1 -1 1
	1 -1 1 -1 1 -1 1 -1

FIGURE 11–34. Walsh functions for Hadamard pulses. Pulses that have Walsh function frequency excitation profiles must be used for the Hadamard spectroscopic imaging method. For an eighth-order Hadamard encoding, all eight of these pulse profiles are required. For a fourth-order Hadamard encoding, only the top four are needed.

equally, so it is less clear that knowledge of the $\mathbf{B}_1$ field is necessary for quantification. However, even an otherwise perfect coil, when loaded asymmetrically, has $\mathbf{B}_1$ inhomogeneities. Thus, it may always be necessary to measure the $\mathbf{B}_1$ characteristics of the radiofrequency coil when signal intensities from two different regions of the sample are to be compared.

The final basic ingredient required to complete the quantification of in vivo metabolites is a reference standard. Any such standard must have well-characterized T1 and T2 times as well as accurately known concentrations of the nuclear species of interest. Two common types of standards are in use at this time. The first standard is the internal water signal. This is particularly convenient for a number of reasons. Water is already present in great quantities, its relaxation characteristics are easily measured and often already known, the signal can be obtained from the same volume as the spectrum so coil inhomogeneities can be ignored, and its concentration is, in principle, known to a reasonable accuracy. One potential drawback of water referencing is that it requires extrapolating signal levels from a relatively accurately known concentration of 100 M protons to the signal levels obtained from metabolites, which are often at concentrations of 10 mM or less. The potential for errors in such a large extrapolation cannot be ignored. Such an extrapolation requires accurate knowledge of the receiver gain settings of the spectrometer. However, it appears that water referencing does provide the simplest, most rapid method of quantification with reasonable levels of accuracy.

The second standard commonly used is the external reference. This avoids many of the problems with water referencing because the typical choice of chemical in the reference is exactly the same as the in vivo metabolite and is of the same order of magnitude in concentration. Referencing to an external standard, despite the potential for increased accuracy in the quantification, does have some disadvantages. First, the standard must be mixed carefully to accurate concentration levels and its relaxation characteristics must be determined beforehand. Also, the placement of the external sample near the patient makes the degree of correction for the inhomogeneities of the transmission and reception characteristics of the coil all the more important. Often, the radiofrequency coils have been carefully designed to fit a certain part of the human body without tolerance for added material. In a head coil, for example, the external reference standard might have to be placed near the edge of the coil. Clearly, in this region of the coil, the $\mathbf{B}_1$ field is much more inhomogeneous than in the center. This necessitates accurate determinations of the $\mathbf{B}_1$ field so that the effect of radiofrequency field inhomogeneities may be correctly accounted for.

To obtain quantitative data, it is important to understand exactly what the spectrometer does as well as how the magnetization reacts to the pulse sequence. Casual use of spectroscopy sequences and data-processing methods can lead to inaccurate values entering the literature.

CONCLUSION

The role of spectroscopy in aiding the clinician in both diagnosis and assessment of treatment of diseases is growing. Widespread use of spectroscopy requires a deeper understanding by the radiologist of both its assets and problems. Unfortunately, a comprehensive look at clinical spectroscopy requires a book of its own. We hope that this chapter provides some of the basics necessary to understand and to evaluate the current literature. The techniques covered are ones currently being used in a rather routine way at sites around the world. Unfortunately, this is neither a comprehensive list nor a critical one. Comparisons of many localization methods can be found in the literature.[26, 56-58] In the end, we need to use what is available on our system but with an understanding of both its possible flaws and advantages.

REFERENCES

1. Maris JM, Chance B: Magnetic resonance spectroscopy of neoplasms. Magn Reson Annu :213–235, 1986.
2. Smith SR, Martin PA, Davies JM, et al: The assessment of treatment response in non-Hodgkin's lymphoma by image guided ^{31}P magnetic resonance spectroscopy. Br J Cancer 61:485–490, 1990.
3. Glaholm J, Leach MO, Collins DJ, et al: In vivo ^{31}P magnetic resonance spectroscopy for monitoring treatment response in breast cancer. Lancet 1:1326–1327, 1989.
4. Bloch F: Nuclear induction. Phys Rev 70:460–474, 1946.
5. Radda GK: The use of NMR spectroscopy for the understanding of disease. Science 233:640–645, 1986.
6. Murphy EJ, Rajagopalan B, Brindle KM, Radda GK: Phospholipid bilayer contribution to ^{31}P NMR spectra in vivo. Magn Reson Med 12:282–289, 1989.
7. Cohen MH, Reif F: Nuclear quadrupole effects in nuclear magnetic resonance. Solid State Phys 5:321–438, 1957.
8. Das TP, Hahn EL: Nuclear quadrupole resonance spectroscopy. Solid State Phys 5(suppl 1), 1958.
9. Jacard G, Wimperis S, Bodenhausen G: Multiple-quantum NMR spectroscopy of S=3/2 spins in the isotropic phase: a new probe for multiexponential relaxation. J Chem Phys 85:6282–6293, 1986.
10. Pekar J, Leigh JS Jr: Detection of biexponential relaxation in sodium-23 facilitated by double-quantum filtering. J Magn Reson 69:582–584, 1986.
11. Pekar J, Renshaw PF, Leigh JS Jr: Selective detection of intracellular sodium by coherence transfer NMR. J Magn Reson 72:159–161, 1987.
12. Moon RB, Richards JH: Determination of intracellular pH by ^{31}P magnetic resonance. J Biol Chem 248:7276–7278, 1973.
13. Bodenhausen G: Multiple quantum NMR. Prog NMR Spectrosc 14:137–173, 1981.
14. Warren WS, Sinton S, Weitekamp DP, Pines A: Selective excitation of multiple quantum coherences in nuclear magnetic resonance. Phys Rev Lett 43:1791–1794, 1979.
15. Ackerman JJH, Grove TH, Wong GG, et al: Mapping of metabolites in whole animals by ^{31}P NMR using surface coils. Nature 283:167–168, 1980.
16. Ahn CB, Cho AH: Analysis of eddy currents in nuclear magnetic resonance imaging. Magn Reson Med 17:149–163, 1991.
17. Ordidge RJ, Cresshull ID: The correction of transient B_0 field shifts following the application of pulsed gradients by phase correction in the time domain. J Magn Reson 69:151–155, 1986.
18. Klose U: In vivo proton spectroscopy in the presence of eddy currents. Magn Reson Med 14:26–30, 1990.
19. Riddle WR, Gibbs SJ, Willcott MR: Removing effects of eddy currents in proton MR spectroscopy. Magn Reson Med 19:501–509, 1992.
20. Hore PJ: Solvent suppression in Fourier transform nuclear magnetic resonance. J Magn Reson 55:283–300, 1983.
21. Singh S, Rutt BK, Henkelman RM: Projection presaturation: a fast and accurate technique for multidimensional spatial localization. J Magn Reson 87:567–583, 1990.
22. Sauter R, Mueller S, Weber H, Localization in in vivo ^{31}P NMR spectroscopy by combining surface coils and slice selective saturation. J Magn Reson 75:167–173, 1987.
23. Haase A: Localization of unaffected spins in NMR imaging and spectroscopy (LOCUS spectroscopy). Magn Reson Med 3:963–969, 1986.
24. Shungu DC, Glickson JD: Sensitivity and localization enhancement in

multinuclear in vivo NMR spectroscopy by outer volume presaturation. Magn Reson Med 30:661–671, 1993.

25. Ernst RR, Bodenhausen G, Wokaun A: Principles of Nuclear Magnetic Resonance in One and Two Dimensions. Oxford: Oxford University Press, 1987, pp 124–131.

26. Bolinger L: A Novel Technique for Nuclear Magnetic Resonance Spectroscopic Imaging Using Hadamard Transforms. Philadelphia: University of Pennsylvania, Ph.D. dissertation, 1989.

27. Garwood M, Schleich T, Ross BD, et al: A modified rotating frame experiment based on a Fourier series windowing function. Application to in vivo spatially localized NMR spectroscopy. J Magn Reson 65:239–251, 1985.

28. Insko EK, Bolinger L: Mapping of the radiofrequency field. J Magn Reson Ser A 103:82–85, 1993.

29. Oh CH, Hilal SK, Cho ZH, Mun IK: Radiofrequency field intensity mapping using a composite spin echo sequence. Magn Reson Imaging 8:21–25, 1990.

30. Lian J, Zhang W, Lowe IJ: A rugged three dimensional NMR technique for B₁ mapping of RF coils. In: Abstracts of the 11th Annual Meeting of the Society of Magnetic Resonance in Medicine, Berlin, Germany, 1992, p 4013.

31. Hoult DI: Rotating frame zeugmatography. J Magn Reson 33:183–197, 1979.

32. Styles P, Scott CA, Radda GK: A method for localizing high resolution NMR spectra from human subjects. Magn Reson Med 2:402–409, 1985.

33. Blackledge MJ, Rajagopalan B, Obehaensli RD, et al: Quantitative studies of human cardiac metabolism by ³¹P rotating frame NMR. Proc Natl Acad Sci USA 84:4283–4287, 1987.

34. Bottomley PA: Selective volume method for performing localized NMR spectroscopy. U.S. Patent 4,480,228, 1984.

35. Bottomley PA, Forster TB, Darrow RD: Depth-resolved surface-coil spectroscopy (DRESS) for in vivo ¹H, ³¹P and ¹³C NMR. J Magn Reson 59:338–342, 1984.

36. Aue WP, Mueller S, Cross TA, Seelig J: Volume-selective excitation. A novel approach to topical NMR. J Magn Reson 56:350–354, 1984.

37. Luyten PR, den Hollender JA: ¹H MR spatially resolved spectroscopy of human tissues in situ. Magn Reson Imaging 4:237–239, 1986.

38. Jensen DJ, Narayana PA, Delayre JL: Pulse sequence design for volume selective excitation in magnetic resonance. Med Phys 14:38–42, 1987.

39. Hasse A, Frahm J, Hanicke W, Matthei D: ¹H NMR chemical shift selective (CHESS) imaging. Phys Med Biol 30:341–345, 1985.

40. Granot J: Selective volume excitation using stimulated echoes (VEST). Applications to spatially localized spectroscopy and imaging. J Magn Reson 70:488–492, 1986.

41. Kimmich R, Hoepfel D: Volume-selective multipulse spin-echo spectroscopy. J Magn Reson 72:379–384, 1987.

42. Frahm J, Merboldt KD, Hanicke W: Localized proton spectroscopy using stimulated echoes. J Magn Reson 72:502–508, 1987.

43. Moonen CTW, Kienlin MV, van Zijl PCM, et al: Comparison of single shot localization methods (STEAM and PRESS) for in vivo proton NMR spectroscopy. NMR Biomed 2:201–208, 1989.

44. Ordidge RJ, Mansfield P, Lohman JAB, Prime SB: Volume selection using gradients and selective pulses. Ann N Y Acad Sci 508:376–385, 1987.

45. Kimmich R, Rommel E, Knuttel A: Theoretical treatment of volume-selective NMR spectroscopy (VOSY) applied to coupled spin systems. J Magn Reson 81:333–338, 1989.

46. Bolinger L, Lenkinski RE: Localization in clinical NMR spectroscopy. In: Berliner LJ, Reuben J, eds. Biological Magnetic Resonance, Volume 11. New York: Plenum Publishing, 1992, pp 1–53.

47. Brown TR, Kincaid BM, Ugurbil K: NMR chemical shift imaging in three dimensions. Proc Natl Acad Sci USA 79:3523–3526, 1982.

48. Haselgrove JC, Subramanian VH, Leigh JS, et al: In vivo one-dimensional imaging of phosphorus metabolites by phosphorus-31 nuclear magnetic resonance. Science 220:1170–1173, 1983.

49. Maudsley AA, Hilal SK, Perman WH, Simon HE: Spatially resolved high resolution spectroscopy by "four-dimensional" NMR. J Magn Reson 51:147–152, 1983.

50. Wang Z, Bolinger L, Subramanian HV, Leigh JS: Errors of Fourier chemical-shift imaging and their corrections. J Magn Reson 92:64–72, 1991.

51. Ordidge RJ, Connelly A, Lohman JAB: Image-selected in vivo spectroscopy (ISIS). A new technique for spatially selective NMR spectroscopy. J Magn Reson 66:283–294, 1986.

52. Ordidge RJ, Bowley RM, McHale G: A general approach to selection of multiple cubic volume elements using ISIS technique. Magn Reson Med 8:323–331, 1988.

53. Bolinger L, Leigh JS: Hadamard spectroscopic imaging (HSI) for multivolume localization. J Magn Reson 80:162–167, 1988.

54. Goelmen G, Walter G, Leigh JS: Hadamard spectroscopic imaging technique as applied to study human calf muscles. Magn Reson Med 25:349–354, 1992.

55. Gonen O, Hu J, Stoyanova R, et al: Hybrid three dimensional (1D-Hadamard, 2D-chemical shift imaging) phosphorus localized spectroscopy of phantom and human brain. Magn Reson Med 33:300–308, 1995.

56. Posse S, Aue WP: ¹H spectroscopic imaging at high resolution. NMR Biomed 2:234–239, 1989.

57. Galloway GJ, Brereton IM, Brooks WM, et al: A comparison of some gradient-encoded volume-selection techniques for in vivo NMR spectroscopy. Magn Reson Med 4:393–398, 1987.

58. Garwood M, Schleich T, Bendall MR: Simulation of selective pulse techniques for localized NMR spectroscopy. J Magn Reson 73:191–212, 1987.

59. Vanderborne K, McCully K, Kahihira H, et al: Metabolic heterogeneity in human calf muscle during maximal exercise. Proc Natl Acad Sci USA 88:5714–5718, 1992.

MRI-Guided Interventions

FERENC A. JOLESZ ■ GARY P. ZIENTARA

Despite the current progress in interventional radiology and minimally invasive therapy, surgery remains a mostly invasive field. Diagnostic radiology has benefited most from the advances in high-technology devices, electronics, and computers. At the same time, these advances have only minimally influenced conventional surgical practices. Nevertheless, new concepts and terminologies such as image-guided therapy, computer-assisted surgery, surgical robotics, and telesurgery have emerged. These potential new approaches to surgery may use advanced imaging modalities and computers to improve or complement the surgeon's ability to perform procedures, but their implementation does not necessarily guarantee that the invasive perception of surgery will be altered. The vision of image-guided, computer-assisted, minimally invasive therapy is a relatively new concept. This approach takes advantage of intraoperative imaging to improve essential features of surgery such as localization and targeting, planning, and optimizing access routes. Image guidance can also be used to monitor and control thermal ablative procedures and delivery of drugs.

Why do we need image guidance for minimally invasive surgery? The main reason is the significant reduction of the surgical or operational field associated with most minimally invasive operative procedures. Surgeons try to reduce the operative trauma by exposing and isolating the smallest segment of the anatomy possible while still allowing access to the target volume. This reduced exposure usually results in "keyhole" vision, which allows us to see only a well-defined but spatially limited area. The use of images to complement this narrowly focused direct visualization is quite important. The role of the radiologist is to cleverly use imaging modalities such as computed tomography (CT), ultrasonography, and magnetic resonance imaging (MRI) to provide a more complete anatomic definition and to display the intraoperative images to assist the interventional radiologist, endoscopist, or surgeon.

Direct visibility of the exposed anatomy is restricted to the surfaces. Surgeons, with or without the use of microscopes or endoscopes, cannot see beyond and below the surfaces because of the reflection of visible light. To overcome this limitation, imaging modalities have been used to help surgeons to expand their vision beyond the margins of their operational volume and beyond the exposed surfaces. The various imaging modalities can be distinguished by comparing their ability to represent the body as a three-dimensional (3D) structure, to delineate the anatomy, and to monitor dynamic changes in real time. MRI is potentially a real-time monitoring device. It can provide the best tissue characterization of any existing imaging modality. MRI parameters have some specific properties, such as sensitivity to temperature changes (which can be exploited for imaging thermal interventions) and flow sensitivity (which is applicable for vascular interventions). MR images are multiplanar and volumetric; isotropically sampled data sets can be collected.

The features of interventional MRI, which are consistent with most of the requirements for ideal image guidance, are the following:

1. *Real-time or near real-time image display.* The definition of real time depends on the time constants of the physical or physiologic changes that are monitored. The temporal resolution requirement for imaging mechanical motions of the heart (subsecond) is different from that for diffusion or injected contrast materials or temperature (second), and both are different from the requirements for imaging dynamic, thermally induced changes during interstitial laser treatment or cryotherapy (seconds to minute).

2. *Volumetric imaging.* Images have to encompass the 3D space and should be available in any plane within that volume. Isotropic or close to isotropic sampling of the voxels and the entire image volume is necessary to allow the viewer to appreciate the anatomic complexity.

3. *Interactive display and manipulation of volumetric image data.* Independently from the type of display (multiplanar two-dimensional [2D], 3D, or stereoscopic with or without virtual reality technologies), the user should interactively influence the manifestation of the data set. Interactive scan plane orientation or

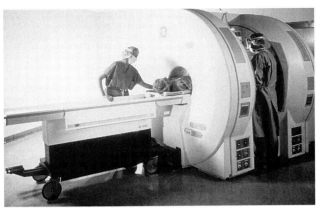

FIGURE 12–1. Interventional MRI system, 0.5-T General Electric (GE) Medical Systems Signa MRT, specifically designed to provide physician access to the patient.

viewing angle selection is essential for evaluation of 3D space. Manipulation, removal, or reinsertion of various components of the images (tissue types or anatomic parts) is necessitated by the limitations of visibility (overlapping tissue layers or organs) and access (surgical simulation).

4. *Freedom of navigation within the operational volume.* Physical limitations restricting the surgeon within the real body can be overcome by displaying the virtual data and freely moving within its space. Free navigation within the anatomic space can simulate surgical access routes and allows alternative viewing positions. The operator can learn the entirety of the operational volume within which procedures will be accomplished.

5. *Integration of imaging with therapy.* If these imaging requirements are fulfilled, MRI guidance for interventional or surgical procedures becomes feasible. The most important requirement is not the imaging itself, however, but the integration of the imaging system with the therapy and surgery components.

Target definition for biopsy and minimally invasive interventions requires image guidance. MRI should be used for every step in this process: detecting the target, guiding and localizing for biopsy, and monitoring the minimally invasive tissue ablations. MRI control of energy delivery during thermal ablation by an automated feedback mechanism is a good example for the integration of imaging with therapy devices.[1]

INTERVENTIONAL MRI

The most versatile imaging technique, MRI is exemplary for image guidance of therapy and surgery. Unfortunately, the cylindrical configuration of conventional MRI systems using a superconducting magnet excludes direct contact with the patient. The most obvious solution to overcome this problem is to image the patient with an open configuration magnet that allows full access to the patient. Open configuration, low-field MRI systems (Toshiba, Siemens) have been developed primarily as the result of resistive magnet

design and without much consideration of potential interventional use. Nevertheless, they allow access to the patient, and some direct control of interventional procedures is feasible in such systems.[2] The first superconductive open magnet system specifically designed for interventional use, the 0.5-T General Electric (GE) Signa MRT, has been developed by General Electric Medical Systems (Milwaukee, WI) and is being tested at the Brigham and Women's Hospital in Boston.[3] Unlike a horizontal gap magnet, the vertical gap configuration of this system is well suited for interventional work because it allows the physician full access to the exposed anatomy of the patient (Fig. 12–1). The surgeon can perform various procedures while standing or sitting between the two static magnet "doughnuts" of the magnet system. The patient in the magnet can be erect, sitting, or lying either parallel or perpendicular to the bore axis.

A notable engineering feature of the GE system is the lack of gradient coils within the open part of the system. These coils are concealed within the doughnuts, where they can provide the necessary spatial gradients within the imaged volume without precluding direct access. In conventional clinical MRI systems, the patient is surrounded not only by the magnetic gradient coils but also by the head or body radiofrequency (RF) transmit-receive coil. The open magnet has no fixed geometric body or head RF coil. Rather, the open magnet system is accompanied by a set of RF coils, each of which is specifically designed for imaging a particular body part. These RF coils are flexible and therefore adapt perfectly to the shape of the anatomic region under investigation. They are integrated into the surgical drape, can be sterilized, and allow full access to the image volume (Fig. 12–2). Optimal coil design for a particular anatomic region can significantly improve image quality; therefore, individual coil development is strategically important for interventional MRI.

The interventional MRI suite is the result of a "cross-fertilization" between an operating room, an interventional radiology suite, and a conventional MRI unit. Because MRI guidance may be provided during endo-

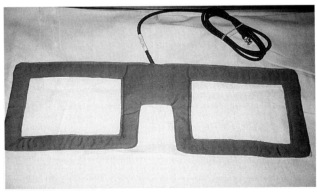

FIGURE 12–2. Flexible radiofrequency (RF) coil used with the GE Signa MRT interventional MRI system. Flexible RF coils are designed to be integrated into the surgical drape and allow full unimpaired access to the tissue of interest, as needed in MRI-guided therapies and biopsies.

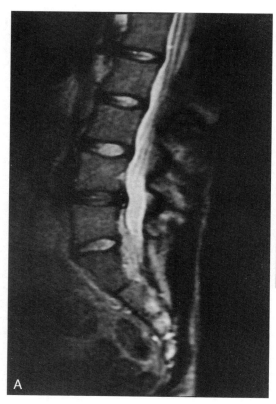

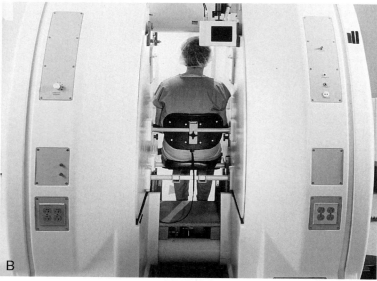

FIGURE 12–3. Lumbosacral spine MRI *(A)* with the patient in the sitting position within the GE Signa MRT interventional MRI system *(B)*. (*A* and *B* courtesy of Amir A. Zamani, MD, and Carl S. Winalski, MD, Department of Radiology, Brigham and Women's Hospital, Boston, MA.)

scopic, laparoscopic, or open surgical procedures, this area must be equipped as an operating room. Because most of the planned procedures are minimally invasive, the suite more resembles a day surgery unit. In addition, the computing facilities, display devices, and integrated therapy systems contribute to making the interventional MRI suite a unique working environment.

The interventional MRI system should have similar imaging characteristics (static field homogeneity, gradient strength, and linearity) and perform well as an imaging system. Image quality must be comparable to that quality (resolution, signal-to-noise ratio) obtained on diagnostic systems at the same field strength. The open configuration, the special gradient coils, and the flexible RF coils should be capable of diagnostic quality images. While larger anatomic regions like the abdomen are imaged, the flexible RF coils cannot provide uniform signal intensity, and without a surrounding body coil an entire cross section of the abdomen cannot be obtained. Furthermore, the homogeneous magnetic field volume does not necessarily extend to include the entire body volume within the open superconducting magnets. These characteristics do not necessarily represent deficiencies if the primary application of the system is interventional and not diagnostic. MRI interventional procedures should follow an appropriate diagnostic work-up that encompasses larger anatomic volumes. During the course of the biopsy or other interventions, however, imaging should be limited to a well-defined target volume. Optimization of the flexible RF coils for the target organ, or only one part of it, can provide a high-resolution road map for the interventional process.

A unique feature of open configuration magnets is the potential to obtain functional musculoskeletal images (Fig. 12–3). This unique opportunity can be expected to improve the clinical diagnosis of various joint diseases. Maybe the most important diagnostic use of a vertically open configuration magnet is in imaging the lumbosacral spine. Conventional spine images are taken with the patient in the neutral, supine position when the weight of the body is not loading the intervertebral disks. Images taken under gravity conditions may well improve the diagnostic potential of MRI for evaluating low back pain.

The major goal of interventional MRI is to provide image guidance for surgical and interventional procedures. The systematic approach should address the main components of the process: imaging, localization, improved access, and control of energy delivery for therapy. Research activities should concentrate on these major issues before this new type of image guidance is accepted for extensive clinical trials.

DYNAMIC MRI

MRI-guided therapy is accomplished by using imaging methods that pulse, acquire, reconstruct, and display a series of images dynamically. Dynamic MRI differs from standard MRI in that a large number of images are formed successively and rapidly, by continually updating or reacquiring image data.

The imaging requirements of interventional[4, 5] and functional[6, 7] MRI have driven the evolution of dynamic MRI methods during the past several years. Clinical applications, such as MR cardiac angiography, have also presented a challenge for dynamic MRI to overcome cardiac and respiratory physiologic motion. Interventional MRI poses perhaps the greatest demands on the temporal and spatial resolution of imaging technology because of a combination of factors: the changing orientation of the imaging plane; surgical and therapeutic events occurring within the field of view (FOV); physiologic motion near and within the FOV; intensity changes in the FOV due to contrast agents or therapy; and the need for 3D volume information to safely and effectively apply and monitor therapies. These particular imaging needs of interventional MRI are not entirely satisfied, but research is progressing.

Dynamic MRI methods are classified in the two major categories: nonadaptive and adaptive. Nonadaptive dynamic MRI methods include four general categories of methods, all designed with the goal of increasing MRI temporal resolution: 1) fast pulse sequences, 2) reduced k-space sampling without using prior knowledge, 3) reduced k-space sampling exploiting prior knowledge, and 4) reduced k-space sampling using model-based reconstruction.

Fast pulse sequences attempt to rapidly manipulate magnetic field gradients and RF pulses to acquire as much spatially encoded information as possible in a short period, with sensitivity to different physical properties (T1 relaxation, T2 relaxation, susceptibility, diffusion, chemical shift). Fast pulse sequence methods include fast spin-echo methods such as rapid acquisition with relaxation enhancement (RARE),[8–10] fast low-flip-angle gradient-recalled echo techniques,[11, 12] BURST,[13] gradient- and spin-echo (GRASE) imaging,[14] echo-planar imaging,[15–17] and spiral scan methods.[18, 19] Fast pulse sequence methods may suffer from low tissue contrast or reduced spatial resolution or low signal-to-noise ratio.

Reduced k-space sampling methods include Fourier-encoded keyhole imaging,[20–22] MR fluoroscopy,[23–25] spiral scan methods, and random k-space sampling methods. During keyhole imaging,[20–22] high spatial frequency data are acquired once from a baseline image. After changes in the FOV occur, only the lower spatial frequency data are dynamically acquired because, it is assumed, no change occurs in the underlying morphology that is responsible for the high spatial frequency variation in the image. MR fluoroscopy[23–25] combines a fast MR pulse sequence and data acquisition techniques with specialized hardware for image reconstruction. Images acquired using reduced k-space sampling may suffer from reduced spatial resolution, artifacts, or low tissue contrast or may be restricted to a small FOV.

A reduced k-space sampling method that advantageously exploits prior knowledge for acquiring data efficiently has been developed, requiring training sets of images displaying the same anatomy.[26] A constrained reconstruction method based on superresolution techniques that exploits prior knowledge has been investigated,[27] and results for limited applications have been published.[28]

One common application of dynamic MRI has been investigation of changes after bolus injection of contrast agents for characterizing tumors, mainly in the brain[29–31] and liver.[32–34] Dynamic MRI has also been used for studies of heart,[35] gastrointestinal tract,[36] and upper airway[37] motion and for imaging of cerebral function.[7] In a novel application, changes induced by heating and cooling were imaged to monitor the progress of thermal damage in tissue.[38, 39] These dynamic studies have employed echo-planar imaging,[38] low-flip-angle gradient-echo techniques,[37] or rapid acquisition with relaxation enhancement techniques,[39] with temporal resolution ranging from about one image per minute to five images per second.

Although advances have been made in designing nonadaptive imaging methods, research is in the initial stages in the design of methods that reduce redundancy in data acquisition. Because the maximal MR data acquisition rate of fast nonadaptive imaging techniques is being approached, dynamically adaptive MRI methods that minimize redundancy in data acquisition are growing in importance. Adaptive methods have the potential to provide the spatial and temporal resolution that will be required by more demanding applications of dynamic MRI such as interventional MRI.

Adaptive MRI methods are distinguished as those in which the image data acquisition strategy is modified dynamically depending on information obtained from the current and most recently acquired images. By this definition, no methods currently in common use are strictly adaptive, but several methods do attempt to obtain information about the motion that would normally cause image artifacts and apply corrections during postprocessing.[40, 41] Respiratory-ordered phase encoding (ROPE)[42] adapts to prior knowledge of the respiration pattern and reorders the phase-encoding steps of a sequence; however, the method has only limited application.

Adaptive imaging methods can be implemented by modifying the spatial encoding of the FOV, by changing the algorithm by which the spatial-encoding order is enacted during the pulse sequence, or by a combination of these two. When spatial encoding is optimized to the best estimate of the current FOV, then additional computations are necessary before each image acquisition. If the algorithm by which the spatial-encoding order is enacted during the pulse sequence is dynamically modified, one or more acquired data sets need to be analyzed immediately after acquisition. Adaptive methods can be implemented in the context of fast pulse sequences such as echo-planar or fast gradient-echo pulse sequences, which in present use do not exploit known redundancy in data acquisition.

Three dynamically adaptive MRI methods are wavelet transform–encoded MRI,[43] singular value decomposition–encoded MRI,[44] and adaptive Fourier transform–encoded MRI (Panych LP, Jolesz FA, unpublished observations). Wavelet transform– and singular value decomposition–encoding techniques are fundamentally different from standard Fourier transform MRI because they use spatially selective RF excitations to encode data in an alternative orthogonal basis set. In both methods, prior image information is exploited to reduce redundancy in data acquisition. The multiresolution structure of the wavelet transform–encoded data can adaptively locate and selectively resolve regions of change in an image.[43] Singular value decomposition–encoded MRI provides near-optimal spatial encoding.[44] Singular value decomposition–encoded MRI is suitable for a multiresolution adaptation as well as keyhole updating method analogous to that employed in keyhole Fourier MRI. Adaptive Fourier transform–encoded MRI differs from standard Fourier MRI in that the necessity of reacquiring data in k-space is determined dynamically, minimizing oversampling.

SURGICAL PLANNING AND INTRAOPERATIVE GUIDANCE

Dynamic MRI methods and navigational aids (as discussed in a later section) provide the fundamental imaging tools for surgical navigation and therapy targeting and monitoring in an interventional MRI system. Complementary to these physics and electronics aids are the computation and display-based capabilities of surgical planning and intraoperative guidance. These tools enhance the surgeon's ability to plan and perform an intervention through the preoperative and intraoperative use of computer-generated displays of specially processed 3D images. A realistic 3D environment is created for the physician, containing the patient's relevant anatomy that can be reoriented, redrawn, specially displayed, and interactively manipulated to explore and rehearse an interventional procedure.

Cross-sectional 2D images are useful for diagnostic purposes. In general, even without a 3D perspective, the radiologist can still establish the diagnosis. If 3D imaging provides an additional advantage for diagnosis, as in complex spine or pelvic fractures, time is usually ample to obtain 3D reconstructions. Similarly, 3D image reconstruction for surgical planning, simulation, and intraoperative guidance occurs during the preoperative phase, and the time required for reconstruction of the cross-sectional images is more or less irrelevant. If 3D images are to be obtained intraoperatively, however, image processing must be real-time or near real-time. In both cases significant computational resources are required. Yet, practical methods for surgical planning and intraoperative guidance can increase the use of minimally invasive therapies and therefore reduce the length of recovery for the patient.

The computer methods required for 3D planning and guidance are generally applied in a sequence of steps: 1) image segmentation, 2) rendering, 3) registration of imaged anatomy with the patient's anatomy, 4) display, and 5) interaction of the surgeon with the displayed information.

The segmentation of the images is a computational process initiated by identification or selection of different tissue classes. This first step, if automated, requires high-performance computers and high-speed computation to allow almost immediate display of the color-coded digital anatomy. Segmentation is followed often by interactive identification of anatomic regions. This can be performed manually or automatically by warping acquired image data to a generic anatomic atlas. The 3D rendering of the data, the creation of a computer display representation of the anatomy, follows, using various techniques.[45–49]

After these initial steps of segmentation and rendering, 3D images must be accurately matched with the orientation of intraoperative images on a computer display or projected onto the patient's corresponding anatomic region to be used for localization (enhanced reality). Accurate determination of the geometric transformation to match images correctly to the patient or patient's images, known as registration, is extremely important for many image-guided procedures. Without accurate registration, images cannot provide an exact road map for procedures.[50, 51]

Although surgeons cannot move freely within the anatomic boundaries of the human body, interventionalists who use interactive virtual reality and enhanced reality displays for surgical planning can navigate freely or move within a virtual data set formed from the 3D segmented, processed, and rendered images. Surgical or interventional tools (needles, forceps, knives) can be tracked within the image space, and their position can serve as the reference for acquiring various image planes, choosing view angles, or performing not only real but also virtual manipulations.[51, 52] These concepts are new for diagnostic radiologists, who are accustomed to fixed image planes and projections and do not usually need to relate the reference frame of one image set to the other.

NAVIGATION AND TARGETING DURING INTERVENTIONAL MRI

Localization in diagnostic radiology is based on anatomic relationships. Stereotactic procedures, with and without the use of frames, require establishment of reference frames, assessment of the correspondence between them, and knowledge of a tool's position in relationship to the anatomy within which they are used.[51–58]

Traditionally, stereotactic methods have been used only by neurosurgeons, but the current trend is to use the same principles for accurately localizing biopsy specimens throughout the entire body.[59] Minimally invasive therapies that remove or ablate tumors in situ minimize the available material for pathologic study and destroy the original anatomic landmarks, especially tumor margins. The only solution is to define the biology of the tumor and localize its exact extent in a series of precise biopsies under image guidance. That is the main reason that the stereotactic approach to tumor diagnosis and treatment is so important.[60] The use of imaging systems, especially MRI, is the only way to resolve the conflict between the need for correct pathologic samples and minimally invasive approaches. We should use the best available imaging modalities, or their combination, to identify the target and define its spatial extent. Image fusion techniques can improve target definition and characterization. The combination of MRI with CT, positron emission tomography, single photon emission computed tomography, or angiography can be extremely helpful for full characterization and definition of the tumors.[59, 61–64]

The knowledge of instrument position is important for registration and stereotactic approaches. Sensor-detectable attachments to instruments can serve as registration aids, and the positional information they provide is needed for computations that define the trajectories. In the open magnet system, we can use a frameless stereotactic method for localization and targeting. This method was originally developed for neurosurgery[52, 56] and implemented at the Brigham and Women's Hospital in Boston in the conventional closed 1.5-T Signa systems. The basic concept is that a tool or instrument (in the case of biopsy, the needle holder) can be localized by attaching two flashing, light-emitting diodes (LEDs) to its surface (Fig. 12–4). These LEDs produce invisible infrared beams detected by three sensors (approximately 1 m from the LEDs) and localized by simple triangulation. By this tracking method, the interventional MRI console computer has continuous information about the instrument tip position and about alignment of the instrument's axis within the space.

This optical tracking concept can be used in the open magnet for interactive image plane acquisition. The optical localizing device, PIXSYS (PIXSYS, Inc., Boulder, CO), an integral part of the GE Signa MRT system, allows tracking of any tool or instrument if a direct optical link can be established between the LEDs and the sensors located above the imaging field. In one method, images can be generated centered on the position of the instrument tip in the conventional axial-coronal-sagittal plane. In another method, a tool can be used in the fashion of an ultrasound transducer, and images can be generated along the axis of the optically tracked tool.

A great advantage in this application is that image planes that are defined by the instrument axis using PIXSYS can be changed without moving the tool itself. Using audio communication with the technologist, the physician can request images in the 0° plane, the 90° plane, or any plane perpendicular to the axis of the tool (see Fig. 12–4). Positioning the optically tracked tools and selecting the related image planes provide an interactive way to localize targets, define trajectories, and review alternative access routes. During biopsy, for example, if the defined plane includes both the entry and target point and review of the anatomy shows no problem, the needle can be advanced to the target.

This one-step localization and targeting using image guidance is the essential feature of frameless stereotaxy. In the open magnet using the PIXSYS, there is no need for several steps to register images with the patient's anatomy, to define trajectories, and to perform a biopsy. In this simplified process, we interactively scan through the image volume, using the instrument and attached LEDs, until the appropriate image or trajectory is found. When the instrument is a biopsy needle holder, for example, target localization is immediately followed by advancement of the needle, which is also continuously visible in images. Because the needle holder is localized during biopsy, the images will be in the same plane as the needle (although some distortion due to bending of the biopsy needle is possible).

Tumors may be located by interactive image plane acquisition and targeting using a needle icon (Fig. 12–5). Review of the orthogonal planes related to the axis of the needle gives an appreciation of anatomy around the needle path. The planned advancement or anticipated trajectory of the needle can be used for targeting and later for comparing the actual path of the needle with the planned trajectory. The near real-time imaging during needle advancement not only offers an opportunity for trajectory correction but also replaces the depth measurement that is necessary for nonmonitored cross-sectional biopsies. Most of the images during tissue biopsy are acquired using a gradient-echo sequence repeated every 1 to 2 seconds, which represents sufficient temporal resolution.

Needle placement for image-guided laser decompression of the intervertebral disk is shown in Figure 12–6. In this case, localizing images of the intervertebral space are taken by interactively manipulating the image plane through the hand-held needle holder. These are aligned when the needle icon's path goes through the disk space. The next step is to acquire the perpendicular image while the position of the needle holder remains unchanged. The images in the perpendicular plane clearly demonstrate that the path of the needle is safe and not obstructed by bony elements or neural structures, ensuring the patient's safety, proper laser positioning, and effective therapy.

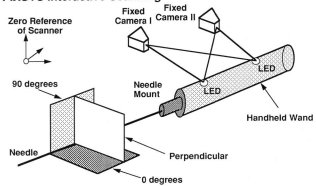

PIXSYS Interactive Scanning

FIGURE 12–4. Schematic description of the optical tracking system used in the GE Signa MRT interventional MRI system. The tracking system defines the MRI plane relative to a hand-held instrument such as a biopsy needle. Shown here are diagrammatic representations of imaging planes at 0°, 90°, and perpendicular to the instrument's axis. (Courtesy of Stuart G. Silverman, MD, Department of Radiology, Brigham and Women's Hospital, Boston, MA.)

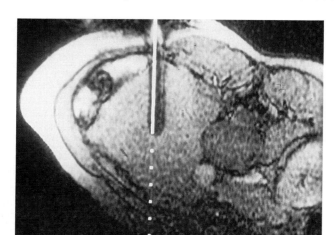

FIGURE 12–5. MRI-guided needle biopsy of a retroperitoneal leiomyosarcoma on the GE Signa MRT interventional MRI system. Needle icon *(solid white line)* superimposed on the image during the intervention indicates the current location of the biopsy needle, determined by the PIXSYS infrared beam tracking system with LEDs affixed to the biopsy needle holder. The MRI appearance of the needle is the region of signal void along the axis of the needle icon. The trajectory of the needle is predicted by the dotted white line superimposed on the image. (Courtesy of Stuart G. Silverman, MD, Department of Radiology, Brigham and Women's Hospital, Boston, MA.)

The PIXSYS tracking method described earlier is appropriate only for rigid instruments that are at least partially outside the body where the instrument-fixed LEDs can be tracked by the sensors. Tracking the tip of flexible devices (catheters, drains, flexible endoscopes) is not possible using optical methods. An MRI-specific method, developed by Dumoulin and co-workers[65] can be used for tracking flexible devices or instruments within the MRI system. A small wire loop attached to the tip of the catheter or other flexible device acts as an RF receiver coil and picks up the spatially specific RF of surrounding tissue during successive orthogonal readout magnetic field gradient pulses. Advancement of the device tip can then be displayed within a previously acquired image plane by this MRI tip-tracking method. Also, the tip position can be used to dynamically select the image plane.

Improvements in surgical strategies are directly related to optimizing access routes and controlling the spatial extent of destructive energies used for therapy. Various devices employed in MRI-guided interventions (including surgical robots, computer-assisted interven-

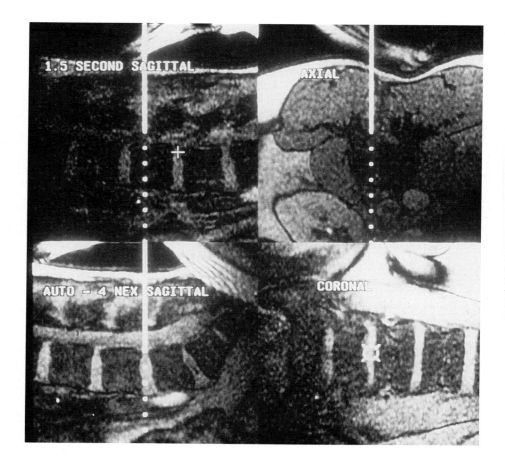

FIGURE 12–6. Planned needle trajectory for MRI-guided laser decompression of the intervertebral disk. Sagittal, axial, and coronal MR images are centered at the needle tip. Needle icon *(solid white line or circle)* is superimposed on the image during the intervention and indicates the current location of the needle; the possible continued trajectory of the needle is displayed as the dotted white line. (Courtesy of Stuart G. Silverman, MD, Department of Radiology, Brigham and Women's Hospital, Boston, MA.)

tional tools, energy delivery devices) are greatly dependent on image-derived information for feedback control of their actions.

MRI-GUIDED THERMAL THERAPY

Image guidance is a general concept, applicable to a variety of controlled interventional procedures and capable of revolutionizing the field of therapy. Interactive control of destructive energy deposition has been until now an unresolved problem in tumor treatment. This is especially true in the case of thermal ablative procedures such as interstitial laser surgery, cryotherapy, and focused ultrasound. Previously, direct measurement or mapping of tissue temperature distribution has been possible only with multiple temperature measuring probes. Thermocouples or temperature-sensitive fiberoptic devices were introduced into the tissue invasively at a finite number of locations. The few temperature-sensitive probes that could be implanted in this procedure were usually insufficient to provide precise monitoring of the spatiotemporal heat distribution.

MRI can provide the information necessary for the planning, monitoring, and control of thermal therapies, ensuring the role of thermal therapies as important tools in the future of interventional MRI. Notably, no conventional imaging modality except MRI can signal the end point of thermal procedures, the phase transition, which is consistent with lethal and irreversible tissue damage. Adequate monitoring of tissue temperature and temperature-induced tissue changes is necessary for safe, controlled energy deposition and the safe and effective use of thermal therapies.

The role of MRI is twofold in imaging thermal surgery: 1) to restrict energy deposition to the target tissue by demonstrating transient temperature elevations in the surrounding normal tissue and 2) to signal the irreversible phase transition (cell necrosis) within the target volume. MRI-visible reversible changes within tissue and irreversible phase transitions within the tumor tissue provide important information that can be used to control (terminate or continue) energy deposition. Therefore, MRI can provide the needed feedback control for thermal ablations.[1]

Research is progressing in the application of MRI to the planning, monitoring, and control of a variety of thermal therapies: hyperthermia, interstitial laser surgery, cryotherapy, and focused ultrasound.

Hyperthermia is based on slight temperature elevation (about 41°C), which requires exact 3D temperature maps to achieve homogeneous treatment of solid tumors. Temperature-sensitive MRI sequences may fulfill this requirement.[39, 65–74]

The temperature sensitivity of various MRI parameters (T1, diffusion, chemical shift) can also be exploited for detecting temperature changes within a critical temperature range. As opposed to hyperthermia, thermal surgery uses temperatures higher than 56°C to 60°C. At that temperature, proteins are denatured and the resulting thermal coagulation causes irreversible tissue damage. Appropriate MRI sequences can demonstrate the normal margins surrounding thermal lesions where the temperature elevation is still too low to cause cell necrosis yet is MRI visible and, most importantly, can differentiate tissue phase transitions. However, accurate temperature mapping is not possible by MRI above 50°C because the tissue undergoes severe metabolic, physiologic, and structural changes above that temperature.

A typical high-temperature ablative procedure is interstitial laser surgery. This method can be a direct continuation of a biopsy because optical fibers can be introduced through a biopsy needle. Both experimental and clinical interstitial laser therapy has been controlled by continuous MRI monitoring of the thermally induced changes during energy delivery. MRI-guided laser treatment of brain and liver tumors has been tested in Europe at several institutions.[75–91]

Cryotherapy is a cold thermal method that uses biopsy-like targeting as a first step before a freezing probe is introduced into the tumor. The frozen tissue is clearly visible on MR images because the tissue water changes to solid ice crystals during the process. The ice crystals give no measurable MR signal: the expanding freezing zone is represented in MR images by an increasing area of signal void.[91–95]

The most promising thermal ablative method is focused ultrasound heating. As opposed to interstitial laser surgery and cryotherapy just described, focused ultrasound heating does not involve an invasive probe. The focused ultrasound beam is targeted by positioning a transducer outside the body and causing a tissue-killing energy dose to develop at a focal point within the body without causing any damage to surrounding or intervening tissue. This technique does not require skin incision, and spatial control is achieved by the motion of the transducer.[4, 5, 96–99] Among currently available image guidance systems, only MRI promises to provide the temperature sensitivity required for monitoring focused ultrasound therapy.

MRI-guided focused ultrasound therapy is tumor ablation for the future. Because focused ultrasound heating can be performed within the MRI system, the extent of heat deposition can be monitored and controlled by MRI. At Brigham and Women's Hospital in Boston, the MR-compatible focused ultrasound transducers have been installed within the table of the conventional 1.5-T GE Signa system.[5] The transducer can advance in all directions by a hydraulic mechanism controlled from a computer workstation. Relatively low energies indicate that a slight but MRI-detectable temperature elevation occurs at the focal point. Images acquired using temperature-sensitive MRI sequences localize the focal area within the tissue (Fig. 12–7). This initial heat deposition causes no irreversible tissue damage and can therefore be utilized for targeting. The focal point can be moved to the desired target location without making any permanent changes. When targeting is completed, the energy level is increased and the resulting higher temperature (60°C to 90°C) causes denaturing of the cellular proteins. This type of energy delivery is safe and accurate within a

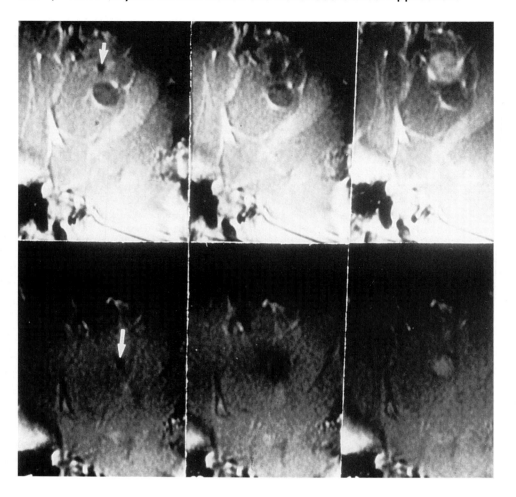

FIGURE 12–7. Rabbit thigh muscle MRI time series *(left to right)* during focused ultrasound pulsing, displaying MRI-detectable temperature elevation and necrosis. The top and bottom rows of images represent equivalent time series for different individual focal positions. Focused ultrasound pulses are applied immediately before acquisition of the leftmost images, and the low-dose focal point appears as a hypointense region *(see arrows)*. A low-dose focused pulse can be used for localizing the focal point and targeting before applying the ablative therapeutic energy pulse. After 15 seconds of focused ultrasound application *(center images)*, the affected focus increases in size. After a few minutes *(rightmost images)*, the affected tissue region becomes hyperintense, indicating necrosis, still MRI visible. (Courtesy of Kullervo H. Hynynen, PhD, Department of Radiology, Brigham and Women's Hospital, Boston, MA.)

few millimeters. In focused ultrasound heating trials using rabbit brain, we have been able to induce lesions as small as 1 mm (Fig. 12–8). The spatial resolution of MRI systems, therefore, is comparable to the accuracy of the focused ultrasound system, which is as accurate as the hand of any good surgeon.

MRI-guided focused ultrasound heating is a good example of integrating therapeutic devices with imaging systems. This integration is a prerequisite of image-guided therapy: both localization and feedback control of the energy disposition call for a fully integrated system.

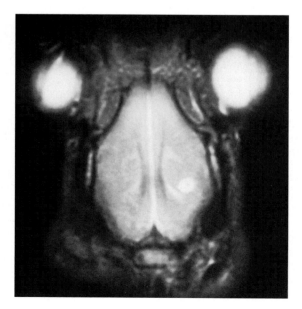

FIGURE 12–8. Rabbit brain MR image displaying MRI-detectable focused ultrasound target of 1-mm-diameter tissue (created lesion) appearing hyperintense after 4 days. This experimental result illustrates the high precision of spatial selectivity of the ablative therapy possible with MRI-guided focused ultrasound ablation therapy. (Courtesy of Kullervo H. Hynynen, PhD, Department of Radiology, Brigham and Women's Hospital, Boston, MA.)

CONCLUSIONS

We are entering a new area of medical applications of high technology. As just described, a wide range of methods, instrumentation, imaging systems, and therapies are being identified and characterized. There are still unresolved problems, and no one has yet tested the clinical efficacy of the techniques under trial. Rather, the few cases already performed contribute to a feasibility study. The scientific, technologic, and medical pathway to the future of interventional MRI and minimally invasive surgery is becoming clearer.

MRI-guided intervention is an interdisciplinary field. Not only radiologists but also surgeons, computer scientists, engineers, and physicists are contributing to the development of this exciting new field. There is also a need for strong collaboration between academic sites and industry. Our ultimate goal is to take these superb technologies—the MRI, the therapy systems, and the computers—into the operating room of the next century.

REFERENCES

1. Wyman DR, Wilson BC, Malone DE: Medical imaging systems for feedback control of interstitial laser photocoagulation. Proc IEEE 80:890–902, 1992.
2. Gronemeyer DH, Kaufman L, Rothschild P, Seibel RM: New possibilities and aspects of low-field magnetic resonance tomography. Radiol Diagn (Berlin) 30:519–527, 1989.
3. Schenck JF, Jolesz FA, Roemer PB, et al: Superconducting open configuration MRI system for image-guided therapy. Radiology 195:805–814, 1995.
4. Cline HE, Schenck JF, Hynynen K, et al: MR-guided focused ultrasound surgery. J Comput Assist Tomogr 16:956–965, 1992.
5. Cline HE, Schenck JF, Watkins RD, et al: Magnetic resonance guided thermal surgery. Magn Reson Med 30:98–106, 1993.
6. Ogawa S, Lee TM, Nayak AS, Glynn P: Oxygenation-sensitive contrast in magnetic resonance image of rodent brain at high magnetic fields. Magn Reson Med 14:68–78, 1990.
7. Belliveau JW, Kennedy DN, McKinstry RC, et al: Functional mapping of the human visual cortex by magnetic resonance imaging. Science 54:716–718, 1991.
8. Hennig J, Nauerth A, Friedburg H: RARE imaging: a fast imaging method for clinical MR. Magn Reson Med 3:823–833, 1986.
9. Hennig J, Friedburg H: Clinical applications and methodological developments of the RARE technique. Magn Reson Imaging 6:391–395, 1988.
10. Melki PS, Mulkern RV, Panych LP, Jolesz FA: Comparing the FAISE method with conventional dual-echo sequences. J Magn Reson Imag 1:319–326, 1991.
11. Haase A, Frahm J, Matthaei D: FLASH imaging: rapid NMR imaging using low flip angle pulses. J Magn Reson Imaging 67:258–266, 1986.
12. Haase A: Snapshot flash MRI: application to T1, T2, and chemical shift imaging. Magn Reson Med 13:77–79, 1990.
13. Duyn JH, van Gelderen P, Liu G, Moonen CT: Fast volume scanning with frequency-shifted BURST MRI. Magn Reson Med 32:429–432, 1994.
14. Oshio K, Feinberg DA: GRASE (gradient- and spin-echo) imaging: a novel fast MRI technique. Magn Reson Med 20:344–349, 1991.
15. Mansfield P: Multiplanar image formation using NMR spin echoes. J Phys C 10:L55–L58, 1977.
16. Mansfield P, Pykett I: Biological and medical imaging by NMR. J Magn Reson 29:355–373, 1978.
17. Cohen MS, Weisskoff RM: Ultra-fast imaging. Magn Reson Imaging 9:1–37, 1991.
18. Ordidge P, Howesman A, Coxon R, et al: Snapshot imaging at 0.5 T using echo-planar techniques. Magn Reson Med 10:227–240, 1989.
19. Rzedzian R, Pykett I: Instant images of the human heart using a new, whole-body MR imaging system. AJR 149:245–250, 1987.
20. van Vaals JJ, Brummer ME, Dixon WT: "Keyhole" method for accelerating imaging of contrast agent uptake. J Magn Reson Imaging 3:671–675, 1993.
21. Brummer ME, Dixon WT, Gerety B, Tuithof T: Composite k-space windows (keyhole techniques) to improve temporal resolution in a dynamic series of images following contrast administration. In: Conference Abstracts. Berkeley, CA: Society of Magnetic Resonance in Medicine, 1992, p 4236.
22. Chenevert TL, Pipe JG: Dynamic 3D imaging at high temporal resolution via reduced k-space sampling. In: Conference Abstracts. Berkeley, CA: Society of Magnetic Resonance in Medicine, 1993, p 1262.
23. Riederer SJ, Tasciyan T, Farzaneh F, et al: MR fluoroscopy: technical feasibility. Magn Reson Med 8:1–15, 1988.
24. Wright RC, Riederer SJ, Farzaneh F, et al: Real-time MR fluoroscopic data acquisition and image reconstruction. Magn Reson Med 12:407–415, 1989.
25. Holsinger AE, Wright RC, Riederer SJ, et al: Real-time interactive magnetic resonance imaging. Magn Reson Med 14:547–553, 1990.
26. Cao Y, Levin DN: Feature-recognizing MRI. Magn Reson Med 30:305–317, 1993.
27. Haacke EM, Liang Z-P, Izen SH: Constrained reconstruction: a superresolution, optimal signal-to-noise alternative to the Fourier transform in magnetic resonance imaging. Med Phys 16:388–397, 1989.
28. Constable RT, Henkelman RM: Data extrapolation for truncation artifact removal. Magn Reson Med 17:108–118, 1991.
29. Nagele T, Petersen D, Klose U, et al: Dynamic contrast enhancement of intracranial tumors with snapshot-FLASH MR. Am J Neuroradiol 14:89–98, 1993.
30. Gowland P, Mansfield P, Bullock P, et al: Dynamic studies of gadolinium uptake in brain tumors using inversion-recovery echo-planar imaging. Magn Reson Med 26:241–258, 1992.
31. Bullock PR, Mansfield P, Gowland P, et al: Dynamic imaging of contrast enhancement in brain tumors. Magn Reson Med 19:293–298, 1991.
32. Yamashita Y, Yoshimatsu S, Sumi M, et al: Dynamic MR imaging of hepatoma treated by transcatheter arterial embolization therapy. Acta Radiol 34:303–308, 1993.
33. Yoshida H, Itai Y, Ohtomo K, et al: Small hepatocellular carcinoma and cavernous hemangioma: differentiation with dynamic FLASH MR imaging with Gd-DPTA. Radiology 171:339–342, 1989.
34. Ward J, Martinez D, Chalmers AG, et al: Rapid dynamic contrast-enhanced magnetic resonance imaging of the liver and portal vein. Br J Radiol 66:214–222, 1993.
35. Rzedzian RR, Pykett IL: Instant images of the human heart using a new, whole-body imaging system. AJR 149:245–250, 1987.
36. Stehling MK, Evans DF, Lamon G, et al: Gastrointestinal tract: dynamic MR studies with echo-planar imaging. Radiology 171:41–46, 1989.
37. Shellock FG, Schatz CJ, Julien PM, et al: Dynamic study of the upper airway with ultrafast spoiled GRASS MR imaging. J Magn Reson Imaging 2:103–107, 1992.
38. Bleier AR, Jolesz FA, Cohen MS, et al: Real-time magnetic resonance imaging of laser heat deposition in tissue. Magn Reson Med 21:132–137, 1991.
39. Matsumoto R, Oshio K, Jolesz FA: Monitoring of laser and freezing-induced ablation in the liver with T1-weighted MR imaging. J Magn Reson Imaging 2:555–562, 1991.
40. Ehman RL, Felmlee JP: Adaptive technique for high-definition MR imaging of moving structures. Radiology 173:255–263, 1989.
41. Xiang QS, Henkelman RM: Dynamic image reconstruction: MR movies from ghosts. J Magn Reson Imaging 2:679–685, 1992.
42. Bailes DR, Gilderdale DJ, Bydder GM, et al: Respiratory ordered phase encoding (ROPE): a method for reducing respiratory motion artifacts in MR imaging. J Comput Assist Tomogr 9:835–838, 1985.
43. Panych LP, Jakab PD, Jolesz FA: An implementation of wavelet-encoded MRI. J Magn Reson Imaging 3:649–655, 1993.
44. Zientara GP, Panych LP, Jolesz FA: Dynamically adaptive MRI with encoding by singular value decomposition. Magn Reson Med 32:268–274, 1994.
45. Cline HE, Lorensen WE, Kikinis R, Jolesz FA: 3-D segmentation of MR images of the head using probability and connectivity. J Comput Assist Tomogr 14:1037–1045, 1990.
46. Cline HE, Lorensen WE, Souza SP, et al: 3D surface rendered MR images of the brain and its vasculature. J Comput Assist Tomogr 15:344–351, 1991.
47. Kikinis R, Jolesz FA, Gerig G, et al: 3D morphometric and morphologic information derived from clinical brain MR images. In: Proceedings of the NATO Advanced Study Institute Series F: Computer and Systems Sciences, Volume 60. New York: Springer-Verlag, 1990, pp 441–454.
48. Kikinis R, Shenton M, Jolesz FA, et al: Routine quantitative analysis of brain and cerebrospinal fluid spaces with MR imaging. J Magn Reson Imaging 2:619–629, 1992.
49. Vannier MW, Butterfield RL, Jordan D, et al: Multispectral analysis of magnetic resonance images. Radiology 154:221–224, 1985.
50. Levin DN, Pelizzari CA, Chen GTY, et al: Retrospective geometric correlation of MR, CT, and PET images. Radiology 169:817–823, 1988.
51. Zinreich SJ, Tebo SA, Long DM, et al: Frameless stereotaxic integration of CT imaging data: accuracy and initial applications. Radiology 168:735–742, 1993.
52. Bucholz RD, McDurmont L, Smith K, Heilbrun P: Use of optical digitizer in resection of supratentorial tumors. In: Proceedings of The International Society for Optical Engineering, 1993, pp 312–322.
53. Andoh K, Nakamae H, Ohkoshi T, et al: Technical note: enhanced MR-guided stereotaxic brain surgery with the patient under general anesthesia. Am J Neuroradiol 12:135–138, 1991.
54. Apuzzo ML, Sabshin JK: Computer tomographic guidance stereotaxis in the management of intracranial mass lesions. Neurosurgery 12:277–285, 1983.

55. Ehricke HH, Schad LR, Gademan G, et al: Use of MR angiography for stereotactic planning. J Comput Assist Tomogr 16:35–40, 1992.

56. Heilbrun MP, McDonald P, Wiker C, et al: Stereotactic localization and guidance using a machine vision technique. Stereotact Funct Neurosurg 58:94–98, 1992.

57. Kelly PK, Ball BA, Goerss S, et al: Computer-assisted stereotaxic laser resection of intra-axial brain neoplasms. J Neurosurg 64:427–439, 1986.

58. Thomas DG, Davis CH, Ingram S, et al: Stereotaxic biopsy of the brain under MR imaging control. Am J Neuroradiol 7:161–163, 1986.

59. Lufkin R, Duckwiler G, Spickler E, et al: MR body stereotaxis: an aid for MR guided biopsies. J Comput Assist Tomogr 12:1088–1089, 1988.

60. Jolesz FA, Shtern F: The operating room of the future: Report of the National Cancer Institute Workshop, "Imaging-Guided Stereotactic Tumor Diagnosis and Treatment." Invest Radiol 27:326–328, 1992.

61. Holman BL, Zimmerman RE, Johnson KA, et al: Computer-assisted superimposition of magnetic resonance and high-resolution technetium-99m-HMPAO and thallium-201 SPECT images of the brain. J Nucl Med 32:1478–1484, 1991.

62. Hu X, Tan KK, Levin DN, et al: Three-dimensional magnetic resonance images of the brain: application to neurosurgical planning. J Neurosurg 72:433–440, 1990.

63. Koutrouvelis PG, Louie A, Lang E, et al: A three dimensional stereotactic device for computed tomography–guided invasive diagnostic and therapeutic procedures. Invest Radiol 28:845–847, 1993.

64. Levin DN, Hu X, Tan KK, et al: The brain: integrated three-dimensional display of MR and PET images. Radiology 172:783–789, 1989.

65. Dumoulin CL, Souza SP, Darrow RD: Real-time position monitoring of invasive devices using magnetic resonance. Magn Reson Med 29:411–415, 1993.

66. Delannoy J, Chen CN, Turner R, et al: Noninvasive temperature imaging using diffusion MRI. Magn Reson Med 19:333–339, 1991.

67. Dickinson RJ, Hall AS, Hind AJ, Young IR: Measurement of changes in tissue temperature using MR imaging. J Comput Assist Tomogr 10:468–472, 1986.

68. LeBihan D, Delannoy J, Levin RL: Temperature mapping with MR imaging of molecular diffusion: application to hyperthermia. Radiology 171:853–857, 1989.

69. Moran D, Leroy-Willig A, Malgouyres A, et al: Simultaneous temperature and regional blood volume measurements in human muscle using an MRI fast diffusion technique. Magn Reson Med 29:371–377, 1993.

70. Panych LP, Hrovat MI, Bleier AR, Jolesz FA: Effects related to temperature changes during MR imaging. J Magn Reson Imaging 2:69–74, 1992.

71. Parker DL, Smith V, Sheldon P, et al: Temperature distribution measurements in two-dimensional NMR imaging. Med Phys 10:321–325, 1983.

72. Young IR, Hand JW, Oatridge A, et al: Further observations on the measurement of tissue T_1 to monitor temperature in vivo by MRI. Magn Reson Med 31:342–345, 1994.

73. Prior MV, Young IR, Hand JW: Modeling and observation of temperature changes in vivo using MRI. Magn Reson Med 32:358–369, 1994.

74. Zhang Y, Samulski TV, Joines WT, et al: On the accuracy of noninvasive thermometry using molecular diffusion magnetic resonance imaging. Int J Hyperthermia 8:263–274, 1992.

75. Jolesz FA, Bleier AR, Jakab P, et al: MR imaging of laser-tissue interactions. Radiology 168:249–253, 1988.

76. Anzai Y, Lufkin R, Castro D, et al: MR imaging-guided interstitial Nd:YAG laser phototherapy: dosimetry study of acute tissue damage in an in vivo model. J Magn Reson Imaging 1:553–559, 1991.

77. Anzai Y, Lufkin RB, Hirschowitz S, et al: MR imaging: histopathologic correlation of thermal injuries induced with interstitial Nd:YAG laser irradiation in the chronic model. J Magn Reson Imaging 2:671–678, 1992.

78. Anzai Y, Lufkin RB, Saxton RE, et al: Nd:YAG interstitial laser phototherapy guided by magnetic resonance imaging in an ex vivo model: dosimetry of laser-MR-tissue interaction. Laryngoscope 101:755–760, 1991.

79. Ascher PW, Justich E, Schrottner O: A new surgical but less invasive treatment of central brain tumors: preliminary report. Acta Neurochir 52:78–80, 1991.

80. Ascher PW, Justich E, Schrottner O: Interstitial thermotherapy of central brain tumors with the Nd:YAG laser under real-time monitoring by MRI. J Clin Laser Med Surg 9:79–83, 1991.

81. Bettag M, Ulrich F, Schober R, et al: Laser-induced interstitial thermotherapy in malignant gliomas. Adv Neurosurg 22:253–257, 1992.

82. Castro DJ, Lufkin RB, Saxton RE, et al: Metastatic head and neck malignancy treated using MRI guided interstitial laser phototherapy: an initial case report. Laryngoscope 102:26–32, 1992.

83. El-Ouahabi A, Guttmann C, Hushek S, et al: MRI-guided interstitial laser therapy in a rat malignant glioma model. Lasers Surg Med 13:503–510, 1993.

84. Fan M, Ascher PW, Shcrottner O, et al: Interstitial 1.06 Nd:YAG laser thermotherapy for brain tumors under real-time monitoring of MRI: experimental study and phase I clinical trial. J Clin Laser Med Surg 10:355–361, 1992.

85. Gewiese B, Beuthan J, Fobbe F, et al: Magnetic resonance imaging–controlled laser-induced interstitial thermotherapy. Invest Radiol 29:345–351, 1994.

86. Higuchi N, Bleier AR, Jolesz FA, et al: MRI of the acute effects of interstitial Nd:YAG laser irradiation on tissues. Invest Radiol 27:814–821, 1992.

87. Kahn T, Furst G, Ulrich F, et al: MRI-guided laser-induced interstitial thermotherapy in cerebral neoplasms. J Comput Assist Tomogr 18:519, 1994.

88. Matsumoto R, Jolesz FA, Selig AM, Colucci VM: Interstitial Nd:YAG laser ablation in normal rabbit liver: trial to maximize the size of laser-induced lesions. Lasers Surg Med 12:650–658, 1992.

89. Tracz RA, Wyman DR, Little PB, et al: Magnetic resonance imaging of interstitial laser photocoagulation in brain. Lasers Surg Med 12:165–173, 1992.

90. Tracz RA, Wyman DR, Little PB, et al: Comparison of magnetic resonance images and histopathological findings of lesions induced by interstitial laser photocoagulation in the brain. Lasers Surg Med 13:45–54, 1993.

91. Charnley RM, Doran UJ, Morris DL: Cryotherapy for liver metastases: a new approach. Br J Surg 76:1040–1041, 1989.

92. Gilbert JC, Rubinsky B, Roos MS, et al: MRI-monitored cryosurgery in rabbit brain. Magn Reson Imaging 11:1155–1164, 1993.

93. Matsumoto R, Selig AM, Colucci VM, Jolesz FA: MR monitoring during cryotherapy in the liver: predictability of histologic outcome. J Magn Reson Imaging 3:770–776, 1993.

94. Onik G, Gilbert J, Hoddick W, et al: Sonographic monitoring of hepatic cryosurgery in an experimental animal model. AJR 144:1043–1047, 1986.

95. Rubinsky B, Gilbert JC, Onik GM, et al: Monitoring cryosurgery in the brain and prostate with proton NMR. Cryobiology 30:191–199, 1993.

96. Billard BE, Hynynen K, Roemer RB: Effects of physical parameters on high temperature ultrasound hyperthermia. Ultrasound Med Biol 16:409–420, 1990.

97. Darkazanli A, Hynynen K, Unger EC, Schenck JF: On-line monitoring of ultrasonic surgery with MR imaging. J Magn Reson Imaging 3:509–514, 1993.

98. Foster RS, Bihrle R, Sanghvi NT, et al: High-intensity focused ultrasound in the treatment of prostatic disease. Eur Urol 23:29–33, 1993.

99. Hynynen K, Darkazanli A, Unger E, Schenck JF: MRI-guided noninvasive ultrasound surgery. Med Phys 20:107–116, 1992.

Bioeffects and Safety of MR Procedures

FRANK G. SHELLOCK ▪ EMANUEL KANAL

During the performance of magnetic resonance (MR) procedures, the patient is exposed to three different forms of electromagnetic radiation: 1) a static magnetic field, 2) gradient magnetic fields, and 3) radiofrequency (RF) electromagnetic fields. Each of these may cause significant bioeffects if applied at sufficiently high exposure levels.

Numerous investigations have been conducted to identify potentially adverse bioeffects related to MR procedures.[1-83] Although none of these investigations have determined the presence of any substantial or unexpected hazards, the data are not comprehensive enough to assume absolute safety. In addition to bioeffects related to exposure to the electromagnetic fields used for MR procedures, there are several areas of health concern for both the patient and the health care practitioner with respect to the clinical use of MR procedures.

In this chapter, we discuss the bioeffects of static, gradient, and RF electromagnetic fields with an emphasis on the data that pertain to MR procedures; describe and summarize the investigations that specifically apply to MR procedures; and provide an overview of other safety considerations and patient-related aspects of this imaging technique.

BIOEFFECTS OF STATIC MAGNETIC FIELDS

GENERAL BIOEFFECTS OF STATIC MAGNETIC FIELDS

Data are scarce concerning the effects of high-intensity static magnetic fields on humans. Some of the original investigations on humans exposed to static magnetic fields were performed by Vyalov,[84, 85] who studied workers involved in the permanent magnet industry. These subjects were exposed to static magnetic fields ranging from 0.0015 to 0.35 T and reported feelings of headache, chest pain, fatigue, vertigo, loss of appetite, insomnia, itching, and other, more nonspecific ailments.[84, 85] Of note is that exposure to other potentially hazardous environmental working conditions (e.g., elevated room temperature, airborne metal-

lic dust, and chemicals) may have been partially responsible for the reported symptoms in these study subjects. Because this investigation lacked an appropriate control group, it is difficult to ascertain if there was a definite correlation between the exposure to the static magnetic field and the reported abnormalities. Subsequent studies performed with more scientific rigor have not substantiated many of these findings.[86-89]

TEMPERATURE EFFECTS

Conflicting reports exist regarding the effect of static magnetic fields on body and skin temperatures of mammals. Some studies have shown that static magnetic fields either increase or both increase and decrease tissue temperature, depending on the orientation of the organism in the static magnetic field.[19, 66] Other researchers have stated that static magnetic fields have no effect on skin and body temperatures of mammals.[55, 61, 88, 90]

None of the investigators who identified a static magnetic field effect on temperatures proposed a plausible mechanism for this response, nor has this work been substantiated. In addition, studies that reported static magnetic field–induced skin or body temperature changes used either laboratory animals that are known to have labile temperatures or instrumentation that may have been affected by the static magnetic fields.[19, 66]

In one investigation, it was indicated that exposure to a 1.5-T static magnetic field does not alter skin and body temperatures in humans.[90] This study was performed using a special fluoroptic thermometry system demonstrated to be unperturbed by high-intensity static magnetic fields. Therefore, skin and body temperatures of humans are believed to be unaffected by exposure to static magnetic fields of up to 1.5 T.[55, 61]

ELECRICAL INDUCTION AND CARDIAC EFFECTS

An induced biopotential may be observed during exposure to static magnetic fields and is caused by blood, a conductive fluid, flowing through a magnetic field. The induced biopotential is exhibited by an augmentation of T wave amplitude as well as by other, nonspecific waveform changes that are apparent on the electrocardiogram (ECG) and have been observed at static magnetic field strengths as low as 0.1 T.[86, 91, 92]

The increase in T wave amplitude is directly related to the intensity of the static magnetic field, such that at low static magnetic field strengths the effects are not as predominant as those at higher field strengths. The most marked effect on the T wave is believed to be caused when the blood flows through the thoracic aortic arch. This T wave amplitude change can be significant enough to falsely trigger the RF excitation during cardiac-gated MR procedures.

Other portions of the ECG may also be altered by the static magnetic field, and this varies with the placement of the recording electrodes. Alternate lead positions can be used to attenuate the static magnetic field–induced ECG changes to facilitate cardiac-gating studies.[93] Once the patient is no longer exposed to the static magnetic field, these ECG voltage abnormalities revert to normal.

Because no circulatory alterations appear to coincide with these ECG changes, no biologic risks are believed to be associated with this effect, which occurs in conjunction with static magnetic field strengths of up to 2.0 T.[86, 91, 92]

NEUROLOGIC EFFECTS

Theoretically, electrical impulse conduction in nerve tissue may be affected by exposure to static magnetic fields; however, this area in the bioeffects literature contains contradictory information. Some studies have reported remarkable effects on both the function and the structure of those portions of the central nervous system that were associated with exposure to static magnetic fields, whereas others have failed to show any significant changes.* Further investigations of potential unwanted bioeffects are needed because of the relative lack of clinical studies in this field that are directly applicable to MR procedures. At present, exposures to static magnetic fields of up to 2.0 T do not appear to significantly influence bioelectrical properties of neurons in humans.[97–99]

In summary, there is no conclusive evidence of irreversible or hazardous biologic effects related to acute, short-term exposures of humans to static magnetic fields of strengths up to 2.0 T. However, as of 1994, several 3.0- and 4.0-T whole-body MR systems are in use at various research sites around the world. A preliminary study has indicated that workers and volunteer subjects exposed to a 4.0-T MR system have experienced vertigo, nausea, headaches, a metallic taste in their mouths, and magnetophosphenes (which are visual flashes; see subsequent section on bioeffects of gradient magnetic fields).[50] Therefore, considerable research is required to study the mechanisms responsi-

ble for these bioeffects and to determine possible means, if any, to avoid them.

CRYOGEN CONSIDERATIONS

All superconductive MR systems in clinical use today use liquid helium. Liquid helium, which maintains the magnet coils in their superconductive state, achieves the gaseous state (boiloff) at approximately −268.93°C (4.22 K).[99] If the temperature within the cryostat rises precipitously, the helium enters the gaseous state. In such a situation, the marked increase in volume of the gaseous versus the liquid cryogen (with gas/liquid volume ratios of 760:1 for helium and 695:1 for nitrogen) dramatically raises the pressure within the cryostat.[99] A pressure-sensitive carbon "pop-off" valve will give way, sometimes with a rather loud popping noise, followed by the rapid (and loud) egress of gaseous helium as it escapes from the cryostat. In normal situations, this gas should be vented out of the imaging room and into the external atmosphere. It is possible, however, that during venting some helium gas might accidentally be released into the ambient atmosphere of the imaging room.

Gaseous helium is considerably lighter than air. If any helium gas is inadvertently released into the imaging room, the dimensions of the room, its ventilation capacity, and the total amount of gas released determine whether the helium gas reaches the patient or health care practitioner who is in the lower part of the room.[99] Helium vapor looks like steam and is entirely odorless and tasteless, but it may be extremely cold. Asphyxiation and frostbite are possible if a person is exposed to helium vapor for a prolonged time. In a system quench, a considerable quantity of helium gas may be released into the imaging room. This might secondarily cause difficulty in opening the room door because of the pressure differential produced. In such a circumstance, the first response should be to evacuate the area until the offending helium vapor is adequately removed from the room environment and safely redirected to an outside environment away from patients, pedestrians, or temperature-sensitive material.[99]

Better cryostat design and insulation have allowed the use of only liquid helium in many of the newer superconducting magnets. However, a great number of magnets still in clinical use utilize liquid nitrogen as well. Liquid nitrogen within the cryostat acts as a buffer between the liquid helium and the outside atmosphere, boiling off at 77.3 K. In the event of an accidental release of liquid nitrogen into the ambient atmosphere of the imaging room, there is a potential for frostbite, similar to that encountered with gaseous helium release. Gaseous nitrogen has roughly the same density as air and is certainly much less buoyant than gaseous helium.

In the event of an inadvertent venting of nitrogen gas into the imaging room, the gas could easily settle near floor level and the amount of nitrogen gas within the room would continue to increase until venting

---

*References 14, 20, 34, 68, 76–79, 94–99.

ceased. The total concentration of nitrogen gas contained within the room would be determined on the basis of the total amount of the gas released into the room, the dimensions of the room, and its ventilation capacity (the existence and size of other routes of egress, e.g., doors, windows, ventilation ducts, and fans). A pure nitrogen environment is exceptionally hazardous, and unconsciousness generally results as quickly as 5 to 10 seconds after exposure.[99] It is imperative that all patients and health care personnel evacuate the area as soon as it is recognized that nitrogen gas is being released into the imaging room, and they should not return until appropriate corrective measures have been taken to clear the gas from the room.[99]

Dewar (cryogen storage containers) storage should also be within a well-ventilated area, lest normal boiloff rates increase the concentration of inert gas within the storage room to a dangerous level (Gray JE, personal communication, 1989). At least one reported death has occurred in an industrial setting during the shipment of cryogens (Gray JE, personal communication, 1989), although to our knowledge no such fatality has occurred in the medical community. There is one report of a sudden loss of consciousness of unexplained cause by an otherwise healthy technologist (with no prior or subsequent similar episodes) passing through a cryogen storage area where multiple Dewar tanks were located (Aisen A, personal communication, 1989). Although there is no verification of ambient atmospheric oxygen concentration to confirm any relationship to the cryogens per se, the history is strongly suggestive of such a relationship.

Cryogens present a potential concern for clinical MR systems despite an overwhelmingly safe record during the past 7 or more years of service.[99] Proper handling and storage of cryogens, as well as the appropriate behavior in the presence of possible leaks, should be emphasized at each site. An oxygen monitor with an audible alarm, situated at an appropriate height within each imaging room, should be a mandatory minimal safety measure for all sites; automatic linking to and activation of an imaging room ventilation fan system when the oxygen monitor registers below 18% or 19% should be considered at each magnet installation.[99]

ELECTRICAL CONSIDERATIONS OF A QUENCH

In addition to the potential for cryogen release, there is a concern about the currents that may be induced in conductors (such as biologic tissues) near the rapidly changing magnetic field associated with a quench.[99] In one study, physiologic monitoring of a pig and monitoring of the environment were performed during an intentional quench from 1.76 T. Apparently, no substantial effect occurred on the blood pressure, pulse, temperature, and electroencephalographic (EEG) and ECG measurements of the pig during or immediately after the quench.[5] Although such a single observation does not prove safety for humans undergoing exposure to a quench, the data suggest that the experi-

ence would be similar and that there would be no deleterious electrical effects on humans undergoing a comparable experience and exposure.

BIOEFFECTS OF GRADIENT MAGNETIC FIELDS

MR procedures expose the human body to rapid variations of magnetic fields due to the transient application of magnetic field gradients during the imaging sequence. Gradient magnetic fields can induce electrical fields and currents in conductive media (including biologic tissue) according to Faraday's law of induction. The potential for interaction between gradient magnetic fields and biologic tissue is inherently dependent on the fundamental field frequency, the maximal flux density, the average flux density, the presence of harmonic frequencies, the waveform characteristics of the signal, the polarity of the signal, the current distribution in the body, and the electrical properties and sensitivity of the particular cell membrane.[97–99]

For animals and human subjects, the induced current is proportional to the conductivity of the biologic tissue and the rate of change of the magnetic flux density.[98–101] In theory, the largest current densities will be produced in peripheral tissues (i.e., at the greatest radius) and will linearly diminish toward the body's center.[98–101] The current density will be enhanced at higher frequencies and magnetic flux densities and will be further accentuated by a larger tissue radius with a greater tissue conductivity. Current paths are affected by differences in tissue types, such that tissues with low conductivity (e.g., adipose and bone) will change the pattern of the induced current.

Bioeffects of induced currents can be due either to the power deposited by the induced currents (thermal effects) or to direct effects of the current (nonthermal effects). Thermal effects due to switched gradients used in MR procedures are negligible and are not believed to be clinically significant.[96, 98, 99]

Possible nonthermal effects of induced currents are stimulation of nerve or muscle cells, induction of ventricular fibrillation, increased brain mannitol space, epileptogenic potential, stimulation of visual flash sensations, and bone healing.[98–103] The threshold currents required for nerve stimulation and ventricular fibrillation are known to be much higher than the estimated current densities that will be induced with routine clinical MR procedures.[96–100]

For the sake of discussion and comparison, let us use the approximation of 1 for a dB/dt of 1.0 T/s as a reasonably expectable current density that will be experienced due to gradient magnetic fields typically used in clinical MR procedures. The MR systems used at the present time can be expected to routinely produce current densities of approximately 3 $\mu A/cm^2$, which is below the level at which biologic effects can be expected. By comparison, 15 to 100 $\mu A/cm^2$ is needed to produce tetanic contractions of the skeletal muscles involved in breathing, whereas 0.2 to 1.0 mA/cm^2 appears to be the threshold current density required to produce ventricular fibrillation in the human heart (at frequency ranges of 20 to 200 Hz for sinusoidal voltages). The shorter the stimulus duration, the greater the threshold required to produce cardiac fibrillation. This can be approximated by an inverse square root ratio between the amplitude of the stimulus and the shock duration necessary to elicit cardiac fibrillation. The current densities required to elicit extrasystoles in guinea pig hearts have been reported to be three to five times less than that required to produce fibrillation. In addition, cardiac thresholds are significantly greater than those necessary to elicit neuromuscular excitations.

Seizure induction thresholds seem to be even higher, when to elicit a convulsive seizure, current densities of roughly 3 mA/cm^2 (and sustained for 300 ms) would be required. Animal data suggest that current densities of approximately 1 A/cm^2 would be needed to induce reversible nerve damage. This is roughly a millionfold lower than those induced by routine MR procedures today.

Mathematic calculations suggest that the threshold currents required to induce ventricular fibrillation in a healthy heart are significantly greater than those that are achieved during routine MR procedures today. Similar statements can be made concerning present-day (non–echo-planar) MR techniques and hardware capabilities and peripheral nerve stimulation, muscular contraction, or seizures.

The production of magnetophosphenes is considered to be one of the most sensitive physiologic responses to gradient magnetic fields.[96–99] Magnetophosphenes are supposedly caused by electrical stimulation of the retina and are completely reversible with no associated health effects.[96–99] These have been elicited by current densities of roughly 17 μA/cm^2. Although we know of no reported cases of magnetophosphenes for fields of 1.95 T or less, magnetophosphenes have been reported in volunteers working in and around a 4.0-T research system.[50] In addition, a metallic taste and symptoms of vertigo seem to be reproducible and associated with rapid motion within the static magnetic field of these 4.0-T systems.[50]

Time-varying, extremely low frequency magnetic fields have been demonstrated to be associated with multiple effects, including clustering and altered orientation of fibroblasts, as well as increased mitotic activity of fibroblast growth, altered DNA synthesis, and reduced fentanyl-induced anesthesia.[49, 64, 99] Possible effects in many other organisms, including humans, have also been mentioned.[99] Although there have been no studies to conclusively demonstrate carcinogenic effects from exposure to time-varying magnetic fields of various intensities and durations, several reports suggest that an association between the two is still plausible.[104–106]

NEURAL STIMULATION AND ECHO-PLANAR MR SYSTEMS

Any discussion of the gradient magnetic fields used for MR procedures and their secondary induced voltages is incomplete without bringing up the gradient strengths and rise time capabilities of the MR systems used for echo-planar techniques.[11] The direction in which the entire MR industry is heading is one in which there is a marked advance in the peak gradient amplitudes and rise times to maximal amplitude capabilities of the gradient magnetic field subsystems of the MR systems. Only a few years ago, many of these systems would have had 1 Gs/cm (1 mT/m) maximal gradient amplitudes with 600- or 700-μs rise times; today it is not uncommon to find clinical MR systems with 15 G/cm or more maximal gradient magnetic field strengths and 300- to 500-μs rise times.[11]

In addition, with the development and infusion into the MR industry of echo-planar technology and hardware, 23 to 25 G/cm and less than 100-μs rise times are now the range of the hardware specifications for systems to be imminently delivered to clinical MR sites. Therefore, the potential for exposing patients to considerably increased levels of induced voltages will soon be created. Several investigators using MR systems from various manufacturers have already reported what is believed to represent direct stimulation of peripheral muscle in the form of uncontrolled, involuntary contractions of skeletal muscle or twitching in human subjects induced from echo-planar imaging sequences.[12, 98] The threshold for these gradient magnetic field–induced bioeffects has been observed at and above 60 T/s.[98] The bioeffects have included sensory stimulation in the form of creeping sensations along the back or twitching along the bridge of the nose or feelings like electrical shocks and have ranged from imperceptible to painful sensations. The positioning of the subject or patient seems also to play a role in the severity of the response to stimulation. Of additional note is that cardiac and respiratory function at gradient dB/dt values of up to 60 T/s have been found to be unaffected in anesthetized rabbits.[14]

BIOEFFECTS OF RADIOFREQUENCY ELECTROMAGNETIC FIELDS

GENERAL BIOEFFECTS OF RADIOFREQUENCY ELECTROMAGNETIC FIELDS

As a result of resistive losses, RF radiation is capable of generating heat in tissues. Therefore, the main bioeffects associated with exposure to RF radiation are related to the thermogenic qualities of this electromagnetic field.[96–99, 107–116] Exposure to RF radiation may also cause athermal, field-specific alterations in biologic systems that are produced without a significant increase in temperature.[108–114] This topic is somewhat controversial, owing to assertions concerning the role of electromagnetic fields in producing cancer and developmental abnormalities, along with the concomitant ramifications of such effects.[108–114]

A report from the U.S. Environmental Protection Agency claimed that the existing evidence on this issue is sufficient to demonstrate a relationship between low-level electromagnetic field exposures and the development of cancer.[106] No specific studies have been performed to study potential athermal bioeffects of MR procedures. Those interested in a thorough review of this topic, particularly as it pertains to MR procedures, are referred to the extensive article written by Beers.[113]

With regard to RF power deposition concerns, investigators have typically quantified exposure to RF radiation by means of determining the specific absorption rate (SAR).[108–112, 115–119] The SAR is the mass normalized rate at which RF power is coupled to biologic tissue and is indicated in units of watts per kilogram. Measurements or estimates of SAR are not trivial, particularly in human subjects, and there are several methods of determining this parameter for RF energy dosimetry.[108–112, 119]

The SAR that is produced during MR procedures is a complex function of numerous variables, including the frequency (which, in turn, is determined by the strength of the static magnetic field), type of RF pulse (e.g., 90° or 180°), repetition time, pulse width, type of RF coil used, volume of tissue within the coil, resistivity of the tissue, and configuration of the anatomic region imaged, as well as other factors.[96–99] The RF power used during MR procedures is typically expressed as both "whole-body averaged" and "local SAR" to distinguish between the relative concentration of RF energy specific to an anatomic area. The actual increase in tissue temperature caused by exposure to RF radiation is dependent on the subject's thermoregulatory system (e.g., skin blood flow, skin surface area, and sweat rate).[97–99]

The efficiency and absorption pattern of RF energy are mainly determined by the physical dimensions of the tissue in relation to the incident wavelength.[108–112] Therefore, if the tissue size is large relative to the wavelength, energy is predominantly absorbed on the surface; if it is small relative to the wavelength, there is little absorption of RF power.[108–112] Because of the above relationship between RF energy and physical dimensions, studies designed to investigate the effects of exposure to RF radiation during MR procedures that are intended to be applicable to the clinical setting require tissue volumes and anatomic shapes comparable to that of human subjects. Of additional note is that no laboratory animal sufficiently mimics or simulates the thermoregulatory system or responses of humans. For these reasons, results obtained in laboratory animal experiments cannot simply be "scaled" or extrapolated to humans.[110–112, 119]

MR AND EXPOSURE TO RF RADIATION

Few quantitative data have been previously available on thermoregulatory responses of humans exposed to RF radiation before the studies performed with MR. The few studies that existed did not directly apply to MR procedures because these investigations examined either thermal sensations or therapeutic applications of diathermy, usually involving only localized regions of the body.[108, 109, 110, 114]

Several studies of RF power absorption during MR procedures have been performed and have yielded useful information about tissue heating in humans.[28, 58–60, 62, 63, 65] During MR procedures, tissue heating results primarily from magnetic induction with a negligible contribution from the electrical fields, so that ohmic heating is greatest at the surface of the body and approaches zero at the center of the body. Predictive calculations and measurements obtained in phantoms and human subjects exposed to MR support this pattern of temperature distribution.[58–60, 115, 116]

Although one paper reported significant temperature rises in internal organs produced by MR,[65] this study was conducted on anesthetized dogs and is unlikely to be applicable to conscious adult humans because of factors related to the physical dimensions and dissimilar thermoregulatory systems of these two species. However, these data may have important implications for the use of MR procedures in pediatric patients because this population is typically sedated or anesthetized for MR procedures.

An investigation using fluoroptic thermometry probes that are unperturbed by electromagnetic fields[117] demonstrated that human subjects exposed to MR at SAR levels up to 4.0 W/kg (i.e., 10 times higher than the level recommended by the U.S. Food and Drug Administration [FDA]) have no statistically significant increases in body temperatures and elevations in skin temperatures that are not believed to be clinically hazardous.[62] These results imply that the suggested exposure level of 0.4 W/kg for RF radiation during MR procedures is too conservative for individuals with normal thermoregulatory function.[62] Additional studies are needed, however, to assess physiologic responses of patients with conditions that may impair thermoregulatory function (e.g., elderly patients; patients with underlying conditions such as fever, diabetes, cardiovascular disease, or obesity; and patients taking medications that affect thermoregulation such as calcium blockers, β-blockers, diuretics, or vasodilators) before subjecting them to procedures that require high SARs.

TEMPERATURE-SENSITIVE ORGANS

Certain human organs that have reduced capabilities for heat dissipation, such as the testis and eye, are particularly sensitive to elevated temperatures. Therefore, these are primary sites of potential harmful effects if RF radiation exposures during MR procedures are excessive. Laboratory investigations have demonstrated detrimental effects on testicular function (e.g., a reduction or cessation of spermatogenesis, impaired sperm motility, and degeneration of seminiferous tubules), caused by RF radiation–induced heating from exposures sufficient enough to raise scrotal or testicular tissue temperatures to 38°C to 42°C.[118]

Scrotal skin temperatures (i.e., an index of intratesticular temperature) were measured in volunteer subjects undergoing MR procedures at a whole-body–averaged SAR of 1.1 W/kg.[63] The largest change in scrotal skin temperature was 2.1°C, and the highest scrotal skin temperature recorded was 34.2°C.[63] These temperature changes were below the threshold known to impair testicular function. However, excessively heating the scrotum during MR procedures could exacerbate certain preexisting disorders associated with increased scrotal or testicular temperatures (e.g., acute febrile illnesses and varicocele) in patients who are already oligospermic and could lead to possible temporary or permanent sterility.[63] Therefore, additional studies designed to investigate these issues are needed, particularly if patients are scanned at whole-body–averaged SARs higher than those previously evaluated.

Dissipation of heat from the eye is a slow and inefficient process owing to its relative lack of vascularization. Acute near-field exposures of RF radiation to the eyes or heads of laboratory animals have been demonstrated to be cataractogenic as a result of the thermal disruption of ocular tissues if the exposure is of a sufficient intensity and duration.[108, 110] An investigation conducted by Sacks and associates[53] revealed no discernible effects on the eyes of rats produced by MR procedures at exposures that far exceeded typical clinical imaging levels. However, it may not be acceptable to extrapolate these data to human subjects in view of the coupling of RF radiation to the anatomy and tissue volume of the laboratory rat eyes compared with those of humans.

Corneal temperatures have been measured in patients undergoing MR procedures of the brain using a send-receive head coil at local SARs up to 3.1 W/kg.[59] The largest corneal temperature change was 1.8°C, and the highest temperature measured was 34.4°C. Because the temperature threshold for RF radiation–induced cataractogenesis in animal models has been demonstrated to be between 41°C and 55°C for acute, near-field exposures, it does not appear that MR procedures using a head coil have the potential to cause thermal damage in ocular tissue.[59] The effect of MR procedures at higher SARs and the long-term effects of MR procedures on ocular tissues remain to be determined.

RF Radiation and "Hot Spots"

Theoretically, RF radiation hot spots caused by an uneven distribution of RF power may arise whenever current concentrations are produced in association with restrictive conductive patterns. It has been suggested that RF radiation hot spots may generate thermal hot spots under certain conditions during MR procedures.[98] Because RF radiation is absorbed mainly by peripheral tissues, thermography has been used to study the heating pattern associated with MR procedures at high whole-body SARs.[57] This study demonstrated no evidence of surface thermal hot spots related to MR procedures in humans. The thermoregulatory system apparently responds to the heat challenge by distributing the thermal load, producing a "smearing" effect of the surface temperatures. However, the possibility exists that internal thermal hot spots may develop from MR procedures.[59]

GUIDELINES FOR MR DEVICES

In 1988, MR diagnostic devices were reclassified by the FDA from class III, in which premarket approval is required, to class II, which is regulated by performance standards, as long as the devices are within the "umbrella" of defined limits addressed in the following.[107] Subsequent to this reclassification, new devices had only to demonstrate that they were "substantially equivalent" to any class II device that was brought to market using the premarket notification process (510[k]) or, alternatively, to any of the devices described by the 13 MR system manufacturers that had petitioned the FDA for such a reclassification.

Four areas relating to the use of MR systems have been identified for which safety guidelines have been issued by the FDA. These include the static magnetic field, the gradient magnetic fields, the RF power of the examination, and the acoustic considerations. Excerpts from the FDA Safety Parameter Action Levels are as follows[107]:

Static magnetic field—Static magnetic field strengths not exceeding 2.0 T are below the level of concern for the static magnetic field. Should the static magnetic field strength exceed 2.0 T, additional evidence of safety must be provided by the sponsor.

Gradient magnetic field—Limit patient exposure to time-varying magnetic fields with strengths less than those required to produce peripheral nerve stimulation or other effects. There are three alternatives:

1. Demonstrate that the maximum dB/dt of the system is 6 T/sec or less.
2. Demonstrate that for axial gradients, dB/dt < 20 T/sec for p ≥ 120 msec, or dB/dt < (2,400/p) T/sec for 12 msec < p < 120 msec, or dB/dt < 200 T/sec for p ≤ 12 msec (p equals the width in microseconds of a rectangular pulse or the half period of a sinusoidal dB/dt pulse). For transverse gradients, dB/dt is considered to be below the level of concern when it is less than three times the above limits for axial gradients.
3. Demonstrate with valid scientific evidence that the rate of change of magnetic field for the system is not sufficient to cause peripheral nerve stimulation by an adequate margin of safety (at least a factor of three).

The parameter dB/dt must be lower than that of either of the two levels of concern by presentation of valid scientific measurement of calculational evidence sufficient to demonstrate that the time rate of magnetic field change (dB/dt) is of no concern.

RF power deposition—Options to control the risk of systemic thermal overload and local thermal injury caused by RF energy absorption are as follows:

1. If the specific absorption rate is 0.4 W/kg or less for the whole body and 8.0 W/kg or less spatial peak in any 1 gram of tissue, and if the specific absorption rate is 3.2 W/kg or less averaged over the head, then it is below the level of concern.
2. If exposure to RF magnetic fields is insufficient to produce a core temperature increase of 1°C and localized heating to no greater than 38°C in the head, 39°C in the trunk, and 40°C in the extremities, then it is considered to be below the level of concern.

The parameter RF heating must be below either of the

two levels of concern by presentation of valid scientific measurement or calculational evidence sufficient to demonstrate that RF heating effects are of no concern.

Acoustic noise levels—The acoustic noise levels associated with the device must be shown to be below the level of concern established by pertinent federal regulatory or other recognized standards-setting organizations. If the acoustic noise is not below the level of concern, the sponsor must recommend steps to reduce or alleviate the noise perceived by the patient.

Guidelines relating to the magnetic field gradients are currently undergoing revision, which is particularly relevant for echo-planar imaging.

MR PROCEDURES AND ACOUSTIC NOISE

The acoustic noise produced during MR procedures represents a potential risk to patients. Acoustic noise is associated with the activation and deactivation of electrical current that induces vibrations of the gradient coils. This repetitive sound is enhanced by higher gradient duty cycles and sharper pulse transitions. Acoustic noise is thus likely to increase with decreases in section thicknesses and decreased fields of view, repetition times, and echo times.

Gradient magnetic field–related noise levels measured on several commercial MR systems were in the range of 65 to 95 dB, which is considered to be within the recommended safety guidelines set forth by the FDA.[107] However, there have been reports that acoustic noise generated during MR procedures has caused annoyance in patients, interference with oral communication, and reversible hearing loss in patients who did not wear ear protection.[9, 28, 120, 121] One study of patients undergoing an MR procedure without earplugs reported temporary hearing loss in 43% of the subjects.[9] Furthermore, significant gradient coil–induced noise may produce permanent hearing impairment in certain patients who are particularly susceptible to the damaging effects of relatively loud noises.[9, 120]

The safest and least expensive means of preventing problems associated with acoustic noise during MR procedures is to encourage the routine use of disposable earplugs.[9, 28, 120] The use of hearing protection has been demonstrated to successfully avoid the potential temporary hearing loss that can be associated with clinical MR procedures.[9, 98, 120] MR-compatible headphones that significantly muffle acoustic noise are also available.

An acceptable alternative strategy for reducing sound levels during MR procedures is to use an "antinoise" or destructive interference technique that not only effectively reduces noise but also permits better oral communication.[122] This technique consists of a real-time Fourier analysis of the noise emitted from the MR system.[122] A signal possessing the same physical characteristics but opposite phase than the sound generated by the system is produced. The two opposite-phase signals are then combined, resulting in a cancellation of the repetitive noise, while allowing other sounds such as music and voice to be transmitted to the patient. One investigation demonstrated no significant degradation of image quality when MR procedures are performed with systems that use this antinoise method.[122] Although this technique has not yet found widespread clinical application, it has considerable potential for minimizing acoustic noise and its associated problems.

INVESTIGATIONS OF BIOLOGIC EFFECTS OF MR PROCEDURES

Investigations performed to specifically study the potential bioeffects of MR procedures are summarized in Table 13–1.[1-83] The results of these studies have been predominantly negative, supporting the widely held view that there are no significant health risks associated with the use of this imaging modality. Experiments that yielded positive results either identified possible, nonspecific biologic responses, determined short-term biologic changes that were not considered to be deleterious, or found bioeffects that require further substantiation.

When perusing these studies, the reader should note that the dosimetric aspects of the exposure or exposures to static, gradient, or RF electromagnetic fields were quite variable and include those that exceeded clinical exposures, simulated clinical exposures, or involved low-level, chronic exposures. In certain cases, the effects of only one of the electromagnetic fields used for MR procedures were evaluated. Theoretically, the possibility exists that the combination of static, gradient, and RF electromagnetic fields may produce some unusual or unpredictable bioeffects that are unique to MR procedures.

"Window" effects are often present with respect to biologic changes that occur in response to electromagnetic radiation. Window effects are those biologic changes associated with a specific spectrum of electromagnetic radiation that are not observed at levels below or above this range.[108, 119] Both field strength and frequency windows have been reported in the literature.[108, 119] Virtually all of the experiments conducted on MR bioeffects have been performed at specific windows, and the results cannot be assumed to apply to all of the various field strengths or frequencies used for clinical MR procedures.

A variety of different biologic systems were also used for these experiments. As previously mentioned, because the coupling of electromagnetic radiation to biologic tissues is highly dependent on subject size, anatomic factors, duration of exposure, the sensitivity of the involved tissues, and myriad other variables, studies performed on laboratory preparations may not be extrapolated or directly applicable to humans or to the clinical use of MR procedures. Therefore, a cautionary approach to the interpretation of the results of these studies is advisable.

ELECTRICALLY, MAGNETICALLY, OR MECHANICALLY ACTIVATED IMPLANTS AND DEVICES

The FDA requires labeling of MR systems to indicate that the device is contraindicated for patients who have

Text continued on page 404

TABLE 13–1. SUMMARY OF MR BIOEFFECTS STUDIES

STUDY DESCRIPTION	RESULTS	REFERENCE
2.0 T Clinical imaging conditions Rats Studied effect of MRI on blood-brain barrier permeability	"No MRI-induced difference was detected."	Adzamli et al[1]
1.5 T Exposure to RF radiation in excess of clinical imaging conditions Sheep Studied RF radiation–induced heating	"For exposure periods in excess of standard clinical imaging protocols the temperature increase was insufficient to cause adverse thermal effects."	Barber et al[2]
0.5 and 1.5 T Clinical imaging conditions Humans Studied effect of MRI on the electroencephalogram and evaluated neuropsychologic status	"No measurable influence of MRI on cognitive functions."	Bartels et al[3]
0.04 T Clinical imaging conditions Humans Studied effects of MRI on cognition	"MRI did not cause any cognitive deterioration."	Besson et al[4]
1.6 T Quenched magnet Pigs Studied effect of quenching a magnet	"Our findings, which in the circumstances of this experiment, suggested that the risks are small."	Bore et al[5]
MRI gradient-induced electrical fields Dogs Studied bioeffects at high MRI gradient-induced fields	"As the strength of MRI gradient-induced fields increases, biological effects in order of increasing field and severity include stimulation of peripheral nerves, nerves of respiration and finally, the heart."	Bourland et al[6]
0.38 T Static magnetic field only Deoxygenated erythrocytes Studied orientation of sickled erythrocytes	"Further studies are needed to assess possible hazards of MRI of sickle cell disease."	Brody et al[7]
0.35 and 1.5 T Clinical imaging conditions Humans with sickle cell disease Studied effects of MRI on patients with sickle cell disease	"No change in sickle cell blood flow during MR imaging in vivo."	Brody et al[8]
0.35 T Clinical imaging conditions Humans Studied effects of noise during MRI on hearing	"Noise generated by MR imaging may cause temporary hearing loss, and earplugs can prevent this."	Brummett et al[9]
Varying gradient fields Humans Studied neural stimulation threshold with varying oscillations and gradient field strength	"The threshold decreases with the number of oscillations and increases with frequency. The repeatable threshold of 63 T/s (1270 Hz) remains constant from 32 oscillations (25.6 msec) to 128 oscillations (102.4 msec)."	Budinger et al[10]
0.15 T Simulated imaging conditions HL60 promyelocytic cells Studied effect of MRI of Ca^{2+}	"Results demonstrate that time-varying magnetic fields associated with MRI procedures increase Ca^{++}."	Carson et al[11]
Gradient magnetic fields up to 66 T/s in dogs and 61 T/s in humans Dogs and humans Studied physiologic responses to large amplitude time-varying magnetic fields	Dogs—"no motion, twitch, or ECG abnormalities." Humans—brief minimal muscular twitches observed on various parts of the body due to magnetic stimulation.	Cohen et al[12]
0.5 and 1.0 T Simulated imaging conditions Cultured human blood cells Studied effects of static magnetic fields and line scan imaging on human blood cells	"Neither treatment had any significant effect on any of the parameters measured."	Cooke and Morris[13]
4.7 T Exposures to static and RF electromagnetic fields Isolated rabbit hearts Studied effects on cardiac excitability and vulnerability	No measurable effect on strength interval relationship or ventricular vulnerability.	Doherty et al[14]

TABLE 13–1. SUMMARY OF MR BIOEFFECTS STUDIES *Continued*

STUDY DESCRIPTION	RESULTS	REFERENCE
Gradient magnetic fields only Sinusoidal gradients at a frequency of 1.25 kHz with amplitudes up to 40 mT/min for a z coil and 25 mT/min for an x coil Humans Studied physiologic effects, physiologic responses	Observed peripheral muscle stimulation, no extrasystoles or arrhythmias.	Fischer[15]
0.3, 0.5, and 1.5 T Simulated imaging conditions and static/RF and gradient fields separately Rats Studied blood-brain barrier permeability	"Increased brain mannitol associated with gradient fluid flux may reflect increase in blood-brain barrier permeability or blood volume in brain."	Garber et al[16]
2.2–2.7 T Simulated imaging conditions Mouse cells Studied oncogenic and genotoxic effects of MRI	"Data clearly mitigate against an association between exposure to MR imaging modalities and both carcinogenic and genotoxic effects."	Geard et al[17]
60 T/s Gradient magnetic fields only Humans Studied effects of gradient magnetic fields on cardiac and respiratory function	"No changes were observed."	Gore et al[18]
0.1–1.5 T Static magnetic field only Humans Studied effects of static magnetic fields on temperature	Temperatures increased or decreased depending on field strength of magnet.	Gremmel et al[19]
2.11 T Static magnetic field only Isolated rat hearts Studied effect of static magnetic field on cardiac muscle contraction	"Static magnetic fields used in NMR imaging do not constitute any hazard in terms of cardiac contractility."	Gulch and Lutz[20]
2.0 T RF at 90 MHz Simulated imaging conditions Phantom Capuchin monkey Studied temperature changes in phantom and monkey brain during high RF power exposures	"Blood flowing through the brain used the body as a heat sink."	Hammer et al[21]
0.35 T Simulated imaging conditions Mice Studied teratogenic effects of MRI	"Prolonged midgestional exposure failed to reveal any overt embryotoxicity or teratogenicity." "Slight but significant reduction in fetal crown-rump length after prolonged exposure justified further study of higher MRI energy levels."	Heinrichs et al[22]
1.5 T Static magnetic field only Humans Studied effect of static magnetic field on somatosensory evoked potentials	"Short-term exposure to 1.5 T static magnetic field does not affect SEPs in human subjects."	Hong and Shellock[23]
0.15 T Simulated imaging conditions Rats Studied effects on cognitive processes	"MRI procedure has no significant effect on spatial memory processes in rats."	Innis et al[24]
2.0 T Static magnetic field only Humans Studied effect of static magnetic field on cardiac rhythm	Cardiac cycle length was significantly increased but this is probably harmless in normal subjects; safety in dysrhythmic patients remains to be determined.	Jehenson et al[25]
1.5 T Simulated imaging conditions Frog embryo Studied effect of MRI on embryogenesis	"No adverse effects of MRI components on development of this vertebrate *(Xenopus laevis)*."	Kay et al[26]
2.3, 4.7, and 10 T Static magnetic fields only Physiologic solutions (2.3 and 4.7 T) and mathematic modeling (10 T) Studied hydrostatic pressure and electrical potentials across vessels in presence of static magnetic fields	"A 10-T magnetic field changes vascular pressure in a model of the human vasculature by less than 0.2%."	Keltner et al[27]

Table continued on following page

TABLE 13–1. SUMMARY OF MR BIOEFFECTS STUDIES *Continued*

STUDY DESCRIPTION	RESULTS	REFERENCE
1.5 T Clinical imaging conditions Humans Studied physiologic changes during high-field-strength MRI	"Temperature changes and other physiologic changes . . . were small and of no clinical concern."	Kido et al[28]
1.5 T Simulated imaging conditions Rats Studied effects of MRI on receptor-mediated activation of pineal gland indole biosynthesis	"Strong magnetic fields and/or radiofrequency pulsing used in MRI inhibited beta-adrenergic activation of the gland."	LaPorte et al[29]
3.5–12 kT/s Gradient magnetic fields only Mice Studied effect of gradient magnetic fields on pregnancy and postnatal development	"No significant difference between the litter numbers and growth rates of the exposed litters compared with controls."	McRobbie and Foster[30]
Various strong magnetic fields Gradient magnetic fields only Anesthetized rats Studied cardiac response to gradient magnetic fields	"The types of pulsed magnetic fields used in the present study did not affect the cardiac cycle of anesthetized rats."	McRobbie and Foster[31]
1.89 T Simulated imaging sequence Rats Studied taste aversion in rats to evaluate possible toxic effects of MRI	"Rats exposed to MRI did not display any aversion to the saccharin solution."	Messmer et al[32]
1.89 T Simulated imaging sequence Mouse spleen cells Studied possible interaction between ionizing radiation and MRI on damage to normal tissue	"For the normal tissues studied, MR imaging neither increases radiation damage nor inhibits repair."	Montour et al[33]
0–2.0 T Clinical imaging conditions Humans Studied the extent of changes of the brain stem evoked potentials with MRI	"Routine MRI examinations do not produce pathological changes in auditory evoked potentials."	Muller and Hotz[34]
1.5 T Simulated MRI Humans Studied effect of MRI on somatosensory and brain stem auditory-evoked potentials	"It may be assumed that MRI causes no lasting changes."	Niemann et al[35]
0.75 T Static magnetic field only Hamster cells Studied effect of static magnetic field on DNA synthesis and survival of mammalian cells irradiated with fast neutrons	"Presence of the magnetic field either during or subsequent to fast-neutron irradiation does not affect the neutron-induced radiation damage or its repair."	Ngo et al[36]
1.89 T Static magnetic field only Mice Studied effects of long-term exposure to a static magnetic field	"No consistent differences found in gross and microscopic morphology, hematocrit and WBCs, plasma creatine phosphokinase, lactic dehydrogenase, cholesterol, triglyceride, or protein concentrations in magnet groups compared to two control groups."	Osbakken et al[37]
0.15 T Simulated imaging conditions Rats Studied effects of MRI on behavior of rats	"Results fail to provide any evidence for short or long term behavioral changes in animals exposed to MRI."	Ossenkopp et al[38]
0.15 T Simulated imaging conditions Rats Studied effect of MRI on murine opiate analgesia levels	"NMRI procedure alters both day and night time responses to morphine."	Ossenkopp et al[39]
1.0 T Static magnetic field only Mice Studied effect of static magnetic field on in vivo bone growth	"Results suggest that exposure to intense magnetic fields does not alter physiological mechanisms of bone mineralization."	Papatheofanis and Papatheofanis[40]

TABLE 13–1. SUMMARY OF MR BIOEFFECTS STUDIES *Continued*

STUDY DESCRIPTION	RESULTS	REFERENCE
2.35 T Static and gradient magnetic fields only Nematodes Studied toxic effects of static and gradient magnetic fields	"Static magnetic fields have no effect on fitness of test animals." "Time-varying magnetic fields cause inhibition of growth and maturation." "Combination of pulsed magnetic field gradients in a static uniform magnetic field also has a detrimental effect on the fitness of the test animals."	Peeling et al[41]
2.35 T Simulated imaging conditions Mice Studied the effect of MRI on tumor development	"Immune response may be enhanced following MRI exposure, as indicated by the longer latency and smaller sizes of tumors in animals receiving MRI exposure."	Prasad et al[42]
4.5 T Simulated imaging conditions Mice Studied effects of MRI on mouse testes epididymes	"Little, if any, damage to male reproductive tissues from . . . high intensity MRI exposure."	Prasad et al[43]
0.7 T Simulated imaging conditions Mouse bone marrow cells Studied the cytogenic effects of MRI	"NMR exposure causes no adverse cytogenic effects."	Prasad et al[44]
0.15 T Simulated imaging conditions Mice Studied effects of MRI on the immune system	"MR exposure has no adverse effect on the immune system, as evidenced by natural killer cell activity."	Prasad et al[45]
2.35 T Simulated imaging conditions Human peripheral blood mononuclear cells Studied effect of MRI on natural killer cell toxicity of peripheral blood mononuclear cells with and without interleukin-2	"In neither case was cytotoxicity affected by prior exposure to MR imaging."	Prasad et al[46]
0.15 and 4.0 T Simulated imaging conditions Fertilized frog eggs Studied effect of MRI on developing embryos	"No adverse effect on early development."	Prasad et al[47]
0.7 T Simulated imaging conditions Frog spermatozoa, fertilized eggs, and embryos Studied effects of MRI on development	"NMR exposure, at the dose used, does not cause detectable adverse effects in this amphibian."	Prasad et al[48]
0.15 T Exposed separately to static, gradient, and RF electromagnetic fields Mice Studied separate effects of static, gradient, and RF electromagnetic fields on morphine-induced analgesia in mice	"Time-varying, and to a lesser extent the RF, fields associated with the MRI procedure inhibit morphine-induced analgesia in mice."	Prato et al[49]
4.7 T Clinical imaging conditions Humans Studied bioeffects of 4.7-T scanner	"Mild vertigo." "Headaches, nausea." "Magnetophosphenes." "Metallic taste in mouth."	Redington et al[50]
0.04 T Clinical imaging conditions Humans Follow-up study	"Average follow-up time was 6 months . . . none of the 35 deaths recorded was unexpected." "Using the magnetic field and radiofrequency levels currently in operation . . . we believe NMRI to be a safe, non-invasive method of whole-body imaging."	Reid et al[51]
4.0 T RF at 8–170 MHz No gradient magnetic fields Humans Studied response of human auditory system to RF pulses	"In accordance with the used RF modulation envelope three distinct chirps per sequence could be resolved." "RF induced auditory noise is usually completely masked by noise from simultaneously switched gradient fields."	Roschmann[52]

Table continued on following page

TABLE 13–1. SUMMARY OF MR BIOEFFECTS STUDIES *Continued*

STUDY DESCRIPTION	RESULTS	REFERENCE
2.7 T Simulated imaging conditions Rats Studied effects of MRI on ocular tissues	"There were no discernable effects on the rat eye."	Sacks et al[53]
0.35 T Simulated imaging conditions Hamster ovary cells Studied effects of MRI on observable mutations and cytotoxicity	"NMR imaging caused no detectable genetic damage and does not affect cell viability."	Schwartz and Crooks[54]
1.5 T Static magnetic field only Humans Studied effect of static magnetic field on body temperature	"No effect on body temperature of normal human subjects."	Shellock et al[55]
1.5 T Clinical imaging conditions Humans Studied temperature, heart rate, and blood pressure changes associated with MRI	"MR imaging . . . not associated with any temperature or hemodynamic related deleterious effects."	Shellock and Crues[56]
1.5 T Clinical imaging conditions Humans Studied thermal effects of MRI of the spine	"No surface hot spots." "Temperature effects were well-below known thresholds for adverse effects."	Shellock et al[57]
1.5 T Clinical imaging conditions Humans Studied possible hypothalamic heating produced by MRI of the head	"There was probably no direct hypothalamic heating produced by clinical MRI of the head."	Shellock et al[58]
1.5 T Clinical imaging conditions Humans Studied effect of MRI on corneal temperatures	"MR imaging . . . causes relatively minor increases in corneal temperature that do not appear to pose any thermal hazard to ocular tissue."	Shellock and Crues[59]
1.5 T Clinical imaging conditions Humans Studied temperature changes associated with MRI of the brain	"No significant increases in average body temperature." "Observed elevations in skin temperatures were physiologically inconsequential."	Shellock and Crues[60]
1.5 T Static magnetic field only Humans Studied effects of static magnetic field on body and skin temperatures	"There were no statistically significant changes in body or any of the skin temperatures recorded."	Shellock et al[61]
1.5 T Clinical imaging conditions Humans Studied effect of MRI performed at high specific absorption rates	"Recommended exposure to RF radiation during MR imaging of the body for patients with normal thermoregulatory function may be too conservative."	Shellock et al[62]
1.5 T Clinical imaging conditions Humans Studied effect of MRI on scrotal skin temperature	"Absolute temperature is below threshold known to affect testicular function."	Shellock et al[63]
0.15 T Simulated imaging conditions Anesthetized rats Studied effect of MRI on blood-brain barrier permeability	"These findings raise the possibility that exposure to clinical MRI procedures may also temporarily alter the central blood-brain permeability in human subjects."	Shivers et al[64]
1.5 T Simulated imaging conditions Anesthetized dogs Studied effect of MRI performed at high specific absorption rates	"These findings argue for continued caution in the design and operation of imagers capable of high specific absorption rates."	Shuman et al[65]

TABLE 13–1. SUMMARY OF MR BIOEFFECTS STUDIES *Continued*

STUDY DESCRIPTION	RESULTS	REFERENCE
0.4–8.0 T Static magnetic field only Mice Studied effect of static magnetic field on temperature	"Observed a field-induced increase in temperature."	Sperber et al[66]
0.4–1.0 T Static magnetic field only Humans Studied the effects of static magnetic fields on tissue perfusion	"Neither at the skin of the thumb nor at the forearm were the changes in local blood flow attributable to the magnetic fields applied."	Stick et al[67]
0.4 T Static magnetic field only Humans Studied magnetic field–induced changes in auditory evoked potentials	"Strong steady magnetic fields induce changes in human auditory evoked potentials."	Stojan et al[68]
0.15 T Clinical imaging conditions Humans Studied effect of MRI on cognitive functions	"No significant effect upon cognitive functions assessed."	Sweetland et al[69]
0.6 T/s Gradient magnetic field only Mice Studied effect of gradient magnetic fields on the analgesic properties of specific opiate antagonists	"Results indicate that the time-varying fields associated with MRI have significant inhibitory effects on analgesic effects of specific myopiate-directed ligands."	Teskey et al[70]
0.15 T Simulated imaging conditions Rats Studied effects of MRI on survivability and long-term stress reactivity levels	"Results fail to provide any evidence for changes in survivability and long-term reactivity levels in rats exposed to MRI."	Teskey et al[71]
0.01 and 1.0 T Simulated imaging conditions and static magnetic field only *Escherichia coli* Studied effect of MRI and static magnetic field on various properties of *E. coli*	"No mutations or lethal effects observed."	Thomas and Morris[72]
1.5 T Simulated imaging conditions Mice Studied the potential effects of MRI fields on eye development	"These data suggest a potential for MRI teratogenicity in a strain of mouse predisposed to eye malformations."	Tyndall and Sulik[73]
1.5 T Simulated imaging conditions C57BL/6J mouse Studied combined effects of MRI and x-irradiation on the developing eye of the mouse	"Results . . . suggested that the MRI techniques employed for this investigation did not enhance teratogenicity of X-irradiation on eye malformations produced in the C57BL/6J mouse."	Tyndall[74]
0.35 and 1.5 T Clinical imaging conditions Humans Studied effects of MRI on temperature	"No significant changes in central or peripheral temperatures resulting from the application of static or dynamic or radiofrequency."	Vogl et al[75]
0.35 T Static magnetic field only Humans Studied effect of static magnetic field on auditory evoked potentials	"Magnetically induced shift may be explained by changes in electric capacities of the magnetically exposed biological system."	Von Klitzing[76]
0.2 T Static magnetic field only Humans Studied effect of static magnetic field on power intensity of EEG	"The increased control values following on inverted magnetic flux vector point to a reversible alteration of brain function induced by a static magnetic field."	Von Klitzing[77]
0.2 T Static magnetic field only Humans Studied encephalomagnetic fields during exposure to static magnetic field	"Exposure to static magnetic fields as used in NMR-equipment generates a new encephalomagnetic field in human brain."	Von Klitzing[78]
1.5 and 4.0 T Static magnetic fields only Rats Studied effect of magnetic field on behavior	"At 4 T . . . in 97% of the trials the rats would not enter the magnet."	Weiss et al[79]

Table continued on following page

TABLE 13–1. SUMMARY OF MR BIOEFFECTS STUDIES *Continued*

STUDY DESCRIPTION	RESULTS	REFERENCE
0.16 T Static and gradient magnetic fields only Anesthetized rats and guinea pigs Studied effects of static and gradient magnetic fields on cardiac function of rats and guinea pigs	"No change in blood pressure, heart rate, or ECG."	Willis and Brooks[80]
0.3 T Static magnetic field only Mouse sperm cell Studied effect of static magnetic field on spermatogenesis	"Acute and subacute exposure to static magnetic fields associated with diagnostic MR imaging devices is unlikely to have any significant adverse effect on spermatogenesis."	Withers et al[81]
0.35 T Simulated imaging conditions Hamster ovary cells Studied effect of MRI on DNA and chromosomes	"The conditions used for NMR imaging do not cause genetic damage which is detectable by any of these methods."	Wolff et al[82]
Varying gradient fields Humans Studied the effects of time-varying gradient fields on peripheral nerve stimulation using trapezoidal and sinusoidal pulse trains	"The thresholds of trapezoidal pulses were higher than those of sinusoidal pulses by 11% and 30% respectively, at equivalent power level."	Yamagata et al[83]

electrically, magnetically, or mechanically activated implants because electromagnetic fields produced by the system may interfere with the operation of these devices.[107] Therefore, patients with internal cardiac pacemakers, implantable cardiac defibrillators, cochlear implants, neurostimulators, bone growth stimulators, implantable electronic drug infusion pumps, and other similar devices that could be adversely affected by the electromagnetic fields used for MR procedures should not be examined by this diagnostic technique.[120, 123–126] Prior ex vivo testing of certain of these implants and devices may indicate that they are, in fact, MR compatible. For example, it is acceptable to perform MR procedures on patients who have certain types of EEG electrodes in place (see Table 13–2).

The associated risks of scanning patients with cardiac pacemakers are related to the possibility of movement, reed switch closures or damage, programming changes, inhibition, reversion to an asynchronous mode of operation, electromagnetic interference, and induced currents in lead wires.[120, 123, 124, 126] At least one patient with a pacemaker has been scanned by an MR procedure without incident.[125] A letter to the editor indicated that a patient who was not pacemaker dependent underwent an MR procedure by having his pacemaker "disabled" during the procedure. Although this patient sustained no apparent discomfort and the pacemaker was not damaged, routinely performing this type of maneuver on patients with pacemakers is not advised because of the potential of encountering the aforementioned hazards. An MR-related death of a patient with a pacemaker has been reported.[99]

Of particular concern is the possibility that the pacemaker lead wires or other similar intracardiac wire configuration could act as an antenna in which the gradient or RF electromagnetic fields may induce sufficient current to cause fibrillation, a burn, or other potentially dangerous event.[99, 120, 123, 124, 126] Because of this theoretically deleterious and unpredicted effect,

patients with residual external pacing wires, temporary pacing wires, Swan-Ganz thermodilution catheters, or any other type of internally or externally positioned conductive wire or similar device should not undergo MR procedures because of the possible associated risks.[99, 120, 127]

Some types of cochlear implants employ a relatively high-field-strength cobalt samarium magnet used in conjunction with an external magnet to align and retain an RF transmitter coil on the patient's head, whereas other types of cochlear implants are electronically activated.[128] Consequently, MR procedures are strictly contraindicated in patients with these implants because of the possibility of injuring the patient or damaging or altering the operation of the cochlear implant.

Because there is a potential for demagnetizing implants that involve magnets (e.g., dental implants, magnetic sphincters, magnetic stoma plugs, magnetic ocular implants, and other similar devices) that may necessitate surgery to replace the damaged implant, these implants should be removed from the patient before an MR procedure, if possible.[128–130] Otherwise, an MR procedure should not be performed on a patient with a magnetically activated implant or device. A patient with any other similar electrically, magnetically, or mechanically activated implant or device should be excluded from examination by MR procedures unless the particular implant or device has been previously demonstrated to be unaffected by the magnetic and electromagnetic fields.[120]

PATIENTS WITH METALLIC IMPLANTS, MATERIALS, AND FOREIGN BODIES

MR procedures are contraindicated for patients who have certain ferromagnetic implants, materials, or foreign bodies, primarily because of the possibility of movement or dislodgement of these objects.[97-99] Other problems may also occur in patients with ferromagnetic implants, materials, or foreign bodies who undergo MR procedures, including the induction of electrical current in the object, excessive heating of the object, and misinterpretation of an artifact produced by the presence of the object as an abnormality.[97, 99, 131-134] These latter potentially hazardous situations, however, are encountered infrequently or are insignificant in comparison with movement or dislodgement of a ferromagnetic implant or foreign body by the magnetic fields.

Numerous investigations have evaluated the ferromagnetic qualities of a variety of metallic implants, materials, or foreign bodies by measuring deflection forces or movements associated with the static magnetic fields used for MR procedures.[134-153] These studies were conducted to determine the relative risk of performing an MR procedure on a patient with a metallic object with respect to whether the magnetic attraction was strong enough to produce movement or dislodgement.

A variety of factors require evaluation when establishing the relative risk of performing an MR procedure on a patient with a ferromagnetic implant, material, device, or foreign body, such as the strength of the static and gradient magnetic fields, the relative degree of ferromagnetism of the object, the mass of the object, the geometry of the object, the location and orientation of the object in situ, and the length of time the object has been in place.[98, 99] Each of these factors should be considered before allowing a patient who has a ferromagnetic object to enter the electromagnetic environment of the MR system.

Table 13–2 provides a comprehensive summary of information pertaining to biomedical implants, materials, and devices evaluated for compatibility with MR systems. If a patient is identified to have an implant or foreign body during pre-MR screening, this compilation of implants, materials, or foreign bodies tested for ferromagnetism should be consulted to determine whether the object is safe (i.e., there are no or only insignificant associated deflection forces associated with the object).

ANEURYSM AND HEMOSTATIC CLIPS. Of the different aneurysm and vascular clips studied and reported in the literature, many of the aneurysm clips and none of the vascular clips were found to be ferromagnetic. If there is no definitive information available related to the ferromagnetic qualities of an aneurysm clip, the patient should not undergo an MR procedure. Therefore, only patients who have nonferromagnetic aneurysm clips (i.e., the clips were tested independently before being placed in the patient) should be exposed to the magnetic fields used for MR procedures. Any patient with one of the previously tested hemostatic clips may safely undergo an MR procedure.

CAROTID ARTERY VASCULAR CLAMPS. Each of the carotid artery vascular clamps evaluated for ferromagnetism exhibited deflection forces. However, only the Poppen-Blaylock clamp was considered to be contraindicated for patients undergoing MR procedures because of the significant ferromagnetism shown by this object. The other carotid artery vascular clamps are believed to be safe for MR procedures because of the minimal deflection forces relative to their use in an in vivo application (i.e., the deflection forces are insignificant and, therefore, there is little possibility of significant movement or dislodgement of the implant).

DENTAL DEVICES AND MATERIALS. Various dental devices and materials have been tested for ferromagnetism. Although many of them demonstrated deflection forces, only a few of these pose a possible risk to patients undergoing MR procedures because they are magnetically activated devices.

HEART VALVES. Many of the commercially available heart valve prostheses have been tested for ferromagnetism. The majority of these displayed measurable deflection forces, but the deflection forces were relatively insignificant compared with the force exerted by the beating heart. Therefore, patients with these heart valve prostheses may safely undergo MR procedures.

INTRAVASCULAR COILS, FILTERS, AND STENTS. Less than half of the different intravascular coils, filters, and stents tested were ferromagnetic.[145, 152] These ferromagnetic devices are usually attached firmly into the vessel wall at approximately 6 weeks after introduction.[152] Therefore, it is unlikely that any of them would become dislodged by attraction from magnetic forces presently used for MR procedures after a suitable time has elapsed (i.e., for the coils, filters, and stents that have ferromagnetic qualities). Patients with intravascular coils, filters, or stents in which there is a possibility that the device is not properly positioned or held firmly in place should not undergo MR procedures.

OCULAR IMPLANTS. Various ocular implants have been evaluated for ferromagnetism. Of these, the Fatio eyelid spring and retinal tack made from martensitic stainless steel displayed measurable deflection forces. Although it is unlikely that the associated deflection forces would cause movement or dislodgement of these implants, it is possible that a patient with one of these implants would be uncomfortable or sustain a minor injury during MR procedures. Lens implants are typically made from nonferromagnetic materials such as certain forms of plastic, but details must be known about these implants before conducting MR procedures to determine that they are not held in place using a ferromagnetic suture material or other potentially hazardous means.

ORTHOPEDIC IMPLANTS, MATERIALS, AND DEVICES. Most orthopedic implants, materials, and devices tested for ferromagnetism have been demonstrated to be made from nonferromagnetic materials. Therefore, patients with these particular orthopedic implants, materials, and devices may be imaged safely by MR procedures. The Perfix interference screw used for reconstruction of the anterior cruciate ligament, although composed of ferromagnetic material, does not pose a hazard to the patient undergoing an MR procedure because of the significant force that holds it in place in vivo. However, the resulting artifact pre-

Text continued on page 421

TABLE 13–2. METALLIC IMPLANTS, MATERIALS, DEVICES, AND OBJECTS TESTED FOR MOVEMENT/ DEFLECTION FORCES DURING EXPOSURE TO STATIC MAGNETIC FIELDS

METALLIC IMPLANT, MATERIAL, DEVICE, OR OBJECT*	MOVEMENT/ DEFLECTION	HIGHEST FIELD STRENGTH† (T)	REFERENCE
Aneurysm and Hemostatic Clips			
Downs multi-positional (17-7PH)	Yes	1.39	154
Drake (DR 14, DR 21) Edward Weck Triangle Park, NJ	Yes	1.39	148, 154
Drake (DR 16) Edward Weck	Yes	0.147	154
Drake (301 SS) Edward Weck	Yes	1.5	138, 148
Gastrointestinal anastomosis clip Auto Suture SGIA (SS) United States Surgical Corporation Norwalk, CT	No	1.5	138
Heifetz (17-7PH) Edward Weck	Yes	1.89	139, 155
Heifetz (Elgiloy) Edward Weck	No	1.89	139, 148, 155
Hemoclip No. 10 (316L SS) Edward Weck	No	1.5	138
Hemoclip (tantalum) Edward Weck	No	1.5	138
Housepian	Yes	0.147	154
Kapp (405 SS) V. Mueller	Yes	1.89	139, 148
Kapp, curved (404 SS) V. Mueller	Yes	1.39	154
Kapp, straight (404 SS) V. Mueller	Yes	1.39	154
Ligaclip No. 6 (316L SS) Ethicon, Inc. Somerville, NJ	No	1.5	138
Ligaclip (tantalum) Ethicon	No	1.5	138
Mayfield (301 SS) Codman Randolph, MA	Yes	1.5	138
Mayfield (304 SS) Codman	Yes	1.89	139
McFadden (301 SS) Codman	Yes	1.5	138, 148
Olivecrona	No	1.39	154
Pivot (17-7PH)	Yes	1.89	139
Scoville (EN58J) Downs Surgical, Inc Decatur, GA	Yes	1.89	139, 148
Stevens (50-4190, silver alloy)	No	0.15	156
Sugita (Elgiloy) Downs Surgical	No	1.89	139, 148
Sundt-Kees (301 SS) Downs Surgical	Yes	1.5	138, 148
Sundt-Kees Multi-Angle (17-7PH) Downs Surgical	Yes	1.89	139, 148
Surgiclip, Auto Suture M-9.5 (SS) United States Surgical Corporation	No	1.5	138
Vari-Angle (17-7PH) Codman	Yes	1.89	139

TABLE 13–2. METALLIC IMPLANTS, MATERIALS, DEVICES, AND OBJECTS TESTED FOR MOVEMENT/ DEFLECTION FORCES DURING EXPOSURE TO STATIC MAGNETIC FIELDS *Continued*

METALLIC IMPLANT, MATERIAL, DEVICE, OR OBJECT*	MOVEMENT/ DEFLECTION	HIGHEST FIELD STRENGTH† (T)	REFERENCE
Vari-Angle McFadden (MP35N) Codman	No	1.89	139, 148
Vari-Angle Micro (17-7PM SS) Codman	Yes	0.15	148, 156
Vari-Angle Spring (17-7PM SS) Codman	Yes	0.15	148, 156
Yasargil (316 SS) Aesculap	No	1.89	139
Yasargil (Phynox) Aesculap	No	1.89	148
Biopsy Needles ASAP 16, automatic 16 gauge, core biopsy system, 19 cm length (304 SS) Microvasive Watertown, MA	Yes	1.5	NA
Biopty-cut, biopsy needle, 14 gauge, 10 cm length (304 SS) C. R. Bard, Inc. Covington, GA	Yes	1.5	NA
Biopty-cut, biopsy needle, 16 gauge, 16 cm length (304 SS) C. R. Bard, Inc.	Yes	1.5	NA
Biopty-cut, biopsy needle, 18 gauge, 18 cm length (304 SS) C. R. Bard, Inc.	Yes	1.5	NA
Lufkin aspiration cytology needle, 20 gauge, 5 cm length E-Z-EM, Inc. Westbury, NY	No	1.5	157
Ultra-Core, biopsy needle, 16 gauge, 16 cm length (304 SS) Gainesville, FL	Yes	1.5	NA
Carotid Artery Vascular Clamps Crutchfield (SS) Codman	Yes‡	1.5	158
Kindt (SS) V. Mueller	Yes‡	1.5	158
Poppen-Blaylock (SS) Codman	Yes	1.5	158
Salibi (SS) Codman	Yes‡	1.5	158
Selverstone (SS) Codman	Yes‡	1.5	158
Dental Devices and Materials Brace band (SS) American Dental Missoula, MT	Yes‡	1.5	138
Brace wire (chrome alloy) Ormco Corporation San Marcos, CA	Yes‡	1.5	138
Castable alloy Golden Dental Products, Inc. Golden, CO	Yes‡	1.5	159
Cement-in Keeper Solid State Innovations, Inc. Mt. Airy, NC	Yes‡	1.5	159
Dental amalgam	No	1.39	154
Gutta percha points	No	1.5	NA

Table continued on following page

TABLE 13–2. METALLIC IMPLANTS, MATERIALS, DEVICES, AND OBJECTS TESTED FOR MOVEMENT/ DEFLECTION FORCES DURING EXPOSURE TO STATIC MAGNETIC FIELDS *Continued*

METALLIC IMPLANT, MATERIAL, DEVICE, OR OBJECT*	MOVEMENT/ DEFLECTION	HIGHEST FIELD STRENGTH† (T)	REFERENCE
GDP Direct Keeper, preformed post Golden Dental Products, Inc. Golden, CO	Yes‡	1.5	159
Indian Head Real Silver Points Union Broach Company, Inc. New York, NY	No	1.5	NA
Keeper, preformed post Parkell Products, Inc. Farmingdale, NY	Yes‡	1.5	154
Magna-Dent, large indirect keeper Dental Ventures of America Yorba Linda, CA	Yes‡	1.5	154
Palladium clad magnet Parkell Products, Inc.	Yes	1.5	129
Palladium/palladium keeper Parkell Products, Inc.	Yes‡	1.5	129
Palladium/platinum casting alloy Parkell Products, Inc.	Yes‡	1.5	129
Permanent crown (amalgam) Ormco Corporation	No	1.5	138
Stainless steel clad magnet Parkell Products, Inc.	Yes	1.5	129
Stainless steel keeper Parkell Products, Inc.	Yes‡	1.5	129
Silver point Union Broach Company, Inc. New York, NY	No	1.5	138
Titanium clad magnet Parkell Products, Inc.	Yes	1.5	129
Halo Vests Ambulatory Halo System AOA Company Greenwood, SC	No	1.5	160
Bremer standard halo crown and vest Bremmer Medical Company Jacksonville, FL	No	1.0	161
Bremmer halo system, MR compatible Bremmer Medical Company	No	1.0	161
EXO adjustable collar Florida Manufacturing Company Daytona, FL	Yes§	1.0	161
Guilford cervical orthosis Guilford & Son, Ltd. Cleveland, OH	Yes§	1.0	161
Guilford cervical orthosis, modified Guilford & Son, Ltd.	No	1.0	161
MR-compatible halo vest and cervical orthosis Lerman & Son Company Beverly Hills, CA	No	1.5	NA
Philadelphia collar Philadelphia Collar Company Westville, NJ	No	1.0	161
PMT halo cervical orthosis PMT Corporation Chanhassen, MN	No	1.0	161
PMT halo cervical orthosis with graphite rods and halo ring PMT Corporation	No	1.0	161

TABLE 13–2. METALLIC IMPLANTS, MATERIALS, DEVICES, AND OBJECTS TESTED FOR MOVEMENT/ DEFLECTION FORCES DURING EXPOSURE TO STATIC MAGNETIC FIELDS *Continued*

METALLIC IMPLANT, MATERIAL, DEVICE, OR OBJECT*	MOVEMENT/ DEFLECTION	HIGHEST FIELD STRENGTH† (T)	REFERENCE
S.O.M.I. cervical orthosis US. Manufacturing Company Pasadena, CA	Yes§	1.0	161
Heart Valve Prostheses Beall Coratomic, Inc Indiana, PA	Yes‡	2.35	162
Bjork-Shiley (convex/concave) Shiley, Inc. Irvine, CA	No	1.5	138
Bjork-Shiley (universal/spherical) Shiley, Inc.	Yes‡	1.5	138
Bjork-Shiley, model MBC Shiley, Inc.	Yes‡	2.35	163
Bjork-Shiley, model 22 MBRC 11030 Shiley, Inc.	Yes‡	2.35	163
CarboMedics Heart Valve Prosthesis, aortic, reduced, model R500, size 19 CarboMedics Austin, TX	No	1.5	NA
CarboMedics Heart Valve Prosthesis, aortic, reduced, model R500, size 21 CarboMedics	No	1.5	NA
CarboMedics Heart Valve Prosthesis, aortic, reduced, model R500, size 23 CarboMedics	No	1.5	NA
CarboMedics Heart Valve Prosthesis, aortic, reduced, model R500, size 25 CarboMedics	No	1.5	NA
CarboMedics Heart Valve Prosthesis, aortic, reduced, model R500, size 27 CarboMedics	No	1.5	NA
CarboMedics Heart Valve Prosthesis, aortic, reduced, model R500, size 29 CarboMedics	No	1.5	NA
CarboMedics Heart Valve Prosthesis, aortic, standard, model 500, size 31 CarboMedics	No	1.5	NA
CarboMedics Heart Valve Prosthesis, mitral, standard, model 700, size 23 CarboMedics	No	1.5	NA
CarboMedics Heart Valve Prosthesis, mitral, standard, model 700, size 25 CarboMedics	No	1.5	NA
CarboMedics Heart Valve Prosthesis, mitral, standard, model 700, size 27 CarboMedics	No	1.5	NA
CarboMedics Heart Valve Prosthesis, mitral, standard, model 700, size 29	No	1.5	NA
CarboMedics Heart Valve Prosthesis, mitral, standard, model 700, size 31 CarboMedics	No	1.5	NA
CarboMedics Heart Valve Prosthesis, mitral, standard, model 700, size 33 CarboMedics	No	1.5	NA
Carpentier-Edwards model 2650 American Edwards Laboratories Santa Ana, CA	Yes‡	2.35	163
Carpentier-Edwards (porcine) American Edwards Laboratories	Yes‡	2.35	163

Table continued on following page

TABLE 13–2. METALLIC IMPLANTS, MATERIALS, DEVICES, AND OBJECTS TESTED FOR MOVEMENT/ DEFLECTION FORCES DURING EXPOSURE TO STATIC MAGNETIC FIELDS *Continued*

METALLIC IMPLANT, MATERIAL, DEVICE, OR OBJECT*	MOVEMENT/ DEFLECTION	HIGHEST FIELD STRENGTH† (T)	REFERENCE
Hall-Kaster, model A7700 Medtronic, Inc. Minneapolis, MN	Yes‡	1.5	138
Hancock I (porcine) Johnson & Johnson Anaheim, CA	Yes‡	1.5	138
Hancock II (porcine) Johnson & Johnson	Yes‡	1.5	138
Hancock extracorporeal, model 242R Johnson & Johnson	Yes‡	2.35	163
Hancock extracorporeal, model M 4365-33 Johnson & Johnson	Yes‡	2.35	163
Hancock Vascor, model 505 Johnson & Johnson	No	2.35	163
Ionescu-Shiley, Universal ISM	Yes‡	2.35	163
Lillehi-Kaster, model 300S Medical, Inc. Inner Grove Heights, MN	Yes‡	2.35	162
Lillehi-Kaster, model 5009 Medical, Inc.	Yes‡	2.35	163
Medtronic Hall Medtronic, Inc. Minneapolis, MN	Yes‡	2.35	163
Medtronic Hall, model A7700-D-16 Medtronic, Inc.	Yes‡	2.35	163
Omnicarbon, model 35231029 Medical Inc.	Yes‡	2.35	163
Omniscience, model 6522 Medical, Inc.	Yes‡	2.35	163
Smeloff-Cutter Cutter Laboratories Berkeley, CA	Yes‡	2.35	138
Starr-Edwards, model 1260 American Edwards Laboratories	Yes‡	2.35	162
Starr-Edwards, model 2320 American Edwards Laboratories	Yes‡	2.35	162
Starr-Edwards, model 2400 American Edwards Laboratories	No	1.5	138
Starr-Edwards, model Pre 6000 American Edwards Laboratories	Yes‡	2.35	162
Starr-Edwards, model 6518 American Edwards Laboratories	Yes‡	2.35	163
St. Jude St. Jude Medical, Inc. St. Paul, MN	No	1.5	138
St. Jude, model A 101 St. Jude Medical, Inc.	Yes‡	2.35	163
St. Jude, model M 101 St. Jude Medical, Inc.	Yes‡	2.35	163
Intravascular Coils, Filters, and Stents Amplatz IVC filter Cook, Inc. Bloomington, IN	No	4.7	152
Cook occluding spring embolization coil MWCE-33-5-10 Cook, Inc.	Yes‡‖	1.5	NA
Cragg nitinol spiral filter	No	4.7	152

TABLE 13–2. METALLIC IMPLANTS, MATERIALS, DEVICES, AND OBJECTS TESTED FOR MOVEMENT/DEFLECTION FORCES DURING EXPOSURE TO STATIC MAGNETIC FIELDS *Continued*

METALLIC IMPLANT, MATERIAL, DEVICE, OR OBJECT*	MOVEMENT/ DEFLECTION	HIGHEST FIELD STRENGTH† (T)	REFERENCE
Flower embolization microcoil (platinum) Target Therapeutics San Jose, CA	No	1.5	164
Gianturco embolization coil Cook, Inc.	Yes‡‖	1.5	152
Gianturco bird nest IVC filter Cook, Inc.	Yes‡‖	1.5	152, 165
Gianturco zig-zag stent Cook, Inc.	Yes‡‖	1.5	152
Greenfield vena cava filter (stainless steel), Meditech Watertown, MA	Yes‡‖	1.5	152, 166
Greenfield vena cava filter (titanium alloy) Ormco Glendora, CA	No	1.5	152
Gunther IVC filter William Cook Europe	Yes‡‖	1.5	152
Hilal embolization microcoil Cook, Inc.	No	1.5	164
IVC venous clip (Teflon) Pilling Co.	No	1.5	NA
Maas helical IVC filter Medinvent Lausanne, Switzerland	No	4.7	152
Maas helical endovascular stent Medinvent	No	4.7	152
Mobin-Uddin IVC/umbrella filter American Edwards Santa Ana, CA	No	4.7	152
New retrievable IVC filter Thomas Jefferson University Philadelphia, PA	Yes‡‖	1.5	152
Palmaz endovascular stent Johnson & Johnson, Interventional Warren, NJ	No	1.5	NA
Palmaz endovascular stent Ethicon	Yes‡‖	1.5	152
Strecker stent (tantalum) Meditech	No	1.5	167
Ureteral stent	No	1.5	NA
Ocular Implants			
Clip 50, double tantalum clip Mira, Inc.	No	1.5	168
Clip 51, single tantalum clip Mira, Inc.	No	1.5	168
Clip 52, single tantalum clip Mira, Inc.	No	1.5	168
Clip 250, double tantalum clip Mira, Inc.	No	1.5	168
Double tantalum clip Storz Instrument Co.	No	1.5	168
Double tantalum clip, style 250 Storz Instrument Co.	No	1.5	168
Fatio eyelid spring/wire	Yes	1.5	140
Gold eyelid spring	No	1.5	NA

Table continued on following page

**TABLE 13–2. METALLIC IMPLANTS, MATERIALS, DEVICES, AND OBJECTS TESTED FOR MOVEMENT/
DEFLECTION FORCES DURING EXPOSURE TO STATIC MAGNETIC FIELDS** *Continued*

METALLIC IMPLANT, MATERIAL, DEVICE, OR OBJECT*	MOVEMENT/ DEFLECTION	HIGHEST FIELD STRENGTH† (T)	REFERENCE
Intraocular lens implant, Binkhorst, iridocapsular lens, platinum-iridium loop	No	1.5	169
Intraocular lens implant, Binkhorst, iridocapsular lens, titanium loop	No	1.0	169
Intraocular lens implant Worst, platinum clip lens	No	1.0	169
Retinal tack (303 SS) Bascom Palmer Eye Institute	No	1.5	170
Retinal tack (titanium alloy) Coopervision Irvine, CA	No	1.5	170
Retinal tack (303 SS) Duke	No	1.5	170
Retinal tack (cobalt/nickel) Grieshaber Fallsington, PA	No	1.5	171
Retinal tack, Norton staple (platinum/ rhodium) Norton	No	1.5	170
Retinal tack (aluminum textraoxide) Ruby	No	1.5	170
Retinal tack (SS-martensitic) Western European	Yes	1.5	170
Single tantalum clip	No	1.5	168
Troutman magnetic ocular implant	Yes	1.5	NA
Unitech round wire eye spring	Yes	1.5	NA
Orthopedic Implants, Materials, and Devices			
AML femoral component bipolar hip prosthesis Zimmer Warsaw, IN	No	1.5	138
Cervical wire, 18 gauge (316L SS)	No	0.3	172
Charnley-Muller hip prosthesis, Protasyl-10 alloy	No	0.3	NA
Cortical bone screw, large (titanium, Ti-6Al 4V alloy) Zimmer	No	1.5	173
Cortical bone screw, small (titanium, Ti-6Al-4V alloy) Zimmer	No	1.5	173
Cotrel rods with hooks (316L SS)	No	0.3	172
Cotrel rod (SS-ASTM, grade 2)	No	1.5	NA
DTT, device for transverse traction (316L SS)	No	0.3	172
Drummond wire (316L SS)	No	0.3	172
Endoscopic noncannulated interference screw (titanium) Acufex Microsurgical Norwood, MA	No	1.5	173
Fixation staple (cobalt chromium alloy, ASTM F 75) Richards Medical Company Memphis, TN	No	1.5	173

TABLE 13-2. METALLIC IMPLANTS, MATERIALS, DEVICES, AND OBJECTS TESTED FOR MOVEMENT/ DEFLECTION FORCES DURING EXPOSURE TO STATIC MAGNETIC FIELDS *Continued*

METALLIC IMPLANT, MATERIAL, DEVICE, OR OBJECT*	MOVEMENT/ DEFLECTION	HIGHEST FIELD STRENGTH† (T)	REFERENCE
Halifax clamps American Medical Electronics Richardson, TX	No	1.5	NA
Harrington compression rod with hooks and nuts (316L SS)	No	0.3	172
Harrington distraction rod with hooks (316L SS)	No	0.3	172
Harris hip prosthesis Zimmer	No	1.5	138
Jewett nail Zimmer	No	1.5	138
Kirschner intermedullary rod Kirschner Medical Timonium, MD	No	1.5	138
"L" rod (cobalt-nickel) Richards Medical Company	No	1.5	NA
Luque wire	No	0.3	172
Moe spinal instrumentation Zimmer	No	1.5	NA
Perfix interence screw (17-4 stainless steel, Al 630-Cr_{17}) Instrument Makar Okemos, MI	Yes	1.5	173
Rusch rod	No	1.5	NA
Spinal L-rod DePuy Warsaw, IN	No	1.5	NA
Stainless steel plate Zimmer	No	1.5	138
Stainless steel screw Zimmer	No	1.5	138
Staple plate, large, Zimaloy Zimmer	No	1.5	173
Stainless steel mesh Zimmer	No	1.5	138
Stainless steel wire Zimmer	No	1.5	138
Synthes AO DCP 2, 3, 4, 5 hole plate	No	1.5	NA
Zielke rod with screw, washer, and nut (316L SS)	No	0.3	172
Otologic Implants Austin tytan piston (titanium) Treace Medical Nashville, TN	No	1.5	141
Berger "V" bobbin ventilation tube (titanium) Richards Medical Company Memphis, TN	No	1.5	141
Cochlear implant 3M/House	Yes	0.6	174
Cochlear implant 3M/Vienna	Yes	0.6	174
Cochlear implant Nucleus Mini 20-channel Cochlear Corporation Englewood, CO	Yes	1.5	175

Table continued on following page

TABLE 13–2. METALLIC IMPLANTS, MATERIALS, DEVICES, AND OBJECTS TESTED FOR MOVEMENT/DEFLECTION FORCES DURING EXPOSURE TO STATIC MAGNETIC FIELDS *Continued*

METALLIC IMPLANT, MATERIAL, DEVICE, OR OBJECT*	MOVEMENT/ DEFLECTION	HIGHEST FIELD STRENGTH† (T)	REFERENCE
Cody tack	No	0.6	174
Ehmke hook stapes prosthesis (platinum) Richards Medical Company	No	1.5	141
Fisch piston (Teflon, stainless steel) Richards Medical Company	No	1.5	175
House single loop (ASTM-318-76 grade 2 stainless steel) Storz St. Louis, MO	No	1.5	141
House single loop (tantalum) Storz	No	1.5	141
House double loop (tantalum) Storz	No	1.5	141
House double loop (ASTM-318-76 grade 2 stainless steel) Storz	No	1.5	141
House-type incus prosthesis	No	0.6	NA
House-type wire loop stapes prosthesis (316L SS) Richards Medical Company Memphis, TN	No	1.5	141, 175
House-type stainless steel piston and wire (ASTM-318-76 grade 2 stainless steel) Xomed-Treace Inc.	No	1.5	141
House wire (tantalum) Otomed	No	0.5	176
House wire (stainless steel) Otomed	No	0.5	176
McGee piston stapes prosthesis (316L SS) Richards Medical Company	No	1.5	141, 175
McGee piston stapes prosthesis (platinum/316L SS) Richards Medical Company	No	1.5	141, 175
McGee piston stapes prosthesis (platinum/$Cr_{17}Ni_4$ SS) Richards Medical Company	Yes	1.5	175
McGee shepherd's crook stapes prosthesis (316L SS) Richards Medical Company	No	1.5	141
Plasti-pore piston (316L SS/plasti-pore material) Richards Medical Company	No	1.5	141, 175
Platinum ribbon loop stapes prosthesis (platinum) Richards Medical Company	No	1.5	141
Reuter bobbin ventilation tube (316L SS) Richards Medical Company	No	1.5	141
Richards bucket handle stapes prosthesis (316L SS) Richards Medical Company	No	1.5	141, 175
Reuter drain tube	No	1.5	140
Richards Plasti-pore with Armstrong-style platinum ribbon	No	1.5	140

TABLE 13–2. METALLIC IMPLANTS, MATERIALS, DEVICES, AND OBJECTS TESTED FOR MOVEMENT/ DEFLECTION FORCES DURING EXPOSURE TO STATIC MAGNETIC FIELDS *Continued*

METALLIC IMPLANT, MATERIAL, DEVICE, OR OBJECT*	MOVEMENT/ DEFLECTION	HIGHEST FIELD STRENGTH† (T)	REFERENCE
Richards platinum Teflon piston 0.6 mm (Teflon, platinum) Richards Medical Company	No	1.5	175
Richards platinum Teflon piston 0.8 mm (Teflon, platinum) Richards Medical Company	No	1.5	175
Richards piston stapes prosthesis (platinum/fluoroplastic) Richards Medical Company	No	1.5	141
Richards shepherd's crook (platinum) Richards Medical Company	No	0.5	176
Richards Teflon piston (Teflon) Richards Medical Company	No	1.5	175
Robinson-Moon-Lippy offset stapes prosthesis (ASTM-318-76 grade 2 stainless steel) Storz	No	1.5	141
Robinson-Moon offset stapes prosthesis (ASTM-318-76 grade 2 stainless steel) Storz	No	1.5	141
Robinson incus replacement prosthesis (ASTM-318-76 grade 2 stainless steel)	No	1.5	141
Robinson stapes prosthesis (ASTM-318-76 grade 2 stainless steel) Storz	No	1.5	141
Ronis piston stapes prosthesis (316L SS/fluoroplastic) Richards Medical Company	No	1.5	141
Schea cup piston stapes prosthesis (platinum/fluoroplastic) Richards Medical Company	No	1.5	141, 175
Schea malleus attachment piston (Teflon) Richards Medical Company	No	1.5	175
Schea stainless steel and Teflon wire prosthesis (Teflon, 316L SS) Richards Medical Company	No	1.5	175
Scheer piston stapes prosthesis (316L SS/fluoroplastic) Richards Medical Company	No	1.5	141
Scheer piston (Teflon, 316L SS) Richards Medical Company	No	1.5	175
Schuknecht Gelfoam and wire prosthesis, Armstrong style (316L SS) Richards Medical Company	No	1.5	177
Schuknecht piston stapes prosthesis (316L SS/fluoroplastic) Richards Medical Company	No	1.5	141
Schuknecht tef-wire incus attachment (ASTM-318-76 grade 2 stainless steel) Storz	No	1.5	141, 175
Schuknecht tef-wire malleus attachment (ASTM-318-76 grade 2 stainless steel) Storz	No	1.5	141, 175
Schuknecht teflon wire piston 0.6 mm (Teflon, 316L SS) Richards Medical Company	No	1.5	175
Schuknecht Teflon wire piston, 0.8 mm (Teflon, 316L SS) Richards Medical Company	No	1.5	175

Table continued on following page

TABLE 13–2. METALLIC IMPLANTS, MATERIALS, DEVICES, AND OBJECTS TESTED FOR MOVEMENT/ DEFLECTION FORCES DURING EXPOSURE TO STATIC MAGNETIC FIELDS *Continued*

METALLIC IMPLANT, MATERIAL, DEVICE, OR OBJECT*	MOVEMENT/ DEFLECTION	HIGHEST FIELD STRENGTH† (T)	REFERENCE
Sheehy incus replacement (ASTM-318-76 grade 2 stainless steel) Storz	No	1.5	141
Sheehy incus strut (316L SS) Richards Medical Company	No	1.5	175
Sheehy-type incus replacement strut (Teflon, 316L SS) Richards Medical Company	No	1.5	141
Silverstein malleus clip ventilation tube (Teflon, 316L SS) Richards Medical Company	No	1.5	175
Spoon bobbin ventilation tube (316L SS) Richards Medical Company	No	1.5	141
Tantalum wire loop stages prosthesis (tantalum) Richards Medical Company	No	1.5	141, 175
Tef-platinum piston (platinum) Xomed-Treace Inc.	No	1.5	141
Total ossibular replacement prosthesis (TORP) (316L SS) Richards Medical Company	No	1.5	175
Trapeze ribbon loop staples prosthesis (platinum) Richards Medical Company	No	1.5	141
Williams microclip (316L SS) Richards Medical Company	No	1.5	141
Xomed stapes (ASTM-318-76 grade 2 stainless steel) Xomed-Treace Inc.	No	1.5	141
Xomed ceravital partial ossicular prosthesis	No	1.5	NA
Xomed Baily stapes implant	No	1.5	140
Xomed stapes prosthesis, Robinson-style Richards Medical Company	No	1.5	140
Patent Ductus Arteriosus (PDA), Atrial Septal Defect (ASD), and Ventricular Septal Defect (VSD) Occluders			
Rashkind PDA Occlusion Implant, 12 mm, lot no. 07IC1391 (304V SS) C. R. Bard, Inc. Billerica, MA	Yes‡	1.5	NA
Rashkind PDA Occlusion Implant, 17 mm, lot no. 514486 (304 V SS) C. R. Bard, Inc.	Yes	1.5	NA
Lock Clamshell Septal Occlusion Implant, 17 mm, lot no. 07BCO321 (304 V SS) C. R. Bard, Inc.	Yes	1.5	NA
Lock Clamshell Septal Occlusion Implant, 23 mm, lot no. 07CC1903 (304 V SS) C. R. Bard, Inc.	Yes	1.5	NA
Lock Clamshell Septal Occlusion Implant, 28 mm, lot no. 07BC1557 (304 V SS) C. R. Bard, Inc.	Yes	1.5	NA

TABLE 13–2. METALLIC IMPLANTS, MATERIALS, DEVICES, AND OBJECTS TESTED FOR MOVEMENT/ DEFLECTION FORCES DURING EXPOSURE TO STATIC MAGNETIC FIELDS *Continued*

METALLIC IMPLANT, MATERIAL, DEVICE, OR OBJECT*	MOVEMENT/ DEFLECTION	HIGHEST FIELD STRENGTH† (T)	REFERENCE
Lock Clamshell Septal Occlusion Implant, 33 mm, lot no. 07ACI785 (304 V SS) C. R. Bard, Inc.	Yes	1.5	NA
Lock Clamshell Septal Occlusion Implant, 40 mm, lot no. 07ACI785 (304 V SS) C. R. Bard, Inc.	Yes	1.5	NA
Bard Clamshell Septal Umbrella, 17 mm, lot no. 09ED1230 (MP35n) C. R. Bard, Inc.	No	1.5	NA
Bard Clamshell Septal Umbrella, 23 mm, lot no. 09ED1232 (MP35n) C. R. Bard, Inc.	No	1.5	NA
Bard Clamshell Septal Umbrella, 28 mm, lot no. 09ED1233 (MP35n) C. R. Bard, Inc.	No	1.5	NA
Bard Clamshell Septal Umbrella, 33 mm, lot no. 09ED1234 (MP35n) C. R. Bard, Inc.	No	1.5	NA
Bard Clamshell Septal Umbrella, 40 mm, lot no. 09ED1231 (MP35n) C. R. Bard, Inc.	No	1.5	NA
Pellets and Bullets			
BBs (Daisy)	Yes	1.5	NA
BBs (Crosman)	Yes	1.5	NA
Bullet, .330 inch (copper, plastic, lead) Glaser	No	1.5	143
Bullet, .39 inch (Teflon, bronze) North American Ordinance	No	1.5	143
Bullet, 7.62 × 34 mm (copper, steel) Norinco	Yes	1.5	143
Bullet, .317 inch (copper, lead) Cascade	No	1.5	143
Bullet, .317 inch (lead) Remington	No	1.5	143
Bullet, .317 inch (aluminum, lead) Winchester	No	1.5	143
Bullet, 9 mm (copper, lead) Remington	No	1.5	143
Bullet, .330 inch (copper, nickel, lead) Winchester	Yes	1.5	143
Bullet, .317 inch (nylon, lead) Smith & Wesson	No	1.5	143
Bullet, .317 inch (nickel, copper, lead) Winchester	No	1.5	143
Bullet .45 inch (steel, lead) Evansville Ordinance	Yes	1.5	143
Bullet, .317 inch (steel, lead) Fiocchi	No	1.5	143
Bullet, .317 inch (copper, lead) Hornady	No	1.5	143
Bullet, 9 mm (copper, lead) Norma	Yes	1.5	143
Bullet, .317 inch (bronze, plastic) Patton-Morgan	No	1.5	143

Table continued on following page

TABLE 13–2. METALLIC IMPLANTS, MATERIALS, DEVICES, AND OBJECTS TESTED FOR MOVEMENT/ DEFLECTION FORCES DURING EXPOSURE TO STATIC MAGNETIC FIELDS *Continued*

METALLIC IMPLANT, MATERIAL, DEVICE, OR OBJECT*	MOVEMENT/ DEFLECTION	HIGHEST FIELD STRENGTH† (T)	REFERENCE
Bullet, .317 inch (copper, lead) Patton-Morgan	No	1.5	143
Bullet, .45 inch (copper, lead) Samson	No	1.5	143
Shot, 12 gauge, size: 00 (copper, lead) Federal	No	1.5	143
Shot, 7½ (lead)	No	1.5	143
Shot, 4 (lead)	No	1.5	143
Shot, 00 buckshot (lead)	No	1.5	143
Penile Implants			
Penile implant, AMS 700, CX Inflatable	No	1.5	178
Penile implant, AMS Hydroflex self-contained	No	1.5	NA
Penile implant, AMS Malleable 600 American Medical Systems Minnetonka, MN	No	1.5	178
Penile implant Duraphase	Yes	1.5	NA
Penile implant, Flexi-Flate Surgitek, Medical Engineering Corporation Racine, WI	No	1.5	178
Penile implant, Flexi-Rod (Standard) Surgitek, Medical Engineering Corporation	No	1.5	178
Penile implant, Osmond, external	No	1.5	NA
Penile implant, Flex-Rod II (Firm) Surgitek, Medical Engineering Corporation	No	1.5	178
Penile implant, Jonas Dacomed Corporation Minneapolis, MN	No	1.5	178
Penile implant, Mentor Flexible Mentor Corporation	No	1.5	178
Penile implant, Mentor Inflatable Mentor Corporation	No	1.5	178
Penile implant, OmniPhase Dacomed Corporation	Yes	1.5	178
Penile implant, Uniflex 1000	No	1.5	NA
Vascular Access Ports			
Button (polysulfone polymer, silicone) Infusaid Inc. Norwood, MA	No	1.5	142
Dome Port (titanium) Davol, Inc., a subsidiary of C. R. Bard, Inc. Cranston, RI	No	1.5	142
Dual MicroPort (polysulfone polymer, silicone) Infusaid, Inc. Norwood, MA	No	1.5	142
Dual MacroPort (polysulfone polymer, silicone) Infusaid, Inc.	No	1.5	142
Groshung catheter	Yes‡	1.5	NA
Hickman Port (316L SS) Davol, Inc.	Yes‡	1.5	142

TABLE 13–2. METALLIC IMPLANTS, MATERIALS, DEVICES, AND OBJECTS TESTED FOR MOVEMENT/ DEFLECTION FORCES DURING EXPOSURE TO STATIC MAGNETIC FIELDS *Continued*

METALLIC IMPLANT, MATERIAL, DEVICE, OR OBJECT*	MOVEMENT/ DEFLECTION	HIGHEST FIELD STRENGTH† (T)	REFERENCE
Hickman Port, pediatric (titanium) Davol, Inc.	No	1.5	142
Hickman subcutaneous port (SS, titanium, plastic components) Davol, Inc.	No	1.5	NA
Implantofix II (polysulfone) Burron Medical, Inc. Bethlehem, PA	No	1.5	142
Infusaid, model 350 (titanium) Infusaid, Inc.	No	1.5	142
Infusaid, model 600 (titanium) Infusaid, Inc.	No	1.5	142
Lifeport, model 6013 (Delrin) Strato Medical Corporation Beverly, MA	No	1.5	142
Lifeport, model 1013 (titanium) Strato Medical Corporation	No	1.5	142
MacroPort (polysulfone polymer, silicone) Infusaid, Inc.	No	1.5	142
Mediport Cormed	No	1.5	NA
MicroPort (polysulfone polymer, silicone) Infusaid, Inc.	No	1.5	142
MRI Port (Delrin plastic, silicone) Davol, Inc.	No	1.5	142
Norport-AC (titanium) Norfolk Medical Skokie, IL	No	1.5	142
Norport-DL (316L SS) Norfolk Medical	No	1.5	142
Norport-LS (titanium) Norfolk Medical	No	1.5	142
Norport-LS (316L SS) Norfolk Medical	No	1.5	142
Norport-LS (polysulfone) Norfolk Medical	No	1.5	142
Norport-PT (titanium) Norfolk Medical	No	1.5	142
Norport-SP (polysulfone, silicone rubber, Dacron) Norfolk Medical	No	1.5	142
PeriPort (polysulfone, titanium) Infusaid, Inc.	No	1.5	142
Port-A-Cath, P.A.S. Port Portal (titanium) Pharmacia Deltec St. Paul, MN	No	1.5	142
Port-A-Cath, Titanium Dual Lumen Portal (titanium) Pharmacia Deltec	No	1.5	142
Port-A-Cath, Titanium Peritoneal Portal (titanium) Pharmacia Deltec	No	1.5	142
Port-A-Cath, Titanium Venous Low Profile Portal (titanium) Pharmacia Deltec	No	1.5	142

Table continued on following page

TABLE 13–2. METALLIC IMPLANTS, MATERIALS, DEVICES, AND OBJECTS TESTED FOR MOVEMENT/ DEFLECTION FORCES DURING EXPOSURE TO STATIC MAGNETIC FIELDS *Continued*

METALLIC IMPLANT, MATERIAL, DEVICE, OR OBJECT*	MOVEMENT/ DEFLECTION	HIGHEST FIELD STRENGTH† (T)	REFERENCE
Port-A-Cath, Titanium Venous Portal (titanium) Pharmacia Deltec	No	1.5	142
Port-A-Cath, Venous Portal (316L SS)	No	1.5	142
Porto-cath Pharmacin, NUTECH Pharmacia Deltec	No	1.5	142
Q-Port (316L SS) Quinton Instrument Company Seattle, WA	Yes‡	1.5	142
S.E.A. (titanium) Harbor Medical Devices, Inc. Boston, MA	No	1.5	142
Snap-Lock (titanium, polysulfone polymer, silicone) Infusaid, Inc.	No	1.5	142
Synchromed, model 8500-1 (titanium, thermoplastic, silicone) Medtronic, Inc. Minneapolis, MN	No	1.5	142
Triple Lumen Arrow	No	1.5	NA
Vasport (titanium/fluoropolymer) Gish Biomedical, Inc. Santa Ana, CA	No	1.5	142
Miscellaneous			
Artificial urinary sphincter, AMS 800 American Medical Systems	No	1.5	138
Biosearch endo-feeding tube	No	1.5	NA
Breast implant (inflatable) Inflall, 3101198 Model Heyerschultzz	Yes	1.5	NA
Cerebral ventricular shunt tube connector, Accu-Flow, straight Codman Randolph, MA	No	1.5	138
Cerebral ventricular shunt tube connector, Accu-Flow, right angle Codman	No	1.5	138
Cerebral ventricular shunt tube connector, Accu-Flow, T connector Codman	No	1.5	138
Cerebral ventricular shunt tube connector (type unknown)	Yes	0.147	154
Contraceptive diaphragm, All Flex Ortho Pharmaceutical Raritan, NJ	Yes‡	1.5	138
Contraceptive diaphragm, flat spring Ortho Pharmaceutical	Yes‡	1.5	138
Contraceptive diaphragm, Koroflex Young Drug Products Piscataway, NJ	Yes‡	1.5	138
EEG electrodes, Pediatric E-5-GH (gold plated silver) Grass Company Quincy, MA	No	0.3	179
EEG electrodes, Adult E-6-GH (gold plated silver) Grass Company	No	0.3	179

TABLE 13–2. METALLIC IMPLANTS, MATERIALS, DEVICES, AND OBJECTS TESTED FOR MOVEMENT/DEFLECTION FORCES DURING EXPOSURE TO STATIC MAGNETIC FIELDS *Continued*

METALLIC IMPLANT, MATERIAL, DEVICE, OR OBJECT*	MOVEMENT/ DEFLECTION	HIGHEST FIELD STRENGTH† (T)	REFERENCE
Endotracheal tube with metal ring marker Trachmate	No	1.5	NA
Forceps (titanium)	No	1.39	154
Hakim valve and pump	No	1.39	154
Intraflex feeding tube, tungstun weight, plastic	No	1.5	NA
Intrauterine contraceptive device (IUD), Copper T Searle Pharmaceuticals Chicago, IL	No	1.5	180
Intrauterine contraceptive device, Lippes loop, plastic	No	1.5	NA
Intrauterine contraceptive device, Perigard Gyne Pharmaceuticals	No	1.5	NA
Mercury Duotube-feeding	No	1.5	NA
Mitek anchor	No	1.5	NA
Shunt valve, Holter type The Holter Company Bridgeport, PA	Yes‡	1.5	181
Shunt valve, Holter-Hausner type Holter-Hausner, Inc. Bridgeport, PA	No	1.5	181
Swan-Ganz thermodilution catheter American Edwards Laboratories Irvine, CA	No¶	1.5	127
Tantalum powder	No	1.39	154
Tissue expander with magnetic port McGhan Medical Corporation Santa Barbara, CA	Yes	1.5	130
Vascular marker, O ring washer (262 SS) PIC Design Middlebury, CT	Yes‡	1.5	NA
Vitallium implant	No	1.5	NA
Winged infusion set, MRI compatible E-Z-EM, Inc.	No	1.5	182

*Manufacturer information provided if known, with city and state given at first mention. SS = stainless steel; NA = not applicable. These implants, materials, devices, or objects were tested for ferromagnetism by F. Shellock or E. Kanal; however, the data have not been published. Methods for testing these implants, materials, devices, or objects are described in references 138 and 173.

†Highest field strength refers to the highest static magnetic field that was used for the evaluation of deflection force or movement of the various metallic implants, materials, devices, or objects tested.

‡Denotes the metallic implants, materials, devices, or objects that were considered to be safe for MR procedures despite being attracted by the static magnetic fields. For example, certain prosthetic heart valves were attracted by the static magnetic field but the deflection forces were considered to be less than the force exerted on the valves by the beating heart.

§These halo vests are known to have ferromagnetic components; however, the deflection force or amount of attraction was not determined. Refer to specific information on halo vests regarding additional details for these devices.

‖Ferromagnetic coils, filters, and stents typically become firmly incorporated into the vessel wall several weeks after placement, and, therefore, it is highly unlikely that they will be moved or dislodged by attraction to the static magnetic fields of an MR system. It is recommended that coils, filters, and stents marked as ‡‖ in the deflection column have a minimal 6-wk wait after placement to ensure firm implantation into vessel wall before an MR procedure.

¶Although there is no magnetic field deflection associated with the triple-lumen thermodilution Swan-Ganz catheter, there has been a report of a catheter "melting" in a patient. Therefore, this catheter is considered a relative contraindication for MR procedures.

cludes diagnostic assessment of the knee using an MR procedure.

OTOLOGIC IMPLANTS. The cochlear implants evaluated for ferromagnetism are considered to be contraindicated for patients referred for MR procedures. Besides being attracted by static magnetic fields, these implants are also electronically or magnetically activated. Only one of the remaining tested otologic implants has associated deflection forces. This implant, the McGee stapedectomy piston prosthesis composed of platinum and $^{17}Cr-^4Ni$ stainless steel, was made on a limited basis during mid-1987 and was recalled by the manufacturer. Patients with this otologic implant were issued warning cards that instructed them to not be examined by MR procedures because of the possibility of moving or dislodging the stapedectomy piston prosthesis, which would require surgery to reposition it.

PELLETS, BULLETS, AND SHRAPNEL. Most of the pellets and bullets previously tested for ferromagnetism are composed of nonferromagnetic materials.[143, 145] Ammunition found to be ferromagnetic typically came from foreign countries or was used by the military. Pellets, bullets, and shrapnel may be contaminated with ferromagnetic materials; these objects represent relative contraindications for MR procedures. Patients with these foreign bodies should be evaluated on an individual basis with respect to whether the object is positioned near a vital neural, vascular, or soft tissue structure. This may be assessed by taking a careful history and using plain film radiography to determine the location of the foreign body so that a decision can be made about the safety of an MR procedure.

PENILE IMPLANTS AND ARTIFICIAL SPHINCTERS. One of the penile implants tested for ferromagnetism displayed significant deflection forces. Although it is unlikely that this implant, the Dacomed Omniphase, would cause serious injury to a patient undergoing an MR procedure, it would undoubtedly be uncomfortable for the patient. Artificial sphincters that have been tested are made from nonferromagnetic materials. However, at least one artificial sphincter undergoing clinical trials has a magnetic component and, therefore, patients with this device should not undergo an MR procedure.

VASCULAR ACCESS PORTS. Of the various vascular access ports tested for ferromagnetism, two showed measurable deflection forces, but the forces were believed to be insignificant relative to the in vivo application of these implants.[142] Therefore, it is considered safe to perform an MR procedure on a patient who may have one of these previously tested vascular access ports. The exception to this is any vascular access port that is programmable or electronically activated.

MISCELLANEOUS. Various types of other metallic implants, materials, objects, devices, and foreign bodies have also been tested for ferromagnetism. Of these, the cerebral ventricular shunt tube connector (type unknown) and tissue expander that is magnetically activated exhibited deflection forces that may pose a risk to patients during MR procedures. An O ring washer used as a vascular marker also showed ferromagnetism, but the deflection force was determined to be minimal relative to the in vivo use of this device.

Each of the contraceptive diaphragms tested for ferromagnetism displayed significant deflection forces. However, we have performed MR procedures on patients with these devices who did not complain of any sensation related to movement of these objects. Therefore, scanning patients with diaphragms is not believed to be considered to be physically hazardous to patients.

According to the information on policies, guidelines, and recommendations for MR safety and management of patients issued by the Society for Magnetic Resonance Imaging Safety Committee,[120] patients with electrically, magnetically, or mechanically activated or electrically conductive devices should be excluded from MR procedures unless the particular device has been previously shown (usually by ex vivo testing procedures) to be unaffected by the electromagnetic fields used for MR procedures and there is no possibility of injuring the patient or damaging the implant or device.

During the screening process for MR procedures, patients with these objects should be identified before their examination and before being exposed to the electromagnetic fields used for this imaging technique. Patients who have untested objects should not be allowed to undergo MR procedures.

SCREENING PATIENTS WITH METALLIC FOREIGN BODIES

Patients may present for MR procedures with a history of metallic foreign bodies such as slivers, bullets, shrapnel, or other types of metallic fragments. The relative risk of scanning these patients is dependent on the ferromagnetic properties of the object, the geometry and dimensions of the object, and the strength of the static and gradient magnetic fields of the MR system. Also important is the strength with which the object is fixed within the tissue and whether it is positioned in or adjacent to a potentially hazardous site of the body such as a vital neural, vascular, or soft tissue structure.[98]

A patient who encounters the static magnetic field of an MR system with an intraocular metallic foreign body is at a particular risk for significant eye injury. The single reported case of a patient who experienced a vitreous hemorrhage resulting in blindness underwent an MR procedure with a 0.35-T scanner and had an occult intraocular metal fragment that was 2.0 × 3.5 mm dislodge during the procedure.[183] This incident emphasizes the importance of adequately screening patients with suspected intraocular metallic foreign bodies before MR procedures.

Research has demonstrated that intraocular metallic fragments as small as 0.1 × 0.1 × 0.1 mm are detected by using standard plain film radiographs.[184] Although thin slice (i.e., ≤3 mm) computed tomography has been demonstrated to detect metallic foreign bodies as small as approximately 0.15 mm, it is unlikely that a metallic fragment of this size would be dislodged during an MR procedure, even with a static magnetic field up to 2.0 T.[184] Metallic fragments of various sizes and dimensions ranging from 0.1 × 0.1 × 0.1 mm to 3.0 × 1.0 × 1.0 mm have been examined to determine if they were moved or dislodged from the eyes of laboratory animals during exposure to a 2.0-T MR system.[184] Only the largest fragment (3.0 × 1.0 × 1.0 mm) rotated, but it did not cause any discernable damage to the ocular tissue.[184] Therefore, the use of plain film radiography may be an acceptable technique for identifying or excluding an intraocular metallic foreign body that represents a potential hazard to the patient undergoing an MR procedure.[120]

Patients suspected of having an intraocular metallic foreign body (e.g., a metal worker exposed to metallic slivers with a history of an eye injury) should have plain film radiographs of the orbits to rule out the presence of a metallic fragment before exposure to the static magnetic field. If a patient with a suspected ferromagnetic intraocular foreign body has no symptoms and a plain film series of the orbits does not demonstrate a radiopaque foreign body, the risk of performing an MR procedure is minimal.[120]

Each MR facility should establish a standardized policy for screening patients with suspected foreign bodies. The policy should include guidelines as to which patients require work-up by radiographic procedures and the specific procedure to be performed (e.g., number and type of views, position of the anatomy), and each case should be considered on an individual basis. These precautions should be taken with regard to patients referred for MR procedures in any type of system regardless of the field strength, the magnet type, and the presence or absence of magnetic shielding.[120]

MR PROCEDURES DURING PREGNANCY

Although an MR procedure is not believed to be hazardous to the fetus, only a few investigations have examined its teratogenic potential. By comparison, thousands of studies have been performed to examine the possible hazards of ultrasound during pregnancy, and controversy still exists concerning the safe use of this nonionizing radiation imaging technique.

Most of the earliest studies conducted to determine possible unwanted bioeffects during pregnancy showed negative results.[17, 22, 26, 31, 41, 47, 82] More recently, one study examined the effects of an MR procedure on mice exposed during midgestation.[22] No gross embryotoxic effects were observed, but there was a reduction in crown-rump length.[22] In another study performed by Tyndall and Sulik,[74] exposure to the electromagnetic fields used for a simulated clinical MR procedure caused eye malformations in a genetically prone mouse strain.

A variety of mechanisms exist that could produce deleterious bioeffects with respect to the developing fetus and the use of electromagnetic fields during MR procedures.* In addition, it is well known that cells undergoing division, as in the case of the developing fetus during the first trimester, are highly susceptible to damage from different types of physical agents. Therefore, because of the few data available at the present time, a cautionary approach is recommended for the use of MR procedures in pregnant patients.

According to the Safety Committee of the Society for Magnetic Resonance Imaging[120] (this information has also been adopted by the American College of Radiology), MR procedures are indicated for use in pregnant women if other nonionizing forms of diagnostic imaging are inadequate or if the examination provides important information that would otherwise require exposure to ionizing radiation. Pregnant patients should be informed that there has been no indication that the use of MR procedures during pregnancy has produced deleterious effects. However, as noted by the FDA, the safety of MR procedures during pregnancy has not been proved.[107]

Patients who are pregnant or suspect they are pregnant must be identified before undergoing MR procedures to assess the risks versus the benefits of the examination. Because there is a high spontaneous abortion rate in the general population during the first trimester of pregnancy (i.e., >30%), particular care should be exercised with the use of MR procedures during the first trimester because of associated potential medicolegal implications related to spontaneous abortions.

MR PROCEDURES AND CLAUSTROPHOBIA, ANXIETY, AND PANIC DISORDERS

Claustrophobia and a variety of other psychologic reactions, including anxiety and panic disorders, may be encountered by as many as 5% to 10% of patients undergoing MR procedures. These sensations originate from several factors, including the restrictive dimensions of the interior of the scanner, the duration of the examination, the gradient-induced noises, the ambient conditions within the bore of the scanner, and so on.[185–193]

Fortunately, adverse psychologic responses to MR procedures are usually transient. However, two patients with no prior history of claustrophobia have been reported who tolerated MR procedures with great difficulty and had persistent claustrophobia that required long-term psychiatric treatment.[186] Because adverse psychologic responses to MR procedures typically delay or require cancellation of the examination, several techniques have been developed and may be used to avert these problems[120, 185–193]:

1. Brief the patient concerning the specific aspects of the MR procedure, including the level of gradient-induced noise to expect, the internal dimensions of the scanner, and the length of the examination.
2. Allow an appropriately screened relative or friend to remain with the patient during the examination.
3. Use headphones with calming music to decrease the acoustic noise created by the gradient coils and to serve as a distraction.
4. Maintain physical or verbal contact with the patient throughout the examination.
5. Place the patient in a prone position with the chin supported by a pillow. In this position, the patient is able to visualize the opening of the bore and thus alleviate the closed-in feeling. An alternative method to reduce claustrophobia is to place the subject feet-first instead of head-first into the MR system.

---

*References 86, 88, 89, 102, 108, 109, 118.

6. Use MR system–mounted mirrors. Mirror or prism glasses within the scanner allow the patient to see out of the system.

7. Use a large light at either end of the scanner to decrease the anxiety of being in a long dark enclosure.

8. Use a blindfold on the patient so that he or she is unaware of the close surroundings.

9. Use relaxation techniques such as controlled breathing and mental imagery.[194] Also, several case reports have shown hypnotherapy to be successful in reducing MR-related claustrophobia and anxiety.

10. Use psychologic desensitization techniques before the procedure.

Several investigators have attempted to compare the effectiveness of some of the previously mentioned techniques in reducing MR-induced anxiety or claustrophobia.[187, 188, 191] One such study demonstrated that providing detailed information about the examination in addition to relaxation exercises successfully reduced the anxiety level of a group of patients both before and during MR procedures.

MONITORING PHYSIOLOGIC PARAMETERS DURING MR PROCEDURES

Because the typical MR system is constructed so that the patient is placed inside a cylindrical structure, routine observations and monitoring of vital signs are not trivial tasks. Conventional monitoring equipment was not designed to operate in the MR environment where static, gradient, and RF electromagnetic fields can adversely affect the operation of these devices. Fortunately, MR-compatible monitors have been developed and are commonly used in inpatient and outpatient MR sites.[195–203]

Physiologic monitoring is required for the safe use of MR procedures in patients who are sedated, anesthetized, comatose, critically ill, or unable to communicate with the system operator. All of these categories of patients should be routinely monitored during MR procedures and, considering the current availability of MR-compatible monitors, there is no reason to exclude these types of patients from MR procedures. Every physiologic parameter that can be obtained under normal circumstances in the intensive care unit or operating room can be monitored during MR procedures, including heart rate, systemic blood pressure, intracardiac pressure, end-tidal carbon dioxide, oxygen saturation, respiratory rate, skin blood flow, and temperature.[196–203] Table 13–3 lists examples of MR-compatible monitors that have been successfully tested and operated at field strengths of up to 1.5 T. In addition, there are now MR-compatible ventilators for patients who require ventilatory support.

Monitors that contain ferromagnetic components (e.g., transformers or outer casings) can be strongly attracted by mid- and high-field MR systems, posing a serious hazard to patients and possible damage to the

TABLE 13–3. EXAMPLES OF MR-COMPATIBLE MONITORS*

DEVICE AND MANUFACTURER	MONITORING FUNCTION	DEVICE AND MANUFACTURER	MONITORING FUNCTION
MR-Compatible Pulse Oximeter Invivo Research, Inc. Orlando, FL	Oxygen saturation, heart rate	Laserflow Blood Perfusion Monitor Vasomed, Inc. St. Paul, MN	Cutaneous blood flow
MRI Fiber-optic Pulse Oximeter Nonin Medical Inc. Plymouth, MN	Oxygen saturation, heart rate	Medpacific LD 5000 Laser-Doppler Perfusion Monitor Medpacific Corporation Seattle, WA	Cutaneous blood flow
MR-Compatible Pulse Oximeter Patient Monitoring System Magnetic Resonance Equipment Corporation Bay Shore, NY	Oxygen saturation, heart rate	Respiratory Rate Monitor, Models 515 and 525 Biochem International Waukesha, WI	Respiratory rate, apnea
Omega 1400 Invivo Research, Inc. Orlando, FL	Blood pressure, heart rate	MicroSpan Capnometer 8800 Biochem International Waukesha, WI	Respiratory rate, end-tidal carbon dioxide, apnea
Omni-Trak 3100 MRI Vital Signs Monitor Invivo Research, Inc. Orlando, FL	Heart rate, ECG, oxygen saturation, respiratory rate, gas exchange, blood pressure	Aneuroid Chest Bellows Coulborun Instruments Allentown, Pennsylvania	Respiratory rate
MR Equipment Vital Signs Monitor† Model 6500 Bay Shore, NY	Heart rate, ECG, oxygen saturation, respiratory rate, gas exchange, blood pressure	Fluoroptic Thermometry System, Model 3000 Luxtron Santa Clara, CA	Temperature

*Note that these devices may require modifications to make them MR-compatible, and none of them should be positioned closer than 8 feet from the entrance of the bore of a 1.5-T MR system. Also, monitors with metallic cables, leads, probes, or other similar interfaces with patients may cause mild to moderate imaging artifacts if placed near the imaging area of interest. Consult manufacturers to determine additional information related to compatibility with specific MR systems.
†This multiparameter monitoring device has not received FDA recognition as of August 1994.

systems. Because the intensity of standard static magnetic field falls off as the third power of the distance from the magnet, simply placing the monitor a suitable distance from the system is sufficient to protect the operation of the device and to help prevent it from becoming a potential projectile.[200, 203] If monitoring equipment is not placed in a permanently fixed position, instructions should be given to all appropriate personnel regarding the hazards of moving this equipment too close to the MR system.[200, 203]

In addition to being influenced by the static magnetic field, monitors may be adversely affected by electromagnetic interference from the gradient and RF pulses from the MR system.[200, 203] In these instances, increasing the length of the patient-monitor interface and positioning the equipment outside the RF-shielded room (e.g., the control room) will enable the monitor to operate properly. It is usually necessary to position all monitors with cathode-ray tubes at a location in the magnetic fringe field such that the display is not "bent" or distorted.

Certain monitors emit spurious electromagnetic noise that can result in moderate to severe imaging artifacts.[200, 203] These monitors can be modified to work during MR procedures by adding RF-shielded cables, using fiberoptic transmission of the signals (which is becoming increasingly the method of choice in the MR procedure environment), or using special outer casing. Also, special filters may be added to the monitor to inhibit electromagnetic noise.

Of further concern is the fact that some monitoring equipment can be potentially harmful to patients if special precautions are not followed.[200, 203–206] A primary source of adverse MR system and physiologic monitor interactions has been the interface that is used between the patient and the equipment because this usually requires a conductive cable or other device. The presence of a conductive material in the immediate MR system area is a safety concern because of the potential for monitor-related burns. For example, there has been a report of an accident involving an anesthetized patient who sustained a third-degree burn of the finger associated with using a pulse oximeter during an MR procedure.[205] Investigation of this incident revealed that the cable leading from the pulse oximeter to the finger probe may have been looped during the procedure and the gradient or RF magnetic fields induced sufficient current to heat the finger probe excessively, resulting in the burn.[205] This problem may also occur with the use of ECG lead wires or any other cable that may be looped or form a conductive loop that contacts the patient.

Therefore, the following procedures are recommended to prevent potential monitor-related accidents from occurring:

1. Monitoring equipment should be used only by trained personnel.

2. All cables and lead wires from monitoring devices that come into contact with the patient (e.g., the monitor-patient interface) should be positioned so that no conductive loops are formed.

3. Monitoring devices that do not appear to operate properly during the procedure should be immediately removed from the patient and the magnetic environment.

The following is a brief description of some of the techniques of monitoring various physiologic parameters.

MONITORING BLOOD PRESSURE. Noninvasive blood pressure monitors typically use the oscillometric technique for measuring blood pressure with a pressure transducer connected to a pressure cuff by a pneumatically filled hose. Certain monitors (e.g., Omega 1400, Invivo Research Laboratories, Orlando, FL) have adjustable audible and visual alarms as well as a strip-chart recorder.

Occasionally, the cuff inflation tends to disturb lightly sedated patients, especially pediatric patients, which may cause them to move and may result in distorted MR images. For this reason, the noninvasive blood pressure monitor may not be the optimal instrument for obtaining vital signs in all patients. Direct pressure monitoring of systemic or intracardiac pressures, if necessary, can be accomplished by using a fiberoptic pressure transducer made entirely of plastic.

MONITORING RESPIRATORY RATE, OXYGENATION, AND GAS EXCHANGE. Monitoring of respiratory parameters of sedated or anesthetized patients during MR procedures is particularly important because the medications used for these procedures may produce complications of respiratory depression. Therefore, as a standard of care, a pulse oximeter, capnograph, or capnometer should always be used to monitor patients who are sedated or anesthetized during MR procedures.

The respiratory monitors used successfully on sedated pediatric or adult patients (e.g., model 515 Respiration Monitor and model 8800 Capnometer, Biochem International, Waukesha, WI) are relatively inexpensive and can be modified for use during MR procedures by simply lengthening the plastic tubing interface to the patient so that the monitors can be placed at least 8 feet from the unshielded MR system.

Pulse oximeters are used to record oxygen saturation and heart rate. Commercially available, modified pulse oximeters using hard wire cables have been previously used to monitor sedated and anesthetized patients during the procedure and the recovery period with moderate success. These pulse oximeters tend to work intermittently during MR procedures, owing to interference from the gradient or RF electromagnetic fields. In certain instances, patients have been burned, presumably as a result of excessive current being induced in inappropriately looped conductive cables attached to the probes of the pulse oximeters.[204–206]

Newly developed portable fiberoptic pulse oximeters are available for use during MR procedures[207] (see Table 13–3). Using fiberoptic technology to obtain and transmit physiologic signals from patients undergoing MR procedures has been demonstrated to be a technique that does not have any associated MR-related electromagnetic interference. It is physically impossible for a patient to be burned when this fiberoptic monitor is used during an MR procedure because there are no conductive pathways formed by any metallic materials.

MONITORING CUTANEOUS BLOOD FLOW. Cutaneous blood flow can be monitored during MR procedures by means of the laser Doppler velocimetry technique. This noninvasive measurement technique uses laser light that is delivered to and detected from the region of interest by flexible, graded-index fiberoptic light wires. The Doppler broadening of laser light scattered by moving red blood cells within the tissue is analyzed in real time by an analog processor that indicates instantaneous blood velocity and the effective blood volume and flow. A small circular probe can be attached to any available skin surface of the patient. Areas with a relatively high cutaneous blood flow (e.g., hand, finger, foot, toe, or ear) yield the best results.

Tracings obtained by laser Doppler velocimetry can be used to determine the patient's heart rate, respiratory rate, and cutaneous blood flow. An audible signal may be activated to permit the operator to hear blood flow changes during monitoring. This technique of continuous physiologic monitoring is particularly useful when there is concern about disturbing a sedated patient because it is easily tolerated.

MONITORING HEART RATE. Monitoring the ECG during an MR procedure is typically required for cardiac imaging, for gating to reduce imaging artifacts from the physiologic motion of cerebrospinal fluid in the brain and spine, and for determining the patient's heart rate. Artifacts caused by the static, gradient, and RF electromagnetic fields may severely distort the ECG, making determination of cardiac rhythm during a procedure extremely difficult and unreliable. Although sophisticated filtering techniques can be used to attenuate the artifacts from the gradient and RF fields, the static magnetic field produces an augmentation of the T wave and other nonspecific waveform changes that are in direct proportion to the strength of the field, which cannot be easily counterbalanced.

In some instances, static magnetic field–induced augmented T waves have a higher amplitude than the R waves, resulting in false triggering and an inaccurate determination of the beats per minute. ECG artifacts can be minimized during MR procedures by using special filters, using ECG electrodes with minimal metal, selecting lead wires with minimal metal, twisting or braiding the lead wires, and using special lead placements.[202]

The previously mentioned pulse oximeters may also be used to accurately record heart rate during MR procedures. These devices have probes that may be attached to the finger, toe, or earlobe of the patient.

SAFETY CONSIDERATIONS OF CONTRAST AGENTS

Although the first intravenous MR contrast agent was introduced into the clinical arena only in mid-1988, there are now three different contrast agents available. Throughout the United States, roughly one third of all MR procedures require use of contrast agents. Therefore, it is important to be familiar with the safety aspects of using these medications that are so ubiquitous in the clinical MR environment.[208–210]

The three MR contrast agents approved for intravenous administration by the FDA are gadolinium diethylenetriaminepentaacetic acid (Gd-DTPA, gadopentetate dimeglumine injection; Magnevist, Berlex Laboratories, Wayne, NJ), gadodiamide injection (Omniscan, Nycomed Salutar, Oslo, Norway), and gadoteridol injection (ProHance, Bracco, Princeton, NJ). In addition, another agent approved internationally is gadoterate meglumine (Gd-DOTA; Dotarem, Guebet Laboratories, Aulnay-sous-Bois, France).

All of these contrast agents are based on the element gadolinium and have similar mechanisms of action, biodistribution, and half-lives.[209–212] Drug equilibration and physiologic biodistribution for each of the agents are in the extracellular fluid space, with biologic elimination half-lives of roughly 1.5 hours.[209]

Gadolinium-based MR contrast agents are paramagnetic substances and therefore develop a magnetic moment when placed in a magnetic field. The relatively large magnetic moment produced by a paramagnetic agent results in a relatively large local magnetic field that can enhance the relaxation rates of water protons in the vicinity of the contrast agent. When placed in a magnetic field, gadolinium-based contrast agents decrease the T1 and T2 relaxation times in tissues where they accumulate (although the T1 relaxation time is affected mainly at the dosages used in the clinical setting), with the purpose of improving image contrast between two adjacent tissue compartments, thus showing a more conspicuous abnormality, if one exists.[209]

Free gadolinium ion is toxic, with a markedly prolonged biologic half-life of several weeks. The predominant uptake and excretion of gadolinium are by the kidneys and liver. However, gadolinium ion is chelated to another structure that restricts the ion, which markedly decreases its toxicity and alters its pharmacokinetics.[209] In fact, this chelation also decreases the ability of the gadolinium ion to accomplish its task of T1 shortening. The science of MR contrast agent design and development is often a tricky act of decreasing toxicity while not overly decreasing the T1 relaxivity.

As noted earlier, the chelating process also alters the pharmacokinetics of the agent. For example, chelating the gadolinium ions allows for approximately a 500-fold increase in the rate of renal excretion of the substance.[211–214] In each case, the chelating substance is what makes these various contrast agents differ from one another.

In the case of Magnevist, the chelating agent is the DTPA molecule. In the case of Omniscan it is DTPA-bis(methylamide) (DTPA-BMA), and in the case of ProHance it is the HP-DO$_3$A molecule. Magnevist has a linear structure and is an ionic compound; Omniscan has a linear structure and is nonionic; ProHance is also nonionic and possesses a macrocyclic ring structure.

Despite the marked differences in these chelating molecules, their ionic versus nonionic nature, and their linear versus ring-like molecular structure, these agents appear to have remarkably similar effectiveness and safety profiles. Some differences exist, both theoretically as well as on paper, and it is these differences on which we will elaborate.

Multiple studies have documented the high safety index of the contrast agents used in MR procedures, especially when compared with iodinated contrast media used for computed tomography.[210, 215–231] However, from a safety standpoint, it is inappropriate to compare ionic and nonionic MR contrast agents to ionic and nonionic contrast agents used in computed tomography because of the drastically different osmotic loads associated with each of these drugs.

The LD_{50} (i.e., the 50% lethal dose—the term used to denote the dose of an agent that, when administered to test animals, results in rapid death of half of the population of the recipients) of these agents, as studied in rodents, is quite high: it is the highest for Omniscan (>30 mmol/kg), next highest for ProHance (12 mmol/kg), and lowest for Magnevist (6 to 7 mmol/kg). In all cases, the LD_{50} is generally in excess of about 300, 120, and 60 times the typical diagnostic dose of 0.1 mmol/kg.[209, 232] Data also suggest that there are fewer acute cardiodepressive effects from the nonionic drugs (specifically, ProHance was used in one study) than from the ionic agent, Magnevist, when injected rapidly and into a central vein.[233] This may have limited clinical applicability, however, because contrast agents used in MR procedures are typically injected into peripheral veins, with only small total volumes being administered.[209]

ADVERSE EVENTS RELATED TO THE USE OF CONTRAST AGENTS

The frequency of adverse reactions of all types for each of the contrast agents used in MR procedures ranges from 2% to 4%.[210, 225, 234] The most common reactions are nausea, emesis, hives, headaches, and local injection site symptoms, such as irritation, focal burning, or a cool sensation. With the use of Magnevist, transient elevations have also been reported in serum bilirubin (3% to 4% of patients), and with both Magnevist and Omniscan a transient elevation in iron (15% to 30% of patients); these elevations seem to reverse spontaneously within 24 to 48 hours.[210, 235] No such alterations in blood chemistry have been reported with the use of ProHance. Of special note is that there are no known contraindications for Magnevist, Omniscan, and ProHance.

The MR contrast agent that has had FDA approval the longest, and therefore the one for which there is the most clinical experience and information, is Magnevist. There have been approximately 5.7 million doses administered worldwide since its approval in June 1988. This compares with approximately 150,000 total administered doses for ProHance since its FDA approval in November 1992 and approximately 100,000

doses for Omniscan since its FDA approval in January 1993. There have been rare reported incidents of laryngospasm and anaphylactoid reactions (requiring interventional therapy with epinephrine) associated with the administration of each of these agents (Reich L, personal communication, 1993).[234–243]

It may well be advisable to continue a prolonged observation period of all patients with a history of allergy or drug reaction. As stated in the package insert for Magnevist, for example: "The possibility of a reaction, including serious, fatal, anaphylactoid, or cardiovascular reactions or other idiosyncratic reactions should always be considered especially in those with a known clinical history of asthma or other allergic respiratory disorders."

Delayed reactions of hypertension, vasovagal responses, and syncope have also been reported with the use of MR contrast agents. Accordingly, the product inserts for these drugs advise that all patients should be observed for several hours after drug administration.

SPECIFIC ADVERSE EVENTS. The specific adverse events associated with the use of MR contrast agents vary to a minor degree.[234–248] The vast majority of these adverse events occur at a frequency of less than 1%. An anaphylactoid reaction is one that involves respiratory, cardiovascular, and cutaneous (and possibly gastrointestinal or genitourinary) manifestations.[244] This is not to say that all events that have such symptoms are by definition anaphylactoid. However, it becomes more difficult to make the diagnosis of anaphylaxis in the absence of such symptoms, especially the classic triad of upper airway obstructive symptoms, decreased blood pressure (or other similar severe cardiovascular symptoms), and cutaneous manifestations, such as urticaria.

As defined by the FDA, a "serious reaction" is one in which an adverse experience from a drug proves fatal or life threatening, is permanently disabling, requires inpatient hospitalization, or is an overdose (FDA docket 85D-0249). A life-threatening reaction in FDA terminology is one in which the initial reporter (i.e., the individual initially reporting the incident) believes that the patient was at immediate risk of death from the event. In consideration of this information, one may now understand how the interpretation of an adverse event may differ from that designated by the FDA.

Magnevist. As of June 1993, there have been 13 anaphylactoid reactions with Magnevist, for an estimated anaphylactoid reaction rate of 1:450,000 (Gifford L, personal communication, 1993). One of the patients who had an anaphylactoid reaction died, and another patient suffered brain damage (at the time of this writing the patient is still in a coma) subsequent to administration of this agent. In each case, there was a history of respiratory difficulty or allergic respiratory problem, such as asthma. The current package insert for Magnevist warns that caution should be exercised when administering this contrast agent to patients with known allergic respiratory disease.

The total reported frequency of adverse reactions to Magnevist of any kind is 2.4%, based on a retrospective review of 15,496 patients (Gifford L, personal communication, 1993). Of these cases, only two reactions were labeled serious by FDA standards. In one of these cases, one patient being evaluated for metastatic disease died of herniation from an intracranial tumor within 24 hours of the contrast-enhanced MR study. Because of the design of the present review process, this temporal association is sufficient to have the case reported as "associated" with Magnevist administration, regardless of any perceived, or real, causal relationship. The second serious reaction in this series of patients occurred in a patient who was undergoing evaluation for vertigo and had an acute progression of vertigo after administration of Magnevist. Seizures occurring after administration of this drug have been reported.[248] In at least one case, Magnevist injection was believed to induce a seizure in a patient with a history of grand mal seizures (see product insert information for Magnevist).

Mild elevations in serum chemistry assay results are associated with the use of Magnevist, which suggests that there may be a component of mild hemolysis in some unknown manner associated with the use of this drug. However, this association is not definite and there is no evidence demonstrating increased hemolysis as a result of Magnevist being administered to patients with hemolytic anemias.

On the package insert, the FDA has stated concern regarding the use of Magnevist, as well as the other gadolinium-based agents, in patients with sickle cell anemia. The enhancement of magnetic moment by Magnevist, Omniscan, or ProHance may potentiate sickle erythrocyte alignment. This information was based on in vitro studies that showed that deoxygenated sickle erythrocytes align perpendicularly to a magnetic field and, therefore, vaso-occlusive complications may result in vivo. However, there have been no studies performed to assess the effect of the use of these MR contrast agents in patients with sickle cell anemia and other forms of hemoglobinopathies. In addition, there has been no report of sickle crisis precipitated by the administration of any of these drugs.

Of the three MR contrast agents, Magnevist has the highest osmolality, measuring 1960 mmol/kg, or roughly six to seven times that of plasma (approximately 285 mmol/kg).[249] Doses greater than or equal to double that used in the United States (i.e., doses of up to 0.5 mmol/kg) have already been investigated in the clinical setting[235, 250–252] and have been used for some time in Europe, with no apparent significant deleterious effects.[253]

Of note is that because the osmolality of Magnevist is approximately six to seven times the osmolality of plasma, one might expect local irritative reactions as a possible adverse response with the use of this relatively hyperosmolar substance. Indeed, there has been at least one incident of possible phlebitis requiring hospitalization that was related temporally to the administration of an intravenous dose of Magnevist (LaFlore J, personal communication, 1990). The mechanisms behind this are still unclear, although objective studies have demonstrated that tissue sloughing can occur as a result of extravasation of Gd-DTPA.[245, 246]

There have also been several cases of erythema, swelling, and pain localized to the site of administration and proximally that were of delayed onset, usually appearing between 1 and 4 days after intravenous administration of Gd-DTPA. This typically progressed for several days, plateaued, and then resolved over several more days.[247] Nevertheless, severe adverse local reactions to even considerable quantities (>10 mL) of Magnevist extravasation seem to be quite rare at best.

Interestingly, Magnevist is the only one of the three MR contrast agents approved in the United States that has a package insert that recommends a slow intravenous administration at a rate not to exceed 10 mL/min. The FDA has approved rapid bolus intravenous administration of Omniscan and ProHance. Nevertheless, studies have been performed with rapid intravenous administration of Magnevist and have indicated that there was no significant difference in the incidence of adverse effects compared with the slow intravenous administration of this drug.[223, 235, 247]

Omniscan. Omniscan is the most recently FDA-approved MR contrast agent, and there are relatively few data available related to the safety aspects of this drug. Of the estimated 100,000 doses that have been distributed, there have been 28 reports of adverse reactions of any type, of which 20 were nausea and emesis. A single case of laryngospasm was successfully treated with epinephrine, and a single case has been reported of a patient who had a history of seizure disorder experiencing a seizure after receiving Omniscan. There have been no reports of hospitalizations or permanent disabilities related to the use of Omniscan (Reich L, personal communication, 1993).

Omniscan has an osmolality of 789 mmol/kg.[249] The manufacturer of Omniscan is in the process of applying for approval of higher total dose administration for specified entities where this might be of clinical significance and benefit (Reich L, personal communication, 1993).

ProHance. ProHance was approved for use 2 months before the release of Omniscan; therefore, there is also a relative lack of postmarket safety data concerning this agent. Of the estimated 150,000 doses administered, there have been no deaths associated with the use of ProHance. Ten anaphylactoid reactions have occurred, of which five required hospitalization or ended in permanent disabilities (Rogan R, personal communication, 1993).

At this time, ProHance is the only MR contrast agent with FDA approval to be administered for specific clinical indications up to a total dose of 0.3 mmol/kg, or a total of three times the "standard" dose for each of the other two FDA-approved MR contrast agents. The relatively low osmolality of ProHance (630 mmol/kg) may be one of the major factors that permits use of higher doses of this agent to be used without significant deleterious effects on the patient.[42] However, this is purely speculation. Here, too, total adverse effects of any type seem to be less than 4%, with nausea and taste disturbance each having a frequency of roughly

1.4% and all other adverse reactions being less than 1% each (Olukoton AY, Rogan R, personal communication, 1993).

The lower osmolality of ProHance compared with that of Magnevist was the subject of an investigation into the effect of extravasation of these agents in the rat model.[39] The findings indicated that extravasation of Magnevist was associated with more necrosis, hemorrhage, and edema compared with ProHance, although the authors of this report cautioned about extrapolating the results of their study to contrast agent extravasation in humans.

ADMINISTRATION OF MR CONTRAST AGENTS TO PATIENTS WITH RENAL FAILURE

As previously indicated, toxicity may result from the dissociation of the gadolinium ion from its chelate. After intravenous administration of gadolinium-based contrast agents, intravascular copper and zinc (normally found in small amounts within the blood stream), which have a competing affinity for the DTPA chelate, will displace some of the gadolinium from the chelating molecule, such as DTPA, which will be released as free gadolinium ion (Gd^{3+}). Although gadolinium is a highly toxic substance, the total concentration of the released free gadolinium is quite low and is cleared rapidly, allowing a low concentration of free ion to be maintained. In fact, in patients with normal renal function, the rate of dissociation is lower than that of clearance, thus preventing any accumulation phenomenon from occurring.[214] It is also believed that the macrocyclic molecules tend to bind the gadolinium more tightly than do the linear ones.[212, 254]

As new physiologic sources of copper and zinc ions are "leaked" into the intravascular space in an attempt to reestablish their concentration equilibrium, they also displace more gadolinium from its chelate. This cycle continues until all the gadolinium chelate is cleared from the body by glomerular filtration. For this reason, there is concern about the level of free gadolinium ion in cases of renal failure, as there is in patients with a decreased rate of renal clearance of all such substances from the body.

The safety of administering MR contrast agents to patients with impaired renal function, or even overt renal failure, has not been clearly established, although several studies suggest that they should be well tolerated.[219, 235, 255–259] There is a theoretic concern that decreasing the rate of clearance of the gadolinium chelate from the body might serve to increase the concentration of free gadolinium within the body, but data suggest that, for a given level of renal function, administration of lower volume doses may be safer than administering standard doses of iodine-based contrast agents to that same patient.[255] Similarly, the safety of administering one of the MR contrast agents to patients with elevated levels of copper (e.g., patients with Wilson's disease) or zinc has not been firmly established and will likely depend on factors such as the glomerular filtration rate and renal clearance rates,

as well as the blood copper levels, of those patients.[214] It has also been shown that Magnevist is dialyzable, with more than 95% of the administered dose being removed by the third dialysis treatment.[28, 52]

CHRONIC AND REPEATED ADMINISTRATION OF MR CONTRAST AGENTS

There is concern related to the total storage or accumulation of the MR contrast agents, or even free gadolinium ion, after multiple doses are administered throughout a patient's lifetime. The amount of detectable drug still in the liver, kidneys, and bone days after administration seems to be higher in the case of Omniscan than for Magnevist,[210] and these both seem to be higher than the level for ProHance.[212, 254] Currently, there are no data available regarding the safety of long-term cumulative exposure to low doses of free gadolinium ion. Therefore, there may be a clinical limitation regarding the number of times a patient is scanned safely with gadolinium-based contrast agents. As of now, however, this question remains unanswered and is a topic that warrants investigation.

USE OF MR CONTRAST AGENTS DURING PREGNANCY AND LACTATION

Magnevist has been shown to cross the placenta and appear within the fetal bladder only moments after intravenous administration. It is assumed that the other MR contrast agents behave in a similar fashion and cross the blood-placenta barrier easily. From the fetal bladder, these contrast agents would then be excreted into the amniotic fluid and subsequently swallowed by the fetus. This will then be filtered and excreted in the urine of the fetus, with the entire cycle being repeated innumerable times.

There are no data available to assess the rate of clearance of MR contrast agents from the amniotic fluid cycle. Therefore, we believe that there is no information to support the safety of the use of MR contrast agents in pregnant women. Our conservative approach is to recommend against the administration of any of the MR contrast agents to a pregnant patient until more data become available. Pregnant patients should receive these drugs only if the potential benefit justifies the potential risk to the fetus. In any case, should it be decided to administer such agents to pregnant patients to facilitate MR, the patient should be provided written informed consent that stipulates specifically that the risk associated with the use these drugs during pregnancy is unknown.

Magnevist has been shown to be excreted in low concentrations (i.e., 0.011% of the total dose) in human breast milk over approximately 33 hours.[260, 261] The concentration of this contrast agent in breast milk peaks at approximately 4.75 hours and decreases to less than a fifth of this level (down to less than 1 μmol/L) 22 hours after the injection.[260, 261] For this reason and as an extra precaution, we recommend that nursing mothers express their breasts and not breast feed their infants for 36 to 48 hours after the administration of an MR contrast agent to ensure that the nursing child does not receive the drug in any notable quantity by mouth. However, it should be noted that the LD_{50} of gadolinium chloride or gadolinium acetate (which easily release free gadolinium ions) when given intravenously is approximately 1000 times lower if taken orally because of the low absorption of gadolinium from the gastrointestinal tract.[262] This supports other data that have demonstrated that 99.2% of orally administered Magnevist was fecally excreted and not absorbed.[263]

REFERENCES

1. Adzamli IK, Jolesz FA, Blau M: An assessment of blood-brain barrier integrity under MRI conditions: brain uptake of radiolabeled Gd-DTPA and In-DTPA-IgG. J Nucl Med 30:839, 1989. Abstract.
2. Barber BJ, Schaefer DJ, Gordon CJ, et al: Thermal effects of MR imaging: worst-case studies in sheep. AJR 155:1105–1110, 1990.
3. Bartels MV, Mann K, Matejcek M, et al: Magnetresonanztomographie und Sicherheit: Elektroenzephalographische und neuropsychologische Befunde vor und nach MR-Untersuchungen des Gehirns. Fortschr Rontgenstr 145:383–385, 1986.
4. Besson J, Foreman EI, Eastwood LM, et al: Cognitive evaluation following NMR imaging of the brain. J Neurol Neurosurg Psychiatry 47:314–316, 1984.
5. Bore PJ, Galloway GJ, Styles P, et al: Are quenches dangerous? Magn Reson Imaging 3:112–117, 1986.
6. Bourland JD, Nyenhuis JA, Mouchawar GA, et al: Physiologic indicators of high MRI gradient-induced fields. In: Book of Abstracts. Berkeley, CA: Society of Magnetic Resonance in Medicine, 1990, p 1276.
7. Brody AS, Sorette MP, Gooding CA, et al: Induced alignment of flowing sickle erythrocytes in a magnetic field. A preliminary report. Invest Radiol 20:560–566, 1985.
8. Brody AS, Embury SH, Mentzer WC, et al: Preservation of sickle cell blood flow patterns during MR imaging. An in vivo study. AJR 151:139–141, 1988.
9. Brummett RE, Talbot JM, Charuhas P: Potential hearing loss resulting from MR imaging. Radiology 169:539–540, 1988.
10. Budinger TF, Fischer H, Hentschel D, et al: Physiological effects of fast oscillating magnetic field gradients. J Comput Assist Tomogr 15:909–914, 1991.
11. Carson JJL, Prato FS, Drost DJ, et al: Time-varying fields increase cytosolic free Ca^{2+} in HL-60 cells. Am J Physiol 259:C687–C692, 1990.
12. Cohen MS, Weisskoff R, Rzedzian R, et al: Sensory stimulation by time-varying magnetic fields. Magn Reson Med 14:409–414, 1990.
13. Cooke P, Morris PG: The effects of NMR exposure on living organisms. II. A genetic study of human lymphocytes. Br J Radiol 54:622–625, 1981.
14. Doherty JU, Whitman GJR, Robinson MD, et al: Changes in cardiac excitability and vulnerability in NMR fields. Invest Radiol 20:129–135, 1985.
15. Fischer H: Physiological effects of fast oscillating magnetic field gradients. Radiology 173(P):382, 1989. Abstract.
16. Garber HJ, Oldendorf WH, Braun LD, et al: MRI gradient fields increase brain mannitol space. Magn Reson Imaging 7:605–610, 1989.
17. Geard CR, Osmak RS, Hall EJ, et al: Magnetic resonance and ionizing radiation: a comparative evaluation in vitro of oncogenic and genotoxic potential. Radiology 152:199–202, 1984.
18. Gore JC, McDonnell MJ, Pennock JM: An assessment of the safety of rapidly changing magnetic fields in the rabbit: implications for NMR imaging. Magn Reson Imaging 1:191–195, 1982.
19. Gremmel H, Wendhausen H, Wunsch F: Biologische Effekte statischef Magnetfelder bei NMR-Tomographie am Menschen. Wiss. Radiologische Klinik, Christian-Albrechts-Universität, Kiel, Germany, 1983.
20. Gulch RW, Lutz O: Influence of strong static magnetic fields on heart muscle contraction. Phys Med Biol 31:763–769, 1986.
21. Hammer BE, Wadon S, Mirer SD, et al: In vivo measurement of RF heating in capuchin monkey brain. In: Book of Abstracts. Berkeley, CA: Society of Magnetic Resonance in Medicine, 1991, p 1278.
22. Heinrichs WL, Fong P, Flannery M, et al: Midgestational exposure of pregnant BALB/c mice to magnetic resonance imaging conditions. Magn Reson Imaging 6:305–313, 1988.
23. Hong CZ, Shellock FG: Short-term exposure to a 1.5 tesla static magnetic field does not affect somato-sensory–evoked potentials in man. Magn Reson Imaging 8:65–69, 1989.
24. Innis NK, Ossenkopp KP, Prato FS, et al: Behavioral effects of exposure to nuclear magnetic resonance imaging: II. Spatial memory tests. Magn Reson Imaging 4:281–284, 1986.
25. Jehenson P, Duboc D, Lavergne T, et al: Change in human cardiac rhythm by a 2-T static magnetic field. Radiology 166:227–230, 1988.
26. Kay HH, Herfkens RJ, Kay BK: Effect of magnetic resonance imaging on Xenopus laevis embryogenesis. Magn Reson Imaging 6:501–506, 1988.
27. Keltner JR, Roos MS, Brakeman PR, et al: Magnetohydrodynamics of blood flow. Magn Reson Med 16:139–149, 1990.
28. Kido DK, Morris TW, Erickson JL, et al: Physiologic changes during high field strength MR imaging. Am J Neuroradiol 8:263–266, 1987.
29. LaPorte R, Kus L, Wisniewski RA, et al: Magnetic resonance imaging (MRI) effects on rat pineal neuroendocrine function. Brain Res 506:294–296, 1990.
30. McRobbie D, Foster MA: Cardiac response to pulsed magnetic fields with regard to safety in NMR imaging. Phys Med Biol 30:695–702, 1985.
31. McRobbie D, Foster MA: Pulsed magnetic field exposure during pregnancy and implications for NMR foetal imaging: a study with mice. Magn Reson Imaging 3:231–234, 1985.
32. Messmer JM, Porter JH, Fatouros P, et al: Exposure to magnetic resonance imaging does not produce taste aversion in rats. Physiol Behav 40:259–261, 1987.
33. Montour JL, Fatouros PP, Prasad UR: Effect of MR imaging on spleen colony formation following gamma radiation. Radiology 168:259–260, 1988.
34. Muller S, Hotz M: Human brainstem auditory evoked potentials (BAEP) before and after MR examinations. Magn Reson Med 16:476–480, 1990.
35. Niemann G, Schroth G, Klose U, et al: Influence of magnetic resonance imaging on somatosensory potential in man. J Neurol 235:462–465, 1988.
36. Ngo FQH, Blue JW, Roberts WK: The effects of a static magnetic field on DNA synthesis and survival of mammalian cells irradiated with fast neutrons. Magn Reson Med 5:307–317, 1987.
37. Osbakken M, Griffith J, Taczanowsky P: A gross morphologic, histologic, hematologic, and blood chemistry study of adult and neonatal mice chronically exposed to high magnetic fields. Magn Reson Med 3:502–517, 1986.
38. Ossenkopp KP, Kavaliers M, Prato FS, et al: Exposure to nuclear magnetic imaging procedure attenuates morphine-induced analgesia in mice. Life Sci 37:1507–1514, 1985.
39. Ossenkopp KP, Innis NK, Prato FS, et al: Behavioral effects of exposure to nuclear magnetic resonance imaging: I. Open-field behavior and passive avoidance learning in rats. Magn Reson Imaged 4:275–280, 1986.
40. Papatheofanis FJ, Papatheofanis BJ: Short-term effect of exposure to intense magnetic fields on hematologic indices of bone metabolism. Invest Radiol 24:221–223, 1989.
41. Peeling J, Lewis JS, Samoiloff MR, et al: Biological effects of magnetic fields on the nematode Panagrellus redivivus. Magn Reson Imaging 6:655–660, 1988.
42. Prasad N, Kosnik LT, Taber KH, et al: Delayed tumor onset following MR imaging exposure. In: Book of Abstracts. Berkeley, CA: Society of Magnetic Resonance in Medicine, 1990, p 275.
43. Prasad N, Prasad R, Bushong SC, et al: Effects of 4.5 T MRI exposure on mouse testes and epididymes. In: Book of Abstracts. Berkeley, CA: Society of Magnetic Resonance in Medicine, 1990, p 606.
44. Prasad N, Bushong SC, Thornby JI, et al: Effect of nuclear resonance on chromosomes of mouse bone marrow cells. Magn Reson Imaging 2:37–39, 1984.
45. Prasad N, Lotzova E, Thornby JI, et al: Effects of MR imaging on murine natural killer cell cytotoxicity. AJR 148:415–417, 1987.
46. Prasad N, Lotzova E, Thornby JI, et al: The effect of 2.35-T MR imaging on natural killer cell cytotoxicity with and without interleukin-2. Radiology 175:251–263, 1990.
47. Prasad N, Wright DA, Ford JJ, et al: Safety of 4-T MR imaging: a study of effects of developing frog embryos. Radiology 174:251–253, 1990.
48. Prasad N, Wright DA, Forster JD: Effect of nuclear magnetic resonance on early stages of amphibian development. Magn Reson Imaging 1:35–38, 1982.
49. Prato FS, Ossenkopp KP, Kavaliers M, et al: Attenuation of morphine-induced analgesia in mice by exposure to magnetic resonance imaging: separate effects of the static, radiofrequency and time-varying magnetic fields. Magn Reson Imaging 5:9–14, 1987.
50. Redington RW, Dumoulin CL, Schenck JL, et al: MR imaging and bioeffects in a whole body 4.0 Tesla imaging system. In: Book of Abstracts. Berkeley, CA: Society of Magnetic Resonance Imaging, 1988, p 20.
51. Reid A, Smith FW, Hutchison JMS: Nuclear magnetic resonance imaging and its safety implications: follow-up of 181 patients. Br J Radiol 55:784–786, 1982.
52. Roschmann P: Human auditory system response to pulsed radiofrequency energy in RF coils for magnetic resonance at 2.4 to 170 MHz. Magn Reson Med 21:197–215, 1991.
53. Sacks E, Worgul BV, Merriam GR, et al: The effects of nuclear magnetic resonance imaging on ocular tissues. Arch Ophthalmol 104:890–893, 1986.

54. Schwartz JL, Crooks LE: NMR imaging produces no observable mutations or cytotoxicity in mammalian cells. AJR 139:583–585, 1982.

55. Shellock FG, Schaefer DJ, Gordon CJ: Effect of a 1.5 T static magnetic field on body temperature of man. Magn Reson Med 3:644–647, 1986.

56. Shellock FG, Crues JV: Temperature, heart rate, and blood pressure changes associated with clinical MR imaging at 1.5 T. Radiology 163:259–262, 1987.

57. Shellock FG, Schaefer DJ, Grundfest W, Crues JV: Thermal effects of high-field (1.5 tesla) magnetic resonance imaging of the spine. Clinical experience above a specific absorption rate of 0.4 W/kg. Acta Radiol Suppl 369:514–516, 1986.

58. Shellock FG, Gordon CJ, Schaefer DJ: Thermoregulatory responses to clinical magnetic resonance imaging of the head at 1.5 tesla. Lack of evidence for direct effects on the hypothalamus. Acta Radiol Suppl 369:512–513, 1986.

59. Shellock FG, Crues JV: Corneal temperature changes associated with high-field MR imaging using a head coil. Radiology 167:809–811, 1986.

60. Shellock FG, Crues JV: Temperature changes caused by MR imaging of the brain with a head coil. Am J Neuroradiol 9:287–291, 1988.

61. Shellock FG, Schaefer DJ, Crues JV: Exposure to a 1.5-T static magnetic field does not alter body and skin temperatures of man. Magn Reson Med 11:371–375, 1989.

62. Shellock FG, Schaefer DJ, Crues JV: Alterations in body and skin temperatures caused by MR imaging: is the recommended exposure for radiofrequency radiation too conservative? Br J Radiol 62:904–909, 1989.

63. Shellock FG, Rothman B, Sarti D: Heating of the scrotum by high-field-strength MR imaging. AJR 154:1229–1232, 1990.

64. Shivers RR, Kavaliers M, Tesky CJ, et al: Magnetic resonance imaging temporarily alters blood-brain barrier permeability in the rat. Neurosci Lett 76:25–31, 1987.

65. Shuman WP, Haynor DR, Guy AW, et al: Superficial and deep-tissue increases in anesthetized dogs during exposure to high specific absorption rates in a 1.5-T MR imager. Radiology 167:551–554, 1988.

66. Sperber D, Oldenbourg R, Dransfeld K: Magnetic field induced temperature change in mice. Naturwissenschaften 71:100–101, 1984.

67. Stick VC, Hinkelmann ZK, Eggert P, et al: Beeinflussen starke statische Magnetfelder in der NMR-Tomographie die Gewebedurchblutung? (Strong static magnetic fields of NMR: Do they affect tissue perfusion?) Fortschr Rontgenstr 154:326–331, 1991.

68. Stojan L, Sperber D, Dransfeld K: Magnetic-field-induced changes in the human auditory evoked potentials. Naturwissenschaften 75:622–623, 1988.

69. Sweetland J, Kertesz A, Prato FS, et al: The effect of magnetic resonance imaging on human cognition. Magn Reson Imaging 5:129–135, 1987.

70. Teskey GC, Prato FS, Ossenkopp KP, et al: Exposure to time varying magnetic fields associated with magnetic resonance imaging reduces fentanyl-induced analgesia in mice. Bioelectromagnetics 9:167–174, 1988.

71. Teskey GC, Ossenkopp KP, Prato FS, et al: Survivability and long-term stress reactivity levels following repeated exposure to nuclear magnetic resonance imaging procedures in rats. Physiol Chem Phys Med NMR 19:43–49, 1987.

72. Thomas A, Morris PG: The effects of NMR exposure on living organisms. I. A microbial assay. Br J Radiol 54:615–621, 1981.

73. Tyndall DA, Sulik KK: Effects of magnetic resonance imaging on eye development in the C57BL/6J mouse. Teratology 43:263–275, 1991.

74. Tyndall DA: MRI effects on the teratogenicity of X-irradiation in the C57BL/6J mouse. Magn Reson Imaging 8:423–433, 1990.

75. Vogl T, Krimmel K, Fuchs A, et al: Influence of magnetic resonance imaging on human body core and intravascular temperature. Med Phys 15:562–566, 1988.

76. Von Klitzing L: Do static magnetic fields of NMR influence biological signals. Clin Phys Physiol Measure 7:157–160, 1986.

77. Von Klitzing L: Static magnetic fields increase the power intensity of EEG of man. Brain Res 483:201–203, 1989.

78. Von Klitzing L: A new encephalomagnetic effect in human brain generated by static magnetic fields. Brain Res 540:295–296, 1991.

79. Weiss J, Herrick RC, Taber KH, et al: Bio-effects of high magnetic fields: a study using a simple animal model. Magn Reson Imaging 8(S1):166, 1990.

80. Willis RJ, Brooks WM: Potential hazards of NMR imaging. No evidence of the possible effects of static and changing magnetic fields on cardiac function of the rat and guinea pig. Magn Reson Imaging 2:89–95, 1984.

81. Withers HR, Mason KA, Davis CA: MR effect on murine spermatogenesis. Radiology 156:741–742, 1985.

82. Wolff S, Crooks LE, Brown P, et al: Tests for DNA and chromosomal damage induced by nuclear magnetic resonance imaging. Radiology 136:707–710, 1980.

83. Yamagata H, Kuhara S, Eso Y, et al: Evaluation of dB/dt thresholds for nerve stimulation elicited by trapezoidal and sinusoidal gradient fields in echo-planar imaging. In: Book of Abstracts. Berkeley, CA: Society of Magnetic Resonance in Medicine, 1991, p 1277.

84. Vyalov AM: Magnetic fields as a factor in the industrial environment. Vestn Akad Med Nauk 8:72–79, 1967.

85. Vyalov AM: Clinico-hygienic and experimental data on the effect of magnetic fields under industrial conditions. In: Kholodov Y, ed. Influence of Magnetic Fields on Biological Objects. Moscow, 1971. Translated by the Joint Publications Research Service, 1974, pp 20–35, 63–38.

86. Barnothy MF: Biological Effects of Magnetic Fields, Volumes 1 and 2. New York: Plenum Publishing, 1964 and 1969.

87. Persson BR, Stahlberg F: Health and Safety of Clinical NMR Examinations. Boca Raton, FL: CRC Press, 1989.

88. Tenforde TS: Magnetic Field Effects on Biological Systems. New York: Plenum Publishing, 1979.

89. Michaelson SM, Lin JV: Biological Effects and Health Implications of Radiofrequency Radiation. New York: Plenum Publishing, 1987.

90. Tenforde TS: Thermoregulation in rodents exposed to high-intensity stationary magnetic fields. Bioelectromagnetics 7:341–346, 1986.

91. Beischer DE, Knepton J: Influence of strong magnetic fields on the electrocardiogram of squirrel monkey (Saimiri sciures). Aeroscope Med 35:939–944, 1964.

92. Tenforde TS, Gaffey CT, Moyer BR, et al: Cardiovascular alterations in Macaca monkeys exposed to stationary magnetic fields. Experimental observations and theoretical analysis. Bioelectromagnetics 4:1–9, 1983.

93. Dimick RM, Hedlund LW, Herfkens RJ, et al: Optimizing electrocardiographic electrode placement for cardiac-gated magnetic resonance imaging. Invest Radiol 22:17–22, 1987.

94. Abdullakhozhaeva MS, Razykov SR: Structural changes in central nervous system under the influence of a permanent magnetic field. Bull Exp Biol Med 102:1585–1587, 1986.

95. Hong CZ: Static magnetic field influence on human nerve function. Arch Phys Med Rehabil 68:162–164, 1987.

96. Budinger TF: Nuclear magnetic resonance (NMR) in vivo studies: known thresholds for health effects. J Comput Assist Tomogr 5:800–811, 1981.

97. Shellock FG, Crues JV: MRI: safety considerations in magnetic resonance imaging. MRI Decisions 2:25–30, 1988.

98. Shellock FG, Kanal E: Magnetic Resonance: Bioeffects, Safety, and Patient Management. New York: Raven Press, 1994.

99. Kanal E, Talagala L, Shellock FG: Safety considerations in MR imaging. Radiology 176:593–606, 1990.

100. Reilly JP: Peripheral nerve stimulation by induced electric currents: exposure to time-varying magnetic fields. Med Biol Eng Comput 27:101–112, 1989.

101. Bernhardt J: The direct influence of electromagnetic fields on nerve- and muscle cells of man within the frequency range of 1 Hz to 30 MHz. Radiat Environ Biophys 16:309–323, 1979.

102. Adey WR: Tissue interactions with nonionizing electromagnetic fields. Physiol Rev 61:435–514, 1981.

103. Watson AB, Wright JS, Loughman L: Electrical thresholds for ventricular fibrillation in man. Med J Aust 1:1179–1182, 1973.

104. Modan B: Exposure to electromagnetic fields and brain malignancy: a newly discovered menace? Am J Ind Med 13:625–627, 1988.

105. Brown HD, Chattopadhyay SK: Electromagnetic-field exposure and cancer. Cancer Biochem Biophys 9:295–342, 1988.

106. Pool R: Electromagnetic fields: the biological evidence. Science 249:1378–1381, 1990.

107. FDA: Magnetic resonance diagnostic device; panel recommendation and report on petitions for MR reclassification. Fed Regist 53:7575–7579, 1988.

108. Biological Effects and Exposure Criteria for Radiofrequency Electromagnetic Fields. Bethesda, MD: National Council on Radiation Protection and Measurements, 1986. NCRP report no. 86.

109. Erwin DN: Mechanisms of biological effects of radiofrequency electromagnetic fields: an overview. Aviat Space Environ Med 59(suppl 11):A21–A31, 1988.

110. Gordon CJ: Thermal physiology. In: Biological Effects of Radiofrequency Radiation. Washington, DC: US Government Publishing Office, 1984, pp 4-1–4-28. Environmental Protection Agency publication EPA-600/8-830-026A.

111. Gordon CJ: Normalizing the thermal effects of radiofrequency radiation: body mass versus total body surface area. Bioelectromagnetics 8:111–118, 1987.

112. Gordon CJ: Effect of radiofrequency radiation exposure on thermoregulation. In: ISI Atlas of Science, Plants and Animals, Volume 1. Philadelphia: Institute for Scientific Information, 1988, pp 245–250.

113. Beers J: Biological effects of weak electromagnetic fields from 0 Hz to 200 MHz: a survey of the literature with special emphasis on possible magnetic resonance effects. Magn Reson Imaging 7:309–331, 1989.

114. Coulter JS, Osbourne SL: Short wave diathermy in heating of human tissues. Arch Phys Ther 17:679–687, 1936.

115. Bottomley PA, Edelstein WA: Power disposition in whole body NMR imaging. Med Phys 8:510–512, 1981.

116. Bottomley PA, Redington RW, Edelstein WA, et al: Estimating radiofrequency power disposition in body NMR imaging. Magn Reson Med 2:336–349, 1985.

117. Wickersheim KA, Sun MH: Fluoroptic thermometry. Med Electronics February:84–91, 1987.

118. Berman E: Reproductive effects. In: Biological Effects of Radiofrequency Radiation. Washington, DC: US Government Printing Office, 1984. Environmental Protection Agency publication EPA-600/8-83-026A.

119. Michaelson SM, Lin JC: Biological Effects and Health Implications of Radiofrequency Radiation. New York: Plenum Press, 1991.

120. Shellock FG, Kanal E: Policies, guidelines, and recommendations for MR imaging safety and patient management. SMRI Safety Committee. J Magn Reson Imaging 1:97–101, 1991.

121. Hurwitz R, Lane SR, Bell RA, et al: Acoustic analysis of gradient-coil noise in MR imaging. Radiology 173:545–548, 1989.

122. Goldman AM, Grossman WE, Friedlander PC: Reduction of sound levels with antinoise in MR imaging. Radiology 173:549–550, 1989.

123. Hayes DL, Holmes DR, Gray JE: Effect of 1.5 tesla nuclear magnetic resonance imaging scanner on implanted permanent pacemakers. J Am Coll Cardiol 10:782–786, 1987.

124. Gangarosa RE, Minnis JE, Nobbe J, et al: Operational safety issues in MRI. Magn Reson Imaging 5:287–292, 1987.

125. Alagona P, Toole JC, Maniscalco BS, et al: Nuclear magnetic resonance imaging in a patient with a DDD pacemaker. PACE Pacing Clin Electrophysiol 12:619, 1989.

126. Edelman RR, Shellock FG, Ahladis J: Practical MRI for the technologist and imaging specialist. In: Edelman RR, Hesselink J, eds. Clinical Magnetic Resonance Imaging, Philadelphia: WB Saunders, 1990, pp 39–73.

127. ECRI. Health Devices Alert. A new MRI complication? May 27:1, 1988.

128. Dormer KJ, Richard GJ, Hough JVD, et al: The use of rare-earth magnet couplers in cochlear implants. Laryngoscope 91:1812–1820, 1981.

129. Shellock FG: Ex vivo assessment of deflection forces and artifacts associated with high-field MRI of ''mini-magnet'' dental prostheses. Magn Reson Imaging 7(suppl 1):IT-03, 1989. Letter.

130. Liang MD, Narayanan K, Kanal E: Magnetic ports in tissue expanders: a caution for MRI. Magn Reson Imaging 7:541–542, 1989.

131. Lund G, Nelson JD, Wirtschafter JD, et al: Tatooing of eyelids: magnetic imaging artifacts. Ophthalmic Surg 17:550–553, 1986.

132. Sacco DA, Steiger DA, Bellon EM, et al: Artifacts caused by cosmetics in MR imaging of the head. AJR 148:1001–1004, 1987.

133. Jackson JG, Acker JD: Permanent eyeliner and MR imaging. AJR 149:1080, 1987. Letter.

134. Pusey E, Lufkin RB, Brown RKJ, et al: Magnetic resonance imaging artifacts: mechanism and clinical significance. Radiographics 6:891–911, 1986.

135. Buchli R, Boesiger P, Meier D: Heating effects of metallic implants by MRI examinations. Magn Reson Med 7:255–261, 1988.

136. Davis PL, Crooks L, Arakawa M, et al: Potential hazards in NMR imaging: heating effects of changing magnetic fields and RF fields on small metallic implants. AJR 137:857–860, 1981.

137. Shellock FG, Crues JV: High-field MR imaging of metallic biomedical implants: an in vitro evaluation of deflection forces and temperature changes induced in large prostheses. Radiology 165:150, 1987. Letter.

138. Shellock FG, Crues JV: High-field MR imaging of metallic biomedical implants: an ex vivo evaluation of deflection forces. AJR 151:389–392, 1988.

139. Dujovny M, Kossovsky N, Kossowsky R, et al: Aneurysm clip motion during magnetic resonance imaging: in vivo experimental study with metallurgical factor analysis. Neurosurgery 17:543–548, 1985.

140. Shellock FG, Schatz CJ, Shelton C, et al: Ex vivo evaluation of 9 different ocular and middle-ear implants exposed to a 1.5 Tesla MR scanner. Radiology 177(P):271, 1990. Abstract.

141. Shellock FG, Schatz CJ: High-field strength MRI and otologic implants. Am J Neuroradiol 12:279–281, 1991.

142. Shellock FG, Meeks T: Ex vivo evaluation of ferromagnetism and artifacts for implantable vascular access ports exposed to a 1.5 T MR scanner. J Magn Reson Imaging 1:243, 1991. Abstract.

143. Teitelbaum GP, Yee CA, Van Horn DD, et al: Metallic ballistic fragments: MR imaging safety and artifacts. Radiology 175:855–859, 1990.

144. Shellock FG: MR imaging of metallic implants and materials: a compilation of the literature. AJR 151:811–814, 1988.

145. Shellock FG, Curtis JS: MR imaging and biomedical implants, materials, and devices: an updated review. Radiology 180:541–550, 1991.

146. Holtas S, Olsson M, Romner B, et al: Comparison of MR imaging and CT in patients with intracranial aneurysm clips. Am J Neuroradiol 9:891–897, 1988.

147. Huttenbrink KB, Gross-Nobis W: Experimentelle Untersuchungen und theoretische Betrachtungen uber das Verhalten von Stapes-Metall-Prothesen im Magnetfeld eines Kernspintomographen. (Experimental studies and theoretical considerations on behavior of stapes metal prostheses in the magnetic field of a nuclear magnetic resonance tomograph.) Laryngol Rhinol Otol 66:127–130, 1987.

148. Becker R, Norfray JF, Teitelbaum GP, et al: MR imaging in patients with intracranial aneurysm clips. Am J Neuroradiol 9:885–889, 1988.

149. Randall PA, Kohman LJ, Scalzetti EM, et al: Magnetic resonance imaging of prosthetic cardiac valves in vitro and in vivo. Am J Cardiol 62:973–976, 1988.

150. Romner B, Olsson M, Ljunggren B, et al: Magnetic resonance imaging and aneurysm clips. J Neurosurg 70:426–431, 1989.

151. Augustiny N, von Schulthess GK, Meier D, et al: MR imaging of large nonferromagnetic metallic implants at 1.5 T. J Comput Assist Tomogr 11:678–683, 1987.

152. Teitelbaum GP, Bradley WG, Klein BD: MR imaging artifacts, ferromagnetism, and magnetic torque of intravascular filters, stents, and coils. Radiology 166:657–664, 1988.

153. Yuh WTC, Hanigan MT, Nerad JA, et al: Extrusion of a magnetic eye implant after MR examination: a potential hazard to the enucleated eye. J Magn Reson Imaging 1:711–713, 1991.

154. New PFJ, Rosen BR, Brady TJ, et al: Potential hazards and artifacts of ferromagnetic and nonferromagnetic surgical and dental materials and devices in nuclear magnetic resonance imaging. Radiology 147:139–148, 1983.

155. Brown MA, Carden JA, Coleman RE, et al: Magnetic field effects on surgical ligation clips. Magn Reson Imaging 5:443–453, 1987.

156. Barrafato D, Henkelman RM: Magnetic resonance imaging and surgical clips. Can J Surg 27:509–512, 1984.

157. Teitelbaum GP, Lin MCW, Watanabe AT, et al: Ferromagnetism and MR imaging: safety of carotid vascular clamps. AJNR 11:267–272, 1990.

158. Hathout G, Lufkin RB, Jabour B, et al: MR-guided aspiration cytology in the head and neck at high field strength. J Magn Reson Imaging 2:93–94, 1992.

159. Gegauff A, Laurell KA, Thavendrarajah A, et al: A potential MRI hazard: forces on dental magnet keepers. J Oral Rehabil 17:403–410, 1990.

160. Shellock FG, Slimp G: Halo vest for cervical spine fixation during MR imaging. AJR 154:631–632, 1990.

161. Clayman DA, Murakami ME, Vines FS: Compatibility of cervical spine braces with MR imaging. A study of nine nonferrous devices. AJNR 11:385–390, 1990.

162. Soulen RL, Budinger TF, Higgins CB: Magnetic resonance imaging of prosthetic heart valves. Radiology 154:705–707, 1985.

163. Hassler M, Le Bas JF, Wolf JE, et al: Effects of magnetic fields used in MRI on 15 prosthetic heart valves. J Radiol 67:661–666, 1986.

164. Marshall MW, Teitelbaum GP, Kim HS, et al: Ferromagnetism and magnetic resonance artifacts of platinum embolization microcoils. Cardiovasc Intervent Radiol 14:163–166, 1991.

165. Watanabe AT, Teitelbaum GP, Gomes AS, et al: MR imaging of the bird's nest filter. Radiology 177:578–579, 1990.

166. Leibman CE, Messersmith RN, Levin DN, et al: MR imaging of inferior vena caval filter: safety and artifacts. AJR 150:1174–1176, 1988.

167. Teitelbaum GP, Raney M, Carvlin MJ, et al: Evaluation of ferromagnetism and magnetic resonance imaging artifacts of the Strecker tantalum vascular stent. Cardiovasc Intervent Radiol 12:125–127, 1989.

168. Shellock FG, Myers SM, Schatz CJ: Ex vivo evaluation of ferromagnetism determined for metallic scleral ''buckles'' exposed to a 1.5 T MR scanner. Radiology 185(P):288–289, 1992.

169. de Keizer RJ, Te Strake L: Intraocular lens implants (pseudophakoi) and steelwire sutures: a contraindication for MRI? Doc Ophthalmol 61:281–284, 1984.

170. Albert DW, Olson KR, Parel JM, et al: Magnetic resonance imaging and retinal tacks. Arch Ophthalmol 108:320–321, 1990.

171. Joondeph BC, Peyman GA, Mafee MF, et al: Magnetic resonance imaging and retinal tacks. Arch Ophthalmol 105:1479–1480, 1987. Letter.

172. Lyons CJ, Betz RR, Mesgarzadeh M, et al: The effect of magnetic resonance imaging on metal spine implants. Spine 14:670–672, 1989.

173. Shellock FG, Mink JH, Curtin S, et al: MRI and orthopedic implants used for anterior cruciate ligament reconstruction: assessment of ferromagnetism and artifacts. J Magn Reson Imaging 2:225–228, 1992.

174. Mattucci KF, Setzen M, Hyman R, et al: The effect of nuclear magnetic resonance imaging on metallic middle ear prostheses. Otolaryngol Head Neck Surg 94:441–443, 1986.

175. Applebaum EL, Valvassori GE: Further studies on the effects of magnetic resonance fields on middle ear implants. Ann Otol Rhinol Laryngol 99:801–804, 1990.

176. White DW: Interaction between magnetic fields and metallic ossicular prostheses. Am J Otol 8:290–292, 1987.

177. Leon JA, Gabriele OF: Middle ear prothesis: significance in magnetic resonance imaging. Magn Reson Imaging 5:405–406, 1987.

178. Shellock FG, Crues JV, Sacks SA: High-field magnetic resonance imaging of penile prostheses: in vitro evaluation of deflection forces and imaging artifacts. Presented at the Annual Meeting of the Society of Magnetic Resonance in Medicine, Berkeley, CA, 1987, p 915. Abstract.

179. Lufkin R, Jordan S, Lylcyk M: MR imaging with topographic EEG electrodes in place. AJNR 9:953–954, 1988.

180. Mark AS, Hricak H: Intrauterine contraceptive devices: MR imaging. Radiology 162:311–314, 1987.

181. Go KG, Kamman RL, Mooyaart EL: Interaction of metallic neurosurgical implants with magnetic resonance imaging at 1.5 tesla as a cause of image distortion and of hazardous movement of the implant. Clin Neurosurg 91:109–115, 1989.

182. To SYC, Lufkin RB, Chiu L: MR-compatible winged infusion set. Comput Med Imaging Graphics 13:469–472, 1989.

183. Kelly WM, Pagle PG, Pearson A, et al: Ferromagnetism of intraocular foreign body causes unilateral blindness after MR study. Am J Neuroradiol 7:243–245, 1986.

184. Williams S, Char DH, Dillon WP, et al: Ferrous intraocular foreign bodies and magnetic resonance imaging. Am J Ophthalmol 105:398–401, 1988.

185. Flaherty JA, Hoskinson K: Emotional distress during magnetic resonance imaging. N Engl J Med 320:467–468, 1989.

186. Fishbain DA, Goldberg M, Labbe E, et al: Long-term claustrophobia following magnetic resonance imaging. Am J Psychiatry 145:1038–1039, 1988.

187. Quirk ME, Letendre AJ, Ciottone RA, et al: Anxiety in patients undergoing MR imaging. Radiology 170:463–466, 1989.

188. Quirk ME, Letendre AJ, Ciottone RA, et al: Evaluation of three psychological interventions to reduce anxiety during MR imaging. Radiology 173:759–762, 1989.

189. Hricak H, Amparo EG: Body MRI: alleviation of claustrophobia by prone positioning. Radiology 152:819, 1984. Letter.

190. Weinreb JC, Maravilla KR, Peshock R, et al: Magnetic resonance imaging: improving patient tolerance and safety. AJR 143:1285–1287, 1984.

191. Klonoff EA, Janata JW, Kaufman B: The use of systematic desensitization to overcome resistance to magnetic resonance imaging (MRI) scanning. J Behav Ther Exp Psychiatry 17:189–192, 1986.

192. Granet RB, Gelber LJ: Claustrophobia during MR imaging. N J Med 87:479–482, 1990.

193. Phelps LA: MRI and claustrophobia. Am Fam Physician 42:930, 1990. Letter.

194. McGuinness TP: Hypnosis in the treatment of phobias: a review of the literature. Am J Clin Hypnosis 26:261–272, 1984.

195. Karlik SJ, Heatherley T, Pavan F, et al: Patient anesthesia and monitoring at a 1.5 T MRI installation. Magn Reson Med 7:210–221, 1988.

196. Barnett GH, Ropper AH, Johnson KA: Physiological support and monitoring of critically ill patients during magnetic resonance imaging. J Neurosurg 68:244–250, 1988.

197. Dunn V, Coffman CE, McGowan JE, et al: Mechanical ventilation during magnetic resonance imaging. Magn Reson Imaging 3:169–172, 1985.

198. McArdle CB, Nicholas DA, Richardson CJ, et al: Monitoring of the neonate undergoing MR imaging: technical considerations. Radiology 159:223–226, 1986.

199. Roth JL, Nugent M, Gray JE, et al: Patient monitoring during magnetic resonance imaging. Anesthesiology 62:80–83, 1985.

200. Shellock FG: Monitoring during MRI. An evaluation of the effect of high-field MRI on various patient monitors. Med Electronics September:93–97, 1986.

201. Shellock FG: Monitoring sedated patients during MRI. Radiology 177:586, 1990. Letter.

202. Wendt RE, Rokey R, Vick GW, et al: Electrocardiographic gating and monitoring during NMR imaging. Magn Reson Imaging 6:89–95, 1988.

203. Holshouser BA, Hinshaw DB, Shellock FG: Sedation, anesthesia, and physiologic monitoring during MRI. In. Hasso AN, Stark DD, eds. Categorical Course Syllabus, Spine and Body Magnetic Resonance Imaging. American Roentgen Ray Society, 1991.

204. Kanal E, Applegate GR: Thermal injuries/incidents associated with MR imaging devices in the US: a compilation and review of the presently available data. In: Book of Abstracts. Society of Magnetic Resonance Imaging, 1990, p 274.

205. Shellock FG, Slimp G: Severe burn of the finger caused by using a pulse oximeter during MRI. AJR 153:1105, 1989.

206. Kanal E, Shellock FG: Burns associated with clinical MR examinations. Radiology 175:585, 1990. Letter.

207. Shellock FG, Myers SM, Kimble K: Monitoring heart rate and oxygen saturation during MRI with a fiber-optic pulse oximeter. AJR 158:663–664, 1992.

208. Runge V: Clinical application of magnetic resonance contrast media in the head. In: Runge V, ed. Contrast Media in Magnetic Resonance Imaging: A Clinical Approach. Philadelphia: JB Lippincott, 1992.

209. Oksendal A, Hals P: Biodistribution and toxicity of MR imaging contrast media. J Magn Reson Imaging 3:157–165, 1993.

210. Harpur E, Worah D, Hals P, et al: Preclinical safety assessment and pharmacokinetics of gadodiamide injection, a new magnetic resonance imaging contrast agent. Invest Radiol 28(suppl):S280, 1993.

211. Tweedle M, Eaton S, Eckelman W, et al: Comparative chemical structure and pharmacokinetics of MRI contrast agents. Invest Radiol 23(suppl 1):S236, 1988.

212. Tweedle M: Physiochemical properties of gadoteridol and other magnetic resonance contrast agents. Invest Radiol 27(suppl 1):S2–S6, 1992.

213. Chang C: Magnetic resonance imaging contrast agents. Design and physiochemical properties of gadodiamide. Invest Radiol 28(suppl 1):S21–S27, 1993.

214. Cacheris W, Quay S, Rocklage S: The relationship between thermodynamics and the toxicity of gadolinium complexes. Magn Reson Imaging 8:467–481, 1990.

215. Felix R, Schorner W: Intravenous contrast media in MRI: clinical experience with gadolinium-DTPA over four years. Presented at the Second European Congress of NMR in Medicine and Biology, Berlin, 1988.

216. Niendorf H, Ezumi K: Magnevist (Gd-DTPA): tolerance and safety after 4 years of clinical trials in more than 7000 patients. Presented at the Second European Congress of NMR in Medicine in Biology, Berlin, 1988.

217. Niendorf H, Valk J, Reiser M: First use of Gd-DTPA in pediatric MRI. Presented at the Second European Congress of NMR in Medicine and Biology, Berlin, 1988.

218. Ball WJ, Nadel S, Zimmerman R, et al: Phase III multicenter clinical investigation to determine the safety and efficacy of gadoteridol in children suspected of having neurologic disease. Radiology 186:769–774, 1993.

219. Niendorf H, Haustein J, Cornelius I, et al: Safety of gadolinium-DTPA: extended clinical experience. Magn Reson Med 22:222–228, 1991.

220. Sullivan M, Goldstein H, Sansone K, et al: Hemodynamic effects of Gd-DTPA administered via rapid bolus or slow infusion: a study in dogs. Am J Neuroradiol 11:537–540, 1990.

221. Goldstein H, Kashanian F, Blumetti R, et al: Safety assessment of gadopentetate dimeglumine in US clinical trials. Radiology 174:17–23, 1990.

222. Hajek P, Sartoris D, Gylys-Morin V, et al: The effect of intra-articular gadolinium-DTPA on synovial membrane and cartilage. Invest Radiol 25:179–183, 1990.

223. Kashanian F, Goldstein H, Blumetti R, et al: Rapid bolus injection of gadopentetate dimeglumine: absence of side effects in normal volunteers. Am J Neuroradiol 11:853–856, 1990.

224. Brasch R: Safety profile of gadopentetate dimeglumine. MRI Decisions 3:13–19, 1989.

225. McLachlan S, Lucas M, DeSimone D, et al: Worldwide safety experience with gadoteridol injection (ProHance). In: Book of Abstracts. Berkeley, CA: Society of Magnetic Resonance in Medicine, 1992, 1426.

226. A Two Year Report on the Safety and Efficacy of Magnevist (Gadopentate Dimeglumine) Injection. Wayne, NJ: Berlex Laboratories, 1990.

227. DeSimone D, Morris M, Rhoda C, et al: Evaluation of the safety and efficacy of gadoteridol injection (a low osmolal MR contrast agent): clinical trials report. Invest Radiol 26(suppl 1):S212–S216, 1991.

228. Carvlin M, DeSimone D, Meeks M: Phase II clinical trial of gadoteridol injection, a low osmolal magnetic resonance imaging contrast agent. Invest Radiol 27:S16–S21, 1992.

229. Runge V, Bradley W, Brant-Zawadski M, et al: Clinical safety and efficacy of gadoteridol: a study in 411 patients with suspected intracranial and spinal disease. Radiology 181:701–709, 1991.

230. McLachlan S, Eaton S, DeSimone D: Pharmacokinetic behavior of gadoteridol injection. Invest Radiol 27(suppl 1):S12–S15, 1992.

231. Soltys R: Summary of preclinical safety evaluation of gadoteridol injection. Invest Radiol 27(suppl 1):S7–S11, 1992.

232. Weinmann HJ, Gries H, Speck U: Gd-DTPA and low osmolar Gd chelates. In: Runge V, ed. Enhanced Magnetic Resonance Imaging. St. Louis: CV Mosby, 1989.

233. Muhler A, Saeed M, Brasch R, Higgins C: Hemodynamic effects of bolus injection of gadodiamide injection and gadopentetate dimeglumine as contrast media at MR imaging in rats. Radiology 183:523–528, 1992.

234. LaFlore J, Goldstein H, Rogan R, et al: A prospective evaluation of adverse experiences following the administration of Magnevist (gadopentetate dimeglumine) injection. In: Book of Abstracts. Berkeley, CA: Society of Magnetic Resonance in Medicine, 1989, p 1067.

235. Niendorf H, Dinger J, Haustein J, et al: Tolerance data of Gd-DTPA: a review. Eur J Radiol 13:15–20, 1991.

236. Takebayashi S, Sugiyama M, Nagase M, Matsubara S: Severe adverse reaction to IV gadopentetate dimeglumine. AJR 14:912–913, 1990.

237. Shellock FG, Hahn P, Mink JH, Itskovich E: Adverse reaction to intravenous gadoteridol. Radiology 189:1–2, 1993.

238. Salonen O: Case of anaphylaxis and four cases of allergic reaction following Gd-DTPA administration. J Comput Assist Tomogr 14:912–913, 1990.

239. Tishler S, Hoffman JC: Anaphylactoid reactions to IV gadopentetate dimeglumine. Am J Neuroradiol 11:1167, 1990.

240. Weiss K: Severe anaphylactoid reaction after IV Gd-DTPA. Magn Reson Imaging 8:817–818, 1990.

241. Tardy B, Guy C, Barral G, et al: Anaphylactic shock induced by intravenous gadopentetate dimeglumine. Lancet 339:494, 1992.

242. Omohundro J, Elderbrook M, Ringer T: Laryngospasm after administration of gadopentetate dimeglumine. J Magn Reson Imaging 1:729–730, 1992.

243. Chan C, Bosanko C, Wang A: Pruritus and paresthesia after IV administration of Gd-DTPA. Am J Neuroradiol 10:S53, 1989.

244. American College of Radiology: Manual on Iodinated Contrast Media. Reston, VA: American College of Radiology, 1991.

245. McAlister W, McAlister V, Kissane J: The effect of Gd-dimeglumine on subcutaneous tissues: a study with rats. Am J Neuroradiol 11:325–327, 1990.

246. Cohan RH, Leder RA, Herzberg AJ, et al: Extravascular toxicity of two magnetic resonance contrast agents. Preliminary experience in the rat. Invest Radiol 26:224–226, 1991.

247. Kanal E, Applegate G, Gillen C: Review of adverse reactions, including anaphylaxis, in 5260 cases receiving gadolinium-DTPA by bolus injection. Radiology 177(P):159, 1990.

248. Harbury O: Generalized seizure after IV gadopentetate dimeglumine. Am J Neuroradiol 12:666, 1991.

249. Watson A, Rocklage S, Carvlin M: Contrast media: In: Stark D, Bradley W, eds. Magnetic Resonance Imaging. St. Louis: CV Mosby, 1991.

250. Niendorf H, Haustein J, Louton T, et al: Safety and tolerance after intravenous administration of 0.3 mmol/kg Gd-DTPA. Invest Radiol 26:S221–S223, 1991.

251. Niendorf H, Laniado M, Semmler W, et al: Dose administration of gadolinium-DTPA in MR imaging of intracranial tumors. Am J Neuroradiol 8:803–815, 1987.

252. Haustein J, Bauer W, Hibertz T, et al: Double dosing of Gd-DTPA in MRI of intracranial tumors. In: Book of Abstracts. Berkeley, CA: Society of Magnetic Resonance in Medicine, 1990, p 258.
253. Leander P, Allard M, Caille J, Golman K: Early effect of gadopentetate and iodinated contrast media on rabbit kidneys. Invest Radiol 27:922–926, 1992.
254. Wedeking P, Kumar K, Tweedle M: Dissociation of gadolinium chelates in mice: relationship to chemical characteristics. Magn Reson Imaging 10:641–648, 1992.
255. Haustein J, Niendorf H, Louton T: Renal tolerance of Gd-DTPA—a retrospective evaluation of 1,171 patients. Magn Reson Imaging 8(S1):43, 1990.
256. Frank J, Choyke P, Girton M, et al: Gadopentetate dimeglumine clearance in renal insufficiency in rabbits. Invest Radiol 25:1212–1216, 1990.
257. Haustein J, Niendorf H, Krestin G, et al: Renal tolerance of gadolinium-DTPA/dimeglumine in patients with chronic renal failure. Invest Radiol 27:153–156, 1992.
258. Runge V, Rocklage S, Niendorf H, et al: Discussion: gadolinium chelates. Berkeley, CA: Society of Magnetic Resonance in Medicine Workshop on Contrast Enhanced Magnetic Resonance, 1991, pp 229–232.
259. Lackner K, Krahe T, Gotz R, Haustein J: The dialysability of Gd-DTPA. In: Bydder G, Felix R, Bucheler E, eds. Contrast Media in MRI. Bussum, Netherlands: Medicom Europe, 1990, pp 321–326.
260. Schmiedl U, Maravilla K, Gerlach R, Dowling C: Excretion of gadopentetate dimeglumine in human breast milk. AJR 154:1305–1306, 1990.
261. Rofsky N, Weinreb J, Litt A: Quantitative analysis of gadopentetate dimeglumine excreted in breast milk. J Magn Reson Imaging 3:131–132, 1993.
262. Nell G, Rummel W: Pharmacology of intestinal permeation. In: Csaky T, ed. Handbook of Experimental Pharmacology, Volume 70, Part II. Berlin: Springer-Verlag, 1984, p 489.
263. Weinmann H, Brasch R, Press W, Wesbey G: Characteristics of gadolinium-DTPA complex: a potential NMR contrast agent. AJR 142:619–624, 1984.

14

Instrumentation

ECKART STETTER

SYSTEM OVERVIEW

In principle, a magnetic resonance imaging (MRI) system is quite simple, consisting of a large main magnet and smaller auxiliary field coils (gradient coils), radiofrequency (RF) antennas (transmitter and receiver coils), associated electronics, and a computer to process the data from the imaging experiment. However, in practice, MRI systems are quite complex, and careful attention must be paid to the design of all components to ensure consistent, high-quality images.

In this chapter, I attempt to present a balanced view of MRI instrumentation, giving an overview of the various components as well as more technical details essential to a full understanding of the system.

An MRI system has many similarities to the nuclear magnetic resonance (NMR) spectrometers, applied to chemical analysis, that have been in use for decades. In addition, MRI systems use magnetic field gradient coils and associated power supplies, as well as an image processor for reconstruction and display of images. The system must obviously be scaled to the size of a patient, rather than of test tubes, as are most spectrometers. The basic components of an MRI system using a superconducting magnet are shown in Figure 14–1. These components can be summarized as follows.

MAIN MAGNET. The main magnet generates a stable magnetic field to align the nuclei in the patient's tissues. This magnet has a large opening, called the *bore*, containing additional hardware (shim, gradient, RF coils). The open bore that remains after placement of this hardware must be large enough to hold the patient comfortably (typically 60 cm in diameter).

SHIM SYSTEM. The shim, placed within the magnet bore, guarantees the homogeneity of the main magnetic field throughout the imaging volume. In most cases the shim consists of a manifold of iron sheets distributed appropriately to make the field homogeneous. In addition, special shim coils wound on the bore tube surface and driven by a set of power supply units are used to further improve homogeneity.

GRADIENT COILS. The gradient coils are mounted on a cylinder that is concentrically placed within the magnet bore. There are three sets of windings, designed to generate a linear magnetic field gradient along three orthogonal axes (x, y, z). The strength of the gradient field is proportional to the strength of the applied electrical current.

RADIOFREQUENCY COILS. The RF coils are placed inside the gradient coils. The RF transmitter coil converts the electrical power from a power transmitter into an oscillating magnetic field (the RF pulse) to excite the tissue nuclei. A receiver coil detects the minute MR signal, which is then amplified by preamplifiers and amplifiers and forwarded to the receiver.

PULSE SEQUENCE CONTROLLER. The pulse sequence controller acts as the chief operating officer for the MR system. It uses the user-defined pulse sequence as a blueprint for running the signal measurement procedure. It ensures the correct timing and amplitudes of the gradient pulses using digital-to-analog converters and generates an RF pulse with the correct amplitude and phase using a *modulator*. A *synthesizer* acts as a central clock. The analog-to-digital converter (ADC) translates the MR signal into digital numbers that can be used directly by the computer.

IMAGE PROCESSOR. Data acquired during the imaging process are fed into the image processor, which reconstructs them as a set of two-dimensional images. The images are copied into the video memory of the console monitor.

HOST PROCESSOR. The host processor manages interactions between the various subsystems.

MAGNETS

TYPES OF MAGNETS

Several types of magnets are in routine clinical use. These can be categorized as *permanent, resistive,* and *superconducting.* Permanent magnets consist of material that is strongly magnetized. Such materials are said to have a high *magnetic remanence.* Resistive magnets are electromagnets, consisting of an air core or iron yoke wrapped with loops of wire in a configuration that produces a uniform magnetic field. Commercial permanent and resistive yoke-type magnets have a vertical magnetic field in most cases. Like electromagnets, superconducting magnets consist of loops of wire wrapped around a support structure. However, once

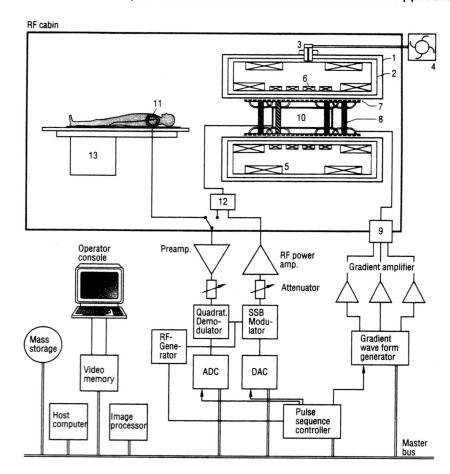

FIGURE 14–1. Overview of an MRI system. Magnet components: 1 = vacuum container; 2 = cryoshield; 3 = cold head; 4 = compressor; 5 = superconducting shield coil; 6 = superconducting field coil; 7 = shim system; 8 = gradient coil set; 9 = RF filters; 10 = RF coil; 11 = (optional) local RF coil; 12 = transmit-receive switch; 13 = couch for patient. (From Morneburg H, ed: Bildgebende Systeme für die medizinische Diagnostik. 3rd ed. Munich: Publicis MCD Verlag, 1995.)

powered up by an electrical current, these magnets remain at full strength without any additional input of electrical power. Schematics of the magnets are shown in Figure 14–2, and their characteristics are summarized in Table 14–1. There are significant differences in attainable field strength, homogeneity, field stability, and siting requirements for the different types of magnets.

Field Strength

For a permanent magnet, the attainable field strength within the imaging volume is determined by the amount of energy needed to produce the desired field inside the accessible volume versus the amount of energy that can be stored in the permanent magnetic material. Practical permanent magnet design is a compromise between an extremely large amount of a fairly inexpensive material with a modest magnetic remanence and a smaller amount of more expensive material having a high remanence.

Resistive magnets are limited in field strength by electrical power requirements. The available power in most clinical installations does not usually exceed 100 kW, which currently limits the maximal field strength for whole-body systems to 0.3 T for iron core resistive magnets. On the other hand, superconducting whole-body MR systems have been constructed with field strengths up to 4 T. The attainable field strength of superconducting magnets is limited by the current-carrying capacity of the superconducting wire and by the physical forces generated at these large field strengths.

Homogeneity

The usable imaging volume in a magnet is determined by magnetic field homogeneity over this region. A large magnet is required to produce a homogeneous field over a large region. This is best accomplished with superconducting magnets, which can produce usable fields of view up to 50 cm. The usable imaging volume for permanent and resistive magnets is usually smaller than that for superconducting magnets. The Fourier transform imaging process is much more tolerant of main field inhomogeneities than is spectroscopy. In most in vivo spectroscopy, the magnet is reshimmed to optimize homogeneity for each individual volume of interest (e.g., brain, kidney). This reshimming is not necessary for imaging unless spectroscopic imaging methods are to be applied (including use for fat suppression).

Field Stability

MRI requires a stable main magnetic field. Any temporal variation in the field produces phase errors and results in image artifacts. Simulations show that field

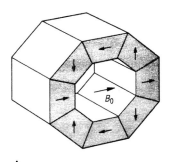
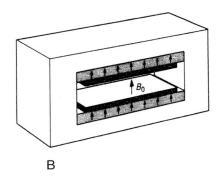

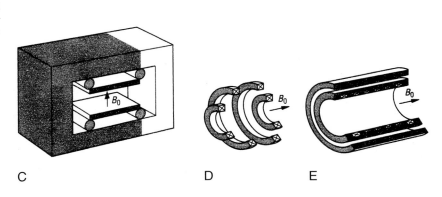

FIGURE 14–2. Various types of magnets: *(A)* permanent magnet (ring type); *(B)* permanent magnet (yoke type); *(C)* resistive magnet (yoke type, part of the yoke can be omitted to get an open C-shaped magnet); *(D)* resistive magnet (air core); *(E)* superconducting (air core) magnet. (*A* to *E* from Morneburg H, ed: Bildgebende Systeme für die medizinische Diagnostik. 3rd ed. Munich: Publicis MCD Verlag, 1995.)

TABLE 14–1. MAGNET TYPES FOR MRI SYSTEMS

TECHNICAL CHARACTERISTICS	SUPERCONDUCTING	RESISTIVE AIR CORE	RESISTIVE IRON YOKE	PERMANENT YOKE	PERMANENT RING
Field strength	High (≤4 T)	Limited (≤0.3 T)	Limited (≤0.4 T)	Limited (≤0.2 T)	Limited (≤0.2 T)
Field direction	Axial	(Mostly) axial	Vertical	Vertical	Vertical or transverse
Homogeneity and effective volume	Good (<5 ppm over 50 cm dsv*)	Medium (<40 ppm over 40 cm dsv*)	Medium (<40 ppm over 35 cm dsv*)	Medium (<40 ppm over 35 cm dsv*)	Medium (<40 ppm over 35 cm dsv*)
Stability	Good	Depending on power supply	Depending on power supply	Depending on temperature	Depending on temperature
Shielding of external interferences	Significant	None	Low	Low	Low
Gradient eddy fields (time constant τ)	Large (needs compensation or active shielded (AS) gradients, τ ≈ 200 ms)	Low (depending on former design, τ ≈ 20 ms)	Medium (anisotropic, needs compensation or AS gradients, τ ≈ 20 ms)	Medium (anisotropic, needs compensation or AS gradients, τ ≈ 20 ms)	Low (short τ)
Fringe field extension	Large, usually needs shielding	Medium	Low to medium	Low to medium	Low to medium
Emergency shutdown (time)	By emergency quench (some seconds)	Immediate by power off	Immediate by power off	Not possible	Not possible
Dimensions	Quite large, 1.8 m dsv × 1.7 m	Large, 1.5 m dsv × 1.5 m	Medium to large, 1.2–2.5 m × 1.5 m × 1.7 m	Medium to large, 1.2–2.5 m × 1.5 m × 1.7 m	Medium to large, 1.4 m dsv × 1.5 m
Weight (tons)	Large (4–6)	Medium (1.5)	Extremely large (10–20)	Extremely large (10–50)	Large (6)
Costs and expenses					
Purchase price	High	Low	Low	Medium	Medium to high
Energy usage	None except refrigerator	High (>60 kW)	Medium (10–20 kW)	None	None
Cooling	Needs 0.1–0.3 L/h liquid helium	Needs much cooling water	Needs cooling water	None	None

*dsv = diameter of spherical volume.

variations having a magnitude of only a few ten billionths of a tesla, resulting in phase errors as small as 3°, can produce visible artifacts. Because of fluctuations in the power supply, resistive magnets have difficulty producing the required level of stability. In contrast, this degree of stability is readily achieved by superconducting magnets and by permanent magnets, especially if the latter are in a temperature-stabilized environment.

Superconducting magnets have an additional benefit in that they intrinsically shield against external magnetic field interference, such as that produced by moving cars or alternating current power lines. These magnets can tolerate external field interference on the order of one millionth of a tesla (1 μT) without significantly affecting image quality.

SUPERCONDUCTING MAGNETS

Because superconducting magnets are mostly applied for MRI systems, I now consider the technical factors involved in the construction and operation of such magnets in some detail. Further details on the construction and basic physics of superconducting magnets are available elsewhere.[1]

Construction, Field Strength, and Homogeneity

Superconductors have no resistance to electrical current. By constructing magnets from superconducting materials, large, stable magnetic fields can be generated. There are several important considerations in the choice of superconducting material. First, the superconducting wire material must be capable of carrying large currents needed to produce strong magnetic fields. In addition, it must be possible to keep the material in a superconducting state. Therefore, the critical temperature of the material (i.e., the temperature above which the material develops resistance and is no longer superconducting) must be higher than the boiling point of an appropriate coolant such as liquid helium, which is 4.2° above absolute zero at atmospheric pressure. Another option would be to use a refrigerator that is able to keep the superconducting wire at the required low temperatures. Finally, the material must have the appropriate physical properties (e.g., ductility, flexibility) to permit it to be drawn out as a wire and formed into the correct configuration. This excludes the use of so-called high-temperature superconducting wire at this time.

The most frequently used material is titanium-niobium. A multifilament wire composed of approximately 30 titanium-niobium strands, of 0.1 mm diameter each, is embedded in a copper matrix (about 2 mm in diameter) for stability. Such a wire can carry currents of up to 700 A. The wire is wound around a cylindrical core, and the number of windings is determined by the required field strength. An unshielded 2-T magnet typically uses nearly 40 miles of wire.

The magnet is divided into several subcoils, and the number of windings in each is calculated to maximize homogeneity in a central spherical volume of 50 cm diameter. The best possible homogeneity that can be achieved over a 50-cm central sphere is approximately 2 ppm and in practice is typically much worse, for example, 150 ppm, because of unavoidable tolerances in the construction of the magnet. Therefore, the magnet must be shimmed. To avoid spatial distortion and to allow spectroscopic imaging (e.g., for fat suppression) at least locally, the magnet homogeneity over the usable volume should be better than 10 ppm.

Cryostat

The superconducting windings are bathed in liquid helium. To insulate these windings from the higher temperature of the outside environment and prevent boiloff of the helium, the magnet is contained within a Dewar called the *cryostat*.

The cryostat must have excellent thermal insulating characteristics. The amount of insulation can be calculated, based on the allowable rate of evaporation and the surface area of the helium tank. A cross section of a cryostat is shown in Figure 14–3, which illustrates the measures that must be taken to ensure low heat transfer between the outside environment and the magnet windings. Care must be taken to prevent any kind of thermal energy from penetrating to the helium. This protection is accomplished by two heat radiation shields and superinsulating foil. The radiation shields are kept at constant temperature (20 K and 70 K, approximately) by a refrigerator. Convection of heat energy is avoided by maintaining the entire Dewar in a high vacuum. The components of the cryostat are suspended on thin, strong plastic rods that are poor conductors of heat. These design measures insulate the cryogen container so well that the evaporation rate of liquid helium is generally less than 0.1 L/h. Therefore, cryogen refill is necessary only every 3 to 6 months. At the top of the cryostat is an insulated service access that allows liquid helium to be refilled and power cables to be attached. Some systems are designed to reliquefy cryogen boiloff and require no refill.

Ramping and Quenching

Superconducting magnets must be initially powered up (*ramped*) to full field strength but then maintain the magnetic field for years without additional power input. For the initial ramping procedure, the magnet is first cooled to the point that the windings become superconducting, and then an electrical current is induced within the windings by connecting them to a power supply. This procedure is explained by a simplified circuit diagram shown in Figure 14–4. The superconducting switch, when cooled to the temperature of liquid helium, short-circuits the magnet windings. To bring the magnet to full field strength, this switch is first inactivated by heating it above its critical temperature so that it develops electrical resistance. It is then possible to induce a current in the magnet windings

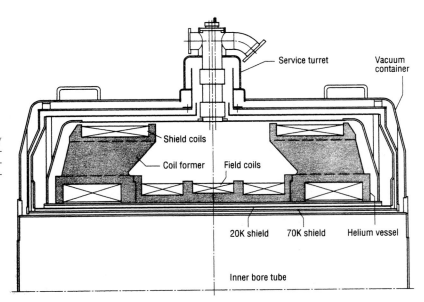

FIGURE 14–3. Cross section through an actively shielded superconducting magnet. (From Morneburg H, ed: Bildgebende Systeme für die medizinische Diagnostik. 3rd ed. Munich: Publicis MCD Verlag, 1995.)

by applying a voltage across the terminals of this switch. Once the desired magnet field strength is attained, the heater is shut off, so that the switch returns to being a superconductor. As a result, the current can now flow through the magnet windings, including the switch, without any resistance. Then the power supply is disconnected. Controlled discharging of the energy stored in the magnetic field (approximately 7 MJ for an unshielded 2-T magnet), which might be needed for servicing, is performed by reversing this procedure.

A *quench* represents the sudden loss of superconductivity, either spontaneous or caused by external influences. The magnet can be quenched in an emergency by heating the superconducting coils locally. More often, quenches result from negligence, as when liquid helium levels are allowed to drop too low. The quench may begin in one region of the windings but rapidly spreads to other regions as the portion of the windings that is no longer superconducting generates heat because of electrical resistance. The rate of loss of magnetic field strength is determined by the resistance, self-inductance, and mutual inductance of the coil windings. To slow the quench, so-called *quench protection diodes* are connected in parallel with the windings to provide an alternative low-resistance pathway for the rapidly discharging electrical current and thereby reduce the voltage across the windings, which might destroy the insulation of the wires. The heat produced by the quench causes the liquid helium to boil off. To prevent asphyxiation in the magnet enclosure resulting from release of gaseous helium, the helium gas is vented to the outside environment.

Fringe Field Shielding

If limited space is available for siting, it is necessary to provide adequate shielding from the fringe field of the magnet. Magnetic shielding using ferromagnetic iron plates can be placed around the magnet room[2] or directly on the magnet. In either case, a large mass of iron is necessary for effective shielding. One may assume that the required mass of iron is similar in both cases; although the required thickness of shielding material is less for room shielding, the surface area to be shielded is larger than that for self-shielding.

Magnetic shielding affects the homogeneity of the magnet. The tighter and more eccentric the distribution of the shielding, the more difficult it is to shim the magnet properly. Room shielding has the drawback of being dependent on the structure of the building and therefore has to be designed individually for each site. Sometimes, an incomplete magnetic shield is adequate —for instance, to shield an adjoining waiting area from the 0.5-mT cardiac pacemaker zone.

The fringe field can also be reduced by *active shielding*. This method has become quite popular. It uses an opposing current-carrying winding that is external to the magnet to decrease fringe fields. Superconducting active shields are incorporated directly into the cryostat. Although active shielding increases the physical size of the magnet, the weight is much reduced compared with the weight involved in shielding

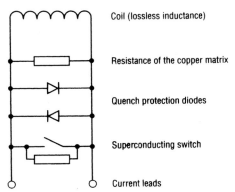

FIGURE 14–4. Simplified circuitry of a superconducting magnet. (From Morneburg H, ed: Bildgebende Systeme für die medizinische Diagnostik. 3rd ed. Munich: Publicis MCD Verlag, 1995.)

with ferromagnetic materials. Active shields compensate the so-called dipole field of the magnet; without the shield, the dipole magnetic field decreases only by the cube of the distance and extends many feet in each direction from the magnet. With active shielding, the dipole field is eliminated, leaving only a quadrupole field. This latter magnetic field decreases by the fifth power of distance and therefore extends for only a few feet from the magnet (see Table 14–3).

Shimming

Shimming is the process by which magnetic field inhomogeneities are eliminated. These inhomogeneities may arise from imperfections in the magnet itself or may be due to ferromagnetic materials in the magnet environment. Correction of these magnetic field inhomogeneities may be accomplished by passive shimming, using iron plates placed inside the magnet bore, or by active shimming, using special coil windings that act as electromagnets.

Shimming is accomplished by using a special probe to measure the magnetic field strength at multiple points along the spherical surface of the 50-cm imaging volume. A mathematic method, based on spherical harmonics expansion, is used to determine the shim coefficients needed to correct the magnetic field inhomogeneities.

PASSIVE SHIMMING. Field inhomogeneity is corrected by placing sheets of iron inside the magnet.[3] Preferably one uses a standard configuration of iron plate positions. The number of iron sheets to be placed at each location is computed by a special shim program. Shimming with iron has the advantage that the iron can be placed in a large number of different configurations, which allows correction of high-order magnetic field inhomogeneities. It is cheap and does not need an expensive high-precision power supply. However, if one needs high or adjustable homogeneity, active magnetic field shimming is necessary.

ACTIVE MAGNETIC FIELD SHIMMING. For this purpose a set (5 to 12) of current-carrying windings are arranged on a cylindrical tube within the magnet bore. These windings are configured so that each generates a magnetic field correction approximating one of the spherical harmonics expansion coefficients. These windings must be designed to avoid magnetic interactions between them, as well as between them and the magnet and gradient coils. The linear gradients used for imaging (see section on gradients) can be used as first-order shims as well, so the active shim coil needs to compensate only for the higher order (order ≥ 2) field inhomogeneities.

CRITERIA FOR SELECTING MAGNETIC FIELD STRENGTH

It has been shown that the signal-to-noise (S/N) ratio increases at least linearly with the strength of the main magnetic field (B_0).[4] One might therefore assume that image quality and other system performance data like speed would continue to improve at arbitrarily high magnetic field strengths. However, other factors, some of which I now review, limit the improvement in image quality at high fields.[5] These factors are related to chemical shift artifact, RF characteristics such as power deposition, T1 relaxation times, and safety (Table 14–2).

Chemical-Shift Artifact

Chemical shift represents the shift in resonance frequency caused by the magnetic shielding effect of the electron cloud that surrounds the nucleus. In MR images, this magnetic shielding, which is different for fat and water protons, produces a difference in their resonance frequencies of approximately 3.5 ppm of the resonance frequency. As a result, as discussed in more detail in Chapter 3, the effect of chemical shift is to produce an artifactual shift in the position of fat relative to water along both the slice-selection and frequency-encoding directions. Because chemical shift is proportional to magnetic field strength, chemical-shift artifact is most serious with high-field systems.

Along the frequency-encoding axis, chemical-shift artifact can be compensated for by using a stronger readout gradient (Fig. 14–5). However, this solution results in an increased signal bandwidth and, consequently, more image noise. Along the slice-selection axis, chemical-shift artifact is more easily controlled. The slice-selection gradient can be increased, resulting in a proportional reduction in chemical-shift artifact. To maintain the slice thickness, the increase in gradient strength necessitates an increase in the bandwidth of the RF pulse, which can be accomplished by reducing the RF pulse duration. The main drawback of this approach is greater peak and average RF power deposition.

Main Field Inhomogeneity

Like chemical shift, magnetic field inhomogeneities increase with field strength. These inhomogeneities produce signal loss because of dephasing (T2* effect) as well as geometric distortion. Field distortions related to variations in the magnetic susceptibility of the pa-

TABLE 14–2. FACTORS IN THE SELECTION OF FIELD STRENGTH IN PROTON MRI

CAUSE	EFFECT
Chemical shift	Image shift between tissue containing water and that containing fat
Inhomogeneity of the main field	Spatial distortion
RF eddy currents (skin effect)	Lack of image uniformity
RF loss	Rise in patient's temperature
T1 time dependence on field	Changed contrast-to-noise ratio
Fringe field	Attraction of ferromagnetic objects at a given distance from the main magnet, interference with cardiac pacemakers and other devices

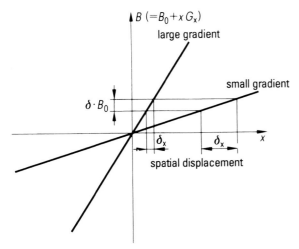

FIGURE 14–5. Fat-water shifts as a function of the field gradient. (From Morneburg H, ed: Bildgebende Systeme für die medizinische Diagnostik. 3rd ed. Munich: Publicis MCD Verlag, 1995.)

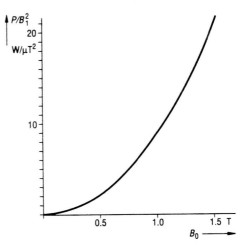

FIGURE 14–6. RF pulse power required per square of B_1 field for a given B_0 (average experimental results for a 75-kg patient in a circularly polarized whole-body transmit resonator). (From Morneburg H, ed: Bildgebende Systeme für die medizinische Diagnostik. 3rd ed. Munich: Publicis MCD Verlag, 1995.)

tient (e.g., at air-tissue interfaces) also increase with field strength. To overcome the distortions caused by main field inhomogeneities, the magnetic field gradients used on higher field systems must be stronger than those used on lower field systems.

Radiofrequency Power Deposition

If the frequency dependence of tissue conductivity and power loss in the RF coil is disregarded, the amount of transmitted RF power required to produce a given flip angle excitation increases as the square of the resonance frequency. Therefore, RF power deposition increases with field strength. The problem is worsened by the larger RF pulse bandwidths generally used at high field strengths. RF power deposition heats the body much as a microwave oven heats a frozen dinner.

For safety reasons, some countries have established regulations for power deposition, represented by the specific absorption rate. The specific absorption rate is the allowable amount of RF power deposition per kilogram of body weight (see Chapter 13). Figure 14–6 shows the experimentally determined RF power deposition for an average patient as a function of field strength. Within these guidelines, one finds that excess power deposition can limit the repetition time (TR) at field strengths above 1.5 T, for example, for a two-echo spin-echo pulse sequence using RF pulses of 0.5 ms effective duration.

Radiofrequency Penetration

The RF (B_1) field induces electrical currents within the patient's tissues. These RF-induced *eddy currents* (to be differentiated from gradient-induced eddy currents in the magnet structures, discussed further on) oppose the RF field and reduce penetration of the RF pulse into deep tissues. This so-called skin effect,[6] which is frequency dependent, causes the RF excitation to be

nonuniform throughout the imaging volume and can result in prominent shading artifacts at high field strengths.

T1 Relaxation

As discussed in Chapter 1, T1 relaxation times increase with field strength.[7] For a given TR, this increase results in greater saturation of the nuclear magnetization and therefore reduced signal intensity. Consequently, the actual increase in S/N ratio is less than proportional to field strength (Fig. 14–7).

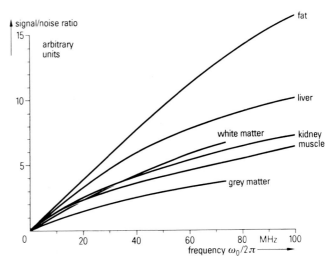

FIGURE 14–7. S/N ratio as a function of B_0 (constant receiver bandwidth assumed). Increase in the S/N ratio with the field, taking into consideration the dependence of the T1 relaxation time on the field strength B_0 for a constant TR. (From Morneburg H, ed: Bildgebende Systeme für die medizinische Diagnostik. 3rd ed. Munich: Publicis MCD Verlag, 1995.)

TABLE 14–3. SAFETY DISTANCE (IN METERS) FROM CENTER OF MAGNET

B_0 (T)	0.5-mT LINE (RADIAL) (m)	0.5-mT LINE (AXIAL) (m)
0.5*	6.5	8.3
1.0*	8.2	10.5
1.5*	9.4	12.0
2.0*	10.3	13.1
Actively shielded magnets		
1.0†	2.4	4.3
1.5†	2.8	4.8

*Magnets having a 1.05-m bore and a length of 2.30 m.
†Magnets having a 0.90-m bore and 1.9-m length.

Safety

High-field magnets have several potential safety problems. In practice, the most important possible hazard comes from the fact that magnets exert strong forces on ferromagnetic objects inadvertently brought nearby. If these objects are fully saturated (fully magnetized), which depends on the shape and composition of the object, the attractive forces increase linearly with field strength. Finally, fringe fields increase with field strength. Table 14–3 shows the distance of the 0.5-mT line (pacemaker restriction) for magnets of the same size but different field strengths. Various electronic devices are also sensitive to weak magnetic fields (Table 14–4). Magnetic shielding can reduce siting problems considerably (see last two lines in Table 14–3).

GRADIENTS

The gradient coils are configured to produce highly linear magnetic field gradients within the imaging volume. A schematic drawing of gradient coil windings suitable for cylindrical magnets with an axial field is shown in Figure 14–8. In most applications, the gradient waveform is trapezoidal. A trapezoidal gradient is designed to increase (ramp up) from zero to a plateau value determined by the pulse sequence. The gradient stays at the plateau value for a certain time and then rapidly decreases (ramps down) to zero. The coils and power supply are designed for strong amplitudes and rapid ramping. Echo-planar and hybrid imaging systems sometimes use oscillating, sinusoidal gradients, which permit even more rapid switching without re-

TABLE 14–4. SENSITIVITY OF VARIOUS DEVICES TO STATIC MAGNETIC FIELDS

Magnetic data storage devices (disks, tapes, and so on)	3 mT
Screened video monitors	3 mT
Video monitors (monochrome)	1 mT
Cardiac pacemakers and other electronic implants	0.5 mT
X-ray equipment	0.2 mT
Image intensifiers	50 μT
Photo multipliers	50 μT
Earth's magnetic field (for comparison)	50 μT

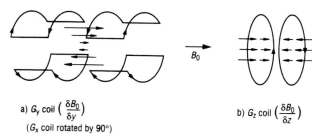

a) G_y coil $\left(\dfrac{\delta B_0}{\delta y} \right)$
(G_x coil rotated by 90°)

b) G_z coil $\left(\dfrac{\delta B_0}{\delta z} \right)$

FIGURE 14–8. Simplified design of windings of gradient coils for axial magnets. (From Morneburg H, ed: Bildgebende Systeme für die medizinische Diagnostik. 3rd ed. Munich: Publicis MCD Verlag, 1995.)

quiring extremely high voltages directly from the power supply (see Chapter 10).

POWER SUPPLY

The power supply ultimately limits the possible maximal gradient amplitude. The gradient power requirements for a given gradient strength and minimal switching time depend on a number of design assumptions but in general increase by the fourth to fifth power of the gradient coil radius. Although current requirements can be reduced by increasing the number of windings in the gradient coil, this increases the coil inductance and requires a correspondingly high voltage to allow rapid switching. Typical current requirements are in the range of 200 to 300 A. To meet this requirement with rapid gradient switching, the power supply must be able to support current changes at rates of 300 kA/s and more. This means for a typical coil inductance of 1 mH minimal voltages of 300 V plus some surplus to compensate for resistive losses of coils and leads. In addition, the power supply must be extremely precise, have minimal electronic noise, and have minimal current instability (ripple). High gradient stability (less than a few hundred thousandths of maximal gradient strength) is essential because the gradient determines the sampled point in the spatial frequency domain,[8] and instabilities lead to image artifacts such as smearing in the phase-encoding direction.

EDDY CURRENTS

As the gradients switch amplitudes during the imaging process, the changing magnetic field induces time-varying currents in nearby conducting materials. In particular, they induce electrical currents in the wall of the magnet Dewar (cryoshield). These eddy currents themselves create a time-varying magnetic field in the same distribution as that produced by the gradient coils but with opposite direction (Fig. 14–9). The net effect of the gradient-induced eddy currents is to oppose and weaken the gradient magnetic field.

Eddy currents increase with the gradient amplitude and the rate of change of that amplitude. Once the gradient reaches a stable, plateau value, the eddy cur-

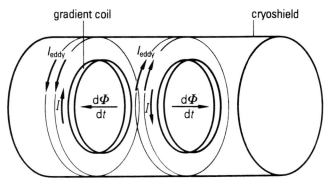

FIGURE 14–9. Eddy currents generated by a pulsed gradient field.

rents begin to decay. The decay of the eddy currents can be approximated mathematically by an exponential function, with a time constant that is generally determined by the conductivity and effective inductance of the cryoshield.

Without any compensation for eddy currents, a square current pulse produces a distorted gradient waveform, rather than the expected trapezoidal waveform (Fig. 14–10A). The distorted gradient pulse produces image artifacts, such as blurring and spatial misregistration.

Eddy current suppression can be obtained by precompensating the driving current for the gradients (Fig. 14–10B). Basically, the driving current is dynamically modified so that the gradient magnetic field, when added to the opposing field generated by the eddy currents, always produces a net magnetic field of the proper strength and pulse shape.

However, as can be seen in Figure 14–9, the distribution of the eddy currents differs from the gradient coil current distribution. This deviation is primarily along the radial direction but also occurs along the long axis of the magnet. Because the spatial distribution of the eddy current–induced magnetic fields differs slightly from that of the gradient-induced magnetic fields, precompensation of the driving current does not perfectly eliminate eddy fields at every point in space. This problem can be minimized by proper consideration of the design of the gradient coil. However, the eddy

currents decay over time, and this *dynamic nonlinearity* cannot be completely compensated for in the design of the gradient coil or in precompensation of the driving for the gradients. Because more sophisticated pulse sequences may be sensitive to higher order field distortions (i.e., the result may be inconsistent image quality), active shielded gradients are used to avoid dynamic nonlinearity.

ACTIVE GRADIENT SHIELDING

Eddy current effects can be largely eliminated by imposing shielding coils between the gradient coil and the cryostat (active shielding). In effect, the active shield is a second set of gradient coils mounted concentrically around the imaging gradient coils.[9] Current flow in the active shield is opposite to that of the imaging gradient coils; this shielding current is switched on and off in synchrony with the imaging gradients. The effect of the active shield is to counteract the magnetic field of the imaging gradient in the vicinity of the cryoshield and thereby to eliminate eddy currents and especially occurrence of dynamic field distortions of higher spatial order. This benefit outweighs certain disadvantages of active shielding gradients such as higher complexity (cost) and power requirements.

CRITERIA FOR REQUIRED GRADIENT STRENGTH

The cost of a gradient system increases considerably with the level of performance capability. In particular, power requirements become a limitation at higher gradient amplitudes. Therefore, a compromise must be reached between unlimited, expensive gradient capabilities and practical requirements for MRI. The essential question is as follows: How strong a gradient is needed to achieve the desired level of spatial and contrast resolution, which depends on pulse sequence timing parameters[10] and consequently the speed of the imaging process.

In addition, for many applications newer techniques such as fast gradient-echo sequences, fast spin-echo techniques, and echo-planar methods, frequently combined with flow compensation, are quite useful. These generally impose even higher demands on the gradient system.

For a simple approach, consider the least complex pulse sequence that is of practical usefulness, a spin-warp gradient-echo sequence as shown in Figure 14–11, which gives a two-dimensional image. In this case the gradients are used only to spatially encode the NMR signal, that is, make the excitation selective in one dimension (z), do a phase encoding in the second dimension (y), and frequency encode in the third dimension (x). As the switching time t_g is not negligible with respect to the selection, phase-encoding, and readout (frequency-encoding) period, it has to be taken into consideration as well. For simplicity we assume a minimal t_g independent of the gradient ampli-

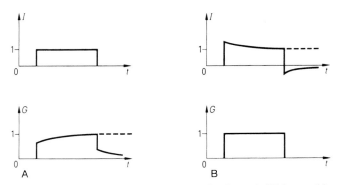

FIGURE 14–10. Current and gradient pulse form. *A*, Without eddy current compensation. *B*, With eddy current compensation. (*A* and *B* from Morneburg H, ed: Bildgebende Systeme für die medizinische Diagnostik. 3rd ed. Munich: Publicis MCD Verlag, 1995.)

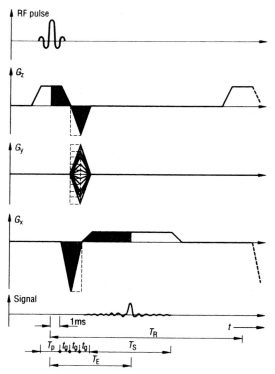

FIGURE 14–11. Gradient-echo pulse sequence including gradient switching times. For proper echo refocusing the shaded areas of positive and negative gradient pulse lobes must be equal. (From Morneburg H, ed: Bildgebende Systeme für die medizinische Diagnostik. 3rd ed. Munich: Publicis MCD Verlag, 1995.)

tude. In this way, the slice thickness and in-plane resolution (pixel size) can easily be adjusted by the gradient strength without need to change the sequence timing. For such a sequence the echo time (TE) is calculated as

$$TE = 0.5T_p + 3t_g + 0.5T_s \qquad (1)$$

where T_p is the time of the selective pulse and T_s is the readout time. Because the image noise N is inversely proportional to the square root of T_s, it is given by

$$N = 1/\sqrt{2TE - T_p - 6t_g} \qquad (2)$$

On the other hand, the image contrast ΔS depends strongly on TE, assuming the simple approximation for the NMR signal strength as a function of spin density ρ, relaxation times T1 and T2, and TR:

$$S = const \times \rho \times \exp(-TE/T2)[1 - \exp(-TR/T1)] \qquad (3)$$

Hence the contrast is

$$\Delta S = const\{\rho' \exp(-TE/T2')[1 - \exp(-TR/T1')] - \rho'' \exp(-TE/T2'')[1 - \exp(-TR/T1'')]\} \qquad (4)$$

From Equations 2 and 4 one can calculate the contrast-to-noise ratio as a function of TE for different T_p and t_g values at given TR and tissue parameters (ρ, T1, T2).[11] An example is shown in Figure 14–12. It is obvious that by reducing T_p (the lower boundary is given by the RF power limitations; see next section) and especially t_g, the contrast-to-noise ratio can be significantly improved.

When the sequence timing has been settled (i.e., optimized using the foregoing considerations), the gradient strength necessary for a certain desired spatial resolution can be calculated:

$$G_x = \frac{2\pi}{\gamma T_s \Delta x}, \quad G_x' = -0.5G_x\left(\frac{T_s}{t_g} + 1\right) \qquad (5)$$

$$G_y = \frac{\pi}{\gamma T_\varphi \Delta y}, \quad \text{here } T_\varphi = t_g \qquad (6)$$

$$G_z = \frac{\Delta\omega_p}{\gamma\Delta z}, \quad G_z' = -0.5G_z\left(\frac{T_p}{t_g} + 1\right) \qquad (7)$$

where Δx is the pixel dimension in the readout direction, Δy is the pixel dimension in the phase-encoding direction, Δz is the slice thickness, T_φ is the phase-encoding time, and $\Delta\omega_p$ is the selective pulse bandwidth.

An example is given in Table 14–5. As shown in Chapters 4 and 10, there are many extensions of the basic principle demonstrated here.

Gradient motion refocusing should be mentioned in this context. This technique applies additional positive and negative gradient pulses before the signal data acquisition so that the first moment of the gradient pulse sequence vanishes at the center of the readout interval:

$$\int_0^{TE} G(t')t' \, dt' = 0 \qquad (8)$$

Of course, these pulses should take as little time as possible, which means that the gradient has to be strong and the switching time has to be short.

Another application is echo-planar imaging (see Chapter 10). This sequence creates a burst of gradient echoes that are all differently phase encoded through a constant or periodically blipped phase-encoding gradient by rapidly reversing the readout gradient. Data for one image can be acquired in a single shot. To get enough signal and avoid spatial resolution degrada-

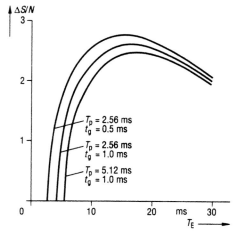

FIGURE 14–12. Contrast-to-noise ratio as a function of TE for gray and white brain matter at various RF pulse times and gradient switching times. (From Morneburg H, ed: Bildgebende Systeme für die medizinische Diagnostik. 3rd ed. Munich: Publicis MCD Verlag, 1995.)

TABLE 14–5. GRADIENT STRENGTH FOR A GIVEN PULSE SEQUENCE (SEE FIG. 14–11) AND DESIRED SPATIAL RESOLUTION

PARAMETER	TIMING	BANDWIDTH	VOXEL SIZE	GRADIENT	REPHASE GRADIENT
Ramp time	t_g = 1 ms				G'_z = −13.94 mT/m
Selective pulse	T_p = 2.56 ms	$\Delta\omega_p/2\pi$ = 1 kHz	Δz = 3 mm	G_z = 7.83 mT/m	G'_x = −13.27 mT/m
Readout	T_s = 7.68 ms	Per pixel = 130 Hz	Δx = 1 mm	G_x = 3.06 mT/m	
Phase encode	T_φ = 1 ms		Δy = 1 mm	G_y = 11.74 mT/m	
Echo time	TE = 8.12 ms				

tion, one has to complete the data sampling in a time not much longer than T2 or T2*. By applying Equation 5, one can easily see that echo-planar imaging needs extremely high gradients and short switching times.

In summary, for a standard MRI system doing routine high-quality clinical imaging, gradients of 10 to 15 mT/m at a rise time of 0.5 to 1 ms might be satisfactory. An MRI system capable of performing advanced and fast imaging methods might well require a high-power gradient subsystem delivering gradients of even more than 25 mT/m at switching times less than 0.25 ms. The technologic development of coil and power amplifier design is on the way to making these features commercially available. On the other hand, it has been found[12] that such gradient systems can expose the patient to high field change rates, which may result in peripheral nerve stimulations (see Chapter 13). This effect may limit further improvements of gradient systems because they would not be applicable to patients.

RADIOFREQUENCY SYSTEM

In this section, we consider some rather technical aspects involved in the design of the RF system. Clinical imaging specialists interested in a more basic discussion of the RF system are referred to Chapter 1 and, for considerations related to pulse sequence design, Chapter 4.

The coils used to transform electrical signals to high-frequency magnetic (B_1) fields (transmit coils) or to convert these fields to electrical signals (receive coils) represent the heart of the RF system.

COILS AND RESONATORS

Coils and resonators, types of RF antennas, are components of the MR system that directly interact with the object to be imaged.

Antenna Characteristics

A coil can be characterized by the spatial distribution of the magnetic field per current through the coil winding $B_i(r)$. Because of reciprocity rules, the peak output voltage ($\hat{u}$) induced by a sample of volume v_{sample} with magnetization M rotating with ω_0[13] can be written as

$$\hat{u} = \omega_0 \int_{v_{sample}} \mathbf{MB}_i \, dV \qquad (9)$$

As a result, the received output power (short circuit at the coil outputs) is

$$P = \tfrac{1}{2}\hat{u}^2/R \qquad (10)$$

where R is the impedance of the matched coil.

Matching

The term *matching* may have multiple connotations in MR instrumentation. For example, a maximum of half the output is available when the coil has been matched to subsequent components; hence a matching circuit (employing impedance transformers) is typically used (Fig. 14–13). In addition, the useful signal output rises with the matching of the spatial coil field distribution to the distribution of the magnetization and falls with the resistive loss. This expression of matching is to be understood in a general manner, that is, not only that the sample volume should correspond to the sensitive volume of the antenna but also that the vectors M and B_i should be parallel. Given an antenna whose B_1 field is perpendicular to B_0 and is circularly polarized, it should theoretically be superior to any other configuration because of the nuclear magnetization precession M about the B_0 direction.

Noise Sources

In addition to signal loss, resistance (R) may be a source of undesirable noise. The resistance may be divided into the resistance induced by the sample and that caused by the coil:

$$R = R_{sample} + R_{coil} \qquad (11)$$

The R_{sample} is strongly dependent on the shape of the

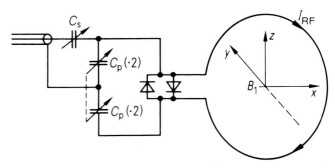

FIGURE 14–13. Surface coil with symmetric matching network. (From Morneburg H, ed: Bildgebende Systeme für die medizinische Diagnostik. 3rd ed. Munich: Publicis MCD Verlag, 1995.)

object to be measured and the distribution of conductive material therein. Generally, this loss in useful signal caused by the subject of measurement (the patient) and the noise it generates are unavoidable. R_{coil}, on the other hand, can be optimized:

$$R_{coil} = \frac{\omega_0 \int_{vcoil} B_i^2 \, dV}{2\mu_0 Q_0} \qquad (12)$$

where $Q\emptyset$ is the unloaded quality factor of the coil. The quality factor is a general measure of the efficiency of the coil.

With the definition of the filling factor (η),

$$\eta = \int_{vsample} B_i^2 \, dV / \int_{vcoil} B_i^2 \, dV \qquad (13)$$

that is, the fraction of the field energy penetrating the sample in relation to total field energy produced, it follows that

$$R_{coil} = \omega_0 \int_{vsample} B_i^2 \, dV / 2\mu_0 \eta Q_0 \qquad (14)$$

Coil losses therefore increase with sample volume and decrease with the (unloaded) Q_0 and the filling factor.

The Optimal MR Antenna

In consequence, the following goals are set for an optimized MR antenna:

1. Field distribution should be homogeneous across the measurement volume to ensure spatially uniform excitation.
2. The filling factor (volume of the sample/volume of the coil) should be large.
3. The direction of polarization should be perpendicular to the main field and whenever possible circular.
4. Coil losses should be minimal compared with the losses induced by the subject to be measured; that is, the unloaded Q_0 should be much better than the Q when the patient is in the coil.

Goals 1 and 2 may occasionally prove counterproductive in medical practice, namely when a portion of

the body that cannot be surrounded by a coil is to be imaged. For these cases, surface coils are used; that is, the homogeneity of the B_1 field is sacrificed in favor of a large filling factor. Newer designs try to recombine goals 1 and 2 even for surface coils by applying a set of two to four coils (array coil) simultaneously.[14] This, of course, requires a corresponding number of independent RF receivers whose NMR signals are separately processed. The resulting images are added together after the noise from the respective insensitive (signal-free) regions has been suppressed. This is a rather expensive technology, although it gives an impressive improvement of image quality for body field-of-view applications.

ANTENNAS WITH HOMOGENEOUS FIELD DISTRIBUTION

Coils and resonators must surround the subject to be measured to generate a homogeneous B_1 field within it.

A suitable configuration would be a solenoid arranged coaxially to the axis of the body. Given that B_1 and B_0 should ideally be perpendicular to each other, this type of coil configuration is limited to use with yoke magnets (see Fig. 14–2). The self-resonance frequency of a solenoid having a diameter corresponding to the size of a human body is relatively low (<10 MHz). At high frequencies, as used with axial superconducting magnets, it is necessary to find cylindrical structures that generate a homogeneous field that is polarized in the direction perpendicular to the axis of the magnet. A sufficiently long tube, subjected to a current distribution $J(\phi)$,

$$J(\phi) = \hat{J} \sin(\phi) \qquad (15)$$

as shown in Figure 14–14A and B, generates the desired field distribution.[15] Implementing this current distribution is not a simple matter. The current density is simulated for several angles with discrete conductor

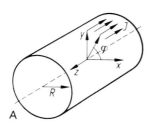
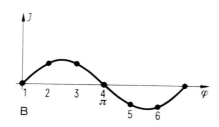

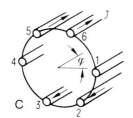
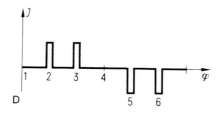

FIGURE 14–14. RF antenna with homogeneous B_1 field. *A,* Hollow tube with current density distribution in longitudinal direction. *B,* Ideal current distribution. *C,* Resonant conductors arranged as a discrete hollow tube. *D,* Current distribution in a discrete hollow tube for a nearly homogeneous B_1 field. (*A* to *D* from Morneburg H, ed: Bildgebende Systeme für die medizinische Diagnostik. 3rd ed. Munich: Publicis MCD Verlag, 1995.)

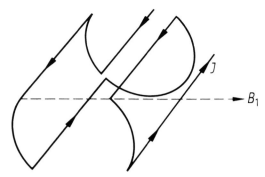

FIGURE 14–15. Saddle coil for low frequencies and small coil dimensions. (From Morneburg H, ed: Bildgebende Systeme für die medizinische Diagnostik. 3rd ed. Munich: Publicis MCD Verlag, 1995.)

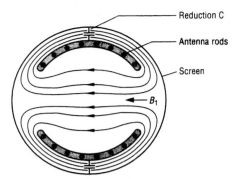

FIGURE 14–17. Cross section of a whole-body antenna using the transmission line resonance principle suitable for high frequencies. (From Morneburg H, ed: Bildgebende Systeme für die medizinische Diagnostik. 3rd ed. Munich: Publicis MCD Verlag, 1995.)

paths (Fig. 14–14C and D). The conductors at $\phi = 0$ and 2π may be eliminated, because they do not carry any current. If the wire rods are connected in the manner shown in Figure 14–15, the result is a saddle coil that can be used in situations in which the frequency is not too high nor the diameter too large (up to 30 cm at approximately 25 MHz).

At higher frequencies and larger diameters (whole-body antennas), the length of the conductors is no longer short compared with the RF wavelength, so the desired current distribution can no longer be achieved with a saddle coil.

At this point, the $\lambda/2$ transmission line resonator principle becomes of interest. If a wave having the length $\lambda = 2\pi c/\omega_0$ (c is the velocity of wave propagation) is generated on a double transmission line (Fig. 14–16A) and the line is $\lambda/2$ long, a resonance or standing wave is produced. Its current distribution is shown in Figure 14–16B, which results in the corresponding B1 field distribution. The circuit can be shortened symmetrically by adding capacitances, so that a nearly uniform current distribution is created in the longitudinal direction (Fig. 14–16C and D). Such resonance conductors can be configured as a hollow tube.

A cross section of such a configuration is shown in Figure 14–17. The sections of the conductors are composed of rods having adjustable capacitors connected between the antenna and ground (exterior shielding). This $\lambda/2$ resonator[16] can be used as a transmit-receive antenna for whole-body MRI up to more than 63 MHz.

Alderman and Grant[17] have developed a variation of this principle (Fig. 14–18). It is used primarily for head imaging antennas as well as for extremities (knee, feet), because the structure is open on two sides and is therefore more pleasant for the patient.

Quadrature (Circularly Polarized) Coils

A circularly polarized B1 field can be generated with the antennas described in the preceding paragraphs by joining pairs of resonators via a power divider and a phase shifter in such a way that a rotating high-frequency field is generated within the antenna. Inversely, the voltages, induced in the resonators by the precessing magnetization and shifted by 90°, are forwarded to the preamplifier via a summation network. This configuration requires only half the RF output to

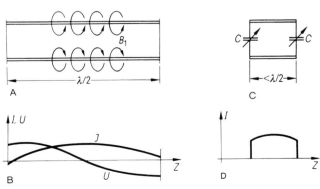

FIGURE 14–16. A $\lambda/2$ (1/2 wavelength) resonator (antenna). A, Conductor configuration. B, Current distribution. C, Electrically shortening the conductors by applying a capacitance load to the ends. D, Current distribution with shortened conductors. (A to D from Morneburg H, ed: Bildgebende Systeme für die medizinische Diagnostik. 3rd ed. Munich: Publicis MCD Verlag, 1995.)

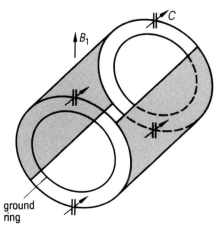

FIGURE 14–18. Variation of the conductor resonance principle according to Alderman and Grant.[17] (From Morneburg H, ed: Bildgebende Systeme für die medizinische Diagnostik. 3rd ed. Munich: Publicis MCD Verlag, 1995.)

generate a rotating B_1 field and results in an S/N ratio that is improved by the $\sqrt{2}$ (40%)[18] if the Q of the antenna under load conditions corresponds to that of a comparable, linearly polarized configuration. Unfortunately, because a cross section of the human body is more elliptic (i.e., the coils are not evenly loaded), the advantages of circular polarization may not be fully realized in practice.

SURFACE COILS

As the name indicates, these coils are used for imaging organs that are located close to the surface of the patient's body. They are placed on the patient directly over the position in which the organ is located. The coil must be oriented so that the B_1 field is perpendicular to B_0. In the simplest case, the coil comprises a single wire ring that is tuned to resonance at ω_0 via variable capacitors (see Fig. 14–13). The field distribution of a current-carrying circular loop with a radius of r is described along the y axis of the coil by the following equation:

$$B_i(y) = \mu_0 r^2 / [2(r^2 + y^2)^{3/2}] \qquad (16)$$

According to this equation, the sensitivity along the coil axis decreases with increasing distance from the coil plane. The maximal sensitivity and the effective penetration depth ("break-even" distance when comparing the S/N ratio of a surface coil with that of a volume coil) depend strongly on the radius of the surface coil. Depending on the imaging objective, it is possible to trade sensitivity for the magnitude of the useful volume by varying the dimensions of the coil.

In some cases the configuration of the coil windings can also be adapted to the surface of the human body (e.g., the female breast). Surface coils are generally used only to receive MR signals because of the inhomogeneity of the field distribution; for instance, a 180° excitation may be generated near the surface, whereas at some distance away the tissues experience only a 90° flip. For this reason, the typical MRI configuration uses the whole-body resonators for more uniform excitation and uses the surface coil for a receiving antenna.

Figure 14–19 shows several examples of surface coils.

Decoupling

When the body resonator is used for excitation, the surface coil must not oscillate during the transmit phase, or the distribution of the transmitter field will be distorted. This interaction between the transmit and receive coils is called *coupling*. In the simplest case, decoupling is achieved via "detuning" diodes, which are illustrated in Figure 14–13. These diodes are switched into the conductive state by the induced voltage during RF transmission and thus detune the coil off-resonance.

ARRAY COILS

As already mentioned, a set of two, four, or more coils can be applied to an object of interest that is large enough that it cannot be wrapped in a single surface coil.[14] Examples are linear coil arrays to image the spine from the neck to the lumbar region and two-by-two arrays that fit around the abdomen, which are useful for performing, for example, liver studies. To take the full S/N ratio advantage of each of the coil elements it is necessary to magnetically decouple the coil elements (e.g., by slightly overlapping them) so that the noise for each coil is uncorrelated with the noise from adjacent coils, and to connect these to individual receiver channels. This is the configuration of so-called phased-array coils. The individual coil elements can be linear or quadrature, the latter giving a better S/N ratio. Each individual NMR signal has to be processed to a final image before the data can be assembled to a complete image of the region covered by the array. If one just added the signals from the coils together, the gain in S/N ratio would be gone. Figure 14–20 demonstrates the performance of a four-channel body array in comparison with the circularly polarized body coil. The S/N ratio advantage is clearly visible. At least at sites where abdomen or whole-spine imaging is done frequently, the reasonable cost for an array coil extension can be justified.

TRANSMIT AND RECEIVE SYSTEM

The RF electronics of an MR system are designed to generate the pulsed RF output needed for MR and to prepare the signals picked up by the antenna for image processing. The signal paths are illustrated in Figure 14–21.

Transmit Path

The RF pulses required for MR are first digitally synthesized as a series of complex numbers by the sequence-controlling unit. The magnitude of a complex numeric value represents the momentary amplitude, and the phase determines the direction of the B_1 field in the rotating coordinate system.

The series of complex numbers is converted to voltages by two digital-to-analog converters. The bandwidth and the length of the programmed pulse form are determined by the sample clock and the number of data points. The signals are fed into the modulator via two low-pass filters, which suppress any undesirable harmonics caused by the digital generation of the pulse. The function of the modulator corresponds to the transformation from the rotating coordinate system (the phase at the resonance frequency) to the laboratory coordinate system (what the coil actually "sees"). It multiplies the (generally) complex pulse form (the audio frequency signal) $F(t)$ by the complex (quadrature) carrier signal $e^{i\omega_0 t}$. The real portion of the product appears at the output of the modulator and is fed to the RF power transmitter. This type of modulator is frequently referred to as a single-sideband modulator because only one sideband of the amplitude-modulated RF shows up on the output and the other sideband and the carrier signal are sup-

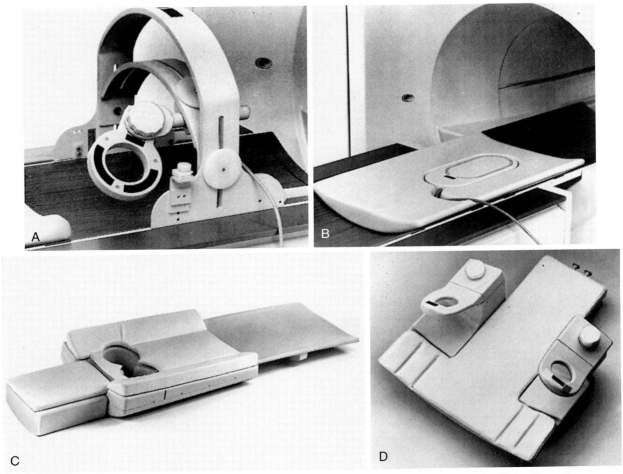

FIGURE 14–19. Examples of surface coils: *(A)* coil for small regions near the surface; *(B)* (lumbar) spine coil; *(C)* female breast (mamma) coil; *(D)* pair of shoulder coils. (*A* to *D* from Morneburg H, ed: Bildgebende Systeme für die medizinische Diagnostik. 3rd ed. Munich: Publicis MCD Verlag, 1995.)

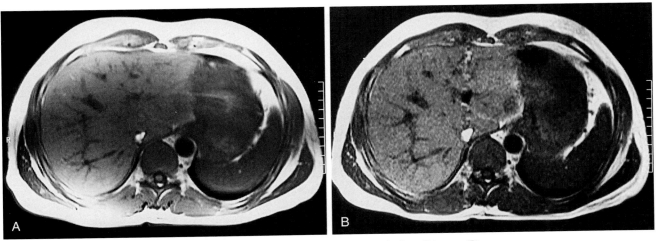

FIGURE 14–20. Array coil image *(A)* versus body coil image *(B)*.

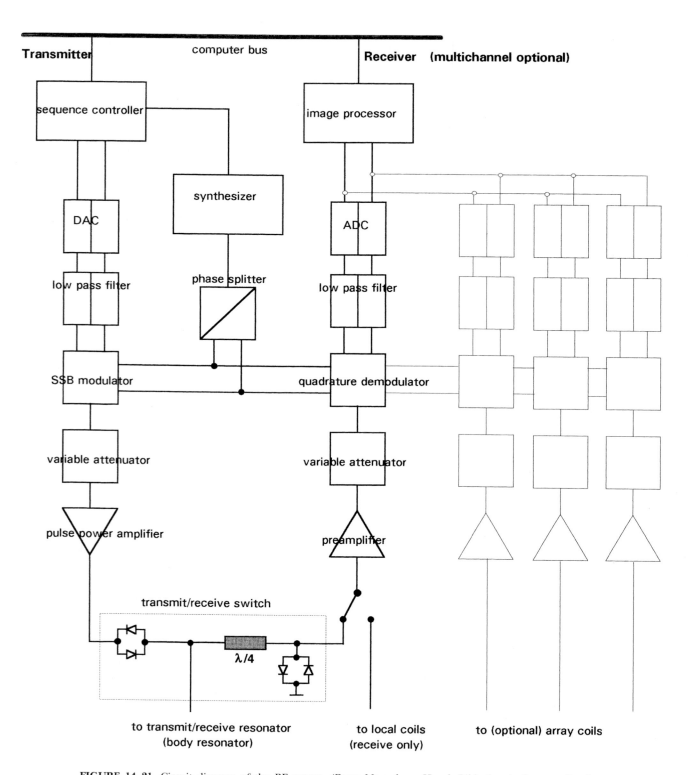

FIGURE 14–21. Circuit diagram of the RF system. (From Morneburg H, ed: Bildgebende Systeme für die medizinische Diagnostik. 3rd ed. Munich: Publicis MCD Verlag, 1995.)

pressed. In newer systems, the modulation is done digitally (digital RF system).

Radiofrequency Power Transmitter

The RF final stage must amplify the pulse so that a B_1 field of sufficient strength is generated in the subject surrounded by the resonator. This field must fulfill the following requirements:

$$B_1 = \alpha/\gamma t_p \qquad (17)$$

where α is the desired flip angle of magnetization and t_p is the effective duration of the B_1 field.

This expression applies to a circularly polarized B_1 field. For a 180° pulse of 1 ms duration B_1 is 11.8 μT. If the RF field is linearly polarized, twice the B_1 amplitude is required for the same flip angle. The power needed depends on the losses in the object being measured as well as in the resonator and its connecting lines. Although in principle it is possible to calculate the power needed for simple lossy objects (like a cylinder filled with conductive water doped with salt), the power requirements are usually deduced from experimental experience because the human body cannot easily be described mathematically. It has been found that approximately 15 kW of peak power is quite sufficient at 63 MHz to allow an effective pulse duration of 0.5 ms or less in most patients when a circularly polarized transmit antenna is used. At a given B_1 the peak power requirements go with the square of B_0. However, the average available output power may be considerably lower.

Mean power is governed by how much the patient's safety would be affected by the absorbed RF power (heating effect) and is enforced through regulations for medical equipment. Thermal dimensioning and the power supply for the final stage are designed for the continuous-output power needs; the energy for a high-output pulse or series of pulses may be taken from a capacitor battery that is recharged during off times.

Receive Path

The receiving channel is shown in the right half of Figure 14–21. The MR signals from the receiver coil are raised to a sufficient level by the preamplifier so that line attenuation and input noise from the following stage are negligible. After further amplification, the signal is demodulated.

Demodulator

The function of the demodulator is inverse to that of the modulator, namely transformation of the laboratory coordinate system into the coordinate system that rotates with ω_0. This is done through multiplication of the RF NMR signal with the quadrature reference signal from the synthesizer $e^{i\omega_0 t}$. At the two outputs of this circuit, which is called a quadrature demodulator, signals representing the magnetization components in the rotating frame M_x and M_y appear. The circuit can

distinguish between frequencies greater and smaller than ω_0 (upper and lower sidebands); therefore, the output bandwidth is half of the input bandwidth. This feature improves the S/N ratio by $\sqrt{2}$ in comparison with simple phase-sensitive rectifiers.[19]

The output signals of the demodulator pass through a pair of low-pass filters that cut off all frequencies that exceed half the sampling (Nyquist) frequency. Finally, two ADCs convert them into a sequence of complex numbers suitable for digital image processing. As with the modulator, quadrature demodulation can be realized digitally; that is, the RF signal (eventually mixed down to a more convenient low or intermediate frequency) is first analog-to-digital converted and then multiplied with $e^{i\omega_0 t}$ and filtered digitally.

Signal Levels

To specify the necessary total receiver gain and dynamic range—that is, the signal limit divided by noise—the expected S/N ratio and input voltage at the preamplifier should be known. As discussed in the section on pulse output, any assumption is valid only to a certain extent because the human body cannot be described by a simple mathematic model. Similarly, coil characteristics cannot be calculated exactly. Therefore, one must rely on the results of empirical studies to design a practical receiver system as well. If the antenna impedance is matched to the actual line impedance R_L via tuning circuits, the noise voltage (U_N) at the input of the preamplifier (input impedance Z_i) is always the same regardless of the coil load.

$$U_N = (4kTR_L\Delta\omega_s/2\pi 10^{F/10dB})^{1/2}|Z_i|/(R_L + |Z_i|) \qquad (18)$$

where F is the noise figure of the preamplifier in decibels. The total gain of the receive channel consists of the gain of the individual components minus the attenuation values of both the attenuator and the cables. The antenna and preamplifier noise, which is dependent on the input bandwidth $\Delta\omega_s$, should be sufficiently higher than the frequency-independent ADC quantization noise $U_{LSB}/\sqrt{12}$. Therefore, for the smallest commonly used bandwidth, U_o/U_i must be

$$\frac{U_o}{U_i} > \frac{U_{LSB}}{\sqrt{12}U_N} \qquad (19)$$

Dynamic Range

The size of a useful signal depends largely on the type of MRI sequence performed, especially on the volume excited. At 63 MHz, the dynamic range of the MR signal may be substantially higher than 100 dB. This means that the S/N gain resulting from the excitation of a large volume (e.g., for three-dimensional imaging) cannot be fully realized with conventional 16-bit ADCs. The adaptability of the preamplifier, as well as the variable attenuation elements in the intermediate amplifier, still allows the processing of high-input signals, for example, with thick slices and with nonselective excitation, as well as low-input signals with thin slices or low-flip-angle sequence even if the MR signal dynamic range exceeds the capabilities of the ADC.

Transmit-Receive Switch

The transmit-receive switch is the link between the RF resonator and the RF pulse transmitter or the pre-amplifier. It must make possible the path from the transmitter to the antenna during the RF pulse and at the same time protect the sensitive preamplifier from the high pulse power. In the receive mode, the weak MR signal must reach the preamplifier with as little attenuation as possible, and the noise of the RF power amplifier must be kept out of the antenna circuit. Figure 14–21 (bottom) shows a simplified diagram of the switch, which automatically switches between transmit and receive without additional control circuitry. The antiparallel pair of diodes in the transmit cable do not conduct during the receive mode. This feature prevents noise generated by the power section from reaching the preamplifier while preventing the MR signal from disappearing into the transmitter. In the transmit mode, the voltages are high enough to switch on the diodes, so that the power reaches the antenna (resonator) with practically no loss. The pair of diodes at the preamplifier input also conduct. The quarter-wavelength cable connected in front of the diodes transforms the short circuit to a high impedance at the input of the antenna. In the receive mode, the impedance of the diodes is high, and the signal reaches the preamplifier virtually unattenuated by the $\lambda/4$ line. The circuit contains other adjustable components that neutralize the diode capacitance.

RADIOFREQUENCY ROOM SHIELDING

Effective antenna shielding against RF interference is essential because of the extreme sensitivity of the receiving system to high-frequency fields. Antenna sensitivity, self-shielding capacity (a function of the length and diameter of the antenna resonator relative to wavelength λ), and estimates of the intensity of possible RF interference (e.g., short-wave broadcasting stations) must all be included when considering the required attenuation factor.

Experience has shown that the shielding factor should be more than 90 dB for almost all practical siting cases.

SUBJECT-DEPENDENT SYSTEM CALIBRATIONS

After the patient has been positioned, the parameters that are influenced by the subject to be measured must be calibrated before the measurement can be started. Calibration procedures for an MR examination are performed as follows after positioning the patient:

1. Adjustment of antennas (coil tuning)
2. Checking and setting the MR center frequency (frequency adjustment)
3. Pulse amplitude calibration (transmitter adjustment)
4. Automatic shim, especially the linear gradients (optional, only if extremely high homogeneity is required, e.g., for spectral saturation purposes)
5. Selection of measurement parameters (or pulse sequence)
6. Setting of the receiver gain (receiver adjustment)

Steps 1 to 4 must be repeated only if the patient has been moved to another position. The selection of measurement parameters (step 5) may initially be performed earlier in this sequence. A receiver adjustment (step 6) is repeatedly required as soon as sequence parameters are changed.

Step 1 can be omitted in certain cases when coil load does not change much from patient to patient (e.g., in the head coil or fixed tune coils). Which steps of the adjustments have to be performed is generally under automatic control of the MR system so the technician does not need to be concerned about them.

ANTENNA ADJUSTMENT (COIL TUNING)

The transmit-receive coil impedance, which is dependent on the size and position of the patient, must first be matched to the impedance of the transmission line. With the help of a fully automatic control system, the capacitors of the matching network are set so that there is minimal reflection of the RF power fed into the antenna.

SETTING THE CENTER FREQUENCY (FREQUENCY ADJUSTMENT)

The next step is the determination of the MR frequency. This would seem to be a superfluous step when dealing with the stability of superconducting magnets, but the frequency changes by tens of hertz from patient to patient because of varying susceptibility. A variation in resonance would cause a noticeable shift in the image corresponding to the gradient strength employed. Resonance frequency can be determined by a simple MR experiment, namely the excitation and readout of a free induction decay, which is Fourier transformed to find the resonance frequency from the peak signal position in the spectrum. The synthesizer is then readjusted accordingly.

PULSE AMPLITUDE CALIBRATION (TRANSMITTER ADJUSTMENT)

Because the degree of efficiency of the transmission antenna, expressed in generated B_1 field per square root of the RF power input, is strongly dependent on the subject of the examination, the pulse amplitude must be adjusted. This adjustment determines the RF output necessary to flip the nuclear magnetization by

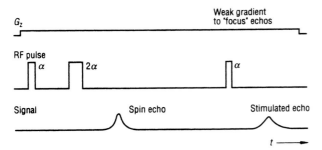

FIGURE 14–22. Pulse sequence used to calibrate the RF transmitter amplitude. (From Morneburg H, ed: Bildgebende Systeme für die medizinische Diagnostik. 3rd ed. Munich: Publicis MCD Verlag, 1995.)

an angle of α by using a pulse of the length t_p. A practical method makes use of the relationship between the primary echo and stimulated-echo signal occurring when using a three-pulse (α-2α-α) sequence[20] as shown in Figure 14–22. In this case,

$$S \text{ (stimulated echo)}/S \text{ (primary echo)} = \cos \alpha/2 \quad (20)$$

The nutation angle α can immediately be calculated from this equation (as long as $0° < \alpha < 360°$). With use of the applied pulse length t_p and the transmitter amplitude determined during calibration, the RF amplitude required for any flip angle for any other pulse form may be calculated.

AUTOMATIC SHIM OF THE LINEAR GRADIENTS

The following method allows an immediate determination of the gradient offset necessary for creating optimal homogeneity inside the object of interest.[21] For this purpose a gradient-echo pulse sequence according to Figure 14–23 is used. If there is an inappropriate bias of the gradient used in the sequence, the echo maximum is shifted away by Δt from the center of the readout interval because the echo maximum

occurs at a time when the integral of the gradient is zero. From Δt and the gradient pulse G applied in the sequence the necessary correction G_{offset} can be calculated:

$$G_{offset} = -\frac{\Delta t \, G}{TE + \Delta t} \quad (21)$$

To compensate for small imperfections of the gradient pulse shape, the sequence is repeated with the inverse gradient pulse and the average of the resulting G_{offset} is taken. This procedure is repeated for all three gradient directions.

RECEIVER GAIN (RECEIVER ADJUSTMENT)

The last step in the calibration process is the adjustment of receiver gain with respect to the maximal MR signal occurring during imaging. This adjustment, discussed in Chapter 3, is important because inappropriate signal levels may introduce image distortion if the ADC is overloaded or increased noise if the ADC is underloaded. The same pulse sequence is used for the receiver adjustment as for imaging, except that the phase-encoding gradient is not switched on to find the MR signal at its maximum. For this reason, the pulse sequence parameters must be selected before this step. If no overload has occurred, the resulting measurement data can be used to calculate the amplifier settings necessary for proper modulation of the receiving components. If this is not the case, the calibration measurement must be repeated using reduced total gain.

REFERENCES

1. Wilson MN: Superconducting Magnets. Oxford, UK: Clarington Press, 1983.
2. Oxford Magnet Technology: Magnets in Clinical Use. Oxford, UK: OMT Publishing, 1983.
3. Hoult DI, Lee D: Shimming a superconducting imaging magnet with steel. Rev Sci Instrum 56:131, 1985.
4. Hoult DI, Chen CN, Sank VJ: The field dependence of NMR imaging. II. Arguments concerning an optimal field strength. Magn Reson Med 3:730, 1986.
5. Loeffler W, Oppelt A, von Wulfen H, Zimmermann B: An approach for selecting the best field strength for proton imaging. In: Proceedings of the Third Annual Meeting of the Society of Magnetic Resonance in Medicine, New York, August 1984, p 483.
6. Bottomley PA, Andrew ER: RF magnetic field penetration, phase shift and power dissipation in biological tissue: Implications for NMR imaging. Phys Med Biol 23:630, 1978.
7. Bottomley PA, Foster TH, Argersinger RE, Pfeifer LM: A review of normal tissue hydrogen NMR relaxation times and relaxation mechanisms from 1–100 MHz: dependence on tissue type, NMR frequency, temperature, species, excision, and age. Med Phys 11:425, 1984.
8. Ljunggren S: A simple graphical representation of Fourier based imaging methods. J Magn Reson 54:33, 1983.
9. Mansfield P, Chapman B: Active magnetic screening of gradient coils in NMR imaging. J Magn Res 66:573, 1986.
10. Stetter E, Oppelt A: Image quality in NMR tomography. In: Proceedings of the World Congress on Medicine, Physics and Biomedical Engineering, Hamburg, September 1982, paper 24.10.
11. Wehrli FW, McFall JR, Glover GH, et al: The dependence of nuclear magnetic resonance (NMR) image contrast on intrinsic and pulse sequence timing parameters. Magn Reson Imaging 2:3, 1984.
12. Budinger TF, Fischer H, Hentschel D, et al: Physiological effects of fast oscillating magnetic field gradients. J Comput Assist Tomogr 15:909, 1991.

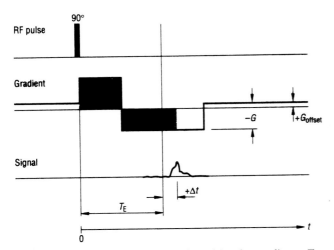

FIGURE 14–23. Pulse sequence used to shim the gradient offset. (From Morneburg H, ed: Bildgebende Systeme für die medizinische Diagnostik. 3rd ed. Munich: Publicis MCD Verlag, 1995.)

13. Hoult DI, Lauterbur PC: The sensitivity of the Zeugmatographic experiment involving human samples. J Magn Reson 34:425, 1979.
14. Roemer PB, Edelstein WA, Hayes CE, et al: The NMR phased array. Magn Reson Med 16:192, 1990.
15. Hayes CE: Radiofrequency coil for NMR. European Patent Application No. 0 151 745, 1985.
16. Krause N: Hochfrequenzfeldeinrichtung für eine Kernresonanzapparatur. German Patent Application No. 32 33 432, 1983.
17. Alderman D, Grant D: An efficient decoupler coil design which reduces heating in conductive samples in superconducting spectrometers. J Magn Reson 36:447, 1979.
18. Hoult DI, Chen CN, Sank VJ: Quadrature detection in the laboratory frame. Magn Reson Med 1:339, 1984.
19. Hoult DI: The NMR receiver: a description and analysis of design. Prog NMR Spectrosc 2:4, 1978.
20. van der Meulen P, van Yperen GH: A novel method for rapid pulse angle optimisation. In: Proceedings of the Society for Magnetic Resonance in Medicine, Montreal, August 1986.
21. Manabe A: Multiple angle projection shim (MAP shim): in vivo shim adjustment up to 2nd order with 0.2 second sequence time. In: Proceedings of the Second Annual Meeting of the Society of Magnetic Resonance, San Francisco, August 1994.

PART II

BRAIN

Brain: Indications, Techniques, and Atlas

MICHAEL V. KLEIN ▪ JOHN R. HESSELINK

Magnetic resonance imaging (MRI) is a dynamic and flexible technology that allows one to tailor each study to the anatomic part of interest and to the disease process. With its dependence on the more biologically variable parameters of proton density, longitudinal relaxation time (T1), and transverse relaxation time (T2), variable image contrast can be achieved by using different pulse sequences and by changing the imaging parameters. Signal intensities on T1-, T2-, and proton density–weighted images relate to specific tissue characteristics. For example, the changing chemistry and physical structure of hematomas over time directly affect the signal intensity on MR images, providing information about the age of the hemorrhage. Moreover, with MRI's multiplanar capability, the imaging plane can be optimized for the anatomic area being studied and the relationship of lesions to eloquent areas of the brain can be defined more accurately.[1] Flow-sensitive pulse sequences and MR angiography yield data about blood flow, as well as displaying the vascular anatomy. Even brain function can be investigated by having a subject perform specific mental tasks and noting changes in regional cerebral blood flow and oxygenation. Finally, MR spectroscopy has enormous potential for providing information about the biochemistry and metabolism of tissues. As an imaging technology, MRI has advanced considerably in the past 10 years, and it continues to evolve as new capabilities are developed.

CLINICAL INDICATIONS

As imaging techniques of the brain, MRI and computed tomography (CT) are both competitive and complementary. In general, CT performs better in cases of trauma and emergent situations. It provides better bone detail and has high sensitivity for acute hemorrhage. Supporting equipment and personnel can be brought directly into the scan room. Scanning in CT is fast. Single scans can be done in 1 second, so that even with uncooperative patients, adequate scans can usually be obtained. CT is far more sensitive than MRI for subarachnoid hemorrhage, and it is also more sensitive for detecting intracranial calcifications.

MRI, on the other hand, functions best as an elective outpatient procedure. Proper screening of patients, equipment, and personnel for ferromagnetic materials, pacemakers, and so on is mandatory to avoid possible catastrophe in the magnet room (see Chapter 13). If proper precautions are in place, emergency studies can be done, but the setup time is longer and the imaging also requires more time. With conventional MRI systems, most pulse sequences take a minimum of 2 minutes. At this time, echo-planar capability is not standard on most systems, but this advanced technology can acquire subsecond MR images.

Because of its high sensitivity for brain water, MRI is generally more sensitive for detecting brain abnormalities during the early stages of disease. For example, in cases of cerebral infarction,[2] brain tumors, or infections,[3] the MR image will become positive earlier than a CT scan. When early diagnosis is critical for favorable outcomes, such as in suspected herpes encephalitis, MRI is the imaging procedure of choice.[4] MRI is exquisitely sensitive for detecting white matter disease, such as multiple sclerosis,[5] progressive multifocal leukoencephalopathy,[6] leukodystrophy,[7] and postinfectious encephalitis.[8] Patients with obvious white matter abnormalities on MR images may have an entirely normal CT scan. Other clinical situations in which MRI discloses abnormalities earlier and more definitively than CT are temporal lobe epilepsy,[9] nonhemorrhagic brain contusions, and traumatic shear injuries.[10]

In general, nonenhancing disease processes are much more apparent with MRI than with CT. When the blood-brain barrier is damaged, enhancement occurs with both gadolinium and iodinated contrast agents on MR images and CT scans, respectively. As a rule, the degree of enhancement is greater on MR images.

For evaluating posterior fossa disease, MRI is preferable to CT. The CT scans are invariably degraded by streaking artifacts from the bones at the skull base. In conjunction with gadolinium enhancement, MRI can reliably detect intracanalicular acoustic neuromas[11] and other schwannomas arising along the cranial nerves within the basal cisterns and foramina of the skull base. Similarly, MRI has largely supplanted CT for imaging the sella turcica and pituitary gland.[12]

The value of MRI for defining congenital malformations is unquestioned. The multiplanar display of anatomy gives important information about the corpus callosum and posterior fossa structures.[13] The superior gray and white contrast allows accurate assessment of myelination.[14]

The phenomenon of flow void within arteries on spin-echo (SE) images, the high sensitivity for chronic hemorrhage and hemosiderin deposition,[15] and the capability of MR angiography give MRI distinct advantages over CT for imaging vascular disease. Vascular stenoses or occlusions, aneurysms,[16] and arteriovenous malformations[17] can be imaged without use of intravenous contrast media. In cases of cryptic vascular malformations and cavernous angiomas, where the angiogram and CT scan are often negative, MRI may reveal small deposits of hemosiderin from prior small hemorrhages.[18]

Along with the function of MRI as a primary imaging procedure, there are indications for MRI as a secondary procedure after the disease has already been demonstrated by CT. In patients with solitary lesions on CT scans, in whom the diagnosis of metastatic disease, abscess, or multiple sclerosis would be strengthened by the finding of additional lesions, MRI may resolve the issue. Similarly, in a patient with brain metastases in whom none of the lesions account for the patient's signs or symptoms, MRI can help evaluate the particular anatomic area of interest. A potential problem in both of these circumstances is the nonspecificity of white matter hyperintensities, and contrast MRI may be necessary to clarify the situation.

IMAGING TECHNIQUES

MRI of the brain has evolved to a point where standard protocols can be set to handle most clinical situations (see Appendix I). Nonetheless, protocols need to be modified in special cases and as software upgrades and new imaging capabilities are added to MRI systems. To properly select a technique, an understanding of the interrelationships of the imaging parameters is required. Signal-to-noise (S/N) ratio and spatial resolution must be balanced against scan time, and compromises must often be made. In addition to the standard parameters, multiple options are available for motion and artifact reduction, and one must know when to use them and be aware of how they limit other parameters. Gradient-echo techniques allow for fast scanning and flow imaging. Finally, decisions must be made about the use of gadolinium-based contrast agents for MRI. The MRI principles of contrast, pulse sequence design, fast scanning, artifacts, and paramagnetic enhancement are covered in detail in Part I of this book. The following overview is intended to guide the physician with MRI techniques.

The scan parameters include repetition time (TR), echo time (TE), matrix size, field of view (FOV), slice thickness, and number of excitations (NEX). The TR and TE are the only parameters that affect the T1 and T2 weighting of SE images. A long TR and a long TE (TR > 1500 ms, TE > 60 ms) provide T2 weighting, whereas a short TR and a short TE (TR < 1000 ms, TE < 30 ms) result in T1-weighted images. The T2-weighted sequence is usually employed as a dual-echo sequence. The first or shorter echo (TE < 30 ms) is proton density weighted, or a mixture of T1 and T2 weighting. In the literature, the proton density–weighted image is also referred to as a mixed T1/T2–weighted image, as the balanced image, or simply as the first echo image. This image is helpful for evaluating periventricular disease, such as multiple sclerosis, because the hyperintense plaques are contrasted to the lower signal intensity cerebrospinal fluid (CSF).

The TR, matrix size, and NEX are the only parameters that affect scan time. Increasing any one of these parameters increases the minimal scan time. Spatial resolution is determined by matrix size, FOV, and slice thickness. Increasing matrix size or decreasing FOV and slice thickness increases spatial resolution, but at the expense of either decreased S/N ratio or increased scan time. To obtain images of high resolution with a high S/N ratio requires longer scan times. All of the scan parameters affect the S/N ratio. The signal within an image can be improved by increasing TR, FOV, slice thickness, and NEX or by decreasing TE and matrix size. The most direct way to increase signal intensity is by increasing NEX, but one must keep in mind that increasing NEX from 2 to 4, for example, doubles the scan time but increases the signal intensity by only $\sqrt{2}$.[19] Finally, TE does not affect scan time; however, it does determine the maximal number of slices in multislice mode. Increasing the TE or shortening the TR decreases the number of slices that can be obtained with one pulse sequence.

Conventional SE has been the workhorse for imaging the central nervous system. It provides good tissue contrast and has high sensitivity for abnormalities. The fast spin-echo (FSE) sequence is based on the original Carr-Purcell-Meiboom-Gill (CPMG) echo train. In 1986, Hennig and colleagues[20] proposed the rapid acquisition with relaxation enhancement (RARE) sequence, and all FSE methods are based on that sequence. For FSE, the initial 90° radiofrequency (RF) pulse is followed by multiple 180° RF pulses to generate a series of echoes. An echo train is produced, but unlike in the Carr-Purcell-Meiboom-Gill sequence, each echo is acquired with a different phase-encoding gradient. Pulse sequence variables unique to FSE include echo train length, echo spacing, and effective TE. Compared with conventional SE, FSE sequences are faster and yield higher S/N ratios. The primary disadvantages of FSE are increased fat signal intensity on T2-weighted images and decreased sensitivity for magnetic susceptibility. The reader is referred to Part I for further details on the FSE technique.

Studies have shown that T2-weighted images are most sensitive for detecting brain disease, so patients with suspected intracranial disease should be screened with a T2-weighted SE or FSE sequence (TR 3400 ms, effective TE 17/102 ms). The axial plane is commonly used because of our familiarity with the anatomy from CT. As outlined in Appendix I, the other scan parameters include a 256 × 256 matrix, 1 NEX, 22-cm FOV, and 5-mm slice thickness for a scan time of less than 4 minutes and a voxel size of 5 × 0.86 × 0.86 mm. A 2.5-mm interslice gap prevents RF interference between slices.[21]

If an abnormality is found, additional scans help characterize the lesion. Nonenhanced T1-weighted images are needed only if the preliminary scans suggest hemorrhage, lipoma, or dermoid. Otherwise, contrast medium–enhanced scans are recommended. Gadolinium-based contrast agents for MRI are paramagnetic and have demonstrated excellent biologic tolerance. No significant complications or side effects have been reported. The agent is injected intravenously at a dose of 0.1 mmol/kg. The gadolinium contrast agents do not cross the intact blood-brain barrier. If the blood-brain barrier is disrupted by a disease process, the contrast agent diffuses into the interstitial space and shortens the T1 relaxation time of the tissue, resulting in increased signal intensity on T1-weighted images.[22] The scans should be acquired between 3 and 30 minutes after injection for optimal results.

Enhancement with contrast medium is especially helpful for extra-axial tumors because they tend to be isointense to brain on plain scans, but it also identifies areas of blood-brain barrier breakdown associated with intra-axial lesions. Gadolinium enhancement is essential for detecting leptomeningeal inflammatory and neoplastic processes. Contrast scans are obtained routinely in patients with symptoms of pituitary adenoma (e.g., elevated prolactin, growth hormone) or acoustic neuroma (sensorineural hearing loss). To screen for brain metastases in patients with a known primary tumor, contrast medium–enhanced T1-weighted images alone are probably sufficient.[23]

Gadolinium does not enhance rapidly flowing blood. If vascular structures are not adequately seen on a plain scan, the positive contrast provided by gradient-echo techniques or MR angiography may be helpful to confirm or disprove a suspected carotid occlusion or cerebral aneurysm, to evaluate the integrity of the venous sinuses, and to assess the vascularity of lesions. Gradient-echo imaging also enhances the magnetic

susceptibility effects of acute and chronic hemorrhage, making them easily observable, even on low-field and mid-field MR systems. Finally, using lower flip angles, gradient-echo sequences are efficient for obtaining a few T2-weighted images of a focal area.

Although the axial plane is the primary plane for imaging the brain, the multiplanar capability of MRI allows one to select the optimal plane to visualize the anatomy of interest. Coronal views are good for parasagittal lesions near the vertex and lesions immediately above or below the lateral ventricles (corpus callosum or thalamus), temporal lobes, sella, and internal auditory canals. The coronal plane can be used as the primary plane of imaging in patients with temporal lobe seizures. Sagittal views are useful for midline lesions (sella, third ventricle, corpus callosum, pineal region), and for the brain stem and cerebellar vermis.

As outlined in the protocols, scan techniques are slightly different for the sella and cerebellopontine angle. For the sella, the plain and enhanced scans are obtained in the coronal and sagittal planes using a smaller FOV and thin (3 mm or less) contiguous or overlapping sections. For patients with a sensorineural hearing loss or suspected acoustic neuroma, enhanced scans with T1 weighting are obtained through the internal auditory canals, again using thin overlapping sections.

Specialized techniques for reducing motion and artifacts on the images also have applications for brain imaging. Gradient motion rephasing or flow compensation techniques effectively reduce ghost artifacts resulting from CSF flow. They should be used for T2-weighted SE imaging (not compatible with FSE sequences) and gradient-echo acquisitions, but not for T1-weighted imaging because they increase the signal from CSF. Flow compensation techniques do not contribute to specific absorption rate (a measure of power deposition), but the extra gradient pulses lengthen the minimal TE, and gradient heating may limit the number of slices, the minimal FOV, and the slice thickness.[24] Cardiac gating also reduces artifacts from CSF pulsations, resulting in superior object contrast and resolving power in the temporal lobes, basal ganglia, and brain stem.[25]

Saturation techniques use extra RF pulses to eliminate artifacts from moving tissues outside the imaging volume, such as from swallowing or respiratory motion, and from unsaturated protons that enter the imaging volume through vascular channels.[26] Saturation techniques should be used for T1-weighted imaging of the sella and internal auditory canals. The extra RF pulses increase the specific absorption rate and take time, lengthening the minimal TR or decreasing the maximal number of slices in a multislice mode.

Methods for eliminating wraparound or aliasing should be prescribed for imaging small anatomic areas, such as the sella and internal auditory canals, with smaller FOVs. The "no phase wrap" option is most effective in the anteroposterior direction for sagittal and axial scans.

ATLAS

The brain images were obtained by using a 1.5-T MR scanner. Pulse sequences and other pertinent scan parameters were as follows:

- **Sagittal T1-weighted images**
  Inversion recovery, TI 708 ms, TR 1500 ms, TE 25 ms, FOV 24 cm, slice thickness 5 mm, matrix 256 × 256, NEX 2
- **Coronal T1-weighted images**
  Inversion recovery, TI 708 ms, TR 1500 ms, TE 25 ms, FOV 24 cm, slice thickness 5 mm, matrix 256 × 256, NEX 2
- **Axial T2-weighted images**
  FSE, echo train 8, TR 3400 ms, TE 102 ms, FOV 22 cm, slice thickness 5 mm, matrix 256 × 256, NEX 2
- **Axial brain stem T2-weighted images**
  FSE, echo train 8, TR 2500 ms, TE 108 ms, FOV 16 cm, slice thickness 4 mm, matrix 256 × 256, NEX 4

Image labels in *italics* indicate locations of structures that lack contrast from the surrounding brain, such as brain stem nuclei and small fiber tracts.[27, 28]

SAGITTAL T1 WEIGHTED

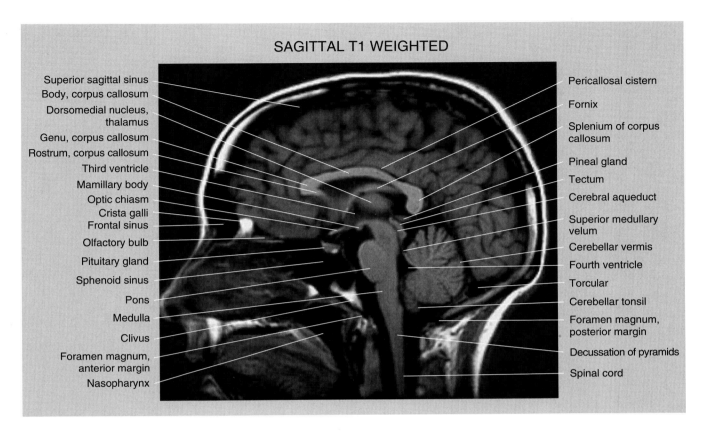

Superior sagittal sinus
Body, corpus callosum
Dorsomedial nucleus, thalamus
Genu, corpus callosum
Rostrum, corpus callosum
Third ventricle
Mamillary body
Optic chiasm
Crista galli
Frontal sinus
Olfactory bulb
Pituitary gland
Sphenoid sinus
Pons
Medulla
Clivus
Foramen magnum, anterior margin
Nasopharynx

Pericallosal cistern
Fornix
Splenium of corpus callosum
Pineal gland
Tectum
Cerebral aqueduct
Superior medullary velum
Cerebellar vermis
Fourth ventricle
Torcular
Cerebellar tonsil
Foramen magnum, posterior margin
Decussation of pyramids
Spinal cord

SAGITTAL T1 WEIGHTED

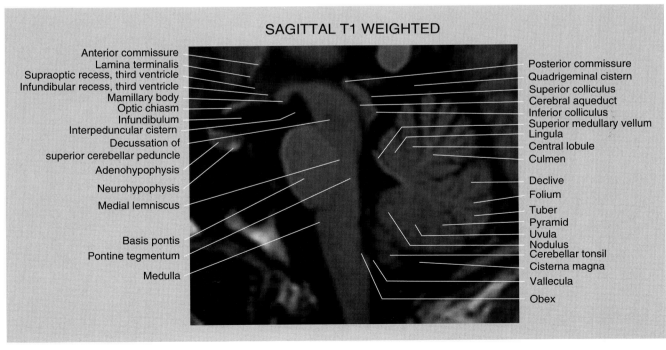

Anterior commissure
Lamina terminalis
Supraoptic recess, third ventricle
Infundibular recess, third ventricle
Mamillary body
Optic chiasm
Infundibulum
Interpeduncular cistern
Decussation of superior cerebellar peduncle
Adenohypophysis
Neurohypophysis
Medial lemniscus
Basis pontis
Pontine tegmentum
Medulla

Posterior commissure
Quadrigeminal cistern
Superior colliculus
Cerebral aqueduct
Inferior colliculus
Superior medullary vellum
Lingula
Central lobule
Culmen
Declive
Folium
Tuber
Pyramid
Uvula
Nodulus
Cerebellar tonsil
Cisterna magna
Vallecula
Obex

SAGITTAL T1 WEIGHTED

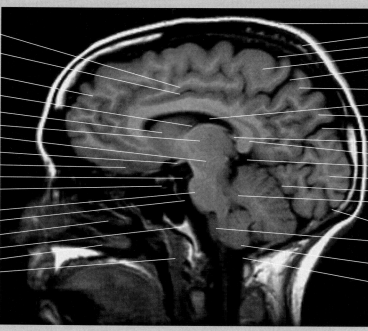

Cingulate gyrus
Cingulate sulcus
Frontal lobe
Caudothalamic groove
Head, caudate nucleus
Thalamus
Red nucleus
Optic chiasm
Gyrus rectus
Oculomotor nerve (III)
Internal carotid artery, cavernous portion
Pons
Prepontine cistern
Middle turbinate
Clivus
Inferior turbinate
Longus colli and Longus capitis muscles

Scalp
Diploë
Central sulcus
Paracentral lobule
Marginal branch of cingulate sulcus
Superior parietal lobule
Lateral ventricle
Precuneus
Parieto-occipital fissure
Crus, fornix
Splenium of corpus callosum
Quadrigeminal cistern
Occipital lobe
Tentorium cerebelli
Superior cerebellar peduncle (brachium conjunctivum)
Calcarine fissure
Inferior olive of medulla oblongata
Cerebellar tonsil
Cisterna magna

SAGITTAL T1 WEIGHTED

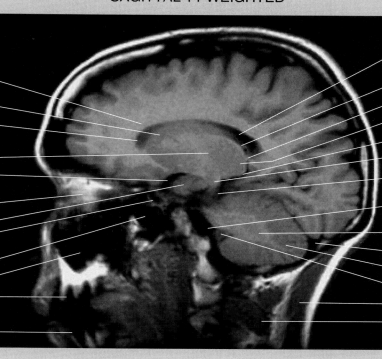

Corpus callosum
Caudate nucleus
Anterior horn of lateral ventricle
Thalamus
Sylvian fissure with middle cerebral artery
Orbital fat
Uncus
Internal carotid artery, cavernous portion
Sphenoid sinus
Maxillary sinus
Maxillary teeth
Mandibular teeth

Lateral ventricle
Stria medullaris thalami
Fornix
Pulvinar
Ambient wing cistern
Cerebral peduncle
Edge of tentorium cerebelli in ambient cistern
Cerebellopontine angle cistern
Corpus medullare
Transverse sinus
Cerebellar hemisphere
Cranial nerves VII and VIII
Trapezius muscle
Inferior oblique muscle

SAGITTAL T1 WEIGHTED

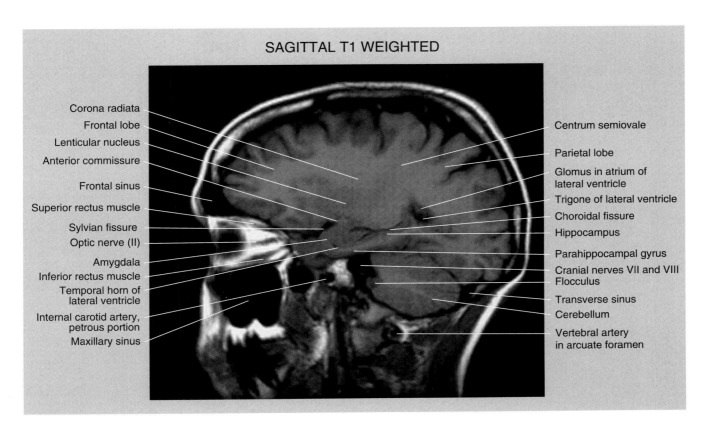

Corona radiata
Frontal lobe
Lenticular nucleus
Anterior commissure
Frontal sinus
Superior rectus muscle
Sylvian fissure
Optic nerve (II)
Amygdala
Inferior rectus muscle
Temporal horn of
lateral ventricle
Internal carotid artery,
petrous portion
Maxillary sinus

Centrum semiovale
Parietal lobe
Glomus in atrium of
lateral ventricle
Trigone of lateral ventricle
Choroidal fissure
Hippocampus
Parahippocampal gyrus
Cranial nerves VII and VIII
Flocculus
Transverse sinus
Cerebellum
Vertebral artery
in arcuate foramen

SAGITTAL T1 WEIGHTED

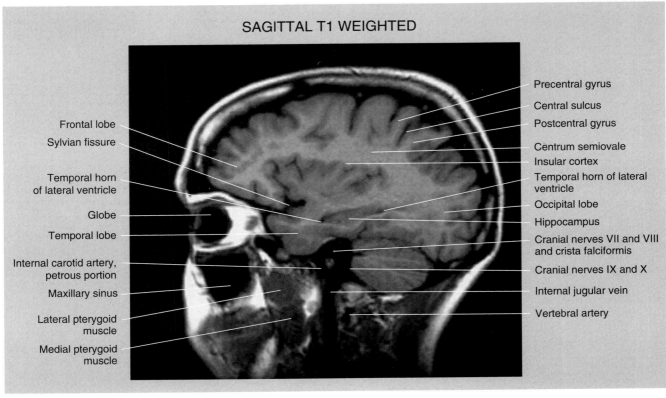

Frontal lobe
Sylvian fissure
Temporal horn
of lateral ventricle
Globe
Temporal lobe
Internal carotid artery,
petrous portion
Maxillary sinus
Lateral pterygoid
muscle
Medial pterygoid
muscle

Precentral gyrus
Central sulcus
Postcentral gyrus
Centrum semiovale
Insular cortex
Temporal horn of lateral
ventricle
Occipital lobe
Hippocampus
Cranial nerves VII and VIII
and crista falciformis
Cranial nerves IX and X
Internal jugular vein
Vertebral artery

SAGITTAL T1 WEIGHTED

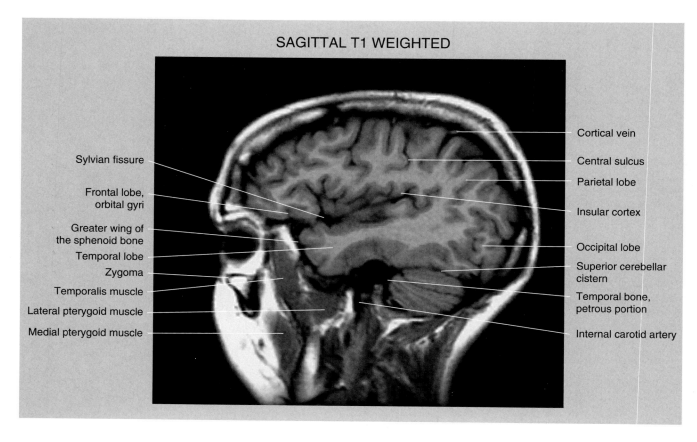

Sylvian fissure

Frontal lobe, orbital gyri

Greater wing of the sphenoid bone

Temporal lobe

Zygoma

Temporalis muscle

Lateral pterygoid muscle

Medial pterygoid muscle

Cortical vein

Central sulcus

Parietal lobe

Insular cortex

Occipital lobe

Superior cerebellar cistern

Temporal bone, petrous portion

Internal carotid artery

SAGITTAL T1 WEIGHTED

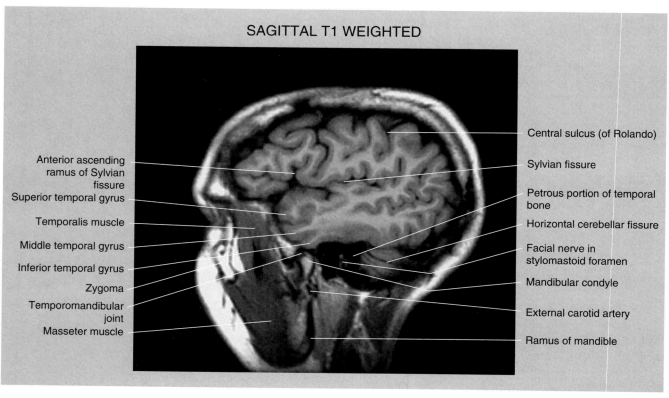

Anterior ascending ramus of Sylvian fissure

Superior temporal gyrus

Temporalis muscle

Middle temporal gyrus

Inferior temporal gyrus

Zygoma

Temporomandibular joint

Masseter muscle

Central sulcus (of Rolando)

Sylvian fissure

Petrous portion of temporal bone

Horizontal cerebellar fissure

Facial nerve in stylomastoid foramen

Mandibular condyle

External carotid artery

Ramus of mandible

CORONAL T1 WEIGHTED

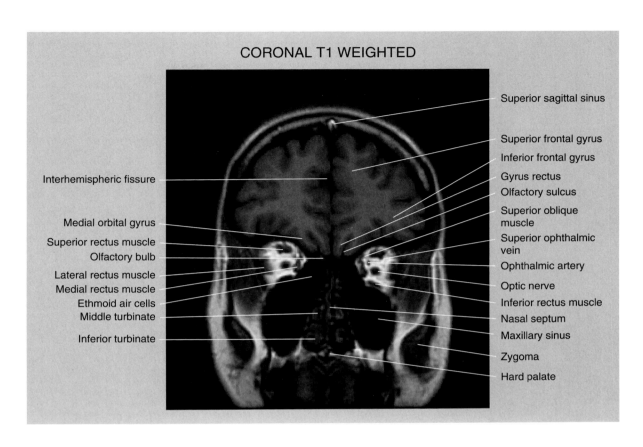

Interhemispheric fissure

Medial orbital gyrus
Superior rectus muscle
Olfactory bulb
Lateral rectus muscle
Medial rectus muscle
Ethmoid air cells
Middle turbinate
Inferior turbinate

Superior sagittal sinus

Superior frontal gyrus
Inferior frontal gyrus
Gyrus rectus
Olfactory sulcus
Superior oblique muscle
Superior ophthalmic vein
Ophthalmic artery
Optic nerve
Inferior rectus muscle
Nasal septum
Maxillary sinus
Zygoma
Hard palate

CORONAL T1 WEIGHTED

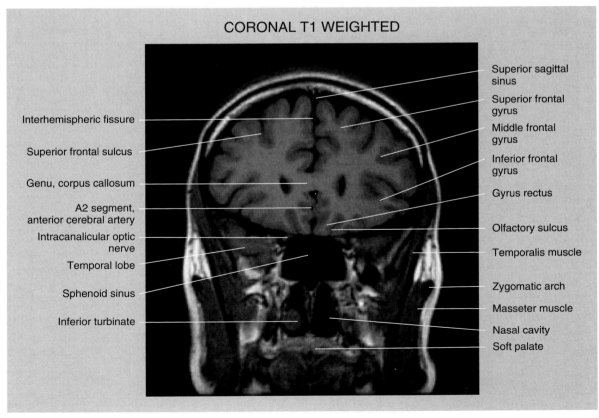

Interhemispheric fissure

Superior frontal sulcus

Genu, corpus callosum

A2 segment, anterior cerebral artery
Intracanalicular optic nerve
Temporal lobe

Sphenoid sinus

Inferior turbinate

Superior sagittal sinus

Superior frontal gyrus

Middle frontal gyrus

Inferior frontal gyrus

Gyrus rectus

Olfactory sulcus

Temporalis muscle

Zygomatic arch

Masseter muscle

Nasal cavity
Soft palate

CORONAL T1 WEIGHTED

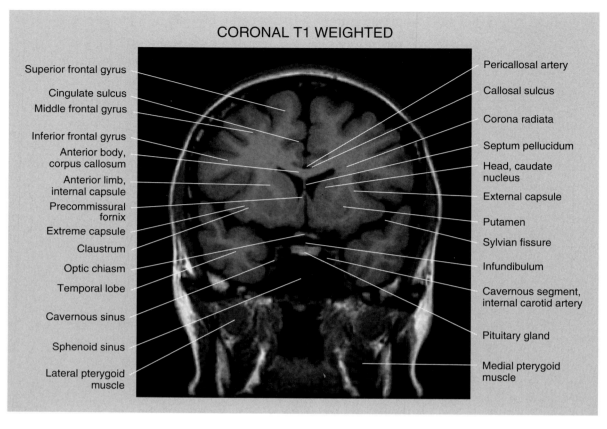

Superior frontal gyrus
Cingulate sulcus
Middle frontal gyrus
Inferior frontal gyrus
Anterior body, corpus callosum
Anterior limb, internal capsule
Precommissural fornix
Extreme capsule
Claustrum
Optic chiasm
Temporal lobe
Cavernous sinus
Sphenoid sinus
Lateral pterygoid muscle

Pericallosal artery
Callosal sulcus
Corona radiata
Septum pellucidum
Head, caudate nucleus
External capsule
Putamen
Sylvian fissure
Infundibulum
Cavernous segment, internal carotid artery
Pituitary gland
Medial pterygoid muscle

CORONAL T1 WEIGHTED

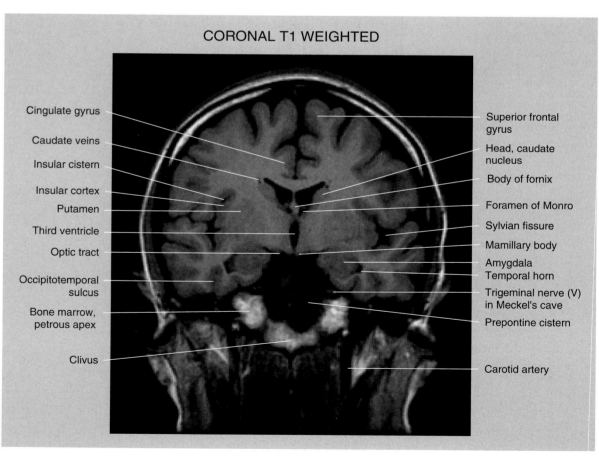

Cingulate gyrus
Caudate veins
Insular cistern
Insular cortex
Putamen
Third ventricle
Optic tract
Occipitotemporal sulcus
Bone marrow, petrous apex
Clivus

Superior frontal gyrus
Head, caudate nucleus
Body of fornix
Foramen of Monro
Sylvian fissure
Mamillary body
Amygdala
Temporal horn
Trigeminal nerve (V) in Meckel's cave
Prepontine cistern
Carotid artery

CORONAL T1 WEIGHTED

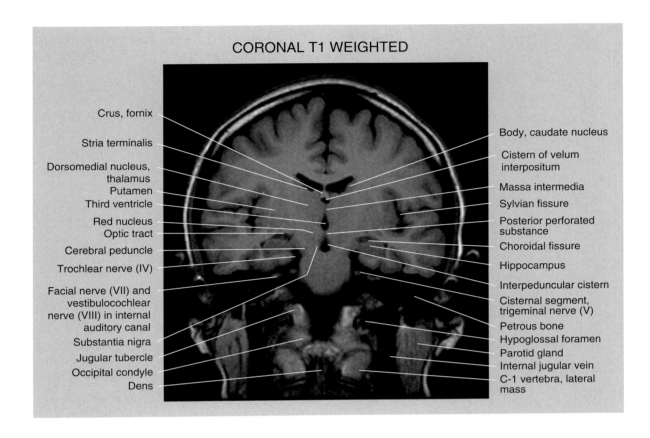

Crus, fornix

Stria terminalis

Dorsomedial nucleus, thalamus

Putamen

Third ventricle

Red nucleus

Optic tract

Cerebral peduncle

Trochlear nerve (IV)

Facial nerve (VII) and vestibulocochlear nerve (VIII) in internal auditory canal

Substantia nigra

Jugular tubercle

Occipital condyle

Dens

Body, caudate nucleus

Cistern of velum interpositum

Massa intermedia

Sylvian fissure

Posterior perforated substance

Choroidal fissure

Hippocampus

Interpeduncular cistern

Cisternal segment, trigeminal nerve (V)

Petrous bone

Hypoglossal foramen

Parotid gland

Internal jugular vein

C-1 vertebra, lateral mass

CORONAL T1 WEIGHTED

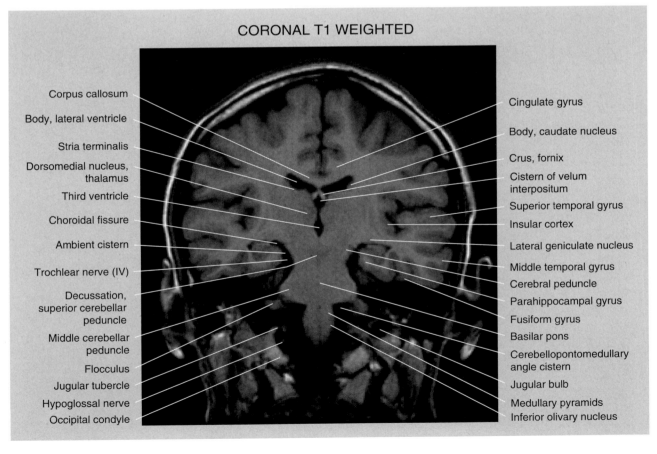

Corpus callosum

Body, lateral ventricle

Stria terminalis

Dorsomedial nucleus, thalamus

Third ventricle

Choroidal fissure

Ambient cistern

Trochlear nerve (IV)

Decussation, superior cerebellar peduncle

Middle cerebellar peduncle

Flocculus

Jugular tubercle

Hypoglossal nerve

Occipital condyle

Cingulate gyrus

Body, caudate nucleus

Crus, fornix

Cistern of velum interpositum

Superior temporal gyrus

Insular cortex

Lateral geniculate nucleus

Middle temporal gyrus

Cerebral peduncle

Parahippocampal gyrus

Fusiform gyrus

Basilar pons

Cerebellopontomedullary angle cistern

Jugular bulb

Medullary pyramids

Inferior olivary nucleus

CORONAL T1 WEIGHTED

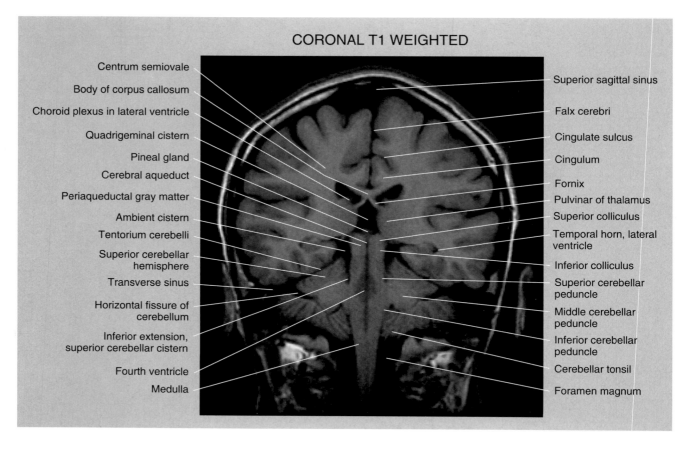

Centrum semiovale

Body of corpus callosum

Choroid plexus in lateral ventricle

Quadrigeminal cistern

Pineal gland

Cerebral aqueduct

Periaqueductal gray matter

Ambient cistern

Tentorium cerebelli

Superior cerebellar hemisphere

Transverse sinus

Horizontal fissure of cerebellum

Inferior extension, superior cerebellar cistern

Fourth ventricle

Medulla

Superior sagittal sinus

Falx cerebri

Cingulate sulcus

Cingulum

Fornix

Pulvinar of thalamus

Superior colliculus

Temporal horn, lateral ventricle

Inferior colliculus

Superior cerebellar peduncle

Middle cerebellar peduncle

Inferior cerebellar peduncle

Cerebellar tonsil

Foramen magnum

CORONAL T1 WEIGHTED

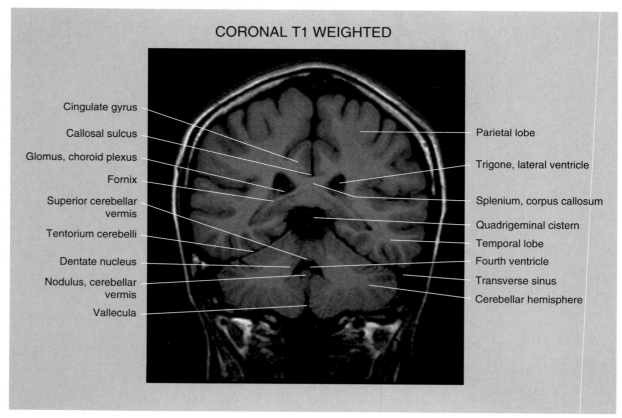

Cingulate gyrus

Callosal sulcus

Glomus, choroid plexus

Fornix

Superior cerebellar vermis

Tentorium cerebelli

Dentate nucleus

Nodulus, cerebellar vermis

Vallecula

Parietal lobe

Trigone, lateral ventricle

Splenium, corpus callosum

Quadrigeminal cistern

Temporal lobe

Fourth ventricle

Transverse sinus

Cerebellar hemisphere

AXIAL T2 WEIGHTED

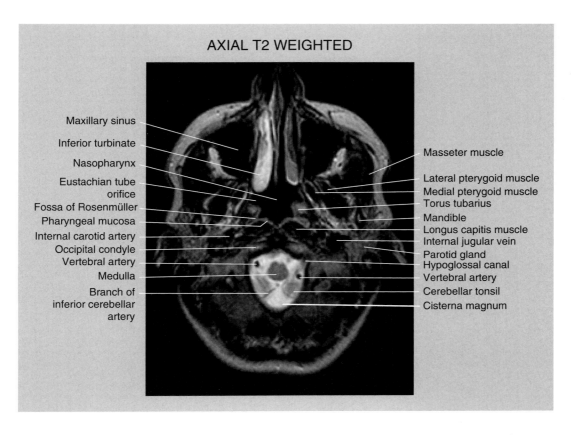

Maxillary sinus
Inferior turbinate
Nasopharynx
Eustachian tube orifice
Fossa of Rosenmüller
Pharyngeal mucosa
Internal carotid artery
Occipital condyle
Vertebral artery
Medulla
Branch of inferior cerebellar artery

Masseter muscle
Lateral pterygoid muscle
Medial pterygoid muscle
Torus tubarius
Mandible
Longus capitis muscle
Internal jugular vein
Parotid gland
Hypoglossal canal
Vertebral artery
Cerebellar tonsil
Cisterna magnum

AXIAL T2 WEIGHTED

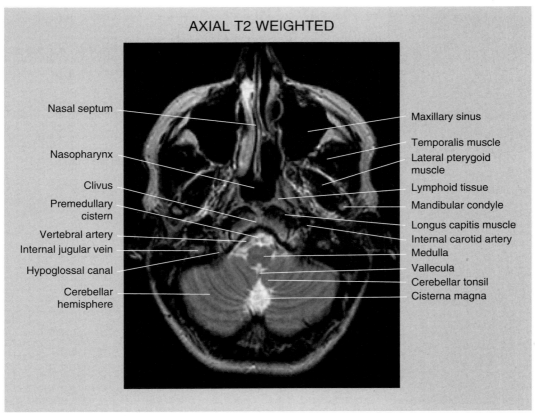

Nasal septum
Nasopharynx
Clivus
Premedullary cistern
Vertebral artery
Internal jugular vein
Hypoglossal canal
Cerebellar hemisphere

Maxillary sinus
Temporalis muscle
Lateral pterygoid muscle
Lymphoid tissue
Mandibular condyle
Longus capitis muscle
Internal carotid artery
Medulla
Vallecula
Cerebellar tonsil
Cisterna magna

AXIAL T2 WEIGHTED

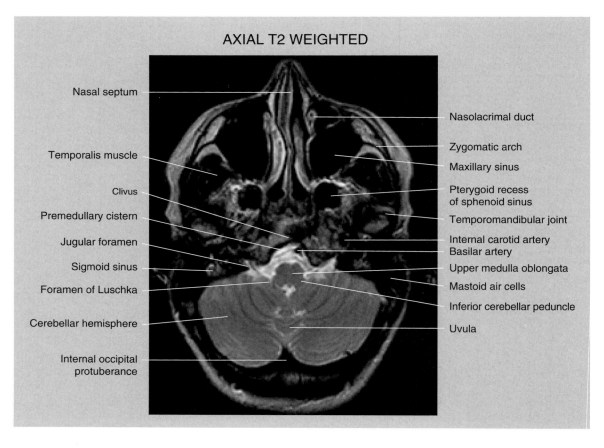

Nasal septum

Temporalis muscle

Clivus

Premedullary cistern

Jugular foramen

Sigmoid sinus

Foramen of Luschka

Cerebellar hemisphere

Internal occipital protuberance

Nasolacrimal duct

Zygomatic arch

Maxillary sinus

Pterygoid recess of sphenoid sinus

Temporomandibular joint

Internal carotid artery
Basilar artery

Upper medulla oblongata

Mastoid air cells

Inferior cerebellar peduncle

Uvula

AXIAL T2 WEIGHTED

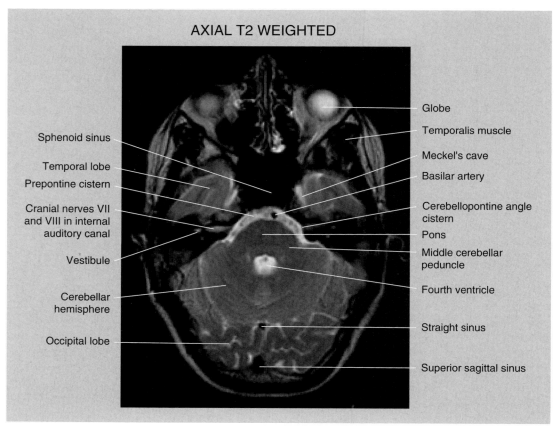

Sphenoid sinus

Temporal lobe

Prepontine cistern

Cranial nerves VII and VIII in internal auditory canal

Vestibule

Cerebellar hemisphere

Occipital lobe

Globe

Temporalis muscle

Meckel's cave

Basilar artery

Cerebellopontine angle cistern

Pons

Middle cerebellar peduncle

Fourth ventricle

Straight sinus

Superior sagittal sinus

AXIAL T2 WEIGHTED

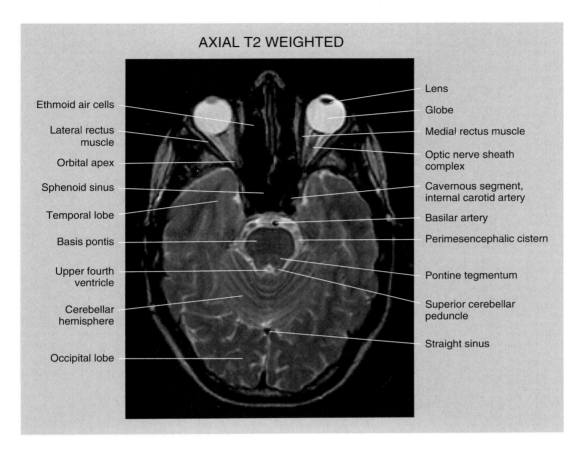

Ethmoid air cells
Lateral rectus muscle
Orbital apex
Sphenoid sinus
Temporal lobe
Basis pontis
Upper fourth ventricle
Cerebellar hemisphere
Occipital lobe

Lens
Globe
Medial rectus muscle
Optic nerve sheath complex
Cavernous segment, internal carotid artery
Basilar artery
Perimesencephalic cistern
Pontine tegmentum
Superior cerebellar peduncle
Straight sinus

AXIAL T2 WEIGHTED

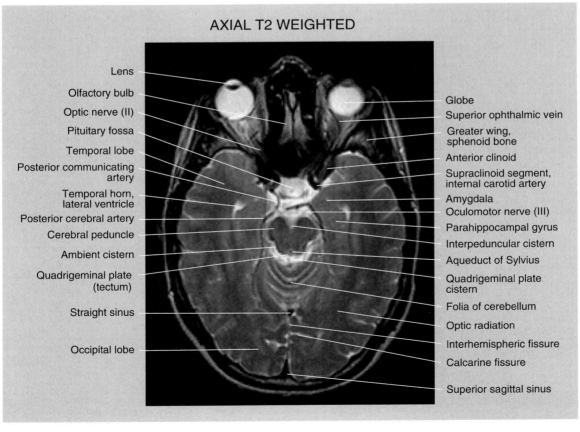

Lens
Olfactory bulb
Optic nerve (II)
Pituitary fossa
Temporal lobe
Posterior communicating artery
Temporal horn, lateral ventricle
Posterior cerebral artery
Cerebral peduncle
Ambient cistern
Quadrigeminal plate (tectum)
Straight sinus
Occipital lobe

Globe
Superior ophthalmic vein
Greater wing, sphenoid bone
Anterior clinoid
Supraclinoid segment, internal carotid artery
Amygdala
Oculomotor nerve (III)
Parahippocampal gyrus
Interpeduncular cistern
Aqueduct of Sylvius
Quadrigeminal plate cistern
Folia of cerebellum
Optic radiation
Interhemispheric fissure
Calcarine fissure
Superior sagittal sinus

AXIAL T2 WEIGHTED

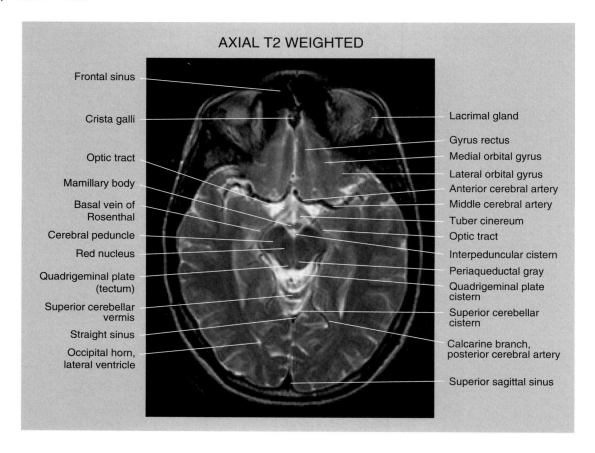

Frontal sinus

Crista galli

Optic tract

Mamillary body

Basal vein of Rosenthal

Cerebral peduncle

Red nucleus

Quadrigeminal plate (tectum)

Superior cerebellar vermis

Straight sinus

Occipital horn, lateral ventricle

Lacrimal gland

Gyrus rectus

Medial orbital gyrus

Lateral orbital gyrus

Anterior cerebral artery

Middle cerebral artery

Tuber cinereum

Optic tract

Interpeduncular cistern

Periaqueductal gray

Quadrigeminal plate cistern

Superior cerebellar cistern

Calcarine branch, posterior cerebral artery

Superior sagittal sinus

AXIAL T2 WEIGHTED

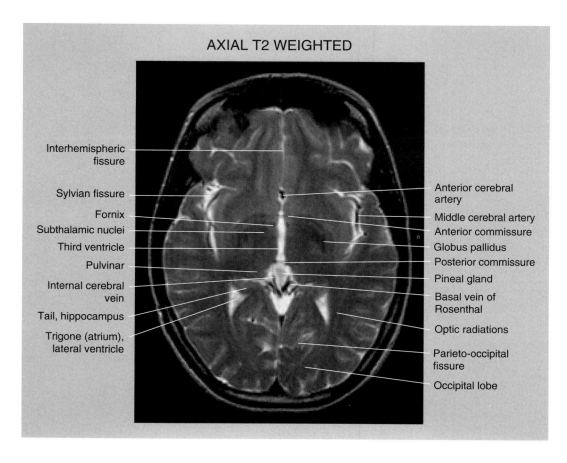

Interhemispheric fissure

Sylvian fissure

Fornix

Subthalamic nuclei

Third ventricle

Pulvinar

Internal cerebral vein

Tail, hippocampus

Trigone (atrium), lateral ventricle

Anterior cerebral artery

Middle cerebral artery

Anterior commissure

Globus pallidus

Posterior commissure

Pineal gland

Basal vein of Rosenthal

Optic radiations

Parieto-occipital fissure

Occipital lobe

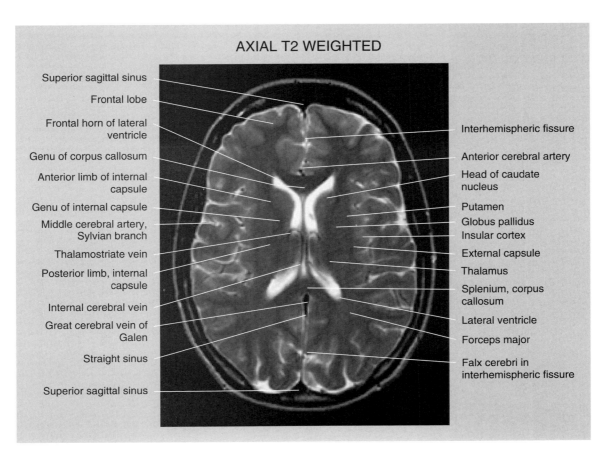

AXIAL T2 WEIGHTED

Interhemispheric fissure
Cingulate gyrus
Anterior limb, internal capsule
Fornix
Posterior limb, internal capsule
Insular cortex
Dorsomedial nucleus, thalamus
Pulvinar
Corpus callosum, splenium
Glomus in trigone, lateral ventricle
Straight sinus
Diploë, occipital bone

Frontal lobe
Frontal horn, lateral ventricle
Pericallosal artery
Head of caudate nucleus
Putamen
Globus pallidus
Foramen of Monro
Third ventricle
Internal cerebral vein in velum interpositum
Vein of Galen
Superior sagittal sinus

AXIAL T2 WEIGHTED

Superior sagittal sinus
Frontal lobe
Frontal horn of lateral ventricle
Genu of corpus callosum
Anterior limb of internal capsule
Genu of internal capsule
Middle cerebral artery, Sylvian branch
Thalamostriate vein
Posterior limb, internal capsule
Internal cerebral vein
Great cerebral vein of Galen
Straight sinus
Superior sagittal sinus

Interhemispheric fissure
Anterior cerebral artery
Head of caudate nucleus
Putamen
Globus pallidus
Insular cortex
External capsule
Thalamus
Splenium, corpus callosum
Lateral ventricle
Forceps major
Falx cerebri in interhemispheric fissure

AXIAL T2 WEIGHTED

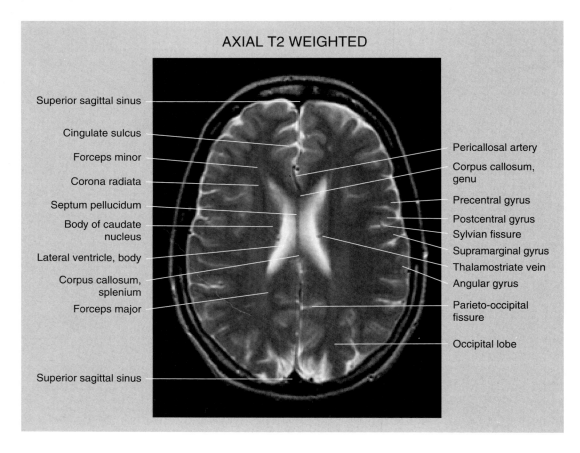

Superior sagittal sinus

Cingulate sulcus

Forceps minor

Corona radiata

Septum pellucidum

Body of caudate nucleus

Lateral ventricle, body

Corpus callosum, splenium

Forceps major

Superior sagittal sinus

Pericallosal artery

Corpus callosum, genu

Precentral gyrus

Postcentral gyrus

Sylvian fissure

Supramarginal gyrus

Thalamostriate vein

Angular gyrus

Parieto-occipital fissure

Occipital lobe

AXIAL T2 WEIGHTED

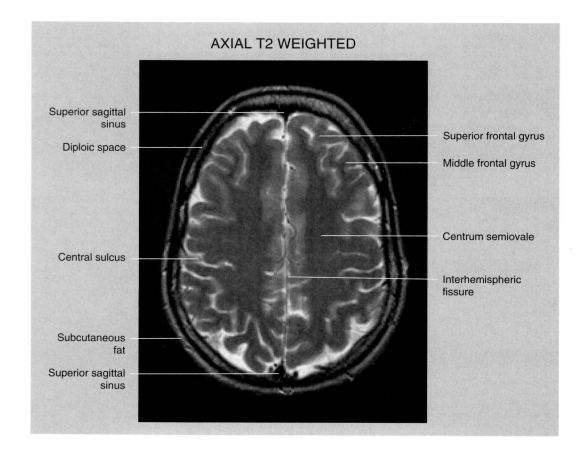

Superior sagittal sinus

Diploic space

Central sulcus

Subcutaneous fat

Superior sagittal sinus

Superior frontal gyrus

Middle frontal gyrus

Centrum semiovale

Interhemispheric fissure

AXIAL T2 WEIGHTED

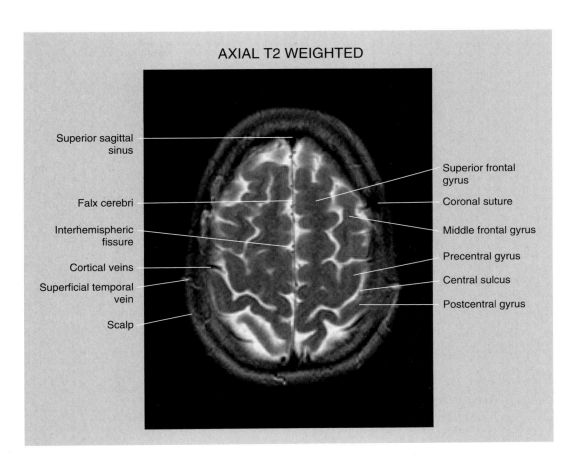

Superior sagittal sinus

Falx cerebri

Interhemispheric fissure

Cortical veins

Superficial temporal vein

Scalp

Superior frontal gyrus

Coronal suture

Middle frontal gyrus

Precentral gyrus

Central sulcus

Postcentral gyrus

AXIAL BRAIN STEM T2 WEIGHTED

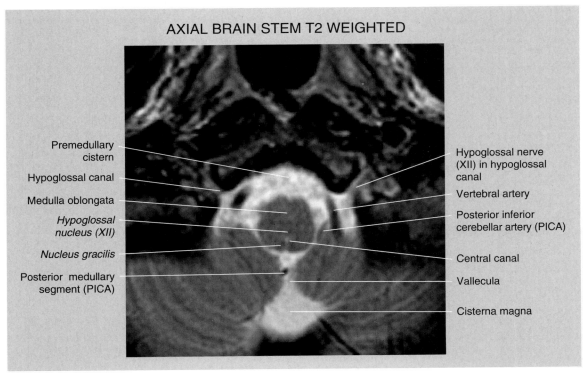

Premedullary cistern

Hypoglossal canal

Medulla oblongata

Hypoglossal nucleus (XII)

Nucleus gracilis

Posterior medullary segment (PICA)

Hypoglossal nerve (XII) in hypoglossal canal

Vertebral artery

Posterior inferior cerebellar artery (PICA)

Central canal

Vallecula

Cisterna magna

AXIAL BRAIN STEM T2 WEIGHTED

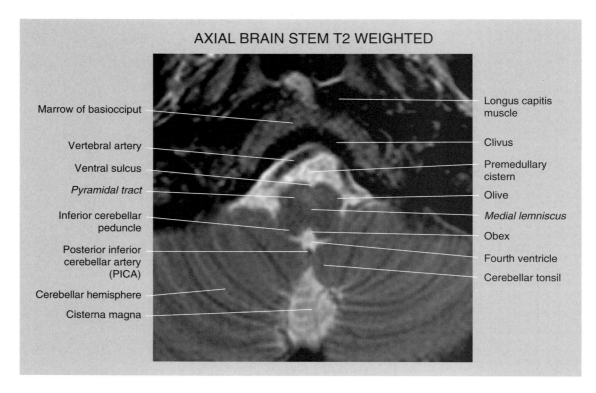

Marrow of basiocciput

Vertebral artery

Ventral sulcus

Pyramidal tract

Inferior cerebellar peduncle

Posterior inferior cerebellar artery (PICA)

Cerebellar hemisphere

Cisterna magna

Longus capitis muscle

Clivus

Premedullary cistern

Olive

Medial lemniscus

Obex

Fourth ventricle

Cerebellar tonsil

AXIAL BRAIN STEM T2 WEIGHTED

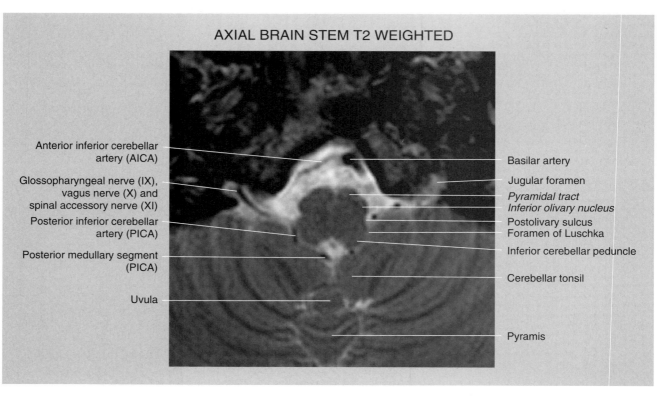

Anterior inferior cerebellar artery (AICA)

Glossopharyngeal nerve (IX), vagus nerve (X) and spinal accessory nerve (XI)

Posterior inferior cerebellar artery (PICA)

Posterior medullary segment (PICA)

Uvula

Basilar artery

Jugular foramen

Pyramidal tract
Inferior olivary nucleus

Postolivary sulcus
Foramen of Luschka

Inferior cerebellar peduncle

Cerebellar tonsil

Pyramis

AXIAL BRAIN STEM T2 WEIGHTED

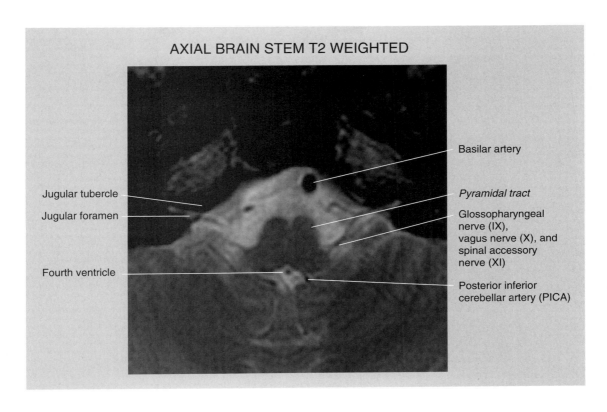

Jugular tubercle

Jugular foramen

Fourth ventricle

Basilar artery

Pyramidal tract

Glossopharyngeal nerve (IX), vagus nerve (X), and spinal accessory nerve (XI)

Posterior inferior cerebellar artery (PICA)

AXIAL BRAIN STEM T2 WEIGHTED

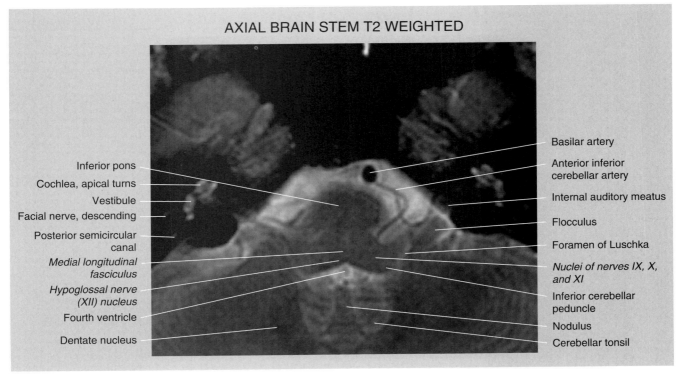

Inferior pons

Cochlea, apical turns

Vestibule

Facial nerve, descending

Posterior semicircular canal

Medial longitudinal fasciculus

Hypoglossal nerve (XII) nucleus

Fourth ventricle

Dentate nucleus

Basilar artery

Anterior inferior cerebellar artery

Internal auditory meatus

Flocculus

Foramen of Luschka

Nuclei of nerves IX, X, and XI

Inferior cerebellar peduncle

Nodulus

Cerebellar tonsil

AXIAL BRAIN STEM T2 WEIGHTED

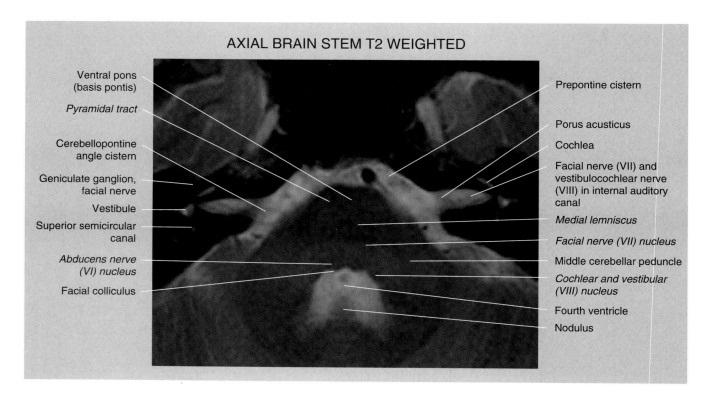

Ventral pons (basis pontis)

Pyramidal tract

Cerebellopontine angle cistern

Geniculate ganglion, facial nerve

Vestibule

Superior semicircular canal

Abducens nerve (VI) nucleus

Facial colliculus

Prepontine cistern

Porus acusticus

Cochlea

Facial nerve (VII) and vestibulocochlear nerve (VIII) in internal auditory canal

Medial lemniscus

Facial nerve (VII) nucleus

Middle cerebellar peduncle

Cochlear and vestibular (VIII) nucleus

Fourth ventricle

Nodulus

AXIAL BRAIN STEM T2 WEIGHTED

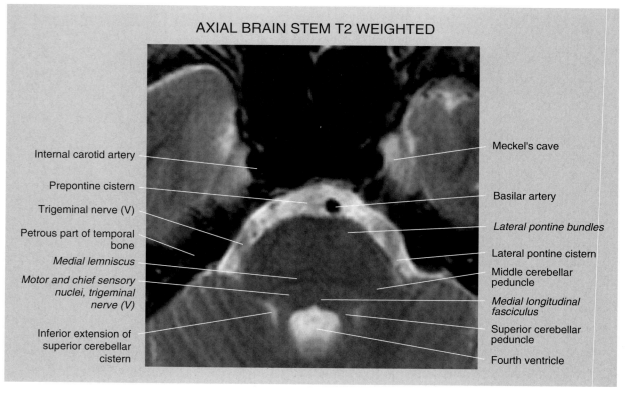

Internal carotid artery

Prepontine cistern

Trigeminal nerve (V)

Petrous part of temporal bone

Medial lemniscus

Motor and chief sensory nuclei, trigeminal nerve (V)

Inferior extension of superior cerebellar cistern

Meckel's cave

Basilar artery

Lateral pontine bundles

Lateral pontine cistern

Middle cerebellar peduncle

Medial longitudinal fasciculus

Superior cerebellar peduncle

Fourth ventricle

AXIAL BRAIN STEM T2 WEIGHTED

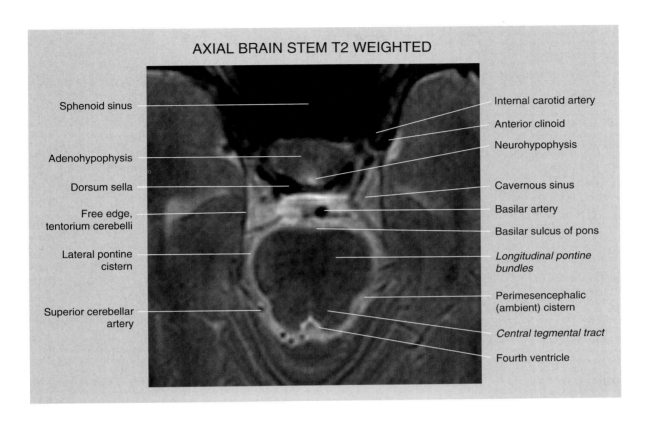

Sphenoid sinus

Adenohypophysis

Dorsum sella

Free edge, tentorium cerebelli

Lateral pontine cistern

Superior cerebellar artery

Internal carotid artery

Anterior clinoid

Neurohypophysis

Cavernous sinus

Basilar artery

Basilar sulcus of pons

Longitudinal pontine bundles

Perimesencephalic (ambient) cistern

Central tegmental tract

Fourth ventricle

AXIAL BRAIN STEM T2 WEIGHTED

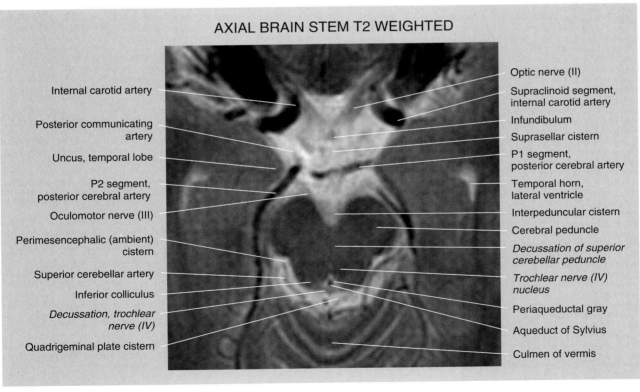

Internal carotid artery

Posterior communicating artery

Uncus, temporal lobe

P2 segment, posterior cerebral artery

Oculomotor nerve (III)

Perimesencephalic (ambient) cistern

Superior cerebellar artery

Inferior colliculus

Decussation, trochlear nerve (IV)

Quadrigeminal plate cistern

Optic nerve (II)

Supraclinoid segment, internal carotid artery

Infundibulum

Suprasellar cistern

P1 segment, posterior cerebral artery

Temporal horn, lateral ventricle

Interpeduncular cistern

Cerebral peduncle

Decussation of superior cerebellar peduncle

Trochlear nerve (IV) nucleus

Periaqueductal gray

Aqueduct of Sylvius

Culmen of vermis

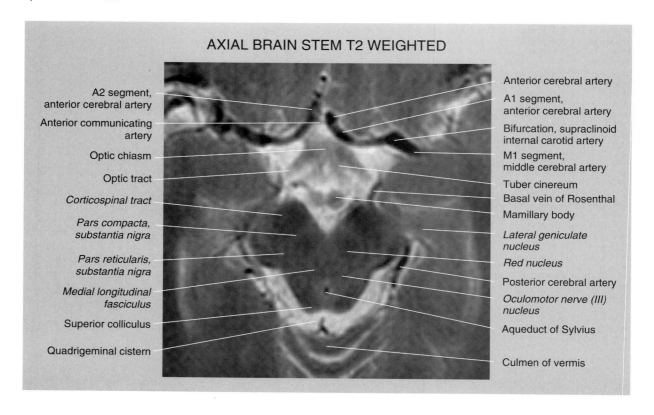

AXIAL BRAIN STEM T2 WEIGHTED

A2 segment, anterior cerebral artery
Anterior communicating artery
Optic chiasm
Optic tract
Corticospinal tract
Pars compacta, substantia nigra
Pars reticularis, substantia nigra
Medial longitudinal fasciculus
Superior colliculus
Quadrigeminal cistern

Anterior cerebral artery
A1 segment, anterior cerebral artery
Bifurcation, supraclinoid internal carotid artery
M1 segment, middle cerebral artery
Tuber cinereum
Basal vein of Rosenthal
Mamillary body
Lateral geniculate nucleus
Red nucleus
Posterior cerebral artery
Oculomotor nerve (III) nucleus
Aqueduct of Sylvius
Culmen of vermis

REFERENCES

1. Iwasaki S, Nakagawa H, Fukusumi A, et al: Identification of pre- and postcentral gyri on CT and MR images on the basis of the medullary pattern of cerebral white matter. Radiology 179:207–213, 1991.
2. Bryan RN: Imaging of acute stroke. Radiology 177:615–616, 1990.
3. Schroth G, Kretzschmar K, Gawehn J, Voigt K: Advantage of MRI in the diagnosis of cerebral infections. Neuroradiology 29:120–126, 1987.
4. Schroth G, Gawehn J, Thron A, et al: Early diagnosis of herpes simplex encephalitis by MRI. Neurology 37:179–183, 1987.
5. Simon JH: Neuroimaging of multiple sclerosis. Neuroimaging Clin North Am 3:229–246, 1993.
6. Whiteman JLH, Post MJD, Berger JR, et al: Progressive multifocal leukoencephalopathy in 47 HIV-seropositive patients: neuroimaging with clinical and pathologic correlation. Radiology 187:233–240, 1993.
7. Lee BCP: Magnetic resonance imaging of metabolic and primary white matter disorders in children. Radiol Clin North Am 3:267–289, 1993.
8. Galdemeyer KS, Smith RR, Harris TM, Edwards MK: MRI in acute disseminated encephalomyelitis. Neuroradiology 36:216–220, 1994.
9. Bronen R: Epilepsy: the role of MR imaging. AJR 159:1165–1174, 1992.
10. Hesselink JR, Dowd CF, Healy ME, et al: MR imaging of brain contusions: a comparative study with CT. AJNR 9:269–278, 1988.
11. Daniels DL, Millen SJ, Meyer GA, et al: MR detection of tumor in the internal auditory canal. AJNR 8:249–252, 1987.
12. Elster AD: Modern imaging of the pituitary. Radiology 187:1–14, 1993.
13. Barkovich AJ: Pediatric Neuroimaging. 2nd ed. New York: Raven Press, 1995, pp 177–276.
14. Byrd SE, Darling CF, Wilczynski MA: White matter of the brain: maturation and myelination on magnetic resonance in infants and children. Neuroimaging Clin North Am 3:247–266, 1993.
15. Gomori JM, Grossman RI, Goldberg HI, et al: Intracranial hematomas: imaging by high field MR. Radiology 157:87–93, 1985.
16. Ross JS, Masaryk TJ, Modic MT, et al: Intracranial aneurysms: evaluation by MR angiography. AJNR 11:449–456, 1990.
17. Smith HJ, Strother CM, Kikuchi Y, et al: MR imaging of the supratentorial intracranial AVMs. AJNR 9:225–235, 1988.
18. Gomori JM, Grossman RI, Goldberg HI, et al: Occult cerebral vascular malformations: high-field MR imaging. Radiology 158:707–713, 1986.
19. Wehrli FW, MacFall JR, Glover GH, et al: The dependence of nuclear magnetic resonance (NMR) image contrast in intrinsic and pulse sequence timing parameters. Magn Reson Imaging 2:3–16, 1984.
20. Hennig J, Naureth A, Friedburg H: RARE imaging: a fast imaging method for clinical MR. Magn Reson Med 8:823–833, 1986.
21. Hesselink JR, Berthoty DP: MR parameters must be chosen judiciously to optimize brain studies. Diagn Imaging 10:163–167, 1988.
22. Carr DH, Brown J, Bydder GM, et al: Intravenous chelated gadolinium as a contrast agent in NMR imaging of cerebral tumours. Lancet 1:484–486, 1984.
23. Hesselink JR, Healy ME, Press GA, Brahme FJ: Benefits of Gd-DTPA for MR imaging of intracranial abnormalities. J Comput Assist Tomogr 12:266–274, 1988.
24. Haacke EM, Lenz GW: Improving MR image quality in the presence of motion by using rephasing gradients. AJR 148:1251–1255, 1987.
25. Enzmann DR, Rubin JB, O'Donahue JO, et al: Use of cerebrospinal fluid gating to improve T2-weighted images. Part 2. Temporal lobes, basal ganglia and brain stem. Radiology 162:768–773, 1987.
26. Frahm J, Merboldt K-D, Hanicke W, Haase A: Flow suppression in rapid FLASH NMR images. Magn Reson Med 4:372–377, 1987.
27. Truwit CL, Lempert TE: High Resolution Atlas of Cranial Neuroanatomy. Baltimore: Williams & Wilkins, 1994.
28. Schnitzlein HN, Murtagh FR: Imaging Anatomy of the Head and Spine. Baltimore: Urban & Schwarzenburg, 1990.

Developmental Disorders

GARY A. PRESS

As a rule, the different categories of congenital malformations of the central nervous system (CNS) reflect the time at which a noxious agent disrupted the normal sequence of neural development rather than the nature of the noxious agent itself. Accordingly, Volpe[1] arranged many congenital CNS disorders according to the time of onset of the morphologic derangement. This classification was later expanded to include several important conditions formerly omitted: cerebellar malformations, congenital vascular malformations, congenital tumors, and secondarily acquired congenital abnormalities.[2] A portion of the complete classification including all of the primary brain malformations is presented in Table 16–1. The etiology and time of insult of several congenital deformities (e.g., corpus callosum dysgenesis, schizencephaly) remain controversial.

TECHNIQUE

At no other time are we made more acutely aware of the need to minimize motion of a patient than when magnetic resonance imaging (MRI) is performed in the pediatric age group. During the second through fourth years of life, patients tend to be especially uncooperative and require sedation. Younger infants may often be examined merely by employing a pacifier, or by withholding food until they are quite hungry, feeding them, and then performing the examination during a postprandial nap. Older children may be surprisingly cooperative, especially after a brief, nonthreatening introduction to the machine. Parental presence by or partly in the scanner during the examination is most helpful.

When pharmacologic restraint is required, oral chloral hydrate, 75 mg/kg initial dose, given 30 minutes before the examination, supplemented by an additional 25 mg/kg if the patient is not asleep in 30 minutes, is most effective. A maximal total dose of 2000 mg may be administered. This regimen combined with sleep deprivation was successful on the first attempt in 90% of 3000 sedation attempts in one series.[3]

For the remaining 10% of patients who fail to respond to chloral hydrate sedation, pentobarbital (Nembutal), 5 to 6 mg/kg as an initial dose given intravenously or intramuscularly, supplemented by an additional 2 to 3 mg/kg if not asleep in 30 minutes, can be useful. A maximal total dose of 200 mg of pentobarbital may be administered. This drug is also useful for patients who weigh too much (more than 25 kg) to receive an adequate dose of oral chloral hydrate within the 2000-mg maximal total dose guideline.

Rarely, a pediatric patient requires general anesthesia during an MRI study. Considerable effort and coordination between the anesthesiologists and the MRI staff is required in such instances. At my institution, a respirator without ferrous components is placed immediately adjacent to the scanner (1.5 T); connecting the respirator to the patient are 6-foot-long plastic hoses introduced into the bore of the magnet from the foot of the scanning table. The patient is closely monitored during the study by two anesthesiologists, one of whom remains in the scanning room at all times. All monitoring is performed with nonferrous devices.

Selection of imaging parameters for evaluation of congenital CNS malformations is straightforward.[4] Because morphologic information is often paramount, T1-weighted sequences that provide excellent parenchyma–cerebrospinal fluid (CSF) contrast can be employed alone for most patients. Assessing the progress of myelination is best performed using T1-weighted (or inversion recovery [IR]) images for patients from 29 weeks' gestation to 6 months of age (see later section on myelination). In older patients, T2-weighted images are also useful for the detection of parenchymal abnormalities (tumors, heterotopias) associated with the neurocutaneous syndromes.

STAGES OF BRAIN DEVELOPMENT

A brief review of the stages of normal development of the CNS will facilitate understanding the MRI appearance of congenital CNS malformations. The devel-

TABLE 16–1. CLASSIFICATION OF CONGENITAL CEREBRAL AND CEREBELLAR MALFORMATIONS

DISORDER	TIME OF ONSET (GESTATIONAL AGE)*
Dorsal induction, primary neurulation/ neural tube defects	(3–4 wk)
Craniorachischisis totalis	3 wk
Anencephaly	4 wk
Myeloschisis	4 wk
Encephalocele	4 wk
Myelomeningocele	4 wk
Chiari malformation	4 wk
Hydromyelia	4 wk
Ventral induction	(5–10 wk)
Atelencephaly	5 wk
Holoprosencephaly	5–6 wk
Septo-optic dysplasia	6–7 wk
Agenesis of the septum pellucidum	6 wk
Diencephalic cyst	6 wk
Cerebral hemihypoplasia or aplasia	6 wk
Lobar hypoplasia or aplasia	6 wk
Hypoplasia or aplasia of the cerebellar hemispheres	6–8 wk
Hypoplasia or aplasia of the vermis	6–10 wk
Dandy-Walker syndrome or variant	7–10 wk
Craniosynostosis	6–8 wk
Neuronal proliferation, differentiation, and histogenesis	(2–5 mo)
Micrencephaly	2–4 mo
Megalencephaly	2–4 mo or later
Unilateral megalencephaly	2–4 mo or later
Neurofibromatosis	5 wk–6 mo
Tuberous sclerosis	5 wk–6 mo
Sturge-Weber syndrome	5 wk–6 mo
von Hippel–Lindau disease	5 wk–6 mo
Ataxia-telangiectasia	5 wk–6 mo
Other neurocutaneous syndromes	5 wk–6 mo
Congenital vascular malformations	2–3 mo
Congenital tumors of the nervous system	2–5 mo
	4 mo
Aqueduct stenosis	2–6 mo
Colpocephaly	3–4 mo
Porencephaly	3–4 mo
Multicystic encephalopathy	3 mo or later
Hydranencephaly	
Migration	(2–5 mo)
Schizencephaly	2 mo
Lissencephaly	3 mo
Pachygyria	3–4 mo
Polymicrogyria	5 mo
Neuronal heterotopias	5 mo
Anomalies of the corpus callosum	3–5 mo
Myelination	(7 mo gestation–18 mo of age)
Hypomyelination	Variable
Retarded myelination	Variable
Accelerated myelination	Variable

*Numbers in parentheses indicate an inclusive time period. Numbers without parentheses are more focal time points.

Modified from van der Knapp MS, Valk J: Classification of congenital abnormalities of the CNS. AJNR 9:315–326, 1988.

opmental stages occur serially or concurrently at well-defined fetal and postnatal ages; unique patterns of congenital abnormalities may result from disruption of any one of the stages.[2, 5]

DORSAL INDUCTION

Dorsal induction occurs during the third and fourth weeks of gestation. This stage has three phases, only the first of which concerns us in this discussion. During the first (neurulation) phase the neural tube is formed, which ultimately gives rise to the brain and spinal cord. The second (canalization) and third (retrogressive differentiation) phases apply only to the caudal neural tube and are not described further in this chapter.

During the neurulation phase, the embryonic ectoderm dorsal to the cellular notochord is induced to thicken and form a neural plate. The ectoderm of the plate (neuroectoderm) invaginates along its central axis to form the neural groove with neural folds created along each side of the groove. Fusion of the neural folds in the midline begins in the thoracic region and then progresses toward both ends to form the neural tube. The interaction between the forming neural tube and the adjacent mesoderm produces the meningeal coverings, vertebrae, and skull.

VENTRAL INDUCTION

Occurring between the 5th and 10th weeks of gestation, the major events of ventral induction result in formation of the brain and the face. Initially, the prechordal mesoderm at the cephalic end of the embryo induces the formation of the prosencephalon, mesencephalon, rhombencephalon, and facial structures. The prosencephalon divides into the telencephalon and diencephalon, while the rhombencephalon divides into the metencephalon and myelencephalon. By dividing into halves, the telencephalon forms two hemispheres and two lateral ventricles. Subsequent opercularization results in formation of the sylvian fissures and temporal lobes. The two hemispheres are then joined by the corpus callosum. The cerebellum forms also during this stage from the dorsal part of the metencephalon. The successful completion of the first two stages of cerebral development results in the brain lying within an intact calvaria with a complete face. Hereafter, the brain grows by neuronal proliferation.

NEURONAL PROLIFERATION, DIFFERENTIATION, AND HISTOGENESIS

After the successful formation of the external form of the brain by ventral induction, three processes (neuronal proliferation, differentiation, and histogenesis) become operative simultaneously between 8 and 20 weeks of gestation and continue into the postnatal period. In the normal embryo, beginning at the seventh week of gestation, neuroblasts are generated in the proliferative zones situated along the ependymal surface of the developing brain (germinal matrix). Shortly after the beginning of this stage, the germinal matrix separates from the more superficial cellular layer so that an intervening zone of low cell density is formed that will become the white matter of the brain.

Derangements of neuronal proliferation, differentiation, and histogenesis result in tumors of remains of embryonic neural cells, such as hamartomas, craniopharyngiomas, and medulloblastomas. Moreover, although the precise origin and onset of the various neurocutaneous syndromes remain unknown, several authors believe that abnormal neuronal proliferation, differentiation, and histogenesis may be responsible.[2]

MIGRATION

This highly complex and lengthy (8 to 20 weeks of gestation) stage is vulnerable to many possible insults. During this period, neuroblasts formed in the germinal matrix migrate from the ventricular wall through the white matter to form the superficial cortex and deep nuclei of the basal ganglia. Moreover, in this stage, the cerebellar cortex and nuclei are formed. The sequence of appearance of the surface sulci is provided in Table 16–2.[6]

By 28 to 32 weeks of gestation, the surface of the cerebral cortex amounts to 10% to 11% (180 cm²) of that of the adult brain.[7] The further vast increase in cortical surface area is accomplished by an increase in the size and complexity of the gyri. By 8 to 16 weeks' postnatal age, the surface of the cortex measures 44% (724 cm²) that of the adult, whereas at 2 years' postnatal age, it lies within the limits of variation observed in adults (1635 cm²). In the adult, the intrasulcal component of the surface of the cortex is approximately 65%.[7]

MYELINATION

The process of normal myelination as visualized on MR images has been described in detail[8–10] (Table 16–3; Figs. 16–1 through 16–7). The initial phase of myelination is detected most sensitively on T1-weighted and IR pulse sequences; increased signal intensity of the myelinating white matter is possibly due to T1 shortening by the components of the developing myelin sheaths.[8–10] This early phase of myelination occurs from 29 weeks of gestation to 6 months postnatal age. Beyond this age, the further maturation of myelin may be followed on T2-weighted images. On these images, mature myelinated white matter has decreased signal intensity, explained by the decrease in water content of the brain over the first 2 years of life. T2-

TABLE 16–2. SEQUENCE OF APPEARANCE OF CEREBRAL SULCI

NAME OF SULCUS	TIME OF APPEARANCE (GESTATIONAL WEEK)
Sylvian fissure	14
Calcarine, rolandic	16–20
Superior temporal and pre- and postcentral	23–25
Remainder of sulci	26–30

From Larroche JC: Development of the nervous system in early life. Part II. The development of the central nervous system during intrauterine life. In: Falkner F, ed. Human Development. Philadelphia: WB Saunders, 1966, pp 257–276.

TABLE 16–3. AGES WHEN CHANGES OF MYELINATION APPEAR*

ANATOMIC REGION	T1-WEIGHTED IMAGES	T2-WEIGHTED IMAGES
Middle cerebellar peduncle	Birth	Birth–2 mo
Cerebellar white matter	Birth–4 mo	3–5 mo
Posterior limb internal capsule		
Anterior portion	Birth	4–7 mo
Posterior portion	Birth	Birth–2 mo
Anterior limb internal capsule	2–3 mo	7–11 mo
Genu corpus callosum	4–6 mo	5–8 mo
Splenium corpus callosum	3–4 mo	4–6 mo
Occipital white matter		
Central	3–5 mo	9–14 mo
Peripheral	4–7 mo	11–15 mo
Frontal white matter		
Central	3–6 mo	11–16 mo
Peripheral	7–11 mo	14–18 mo
Centrum semiovale	2–4 mo	7–11 mo

*Observations were made at 1.5 T using T1-weighted sequence (600/20) and T2-weighted sequence (2500/70).
From Barkovich AJ, Kjos BO, Jackson DE Jr, Norman D: Normal maturation of the neonatal and infant brain: MR imaging at 1.5 T. Radiology 166:173–180, 1988.

weighted images correlate best with the development of myelination as demonstrated with histochemical methods.[10]

Normal CNS myelination begins during the fifth fetal month with the myelination of the cranial nerves and continues throughout life.[10] On T1-weighted or IR images, at 29 weeks after conception, immature (early) myelin is found in the brain stem and cerebral peduncles. Between 29 and 36 weeks, myelination progresses to the level of the posterior limb of the internal capsule. Early myelin is seen in the corona radiata by 37 weeks and in the centrum semiovale by 42 weeks.

At birth in normal infants, only the dorsal pons, portions of the superior and inferior cerebellar peduncles, and the ventrolateral thalamus have mature myelin and appear as regions of relatively decreased signal intensity on T2-weighted images. Mature myelin is present within the precentral gyrus within the first 2 postnatal months. Mature myelin may be detected within the deep white matter of the cerebellar hemispheres between 3 and 5 months postnatally on T2-weighted images. Myelin within the white matter of the corpus callosum, internal capsule, corona radiata, and centrum semiovale matures during the first 4 to 11 months postnatally. The subcortical white matter matures last, with myelination proceeding from the occipital region anteriorly to the frontal lobes from 11 to 18 months postnatally.[10]

DEVELOPMENTAL ANOMALIES

DISORDERS OF DORSAL INDUCTION

These disorders include malformation of the meningeal coverings, vertebrae, and skull. Cephaloceles, an-

Text continued on page 491

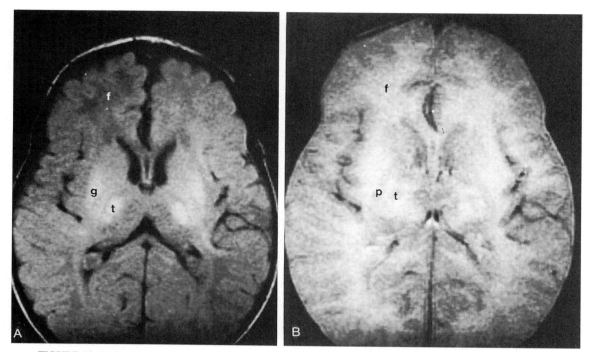

FIGURE 16–1. Normal myelination: 15-day-old male infant. Axial T1-weighted image *(A)* demonstrates normal early myelination as high signal intensity within the basal ganglia (g) and ventrolateral thalami (t) at this level. Low signal intensity persists in the nonmyelinated forceps minor (f). On a corresponding T2-weighted image *(B)*, the maturation of the white matter is manifested as a decrease in signal intensity. In this subject, subtle low signal intensity is seen in the posterior limb of the internal capsule (p) and ventrolateral thalami (t) only. The remainder of the white matter including the forceps minor (f) retains high signal intensity at this level.

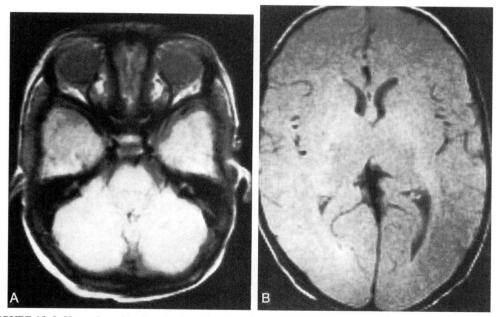

FIGURE 16–2. Normal myelination: 15-day-old male infant. Axial T1-weighted *(A to C)* and T2-weighted *(D to F)* images. Mild hyperintensity within the dorsal pons, posterior limbs of the internal capsule, optic radiations, and centrum semiovale *(A to C)* represents normal early myelination. Subcortical white matter remains hypointense (nonmyelinated). T2-weighted images *(D to F)* at same levels demonstrate that hypointensity is restricted to the dorsal pons, the posterior limb of the internal capsule, the ventrolateral region of the thalamus, and the paracentral region of the cortex corresponding to mature myelin in these areas.

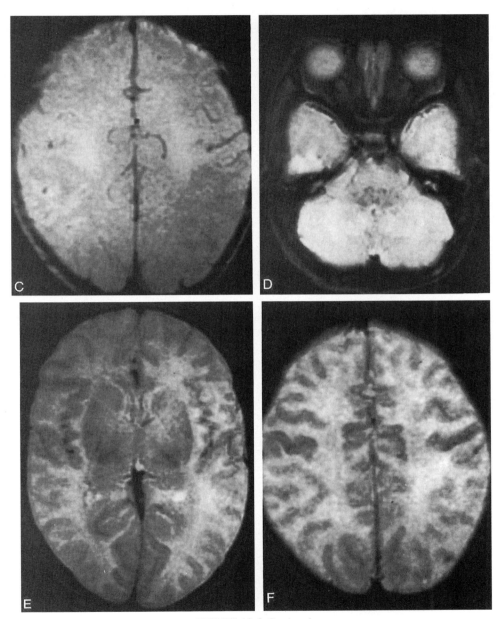

FIGURE 16–2 *Continued*

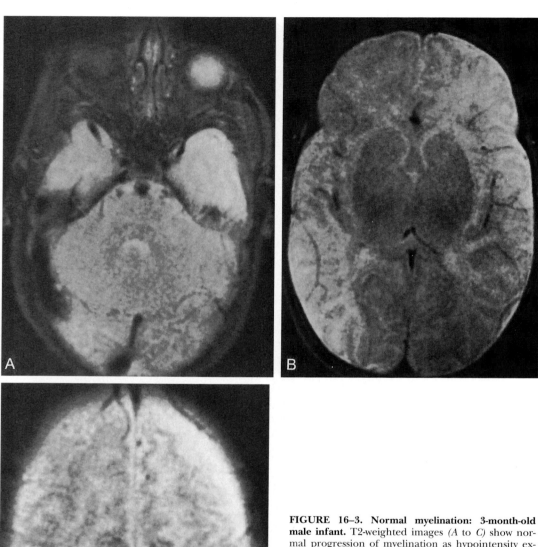

FIGURE 16–3. Normal myelination: 3-month-old male infant. T2-weighted images *(A to C)* show normal progression of myelination as hypointensity extending throughout the pons and into the dorsal aspect of the middle cerebellar peduncles (compare with Fig. 16–2D). Supratentorial regions remain relatively unchanged (compare with Fig. 16–2E and F).

FIGURE 16–4. Normal myelination: 5-month-old-female infant. T1-weighted images *(A to C)* show hyperintensity within deep white matter of cerebellar hemispheres, genu and splenium of the corpus callosum, internal and external capsules, and forceps major and minor. There is increased arborization within the centrum semiovale and subcortical white matter, most notably in the occipital and paracentral regions (compare with Figs. 16–1A and 16–2A to C). On T2-weighted images at the corresponding levels *(D to F)*, maturation of myelin is seen as hypointensity within deep white matter of the cerebellum, entire posterior limb of the internal capsule, and splenium of the corpus callosum (compare with Figs. 16–1B, 16–2D to F, and 16–3A to C). Centrum semiovale and subcortical white matter are normally hyperintense at this age. Overall, the progress of normal myelination from birth to 6 months may be followed best on T1-weighted images.[8–10]

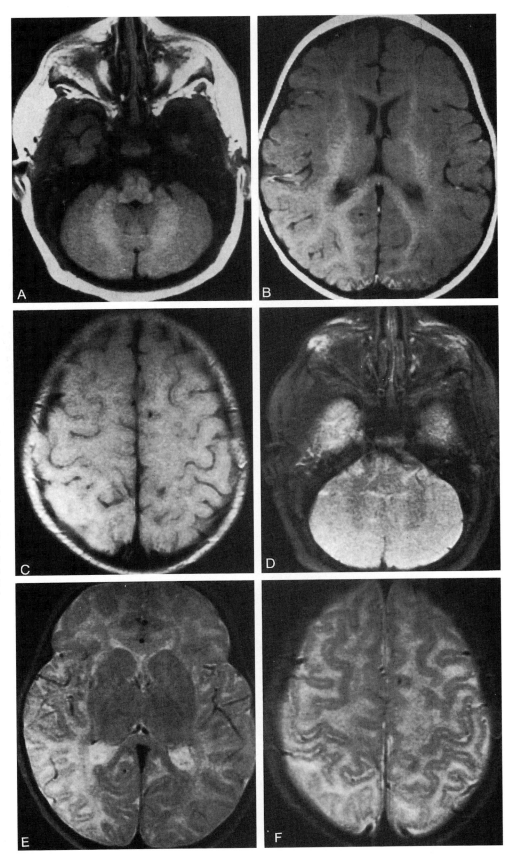

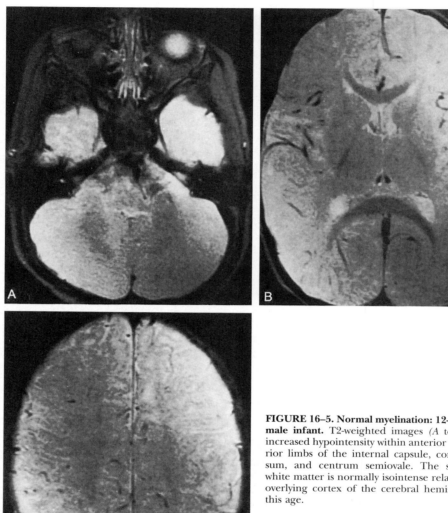

FIGURE 16–5. Normal myelination: 12-month-old male infant. T2-weighted images *(A to C)* show increased hypointensity within anterior and posterior limbs of the internal capsule, corpus callosum, and centrum semiovale. The subcortical white matter is normally isointense relative to the overlying cortex of the cerebral hemispheres at this age.

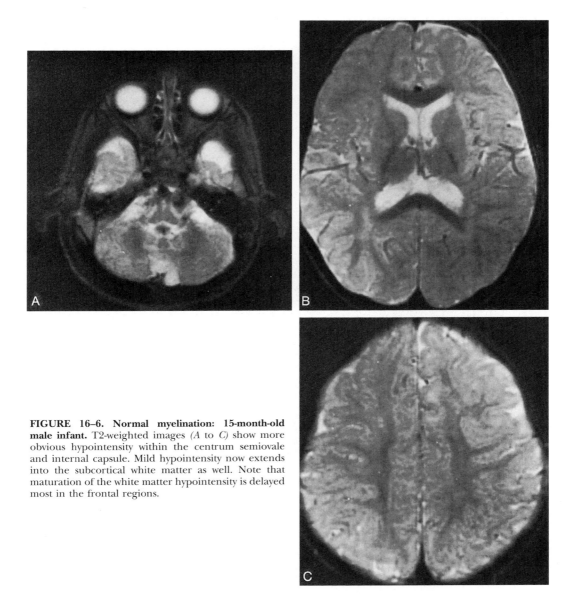

FIGURE 16–6. Normal myelination: 15-month-old male infant. T2-weighted images *(A to C)* show more obvious hypointensity within the centrum semiovale and internal capsule. Mild hypointensity now extends into the subcortical white matter as well. Note that maturation of the white matter hypointensity is delayed most in the frontal regions.

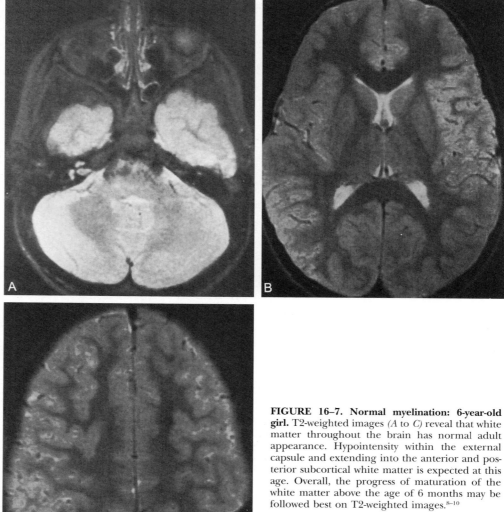

FIGURE 16–7. Normal myelination: 6-year-old girl. T2-weighted images *(A to C)* reveal that white matter throughout the brain has normal adult appearance. Hypointensity within the external capsule and extending into the anterior and posterior subcortical white matter is expected at this age. Overall, the progress of maturation of the white matter above the age of 6 months may be followed best on T2-weighted images.[8–10]

encephaly, and myelomeningoceles are manifestations of aberrant dorsal induction.

Cephaloceles

A defect in the dura and cranium with associated extracranial herniation of intracranial structures is known as a cephalocele. When only the leptomeninges (pia and arachnoid) and CSF herniate extracranially, a meningocele is formed. Parenchymal herniation together with the meninges creates an encephalocele (Fig. 16–8). Herniation of meninges, brain, and ventricles together is called an encephalocystomeningocele.[11]

In North America and Europe, the large majority (71%) of cephaloceles occur in the occipital region (see Fig. 16–8). Other common locations include the parietal (10%), frontal (9%), nasal (9%) (Fig. 16–9), and nasopharyngeal (1%) regions. Interestingly, nasal cephaloceles are reported to be the most common form in Southeast Asia.[12] Within the same geographic area (Australia), nasal cephaloceles occur far less frequently in whites (2%) than in aboriginal Australians (50%). The geographic and racial variations in the prevalence of the different types of cephaloceles suggest that cephaloceles may be caused by genetic defects; moreover, different types of genetic defects may result in different kinds of cephaloceles.[13]

The incidence of cephaloceles is between 0.8 and 3.0 per 10,000 births.[13] The majority of cephaloceles occur in isolation and not as a manifestation of a syndrome.

Cephaloceles may result from defective tissue induction (simultaneously causing both parenchymal and calvarial abnormalities), defective formation of the endochondral portion of the calvaria, or constriction of the fetal head by in utero bands. The last cause usually results in a "nonanatomic" site of presentation (e.g., lateral parietal bone).

Patients with cephaloceles may present with micro-cephaly and a skin-covered sac protruding from the skull.[4] Symptoms depend on the location of the cephalocele and the volume of protruding brain. Poor motor coordination may be seen in patients with low occipital encephaloceles; visual problems may be detected in those with high occipital encephaloceles; sensory and speech disturbances may be present in patients with parietal encephaloceles. An association with facial anomalies is a unique feature of sphenoethmoid cephaloceles. Midline clefts of the upper lips and nose, optic nerve dysplasias, and dysgenesis of the corpus callosum occur in 40% to 60% of patients with sphenoethmoid cephaloceles.

Typical MR findings in patients with cephaloceles include (see Figs. 16–8 and 16–9)

1. Microcephaly and a cranial defect through which protrudes a variable amount of meninges, CSF, and brain, contained by a skin-covered sac. The subcutaneous fat of the sac lining is continuous with that of the scalp (see Fig. 16–8).

2. There may be torquing and displacement of the parenchyma within both the cranium and the hernia sac. Portions of the ventricles within the sac are commonly more dilated than those that remain within the cranial cavity. Arterial supply herniates along with the brain into the sac. Azygous anterior cerebral arteries may accompany a frontal encephalocele. Large veins drain blood through the cranial defect from the sac contents to the intracranial sinuses.

3. Nests of disorganized neuroglial tissue may line the walls of the sac.

Chiari Malformations

Controversy exists in the classification of Chiari malformations. Because myelomeningoceles, Chiari malformations, and hydromyelia are so often associated with one another, they are considered by some to be

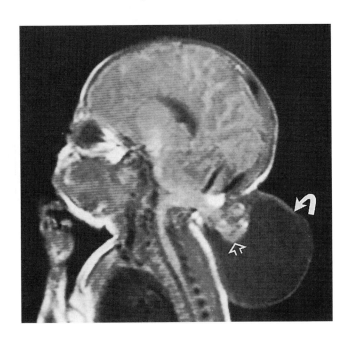

FIGURE 16–8. Inferior occipital myelomeningoencephalocele: neonate. T1-weighted sagittal image demonstrates the inferior cerebellum, medulla, and high cervical spinal cord *(open arrow)* protruding through a cranial defect into a skin-covered, CSF-filled sac *(curved arrow)*.

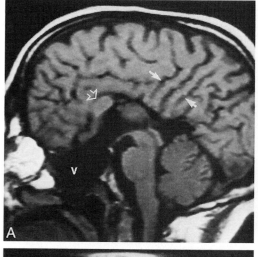
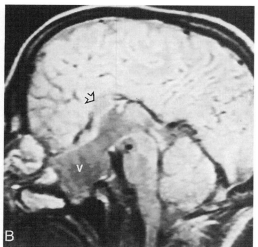
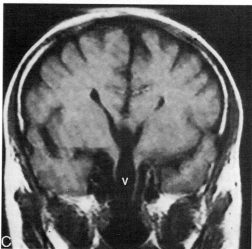

FIGURE 16–9. Sphenoethmoid meningoencephalocele and partial agenesis of corpus callosum: neonate. T1-weighted *(A)* and proton density–weighted *(B)* midline sagittal images demonstrate herniation of enlarged inferior (chiasmatic and infundibular) recesses of third ventricle (V) through a defect in the region of the cribriform plate, fovea ethmoidalis, and planum sphenoidale. The inferior aspect of the hernia sac presents in the nasopharynx. T1-weighted coronal image *(C)* confirms herniation of the enlarged third ventricle. Agenesis of the corpus callosum posterior to a rudimentary genu *(open arrow)* is also noted in *A* and *B*. Observe that the medial sulci of the posterior portion of the hemisphere *(solid arrows, A)* are radially arranged perpendicular to the narrow inferior margin of the hemisphere.

different components of a single clinical syndrome[2, 14]; others consider them to be unrelated anomalies of the hindbrain.[11, 15]

The scheme used to classify the Chiari malformations is based on the research of Hans Chiari, published in 1891. His work on infant cadavers revealed three "distinct" forms of hindbrain abnormality:

Type I. The cerebellar tonsils extend through the foramen magnum and into the cervical canal. The fourth ventricle is normal or nearly normal in position (Figs. 16–10 and 16–11).

Type II. This malformation is almost always associated with a meningomyelocele and hydrocephalus. Affected patients demonstrate displacement of the vermis and tonsils into the spinal canal, accompanied by caudal displacement of the brain stem and elongation of the fourth ventricle. Additional important supratentorial abnormalities (described later) are also seen (Figs. 16–12 to 16–14).

Type III. This is a much rarer malformation characterized by a large, high cervical meningoencephalocele containing the medulla and the cerebellum.

Proposed Cause of Chiari Malformation

Although somewhat complex, a unified theory addresses the development of the Chiari II malformation[16, 17] and ties together the spinal, infratentorial, and supratentorial abnormalities that are manifest in affected patients. (Mikulis and associates[18] have proposed extending this theory to the genesis of the Chiari I malformation.) A brief review of this theory will help the practicing radiologist to recall in detail the disparate anomalies encountered in Chiari II malformation, encouraging accuracy in diagnosis.

Using a mouse model with a sacral neural tube defect, McLone and Knepper[16] have proposed that the intracranial manifestations of the Chiari II malformation may result from a lack of distention of the primitive ventricular system (telencephalic vesicles, or neurocele). Such a lack of distention of the primitive central cavity of the CNS may result from failure to transiently occlude the developing neurocele at a crucial time during development. Alternatively, lack of distention of the neurocele may result from excessive "ventricular" fluid loss from the central cavity of the developing CNS through a neural tube defect (e.g., myelomeningocele).

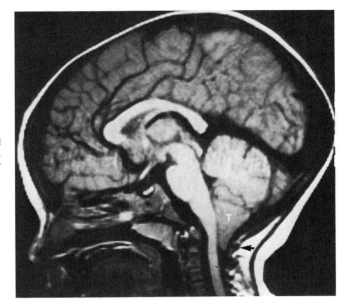

FIGURE 16–10. Chiari I malformation: 2-year-old boy. Midline sagittal T1-weighted image demonstrates a low position of peg-like tonsils (T). The inferior aspect of the tonsils reaches the level of the posterior arch of C-1 *(arrow)*. The cisterna magna is effaced.

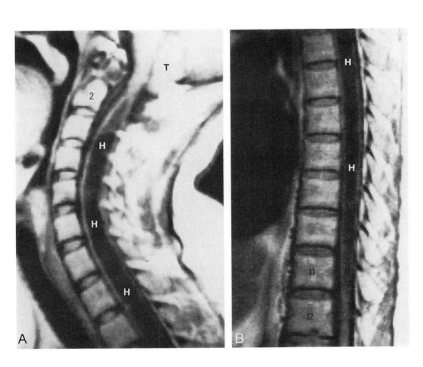

FIGURE 16–11. Chiari I malformation and hydromyelia: 12-year-old girl. Midline sagittal T1-weighted images at the level of the cervical *(A)* and low thoracic *(B)* spine. Tonsillar (T) herniation below the level of the foramen magnum is evident *(A)*. Hydromyelia (H) expands the spinal cord from C-2 *(A)* through T-11 and T-12 *(B)*.

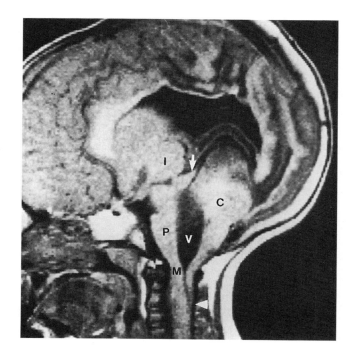

FIGURE 16–12. Chiari II malformation: 6-year-old girl. Midline sagittal T1-weighted image demonstrates marked elongation of the cerebellum (C) and fourth ventricle (V). The surface of the inferior vermis is smooth. There is caudal displacement of the medulla (M), vermis, and tonsils into the cervical spinal canal *(arrowhead)* through an enlarged foramen magnum. The superior and inferior colliculi *(arrow)* are fused and form a peak posteriorly. The sylvian aqueduct is not seen. The massa intermedia (I) is large and the posterior aspect of the corpus callosum is quite thin. P = pons.

FIGURE 16–13. Chiari II malformation: 10-year-old boy. Coronal T1-weighted *(A)* and axial proton density–weighted *(B)* images demonstrate that the posterior fossa is small and the tentorial leaves *(arrows)* are hypoplastic, inserting low, near the foramen magnum. Upward bulging of the cerebellar vermis (Ve) through the wide tentorial incisura forms a pseudomass between the temporal lobes (T).

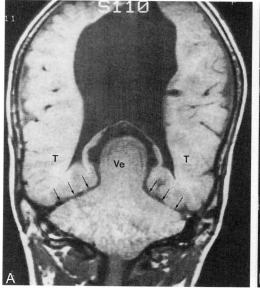

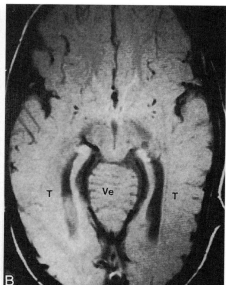

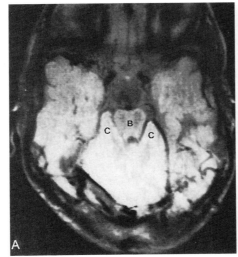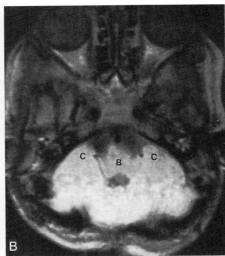

FIGURE 16–14. Chiari II malformation: 5-year-old boy. Axial proton density–weighted images (A and B) demonstrate that the medial portions of the cerebellar hemispheres (C) migrate forward into the prepontine and premedullary cisterns enveloping the brain stem (B).

In the absence of the inductive effect of the pressure and volume of a distended ventricular system, the surrounding mesenchyme and endochondral bone forming the base of the skull grow inadequately. The posterior fossa then develops with a significantly reduced capacity.

The development of the cerebellum and brain stem within the confines of a small posterior fossa then results in downward herniation of components of the brain stem and lower vermis through an enlarged foramen magnum into the upper cervical spinal canal. Simultaneously, there is upward herniation of the upper vermis through a widened, dysplastic tentorium cerebelli. These are some of the major infratentorial anomalies encountered in the Chiari II malformation.[16]

In the supratentorial space, the absence of the distended ventricular system leads to additional manifestations of Chiari II malformation. Close approximation of the thalami leads to a large massa intermedia. Inadequate ventricular distention results in a failure of support for migrating neuroblasts; this leads to a high frequency of migration defects, including dysgenesis of the corpus callosum, cortical heterotopia, and polygyria. Absence of the inductive effect of the distended ventricles also results in a failure of collagen formation and ossification of the cranial vault, leading to lückenschädel. These are some of the major supratentorial anomalies encountered in the Chiari II malformation.

According to the mechanism of McLone and Knepper,[16] the hydrocephalus encountered in Chiari II malformation represents the result (not the cause) of the hindbrain anomaly. The maldevelopment of the posterior fossa and contents in Chiari II malformation may lead to the hydrocephalus in one or more of a number of ways, including 1) occlusion of the cerebral aqueduct, 2) obstruction of the fourth ventricle outlets, 3) obliteration of the subarachnoid spaces surrounding the brain tissue at the level of the foramen magnum, and 4) obstruction to ascent of CSF at the level of the tentorium cerebelli, owing to upward herniation of the contents of the posterior fossa.

Mikulis and associates[18] have postulated that the pathogenesis of the Chiari I malformation might also be explained by the McLone and Knepper theory and represent a less severe manifestation of the same operative mechanism—failure to occlude transiently the developing neurocele (but without a dorsal myeloschisis).

Normal Position of the Cerebellar Tonsils Varies with Age

Location of the inferior aspect of the cerebellar tonsils excessively below the opening of the foramen magnum is the key indicator of the presence of a Chiari I malformation. However, the position of the cerebellar tonsils relative to the foramen magnum varies with age. Therefore, a single standard measurement cannot be used in all cases but must be "tailored" to the patient's age.

On the basis of a study of 221 patients aged 5 months to 89 years, who were considered not to have disorders that would affect tonsillar position, the 95% confidence limits for tonsillar position as a function of age were determined.[18] The results of this study are presented in Table 16–4. For example, the location of the tonsils more than 4 mm below the level of the foramen magnum (as measured on sagittal T1-

TABLE 16–4. POSITION OF CEREBELLAR TONSILS ACCORDING TO AGE

AGE RANGE (Y)	GREATEST NORMAL DISTANCE BELOW FORAMEN MAGNUM (95% CONFIDENCE LIMIT IN MM)
0–9	6
10–29	5
30–79	4
80–89	3

Data from Mikulis DJ, Diaz O, Egglin TK, Sanchez R: Variance of the position of the cerebellar tonsils with age: preliminary report. Radiology 183:725–728, 1992.

weighted MR images) is considered abnormal in individuals between 30 and 79 years of age.[18]

Another interesting result of Mikulis and associates' study is that in individuals younger than age 29 years the position of the cerebellar tonsils averaged from 0.4 to 1.5 mm below the foramen magnum. In older persons, the average position of the cerebellar tonsils was at or above the level of the foramen magnum.

Ethnic (genetic?) differences in the range of normal tonsillar position have been encountered, however. For example, in one study of 50 healthy Japanese subjects,[19] the tonsils were located at or above the foramen magnum in all instances.

Chiari I Malformation

CLINICAL MANIFESTATIONS AND CRITERIA FOR DIAGNOSIS. Although patients with tonsils greater than 12 mm below the level of the foramen magnum were invariably symptomatic in one series,[20] approximately 30% of patients with tonsils herniating 5 to 10 mm below the foramen magnum were asymptomatic. Therefore, mere detection of tonsillar ectopia does not indicate the presence of symptoms, and the presence of tonsillar herniation may be discovered only when an MRI examination is performed for an unrelated reason. A careful clinical assessment remains the foundation for the diagnosis and management of patients with Chiari I malformation.

Syringomyelia (see Fig. 16–11) has been reported in 20% to 73% of cases[4, 20, 21] of patients with Chiari I deformity, whereas the frequency of associated skeletal anomalies varies between 23% and 45%.[20]

Patients with Chiari I malformation may present either with symptoms of syrinx or with symptoms of hindbrain compression. Patients with Chiari I malformation and a syrinx nearly always present with symptoms referable to the syrinx: central cord syndrome, impaired sensation, pain, backache, scoliosis, spasticity, and weakness.[20]

Patients with symptoms of hindbrain compression have a greater average degree of tonsillar herniation than those with other clinical presentations. Symptoms and signs of hindbrain compression include headache, neckache, weakness, numbness, oscillating vision, apnea, sudden death, dysphagia, cranial nerve palsies, and incontinence.

A female predominance of the malformation has been observed,[20] with a female-to-male ratio of approximately 3:2.

CNS MRI MANIFESTATIONS. This malformation combines cervicomedullary and craniovertebral anomalies. In such patients, MRI reveals a low position (5 mm or greater herniation) of at least one cerebellar tonsil below the foramen magnum.[20] The inferior aspect of the tonsils may be at the level of the posterior arch of C-1 or C-2 (see Figs. 16–10 and 16–11). The inferior aspect of the cerebellar hemispheres may be drawn slightly toward the foramen magnum; the fourth ventricle may be normal or slightly elongated craniocaudally. The cisterna magna is extremely small or

nonexistent. Hydromyelia is frequently seen (see Fig. 16–11).

Associated craniovertebral anomalies include basilar impression (25%), atlanto-occipital fusion (10%), and Klippel-Feil anomaly (10%)[11] (see Chapter 41).

Chiari II Malformation

CLINICAL MANIFESTATIONS AND CRITERIA FOR DIAGNOSIS. This complex deformity is characterized by an elongated, small cerebellum and brain stem and caudal displacement of the medulla, parts of the cerebellum, and pons through an enlarged foramen magnum into the cervical spinal canal. Maldevelopment of the telencephalon, diencephalon, mesencephalon, and upper cervical canal often accompanies the rhombencephalic deformity of the Chiari II malformation.

The Chiari II malformation is nearly always accompanied by a myelomeningocele (see Chapter 41) and hydrocephalus.[22] The deformity occurs in 2 to 3 per 1000 births.[4]

Although most cases are sporadic, a higher frequency is encountered in families with a history of neural tube defects.

Patients present with sensory and motor deficits of the lower extremities owing to the accompanying myelomeningocele. Hydrocephalus often causes raised intracranial pressure and requires shunting in 90% of patients. Nevertheless, normal intelligence is also present in 90% of patients.

CNS MRI MANIFESTATIONS. A review of 24 patients with Chiari II malformation[22] revealed the following characteristic MRI manifestations.

Rhombencephalon and Spinal Cord. The surface of the cerebellar vermis was unusually smooth on sagittal images, owing to dorsocaudal angulation of the surface sulci and fissures (see Fig. 16–12). Both inferior and superior lobules were so affected. The cerebellar dysplasia accompanying a Chiari II malformation represents a spectrum varying from heterotopias and heterotaxias to marked cerebellar and brain stem dysgenesis. Upward bulging of the cerebellum occurs through a wide tentorial incisura that inserts low near the foramen magnum (see Fig. 16–13). Medial portions of the cerebellar hemispheres migrate forward into the prepontine or premedullary cisterns, enveloping the brain stem (see Fig. 16–14). The fourth ventricle elongates and descends into the spinal canal along the posterior surface of the medulla. Varying amounts of the inferior cerebellar hemispheres and the tonsils herniate through the wide foramen magnum and appear as a peg or tongue of tissue below the C-1 ring, behind the spinal cord and medulla. From posterior to anterior in a sagittal MR image one sees a sequence of protrusions: of cerebellum behind fourth ventricle, ventricle behind medulla, and medulla behind spinal cord. In 20% to 83% of patients with Chiari II malformation, hydromyelia is also seen.[22]

Telencephalon. Small, closely spaced gyral folds, or stenogyria, may be seen in the cerebral hemispheres. This histologically normal cerebral cortex is different

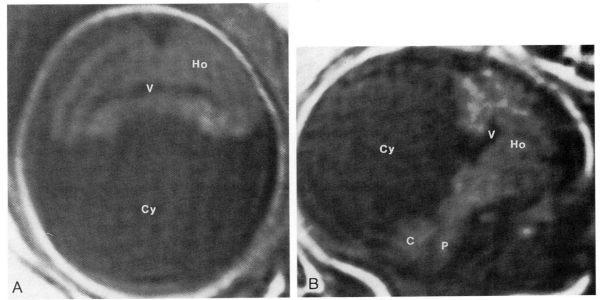

FIGURE 16–15. Alobar holoprosencephaly at 33 weeks' gestation (in utero). Axial T1-weighted image *(A)* shows a single, unlobed holoprosencephalon (Ho) with monoventricle (V) anterior to a large dorsal cyst (Cy). Falx cerebri, septum pellucidum, and corpus callosum are absent. Sagittal T1-weighted image *(B)* shows that a dorsal cyst communicates with the ventricle. P = pons; C = cerebellum.

from polymicrogyria, in which the cellular layers of the cortex are deficient. Anteroinferior pointing of the frontal horns may be noted often in the coronal plane. Partial agenesis of the corpus callosum was seen in one third of the patients in this series.[22] Severe callosal dysplasia may be associated with mental retardation.

Diencephalon. Enlargement of the massa intermedia may be identified in 75% to 90% of patients (see Fig. 16–12). The third ventricle is most often normal or mildly dilated in patients with Chiari II malformation.

Mesencephalon. Nonvisualization of the sylvian aqueduct on sagittal images occurs in the majority of patients with Chiari II malformation (see Fig. 16–12). The explanation—whether aqueduct occlusion is present and whether it is primary or secondary due to external compression—remains controversial. The two inferior colliculi may be elongated sagittally, or the superior and inferior colliculi may be fused into a single collicular mass. Some authors[23] believe that there is an association between the degree of tectal elongation, compression of the brain stem by the dilated ventricles, and narrowing of the aqueduct.

Mesoderm. Scalloping of the clivus (basiocciput only) and of the petrous bone was seen in 79% of patients in one series.[22] These changes are, however, a result from pressure by the adjacent cerebellum.

DISORDERS OF VENTRAL INDUCTION

Holoprosencephaly

The disorders of ventral induction affect formation of the forebrain and face; variable failure of normal separation of the primitive forebrain into individual cerebral hemispheres is associated with typical facial anomalies. Three points along the spectrum of disease from most to least severe are alobar, semilobar, and lobar holoprosencephaly.

In alobar holoprosencephaly, MRI reveals a single, unlobed holoprosencephalon with a monoventricle[24] (Fig. 16–15). No interhemispheric fissure, falx, septum pellucidum, or corpus callosum is present. The thalami are fused into a single midline mass. This central gray matter mass indents the inferior aspect of the monoventricle, imparting a horseshoe shape. The membranous roof of the third ventricle may balloon into a dorsal cyst or sac-like structure that lies either above or above and below the tentorial incisura[24a] (see Fig. 16–15). There is absence of the straight, superior, and inferior sagittal sinuses and internal cerebral veins. Increased incidence of azygous anterior cerebral arteries and of hypoplastic middle cerebral arteries accompanies alobar holoprosencephaly.

In semilobar holoprosencephaly (Fig. 16–16), MRI reveals partial development of the posterior interhemispheric fissure, falx, and associated dural sinuses. There may be partial separation of the occipitotemporal lobes and partial differentiation of the temporooccipital horns from the monoventricle (see Fig. 16–16). There is often partial cleavage of the diencephalon into two thalami with formation of a rudimentary third ventricle. A rudimentary corpus callosum may also be present.

In lobar holoprosencephaly, MRI reveals more normal cerebral hemispheres and thalami. There remains only partial fusion of the two frontal lobes with local continuity of the gyri and underlying white matter across the midline beneath a shallow interhemispheric fissure.[4] The temporal and occipital horns are well formed, and the bodies of the lateral ventricles are

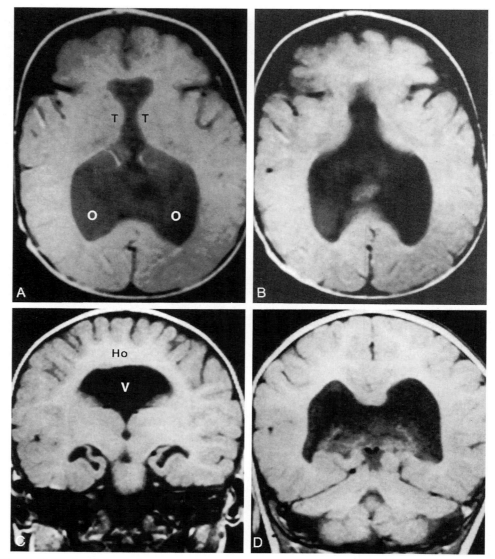

FIGURE 16–16. Semilobar holoprosencephaly: 10-month-old male infant. Axial T1-weighted images show absence of the septum pellucidum *(A and B)* and absence of the anterior interhemispheric fissure superiorly *(B)*. Continuity of the gray and white matter across the midline is seen *(B)*. Nevertheless, partial formation of separate hemispheres is evident, with presence of interhemispheric fissure posteriorly *and* anteriorly at the level of the frontal horns *(A)*, partial formation of occipital horns (O), and separate thalami (T). Coronal T1-weighted sections *(C and D)* emphasize the continuity of the holoprosencephalon (Ho) and the ventricle (V) across the midline. There is partial formation of the temporal horns as well *(C)*.

narrow. The septum pellucidum remains absent, and the frontal horns maintain a squared-off appearance.

The incidence of holoprosencephaly is approximately 1 in 16,000 births. Most cases are sporadic. Most patients with alobar and semilobar forms present at birth with characteristic facial anomalies, including microcephaly, hypotelorism, and one of cyclopia, ethmocephaly, cebocephaly, or absent premaxillary segment.[11] Poikilothermia, apneic spells, motor and mental retardation, and reduced life expectancy are part of the clinical spectrum.

Septo-optic Dysplasia

In this disorder (also known as De Morsier's syndrome), development of the midline telencephalic structures is defective. The etiologic insult may occur during the fifth to seventh weeks of gestation at the time of differentiation of the optic vesicle and of the commissural plate (necessary for the subsequent development of the septum pellucidum and the midline anterior hippocampal and callosal structures). MRI may reveal optic nerve hypoplasia, dilatation of the suprasellar cistern and anterior third ventricle, absence of the septum pellucidum, flattening of the roof of the frontal horns, and dysplasia of the corpus callosum and fornix (Fig. 16–17). Additional features reported in patients with septo-optic dysplasia include mild to moderate lateral ventricular dilatation, schizencephalic defects, and falx hypoplasia.[25-27] Pituitary and hypothalamic insufficiency is recognized clinically in these patients.

Dysplasias of the Posterior Fossa

Dysplasias of the posterior fossa often involve agenesis or hypoplasia of the cerebellar vermis or hemispheres and formation of posterior fossa CSF collections that may or may not communicate with the fourth ventricle. The size of the posterior fossa in affected patients is variable; the posterior fossa may be enlarged by expansion of a cyst, may be of normal size, or may be smaller than normal depending on the malformation and time of insult to the developing CNS.

Cystic Malformations of the Cerebellum and Posterior Fossa

A classification of posterior fossa cysts and cyst-like malformations based on the results of multiplanar MRI has been promulgated.[28] In this classification, the Dandy-Walker malformation, Dandy-Walker variant, and mega–cisterna magna represent a continuum of developmental abnormalities of the posterior fossa. One author has proposed that these terms be abandoned and replaced by a single entity called the Dandy-Walker complex.[28] Nevertheless, others continue to delineate individual patients according to the severity of abnormalities and use these terms that have been widely accepted for many years.[29] In this chapter, posterior fossa cystic malformations are described us-

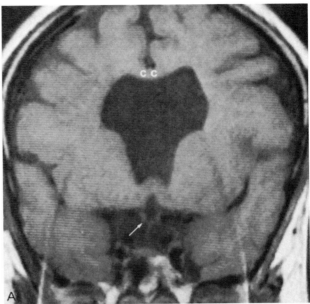

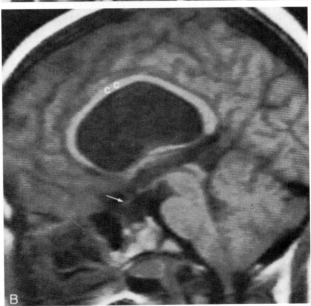

FIGURE 16–17. Septo-optic dysplasia in a child. Coronal *(A)* and midline sagittal *(B)* T1-weighted images demonstrate absence of the septum pellucidum, dilatation of the suprasellar cistern, and hypoplasia of the optic chiasm and optic tracts *(arrows)*. Moderate dilatation of the lateral ventricles and thinning of the corpus callosum (cc) are evident.

ing a middle-of-the-road approach, incorporating the terms *Dandy-Walker malformation, Dandy-Walker variant,* and *mega–cisterna magna* as landmarks along a spectrum of posterior fossa cystic malformations known as the Dandy-Walker complex.

One of the tenets of a classification system based on the findings of MRI is that an insult occurs to both the developing cerebellar hemispheres and the developing fourth ventricular roof in patients with cystic malformations of the posterior fossa[28]; the severity of the insult determines where the affected brain lies on the continuum of developmental abnormality encountered in these malformations.

The classic Dandy-Walker malformation (Fig. 16–18) involves complete or partial agenesis of the vermis; cystic dilatation of the fourth ventricle; and enlargement of the posterior fossa associated with upward displacement of the lateral sinuses, tentorium, and torcular.[29] Hypoplasia of the cerebellar hemispheres, although not often emphasized in the literature, is also seen frequently and may be severe.[28] In such patients, the insult to the developing cerebellum and developing fourth ventricular roof is presumed to be severe and diffuse.

In other patients with less severe involvement of the developing fourth ventricular roof and predominant involvement of the developing cerebellum, the result is cerebellar hypoplasia (hemispheric and/or vermian) without marked expansion of the posterior fossa, a condition that has been labeled the Dandy-Walker variant.

If instead the insult involves mainly the developing fourth ventricular roof, the result is a large retrocerebellar CSF collection that communicates with the fourth ventricle, an expanded posterior fossa, and relatively minor cerebellar or vermian hypoplasia. These are the features of the classic mega–cisterna magna (Fig. 16–19).

Two additional causes of large posterior fossa CSF

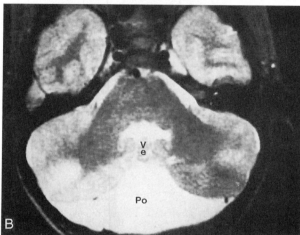

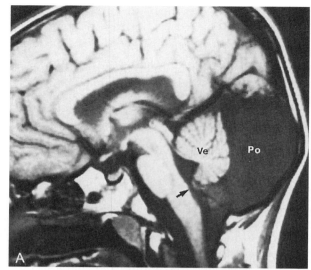

FIGURE 16–19. Mega–cisterna magna: 11-year-old boy. Sagittal T1-weighted (A) and axial T2-weighted (B) images demonstrate a large CSF space (Po) posterior to an intact but small (possibly hypoplastic) vermis (Ve) and hemispheres of the cerebellum. The fourth ventricle and CSF space appear to communicate through the foramen of Magendie (arrow). The superior aspect of the cyst lies at or above the level of the torcular Herophili.

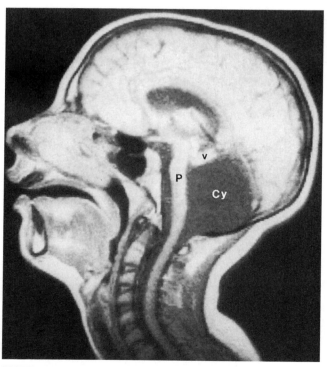

FIGURE 16–18. Dandy-Walker malformation: 5-year-old girl. Midline sagittal T1-weighted image demonstrates near-complete agenesis of the vermis; only the superior lobules (v) are preserved and displaced upward to lie posterior to the tectal plate. There is continuity between the fourth ventricle and the large posterior fossa cyst (Cy). The sagittal diameter of the pons (P) is abnormally small in this patient. Hydrocephalus was relieved by placement of a CSF shunt catheter (not shown) before MRI.

collections are thought to be unrelated to the Dandy-Walker continuum: 1) discrete posterior fossa CSF collections clearly separated from and not in communication with the fourth ventricle or vallecula (Fig. 16–20) (i.e., arachnoid cysts) and 2) posterior cerebellar and vermian atrophy, associated with degenerative disorders that cause an ex vacuo enlargement of the CSF spaces within the posterior fossa after previously normal development.

A "small" cerebellar vermis or hemispheres may result either from stunted development (hypoplasia or agenesis) or from shrinkage of a previously normally formed cerebellum (atrophy). When vermian or cerebellar lobules are absent, or there is diminished size of the hemispheres or vermis *without* enlargement of the sulci or fissures between the folia, a state of hypoplasia or agenesis may be said to exist. On the other hand, if all of the cerebellar lobules are present but

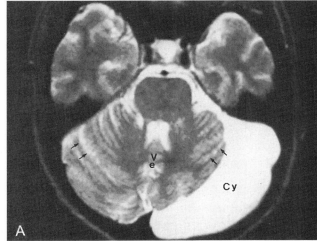

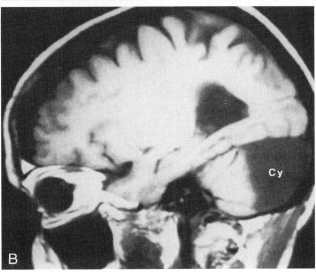

FIGURE 16–20. Arachnoid cyst: 45-year-old woman. Axial T2-weighted *(A)* and paramidline sagittal T1-weighted *(B)* images demonstrate that unilateral posterior fossa CSF collection (Cy) displaces cerebellar hemispheres and vermis (Ve) from left to right. Sulci *(arrows)* of left cerebellar hemisphere are effaced when compared with those on the right side. Subtle thinning of overlying left occipital bone is evident.

the cerebellum is small and the fissures between the lobules and folia are enlarged, a state of atrophy may be said to exist (as opposed to hypoplasia). Some patients with cerebellar or vermian atrophy will have an enlarged cisterna magna that may *appear* similar to patients with mega–cisterna magna on the basis of developmental hypoplasia of the roof of the fourth ventricle (proposed Dandy-Walker mechanism). Nevertheless, these two distinct groups of patients can be differentiated, because those with mega–cisterna magna on the basis of atrophy of the cerebellum demonstrate thin cerebellar cortex, small folia, and enlarged sulci and fissures between the folia.[28] These findings are not present in patients with the hypoplasia of the cerebellum associated with the Dandy-Walker continuum.

DANDY-WALKER COMPLEX. This complex represents a continuum of developmental abnormality including patients with classic Dandy-Walker malformation, Dandy-Walker variant, and mega–cisterna magna.

Dandy-Walker Malformation. A classic triad of findings characterizes this disorder (see Fig. 16–18): 1) hypoplasia of the cerebellar vermis (and hemispheres);

2) expansion of the fourth ventricle to form a posterior fossa cyst; and 3) enlargement of the posterior fossa associated with upward displacement of the lateral sinuses, tentorium, and torcular.[29]

This malformation occurs in 1 in 25,000 to 30,000 births[30] and accounts for 14% of cystic malformations of the posterior fossa.[29] Most cases are sporadic.[11] A large majority (80%) of patients present with hydrocephalus in early life (when younger than 3 months of age). The degree of hydrocephalus is variable and does not correlate with the size of the posterior fossa cyst. The level of obstruction to flow of the CSF is variable and may occur at the aqueduct of Sylvius, fourth ventricular outlet foramina, incisura, or elsewhere.[29]

The reported mental development in patients with Dandy-Walker malformation is variable, with more recent series tending toward greater optimism. For example, mental development was normal in 75% in one report.[31] In another series, 73% had normal intellect, whereas 11% had moderate developmental delay, and the remaining 16% had a severe delay.[32] Many patients have some motor deficit as well. The severity of the clinical symptoms does not appear to correlate with the severity of the hindbrain deformity.[28] Nevertheless, the more severe degree of developmental delay does appear to correlate with the presence of supratentorial anomalies (e.g., heterotopic gray matter or dysgenesis of the corpus callosum with interhemispheric cyst).[28]

Patients with hydrocephalus usually require cystoperitoneal and/or ventriculoperitoneal shunting. Associated anomalies include Klippel-Feil syndrome, polydactyly, syndactyly, and cleft palate. There is also an association between Dandy-Walker malformation and other cerebral anomalies.

In 25% of patients with Dandy-Walker malformation, the vermis is completely absent.[29] Partial aplasia of the posterior vermis involving five lobules (the declive, folium, tuber, pyramis, and uvula) is seen in the remaining 75%. The superior vermis may be displaced upward into the cistern of the velum interpositum or may lie posterior to the tectal plate (see Fig. 16–18). The cerebellar hemispheres are hypoplastic and may be displaced anterolaterally against the petrous pyramids. Disorganization and heterotopias of the cerebellar cortex may be present.[29] The brain stem usually appears small as a result of accompanying hypoplasia. The aqueduct may be partially narrowed or occluded.

There is marked dilatation of the fourth ventricle, which forms a cyst posterior to the cerebellar hemispheres that are displaced anteriorly (see Fig. 16–18). The cyst expands the posterior fossa, creating a dolichocephalic configuration. The lambdoid sutures may be widened and separated preferentially.[29] There is often pressure erosion of the petrous pyramids. The tentorium inserts above the lambdoid suture (the reverse of the normal situation). Although the falx cerebri is normal, the falx cerebelli is absent,[29] or inconsistently present, displaced, and elongated[28] in patients with the Dandy-Walker malformation. The exit foramina of the fourth ventricle may be open or occluded. The degree of cerebellar hypoplasia in the Dandy-Walker malformation appears unrelated to the size of the cyst.[28]

Hydrocephalus occurs in almost all cases; the exact site of obstruction to CSF flow is variable. Shunting of the cyst may relieve the hydrocephalus. Shunting of the lateral ventricles may also be necessary in patients with occlusion of the aqueduct.

Other cerebral anomalies associated with Dandy-Walker malformation include dysplasia (neuronal heterotopias, polymicrogyria, agyria, schizencephaly, and lipomas of the cerebral and cerebellar hemispheres [20% to 25%]), dysgenesis of the corpus callosum (15% to 25%), and holoprosencephaly (10% to 25%).

Dandy-Walker Variant. In patients with less severe insult to the developing fourth ventricular roof and predominant involvement of the developing cerebellum, the result is cerebellar hypoplasia (hemispheric and/or vermian) without marked expansion of the posterior fossa, a condition that has been labeled the Dandy-Walker variant.[29] Such patients have variable enlargement of the fourth ventricle with open communication between the posteroinferior fourth ventricle and cisterna magna through an enlarged vallecular cistern. Hydrocephalus may or may not be present.

These patients may present with an enlarging head owing to hydrocephalus or with developmental delay.[29] This condition is more common than true Dandy-Walker malformation; the Dandy-Walker variant accounts for nearly one third of posterior fossa cystic malformations according to one investigator.[33]

Associated supratentorial anomalies are similar to those encountered in the Dandy-Walker malformation and include dysgenesis of the corpus callosum, gray matter heterotopias, malformations of the cerebral gyri, holoprosencephaly, and diencephalic cysts.

The MRI findings in Dandy-Walker variant are similar to those in classic Dandy-Walker malformation but differ in severity. The fourth ventricle is enlarged but better formed; the tentorium is elevated in only 10% of cases; the hypoplasia of the cerebellar vermis and hemispheres tends to be less severe. The brain stem is usually normal in appearance.[29, 34]

Mega–Cisterna Magna. In patients with a relatively minor insult to the developing cerebellum, and dominant involvement of the developing fourth ventricular roof, the result is an enlarged posterior fossa with a large retrocerebellar CSF collection that communicates with a relatively normal-appearing fourth ventricle, and relatively minor cerebellar or vermian hypoplasia (see Fig. 16–19). These are the features of the classic mega–cisterna magna.[28] This condition accounts for approximately one half of the cystic malformations of the posterior fossa.[33]

The size of the mega–cisterna magna is variable. The cisterna magna may extend above the vermis to the straight sinus. There may be interruption or fenestration of the straight sinus.[29] The cerebellar vermis often appears intact or with minimal signs of hypoplasia.

These patients present with hydrocephalus or with developmental delay. The mental retardation is due to occasional associated supratentorial anomalies, including dysgenesis of the corpus callosum, diencephalic cysts, and holoprosencephaly.[29] One report found that patients with classic Dandy-Walker malformation may be impossible to differentiate from those with Dandy-Walker variant or mega–cisterna magna on clinical grounds.[28]

POSTERIOR FOSSA ARACHNOID CYST. Posterior fossa CSF collections without demonstrable communication with the fourth ventricle and no evidence of cerebellar atrophy are known as arachnoid cysts[28] (see Fig. 16–20). Pathologically, these collections lie between layers of pia-arachnoid and are lined by arachnoid cells and collagen.[29] The fourth ventricle and vermis and cerebellar hemispheres are normally formed but are displaced by the cyst. No supratentorial or systemic abnormalities accompany the posterior fossa cyst.

Affected patients present with hydrocephalus and compression of the brain stem and cerebellum. Truncal ataxia and headache occur. Age at presentation varies from the first few months of life through adulthood. These lesions are sporadic. Many arachnoid cysts are discovered by use of MRI when they are small and asymptomatic as incidental findings in patients studied for unrelated reasons. Hydrocephalus is treated with cystoperitoneal shunting or fenestration.

MRI reveals a nonenhancing mass with signal intensity similar to that of CSF. There are no mural nodules or calcifications. Arachnoid cysts are unilocular, round, oval, or crescentic and are usually situated in the cerebellopontine angle cistern, quadrigeminal plate cistern, or posterior to the vermis. Occasional cysts lie in the prepontine or interpeduncular cisterns.[29]

The differential diagnosis of posterior fossa arachnoid cysts includes the Dandy-Walker continuum and inflammatory and enterogenous cysts. Benign (dermoid, epidermoid) and malignant (hemangioblastoma, pilocytic astrocytoma) tumors should also be considered.[35]

Cerebellar Agenesis or Hypoplasia

Agenesis of the cerebellum is most uncommon and has been described in a heterogeneous group of patients (Fig. 16–21). Other severe anomalies may be associated (anencephaly, amyelia). A survey of 12 cases of "agenesis of the cerebellum"[36] revealed small remnants of cerebellar tissue in several instances. In affected patients, related structures, including the pontine nuclei, inferior olives, and cerebellar peduncles, are either hypoplastic or malformed. Absence of one cerebellar hemisphere occurs more frequently; anomalies of the contralateral inferior olive and pons may take the form of atrophy rather than maldevelopment.

Total or partial agenesis of the vermis may also occur. The cerebellar hemispheres may be fused to one another[37] or separated by a wide CSF-filled cleft[38] in the region of absent vermal parenchyma.

The most common lesion is partial agenesis of the vermis. In all instances of partial agenesis, the anterosuperior portion of the vermis is preserved, presumably because fusion of the vermis proceeds from rostral to caudal during the second month of gestation.[39]

Hypoplasia of the vermis may be regionally localized (e.g., posterior vermis in a subset of patients with autism[40]; Fig. 16–22). Quantitative analyses of MRI data[41] have revealed two different subtypes of autistic patients based on the presence of vermian hypoplasia or hyperplasia as seen on MR images. Diffuse hypoplasia of the vermis may be seen in other disorders (e.g., Down's syndrome).[42] There are no reports of hypoplasia involving *only* anterosuperior vermal regions. In all reported cases, vermal hypoplasia is accompanied also by hypoplasia of the cerebellar hemispheres.

In patients with cerebellar or vermal agenesis or hypoplasia, MRI reveals variable-sized remnants of cerebellar tissue associated with hypoplastic or absent cerebellar peduncles and brain stem (see Fig. 16–21). Ex vacuo dilatation of the retrocerebellar CSF space usually accompanies these deformities.

DISORDERS OF NEURONAL PROLIFERATION, DIFFERENTIATION, AND HISTOGENESIS

Neurofibromatosis

On the basis of genetic studies, two distinct variants of neurofibromatosis have been identified: neurofi-

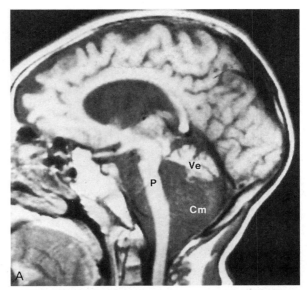
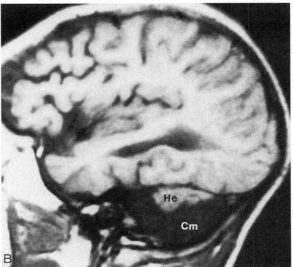

FIGURE 16–21. Marked generalized cerebellar hypoplasia: 6-year-old girl. Sagittal T1-weighted images (A and B) demonstrate that cerebellar vermis (Ve) and hemispheres (He) are quite small with a relatively smooth surface suggesting hypoplasia. The brain stem is diminutive also. Ex vacuo dilatation of the cisterna magna (Cm) is seen. P = pons.

bromatosis 1 (NF-1), previously known as von Recklinghausen's neurofibromatosis, has been localized to chromosome 17; neurofibromatosis 2 (NF-2), previously known as bilateral acoustic neurofibromatosis, has been localized to chromosome 22. The incidence and inheritance, clinical manifestations and diagnostic criteria, and CNS manifestations of these disorders are also unique and are described separately.

For the practicing radiologist, the key distinction between these two forms of neurofibromatosis lies in the tendency for patients with NF-1 to develop intracranial neoplasms involving primary CNS components (i.e., astrocytes and neurons), whereas intracranial neoplasms involving the coverings of the CNS (meninges and Schwann cells) tend to develop in those with

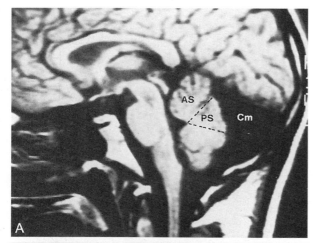

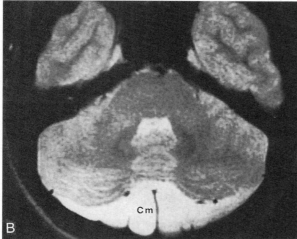

FIGURE 16–22. Focal hypoplasia of cerebellar vermis in autism: 22-year-old man. Sagittal T1-weighted *(A)* and axial T2-weighted *(B)* images demonstrate focal hypoplasia of posterosuperior (PS) lobules (declive, folium, and tuber) of the vermis. Anterosuperior (AS) vermal lobules are normal in size. Ex vacuo dilatation of the cisterna magna (Cm) is seen.

NF-2. Tables 16–5 and 16–6 conveniently summarize the differences between NF-1 and NF-2.[43]

Neurofibromatosis 1

INCIDENCE AND INHERITANCE. NF-1 accounts for more than 90% of all cases of neurofibromatosis and is the most common neurocutaneous syndrome.[43] It achieves a penetrance of almost 100%. The expressivity of NF-1 is highly variable, however.[44] A significant spontaneous mutation rate is encountered: approximately 50% of patients with NF-1 have no family history of this disorder.

CLINICAL MANIFESTATIONS AND CRITERIA FOR DIAGNOSIS. The National Institutes of Health Consensus Development Conference proposed criteria for the diagnosis of NF-1.[45] According to these criteria, the presence of two or more of the following establishes the diagnosis of NF-1:

1. Six or more café au lait spots greater than 5 mm in diameter

2. Two or more neurofibromas of any type or one plexiform neurofibroma

3. Axillary or inguinal region freckling

4. Glioma of the optic nerve

5. Two or more iris hamartomas (Lisch nodules)

6. The presence of a distinctive bony lesion, including sphenoid dysplasia, pseudarthrosis, or thinning of long bone cortex

7. Family history of NF-1 in a first-degree relative

The somatic abnormalities encountered in this disorder, including the cutaneous findings and the tumors at many sites, become more common with increasing age. The external signs of this disorder are often absent in extremely young patients.

TABLE 16–5. NEUROFIBROMATOSIS TYPE 1

SYNONYMS
NF-1, von Recklinghausen's disease (obsolete: "peripheral" neurofibromatosis)

INCIDENCE
1:2000–3000 (>90% of all NF cases)

INHERITANCE
Autosomal dominant
High penetrance, variable expressivity
Chromosome 17

CLINICAL
Prominent cutaneous manifestations

CNS LESIONS IN 15%–20%
Brain: lesions of neurons, astrocytes
  Optic nerve glioma
  Nonoptic gliomas (usually low-grade astrocytomas)
  Non-neoplastic "hamartomatous" lesions
    Basal ganglia
    White matter
Spinal cord/roots/peripheral nerves
  Non-neoplastic "hamartomatous" cord lesions
  Cord astrocytoma
  Neurofibromas of spinal or peripheral nerves
    Scattered
    Plexiform
Osseous or dural lesions
  Hypoplastic sphenoid wing
  Sutural defects
  Kyphoscoliosis
  Dural ectasia
  Meningoceles
Ocular or orbital manifestations
  Optic nerve glioma
  Lisch nodules in iris
  Buphthalmos (cow eye or macrophthalmia)
  Retinal phakomas
  Plexiform neurofibroma (cranial nerve V_1 most common)
Vascular lesions
  Progressive cerebral arterial occlusions
  Aneurysms
  Vascular ectasia
  Arteriovenous fistulas, malformations

NON-CNS LESIONS
Visceral, endocrine tumors
Musculoskeletal lesions (outside skull, spine)
  "Ribbon ribs"
  Tibial bowing
  Pseudarthroses
  Focal overgrowth of digit, ray, or limb

From Osborn AG: Posterior fossa malformations and cysts. In: Diagnostic Neuroradiology—A Text-Atlas. St. Louis: Mosby–Year Book, 1994, pp 59–71.

TABLE 16–6. NEUROFIBROMATOSIS TYPE 2

SYNONYMS
NF-2, bilateral acoustic schwannomas (obsolete: "central" neurofibromatosis)

INCIDENCE
1:50,000

INHERITANCE
Autosomal dominant
Chromosome 22

CLINICAL
Cutaneous manifestations rare

CNS LESIONS IN ~100%
Brain: lesions of Schwann cells, meninges
   Cranial nerve VIII schwannomas most common (bilateral acoustic schwannomas diagnostic for NF-2; multiple schwannomas of other cranial nerves highly suggestive of NF-2)
   Meningiomas; often multiple
   Non-neoplastic intracranial calcifications (especially choroid plexus)
Spinal cord or roots
   Cord ependymomas
   Multilevel, bulky schwannomas of exiting roots
   Meningiomas
Spine
   Secondary changes (expansion, erosion secondary to cord or root tumors)

From Osborn AG: Posterior fossa malformations and cysts. In: Diagnostic Neuroradiology—A Text-Atlas. St. Louis: Mosby–Year Book, 1994, pp 59–71.

CNS MRI MANIFESTATIONS

High-Signal-Intensity White Matter Lesions on T2-Weighted Images. A review of the MR images obtained in 43 patients with NF-1[46] revealed foci of high signal intensity on T2-weighted images within the white matter in 34 patients (79%); the lesions occurred without corresponding neurologic deficits (Fig. 16–23). This is the most common MRI manifestation of NF-1. These lesions do not occur in NF-2.

Such lesions have been noted primarily in the cerebellar peduncles, followed by the brain stem (pons > midbrain > medulla) and, less frequently, the cerebral peduncles and cerebral white matter.[47] Most of these lesions demonstrate no mass effect or enhancement on postgadolinium T1-weighted images.[46, 47] They are characteristically multiple and do not correspond to abnormalities on computed tomographic (CT) scans. They are isointense (and invisible) on T1-weighted images. Maximal lesion diameter was reported to be 25 mm in one series.[46] These lesions occur most commonly in younger patients and are rarely seen in patients older than 20 years of age.[47] Younger patients have been observed to have a temporary increase in either the size or the number of these white matter lesions, which resolve in later life. Progression of such lesions in a child older than 10 years is suggestive of neoplasm and worthy of close clinical and MRI follow-up.[46]

Although the exact nature of these lesions remains unclear, foci of heterotopia, hamartomas, or benign or malignant proliferation of glial cells or neurons would not be expected to cause age-related reversible signal intensity abnormalities as seen in these white matter lesions. Therefore, one group[46] has proposed that focal formation of chemically abnormal myelin that is subsequently broken down and replaced by more normal, stable myelin may explain this unusual manifestation of NF-1. In fact, histopathologic findings in three patients with NF-1[47a] revealed intramyelinic spongiotic or vacuolar change; these authors proposed that fluid-filled vacuoles explain the occurrence of high signal intensity on T2-weighted images.

Their lack of mass effect and isointensity on T1-weighted images help to distinguish these benign lesions from parenchymal gliomas in most instances. The latter often cause mass effect and are *hypointense* on T1-weighted images.

High-Signal-Intensity Basal Ganglia Lesions on T1-Weighted Images. Basal ganglia lesions characterized by increased signal intensity on T1-weighted images (Fig. 16–24) have been reported in a significant number of patients with NF-1 (10 of 53 patients in one series[47]). Such lesions often involve the globus pallidus and internal capsules in a bilateral and symmetric fashion and extend across the anterior commissure, resulting in a "dumbbell" configuration. Corresponding foci of increased signal intensity on T2-weighted images were smaller and less prominent. In seven affected patients,[48] these lesions did not exhibit mass effect, edema, or enhancement with gadolinium diethylenetriaminepentaacetic acid (Gd-DTPA). In another series, globus pallidus lesions in 17 patients "were occasionally associated with mass effect."[47]

The cause of these (T1-weighted) high-signal-intensity lesions is the subject of controversy. Neuropathologic studies support speculation that inclusion of Schwann cells, melanocytes, or microcalcifications within heterotopic or hamartomatous lesions of the basal ganglia may be responsible for the demonstrated high signal intensity on T1-weighted MR images.[47a, 48]

Optic Nerve and Chiasmal Gliomas. These lesions (Fig. 16–25) occurred in 36% (19 of 53) of patients with NF-1 in one series.[47] Such tumors are generally of low histologic grade, but there is variability; some may be high-grade malignancies and demand appropriately aggressive therapies.

These tumors may be confined to a single optic nerve or may spread to involve both optic nerves and the optic chiasm. Occasional lesions involve the optic tracts, to the level of the lateral geniculate bodies and beyond into the optic radiations either unilaterally or symmetrically. Enlargement of the affected region(s) accompanied by high signal intensity on T2-weighted images is commonly seen. Some of these lesions demonstrate enhancement after administration of Gd-DTPA.

Other Parenchymal Gliomas. MRI features of these lesions in patients with neurofibromatosis include mass effect and decreased signal intensity on T1-weighted images and slightly heterogeneous increased signal intensity with variable surrounding edema on T2-weighted images. Homogeneous increased signal intensity is seen on T2-weighted images in tumor cysts.

Parenchymal (nonoptic) gliomas were seen in 15% (8 of 53) of patients with NF-1 in one series.[47]

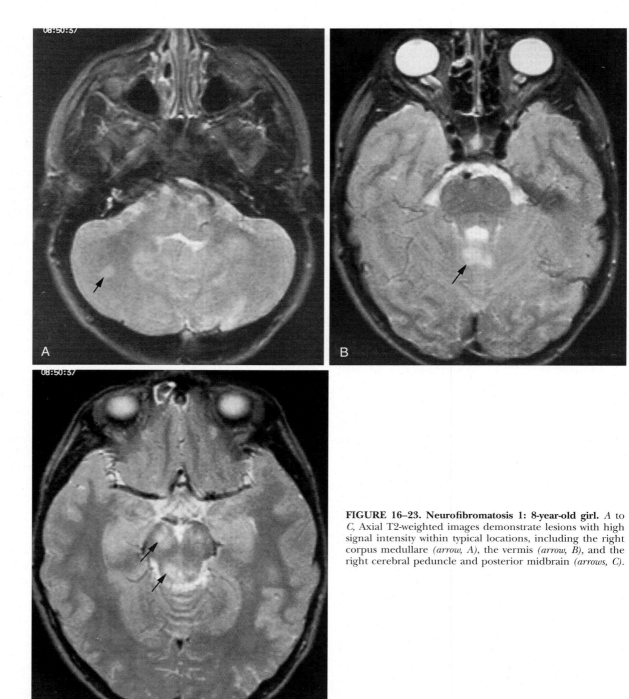

FIGURE 16–23. Neurofibromatosis 1: 8-year-old girl. *A* to *C,* Axial T2-weighted images demonstrate lesions with high signal intensity within typical locations, including the right corpus medullare *(arrow, A),* the vermis *(arrow, B),* and the right cerebral peduncle and posterior midbrain *(arrows, C).*

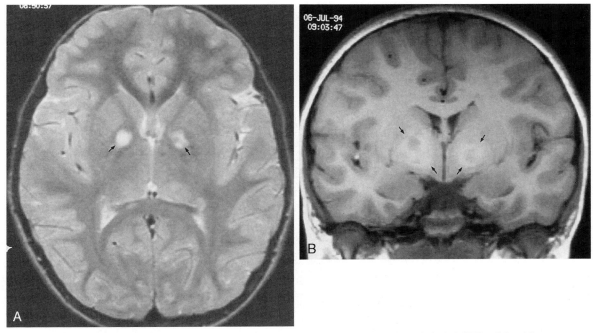

FIGURE 16–24. Neurofibromatosis 1: 8-year-old girl (same patient as in Fig. 16–23). Axial T2-weighted image *(A)* shows foci of hyperintensity within the globus pallidus on each side *(arrows)*. Coronal T1-weighted image *(B)* demonstrates lesions that are mildly hyperintense peripherally and hypointense centrally. The cause of the T1-weighted hyperintensity within such lesions is the subject of controversy (see text).

Plexiform Neurofibromas. Extracranial neurofibromas commonly grow into the orbit along the first (ophthalmic) division of the trigeminal nerve or progress along the course of small and often unidentified nerves into the confines of the skull, thereby distorting or compressing the brain[49] (Fig. 16–26). Intraorbital extension may compromise coordination of the extraocular muscles or result in exophthalmos. Retro-orbital extension involving the cavernous sinus is frequently seen.

These tumors contain a combination of Schwann cells, neurons, and collagen arranged in tortuous, worm-like cords. They are unencapsulated, locally aggressive lesions that tend to infiltrate and separate the normal nerve fascicles.

Plexiform neurofibromas were seen on cranial MR images in 34% (18 of 53) of patients with NF-1.[47]

Sphenoid Dysplasia. Dysplasia of the greater sphenoid wing was demonstrated in 4% (2 of 53) of patients with NF-1.[47] Affected patients may present with pulsatile exophthalmos or anophthalmos, owing to herniation of the anterior temporal lobe into the posterior orbit.

SPINAL MANIFESTATIONS. MRI of the entire spine (T1 weighted with gadolinium) was performed in 28 patients with NF-1 in one series.[50] Only one patient had a biopsy-proven, low-grade astrocytoma. Three additional patients had findings suggestive of intramedullary disease; the frequency of subtle intramedullary lesions (hamartomas of the spine) may have been underestimated in this study because (due to time constraints) no T2-weighted images were obtained.[50]

Intradural, extramedullary disease was found in 5 of 28 patients with NF-1.[50] A total of 23 masses consistent with neurofibromas were detected throughout the spine in these patients; a predominance of the masses was noted in the lumbar spine. One of the 28 patients had cervical extradural masses consistent with neurofibromas. No clinical symptoms related to lesion location were noted in the five patients with intradural, extramedullary masses; in one patient with extradural masses; or in three patients with possible intramedullary masses in this series.[50]

Bony abnormalities were found in 16 of the 28 patients. The abnormalities included 1) enlarged neural foramina due to neurofibromas, dural ectasia, or arachnoid cyst; 2) posterior vertebral body scalloping secondary to dural ectasia or arachnoid cyst; and 3) scoliosis.

Neurofibromatosis 2

INCIDENCE AND INHERITANCE. NF-2 accounts for less than 10% of all cases of neurofibromatosis. It is an autosomal dominant disorder localized to a gene linked to chromosome 22. This disorder has an incidence of approximately 1 in 50,000 live births.[43]

CLINICAL MANIFESTATIONS AND CRITERIA FOR DIAGNOSIS. NF-2 may be diagnosed in individuals who have either of the following abnormalities:

1. Bilateral acoustic neurinomas seen by CT or MRI *or*
2. A first-degree relative with NF-2 *and* either a unilateral acoustic neurinoma *or* at least two of the following:

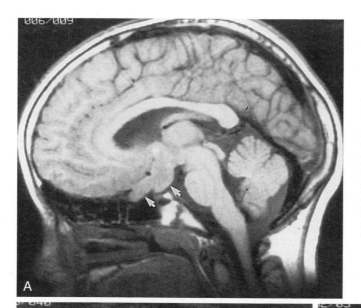

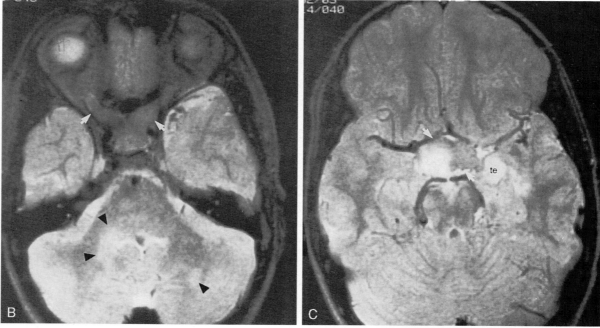

FIGURE 16–25. Neurofibromatosis 1: 7-year-old girl. Midline sagittal T1-weighted image *(A)* shows a mass *(arrows)* extending within the suprasellar cistern, optic chiasm, hypothalamus, and anterior third ventricle. Axial T2-weighted image *(B)* reveals tumor enlarging intracranial optic nerves bilaterally. Axial T2-weighted image *(C)* shows a large astrocytoma of mixed signal intensity filling the suprasellar cistern *(arrows)* and extending into the left temporal lobe (te). The areas of high signal intensity within the right middle cerebellar peduncle and left corpus medullare *(arrowheads, B)* are common in NF-1; their pathologic nature is unclear.

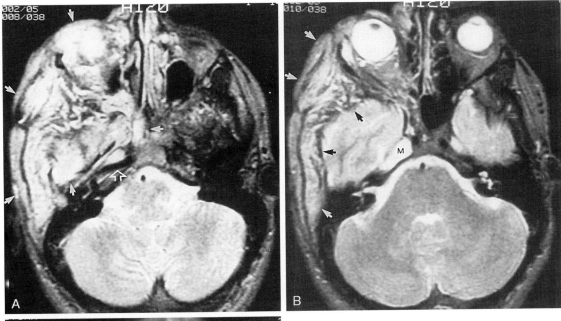

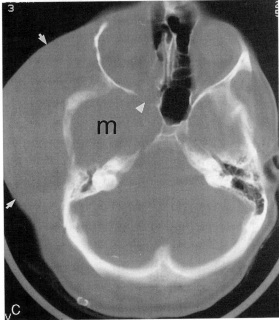

FIGURE 16–26. Neurofibromatosis 1: 30-year-old man. Axial T2-weighted images *(A and B)* show a large facial plexiform neurofibroma with heterogeneous signal intensity *(solid arrows)*. Tumor extends within the infratemporal fossa and temporal fossa and penetrates the orbital septum inferiorly to access the inferolateral aspect of the right orbit. Infiltration of the orbit and extraocular muscles is associated with medial deviation of the right globe. The right globe is also larger than the left globe; such unilateral macro-ophthalmia ("cow eye" or buphthalmos) occurs occasionally in NF-1. Enlargement of the right gasserian ganglion indicates extension into Meckel's cave (M in *B*). There is posterior deviation of the right internal carotid artery *(open arrow* in *A)* within the carotid canal. Axial bone window from an earlier CT examination *(C)* demonstrates sphenoid dysplasia with thinning of lateral orbital process of the greater sphenoid wing; the superior ophthalmic fissure is widened *(arrowhead)*. Enlargement of the middle cranial fossa (m) is also seen. The plexiform neurofibroma *(arrows)* extends outward far beyond the normal lateral convex curvature of the face seen on the left side. The MRI examination was performed after partial resection of this bulky extracranial mass.

a. Neurofibroma
b. Meningioma
c. Glioma
d. Schwannoma
e. Juvenile posterior subcapsular lenticular opacity

Because cutaneous and ocular manifestations are absent in most patients with NF-2, a later age at presentation (second through fourth decades of life) is common. Moreover, the radiologist may be the first to obtain objective (MRI or CT) evidence of NF-2 in many patients.[49] It therefore places an important burden on the practicing radiologist to be aware of the key CNS findings in this disorder[43] (see Table 16–6).

CNS MRI MANIFESTATIONS

Bilateral Acoustic Neurinomas. A review of the MR images obtained in 11 patients with NF-2[47] revealed neurinomas of the acoustic nerves that enlarged the seventh and eighth cranial nerve complexes in 10 patients (91%) (Fig. 16–27). These tumors generally cause enhancement of the affected nerves and erosion of the walls of the internal auditory canals. Small tumors may be detected solely by their enhancement on T1-weighted MR images after administration of Gd-DTPA.

Other Cranial Neurinomas. Seventeen cranial nerve tumors other than acoustic neurinomas were detected in 8 of 11 patients (73%) with NF-2 in one series.[47] Cranial nerves V, X, XI, and XII were most often involved (Fig. 16–28; see Fig. 16–27). Nodular enlarge-ment or fusiform thickening of the involved nerve is accompanied by enhancement after Gd-DTPA administration in most cases.

Meningiomas. Twelve meningiomas were detected in 6 of 11 patients (55%) with NF-2.[47] More than one meningioma was present in four patients. Seven of the meningiomas detected were dura-based lesions, whereas five were intraventricular masses (see Fig. 16–28).

No optic gliomas or "high-intensity white matter lesions" (both of which are seen often in NF-1) were detected in any of the 11 patients with NF-2 reported in one series.[47]

SPINAL MANIFESTATIONS. All nine patients with NF-2 had an abnormal MRI examination of the spine in one series.[50] In this series, MRI included only T1-weighted gadolinium-enhanced sequences. Owing to time constraints, no T2-weighted images were obtained.

Five patients had a total of eight enhancing intramedullary masses; intramedullary masses in the cervical region outnumbered thoracic region masses. Pathologic analysis available in five of the masses revealed ependymoma. Syringomyelia can be associated with intramedullary masses in patients with NF-2.[50]

All nine patients had enhancing, intradural, extramedullary masses consistent with schwannomas or meningiomas (Fig. 16–29; see Fig. 16–28). An average of 12 masses (range 2 to 34) was present in each patient.

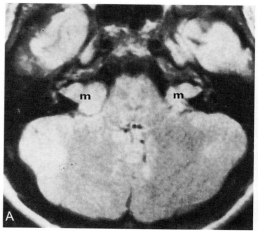

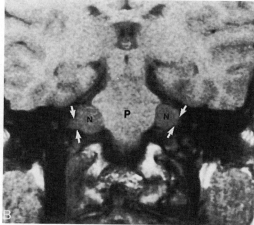

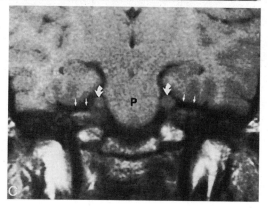

FIGURE 16–27. Neurofibromatosis 2: 17-year-old girl. Axial proton density–weighted image *(A)* demonstrates bilateral fifth and eighth cranial nerve neurinomas seen as single large masses (m) within both cerebellopontine angle cisterns. Coronal T1-weighted images *(B* and *C)* distinguish hypointense *(B)* eighth cranial nerve tumors (N) widening internal auditory canals *(large straight arrows)* and compressing the pons (P) from slightly hypointense *(C)* neurinomas of cisternal portions of fifth cranial nerves *(curved arrows)*, cut in cross section above roofs of internal auditory canals *(small straight arrows)* on slightly more anterior section.

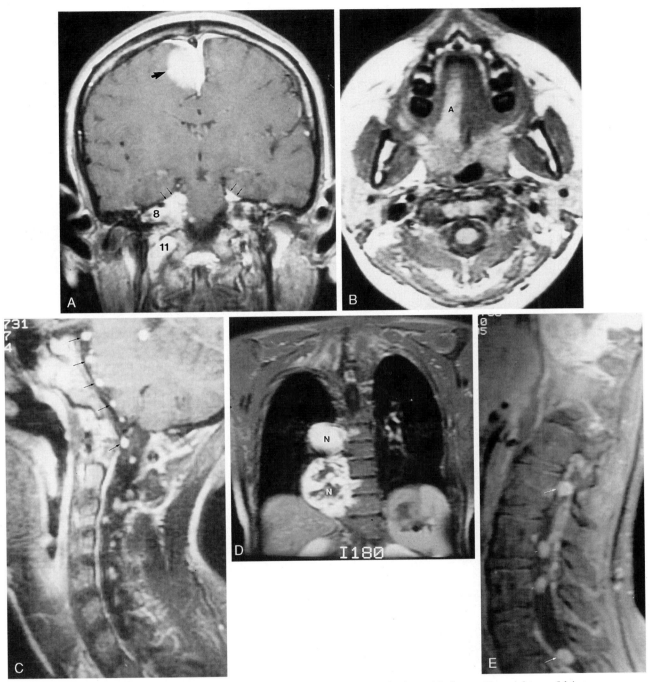

FIGURE 16–28. Neurofibromatosis 2: 20-year-old woman. Large meningioma *(single arrow)* in a right parafalcine location enhances uniformly on a postgadolinium T1-weighted coronal image *(A)*. Bilateral fifth cranial nerve tumors are detected *(small double arrows)* as well. Enlargement and excessive enhancement of the right acoustic nerve (8) and hypoglossal nerve (11) are displayed. In this patient, denervation atrophy of the right side of the tongue and tongue fasciculations were noted clinically and ascribed to the right hypoglossal neurinoma. An axial pregadolinium T1-weighted image *(B)* demonstrates increased signal intensity within the right side of the musculature of the tongue, representing fatty replacement, owing to denervation atrophy (A in *B*). Numerous additional enhancing, intradural, extramedullary masses *(arrows)* consistent with schwannomas or meningiomas are seen on a paramidline sagittal T1-weighted image *(C)*, including the posterior fossa and the cervical spine. Coronal, postgadolinium T1-weighted image *(D)* demonstrates enhancing paraspinal lesions (N) in the middle to low thoracic region, likely representing schwannomas. Sagittal, postgadolinium fat suppression image *(E)* shows numerous additional enhancing, extramedullary masses *(arrows)* in the lumbar region, several of which extend into and enlarge the neural foramina.

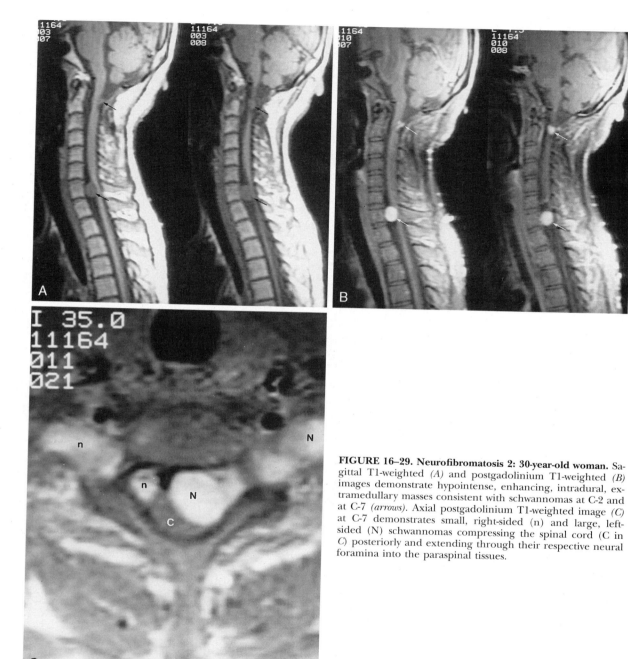

FIGURE 16–29. Neurofibromatosis 2: 30-year-old woman. Sagittal T1-weighted *(A)* and postgadolinium T1-weighted *(B)* images demonstrate hypointense, enhancing, intradural, extramedullary masses consistent with schwannomas at C-2 and at C-7 *(arrows)*. Axial postgadolinium T1-weighted image *(C)* at C-7 demonstrates small, right-sided (n) and large, left-sided (N) schwannomas compressing the spinal cord (C in *C*) posteriorly and extending through their respective neural foramina into the paraspinal tissues.

The masses were slightly more common in the thoracic and lumbar regions. Masses of multiple histologies were present in several patients.

No clinical symptoms related to lesion location were noted in three of five patients with intramedullary masses, and in six of nine patients with intradural, extramedullary masses in this series.[50] The remaining patients in this group with NF-2 had neurologic symptoms that correlated with the MRI findings.

Four of nine patients with NF-2 had associated bony abnormalities.[50] The abnormalities included enlarged neural foramina (see Figs. 16–28 and 16–29) due to masses in three patients and posterior vertebral body scalloping also secondary to a mass in one patient. Dural ectasia was not seen in the NF-2 group.

Sturge-Weber Syndrome

Encephalotrigeminal angiomatosis is a phakomatosis that includes the following clinical characteristics: a facial vascular nevus in the territory of the ophthalmic division of the trigeminal nerve, seizures, dementia, hemiplegia, hemianopsia, and buphthalmos or glaucoma.[51] Intraparenchymal calcification, parenchymal volume loss, engorgement of deep veins, and leptomeningeal and choroid plexus angiomas are seen at pathologic examination.[14] The incidence of Sturge-Weber syndrome is 1 per 1000 patients in mental institutions. It appears sporadically.[4]

In patients with Sturge-Weber syndrome, MRI reveals the following (Figs. 16–30 and 16–31).

ATROPHY. Unilateral or bilateral parenchymal volume loss may be associated with hemicranial atrophy[51] (see Fig. 16–30). Thickened cortex and decreased convolutions in regions of parenchymal atrophy may represent disturbed neuronal proliferation and migration as a consequence of abnormal cerebral venous blood flow[51] (Fig. 16–32; see Fig. 16–30).

CALCIFICATION. Regions of hypointensity on T2-weighted images were seen at the cortical-subcortical junction in areas of known parenchymal calcification detected on CT scans (see Fig. 16–30). MRI with spin-echo sequences continually underestimated the severity and extent of parenchymal calcification in this[51] and other[52] disorders. MRI with gradient-echo acquisition proved to be more sensitive than spin-echo MRI for the detection of intraparenchymal calcification.[53]

VASCULAR ANOMALIES. In one small series,[51] no superficial regions of flow-related signal void, thrombosis, or other direct evidence suggested the presence of leptomeningeal angiomas. Nevertheless, a paucity of superficial cortical veins and engorgement and tortuosity of subependymal and medullary veins were seen on the affected side, providing important indirect evidence of abnormal cerebral hemodynamics (see Fig. 16–30). Enlarged and calcified choroid plexus lesions, hyperintense on T2-weighted images, are reported to represent angiomatous involvement.[51, 54]

ACCELERATED MYELINATION. In three infants younger than age 9 months, MRI demonstrated accelerated myelination; affected white matter had prematurely decreased signal intensity on T2-weighted images[51, 55] and had increased signal intensity on IR images[55] (see Fig. 16–32). Ischemia of the brain parenchyma underlying the leptomeningeal angioma may lead to a hypermyelinative state once myelin begins to be laid down.[55]

Tuberous Sclerosis

This is a rare heredofamilial disease with the classic clinical triad of adenoma sebaceum (30% to 85% of cases), seizures (80%), and mental retardation (50% to 80%). Hyperpigmented nevi (83%), shagreen patches, subungual fibromas, rhabdomyomas and sarcomas of the heart, and angiomyolipomas of the kidney (80%) may also be seen.[4] Its incidence varies from 1 in 20,000 to 1 in 500,000 persons. The disorder is inherited in autosomal dominant fashion in 20% to 50% of cases; a genetic mutation is believed to be responsible for the remainder.

The diagnostic features of tuberous sclerosis have been divided into primary and secondary criteria.[56]

The presence of any one of the following primary criteria establishes the diagnosis of tuberous sclerosis[44, 56]:

1. Adenoma sebaceum
2. Ungual fibroma
3. Cerebral cortical hamartomas (so-called tubers)
4. Subependymal hamartomas
5. Fibrous forehead plaque

The presence of two or more of the following secondary features also indicates a firm diagnosis of tuberous sclerosis[44, 56]:

1. Infantile spasms (hypsarrhythmia)
2. Hypopigmented macules
3. Shagreen patch
4. Retinal hamartoma
5. Bilateral renal cysts or angiomyolipomas
6. Cardiac rhabdomyoma
7. First-degree relative with tuberous sclerosis

The diagnosis of tuberous sclerosis can also be firmly established by imaging criteria.[44] The presence of one of the following features on CT or MRI scans is diagnostic of tuberous sclerosis:

1. Multiple subependymal nodules, especially with calcification
2. Multiple cortical abnormalities with calcification and subcortical white matter edema

A diagnosis of tuberous sclerosis may be suspected (but not established) when CT or MRI scans reveal any one (or more) of the following:

1. An intraventricular tumor consistent with a subependymal giant cell astrocytoma
2. Focal wedge-shaped calcifications in the cerebral or cerebellar cortex
3. Multiple cortical or subcortical foci of edema

The hamartomas of tuberous sclerosis are histologically benign masses that appear in two characteristic locations: 1) superficially within the cerebral cortex

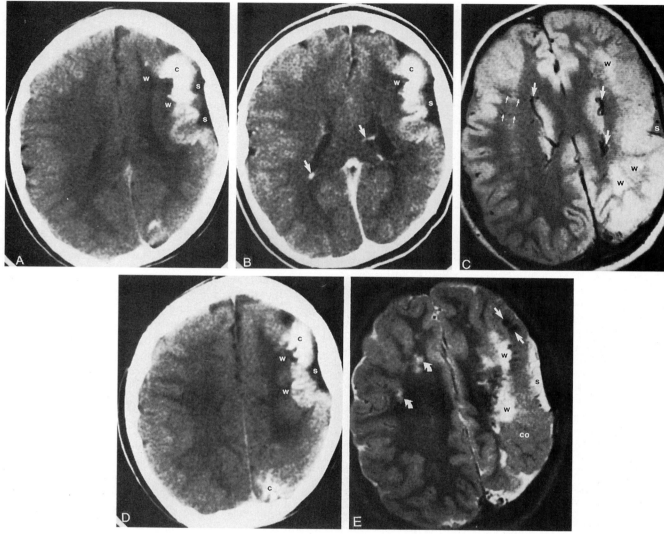

FIGURE 16–30. Sturge-Weber syndrome: 6-year-old boy. Noncontrast *(A)* and postcontrast *(B)* axial CT sections demonstrate prominent subarachnoid spaces (s) overlying atrophic left frontal lobe. Cortical calcification (c) and hypodense white matter (w) of the forceps minor are well shown. Proton density–weighted axial MRI section *(C)* at the same level shows high signal intensity within the subcortical and periventricular white matter of the left frontal and parietal lobes (w). In addition, dilated medullary veins *(small arrows, C)* and subependymal veins *(large arrows, B and C)* are more obvious with MRI. A paucity of superficial cortical veins is seen overlying the left hemisphere. No evidence of calcification is detected by MRI at this level. Noncontrast CT section *(D)* at a slightly higher level detects calcification (c) within the left occipital and frontal cortex. On corresponding T2-weighted MRI section *(E)*, two nonspecific foci of hypointensity measuring less than 5 mm in diameter *(arrows)* are the only findings suggesting calcification. MRI, however, shows best the thickened cortex (co) overlying the left parietal lobe (compare with *D*). MRI also demonstrates abnormally high signal intensity within the white matter of the right frontal lobe *(curved arrows)*, which appeared normal on CT scans (compare with *D*). Dilated subarachnoid spaces (s) and abnormal white matter (w) within the left centrum semiovale are also seen.

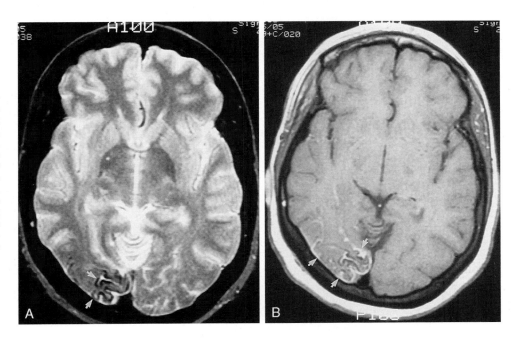

FIGURE 16–31. Sturge-Weber syndrome: 34-year-old woman. Dystrophic cortical and subcortical calcification in the right occipital lobe is well demonstrated on an axial T2-weighted image *(A)* as gyriform regions of hypointensity *(arrows)*. Sulci of the right occipital lobe appear slightly larger than contralateral sulci, reflecting ipsilateral atrophy. Corresponding postcontrast axial T1-weighted image *(B)* shows gyriform enhancement within the affected lobe *(arrows)*.

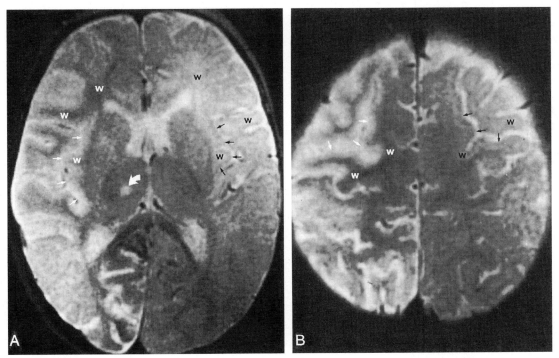

FIGURE 16–32. Sturge-Weber syndrome: 5-month-old female infant. Axial T2-weighted images show abnormal thickening and high signal intensity affecting the insular cortex *(white arrows, A)* and cortex of the high right frontal lobe *(white arrows, B)*. Compare with the normal cortex *(black arrows, A and B)* on the left side. White matter within the right forceps minor and beneath the thickened cortex (white w, *A and B*) has low signal intensity, unusual in a patient only 5 months of age. Compare with normal white matter (black w, *A and B*) on the left side. A focal lesion *(curved arrow, A)* is also detected within the right thalamus.

(tubers) or 2) deep in a subependymal location, along the lateral borders of the ventricles in the striatothalamic groove between the caudate nucleus and the thalamus.[44] Hamartomas in both locations contain unusual large cells of both neuronal and astrocytic differentiation, gliosis (astrocytosis), and demyelination. The hamartomas in the subependymal region calcify more frequently and to a greater degree than those in the cortex. Less than 20% of patients have cerebellar hamartomas.

A minority (5% to 15%) of individuals with tuberous sclerosis will develop a giant cell astrocytoma in the subependymal surface of the caudate nucleus near the foramen of Monro. Such tumors are benign and slow-growing lesions that are believed to arise from a preexisting hamartoma. The lesions may cause mechanical obstruction of the lateral ventricle and result in hydrocephalus.

CNS MRI MANIFESTATIONS. In patients with tuberous sclerosis, MRI reveals the following (Figs. 16–33 and 16–34).

Subependymal Nodules. When the calcifications are large enough, these lesions may be seen as focal signal voids, owing to shortening of both T1 and T2 (see Fig. 16–34). Other lesions may be hyperintense on T2-weighted images, owing to a predominance of gliosis and demyelination (prolongation of both T1 and T2). Enhancement of subependymal nodules can occur after gadolinium administration, making it more difficult to distinguish between a small, early subependymal giant cell astrocytoma and a subependymal hamartomatous nodule. Subependymal nodules are often bilateral and asymmetric.

Cortical Tubers. MRI reveals such lesions as enlarged gyri with abnormal signal intensity (see Figs. 16–33 and 16–34). The MRI appearance of cortical tubers varies with age and the degree of myelination of the white matter. In neonates and young children, the lesions are hyperintense relative to nonmyelinated white matter on T1-weighted images and hypointense on T2-weighted images. In older children and adults, cortical tubers are isointense to hypointense relative to myelinated white matter on T1-weighted images; on T2-weighted images the lesions are hyperintense relative to both gray and white matter in this age group.[43] Cortical tubers are visualized in the cortex, the subcortical white matter, or both. Cortical tubers do not enhance after gadolinium administration in 95% of lesions.

Cortical Heterotopias. Owing to associated deranged neuroblast migration, focal islands of gray matter with cortex-like signal intensity on T1- and T2-weighted images may remain within the white matter of the hemispheres. Such lesions do not enhance after gadolinium administration.

Giant Cell Astrocytomas. These lesions almost always present as larger masses with intraventricular extension within or near the foramen of Monro (see Figs. 16–33 and 16–34). They are often heterogeneous in signal intensity on both T1- and T2-weighted images, may contain one or several focal calcifications or cystic areas, and often obstruct one or both lateral ventricles.

These benign neoplasms enhance after gadolinium administration.

Hydrocephalus. Tubers (or giant cell astrocytomas) located subependymally may restrict egress of CSF from the lateral or third ventricles by compressing the foramen of Monro or the aqueduct of Sylvius, respectively.

The MRI findings correlate well with the severity of mental impairment and seizures.[56a]

Von Hippel–Lindau Disease

Von Hippel–Lindau disease comprises disseminated capillary angiomas in the skin and viscera with, at times, cyst formation. The tumors in the CNS are called capillary hemangioblastomas; lesions are found most frequently in the cerebellum (36% to 60% of cases),[57] brain stem, or spinal cord (<5%). Tumors of the retina are also characteristic (>50%). Hemangioblastomas rarely occur in the cerebral hemispheres. Associated visceral lesions include renal cell carcinoma (25% to 38%) and pheochromocytoma (>10%). The disease has autosomal dominant inheritance with nearly 100% penetrance. Both sexes are affected equally.[14, 57]

The gene for von Hippel–Lindau disease has been mapped to chromosome 3p25-p26.[58, 58a] Patients may now be diagnosed by using DNA markers in the presymptomatic phase of their disease.

Clinical manifestations of patients with von Hippel–Lindau disease include increased intracranial pressure, cerebellar dysfunction, subarachnoid hemorrhage, and polycythemia (secondary to hemangioblastoma, renal cell carcinoma, or pheochromocytoma). Cysts may be present in the liver, spleen, pancreas, kidneys, adrenals, omentum, mesentery, epididymis, lung, and bone. The most common causes of death are cerebellar hemangioblastoma and renal cell carcinoma.[58b]

Diagnostic criteria include any one of the following[59]: 1) more than one hemangioblastoma of the CNS; 2) one CNS hemangioblastoma and one (or more) visceral manifestation; and 3) one CNS or other visceral manifestation of the disease and a positive family history of the disease.

During a 2-year study,[57] MRI of the head, spine, and abdomen was used for screening and follow-up of 26 members of nine families with the disease. Lesions causing significant morbidity and mortality (cerebellar and spinal cord hemangioblastomas, renal cell carcinoma, and pheochromocytoma) were correctly depicted with MRI, sometimes before the lesions could be seen with other imaging modalities.

In most cases the intracranial tumor consists of a vascular nodule incorporated into the wall of a cyst situated at the surface of the cerebellum (Fig. 16–35). The tumor may be completely solid in 20% of cases. The tumor is often within the posterolateral aspect of the cerebellar hemisphere; the vermis may also be involved on occasion.

Cerebellar and spinal cord hemangioblastomas have a characteristic appearance on MR images (see Figs. 16–35 and 16–36). The vascular mural nodule is hyperintense compared with normal parenchyma on T2-

Text continued on page 521

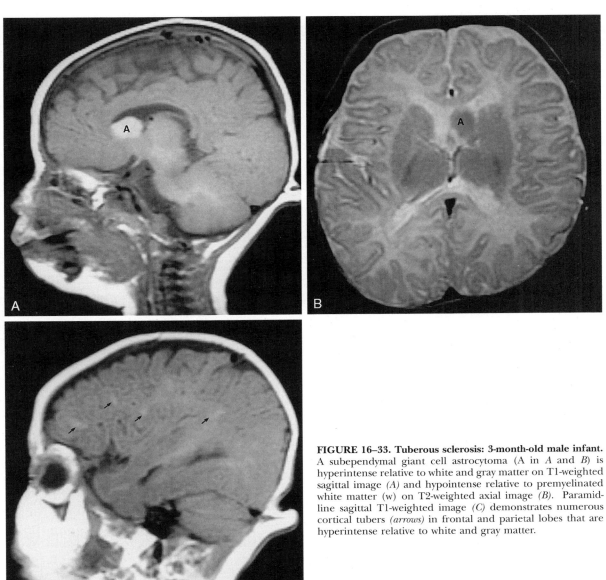

FIGURE 16–33. Tuberous sclerosis: 3-month-old male infant. A subependymal giant cell astrocytoma (A in *A* and *B*) is hyperintense relative to white and gray matter on T1-weighted sagittal image *(A)* and hypointense relative to premyelinated white matter (w) on T2-weighted axial image *(B)*. Paramidline sagittal T1-weighted image *(C)* demonstrates numerous cortical tubers *(arrows)* in frontal and parietal lobes that are hyperintense relative to white and gray matter.

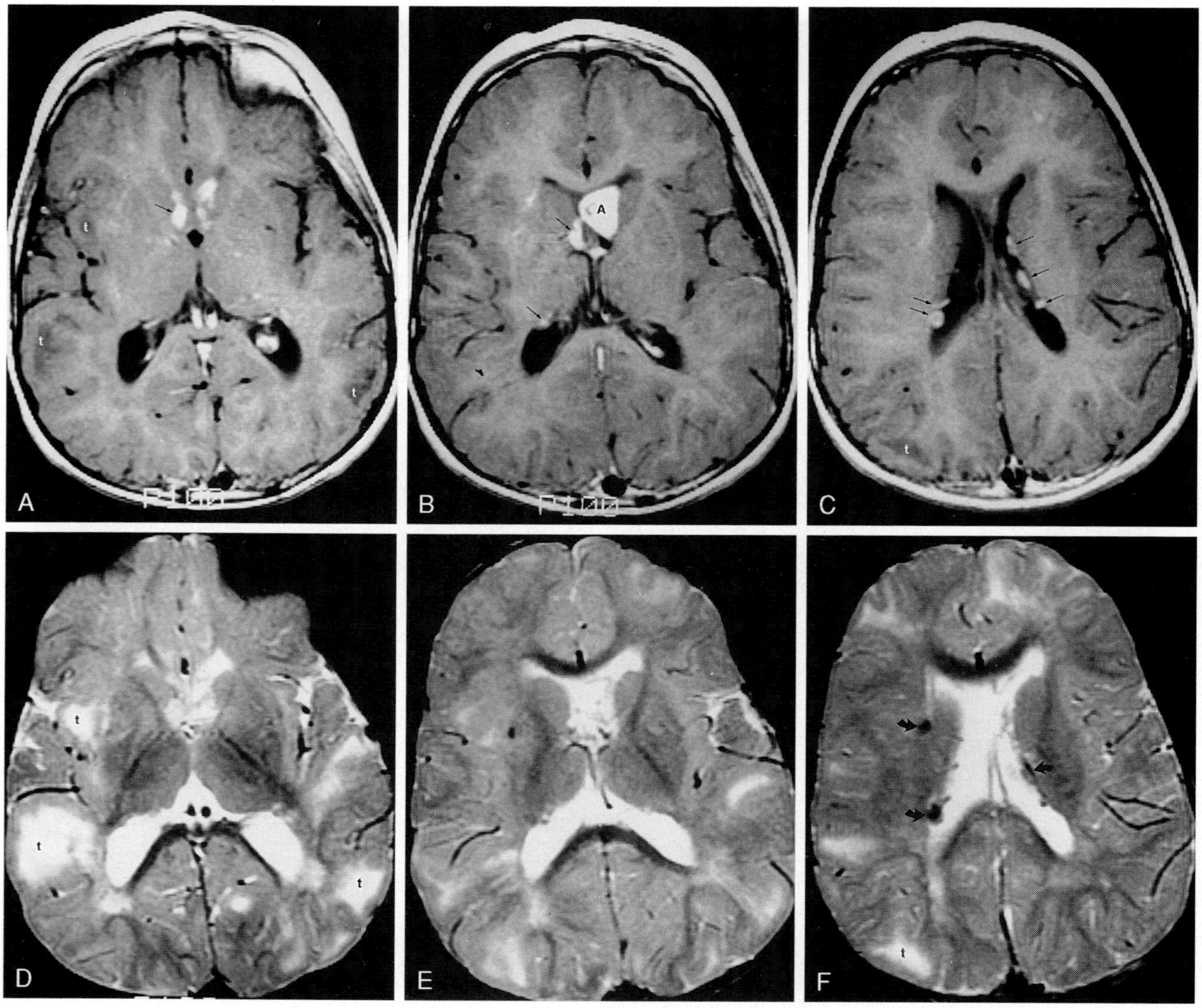

FIGURE 16–34. Tuberous sclerosis: 15-year-old boy. Numerous benign cortical tubers (t) are hypointense on postcontrast T1-weighted axial images *(A to C)* and hyperintense on T2-weighted axial images *(D to F)*. Multiple enhancing subependymal nodules are also seen *(arrows, A to C)*; three of these lesions *(curved arrows)* are hypointense relative to white matter on a T2-weighted image *(F)* owing to calcification. The large enhancing subependymal mass *(A)* in the vicinity of the left foramen of Monro is much more readily seen on the axial T1-weighted postcontrast image *(B)* than on the corresponding T2-weighted image *(E)* in which its hyperintense signal pattern is obscured by the adjacent hyperintense signal pattern of the CSF within the left frontal horn. This large mass was a subependymal giant cell astrocytoma.

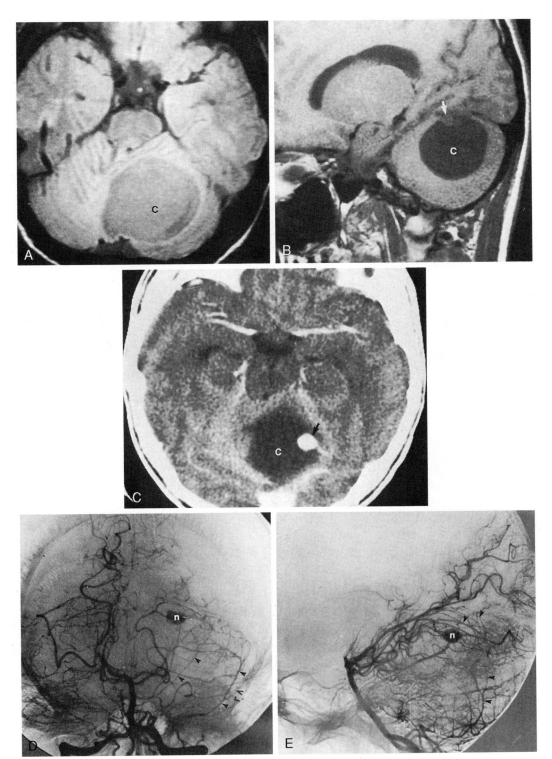

FIGURE 16–35. Von Hippel–Lindau disease and cerebellar hemangioblastoma: 32-year-old man. Axial proton density–weighted image *(A)* and paramidline sagittal T1-weighted image *(B)* demonstrate large cystic component of tumor (c). The cyst is hypointense relative to cortex on both images. Tumor nodule *(B, arrow)*, isointense relative to cortex, is sectioned at the top of the cyst. Axial postcontrast CT image *(C)* shows that the tumor nodule *(arrow)* enhances brightly. The brain stem is effaced *(A and C)*. Anteroposterior and lateral subtraction views of left vertebral artery injection *(D and E)* demonstrate well the vascular tumor nodule (n) and stretching of cerebellar arteries *(arrowheads)* around the avascular mass (cyst).

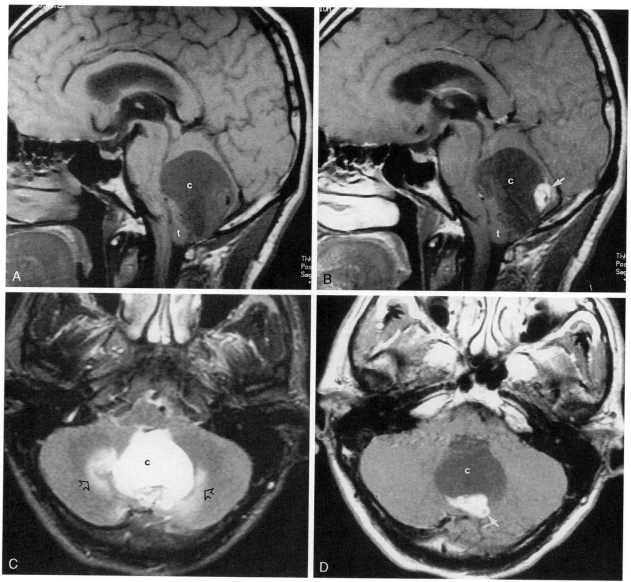

FIGURE 16–36. Von Hippel–Lindau disease and cerebellar hemangioblastoma: 25-year-old man. T1-weighted midline sagittal images before *(A)* and after *(B)* gadolinium administration show the brain stem flattened against the clivus by the large cystic component of tumor (c). The fourth ventricle is effaced. Tonsillar herniation (t) is present. The solid tumor nodule *(arrow, B)* enhances and is more readily seen than on the precontrast study *(A)*. Axial T2-weighted image *(C)* shows that the cystic portion of tumor lies in the vermis and extends into both cerebellar hemispheres. Surrounding hyperintense edema *(open arrows)* is seen. Enhancing tumor nodule *(arrow)* is seen well on a T1-weighted axial postcontrast image *(D,* performed at same level as *C)*. Mild hydrocephalus was present in this patient, owing to compression of the fourth ventricle.

weighted images and hypointense to isointense on T1-weighted images. The tumoral cyst has a relatively high protein content and, therefore, often appears slightly hyperintense compared with normal CSF on both T1- and T2-weighted images. Detection of associated tumoral vessels as regions of serpentine signal void may help to differentiate hemangioblastomas from other cystic neoplasms, such as cystic astrocytoma and medulloblastoma.

DISORDERS OF MIGRATION

Disorders of migration are characterized by abnormalities of the cerebral cortex: the cortical mantle may appear too thick, too flat, or too folded.[24] Often bilateral and symmetric, the neuronal migration abnormalities may be distinguished from the predominantly unilateral, acquired intrauterine insults caused by infection or infarction. The earlier the disturbance of neuroblast migration, the more severe and generalized is the resulting cerebral deformity.

Lissencephaly

The most severe form of migrational disorder is associated with a smooth brain having no gyri. In most cases, however, regions of broad, flattened gyri (pachygyria) may be seen in the same hemisphere.[60] Lissencephaly occurs in association with abnormalities in other parts of the body as part of a syndrome (e.g., Miller-Dieker) or as an isolated abnormality. It may be inherited (autosomal recessive) or may occur spontaneously. The most severely affected patients with lissencephaly are decerebrate. All have mental retardation. Seizures develop by the age of 1 year; death ensues by the age of 2 years. Microscopically, the cortex has only four layers; in contrast, normal cortex has six layers. The cortex is thickened in this disorder due to arrest of the later waves of migrating neuroblasts. Accordingly, the white matter becomes reduced in size and the cortical surface remains devoid of gyri.

On axial MR images, there is micrencephaly, with the cerebral hemispheres taking on an hourglass contour because the brain fails to develop opercula (Fig. 16–37). The insular cortex remains superficial, and the middle cerebral arteries course within shallow sylvian grooves. The claustrum and the extreme capsule are often absent. Other findings include atrophy of the corpus callosum, heterotopic nodules of gray matter near the lateral ventricles, and mild dilatation of the lateral ventricles with accentuation in the region of the atria and occipital horns (colpocephaly).[4, 60, 61]

Pachygyria

Pachygyria is a rare disorder occurring sporadically. The severity of clinical symptoms varies with the degree of morphologic derangement. The most severely affected patients may have a lack of awareness of the environment and severe mental retardation. Seizures may develop in childhood. Patients with pachygyria

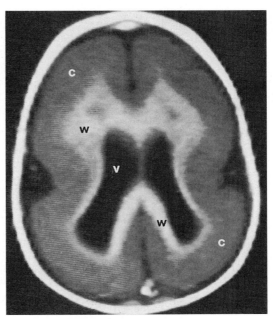

FIGURE 16–37. Lissencephaly: neonate. Axial T1-weighted image demonstrates a smooth brain surface with an hourglass configuration. The white matter (w) is reduced in thickness from premature arrest of later waves of migrating neuroblasts. Accordingly, the cortex (c) is thickened. Mild dilatation of the lateral ventricles (v) with posterior predominance is seen.

have a longer survival than those with lissencephaly. This anomaly may occur without associated agyria.

MRI demonstrates abnormally broad and thickened gyri separated by shallow sulci (Fig. 16–38). All or only a part of the brain may be involved. The gray matter–white matter interface is abnormally smooth with incomplete digitations.[4]

Polymicrogyria

The final waves of neurons migrate to the cortex during the fifth to sixth month of fetal gestation; these neurons form the most superficial cortical layers. If these migrating neurons do not distribute normally at their final destination, an imbalance of growth rates may occur between cortical layers. Such an imbalance causes the formation of numerous small gyri (polymicrogyria).[14] The affected gyri may involve large areas of both hemispheres or be restricted to smaller regions in one or both hemispheres. Even at autopsy, polymicrogyria may be mistaken for pachygyria because the multiple small gyri have fused surfaces that are not exteriorized by sulci. This is a potential pitfall in imaging diagnosis.

Patients with small foci of polymicrogyria may be asymptomatic, but those with extensive regions are often retarded and have other neurologic deficits.

Heterotopic Gray Matter

Regions of heterotopic gray matter are islands of neurons located anywhere from the subependymal region to the cortex that result from arrested neuroblast

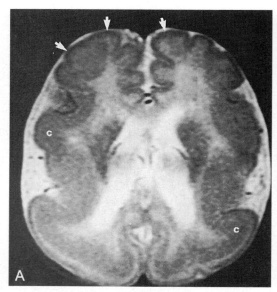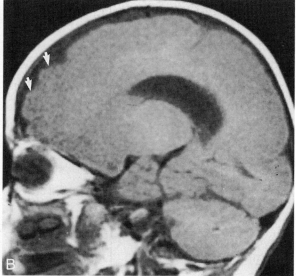

FIGURE 16–38. Pachygyria: neonate. Axial T2-weighted *(A)* and sagittal T1-weighted *(B)* images demonstrate that frontal gyri *(arrows)* are abnormally broad and separated by shallow sulci. Posterior hemispheres are nearly agyric. Cortex (c) is abnormally thick, especially posteriorly, best seen on the T2-weighted image *(A)*.

migration. Three broad clinical classes of heterotopias may be differentiated[62]:

1. Subependymal heterotopias (Fig. 16–39). Such patients have milder symptoms, including mixed partial complex and tonic-clonic seizures. Their mental development and motor function are most often normal.

2. Focal subcortical heterotopias (Fig. 16–40). The severity of symptoms encountered in affected patients varies with the quantity of neurons that have been arrested during the migration phase. Those with larger and thicker islands of subcortical neurons may have moderate to severe developmental delay and hemiplegia; normal mental development and normal motor function may be seen in patients with smaller, thinner zones of involvement.

3. Diffuse gray matter heterotopias. In affected patients, the migration of a variable thickness layer of neurons has been arrested before reaching the cerebral cortex. A band of heterotopic neurons becomes isolated within the white matter, giving the appearance of a "double cortex." Such patients generally have moderate to severe developmental delay and refractory seizure disorder beginning at an early age.[62]

Heterotopias have signal intensity properties similar to those of gray matter on all image sequences. Subependymal heterotopias appear as multiple, small (often <5 mm) smooth and rounded masses that bulge into the adjacent lateral ventricle creating a nodular-appearing inner surface (see Fig. 16–39). Differentiation of subependymal heterotopias from subependymal hamartomas of tuberous sclerosis depends on noticing differences in shape, signal intensity, and enhancement properties[62] (Table 16–7).

Subcortical heterotopias typically form nodular masses that may range from several millimeters to as large as 10 cm in maximal diameter. Thinning of the

cortex may occur, and there may be a decrease in depth of the sulci overlying larger subcortical heterotopias. Heterotopias may occur as isolated derangements or be associated with other migrational abnormalities.[24]

Diffuse gray matter heterotopias may appear as an annular band of gray matter deep to the cerebral cortex; an intervening layer of normal-appearing white matter is present. The condition of the overlying cortex varies with the thickness of the abnormal subcortical band: a thick band frequently underlies cortex that is pachygyric, whereas a thin band may underlie a normal-appearing cortex of normal thickness, with normal sulcal depth.

MRI may detect heterotopias missed by CT before and after intravenous administration of contrast medium.[63]

Schizencephaly

Schizencephaly refers to full-thickness clefts within the cerebral hemispheres. On pathologic examination, an infolding of gray matter is found along the cleft from the cortex to the ventricles and a fusion of the

TABLE 16–7. DIFFERENTIATION OF SUBEPENDYMAL HAMARTOMA AND SUBEPENDYMAL HETEROTOPIA

FACTOR	SUBEPENDYMAL HAMARTOMA	SUBEPENDYMAL HETEROTOPIA
Shape	Irregular, elongated	Smooth, rounded
Signal intensity	Isointense to hypointense relative to white matter	Isointense relative to gray matter
Postcontrast enhancement	Occasionally	Never

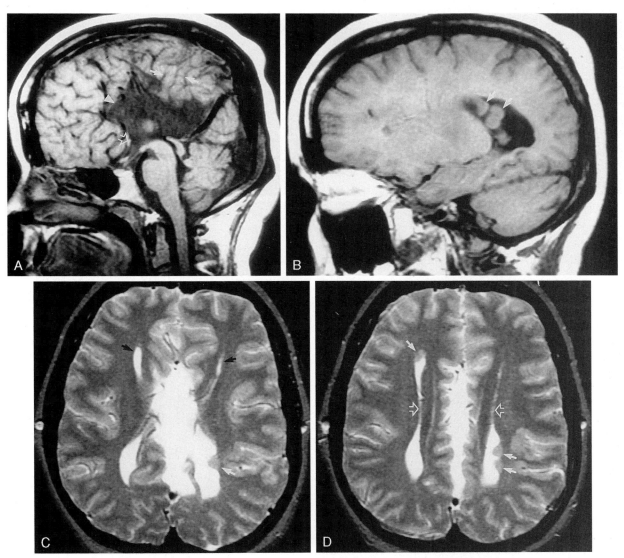

FIGURE 16–39. Callosal agenesis and associated subependymal heterotopias: 31-year-old woman. Midline sagittal T1-weighted image *(A)* shows absence of the entire corpus callosum. The sulci *(solid arrows)* along the medial aspect of the hemisphere are arranged radially, perpendicular to the inferior margin of the hemisphere. The anterior commissure *(open arrow)* is intact. There is continuity of the third ventricle with the anterior interhemispheric fissure *(arrowhead)*. Left paramidline sagittal T1-weighted image *(B)* through dilated lateral ventricular atrium shows subependymal heterotopias *(arrows)* isointense relative to gray matter, bulging into the lumen of the ventricle. Axial T2-weighted image *(C)* through the level of the lateral ventricles shows that frontal horns *(black arrows)* are widely separated and convex laterally (as opposed to concave as in normal subjects); the interhemispheric fissure is dilated; a subependymal heterotopia *(white arrow)* bulges into the lumen of the left ventricular trigone. Axial T2-weighted image *(D)* shows additional subependymal heterotopias *(solid arrows)* isointense relative to gray matter indenting the right frontal horn and posterior body of the left lateral ventricle. The characteristic parallel lateral ventricles *(open arrows)* are well seen.

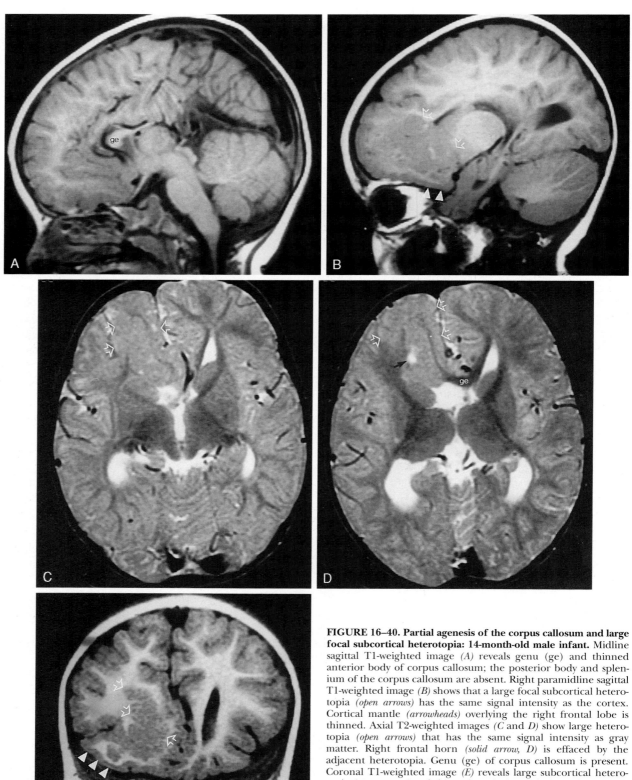

FIGURE 16–40. Partial agenesis of the corpus callosum and large focal subcortical heterotopia: 14-month-old male infant. Midline sagittal T1-weighted image *(A)* reveals genu (ge) and thinned anterior body of corpus callosum; the posterior body and splenium of the corpus callosum are absent. Right paramidline sagittal T1-weighted image *(B)* shows that a large focal subcortical heterotopia *(open arrows)* has the same signal intensity as the cortex. Cortical mantle *(arrowheads)* overlying the right frontal lobe is thinned. Axial T2-weighted images *(C and D)* show large heterotopia *(open arrows)* that has the same signal intensity as gray matter. Right frontal horn *(solid arrow, D)* is effaced by the adjacent heterotopia. Genu (ge) of corpus callosum is present. Coronal T1-weighted image *(E)* reveals large subcortical heterotopia *(open arrows)* and thinned cortical mantle *(arrowheads)* overlying the right frontal lobe.

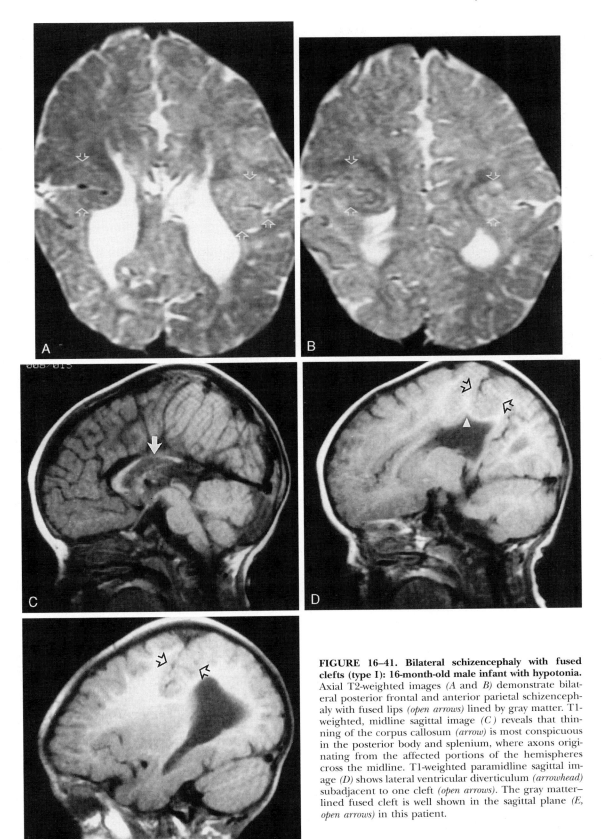

FIGURE 16–41. Bilateral schizencephaly with fused clefts (type I): 16-month-old male infant with hypotonia. Axial T2-weighted images *(A* and *B)* demonstrate bilateral posterior frontal and anterior parietal schizencephaly with fused lips *(open arrows)* lined by gray matter. T1-weighted, midline sagittal image *(C)* reveals that thinning of the corpus callosum *(arrow)* is most conspicuous in the posterior body and splenium, where axons originating from the affected portions of the hemispheres cross the midline. T1-weighted paramidline sagittal image *(D)* shows lateral ventricular diverticulum *(arrowhead)* subadjacent to one cleft *(open arrows)*. The gray matter–lined fused cleft is well shown in the sagittal plane *(E, open arrows)* in this patient.

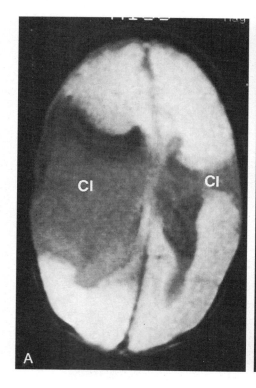

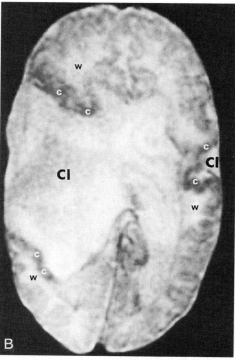

FIGURE 16–42. Schizencephaly with open clefts (type II): 4-month-old infant. Proton density–weighted *(A)* axial image shows full-thickness clefts (Cl) within both hemispheres. T2-weighted image *(B)* at a slightly higher level shows that the cortex (c) lining both clefts has lower signal intensity than underlying white matter (w), as expected in a subject of this age.

cortical pia and ventricular ependyma forms a pial-ependymal seam (Figs. 16–41 and 16–42). An ischemic episode occurring during the seventh week of gestation has been proposed as the underlying cause of these anomalies.[64]

Patients with unilateral schizencephaly and a small cleft often have normal intellect, although they may be hemiplegic. Those with large, unilateral clefts have a high frequency of moderate to severe developmental delay. Those with bilateral clefts also present with moderate to severe developmental delay and delayed language and motor skills.[62]

MRI may reveal two varieties of schizencephaly: type I with fusion of the cleft lips and type II with open clefts allowing communication between the sylvian subarachnoid space and the lateral ventricles. Associated findings include 1) abnormal cortex (pachygyria) flanking and lining the cleft, 2) lateral ventricular diverticulum subjacent to the cleft, 3) hypoplastic sylvian vessels ipsilateral to the cleft, 4) absence of the septum pellucidum, 5) thinning of the corpus callosum, and 6) small pyramidal tracts owing to axonal loss.[65] MRI proved to be more accurate than cranial ultrasonography and CT in the depiction of the pathoanatomy in two neonates with schizencephaly.[65]

Anomalies of the Corpus Callosum

The numerous disorders of formation of the corpus callosum include partial or complete callosal agenesis, lipomas of the interhemispheric fissure, and callosal atrophy or "hypoplasia" (Figs. 16–43 and 16–44; see Figs. 16–39 and 16–40). Evidence suggests that partial or complete callosal agenesis is caused by insults that arrest formation of callosal embryologic precursors

(lamina reuniens, sulcus medianus telencephali medii, massa commissuralis) between 8 and 13 weeks of gestation.[66] Lipomas and sphenoidal encephaloceles probably occur as a result of faulty dysjunction of neuroectoderm and cutaneous ectoderm at the anterior neuropore.[66] A complete but atrophic corpus callosum results from an insult to the cortex or white matter after formation of the corpus callosum is complete (at 18 to 20 weeks of gestation).

The incidence of callosal agenesis is not known. It has been observed in 0.7% of pneumoencephalograms. Most cases are sporadic; males and females are affected with equal frequency. Clinically, most patients with complete agenesis are asymptomatic. Careful examination may reveal that learning and memory are not shared between the hemispheres (cerebral disconnection syndrome).[4] When symptoms (seizures, developmental delay) are present, they are often related to concurrent migrational disorders, not to the callosal anomaly itself.

In patients with callosal agenesis, MRI demonstrates the following (see Figs. 16–43 and 16–44).

PARENCHYMAL AND VASCULAR ANOMALIES. Midline sagittal images reveal the partial or complete absence of the corpus callosum and, possibly, the concurrent absence of the hippocampal and anterior commissures (see Fig. 16–43). Because the axons from the hemispheres do not cross in the commissure, they course sagittally instead to establish paired bundles along the medial aspects of the lateral ventricles known as the bundles of Probst (see Fig. 16–43). The parieto-occipital and calcarine sulci fail to intersect. Like the other sulci of the medial hemisphere, they become radially oriented perpendicular to the narrow inferior margin of the hemisphere (see Figs. 16–39 and 16–43). Abnormal formation

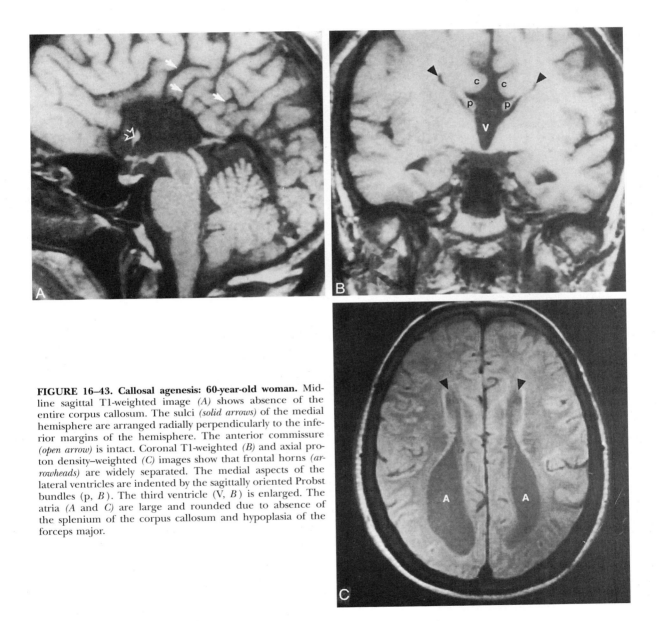

FIGURE 16–43. Callosal agenesis: 60-year-old woman. Midline sagittal T1-weighted image *(A)* shows absence of the entire corpus callosum. The sulci *(solid arrows)* of the medial hemisphere are arranged radially perpendicularly to the inferior margins of the hemisphere. The anterior commissure *(open arrow)* is intact. Coronal T1-weighted *(B)* and axial proton density–weighted *(C)* images show that frontal horns *(arrowheads)* are widely separated. The medial aspects of the lateral ventricles are indented by the sagittally oriented Probst bundles (p, *B*). The third ventricle (V, *B*) is enlarged. The atria *(A and C)* are large and rounded due to absence of the splenium of the corpus callosum and hypoplasia of the forceps major.

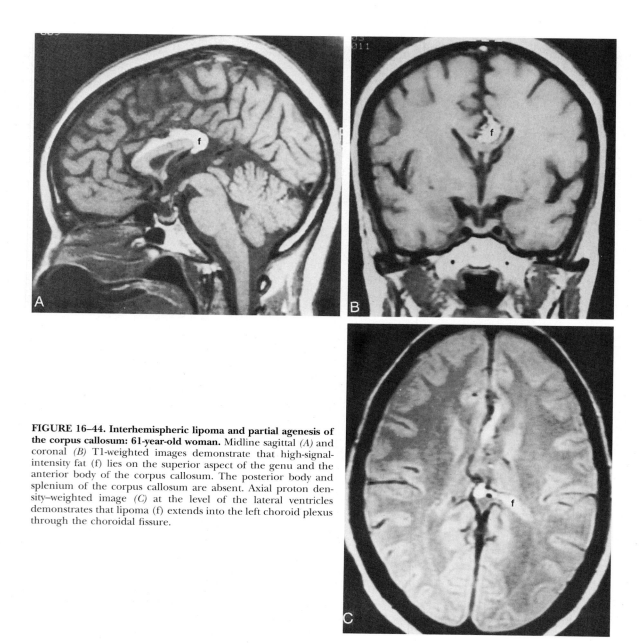

FIGURE 16–44. Interhemispheric lipoma and partial agenesis of the corpus callosum: 61-year-old woman. Midline sagittal *(A)* and coronal *(B)* T1-weighted images demonstrate that high-signal-intensity fat (f) lies on the superior aspect of the genu and the anterior body of the corpus callosum. The posterior body and splenium of the corpus callosum are absent. Axial proton density–weighted image *(C)* at the level of the lateral ventricles demonstrates that lipoma (f) extends into the left choroid plexus through the choroidal fissure.

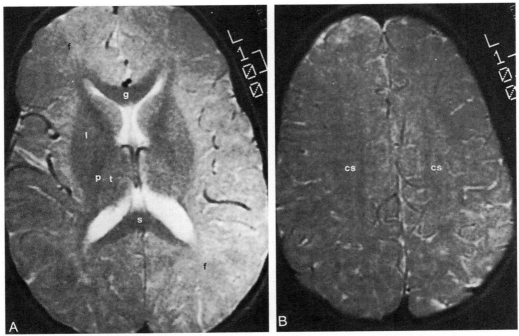

FIGURE 16–45. Delayed myelination in a patient with developmental and speech delay: 4-year-old girl. Axial T2-weighted images (*A* and *B*) demonstrate that mature myelin within the genu (g) and splenium (s) of the corpus callosum, posterior limb of the internal capsule (p), and lentiform nucleus (l) has decreased signal intensity. White matter of the forceps minor and major (f) and centrum semiovale (cs) remains isointense relative to the cortex indicating delayed myelination in these areas. (Myelination of all white matter tracts should be completed by 2 years postnatally.[10])

of the cerebral cortex with agyria, pachygyria, polymicrogyria, and gray matter heterotopias may be seen (see Figs. 16–39 and 16–40). Lateral separation of the pericallosal arteries and internal cerebral veins may be caused by a high third ventricle or interhemispheric cyst. Azygous anterior cerebral arteries may be seen.

VENTRICULAR AND CSF SPACE ANOMALIES. The small frontal horns are widely separated with concave medial borders and sharply angled lateral peaks (see Fig. 16–43). The medial walls of the frontal horns diverge, forming an angle that opens anteriorly. The third ventricle is large and may have a high position. A variably large interhemispheric cyst may spread the hemispheres and may communicate freely with the third ventricle or may consist of multiple poorly or noncommunicating lobules. The atria are large and rounded secondary to absence of the splenium and hypoplasia of the forceps major.

INTERHEMISPHERIC LIPOMAS. Forty percent of patients with these rare lesions have callosal agenesis[67] (see Fig. 16–44). Lipomas appear as variably asymmetric masses of fat within the interhemispheric fissure, usually adjacent to the genu. The lesion may extend to the choroid plexus unilaterally or bilaterally through the choroidal fissure. The pericallosal arteries course through the lipoma.

DISORDERS OF MYELINATION

The early landmarks of normal myelination have been discussed (see earlier section on myelination and Figs. 16–1 to 16–7). Many reports have described delayed myelination in association with hydrocephalus,[68] presumed rubella infection,[66] periventricular leukomalacia,[69, 70] and cerebral palsy.[66] In one series including 33 infants[71] with delayed myelination, hydrocephalus was detected also in 9; bronchopulmonary dysplasia in 14; infarction and/or cerebral atrophy in 18; and respiratory insufficiency requiring assisted ventilation in 25. In a group with normal myelination, no infants with these problems were seen.

Preliminary results indicate that delay in myelination observed by MR methods may have prognostic implications.[71] In a small series of 13 infants with initial delayed myelination who had repeated MRI in the first year of life, the condition persisted in 11 infants. Seven infants proceeded to have developmental delay[71] (Fig. 16–45).

Myelination delay has been reported also in patients with nonketotic hyperglycinemia, a heritable disorder of amino acid metabolism in which large quantities of glycine accumulate in plasma, urine, and CSF.[72] Onset of this disease occurs most often in early infancy. Clinical manifestations include seizures, abnormal muscle tone and reflexes, and pronounced developmental delay. Death ensues usually before the age of 5 years.[72] When assessed using T2-weighted images, decreased or absent myelination within supratentorial white matter tracts was detected in four patients with nonketotic hyperglycinemia older than 10 months in age. Myelination of the brain stem and cerebellum was normal (Fig. 16–46). Abnormalities shown by MRI correlate

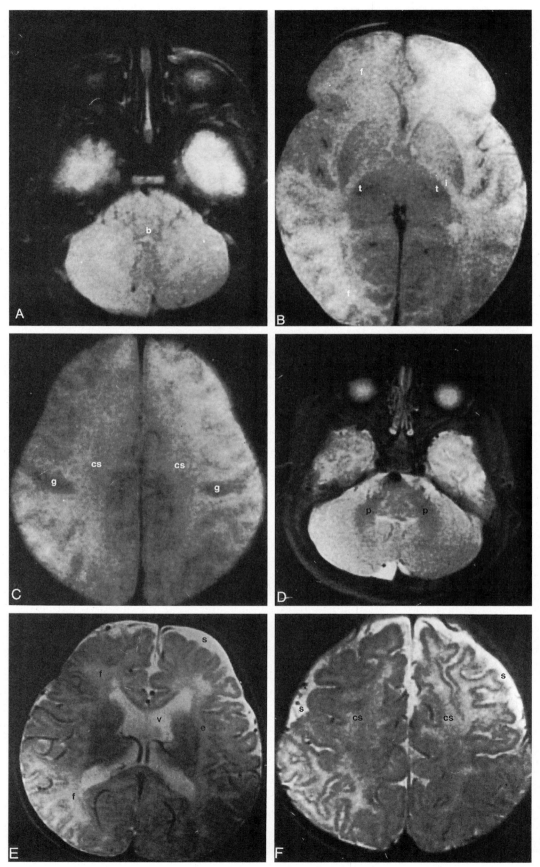

FIGURE 16–46 *See legend on opposite page*

FIGURE 16–46. Patient with nonketotic hyperglycinemia and abnormal progress of myelination. *A* to *C*, Initial (8 days postnatal) axial T2-weighted images demonstrate normal myelination of the brain as decreased signal intensity limited to the dorsal brain stem (b), ventrolateral thalami (t), and paracentral gyri of the cortex (g). The forceps major and minor (f), internal capsule (i), and centrum semiovale (cs) are not myelinated at this age and appear hyperintense relative to the cortex, as expected.[10] *D* to *F*, Follow-up (10 months postnatal) axial T2-weighted images demonstrate interval dilatation of ventricles (v) and subarachnoid spaces overlying the hemispheres (s) compatible with moderate volume loss (compare with *B* and *C*). Decreased signal intensity within the entire brain stem, middle cerebellar peduncles (p), and deep white matter of the cerebellum reflects normal interval progression of myelination in these regions *(D)*. However, white matter within forceps major and minor (f), external capsule (e), and centrum semiovale (cs) remains distinctly brighter than the cortex and basal ganglia (*E* and *F*), indicating delayed myelination in these areas. (The cortex, underlying white matter, and basal ganglia regions should appear essentially isointense in a normal 10-month-old infant.[10])

---

well with known pathologic findings in patients with nonketotic hyperglycinemia.

Accelerated myelination has been detected on MR images in three infants younger than the age of 5 months with Sturge-Weber syndrome.[51, 55] MRI findings in such patients are described earlier in this chapter (see Fig. 16–32).

REFERENCES

1. Volpe JJ: Neurology of the Newborn. 2nd ed. Philadelphia: WB Saunders, 1987.
2. van der Knapp MS, Valk J: Classification of congenital abnormalities of the CNS. AJNR 9:315–326, 1988.
3. Boyer RS: Sedation in pediatric neuroimaging: the science and the art. AJNR 13:777–783, 1992.
4. Naidich TP, Zimmerman RA: Common congenital malformations of the brain. In: Brant-Zawadzki M, Norman D, eds. Magnetic Resonance Imaging of the Central Nervous System. New York: Raven Press, 1987, pp 131–150.
5. Volpe JJ: Normal and abnormal human brain development. Clin Perinatol 4:3–30, 1977.
6. Larroche JC: Development of the nervous system in early life. Part II. The development of the central nervous system during intrauterine life. In: Falkner F, ed. Human Development. Philadelphia: WB Saunders, 1966, pp 257–276.
7. Scammon RE, Hesdorffer MB: Growth of the human nervous system; indices of relation of cerebral volume to surface in developmental period. Proc Soc Exp Biol Med 33:418–421, 1935.
8. McArdle CB, Richardson CJ, Nicholas DA, et al: Developmental features: MR imaging. I. Gray-white matter differentiation and myelination. Radiology 162:223–229, 1987.
9. McArdle CB, Richardson CJ, Hayden CK, et al: Abnormalities of the neonatal brain: MR imaging. II. Hypoxic-ischemic brain injury. Radiology 163:395–403, 1987.
10. Barkovich AJ, Kjos BO, Jackson DE Jr, Norman D: Normal maturation of the neonatal and infant brain: MR imaging at 1.5 T. Radiology 166:173–180, 1988.
11. Byrd S, Naidich TP: Common congenital brain abnormalities. Radiol Clin North Am 26:755–772, 1988.
12. Friede RL: Developmental Neuropathology. New York: Springer-Verlag, 1975.
13. Naidich TP, Altman NR, Braffman BH, et al: Cephalocoeles and related malformations. AJNR 13:655–690, 1992.
14. Larroche JC: Malformations of the nervous system. In: Adams JH, Carsellis JAN, Ducken LW, eds. Greenfield's Neuropathology. 4th ed. New York: John Wiley & Sons, 1985.
15. Zimmerman RA, Bilaniuk LT: Pediatric central nervous system. In: Stark DD, Bradley WG Jr, eds. Magnetic Resonance Imaging. St. Louis: CV Mosby, 1988, pp 683–714.
16. McLone DG, Knepper PA: The cause of Chiari malformation: a unified theory. Pediatr Neurosci 15:1–12, 1989.
17. McLone DG, Naidich TP: Developmental morphology of the subarachnoid space, brain vasculature, and contiguous structures and the cause of the Chiari II malformation. AJNR 13:463–482, 1992.
18. Mikulis DJ, Diaz O, Egglin TK, Sanchez R: Variance of the position of the cerebellar tonsils with age: preliminary report. Radiology 183:725–728, 1992.
19. Ishikawa M, Kikuchi H, Fujisawa I, Yonekawa Y: Tonsillar herniation on MR imaging. Neurosurgery 22:77–80, 1988.
20. Elster AD, Chen MYM: Chiari I malformations: clinical and radiologic reappraisal. Radiology 183:347–353, 1992.
21. Spinos E, Lasler DW, Moody DM, et al: MR evaluation of Chiari I malformations at 0.15 T. AJNR 6:203–208, 1985.
22. Wolpert SM, Anderson M, Scott RM, et al: Chiari II malformation: MR imaging evaluation. AJNR 8:783–792, 1987.
23. Emery JL: Deformity of the aqueduct of Sylvius in children with hydrocephalus and meningomyelocele. Dev Med Child Neurol (Suppl) 16(32):40–48, 1974.
24. Zimmerman RA: Congenital abnormalities. Syllabus for the Categorical Course on MR. Reston, VA: American College of Radiology, 1985.
24a. Oba H, Barkovich AJ: Holoprosencephaly: an analysis of callosal formation and its relation to development of the interhemispheric fissure. AJNR 16:453–460, 1995.
25. Arrington JA, Martinez CR, Kaffenberger DA, et al: Associated intracranial abnormalities with septo-optic dysplasia: evaluation with CT and MRI. AJNR 8:951, 1987. Abstract.
26. Barkovich AJ, Fram EK, Norman D: Septo-optic dysplasia: MR imaging. Radiology 171:189–192, 1989.
27. Barkovich AJ, Normal D: Absence of the septum pellucidum: a useful sign in the diagnosis of congenital brain malformations. AJNR 9:1107–1114, 1988.
28. Barkovich AJ, Kjos BO, Normal D, Edwards MS: Revised classification of posterior fossa cysts and cystlike malformations based on the results of multiplanar MR imaging. AJNR 10:977–988, 1989.
29. Altman NR, Naidich TP, Braffman BH: Posterior fossa malformations. AJNR 13:691–724, 1992.
30. Hirsch JF, Pierre-Kahn A, Renier D, et al: The Dandy-Walker malformation. J Neurosurg 61:515–522, 1984.
31. Golden JA, Rorke LB, Bruce DA: Dandy-Walker syndrome and associated anomalies. Pediatr Neurosci 13:38–44, 1987.
32. Maria BL, Zinreich SJ, Carson BC, et al: Dandy-Walker syndrome revisited. Pediatr Neurosci 13:45–51, 1987.
33. Raybaud C: Cystic malformations of the posterior fossa: abnormalities associated with development of the roof of the fourth ventricle and adjoining meningeal structures. J Neuroradiol 9:103–133, 1982.
34. Naidich TP, Radkowski MA, Bernstein RA, Tan WS: Congenital malformations of the posterior fossa. In: Taveras JM, Ferruci JT, eds. Radiology. Philadelphia: JB Lippincott, 1986, pp 1–17.
35. Osborn AG: Posterior fossa malformations and cysts. In: Diagnostic Neuroradiology—A Text-Atlas. St. Louis: Mosby–Year Book, 1994, pp 59–71.
36. Macchi G, Bentivoglio M: Agenesis or hypoplasia of cerebellar structures. In: Vinkin PJ, Bruyn GW, eds. Congenital Malformations of the Brain and Skull. Amsterdam: North Holland Publishing, 1977, pp 367–393.
37. DeMorsier G: Etudes sur les dysraphies cranio-encephaliques: II. Agenesie du vermis cerebelleux-dysraphie rhombocephalique mediane (rhomboschisis). Monatsschr Psychiatr Neurol 129:321–344, 1955.
38. Joubert M, Eisenring JJ, Robb JP, Andermann F: Familial agenesis of the cerebellar vermis. A syndrome of episodic hyperpnea, abnormal eye movements, ataxia and retardation. Neurology 19:813–825, 1969.
39. Press GA, Murakami J, Courchesne E, et al: The cerebellum in sagittal plane: anatomic-MR correlation. Part 2. The cerebellar hemispheres. AJNR 10:667–676, 1989.
40. Courchesne E, Yeung-Courchesne R, Press GA, et al: Hypoplasia of cerebellar vermal lobules VI and VII in infantile autism. N Engl J Med 318:1349–1954, 1988.
41. Courchesne E, Saitoh O, Yeung-Courchesne R, et al: Abnormality of cerebellar vermian lobules VI and VII in patients with infantile autism: identification of hypoplastic and hyperplastic subgroups with MR imaging. AJNR 162:123–130, 1994.
42. Benda CE: Down's Syndrome. Mongolism and Its Management. New York: Grune & Stratton, 1969, pp 134–166.
43. Osborn AG: Disorders of histogenesis: neurocutaneous syndromes. In: Diagnostic Neuroradiology—A Text-Atlas. St. Louis: Mosby–Year Book, 1994, pp 72–111.
44. Smirniotopoulos JG, Murphy FM: The phakomatoses. AJNR 13:725–746, 1992.
45. Neurofibromatosis. Conference statement. National Institutes of Health Consensus Development Conference. Arch Neurol 45:575–578, 1988.

46. Sevick RJ, Barkovich AJ, Edwards MSB, et al: Evolution of white matter lesions in neurofibromatosis type 1: MR findings. AJR 159:171–175, 1992.
47. Aoki S, Barkovich AJ, Nishimura K, et al: Neurofibromatosis types 1 and 2: cranial MR findings. Radiology 172:527–534, 1989.
47a. DiPaolo DP, Zimmerman RA, Rorke LB, et al: Neurofibromatosis type I: pathologic substrate of high-signal-intensity foci in the brain. Radiology 195:721–724, 1995.
48. Mirowitz SA, Sartor K, Gado M: High-intensity basal ganglia lesions on T1-weighted MR images in neurofibromatosis. AJNR 10:1159–1163, 1989.
49. Barkovich AJ: Pediatric Neuroimaging. New York: Raven Press, 1990.
50. Egelhoff JC, Bates DJ, Ross JS, et al: Spinal MR findings in neurofibromatosis types 1 and 2. AJNR 13:1071–1077, 1992.
51. Chamberlain MC, Press GA, Hesselink JR: MR and CT in three cases of Sturge-Weber syndrome: a prospective comparison. AJNR 10:491–496, 1989.
52. Oot RF, New PJF, Pile-Spellman J, et al: The detection of intracranial calcifications by MR. AJNR 7:801–809, 1986.
53. Atlas SW, Grossman RI, Hackney DB, et al: Calcified intracranial lesions: detection with gradient-echo acquisition rapid MR imaging. AJNR 9:253–259, 1988.
54. Stimac GK, Solomon MA, Newton TH: CT and MR of angiomatous malformations of the choroid plexus in patients with Sturge-Weber disease. AJNR 7:629–632, 1986.
55. Jacoby CG, Yuh WTC, Afifi AK, et al: Accelerated myelination in early Sturge-Weber syndrome demonstrated by MR imaging. J Comput Assist Tomogr 11:226–231, 1987.
56. Gomez MR: Diagnostic criteria. In: Gomez MR, ed. Tuberous Sclerosis. 2nd ed. New York: Raven Press, 1985, pp 9–20.
56a. Shepherd CW, Houser OW, Gomez MR: MR findings in tuberous sclerosis complex and correlation with seizure development and mental impairment. AJNR 16:149–155, 1995.
57. Sato Y, Waziri M, Smith W, et al: Hippel-Lindau disease: MR imaging. Radiology 166:241–246, 1988.
58. Crossey PA, Maher ER, Jones MH, et al: Genetic linkage between von Hippel–Lindau disease and three microsatellite polymorphisms refines the localization of the vHL locus. Hum Mol Genet 2:279–282, 1993.
58a. Choyke PL, Glenn GM, Walther MM, et al: von Hippel–Lindau disease: genetic, clinical and imaging features. Radiology 194:629–642, 1995.
58b. Choyke PL, Glenn GM, Walther MM, et al: The natural history of renal lesions in von Hippel-Lindau disease: a serial CT study in 28 patients. AJR 159:1229–1234, 1992.
59. Huson SM, Harper PS, Hourihan MD, et al: Cerebellar hemangioblastoma and von Hippel–Lindau disease. Brain 109:1297–1310, 1986.
60. Byrd SE, Bohan TP, Osborn RE, Naidich TP: The CT and MR evaluation of lissencephaly. AJNR 9:923–927, 1988.
61. Lee BCP, Engel M: MR of lissencephaly. AJNR 9:804, 1988.
62. Barkovich AJ, Gressens P, Evrard P: Formation, maturation, and disorders of brain neocortex. AJNR 13:423–446, 1992.
63. Dunn V, Mock T, Bell WE, Smith W: Detection of heterotopic grey matter in children by magnetic resonance imaging. Magn Reson Imaging 4:33–39, 1986.
64. Barkovich AJ, Norman D: MR imaging of schizencephaly. AJNR 9:297–302, 1988.
65. Chamberlain MC, Press GA, Bejar RF: Neonatal schizencephaly: comparison of brain imaging. Pediatr Neurol 6:382–387, 1990.
66. Barkovich AJ, Norman D: Anomalies of the corpus callosum: correlation with further anomalies of the brain. AJNR 9:493–501, 1988.
67. Dean B, Drayer BP, Beresini DC, Bird CR: MR imaging of pericallosal lipoma. AJNR 9:929–931, 1988.
68. Johnson MA, Pennock JM, Bydder GM, et al: Clinical NMR imaging of the brain in children: normal and neurologic disease. AJR 141:1005–1018, 1983.
69. Dubowitz LM, Bydder GM, Mushin J: Developmental sequence of periventricular leukomalacia: correlation of ultrasound, clinical and nuclear magnetic resonance functions. Arch Dis Child 60:349–355, 1985.
70. Wilson DA, Steiner RE: Periventricular leukomalacia: evaluation with MR imaging. Radiology 160:507–511, 1986.
71. McArdle CB: MRI helps detect injury in neonatal, infant brain. Diagn Imaging 9:272–278, 1987.
72. Press GA, Barshop BA, Haas RH, et al: Abnormalities of the brain in nonketotic hyperglycinemia: MR manifestations. AJNR 10:315–321, 1989.

Supratentorial Brain Tumors

RICHARD J. HICKS

In the diagnostic work-up of intracranial tumors, the primary goals of the imaging studies are to detect the abnormality, localize and determine its extent, characterize the lesion, and provide a list of differential diagnoses or, if possible, the specific diagnosis. Correlative studies have proved that magnetic resonance imaging (MRI) is more sensitive than computed tomography (CT) for detecting intracranial masses.[1, 2] Moreover, the multiplanar capability of MRI assists in determining the anatomic site of origin of lesions and demarcating extension into adjacent compartments and brain structures. The superior contrast resolution of MRI displays the different components of lesions more clearly. MRI can assess the vascularity of lesions without contrast medium infusion. CT does detect calcification better than MRI, which is often useful in differential diagnosis. Gradient-echo techniques have increased the sensitivity of MRI to calcifications.

When going through the exercise of differential diagnosis, localization of the mass to a specific region is important, because most tumors occur in certain locations and not in others. First, is the lesion intra-axial or extra-axial? In what region of the brain is it located? Is it a solitary process or a multifocal process? Once the location of a mass has been determined, then the internal texture, enhancement features, and clinical setting help narrow the list of possibilities.

Several different gadolinium-containing compounds (gadopentetate dimeglumine, gadoteridol, gadiodamide) can be used to increase the sensitivity and specificity of MRI. These substances act as a blood-brain barrier contrast agent like iodinated agents for CT. They do not cross the intact blood-brain barrier, but when the barrier is absent or deficient, gadolinium agents enter the interstitial space to produce enhancement (increased signal intensity) on T1-weighted images.

Although the enhancement patterns are not tumor specific, the additional information is often helpful for diagnosis. Lesions can be characterized as enhancing or nonenhancing and homogeneous or heterogeneous, and necrotic and cystic components are seen more clearly. In enhancing lesions the margins of enhancement may provide a gross measure of tumor extension.[3–5] Contrast MRI is particularly valuable for extra-axial tumors because they tend to be isointense relative to the brain on plain scans.[6, 7]

Any intracranial structures without a blood-brain barrier are normally enhanced and should not be confused with disease. Enhancement is routinely seen in the pituitary gland, infundibulum, and choroid plexus. Slowly flowing blood within cortical veins and the cavernous sinuses enhances, whereas more variable enhancement is seen in the superior sagittal and transverse sinuses. In the unoperated brain, only limited dural enhancement is apparent with MRI, unlike the case with CT.

CLASSIFICATION OF BRAIN TUMORS

Neurons and neuroglia are the two tissues that make up the central nervous system. Neuroglia consists of astrocytes, oligodendrocytes, microglia, ependyma, and choroid epithelium. The vast majority of brain tumors arise from the neuroglia and are included under the broad term of *gliomas*. Added to the list of primary brain tumors are tumors arising from the pineal body (pineoblastoma and pineocytoma), meningothelium (meningioma), germ cell tumors, and lymphoma. Dermoid, epidermoid, lipoma, colloid cyst, and arachnoid cyst are considered to be of maldevelopmental origin. Metastatic tumors represent secondary malignancies of the brain and its coverings. The current International Histologic Classification of Central Nervous System Tumors drafted in 1990 by the World Health Organization is presented in a simplified format in Table 17–1.

CEREBRAL GLIOMAS

In its broadest sense the term glioma includes tumors of both neuroglial and neuronal origins. Gliomas account for 40% to 50% of all primary and metastatic intracranial tumors.[8] Precise relative frequencies of the different types of glioma vary between studies based

TABLE 17–1. CLASSIFICATION OF CENTRAL NERVOUS SYSTEM TUMORS

TUMORS OF NEUROEPITHELIAL TISSUE

Astrocytic Tumors
Astrocytoma
Anaplastic (malignant) astrocytoma
Glioblastoma
Pilocytic astrocytoma
Pleomorphic xanthoastrocytoma
Subependymal giant cell astocytoma

Oligodendroglial Tumors
Oligodendroglioma

Ependymal Tumors
Ependymoma
Subependymoma

Mixed Gliomas
Oligoastrocytoma

Choroid Plexus Tumors
Choroid plexus papilloma
Choroid plexus carcinoma

Neuroepithelial Tumors of Uncertain Origin
Gliomatosis cerebri

Neuronal and Mixed Neuronal-Glial Tumors
Gangliocytoma
Ganglioglioma
Dysembryoplastic neuroepithelial tumor
Central neurocytoma

Pineal Parenchymal Tumors
Pineocytoma
Pineoblastoma

Embryonal Tumors
Neuroblastoma
Primitive neuroectodermal tumors
Medulloblastoma

TUMORS OF THE MENINGES

Tumors of Meningothelial Cells
Meningioma

Mesenchymal, Nonmeningothelial Tumors
Hemangiopericytoma
Meningeal sarcomatosis

LYMPHOMAS AND HEMATOPOIETIC NEOPLASMS
Malignant lymphoma
Granulocytic sarcoma

GERM CELL TUMORS
Germinoma
Embryonal carcinoma
Choriocarcinoma
Teratoma

CYSTS AND TUMOR-LIKE LESIONS
Rathke's cleft cyst
Epidermoid cyst
Dermoid cyst
Colloid cyst

METASTATIC TUMORS

Modified from Kleihues P, Burger PC, Scheithauer BW: Histologic Typing of Tumours of the Central Nervous System. Berlin: Springer-Verlag, 1993.

on autopsy and biopsy populations, but glioblastoma is consistently the most common type, constituting 55% of intracranial gliomas in one study. In this same group, the incidence of astrocytoma was 20%; ependymoma, 6%; medulloblastoma, 6%; oligodendroglioma, 5%; and choroid plexus papilloma, 2%.[9] Intracranial gliomas are more commonly seen in men, with a pre-ponderance of 3:2.[9] The peak occurrence is during middle adult life, when patients present with seizures or symptoms related to the location of the gliomas and the brain structures involved. Gliomas occur predominantly in the cerebral hemispheres, but the brain stem and cerebellum are frequent locations of gliomas in children, and these tumors are also found in the spinal cord.

ASTROCYTOMA

Astrocytomas are a large and heterogeneous group of tumors demonstrating a wide range of biologic behavior. Astrocytomas are graded 1 to 4 according to the degree of anaplasia present. However, anaplasia is often a localized phenomenon within the tumor, and grading thus becomes dependent on the tissue sample obtained. Deeper, less accessible portions of a tumor may be more anaplastic than the periphery, and anaplasia may progress within a tumor with time.

Astrocytoma, as a more specific term, is applied to grade 1 and 2 tumors that can be further divided into fibrillary and pilocytic types. These are usually slowly growing tumors but are poorly demarcated from adjacent structures. This often results in incomplete surgical resection and a tendency to recur. These tumors often have cystic components, and calcifications are not uncommon. Fibrillary astrocytoma is the most frequent variant of astrocytoma. It can occur as a diffuse, infiltrative form with an anaplastic tendency in the cerebral hemispheres of adults. Pilocytic astrocytomas are more circumscribed, expand into surrounding brain slowly, and only rarely demonstrate anaplasia. They usually involve midline structures and are more commonly seen in children and young adults. The third ventricle and optic chiasm are frequent sites of involvement.

Anaplastic astrocytomas are grade 3 tumors that tend to progress and ultimately transform into the grade 4 glioblastoma multiforme. Glioblastomas usually occur late in adult life, with a peak occurrence between 45 and 60 years. They are the most common form of cerebral glioma. These rapidly growing tumors are highly cellular, often provoke a large amount of edema, and usually contain areas of necrosis. The frontal lobes are a common site of involvement, and extension contralaterally through the corpus callosum may give rise to a "butterfly" pattern. Glioblastomas may become adherent to overlying dura but seldom penetrate it. Infiltration of the ependyma is frequent and may lead to dissemination through cerebrospinal fluid (CSF) pathways. Extraneural metastases occur rarely. Prognosis continues to be dismal, with an almost 90% mortality after 2 years.[9]

Multicentricity of gliomas may be noted in 4% to 6% of cases.[9] This usually takes the form of a small focus of tumor a short distance away from the main lesion, but rarely the tumors may be widely separated. Multicentricity is almost exclusively seen in glioblastomas and when seen in lower grade astrocytomas usually denotes progression to a malignant phase.

Gliomatosis cerebri is an unusual condition in which there is diffuse infiltration of the brain with neoplastic glial cells involving several cerebral lobes. The diagnosis usually requires neuroimaging to document the extent of involvement. Gliomatosis cerebri usually presents in the second and third decades with nonspecific personality and mental changes and may represent an extreme example of diffuse fibrillary astrocytoma. Foci of dedifferentiation to glioblastoma multiforme may be present, and the lesion behaves like a grade 3 to 4 astrocytoma.

OLIGODENDROGLIOMA

This slowly growing tumor arises in the cerebral hemispheres with a frontal lobe predominance. Calcifications are frequently seen by CT. Although most oligodendrogliomas are relatively benign lesions, there is also a more aggressive form with a tendency to recur and the ability to disseminate by way of CSF pathways. It is difficult to predict the biologic behavior of the tumor on the basis of its histologic picture.

EPENDYMOMA

These tumors arising from the ventricular lining are more commonly seen in children and are discussed in Chapter 19 on brain stem and cerebellar lesions.

GANGLIOCYTOMA AND GANGLIOGLIOMA

These tumors contain neuronal elements along with varying amounts of glial tissue. Gangliocytomas (ganglioneuromas) contain neoplastic but mature ganglion cells with a small amount of glial elements; the glial elements predominate in gangliogliomas. In practice, the tumors are difficult to separate pathologically and share similar biologic behavior. They are slowly growing, circumscribed lesions occurring most often in children and young adults. Both of these neuronal tumors frequently contain calcifications and cysts. The temporal lobe is the most often affected site, and seizures are a common feature at presentation. The tumors are often relatively small at the time of discovery.

MRI FEATURES OF GLIOMAS

These intra-axial tumors demonstrate high signal intensity on T2-weighted images and low signal intensity on T1-weighted images, unless hemorrhage or calcifications are present. Subacute hemorrhage (methemoglobin) exhibits increased T1 and T2 signal intensity, whereas acute hemorrhage (deoxyhemoglobin) and chronic hemorrhage (hemosiderin) show decreased signal intensity on T2-weighted sequences. Calcification, if apparent by MRI, is most often seen as an area of decreased signal intensity, which is better appreciated on T2-weighted than T1-weighted images.

Rarely, calcification may have increased signal intensity on T1-weighted images. Gliomas infiltrate along white matter tracts, and the deeper lesions have a propensity to extend across the corpus callosum into the opposite hemisphere (Fig. 17–1). Most are quite large at the time of clinical presentation. Most gliomas are infiltrative lesions, and microscopic fingers of tumor usually extend for variable distances beyond the area of enhancement.

Low-grade astrocytomas (grades 1 and 2) tend to be well defined and nonhemorrhagic and demonstrate little mass effect, vasogenic edema, or heterogeneity.[10] Enhancement of lower grade gliomas is variable, but more gliomas in general enhance with MRI than CT.[3] The pilocytic form of low-grade astrocytoma tends to be sharply demarcated, smoothly marginated, and cystic (Fig. 17–2). Although pilocytic astrocytomas are considered relatively benign, they often demonstrate moderate enhancement, and a significant number have a much more aggressive course. Unfortunately, the initial imaging features cannot predict the biologic behavior of these tumors.[11–13]

Anaplastic astrocytomas (grade 3) are less well defined and demonstrate moderate amounts of mass effect, heterogeneity, and edema. Virtually all display some degree of enhancement. Glioblastomas (grade 4) are poorly defined and often have considerable mass effect, vasogenic edema, and heterogeneity as well as more commonly showing evidence of hemorrhage[10] (Figs. 17–3 and 17–4). Irregular ring enhancement with nodularity and nonenhancing necrotic foci is typical of glioblastoma.[14]

Gliomatosis cerebri exhibits diffuse, poorly defined, variable degrees of T2 hyperintensity in the cerebral hemispheres with variable amounts of swelling. In one study, eight of nine cases demonstrated enhancement, all crossed midline, and MRI was more sensitive than CT for detecting lesions and their extent.[15]

Oligodendrogliomas tend to be relatively superficial in location (cortical and subcortical), are round or oval, and are frequently sharply demarcated without edema. Approximately 40% are calcified as seen by CT or MRI, and enhancement may be noted.[16, 17] They may be difficult to differentiate from low-grade astrocytoma, ganglioglioma, and neurocytoma, but astrocytomas tend to be deeper and more infiltrative.

Gangliogliomas and gangliocytomas have no specific imaging features but should be included in the differential diagnosis of temporal lobe lesions, particularly if calcified or cystic. Enhancement is relatively common, especially in the solid forms of these tumors[18, 19] (Fig. 17–5).

UNUSUAL GLIAL, NEURONAL, AND MIXED TUMORS

Pleomorphic Xanthoastrocytoma

Pleomorphic xanthoastrocytomas are superficially located astrocytic neoplasms characterized histologically by marked cellular pleomorphism and frequent xanthomatous change. Despite the marked pleomor-

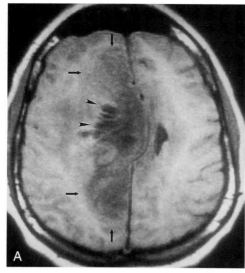

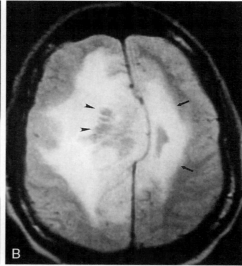

FIGURE 17–1. Grade 1 infiltrating astrocytoma (butterfly glioma). *A,* T1-weighted image shows the heterogeneous hypointense mass in the medial right hemisphere *(arrows)* with subfalcial herniation. Several small cysts are present *(arrowheads).* *B,* Proton density–weighted image reveals extensive involvement of the right hemisphere with tumor and contralateral spread through the corpus callosum *(arrows).* Areas of lesser signal intensity *(arrowheads)* represent small cysts.

FIGURE 17–2. Grade 2 pilocytic astrocytoma. *A,* Gadolinium-enhanced T1-weighted image demonstrates well-defined enhancing mass posteriorly with cystic area anteriorly. *B,* T2-weighted image reveals edema anterior to cyst *(white arrow).* Demarcation between cystic and solid portions is limited with this sequence *(black arrows).*

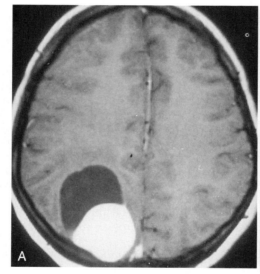

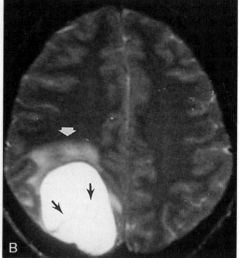

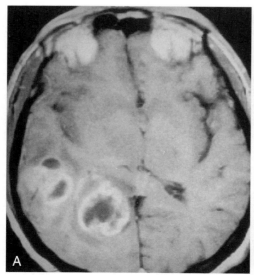

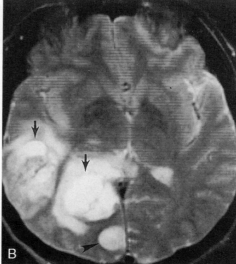

FIGURE 17–3. Multicentric glioblastoma multiforme (grade 4 astrocytoma). *A,* Gadolinium-enhanced T1-weighted image reveals two irregular ring-enhancing masses typical in appearance for glioblastoma. The atrium of the right lateral ventricle is effaced. *B,* T2-weighted image demonstrates surrounding edema and hyperintense necrotic or cystic areas *(arrows).* The right occipital lesion *(arrowhead)* was not biopsied.

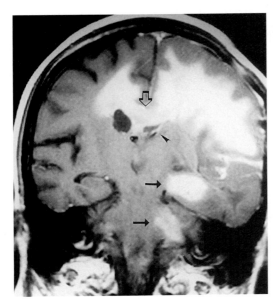

FIGURE 17–4. Metastatic glioblastoma. Gadolinium-enhanced T1-weighted image shows extension of large enhancing left fronto-temporal mass through the corpus callosum *(open arrow)* into the contralateral hemisphere. Ependymal enhancement is present in the frontal horn of the left lateral ventricle *(arrowhead)*, and left medial temporal and pontine metastases *(solid arrows)* are apparent.

phism, few mitotic figures are present and necrosis is absent unless the rare transformation into a malignant form has occurred.[20] They are most commonly found in adolescents or young adults who present with seizures. The biologic behavior of the tumor is less aggressive than suggested by the microscopic appearance. Although these lesions were initially considered to be benign, recurrences can occur and may be associated with malignant transformation.

By MRI these tumors are seen as peripherally located, partially cystic masses, most often within the temporal lobes, but occasionally in the frontal and parietal lobes. A site of dural attachment is frequently present. They are usually isointense relative to gray matter on T1-weighted images and mildly hyperintense on T2-weighted images (Fig. 17–6). Enhancement of the solid portion can be seen. In a series of six cases, the only lesion that incited edema was a more aggressive tumor that recurred.[21] All six tumors in this series demonstrated enhancement, but only two were cystic. Calcifications are not frequent.[22] The appearance is nonspecific and may mimic ganglion cell neoplasms, pilocytic astrocytomas, meningiomas, oligodendrogliomas, and inflammatory masses.

Dysembryoplastic Neuroepithelial Tumors

Patients with these uncommon masses usually present during the first two decades of life with partial complex seizures. These tumors most commonly occur in the temporal lobes as a multinodular intracortical mass. Histology reveals the tumors to contain predominantly oligodendrocytes with a few scattered neurons. An astrocytic component may be seen as well.[20] These slow-growing tumors are usually only several centimeters in diameter at presentation. The biologic behavior and prognosis for dysembryoplastic neuroepithelial tumors remain uncertain.

MRI shows these well-marginated cortical lesions to be hypointense relative to gray matter on T1-weighted images, hypointense to hyperintense on proton density–weighted images, and hyperintense on T2-weighted images.[23] Peritumor edema is absent. Approximately 80% of dysembryoplastic neuroepithelial tumors will be found in the temporal lobes. Most lesions demonstrate minimal to no enhancement. Calcifications are rare. Ganglioglioma and low-grade astrocytoma are usually included in the MRI differential diagnosis.

Central Neurocytoma

Central neurocytoma is a benign primary neoplasm that most commonly occurs in the lateral and third ventricles of young adults. The tumors are often attached to the septum pellucidum within the body

FIGURE 17–5. Ganglioglioma. *A,* The peripherally enhancing mass *(arrows)* is difficult to differentiate from the hyperintense cyst anteriorly on this gadolinium-enhanced T1-weighted image. The cyst was semisolid at surgery. No hemorrhage was found, and the hyperintensity is presumably related to a high protein concentration. *B,* T2-weighted image shows edema *(arrowheads)* extending from the lesion *(arrows)*. A hypointense rim is seen about the solid portion of the lesion.

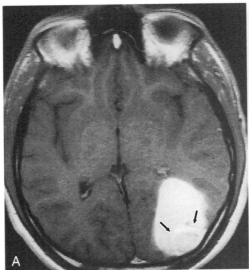
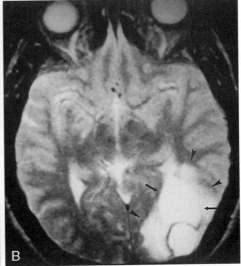

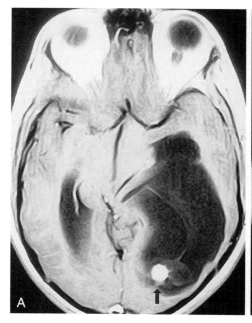 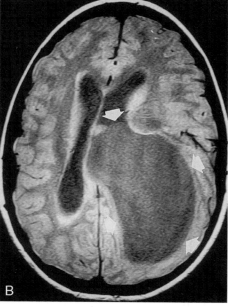

FIGURE 17–6. Pleomorphic xanthoastrocytoma. A, An enhancing nodule (arrow) is present in the atrium of the left lateral ventricle on this gadolinium-enhanced T1-weighted image. A septum in the ventricle is also apparent. B, The extent of the mass (arrows) is better depicted on this spin density–weighted fast spin-echo image. This atypical intraventricular presentation of pleomorphic xanthoastrocytoma is seen to be mildly hyperintense relative to CSF.

or frontal horn of the lateral ventricles. The presenting symptoms are usually those of headache and increased intracranial pressure. Histology demonstrates a small cell neoplasm with a fine fibrillar background and absent mitoses. The appearance may mimic an oligodendroglioma, especially when calcifications are present. Most tumors previously reported as intraventricular oligodendrogliomas actually represent neurocytomas.[20] Even though excisions are often subtotal, patients with these slowly growing tumors generally have an excellent prognosis.

The masses are most often oval, sharply demarcated, and lobulated. A heterogeneous appearance is typical by MRI. The major part of the tumor is isointense relative to gray matter on both T1- and T2-weighted images. Visualization of small T2 hyperintense cysts is frequent, with large cysts more rarely seen[24] (Fig. 17–

7). The calcifications that are so often present histologically are frequently overlooked with MRI, so that CT may play an important role in differential diagnosis. Mild to moderate enhancement may be seen. Although these tumors are usually noninvasive, extraventricular extension has been noted in two cases of anaplastic central neurocytoma.[25] The appearance by MRI may be shared with meningioma, oligodendroglioma, choroid plexus papilloma, and colloid cyst. More marked enhancement is typically seen with choroid plexus papilloma and meningioma, whereas intraventricular oligodendrogliomas are often larger and contain coarser calcifications.

Subependymal Giant Cell Astrocytoma

These circumscribed, largely intraventricular tumors are usually found in young patients with tuberous scle-

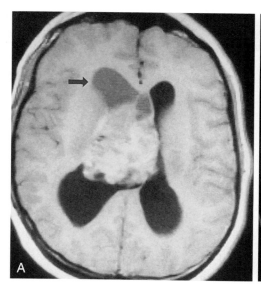 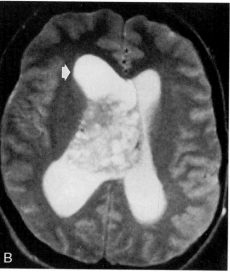

FIGURE 17–7. Central neurocytoma. A, A heterogeneous, enhancing mass is shown within the body of the right lateral ventricle, attached to the septum pellucidum, on this gadolinium-enhanced T1-weighted image. The hyperintensity of CSF within the ventricle anterior to the mass (arrow) is likely secondary to obstruction. B, Marked heterogeneity of the tumor is noted on the T2-weighted image. Although areas of relative hypointensity are present within the mass, the calcifications shown by CT cannot be reliably diagnosed by MRI in this case. Again seen is hyperintense CSF anterior to the mass (arrow).

rosis. Because tuberous sclerosis may be incompletely expressed as a syndrome, and because the findings may rarely be limited to the central nervous system, these tumors can present in patients without an established diagnosis of tuberous sclerosis. These masses are limited to the region of the foramen of Monro and usually present as increased intracranial pressure or are found during evaluation of an asymptomatic patient with tuberous sclerosis. The histologic appearance is variable but usually consists of large tumor cells without incorporated normal brain parenchyma as seen in diffuse or fibrillary astrocytomas.[20] Calcifications are common and may be coarse.

Evaluation with MRI reveals a usually large, bulky mass at the foramen of Monro. The margins are well defined, with infiltration of the adjacent brain parenchyma occurring infrequently. Variable signal intensity is present on T1-weighted images; hyperintensity predominates on spin density–weighted images. The masses may become hypointense relative to CSF on heavily T2-weighted images. Enhancement is usually present. Calcifications may be seen as areas of decreased signal intensity.

LYMPHOMA

Primary malignant lymphoma is a non-Hodgkin lymphoma that occurs in the brain in the absence of systemic involvement. These tumors are highly cellular and grow rapidly. About 70% represent large cell variants of the B cell type. Favorite sites include the deeper, often subependymal parts of the frontal and parietal lobes, basal ganglia, and hypothalamus. Primary lymphoma is multicentric within the brain at the time of presentation in about 25% of cases.[9] Formerly rare lesions that represented less than 1% of intracranial neoplasms, they are now being seen with increasing frequency in immunocompromised hosts. Most now occur in patients with acquired immunodeficiency syndrome (AIDS) or in organ transplant recipients who are taking immunosuppressant drugs. Primary lymphomas found in immunocompromised patients are more frequently multicentric and demonstrate larger areas of necrosis. Cerebral lymphomas are radiosensitive and respond dramatically to corticosteroid therapy, but local recurrences and seeding through CSF pathways are common and 5-year survivals are rare.

Secondary involvement of the central nervous system with lymphoma occurs much less commonly than the primary type and is seen almost exclusively with non-Hodgkin's lymphoma. It usually presents as leptomeningeal disease. Dural disease is less common, and the spinal canal is affected more often with dural deposits than is the cranial cavity.

Leukemic extension to the central nervous system may result in leptomeningeal infiltration, hemorrhage from impaction of leukemic cells in the cerebral white matter, and, more rarely, solid extra-axial masses of chloroma (granulocytic sarcoma).

MRI FEATURES OF LYMPHOMAS

Lymphomas typically appear as homogeneous, slightly high signal intensity to isointense, well-demarcated masses deep within the brain on T2-weighted images. The observed mild T2 prolongation is probably related to dense cell packing within these tumors, leaving relatively little interstitial space for accumulation of water. They are usually slightly hypointense relative to parenchyma on T1-weighted images. Intense, homogeneous enhancement is usually seen. Lymphomas tend to occur in deep locations adjacent to the corpus callosum or ependyma.[26, 27] Multiple lesions may be seen in up to 50% of patients[28] (Fig. 17–8). Most lymphomas have only a small amount of associated edema and mass effect, features that help distinguish them from metastases and glioblastomas.

The pattern is modified somewhat in patients with AIDS. Multiplicity is more common, as is moderate edema and mass effect[29] (Fig. 17–9). Moreover, the lymphomas exhibit more aggressive behavior and readily outgrow their blood supply. As a result, heterogeneous lesions with central necrosis and ring enhancement are often seen in lymphomatous masses in patients with AIDS.

METASTATIC DISEASE

Metastatic disease accounts for 15% to 25% of intracranial tumors,[8] and cerebral metastases occur in about 5% of all patients with fatal malignancies.[9] Metastases to the head can occur in three different patterns or locations: the skull and dura, brain parenchyma, and meninges (carcinomatous meningitis). Any tumors that metastasize to bone are also prone to involve the skull. Breast and prostate are the most common primary source for calvarial metastases, which often occur without associated brain lesions. Cranial nerve deficits may result from skull base involvement. Epidural metastases are usually associated with overlying calvarial tumor, but metastases to the dura itself can occur without involvement of bone. Dural metastases may lead to subdural deposits of tumor and are particularly seen with breast carcinoma. Extension through the dura to involve adjacent brain is rare.

Metastases to the brain parenchyma occur by hematogenous spread, and multiple lesions are found in 70% of cases. The most common primary lesions are lung tumors, breast tumors, and melanoma, in that order of frequency. Other potential sources include the gastrointestinal tract, kidney, and thyroid. Metastases from other sites are uncommon. Clinical symptoms are nonspecific and no different from those of primary tumors. The most common site of involvement is the corticomedullary junction of the cerebrum and cerebellum. Associated edema is usually extensive.

Extension of tumor through the cortex or ependyma can lead to leptomeningeal seeding and carcinomatous meningitis. This occurrence is most frequently associated with adenocarcinoma. As previously noted,

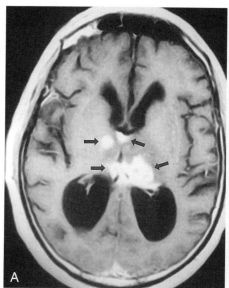

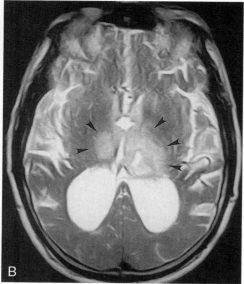

FIGURE 17–8. Primary lymphoma. *A,* Multiple areas of enhancing periventricular tumor *(arrows)* are present in the thalami and basal ganglia on this gadolinium-enhanced T1-weighted image. *B,* The tumor *(arrowheads)* is shown to be mildly hyperintense relative to brain but hypointense relative to CSF on this fast spin-echo T2-weighted image. Note the paucity of associated edema and mass effect.

FIGURE 17–9. Atypical lymphoma associated with AIDS. *A,* The enhancing basal ganglia mass on this gadolinium-enhanced T1-weighted image is surrounded by more edema *(arrows)* and has more mass effect than usually seen in lymphoma (see Fig. 17–8). Near-complete effacement of the frontal horn of the left lateral ventricle is present. *B,* The full extent of edema is shown on this T2-weighted image. The central portion of the mass is more heterogeneous than usual for lymphoma.

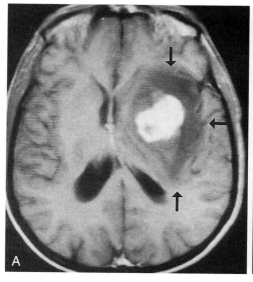

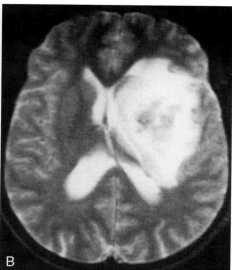

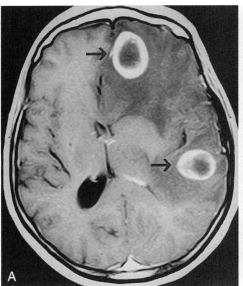

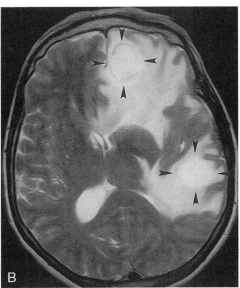

FIGURE 17–10. Metastatic disease. *A,* Two ring-enhancing masses *(arrows)* with a large amount of associated edema representing metastatic breast carcinoma are shown on this gadolinium-enhanced T1-weighted image. The regular margins are in contrast to those often seen with glioblastoma (see Fig. 17–3). *B,* The metastases *(arrowheads)* become more difficult to separate from the edema on this fast spin-echo T2-weighted image.

carcinomatous meningitis can also be seen with secondary lymphoma.

MRI FEATURES OF METASTATIC DISEASE

Metastases are most commonly imaged as multiple lesions within the cerebral and cerebellar hemispheres, with a tendency to occur at the gray matter–white matter interface. These lesions are usually hypointense to isointense relative to brain parenchyma on T1-weighted images and hyperintense on T2-weighted images (Fig. 17–10). Metastatic adenocarcinoma, espe-

cially with gastrointestinal primary lesions, may be isointense on T2-weighted images so that their detection is dependent on surrounding T2-hyperintense edema or contrast medium–enhanced T1-weighted images[30, 31] (Fig. 17–11). Metastatic melanoma is also unusual in that it may demonstrate increased T1 signal intensity on nonenhanced scans due to hemorrhage or the paramagnetic effects of melanin[32, 33] (Fig. 17–12).

Nonenhanced MRI has not proved superior to enhanced CT, but controlled clinical trials have shown that enhanced MRI is superior to enhanced CT for detecting cerebral metastases.[34–36] Moderate to marked enhancement is the rule—nodular for smaller lesions and ring-like with central nonenhancing areas for the larger ones. T2-weighted images demonstrate the sur-

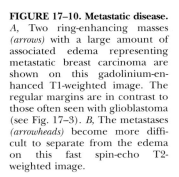

FIGURE 17–11. Atypical metastases. These bilateral metastases *(arrowheads)* from carcinosarcoma of the lung are largely isointense with white matter. Except for the small eccentric areas of higher signal intensity, these lesions could be overlooked without gadolinium-enhanced T1-weighted images.

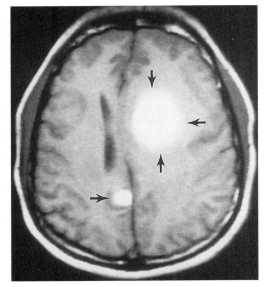

FIGURE 17–12. Metastatic malignant melanoma. Hyperintense lesions *(arrows)* are evident on this nonenhanced T1-weighted image, due to the presence of hemorrhage or paramagnetic melanin.

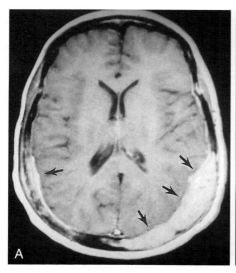
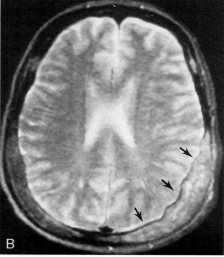

FIGURE 17–13. Calvarial metastases. *A,* Abnormal enhancement *(arrows)* is present within the diploë on this gadolinium-enhanced T1-weighted image. There is expansion of the left parietal bone, affecting the inner table more than the outer table. *B,* Heterogeneous hyperintensity *(arrows)* persists within the calvaria on this T2-weighted image. The right parietal lesion is no longer imaged on this more superior section.

rounding edema, which is often marked. Enhancement with edema helps in distinguishing metastases from other benign lesions commonly present on MR images. Nonenhancing white matter lesions recognized on T2-weighted images in cancer patients have a low probability of representing metastatic disease.[37] Given the data supporting resection of solitary, and occasionally multiple, cerebral metastases,[38] contrast medium–enhanced MRI plays an important role in the evaluation of these patients. Whether high-dose gadolinium enhancement[39] or magnetization transfer contrast MRI[40] will become a standard addition to this work-up remains to be seen.

Skull metastases are visualized on T2-weighted and proton density–weighted images as slightly hyperintense masses that have replaced the normal diploic space and cortical bone. They can also be seen on T1-weighted images, particularly in the skull base, because the lower signal intensity tumor replaces the higher signal intensity marrow fat. Gadolinium-enhanced T1-weighted images are better for subtle diploic metastases than are nonenhanced images but become more limited as tumor extends into fat-containing areas[41] (Fig. 17–13). The addition of fat saturation pulses or short-tau inversion recovery sequences helps in these areas.

Carcinomatous meningitis is best imaged with enhanced T1-weighted scans and is displayed as multiple nodular or linear areas of increased signal intensity involving the meninges and ependymal surfaces (Fig. 17–14). Occasionally, the tumor deposits may also be hyperintense relative to CSF on proton density–weighted images and hypointense relative to CSF on T2-weighted images. Although enhanced MRI has proved more sensitive than enhanced CT, CSF cytology remains the most sensitive diagnostic tool.[42]

MENINGIOMA

Meningiomas account for 15% of all intracranial tumors[9] and are the most common extra-axial tumor.

They originate from the dura or arachnoid and occur in middle-aged adults. Women are affected twice as often as men. Clinical symptoms are usually nonspecific, consisting of headache, visual impairment, and seizures, but focal weakness or numbness in an opposite extremity may be present if the mass compresses the brain around the rolandic fissure.

Meningiomas are well-differentiated, benign, and encapsulated lesions that indent the brain as they enlarge. They grow slowly and may be present for many years before producing symptoms. The histologic picture shows cells of uniform size that tend to form whorls or psammoma bodies; these latter structures are responsible for the typical calcifications. Hemor-

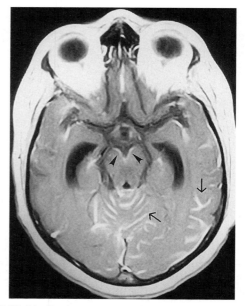

FIGURE 17–14. Carcinomatous meningitis. Pronounced enhancement is demonstrated within multiple cerebral sulci and cerebellar fissures *(arrows)* on this gadolinium-enhanced image of a patient with metastatic breast carcinoma. Enhancing tumor is seen along the surface of the midbrain in the interpeduncular fossa *(arrowheads).*

rhage or cyst formation is rare. On rare occasions, a meningioma exhibits malignant and invasive features of hemangiopericytoma.

The parasagittal region is the most frequent site for meningiomas, followed by the sphenoid wings, parasellar region, olfactory groove, cerebellopontine angle, and, rarely, the intraventricular region. These tumors arise from cells in the arachnoid villi, and this correlates with their typical locations. Meningiomas may induce an osteoblastic reaction in the adjacent bone, resulting in a characteristic focal hyperostosis. They are also hypervascular, receiving their blood supply predominantly from dural vessels. A prominent and persistent vascular blush is a classic sign on angiograms. Those that are accessible can be completely cured with surgical excision. Meningiomas at the skull base may invade the bone and adjacent cavernous sinuses and incorporate cranial nerves and major vascular structures as they grow, rendering them unresectable. Meningiomas are usually mass-like but the "en plaque" form spreads superficially along the dura. Multiple meningiomas can occasionally be seen, particularly in association with neurofibromatosis type 2.

Intraventricular meningiomas arise from arachnoid cells in the tela choroidea or choroid plexus. These tumors usually occur in the lateral ventricles, and there is a distinct preference for involvement of the left lateral ventricle (Fig. 17–15). Tumors in the third or fourth ventricle occur infrequently.

A pure intraosseous meningioma without underlying dural involvement occurs with great rarity and is probably due to ectopic rests of arachnoid cells. Other ectopic locations include the orbit, temporal bone, and extracranial regions such as the nasal cavity and paranasal sinuses.

MRI FEATURES OF MENINGIOMAS

Initially there was concern that MRI would miss many significant meningiomas, but with more experience and the use of multiple imaging sequences this has not proved to be the case. Comparison of studies performed at or below 0.5 T[1, 43] with those performed with high-field-strength imagers[44] shows an advantage for the higher field systems in meningioma detection. T1-weighted images often provide the best depiction of anatomic distortion and white matter buckling indicative of an extra-axial mass. Most meningiomas are relatively isointense to central nervous system parenchyma on nonenhanced T1-weighted images and hyperintense relative to white matter on T2-weighted images, particularly at higher field strengths, but there can be considerable variation in the appearance on T2-weighted images. Occasionally, a densely calcified meningioma is encountered that is distinctly hypointense on all pulse sequences. The different histopathologic types of meningioma may account for some of these variations. In one study, meningiomas that were hyperintense relative to cortex on T2-weighted images were syncytial and angioblastic lesions, whereas hypointense meningiomas were fibroblastic or transitional.[45] The presence of edema also correlated with the syncytial and angioblastic meningiomas, whereas MRI evidence of calcification was most commonly seen with the fibroblastic and transitional types. At 1.5 T, a heterogeneous internal texture was noted in all but the smallest meningiomas.[44] The mottled pattern is likely due to a combination of flow void from vascularity, focal calcification, small cystic foci, and entrapped CSF spaces. Hemorrhage is not a common feature. An interface between the brain and lesion can often be

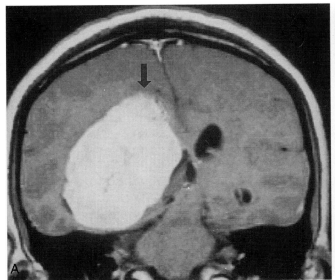
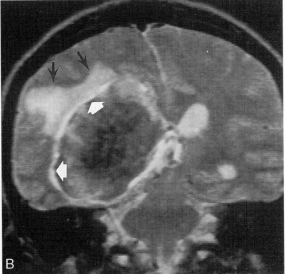

FIGURE 17–15. Intraventricular meningioma. *A,* A homogeneously enhancing mass is demonstrated within the expanded atrium of the right lateral ventricle on this gadolinium-enhanced T1-weighted image. The more irregular margin superiorly *(arrow)* suggests parenchymal invasion. *B,* A thin rim of higher signal intensity CSF *(white arrows)* surrounds the predominantly hypointense mass on this T2-weighted image. Edema *(black arrows)* extends peripherally from a portion of the tumor.

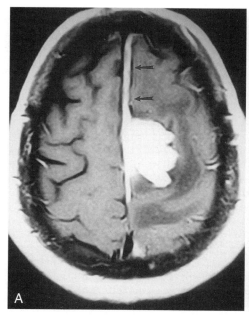

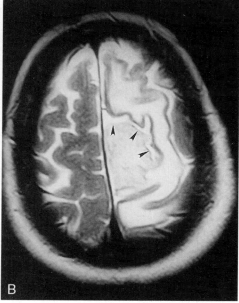

FIGURE 17–16. Parasagittal meningioma. *A,* Intensely, homogeneously enhancing lobulated mass arises from the falx on this gadolinium-enhanced T1-weighted image. Thick, dural "flare" or "tail" of enhancement *(arrows)* extends along falx anteriorly and posteriorly. *B,* Meningioma is shown to be mildly hyperintense relative to brain parenchyma on this fast spin-echo T2-weighted image. A hyperintense cleft *(arrowheads)* is present about the extra-axial mass with edema present in the adjacent gyrus.

identified; this may be related to a CSF cleft, a vascular rim, or a dural margin (Figs. 17–16 and 17–17). MRI has special advantages over CT in assessing venous sinus involvement and arterial encasement.

Meningiomas show intense enhancement with gadolinium and are sharply circumscribed.[46] They have a characteristic broad base of dural attachment, but at times this is evident only with imaging in sagittal or coronal planes. An enhancing dural "tail" may be seen in up to 60% of meningiomas. Whether this

represents benign reactive changes to the adjacent tumor[47, 48] or microscopic infiltration of tumor[49] remains uncertain. Although most commonly seen with meningioma, it can also be present with dural metastases and nonmeningiomatous malignant lesions as well.[50] Associated hyperostosis may result in thickening of low-signal-intensity bone as well as diminished signal from the diploic spaces. Although meningiomas are not invasive, vasogenic edema is present in the adjacent brain in 30% of cases; rarely, this edema is extensive enough to mimic glioblastoma and metastatic disease.

Meningiomas in pediatric patients are unusual and associated with neurofibromatosis in 25% of cases. Pediatric meningiomas are more commonly seen in the posterior fossa or unusual sites such as intraventricular and intraparenchymal. Hyperintensity on proton density–weighted and T2-weighted images is the rule.[51]

Ossification or bony metaplasia of the falx has a distinctive appearance by MRI that should not be misinterpreted as a meningioma. Ossification has a central area of fatty marrow that is of high signal intensity on T1-weighted images and isointense or of low signal intensity on T2-weighted images. The peripheral rim of cortical bone is hypointense on all sequences.

HEMANGIOPERICYTOMA

Hemangiopericytoma, and its relationship to angioblastic meningiomas, remain a controversial topic among pathologists. Angioblastic meningiomas demonstrate rapid and aggressive growth and high cellularity, features similar to those of the extracranial soft tissue hemangiopericytoma. As a result, these lesions are considered by the World Health Organization International Histologic Classification of Central Nervous System Tumours (see Table 17–1) to represent a mes-

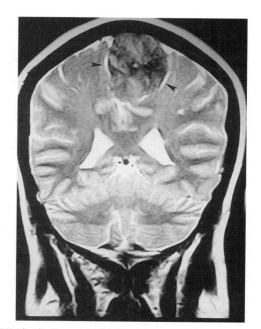

FIGURE 17–17. Parasagittal T2-weighted hypointense meningioma. A heterogeneous but predominantly hypointense extra-axial mass is revealed on this fast spin-echo T2-weighted image. A hyperintense cleft *(arrowheads)* is present between the meningioma and adjacent brain. Note the absence of associated edema.

enchymal, nonmeningothelial tumor, whereas others continue to include them as a subtype of meningioma. Regardless of nomenclature, these tumors exhibit a strong tendency for recurrence and a greater propensity to metastasize.

Hemangiopericytomas share many of the imaging features of meningiomas. They more commonly exhibit heterogeneous T2 hyperintensity than do meningiomas. Diffuse but heterogeneous enhancement is seen with gadolinium, and multiple flow voids are usually present within the mass. Calcification is infrequent.[52]

MENINGEAL SARCOMA

Meningeal sarcomas constitute a rare group of neoplasms. In contradistinction to meningiomas, these tumors are more common in infants and children. Sarcomas usually form large masses separated from the brain with a dural attachment. There may be secondary involvement of the brain, but in some instances the sarcomas arise within the brain substance. Leptomeningeal spread is not infrequent. There may be an association with prior radiation therapy.

PINEAL REGION TUMORS

Tumors in the pineal region are classified into three major groups based on their origin: germ cell, pineal parenchymal, and parapineal. The parapineal lesions include gliomas of the tectum and posterior third ventricle (Fig. 17–18), meningiomas arising within the quadrigeminal cistern, and developmental cysts (epidermoid, dermoid, arachnoid cyst). These parapineal masses are discussed elsewhere under the individual entities. True pineal parenchymal tumors occur less often than the germ cell tumors. Astrocytes are also present within the pineal and may give rise to pineal astrocytomas. The clinical expression of these tumors is usually related to compression of adjacent structures, with hydrocephalus due to aqueductal obstruction being a common presentation.

GERMINOMA

This least-differentiated of the germ cell tumors is also the most common intracranial germ cell tumor, the most frequent type of pineal mass, and the most frequently encountered suprasellar germ cell tumor. Germinomas probably account for more than 50% of the neoplasms arising in or near the pineal gland.[9] Pineal germinomas have also been referred to as pinealomas, and suprasellar germinomas have been called ectopic pinealomas. Most germinomas appear in the second and third decades of life with an overwhelming male predominance. They may present as Parinaud's syndrome (paralysis of upward gaze due to compression of the third cranial nerve nucleus), but often the symptoms are nonspecific. Suprasellar lesions may present as hypothalamic disturbances. Germinomas are histologically malignant and infiltrative and are prone to spread through CSF pathways but are highly radiosensitive.

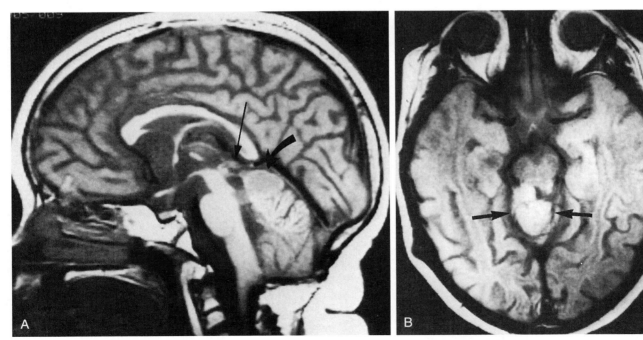

FIGURE 17–18. Exophytic tectal glioma. *A*, T1-weighted sagittal image (spin echo, 600/25) discloses a pineal region mass *(curved arrow)* that is distinct from a normal pineal gland *(long arrow)*. *B*, The lesion *(arrows)* is slightly hyperintense on a proton density–weighted image (spin echo, 2000/70). Surgery revealed a glioma arising from the quadrigeminal plate with a large exophytic component occupying the quadrigeminal cistern.

EMBRYONAL CARCINOMA

Embryonal carcinoma, yolk sac carcinoma (endodermal sinus tumor), and choriocarcinoma represent types of more differentiated germ cell tumors that may arise in the pineal region. All three are rare, with choriocarcinoma being the least common. All tend to be highly malignant with frequent metastases and a more dismal prognosis than germinomas.

TERATOMA

These tumors are composed of well-differentiated tissues from all three germinal layers. The most common intracranial location is the pineal region. They share a male predominance with germinomas but occur at an earlier age, being found most often during the first two decades of life. Complete excision of mature teratomas is associated with a good prognosis, but the presence of immature elements may predict a less favorable course.

PINEOBLASTOMA

This malignant tumor of primitive pinealocytes is most often seen in children, and, like most pineal germ cell tumors, it also exhibits a male predominance. The histologic picture and biologic behavior are similar to those of medulloblastoma (primitive neuroectodermal tumor). These tumors are often ill defined and are uniformly associated with ventricular and leptomeningeal spread. Symptoms are usually from obstruction of CSF pathways or invasion of adjacent brain. Pineoblastoma may be seen in association with retinoblastoma (trilateral retinoblastoma).

PINEOCYTOMA

This slowly growing tumor of mature pinealocytes can present at any age and affects both sexes equally. It is usually well defined, and CSF seeding is infrequent. Pineocytoma cells may further differentiate into astrocytes or neurons; those that do not demonstrate differentiation behave similarly to pineoblastomas.

MRI FEATURES OF PINEAL REGION TUMORS

Because of the infrequent occurrence of these tumors, our knowledge of the MRI characteristics of the various pineal region tumors is still evolving. Particularly with the rarer, more differentiated germ cell tumors, only a handful of cases have been reported.[53, 54] Sagittal images are invaluable for evaluating these masses because they provide excellent depiction of their relationship to the aqueduct, midbrain, and posterior third ventricle and help establish the pineal

region origin of the mass. Tumor markers assist in differentiating the germ cell tumors. Elevation of β-human chorionic gonadotropin is seen in choriocarcinoma and germ cell tumors, and elevation of α-fetoprotein with a normal β-human chorionic gonadotropin occurs in malignant germ cell tumors (often endodermal sinus tumor). Elevation of both β-human chorionic gonadotropin and α-fetoprotein levels can be seen with embryonal cell carcinoma, malignant teratomas, and mixed germ cell tumors.[53]

Germinomas are usually seen as a mass invading the tectum, isointense relative to white matter on T1-weighted images, and slightly hyperintense on T2-weighted images (Fig. 17–19). Both small cysts within the mass and a homogeneous appearance have been noted. Intense, homogeneous enhancement has been present, and seeding of tumor to the anterior third ventricle is common. Endodermal sinus tumor and choriocarcinoma demonstrate more heterogeneity on T2-weighted images, and both are seen to be invasive. This heterogeneity in choriocarcinoma is due in part to areas of hemorrhage. Teratomas also are more heterogeneous on T2-weighted sequences but exhibit more T2 hyperintensity than do germinomas and embryonal carcinomas. Invasion of adjacent structures, a lack of fat, and a larger size at presentation serve to signal the malignant teratomas.[54a]

Pineocytomas demonstrate a cyst-like pattern of homogeneously decreased T1 signal intensity and homogeneously increased T2 signal intensity. Pineoblastomas have the expected aggressive appearance of a lobulated, heterogeneous, invasive, and enhancing mass (Fig. 17–20). A larger size at presentation than most of the other pineal region masses is common: two of three were greater than 4 cm in diameter in one study.[53]

BENIGN CYSTIC MASSES

Differentiating among the wide variety of benign cystic intracranial masses has become easier with the ability to demonstrate different signal intensities with MRI.

ARACHNOID CYST

Arachnoid cysts are relatively common masses of uncertain origin. They may be related to prior leptomeningitis or trauma. Alternatively, they may represent an aberration of CSF flow resulting from splitting of the arachnoid membrane during development. These cysts are located in the subdural space or in a split in the arachnoid. Although benign, they slowly grow as they accumulate fluid. Remodeling of the adjacent skull is an important clue for a benign, expansile process. Approximately 50% of intracranial arachnoid cysts are related to the sylvian fissure. They are also commonly seen in the anteroinferior portion of the middle cranial fossa. Other locations include the cere-

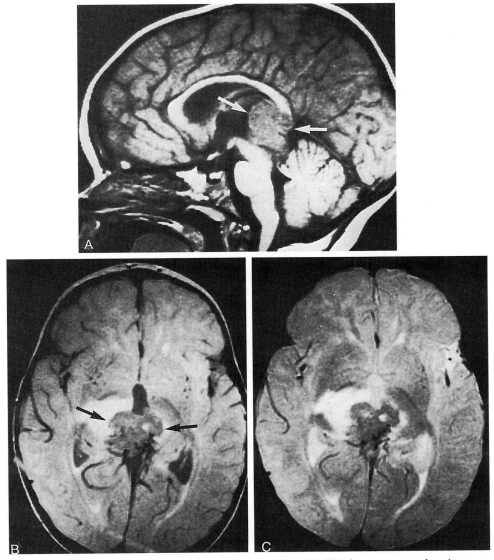

FIGURE 17–19. Germinoma. *A,* T1-weighted scan (spin echo, 600/25) demonstrates a hypointense mass *(arrows)* in the pineal region that compresses the midbrain and elevates the splenium of the corpus callosum. *B* and *C,* The tumor *(arrows)* is essentially isointense relative to brain on proton density– and T2-weighted images (spin echo, 2000/25,70) and is associated with some peritumor edema.

bellopontine angle cistern and the retrocerebellar, suprasellar, and pineal regions.

It is important to differentiate arachnoid cysts from porencephaly and encephalomalacia because they require different therapies. Porencephalic cysts can be decompressed with a ventricular shunt. Arachnoid cysts do not communicate with the ventricular system and, if treatment is indicated, must be resected, marsupialized or directly shunted. In most cases, brain tissue separates the extra-axial cyst from the ventricle. With the large congenital variety, occasionally intrathecal contrast medium is required to establish the diagnosis. The presence of mass effect and the lack of adjacent brain reaction are usually sufficient to differentiate an arachnoid cyst from encephalomalacia, which is an atrophic process associated with gliosis. No therapy is indicated for encephalomalacia.

EPIDERMOID CYST

Epidermoid cysts (primary cholesteatomas) result from inclusion of ectodermal tissue at the time of neural groove closure. They constitute less then 1% of intracranial tumors, and although seen in a wide range of age groups, epidermoids most commonly present during middle adult years.[9] The cerebellopontine angle cistern and parapituitary region are the most common locations, followed by the diploë of the calvaria. They are predominantly extra-axial in location, but the parapituitary lesions are often embedded in the temporal lobe. The lesions vary in size, have an irregularly nodular capsule, and may have a pearly sheen, leading to the name "pearly tumor." They arise from epithelial rests in the basal cisterns, and the interior is usually filled with soft, waxy, or flaky mate-

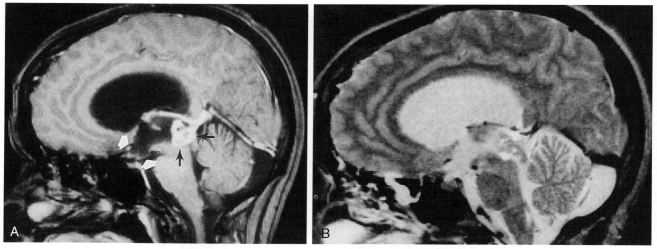

FIGURE 17–20. Pineoblastoma. *A,* A heterogeneously enhancing, slightly lobulated pineal mass *(black arrows)* is revealed by this gadolinium-enhanced T1-weighted image. The tumor has obstructed the aqueduct with resultant hydrocephalus and dilatation of the anterior recesses of the third ventricle *(white arrows). B,* Several small hyperintense cysts are shown within the mass on this T2-weighted image.

rial laden with cholesterol crystals produced by desquamation and breakdown of the keratin lining of the cyst. Rupture of the cyst may result in a granulomatous meningitis. Although almost always benign, they slowly grow into the various crevices found at the base of the brain and may recur if incompletely excised.

DERMOID CYST

Dermoid cysts share a similar origin with epidermoid cysts, but they contain additional dermal elements such as hair, resulting in a more varied histologic and MRI appearance. Additional similarities with epidermoid cysts include a tendency to recur with incomplete excision, and the ability to invoke a chemical meningitis with rupture of the cyst. Dermoid cysts tend to occur in the midline, most commonly in the posterior fossa but also in the pineal region and suprasellar regions, as well as the skull base. They are less common than epidermoid cysts. A dermal sinus may overlie the usually well-defined and sometimes lobulated mass.

GIANT CHOLESTEROL CYST

Giant cholesterol cysts (cholesterol granulomas) involve the petrous apex and usually present as large masses with palsy of the fifth through eighth cranial nerves. They represent an inflammatory response to cholesterol crystals, possibly caused by recurrent episodes of hemorrhage into obstructed and pneumatized petrous apex air cells.[55] The semiliquid cyst material contains both blood degradation products and cholesterol.

COLLOID CYST

Colloid cysts originate from primitive neuroepithelium within the roof of the anterior third ventricle.

They are positioned just posterior to the foramen of Monro between the columns of the fornix. Histologically, they consist of a thin fibrous capsule with an epithelial lining. The cysts contain a mucinous fluid with variable amounts of proteinaceous debris, blood components, and desquamated cells.[9] The contents of the cyst are usually soft but vary in consistency. They vary from less than 1 cm to 3 to 4 cm in diameter and may obstruct the foramina of Monro with resultant hydrocephalus. The cysts may be pendulous, leading to intermittent obstruction and the possibility of sudden death. The classic symptoms are positional headaches related to intermittent obstruction of the foramina of Monro. Although congenital, they usually present during adult life.

PINEAL CYST

These benign, fairly small and relatively common cysts have been recognized with increasing frequency with the advent of MRI.[56] They are almost always of no clinical significance, but it is important to recognize them as a benign lesion to be differentiated from other pineal region masses.

MRI FEATURES AND DIFFERENTIAL DIAGNOSIS OF BENIGN CYSTIC MASSES

Arachnoid cysts are most commonly identified as smooth to somewhat lobulated, homogeneous masses isointense relative to CSF on all sequences (Fig. 17–21). Occasionally, an arachnoid cyst may be mildly hyperintense relative to CSF on both T1- and proton density–weighted sequences due to diminished CSF pulsations or elevated protein content within the cyst. They are not calcified and do not enhance.

An epidermoid cyst may also be isointense relative

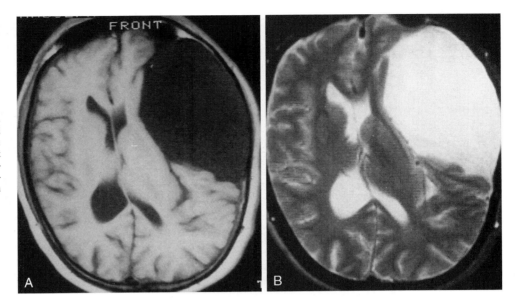

FIGURE 17–21. Arachnoid cyst. *A,* A large, smoothly marginated extra-axial mass, isointense with CSF, is demonstrated in the left frontotemporal region on this T1-weighted image. *B,* The homogeneous cyst remains isointense with CSF on this T2-weighted image.

to CSF on T1- and T2-weighted sequences but are more commonly slightly hyperintense on T1-weighted images and moderately hyperintense and heterogeneous on T2-weighted images (Fig. 17–22). Rarely, an epidermoid cyst may appear bright on a T1-weighted image. The margins are more irregular than those seen with arachnoid cysts, and MRI in particular can document an insinuating pattern of growth. MRI can assess for involvement of vessels and other adjacent structures better than CT, but CT may assist in differential diagnosis by revealing calcifications in 25% of epidermoids.[57] Epidermoid tumors do not enhance after administration of contrast medium.

A dermoid cyst may contain areas of T1 hyperintensity due to fat (Fig. 17–23), helping to differentiate it

from most epidermoid cysts. In addition, the midline location, possible associated calvarial defect, and less lobular margins signal the presence of a dermoid cyst. With rupture, the cyst contents can be seen scattered throughout the cisterns and ventricles (Fig. 17–24).

Giant cholesterol cyst is characteristically seen as an expansile petrous apex mass that is hyperintense on both T1- and T2-weighted images. The T1 hyperintensity separates this lesion from most cases of simple mucosal disease, and the T2 hyperintensity distinguishes this lesion from marrow within the petrous apex.

Colloid cysts do not have a typical MRI appearance but do have a characteristic location in the anterior third ventricle. A discrete rim is usually identified with

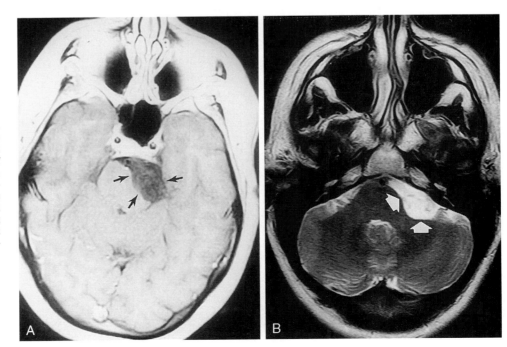

FIGURE 17–22. Epidermoid cyst. *A,* This extra-axial mass is shown to have irregular margins *(arrows)* and mild heterogeneity of signal intensity. No enhancement of the epidermoid cyst is noted on this gadolinium-enhanced T1-weighted image. *B,* The margins appear smoother *(arrows)* at a more inferior level on this fast spin-echo T2-weighted image, but internal heterogeneity remains evident.

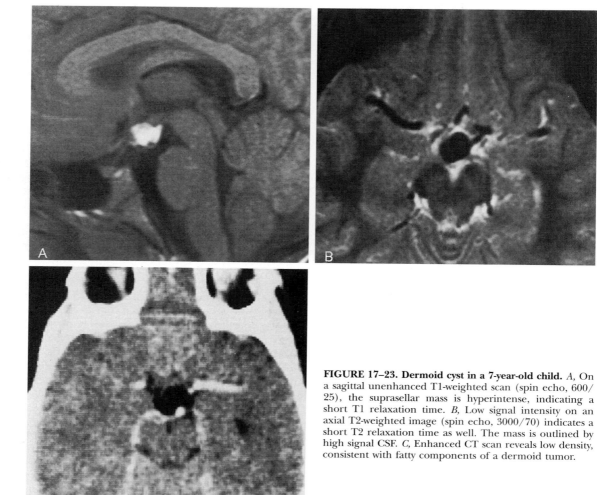

FIGURE 17–23. Dermoid cyst in a 7-year-old child. *A,* On a sagittal unenhanced T1-weighted scan (spin echo, 600/25), the suprasellar mass is hyperintense, indicating a short T1 relaxation time. *B,* Low signal intensity on an axial T2-weighted image (spin echo, 3000/70) indicates a short T2 relaxation time as well. The mass is outlined by high signal CSF. *C,* Enhanced CT scan reveals low density, consistent with fatty components of a dermoid tumor.

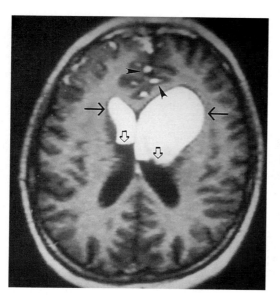

FIGURE 17–24. Ruptured dermoid cyst. High-signal-intensity lipid is seen in the anterior lateral ventricles *(arrows)* and within sulci anteriorly *(arrowheads)* on this T1-weighted image. CSF-lipid levels are present within the lateral ventricles *(open arrows).*

MRI. Variable signal intensities of both the rim and the core on both T1- and T2-weighted images have been noted[58, 59] (Fig. 17–25), likely due to the variable consistency of the cyst contents. Those that are high density on CT scans are usually hypointense on T2-weighted images and slightly hyperintense on T1-weighted images (Fig. 17–26). Colloid cysts may show ring enhancement, owing to either enhancement of the cyst wall or choroid plexus draped around the cyst. In some cases, delayed scans reveal enhancement of the cyst contents.

Pineal cysts are most commonly visualized as well-defined, round masses in the posterior third ventricle, exhibiting slightly increased signal intensity relative to CSF on T1-weighted and proton density–weighted images (Fig. 17–27), and becoming isointense on more heavily T2-weighted images.[56] There rarely have been larger, symptomatic pineal cysts reported in this region.[60] These unusual masses demonstrate a heterogeneous signal intensity pattern that may be indistinguishable from the pattern of a cystic neoplasm.

POSTOPERATIVE IMAGING

An understanding of the range of appearances of the brain and meninges after surgery is crucial to the appropriate interpretation of postoperative MRI studies. Deviations from the expected findings on serial studies may indicate the presence of residual or recurrent tumor, postoperative complications, or radiation necrosis. Contrast medium–enhanced MRI has proved superior to CT for visualization of residual tumor and differentiation of tumor from blood.[61]

Meningeal enhancement after surgery is extremely common, having been seen in 80% of patients in one study.[62] This may be localized to the surgical site or be diffuse. Diffuse meningeal enhancement is often seen in children after ventriculoperitoneal shunting[63] (Fig. 17–28). The smooth, thin, and regular appearance of this benign postoperative meningeal enhancement serves to distinguish it from the more nodular and irregular pattern associated with subarachnoid and dural metastases and meningitis. Ependymal enhancement also suggests tumor or infection. Moderate meningeal enhancement may be noted in the presence of postoperative subdural collections. Benign meningeal postoperative enhancement remains stable.

Parenchymal enhancement may also be present postoperatively and must be separated from hemorrhage and residual tumor. In general, enhancing brain tissue is seen up to 6 months after surgery by MRI and no benign parenchymal enhancement should remain after 1 year.[61, 64] Obtaining the first postoperative MRI study in the first few postoperative days helps to separate tumor from hemorrhage, because only minimal T1-bright methemoglobin is expected in the first 3 days. Widespread enhancement along the resection lines is seen beginning in the second postoperative week, and the pattern is impossible to differentiate from that of residual tumor[61] (Fig. 17–29). During this time period, T1 hyperintense hemorrhage may also be imaged, so that the acquisition of both nonenhanced and enhanced images is imperative. In most patients, benign linear enhancement at the margins of the surgical bed resolves at 2 months but can persist up to 6 months or rarely longer in some patients. Residual tumor is usually more irregular, nodular, or mass-like. Obviously, if the original tumor was nonenhancing, areas of enhancement in the early postoperative period should be benign, but on later studies the possibility of a low-grade glioma dedifferentiating into a higher grade, enhancing lesion must be considered. For this reason, even low-grade gliomas should be followed with gadolinium-enhanced studies.

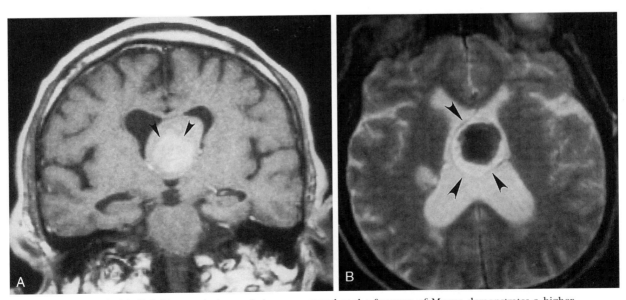

FIGURE 17–25. Colloid cyst. *A,* A rounded mass centered at the foramen of Monro demonstrates a higher signal intensity core *(arrowheads)* on this T1-weighted image. There is only mild dilatation of the lateral ventricles. *B,* The inner core is hypointense, and the periphery *(arrowheads)* is nearly isointense with CSF on this T2-weighted image.

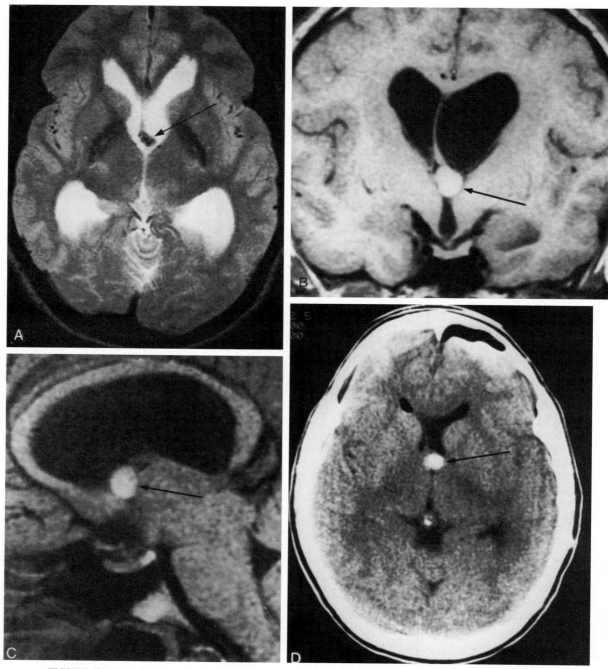

FIGURE 17–26. Colloid cyst. *A,* Axial T2-weighted scan (spin echo, 2800/80) reveals a small hypointense mass *(arrow).* The lateral ventricles are moderately enlarged, but the third ventricle is normal, indicating obstruction at the level of the foramina of Monro. *B* and *C,* Coronal and sagittal T1-weighted images (spin echo, 600/20) confirm the mass *(arrow)* positioned at the foramina of Monro. The mass has slightly higher signal intensity than brain. The left lateral ventricle is larger as a result of asymmetric obstruction of the two foramina. *D,* On a nonenhanced CT scan, obtained after a ventricular shunting procedure, the colloid cyst *(arrow)* is hyperdense relative to brain parenchyma. *(A* to *D* courtesy of George Wesbey, Scripps Memorial Hospital, La Jolla, CA.)

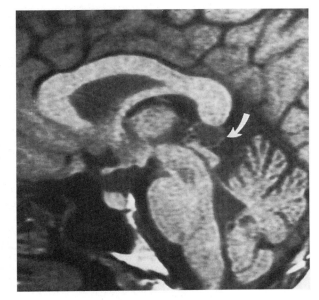

FIGURE 17–27. Pineal cyst. T1-weighted sagittal scan (spin echo, 600/20) demonstrates a low-signal-intensity lesion *(arrow)* within the pineal gland. Its homogeneous texture and smooth margins suggest a benign cyst.

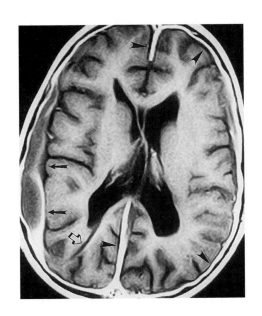

FIGURE 17–28. Benign meningeal enhancement. A smooth, regular pattern of meningeal enhancement *(arrowheads)* is seen in this patient after placement of a ventriculoperitoneal shunt *(open arrow)* on this T1-weighted gadolinium-enhanced image. The magnitude of enhancement is greater than that sometimes seen after shunting, likely due to the presence of a subdural hematoma *(solid arrows)*.

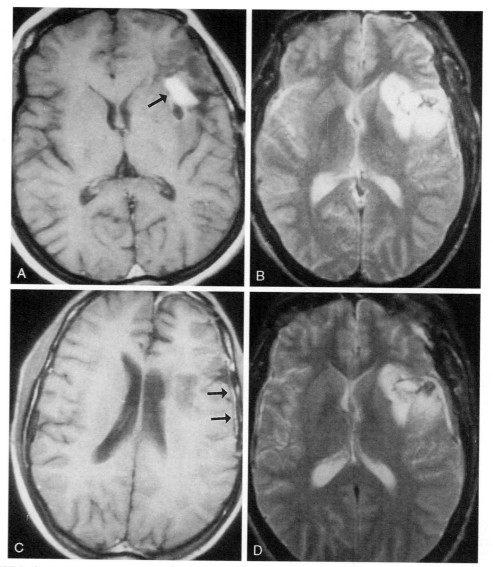

FIGURE 17–29. Normal postoperative appearance. *A,* Enhancement is present within the surgical bed *(arrow)* 4 months after resection of a low-grade glioma on this T1-weighted gadolinium-enhanced image. *B,* A larger area of increased signal intensity representing edema and gliosis is present on the T2-weighted image obtained at the same time. *C,* Surgical bed enhancement has resolved 12 months after surgery on this T1-weighted gadolinium-enhanced image. Benign meningeal enhancement is noted at the craniotomy site *(arrows). D,* The area of increased signal intensity has diminished in size on the 12-month postoperative T2-weighted image. The remaining signal abnormality is consistent with gliosis and encephalomalacia.

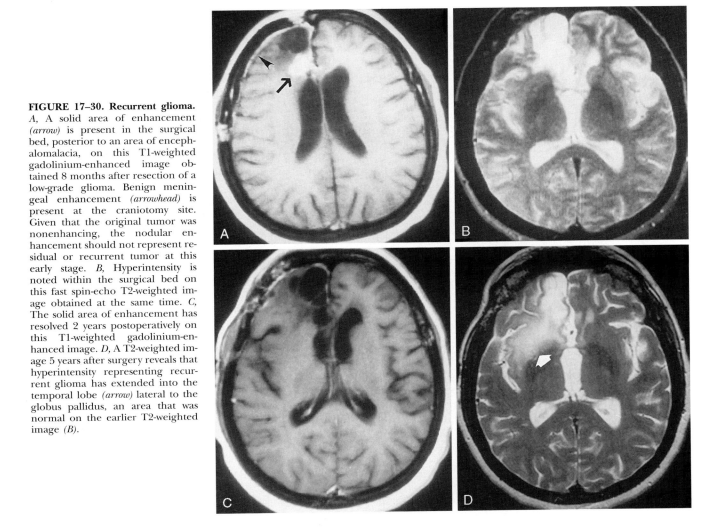

FIGURE 17–30. Recurrent glioma. *A*, A solid area of enhancement *(arrow)* is present in the surgical bed, posterior to an area of encephalomalacia, on this T1-weighted gadolinium-enhanced image obtained 8 months after resection of a low-grade glioma. Benign meningeal enhancement *(arrowhead)* is present at the craniotomy site. Given that the original tumor was nonenhancing, the nodular enhancement should not represent residual or recurrent tumor at this early stage. *B*, Hyperintensity is noted within the surgical bed on this fast spin-echo T2-weighted image obtained at the same time. *C*, The solid area of enhancement has resolved 2 years postoperatively on this T1-weighted gadolinium-enhanced image. *D*, A T2-weighted image 5 years after surgery reveals that hyperintensity representing recurrent glioma has extended into the temporal lobe *(arrow)* lateral to the globus pallidus, an area that was normal on the earlier T2-weighted image *(B)*.

The time course of T2 hyperintense edema adjacent to the operative bed must also be monitored. Increasing amounts of T2 hyperintensity, even without associated enhancement, must be viewed with suspicion (Fig. 17–30).

REFERENCES

1. Bradley WG, Waluch V, Yadley RA, Wycoff RR: Comparison of CT and MR in 400 patients with suspected disease of the brain and cervical spinal canal. Radiology 152:695–702, 1984.
2. Brant-Zawadzki M, Davis PL, Crooks LE, et al: NMR demonstration of cerebral abnormalities: comparison with CT. AJR 140:847–854, 1983.
3. Graif M, Bydder GM, Steiner RE, et al: Contrast-enhanced MR imaging of malignant brain tumors. AJNR 6:855–862, 1985.
4. Schorner W, Laniado M, Neindorf HP, et al: Brain tumors: imaging with gadolinium-DTPA. Radiology 156:681–688, 1985.
5. Hesselink JR, Press GA: MR contrast enhancement of intracranial lesions with Gd-DTPA. Radiol Clin North Am 26:873–887, 1988.
6. Berry I, Brant-Zawadzki M, Osaki L, et al: Gd-DTPA in clinical MR of the brain: 2. Extraaxial lesions and normal structures. AJR 147:1231–1235, 1986.
7. Breger RK, Papke RA, Pojunas KW, et al: Benign extraaxial tumors: contrast enhancement with Gd-DTPA. Radiology 163:427–429, 1987.
8. Rubinstein LJ: Tumors of the Central Nervous System. Washington, DC: Armed Forces Institute of Pathology, 1972.
9. Russell DS, Rubinstein LJ: Pathology of Tumours of the Nervous System. 5th ed. Baltimore: Williams & Wilkins, 1989.
10. Dean BL, Drayer BP, Bird CR, Flom RA, et al: Gliomas: classification with MR Imaging. Radiology 174:411–415, 1990.
11. Strong JA, Hatten HP Jr, Brown MT, et al: Pilocytic astrocytoma: correlation between the initial imaging features and clinical aggressiveness. AJR 161:369–372, 1993.
12. Lee Y-Y, Tassel PV, Bruner JM, et al: Juvenile pilocytic astrocytomas: CT and MR characteristics. AJNR 10:363–370, 1989.
13. Fulham MJ, Melisi JW, Nishimiya J, et al: Neuroimaging of pilocytic astrocytomas: an enigma. Radiology 189:221–225, 1993.
14. Kilgore DP, Breger RL, Daniels DL, et al: Cranial tissues: normal MR appearance after intravenous injection of Gd-DTPA. Radiology 160:757–761, 1986.
15. Shin YM, Chang KH, Han MH, et al: Gliomatosis cerebri: a comparison of MR and CT features. AJR 161:859–862, 1993.
16. Tice H, Barnes PD, Goumnerova L, et al: Pediatric and adolescent oligodendrogliomas. AJNR 14:1293–1300, 1993.
17. Lee Y-Y, Tassel PV: Intracranial oligodendrogliomas: imaging findings in 35 untreated cases. AJNR 10:119–127, 1989.
18. Castillo M, Davis PC, Takei Y, Hoffmann JC: Intracranial ganglioglioma: MR, CT and clinical findings in 18 patients. AJNR 11:109–114, 1990.
19. Altman NR: MR and CT characteristics of gangliocytoma: a rare cause of epilepsy in children. AJNR 9:917–921, 1988.
20. Burger PC, Scheithauer BW: Tumors of the Central Nervous System. Washington, DC: Armed Forces Institute of Pathology, 1994.
21. Tien RD, Cardenas CA, Rajagopalan S: Pleomorphic xanthoastrocytoma of the brain: MR findings in six patients. AJR 159:1287–1290, 1992.
22. Yoshino MT, Lucio R: Pleomorphic xanthoastrocytoma. AJNR 13:1330–1332, 1992.
23. Koeller KK, Dillon WP: Dysembryoplastyic neuroepithelial tumors: MR appearance. AJNR 13:1319–1325, 1992.
24. Goergen SK, Gonzales MF, McLean CA: Intraventricular neurocytoma: radiologic features and review of the literature. Radiology 182:787–792, 1992.

25. Wichman W, Schubiger O, Deimling A, et al: Neuroradiology of central neurocytoma. Neuroradiology 33:143–148, 1991.
26. Schwaighofer BW, Hesselink JR, Press GA, et al: Primary intracranial CNS lymphoma: MR manifestations. AJNR 10:725–729, 1989.
27. Roman-Goldstein SM, Goldman DL, Howieson J, et al: MR of primary CNS lymphoma in immunologically normal patients. AJNR 13:1207–1213, 1992.
28. Tadmor R, Davis KR, Roberson HG, Kleinman GM: Computed tomography in primary malignant lymphoma of the brain. J Comput Assist Tomogr 2:135–140, 1978.
29. Cordoliani Y-S, Derosier C, Pharaboz C, et al: Primary cerebral lymphoma in patients with AIDS: MR findings in 17 cases. AJR 159:841–847, 1992.
30. Carrier DA, Mawad ME, Kirkpatrick JB, Schmid MF: Metastatic adenocarcinoma to the brain: MR with pathologic correlation. AJNR 15:155–159, 1994.
31. Egelhoff JC, Ross JS, Modic MT, et al: MR imaging of metastatic GI adenocarcinoma in brain. AJNR 13:1221–1224, 1992.
32. Woodruff WW Jr, Djang WT, McLendon RE, et al: Intracerebral malignant melanoma: high-field-strength MR imaging. Radiology 165:209–213, 1987.
33. Atlas SW, Grossman RI, Gomori JM, et al: MR imaging of intracranial metastatic melanoma. J Comput Assist Tomogr 11:577–582, 1987.
34. Healy ME, Hesselink JR, Press GA, Middleton MS: Increased detection of intracranial metastases with intravenous Gd-DTPA. Radiology 165:619–624, 1987.
35. Russell EJ, Geremia GK, Johnson CE, et al: Multiple cerebral metastases: detectability with Gd-DTPA-enhanced MR imaging. Radiology 165:609–617, 1987.
36. Davis PC, Hudgins PA, Peterman SB, Hoffman JC: Diagnosis of cerebral metastases: double-dose delayed CT vs. contrast-enhanced MR imaging. AJNR 12:293–300, 1991.
37. Elster AD, Chen MYM: Can nonenhancing white matter lesions in cancer patients be disregarded? AJNR 13:1309–1315, 1992.
38. Patchell RA, Tibbs PA, Walsh JW, et al: A randomized trial of surgery in the treatment of single metastases to the brain. N Engl J Med 322:494–500, 1990.
39. Yuh WTC, Tali ET, Nguyen HD, et al: The effect of contrast dose, imaging time, and lesion size in the MR detection of intracerebral metastasis. AJNR 16:373–380, 1995.
40. Finelli DA, Hurst GC, Gullapalli RP, Bellon EM: Improved contrast of enhancing brain lesions on post-gadolinium, T1-weighted spin echo images with the use of magnetization transfer. Radiology 190:553–559, 1994.
41. West MS, Russell EJ, Breit R, et al: Calvarial and skull base metastases: comparison of nonenhanced and Gd-DTPA-enhanced MR images. Radiology 174:85–91, 1990.
42. Sze G, Soletsky S, Bronen R, Krol G: MR imaging of the cranial meninges with emphasis on contrast enhancement and meningeal carcinomatosis. AJNR 10:969–975, 1989.
43. Zimmerman RD, Fleming CA, Saint-Louis CA, et al: Magnetic resonance imaging of meningiomas. AJNR 6:149–157, 1985.
44. Spagnoli MV, Goldberg HI, Grossman RI, et al: Intracranial meningiomas: high-field MR imaging. Radiology 161:369–375, 1986.
45. Elster AD, Challa VR, Gilbert TH, et al: Meningiomas: MR and histopathologic features. Radiology 170:857–862, 1989.
46. Bydder GM, Kingsley DPE, Brown J, et al: MR imaging of meningiomas including studies with and without Gd-DTPA. J Comput Assist Tomogr 9:690–697, 1985.
47. Tokumaru A, O'uchi T, Eguchi T, et al: Prominent meningeal enhancement adjacent to meningioma on Gd-DTPA-enhanced MR images: histopathologic correlation. Radiology 175:431–433, 1990.
48. Aoki S, Sasaki Y, Machida T, Tanioka H: Contrast-enhanced MR images in patients with meningioma: importance of enhancement of the dura adjacent to the tumor. AJNR 11:935–938, 1990.
49. Goldsher D, Litt AW, Pinto RS, et al: Dural "tail" associated with meningiomas on Gd-DTPA-enhanced MR images: characteristics, differential diagnostic value, and possible implications for treatment. Radiology 176:447–450, 1990.
50. Wilms G, Laemmens M, Marchal G, et al: Prominent dural enhancement adjacent to nonmeningiomatous malignant lesions on contrast-enhanced MR images. AJNR 12:761–764, 1991.
51. Glasier CM, Husain MM, Chadduck W, Boop FA: Meningiomas in children: MR and histopathologic findings. AJNR 14:237–241. 1993.
52. Cosentino CM, Poulton TB, Esguerra JV, Sands SF: Giant cranial hemangiopericytoma: MR and angiographic findings. AJNR 14:253–256, 1993.
53. Tien RD, Barkovich AJ, Edwards MSB: MR imaging of pineal tumors. AJNR 11:557–565, 1990.
54. Nakagawa H, Iwaski S, Kichikawa K, et al: MR imaging of pineocytoma: report of two cases. AJNR 11:195–198, 1990.
54a. Chiechi MV, Smirniotopoulos JG, Mena H: Pineal parenchymal tumors: CT and MR features. J Comput Assist Tomogr 19:509–517, 1995.
55. Greenberg JJ, Oot RF, Wismer GL, et al: Cholesterol granuloma of the petrous apex: MR and CT evaluation. AJNR 9:1205–1214, 1988.
56. Mamourian AC, Towfighi J: Pineal cysts: MR imaging. AJNR 7:1081–1086, 1986.
57. Tampieri D, Melanson D, Ethier R: MR imaging of epidermoid cysts. AJNR 10:351–356, 1989.
58. Maeder PP, Holtas SL, Basibuyuk LN, et al: Colloid cysts of the third ventricle: correlation of MR and CT findings with histology and chemical analysis. AJNR 11:575–581, 1990.
59. Roosen N, Gablen D, Stork W, et al: Magnetic resonance imaging of colloid cysts of the third ventricle. Neuroradiology 29:10–14, 1987.
60. Fleege MA, Miller GM, Fletcher GP, et al: Benign glial cysts of the pineal gland: unusual imaging characteristics with histologic correlation. AJNR 15:161–166, 1994.
61. Forsting M, Albert FK, Kunze S, et al: Extirpation of glioblastomas: MR and CT follow-up of residual tumor and regrowth patterns. AJNR 14:77–87, 1993.
62. Burke JW, Podrasky AE, Bradley WG: Meninges: benign postoperative enhancement on MR images. Radiology 174:99–102, 1990.
63. Hudgins PA, Davis PC, Hoffman JC Jr: Gadopentetate dimeglumine–enhanced MR imaging in children following surgery for brain tumors: spectrum of meningeal findings. AJNR 12:301–307, 1991.
64. Elster AD, DiPersio DA: Cranial postoperative site: assessment with contrast-enhanced MR imaging. Radiology 174:93–98, 1990.

Pituitary Gland and Parasellar Region

BRIAN W. CHONG ■ JAMES A. BRUNBERG

PULSE SEQUENCES AND IMAGING PARAMETERS

Magnetic resonance imaging (MRI) is the preferred modality for imaging the sella and the parasellar regions because of its intrinsic merits of higher spatial resolution, multiplanar capabilities, and absence of ionizing radiation.

For imaging the pituitary gland, MRI parameters are selected to provide maximal signal-to-noise ratio, spatial resolution, and image contrast in the shortest possible time. A sagittal T1-weighted image is used to assess the midline structures. The optimal plane for imaging the contents of the sella is the coronal plane. This plane diminishes the partial volume effects from the carotid arteries, sphenoidal sinus, and suprasellar cistern, which are inherent to the axial plane. For high spatial detail, thin slices (≤3 mm), a fine matrix (256 × 256 to 512 × 256), and a small field of view (16 to 18 cm) are needed. Good signal-to-noise ratio can be obtained with two to four excitations. Any more than four excitations increases the imaging time and the likelihood of movement of the patient. Peripheral gating will diminish flow-related artifact, especially on postcontrast sequences.

The most widely employed pulse sequence is a conventional spin-echo T1-weighted image (short repetition time [TR], short echo time [TE]) in the coronal plane. For difficult cases, a fast spin-echo T2-weighted pulse sequence can be added.[1] Three-dimensional (3D) Fourier transform images have been used to provide results comparable to the conventional spin-echo T1-weighted images.[2, 3] An advantage of 3D Fourier transform imaging is better spatial resolution due to thinner slices, contiguous slices, and isotropic voxel size. A disadvantage is the potential for motion and truncation artifacts in the two dimensions that are phase encoded.

Paramagnetic contrast agents such as the gadolinium complexes are useful adjuncts for defining sellar and parasellar disease. Enhancement will be seen in areas where the blood-brain barrier is absent or not well developed (pituitary gland, infundibulum, median eminence, tuber cinereum, cavernous sinus, and nasopharyngeal mucosa) or where it has been rendered incompetent by tumor or an inflammatory process.[4–10]

Dynamic scans performed after rapid injection of contrast material are useful for visualizing small pituitary adenomas.[7, 11, 12] A coronal, fast multiplanar spoiled gradient-echo sequence using a flip angle of 45°, two excitations, 3-mm thickness, 128 × 192 matrix, TR of 52 ms, and TE of 4 ms can be employed with images obtained at four locations through the sella. Sequential enhancement patterns of the normal pituitary gland and microadenomas are discussed later in this chapter.

ANATOMY

The sella turcica is the bony depression within the sphenoid bone in which the pituitary gland rests. Anteriorly lies the tuberculum sella, and posteriorly is the dorsum sella and brain stem. The sphenoidal sinus is inferior and anterior. Laterally lie the paired cavernous sinuses. The lateral wall of the cavernous sinus is composed of two dural layers: a lateral dural layer (dura propria) and an inner membranous layer. Within the lateral dural wall are cranial nerves III, IV, V1, and V2, some of which may be seen on MR images.[13] Cranial nerve VI lies medially within the sinus, along with the cavernous internal carotid artery, which is immediately above the nerve. The medial wall of the cavernous sinus is much thinner than the lateral wall and can be difficult to separate from the pituitary gland on MR images. The cavernous sinuses extend anteriorly to the level of the orbital fissures and posteriorly to Meckel's cave, where the trigeminal ganglion lies. The venous sinuses are composed of numerous endothelium-lined vascular channels. The two cavernous sinuses interconnect by means of intercavernous channels that encircle the pituitary gland.[14] Above the sella turcica is the suprasellar cistern. This space contains several vital structures, including the optic chiasm, the vascular

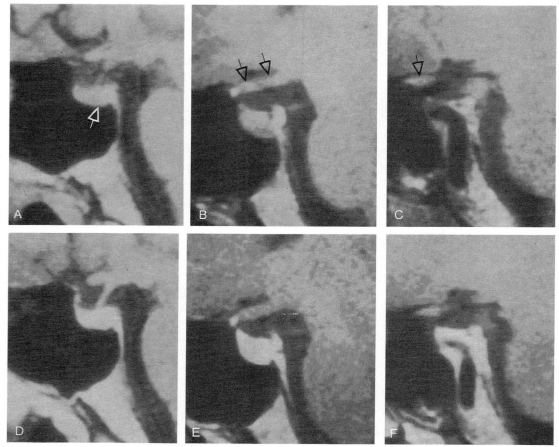

FIGURE 18–1. Normal pituitary gland. T1-weighted images after precontrast and postcontrast enhancement with gadolinium diethylenetriaminepentoacetic acid (Gd-DTPA): precontrast *(A to C)* and postcontrast *(D to F)* sagittal and parasagittal scans, left to right.

anastomosis of the circle of Willis, and the pituitary stalk. The pituitary stalk (infundibulum) passes through the diaphragma sella and into the suprasellar cistern. It extends superiorly, posterior to the chiasm, to insert into the median eminence, the inferior aspect of the hypothalamus. The third ventricle lies immediately above (Fig. 18–1).

In contrast to its diminutive size, the pituitary gland is the focal point of neuroendocrine activity. The normal gland weighs 0.5 to 0.9 g and rests within the saddle-shaped sella turcica. The pituitary gland can be divided into an anterior lobe (adenohypophysis) and a posterior lobe (neurohypophysis) based on embryologic development, adult morphology, and function.[15]

Traditional embryologic thinking that the pituitary gland arises from two distinct sources has been challenged. It has long been thought that the anterior lobe of the gland arose from Rathke's pouch, an epithelial outgrowth from the posterior pharyngeal wall, and that the posterior lobe arose from a neural downgrowth from the hypothalamus. Detailed examination of 4- to 5-week-old embryos suggests that Rathke's pouch may in fact originate near the buccal cavity as a separate vesicle that is not attached to the buccal cavity.[16, 17] In addition, immunohistochemical studies have shown

that some of the anterior pituitary cells can be considered part of the amine precursor uptake and decarboxylation system, which are of neuroectodermal origin, arising from the ventral neural ridge and not from the posterior pharyngeal wall.[18]

The anterior lobe of the pituitary gland (adenohypophysis) can be divided into the pars distalis, the pars tuberalis, and the pars intermedia.[15] The pars distalis forms the bulk of the anterior lobe. The cells of the adenohypophysis are organized geographically by function. Prolactin-secreting cells (lactotrophs) and growth hormone (GH)–secreting cells (somatotrophs) are situated laterally in the gland.[19] Adenomas of these cells are therefore generally situated laterally in the gland. Thyrotrophs, corticotrophs, and gonadotrophs, which secrete, respectively, thyroid-stimulating hormone (TSH), corticotropin (ACTH), and follicle-stimulating hormone (FSH) plus luteinizing hormone (LH), are situated medially, as are adenomas arising from these cells. This medial portion of the pars distalis has been termed the *mucoid wedge* because the hormones that it secretes are glycoproteins. We have been able to demonstrate the mucoid wedge in excised pituitary glands using high-resolution spoiled gradient-recalled acquisition in the steady state (GRASS) T1-weighted MR images of a wedge-shaped area that is of lower

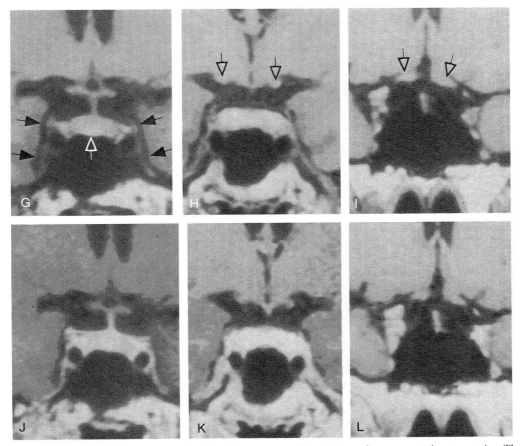

FIGURE 18–1 *Continued* Precontrast *(G to I)* and postcontrast *(J to L)* coronal scans, posterior to anterior. The posterior lobe of the pituitary gland *(open white arrow)* is slightly hyperintense relative to the anterior lobe. The optic chiasm and optic nerves *(open black arrows)* are seen superior and lateral to the pituitary stalk. The well-defined lateral walls of the cavernous sinuses *(black arrows)* have low signal intensity. The medial walls of the cavernous sinuses are thin and not delineated on MR images. The anterior lobe of the pituitary gland, pituitary stalk (infundibulum), median eminence, and cavernous sinuses enhance with contrast medium *(D to F and J to L)*. The carotid arteries are seen as signal voids due to rapidly flowing blood within. *(A to L from Chong BW, Newton TH: Hypothalamic and pituitary pathology. Radiol Clin North Am 31:1147–1183, 1993.)*

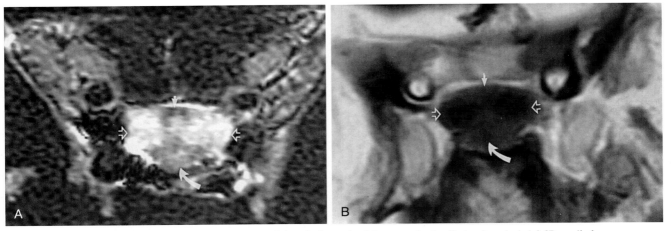

FIGURE 18–2. Postmortem MR images of the pituitary gland in an excised sella turcica. *A,* Axial 3D spoiled GRASS image (SPGR) (TR/TE/flip angle [FA] = 45/6/60°; number of excitations [NEX], 1; field of view [FOV], 18 cm; matrix, 512 × 256; slice thickness [THK], 1.0 mm). *B,* Axial fast spin-echo (FSE) image (echo train, 16; TR/TE = 4000/144; NEX, 4; FOV, 16 cm; matrix, 512 × 256; THK, 3.0 mm). The top of the image is anterior. The mucoid wedge *(white arrow)* is seen anteriorly as an area of decreased signal intensity in *A* and increased signal intensity in *B* relative to the lateral portions of the anterior lobe *(open arrows)*. The lack of bright signal pattern in the posterior pituitary lobe of the pituitary gland *(curved white arrow)* is likely because this is a postmortem specimen.

signal intensity than are the adjacent lateral margins of the anterior lobe (Fig. 18–2).

The pars tuberalis of the adenohypophysis is formed by a thin layer of cells from the pars distalis, which projects upward, surrounding the stalk (infundibulum) and extending as high as the median eminence. Adenomas may arise from this site.[20] The pars tuberalis may also independently maintain normal endocrine function after resection of the anterior lobe. The pars intermedia, between the adenohypophysis and the neurohypophysis, is vestigial in humans. It may also be the site of cystic embryologic remnants of Rathke's cleft. These cysts are usually incidental findings, but they may enlarge and cause symptoms.

The neurohypophysis consists of the pituitary stalk and the posterior lobe. It is the storage and release site for vasopressin (antidiuretic hormone, or ADH) and oxytocin. Both are synthesized in the hypothalamus and are transported to the neurohypophysis within secretory granules. The transport occurs within the axons of neurons in which the hormones are synthesized.[21] Hormones are then released into nearby capillaries by exocytosis in response to nerve impulses originating in the hypothalamus. The posterior lobe of the pituitary gland also contains pituicytes, which are modified glial cells that may function by scavenging substances released at the secretory terminals.[22]

Delivery of hypothalamic releasing hormones to the anterior lobe of the pituitary gland occurs by means of the hypophysial-portal system.[21] The adenohypophysis receives its predominant blood supply indirectly through a proximal portal venous system, the arterial supply of which is from the superior and inferior hypophysial arteries[23, 24] (Fig. 18–3). Venous drainage from the pituitary gland is to the cavernous sinuses. Nerve fibers of the hypothalamus terminate in the median eminence adjacent to the vessels of the proximal capillary network.[21] Hypothalamic hormones are released by exocytosis from the nerve fibers at this location. The hypophysial-portal vessels arise from this capillary network. The portal vessels then terminate on a secondary capillary plexus in the anterior lobe where the hypothalamic hormones stimulate the release of the various hormones synthesized in the adenohypophysis. The lack of a blood-brain barrier at the location where the portal vessels originate and terminate (the median eminence and the pituitary gland) allows passage of neurohormones into the blood stream at these sites.

The posterior pituitary is supplied by the inferior hypophysial artery, which is derived from the meningohypophysial trunk of the internal carotid artery. Venous drainage of the anterior and posterior pituitary is through the inferior hypophysial veins to the dural venous sinuses.

CLINICAL AND IMAGING CORRELATES OF ANATOMY

The unique vascular supply to the pituitary gland and the distinct differences between the supply to the anterior and the posterior lobes have several clinical

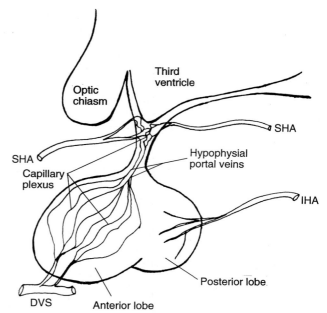

FIGURE 18–3. Vascular anatomy of the pituitary gland. The superior hypophysial artery (SHA), from the supraclinoid internal carotid artery and branches of the anterior and posterior cerebral arteries, gives rise to short terminal arterioles in the region of the median eminence. The arterioles are surrounded by a dense capillary plexus. The capillary plexus drains into the hypophysial portal veins that run along the surface of the pituitary stalk (infundibulum) and terminate in the capillary plexus of the anterior pituitary gland. Venous drainage is to the dural venous sinus (DVS). The posterior pituitary gland receives direct arterial supply from the inferior hypophysial artery (IHA), a branch of the meningohypophysial trunk of the internal carotid artery.

and imaging correlates. Postpartum pituitary necrosis or Sheehan's syndrome has been postulated to be the result of both the lack of a direct arterial supply to the adenohypophysis and adenohypophysial susceptibility to ischemia.[25] The propensity for larger pituitary tumors to infarct and hemorrhage (pituitary apoplexy) may similarly be related to a tenuous and indirect arterial supply.[26]

The lack of a blood-brain barrier in the pituitary gland and in the median eminence explains the normal enhancement of these regions after contrast medium administration. The sequential enhancement pattern of the pituitary gland on dynamic gadolinium-enhanced MRI studies is a direct consequence of flow in regional vessels and of normal parenchymal perfusion. The normal gland first demonstrates enhancement of the posterior lobe followed by the pituitary stalk and then the anterior lobe[12, 27, 28] (see Fig. 18–1). Pituitary adenomas have been shown to enhance in a delayed fashion relative to the normal gland parenchyma.[11, 12] This feature has proved to be useful for the diagnosis of small microadenomas.[7] Delayed imaging, 30 to 60 minutes after contrast medium injection, may mask signal intensity differences between a microadenoma and the remainder of the gland. Alternatively, a reversal of the pattern of enhancement can be seen at this time, when the adenoma may have a higher signal intensity than the normal gland. One report utilizing

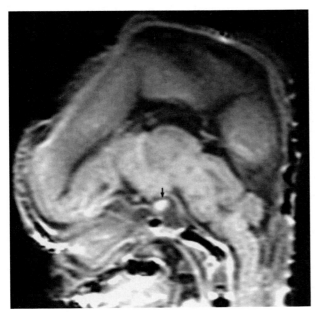

FIGURE 18–4. Postmortem study of 15-week fetus. Sagittal 3D SPGR image (TR/TE/FA = 42/10/45°; NEX, 6; FOV, 8 × 4; matrix, 512 × 512; THK, 0.7). The pituitary gland (arrow) is diffusely bright.

an image acquisition method with 5 to 10 seconds of temporal resolution (compared with 14 to 60 seconds) suggests that macroadenomas may enhance earlier than the normal gland, perhaps due to a direct neovascular arterial supply.[27]

The high signal intensity of the posterior lobe on T1-weighted MR images is a direct consequence of the anatomy and physiology of the gland. The bright signal was initially thought to be secondary to fat. It is now considered to be due to T1 shortening by the phospholipids in the neurosecretory granules in which ADH and oxytocin are transported to the neurohypophysis from the hypothalamus.[29, 30]

The pituitary gland has a varied appearance depending on the age and the endocrinologic status of the patient. We have imaged the glands of formalin-fixed fetuses and demonstrated a diffusely bright gland that is relatively large compared with the rest of the fetal brain as early as 15 weeks' gestational age (Fig. 18–4). The pituitary gland remains bulbous and bright on T1-weighted images from birth to 2 months of age.[31-33] This appearance has been attributed to cellular hypertrophy,[33] to an increase in the number of prolactin cells, to the quantity and activity of the endoplasmic reticulum,[32, 34, 35] and to shortening of T1 relaxation time secondary to an increase in the bound fraction of water molecules related to hormone secretion.[36] With increasing age during childhood, the height of the gland flattens and the anterior lobe decreases in signal intensity on T1-weighted images so that the gland resembles the adult gland in signal intensity. The height of the gland in children younger than 1 year old is 2 to 6 mm.[32] In individuals younger than 10 years old the height is no greater than 6 mm as well. Maximal adult gland height of 10 and 12 mm

is found in pregnant women and in women the first postpartum week, respectively.

The pituitary gland again increases in size and convexity during adolescence, particularly in pubertal females.[37] During pregnancy and lactation, the gland also enlarges and the anterior lobe increases in signal intensity.[38, 39] With precocious puberty the gland also increases in height.[40] In adults, age inversely correlates with pituitary height and cross-sectional area.[41] Physiologic hypertrophy or atrophy of the pituitary gland in response to activity of the hypothalamic-pituitary-gonadal axis is postulated as the explanation for these fluctuations in pituitary size, shape, and signal intensity.[37, 38, 41] In summary, the appearance of the gland on MR images is functionally linked to the maturation of the gland and the degree of pituitary hormonal activity at the time of imaging.

PITUITARY AND HYPOTHALAMIC FUNCTION

The pituitary gland and the hypothalamus are physiologically inseparable and referred to as the hypothalamic-pituitary axis. Both structures interact with each other, as well as with a specific end organ in a negative and positive feedback loop through the release of hormones (Fig. 18–5). The hypothalamus manufactures and secretes various hypothalamic releasing factors that stimulate or inhibit pituitary hormone secretion. Hormones then pass into the blood stream, where they are distributed systemically, eventually reaching target organs, which in turn will increase or decrease produc-

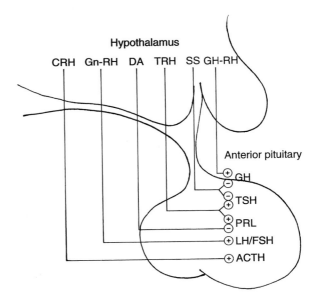

FIGURE 18–5. Hypothalamic releasing factors and their effect on the anterior pituitary hormones. (+) = stimulatory; (−) = inhibitory; CRH = corticotropin-releasing hormone; Gn-RH = gonadotropin-releasing hormone; DA = dopamine; TRH = thyrotropin-releasing hormone; SS = somatostatin; GH-RH = growth hormone-releasing hormone; GH = growth hormone; TSH = thyroid-stimulating hormone; PRL = prolactin; LH = luteinizing hormone; FSH = follicle-stimulating hormone; ACTH = corticotropin.

tion and secretion of a specific hormone. Circulating pituitary hormones and blood levels of end-organ hormones affect the release of neurohormones from the hypothalamus and the pituitary gland. Each hypothalamic neurohormone, corresponding pituitary hormone, and target organ can be discussed in terms of a specific axis.

PROLACTIN AXIS

Dopamine released from the hypothalamus decreases the rate of transcription of the prolactin gene and thereby inhibits production and secretion of prolactin by the pituitary gland. This same effect can be achieved pharmacologically by administration of the dopamine agonist bromocriptine, which is used in the treatment of prolactin-secreting pituitary microadenomas. Several additional medications can interfere with dopamine synthesis or act as dopamine antagonists. Antipsychotics (phenothiazines and butyrophenones) and metoclopramide are recognized dopamine antagonists that increase prolactin production, whereas reserpine and α-methyldopa are antihypertensive agents that deplete catecholamines (including dopamine), resulting in hyperprolactinemia.

The breast is a target organ for prolactin. In conjunction with estrogens, progesterone, glucocorticoids, and insulin, prolactin stimulates breast development. Prolactin also inhibits the production of the gonadotropins LH and FSH, which are required for ovulation. Elevated prolactin secretion normally occurs transiently with pregnancy, suckling, and sexual intercourse. Hyperprolactinemia in females commonly causes amenorrhea and galactorrhea. In males, hyperprolactinemia results in an inhibition of gonadotropin production and a decrease in libido. Because males lack estrogen-dependent breast development, galactorrhea is rare.

CORTICOTROPIN-RELEASING HORMONE–CORTICOTROPIN–CORTISOL AXIS

Corticotropin-releasing hormone (CRH), ACTH, and cortisol interact to effect an integrated response to stress. CRH release from the neurosecretory cells in the hypothalamus is modulated by several neurotransmitters. CRH then activates the sympathetic nervous system and stimulates the biosynthesis and release of ACTH and β-endorphin. ACTH from the adenohypophysis stimulates adrenocortical cortisol production. Cortisol acts on target organs to regulate adaptive responses to stress and in turn inhibits ACTH and CRH release in a negative feedback loop. In this manner the CRH-ACTH-cortisol axis enables an adaptive response to adverse conditions through physiologic mechanisms that maintain energy metabolism and blood pressure.

GH-RELEASING HORMONE–GH AXIS

The hypothalamus produces GH-releasing hormone, which is the major stimulator of GH production and release from the anterior pituitary. Somatostatin inhibits GH release. Several metabolic substrates and peripheral neurohormones stimulate GH release through hypothalamic regulation of GH-releasing hormone, as well as by a direct effect on the pituitary gland. Thyroid hormone and blood glucose levels affect GH secretion. GH is responsible for stimulating somatic growth and regulating metabolism. A deficiency of GH in childhood results in proportional dwarfism, and excess GH after epiphyseal closure causes acromegaly.

Growth is mediated by somatomedins, which are insulin-like growth factors. Synthesis of somatomedins by fibroblasts and in the liver is stimulated by GH. However, somatomedins are only one component of an integrated process of growth that requires the complex orchestration of several hormones.[21]

THYROTROPIN-RELEASING HORMONE–TSH–THYROID HORMONE AXIS

TSH output is regulated by the production and release of thyrotropin-releasing hormone from the hypothalamus as well as of circulating thyroid hormone. TSH regulates the function of the thyroid gland. Circulating plasma levels of TSH vary in a circadian rhythm, most likely secondary to fluctuations in thyrotropin-releasing hormone levels.

HYPOTHALAMIC-PITUITARY-GONADAL AXIS

The hypothalamus synthesizes and secretes gonadotropin-releasing hormone, which in turn regulates LH and FSH production. LH and FSH affect sexual development and regulate the reproductive process in both sexes through their effect on ovarian and testicular function.

VASOPRESSIN-OXYTOCIN AXIS

ADH and oxytocin are synthesized in the hypothalamus. They are bound to specific carrier proteins, transported within axons down the pituitary stalk, and stored in secretory granules in nerve terminals within the posterior pituitary gland. An ADH analogue, 1-desamino-8-D-arginine vasopressin (desmopressin, DDAVP), is routinely used in the management of ADH deficiency.

ADH and desmopressin act on renal collecting ducts to promote the absorption of free water and thereby maintain fluid homeostasis. A lack of ADH results in central diabetes insipidus. Inability of the kidney to respond to ADH is the defect in nephrogenic or peripheral diabetes insipidus. Imaging findings associated with both diseases are discussed later in the chapter. Surgical or traumatic hypophysectomy causes retrograde degeneration of the hypothalamic neurosecretory cells. The resultant loss of posterior pituitary function in the form of diabetes insipidus is usually transient, however, because many hypothalamic neurons terminate on the median eminence. These cells continue to produce and release ADH from this location. This is manifest on MR images by the displacement of the normal bright posterior pituitary signal to the median eminence.

Excess ADH is found in the syndrome of inappropriate ADH secretion (SIADH). This syndrome is characterized by the triad of low plasma osmolality, inappropriately high urine osmolality, and high urine sodium levels. SIADH is treated by restricting water intake. Demeclocycline is a pharmacologic agent that causes a reversible diabetes insipidus and can also be used to treat SIADH.

Oxytocin stimulates myoepithelial cells within the breast to contract and thereby eject milk. In addition, oxytocin causes contraction of uterine smooth muscle and can be administered pharmacologically to augment labor.

PITUITARY PATHOLOGY

Patients with diseases of the pituitary gland present with symptoms of endocrine dysfunction or with symptoms due to mass effect on sellar and parasellar structures. Attention to the clinical presentation of the patient can assist the radiologist in establishing a radiologic diagnosis. Endocrinologically inactive lesions of the pituitary often present as symptoms secondary to mass effect. These symptoms may include diabetes insipidus due to compression of the infundibulum, visual disturbances due to compression of the optic chiasm or optic nerves, or other cranial neuropathy due to direct compression or invasion of the nerves as they traverse the parasellar region.

PITUITARY ADENOMAS

Pituitary tumors arise from epithelial cells of the anterior lobe. They are most commonly histologically benign lesions that have been reported to occur in 3% to 27% of autopsy series.[42, 43] Tumors smaller than 10 mm are defined as microadenomas. Larger tumors are macroadenomas. Pituitary adenomas are also classified as functioning or nonfunctioning adenomas, referring to their ability to secrete hormones.

Nonfunctioning microadenomas may be detected either as an incidental finding on MR images or at autopsy. As macroadenomas, they present as signs and symptoms of compression of adjacent neural structures. Compression on the optic chiasm or the optic nerves causes visual field defects. Mass effects on the hypothalamus or the stalk may result in diabetes insipidus, whereas lateral extension into the cavernous sinus may cause cranial nerve deficits.[44] With extension into the third ventricle, obstruction of the foramen of Monro and hydrocephalus may be the clinical presen-

tation. Hypopituitarism may occur when an adenoma replaces the normal gland or when there is hemorrhage into the tumor. Rapidly progressive visual loss, extraocular movement palsies, or facial sensory loss may herald a malignant tumor of the pituitary gland, in contrast to the generally slowly progressive symptoms associated with a benign adenoma.[45]

Functioning adenomas generally present as well-defined clinical syndromes. Amenorrhea, galactorrhea, and infertility make up the triad of symptoms seen in women with a prolactin-secreting adenoma, the most common functioning adenoma of the pituitary gland.[46] Serum prolactin levels in patients with prolactin-secreting tumors are usually greater than 100 ng/mL (normal < 20 ng/mL).[47] Serum prolactin levels of 20 to 100 ng/mL may reflect a pituitary abnormality or other causes of mild to moderate hyperprolactinemia such as pregnancy, postpartum state, hypothyroidism, renal failure, chest wall injury, breast disease, breast stimulation, or estrogen therapy. Many drugs also cause hyperprolactinemia. These include phenothiazines, antidepressants, haloperidol, methyldopa, reserpine, amphetamines, opiates, and cimetidine (Table 18–1).

Signs and symptoms of hypercortisolism in Cushing's disease are usually present when the tumor is only 1 to 2 mm.[46] Consequently, these tumors may be difficult to diagnose radiologically. If MRI and computed tomography do not demonstrate an adenoma of the pituitary gland, then ectopic sources of ACTH must be excluded in patients with hypercortisolism (Table 18–2). Small cell lung carcinoma, bronchial or intestinal carcinoid, pancreatic islet cell tumor, medullary thyroid carcinoma, and pheochromocytoma are

TABLE 18–1. CAUSES OF HYPERPROLACTINEMIA

Pregnancy
Postpartum state
Hypothyroidism
Renal failure
Chest wall injury
Breast disease
Breast stimulation
Estrogen therapy
Drugs
  Phenothiazines
  Antidepressants
  Haloperidol
  Methyldopa
  Reserpine
  Amphetamines
  Opiates
  Cimetidine

TABLE 18–2. SOURCES OF ECTOPIC CORTICOTROPIN

Small cell lung carcinoma
Bronchial or intestinal carcinoid
Pancreatic islet cell tumor
Medullary thyroid carcinoma
Pheochromocytoma

known ectopic sources of ACTH. Primary hypercortisolism secondary to an ACTH-independent adrenal adenoma or carcinoma must also be excluded. If MRI and computed tomography results are normal and a pituitary adenoma is suspected, petrosal sinus sampling for ACTH levels may be useful.[48, 49]

A GH-secreting pituitary adenoma will cause acromegaly in adults. Patients with acromegaly are often diagnosed late in the course of their disease when the tumors are large. Approximately 10% of pituitary adenomas secrete more than one hormone, most commonly a prolactin- and GH-producing adenoma.[42, 43] Another less common combination is the TSH-, FSH-, and LH-producing adenoma. Another clinical syndrome associated with pituitary adenoma is Nelson's syndrome. In this disorder, ACTH overproduction by a pituitary adenoma occurs in a patient who has been treated for hypercortisolism with adrenalectomy (Fig. 18–6). In this instance the normal feedback mechanism is stopped with removal of the adrenal gland, and the pituitary adenoma continues to secrete ACTH and melanin-stimulating hormone, resulting in hypercortisolism and hyperpigmentation.

Pituitary apoplexy is the result of acute hemorrhagic necrosis of a pituitary adenoma, usually a macroadenoma, with ensuing subarachnoid hemorrhage and mass effect of the hematoma (Fig. 18–7). Symptoms may include the acute onset of headache, with vomiting, ophthalmoplegia, bilateral amaurosis, and decreased level of consciousness.[50] Although approximately 10% of pituitary adenomas will have evidence of hemorrhagic changes at surgery, less than 30% of these patients will have experienced acute symptoms of pituitary apoplexy.[51] Adenomas with hemorrhage tend to be invasive with suprasellar extension. Hemorrhagic changes may occur during pregnancy in a preexisting adenoma, possibly due to acceleration of tumor growth in association with pregnancy. Postpartum pituitary necrosis or Sheehan's syndrome may occur after complicated deliveries when the hyperplastic pituitary gland may be especially vulnerable to circulatory disturbances.[52] Patients present with pituitary insufficiency. Bromocriptine therapy for prolactin-secreting tumors may also increase the incidence of intratumoral hemorrhage.[53]

At MRI 80% to 90% of microadenomas are hypointense relative to the normal gland on T1-weighted images[54] (Fig. 18–8). On T2-weighted images, one third to one half are hyperintense. As many as 40% of normal volunteers have focal hypointensities in their pituitary glands on T1-weighted images.[55] However, these hypointensities tend to be smaller and not as dark as microadenomas. Contrast medium enhancement is required in patients in whom a pituitary tumor cannot be definitely identified on the nonenhanced scans.[3, 12] Adenomas usually enhance in a delayed fashion relative to the normal gland so that scanning immediately or within 15 to 20 minutes after contrast medium injection reveals an adenoma to be hypointense relative to normal pituitary gland parenchyma (see Fig. 18–8). Delayed scans (30 to 60 minutes after contrast medium injection) may mask the difference in signal intensity between the normal gland and the pituitary adenoma. Alternatively, a reversal of signal intensity may be seen at 30 to 60 minutes after contrast medium injection, when the normal gland is hypointense and the adenoma is relatively bright.[7] Dynamic scans obtained after a rapid injection of contrast material may be required to visualize small adenomas[7, 11, 12] (Fig. 18–9).

There exists such a wide range of normal variation in stalk position that deviation of the stalk is not a reliable indirect sign for a pituitary microadenoma.[56] When situated in the lateral lobe of the gland, pituitary adenomas may cause no discernible deviation of the stalk. Cavernous sinus invasion is associated with a higher morbidity and mortality and indicates that the tumor is biologically aggressive.[57] Because the medial dural reflection of the cavernous sinus is extremely thin and cannot be easily seen with MRI, early detection of cavernous sinus invasion may be difficult[56, 58] (Fig. 18–10). The lateral wall of the cavernous sinus is well seen. If tumor is seen to extend to this site, invasion of the sinus can be inferred. Extension of the tumor to surround greater than 50% of the internal carotid artery is considered evidence of cavernous sinus invasion. It is rare for pituitary tumors to constrict or occlude the carotid arteries. Pituitary adenomas may occasionally extend inferiorly to present as a sphenoidal sinus mass.

Areas of cystic degeneration may be seen in macroadenomas as areas of low signal intensity on T1-weighted images and areas of high signal intensity on T2-weighted images. Occasionally, a fluid-fluid level will also be seen.

Areas of hemorrhage may be present within pituitary adenomas, particularly macroadenomas (see Fig. 18–7). In the subacute phase, the hemorrhage is bright on T1- and T2-weighted images, owing to the presence of methemoglobin. In the acute phase, the hemorrhage appears isointense on T1-weighted images and hypointense on T2-weighted images because of deoxyhemoglobin. Residual adenoma may also be identified.[59]

The postoperative pituitary gland has a varied appearance on MR images that depends on the size and extension of the adenoma preoperatively, surgical approach, packing material used, and time interval between the operation and MRI.[60] Postoperative follow-up MRI at 4 to 6 months is recommended. After this period, blood, fluid, debris, and some implant materials have been resorbed.[60] Implanted fat may remain viable indefinitely. Surgical resection and involution of the packing material may result in a smaller and irregularly contoured pituitary gland.[60, 61] Contrast medium administration and fat suppression techniques may be necessary to distinguish between residual tumor and implant material. Correlation with the preoperative appearance of the tumor on MR images and with surgical information such as the nature of the implant material is essential for accurate interpretation of the findings.

METASTASIS

Metastasis to the pituitary gland is more commonly reported in autopsy series than is clinically apparent.

Text continued on page 570

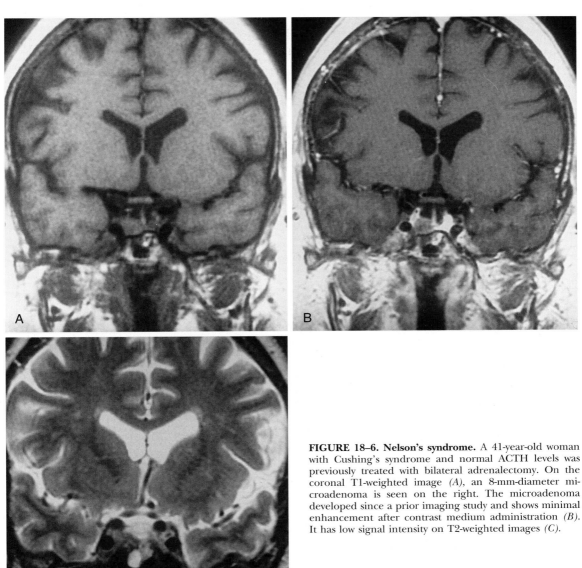

FIGURE 18–6. Nelson's syndrome. A 41-year-old woman with Cushing's syndrome and normal ACTH levels was previously treated with bilateral adrenalectomy. On the coronal T1-weighted image *(A)*, an 8-mm-diameter microadenoma is seen on the right. The microadenoma developed since a prior imaging study and shows minimal enhancement after contrast medium administration *(B)*. It has low signal intensity on T2-weighted images *(C)*.

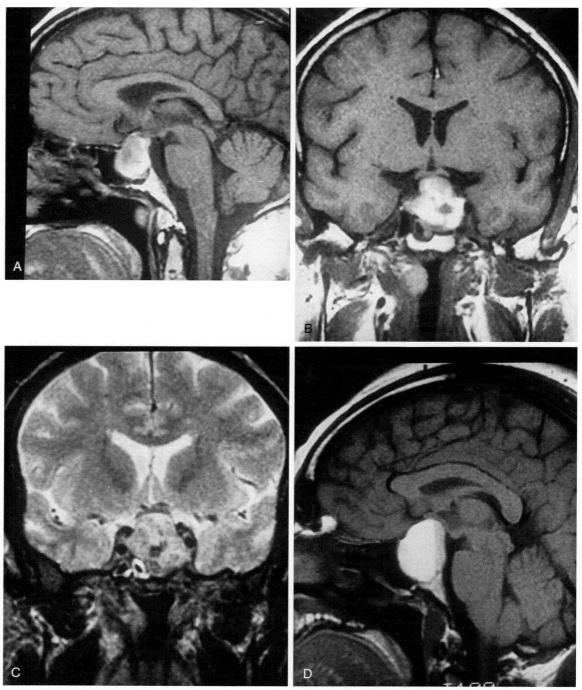

FIGURE 18–7. Hemorrhagic macroadenoma. A 53-year-old man experienced visual blurring and abrupt onset of severe headache. Nonenhanced T1-weighted sagittal *(A)* and coronal *(B)* images demonstrate a mixture of high signal intensity (methemoglobin) and lower signal intensity (adenoma) in an intrasellar and suprasellar mass that elevates and distorts the optic chiasm. On a T2-weighted image *(C)* an admixture of low signal intensity (deoxyhemoglobin) and moderate signal intensity (adenoma and parenchymal edema) is demonstrated. *D,* A 38-year-old patient presented with a history of visual loss and apparent pituitary hemorrhage several months earlier. Sagittal T1-weighted image demonstrates high signal intensity in the anterior portion of the mass with layering of lower signal intensity material posteriorly. At surgery a large cyst was identified with hemosiderin and proteinaceous debris layering posteriorly. Fragments of pituitary adenoma were histologically identified in the cyst wall.

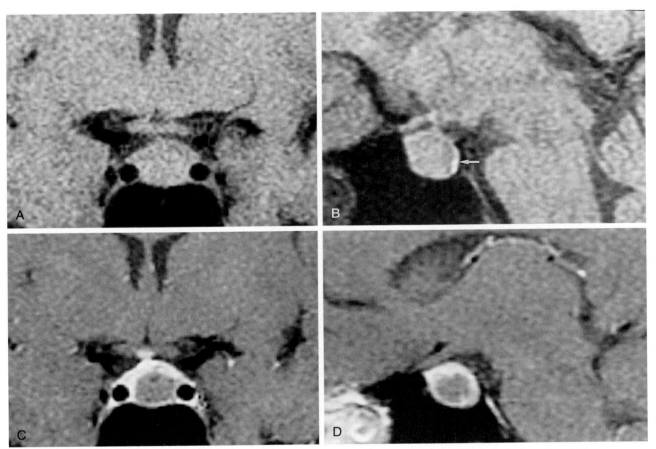

FIGURE 18–8. Nonenhancing pituitary adenoma. T1-weighted images before *(A and B)* and after *(C and D)* contrast enhancement in the coronal *(A and C)* and sagittal *(B and D)* planes. On the nonenhanced images the pituitary gland is enlarged. A small rim of bright posterior lobe of the pituitary gland *(arrow)* is seen on the sagittal nonenhanced images. After intravenous administration of Gd-DTPA, the normal pituitary gland enhances and a central nonenhancing 9-mm microadenoma is more conspicuous than on the nonenhanced images.

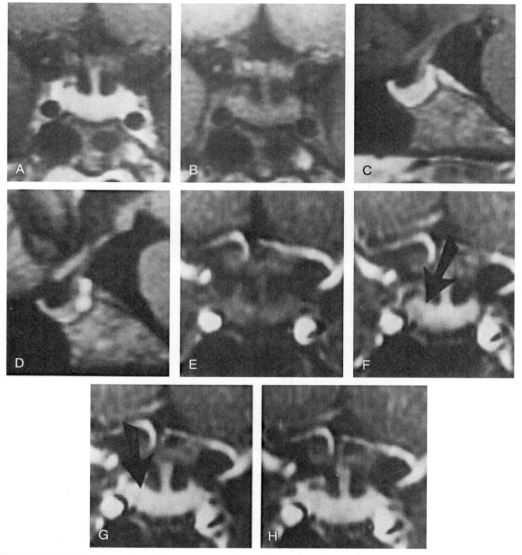

FIGURE 18–9. Pituitary microadenoma seen only on dynamic enhanced MR images. An adenoma is not apparent on routine T1-weighted images before *(B and D)* and after *(A and C)* enhancement. Dynamic scans *(E to H)* obtained at 25-second intervals after rapid intravenous injection of Gd-DTPA demonstrate the microadenoma as a small area of low signal intensity in the right side of the gland *(arrows)*. *(A to H* from Chong BW, Newton TH: Hypothalamic and pituitary pathology. Radiol Clin North Am 31:1147–1183, 1993.)

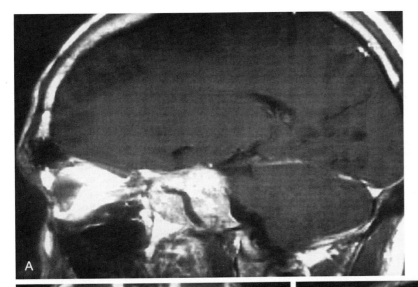

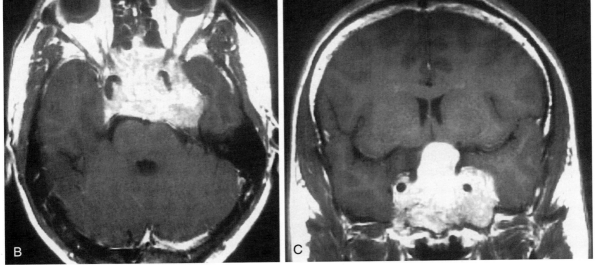

FIGURE 18–10. Pituitary macroadenoma invading both cavernous sinuses. Sagittal *(A)*, axial *(B)*, and coronal *(C)* contrast-enhanced T1-weighted images. There is more extensive invasion of the left cavernous sinus. The serum prolactin level was markedly elevated at 14,000 μg/L (normal level is up to 20 μg/L), a common finding when a prolactinoma has invaded the cavernous sinus.

This is because patients usually die of their malignancy before pituitary function is significantly altered. Diabetes insipidus may be the initial presentation of metastasis to the pituitary gland.[62] The common primary sources of metastatic disease include lung tumors, breast tumors, leukemia, and lymphoma.[63] On MR images, a mass in the pituitary gland may extend to the stalk or the hypothalamus (Fig. 18–11). A metastasis to the pituitary gland may be differentiated from an adenoma by rapid interval growth. Most metastases have a pattern of signal intensity consistent with the tumor of origin and enhance with administration of contrast medium. A primary intrasellar melanoma may be hypointense on both T1- and T2-weighted images because of the paramagnetic effect of melanin causing shortening of both T1 and T2 relaxation.[64]

BENIGN PITUITARY HYPERPLASIA

Relative enlargement of the pituitary gland normally occurs around the time of birth, at puberty, and during pregnancy.[32, 33, 37, 39, 41] Primary pituitary hyperplasia that is not a normal physiologic response results in an enlarged hyperfunctioning gland that mimics an adenoma both clinically and radiologically.[65–69] Secondary pituitary hyperplasia is seen with exogenous estrogen therapy,[70] neoplasms secreting ectopic hypothalamic releasing factors,[66] hypothalamic tumors,[71] and central precocious puberty.[72] Primary hypothyroidism may also cause pituitary gland enlargement due to the stimulatory effects of high circulating levels of thyrotropin-releasing hormone on thyrotrophs in the pituitary gland[73, 74] (Fig. 18–12). There may also be hyperprolactinemia in this condition because thyrotropin-releasing hormone also has a weak stimulatory effect on lactotrophs.

LYMPHOCYTIC HYPOPHYSITIS

Lymphocytic hypophysitis is exclusive to women and occurs during pregnancy or in the postpartum period.

The clinical presentation includes failure of lactation, amenorrhea, headache, visual loss, and hyperprolactinemia.[75] The cause is suspected to be an autoimmune reaction to pituitary antigens released during puerperal involution of the hypophysis,[76] a theory that is supported by the fact that antipituitary antibodies have been described.[77] Ultrastructural features shown by electron microscopy also support an immune mechanism.[78] There is an association with other autoimmune endocrine disorders. Within the adenohypophysis there is diffuse lymphocytic plasma cell infiltration. On MR images there is diffuse homogeneous enlargement of the anterior pituitary gland and infundibulum[79] (Fig. 18–13).

SHEEHAN'S SYNDROME

The pituitary gland enlarges with physiologic hypertrophy of the lactotrophs of the pituitary gland during pregnancy. During this time the gland becomes more susceptible to circulatory disturbances.[52] After complicated deliveries that are associated with hemorrhage and hypotension, postpartum necrosis and hemorrhage of the pituitary gland may occur and result in hypopituitarism. Hemorrhage in the pituitary gland due to Sheehan's syndrome has a similar appearance on MR images to that seen with pituitary apoplexy, except the sella is not enlarged and an adenoma cannot be identified (Fig. 18–14). Patients may also eventually develop a partially or completely empty sella.[80]

EMPTY SELLA

An absent or small, compressed pituitary gland may occur in association with herniated arachnoid and cerebrospinal fluid pulsations transmitted through a thin diaphragma sella or through a large diaphragmatic hiatus. Mechanical pressure causes compression and atrophy of the gland as well as expansion of the sella turcica. The majority of patients are female, and more than 75% are obese.[81] The frequency increases with

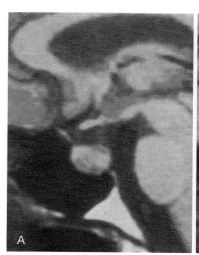
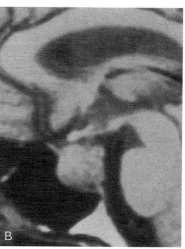

FIGURE 18–11. Carcinoma of the colon metastatic to the pituitary gland. *A*, Sagittal T1-weighted image. The pituitary gland is enlarged, which suggests the possibility of a pituitary adenoma. *B*, Three months later, a follow-up examination demonstrates interval enlargement of the pituitary gland. Enlargement of the gland in this short time interval contradicts the diagnosis of an adenoma. (*A* and *B* from Chong BW, Newton TH: Hypothalamic and pituitary pathology. Radiol Clin North Am 31:1147–1183, 1993.)

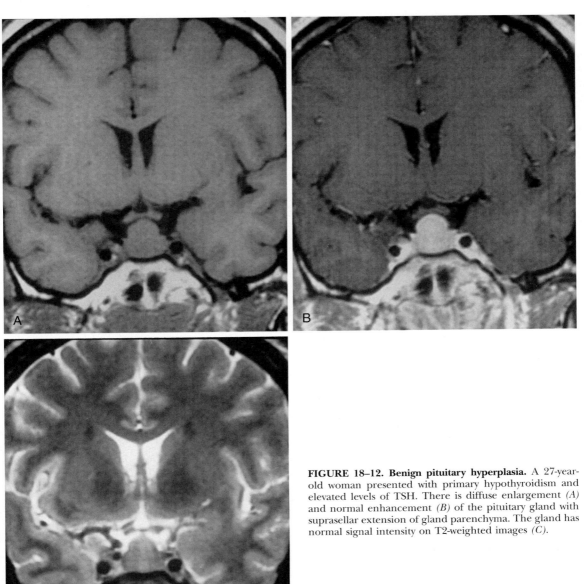

FIGURE 18–12. Benign pituitary hyperplasia. A 27-year-old woman presented with primary hypothyroidism and elevated levels of TSH. There is diffuse enlargement (A) and normal enhancement (B) of the pituitary gland with suprasellar extension of gland parenchyma. The gland has normal signal intensity on T2-weighted images (C).

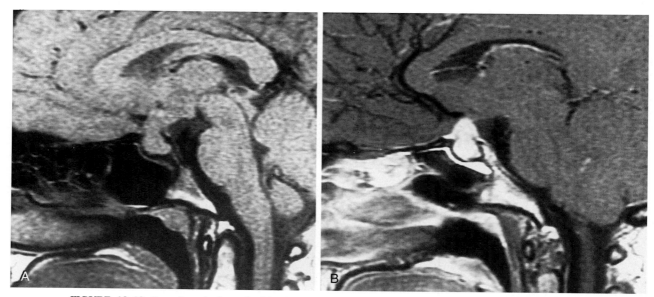

FIGURE 18–13. Lymphocytic hypophysitis. Sagittal T1-weighted images before *(A)* and after *(B)* contrast enhancement. The pituitary gland and stalk (infundibulum) are enlarged and demonstrate homogeneous enhancement.

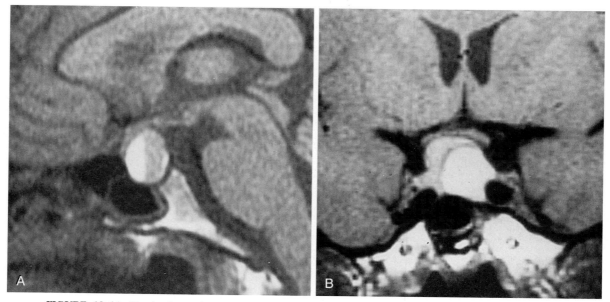

FIGURE 18–14. Sheehan's syndrome. This woman experienced acute headache, visual disturbance, and hypopituitarism in the postpartum period. Sagittal *(A)* and coronal *(B)* nonenhanced MR images demonstrate hemorrhage into the pituitary gland with a fluid-fluid level. The normal gland is displaced superiorly and to the right. *(A* and *B* courtesy of Walter Kucharczyk, MD, Toronto, Ontario, Canada.)

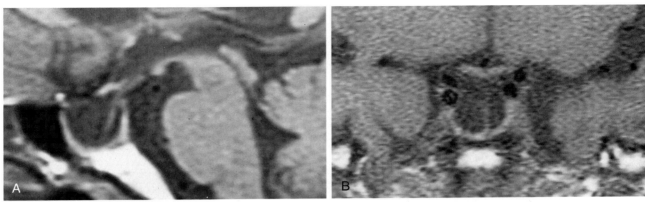

FIGURE 18–15. Empty sella. This was an incidental finding in a patient who was asymptomatic with respect to this finding. Sagittal *(A)* and coronal *(B)* T1-weighted images demonstrate enlargement of the sella, which is filled with cerebrospinal fluid. The gland is flattened along the floor of the sella.

age, likely reflecting the presence of an enlarging diaphragmatic hiatus in older patients. In most instances an empty sella is an incidental finding without symptoms. The absence of symptoms can be explained by the great functional reserve of the pituitary gland. If there is greater than 10% of the gland remaining functionally active, the physiology is undisturbed and the abnormality is clinically inapparent. Symptoms usually occur when patients are between 30 and 59 years of age, are commonly nonspecific, and include headache, memory loss, and dizziness. In severe cases, patients may present with endocrine dysfunction, cerebrospinal fluid rhinorrhea, and visual loss.[82, 83] On T1-weighted sagittal MR images, the pituitary gland is flattened along the floor of the sella turcica (Fig. 18–15). The stalk is midline, which differentiates this entity from a cyst in which the stalk is displaced.[46]

DIABETES INSIPIDUS

Diabetes insipidus is characterized by a disturbance of water balance. Central diabetes insipidus occurs when there is an inadequate amount of ADH secretion due to hypothalamic or pituitary disease. Nephrogenic diabetes insipidus is due to a congenital or acquired inability of the collecting ducts of the kidney to respond to normal amounts of ADH. Regardless of the cause, the result is an inappropriate secretion of excess dilute urine. The majority of cases of central diabetes insipidus are secondary to head injury[84]; approximately 25% of cases are idiopathic. Less common causes include suprasellar and intrasellar neoplasms, Langerhans' cell histiocytosis, and cranial or transsphenoidal surgery.[85]

MRI of the pituitary in patients with diabetes insipidus provides a unique opportunity to observe the functional status of the posterior pituitary gland. As discussed earlier, the normal bright signal of the posterior pituitary gland is likely to be due to phospholipids in the neurosecretory granules that contain ADH and oxytocin. If ADH secretion from the hypothalamic-pituitary axis is not adequate, the bright posterior lobe may not be expected on MR images. In nearly all cases

of central diabetes insipidus the region of high signal intensity on T1-weighted images in the posterior sella is absent[85–87] (Fig. 18–16). With inherited central diabetes insipidus, the presence of the bright posterior pituitary is variable.[88] Although patients with primary (psychogenic) polydipsia may have a clinical presentation that mimics diabetes insipidus, they have a normal bright posterior pituitary.[89]

PITUITARY DWARFISM

Pituitary dwarfism presents clinically as short stature and GH deficiency.[90–92] There is no diabetes insipidus, but in 50% of cases ACTH and TSH levels are also

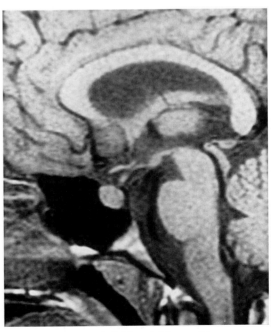

FIGURE 18–16. Diabetes insipidus. A 19-year-old woman presented with idiopathic central diabetes insipidus. There is absence of the posterior pituitary bright spot. The infundibulum was intact, and imaging of the hypothalamus after contrast medium administration was normal.

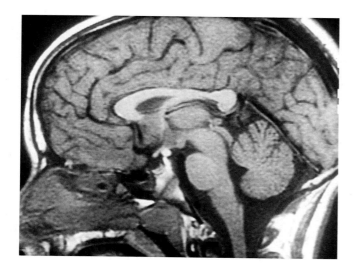

FIGURE 18–17. Congenital pituitary hypoplasia with ectopic posterior pituitary. A 14-year-old boy with pituitary dwarfism had diminished ACTH and TSH production. There is an ectopic posterior pituitary, and the infundibulum cannot be visualized on sagittal or coronal images. The pituitary gland is small.

low. Pituitary dwarfism is postulated to be due to a developmental ischemic event with disruption of the peri-infundibular hypophysial portal system. The pituitary gland is then inaccessible to hypothalamic releasing factors. In 50% of patients with congenital pituitary dwarfism, there is a history of breech delivery or perinatal asphyxia. MRI demonstrates hypoplasia or absence of the infundibulum and absence of the normal bright posterior pituitary signal intensity on T1-weighted images (Fig. 18–17). Instead, the ectopic bright signal pattern of the posterior pituitary is seen in the median eminence where there is continued secretion of posterior lobe hormones. The remaining anterior pituitary gland is small or markedly hypoplastic, as is the sella turcica.

SUPRASELLAR PATHOLOGY

CRANIOPHARYNGIOMAS

Craniopharyngiomas are benign slow-growing tumors that originate from squamous epithelial remnants of Rathke's cleft in the pars tuberalis. Peak incidence is at 5 to 10 years of age,[93] with a smaller peak in the sixth decade. Pediatric patients present with signs and symptoms of increased intracranial pressure, including headache, nausea and vomiting, and papilledema, or with growth failure. Adults usually present with pituitary insufficiency due to compression of the hypothalamus, pituitary stalk, or the gland. Com-

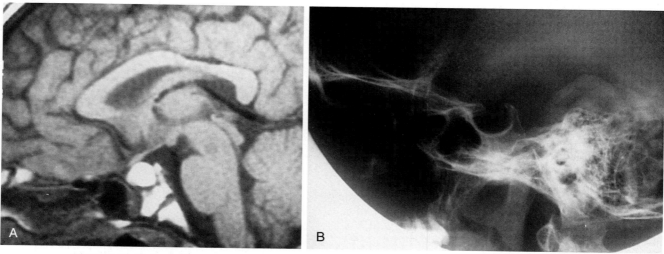

FIGURE 18–18. Intrasellar craniopharyngioma. A 14-year-old boy presented with headache and small stature. Nonenhanced T1-weighted image (A) demonstrates intrasellar contents to be enlarged and of high signal intensity. On plain films (B) there is enlargement of the sella with no abnormal calcification. At surgery there was an intrasellar craniopharyngioma with suprasellar extension.

pression of the chiasm or the optic nerves causes visual disturbances.

Craniopharyngiomas are often both intrasellar and suprasellar.[94] Posterior extension into the prepontine cistern is common. Rarely, the tumor may be isolated within the sella, the optic chiasm, or the third ventricle.[95, 96] Calcification is common, especially in children. The epithelium-lined cysts have variable contents, including keratin, cholesterol, proteinaceous fluid, and desquamated blood cells and blood products. It is not surprising that the appearance at MRI of these tumors is also varied (Fig. 18–18). On T1-weighted images the solid components of the tumor are hypointense.[97] The cystic portions of the tumor are usually slightly hyperintense relative to cerebrospinal fluid. Increased signal intensity on T1-weighted images can be caused by protein concentrations greater than 90 g/L, by the presence of methemoglobin, or by both.[98, 99] Calcified areas in the tumor may appear hypointense on T1-weighted images. On T2-weighted images the solid components are hyperintense. Enhancement of the tumor with gadolinium is heterogeneous and intense.

RATHKE'S CLEFT CYSTS

Rathke's cleft cysts are also derived from Rathke's pouch. They are distinguished from craniopharyngiomas pathologically by the fact that they are lined by a single layer of columnar or cuboidal epithelium, which may be ciliated and contain goblet cells.[43] The cyst may contain mucoid, serous, or cellular debris.[100, 101] In contrast, craniopharyngiomas have thick walls of squamous or basal cells. Rathke's cleft cysts are usually smaller and intrasellar in contrast to craniopharyngiomas. Approximately 70% are both intrasellar and suprasellar.[102] Each entity demonstrates different biologic behavior as well. Rathke's cleft cysts are not invasive and are treated with incision and drainage without recurrence. This is contrasted by the locally aggressive behavior and postsurgical recurrence of craniopharyngiomas.

The MRI appearance of Rathke's cleft cyst reflects the pathologic characteristics. The cyst is most often a well-defined intrasellar mass, although there may a suprasellar component. The smaller cysts usually contain mucus (Fig. 18–19), whereas the larger cysts contain serous fluid (Fig. 18–20). The mucus is bright on T1-weighted images, and thus the appearance may be indistinguishable from that of craniopharyngioma. The larger cysts containing serous fluid are usually isointense relative to cerebrospinal fluid on both T1- and T2-weighted images. Rathke's cleft cysts do not enhance with gadolinium, a feature that distinguishes them from the majority of craniopharyngiomas. A thin rim of enhancing residual pituitary gland may be seen and is not to be confused with enhancing tumor.[103]

CHIASMATIC AND HYPOTHALAMIC GLIOMAS

Gliomas arising from the optic chiasm are distinct from those arising from the hypothalamus in a number

of ways. Chiasmatic gliomas occur predominantly in childhood, especially during the first decade, and represent 15% of pediatric supratentorial tumors.[43] Up to one third of all patients with optic glioma have a history of neurofibromatosis type 1. Even though optic gliomas are generally low-grade astrocytomas, they tend to spread along the optic tracts. In contrast, hypothalamic gliomas are more malignant and invasive tumors that present earlier with disturbances in hypothalamic function, including temperature regulation, appetite, growth failure, and diabetes insipidus, or with SIADH.[104] Patients may also present with monocular or binocular visual disturbances or hydrocephalus. Even so, patients with either optic or hypothalamic gliomas can have long-term survival. The 5- and 10-year survival rates for unresectable hypothalamic-opticochiasmatic tumors are 93% and 74%, respectively.[105]

MRI demonstrates that tumors originating in the chiasm or the hypothalamus tend to be solid tumors that are hypointense or isointense relative to normal brain on T1-weighted images (Fig. 18–21). The tumor may be too large at imaging to discern the exact site of origin, or it may localize to either the chiasm or the hypothalamus, enlarging either structure. On T2-weighted images the tumors are hyperintense regardless of location. T2-weighted images are useful for assessment of spread of tumor along the optic pathways to the lateral geniculate bodies, the optic radiations, and the visual cortex. However, a similar appearance is seen in patients with neurofibromatosis type 1 when there are benign cerebral hamartomas or atypical glial cell rests within the basal ganglia and the optic tracts in similar locations.[106, 107] These lesions of neurofibromatosis may be distinguished by the lack of enhancement after administration of contrast medium and by the absence of interval growth. Rather than spread into the optic tract, tumors that originate in the hypothalamus more commonly invade the adjacent thalamus and the brain stem (Fig. 18–22). They may also obstruct the third ventricle, causing hydrocephalus. Larger tumors may contain necrotic elements. Hemorrhage and calcification are uncommon. Cyst formation is not uncommon for tumors originating in the hypothalamus. Tumors in either location have variable patterns of enhancement.

HAMARTOMAS OF THE TUBER CINEREUM

Tumors in this location are often congenital and are non-neoplastic.[108] Hamartomas consist of hyperplastic hypothalamic glial and neural tissue. These lesions generally grow slowly or do not grow and are not invasive. Histologic variants include lipoma, osteolipoma, and tuberous sclerosis.[109] The pituitary gland is usually normal, but associated pituitary adenoma has been reported.[110] Grossly, hamartomas are sessile or pedunculated masses arising from the tuber cinereum between the infundibular stalk and the mamillary bodies. The mass may be discovered incidentally or may occur in association with precocious puberty secondary to disruption of the normal hypothalamic prepubertal

Text continued on page 580

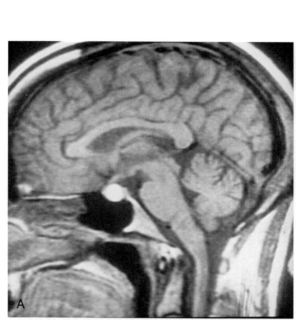

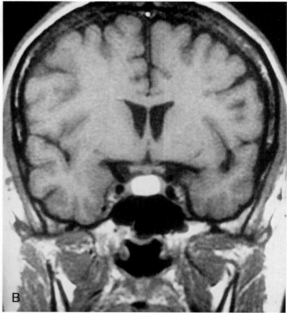

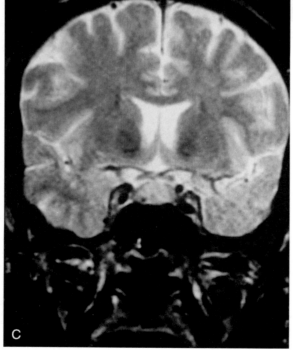

FIGURE 18–19. Rathke's cleft cyst. A 41-year-old woman presented with headache. Sagittal *(A)* and coronal *(B)* nonenhanced images demonstrate enlargement of the pituitary gland due to an intraparenchymal cyst that has high signal intensity on T1-weighted images. The cyst has moderate signal intensity on the T2-weighted image *(C).*

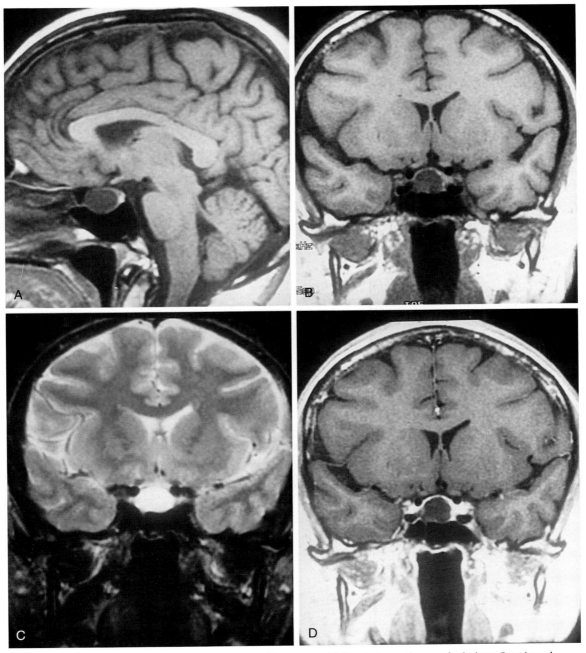

FIGURE 18–20. Rathke's cleft cyst. A 40-year-old woman with headache and normal pituitary function. A nonenhancing cyst, of low signal intensity on T1-weighted images *(A* and *B)* and bright on a T2-weighted image *(C)*, enlarges the sella. The margin of the cyst, predominately thinned pituitary parenchyma, enhances after contrast medium administration *(D)*.

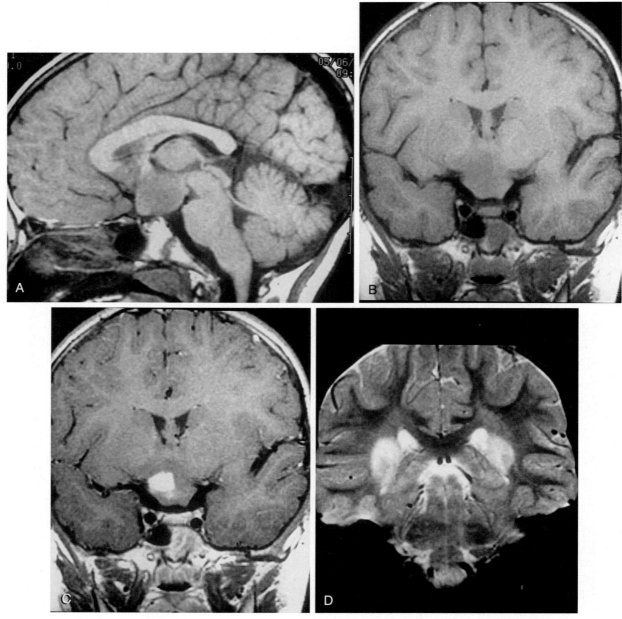

FIGURE 18–21. Optic glioma with spread along the optic tracts. A 5-year-old boy had neurofibromatosis type 1 and optic chiasm glioma. Tumor extends into the hypothalamus *(A and B)*, and a portion of the tumor demonstrates dense enhancement after contrast medium administration *(C)*. The chiasm had high signal intensity on T2-weighted images (not shown). T2-weighted images also demonstrate high signal intensity in the optic radiation surrounding the lateral ventricles *(D)*. There was no mass effect or contrast enhancement of the periventricular alteration.

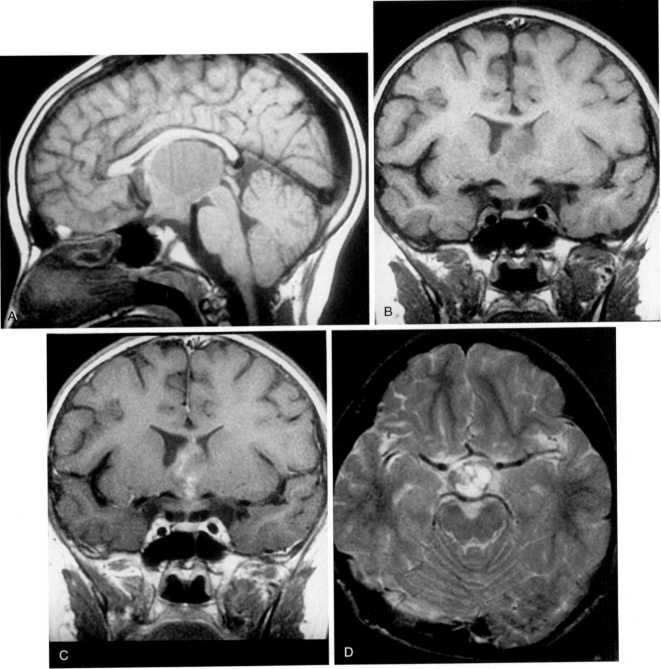

FIGURE 18–22. Hypothalamic glioma. An 8-year-old patient presented with growth failure due to hypothalamic glioma. A partially cystic mass within the hypothalamus effaces the third ventricle and extends inferiorly to involve the chiasm *(A* and *B)*. There is patchy enhancement of the solid portion of the tumor after contrast medium administration *(C)*. The inferior portion of the tumor is of mixed moderate and high signal intensity on a T2-weighted image *(D)*.

inhibition of gonadotropin production. Gelastic seizures, characterized by laughing seizures, intellectual impairment, and even psychiatric disturbances, may be presenting complaints.[111, 112]

On MR images most hypothalamic hamartomas are isointense relative to gray matter on T1-weighted images and hyperintense on T2-weighted images[113] (Fig. 18–23). They do not calcify, nor do they enhance after a contrast agent is administered.

LANGERHANS' CELL HISTIOCYTOSIS

Formerly called histiocytosis X, this disease is characterized by a proliferation of histiocytes.[114] The disease can be multifocal or unifocal; the latter spares the hypothalamic-pituitary axis. The multifocal form presents in childhood with the clinical triad of diabetes insipidus, exophthalmos, and lytic bone lesions. Only 25% of cases present with all three of these components.[46] Visual disturbances and other endocrine dysfunctions, such as delayed puberty, hypothyroidism, hypoadrenalism, and hyperprolactinemia, may also be noted and are secondary to granulomas in the hypothalamus and the pituitary gland.[114]

On MR images there is thickening of an enhancing pituitary stalk[115] (Fig. 18–24). The normal high signal intensity of the posterior lobe is frequently absent. Involvement of the adjacent temporal bone by histiocytosis supports the diagnosis.[115]

CAVERNOUS SINUS AND PARASELLAR PATHOLOGY

TOLOSA-HUNT SYNDROME

The Tolosa-Hunt syndrome consists of painful ophthalmoplegia secondary to an idiopathic granulomatous inflammatory process involving the cavernous sinus.[116] Six clinical criteria characterize the syndrome: 1) steady, gnawing retro-orbital pain; 2) defects in cranial nerves III, IV, or VI or in the first branch of cranial nerve V and less commonly involvement of the optic nerve or the sympathetic fibers around the cavernous carotid artery; 3) a duration of symptoms lasting days to weeks; 4) occasional spontaneous remission; 5) recurrent attacks; and 6) prompt response to steroids.[117] The cause is unknown. The pathologic findings include a granulomatous periarteritis of the cavernous internal carotid artery and the cavernous sinus. The presence of a necrotizing vasculitis with chronic nongranulomatous inflammation has also been reported.[118] These authors have observed an overlap of the pathologic features with those of orbital pseudotumor, implying that they are related histopathologic entities in different locations. Others have described the clinical similarity between the two entities.[119]

Findings at MRI parallel those of orbital pseudotumor to some degree. A mass in the cavernous sinus has a signal intensity on MR images similar to that of the mass seen with orbital pseudotumor—isointense relative to muscle on T1-weighted images and isointense relative to fat on T2-weighted images[120] (Fig. 18–25). The mass may extend to the orbital apex. The cavernous sinus may be enlarged with a convex outer margin. The differential possibilities based on the MRI appearance include meningioma, lymphoma, and sarcoidosis, all of which may be distinguished clinically from Tolosa-Hunt syndrome. Meningioma will not resolve with corticosteroid therapy. Lymphoma and sarcoidosis often have systemic signs and symptoms.

NERVE SHEATH TUMORS

Nerve sheath tumors found in the cavernous sinus and parasellar regions can be divided into schwannomas and plexiform neurofibromas. Schwannomas are also called neurinomas or neurilemmomas. Schwannomas of the trigeminal nerve are much more common than those involving cranial nerves III, IV, and VI.[121] The clinical presentation varies, depending on the exact location of the tumor, whether it is cisternal, cisternocavernous, or cavernous. Cavernous schwanno-

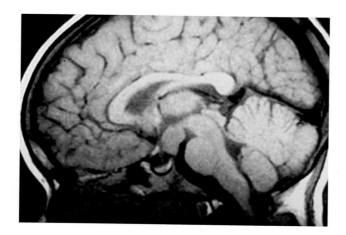

FIGURE 18–23. Hamartoma of the tuber cinereum. A 5-year-old girl presented with precocious puberty. A mass is demonstrated at the floor of the third ventricle, posterior to the infundibulum and involving the mamillary bodies. The lesion did not demonstrate enhancement after contrast medium administration and was isointense relative to gray matter on T2-weighted images.

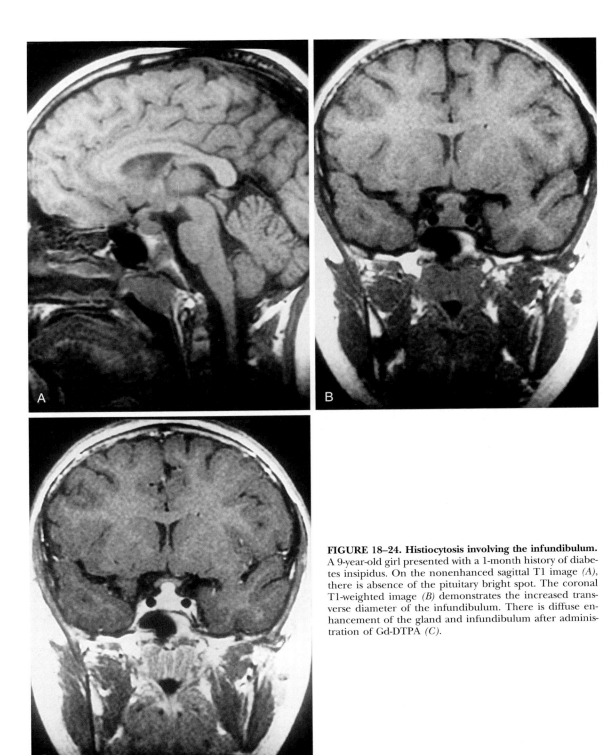

FIGURE 18–24. Histiocytosis involving the infundibulum. A 9-year-old girl presented with a 1-month history of diabetes insipidus. On the nonenhanced sagittal T1 image *(A)*, there is absence of the pituitary bright spot. The coronal T1-weighted image *(B)* demonstrates the increased transverse diameter of the infundibulum. There is diffuse enhancement of the gland and infundibulum after administration of Gd-DTPA *(C)*.

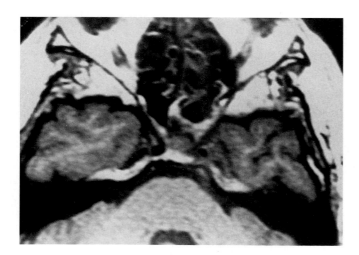

FIGURE 18–25. Tolosa-Hunt syndrome. Axial T1-weighted image demonstrates a low-signal-intensity soft tissue mass filling the left cavernous sinus. (Courtesy of Walter Kucharczyk, MD, Toronto, Ontario, Canada.)

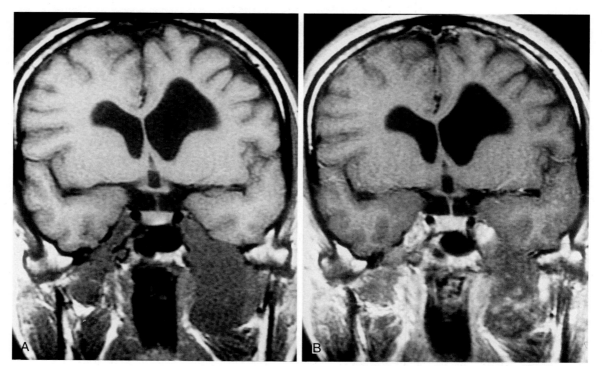

FIGURE 18–26. Schwannoma of cranial nerve V. A 26-year-old patient presented with neurofibromatosis. Bilateral trigeminal schwannomas distend the cavernous sinuses and extend through the foramen ovale into the masticator spaces bilaterally *(A)*. After contrast medium administration there is patchy enhancement of the schwannomas *(B)*.

mas present either with paresis of one or more nerves of the cavernous sinus or as an orbital apex syndrome consisting of pain and diplopia.[122] Schwannomas of the cisternal segment may present with trigeminal pain and sensory loss involving the nerve of origin or symptoms secondary to compression of an adjacent cranial nerve, usually cranial nerves VII or VIII. Cisternocavernous schwannomas may present with signs and symptoms of intracranial hypertension.[121] Schwannomas of the trigeminal nerve may also involve the extracranial portions of the nerve (see also Chapter 19).

The multiplanar capabilities of MRI afford an optimal preoperative assessment of the extent of the tumor.[123] Schwannomas are generally homogeneously hypointense on T1-weighted images and show an increase in signal intensity on T2-weighted images (Fig. 18–26). They enhance strongly in a heterogeneous fashion with administration of contrast medium.

Plexiform neurofibromas are unique to neurofibromatosis type 1. They originate in a peripheral nerve, most commonly the ophthalmic division of cranial nerve V when they involve the head and neck.[124] The tumor then spreads to the intracranial cavity by infiltrating along the nerve to involve the parasellar structures at the skull base. These lesions are ill-defined, infiltrating masses. The tumor can erode bone and expand the neural foramina of the skull base. Plexiform neurofibromas are isointense relative to brain on T1-weighted images, are hyperintense on T2-weighted images, and enhance intensely when a contrast agent is used.

MENINGIOMAS

Meningiomas in the parasellar region arise from the sphenoid wing, the diaphragma sella, the clivus, or the cavernous sinus. The presentation depends on the site of origin and the extent of disease. Signs and symptoms are due to compression of adjacent structures. Cavernous sinus meningiomas may cause multiple cranial nerve palsies. Meningiomas usually show hypointensity or isointensity relative to cortex on T1-weighted images and have variable signal intensity on T2-weighted images (Fig. 18–27). Depending on the presence and degree of tumor calcification, there may be hypointensity on both T1- and T2-weighted images.[123] Meningiomas enhance intensely and rapidly when contrast medium is used[125] (see also Chapter 17).

ANEURYSMS

Aneurysms in the sellar and parasellar regions arise from the cavernous internal carotid artery or the supraclinoid segment of the internal carotid artery. Other sites of origin include the tip of the basilar artery, anterior communicating artery, and posterior communicating artery. Distinction from solid masses is essential for obvious reasons. Other than subarachnoid hemorrhage, the signs and symptoms at presentation are secondary to compression of adjacent structures and usually involve cranial neuropathy. The MRI appearance is characteristic (Fig. 18–28). Signal void within the lumen of the aneurysm on T1- and T2-weighted images is due to rapidly flowing blood. If thrombus is present in the wall or the lumen of the aneurysm, the signal characteristics may include high signal intensity on T1-weighted images in a multilamellated fashion. The presence of low signal intensity in the wall of the aneurysm or in the adjacent brain on spin-echo or gradient-echo images corresponds to

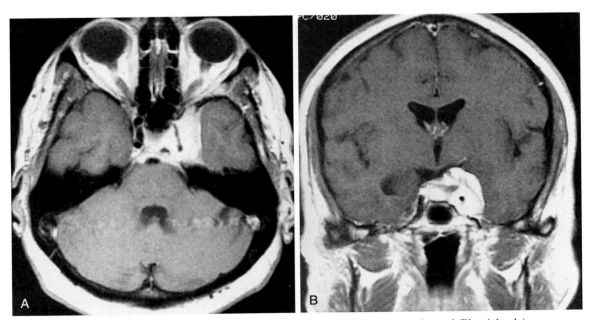

FIGURE 18–27. Parasellar meningioma. Axial *(A)* and coronal *(B)* contrast-enhanced T1-weighted images. There is an intensely enhancing mass adjacent to and involving the left cavernous sinus. The caliber of the ipsilateral cavernous internal carotid artery is narrowed by the tumor.

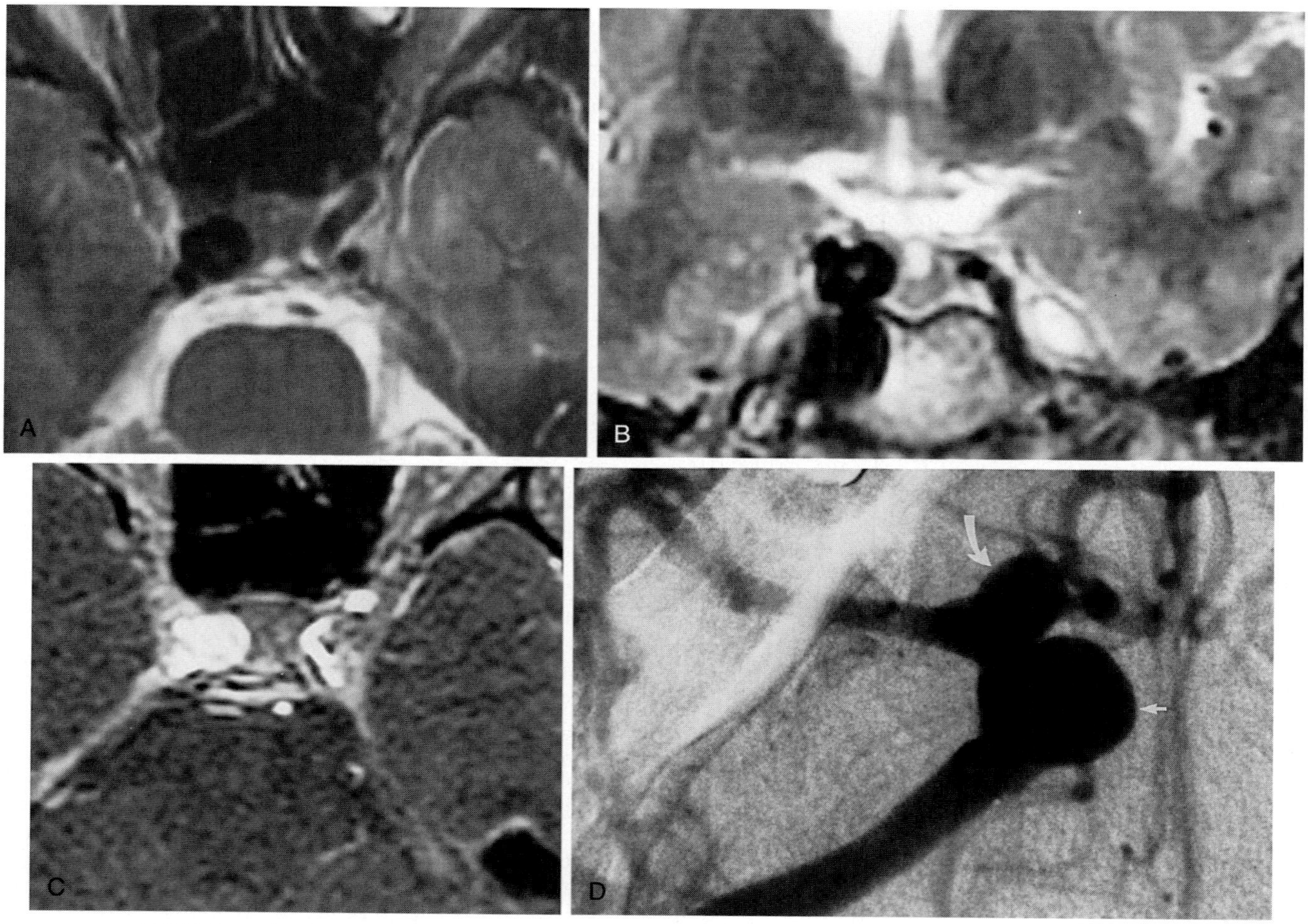

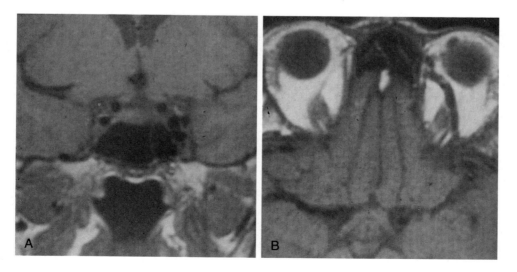

FIGURE 18–28. Cavernous right internal carotid artery aneurysm. Axial *(A)* and coronal *(B)* T2-weighted images, as well as an axial image from a 3D time-of-flight (TOF) MR angiogram *(C)*, demonstrate the aneurysm to similar advantage. Submentovertex projection from a conventional angiogram *(D)* confirms the aneurysm location *(straight arrow)*. The curved arrow indicates a normal vascular loop of the supraclinoid internal carotid artery.

FIGURE 18–29. Carotid-cavernous fistula. Coronal T1-weighted image *(A)* demonstrates multiple signal voids from flowing blood within the vascular channels of the fistulous connection in the left cavernous sinus. Axial T1-weighted image *(B)* shows a dilated superior ophthalmic vein. *(A and B* courtesy of T. Hans Newton, MD, San Francisco, CA.)

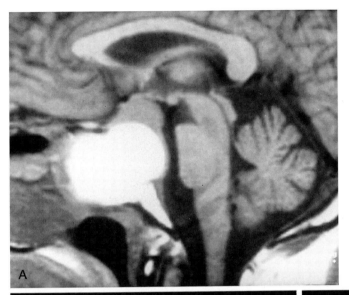

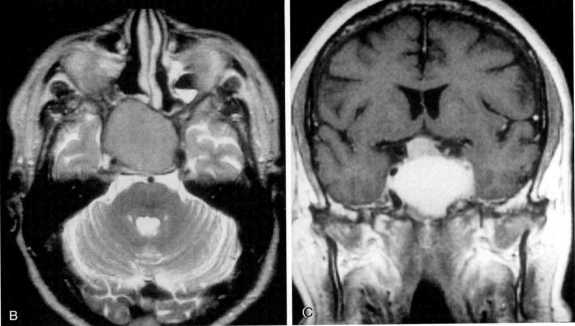

FIGURE 18–30. Sphenoidal sinus mucocele. A 65-year-old man presented with visual alteration. A sphenoidal mucocele and pituitary adenoma are seen. The mucocele has high signal intensity on a T1-weighted image *(A);* it has remodeled and enlarged the sphenoidal sinus. The contents of the mucocele are isointense with cerebral cortex on T2-weighted images *(B).* The adenoma demonstrates diffuse enhancement after contrast medium administration and distorts the optic chiasm *(C).*

hemosiderin deposition. MR angiographic demonstration of aneurysms and their flow patterns is discussed in Chapters 23 and 25.

CAROTID-CAVERNOUS FISTULAS

Most fistulous connections between the cavernous carotid artery and the cavernous sinus are the result of trauma. Spontaneous fistulas may be secondary to congenital or acquired defects in the arterial wall or rupture of an aneurysm of the internal carotid artery.[126] Dural arteriovenous malformations may also involve the cavernous sinus. Patients with carotid-cavernous fistulas present with proptosis, chemosis, visual loss, and occasionally a bruit. The severity of the symptoms depends on the degree of shunting through the fistulous connection. MRI shows dilatation of the cavernous sinus and the superior ophthalmic vein and proptosis (Fig. 18–29). The contralateral venous structures may be dilated if flow is sufficiently high. The pathway of flow is through the intercavernous venous connections and the petrosal venous plexus. The normal signal intensity usually seen in the cavernous sinus is absent, owing to high flow through this structure.

SPHENOIDAL SINUS PATHOLOGY

Inflammatory and infectious disease of the sphenoidal sinus may present as sellar and parasellar masses.

Mucoceles occur in the sphenoidal sinus least frequently. They are more commonly found in the frontal, ethmoidal, and maxillary sinuses, in descending order.[127] They are an accumulation of inspissated mucus due to obstruction of the ostium that drains the sinus that is involved. An infected mucocele is a mucopyocele. On MR images it appears as a well-defined mass that may remodel and expand the sinus (Figs. 18–30 and 18–31). The signal intensity is variable and depends on the contents.[128]

Fungal infection of the sphenoidal sinus may be aggressive and involve sellar and parasellar structures, particularly in the immunocompromised individual (Fig. 18–32). Patients may present with cranial nerve palsies, cavernous sinus thrombosis, internal carotid artery occlusion, and brain abscess.[129] Infections include candidiasis, aspergillosis, histoplasmosis, chromoblastomycosis, and rhinomucormycosis.[130] The mycetomas of fungal sinusitis may be quite hypointense on MR images and subsequently be missed.[131] In contrast, high-attenuation opacification of the sinus is seen by computed tomography, which is superior to MRI for the assessment of the degree of destruction of the bony skull base.

Nonfungal granulomatous disease such as Wegener's granulomatosis and lethal midline granuloma may involve the sphenoidal sinus and spread to the parasellar region.[132, 133] In addition, both primary and secondary neoplasms may involve this area. Squamous cell carcinoma, rhabdomyosarcoma, and plasmacytoma are examples (see also Chapter 33).

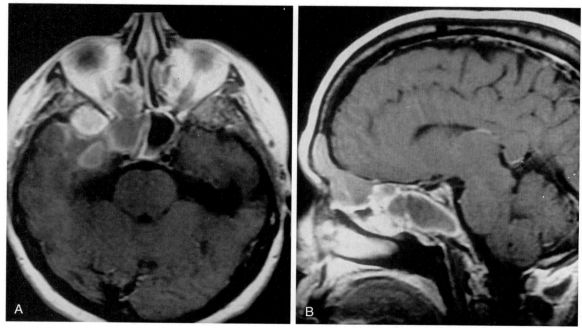

FIGURE 18–31. Sphenoidal mucocele with intracranial extension. A 48-year-old patient presented with a sphenoidal mucocele that extended through the dura and into the right temporal lobe. On axial *(A)* and sagittal *(B)* contrast-enhanced images, there are enhanced membranes surrounding central regions of mucus collection. There was no clinical cerebritis, and there was no histologic evidence of cerebral parenchymal inflammation at the time of surgical resection.

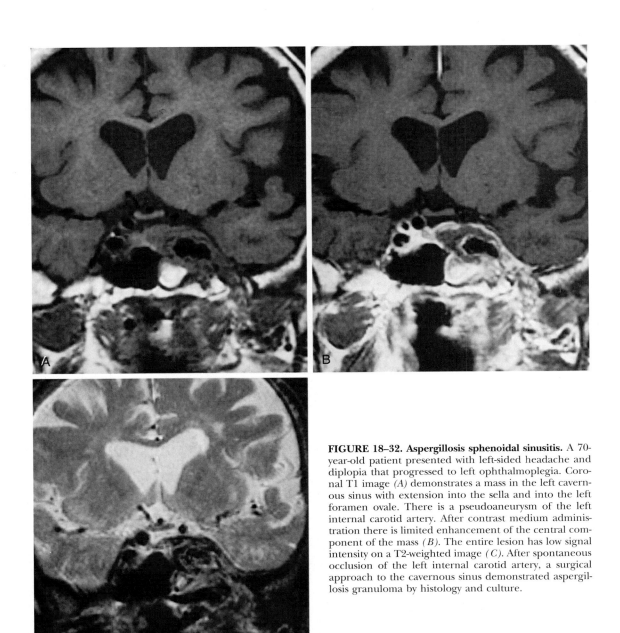

FIGURE 18–32. Aspergillosis sphenoidal sinusitis. A 70-year-old patient presented with left-sided headache and diplopia that progressed to left ophthalmoplegia. Coronal T1 image *(A)* demonstrates a mass in the left cavernous sinus with extension into the sella and into the left foramen ovale. There is a pseudoaneurysm of the left internal carotid artery. After contrast medium administration there is limited enhancement of the central component of the mass *(B)*. The entire lesion has low signal intensity on a T2-weighted image *(C)*. After spontaneous occlusion of the left internal carotid artery, a surgical approach to the cavernous sinus demonstrated aspergillosis granuloma by histology and culture.

REFERENCES

1. Jones KM, Mulkern RV, Schwartz RB, et al: Fast spin-echo MR imaging of the brain and spine: current concepts. AJR 158:1313–1320, 1992.
2. Rao VM, Vinitski S, Barbaria A, Flanders A: Enhanced resolution of the pituitary fossa with 3D fat suppressed gradient echo MRI: pre and post gadolinium enhancement. AJNR 10:892, 1989. Abstract.
3. Stadnik T, Staevenaert A, Beckers A, et al: Pituitary microadenomas: diagnosis with two- and three-dimensional MR imaging at 1.5 T before and after injection of gadolinium. Radiology 176:419–428, 1990.
4. Davis PC, Hoffman JC, Malko JA, Tindall GT: Gadolinium DTPA and MR imaging of pituitary adenoma: a preliminary report. AJNR 8:817–823, 1987.
5. Doppman JL, Frank JA, Dwyer AJ, Oldfield EH: Gadolinium DTPA enhanced MR imaging of ACTH-secreting microadenomas of the pituitary gland. J Comput Assist Tomogr 12:728–733, 1988.
6. Hesselink JR, Press GA: MR contrast enhancement of intracranial lesions with gadolinium DTPA. Radiol Clin North Am 26:873–887, 1988.
7. Dwyer AJ, Frank JA, Doppman JL, Oldfield EH: Pituitary adenomas in patients with Cushing's disease: initial experience with Gd-DTPA–enhanced MR imaging. Radiology 163:421–426, 1987.
8. Steiner E, Imhoff H, Knosp E: Gadolinium-enhanced MR imaging of pituitary adenomas. Radiographics 9:587–598, 1989.
9. Newton DR, Dillon WP, Norman D, Newton TH: Gadolinium-DTPA enhanced MR imaging of pituitary adenomas. AJNR 10:949–953, 1989.
10. Nakamura T, Schorner W, Bittner RC, Felix R: Value of paramagnetic contrast agent gadolinium-DTPA in the diagnosis pf pituitary adenomas. Neuroradiology 30:481–486, 1988.
11. Miki Y, Matsuo M, Nishizawa S, et al: Pituitary adenomas and normal pituitary tissue: enhancement patterns on gadopentate-enhanced MR imaging. Radiology 177:35–38, 1990.
12. Sakamoto Y, Takahashi M, Korogi Y: Normal and abnormal pituitary glands: gadopentate dimeglumine–enhanced MR imaging. Radiology 178:441–445, 1991.
13. Daniels DL, Pech P, Mark L, Pojunas K: Magnetic resonance imaging of the cavernous sinus. AJNR 6:187–192, 1985.
14. Renn WH, Rhoton AL Jr: Microsurgical anatomy of the sellar region. J Neurosurg 43:288–298, 1975.
15. Clemente CD: Gross anatomy of the central nervous system. In: Clemente CD, ed. Gray's Anatomy. 30th American edition. Philadelphia: Lea & Febiger, 1985, pp 1600–1605.
16. Trandafir T, Sipot C, Froicu P: On a possible neural ridge origin of the adenohypophysis. Endocrinologie 28:67–72, 1990.
17. Elster AD: Modern imaging of the pituitary. Radiology 187:1–14, 1993.
18. Takor TT, Pearse AGE: Neuroectodermal origin of avian hypothalamo-hypophyseal complex: the role of the ventral neural ridge. J Embryol Exp Morphol 34:311–325, 1975.
19. Baker BL: Functional cytology of the hypophyseal pars distalis and pars intermedia. In: Greep RO, Astwood EB, Knobil E, et al, eds. Handbook of Physiology. Section 7. Endocrinology. Volume IV. Part 1. The Pituitary Gland and Its Neuroendocrine Control. Washington, DC: American Physiological Society, 1974, pp 45–80.
20. Hamada J, Seto H, Miura M, et al: Suprasellar pituitary adenoma arising from the pars tuberalis: case report. Neurosurgery 27:647–649, 1990.
21. Gill GN: The hypothalamic-pituitary control system. In: West JB, ed. Best and Taylor's Physiological Basis of Medical Practice. 11th ed. Baltimore: Williams & Wilkins, 1985, pp 856–871.
22. Tweedle CD, Hatton GI: Evidence for dynamic interactions between pituicytes and neurosecretory axons in the rat. Neuroscience 5:661–667, 1980.
23. Xuereb GP, Pritchard MML, Daniel PM: The arterial supply and the venous drainage of the human hypophysis cerebri. Q J Exp Physiol 39:199–218, 1954.
24. Xuereb GP, Pritchard MML, Daniel PM: The hypophyseal portal system of vessel in man. Q J Exp Physiol 39:219–227, 1954.
25. Sheehan HL, Stanfield JP: The pathogenesis of postpartum necrosis of the anterior lobe of the pituitary gland. Acta Endocrinol 37:479–510, 1961.
26. Reid RL, Quigley ME, Yen SSC: Pituitary apoplexy: a review. Arch Neurol 42:712–719, 1985.
27. Yuh WT, Fisher DJ, Nguyen HD, Tali ET: Sequential enhancement pattern in normal pituitary gland and in pituitary adenoma. AJNR 15:101–108, 1994.
28. Tien RD: Sequence of enhancement of various portions of the pituitary gland on gadolinium-enhanced MR images: correlation with regional blood supply. AJR 158:651–654, 1992.
29. Kucharczyk J, Kucharczyk W, Berry I, de Groot J: Histochemical characterization and functional significance of the hyperintense signal on MR images of the posterior pituitary. AJNR 9:1079–1083, 1988.
30. Kucharczyk W, Lenkinski RE, Kucharczyk J, Henkelman RM: The effect of phospholipid vesicles on the NMR relaxation of water: an explanation for the appearance of the neurohypophysis? AJNR 11:693–700, 1990.
31. Wolpert SM, Osborne M, Anderson M, Runge VM: The bright pituitary gland: a normal MR appearance in infancy. AJNR 9:1–3, 1989.
32. Cox TD, Elster AD: Normal pituitary gland: changes in shape, size, and signal intensity during the first year of life at MR imaging. Radiology 179:721–724, 1991.
33. Tien RD, Kucharczyk J, Bessette J, Middleton M: MR imaging of the pituitary gland in infants and children: changes in size, shape, and MR signal with growth and development. AJNR 158:1151–1154, 1992.
34. Kovacs K, Horvath E: Cytology. In: Hartman WH, ed. Tumors of the Pituitary Gland. Washington, DC: Armed Forces Institute of Pathology, 1986, pp 16–50.
35. Asa SL, Kovacs K, Laslo FA, et al: Human fetal adenohypophysis: histologic and immunocytochemical analysis. Neuroendocrinology 43:308–316, 1986.
36. Thliveris JA, Currie RW: Observations on the hypothalmo-hypophyseal portal vasculature in the developing human fetus. Am J Anat 157:441–444, 1980.
37. Elster AD, Chen MYM, Williams DW, Key LL: Pituitary gland: MR imaging of physiologic hypertrophy in adolescence. Radiology 174:681–685, 1990.
38. Miki Y, Asato R, Okumura R, et al: Anterior pituitary gland in pregnancy: hyperintensity at MR. Radiology 187:229–231, 1993.
39. Elster AD, Sanders TG, Vines FS, Chen MYM: Size and shape of the pituitary gland postpartum: measurement with MR imaging. Radiology 181:531–535, 1991.
40. Kao SCS, Cook JS, Hansen JR, Simonson TM: MR imaging of the pituitary gland in central precocious puberty. Pediatr Radiol 22:481–484, 1992.
41. Doraiswamy PM, Potts JM, Axelson DA, et al: MR assessment of pituitary gland morphology in healthy volunteers: age- and gender-related differences. AJNR 13:1295–1299, 1992.
42. Kovacs K, Horvath E, Asa SL: Classification and pathology of pituitary tumors. In: Wilkins RH, Rengachary SS, eds. Neurosurgery. New York: McGraw-Hill, 1985, pp 834–842.
43. Russel DS, Rubenstein LF: Pathology of Tumours of the Nervous System. 5th ed. Baltimore: Williams & Wilkins, 1989, pp 809–854.
44. Lee BCP, Deck MDF: Sellar and juxtasellar lesion detection with MR. Radiology 157:143–147, 1987.
45. Juneau P, Schoene WC, Black P: Malignant tumors in the pituitary gland. Arch Neurol 49:555–559, 1992.
46. Kucharczyk W, Montanera WJ: The sellar and paraseller region. In: Atlas SW, ed. Magnetic Resonance Imaging of the Brain and Spine. New York: Raven Press, 1991, pp 625–667.
47. Singer W: Does pituitary stalk compression cause hyperprolactinemia? Endocr Pathol 1:65–67, 1990.
48. Doppman JL, Oldfield LH, Krudy AG, Chrousos GP: Petrosal sinus sampling for Cushing's syndrome: anatomic and technical considerations. Radiology 150:99–103, 1984.
49. Miller DL, Doppman JL: Petrosal sinus sampling: technique and rationale. Radiology 178:37–47, 1991.
50. Brougham M, Heusner AP, Adams RD: Acute degenerative changes in adenomas of the pituitary body—with special reference to pituitary apoplexy. J Neurosurg 7:421–439, 1950.
51. Fraioli B, Esposito V, Palma L, Cantore G: Hemorrhagic pituitary adenomas: clinicopathological features and surgical treatment. Neurosurgery 27:741–748, 1990.
52. Sheehan HL, Stanfield JP: The pathogenesis of postpartum necrosis of the anterior lobe of the pituitary gland. Acta Endocrinol 37:479–510, 1961.
53. Youssem DM, Arrington JA, Zinreich SJ, Kumar AJ: Pituitary adenomas: possible role of bromocriptine in intratumoral hemorrhage. Radiology 170:239–243, 1989.
54. Kucharczyk W, Davis DO, Kelly WM, Sze G: Pituitary adenomas: high resolution MR imaging at 1.5 T. Radiology 161:761–765, 1986.
55. Chong BW, Kucharczyk W, Singer W, George S: Distinguishing focal signal hypointensities in the pituitary glands of normal volunteers from microprolactinomas. AJNR 15:675–677, 1994.
56. Ahmadi H, Larsson EM, Jinkins JR: Normal pituitary gland: coronal MR imaging of infundibular tilt. Radiology 177:389–392, 1990.
57. Wilson CB: Neurosurgical management of large and invasive pituitary tumors. In: Tindall GT, Collins WF, eds. Clinical Management of Pituitary Disorders. New York: Raven Press, 1979, pp 335–342.
58. Scotti G, Yu CY, Dillon WP, et al: MR of cavernous sinus involvement by pituitary adenomas. AJR 151:799–806, 1988.
59. Ostrov SG, Quencer RM, Hoffman JC, et al: Hemorrhage within pituitary adenomas: how often associated with pituitary apoplexy syndrome? AJNR 10:503–510, 1989.
60. Steiner E, Knosp E, Herold CJ, et al: Pituitary adenomas: findings of postoperative MR imaging. Radiology 185:521–527, 1992.
61. Dina T, Feaster SH, Laws ER, et al: MR of the pituitary gland postsurgery: serial MR studies following transsphenoidal resection. AJNR 14:763–769, 1993.
62. Kimmel DW, O'Neill BPP: Systemic cancer presenting as diabetes insipidus. Cancer 52:2355–2358, 1983.

63. Schubiger O, Haller D: Metastasis to the pituitary-hypothalamic axis: an MR study of 7 symptomatic patients. Neuroradiology 34:131–134, 1992.
64. Chappell PM, Kelly WM: Primary intrasellar melanoma simulating hemorrhagic pituitary adenoma. MR and pathologic findings. AJNR 11:1054–1056, 1990.
65. Young WF Jr, Scheithauer BW, Garib H, et al: Cushing's syndrome due to primary multinodular corticotrope hyperplasia. Mayo Clin Proc 63:256–262, 1988.
66. Horvath E: Pituitary hyperplasia. Pathol Res Pract 183:623–625, 1988.
67. Moran A, Asa SL, Kovacs K, et al: Gigantism due to pituitary mammosomatotroph hyperplasia. N Engl J Med 323:322–327, 1990.
68. Peillon F, Dupuy M, Li JY, et al: Pituitary enlargement with suprasellar extension in functional hyperprolactinemia due to lactotroph hyperplasia: a pseudotumoral disease. J Clin Endocrinol Metab 73:1008–1015, 1991.
69. Jay V, Kovacs K, Horvath E, et al: Idiopathic prolactin cell hyperplasia of the pituitary mimicking prolactin cell adenoma: a morphological study in immunocytochemistry, electron microscopy, and in situ hybridization. Acta Neuropathol 82:147–151, 1991.
70. Asscheman H, Gooren LJG, Assies J, et al: Prolactin levels and pituitary enlargement in hormone-treated male-to-female transsexuals. Clin Endocrinol 28:583–588, 1988.
71. Cusimano MD, Kovacs K, Bilbai JM, et al: Suprasellar craniopharyngioma associated with hyperprolactinemia, pituitary lactotroph hyperplasia, and microprolactinoma. J Neurosurg 69:620–623, 1988.
72. Kao SC, Cook JS, Hansen JR, Simonson TM: MR imaging of the pituitary gland in central precocious puberty. Pediatr Radiol 22:481–484, 1992.
73. Atchinson JA, Lee PA, Albright AL: Reversible suprasellar pituitary mass secondary to hypothyroidism. JAMA 262:3175–3177, 1989.
74. Hutchins WW, Crues JV III, Miya P, Pojunas KW: MR demonstration of pituitary hyperplasia and regression after therapy for hypothyroidism. AJNR 11:410, 1990.
75. Quencer RM: Lymphocytic hypophysitis: autoimmune disorder of the pituitary gland. AJNR 1:343–345, 1980.
76. Goudie RB, Pinkerton PH: Anterior hypophysitis and Hashimoto's disease in a young woman. J Pathol Bacteriol 83:584–586, 1962.
77. Bottazzo GF, Pouplard A, Florin-Christiensen A, Doniach D: Antibodies to prolactin secreting cells of human pituitary. Lancet 2:97–101, 1975.
78. Asa SL, Bilbao JM, Kovacs K, et al: Lymphocytic hypophysitis of pregnancy resulting in hypopituitarism: a distinct clinicopathologic entity. Ann Intern Med 95:166–171, 1981.
79. Ahmadi J, Meyers GS, Segall HD, et al: Lymphocytic adenohypophysitis: contrast-enhanced MR imaging in five cases. Radiology 195:30–34, 1995.
80. Dash RJ, Gupta V, Suri S: Sheehan's syndrome: clinical profile, pituitary hormone responses and computed sellar tomography. Aust N Z J Med 23:26–31, 1993.
81. Carmel PW: The empty sella syndrome. In: Wilkins RH, Reganchary SS, eds. Neurosurgery. New York: McGraw-Hill, 1985, pp 884–888.
82. Weisberg LA, Zimmerman EA, Frantz AG: Diagnosis and evaluation of patients with an enlarged sella turcica. Am J Med 61:590–596, 1976.
83. Kaufman R, Tomsak RL, Kaufman BA, et al: Herniation of the suprasellar visual system and the third ventricle into empty sella: morphologic and clinical considerations. AJNR 10:65–76, 1989.
84. Shucart WA, Jackson IMD: Anatomy and physiology of the neurohypophysis. In: Wilkins RH, Reganchary SS, eds. Neurosurgery Update II. New York: McGraw-Hill, 1991, pp 805–811.
85. Tien R, Kucharczyk J, Kucharczyk W: MR imaging of the brain in patients with diabetes insipidus. AJNR 12:533–542, 1991.
86. Fujisawa I, Nishimura K, Asato R, Togashi K: Posterior lobe of the pituitary in diabetes insipidus: MR findings. J Comput Assist Tomogr 11:221–225, 1987.
87. Gudinchet F, Brunelle F, Barth MO, Taviere V: MR imaging of the posterior hypophysis in children. AJNR 10:511–514, 1989.
88. Miyamoto S, Sasaki N, Tanabe Y: Magnetic resonance imaging in familial central diabetes insipidus. Neuroradiology 33:272–273, 1991.
89. Moses AM, Clayton B, Hochhauser L: Use of T1-weighted MR to differentiate between primary polydipsia and central diabetes insipidus. AJNR 13:1273–1277, 1992.
90. Fujisawa I, Kikuchi K, Nishimura K, Togashi K: Transection of the pituitary stalk: development of an ectopic posterior lobe assessed with MR imaging. Radiology 165:487–489, 1987.
91. Kelly WM, Kucharczyk W, Kucharczyk J, Kjos B: Posterior pituitary ectopia: an MR feature of pituitary dwarfism. AJNR 9:453–460, 1988.
92. Kikuchi K, Fujisawa I, Momoi T, et al: Hypothalamic-pituitary function in growth hormone–deficient patients with pituitary stalk transection. J Clin Endocrinol Metab 67:817–823, 1988.
93. Carmel PW, Antunes JL, Chang CH: Craniopharyngiomas in children. Neurosurgery 11:382–389, 1982.
94. Freeman MP, Kessler RM, Allen JH, Price AC: Craniopharyngioma: CT and MR imaging in 9 cases. J Comput Assist Tomogr 11:810–814, 1987.
95. Fukushima T, Hirakawa K, Kimura M, Towanaga M: Intraventricular craniopharyngioma: its characteristics on magnetic resonance imaging and successful total removal. Surg Neurol 33:22–27, 1990.
96. Ikezaki K, Fujii K, Kishikawa T: Magnetic resonance imaging of an intraventricular craniopharyngioma. Neuroradiology 32:247–249, 1990.
97. Karnaze MG, Sartor K, Winthrop JD, Gado MH: Suprasellar lesions: evaluation with MR imaging. Radiology 161:77–82, 1986.
98. Pusey E, Kortman KE, Flannigan BD, Tsuruda J: MR of craniopharyngiomas: tumor delineation and characterization. AJNR 8:439–444, 1987.
99. Ahmadi J, Destian S, Apuzzo MLJ, et al: Cystic fluid in craniopharyngiomas: MR imaging and quantitative analysis. Radiology 182:783–785, 1992.
100. Kucharczyk W, Peck WW, Kelly WM, Norman D: Rathke cleft cysts: CT, MR imaging, and pathological features. Radiology 165:491–495, 1987.
101. Maggio WW, Cail WS, Brookeman JR, Pershing JA: Rathke's cleft cyst: computed tomographic and magnetic resonance imaging appearances. Neurosurgery 21:60–62, 1987.
102. Crenshaw WB, Chew FH: Rathke's cleft cyst. AJR 158:1312, 1993.
103. Hua F, Asato R, Miki Y, et al: Differentiation of suprasellar non-neoplastic cysts from cystic neoplasms by Gd-DTPA MRI. J Comput Assist Tomogr 16:744–749, 1992.
104. Houspian EM, Marquart MD, Behrens M: Optic gliomas. In: Wilkins RH, Rengachary SS, eds. Neurosurgery. New York: McGraw-Hill, 1985, pp 916–920.
105. Rodriguez LA, Edwards MSB, Levin VA: Management of hypothalamic gliomas in children: an analysis of 33 cases. Neurosurgery 26:242–247, 1990.
106. Bognanno JR, Edwards MK, Lee TA, Dunn DW: Cranial MR imaging in neurofibromatosis. AJNR 9:461–468, 1988.
107. Hurst RW, Newman SA, Cail WS: Multifocal intracranial abnormalities in neurofibromatosis. AJNR 9:293–296, 1988.
108. Boyko OB, Curnes JT, Oakes WJ, Burger PC: Hamartomas of the tuber cinereum: CT, MR, and pathological findings. AJNR 12:309–314, 1991.
109. Treip CS: The hypothalamus and the pituitary gland. In: Adams JH, Duchen LW, eds. Greenfield's Neuropathology. 5th ed. New York: Oxford University Press, 1992, pp 1046–1082.
110. Asa SL, Bilbao JM, Kovacs K, Linfoot JA: Hypothalamic neuronal hamartoma associated with pituitary growth hormone cell adenoma and acromegaly. Acta Neuropathol 52:231–234, 1980.
111. Marliani AF, Tampieri D, Melancon D, et al: Magnetic resonance imaging of hypothalamic hamartomas causing gelastic epilepsy. Can Assoc Radiol J 42:335–339, 1991.
112. Cheng K, Sawamura Y, Yamauchi T, Abe H: Asymptomatic large hypothalamic hamartoma associated with polydactyly in an adult. Neurosurgery 32:458–460, 1993.
113. Hubbard AM, Engelhoff JC: MR imaging of large hypothalamic hamartomas in two infants. AJNR 10:1277, 1989.
114. Ober KP, Alexander E Jr, Challa VR, Ferree C: Histiocytosis X of the hypothalamus. Neurosurgery 24:93–95, 1989.
115. Tien RD, Newton TH, McDermott MW, et al: Thickened pituitary stalk on MR images in patients with diabetes insipidus and Langerhans' cell histiocytosis. AJNR 11:703–708, 1990.
116. Tolosa EJ: Periarteritic lesions of the carotid siphon with clinical features of carotid intraclinoid aneurysms. J Neurol Neurosurg Psychiatry 17:300–302, 1954.
117. Hunt WE, Meagher JN, Lefever H: Painful ophthalmoplegia: its relation to indolent inflammation of the cavernous sinus. Neurology 11:56–62, 1961.
118. Campbell RJ, Okazaki H: Painful ophthalmoplegia (Tolosa-Hunt variant): autopsy findings in a patient with necrotizing intracavernous carotid vasculitis and inflammatory disease of the orbit. Mayo Clin Proc 62:520–526, 1987.
119. Kwan EDS, Wolpert SM, Hedges TR III, Laucella M: Tolosa-Hunt syndrome revisited: not necessarily a diagnosis of exclusion. AJNR 8:1067–1072, 1987.
120. Youssem DM, Atlas SW, Grossman RI, Sergott RC: MR imaging of Tolosa-Hunt syndrome. AJNR 10:1181–1184, 1989.
121. Celli P, Ferrante L, Acqui M, et al: Neurinoma of the third, fourth, and sixth cranial nerves: a survey and a report of a new fourth nerve case. Surg Neurol 38:216–224, 1992.
122. Pollack IF, Sekhar LN, Jannetta PJ, Janecka IP: Neurilemomas of the trigeminal nerve. J Neurosurg 70:737–745, 1989.
123. Yuh WTC, Wright DC, Barloon TJ, Schultz DH: MR imaging of primary tumors of trigeminal nerve and Meckel's cave. AJNR 9:665–670, 1988.
124. Osborn AG: Brain tumors and tumor-like masses: classification and differential diagnosis. In: Diagnostic Neuroradiology—A Text-Atlas. St. Louis: Mosby–Year Book, 1994, p 498.
125. Fujii K, Fujita N, Hirabuki N, et al: Neuromas and meningiomas: evaluation of early enhancement with dynamic MR imaging. AJNR 13:1215–1220, 1992.
126. Newton TH, Trost BT: Arteriovenous malformations and fistulas. In: Newton TH, Potts DG, eds. Radiology of the Skull and Brain. St. Louis: CV Mosby, 1974, pp 2490–2565.
127. Delfini R, Missori P, Iannetti G, et al: Mucoceles of the paranasal sinuses

with intracranial and intraorbital extension: report of 28 cases. Neurosurgery 32:901–906, 1993.

128. Van Tassel P, Lee YY, Jing BS, DePena CA: Mucoceles of the paranasal sinuses: MR imaging with CT correlation. AJNR 10:607–612, 1989.

129. Anand V, Alemar G, Griswold JA Jr: Intracranial complications of mucormycosis: an experimental method and clinical review. Laryngoscope 102:656–662, 1992.

130. Malone DG, O'Boynick PL, Ziegler DK, et al: Osteomyelytis of the skull base. Neurosurgery 30:426–431, 1992.

131. Demaerel P, Brown P, Kendall BE, et al: Case report: allergic aspergillosis of the sphenoid sinus: pitfall on MRI. Br J Radiol 66:260–263, 1993.

132. Burlakoff SG, Wong FSH: Wegener's granulomatosis: the great masquerade: a clinical presentation and literature review. J Otolaryngol 22:94–105, 1993.

133. Marsot-Dupuch K, Cabane J, Raveau V, et al: Lethal midline granuloma: impact of imaging studies on the investigation and management of destructive midfacial disease in 13 parients. Neuroradiology 34:155–161, 1992.

Brain Stem, Posterior Fossa, and Cranial Nerves

JOHN F. HEALY

Magnetic resonance imaging (MRI) has revolutionized imaging of the posterior fossa and brain stem. Computed tomography (CT) of the posterior fossa and brain stem is limited by bone and motion artifact. The multiplanar capability, higher spatial and contrast resolution, and lack of artifact make MRI vastly superior to CT, so that MRI is the examination of choice in patients with disorders of these structures.[1-3] Distinguishing intra-axial from extra-axial pathologic processes and precise localization of the tumor site in relationship to adjoining structures are paramount and more important than histologic prediction. However, the histologic picture can often be predicted with a high degree of accuracy if the age of the patient, the exact tumor location, and the imaging characteristics are taken into consideration (Fig. 19–1). Accurate size estimation and lesion location are crucial for surgical planning. Sagittal imaging, in particular, is critical for evaluation of processes that spread to and through the foramen magnum. This area is poorly examined by CT.

Variations in MR signal characteristics and contrast enhancement help to categorize the pathologic tissue. The presence or absence of flow void on spin-echo images, flow-enhanced signal on gradient-echo imaging, and MR angiography graphically demonstrate whether normal or abnormal blood flow is present.

Clinical syndromes can be accurately imaged. Detailed knowledge of the functional anatomy of the midbrain, pons, medulla, cerebellum, and cranial nerves is necessary to adequately investigate patients with symptoms referable to these regions, so that adequate scan protocols and imaging planes are used. Familiarity with the various pathologic conditions that occur in these regions and with the clinical presentations of these diseases[4] and a working familiarity with principles of MRI are necessary to arrive at an accurate differential diagnosis.

The common disease processes seen in the brain stem are infarcts, infection and inflammatory diseases, multiple sclerosis, traumatic injuries, vascular malformations, and primary and secondary tumors. These lesions may all look quite similar on MR images, especially on long repetition time (TR) images on which increased signal intensity is usually seen. Extra-axial disease from either vascular or mass lesions can also be a prominent cause of brain stem or cerebellar symptoms.

Most brain stem lesions are detected by long-TR double-echo scans. Although the T2-weighted image is more sensitive in detecting a pathologic process, the proton density–weighted image will often prove valuable in confirming the presence of disease and in differentiating subtle disease from partial-volume cerebrospinal fluid (CSF) artifact. Multiplanar imaging and the use of gadolinium-enhanced T1-weighted images are of great help in accurately localizing and characterizing a lesion.

Patients with diseases of the brain stem and posterior fossa may present with signs and symptoms caused by compression or destruction of neurologic tissue, evidence of obstructive hydrocephalus, or both. The classic headache of hydrocephalus is persistent, is increased by straining or bending over, is worse in the morning, and may be associated with lethargy, confusion, and vomiting. Patients with diseases involving the brain stem may present with a plethora of cranial neuropathies or with ataxia and paresis owing to interruption of cerebellar and corticospinal pathways. Patients with diseases of the cerebellar hemisphere present with limb ataxia and loss of fine motor coordination. Midline disease involving the vermis presents as truncal ataxia and gait disturbances, and the patients have difficulty with tandem walking and maintaining postural equilibrium.

PULSE SEQUENCES

We investigated patients with posterior fossa and cranial nerve signs and symptoms with a T1-weighted

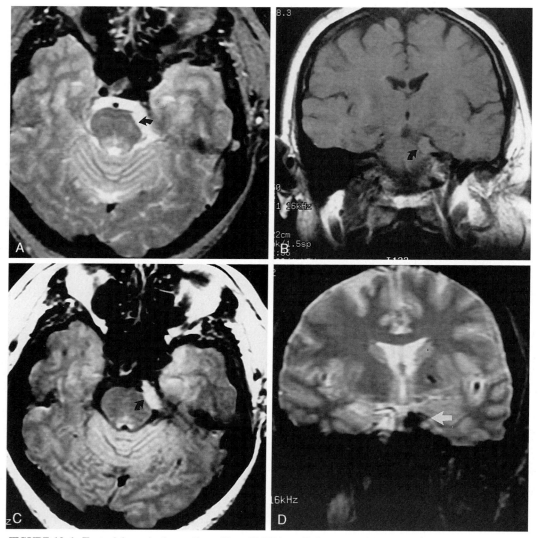

FIGURE 19–1. Tentorial meningioma. Versatility of MRI is well demonstrated in this 47-year-old woman with fifth cranial nerve findings. *A,* T2-weighted axial image shows only flattening of the left side of pons *(arrow)*; the actual lesion is not visible. *B,* T1-weighted coronal image shows lesion in the coronal plane *(arrow)* that appears extra-axial, straddling the tentorial notch. *C,* Axial proton density–weighted postgadolinium image confirms a hemisphere-shaped extra-axial lesion, with broad base on the tentorium *(arrow)* and marked homogeneous enhancement. *D,* Gradient-echo coronal image demonstrates calcification within the mass *(arrow)* evident because of magnetic susceptibility. Thus, multiplanar scanning, different signal characteristics, lack of bone artifact, additional use of gadolinium enhancement and gradient-echo imaging, clinical presentation, and age and sex of patient lead to almost certain histologic diagnosis of meningioma.

sagittal localizer followed by axial fast spin-echo protein density–weighted and T2-weighted images acquired separately with a field of view of 20 cm, 5-mm slice thickness, 2.5-mm gap, 256 × 256 matrix, and 1 NEX (the number of excitations). We try to keep the TR at 3000 ms on the proton density–weighted image to keep CSF intensity of a more intermediate signal intensity than the usual high signal intensity of pathologic changes in the parenchyma. Effective echo time (TE) values of 17 and 104 ms and an echo train of 8 are used. Lack of flow compensation is sometimes a problem on the lower brain slices of the proton density–weighted examination but is rarely a significant problem on the T2–weighted images. Conventional spin-echo images could certainly be substituted for fast spin echo. We consider fast spin-echo and conventional spin-echo imaging to be equivalent in detecting central nervous system (CNS) abnormalities.[5, 6]

We usually acquire axial gradient-echo images with TR of 12 ms, TE of 400 ms, flip angle of 20°, 2 NEX, and 256 × 256 matrix. The 3 minutes invested is trivial and ensures optimal detection of T2 shortening blood products and calcification. The detection of deoxyhemoglobin, hemosiderin, and calcification is limited on spin-echo imaging, especially fast spin-echo.

The use of gadolinium is absolutely essential in evaluating patients with clinical problems referable to the brain stem, posterior fossa, and cranial nerves.[7, 8] We routinely use gadolinium-enhanced T1-weighted images in at least two planes after the acquisition of a nonenhanced T1 weighted image. If a tumor is seen, we recommend postcontrast imaging in all three conventional planes for optimal visualization and localization of the mass and adjacent structures. For skull base lesions involving cranial nerves, we often use fat suppression techniques with gadolinium to suppress high intensity bone marrow signal and better delineate enhancing lesions.

MR angiography is used when indicated and tailored to the particular clinical problem. It is never done without first reviewing the vascular information available on the conventional MR images. The source images are always filmed and reviewed. The anatomy of the brain stem and cranial nerves is often superb on these thin-section source images. Maximal intensity projection algorithm images are routinely displayed in a manner that allows stereoscopic three-dimensional viewing of the vascular anatomy.

For the detection and evaluation of cerebellopontine angle masses,[9, 10] we perform routine fast spin-echo proton density–weighted and T2-weighted axial imaging of the entire brain. Coronal precontrast and coronal and axial postgadolinium sequences are performed using a TR of 600 ms, TE of 25 ms, field of view of 16 cm, 3-mm slice thickness, no gap, 128 × 256 matrix, and 4 NEX. Fat saturation is used if the patient has had previous surgery in the area. Coronal imaging is done from the posterior mastoid area to the pituitary gland. Axial imaging is done from the inferior mastoid to the anterior cerebral arteries. If any abnormalities are seen on the screening long-TR images, a routine postgadolinium examination of the whole brain is done.

CRANIAL NERVES

The anatomy of cranial nerves III through XII is illustrated in Figures 19–2 and 19–3. Cranial nerves I and II are discussed in Chapter 15. The cranial nerve nuclei of the brain stem are located in the tegmentum of the midbrain and pons and the medulla. The spinal sensory nucleus of cranial nerve V extends caudally into the upper cervical spinal cord. All of the cranial nerves exit or enter the ventral or lateral aspects of the brain stem, except for cranial nerve IV, which exits the tectum of the midbrain posteriorly.

Several cranial nerves are often affected in characteristic combinations, owing to their proximity.

1. The nuclei of cranial nerves VI and VII are at the level of the facial colliculi in the pons just beneath the floor of the fourth ventricle.

2. Cranial nerves VII and VIII share a common cisternal segment as they enter the internal auditory canal.

3. The cisternal portions of cranial nerves III and IV pass between the superior cerebellar and posterior cerebral arteries and enter the cavernous sinus.

4. Cranial nerves V and VI may both be involved by lesions of the upper medial portion of the petrous apex.

5. Cranial nerves IX, X, and XI descend through the jugular foramen and carotid sheath in proximity.

Isolated cranial nerve palsies most commonly involve cranial nerves III, VI, or VII.

CRANIAL NERVE I (OLFACTORY)

The olfactory nerve mediates smell by means of the nasal olfactory mucosa, the olfactory bulb, and olfactory tract to the inferior aspect of the medial temporal lobe. Diminished or absent sense of smell may be congenital (Kallmann's syndrome). The most common acquired causes of loss of smell are chronic sinonasal disease, trauma (Fig. 19–4), and compression by tumors. Pediatric tumors in this region include rhabdomyosarcoma, metastatic neuroblastoma, and juvenile angiofibroma. Adult tumors compressing this region are olfactory esthesioneuroblastoma (Fig. 19–5), olfactory groove meningioma, and metastatic disease. MRI findings of acute or chronic contusion and hemorrhage in the gyrus rectus are usually seen in patients with traumatic loss of smell.

CRANIAL NERVE II (OPTIC)

The optic nerve, like the olfactory nerve, is an extension of brain tissue and is thus subject to intra-axial brain disease such as gliomas and multiple sclerosis.[11]

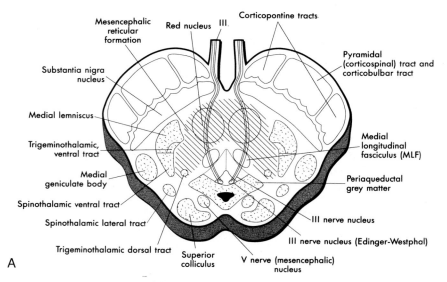

Mesencephalic reticular formation
Red nucleus
III
Corticopontine tracts
Substantia nigra nucleus
Pyramidal (corticospinal) tract and corticobulbar tract
Medial lemniscus
Trigeminothalamic, ventral tract
Medial longitudinal fasciculus (MLF)
Medial geniculate body
Periaqueductal grey matter
Spinothalamic ventral tract
III nerve nucleus
Spinothalamic lateral tract
III nerve nucleus (Edinger-Westphal)
Trigeminothalamic dorsal tract
Superior colliculus
V nerve (mesencephalic) nucleus

A

MIDBRAIN—INFERIOR COLLICULUS

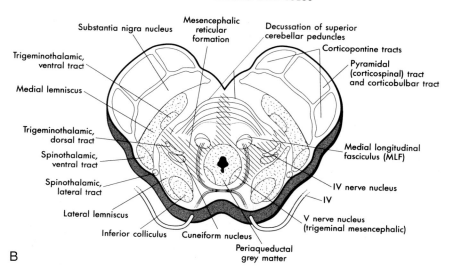

Substantia nigra nucleus
Mesencephalic reticular formation
Decussation of superior cerebellar peduncles
Trigeminothalamic, ventral tract
Corticopontine tracts
Pyramidal (corticospinal) tract and corticobulbar tract
Medial lemniscus
Trigeminothalamic, dorsal tract
Medial longitudinal fasciculus (MLF)
Spinothalamic, ventral tract
Spinothalamic, lateral tract
IV nerve nucleus
IV
Lateral lemniscus
V nerve nucleus (trigeminal mesencephalic)
Inferior colliculus
Cuneiform nucleus
Periaqueductal grey matter

B

UPPER PONS

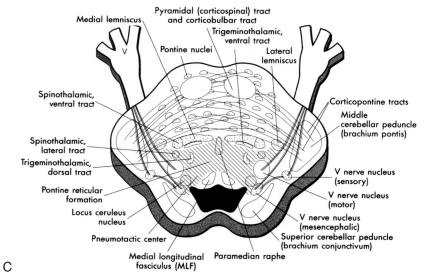

Medial lemniscus
Pyramidal (corticospinal) tract and corticobulbar tract
Trigeminothalamic, ventral tract
Medial lemniscus
Pontine nuclei
Lateral lemniscus
V
Spinothalamic, ventral tract
Corticopontine tracts
Middle cerebellar peduncle (brachium pontis)
Spinothalamic, lateral tract
Trigeminothalamic, dorsal tract
V nerve nucleus (sensory)
V nerve nucleus (motor)
Pontine reticular formation
V nerve nucleus (mesencephalic)
Locus ceruleus nucleus
Superior cerebellar peduncle (brachium conjunctivum)
Pneumotactic center
Paramedian raphe
Medial longitudinal fasciculus (MLF)

C

FIGURE 19–2 *See legend on opposite page*

LOWER PONS

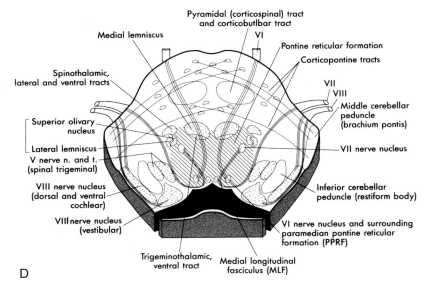

Pyramidal (corticospinal) tract
and corticobutlbar tract

Medial lemniscus

VI

Pontine reticular formation

Corticopontine tracts

Spinothalamic,
lateral and ventral tracts

VII
VIII

Middle cerebellar
peduncle
(brachium pontis)

Superior olivary
nucleus

Lateral lemniscus

V nerve n. and t.
(spinal trigeminal)

VII nerve nucleus

VIII nerve nucleus
(dorsal and ventral
cochlear)

VIII nerve nucleus
(vestibular)

Inferior cerebellar
peduncle (restiform body)

VI nerve nucleus and surrounding
paramedian pontine reticular
formation (PPRF)

Trigeminothalamic,
ventral tract

Medial longitudinal
fasciculus (MLF)

D

UPPER MEDULLA

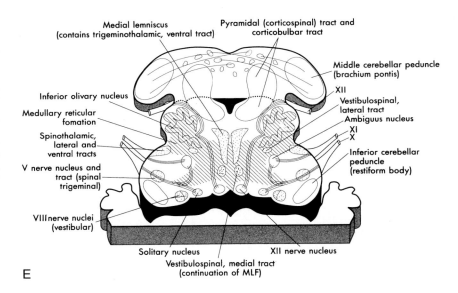

Medial lemniscus
(contains trigeminothalamic, ventral tract)

Pyramidal (corticospinal) tract and
corticobulbar tract

Middle cerebellar peduncle
(brachium pontis)

Inferior olivary nucleus

XII

Medullary reticular
fomation

Vestibulospinal,
lateral tract

Ambiguus nucleus

Spinothalamic,
lateral and
ventral tracts

XI

X

V nerve nucleus and
tract (spinal
trigeminal)

Inferior cerebellar
peduncle
(restiform body)

VIII nerve nuclei
(vestibular)

Solitary nucleus

Vestibulospinal, medial tract
(continuation of MLF)

XII nerve nucleus

E

FIGURE 19–2. **Brain stem anatomy in the axial plane.** *A* to *E,* Diagrammatic representation of brain stem and cranial nerve anatomy. The region of the reticular system is marked by parallel lines, the sensory tracts and nuclei are stippled, and the motor structures are unmarked. The aqueduct *(A and B)* and the fourth ventricle *(C, D, and E)* are the unlabeled black areas posteriorly in the sections. *F,* Sagittal diagram illustrates the levels of the axial sections. (*A* to *F* from Hayman LA: Clinical Brain Imaging: Normal Structure and Functional Anatomy. St. Louis: Mosby–Year Book, 1992, pp 192, 194, 196, 198, 200.)

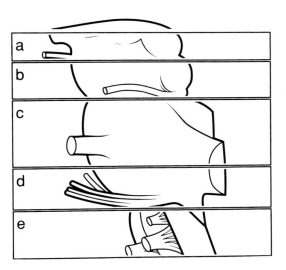

a

b

c

d

e

F

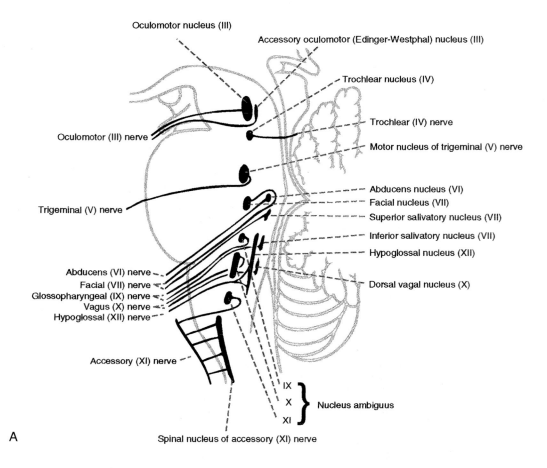

A

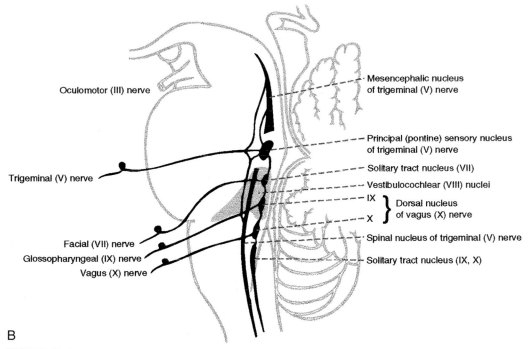

B

FIGURE 19–3. Brain stem anatomy in the sagittal plane. *A,* Sagittal representation of motor and parasympathetic nuclei and nerve roots in the brain stem. *B,* Sagittal diagram of the sensory nuclei and nerve roots. (*A* and *B* modified from Clara M: Das Nervensystem des Menschen. Leipzig: Johann Ambrosius Barth Verlag, 1942.)

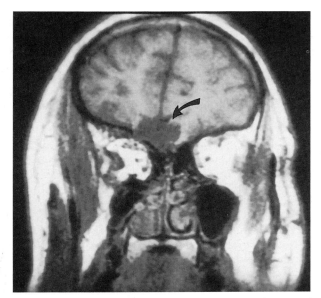

FIGURE 19–4. Post-traumatic anosmia. Post-traumatic anosmia–encephalomalacia *(arrow)* seen in both gyrus recti and olfactory bulbs after closed head injury.

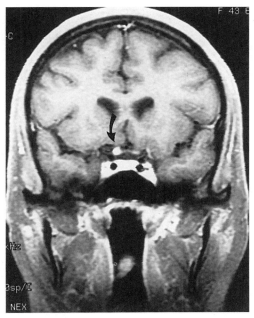

FIGURE 19–6. Multiple sclerosis. Coronal postgadolinium fat-suppressed T1-weighted image reveals abnormal enhancement of the right optic nerve *(arrow)* in this 43-year-old woman with right optic neuritis. Optic nerves were normal on long-TR images (not shown), and only one periventricular white matter hyperintensity was noted.

Optic nerve gliomas usually occur in children and are often associated with neurofibromatosis type 1. Nearly 25% of patients with neurofibromatosis type 1 have optic nerve gliomas. Approximately 20% of these patients have bilateral tumors.

Meningiomas occur in the optic nerve sheath and compress the optic nerve. Other masses in the globe or near the orbital apex may also compress the optic nerve. Optic neuritis may be self-limited but is often related to multiple sclerosis, and white matter lesions elsewhere should be sought on MR images (Fig. 19–6). The optic chiasm and optic radiations can all be affected or compressed by intrinsic CNS disease, and the resulting visual defect should give a clue to the location of the responsible lesion; for example, lesions compressing the optic chiasm from below result in bitemporal hemianopsia with the superior temporal visual

quadrants affected first because the retinal fibers emanating from the lower nasal quadrants are compressed first.

CRANIAL NERVE III (OCULOMOTOR)

The oculomotor nerve innervates four of the six intraocular muscles: the superior rectus, the medial rectus, the inferior rectus, and the inferior oblique. The striated muscle of the levator palpebrae is also innervated by this cranial nerve. The third nerve nucleus is in the paramedian posterior midbrain tegmen-

FIGURE 19–5. Esthesioneuroblastoma. *A,* T1-weighted coronal image reveals a large mass (e) filling the nasal cavity and left ethmoid sinus and invading the left orbit and base of the skull on both sides of the midline. *B,* Gadolinium-enhanced, fat-suppressed T1-weighted image helps define the extent of tumor.

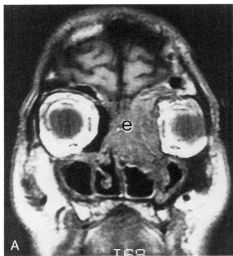
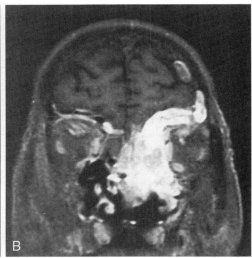

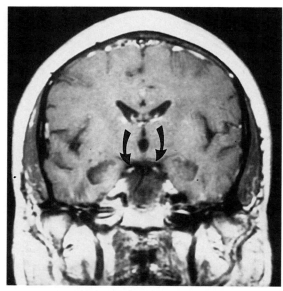

FIGURE 19–7. Sarcoidosis. T1-weighted axial postgadolinium image in a patient with right third nerve dysfunction. Note the cisternal segment of both third nerves enhancing *(arrows)* as they course between flow voids of posterior cerebral *(above)* and superior cerebellar *(below)* arteries.

tum just ventral to the aqueduct at the level of the superior colliculus. Its lower motor neuron fibers extend anteriorly, pass through the red nucleus, and emerge from the midbrain in the interpeduncular cistern to pass between the posterior cerebral and superior cerebellar arteries to enter the dura of the cavernous sinus (Figs. 19–7 and 19–8). The Edinger-Westphal

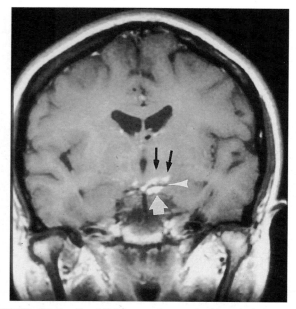

FIGURE 19–8. Coccidioidomycotic meningitis. Gadolinium-enhanced T1-weighted coronal image reveals enhancement *(small arrows)* of basal cisterns. Note flow voids of posterior cerebral artery *(arrowhead)* and superior cerebellar artery *(large arrow)*. Cisternal segment of third cranial nerve runs between these vessels. This patient had left oculomotor neuropathy.

nucleus, situated just posterior to the nucleus of cranial nerve III, supplies parasympathetic fibers running with the third nerve to supply the constrictor pupillae and ciliary muscle.

Cranial neuropathy of the third nerve produces ptosis (drooping of the eyelid) and paralysis of the four extraocular muscles innervated and results in external strabismus caused by unopposed action of the lateral rectus muscle (innervated by the sixth cranial nerve). The patient experiences diplopia on lateral gaze to the affected side. If parasympathetic fibers coursing in the third nerve are involved, dilatation of the pupil results from the paralysis of the constrictor pupillary muscle.

Weber's syndrome, a combination of third nerve palsy and contralateral hemiplegia, indicates a lesion in or near the basal midbrain affecting both the corticospinal tracts and the third nerve fibers as they course ventrally before exiting the brain stem (Fig. 19–9).

Benedikt's syndrome is caused by a lesion involving the third nerve as it courses through the red nucleus in the midbrain. An ipsilateral third nerve paralysis and a contralateral intention tremor result.

A mass lesion can compress the cisternal portion of the third nerve. Specifically, a posterior projecting internal carotid aneurysm or a posterior communicating artery aneurysm can account for a third nerve palsy. Most posterior communicating aneurysms project laterally and posteriorly and can compress the cisternal portion of the third cranial nerve (Figs. 19–10 and 19–11). Parasympathetic fibers from the Edinger-Westphal nucleus are always involved with external compressive lesions. Pure motor third nerve dysfunction without pupil dilatation indicates a noncompressive, usually microvascular, process (e.g., diabetes, atherosclerosis, or hypertension). These incomplete third nerve pareses often resolve spontaneously in several weeks.

CRANIAL NERVE IV (TROCHLEAR)

The trochlear nucleus is situated in the paramedian midbrain tegmentum at the level of the inferior colliculi, just caudal to the third nerve nucleus. However, fibers of the fourth cranial nerve cross to exit from the posterior aspect of the brain stem just beneath the contralateral inferior colliculus. This small cranial nerve has a long cisternal course around the cerebral peduncle to lie lateral to the third cranial nerve in the prepontine cistern between superior cerebellar and posterior cerebral arteries. This 8-cm cisternal segment may be injured during surgery or trauma. The fourth nerve is the only cranial nerve that crosses to innervate the contralateral side and also is the only cranial nerve to exit the dorsal aspect of the brain stem. An isolated fourth nerve palsy causes diplopia in the downward, lateral visual field (e.g., when descending stairs). Nuclear third and fourth cranial neuropathies occur frequently in combination, owing to the proximity of their nuclei in the midbrain.

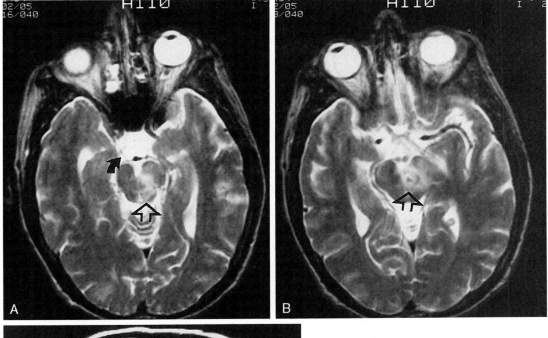

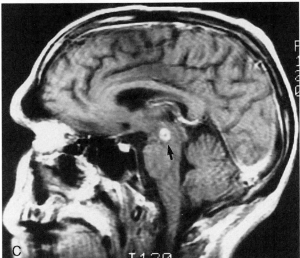

FIGURE 19–9. Toxoplasmosis. *A* and *B*, T2-weighted axial images in patient infected with human immunodeficiency virus. Left third nerve dysfunction and contralateral hemiparesis were noted. Hyperintensity occurs in the area of the third nerve nucleus *(open arrow)* and along the course of the third nerve in the midbrain. The cisternal segment of contralateral third nerve is seen *(curved arrow)*. *C*, Postgadolinium T1-weighted sagittal image shows enhancing lesion *(arrow)* in tegmentum that disappeared on antitoxoplasmosis therapy.

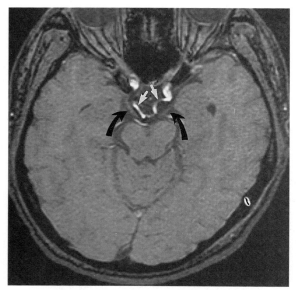

FIGURE 19–10. Posterior communicating artery–third nerve relationship. The relationship of posterior communicating arteries *(straight arrows)* to third nerves *(curved arrows)* is well demonstrated in this 1.5-mm slice of a three-dimensional time-of-flight MR angiogram. Posterior communicating artery aneurysms typically project laterally, posteriorly, and inferiorly and often present with compression of the cisternal segment of the third nerve.

CRANIAL NERVE V (TRIGEMINAL)

The trigeminal nerve arises from several nuclei in the pons and exits the midpons to run through the prepontine cistern into Meckel's cave (an anterior outpouching of the prepontine cistern) and the cavernous sinus. The sensory component of the fifth cranial nerve includes cutaneous sensation for the entire face and much of the scalp, mediated by the ophthalmic, maxillary, and mandibular divisions of the fifth nerve.

The maxillary nerve exits through the foramen rotundum, and the ophthalmic division continues anteriorly through the cavernous sinus to enter the orbit through the superior orbital fissure. In addition to cutaneous innervation of the face, sensation of the mucosa of the paranasal sinuses and the nasopharynx and oropharynx as well as the teeth and the anterior two thirds of the tongue is supplied.

The fifth nerve motor fibers course with the mandibular nerve through the foramen ovale to innervate

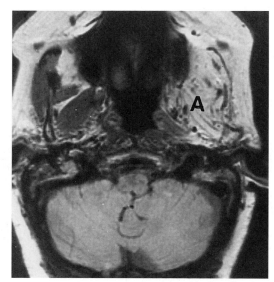

FIGURE 19–12. Denervation atrophy of masticator muscles. T1-weighted axial image reveals fatty infiltration (A) of muscles supplied by the mandibular branch of the left fifth nerve. Adenocystic cancer had spread along the nerve (not shown), causing denervation of masticator muscles. Note normal right masticator muscles.

the muscles of mastication in the infratemporal fossa. Motor dysfunction results in denervation atrophy, seen readily on T1-weighted MR images owing to the characteristic signal changes of fatty replacement in the atrophied muscles (Fig. 19–12). Acute denervation may cause an inflammatory reaction with increased signal intensity on long-TR images and contrast enhancement. This can easily be misinterpreted as infection or tumor (Fig. 19–13). The most common lesion involving the more distal portions of the motor division of the mandibular nerve is a mass lesion originating at the base of the skull (e.g., nasopharyngeal carcinoma, adenoid cystic carcinoma, lymphoma, or metastasis). Perineural spread of these tumors is common.[12-14]

The spinal nucleus of the fifth nerve (pain and temperature) is elongated vertically, extending from the midbrain down to the upper cervical cord level (C-2 to C-4). Thus, a lesion at the upper cervical level may cause a facial neuralgia. A lesion at this level usually symptomatically involves the ophthalmic division of the trigeminal nerve.[15] This region must be evaluated in these patients (Fig. 19–14).

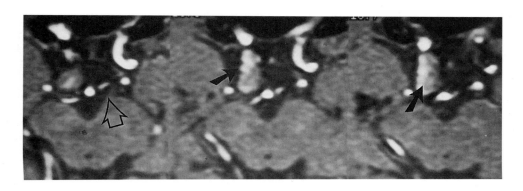

FIGURE 19–11. Posterior communicating artery aneurysm. The patient presented with a headache, right oculomotor palsy, and dilated right pupil. Source images of MR angiogram show flow into the right posterior communicating artery aneurysm *(solid arrows)*. Note the position of the cisternal segment of the normal left third nerve *(open arrow)*.

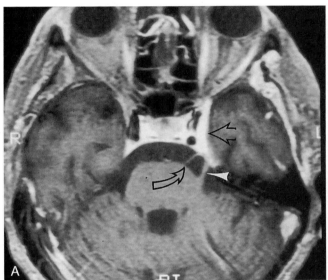

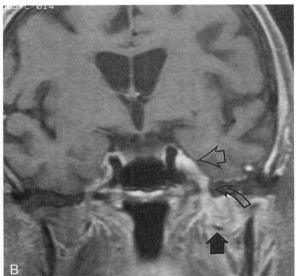

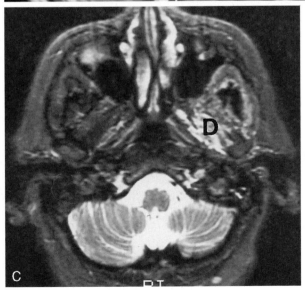

FIGURE 19–13. Hypernephroma metastasis. *A*, Gadolinium-enhanced T1-weighted axial image reveals enhancing mass in left cavernous sinus *(straight arrow)*. Note cisternal segments of the sixth cranial nerve *(curved arrow)* and fifth cranial nerve *(arrowhead)*. *B*, Coronal enhanced T1-weighted image reveals an abnormally enlarged enhancing mandibular branch of the trigeminal nerve widening the cavernous sinus *(straight open arrow)* and extending through the foramen ovale *(curved arrow)* into the enhancing left masticator space *(solid arrow)*. *C*, T2-weighted image shows high signal intensity in the left masticator space (D) secondary to an inflammatory response caused by acute denervation of the motor division of the fifth cranial nerve. There was no tumor in the masticator space.

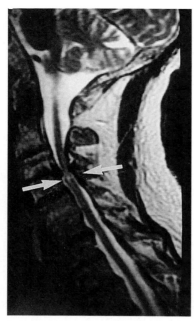

FIGURE 19–14. Lesion of spinal tract of trigeminal nerve. Cervical spine stenosis causing symptoms referable to spinal nucleus and tract of cranial nerve V. Patient had facial numbness and paresthesia as well as Horner's syndrome. Note marked spinal stenosis at C-3 and C-4 and an abnormal bright signal pattern in the cord *(arrows)* at C-3 and C-4.

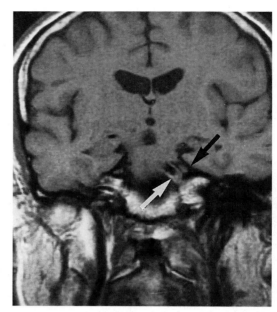

FIGURE 19–15. Tic douloureux: vascular compression of fifth cranial nerve. Coronal T1-weighted image shows the dolichoectatic basilar artery *(white arrow)* compressing the cisternal segment of the fifth cranial nerve *(black arrow)*.

Intrinsic disease or extrinsic compression can affect the cisternal portion of cranial nerve V. Vascular loops or tortuous branches of the vertebrobasilar trunk can transmit vascular pulsations against the fifth nerve trunk, giving rise to trigeminal neuralgia (tic douloureux) (Fig. 19–15). Trigeminal neuralgia is characterized by paroxysms of pain occurring along the second or third sensory divisions of the fifth nerve. High-resolution MRI with thin sections can provide the capability to noninvasively identify tortuous vessels that may visibly impinge on the fifth nerve trunk in affected patients. Source images of MR angiograms may be particularly helpful. Operative intervention that moves tortuous vessels away from the affected nerve may be successful in treating this syndrome. Other cranial nerves can be similarly affected.

Nerve sheath tumors of the fifth nerve are not rare, although they are 10 times less frequent than eighth nerve vestibular neuromas. Patients with fifth nerve neuromas usually present with facial sensory symptoms. These neuromas may form a characteristic dumb-bell configuration if the neuroma is situated in both the posterior and middle cranial fossa. If the neuroma is more peripheral, expansion of the foramen rotundum or ovale may be noted. These tumors more commonly arise from the cisternal segment of the fifth nerve in the pons (Fig. 19–16). They may straddle the incisura, erode the petrous apex, and partially fill or obliterate Meckel's cave, which is a CSF outpouching of the prepontine cistern that extends into the cavernous sinus area. Masses in this area may displace the dural margin of the cavernous sinus outward (Fig. 19–17).

Ophthalmoplegia may result from pressure on or involvement of cranial nerves in the cavernous sinus region and include carotid-cavernous fistula, aneurysm, neuroma, metastasis, and Tolosa-Hunt syndrome (nonspecific inflammatory disease of cavernous sinus).

CRANIAL NERVE VI (ABDUCENS)

Dysfunction of the sixth nerve results in a strabismus in which the globe will not rotate laterally beyond the

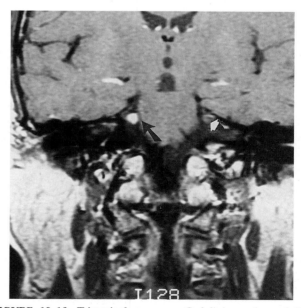

FIGURE 19–16. Trigeminal neuroma. Gadolinium-enhanced T1-weighted coronal image reveals an enlarged enhancing cisternal segment of the right fifth nerve *(black arrow)*. Note the normal size of the nonenhancing left fifth cranial nerve *(white arrow)*.

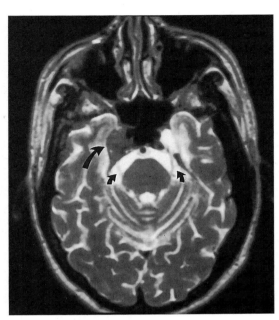

FIGURE 19–17. Metastasis. T2-weighted axial image reveals obliteration of normal CSF-filled Meckel's cave by a mass *(large arrow)* in a patient with facial pain. Note expansion of the convex dural margin by the mass. Note also the cisternal portions of the fifth nerve bilaterally *(small arrows)*.

position of forward gaze. The patient is unable to maintain binocular vision on attempted gaze to the affected side because the lateral rectus is paralyzed. Sixth nerve palsy is frequently a nonspecific, nonlocalizing finding resulting from trauma or hydrocephalus, or it may be associated with microvascular disease (e.g., diabetes, multiple sclerosis, or brain stem masses).

The nucleus of the abducens nerve is in a paramedian location close to the ventral aspect of the fourth ventricle in the pontine tegmentum. The internal genu of the ipsilateral facial (seventh) nerve courses around the sixth nerve nucleus, producing an elevation in the floor of the fourth ventricle called the facial colliculus. Involvement of the sixth nerve nucleus usually produces seventh nerve findings as well (Fig. 19–18). The sixth nerve exits from the ventral aspect of the pontomedullary junction and extends along the clivus to reach the cavernous sinus.

The medial longitudinal fasciculus is located just anterior to the floor of the fourth ventricle and aqueduct and extends from the oculomotor nucleus to the abducens nucleus. Exquisite coordination between the third, fourth, and sixth cranial nerves is mediated through the medial longitudinal fasciculus. Involvement of this coordination center by tumor, multiple sclerosis, infarction, or other pathologic process can cause an intranuclear ophthalmoplegia.[4]

CRANIAL NERVE VII (FACIAL)

The motor nucleus of the seventh nerve is situated in the ventral pons, and its fibers extend posteriorly

toward the floor of the fourth ventricle, course around the sixth nerve nucleus, and then proceed anteriorly to emerge from the brain stem at the lateral aspect of the pontomedullary junction to enter the cerebellopontine angle cistern. The cisternal segment of the seventh nerve enters the internal auditory canal where it becomes the superior-anterior nerve bundle and is accompanied by the three branches of the eighth nerve. The fibers of the seventh nerve progress to the geniculate ganglion within the petrous temporal bone. The geniculate ganglion is a parasympathetic synapse site for sensory neurons receiving taste and cutaneous sensibility. As it exits the stylomastoid foramen, the seventh nerve enters the parotid gland and innervates the muscles of facial expression in addition to the posterior belly of the digastric muscle, the stylohyoid, and the platysma muscles. A lesion of the brain stem nucleus or the peripheral seventh nerve (lower motor neuron) affects all the muscles of the face. In supranuclear cortical lesions, function of the frontalis and orbicularis muscles is maintained.

The solitary nucleus of the seventh nerve in the dorsolateral pons receives special sensory fibers for taste from the anterior two thirds of the tongue. Parasympathetic innervation to the submandibular and sublingual glands and to the lacrimal gland runs with the seventh nerve.

The seventh nerve is vulnerable to mass lesions in the brain stem, lesions within the cerebellopontine angle cistern, and lesions within the petrous bone. Dolichoectasia of the vertebrobasilar vessels may cause hemifacial spasm[16] (Fig. 19–19). The seventh nerve is quite susceptible to trauma, especially as a result of

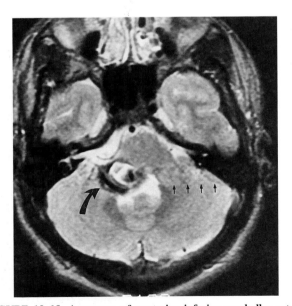

FIGURE 19–18. Aneurysm of posterior inferior cerebellar artery. T2-weighted axial image shows a mass with various signal intensities. Flow void *(large arrow)* is evident on all sequences. Note a motion artifact in the phase-encoding direction *(small arrows)* emanating from the lesion and confirming flow and the vascular nature of lesion. The patient presented with right sixth and seventh nerve dysfunction. Note compression of the right facial colliculus in the floor of the fourth ventricle.

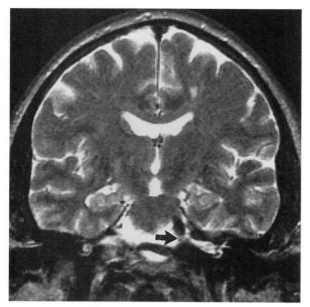

FIGURE 19–19. Hemifacial spasm related to dolichoectasia of vertebro basilar system. T2-weighted coronal image shows ectatic basilar artery *(arrow)* in the cerebellopontine angle cistern in the region of the seventh cranial nerve. The patient had a long history of hypertension.

transverse petrous bone fractures that may sever or contuse the nerve. Inflammatory conditions in the temporal bone can also produce seventh nerve paralysis.[17] Bell's palsy is an uncomplicated seventh nerve palsy that progressively improves. It most likely is a result of viral inflammatory swelling of the facial nerve within the narrow bony confines of the petrous bone.[18, 19]

Ramsay Hunt syndrome is a varicella viral infection with a predilection for the seventh nerve. Patients usually have a vesicular eruption on the surrounding skin. Occasionally, the eighth nerve is involved if the inflammatory response spreads into the internal auditory canal (Fig. 19–20). Gadolinium enhancement may be seen with neuritis, involving the seventh nerve either along its entire course or part of its course.[20]

Seventh nerve neuromas are rare and occur most often in the descending portion of the facial canal within the petrous bone; they may also be found in the internal auditory canal. Unlike acoustic neuromas, seventh nerve neuromas in the internal auditory canal may erode the upper surface of the petrous bone and may extend to the geniculate ganglion region (Fig. 19–21). Compressive symptoms of the seventh nerve may be a late finding if the tumor decompresses into the temporal bone air cavities.

Investigation of seventh nerve palsies should attempt to ascertain the clinical level of the dysfunction. An isolated lower motor neuron seventh nerve palsy affecting only the muscles of facial expression implicates a lesion in the lower stylomastoid foramen or in the parotid gland. Loss of taste in the anterior two thirds of the tongue indicates a more proximal lesion located in the stylomastoid canal above the origin of the chorda tympani. Hyperacusis due to pathologic involvement of the stapedius nerve causes an unpleasant awareness of loud sounds and places the lesion in the upper portion of the facial nerve canal. A loss of lacrimation on the ipsilateral side would localize the pathologic process even more proximally to at least the level of the geniculate ganglion in the petrous bone. Additional findings of either vestibular dysfunction or sensorineural hearing loss would place the lesion more proximally, either in the cistern of the cerebellopontine angle or in the internal auditory canal (see also Chapter 32).

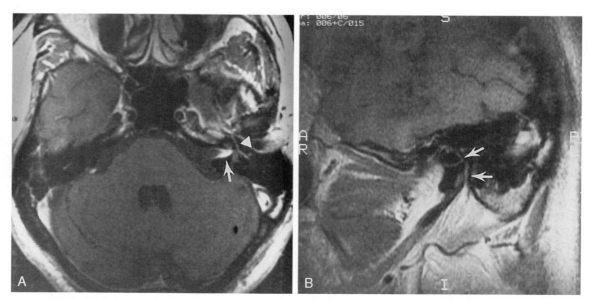

FIGURE 19–20. Ramsay Hunt syndrome. *A,* Axial T1-weighted postgadolinium image reveals enhancement in the left lateral internal auditory canal *(arrow)* and left horizontal petrous portion of facial nerve *(arrowhead).* Note lack of enhancement on the right. *B,* Sagittal image reveals enhancement of the descending facial nerve *(arrows)* in petrous bone.

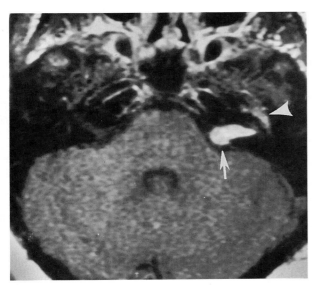

FIGURE 19–21. Facial nerve neuroma. Axial postgadolinium image shows an enhancing internal auditory canal mass with the typical "ice cream cone" appearance of acoustic neuroma at the meatus *(arrow).* However, note enhancement in the region of the geniculate ganglion and horizontal intrapetrous facial nerve *(arrowhead).* A neuroma of the seventh nerve was found at surgery.

CRANIAL NERVE VIII (VESTIBULOCOCHLEAR)

Patients with neurosensory hearing loss should have imaging studies along the entire auditory pathway from the labyrinthine level to the superior temporal gyrus.[21–26] Auditory signals are sent from the inner ear through the cochlear nerve in the internal auditory canal through the cerebellopontine angle to the eighth nerve cochlear nucleus on the ventrolateral pontomedullary junction. In the brain stem, auditory fibers ascend both ipsilaterally and contralaterally in the lateral lemniscus of the brain stem to the inferior colliculus. Postganglionic axons are then transmitted to neurons of the medial geniculate body in the thalamus. The terminal sensory pathway extends from the medial geniculate body to the auditory cortex in the superior temporal gyrus.

The vestibular nerve courses alongside the cochlear nerve and the seventh nerve in the internal auditory canal. It has two divisions, superior and inferior, that penetrate the brain stem at the pontomedullary junction, terminating in the vestibular nuclear complex. Dysfunction is manifested by vertigo, dizziness, unsteadiness, and visceral symptoms such as diarrhea, nausea, and vomiting.

Eighth nerve neuromas constitute 80% to 90% of cerebellopontine angle tumors. Meningiomas constitute about 10% of masses in this region, epidermoids about 5%, and primary malignancies and metastatic disease about 2%. Other tumors (e.g., arachnoid cysts, lateral fourth ventricular ependymomas, and choroid plexus papillomas), infections, and inflammatory diseases are rare in this region (see also Chapter 32).[27]

Acoustic Neuroma

Acoustic neuromas are benign fibrous tumors that arise from the Schwann cells that cover the vestibular portion of the eighth cranial nerve. Schwann cells produce myelin around peripheral nerves. Eighth nerve neuromas make up 10% of all primary intracranial tumors and well over 80% of all cerebellopontine angle tumors. Malignant transformation is rare. Patients with acoustic neuromas present with tinnitus, vertigo, and sensorineural hearing loss. Patients with larger tumors may have fifth or seventh nerve findings, other cranial neuropathies, cerebellar ataxia, and hydrocephalus.

Sophisticated audiologic testing can detect tumors as small as 0.5 mm, but imaging is needed to accurately localize and characterize these tumors. Plain films, tomographic studies, and CT have traditionally been used to demonstrate flaring of the porus acusticus, widening of the internal auditory canal, and amputation of the posterior lip of the internal auditory meatus by the classic funnel-shaped acoustic neuroma extending out of the canal. CT and CT–air cisternography improved the detection and evaluation of cerebellopontine angle tumors. However, MRI is now the imaging modality of choice.[28]

Narrow slice thickness (3 mm or less) and a small field of view (less than 20 cm) are important to give adequate spatial resolution. Most acoustic neuromas are well-defined, uniformly enhancing extra-axial masses centered on the internal auditory canal and forming acute angles with the petrous bone (Fig. 19–22). They may be isointense relative to brain on T1-

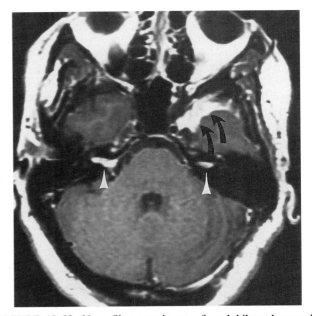

FIGURE 19–22. Neurofibromatosis type 2 and bilateral acoustic neuromas. Postcontrast T1-weighted axial image reveals bilateral acoustic neuromas *(arrowheads).* The right acoustic neuroma has the typical ice cream cone appearance of the cisternal segment of tumor. Tumor is totally intracanalicular on the left and was not seen without gadolinium injection. Note a sphenoid wing meningioma *(arrows).* Meningiomas are common in patients with neurofibromatosis type 2.

weighted images, but a majority have slightly prolonged T1. Most are moderately increased in signal intensity and moderately heterogeneous on T2-weighted images. The signal intensity of small acoustic neuromas is usually close to normal brain. In small tumors, partial-volume effects may result in an uneven or unpredictable signal intensity. More subtle signs of an acoustic neuroma include obscuration of the margins of the seventh and eighth nerves and displacement of CSF signal from the internal auditory canal.[28, 29]

The capillaries of acoustic neuromas do not have a blood-brain barrier, and these tumors markedly enhance with gadolinium. They usually appear more homogeneous after contrast material is administered. Contrast enhancement is greatest at 3 minutes after injection and then declines.

In larger tumors (2 cm) that indent the adjoining cerebellum and cause rotational deformity of the brain stem, hemorrhage and cystic areas are common. Calcification is rare. Cystic areas probably represent necrosis secondary to hemorrhage. Large acoustic neuromas widen the adjacent ipsilateral subarachnoid space in the cerebellopontine angle cistern as they displace the brain stem to the other side. With large tumors, a hypointense rim of vascular flow voids is often present owing to displacement of petrosal veins.

Localization with multiplanar MRI is optimal for planning the surgical approach to these tumors (i.e., suboccipital, translabyrinthine, or transtemporal). The recommended pulse sequences have been outlined previously.[30]

A diagnosis of small intracanalicular acoustic neuromas should be made with caution. Viral, bacterial, and granulomatous infections may enhance with gadolinium and mimic intracanalicular or even cerebellopontine angle acoustic neuromas. Thus, with small enhancing lessons, data points at two different times should be obtained before operative intervention is considered so that there is reasonable proof that there is indeed a growing mass in the canal and not a self-limited process.

There are several possible pitfalls in the MRI evaluation of acoustic neuroma.[31] It is essential that nonenhanced T1-weighted images be obtained before gadolinium images to note high T1 signal intensity that may exist before contrast medium is injected; hemangiomas, vascular malformations, or trauma may bleed and have of increased signal intensity on T1-weighted images owing to presence of methemoglobin. Patients may also have high-signal-intensity lipomas on T1-weighted images.

Postsurgical MRI evaluation of acoustic neuroma is best performed with a baseline scan done soon after surgery with precontrast T1-weighted images and fat-suppressed postgadolinium imaging. Postsurgical enhancement in the internal auditory canal and meninges of the petrous ridge is not uncommon and is usually of no clinical importance. This enhancement should not be misinterpreted as infection or residual or recurring tumor unless sequential scans show

growth. Fat suppression is necessary because surgeons often pack the surgical site with fat.

Ninety percent of patients with neurofibromatosis type 2, a defect on chromosome 22, present with acoustic neuromas, which may be bilateral. Multiple neurofibromas, meningiomas, and gliomas of ependymal origin may be present. Optic gliomas are not seen in this syndrome, and café au lait spots and cutaneous neurofibromas are less prevalent than in neurofibromatosis type 1. Type 2 disease is much less common than type 1 disease, occurring only in 1 in 50,000 births. Less than 10% of patients with eighth nerve neuromas have neurofibromatosis type 2.

Intracranial neurofibromas are unusual except in patients with with neurofibromatosis. Unlike schwannomas, neurofibromas tend to grow within the nerve and entangle the adjacent nerve fibers, making resection difficult. They are more prone to malignant degeneration.

About 5% of acoustic neuromas are associated with arachnoid cysts. When arachnoid cysts are seen in the cerebellopontine angle cistern, a careful search for an acoustic neuroma must be done. Acoustic neuromas are generally somewhat inhomogeneous and have less signal intensity on T2-weighted images than arachnoid cysts. Arachnoid cysts are smoothly marginated and are isointense relative to CSF[32] (Fig. 19–23).

Less than 5% of patients with unilateral neurosensory hearing loss have acoustic neuromas. Vascular disease (e.g., infarcts, superficial siderosis), cochlear disease, multiple sclerosis, petrous bone or brain stem trauma, intrapetrous lesions, and other mass lesions

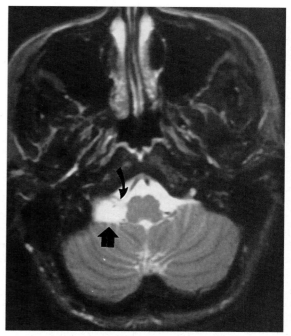

FIGURE 19–23. Arachnoid cyst. T2-weighted axial image reveals a mass *(thick arrow)* isointense relative to CSF. This was true on all sequences. Note anterior displacement of the 9th and 10th nerves *(curved arrow)* in the cerebellopontine angle cistern. The patient had appropriate symptoms.

are other causes of neurosensory hearing loss. Transverse fractures of the petrous bone may sever the cochlear nerve. Multiple sclerosis or an infarct involving the cochlear nucleus and crossing fibers in the trapezoid body of the brain stem may cause sudden unilateral hearing loss.

In the evaluation of eighth cranial nerve findings, the cochlear and the vestibular apparatus must be evaluated. CT and MRI are complementary in this anatomic area. CT evaluates bony erosion as well as abnormal bony productive changes best. MRI better displays soft tissue changes of masses and inflammatory processes.

Cochlear otosclerosis is a cause of sensorineural hearing loss that usually shows lysis and blurring of the bony margins of the cochlea before productive changes are noted. MRI may reveal perivascular enhancement, suggesting an inflammatory process in the cochlea.

Labyrinthine ossificans often occurs after an acute inflammation (e.g., meningitis) and demonstrates marked ossification on CT scans. This dense calcification can be identified on MR images by noting no signal intensity in the region of the membranous labyrinth, where bright signal intensity on long-TR images is normally seen.

Meningioma

Meningiomas occur in the posterior fossa and commonly cause cranial neuropathies (especially involving cranial nerves V, VII, and VIII), mass effect on the cerebellum and brain stem, and hydrocephalus. Meningiomas are the second most common cerebellopontine angle tumor, constituting 10% to 15% of tumors in this region. They occur in middle age and have a 3:1 female predominance. Occasionally, they invade the temporal bone or dural sinuses.

Meningiomas are often isointense or nearly isointense relative to brain on both long- and short-TR images and may be easily overlooked if gradient-echo (increased sensitivity to calcium due to magnetic susceptibility) or postcontrast imaging is not performed. They have a broad-based dural attachment and, in contradistinction to the spherical appearance of acoustic neuromas and their acute-angle relationship to the petrous bone, meningiomas are often hemispheric in appearance and make an obtuse angle with the temporal bone. Although meningiomas can invade the internal auditory canal directly or cause dural reaction in it, the canal is rarely widened and the cisternal portions of the meningiomas are rarely centered on the canal. Visualization of normal seventh and eighth nerve bundles helps differentiate meningioma from acoustic neuroma.[33]

Meningiomas often incite hyperostotic changes in adjacent bones. This can be noted by careful inspection of the petrous bone with MRI, but it is far easier to recognize by CT with bone windows. Vascular pedicles are sometimes seen as flow voids in or adjacent to meningiomas.

A dural tail (contrast enhancement of the dura) is a sign of either tumor infiltration or nonspecific dural fibrotic, vascular, or reactive changes. It is suggestive of, but not diagnostic of, meningioma (Fig. 19–24) and has been seen with neuromas, inflammatory disease, and metastatic disease (see also Chapter 17).

Epidermoid Tumors

Epidermoid tumors, which are sequestered congenital inclusions of ectoderm that form early in fetal life,

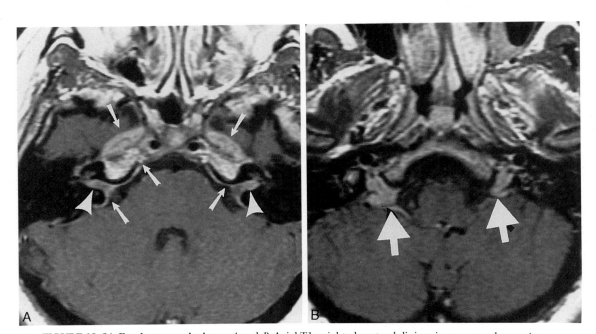

FIGURE 19–24. En plaque meningioma. *A* and *B,* Axial T1-weighted postgadolinium images reveal a contiguous bilateral and symmetric enhancing process *(A, small arrows)* involving dura of petrous apices, Meckel's cave, cavernous sinus, middle cranial fossa, cerebellopontine angle, internal auditory canal *(arrowheads)*, and jugular foramen *(B, large arrows).*

are the third most common lesion in the cerebellopontine angle cistern (Fig. 19–25), representing less than 5% of masses in this location. They tend to spread along CSF spaces but may invaginate or burrow into the adjacent brain. They usually have undulating borders, and sometimes CSF is visible in the interstices of the tumor.

Most epidermoid tumors are nearly isointense with CSF on all pulse sequences. The tumor is frequently best distinguished from CSF by subtle changes in signal intensity on the proton density–weighted image.[34–37] However, asymmetry of the involved cisterns or subtle displacement of adjacent structures must be carefully noted to diagnose epidermoid tumors. A minority (10% to 20%) of epidermoids are bright on T1-weighted images, owing to blood products, protein content, calcium, or fat content. Epidermoids rarely enhance with contrast material. They may seed the CSF pathways with tumor particles. The seeding may be asymptomatic or cause a chemical meningitis, communicating hydrocephalus, or both (see also Chapter 17).[38]

CRANIAL NERVES IX (GLOSSOPHARYNGEAL), X (VAGUS), AND XI (SPINAL ACCESSORY)

Cranial nerves IX, X, and XI are usually clinically involved together. Isolated paresis in only one of these nerves is uncommon. These cranial nerves receive impulses from several common sources, and their functions overlap. They penetrate the jugular foramen in a compact bundle, predisposing to mixed neuropathy in the event of compression or destruction of the base of the skull in this area.[39–40] Patients presenting with

signs of 9th, 10th, and 11th cranial nerve disease should be imaged to the carotid bifurcation.

The ninth cranial nerve supplies cutaneous sensibility and taste to the posterior third of the tongue as well as sensation for the tonsils, pharynx, and soft palate and innervates the parotid gland.

The 10th nerve contains both sensory and motor fibers and involves sensation for the mucosa of the pharynx, larynx, and abdominal viscera. The vagus nerve originates from the medulla in the groove between the inferior cerebellar peduncle and the olive. If lower vagus nerve dysfunction is present (i.e., vocal cord paralysis), images inferior to the aorta-pulmonary window on the left or to the thoracic inlet on the right must be obtained.

The 11th cranial nerve originates from motor cells of the anterior horn gray matter from the first through fifth cervical levels and ascends through the foramen magnum to join its cranial portion and then courses with the 9th and 10th nerves into the jugular foramen. The 11th nerve innervates the trapezius and sternocleidomastoid muscles.

Neuromas of any of the 9th, 10th, or 11th cranial nerves may occur near the jugular foramen and compress the three nerves (Fig. 19–26). They usually displace the flow void of the jugular vein forward, unlike glomus tumors, which usually compress or fill the jugular vein. Schwannomas usually have high signal intensity on T2-weighted images, do not usually have flow voids, and enhance dramatically. Bone erosion from schwannomas is usually smooth and well defined.

Glomus tumors (chemodectoma, paraganglioma) may occur in the jugular foramen.[41, 42] Other locations are the tympanic cavity and carotid bifurcation. This is usually a more vascular tumor than schwannomas on

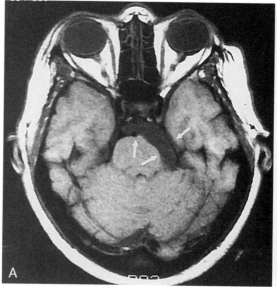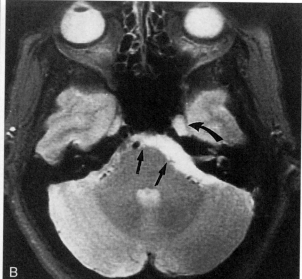

FIGURE 19–25. Epidermoid tumor. *A*, Distortion of left side of pons by mass *(arrows)* nearly isointense relative to CSF is seen on axial T1-weighted image. The mass fills the cerebellopontine angle and prepontine cistern and engulfs the basilar artery. The patient had left fifth nerve numbness. *B*, T2-weighted image shows tumor hyperintense relative to CSF *(straight arrows)*. Note tumor infiltration into left Meckel's cave *(curved arrow)*. Normal right Meckel's cave remains isointense relative to normal CSF in the right cerebellopontine angle cistern.

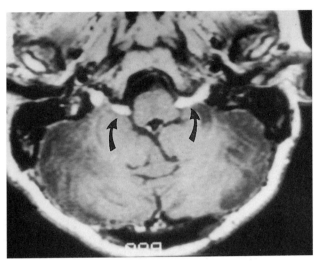

FIGURE 19–26. Bilateral neuromas at jugular foramen. Enhanced T1-weighted axial image shows marked enlargement and marked enhancement of nerve bundles of cranial nerves IX, X, and XI *(curved arrows)* as they leave the medulla and enter the jugular foramen, consistent with bilateral neuromas in a patient with neurofibromatosis type 2.

angiograms or enhanced MR images. However, schwannomas can also be quite vascular. Glomus tumors (chemodectomas) are benign but are locally invasive and recur if not completely excised. Rarely, they are malignant and metastasize. Glomus tumors rarely are catecholamine-secreting tumors. They occur in adults with a 2:1 female predominance and present with pulsating tinnitus and some combination of 7th through 12th cranial neuropathies.

Glomus tumors are inhomogeneous, owing to the many flow voids. They are usually isointense relative to brain on T1-weighted images and have increased signal intensity on T2 weighting. They are vascular on angiograms and enhance dramatically after administration of contrast material. They usually displace the flow void of the carotid artery forward. Jugular vein patency can be assessed with gradient-echo sequences if necessary, but the spin-echo images often demonstrate whether the jugular vein is patent (Fig. 19–27).

Other neoplasms can destroy bone and compress cranial nerves at the skull base in the vicinity of the jugular foramen (e.g., metastasis, chordoma, or sarcoma). Neuromas in the carotid sheath or other mass lesions (e.g., vascular masses) can also compress these nerves in the carotid sheath below the jugular foramen. Carotid body tumors can splay the external and internal carotid arteries and compress the cranial nerves in the carotid sheath (see also Chapter 32).

CRANIAL NERVE XII (HYPOGLOSSAL)

The hypoglossal nerve provides motor function to the tongue, providing innervation to the intrinsic muscles as well as the extrinsic muscles of the tongue: styloglossus, hyoglossus, and genioglossus.

The motor nucleus of the 12th cranial nerve is in the paramedian medulla. Fibers of the hypoglossal nerve exit the brain stem between the pyramid and olive and proceed forward to the hypoglossal canal just above the anterior lateral lip of the foramen magnum. The 12th cranial nerve then descends inferiorly along the carotid sheath just medial to the 9th, 10th, and 11th cranial nerves. A 12th nerve paresis causes wasting and fatty replacement of the ipsilateral tongue muscle, best seen on T1-weighted images. Isolated 12th nerve dysfunction could be caused by a vascular insult, multiple sclerosis (Fig. 19–28), or compression within the medullary cistern or hypoglossal canal caused by a mass lesion. Dysfunction of the 12th nerve results in deviation of the tongue to the affected side, owing to the unopposed action of the contralateral normal genioglossus muscle.

Foramen magnum meningiomas may cause lower cranial neuropathies, brain stem compression, or long tract signs. Symptoms classically mimic multiple sclerosis.

INFECTION

Basal meningeal processes can cause enhancement of the pia and dura of the basal cisterns and posterior fossa. Dural enhancement may be nonspecific and secondary to previous shunting, surgery, head injury, or even lumbar puncture. Lymphomatous or carcinomatous meningitis can have this appearance. Sarcoid, Lyme disease, herpesvirus infections, syphilis, tuberculosis, and other inflammatory processes may also present in this way. Enhancing cranial nerves may or may not be symptomatic. Communicating hydrocephalus may result from malignant or infectious meningitis.

Bacterial and fungal abscesses may involve the brain stem and cerebellum. They may be blood borne, may extend from the adjacent sphenoidal sinuses (Fig. 19–29) or mastoids, or result from open trauma. Inflammatory diseases (i.e., sarcoid), Lyme disease, viral diseases (i.e., herpes), syphilis, and granulomatous infections may all cause cranial neuropathies as well. Immunocompromised individuals, intravenous drug abusers, and diabetic patients are especially prone to CNS infections. Many of our patients with cranial neuropathies are infected with human immunodeficiency virus. Infection may seed along CSF pathways. Enhanced images must be obtained for these individuals or significant pathologic processes will not be demonstrated (see Chapter 20).

CEREBROVASCULAR DISEASE

The cerebellum and brain stem are supplied by the vertebrobasilar system and its branches. The patency of the vertebrobasilar system is usually well evaluated by routine spin-echo imaging. One potential pitfall is the presence of an acute clot in the basilar artery with deoxyhemoglobin of low signal intensity on long-TR images mimicking normal flow void. The clot may be visible but difficult to discern on T1-weighted images

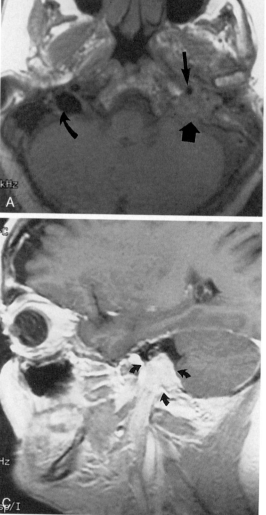
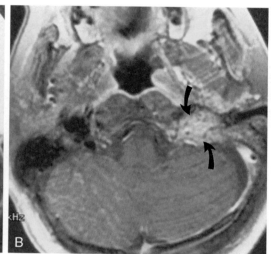

FIGURE 19–27. Glomus jugular tumor. *A,* T1-weighted axial image reveals a heterogeneous soft tissue mass *(wide arrow)* in the left jugular fossa. Note anterior displacement of the left carotid artery flow void *(thin arrow).* Left jugular vein flow void is not seen. Note the normal right carotid and jugular vein *(curved arrow). B,* Postcontrast T1-weighted axial image shows marked tumor enhancement *(arrows).* Note multiple low-signal-intensity flow voids within the tumor. *C,* Postcontrast sagittal T1-weighted image accurately depicts tumor filling the left jugular fossa *(arrows).* (Case courtesy of Sheldon Kleiman, MD, La Jolla, CA.)

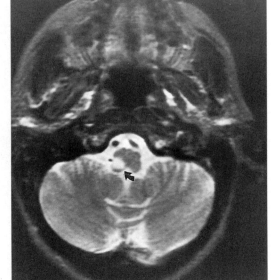

FIGURE 19–28. Multiple sclerosis. T2-weighted axial image with hyperintensity *(arrow)* near the nucleus of the right hypoglossal (12th cranial) nerve in a patient with multiple sclerosis. Ipsilateral hemiatrophy and fatty infiltration of tongue were present (not shown).

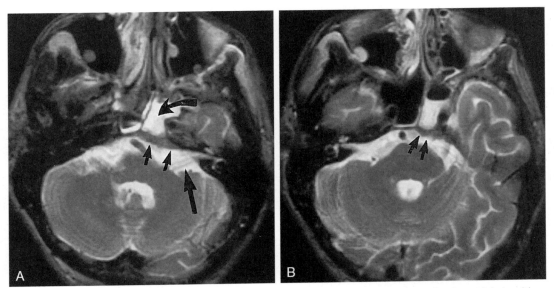

FIGURE 19–29. Epidural abscess. *A* and *B,* Adjoining T2-weighted axial images reveal sphenoidal sinusitis. *Pseudomonas* in the left sphenoidal sinus *(curved arrow)* has eroded into clivus (not shown) and left basilar cisterns *(small arrows).* A 36-year-old patient infected with human immunodeficiency virus presented with multiple left cranial neuropathies. Note left seventh and eighth nerves in the left cerebellopontine angle cistern *(large arrow).*

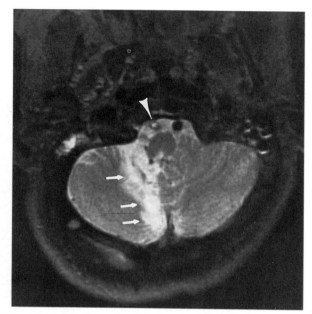

FIGURE 19–30. Posterior inferior cerebellar stroke. Axial T2-weighted image showing abnormal hyperintensity in distribution of the posterior inferior cerebellar artery vascular territory *(small arrows)* and abnormal signal intensity in the right vertebral artery, representing thrombus *(arrowhead)*.

until methemoglobin appears. MR angiography may be of help in selected cases in evaluating the patency of the vertebrobasilar system as well as evaluating possible dissection of the vertebral artery. Vertebral dissections usually take place above the foramen transversarium of C-2 as the vertebral artery courses posteriorly and medially to enter the foramen magnum. Posterior infe-

rior cerebellar artery infarcts are often seen in this clinical setting (see Chapter 23).

Gadolinium enhancement improves the sensitivity and specificity of MRI to acute infarcts. Gradient-echo images are especially sensitive in documenting hemorrhage or patency of vessels.

Many patients with cerebellar infarction have premonitory symptoms of gait disorders, nausea and vomiting, or brain stem symptoms. Patients who do not develop significant mass effect on the fourth ventricle, aqueduct, and brain stem generally have a good prognosis. Patients with extensive mass effect often do poorly.

Cerebellar infarcts often show changes in classic anatomic configurations of the posterior inferior cerebellar artery (80% to 90% of cerebellar infarcts) (Fig. 19–30), the anterior inferior cerebellar artery, or the superior cerebellar artery. Smaller infarcts are usually wedge shaped, extending to the cortical gray matter of the cerebellum. Proton density–weighted images are often valuable both in distinguishing acute infarct (brighter than CSF) from chronic infarct (isointense relative to CSF) and in differentiating small infarcts from normal CSF spaces (e.g., the cisterna magna) (Fig. 19–31).

A classic brain stem infarct is in a paramedian location with a sharp medial border secondary to occlusion of a penetrating branch of the basilar artery (Fig. 19–32). More catastrophic events (e.g., occlusion of the basilar artery itself) may cause infarcts in multiple locations in the brain stem and may demonstrate bilateral findings both clinically and with MRI. Microvascular disease, old multiple sclerosis, and white matter diseases associated with hypertension may show diffusely abnormal signal throughout the brain stem. The

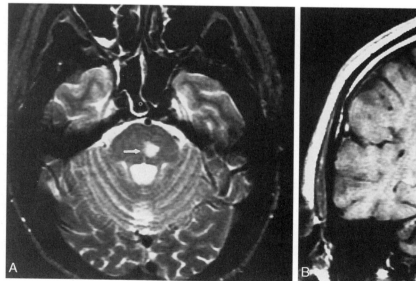

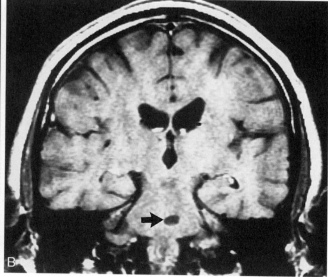

FIGURE 19–31. Pontine infarction. T2-weighted axial image *(A)* and T1-weighted coronal image *(B)* reveal a lesion isointense relative to CSF signal in the left paramedian pons. Note the sharp medial border *(arrow)*. This is the classic location and appearance for pontine stroke resulting from thrombosis of a pontine perforating artery. Flow void was preserved in the basilar artery on all sequences. The fact that it is so clearly seen on T1-weighted image (isointense relative to CSF) suggests that it is an old (more than 30 days) infarct. Note enlargement of the left frontal horn due to a previous basal ganglia infarct (not shown).

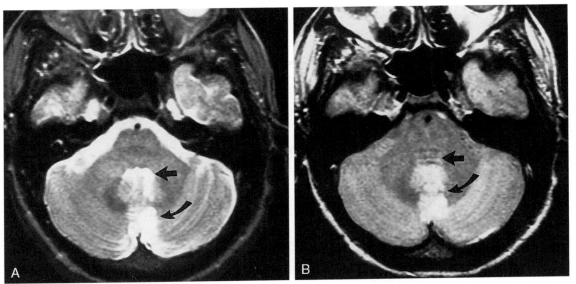

FIGURE 19–32. Vermian infarct. *A*, T2-weighted axial image could be falsely interpreted in this 72-year-old patient as a prominent fourth ventricle *(straight arrow)* and cisterna magna *(curved arrow)*. *B*, Proton density–weighted image, however, reveals a small compressed fourth ventricle *(straight arrow)*. Vermian stroke *(curved arrow)* is now obvious as increased intensity when compared with the lower CSF intensity in Meckel's cave and cerebellopontine angle cisterns.

appearance is similar to a large brain stem infarct, but these patients may be asymptomatic.

The Wallenburg (lateral medullary) syndrome is usually caused by a stroke in the vascular distribution of the posterior inferior cerebellar artery supplying the medulla (Fig. 19–33). Involvement of the nucleus ambiguous affects function in the distribution of the 9th and 10th cranial nerves, causing paralysis of the soft palate and pharyngeal musculature as well as the ipsilateral larynx. Dysarthria and dysphasia result. Involvement of the spinal trigeminal tract and nucleus (cranial nerve V) may alter facial pain and temperature sensation on the affected side. Horner's syndrome may

also be a component of the lateral medullary syndrome owing to interruption of the sympathetic tracts that descend through the lateral medulla to the superior cervical ganglion. Involvement of the vestibular nerve nucleus may cause dizziness, unsteadiness, and ataxia.

Hyponatremia in alcoholic and other poorly nourished patients, especially if corrected too rapidly, may lead to central pontine myelinolysis with devastating clinical consequences (see Chapter 27).

INTRA-AXIAL TUMORS

Intracranial tumors are the third most common malignancy in children.[43, 44] Malignancies of the lymphatic and renal organ systems are more common. More than half of intracranial tumors in the pediatric age group occur in the posterior fossa. In adults, 15% to 20% of intra-axial tumors are infratentorial. Most adult tumors are metastases (Figs. 19–34 and 19–35). Lung, breast, and melanoma metastases are most common.[45–47]

HEMANGIOBLASTOMA

Hemangioblastomas are the most common primary intra-axial tumor of the posterior fossa. They make up 7% of posterior fossa tumors in adults. The peak age at occurrence is the fifth or sixth decade. Polycythemia may be an associated finding.

Most hemangioblastomas occur in the cerebellum, but the medulla and spinal cord may be involved. Syringomyelia may be adjacent to spinal lesions. Supratentorial hemangioblastomas are rare.

The typical hemangioblastoma is a well-demarcated cystic tumor with a superficial vascular tumor nodule

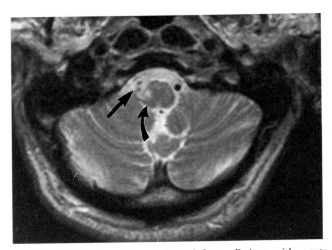

FIGURE 19–33. Lateral medullary infarct. Patient with acute Wallenburg's syndrome after vertebral artery dissection (proved by angiography) during chiropractic manipulation. Infarct *(curved arrow)* is noted in the lateral medulla. No flow void is seen in the right vertebral artery *(straight arrow)*.

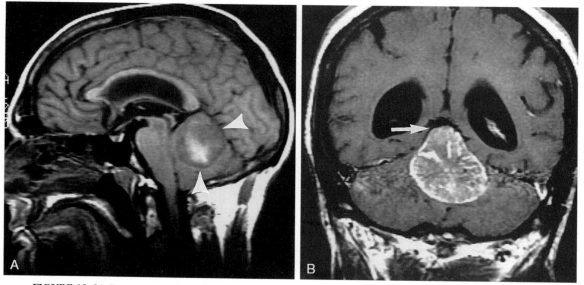

FIGURE 19–34. Lung metastasis. *A,* Sagittal T1-weighted image in a patient presenting with acute hydrocephalus and cerebellar dysfunction. Note high-signal-intensity methemoglobin *(arrowheads)* in the intra-axial metastasis with obliteration of the fourth ventricle and enlargement of the aqueduct and third ventricle. *B,* T1-weighted coronal postgadolinium image reveals enhancement of the lesion and upward herniation through the tentorial notch *(arrow).*

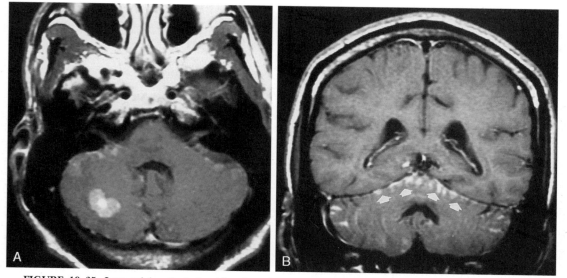

FIGURE 19–35. Intra-axial metastasis with subarachnoid tumor seeding. *A,* Axial T1-weighted postcontrast image demonstrates a right cerebellar hemisphere tumor with minimal mass effect. *B,* Coronal postcontrast T1-weighted image best demonstrates widespread subarachnoid space seeding *(arrows)* manifested by contrast enhancement.

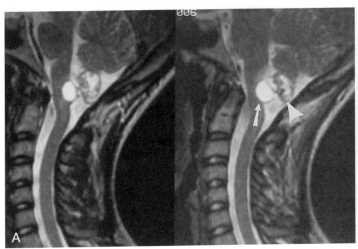

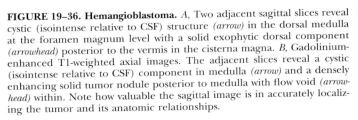

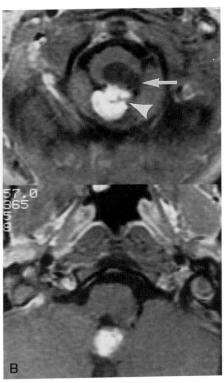

FIGURE 19–36. Hemangioblastoma. *A*, Two adjacent sagittal slices reveal cystic (isointense relative to CSF) structure *(arrow)* in the dorsal medulla at the foramen magnum level with a solid exophytic dorsal component *(arrowhead)* posterior to the vermis in the cisterna magna. *B*, Gadolinium-enhanced T1-weighted axial images. The adjacent slices reveal a cystic (isointense relative to CSF) component in medulla *(arrow)* and a densely enhancing solid tumor nodule posterior to medulla with flow void *(arrowhead)* within. Note how valuable the sagittal image is in accurately localizing the tumor and its anatomic relationships.

situated on a pial surface (Fig. 19–36). However, up to a third may be entirely solid tumors (Fig. 19–37). The nodule enhances markedly and homogeneously with contrast material. Vascular signal voids are often seen in the tumor nodule. Hemorrhage and surrounding edema are unusual. The cyst wall is not involved with tumor and rarely enhances. The cyst contents are often of CSF intensity but may differ if the protein content is elevated.[48, 49]

About 20% of hemangioblastomas are associated with von Hippel–Lindau disease, an autosomal dominant disorder with incomplete penetrance. Forty per-

cent to 60% of patients with von Hippel–Lindau disease have hemangioblastomas. These patients usually present in the third and fourth decades of life, and many have renal cell carcinomas and retinal angiomas. Thus, any patient with a hemangioblastoma should have a funduscopic examination and a renal ultrasound study. Patients with confirmed von Hippel–Lindau disease must have enhanced MRI of the brain and spine to rule out multiple hemangioblastomas. These may not be detected by CT, especially if located low in the posterior fossa or near the craniospinal junction. Multiple hemangioblastomas are seen in 20%

FIGURE 19–37. Hemangioblastoma. *A*, Coronal T2-weighted image reveals a mass of increased signal intensity impressing on the fourth ventricle. The upper margin of the mass is impossible to define because of bright CSF in the fourth ventricle. Note hydrocephalus. *B*, T1-weighted gadolinium-enhanced image shows densely enhancing tumor filling most of the fourth ventricle *(arrow)*. Note flow voids within the mass. Superior and inferior limits of the tumor are clearly seen. The patient had von Hippel–Lindau syndrome.

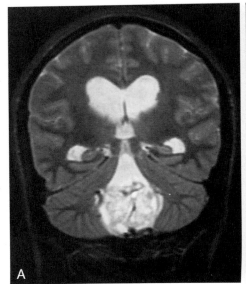

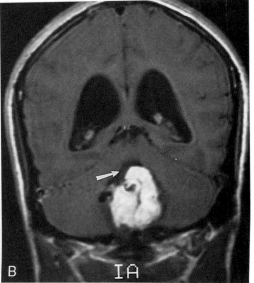

of these patients (Fig. 19–38), who may also have renal and pancreatic cysts and pheochromocytomas.[50]

MEDULLOBLASTOMA

Medulloblastomas make up the vast majority of the group of highly malignant primitive neuroectodermal tumors that also include ependymoblastoma, cerebral neuroblastoma, pinealoblastoma, medulloepithelioma, and other rare varieties. Pathologically, medulloblastomas are homogeneous and hypercellular with round cells that have a high nuclear-to-cytoplasmic ratio. Necrosis, hemorrhage, intratumoral calcium, and cysts are uncommon.[51–54]

Medulloblastomas constitute about 30% of pediatric posterior fossa neoplasms. They usually present with obstructive hydrocephalus or ataxia and gait disturbances. More than half occur in the first decade of life, especially between ages 4 and 8 years. Approximately 30% occur in young adults with a peak in the third decade. Males are affected more than females in a ratio of 3:1. Five-year survival is about 50%. These tumors arise from the remnants of the primitive neu-

roectoderm of the inferior medullary velum in the roof of the fourth ventricle and invade the vermis as well as fill the fourth ventricle and its recesses. They may spread to the lateral recesses of the fourth ventricle and may extend into the cerebellopontine angle cistern or into the cisterna magna. Medulloblastomas have a high tendency (about 30%) to seed the CSF, and thus leptomeningeal metastases are common in the rest of the craniospinal axis.[55] In young adults they have more of a predilection to occur off midline in the cerebellar hemispheres, incite a desmoplastic fibrotic reaction, and are sometimes classified as cerebellar sarcomas. Up to 5% may metastasize outside the CNS, especially to bone.

The typical CT appearance of a medulloblastoma is a midline vermian high-attenuation lesion that encroaches on or fills the fourth ventricle, causes hydrocephalus, and enhances densely and homogeneously with administration contrast material. The high attenuation is due to hypercellularity.

The multiplanar capability of MRI, especially the sagittal plane, gives a more accurate representation of the size and location of medulloblastomas (Fig. 19–39). These median or paramedian tumors appear to

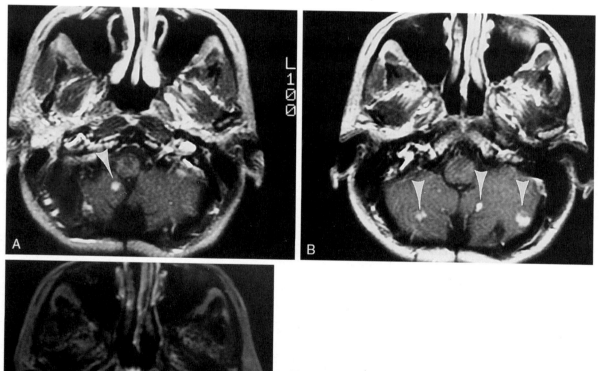

FIGURE 19–38. Hemangioblastoma. *A* and *B*, Gadolinium-enhanced T1-weighted axial images in a sibling of the previous patient show multiple enhancing lesions *(arrowheads)* consistent with hemangioblastomas. *C*, Only one has a cystic component *(arrow)*, best seen on the T2-weighted image.

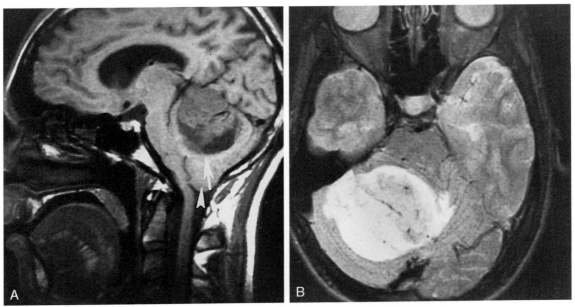

FIGURE 19–39. Medulloblastoma. *A*, Sagittal T1-weighted scan (spin echo, 600/20) demonstrates a lesion in the superior vermis *(arrow)*. The fourth ventricle is compressed, and the brain stem is displaced anteriorly. Note cerebellar herniation below the foramen magnum *(arrowhead)* and upward herniation of tumor through the tentorial notch. *B*, On a T2-weighted axial scan (spin echo, 3000/70), the tumor is hyperintense and has extended into the right cerebellar hemisphere. The signal flow vessels' voids within the lesion indicate the hypervascular nature of the tumor.

invade the adjacent cerebellum and fill the fourth ventricle. They often compress the brain stem but rarely invade the floor of the fourth ventricle. Medulloblastomas are usually homogeneously low to moderate (nearly isointense relative to brain) in signal intensity. Hydrocephalus is usually apparent in the temporal horns and third ventricle. Calcification and hemorrhage are uncommon. Necrosis visible with MRI correlates with increased malignancy and should be noted. These tumors are highly vascular and usually densely enhance with gadolinium. Leptomeningeal enhancement should be searched for both in the brain and in the spine. Radiation therapy or chemotherapy or both are often given prophylactically because of the significant risk of tumor seeding through the CSF pathways.

EPENDYMOMA

Ependymomas constitute about 10% of pediatric CNS tumors and 5% of gliomas in all age groups. The peak age range is 10 to 15 years. Males are affected twice as much as females. The long-term survival rate is about 50%. There is a second age peak in the fourth decade of life.

Two thirds of ependymomas are infratentorial. The atria of the lateral ventricle are the next most common site. Supratentorial ependymomas may be intraparenchymal. Ependymomas usually (70%) arise in the floor of the fourth ventricle, and both infiltrate the surrounding brain and fill the fourth ventricle. They may directly invade the floor of the fourth ventricle and brain stem and present with cranial neuropathies, ocu-

lomotor disturbances, nausea and vomiting, or hydrocephalus.[56] Ependymomas may spread into the basal cisterns through the foramina of Luschka and Magendie. About 10% spread through the foramen magnum to compress the spinal cord. Occasionally, they arise laterally in the foramen of Luschka and spread into the cerebellopontine angle. In these cases the rest of the fourth ventricle may be tumor free.

Ependymomas are moderately malignant tumors and are slowly expansile and infiltrative. They seed by means of the CSF but less frequently than do medulloblastomas. A more malignant subtype is referred to as an ependymoblastoma.

MRI typically shows an irregular, poorly defined infiltrative mass of heterogeneous signal intensity on both T1-weighted and T2-weighted images (Fig. 19–40). The heterogeneity is due to commonly noted intratumoral hemorrhage, necrosis, and dense foci of calcification. Calcification is seen in more than half of ependymomas. Ependymomas, unlike medulloblastomas, are easily separated from the superior vermis but often invade the floor of the fourth ventricle and are frequently attached to the brain stem at surgery. Contrast enhancement is seen in these vascular tumors but is less intense and less homogeneous than that seen in medulloblastomas because of the inhomogeneity of these tumors and the presence of hemorrhage, cysts, necrosis, and calcifications. Subpial coating and nodular intradural enhancement representing CSF seeding should be searched for in both the brain and the spine.[57]

Subependymoma is a noninvasive mixed astrocytic-ependymal tumor arising from cells lying just beneath

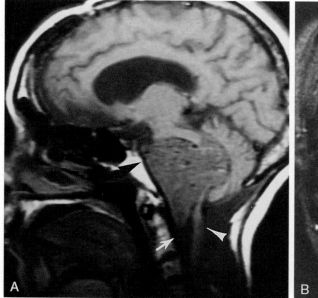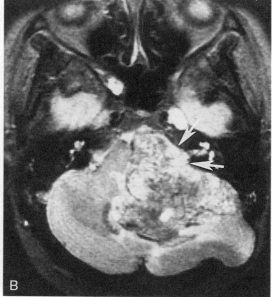

FIGURE 19–40. Ependymoma. *A,* Sagittal T1-weighted image demonstrates a large heterogeneous lesion within the fourth ventricle, extending into the prepontine cistern, flattening the basilar artery against the clivus *(black arrow).* A peg-shaped wedge of tumor *(white arrow)* extends through the foramen magnum anterior to the cord *(arrowhead).* Note the clear cleavage plane with the superior vermis. Low signal intensities within mass correlated with calcifications seen on CT scans. *B,* T2-weighted image shows marked heterogeneity of this lesion and extension through the left foramen of Luschka into the left cerebellopontine angle cistern and prepontine cistern *(arrows).*

the ependyma. Seventy-five percent occur within the fourth ventricle and are often asymptomatic even when they fill the fourth ventricle. These usually occur in men in the sixth or seventh decade.[58]

At MRI, subependymomas are usually solid and homogeneous and often do not enhance after administration of contrast medium. If in the lateral ventricle, they often are in contact with the septum pellucidum.[58a]

CEREBELLAR ASTROCYTOMA

The most common pediatric posterior fossa tumor (slightly more frequent than medulloblastoma), astrocytoma is usually of the juvenile pilocytic type. It is usually hemispheric, presents with hydrocephalus and limb ataxia, and is among the most benign of CNS tumors, having a 80% to 90% 10-year survival. However, late recurrences are not rare, even after 20 years. The peak age at onset is 4 years. There is an increased frequency of these tumors in patients with neurofibromatosis.

Cerebellar astrocytomas are usually sharply demarcated, and the majority are cystic. The cysts are often proteinaceous with a wall of compressed cerebellar tissue and glottic reaction. A mural nodule is usually located laterally. Hemorrhage and seeding through the CSF are rare. These tumors compress adjacent cerebellum and the fourth ventricle but do not enter the fourth ventricle and rarely invade the brain stem unless the tumor has a more aggressive histology. Ten percent to 15% of cerebellar astrocytomas are the

more anaplastic infiltrative fibrillary type. This aggressive type is more common in the adult posterior fossa.

At MRI the majority of cerebellar astrocytomas have large cysts, although they may be solid or have small cysts. They are sharply marginated and hyperintense on T2-weighted images. Homogeneous contrast enhancement is seen in the mural nodule and sometimes in the cyst wall (Fig. 19–41). Calcification is not common (occurring in less than 20%). The cyst fluid may be isointense relative to CSF or have increased signal intensity on T1-weighted images owing to protein content. Occasionally, sedimentation levels or blood products may be seen. Fluid motion within the cyst may be noted.

BRAIN STEM GLIOMA

Brain stem gliomas (astrocytomas) represent about 10% of pediatric and adolescent brain tumors. They are less common in adults. The 5-year survival rate is 20%, and the median survival is 1 to 2 years. Most are of the diffusely infiltrative fibrillary type and are usually quite advanced when discovered. There is a moderate incidence of anaplasia, necrosis, and hemorrhage. The vast majority involve the pons, but involvement of and spread to the midbrain, medulla, cerebellum, and subarachnoid spaces is common.[59–62] Leptomeningeal seeding is unusual. Medullary gliomas may be exophytic laterally or dorsally. Brain stem gliomas present with cranial nerve abnormalities, long tract signs, and gait disturbances. Hydrocephalus is often a late symptom. Rarely is surgery indicated unless the tumor is

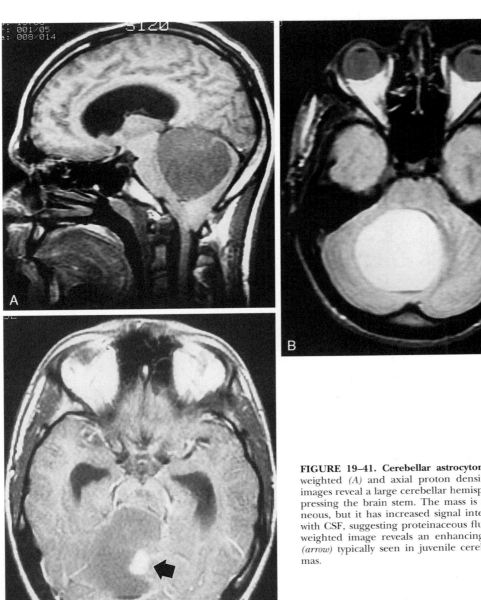

FIGURE 19–41. Cerebellar astrocytoma. Sagittal T1-weighted *(A)* and axial proton density–weighted *(B)* images reveal a large cerebellar hemisphere mass compressing the brain stem. The mass is nearly homogeneous, but it has increased signal intensity compared with CSF, suggesting proteinaceous fluid. *C,* Axial T1-weighted image reveals an enhancing mural nodule *(arrow)* typically seen in juvenile cerebellar astrocytomas.

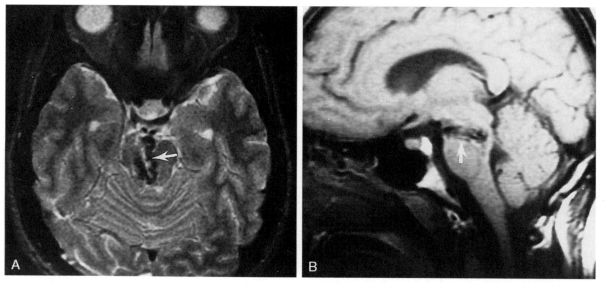

FIGURE 19–42. Brain stem arteriovenous malformation. *A*, T2-weighted axial image demonstrates large flow voids *(arrow)* coursing through the midbrain. *B*, Sagittal T1-weighted image demonstrates vascular malformation *(arrow)* at the junction of the midbrain and pons.

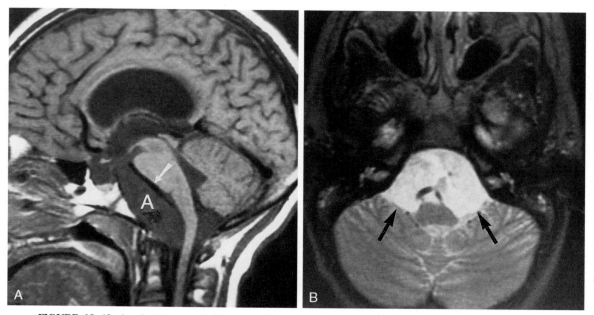

FIGURE 19–43. Arachnoid cyst. *A*, T1-weighted sagittal image demonstrates a large prepontine mass (A) displacing the basilar artery *(arrow)* and brain stem posteriorly. *B*, T2-weighted axial image confirms isointensity relative to CSF. This was true on all sequences. The cystic nature of the mass *(arrows)* is suggested by slight inhomogeneity caused by motion artifact within the cyst.

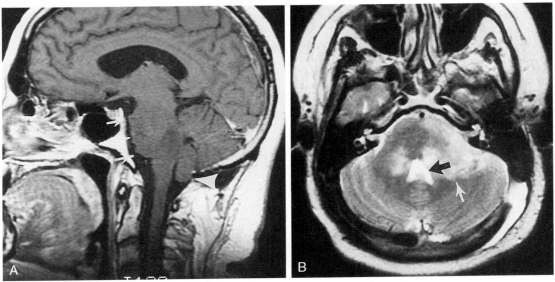

FIGURE 19–44. Brain stem glioma. *A,* Sagittal T1-weighted enhanced image demonstrates a nonenhancing low-attenuation abnormality in the lower pons, an ill-defined anterior border of widened pons *(arrows),* and tonsilar herniation *(arrowhead). B,* T2-weighted axial image shows typical high-signal-intensity abnormality in the pons and both cerebellar peduncles *(white arrow).* Note compression of both sides of the fourth ventricle *(black arrow).*

primarily exophytic or has a large cystic component. The vast majority of these tumors are unresectable and are treated with radiation. MRI is particularly helpful in excluding vascular malformations (Fig. 19–42) and extra-axial masses (Fig. 19–43). These generally have a more favorable prognosis and may be surgically resectable.

MRI is more sensitive and specific than CT because of multiplanar (especially sagittal) imaging and more pronounced differences in tumor signal intensity from normal tissue (Fig. 19–44). Ill-defined hyperintensity is noted on T2-weighted images. CSF spaces clearly outline the brain stem in the sagittal plane and improve detection and accurate localization of these tumors. The brain stem is noted to be widened and the fourth ventricle may be compressed or displaced posteriorly. The normal linear floor of the fourth ventricle be-

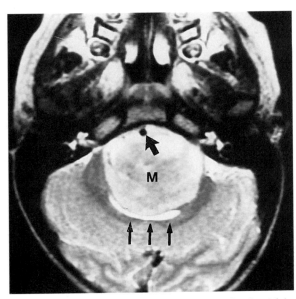

FIGURE 19–45. Brain stem astrocytoma. T2-weighted axial image reveals a large hyperintense mass (M) expanding the brain stem. Note posterior displacement and compression of the fourth ventricle *(thin arrows).* The tumor engulfs the basilar artery *(wide arrow).*

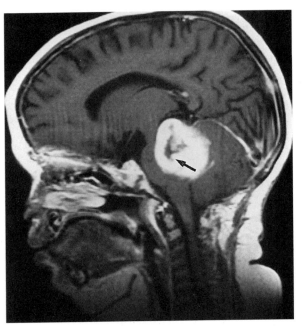

FIGURE 19–46. Brain stem glioma. T1-weighted gadolinium-enhanced sagittal image reveals a large enhancing mass in the dorsal pons and midbrain, extending into the quadrigeminal cistern. Note low signal intensity within tumor *(arrow)* due to tumoral calcification as shown on a CT scan (not shown).

comes convex posteriorly (Fig. 19–45). The borders of the brain stem may be irregular and indistinct. The prepontine cistern may be effaced and the basilar artery encased. Hemorrhage, necrosis, and calcification (Fig. 19–46) are present in some cases. Cysts are not common. More than half of brain stem gliomas enhance, often in an irregular fashion. Spread to the cerebellar peduncles and cerebellum is common.

CHOROID PLEXUS PAPILLOMA

Choroid plexus papillomas are unusual tumors that arise in the ventricles. They are slightly more common in the lateral ventricles than the fourth ventricle, and the vast majority are benign. These well-defined highly vascular masses occur in the ventricle surrounded by CSF. Parenchymal invasion is uncommon and suggests malignant choroid plexus carcinoma. The papillomas occasionally extend out the foramen of Luschka into the cerebellopontine angle cistern. They can cause hydrocephalus by directly obstructing the CSF pathways or cause communicating hydrocephalus secondary to repeated hemorrhages or by increased CSF production.[63]

Choroid plexus papillomas are mildly hyperintense on T2-weighted images, and, like normal choroid plexus, they enhance intensely with contrast medium. Diagnosis is best made by appreciating the mass itself in the ventricle and the associated hydrocephalus. Flow voids are sometimes present.

REFERENCES

1. Bonstelle CT, Kaufman B, Benson JE, et al: Magnetic resonance imaging in the evaluation of the brain stem. Radiology 150:705–712, 1984.
2. Bradley WG Jr: MRI of the brain stem: a practical approach. Radiology 179:319–322, 1991.
3. Peterman SB, Steiner RE, Bydder GM, et al: Nuclear magnetic resonance imaging (NMR), (MRI), of brain stem tumors. Neuroradiology 27:202–207, 1985.
4. Kelly WM: Functional anatomy and cranial neuropathy: neuroimaging perspective. Neuroimaging Clin North Am 3:1–46, 1993.
5. Olson EM, Healy JF, Wong WHM, et al: MR detection of white matter disease of the brain in patients with HIV infection: fast spin-echo vs conventional spin-echo pulse sequences. AJR 162:1199–1204, 1994.
6. Guillaumin BA, Brown FA, Huges DL, et al: Comparison between conventional spin echo (CSE) and fast spin echo (FSE) for the detection and characterization of lesions in the brain and spinal cord. Presented at the Annual Meeting of the American Society of Neuroradiology, St. Louis, 1992, p 36. Abstract.
7. Haughton VM, Rimm AA, Czervionke LF, et al: Sensitivity of Gd-DTPA–enhanced MR imaging of benign extraaxial tumors. Radiology 166:829–833, 1988.
8. Powers TA, Partain CL, Kessler RM, et al: Central nervous system lesion in pediatric patients: Gd-DTPA–enhanced MR imaging. Radiology 169:723–726, 1988.
9. Hasso AN, Smith DS: The cerebellopontine angle. Semin Ultrasound CT MR 10:280–301, 1989.
10. Curati WL, Graif M, Kingsley DPE, et al: Acoustic neuromas: Gd-DTPA enhancement in MR imaging. Radiology 158:447–451, 1986.
11. Albert A, Lee BCP, Saint-Louis L, Deck MDF: MR of optic chiasm and optic pathways. AJNR 7:255–258, 1986.
12. Hutchins LG, Harnsberger HR, Hardin CW, et al: The radiological assessment of trigeminal neuropathy. AJNR 10:1031–1038, 1989.
13. Tien RD, Dillon WP: Herpes trigeminal neuritis and rhombencephalitis on Gd-DPTA–enhanced MR imaging. AJNR 11:413–414, 1990.
14. Daniels DL, Pech P, Pojunas KW, et al: Trigeminal nerve: anatomic correlation with MR imaging. Radiology 159:577–583, 1986.
15. Barakos JA, D'Amour PG, Dillon WP, Newton TH: Trigeminal sensory neuropathy caused by cervical disk herniation. AJNR 11:609, 1990.
16. Tien RD, Wilkins RH: MRA delineation of the vertebral-basilar system in patients with hemifacial spasm and trigeminal neuralgia. AJNR 14:34–36, 1993.
17. Koenig H, Lenz M, Sauter R: Temporal bone region: high-resolution MR imaging using surface coils. Radiology 159:191–194, 1986.
18. Tien RD, Dillon WP, Jackler RK: Contrast-enhanced MR imaging of the facial nerve in 11 patients with Bell's palsy. AJNR 11:735–741, 1990.
19. Daniels DL, Czervionke LF, Millen SJ, et al: MR imaging of facial nerve enhancement in Bell's palsy or after temporal bone surgery. Surgery 171:807–810, 1989.
20. Anderson RE, Laskoff JM: Ramsay Hunt syndrome mimicking intracranialicular acoustic neuroma on contrast-enhanced MR. AJNR 11:409, 1990.
21. Alexander MS, Seltzer S, Harnsberger HR: Sensorineural hearing loss: more than meets the eye? AJNR 14:37–45, 1993.
22. Armington WG, Harnsberger HR, Smoker WRK, Osborn AG: Normal and diseased acoustic pathway: evaluation with MR imaging. Neuroradiology 167:509–515, 1988.
23. Bird CR, Drayer BP: Magnetic resonance imaging of acoustic neuromas. Barrows Neurol Inst Q 3:56–59, 1987.
24. Mulkens TH, Parizel PM, Martin J-J, et al: Acoustic schwannoma: MR findings in 84 tumors. AJNR 160:395–398, 1993.
25. Press GA, Hesselink JR: MR imaging of cerebellopontine angle and internal auditory canal lesions at 1.5 T. AJR 150:1371–1381, 1988.
26. House JW, Waluch V, Jackler RK: Magnetic resonance imaging in acoustic neuroma diagnosis. Ann Otol Rhinol Laryngol 95:16–20, 1986.
27. Smirniotopoulos JG, Yue NC, Rushing EJ: Cerebellopontine angle masses: radiologic-pathologic correlation. Radiographics 13:1131–1147, 1993.
28. Gentry LR, Jacoby CG, Turski PA, et al: Cerebellopontine angle–petromastoid mass lesions: comparative study of diagnosis with MR imaging and CT. Radiology 162:513–520, 1987.
29. Daniels DL, Millen SJ, Meyer GA, et al: MR detection of tumor in the internal auditory canal. AJNR 8:249–252, 1987.
30. Shetter AG, Daspit CP, Medina M: The translabyrinthine approach to acoustic neuromas. Barrows Neurol Inst Q 4:2–6, 1988.
31. Han MH, Jabour BA, Andrews JC, et al: Nonneoplastic enhancing lesions mimicking intracranialicular acoustic neuroma on gadolinium-enhanced MR images. Radiology 179:795–796, 1991.
32. Wiener SN, Pearlstein AE, Eiber A: MR imaging of arachnoid cysts. J Comput Assist Tomogr 11:236–241, 1987.
33. Mikhael MA, Ciric IS, Wolff AP: Differentiation of cerebellopontine angle neuromas and meningiomas with MR imaging. J Comput Assist Tomogr 9:852–856, 1985.
34. Tampieri D, Melanson D, Ethier R: MR imaging of epidermoid cysts. AJNR 10:351–356, 1989.
35. Pei-yi G, Osborn AG, Smirniotopoulos, Harris CP: Radiologic-pathologic correlation of epidermoid tumor of the cerebellopontine angle. AJNR 13:863–872, 1992.
36. Latack JT, Kartush JM, Kemink JL, et al: Epidermoidomas of the cerebellopontine angle and temporal bone: CT and MR aspects. Radiology 157:361–366, 1985.
37. Berger MS, Wilson CB: Epidermoid cysts of the posterior fossa. J Neurosurg 62:214–219, 1985.
38. Hahn FJ, Ong E, McComb RD, et al: MR imaging of ruptured intracranial dermoid. J Comput Assist Tomogr 10:888–889, 1986.
39. Daniels DL, Schenck JF, Foster T, et al: Magnetic resonance imaging of the jugular foramen. AJNR 6:699–703, 1986.
40. Daniels DL, Czervionke LF, Pech P, et al: Gradient recalled echo MR imaging of the jugular foramen. AJNR 9:675–678, 1988.
41. Nelson MD, Kendall BE: Intracranial catecholamine secreting paragangliomas. Neuroradiology 29:277–182, 1987.
42. Olsen WL, Dillon WP, Kelly WM, et al: MR imaging of paragangliomas. AJNR 7:1039–1042, 1986.
43. Zimmerman RA, Bilaniuk LT: Applications of magnetic resonance imaging in disease of the pediatric central nervous system. Magn Reson Imaging 4:11–24, 1986.
44. Barnes PD, Lester PD, Yamanashi WS, et al: Magnetic resonance imaging in childhood intracranial masses. Magn Reson Imaging 4:41–49, 1986.
45. Delattre JY, Krol G, Thaler HT, Posner JB: Distribution of brain metastases. Arch Neurol 45:741–744, 1988.
46. Hasso AN: Infratentorial neoplasms, including the internal auditory canal and cerebellopontine angle regions. Top Magn Reson Imaging 1:37–51, 1989.
47. Bilaniuk LT: Adult infratentorial tumors. Semin Roentgenol 25:155–173, 1990.
48. Lee SR, Sanches J, Mark AS, et al: Posterior fossa hemangioblastoma: MR imaging. Radiology 171:463–468, 1989.
49. Elster AD, Arthur DW: Intracranial hemangioblastomas: CT and MR findings. J Comput Assist Tomogr 12:736–739, 1988.
50. Filling-Katz MR, Choyke PL, Patronaus NJ, et al: Radiologic screening for von Hippel–Lindau disease: the role of Gd-DTPA–enhanced MR imaging of CNS. J Comput Assist Tomogr 13:743–755, 1989.
51. Rollins N, Mendelsohn D, Mulne A, et al: Recurrent medulloblastoma: frequency of tumor enhancement of Gd-DTPA MR imaging. AJNR 11:583–587, 1990.
52. Mueller DP, Moore SA, Sato Y, Yuh WTC: MRI spectrum of medulloblastoma. Clin Imaging 16:250–255, 1992.

53. Meyers SP, Kemp SS, Tarr RW: MR imaging features of medulloblastomas. AJR 158:859–865, 1992.

54. Koci TM, Chiang F, Mehringer CM, et al: Adult cerebellar medulloblastoma: imaging features with emphasis on MR findings. AJNR 14:929–939, 1993.

55. Rippe DJ, Boyko OB, Friedman HS, et al: Gd-DPTA–enhanced MR imaging of leptomeningeal spread of primary intracranial CNS tumor in children. AJNR 11:329–332, 1990.

56. Barloon TJ, Yuh WT, Chiang FL, et al: Lesions involving the fourth ventricle evaluated by CT and MR: a comparative study. MRI 7:635–642, 1989.

57. Spoto GP, Press GA, Hesselink JR, et al: Intracranial ependymoma and subependymoma: MR manifestations. AJNR 11:83–91, 1990.

58. Silverstein JE, Lenchik L, Stanciu MG, Shimkin PM: MR of intracranial subependymoma. J Comput Assist Tomogr 19:264–276, 1995.

58a. Furie DM, Provenzale JM: Supratentorial ependymomas and subependymomas: CT and MR appearance. J Comput Assist Tomogr 19:518–526, 1995.

59. Jelsma RK, Jelsma LF, Johnson GS: Surgical removal of brainstem astrocytoma and hemangioblastomas: report of three cases and review. Surg Neurol 39:494–510, 1993.

60. Kane AG, Robles HA, Smirniotopoulous JG, et al: Radiologic-pathologic correlation diffuse pontine astrocytoma. AJNR 14:941–945, 1993.

61. Hueffle MG, Han JS, Kaufman B, Benson JE: MR imaging of brain stem gliomas. J Comput Assist Tomogr 9:263–267, 1985.

62. Jackson A, Panizza BJ, Hughes D, Reid H: Primary choroid plexus papilloma of the cerebellopontine angle: magnetic resonance imaging, computed tomographic and angiographic appearances. Br J Radiol 65:754–757, 1992.

63. Coates TL, Hinshaw DB, Peckman N, et al: Pediatric choroid plexus neoplasms: MR, CT, and pathologic correlation. Radiology 173:81, 1989.

Infectious and Inflammatory Diseases

SPYROS K. KARAMPEKIOS ■ JOHN R. HESSELINK

In spite of the development of many effective antimicrobial therapies and the general improvement in hygiene and health care systems all over the world, the incidence of central nervous system (CNS) infection has increased significantly in the past 10 years. This can be attributed primarily to the acquired immunodeficiency syndrome (AIDS) epidemic and its devastating effect on the immune system and secondarily to various immunosuppressive agents that are being used in aggressive cancer treatment and in organ transplantations. In the immunocompromised patient, a whole group of life-threatening, opportunistic CNS infections have emerged. Early diagnosis is quite important, so that effective and prompt treatment can be immediately instituted to prevent major brain damage and permanent neurologic complications. Imaging studies play a crucial role in the diagnostic process, along with the history (exposure to infectious agents), host factors (open head trauma, cerebrospinal fluid [CSF] leak, sinusitis, otitis, immune status), physical examination (neurologic signs), and laboratory analysis of CSF.

The brain is relatively protected from infection by the calvaria, the meninges, and the blood-brain barrier. However, a large number of pathogens, including bacteria, viruses, fungi, and parasites, can reach the brain hematogenously or less likely by direct extension from an adjacent infected focus. Once in the intracranial cavity, even weak pathogens may produce a severe inflammatory response that is mainly due to some unique features of the brain, such as the absence of lymphatics, the lack of capillaries in the subarachnoid space, and the existence of perivascular CSF-containing spaces (Virchow-Robin spaces). CSF also acts as an excellent culture medium for dissemination of an infectious process. When an intracranial infection does occur, the precise localization is of great importance, because it narrows the differential diagnosis, sometimes determining the type of the pathogen, more appropriate treatment, and the likely outcome. In a practical approach to differentiate CNS infections, we use some broad categories to localize the lesions by the compartment involved. Some pathogens can in-

vade the brain parenchyma, producing focal (abscess, cyst) or diffuse (encephalitis) lesions; the meninges (meningitis, ependymitis); and the extra-axial spaces (subdural, epidural empyema). We also include a special section dedicated to AIDS-related infections, because they constitute the most common cause of CNS infections and they also present with various manifestations that form an interesting and challenging pattern for diagnosticians.

Magnetic resonance imaging (MRI) is the most sensitive imaging study in detecting focal or diffuse parenchymal infectious lesions, and today it has clearly replaced computed tomography (CT). MRI's optimal contrast resolution, its multiplanar capability, and the absence of signal intensity from the surrounding bone allow an earlier and more exact localization of brain infection, and MRI is proving to be superior for the detection of meningeal inflammation and its related sequelae.[1, 2] Furthermore, intravenous administration of gadolinium-based paramagnetic contrast medium offers more benefits to the patient with no additional risk and increases diagnostic specificity. The pathophysiology of gadolinium enhancement is similar to that of iodinated contrast agents, indicating areas of active blood-brain barrier breakdown and improving detectability of lesions in the brain.[3] However, MRI has proved inferior to CT in the evaluation of some chronic and congenital infections in which calcifications are one of the main findings.

BRAIN ABSCESS

Brain abscess is the most common focal infectious lesion and can be caused by many different types of pathogens, usually bacteria. Brain abscesses frequently arise secondary to hematogenous dissemination of an extracranial site, by direct extension from a contiguous suppurative focus (paranasal sinuses, middle ear, mastoids), or rarely secondary to meningitis. In children the majority of cerebral abscesses are associated with cyanotic heart disease with a right-to-left shunt. In immunocompetent individuals the most frequently encountered pathogens are *Staphylococcus* and *Streptococcus*. In patients with recent history of neurosurgical intervention or contaminated skull fracture, brain abscess is one of the most common and threatening complications and is usually due to *Staphylococcus aureus*.[4] In about 20% of cases the source of infection cannot be found.

When the brain is inoculated with a pathogen, the brain tissue reacts in a predictable way, initially producing an area of local cerebritis. With time, the infectious process continues and a true encapsulated brain abscess is formed. Thus, cerebritis and abscess formation constitute a spectrum of the same process. In the case of brain infection the rate of evolution is slower than acute infarction but faster than neoplasms, and this is an important feature for the differential diagnosis.[5] The evolution of an abscess includes four histopathologic stages, which were described initially in experimental animal studies.[6] This somewhat arbitrary distinction correlates well in humans and follows the CT and MRI findings in serial scans. The four stages include early cerebritis, late cerebritis, early abscess (capsule) formation, and late abscess formation. The rapidity of this infectious process depends on the type of the invading pathogen, the origin of the infection, and the patient's immunocompetence.[7] Patients usually present in the late cerebritis or early abscess stage with clinical manifestations of a rapidly expanding space-occupying lesion rather than symptoms specific for an infection. Most patients have severe headache, drowsiness, confusion, seizures, or focal neurologic deficits. Fever and leukocytosis are common during the invasive phase of an abscess but may resolve as it matures.

Acute cerebritis, the initial phase of a focal cerebral infection, merges into the late cerebritis phase after 4 to 5 days. Areas of necrosis, granulation tissue, and inflammatory cells are produced in the center of the evolving lesion while the abscess capsule has not yet developed. In this area of local cerebritis, vascular congestion, petechial hemorrhage, and brain edema coexist. By the end of the second week the early abscess stage begins with formation of the peripheral, collagenous capsule. With time, more collagen is produced and the capsule becomes complete and thicker, the central tissue becomes necrotic and liquefies, and the surrounding edema decreases. Neurosurgical intervention is preferably delayed until the abscess stage develops because earlier attempts result in incomplete drainage and may cause parenchymal hemorrhage. If left untreated, a brain abscess continues to grow with devastating outcome, such as brain herniation or rupture of the abscess into the ventricular system. With the advent of the new capabilities of neuroimaging (CT and MRI), the prognosis of brain abscesses improved dramatically, owing to early diagnosis and accurate localization of these lesions, rapid detection of postoperative complications, and better monitoring of the response to medical therapy.

IMAGING FEATURES

The MRI features of cerebritis and brain abscess depend on the stage of the infectious process at the time of imaging. The acute cerebritis stage is infrequently seen by MRI because patients usually do not develop any symptoms and do not present until later in the course of the infection. However, when this stage is imaged, MRI reveals an ill-defined area that is slightly hypointense on T1-weighted images. The T1-weighted sequence is also best for demonstrating the early, subtle mass effect (gyral swelling, sulcal obliteration). The focal inflammatory infiltrate exhibits high signal intensity on T2-weighted images, both centrally from inflammation and peripherally from edema. MRI is more sensitive than CT in the early detection of cerebritis because of the superior sensitivity to alterations in tissue water content.[8]

As the infection continues, the infected area increases in size and necrotic debris accumulates centrally, while the collagenous capsule is being formed. The proteinaceous, necrotic fluid of the abscess cavity has signal intensity higher than that of CSF on T1-weighted and proton density–weighted images, similar to fluid in cystic neoplasms. At this stage, mass effect is obvious, manifested by ventricular and cisternal distortion and sulcal effacement. Surrounding vasogenic edema is mildly hypointense on T1-weighted images and hyperintense on T2-weighted images. A moderate degree of vasogenic edema is characteristic of brain abscess.[9]

On T1-weighted images, the abscess capsule stands out as an isointense or slightly hyperintense ring against the hypointense background of the necrotic center and the surrounding edema. On T2-weighted images this ring is consistently and markedly hypointense (Fig. 20–1*A*). There is still some controversy regarding the causes of capsular intensity. Some authors attribute the hyperintensity of the abscess capsule on T1-weighted images to capsular hemorrhage, reflecting paramagnetic effects of methemoglobin. The signal properties of the abscess capsule have been ascribed to paramagnetic hemoglobin degradation products, or free radicals within macrophages. Macrophages are abundant in the capsule, and their activity is highest in the late cerebritis–early abscess phase, exactly when the signal intensity of the capsule on T2-weighted images is particularly low.[10, 11] Another important feature of cerebral abscess is its tendency to grow into the white matter away from the well-vascularized cortex, resulting in an oblong configuration and thickening of the cortical surface of the abscess capsule. The thinner portion of the capsule toward the white matter accounts for the predilection of abscesses to rupture into the ventricles, producing ventriculitis (ependymitis), and, less commonly, into the subarachnoid space.

Contrast medium administration is helpful in the evaluation of brain abscesses. Gadolinium produces mottled, heterogeneous areas of enhancement during the cerebritis stage. As the abscess matures, an enhancing rim develops that is typically smooth, well defined, and thin walled (Fig. 20–1*B*). This ring-like enhancement reflects the damaged blood-brain barrier and ingrowth of vascular granulation tissue. If an abscess ruptures into a ventricle and secondary ependymitis

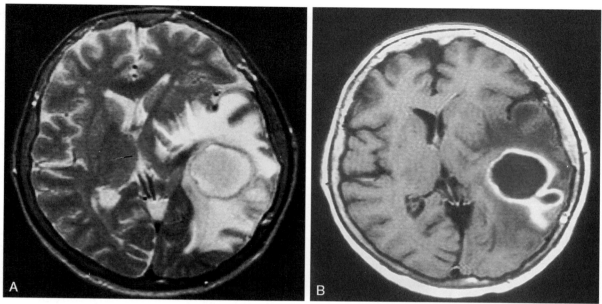

FIGURE 20–1. *Norcadia* **abscess.** *A,* Axial T2-weighted (spin echo [SE], 2500/70) image illustrates the abscess capsule as a hypointense ring, highlighted by areas of increased signal intensity both centrally (necrotic core) and peripherally (edema). Note that the hypointense ring is thinner and less hypointense toward the deep white matter. *B,* Axial postcontrast T1-weighted (SE, 600/20, gadolinium diethylenetriaminepentaacetic acid [Gd-DTPA]) image at the same level shows a ring-enhancing lesion, surrounded by low-signal-intensity vasogenic edema. A satellite lesion (daughter abscess) is seen at the periphery of the abscess.

develops, the ventricular wall enhances, suggesting a poor prognosis (Fig. 20–2). Ring enhancement persists for up to 8 months, and its presence should not be considered as a treatment failure. More reliable signs

of healing are shrinkage of the necrotic center and decrease in capsular hypointensity on T2-weighted images.

Brain abscesses produced by nonpyogenic organisms

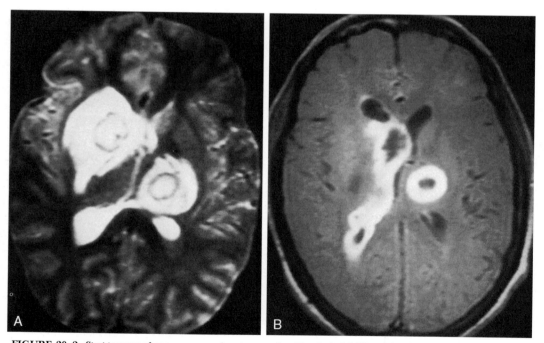

FIGURE 20–2. *Streptococcus* **abscess progressing to ependymitis.** *A,* Axial T2-weighted image demonstrates the abscess capsules as hypointense rings surrounding the necrotic center. There is also a significant amount of peripheral edema. *B,* Axial postcontrast T1-weighted image 1 week later reveals extensive ependymal enhancement of the right lateral ventricle, indicating ependymitis secondary to rupture of an abscess into the ventricular system. (*A* and *B* courtesy of M. Healy, MD, San Antonio, TX.)

(fungi, parasites, mycobacteria) typically occur in patients with defective or suppressed immune systems and are discussed in the section on AIDS-related infections.

MENINGITIS

Meningitis is an acute or chronic inflammation of the pia-arachnoid (leptomeninges) and the adjacent CSF. The two main diagnostic groups are bacterial (purulent) and viral (aseptic) meningitis. They may have an acute, subacute, or chronic presentation and course. The three most frequent bacterial species are *Haemophilus influenzae*, *Neisseria meningitidis*, and *Streptococcus pneumoniae*, accounting for approximately 40% of cases of purulent meningitis in adults. Gram-negative bacillary meningitis caused by *Klebsiella*, *Escherichia coli*, and *Pseudomonas aeruginosa* usually occurs in neonates and immunocompromised patients, as well as in association with head trauma or neurosurgical intervention. Viruses can also produce an acute meningitis (lymphocytic), which typically occurs in children and young adults. The etiology of viral meningitis varies with the season, the patient's age, and the geographic location, although in the majority of cases the offending viruses are enteroviruses (especially echoviruses and coxsackieviruses) and mumps virus. In immunosuppressed patients, adenoviruses and cytomegalovirus (CMV) are often encountered. Patients with viral meningitis have a more gradual onset of symptoms and an indolent course, which is often self-limited with less significant complications than those of bacterial origin.

The clinical signs and symptoms of meningitis are usually characteristic. Patients present with fever, headache, neck stiffness, vomiting, photophobia, and altered consciousness. Almost all patients with viral, and the majority of patients with bacterial, meningitis have a subacute onset of symptoms (1 to 7 days' duration). Patients with an acute presentation (less than 24 hours) constitute a medical emergency that requires immediate institution of antimicrobial therapy.

The outcome of patients with acute purulent meningitis depends on many factors, such as age, underlying health condition, the specific invading organism, and the delay in treatment. The mortality and morbidity of the disease have improved significantly in the past decades but still remain high, with an overall mortality rate ranging from 5% to 15% and existence of severe, persistent neurologic deficits such as seizures, mental retardation, or ataxia in another 10% to 25%.[12] So in patients with acute presentation of meningitis, the first consideration is therapy and not specific diagnosis, whereas in cases with subacute or chronic presentation attention should be focused on identification of the specific organism.

The diagnosis of chronic meningitis is made when clinical symptoms persist and the CSF examination remains abnormal for at least 4 weeks. A large number of infectious and noninfectious agents can cause chronic meningitis, with *Mycobacterium tuberculosis* being the most common. Tuberculous meningitis presents as a long-standing, insidious process, in which vasculitis of the circle of Willis and cerebral infarctions from basal meningeal inflammation predominate. A definitive diagnosis is made on the outcome of CSF cultures. Development of chronic meningitis in immunosuppressed patients can be the result of fungal infection, mainly cryptococcosis, coccidioidomycosis, and blastomycosis. Cryptococcal meningitis is discussed in detail in the section on AIDS-related infections, because it is the most common fungal infection in patients with AIDS.

Another cause of chronic meningitis is spirochetal infection. Neurosyphilis is an easily diagnosed form of secondary syphilis and is caused by *Treponema pallidum*. Most patients present with meningeal infection or parenchymal lesions. Vasculitis, due to inflammatory reaction in the walls of subarachnoid vessels, produces small areas of infarction. Gummas, which are rare intracranial masses of granulation tissue, result from the intense localized reaction of brain tissue and are located near the cerebral convexity. *Borrelia burgdorferi*, the cause of Lyme disease, is another spirochete associated with chronic meningitis or meningoencephalitis and cranial or peripheral neuropathy. Meningitis occurs in the earlier stages of disease from direct spirochetal invasion of the CSF.[13]

Finally, sarcoidosis, a noninfectious granulomatous disease, involves the CNS in approximately 5% of patients. CNS manifestations of neurosarcoidosis include chronic meningitis in the basal cisterns, cranial neuropathy, hypothalamic and pituitary dysfunction, and both intra-axial and extra-axial masses.[14] Other noninfectious causes of chronic meningeal disease are meningeal carcinomatosis, postoperative meningeal irritation, chemical meningitis, Behçet's disease, and subarachnoid hemorrhage.

IMAGING FEATURES

Neuroimaging plays a limited role in the diagnosis of meningitis, which is usually made on a clinical basis by history, physical examination, and laboratory CSF findings. Imaging studies (CT and MRI) are employed in patients in whom complications are suspected, such as vascular thrombosis, brain infarctions, brain abscess, ventriculitis, hydrocephalus, empyemas of epidural or subdural spaces, and subdural effusions. Imaging is also undertaken to confirm the diagnosis of meningitis, to identify possible sources, and to exclude other intracranial diseases. Patients with meningitis, either acute or chronic, usually have a normal nonenhanced MRI study. In more severe chronic cases the CSF may be hyperintense on T1-weighted and proton density–weighted images in the basal cisterns, secondary to obliteration from the inflammatory exudate and meningeal hyperemia.[15] The detection of meningeal disease is much easier after administration of paramagnetic contrast material. On contrast-enhanced MR images normal meningeal enhancement is usually seen in the dural reflections, such as the cavernous sinus and Meckel's cave, and also around the convexity as a thin, discontinuous rim. In cases of acute meningitis, postcontrast MRI reveals diffuse and intense enhancement of the inflamed meninges, which typically occurs over the cerebrum and in the interhemispheric and sylvian fissures (Fig. 20–3). In cases of chronic meningitis of tuberculous, fungal, or sarcoid origin, the enhancement is most prominent in the basal cisterns, where the inflammation is intense and profound. The enhancement is due first to the presence of contrast material in dilated and engorged vessels within vascular granulation tissue and second to leakage of contrast agent from disruption in the blood-meningeal barrier (Fig. 20–4). The term *blood-meningeal barrier* refers to a portion of the blood-brain barrier formed by capillaries of the leptomeninges.[16, 17]

Nonenhanced MRI may also miss meningeal involvement in neurosarcoidosis. Postcontrast MR studies disclose abnormal enhancement of the meninges, typically in the basal cisterns. Involvement of the hypothalamus and the pituitary stalk is a characteristic feature of CNS sarcoidosis, and it may be apparent on MR images as thickening and abnormal enhancement of the hypothalamus and the stalk. The optic chiasm is also commonly affected by sarcoid meningitis, owing to its covering by pia mater. Involvement of the cranial nerves is a complication of sarcoidosis, and MRI can provide evidence of sarcoid infiltration of several nerves (second and seventh the most common) by demonstrating nerve enhancement[18] (Fig. 20–5). An interesting form of meningeal sarcoid results in thick meningeal plaques, often over the convexity. These plaques may mimic meningiomas, in that they remain isointense or hypointense relative to cortex on both T1- and T2-weighted images.[19]

In cases of neurosyphilis the MRI findings display multifocal, small areas of infarction as multiple foci with high signal intensity on T2-weighted images, suggesting the diagnosis of vasculitis.[20] During the early phase of meningovascular involvement there is also widespread thickening of the meninges. Rarely in neurosyphilis, intracranial masses of granulation tissue (gummas) can be seen over the cerebral convexities on postcontrast MR images as enhancing parenchymal nodules indistinguishable from other intra-axial lesions such as gliomas, metastases, and tuberculomas. However, gummas are so rare that when a patient seropositive for *T. pallidum* develops an enhancing intracranial mass, other intra-axial processes, such as a cerebral neoplasm, should be excluded before the possibility of a gumma is entertained.[21]

Contrast-enhanced MRI is much more sensitive than postcontrast CT in the detection of meningeal enhancement, particularly when it occurs near the skull vault.[22, 23] CT is limited by beam-hardening artifacts from the adjacent bone in detecting meningeal enhancement around the convexity, whereas MRI is free of such bone artifacts. Furthermore, MRI has the capability of obtaining scans in any desired plane, another advantage over CT. For example, subtle enhancement of the convexity, the dura, and the tentorium is visualized better on coronal planes. Although more sensitive, postcontrast MRI is no more specific. Any condition that is likely to produce meningeal irritation, such as craniotomy, ventriculoperitoneal shunting, subarachnoid hemorrhage, or meningitis of carcinomatous or chemical origin, may cause meningeal enhancement. Also, abnormal meningeal enhancement is not seen in every case of meningitis, and, therefore, and unremarkable MRI study does not exclude this diagnosis.[24]

COMPLICATIONS OF MENINGITIS

Meningitis may be associated with various and significant complications. First, the exposure of the vessels to the inflammatory exudate may produce vasculi-

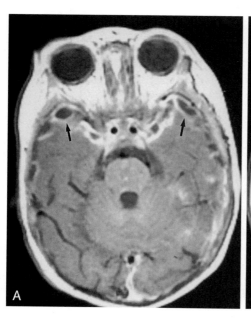
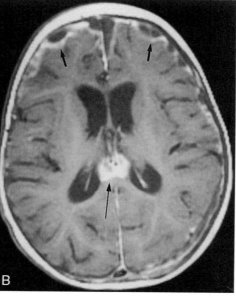

FIGURE 20–3. *Haemophilus influenzae* **meningitis.** *A* and *B*, Contrast-enhanced T1-weighted (SE, 600/20, Gd-DTPA) axial images disclose diffuse enhancement of the basal cisterns, sylvian fissures, and meninges over the temporal and frontal lobes. Also note enhancement within the cisterna velum interpositum *(long arrow).* Multiple CSF loculations *(short arrows)* within the subarachnoid spaces tend to isolate the organisms and make the antibiotic therapy less effective.

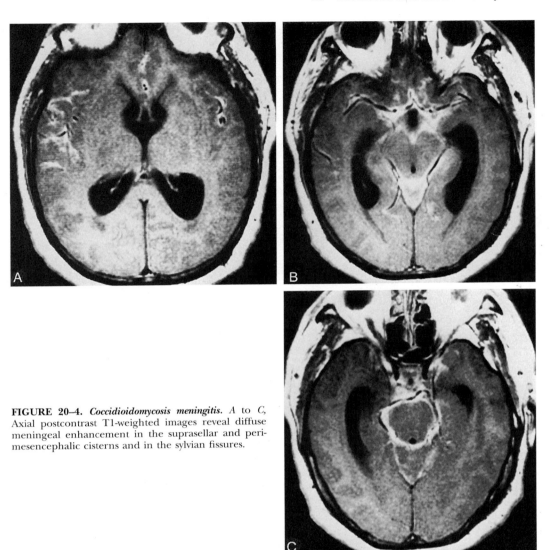

FIGURE 20–4. *Coccidioidomycosis meningitis.* *A* to *C,* Axial postcontrast T1-weighted images reveal diffuse meningeal enhancement in the suprasellar and perimesencephalic cisterns and in the sylvian fissures.

tis and thrombosis, complications most frequently found in patients with tuberculous meningitis. Vascular occlusions result in focal or massive brain infarcts (Fig. 20–6), whereas dural sinus thrombosis (particularly in the superior sagittal sinus) causes multiple hemorrhagic infarcts.[25] Another severe complication of meningitis is brain abscess formation. Ventriculitis and ependymitis may result from direct extension of an abscess, from progression of meningitis, or from an infected intraventricular shunt. In ependymitis, MRI displays increased subependymal signal intensity on proton density–weighted and T2-weighted images that often has a nodular and irregular pattern. On postcontrast scans ependymal enhancement outlines the ventricles. If pyogenic debris fills the ventricles, the CSF exhibits a signal intensity higher than normal on all sequences. For the determination of CSF signal intensity as normal, it is more accurate to compare the intraventricular CSF with the vitreous of the globe and not with CSF in other cisterns because associated meningitis may cause increased signal intensity in the basal cisterns and subarachnoid spaces.[26] Another fre-

quent complication of meningitis is either obstructive or communicating hydrocephalus, which occurs secondary to cellular debris obstructing the CSF pathways or to arachnoid adhesions impairing extraventricular CSF flow and absorption (see Figs. 20–4 and 20–6). Ventricular dilatation may be the only abnormal finding in patients with meningitis and is adequately evaluated with both CT and MRI. Subdural collections can also complicate meningitis and are discussed in the section on extra-axial empyemas.

ENCEPHALITIS

Encephalitis refers to a diffuse parenchymal inflammation of the brain. Even though viruses account for most cases, there are some uncommon nonviral causes of encephalitis, particularly in immunocompromised patients, such as bacteria *(Listeria monocytogenes)*, protozoa *(Toxoplasma)*, or fungi *(Aspergillus).* Viruses usually gain access to the CNS through hematogenous dissemination, although in certain viral

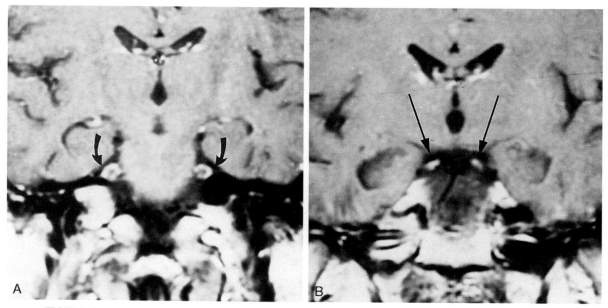

FIGURE 20–5. Meningeal sarcoidosis. *A* and *B,* Contrast-enhanced T1-weighted (SE, 500/15, Gd-DTPA) coronal images demonstrate abnormal perineural enhancement of several cranial nerves, such as the trigeminal *(curved arrows)* and the oculomotor *(straight arrows)* nerves.

infections entry into the CNS occurs by the peripheral nerves. Viral encephalitis is usually acute as a result of primary, direct invasion or may occur from reactivation of a latent virus. The most common causes of viral encephalitis are herpes simplex virus types 1 and 2 (HSV-1 and -2), herpes zoster, arboviruses, and enteroviruses, which produce almost the same inflammatory reaction in brain tissue and appear similar on CT

and MRI.[27] Viral encephalitis in immunosuppressed patients includes infection caused by human immunodeficiency virus (HIV), CMV, and the papovavirus (progressive multifocal leukoencephalopathy) and are discussed separately in the section on AIDS-related infections. Under the group of encephalitis we also include some other encephalitic forms of infection with diffuse and widespread parenchymal involvement.

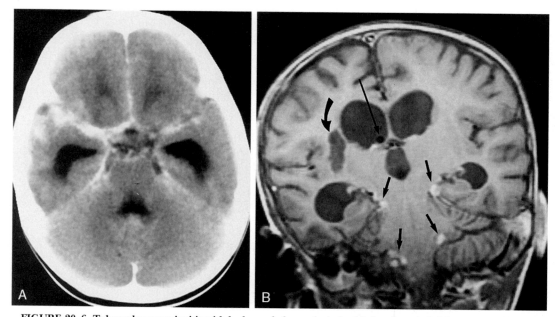

FIGURE 20–6. Tuberculous meningitis with hydrocephalus and cerebral infarction. *A,* Axial contrast-enhanced CT scan shows enhancement within the basal cisterns. The temporal horns are dilated secondary to a communicating hydrocephalus. *B,* Two months later, a Gd-DTPA–enhanced T1-weighted (SE, 600/20) coronal image reveals some residual nodular enhancement of the meninges *(short arrows)* and a large infarct in the putamen *(curved arrow).* The ventricles remain dilated despite a shunt tube in the right lateral ventricle *(long arrow).*

Some forms of encephalitis are described in association with viruses or other nonviral agents that are characterized by long incubation times of months to years followed by rapid, progressive deterioration. The term *slow infection* has been introduced to include a large number of human slow infections and neurologic diseases, such as Creutzfeldt-Jakob disease, kuru, and subacute sclerosing panencephalitis. Other uncommon forms of encephalitis may be seen with Lyme disease (*Borrelia* meningoencephalitis), which has MRI findings similar to those of multiple sclerosis, or with Reye's syndrome, a parainfectious encephalitis of unknown origin affecting the pediatric population and characterized by acute fatty liver and noninflammatory cerebral edema.

Viral pathogens can produce a clinical syndrome of encephalitis indistinguishable one from another. The clinical signs and symptoms are the result of inflammation and destruction of neurons by the virus itself and also sequelae of the development of humoral and cellular immunity to the virus.[28] Patients usually present with fever, headache, seizures, altered consciousness, aphasia, or ataxia. In addition, signs and symptoms of meningeal irritation coexist, because meningeal inflammation often accompanies diffuse brain infections, and so the term *meningoencephalitis* is sometimes more accurate to describe the true pathologic involvement. Particularly in cases of herpetic encephalitis, there are some added, bizarre clinical signs, such as hallucinations, seizures, and personality changes, reflecting the propensity to involve the subfrontal and temporal lobes.

IMAGING OF NONHERPETIC ENCEPHALITIS

In general, the imaging studies reflect the degree of brain involvement, which depends on the specific infecting agent and varies from one person to another. In mild cases, the MRI or CT scan may be entirely negative. The pattern of brain involvement can be focal or diffuse. MR images are most sensitive for detecting the early signs of cortical edema, which is seen as mild hyperintensity on T2-weighted images or thickening of the cortex on T1-weighted images. Severe infections can be associated with breakdown of the blood-brain barrier and enhancement with gadolinium. The enhancing cortex usually has a characteristic serpiginous pattern.

HERPES SIMPLEX VIRUS

HSV-1 accounts for 95% of herpetic encephalitis in adults. The virus usually invades the brain after reactivation of a latent form, which is frequently located in the trigeminal (gasserian) ganglion. The marked predilection for temporal lobe involvement supports the proposed theory that the infection spreads intracranially from the trigeminal ganglion along the meningeal branches of the trigeminal nerve[29] (Fig. 20–7). The resulting necrotizing encepha-

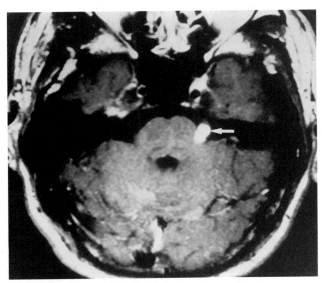

FIGURE 20–7. Herpes simplex trigeminal neuritis. Gadolinium-enhanced T1-weighted (SE, 600/20) coronal image reveals bright enhancement of the cisternal segment of the left trigeminal nerve *(arrow)*. A diagnosis of herpes simplex was made, lending support to the theory that the acute infection is derived from a latent form of the virus in the trigeminal ganglion.

litis rapidly disseminates in the brain, sparing the basal ganglia and producing edema and petechial hemorrhages. Early diagnosis is crucial, owing to the significant mortality rate (approaching 70%), the high incidence of sequelae, and the availability of effective antiviral drugs. Definitive diagnosis of HSV-1 encephalitis is made after isolation of the virus from brain biopsy. However, given the appropriate clinical presentation, with or without MRI or other laboratory diagnostic confirmation, medical treatment (with vidarabine or acyclovir) should be instituted immediately to avoid the devastating and irreversible brain damage.

In the early phase of the infection, HSV-1 encephalitis has a characteristic distribution in the medial temporal and inferior frontal lobes. On MR images the early edematous changes appear as ill-defined areas of low signal intensity on T1-weighted images and high signal intensity on T2-weighted images, usually beginning unilaterally but rapidly progressing to both hemispheres (Fig. 20–8). Variable mass effect and gyral enhancement may occur. Occasionally foci of hemorrhage are visualized as areas of high signal intensity on both T1- and T2-weighted images. Because of its superior sensitivity to increased brain water content and also its multiplanar capability without any bone artifacts, MRI is the imaging modality of choice in detecting early, subtle findings of encephalitis (Fig. 20–9), often demonstrating the possible involvement of the temporal lobes days before CT.[29, 30]

ACUTE DISSEMINATED ENCEPHALOMYELITIS

Acute disseminated encephalomyelitis (ADEM) represents an immune-mediated complication after an an-

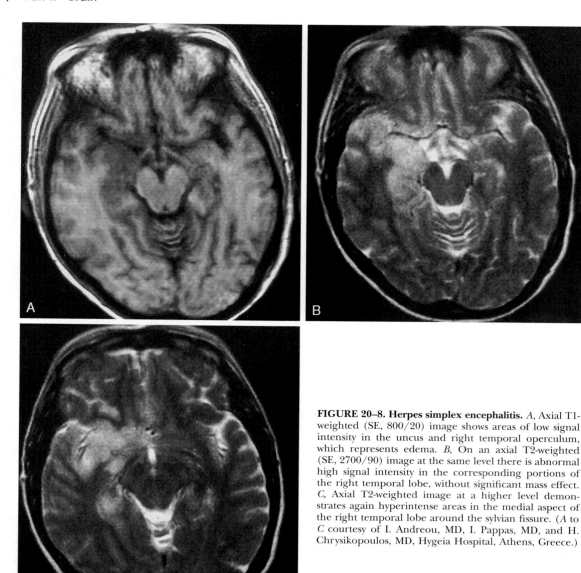

FIGURE 20–8. Herpes simplex encephalitis. *A,* Axial T1-weighted (SE, 800/20) image shows areas of low signal intensity in the uncus and right temporal operculum, which represents edema. *B,* On an axial T2-weighted (SE, 2700/90) image at the same level there is abnormal high signal intensity in the corresponding portions of the right temporal lobe, without significant mass effect. *C,* Axial T2-weighted image at a higher level demonstrates again hyperintense areas in the medial aspect of the right temporal lobe around the sylvian fissure. (*A* to *C* courtesy of I. Andreou, MD, I. Pappas, MD, and H. Chrysikopoulos, MD, Hygeia Hospital, Athens, Greece.)

tecedent viral infection, especially measles, mumps, rubella, or varicella, or a preceding vaccination, more commonly for influenza or rabies. It is a white matter disease that is characterized by a multifocal perivenous demyelination. ADEM was believed to be an uncommon disease but now is discovered more frequently because of the increased sensitivity of MRI to areas of demyelination. T2-weighted images demonstrate patchy, asymmetric areas of increased intensity in cerebral and cerebellar white matter, as well as in the brain stem and spinal cord[31] (Fig. 20–10). Although ADEM is typically a white matter disease, gray matter may be also involved. Because there is no significant mass effect or hemorrhage, the initial nonenhanced T1-weighted images are usually normal.[32, 33] In approximately 25% of patients with ADEM, there is nodular, gyral, or diffuse contrast enhancement due to disrup-

tion of the blood-brain barrier in the early, acute stage of demyelination. A case of ADEM presenting with ring-enhancing lesions in the white matter of cerebrum and cerebellum has also been reported[34] (see also Chapter 27).

CREUTZFELDT-JAKOB DISEASE

Creutzfeldt-Jakob disease is an uncommon dementing illness of older adults with spongiform neuropathologic changes similar to those seen in kuru and caused by a small, nonviral, infectious proteinaceous particle known as a prion. Typically, the patient exhibits a rapidly progressive dementia with significant brain atrophy, and death usually ensures within one year. Both CT and MRI show dramatic, progressive brain atrophy

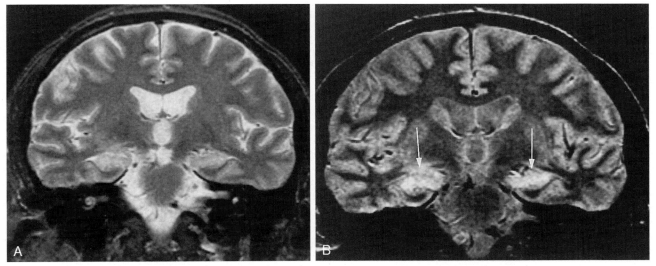

FIGURE 20–9. Herpes simplex encephalitis. *A* and *B*, Coronal T2- and proton density–weighted (SE, 3000/ 20,80) images demonstrate abnormal hyperintensity with the hippocampus bilaterally *(arrows, B)*. The patient was treated promptly with antiviral agents and recovered completely.

with subsequent enlargement of the ventricles and sulci. The value of serial scans is emphasized because progressing brain atrophy seen on imaging studies accompanies the clinical deterioration. Involvement of white matter is unusual in Creutzfeldt-Jakob disease.[35] According to several reports, symmetric areas with hyperintense signal on T2-weighted images were seen in the basal ganglia bilaterally and, in the appropriate clinical setting, are considered a specific sign of Creutzfeldt-Jakob disease[36] (see also Chapter 29).

SUBACUTE SCLEROSING PANENCEPHALITIS

Subacute sclerosing panencephalitis is a progressive and fatal encephalitis that is believed to be a slow viral infection caused by a defective measles virus. It is seen primarily in children after an interval of a few years after measles. Pathologically, there is demyelination of the white matter as well as abnormal findings in the basal ganglia. MRI has proved far more sensitive than CT in demonstrating the lesions of this disorder. On

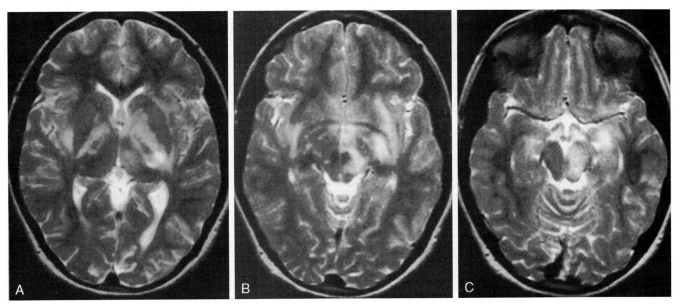

FIGURE 20–10. Acute disseminated encephalomyelitis. *A* to *C*, Sequential axial T2-weighted (fast SE, 3600/ 102) images demonstrate abnormal high signal intensity in the deep gray matter and white matter extending from the level of the basal ganglia *(A)* to the midbrain *(C)*. There is involvement of the left globus pallidus, the left thalamus, the posterior limbs of the internal capsules, the medial portions of the temporal lobe bilaterally, and the left midbrain.

long repetition time (TR), long echo time (TE) images, patchy or diffuse hyperintense areas are demonstrated in the periventricular white matter and basal ganglia bilaterally, which represent demyelination and gliosis. Cortical brain atrophy has been reported in advanced cases[37] (see also Chapter 27).

EXTRA-AXIAL EMPYEMAS

Subdural and epidural empyemas are uncommon purulent collections that develop in the subdural or, less frequently, in the epidural space, and they may occur alone or in combination. The main predisposing conditions are sinusitis, mastoiditis, infection secondary to previous craniotomy, and post-traumatic infection. Rarely, empyemas are secondary to meningitis or to hematogenous spread from a distant infectious focus. Particularly in infants, both sterile subdural effusions and infected subdural empyemas are often seen as a complication of purulent meningitis.[38] Pathophysiologically, pathogens may reach the subdural or the epidural spaces by means of retrograde septic thrombophlebitis through emissary veins or from local dural erosion from an adjacent bone infection.

SUBDURAL EMPYEMA

The outer two layers of meninges, the dura and arachnoid, define a potential subdural space that freely communicates over and between the cerebral hemispheres, but this space is restricted by normal anatomic barriers such as the falx cerebri, tentorium cerebelli, base of the skull, and foramen magnum. Therefore, subdural empyemas may extend throughout the subdural compartments that are enclosed between those barriers, acting as an expanding mass lesion. In the majority of patients who develop subdural empyemas, the source of infection is sinusitis or otitis, with frontal sinusitis accounting for 50% to 80% of the cases.[39] The pathogens that are commonly isolated from subdural empyemas are similar to those from sinusitis or brain abscesses. Therefore, aerobic *Streptococcus, Staphylococcus,* and anaerobic organisms such as *Streptococcus anginosus* are frequently encountered. Polymicrobial empyemas are occasionally found.

Patients present with fever, headache, alteration in mental status, seizures, and focal neurologic deficits. Subdural empyemas secondary to an infected post-traumatic subdural hematoma or to previous craniotomy follow a more prolonged and indolent course, occurring months to years after the original insult. They are characterized by an insidious onset of symptoms of a slowly expanding mass lesion but without signs of systemic infectious disease.[40] The infectious process is limited in the extra-axial compartment because a well-formed membrane after trauma or craniotomy acts as a barrier to the spread of the purulent collection into the brain parenchyma or the cortical veins and dural sinuses. Hence, symptoms in cases of postoperative or post-traumatic subdural empyema are mostly due to mass effect from the purulent collection, in contrast to subdural empyemas in the setting of otorhinologic infections in which the symptoms are related to the dissemination of the infection intracranially and less to the mass effect.

If the subdural empyema remains untreated, rapid clinical deterioration occurs and the mortality is quite high. The overall mortality rate is 10% to 18%, increasing dramatically to 75% when the patient becomes comatose. Even small subdural empyemas may cause severe complications such as vein thrombosis, infarcts, and cerebral abscesses. In most cases, antibiotic therapy alone is not sufficient for satisfactory recovery and neurosurgical intervention is required for drainage and brain decompression.

Imaging Features

Subdural empyema should be considered as a medical emergency, particularly when related to a preceding sinusitis or osteomyelitis. Thus, neuroimaging (CT and MRI) plays a significant role in early diagnosis and successful outcome. Several authors have emphasized the failure of CT to visualize small, crescentic extra-axial collections of fluid, especially when they are located superficially near the inner table of the skull.[41, 42] MRI has become the imaging modality of choice for detecting and defining the extent of subdural empyemas with the greatest accuracy.[25]

With the absence of bone artifacts, the superior morphologic delineation, and the ability to demonstrate views of the brain in coronal and sagittal planes, MRI readily identifies empyemas in the posterior fossa, in the temporal regions, and along the falx cerebri. On T1-weighted and proton density–weighted images, the purulent collections depict signal intensity higher than pure CSF, owing to the increased content of proteins and inflammatory debris, whereas on T2-weighted images the signal intensity approaches that of CSF. In the early stages of an empyema, exactly when the use of MRI is of greatest benefit, long-TR, long-TE sequences are most sensitive for detecting thin lentiform or crescentic fluid collections over the convexity or the interhemispheric fissure. Also, on T2-weighted images, areas of cortex adjacent to the empyema appear thickened and hyperintense and are believed to represent edema or hyperemia secondary to reversible ischemia after vasospasm and venous stasis.[1] MRI can also evaluate the presence of mass effect on the adjacent brain or CSF spaces better than CT, as well as the underlying parenchymal abnormalities such as cerebral edema, brain abscess, or cortical vein and dural sinus thrombosis[43] (Fig. 20–11).

After administration of paramagnetic contrast material (gadolinium), subtle enhancement occurs at the margins of the empyema, which becomes more prominent after time, and is due to formation of a vascular membrane of granulation tissue (Fig. 20–12). This enhancement is similar to that seen on postcontrast CT. By enhanced MRI, in conjunction with the enhancement of the outer membrane (capsule) of the empyema, there is enhancement of the adjacent, displaced,

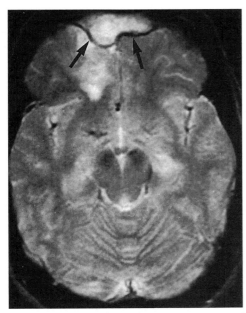

FIGURE 20–11. Subdural empyema. Axial T2-weighted (SE, 2700/90) image shows a subdural collection of fluid with a surrounding black rim of displaced dura *(arrows)*. An area of increased signal intensity is seen within the brain parenchyma next to the empyema representing a focus of cerebritis. (Courtesy of N. Bontozoglou, MD, Evangelismos Hospital, Athens, Greece.)

dural effusions or subdural hematomas. On CT scans, chronic hemorrhagic subdural effusions and empyemas appear similar as hypodense extra-axial collections. By using MRI, subdural hematomas (subacute or chronic) can easily be distinguished owing to the markedly hyperintense signal pattern of extracellular methemoglobin on both T1- and T2-weighted images. Subdural sterile effusions show a signal intensity similar to that of CSF on T1-weighted images, in contrast to the brighter signal intensity of subdural empyemas attributable to the proteinaceous content of the fluid. Also, after contrast medium administration the margins of subdural empyemas enhance, which does not occur in hematomas or subdural effusions.

EPIDURAL EMPYEMA

Epidural empyema refers to a purulent collection that is localized in the potential space between the dura mater and the overlying bones of the skull. Because of the easy spread of infection across the dura through emissary veins, subdural and epidural empyemas often coexist (81% of autopsied cases).[45] In such a case of simultaneous appearance, the neurologic signs are attributed to the subdural empyema. Epidural empyema tends to localize outside the inelastic and firm dura, which limits the growth of the collection, reduces the exerted pressure on the adjacent brain parenchyma, and protects the underlying brain from parenchymal abnormalities. Thus, patients with epidural empyemas have a more insidious and benign clinical course than those with subdural empyemas, with headache and fever often the only clinical clues. Later on, focal neurologic signs and alteration in mental status appear. The etiology, pathogenesis, and bac-

thickened dura mater, which allows accurate localization of the empyema and the distinction between the abscess fluid and the capsule.[44] Occasionally, abnormal enhancement in a concomitant brain abnormality such as brain abscess is seen.

On the basis of signal differences, MRI easily differentiates between subdural empyemas and sterile sub-

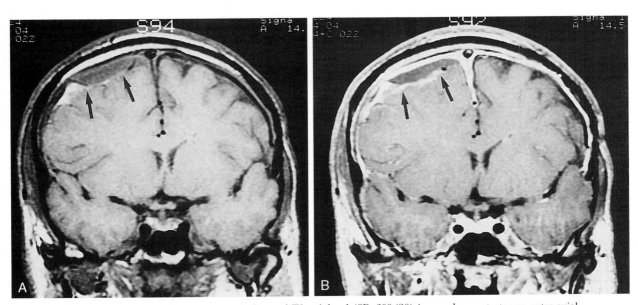

FIGURE 20–12. Subdural empyema. *A,* Coronal T1-weighted (SE, 600/20) image demonstrates an extra-axial, lentiform fluid collection *(arrows)* in the right frontal region with little mass effect on the adjacent brain parenchyma. *B,* Post–gadolinium-enhanced T1-weighted image at the same level shows enhancement at the margins of the empyema *(arrows)*. Note that the purulent fluid collection exhibits higher signal intensity than pure CSF.

teriology of epidural empyemas are similar to those described in the section on subdural empyemas. Frontal sinusitis is the primary preceding condition, although mastoiditis, previous surgery, and trauma are other causes. With early diagnosis and prompt institution of medical or neurosurgical treatment, the prognosis for a patient with an epidural empyema is excellent.

Imaging Features

As with subdural empyemas, MRI is the most sensitive imaging modality for the detection of epidural empyemas.[43, 44] The signal characteristics of these lentiform extra-axial collections are similar to those of subdural empyemas on both T1- and T2-weighted images. Short-TR, short-TE sequences show a hypointense medial rim of thickened, inflamed dura, which enhances profoundly after contrast medium administration, even more than that observed in imaging of subdural empyemas. A moderate degree of mass effect is often present, with sulcal effacement and distortion of the ventricular system. An important imaging feature of epidural empyemas is the normal appearance of the adjacent brain parenchyma, in contrast to subdural empyemas. Other diagnostic clues for an epidural empyema are the presence of a thick hypointense dura on the medial side of the collection and also the presence of osteomyelitis or subgaleal abscess, which makes an epidural empyema more likely.

CYSTIC LESIONS

In the spectrum of focal infectious parenchymal lesions, brain abscesses and cystic lesions are the main representatives. Cystic infections are typically caused by parasitic diseases, which are still an important and not uncommon clinical issue in underdeveloped countries and in patients with defective or suppressed immune status. We review the imaging features of the most frequent parasitic diseases with emphasis on neurocysticercosis. Toxoplasmosis is discussed separately in the section on AIDS-related infections, because it constitutes the most common opportunistic infection in patients with AIDS.

CYSTICERCOSIS

Cysticercosis is the most common parasitic infection of the CNS in immunocompetent individuals and is caused by the larval pork tapeworm *Taenia solium*. Humans ingest the eggs with food contaminated by human or pig feces. In the stomach the eggs release embryos (oncospheres) that enter the intestinal wall and spread hematogenously, invading any human tissue. Once lodged in a tissue, they develop the larvae (cysticerci), which do not move to other sites. Although the distribution of the parasite is worldwide, there are some endemic areas such as parts of Southeast Asia, India, Africa, and Latin America. There is

also an increasing frequency of cysticercosis in North America because of the growing immigrant population. Skeletal muscles and the CNS are most frequently affected by cysticercosis, with CNS infection occurring in 70% to 90% of cases.[46] There are four forms of neurocysticercosis: parenchymal, meningeal (subarachnoid), ventricular, and mixed. Although brain parenchyma is generally considered as the most common site of involvement in neurocysticercosis, certain reports claim that subarachnoid space is more common.[47] Patients present with a broad spectrum of clinical manifestations attributed to the different patterns and anatomic locations of CNS involvement. Epilepsy is the most common clinical sign, and in many cases it represents the primary or sole manifestation of the disease. Furthermore, neurocysticercosis constitutes the main cause of adult-onset seizures in developing countries with poor hygiene, accounting for 50% of epilepsy cases.[48] Other clinical problems include headache, focal neurologic deficits, basal arachnoiditis, hydrocephalus, and symptoms of increase intracranial pressure or dementia.

Parenchymal Form

Neuroimaging (CT and MRI) plays an essential role in the diagnosis of any parasitic disease, along with the history, clinical symptoms, CSF findings, and serologic test results. The appearance of cysticercosis at CT or MRI reflects the pathologic changes of the parasite in the different phases of evolution. In parenchymal cysticercosis, the initial, acute phase of invasion by the larvae causes a mild, focal inflammatory reaction. This

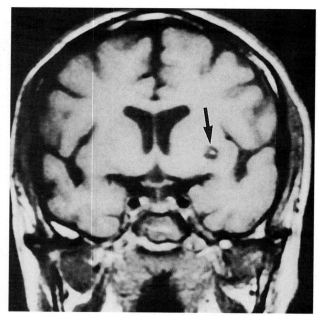

FIGURE 20–13. Parenchymal cysticercosis in viable vesicular stage. Coronal T1-weighted (SE, 550/20) image demonstrates a rounded cystic structure of CSF-equivalent signal intensity in the deep left temporal lobe *(arrow)*. There is no evidence of surrounding edema or mass effect. Note also the presence of the scolex within the cysticercous cyst.

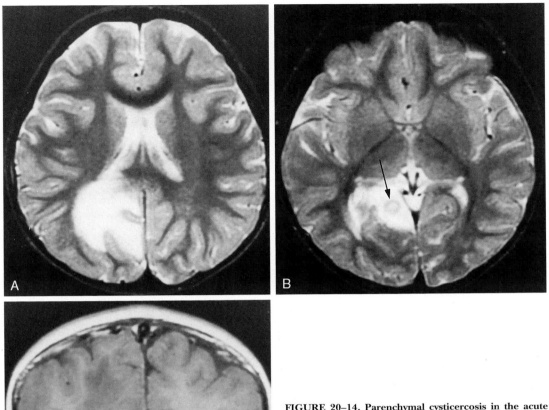

FIGURE 20–14. Parenchymal cysticercosis in the acute degenerating phase. *A* and *B,* Axial T2-weighted (SE, 3000/80) images disclose an acute inflammatory reaction of edema surrounding a cysticercosis cyst that has recently died. The thick wall of the cyst is illustrated in *B (arrow). C,* Gadolinium-enhanced T1-weighted (SE, 600/20) coronal image displays ring-like enhancement of the cyst, surrounded by the hypointense parenchymal edema.

is undetectable on CT scans, but MR images demonstrate a focal, nonenhancing area of edema or a small enhancing focus. In the next stage, 3 to 12 months after infection, larvae (cysticerci) are completely developed, with their bladder full of fluid. At this stage, neuroimaging displays the typical rounded cystic lesions up to 1 to 2 cm in diameter, located peripherally in the cortex or at the gray matter–white matter junction. The cysts contain clear fluid, with signal intensity identical to CSF on all MRI sequences. One of the characteristic features of cysticercosis is that in this stage of cyst formation the larvae are still alive and there is no reaction in the surrounding brain. Therefore, the MR images show no evidence of associated edema or contrast enhancement around the cysts.[49] Also, in this viable stage a small invagination develops along one cystic wall and proliferates, developing the scolex that is pathognomonic for cysticercosis. This

mural nodule can be seen as a focal mural 1- to 2-mm projection that is isointense relative to the brain parenchyma on all pulse sequences (Fig. 20–13). Visualization of the scolex is much easier with MRI than CT, owing to the superior contrast resolution of MRI. Furthermore, MRI has proved more sensitive than CT in the detection of the parenchymal cysts, particularly when they are located near the convexity or in the posterior fossa.[50]

In the next phase the parasites degenerate and die, and so the cysts are no longer tolerated by the immune system, inducing a variable inflammatory reaction of the surrounding neural tissue with marked edema and ring-like enhancement (Fig. 20–14). Thickening of the cyst walls (capsule formation) and accumulation of protein within the cyst also occur. This turbid, cystic content results in shortening of the T1 relaxation time, increasing the signal intensity of the cyst on T1-

weighted images. Therefore, the cysts exhibit a higher signal intensity than CSF on both T1-weighted and proton density–weighted images. On T2-weighted images the cystic fluid becomes indistinguishable from the adjacent edema, whereas the cyst walls and scolex appear as low-intensity structures.[51]

Finally, at the end stage of evolution, the cysts are shrunken and completely mineralized and only punctate foci of calcifications may be seen. CT is superior to MRI in evaluating this final stage of the disease, although specific MRI sequences (gradient-echo) are relatively sensitive to calcified lesions.[52] An important observation is that calcifications occur only in parenchymal cysticercosis and not in the ventricular or subarachnoid forms. It is not known how long the parasite remains in each stage of evolution. It depends partly on the host's defense, but the general concept is that it takes an average of 5 years before the parasite becomes calcified (final stage). It is not uncommon to see patients with multiple lesions at different stages of evolution (Fig. 20–15).

Cisternal Form

Subarachnoid or cisternal cysticercosis is another form of neurocysticercosis, with involvement of the subarachnoid spaces and the adjacent meninges, particularly at the base of the brain. More often, cysts are located in the cerebellopontine angles or the suprasellar region, and they demonstrate different morphologic features than their parenchymal counterparts. They may reach a large size with a racemose configuration. They are multilobular, sterile, and usually without scolices. The cysts are isointense relative to CSF on all pulse sequences, and occasionally the only imaging finding is enlargement or asymmetry of the CSF spaces without evidence of any cyst walls. This form of neurocysticercosis is associated with chronic meningitis and

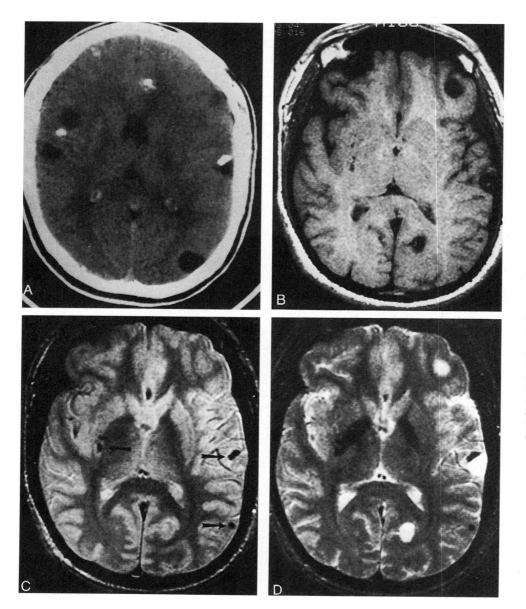

FIGURE 20–15. Parenchymal cysticercosis with multiple lesions at different stages of evolution. *A,* CT scan demonstrates multiple parenchymal lesions. Some are cystic and others are calcified. *B,* T1-weighted (SE, 600/20) image reveals hypointense cystic lesions within the left frontal, temporal, and occipital lobes. Mural nodules, representing the viable scolex, are evident in the temporal and occipital cysts. *C* and *D,* On proton density–weighted and T2-weighted (SE, 3000/30,80) images the cyst fluid follows the CSF signal, which is typical of cysticercosis. The calcifications *(arrows)* are hypointense on both pulse sequences. The calcified lesions represent dead parasites, whereas the cysts contain living larvae.

secondary basal arachnoiditis. The inflammatory lepto-meningeal reaction is profound around the basal cisterns and may result either in communicating hydro-cephalus due to obstruction of CSF pathways or in infarctions due to vasculitis. Therefore, in cases of suspected cisternal cysticercosis, contrast-enhanced MRI should be performed to detect abnormal meningeal enhancement.[53]

Intraventricular Form

Intraventricular cysticercosis occurs in approximately 20% of the cases, and the cysts are more often located in the fourth ventricle, in the aqueduct of Sylvius, or, less frequently, in other ventricular sites. They can migrate within or between ventricles and may be position dependent. Early diagnosis and subsequent treatment are crucial in this form of neurocysticercosis, because it is potentially life threatening by producing an acute, obstructive hydrocephalus. Even though the cystic component is isointense relative to CSF on T1-weighted and proton density–weighted images, the cyst walls and the mural nodule (scolex) are often visible, making the diagnosis obvious (Fig. 20–16). In contrast, the majority of ventricular cysts are not demonstrable on T2-weighted images because the high signal intensity from CSF merges with the cyst fluid, obscuring the walls and the scolex.[54] Sometimes, large fourth ventricular cysts are invisible, because the cyst walls conform to the dilated ventricle. The only clue to the diagnosis may be demonstration of the scolex, or of a high-intensity subependymal reactive rim around the cyst on T2-weighted and proton density–weighted images. After contrast medium administration, the ependymal inflammation enhances in a ring-like pattern.[47, 51]

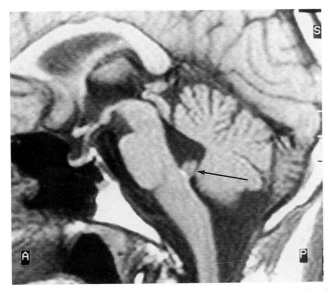

FIGURE 20–16. Intraventricular cysticercosis. Sagittal T1-weighted (SE, 500/20) image shows a fourth ventricular mass, isointense relative to the brain parenchyma, which represents the scolex *(arrow)*. (Courtesy of I. Andreou, MD, I. Pappas, MD, and H. Chrysikopoulos, MD, Hygeia Hospital, Athens, Greece.)

Mixed Form

In cases of subarachnoid and ventricular cysticercosis, MRI has proved far superior to CT in the recognition of the cysts. Small intraventricular cysts can easily be missed using CT without intraventricular contrast material, because they appear the same density as CSF. MRI offers many advantages, including superior contrast resolution to identify the cyst walls and scolices against the ventricular CSF, multiplanar capability to evaluate ventricular distortion better, and optimal visualization of the posterior fossa and fourth ventricle, the most common location of the cysts. In cases of cisternal cysticercosis, contrast-enhanced MRI can demonstrate enhancement in the basal cisterns related to chronic meningitis and also visualizes the cysts better in locations problematic on CT, such the suprasellar cisterns, cerebellopontine angles, and posterior fossa.[1, 46, 55]

HYDATID DISEASE

Hydatid disease is a parasitic infection that results from the ingestion of contaminated dog feces containing eggs of *Echinococcus granulosus*. After the eggs are ingested, they release embryos (oncospheres) in the gastrointestinal tract that spread hematogenously through the portal circulation to human tissues. The embryos transform into cystic larvae, which are called echinococcal or hydatid cysts. The majority of the lesions affect the liver and lungs, although some may reach the brain (2% to 5%). The disease is endemic in many of the sheep- or cattle-raising areas of the world, because the intermediate hosts of the parasite are sheep or cattle. Those endemic areas include the Middle East, Mediterranean countries, and South America. In patients who originate from those geographic areas and who have a large intra-axial cystic lesion in the brain, the diagnosis of hydatid cyst should be included in the differential diagnosis, along with arachnoid cyst, porencephalic cyst, or cystic tumor. Cerebral echinococcosis is more common in infants and children, and it usually occurs supratentorially, preferentially in the parietal lobe. The resultant echinococcal cyst is large, slow growing, single, and unilocular, containing clear fluid. Rarely, the cysts may be multilocular with daughter cysts. Patients with cerebral echinococcosis may present with signs of intracranial hypertension or seizures.

Both CT and MRI demonstrate the hydatid cyst adequately as a spherical thin-walled structure, containing fluid with CSF imaging characteristics (Fig. 20–17). Calcification of the cystic wall may occasionally occur and obviously is better demonstrated by CT.[56] Because of the large size of the cyst there may be severe distortion and shift of the ventricular system and subarachnoid spaces, as well as obstructive hydrocephalus due to obstruction of the CSF pathways. Hydatid cysts are not associated with edema or contrast enhancement, unless cyst rupture and leakage occur and induce an inflammatory reaction in the surrounding neural tis-

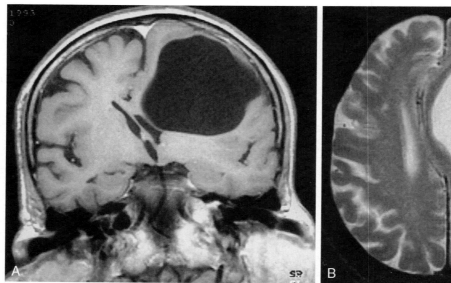
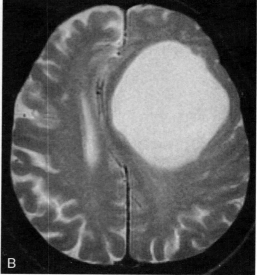

FIGURE 20–17. Hydatid cyst. *A* and *B,* Coronal T1-weighted and axial T2-weighted images demonstrate a large cystic mass in the left frontoparietal region. The cyst appears homogeneous and follows CSF signal intensity on both sequences. Also, because of its enormous size, it produces severe distortion in the ventricular system, which is better appreciated in the coronal scan. Note the absence of any inflammatory reaction in the surrounding brain parenchyma. (*A* and *B* courtesy of S. Trakadas, MD, University of Athens, Athens, Greece.)

sue.[51] Visualization of the rounded cystic lesion, as well as evaluation of the concomitant mass effect, is better with MRI, because it offers the ability for coronal and sagittal views of the brain. Another diagnostic feature of cerebral hydatid disease that has been described is low signal intensity of the cyst wall on T2-weighted images.[57]

PARAGONIMIASIS

Paragonimiasis is a rare parasitic disease that results after the ingestion of freshwater crabs or crayfish contaminated with the lung fluke *Paragonimus westermani.* The disease is endemic in East Asia, West Africa, and Latin America. The primary site of involvement is the lung. Some of the produced larvae may bypass the lungs, and a small percentage (1%) can invade the brain parenchyma, producing arachnoiditis, granulomas, or brain abscesses. In the early stage both CT and MRI demonstrate the granulomas as multiple, conglomerate, ring-enhancing, abscess-like cysts, with a significant amount of surrounding edema. In the chronic stage, granulomas and abscesses are densely calcified. On plain films and CT scans the calcifications have a "soap bubble" appearance (multiple calcified masses with round or oval shapes).[51] On MR images, small calcified foci are easily missed but larger lesions show mixed signal intensity with a peripheral hypointense rim on both T1- and T2-weighted images, representing the conglomeration of calcified ova. A central area of hypointensity on T1-weighted and of hyperintensity on T2-weighted images reflects the soft tissue contents of the chronic granuloma.[58] Also, MRI demonstrates the surrounding inflammatory changes and the associated brain atrophy better than CT does.

OTHER PARASITIC DISEASES

Many other parasites can infect the CNS, resulting in infections such as sparganosis, toxocariasis, schistosomiasis, trichinosis, and amebiasis. They are not discussed separately in this chapter owing to their rare appearance and the nonspecific findings on neuroimaging studies. Additional information on these parasitic diseases can be found elsewhere in the literature.[51]

CONGENITAL INFECTIONS

Congenital infections refer to maternally transmitted infections, which are most frequently caused by the group of TORCH pathogens, which include *Toxoplasma,* others (*Listeria, Treponema*), rubella, cytomegalovirus, and herpes simplex virus (HSV-2). Now, maybe another H should be added to emphasize the common occurrence of HIV in this subgroup of CNS infections. Congenital infections of the brain may produce diffuse, parenchymal inflammation with some unique characteristics, such as microcephaly, brain atrophy, hydrocephalus, neuronal migrational anomalies, and cerebral calcifications. The degree of the destructive brain process and the resultant developmental abnormalities depend on the timing of the infection. The earlier in gestation the CNS involvement occurs, the more profound the brain destruction will be. In cases of congenital infections, in which the prerequisite is involvement of the mother, even in a subclinical form, the causative agents may reach the fetus, either during gestation through a hematogenous-transplacental route or during birth as the fetus passes through the infected birth canal.

TOXOPLASMOSIS

Toxoplasmosis is caused by the parasite *Toxoplasma gondii,* which is typically passed hematogenously through the placenta to the fetus. A large percentage of the population, approaching 50%, has been infected by the parasite sometime in life, but congenital toxoplasmosis occurs only when the mother becomes infected during pregnancy. Infected fetuses have a high frequency (almost 50%) of CNS involvement.[59] Early infection before 20 weeks of gestation is associated with severe, persistent neurologic abnormalities, whereas late infection after 30 weeks is rarely associated with deficits.[60] The most striking clinical symptoms are chorioretinitis, seizures, and developmental delay, with chorioretinitis being the most common single clinical finding in the infected neonate.[61] The clinical signs may be absent initially and develop later in life, with the disorder as presenting seizures, for example.

Neuroimaging of congenital toxoplasmosis may reveal a whole spectrum of findings, such as intracranial calcifications, hydrocephalus, brain atrophy, microcephaly, and neuronal migrational anomalies. Intracranial calcifications constitute a common and characteristic finding and are located in the periventricular area, in the basal ganglia, and in the cerebral hemispheres. Dense, calcified masses in the basal ganglia have been associated with earlier infection (before the 20th week) and greater severity of disease.[60] Obviously, CT is preferable to MRI for detection of those calcifications. Hydrocephalus is adequately evaluated with both CT and MRI and is secondary to aqueductal stenosis. Neural tissue loss produces an ex vacuo expansion of the atria and occipital horns, as well as porencephaly and hydranencephaly. MRI is much better than CT for detecting neuronal migrational anomalies such as pachygyria and also, in older children with some degree of myelination, for the diagnosis of the concomitant demyelinating changes on long-TR, long-TE sequences.

CYTOMEGALOVIRUS INFECTION

CMV is a member of the herpesvirus family, which subclinically infects nearly all the population at some time in life and is the most frequent cause of a congenital viral infection. Congenital infection occurs after primary or secondary (reactivation) maternal infection, and the virus reaches the fetus by the transplacental route. CNS involvement is an important manifestation of the disease, and, as with toxoplasmosis, earlier infection results in poorer outcome with more severe and persistent neurologic sequelae.[62] Clinical symptoms develop in few of the patients with congenital CMV initially, but they become apparent by at least 2 years of age. Symptoms include chorioretinitis, microcephaly, seizures, psychomotor retardation, and sensorineural hearing loss.

CMV produces a diffuse encephalitic infectious process, which results in multifocal destructive changes in the brain that lead to calcifications and microcephaly. The immature cells in the germinal matrix region are the first involved areas in the brain. Necrosis and calcifications of those areas explain the predilection for thick or nodular calcifications in the periventricular area.[63] Intracranial calcifications may also be found in the cortical and subcortical region, as well as in the basal ganglia, so differentiation between congenital infection from CMV or toxoplasmosis is not certain based on imaging criteria alone. CT is probably the more useful imaging modality initially to detect the intracranial calcifications and the presence of brain atrophy, which is manifested by widening of cortical sulci and enlargement of the lateral ventricles (Fig. 20–18). However, MRI has proved far more sensitive than CT in identifying the presence and extent of the additional parenchymal abnormalities, such as infarctions, atrophy, demyelination, neuronal migrational anomalies, and small paraventricular cysts. The presence of paraventricular cysts, usually adjacent to the occipital horns, reflects areas of focal necrosis and gliosis and may represent a specific sign of congenital CMV infection.[64] Accurate evaluation of the parenchymal lesions seemed to correlate well with the subsequent neurologic complications. Thus, MRI is an important and necessary complement to CT to better define the various brain abnormalities and help predict the prognosis.[65]

RUBELLA

Owing to maternal screening methods and systematic immunization, congenital rubella has become quite rare in the developed countries. Rubella virus is transmitted transplacentally during the primary maternal infection, and, as in the other congenital infections, the earlier in gestation the infection occurs, the more severe and extensive is the brain damage. Clinically, the infected neonates have multisystemic involvement with various abnormalities of the heart, eyes, and CNS. Brain involvement typically consists of a meningoencephalitis that may cause brain atrophy, intracranial calcifications (not as common as in the other congenital infections), microcephaly, delayed myelination, and vasculitis. Vasculitis is a unique feature of rubella virus infection. It is a necrotizing angiopathy that involves the leptomeningeal and parenchymal vessels, producing focal areas of destruction in the vessel walls and deposition of microcalcifications in and around the vessels.[63] In cases of congenital rubella encephalitis, CT is able to detect the subtle intracranial calcifications or some areas of low density in the deep white matter, which represent areas of encephalomalacia or demyelination.[66] MRI may miss the calcifications but outperforms CT at identifying the parenchymal developmental anomalies, such as oligogyria/pachygyria, delayed or pathologic myelination, vasculitis, ischemia, or necrosis.[65]

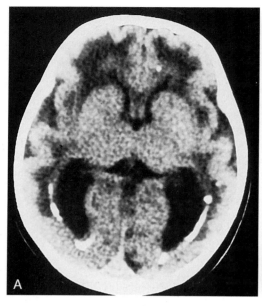

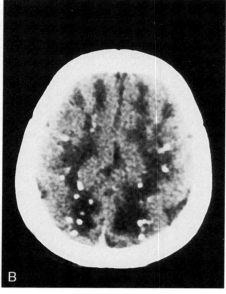

FIGURE 20–18. Congenital CMV encephalitis. *A,* Nonenhanced CT scan shows thick periventricular calcifications lining the walls of the dilated trigones of the lateral ventricles. *B,* CT scan at a higher level shows scattered, punctate calcifications throughout the brain parenchyma.

HERPES SIMPLEX VIRUS INFECTION

Herpes simplex virus is a DNA virus and a member of the herpesvirus family and has two different serotypes, HSV-1 and HSV-2. These serotypes produce the most important acute viral encephalitis in the neonate. In more than 80% of cases of herpes simplex encephalitis, HSV-2 is the causative agent. The infection is most commonly acquired during delivery through an infected birth canal, although hematogenous transmission through the placenta does occur. An explanation for the observed rarity of early transplacental infection is that it causes severe destruction in the fetus, resulting in spontaneous abortions rather than maldevelopment of the CNS.[63] However, if infants survive the early hematogenous infection, the devastating effect of the panencephalitis results in findings similar to those of other placentally transmitted infections, such as microcephaly, cerebral atrophy and necrosis, and intracranial calcifications, but to a greater degree and with more severe neurologic sequelae.

As mentioned earlier, infection during delivery through direct contact with the infected vagina is the origin in the majority of neonatal herpesvirus infections. These infections are divided into three main clinical categories: 1) localized infection of the skin, eyes, and mouth; 2) disseminated infection (occurring 10 to 11 days after birth) with symptoms of severe bacterial sepsis and multiorgan involvement; and 3) isolated CNS involvement (presenting 15 to 25 days after birth) with clinical signs of fever, lethargy, and seizures.[67]

During the initial episode of HSV-2 encephalitis, both CT and MRI have many limitations, and normal imaging does not exclude the diagnosis. Early CT findings are subtle, but with time widespread patchy areas of low-density edema develop diffusely throughout the cerebrum but primarily within the white matter. Eventually, findings of multicystic encephalomalacia be-

come apparent, along with hemorrhagic infarctions and cortical and white matter calcifications. The multifocal edema is demonstrated early on long-TR, long-TE MR images as diffuse areas of high signal intensity in the cerebral hemispheres, basal ganglia, thalami, and cerebellum. The problem that causes confusion on MR images is that at this time in life, normal white matter exhibits high signal intensity due to minimal myelination and high water content, making the differentiation between normal and edematous white matter difficult. Furthermore, the MRI appearance of the encephalitis is harder to appreciate, because the pattern of cerebral edema is diffuse, bilateral, and symmetric. Unlike its adult counterpart, neonatal HSV-2 encephalitis is a panencephalitis without temporal or subfrontal lobe predilection. Thus, for the early diagnosis of this encephalitis, the more reliable MRI sign is not the distribution but the involvement of the gray matter, which causes a loss of gray matter–white matter differentiation on both T1- and T2-weighted images.[68] The encephalitis progresses rapidly; in the intermediate stage, parenchymal or meningeal enhancement may be seen on postcontrast MR images. Within the first 2 to 4 weeks encephalomalacia develops, as well as hemorrhagic foci and intracranial calcifications. Another important and unique imaging finding in HSV-2 encephalitis is a linear, gyriform cortical pattern of increased attenuation on CT scans and hyperintensity on T1-weighted images, overlying abnormal edematous or necrotic white matter or both. The cortical imaging features have been attributed to the presence of microcalcifications and to changes in local vascularity.[68, 69]

HUMAN IMMUNODEFICIENCY VIRUS INFECTION

The majority of cases of HIV infection are transmitted hematogenously through the placenta. Infants infected with HIV are asymptomatic at birth, presenting in time with developmental delay and recurrent infections. At 2 to 3 years of age, a progressive clinical syndrome evolves, manifested by seizures, motor deficits, acquired microcephaly, and behavioral and cognitive decline.[70] Secondary opportunistic infections or CNS tumors, common in adults infected with HIV, are relatively uncommon in the pediatric age group. Neuroimaging displays cerebral atrophy, primarily central, as well as intracranial calcification in the basal ganglia, evaluated better by CT. MRI demonstrates the white matter abnormalities, such as white matter hypoplasia and delayed myelination, better than CT, as well as the presence of the secondary CNS complications of HIV infection.[71]

ACQUIRED IMMUNODEFICIENCY SYNDROME–RELATED INFECTIONS

AIDS is caused by HIV, a member of the lentiviral subfamily of retroviruses, with special lymphotropic and neurotropic properties. A variety of factors, such as genetic susceptibility, coinfection with other viruses, or nutritional habits, may interact with HIV and predispose a patient to disease or determine the course and resultant clinical syndrome.[72] HIV selectively destroys the T helper (T4) lymphocytes, causing a profound defect in cell-mediated immunity and consequent development of multiple opportunistic infections and uncommon malignancies. Also, due to its neurotropism, HIV can attack the neurons directly, damaging the brain and spinal cord with primary manifestations of a subacute encephalitis and a vacuolar myelopathy, respectively.

With the increasing number of patients seropositive for HIV, AIDS has become the leading cause of CNS infections and one of the most common reasons for neuroimaging. At least 10% of all patients with AIDS present initially with neurologic complaints, and more than one third will manifest a clinically apparent neurologic disorder sometime during the course of their disease.[73] However, neurologic impairment may be much more frequent but insidious in the early stages of the disease. It has been reported that in asymptomatic seropositive individuals there are subtle cognitive changes (e.g., reduced speed of information processing, problems in learning and remembering) that can be expressed only by special neuropsychologic tests.[74] On autopsy series, evidence of significant neuropathologic abnormalities has been shown in 75% to 90% of patients with AIDS and usually more than one disease process was present.[75, 76] The CNS infections in the AIDS population share some atypical clinical and imaging characteristics, different from the corresponding picture in individuals with normal immune status. First, the defective immune system makes the nervous system incapable of fighting common pathogens. Therefore, the number of pathogens is large, multiple concurrent microbial agents may be responsible for the infection, and there is minimal inflammatory response of the adjacent neural tissue. Neuroimaging

features in patients with AIDS are based primarily on four different patterns of brain involvement, which include cerebral atrophy, mass lesions, white matter changes, and chronic meningitis.[77] MRI is the imaging modality of choice for the evaluation of CNS infections in patients with AIDS, offering superior contrast resolution, multiplanar capability, and the lack of bone artifacts. In particular, MRI is of great benefit in the detection of white matter abnormalities and posterior fossa disease, and it also has proved more sensitive in detecting the presence and the extent of parenchymal lesions.

The most important and common cerebral infections in patients with AIDS are further analyzed in the following sections.

TOXOPLASMOSIS

Toxoplasmosis is the most common opportunistic brain infection among patients with AIDS and constitutes the most frequent cause of intracranial mass lesions. It is caused by the parasite *T. gondii*, an obligate intracellular protozoan, which invades subclinically (latent form) a large portion of the adult population (up to 70% in some areas). In the immunocompetent patient, clinically apparent infection with *Toxoplasma* results in a benign, self-limited lymphadenopathy with fever and malaise. In patients with AIDS seropositive for *Toxoplasma*, the risk for cerebral toxoplasmosis approaches 30%, and the infection is secondary to reactivation of a latent parasite encysted in the brain.[78, 79] Infection with *Toxoplasma* produces multiple, scattered necrotic and inflammatory brain abscesses, which have a predilection for the corticomedullary junction and the basal ganglia. Focal parenchymal lesions, the most common form of cerebral toxoplasmosis, have three distinct zones and no peripheral capsule. The central zone is necrotic with few organisms, the intermediate zone is hypervascular and contains numerous tachyzoites with pronounced inflammatory reaction, and the peripheral zone has more encysted organisms (bradyzoites). However, in severely immunosuppressed patients, toxoplasmosis may exhibit a more diffuse, necrotizing and fulminant form of encephalitis.[80] Patients may present with clinical symptoms of focal mass effect, such as seizures, focal neurologic deficits, or cranial nerve palsies, as well as more generalized symptoms, such as fever, headache, confusion, or declining mental status.

MRI has proved to be the most sensitive imaging modality for the detection of cerebral toxoplasmosis, by demonstrating lesions in patients with normal CT scans and by delineating the true extent of the disease or displaying more lesions than CT, even compared with delayed, double-dose contrast-enhanced CT.[81, 82] Nonenhanced T1-weighted images show focal areas of mild hypointensity. Postcontrast MR images demonstrate multiple nodular or ring-like enhancing lesions, involving both white and deep gray matter and surrounded by vasogenic edema. The enhancement pattern is similar to that seen on postcontrast CT scans.

Toxoplasma lesions may occur anywhere in the brain parenchyma, supratentorially or infratentorially, although the predominant locations are the basal ganglia and corticomedullary junction. On T2-weighted images, focal lesions exhibit variable signal intensity, ranging from hyperintense (inseparable from the edema), to hypointense or isointense compared with brain parenchyma[83] (Fig. 20–19). Hemorrhagic *Toxoplasma* lesions are uncommon.

The neuroimaging findings with both CT and MRI are not pathognomonic for toxoplasmosis because they can be seen in various infectious or noninfectious diseases, such as brain metastases, intracerebral lymphoma, or Kaposi's sarcoma, or in brain abscesses of nonpyogenic origin (tuberculomas, cryptococcomas). Once toxoplasmosis is suspected by imaging criteria and positive *Toxoplasma* serologic test results, the diagnosis is confirmed empirically by monitoring the response to treatment (sulfadiazine and pyrimethamine) with clinical examination and follow-up CT or MRI. Clinical and radiographic improvement is a reliable indicator of toxoplasmosis and should be evident within 2 to 3 weeks of therapy, manifested by resolution of neurologic abnormalities and a decrease in the size and number of lesions. Typically, the radiographic improvement lags behind the clinical response. Lifelong therapy is recommended to prevent recurrence. If any or all of the lesions fail to respond to therapy, *Toxoplasma* may not be the causative infective agent or there may be another concurrent disease process present. In those cases brain biopsy should be considered.[82, 84]

CRYPTOCOCCOSIS

Cryptococcus neoformans causes the most common CNS fungal infection in patients with AIDS, which in terms of relative frequency ranks third after HIV encephalitis and toxoplasmosis. This yeast-like fungus initially invades the respiratory tract and then spreads hematogenously to other organs, with a special predilection for the CNS. Intracranial cryptococcosis typically produces a basilar chronic meningitis or meningoencephalitis with minimal inflammatory reaction. Fungal invasion can also occur in the distribution of the perforating brain arteries, along the perivascular Virchow-Robin spaces, producing small cystic areas in the brain parenchyma (Fig. 20–20). Another common location for cryptococcal infection is the choroid plexus, where it can cause the formation of mass-like lesions (Fig. 20–21). Rarely, *Cryptococcus* may produce focal parenchymal lesions (cryptococcomas).[85] Cryptococcal meningitis is frequently (in up to 45%) the first manifestation of AIDS, and for unknown reasons, it is more common in patients with AIDS with a history of drug abuse.[86] Once suspected, the diagnosis of cryptococcal infection is confirmed relatively easily. In patients with AIDS and the appropriate insidious clinical syndrome, manifested by fever, headache, stiff neck, vomiting, photophobia, and altered consciousness, the diagnosis of cryptococcal meningitis should be considered. In cases of cryptococcomas, focal signs of seizures or focal neurologic defects predominate. Examination of the CSF is necessary to confirm the diagnosis of cryptococcal meningitis, by demonstrating cryptococcal antigens and ultimately by isolating the causative fungus on CSF cultures. In cases of focal cryptococcomas, CSF examination is usually negative.

Four different patterns of cryptococcosis have been described based on MRI findings: 1) leptomeningeal infection (see Fig. 20–21), 2) focal cryptococcomas, 3) dilated Virchow-Robin spaces in the basal ganglia (see Fig. 20–20) or midbrain, and 4) a mixed form.[87] In cases of cryptococcal meningitis, CT and MRI findings are usually unremarkable, and often the only feature is mild communicating hydrocephalus. The lack of enhancement in the basilar meninges is due to minimal inflammatory reaction of cryptococcosis in patients with AIDS. By performing double-dose contrast-enhanced MRI, a higher frequency of abnormal meningeal enhancement has been described.[88] Focal cryptococcomas are indistinguishable by imaging criteria from other brain abscesses in patients with AIDS, and they present as solid or ring-enhancing lesions on postcontrast MR images. Also, the characteristic soap

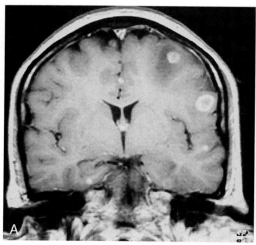
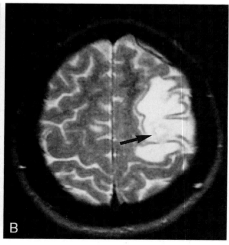

FIGURE 20–19. Toxoplasmosis. *A,* Postcontrast coronal T1-weighted (SE, 600/20, Gd-DTPA) image demonstrates bilateral multiple, scattered nodular or ring-like enhancing lesions, located in the corticomedullary junction. *B,* Axial T2-weighted (SE, 2200/70) image shows one of the *Toxoplasma* lesions in the left parietal lobe *(arrow),* as a focus with signal pattern isointense relative to brain parenchyma, surrounded by a large amount of vasogenic edema.

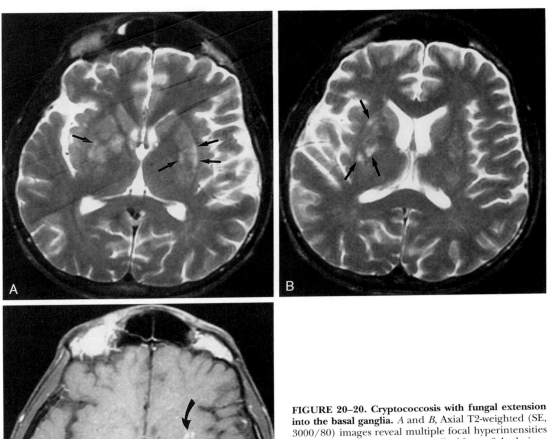

FIGURE 20-20. Cryptococcosis with fungal extension into the basal ganglia. *A* and *B*, Axial T2-weighted (SE, 3000/80) images reveal multiple focal hyperintensities within the basal ganglia bilaterally. Many of the lesions are small and discrete *(arrows)*, representing fungal colonization within dilated perivascular Virchow-Robin spaces. *C*, Gadolinium-enhanced T1-weighted (SE, 600/20) image shows only two punctate areas of contrast enhancement *(curved arrow)*.

bubble appearance, which represents the cystic areas rich in fungi (cryptococcal colonization) along the perivascular Virchow-Robin spaces, is displayed as round areas with signal intensity similar to that of CSF on all sequences and initially without any enhancement after contrast medium administration. These cystic areas are commonly located in the basal ganglia, the periventricular area, or the midbrain, and they are considered to be almost a pathognomonic MRI feature for the early diagnosis of cryptococcosis.[87] Both CT and MRI have the tendency to underestimate the extent of cryptococcosis, or they may fail to recognize the disease. However, MRI has proved much more effective than CT in detecting the dilated Virchow-Robin spaces and cryptococcomas; therefore, MRI should be considered as the imaging modality of choice in patients with suspected cryptococcosis.[89]

OTHER BRAIN ABSCESSES

The patient's immune status is an important indicator for the microbiology of a brain abscess. In patients with AIDS with defective cell-mediated immunity, brain abscesses of bacterial origin are relatively unusual; when they occur, they are often associated with a history of intravenous drug abuse. Common bacteria responsible for brain abscesses in this patient group are *Nocardia asteroides*, *L. monocytogenes*, *Salmonella*, and *E. coli*. *Nocardia* infection almost always invades the lungs as the primary site of infection and produces concomitant multiple brain abscesses.[89a] *Listeria* more often results in meningitis, although single large or disseminated small brain abscesses can be seen.[90]

In immunosuppressed patients, brain abscesses are most frequently caused by nonpyogenic organisms

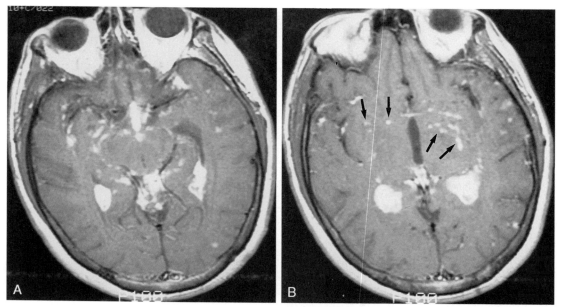

FIGURE 20–21. Cryptococcal meningitis with perivascular Virchow-Robin space involvement and cryptococcomas. *A* and *B*, Gadolinium-enhanced T1-weighted (SE, 600/20) images demonstrate both linear and nodular enhancement of the leptomeninges. The nodules or cryptococcomas are scattered throughout the basal cisterns, quadrigeminal cistern, sylvian fissures, and cortical sulci. Those in the brain parenchyma probably gained access to the brain through the Virchow-Robin spaces. Multiple punctate enhancing areas within the basal ganglia represent cryptococcomas within dilated Virchow-Robin spaces *(arrows, B).* Note the large mass-like cryptococcal lesions in the choroid plexus bilaterally.

(parasites, mycobacteria, fungi) and share almost the same imaging characteristics as the bacterial ones. However, the reduced host response results in some unique features, such as multiplicity or extraparenchymal spread. Toxoplasmosis is the most common cause of brain abscesses in patients with AIDS and has been described previously.

Mycobacterial infection, which experienced a marked decline in developed countries over the past decades, is now back again in epidemic proportions, mostly due to the onset of AIDS. Extrapulmonary dissemination of tuberculosis is more common in patients with AIDS, and CNS involvement may manifest as meningitis, tuberculoma, or brain abscess. In HIV-infected patients, CNS mycobacterial infection is primarily due to *M. tuberculosis,* although there is also an increased incidence of atypical mycobacterial infection, such as *Mycobacterium avium-intracellulare.* Tuberculous brain abscesses contain encapsulated pus with viable tubercle bacilli and differ from the more common tuberculomas (granulomas), which are smaller and contain caseous debris. Their imaging characteristics are similar to those of bacterial abscesses, and occasionally brain biopsy should be considered to obtain the correct diagnosis[90a] (Fig. 20–22). A helpful clue to the diagnosis of tuberculosis is the presence of other associated lesions, such as basal meningitis, multiple granulomas, and deep cerebral infarctions.[91]

Another cause of nonpyogenic brain abscesses in the population with AIDS is fungal infection. The most frequently encountered fungi are *Aspergillus, Mucor,* and *Candida,* because they have large hyphal forms allowing only limited access to the leptomeninges;

therefore, meningitis is relatively uncommon and focal parenchymal lesions are more likely to occur. As previously discussed, cryptococcosis, which results primarily in a chronic meningitis, can also produce focal, mass-like cryptococcomas, which represent brain abscesses. CNS aspergillosis results in single or multiple brain abscesses and is secondary to hematogenous dissemination from the respiratory or gastrointestinal tract or to direct extension from the nasal cavity or the paranasal sinuses. *Aspergillus* can also invade blood vessels, producing hemorrhagic infarctions; in that case the resulting brain abscesses are indistinguishable from other hemorrhagic lesions, such as metastases.[91a] Mucormycosis accounts for about 15% of fungal infections in patients with AIDS and is often associated with uncontrolled diabetes. Initially, *Mucor* infects facial compartments such as the nose, paranasal sinuses, and orbits, and from there it extends directly to the brain.[92] Intracranially, *Mucor* causes brain abscesses; also, like *Aspergillus,* by invading vessels it can lead to thrombosis and cerebral infarctions. Finally, candidiasis is the leading human mycosis causing predominantly oral, esophageal, or renal infection in patients with AIDS, but *Candida* rarely invades the CNS. However, multifocal brain microabscesses due to *Candida albicans* are occasionally seen as multiple enhancing nodules or ring-enhancing lesions by both CT and MRI.[93]

HUMAN IMMUNODEFICIENCY VIRUS ENCEPHALITIS

A neurotropic retrovirus, HIV can cause damage to the nervous system directly, resulting in a subacute

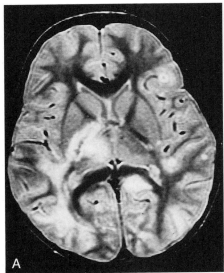
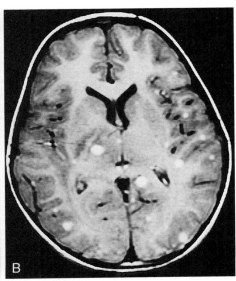

FIGURE 20–22. Multiple cerebral tuberculomas. *A,* Proton density–weighted (SE, 2000/30) axial image displays scattered foci of increased signal intensity within both hemispheres. Separable focal tuberculomas can be identified in the left frontal and parietal lobe as well as in the right occipital lobe. *B,* Axial postcontrast T1-weighted (SE, 600/20, Gd-DTPA) image at the same level reveals multiple nodular or ring-like enhancing tuberculomas throughout the brain parenchyma.

encephalomyelitis with a subtle and gradual clinical course. HIV encephalitis, also known as AIDS encephalopathy or AIDS dementia complex, is the most common CNS complication in AIDS. It has been described in nearly two thirds of all patients with neurologic symptoms and results in a progressive, subacute encephalitis with associated mental impairment, as well as motor and behavioral abnormalities.[25, 94] Patients present with progressive cognitive impairment, memory loss, language difficulties, somnolence, bradykinesia, and diminished concentration. Pathologically, the hallmark of HIV encephalitis is the isolation of multinucleate giant cells, microglial nodules, and demyelination in the deep white matter. Neither CT nor MRI is sensitive enough to detect those typical neuropathologic changes. Thus, despite the presence of diffuse and extensive parenchymal abnormalities seen in brain autopsy specimens in patients with HIV encephalitis, both CT and MRI usually fail to identify the brain abnormalities or grossly underestimate them.[95] Most frequently, the only imaging finding is a progressive, diffuse, nonspecific brain atrophy with a central predominance (ventricular dilatation). In more advanced cases there is variable involvement of white matter, particularly in the periventricular areas and the centrum semiovale. MRI is the most sensitive imaging modality for detecting the demyelinating lesions, which are depicted best on T2-weighted images as large, nearly symmetric, patchy or confluent areas of high signal intensity, without any evidence of mass effect or contrast enhancement[96, 97] (Fig. 20–23). Typically, the MRI findings follow the clinical manifestations of AIDS encephalopathy; therefore, MRI cannot be used to predict which HIV-infected patients will eventually develop dementia[98] (see also Chapter 27).

CYTOMEGALOVIRUS ENCEPHALITIS

A member of the herpesvirus family, CMV exists in a latent form in most of the adult population. After

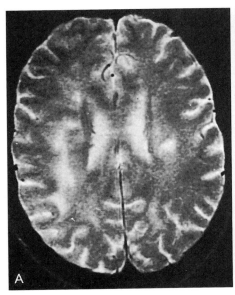
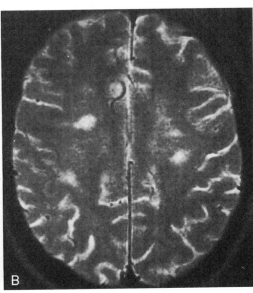

FIGURE 20–23. HIV encephalitis. *A,* T2-weighted image demonstrates multiple lesions in the periventricular white matter, becoming confluent in the right hemisphere. *B,* A higher image reveals more focal abnormalities in the centrum semiovale.

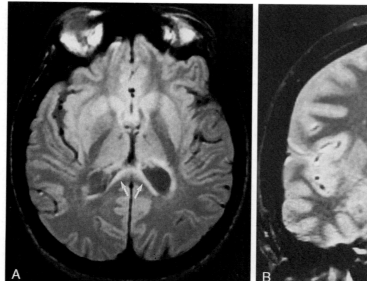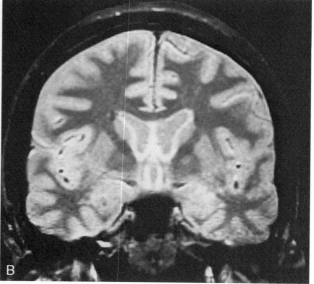

FIGURE 20–24. CMV encephalitis. *A* and *B,* Proton density–weighted (SE, 2700/30) axial and coronal images disclose hyperintensity surrounding the frontal horns and trigones of the lateral ventricles and also involving the splenium of the corpus callosum *(arrows)*.

reactivation in the immunosuppressed host, CMV can produce the following neurologic syndromes: chorioretinitis, encephalitis, myelitis, polyradiculopathy, and peripheral mononeuritis. Neuropathologic changes of CMV encephalitis are found in more than one third of autopsies in patients with AIDS and include areas of necrosis, neuronal loss, and demyelination, most frequently located in the periventricular areas. Also present are accumulations of enlarged cells (microglial nodules) containing the characteristic inclusion bodies of CMV.[99, 100] The pathologic abnormalities of CMV infection involve the gray matter and the ventricular ependyma more than the white matter, differentiating CMV encephalitis from the other viral encephalitides in patients with AIDS, such as HIV encephalitis or progressive multifocal leukoencephalopathy, which show a marked predilection for white matter involvement. Despite the high incidence of CMV encephalitis in autopsy series, the clinical correlation is poor, owing to the insidious and nonspecific clinical course, the insensitive and atypical CSF cultures, and the absence of pathognomonic neuroimaging findings. A good indicator for the diagnosis of CMV encephalitis in patients with AIDS is the high incidence of concurrent CMV retinitis. Retinitis is the most common and readily diagnosed ocular manifestation of CMV, occurring in up to one third of patients with AIDS. Generally, the patients with retinitis have an obvious clinical symptom, such as visual impairment, and characteristic ophthalmoscopic findings.[101, 102]

Brain involvement by CMV results in a necrotizing ventriculoencephalitis or, less commonly, focal parenchymal necrosis (abscess-like formation). CT is usually insensitive in the detection of CMV encephalitis. In advanced cases, CT may show nonspecific brain atrophy and irregular low-density bands in a periventricular distribution, which can enhance after contrast medium administration.[103] MRI is the imaging modality of choice for the evaluation of patients with AIDS with suspected encephalitis, from CMV or any other cause. MRI depicts low signal intensity in the periventricular region on T1-weighted images, whereas on proton density–weighted and T2-weighted images a thick or nodular periventricular hyperintensity is demonstrated, often involving the splenium and the genu of the corpus callosum (Fig. 20–24). After contrast medium administration (gadolinium), irregular subependymal enhancement can be seen, representing the changes of ependymitis.[85, 104] CMV infection usually has a centrifugal spread from the ventricular system, involving diffusely the gray matter and, less frequently, the white matter.

From the onset of the AIDS epidemic, a close and complex relationship of CMV and HIV was observed. Synergism between the two viruses could result in coinfection of the same cells with molecular trans-activation.[105] Therefore, an interaction between CMV and HIV may play a significant role in the pathogenesis of encephalitis in individuals with AIDS. Also, it has been reported that CMV by itself has immunosuppressive properties, which may compromise a patient's natural defense against HIV or other opportunistic infections[106] (see also Chapter 27).

PROGRESSIVE MULTIFOCAL LEUKOENCEPHALOPATHY

Progressive multifocal leukoencephalopathy is a progressive neurologic disorder associated with reactivation of a latent papovavirus infection, specifically the JC virus, that occurs when cell-mediated immunity is impaired. It has been estimated that this disorder affects 3% to 5% of all patients with AIDS and is associated with a rapidly progressive and fatal clinical course.

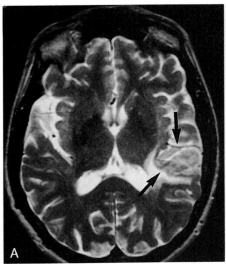 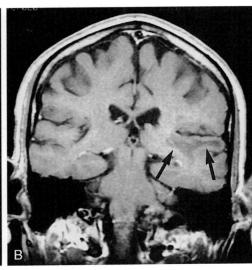

FIGURE 20–25. Progressive multifocal leukoencephalopathy. *A,* Axial T2-weighted (fast SE, 3600/102) image demonstrates an area of high signal intensity in the subcortical white matter of the left posterior temporal lobe *(arrows).* *B,* Postcontrast T1-weighted (SE, 550/20, Gd-DTPA) coronal image discloses low signal intensity in the same region, without any evidence of enhancement or mass effect *(arrows).*

The main target of progressive multifocal leukoencephalopathy is the oligodendrocyte, the myelin-producing cell, which becomes swollen and contains intranuclear inclusion bodies filled with papovavirus-type particles.[107] The resulting demyelination involves the subcortical and deep white matter and produces a rapidly deteriorating neurologic syndrome with altered mental status, limb weakness, visual field deficits, headache, and ataxia. Of note, dementia is not a main feature of this disorder, an important point for differentiating progressive multifocal leukoencephalopathy from HIV encephalitis. The disease is relentlessly progressive, and death ultimately ensues, in the majority of cases (80%), within 6 to 8 months.[108]

Due to its increased sensitivity, MRI can detect white matter abnormalities that are either missed or underestimated by CT, and it can also identify lesions of progressive multifocal leukoencephalopathy even when they are clinically silent.[109] Long TR, long TE sequences reveal bilateral, asymmetric focal areas of high intensity, which become larger and confluent with time and lack any significant associated edema or mass effect (Fig. 20–25). The disorder tends to involve the peripheral white matter, giving the lesions scalloped outer margins. The lesions are predominantly located in the white matter of the parieto-occipital regions, although involvement of the cortical gray matter, basal ganglia, cerebellum, and brain stem has been reported. After contrast medium administration, enhancement has been the exception in imaging of progressive multifocal leukoencephalopathy, although the presence of faint enhancement at the periphery of the lesion is not uncommon.[110, 111]

REFERENCES

1. Bowen BC, Post MJD: Intracranial infection. In: Atlas SW, ed. MRI of the Brain and Spine. New York: Raven Press, 1991, pp 501–538.
2. Davidson HD, Steiner RE: MRI in infections of the CNS. AJNR 6:499–504, 1985.
3. Schroth G, Kretzschmar K, Gawehn J, Voigt K: Advantage of MRI in the diagnosis of cerebral infections. Neuroradiology 29:120–126, 1987.
4. Parker JC, Dyer MC: Neurologic infections due to bacteria, fungi and parasites. In: Doris RL, Robertson DM, eds. Textbook of Neuro-pathology. Baltimore: Williams & Wilkins, 1985, pp 632–703.
5. Enzmann DR, Britt RH, Placone RC: Staging of human brain abscess by CT. Radiology 146:703–708, 1983.
6. Britt RH, Enzmann DR, Yeager AS: Neuropathological and CT findings in experimental brain abscess. J Neurosurg 55:590–603, 1981.
7. Britt RH, Enzmann DR: Clinical stages of human brain abscesses on serial CT scans after contrast infusion. J Neurosurg 59:972–989, 1983.
8. Haimes AB, Zimmerman RD, Morgello S, et al: MRI of brain abscesses. AJR 152:1073–1085, 1989.
9. Yousem DM, Janick PA, Rubin H, et al: Proposed cause for the MR appearance of T_1 hyperintensity in inflammatory lesions and the early conversion to methemoglobin on some hemorrhagic conditions. Radiology 173:330, 1989. Abstract.
10. Zimmerman RD, Weingarten K: Neuroimaging of cerebral abscesses. Neuroimaging Clin North Am 1:1–16, 1991.
11. Dobkin JF, Healton EB, Dickinson PCT, et al: Nonspecificity of ring enhancement in medically cured brain abscesses. Neurology 34:139–144, 1984.
12. McGee ZA, Baringer JR: Acute meningitis. In: Mandell GL, Douglas RG, Bennett JE, eds. Principles and Practice of Infectious Diseases. New York: Churchill Livingstone, 1990, pp 741–755.
13. Pachner AR, Duray P, Steere AC: CNS manifestations of Lyme disease. Arch Neurol 46:790–795, 1989.
14. Delaney P: Neurologic manifestations in sarcoidosis: review of the literature, with a report of 23 cases. Ann Intern Med 87:336–345, 1977.
15. Sze G: Infection and inflammation. In: Bradley WG, Stark DD, eds.: Magnetic Resonance Imaging. 2nd ed. St. Louis: CV Mosby, 1992, pp 670–698.
16. Bilaniuk LT, Zimmerman RA, Brown L, et al: CT in meningitis. Neuroradiology 16:13–14, 1978.
17. Mathews VP, Kuharik MA, Edwards MK, et al: Gd-DTPA–enhanced MRI of experimental bacterial meningitis: evaluation and comparison with CT. AJNR 9:1045–1050, 1988.
18. Seltzer S, Mark AS, Atlas SW: CNS sarcoidosis: evaluation with contrast-enhanced MRI. AJNR 12:1227–1233, 1991.
19. Finelli DA, Christopherson LA, Rhodes RH, et al: Leptomeningeal and calvarial sarcoidosis: CT and MR appearance. J Comput Assist Tomogr 19:639–642, 1995.
20. Holland BA, Perrett LV, Mills CM: Meningo-vascular syphilis: CT and MR findings. Radiology 158:439–442, 1986.
21. Agrons GA, Han SS, Husson MA, Simeone F: MRI of cerebral gumma. AJNR 12:80–81, 1991.
22. Sze G, Saletsky S, Bronen R, Krol G: MRI of the cranial meninges with emphasis on contrast enhancement and meningeal carcinomatosis. AJNR 10:965–975, 1989.
23. Chang KH, Han MH, Roh JK, et al: Gd-DTPA enhanced MRI of the brain in patients with meningitis: comparison with CT. AJNR 11:69–76, 1990.
24. Phillips ME, Ryals TJ, Kambhu SA, Vuh WTC: Neoplastic vs inflammatory meningeal enhancement with Gd-DTPA. J Comput Assist Tomogr 14:536–541, 1990.
25. Sze G, Zimmerman RD: The MRI of infections and inflammatory disease. Radiol Clin North Am 26:839–859, 1988.
26. Barloon TJ, Yuh WTC, Knepper LE, et al: Cerebral ventriculitis: MR findings. J Comput Assist Tomogr 14:272–275, 1990.

27. Jordan J, Enzmann DR: Encephalitis. Neuroimaging Clin North Am 1:17–38, 1991.
28. Hoke CH: Viral encephalitis due to herpes simplex, Togaviridae, Flaviviridae, Bunyaviridae, B virus and HIV. In: Gorbach SL, Bartlett JG, Blacklow NR, eds. Infectious Diseases. Philadelphia: WB Saunders, 1992, pp 1193–1196.
29. Tien RD, Felsberg GJ, Osumi AK: Herpesvirus infections of the CNS: MR findings. AJR 161:167–176, 1993.
30. Schroth G, Gawehn J, Thron A, et al: Early diagnosis of herpes simplex encephalitis by MRI. Neurology 37:179–183, 1987.
31. Kesselring J, Miller DH, Robb SA, et al: Acute disseminated encephalomyelitis. MRI findings and the distinction from multiple sclerosis. Brain 113:291–302, 1990.
32. Atlas SW, Grossman RI, Goldberg HI, et al: MR diagnosis of acute disseminated encephalomyelitis. J Comput Assist Tomogr 10:798–801, 1986.
33. Galdemeyer KS, Smith RR, Harris TM, Edwards MK: MRI in acute disseminated encephalomyelitis. Neuroradiology 36:216–220, 1994.
34. Van der Meyden CH, de Villiers JFK, Middlecote BD, Terblanche J: Gadolinium ring enhancement and mass effect in ADEM. Neuroradiology 36:221–223, 1994.
35. Falcone S, Quencer RM, Bowen B, et al: Creutzfeldt-Jakob disease: focal symmetrical cortical involvement demonstrated by MR imaging. AJNR 13:403–406, 1992.
36. Barboriak DP, Provenzale JM, Boyko OB: MR diagnosis of Creutzfeldt-Jakob disease: significance of high signal intensity of the basal ganglia. AJR 162:137–140, 1994.
37. Tsuchiya K, Yamauchi T, Furui S, et al: MRI vs CT in subacute sclerosing panencephalitis. AJNR 9:943–946, 1988.
38. Silverberg AL, di Nubile MJ: Subdural empyema and cranial epidural abscess. Med Clin North Am 69:361–372, 1985.
39. Kaufman DM, Litman N, Miller MH: Sinusitis: induced empyema. Neurology 33:123–132, 1983.
40. Post EM, Modesti LM: "Subacute" postoperative subdural empyema. J Neurosurg 55:761–765, 1981.
41. Dunker RO, Khakoo RA: Failure of CT scanning to demonstrate subdural empyemas. JAMA 246:1116–1118, 1981.
42. Sadhu VK, Handell SF, Pinto RS, et al: Neuroradiologic diagnosis of subdural empyemas and CT limitations. AJNR 1:39–44, 1980.
43. Weingarten K, Zimmerman RD, Becker RD, et al: Subdural and epidural empyemas. AJR 152:615–621, 1989.
44. Tsuchiya K, Makita K, Furui S, et al: Contrast-enhanced MRI of sub- and epidural empyemas. Neuroradiology 34:494–496, 1992.
45. Moseley IF, Kendall BE: Radiology of intracranial empyemas with special reference to CT. Neuroradiology 26:333–345, 1984.
46. Zee CS, Segall HD, Boswell W, et al: MRI of neurocysticercosis. J Comput Assist Tomogr 12:927–934, 1988.
47. Suss RA, Maravilla KR, Thompson J: MRI of intracranial cysticercosis: comparison with CT and anatomopathologic features. AJNR 7:235–242, 1986.
48. Del Brutto OH, Santibanez R, Noboa CA, et al: Epilepsy due to neurocysticercosis. Analysis of 203 patients. Neurology 42:389–392, 1992.
49. Sze G, Lee SH: Infectious diseases. In: Lee SH, Rao KCVG, Zimmerman RA, eds. Cranial MRI and CT. 3rd ed. New York: McGraw-Hill, 1992, pp 539–588.
50. Martinez HR, Rangel-Guerra R, Elizondo G, et al: MRI in neurocysticercosis. A study of 56 cases. AJNR 10:1011–1019, 1989.
51. Chang KH, Cho SY, Hesselink JR, et al: Parasitic diseases of the central nervous system. Neuroimaging Clin North Am 1:159–178, 1991.
52. Holland BA, Kucharczyk W, Brant-Zawadzki M, et al: MR imaging of calcified intracranial lesions. Radiology 157:353–356, 1985.
53. Teitelbaum GP, Otto RJ, Lin M, et al: MRI of neurocysticercosis. AJNR 10:709–718, 1989.
54. Ginier BL, Poirier VC: MR imaging of intraventricular cysticercosis. AJNR 13:1247–1248, 1992.
55. Chang KH, Lee JH, Han MH, Han MC: The role of contrast-enhanced MR imaging in the diagnosis of neurocysticercosis. AJNR 12:509–512, 1991.
56. Rudwan MA, Khaffaji S: CT of cerebral hydatid disease. Neuroradiology 30:496–499, 1988.
57. Coates R, von Sinner W, Rahm B: MR imaging of an intracerebral hydatid cyst. AJNR 11:1249–1250, 1990.
58. Kadota T, Ishikura R, Tabuchi Y, et al: MR imaging of chronic cerebral paragonimiasis. AJNR 10:S21–S22, 1989.
59. Desmonts G, Couvreur J: Congenital toxoplasmosis: a prospective study of 378 pregnancies. N Engl J Med 290:1110–1116, 1974.
60. Diebler C, Dusser A, Dular O: Congenital toxoplasmosis. Clinical and neuroradiological evaluation of the cerebral lesions. Neuroradiology 27:125–130, 1985.
61. Osborn RE, Byrd SE: Congenital infections of the brain. Neuroimaging Clin North Am 1:105–118, 1991.
62. Stagno S, Pass RF, Cloud G, et al: Primary cytomegalovirus infection in pregnancy. JAMA 256:1904–1908, 1986.
63. Becker LE: Infections of the developing brain. AJNR 13:537–549, 1992.
64. Boesch C, Issakainen J, Kewitz G, et al: MRI of the brain in congenital CMV infection. Pediatr Radiol 19:91–93, 1989.
65. Sugita K, Ando M, Makino M, et al: MRI of the brain in congenital rubella virus and CMV infections. Neuroradiology 33:239–242, 1991.
66. Ishikawa A, Murayama T, Sakuma N, et al: Computed cranial tomography in congenital rubella syndrome. Arch Neurol 39:420–421, 1982.
67. Shaw DWW, Cohen WA: Viral infections of the CNS in children: imaging features. AJR 160:125–133, 1993.
68. Enzmann D, Chang Y, Augustyn G: MR findings in neonatal herpes simplex encephalitis type II. J Comput Assist Tomogr 14:453–457, 1990.
69. Taccone A, Gambano G, Chiorzi M: CT in children with herpes simplex encephalitis. Pediatr Radiol 19:9–12, 1988.
70. Belman AL, Ultmann MH, Horoupian D, et al: Neurological complications in infants and children with AIDS. Ann Neurol 18:560–566, 1985.
71. Chamberlain MC, Press GA, Nichols S, Chase C: Pediatric AIDS: comparative MR and CT brain imaging. Ann Neurol 28:459–465, 1990.
72. McArthur JC: Neurologic manifestations of AIDS. Medicine 66:407–437, 1987.
73. Levy RM, Bredesen DE, Rosenblum ML: Neurological manifestations of the acquired immunodeficiency syndrome (AIDS). Experience at UCSF and review of the literature. J Neurosurg 62:475–495, 1985.
74. Grant I, Atkinson JH, Hesselink JR, et al: Evidence for early CNS involvement in the AIDS and other HIV infections. Studies with neuropsychologic testing and MRI. Ann Intern Med 107:828–836, 1987.
75. Lantos PL, Mclaughlin JE, Scholtz CL, et al: Neuropathology of the brain in HIV infection. Lancet 1:309–311, 1989.
76. DeGirolami U, Smith TW, Henin D, Hauw JJ: Neuropathology of the acquired immunodeficiency syndrome. Arch Pathol Lab Med 114:643–655, 1990. Erratum in Arch Pathol Lab Med 115:33, 1991.
77. Federle MP: A radiologist looks at AIDS: imaging evaluation based on symptom complexes. Radiology 166:553–562, 1988.
78. Grant IH, Gold JWM, Rosenblum ML, et al: Toxoplasma gondii serology in HIV-infected patients: the development of CNS toxoplasmosis in AIDS. AIDS 4:519–523, 1990.
79. McArthur JC: Neurologic complications of HIV infection. In: Gorbach SL, Bartlett JG, Blacklow NR, eds. Infectious Diseases. Philadelphia: WB Saunders, 1992, pp 956–973.
80. Gray F, Gherardi R, Wingate E, et al: Diffuse "encephalitic" cerebral toxoplasmosis in AIDS. J Neurol 236:273–277, 1989.
81. Kupfer MC, Zee CS, Colletti PM, et al: MRI evaluation of AIDS-related encephalopathy: toxoplasmosis vs lymphoma. Magn Reson Imaging 8:51–57, 1990.
82. Mariuz P, Luft BJ: Toxoplasmosis in AIDS. In: Wormser GP, ed. AIDS and Other Manifestations of HIV Infection. 2nd ed. New York: Raven Press, 1992, pp 383–392.
83. Sze G, Brant-Zawadzki MN, Norman D, Newton HT: The neuroradiology of AIDS. Semin Roentgenol 22:42–53, 1987.
84. Cohn JA, McMeeking A, Cohen W, et al: Evaluation of the policy of empiric treatment of suspected Toxoplasma encephalitis in patients with AIDS. Am J Med 86:521–527, 1989.
85. Davenport C, Dillon WP, and Sze G: Neuroradiology of the immunosuppressed state. Radiol Clin North Am 30:611–637, 1992.
86. Chuck SL, Sande MA: Infections with Cryptococcus neoformans in the acquired immunodeficiency syndrome. N Engl J Med 321:794–799, 1989.
87. Tien RD, Chu PK, Hesselink JR, et al: Intracranial cryptococcosis in immunocompromised patients: CT and MR findings in 29 cases. AJNR 12:283–289, 1991.
88. Andreula CF, Burdi N, Carella A: CNS cryptococcosis in AIDS: spectrum of MR findings. J Comput Assist Tomogr 17:438–441, 1993.
89. Mathews VP, Alo PL, Glass JD, et al: AIDS-related CNS cryptococcosis: radiologic-pathologic correlation. AJNR 13:1477–1486, 1992.
89a. LeBlang SD, Whiteman MLH, Post MJD, et al: CNS Nocardia in AIDS patients: CT and MRI with pathologic correlation. J Comput Assist Tomogr 19:15–22, 1995.
90. Wispelwey B, Scheld WM: Brain abscess. In: Mandell GL, Douglas RG, Bennett JE, eds.: Principles and Practice of Infectious Diseases. 3rd ed. New York: Churchill Livingstone, 1990, pp 780–788.
90a. Whiteman M, Espinoza L, Post MJD, et al: Central nervous system tuberculosis in HIV infected patients: clinical and radiographic findings. AJNR 16:1319–1321, 1995.
91. Campi de Castro C, Hesselink JR: Tuberculosis. Neuroimaging Clin North Am 1:119–139, 1991.
91a. Miaux Y, Ribaud P, Williams M, et al: MR of cerebral aspergillosis in patients who have had bone marrow transplantation. AJNR 16:555–562, 1995.
92. Cuadrado LM, Guerrero A, Asenjo JALG, et al: Cerebral mucormycosis in two cases of AIDS. Arch Neurol 45:109–111, 1988.
93. Lipton SA, Hickey WF, Morris JH, et al: Candidal infection in the central nervous system. Am J Med 76:101–108, 1984.
94. Navia BA, Jordan BD, Price RW: The AIDS dementia complex: 1. Clinical features. Ann Neurol 19:517–524, 1986.
95. Post JD, Tate LG, Quencer RM, et al: CT, MR and pathology in HIV encephalitis and meningitis. AJNR 9:469–476, 1988.
96. Chrysikopoulos HS, Press GA, Grafe MR, et al: Encephalitis caused by HIV: CT and MRI manifestations with clinical and pathologic correlation. Radiology 175:185–191, 1990.
97. Flowers CH, Mafee MF, Crowell R, et al: Encephalopathy in AIDS patients: evaluation with MRI. AJNR 11:1235–1245, 1990.

98. McArthur JC, Kumar AJ, Johnson DW, et al: Incidental white matter hyperintensities on magnetic resonance imaging in HIV-1 infection. Multicenter AIDS Cohort Study. J Acquir Immune Defic Syndr 3:252–259, 1990.
99. Wiley CA, Nelson JA: Role of HIV and CMV in AIDS encephalitis. Am J Pathol 133:73–81, 1988.
100. Petito CK, Cho ES, Lemann W, et al: Neuropathology of AIDS: an autopsy review. J Neuropathol Exp Neurol 45:635–646, 1986.
101. Jacobson MA, Mills J: Serious cytomegalovirus disease in the acquired immunodeficiency syndrome (AIDS). Clinical findings, diagnosis, and treatment. Ann Intern Med 108:585–594, 1988.
102. Bloom JN, Palestine AG: The diagnosis of cytomegalovirus retinitis. Ann Intern Med 109:963–969, 1988.
103. Post MJD, Hensley GT, Moskowitz LB, Fischl M: Cytomegalic inclusion virus encephalitis in patients with AIDS: CT, clinical, and pathologic correlation. AJR 146:1229–1234, 1986.
104. Kalayjian RC, Cohen ML, Bonomo RA, Flanigan TP: CMV ventriculoencephalitis in AIDS: a syndrome with distinct clinical and pathologic features. Medicine 72:67–77, 1993.
105. Koval V, Clark C, Vaishnar M, et al: Human CMV inhibits human HIV replication in cells productively infected by both viruses. J Virol 65:6969–6978, 1991.
106. Yarrish RL: CMV infections in AIDS. In: Wormser GP, ed. AIDS and Other Manifestations of HIV Infection. 2nd ed. New York: Raven Press, 1992, pp 249–268.
107. Berger JR, Kaszovitz B, Post MJD, and Dickinson G: PML associated with HIV infection. Ann Intern Med 107:78–87, 1987.
108. Brooks BR, Walker DL: PML. Neurol Clin North Am 2:299–313, 1984.
109. Olsen WL, Longo FM, Mille CM, Norman D: White matter disease in AIDS: findings at MR imaging. Radiology 169:445–448, 1988.
110. Mark AS, Atlas SW: PML in patients with AIDS: appearance on MR images. Radiology 173:517–520, 1989.
111. Hansman Whiteman ML, Post MJD, Berger JR, et al: PML in 47 HIV-seropositive patients: neuroimaging with clinical and pathologic correlation. Radiology 187:233–240, 1993.

Spontaneous and Traumatic Hemorrhage

HEINRICH P. MATTLE ■ ROBERT R. EDELMAN
GERHARD SCHROTH ■ GERALD V. O'REILLY

Spontaneous brain hemorrhage is defined as bleeding into the brain substance by any cause that is of nontraumatic origin. There are many causes of such hemorrhage, but by far the most common is uncontrolled chronic systemic arterial hypertension. Until the advent of computed tomography (CT) in 1972, the diagnosis of spontaneous brain hemorrhage could only be inferred from the angiographic findings of an avascular intracranial mass in a patient presenting with an acute stroke. Unless a ruptured aneurysm or arteriovenous malformation (AVM) was also visualized by angiography, a conclusive antemortem diagnosis of brain hemorrhage was always questionable. Such an avascular mass could also have been the result of an infarction, tumor, or abscess. Since its inception, CT so revolutionized the diagnosis of intracranial disease that it became, and in most hospitals still is, the primary diagnostic tool in the evaluation of a patient presenting with an acute stroke. For the first time, CT made it possible to distinguish by a noninvasive means between an ischemic and a hemorrhagic event in the brain.

However, CT does have significant limitations in its diagnostic capabilities. Small petechial hemorrhages in the brain stem, some hemorrhagic infarctions, and many chronic hematomas may escape detection by CT. This is partly due to low contrast resolution and bone artifacts, which often result in poor definition of posterior fossa structures, and also to partial-volume effects, which tend to lessen sensitivity for the presence of small quantities of blood within an acute infarct. Another issue is that on CT scans, a brain hematoma gradually evolves over several weeks from high density, through an isodense phase, to low density. This change in scan appearance is due to an alteration in tissue density rather than to actual reabsorption of the hematoma. As a consequence, after some months the CT findings of a brain hemorrhage are often indistinguishable from those for an old infarction, even though pathologically there is still evidence of a hematoma in the brain. Finally, CT or even angiography may, in some cases, fail to provide a specific diagnosis of the cause of the original hemorrhage, such as a vascular malformation or a tumor.

Although CT, despite these limitations, remains the diagnostic procedure most useful in the emergency management of an acute stroke patient, magnetic resonance imaging (MRI) may prove to be the ultimate method of refining the diagnosis. Pragmatically, many patients who have suffered a brain hemorrhage are not clinically suitable to undergo MRI in the acute phase, owing to restlessness or the need for life support equipment. Therefore, once the hemorrhagic nature of a lesion is identified by CT, MRI can be used later to increase diagnostic information by more accurately defining the extent of the lesion, assessing the age of its hemorrhagic component, and detecting the presence of any underlying lesion. However, the various MR patterns of brain hemorrhage will need careful evaluation if correct deductions are to be made, because the evolution of hemorrhage is one of the more complex and controversial aspects of MRI. For instance, the impact of petechial hemorrhages detected within infarctions by MRI, but not CT, on the therapeutic application of anticoagulants remains to be determined.

MRI APPEARANCE AND EVOLUTION OF BRAIN HEMORRHAGE

Intracranial hemorrhage has been studied extensively by MRI.[1–25] The biochemical and physiochemical details of hemorrhage are reviewed in depth in Chapter 7 and have also been reviewed by Bradley.[26] In this section the basic concepts involved in interpreting the appearance of brain hemorrhage on MR images are reviewed.

The complex manifestations of hemorrhage on MR images relate to the formation of a series of substances with potent magnetic properties that result from the breakdown of oxyhemoglobin. These substances include deoxyhemoglobin, methemoglobin, ferritin, and hemosiderin. As a result of the magnetic properties of these hemoglobin breakdown products, intracerebral hemorrhage has a variety of appearances on MR images that depend on several factors: 1) pulse sequence; 2) field strength; 3) clot formation and retraction; 4) age of hemorrhage; and 5) state of oxygenation of the hemorrhage, which relates to its location.

INFLUENCE OF PROTEIN CONCENTRATION

Changes of protein concentrations in aqueous solutions alter T1 and T2 relaxation times due to "bound water effects." Water hydration to macromolecules such as proteins shortens T1 and T2 relaxation times. Free water has high frequencies of motion and thus short molecular correlation times. Motion of water in a hydration layer is restricted; it tumbles slower and has longer correlation times. In dilute solutions of protein this effect is minimal. However, in concentrated solutions T1 and even more T2 relaxation times decrease visibly as the protein concentration increases. In hemorrhages, extremely high protein concentrations can occur because of packing and dehydration of red blood cells and because of retraction of the clot matrix. Thus, T1 and T2 of proteinaceous oxyhemoglobin are much less than those of cerebrospinal fluid (CSF) and more like those of brain parenchyma.[27–29] However, the magnetic state of hemorrhage due to hemoglobin breakdown products produces even greater signal changes than alterations of protein concentrations.

MAGNETIC STATES OF MATTER

Matter can exist in several different magnetic states. These states are described in terms of their magnetic susceptibility, which represents the degree to which the presence of a substance tends to attract or repel magnetic lines of force (Fig. 21–1). The magnetic sus-

ceptibility of a substance is predominantly determined by the configuration of the orbital electrons (see Chapter 7). Because of their smaller mass, these electrons have magnetic moments more than a thousand times greater than those of protons. The categories of magnetic susceptibility relevant to interpreting the appearance of hemorrhage on MR images include diamagnetism, paramagnetism, and superparamagnetism.

Most substances, including oxyhemoglobin, are diamagnetic. The orbital electrons in diamagnetic substances are paired, which reduces the effect of their magnetic moments. The paired electrons weakly oppose an applied magnetic field, but to such a minimal extent that the magnetic properties of these electrons have a negligible effect on the appearance of the image. On the other hand, paramagnetic substances, which include all of the previously mentioned hemoglobin breakdown products, have a profound effect on signal intensity. Paramagnetic substances contain unpaired orbital electrons; in the case of hemoglobin breakdown products, the unpaired electrons are localized to iron atoms.

EFFECTS OF PARAMAGNETIC SUBSTANCES ON SIGNAL INTENSITY

The effects of a paramagnetic substance on signal intensity depend on several factors, including the concentration of the paramagnetic substance and the degree to which water molecules have access to it. Depending on the situation, paramagnetic hemoglobin breakdown products can predominantly induce either T2 shortening, resulting in signal loss, or T1 shortening, resulting in signal enhancement.

T2 Shortening

Because paramagnetic molecules have a sizeable magnetic moment, their concentration within a restricted region produces a disturbance in the local magnetic field. The disturbance in magnetic field homogeneity produced by the concentration of these paramagnetic substances is analogous to the effect of placing an iron bar within the bore of the MRI magnet. Examples of paramagnetic substances associated with this phenomenon include intracellular deoxyhemoglobin and intracellular methemoglobin.

Water molecules diffusing past these concentrated paramagnetic centers experience an inhomogeneous field, with resultant rapid dephasing (T2 shortening) and signal loss (Fig. 21–2). This signal loss is seen on T2-weighted images because T2-weighted acquisitions use a long echo time (TE). As the TE is increased there is more time available for the water molecules to diffuse through the inhomogeneous magnetic field, causing further dephasing and greater signal loss.

Ferritin and hemosiderin are categorized as superparamagnetic (see Chapters 6 and 7). Because of their large magnetic moments, these superparamagnetic substances produce marked signal loss at smaller con-

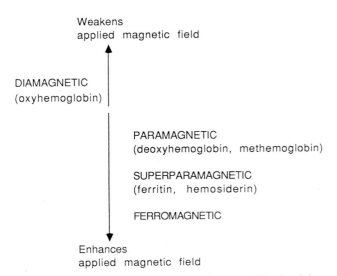

FIGURE 21–1. Magnetic susceptibility of hemoglobin breakdown products.

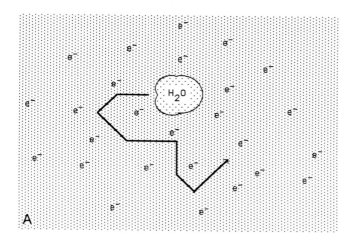

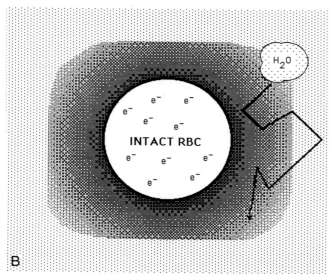

FIGURE 21–2. *A*, When water molecules diffuse through normal brain matter, they experience a homogeneous magnetic field. *B*, When paramagnetic or superparamagnetic substances such as hemoglobin breakdown products concentrate locally after hemorrhage, the homogeneity of the magnetic field in the brain is disturbed. The ensuing local magnetic field inhomogeneity increases dephasing and signal loss when water molecules diffuse past these substances. The signal loss is most pronounced on T2-weighted images because of the long echo time. RBC = red blood cell.

centrations than do intracellular deoxyhemoglobin and methemoglobin.

The superparamagnetic iron-containing cores of ferritin and hemosiderin are largely excluded from contact with water molecules. The same is true for deoxyhemoglobin, because the region of the globin molecule containing paramagnetic iron is hydrophobic and repels water molecules. However, T1 relaxation processes depend on close interaction between water molecules and the paramagnetic center; these interactions decrease with the sixth power of the distance between molecules. As a result, these substances produce only minimal changes in T1 relaxation.

T1 Shortening

Paramagnetic molecules, which are distributed freely in solution, produce quite different alterations in sig-

nal intensity from those just discussed. Extracellular methemoglobin is an example of such a substance. After red blood cell lysis, methemoglobin is released into the extracellular space, where it distributes uniformly in solution and in reduced concentration. The magnetic moments of these unpaired electrons enhance the applied field. If water molecules, through random diffusional processes, come near these paramagnetic centers, they experience fluctuating magnetic fields from the unpaired electrons. These fluctuating magnetic fields promote T1 relaxation in nearby water molecules (dipole-dipole interaction). Although T2 relaxation is also promoted by dipole-dipole interactions, the dominant effect in T1-weighted images is usually an increase in signal intensity, resulting from the T1 shortening.

Because the methemoglobin molecules go into the extracellular space in a relatively uniform distribution and in reduced concentration, they no longer produce a significant degree of magnetic field inhomogeneity. As a result, in contrast to intracellular methemoglobin, the predominant effect of extracellular methemoglobin is to increase the signal from the hematoma.

EVOLUTION OF SIGNAL INTENSITY CHANGES ON MR IMAGES

The appearance of an intracerebral hematoma on MR images follows a well-defined, although somewhat variable, course. The evolution of the signal intensity changes is largely related to the paramagnetic effects described earlier. Table 21–1 summarizes the physical and magnetic properties of hemoglobin breakdown products. However, the appearance of the hemorrhage is strongly dependent on the field strength of the magnet and on the type of pulse sequence used (fast [or turbo] spin echo, spin echo, or gradient echo). Also, the time course discussed in the following sections is only a rough approximation and varies depending on the size of the hemorrhage and other factors. We first consider the appearance of a hematoma on spin-echo images obtained on a high-field (1.5 T) system (Figs. 21–3 and 21–4 and Table 21–2).

Extremely Acute Hematoma (First Few Hours)

Immediately after an intracerebral hemorrhage a liquefied mass occurs within the brain substance. This mass contains oxyhemoglobin but as yet no paramagnetic substances. As a result, the mass appears like any other proteinaceous fluid collection, that is, dark to slightly hyperintense on T1-weighted images and intermediate to bright on T2-weighted images.

Acute Hematoma (Several Hours to Several Days)

During a period of several hours to several days, reduction in the oxygen tension within the hematoma results in the formation of intracellular deoxyhemo-

TABLE 21–1. SUMMARY OF PHYSICAL AND MAGNETIC PROPERTIES OF HEMOGLOBIN BREAKDOWN PRODUCTS*

MOLECULE	IRON FORM	NO. OF UNPAIRED ELECTRONS	DISTRIBUTION	ΔT1	ΔT2
Oxyhemoglobin	Ferrous	1	Intact RBCs	—	—
Deoxyhemoglobin	Ferrous	4	Intact RBCs	—	↓↓
			Lysed RBCs	—	—
Methemoglobin	Ferric	5	Intact RBCs	↓	↓↓
			Lysed RBCs	↓↓	↓
Ferritin	Ferric	~10,000 (insoluble)	Intracellular	—	↓↓
Hemosiderin	Ferric	~10,000 (insoluble)	Intracellular	—	↓↓

*ΔT1, ΔT2 = change produced by molecule in T1 and T2 relaxation times; RBCs = red blood cells.

globin and methemoglobin within intact red blood cells. Because of their distribution, these paramagnetic substances produce T2 shortening, so that the hematoma appears dark (see Fig. 21–3A). The loss of signal is roughly proportional to the square of the magnetic field strength and is most pronounced on images acquired with a long TE (e.g., 90 ms).

As in CT, fluid-fluid levels can be seen in MR images of hematoma. The lower compartment initially contains sedimented red blood cells and appears dark on T2-weighted images owing to the effects of intracellular paramagnetic substances and clot. The upper compartment contains fluid-rich plasma and appears bright on T2-weighted images.

In addition to the region of signal loss associated with the hematoma, on T2-weighted images there is usually a thin rim of increased signal intensity seen surrounding the hematoma, which represents edema.

Subacute Hematoma (Several Days to Several Weeks)

During a period of several days to weeks, there is lysis of red blood cells. Redistribution of methemoglobin into the extracellular space changes the effect of this paramagnetic substance on signal intensity. Now the predominant effect is one of T1 shortening (see Fig. 21–3B to D). This results in signal enhancement, seen on T1-weighted images and also to a lesser extent on T2-weighted images, which begins in the rim of the hematoma and extends inward over time.

There are several reasons why the signal enhancement is seen on T2-weighted images: 1) because of the red blood cell lysis, T2 shortening disappears; 2) osmotic effects draw fluid into the hematoma; and 3) the repetition times (TRs) in general use for T2-weighted images (e.g., 2000 to 2500 ms) are not sufficiently long to completely eliminate T1 contrast effects in the image. As a result of the combination of these effects, the hematoma becomes bright on T2-weighted images.

Edema, of vasogenic type due to leakage of proteinaceous fluid into the intercellular space of the brain tissue, is now visible surrounding the hematoma. This fluid spreads along the fiber tracts, giving the edema an appearance as though fingers ("edema fingers") are reaching into the normal brain tissue.

Sometimes, dark areas persist in the hematoma even after one would have expected red blood cell lysis

to be complete. To some extent, this may represent persistent hyperconcentration of paramagnetic substances such as methemoglobin in portions of the hematoma. However, physical alterations in the structure of the hematoma, such as clot retraction, likely produce significant signal changes as well. It has been demonstrated that the increased hematocrit in retracted blood clots contributes to T2 shortening, independent of any paramagnetic effect.[30] This effect can be shown on images from both high- and low-field systems (see Fig. 21–28).

Chronic Hematoma (Several Weeks to Several Months or More)

During a variable time period, phagocytic cells invade the hemorrhage, beginning at the outer rim and working inward. These phagocytes metabolize the hemoglobin breakdown products and store the iron in the form of particulate ferritin and hemosiderin. In this form, iron is superparamagnetic and produces T2 shortening. The T2 shortening produces signal loss in the rim of the hematoma, which is most pronounced on T2-weighted images but seen to a lesser extent on T1-weighted images (see Fig. 21–3E). Signal loss may be seen in old hematomas for many years, owing to persistent hemosiderin deposition.

USE OF GRADIENT-ECHO PULSE SEQUENCES TO IMPROVE CHARACTERIZATION OF HEMATOMAS

Magnetic susceptibility effects are field strength dependent (see Chapter 7). As a result, T2 shortening is much less pronounced on lower field systems and, in many cases, may be unobservable on low-field images obtained by using spin-echo pulse sequences. To some extent, the problem can be overcome by increasing the TE. Diffusion-related effects, such as T2 shortening, rapidly increase as the TE is lengthened. However, the interpretation of images obtained with a long TE (e.g., >100 ms) may be hampered by a reduction of the signal-to-noise ratio.

This problem may be overcome by using gradient-echo pulse sequences. Gradient-echo pulse sequences differ from spin-echo sequences in that they lack the 180° radiofrequency refocusing pulse. Acute hematomas appear dark on gradient-echo images, even when obtained on a low-field system. On a high-field system,

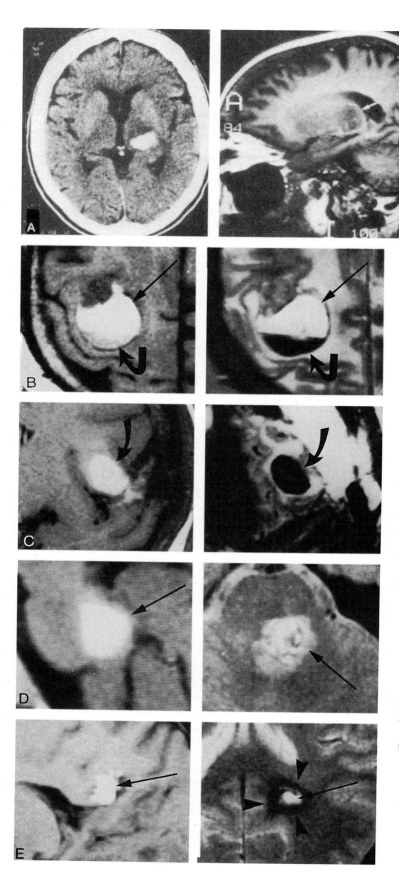

FIGURE 21–3. Temporal changes of hemorrhage on MR images. The evolution of a hematoma on MR images depends on many factors, such as local blood supply, pH, oxygen tension, and hematocrit, as well as on magnetic field strength of the imaging system. All images were obtained at 1.5 T. *A,* Acute hypertensive left thalamic hemorrhage: *left,* unenhanced CT within 12 hours of hemorrhage; *middle,* T1-weighted spin-echo image within 24 hours; and *right,* T2-weighted spin-echo image. Note slight hypointensity of hemorrhage on T1-weighted image and marked hypointensity on T2-weighted image with surrounding bright edema *(arrow).* (From Gomori JM, Grossman RI, Goldberg HI, et al: Intracranial hematomas: imaging by high-field MR. Radiology 157:87–93, 1985.) *B,* Subacute right parietal hemorrhage shows bright signal pattern on T1-weighted image *(left)* owing to extracellular methemoglobin formation. Fluid-fluid level is seen with high intensity in supernatant *(straight arrow)* and decreased signal intensity in clot *(curved arrow).* Signal loss is most pronounced on T2-weighted image *(right).* *C,* Subacute left parietal hemorrhage at later stage than *B* shows complete filling in of bright signal pattern on T1-weighted image *(left),* uniform hypointensity on T2-weighted image *(right)* due to intracellular deoxyhemoglobin and methemoglobin, and perihemorrhage edema *(arrow).* *D,* Late subacute pontine hemorrhage shows bright signal pattern throughout lesion on both T1-weighted *(left)* and T2-weighted *(right)* images. *E,* Chronic left occipital hemorrhage shows a bright signal pattern *(straight arrows)* on T1-weighted *(left)* and T2-weighted *(right)* images. Dark rim *(arrowheads)* is seen on T2-weighted image, representing superparamagnetic ferritin and hemosiderin.

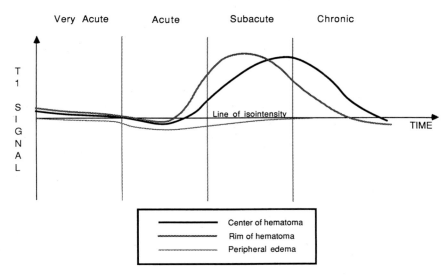

FIGURE 21–4. Evolution of MRI signal intensity of cerebral hematoma.

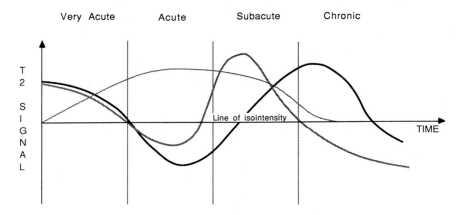

gradient-echo acquisitions improve the sensitivity for the detection of acute, as well as old, hemorrhage[5] (Figs. 21–5 and 21–6). However, the mechanism that causes a hematoma to appear dark on gradient-echo images is different from that proposed for spin-echo images. As we shall now review, spin-echo images are primarily sensitive to the effects of diffusion, whereas gradient-echo images are primarily sensitive to the effects of static magnetic field inhomogeneities.

Diffusion Causes Signal Loss on Spin-Echo Images

Diffusion is a rapid, random motion of molecules. Such diffusional motion through an inhomogeneous magnetic field produces phase shifts, which will vary among water molecules within the same voxel. Because the phase shifts are different, there is signal loss. Furthermore, because of their random motion, the diffusing water molecules experience different amounts of dephasing before and after a 180° radiofrequency refocusing pulse used in the spin-echo pulse sequence. As a result, the signal loss produced by diffusion-related dephasing is irreversible, unlike that produced by static magnetic field inhomogeneities.

The signal loss produced by diffusion increases as the TE is lengthened and is pronounced on spin-echo images acquired with a long TE. However, gradient-echo images are acquired with a much shorter TE than in spin-echo imaging. Because the TE is short, diffusion effects are reduced on gradient-echo images and have a lesser role in producing signal loss.

TABLE 21–2. TIME COURSE OF HEMORRHAGE SIGNAL INTENSITY COMPARED WITH BRAIN IN SPIN-ECHO MR IMAGES

STAGE	T1–WEIGHTED IMAGE	T2–WEIGHTED IMAGE
0–few hours (extremely acute)	Intermediate	Intermediate to bright
Several hours–3 d (acute)	Intermediate to dark	Dark
3 d–3 wk (subacute)	Bright rim	Dark center, bright rim, later bright center
3 wk–several months (chronic)	Bright or dark	Dark rim or completely dark

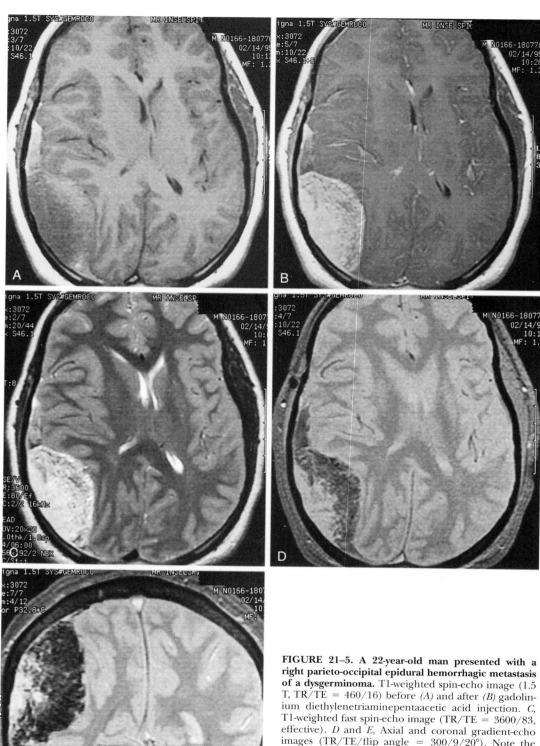

FIGURE 21–5. A 22-year-old man presented with a right parieto-occipital epidural hemorrhagic metastasis of a dysgerminoma. T1-weighted spin-echo image (1.5 T, TR/TE = 460/16) before *(A)* and after *(B)* gadolinium diethylenetriaminepentaacetic acid injection. *C,* T1-weighted fast spin-echo image (TR/TE = 3600/83, effective). *D* and *E,* Axial and coronal gradient-echo images (TR/TE/flip angle = 300/9/20°). Note the hypointensity of the hemorrhagic lesion on the gradient-echo images, mostly due to susceptibility effects.

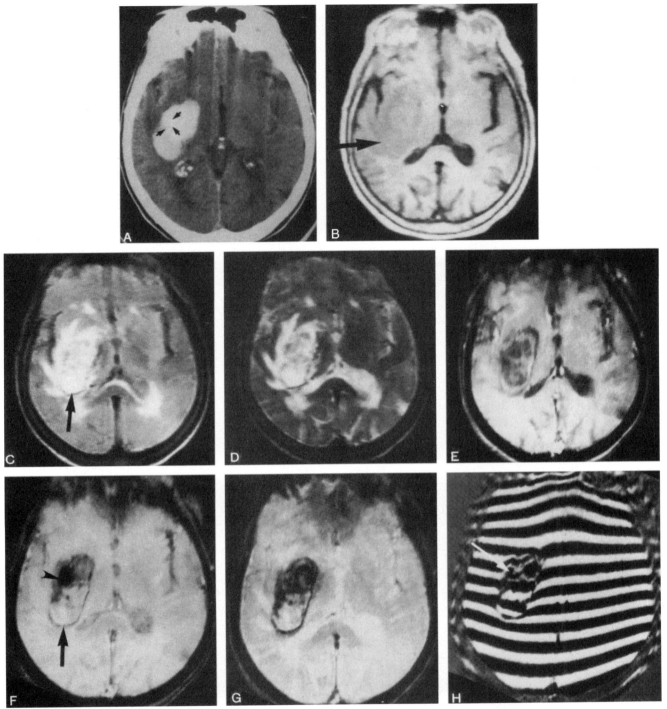

FIGURE 21–6. Acute right putaminal hemorrhage in a patient with history of hypertension. The MR image was obtained 15 hours after the ictus on a 0.6-T system. *A,* CT scan done shortly before MRI shows hyperdense hemorrhage with a more focal region of hyperdensity *(arrows)* of higher attenuation (9H) than rest of hemorrhage. *B,* T1-weighted spin-echo image shows nonspecific lesion *(arrow)* isointense with gray matter. *C,* T2-weighted spin-echo image (TR/TE = 2000/60) shows hyperintense lesion. There is a suggestion of a low-density halo *(arrow)*. Mild central hypointense area is similar in intensity to white matter. Outside the low-density halo there is a hyperintense signal pattern, suggesting vasogenic edema spreading along white fiber tracts. Findings suggest hemorrhage. *D,* A more T2-weighted spin-echo image (TR/TE = 2000/120) shows findings similar to those of *B. E,* T1-weighted gradient-echo image (TR/TE = 100/16) shows hypointensity within the lesion, in contrast to *A. F,* Moderately T2-weighted gradient-echo image (TR/TE = 100/30) shows a definite low-intensity halo *(arrow)*. Also seen is a focal area of marked hypointensity *(arrowhead)* that corresponds to area of increased density on the CT scan in *A. G,* A more T2-weighted gradient-echo image (TR/TE = 100/50) shows a pronounced hypointense halo as well as a markedly hypointense area that is much lower in intensity than white matter. Diagnosis of hemorrhage is unequivocal. *H,* Phase-sensitive zebra-stripe reconstruction susceptibility gradient at the junction of hemorrhage and brain. Also note the focally increased phase shift *(arrow)* in the region of focal hypointensity seen in *E. (A* to *H* from Edelman RR, Johnson K, Buxton R, et al: MR of hemorrhage: a new approach. AJNR 7:751–756, 1986.)

Static Magnetic Field Inhomogeneities Cause Signal Loss on Gradient-Echo Images

Unlike spin-echo images, gradient-echo images are directly sensitive to the effects of static magnetic field inhomogeneities produced by paramagnetic hemoglobin breakdown products. Because of local magnetic field inhomogeneities, water molecules at different positions within a voxel experience different magnetic field strengths, independent of diffusional processes (Fig. 21–7). These static field inhomogeneities result in some spins precessing faster than others. The end result is that the hemoglobin breakdown products, which represent the main source of local field inhomogeneity, produce dephasing and signal loss from surrounding water molecules. Gradient-echo images, acquired without radiofrequency refocusing, are highly sensitive to these effects. However, the dephasing effects of static magnetic field inhomogeneities, unlike diffusion, are constant over time and are eliminated by the radiofrequency refocusing on a spin-echo image. A drawback of gradient-echo imaging is increased sensitivity to susceptibility artifacts.

Boundary Effect

A related point is that the dark rim surrounding a hematoma on T2-weighted gradient-echo images does

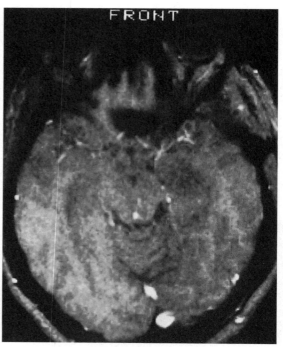

FIGURE 21–8. Axial fast low-angle shot (FLASH) MR image at 1.5 T. Area of signal loss in front of the circle of Willis is not due to hemorrhage but instead represents a magnetic susceptibility effect where the brain adjoins the air-containing sphenoidal sinus.

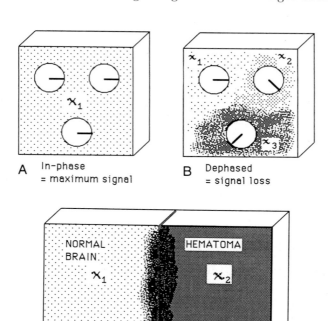

FIGURE 21–7. Signal loss due to intravoxel and intervoxel variations in magnetic susceptibility. *A,* In a voxel with uniform magnetic susceptibility (χ_1), the magnetic field is homogeneous and spins precess in phase. *B,* Within a voxel, variations in magnetic susceptibility (χ_1, χ_2, χ_3) due to paramagnetic hemoglobin breakdown products cause some spins to precess faster than others, leading to dephasing and signal loss. Signal loss is most pronounced on gradient-echo images. *C,* Field inhomogeneity at the boundary between two voxels having different magnetic susceptibilities (χ_1, χ_2) results in signal loss. This explains the dark rim seen at the border between an acute hematoma (higher magnetic susceptibility) and the surrounding brain (lower magnetic susceptibility).

not always represent deposition of hemoglobin breakdown products such as ferritin and hemosiderin. Signal loss can be encountered at the boundary between two regions having different magnetic susceptibilities, even if no paramagnetic substances are located there. For example, one commonly sees this effect on cranial images, where there is signal loss at the surface of the brain adjacent to the paranasal sinuses (Fig. 21–8). This loss of signal is produced by the local field inhomogeneity between a region of higher (brain) and lower (air-containing sinus) magnetic susceptibility. A similar effect is produced at the border between a hematoma (higher susceptibility) and brain (lower susceptibility).

Fast Spin-Echo Imaging

To summarize, the sensitivity to magnetic susceptibility effects of hemorrhage increases from fast spin-echo to routine spin-echo to gradient-echo techniques, from T1 to T2 to T2* weighting, and from lower to higher field strengths. Short echo spacing in fast spin-echo imaging reduces the contribution from various T2 decay mechanisms. Therefore, it has been argued that fast spin-echo imaging is less sensitive than spin-echo imaging to diffusion- and susceptibility-induced signal loss and thus less sensitive to detection of hemorrhage. However, in a series of 15 patients with brain hemorrhages, hemosiderin, deoxyhemoglobin, and iron-containing nuclei had slightly higher signal intensity on fast spin-echo than on spin-echo images, but the differences were not significant. Contrast with the two sequences was comparable and lesion conspicuity was nearly identical.[31] Also, prolongation of the interecho interval is not a clinically useful technique to improve the detection of acute hemorrhage.[32]

Echo-Planar Imaging

Echo-planar imaging is sensitive to the effects of static magnetic field inhomogeneities because the phase-encoding gradient is much weaker than that for standard pulse sequences.[33] The susceptibility artifacts are directed along the phase-encoding gradient rather than along the frequency-encoding direction, as is typical of standard pulse sequences. In principle, echo-planar imaging should be sensitive for detection of blood breakdown products. However, clinical data are missing.

EFFECT OF OXYGENATION ON THE APPEARANCE OF HEMORRHAGE

Signal loss in an acute hematoma is dependent on the formation of deoxyhemoglobin. Deoxyhemoglobin forms only when the intracellular oxygen tension is reduced. Because of the high oxygen tension of CSF, an acute hemorrhage into the subarachnoid space and ventricular system will not usually demonstrate paramagnetic-induced T1 shortening (Fig. 21–9). A hemorrhagic cortical infarction may also show a lesser degree of T2 shortening and signal loss on T2-weighted images, because of the increase in oxygen tension due to "luxury perfusion."[34]

Although acute subarachnoid and intraventricular hemorrhages can be difficult to detect by MRI, such hemorrhages may occasionally be seen as a region of increased signal intensity in the CSF on spin-echo images (see Fig. 21–9). This signal increase, representing T1 shortening, is probably a nonspecific effect of increased protein content. In the latter stages, subarachnoid and intraventricular hemorrhages may demonstrate regions of increased signal intensity due to the formation of extracellular methemoglobin.

EXTRACEREBRAL HEMORRHAGE

An extracerebral hematoma results from such entities as subdural and epidural bleeding, aneurysmal rupture into the subarachnoid space, venous thrombosis, arterial dissection, and musculoskeletal hemorrhage. It shows an MRI pattern of evolution similar to that of an intracerebral hematoma[14] but with one exception. Macrophages, which ingest iron in a hematoma, can transport iron from an extracerebral hematoma more readily than can the phagocytic cells within the brain. This probably relates to the absence of a blood-brain barrier (see Head Trauma and Related Hemorrhages further on). Pituitary hematomas behave like extracerebral hematomas, because the pituitary gland is not separated from the general circulation by a blood-brain barrier. As a result, the

peripheral rim of signal loss, due to storage of iron in the form of ferritin and hemosiderin, is sometimes thin or absent (e.g., see Fig. 21–38).

DIFFERENTIAL DIAGNOSIS OF HEMORRHAGE ON MR IMAGES

Fat, proteinaceous or cholesterol-containing solutions, subacute hemorrhage, metastatic melanoma, and occasionally calcified basal ganglia can all appear bright on T1-weighted images. Flow voids, melanin, calcification, and acute hemorrhage can all appear dark on T2-weighted images. This can lead to considerable diagnostic confusion. Strategies for making this differentiation are presented in the following sections.

Fat Versus Hemorrhage

Signal Intensity Comparisons

Compare the signal intensity of the tissue in question to nearby fat (e.g., subcutaneous fat in the scalp) (Fig. 21–10). If the tissue represents fat, then both regions should have a similar signal intensity on all pulse sequences. Because fat has a moderate T2 relaxation time, it darkens uniformly as the TE is increased. On images obtained with a TE of 80 to 90 ms, fat appears moderately dark. Unlike fat, at least some portions of a subacute hematoma appear bright on T2-weighted images, depending on the hematoma's state of evolution. Although portions of a subacute hematoma may appear dark on a high-field system, the signal intensity is nearly always inhomogeneous. Furthermore, when imaged with a long TE, these portions of the hematoma usually appear darker than scalp fat.

Comparisons between the signal intensities of different tissues can be somewhat difficult when imaging with a surface coil, as in spine imaging. Signal from tissues near the surface coil will appear artifactually enhanced when compared with deeper tissues, owing to the fall off of sensitivity with depth. In this situation, a comparison should be made between tissues that are approximately at the same depth from the coil.

Droplets of oil-based contrast agents that were used for myelography before the advent of water-soluble contrast agents can occasionally be observed in the basal cerebral cisterns, in the temporal horns of the ventricles, or in the lumbar dural sac. Signal comparison and distribution of this "nonbiologic fat" help to differentiate it from blood products.

Chemical-Shift–Selective Saturation

When available, chemical-shift–selective (CHESS) saturation pulses can be used to suppress fat signal intensity (see Chapter 4). These pulses do not alter or suppress the signal intensity of hemorrhage.

Boundary Effect

On spin-echo images, low signal intensity should be sought at borders between the tissue in question and

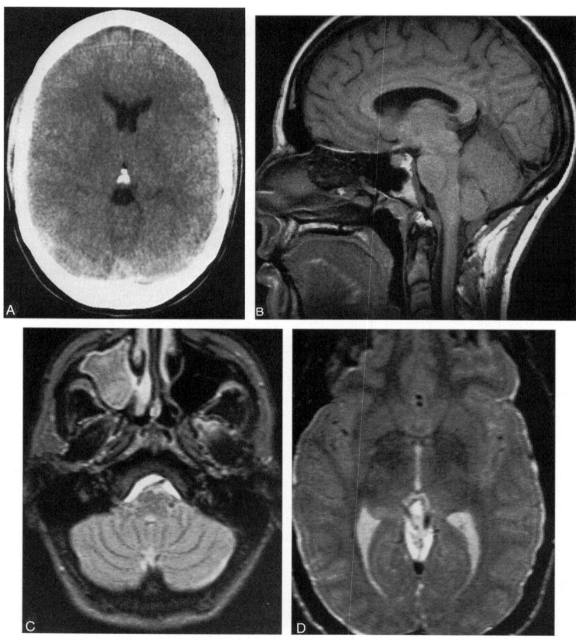

FIGURE 21–9. A 38-year-old woman suffered a subarachnoid hemorrhage 10 days previously. Because subarachnoid blood is dispersed and removed from the CSF within the first days after subarachnoid hemorrhage, the lesion was no longer seen with CT. Although subarachnoid hemorrhage is usually difficult to perceive on MR images, in this case it was clearly demonstrated. *A,* Normal CT scan. In the displayed slice, no blood was visible in the quadrigeminal plate or superior cerebellar cisterns. *B,* Parasagittal T1-weighted spin-echo MR image (1.0 T, TR/TE = 720/26) demonstrating a subarachnoid blood clot isointense relative to brain, anterior to the brain stem, in the inferior and superior cerebellar cisterns, and in the quadrigeminal plate cistern. *C,* Axial T2-weighted spin-echo MR image (TR/TE = 2500/80) demonstrates clot with markedly hyperintense signal anterior to the brain stem. *D,* Axial T2-weighted spin-echo MR image (TR/TE = 2500/80) showing blood as a hyperintense signal pattern in the superior cerebellar cisterns.

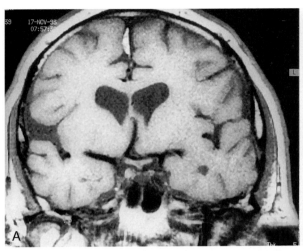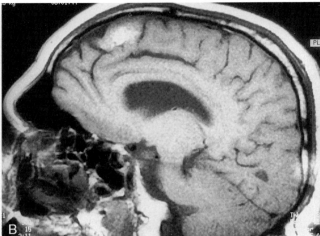

FIGURE 21–10. Calcification of falx in a 54-year-old man. *A* and *B*, T1-weighted coronal and sagittal spin-echo images (1.5 T, TR/TE = 400/20). The calcification contains bone marrow with fat; therefore, the signal intensity is the same as in the diploë between the inner and outer table of the skull.

that of normal surrounding tissue. If the low signal pattern is present on only one side of the lesion, it represents chemical-shift artifact, and the lesion is probably fat. If the low signal pattern, to some degree, is circumferential, it most likely represents magnetic susceptibility artifact from hemorrhage. (Gradient-echo images, such as fast low-angle shot [FLASH] or gradient-recalled acquisition in the steady state [GRASS], can be misleading. Chemical-shift artifacts can surround fatty lesions on gradient-echo images if the TE happens to produce a phase-contrast image [see Chapter 10]).

Proteinaceous Fluid Versus Hemorrhage

Infrequently, a lesion containing highly proteinaceous fluid (e.g., a follicular thyroid cyst) can produce high signal intensity on T1-weighted images, mimicking a subacute hematoma. However, the high signal intensity in such a hematoma usually begins as a thin rim that evolves toward the center of the lesion. A lesion containing proteinaceous fluid tends to be more uniform in appearance. Furthermore, unlike a subacute hematoma, it does not usually have higher than normal magnetic susceptibility and, therefore, would not show signal loss at its interface with normal tissue.

Cholesterol-Containing Cysts Versus Hemorrhage

Colloid cysts of the third ventricle typically show high signal intensity on short TR/TE sequences (Fig. 21–11), which is correlated with high cholesterol content.[35] T2 relaxation may be shortened and rarely prolonged. Such cysts may be confused with subacute hematomas. Cysts in other areas of the cranium may also be filled with cholesterol-rich contents. For example, cholesterol-containing cysts in the hypophysial region may look exactly the same as the hemorrhage

into the pituitary adenoma shown in Figure 21–38, although they do not contain any hemoglobin breakdown products.

Flow Voids Versus Hemorrhage

Blood vessels can also produce signal voids, but these can be evaluated using flow-compensated gradient-echo pulse sequences, which produce increased signal from flowing blood (see Chapter 9).

Melanin Versus Hemorrhage

Within melanin, stable free radicals have been detected that are paramagnetic and decrease both T1 and T2 relaxation times.[36, 37] This effect may make some melanomas appear brighter than the surrounding brain on T1-weighted images and darker on T2-weighted images. These signal characteristics are similar to those of an acute intracerebral hematoma containing intracellular deoxyhemoglobin and intracellular methemoglobin. However, the issue is confused by the high incidence of hemorrhage in melanoma metastases,[36, 37] so that the effects of hemorrhage may dominate those of the free radicals (see Fig. 17–12). This would explain why even an amelanotic melanoma may demonstrate the signal intensity changes characteristic of hemorrhage. Usually additional MRI signs of a tumor are present that allow differentiation of a melanotic metastasis from a primary brain hemorrhage. The differentiation may be further aided by the administration of a contrast agent such as gadolinium diethylenetriaminepentaacetic acid (Gd-DTPA).

Calcification Versus Hemorrhage

Calcification produces local variations in magnetic susceptibility. These susceptibility variations may result in a signal void, which is indistinguishable from the

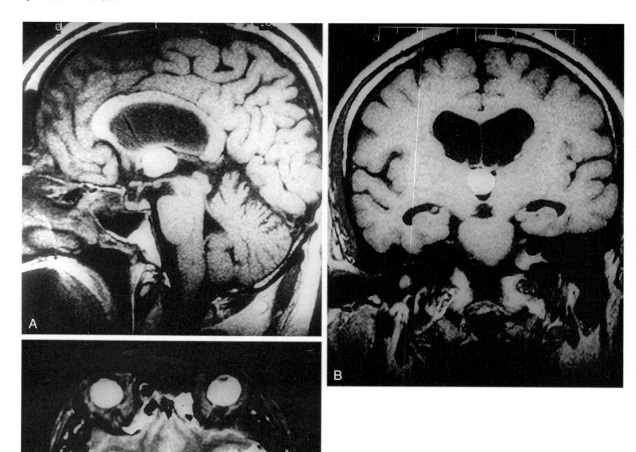

FIGURE 21–11. A 49-year-old man presented with a complaint of tinnitus. *A* to *C*, MRI performed with a 1-T scanner showed a colloid cyst and widening of both lateral ventricles. The cyst is hyperintense on T1-weighted images *(A, B)* and hypointense on T2-weighted images *(C)*. However, the location in the anterosuperior part of the third ventricle is typical for a colloid cyst. Because of its location it causes hydrocephalic widening of the lateral ventricles owing to blockage of CSF outflow through the interventricular foramen of Monro into the third ventricle.

appearance of a subacute hematoma (Fig. 21–12). In an old hematoma, regions of signal loss may persist on T2-weighted images for months or years after the methemoglobin has been absorbed and T1 signal enhancement has disappeared. In this situation, CT may be necessary to differentiate calcification from a hematoma.[38]

Unlike a hematoma, calcification is not usually associated with high signal intensity on MR images. One exception is the infrequent observation of a bright signal within the basal ganglia on T1-weighted images, raising the question of subacute hemorrhage (Fig. 21–13). This appearance has been reported in association with calcification without hemorrhage. Presumably,

these calcifications are hydrated. It has been suggested that the slower motion of water molecules within the hydration layer results in T1 shortening and, therefore, increased signal intensity (diamagnetic effect). On T2-weighted images, these regions may appear dark, presumably representing the susceptibility effect of calcium. This diagnosis is most likely when the bright signal regions are symmetric and have no mass effect (see Fig. 21–13) and when there is no evidence of bright signal on T2-weighted images.[39] Unlike calcification, copper deposition in the gray nuclei in Wilson's disease results generally in a decrease in signal intensity on T1-weighted images and an increase in signal intensity on T2-weighted images.[40, 41]

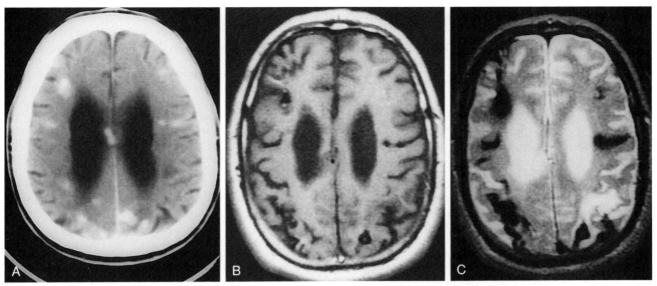

FIGURE 21–12. Multiple cerebral metastases from a cardiac myxoma. *A,* On this CT scan, lesions appear hyperdense. *B,* Axial T1-weighted spin-echo MR image (1.5 T, TR/TE = 400/16). *C,* Axial T2-weighted spin-echo MR image (TR/TE = 2500/90). Lesion is hypointense throughout the area of calcification on both spin-echo MR images. Note that hypointensity is more profound and extensive on the T2-weighted image than on the T1-weighted image. The longer TE of the T2-weighted image permits more dephasing of the spins, which occurs between the lesion and adjacent brain. Angiography (not shown) showed multiple fusiform aneurysms typical of myxoma metastases. (From Mattle HP, Maurer D, Sturzenegger M, et al: Cardiac myxomas: a long term study. J Neurol 242:689–694, 1995. Copyright © 1995 John Wiley & Sons. Reprinted by permission of John Wiley & Sons, Inc.)

GENERAL COMMENTS ON SPONTANEOUS BRAIN HEMORRHAGE

PATHOGENESIS OF BRAIN HEMORRHAGE

Traditional teaching has emphasized that nearly all spontaneous brain hemorrhages are caused by chronic hypertensive damage to penetrating and subcortical arteries and arterioles. A mechanism that can provoke bleeding in these patients is an acute increase in blood flow or pressure leading to vessel rupture. However, even in situations without prior hypertension, acute increases in blood flow or pressure can produce hemorrhage.[42] Examples are 1) acute increases in blood flow after removal or improvement of focal arterial obstructions and 2) reperfusion of ischemic or injured tissue. In the former situation, for example, in migraine[43] or after carotid endarterectomy,[44] bleeding occurs at the site of normal arterioles and capillaries. In the latter situation (e.g., reperfusion after embolic infarction), bleeding takes place in vessels and brain tissues that have suffered ischemic damage. Further mechanisms of brain hemorrhage are increasingly recognized with better diagnostic techniques.[45] These nonhypertensive causes include rupture of vascular malformations and aneurysms, bleeding from abnormally fragile arteries (e.g., arteritis or amyloid angiopathy), hemorrhage with bleeding diathesis, head trauma, bleeding into preexisting lesions such as primary or metastatic tumors or granulomas, and obstruction of blood drainage from the brain, as in venous and sinus thrombosis.

TIME COURSE OF BLEEDING

The period of active bleeding in spontaneous brain hemorrhage is commonly believed to last a fraction of an hour, which generally implies that the active bleeding has ceased by the time the patient arrives at a hospital.[46] Symptoms and signs are maximal in approximately one third of the patients at the outset and in two thirds gradually or smoothly progressive.[47] Unlike in ischemic stroke, a stuttering or stepwise progression is rare. Late progression after hours or days occurs in approximately 3% of patients.[48] Its mechanism is uncertain. Rebleeding is rare. In a study with chromium-labeled red blood cells injected at the time of admission for hypertensive hemorrhage, it was found that patients who died had virtually no evidence of labeling in the original hemorrhage, whereas the Duret hemorrhages in the midbrain, which reflected the postadmission fatal cerebral herniation, were easily labeled.[49] Only occasionally, CT or MRI will show enlargement of the hematoma after admission. The chief mechanism for subsequent worsening is the development of edema and ischemic necrosis around the lesion.[50] However, studies with early CT and repeated CT after neurologic deterioration have shown that polyphasic hematoma expansion occurs and can be the reason for a sudden catastrophic deterioration in a few patients.[51]

ETIOLOGY, LOCATION, AND FREQUENCY

Patients with spontaneous brain hemorrhage tend to be on average a decade younger than patients with

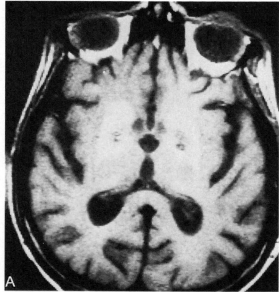

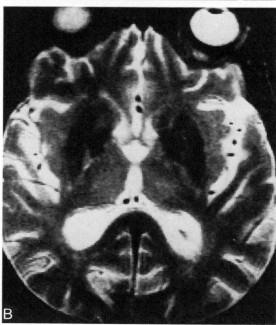

FIGURE 21–13. In this 50-year-old man, CT (not shown) showed extensive basal ganglia calcification. *A,* Axial T1-weighted image (1.5 T, TR/TE = 700/18) demonstrates bright signal surrounding an area of signal loss bilaterally in the basal ganglia. The signal loss is in the globus pallidus. *B,* On the T2-weighted image (TR/TE = 2500/90) there is signal loss in the putamen that is even more marked in the globus pallidus. The symmetry of the lesions helps differentiate them from a hematoma in the subacute stage. The appearance has been on the basis of T1 and T2 shortening due to dipole-dipole interactions between water and calcium.[38] The role of iron, if any, in producing this appearance is uncertain.

ischemic stroke. Hemorrhage accounts for 10% to 13% of all strokes.[52–54] The frequency of underlying causes varies with age. In children, vascular malformations, aneurysms, trauma, and hematologic disorders such as thrombocytopenia, leukemia, and hemophilia account for the majority of cases. Frequency and causes of

brain hemorrhage in young adults are listed in Table 21–3[55]; the causes of intracerebral hemorrhage in adults are summarized in Table 21–4.

Arterial hypertension is the presumed cause in 70% to 90% of nontraumatic brain hemorrhage cases,[52] although the precise frequency depends on whether one examines autopsy specimens, clinical cases, or CT or MRI series. In addition, the incidence of hypertensive intracerebral hemorrhage has been declining in the past decades. In one series, it declined from 78% in the period 1978 to 1981 to 64% in 1986 to 1981.[56] Distribution figures for a study of 100 unselected patients with brain hemorrhage are shown in Table 21–5.[57] When etiology is correlated with the site of brain hemorrhage, hypertensive arteriopathy is the major cause of lenticulocapsular, cerebellar, brain stem, and thalamic hemorrhages. In lobar hemorrhages the causes are much more diverse. They comprise anticoagulant-related hemorrhages, rupture of aneurysms and vascular malformations, intratumoral hemorrhage, cerebral amyloid angiopathy, angiitis, and drug abuse.

CLINICAL PRESENTATION

Spontaneous brain hemorrhage occurs characteristically during physical exertion, and onset during sleep is rare.[58] In 78% there is a focal neurologic deficit[54] depending on the site of the hemorrhage and the disruption of brain tissue. Severe headaches occur in about 40% of patients with brain hemorrhage,[53, 54] as opposed to 5% to 15% in patients with infarction,[54] and seizures occur in 9%.[54] Vomiting is present in 29%, consciousness decreases in 50% to 57%,[53] and coma supervenes in 21%.[54] Decrease of consciousness and coma correlate with either intraventricular extension of the hemorrhage or increased intracranial pressure owing to large hematoma size and transtentorial herniation.

Arterial hypertension is almost always associated.[52, 54] In many instances it occurs as a reflex to maintain

TABLE 21–3. CAUSES AND FREQUENCY OF SPONTANEOUS INTRACEREBRAL HEMORRHAGES IN THE YOUNG

CLINICAL DIAGNOSIS	NO. OF PATIENTS	%
Ruptured AVM	21	29.1
Arterial hypertension	11	15.3
Ruptured saccular aneurysm	7	9.7
Sympathomimetic drug abuse	5	6.9
Tumor	3	4.2
Acute alcohol intoxication	2	2.8
Preeclampsia/eclampsia	2	2.8
Superior sagittal sinus thrombosis	1	1.4
Systemic lupus erythematosus	1	1.4
Moyamoya	1	1.4
Cryoglobulinemia	1	1.4
Undetermined	17	23.6
Total	72	100.0

Adapted from Toffel GJ, Biller J, Adams HP: Nontraumatic intracerebral hemorrhage in young adults. Arch Neurol 44:483–485, 1987. Copyright 1987, American Medical Association.

adequate cerebral perfusion and does not necessarily signify a history of hypertension. Physical signs indicative of previous hypertension include left ventricular hypertrophy and hypertensive retinopathy. Subhyaloid hemorrhages in the ocular fundi are virtually diagnostic of subarachnoid hemorrhage and occur in spontaneous brain hemorrhage only exceptionally.

ETIOLOGY OF HEMORRHAGE BY LOCATION AND ASSOCIATED BRAIN ABNORMALITIES

Although identification of a hematoma is extremely important, it is the underlying cause of the hemorrhage that is critical to treatment of patients. The identification of the cause of a hemorrhage by MRI may preclude the need for invasive diagnostic procedures. In the following sections we review the clinical symptoms and signs and the significance of the location and appearance at MRI of various types of spontaneous brain hemorrhage. Not all brain hematomas have an appearance at MRI or CT that renders a specific diagnosis.

TABLE 21–4. CAUSES OF INTRACEREBRAL HEMORRHAGE

Chronic hypertension
Aneurysms
Bleeding from vascular malformations
  AVM
  Cavernous angioma
  Capillary telangiectasia
  Venous angioma
Abnormally fragile arteries
  Amyloid angiopathy
  Arteritis
Bleeding diathesis
  Warfarin, heparin
  Antiplatelet agents
  Fibrinolysis
  Thrombocytopenia
  Hemophilia
  Leukemia
Drug abuse
Venous and sinus thrombosis
Infective endocarditis, septic emboli
Head trauma
  Primary hemorrhages into contusion site
  Diffuse axonal injuries
  Tear of arteries
  Secondary hemorrhages
Bleeding into preexisting lesions such as primary and metastatic tumors and granulomas
Hemorrhagic stroke, hemorrhage into infarcts
Miscellaneous rare causes
  Migraine
  Medical conditions with acute hypertension such as eclampsia, pheochromocytoma, and glomerulonephritis
  Vasopressor drugs
  After carotid endarterectomy
  On exertion
  Severe dental pain or painful urologic examination
  Exposure to cold weather
  Fat embolism to the brain
  After posterior fossa surgery (supratentorial hemorrhage)
  After occlusion of arteriovenous fistula

TABLE 21–5. DISTRIBUTION OF HEMORRHAGE BY SITE IN 100 UNSELECTED PATIENTS WITH SPONTANEOUS BRAIN HEMORRHAGE

TYPE	NO. OF CASES
Putaminal	34
Lobar	24
Thalamic	20
Cerebellar	7
Pontine	6
Caudate	5
Putaminothalamic	4

From Kase CS, Mohr JP: Supratentorial intracerebral hemorrhage. In: Barnett HJM, Mohr JP, Stein BM, Yatsu FM, eds. Stroke: Pathophysiology, Diagnosis, and Management. Churchill Livingstone, New York, 1986, pp 525–547.

HYPERTENSIVE (DEEP) HEMORRHAGE

More than a century ago, Charcot and Bouchard[59] drew attention to "miliary aneurysms" from brains of patients with hypertensive hemorrhage. Fisher[58] considered them a last link in a pathogenetic chain. Hypertension causes degenerative changes in penetrating arteries in the form of lipid-rich hyaline subintimal material, called lipohyalinosis. The lipohyalinosis disrupts muscle and elastic elements and allows bulging of arterial walls. This process can interrupt blood flow and lead to lacunar infarcts. Alternatively, this process can result in hemorrhage at the site of aneurysmal outpouchings. Once the hemorrhage has started, secondary arterial ruptures at the periphery of the enlarging hematoma follow in avalanche fashion.

By anatomic site of penetrating arteries, hypertensive hemorrhages are located in the basal ganglia, internal capsule, thalamus, or pons or deep in the cerebellum. Furthermore, small cortical perforators can lead to subcortical "slit" hemorrhages oriented parallel to the overlying cortex. Hematomas of less than 1.5 cm in diameter are mostly located in these areas and due to hypertension.[60] Angiography has little role in the evaluation of hypertensive hemorrhage.[61]

Hypertensive hemorrhages, except for petechial hemorrhages in hypertensive encephalopathy, are almost never multiple. Multiple hemorrhages are much more likely due to bleeding diathesis, metastatic tumors, vasculitis, sepsis, cerebral amyloid angiopathy, cerebral venous and sinus occlusion, or trauma.

Putaminal Hemorrhage

Figure 21–6 shows a hypertensive putaminal hemorrhage. Most commonly it arises from a lateral branch of the striate arteries, and if sufficiently large it can extend to adjacent structures. The clinical spectrum reflects the size and the pattern of extension of the hemorrhage. All patients exhibit some form of a motor deficit, in addition to which a sensory disorder and eventually a hemianopsia will ensue from involvement of the optic tract (Fig. 21–14).

Caudate Hemorrhage

The sources of caudate hemorrhages are typically deep penetrating branches of the anterior and middle

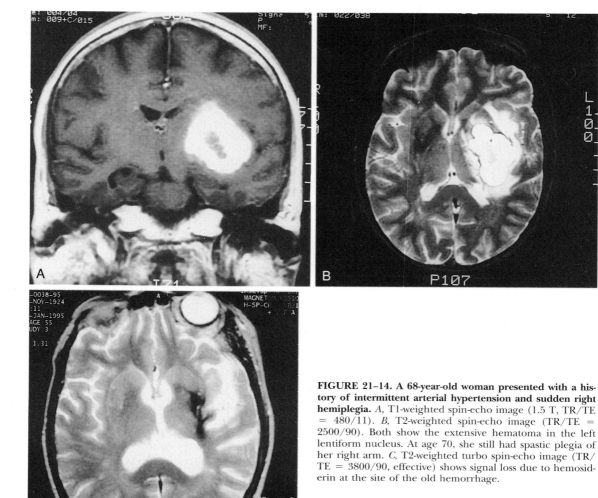

FIGURE 21–14. A 68-year-old woman presented with a history of intermittent arterial hypertension and sudden right hemiplegia. *A*, T1-weighted spin-echo image (1.5 T, TR/TE = 480/11). *B*, T2-weighted spin-echo image (TR/TE = 2500/90). Both show the extensive hematoma in the left lentiform nucleus. At age 70, she still had spastic plegia of her right arm. *C*, T2-weighted turbo spin-echo image (TR/TE = 3800/90, effective) shows signal loss due to hemosiderin at the site of the old hemorrhage.

cerebral arteries.[62] The caudate nucleus also receives its blood supply from ependymal arteries. These vessels are not usually affected by hypertensive vasculopathy but, nonetheless, can be a source of bleeding from an occasional vascular malformation. Hemorrhages occur in the head of the caudate nucleus, and extension into adjacent structures and the lateral ventricle is a common feature[63] (Fig. 21–15).

The clinical picture resembles that of subarachnoid hemorrhage: abrupt onset with headache, vomiting, and temporary behavioral abnormalities. In approximately half the cases, additional clinical features include gaze and contralateral hemiparesis.[63] The outcome in caudate hemorrhage is usually benign. Hydrocephalus can complicate caudate hemorrhage. The hydrocephalus tends to disappear as the hemorrhage resolves, and ventriculoperitoneal shunting is required in most instances only temporarily.[63]

Thalamic Hemorrhage

In the majority of cases, thalamic hemorrhages are due to hypertensive arteriopathy (Fig. 21–16; see also Fig. 21–3A). The clinical presentation reflects again the size and extension of the hematoma.[64, 65] The patients present with a hemisensory syndrome associated with a motor deficit. Usually there is loss of all the sensory modalities over the contralateral limbs, face, and trunk. From a clinical point of view, these findings and the distribution of motor and sensory symptoms do not help to unequivocally differentiate thalamic from putaminal hemorrhage.

Thalamic hematomas have a high rate of intraventricular extension. This or the hemorrhage itself may cause hydrocephalus, requiring emergency ventricular drainage. The outcome of hematomas larger than 3 cm in diameter is bleak.

Brain Stem Hemorrhage

Figure 21–17 shows a brain stem hemorrhage. Most brain stem hemorrhages occur in the pons, which is another classic location for hypertensive hemorrhage. Occasionally, these hemorrhages are due to AVMs and other causes. CT and MRI permit hemorrhages to be

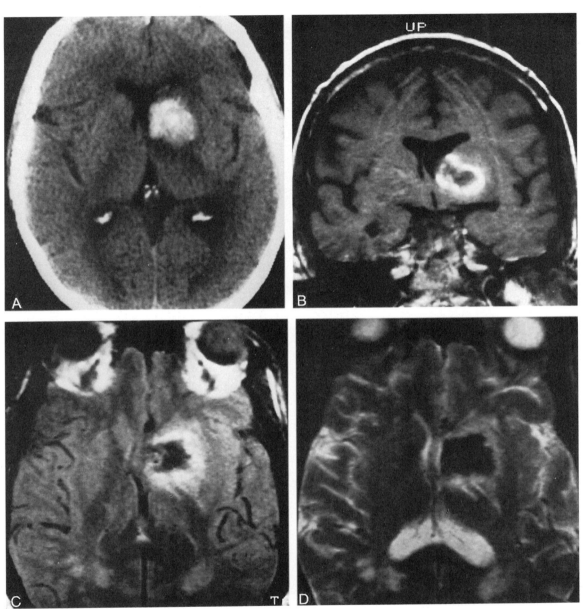

FIGURE 21–15. A 57-year-old man presented with a history of hypertension. *A,* The CT scan shows an acute hemorrhage in the typical location of hypertensive hemorrhages. *B* to *D,* High-field MRI performed 3 days after the bleeding episode shows involvement of the head of the caudate nucleus, anterior limb of the internal capsule, and lentiform nucleus. On the coronal T1-weighted image *(B),* a bright rim (extracellular methemoglobin) surrounds a dark center. The axial proton density–weighted image *(C)* shows a bright rim (extracellular methemoglobin and edema) and a dark center (intracellular methemoglobin and deoxyhemoglobin). The T2-weighted image *(D)* shows more extensive signal loss owing to the prolonged TE and correspondingly greater sensitivity to dephasing effects from concentrated paramagnetic substances. The thin rim with increased signal intensity probably represents edema.

confidently distinguished from ischemic brain stem lesions.[66] Hypertensive brain stem hemorrhages present within minutes, whereas the clinical signs of hemorrhages due to leakage from AVMs evolve gradually over 2 days or more.[67]

Pontine hemorrhages have been categorized according to location.[68–70] They result from rupture of perforating or long circumferential arteries. At the onset of a massive pontine hemorrhage, about one third of the patients complain of severe occipital head-ache[69]; vomiting or motor phenomena, giving a false impression of seizures, may ensue. Focal pontine signs evolve within a few minutes and include quadriplegia, abnormal muscle tone, ophthalmoplegia, pinpoint pupils, and irregular respiration.[71] Massive pontine hemorrhage is almost always fatal. When the patient survives, a so-called locked-in syndrome may occur.

Unilateral hemorrhages limited to the pontine tegmentum cause ipsilateral gaze palsy.[70] Bilateral tegmental hemorrhages cause ophthalmoplegia.[72] Hemor-

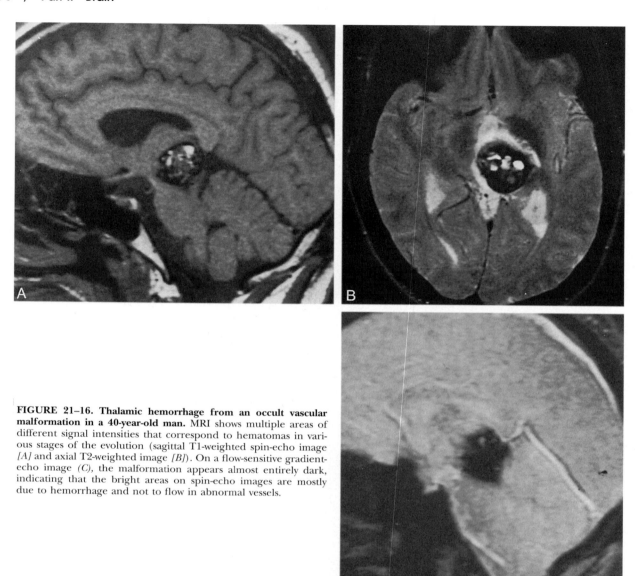

FIGURE 21–16. Thalamic hemorrhage from an occult vascular malformation in a 40-year-old man. MRI shows multiple areas of different signal intensities that correspond to hematomas in various stages of the evolution (sagittal T1-weighted spin-echo image *[A]* and axial T2-weighted image *[B]*). On a flow-sensitive gradient-echo image *(C)*, the malformation appears almost entirely dark, indicating that the bright areas on spin-echo images are mostly due to hemorrhage and not to flow in abnormal vessels.

rhages limited to one side of the basis pontis produce contralateral limb weakness. Small pontine hemorrhages usually have a favorable outcome.

Hematomas in the mesencephalon[73–77] (Fig. 21–18) and medulla oblongata[78] are rare.[79] Their clinical presentation depends on location.[80, 81] Midbrain hemorrhages demonstrate variable combinations of pyramidal tract signs, oculomotor disturbances, cerebellar ataxia, and impaired consciousness. Sudden onset of headache and vertigo with various combinations of medial or lateral medullary involvement characterize medullary hemorrhage.[82] Vascular malformations are a more common cause than hypertension.

Cerebellar Hemorrhage

The leading cause of cerebellar hemorrhage is hypertension, followed by anticoagulant-related hemorrhage[83, 84]; coagulopathies, aneurysms, vascular mal-formations (Fig. 21–19), and cerebral emboli represent other rare causes. Cerebellar hemorrhages commonly arise in the region of the dentate nuclei and seldom in the vermis.[85, 86]

The hemorrhage acts as an acute posterior fossa mass and compresses the brain stem, often leading to necrosis of the tegmentum and acute hydrocephalus[87] (Fig. 21–20). The most constant initial symptoms are occipital headache, dizziness, and inability to stand or walk.[83, 84] A triad of limb ataxia, ipsilateral gaze palsy, and peripheral facial palsy is characteristic.[84] Involvement of the vermis results in severe truncal ataxia. Cerebellar hemorrhage is commonly misdiagnosed as brain stem stroke, labyrinthine disturbance, and subarachnoid hemorrhage.

Because clinical findings cannot reliably distinguish between extrinsic compression and intrinsic lesions of the brain stem, CT and MRI play an important role in their diagnosis. Aside from location and extent of the

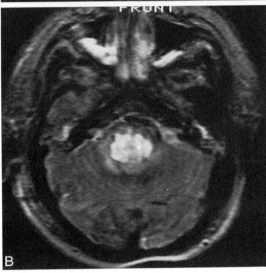

FIGURE 21–17. Pontine hemorrhage. A 57-year-old man presented with a history of hypertension and developed tetraparesis associated with ataxia, bilateral horizontal gaze palsy, and decrease in level of consciousness. The MR image, obtained a few days after the onset of symptoms, shows subacute hemorrhage extending bilaterally into the pontine tegmentum. In the periphery of the hematoma, there is hyperintense signal on both T1-weighted (A) and T2-weighted (B) spin-echo images, whereas the center is still isointense relative to adjacent brain tissue.

hemorrhage, these imaging modalities will show obliteration and displacement of the fourth ventricle, hydrocephalus, effacement of the basal cisterns, and blood in the ventricular system. In medically unstable patients, CT is the imaging modality of choice.

Acute Hypertensive Encephalopathy

In acute hypertensive encephalopathy, nonspecific findings such as focal and diffuse white matter hyperintensities on T2-weighted images are seen, representing reversible edema, irreversible infarction, or preexisting ischemic disease. Hypertensive encephalopathy should be suspected when multiple petechial hemorrhages are visualized.[88] Gradient-echo techniques may be nec-essary to show these petechial hemorrhages, especially on low-field systems (see Chapter 24).

LOBAR HEMORRHAGE

Lobar hemorrhage is defined as a hemorrhage in the cerebral hemisphere, outside the basal ganglia and thalamus (Fig. 21–21). Less than 25% of spontaneous brain hemorrhages are lobar, and hypertensive subcortical bleeding accounts for approximately one third of these.[53, 89] Apart from hypertension, the causes of lobar hemorrhage include the rupture of an aneurysm or vascular malformation; bleeding from abnormally fragile arteries (e.g., amyloid angiopathy, arteritis)[90]; hemorrhage due to a bleeding diathesis, anticoagulant therapy, or drug abuse; bleeding into a preexisting lesion such as a primary or metastatic tumor; and bleeding associated with endocarditis[91] (see Table 21–4). Rarely, these entities bleed in deep structures, where hypertensive hematomas are usually found, resulting in diagnostic confusion.

The causes of lobar hemorrhage also vary with age. In the elderly, the most common cause is chronic hypertension, and only occasionally is amyloid angiopathy the cause. Berry aneurysm rupture producing an intracerebral hematoma is more often seen in middle-aged adults (see Table 21–4). The frequency of causes of lobar hemorrhages from five clinical series is given in Table 21–6.[92–95] The leading causes of brain hemorrhage in young adulthood are ruptured vascular malformations and hypertension (see Table 21–3). In children, vascular malformations and hematologic disorders such as leukemia or thrombocytopenia account for the majority of cases. The clinical presentation depends on the location and size of the hematoma.[94]

Hemorrhage from Aneurysms

It is estimated that there are more than 28,000 cases of aneurysmal subarachnoid hemorrhage in North America each year[96] (Fig. 21–22). About 60% of patients also have an associated brain hemorrhage because the ruptured aneurysm had embedded itself in the adjacent brain parenchyma.[97] The subarachnoid location of a ruptured aneurysm will determine the site of origin of a hematoma, most of which are found in the frontal and temporal lobes. The finding of a

TABLE 21–6. CAUSES AND FREQUENCIES OF LOBAR CEREBRAL HEMORRHAGE IN 213 PATIENTS IN FIVE CLINICAL SERIES

CAUSE	NO. OF PATIENTS	%
Hypertension	79	37
Bleeding diathesis	27	13
Neoplasms	9	4
Vascular malformations, aneurysms	40	19
Other	13	6
Unknown	45	21

Data from references 89 and 92 through 95.

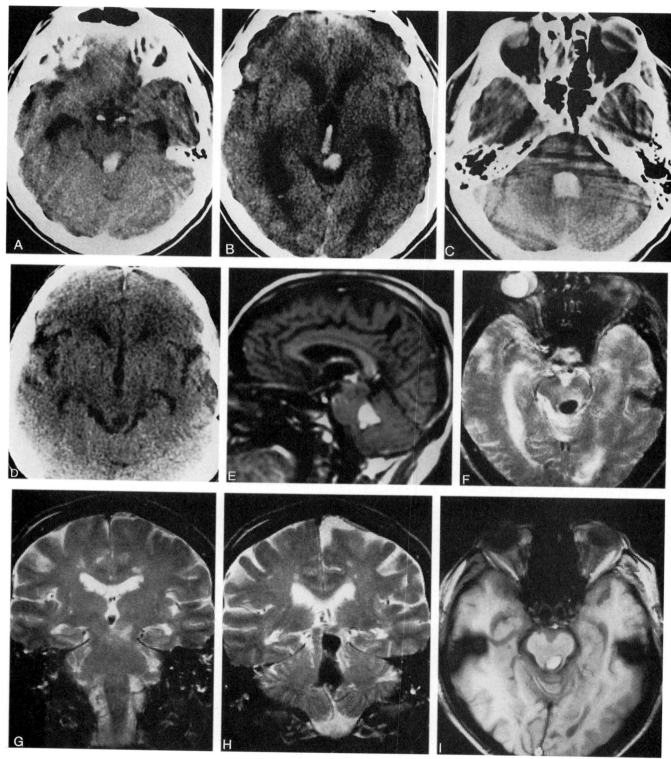

FIGURE 21–18. *See legend on opposite page*

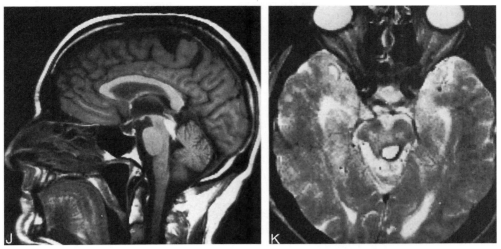

FIGURE 21–18. A 64-year-old man presented with midbrain hemorrhage of unknown etiology. On a CT scan, a mesencephalic hematoma around the aqueduct *(A)* with breakthrough into the third *(B)* and fourth *(C)* ventricle is seen. Four weeks later the CT scan *(D)* demonstrates hypodensity at the site of the original hematoma. Four days after the ictus, The sagittal T1-weighted spin-echo MR image *(E)* demonstrates bright blood in the posterior part of the third ventricle and in the fourth ventricle. The T2-weighted MR images show dark blood in the mesencephalic tegmentum *(F)*, in the third ventricle *(G)*, and in the fourth ventricle *(H)*. Three weeks later, on the axial and sagittal T1-weighted spin-echo images, blood in the midbrain, appearing bright, is still present *(I and J)* but is no longer seen in the ventricles *(J)*. On the T2-weighted spin-echo image *(K)* blood now appears bright, owing to red blood cell lysis and increased water content as a consequence of osmotic effects.

hematoma in the precallosal or septal area is characteristic of a ruptured anterior communicating artery aneurysm. An anterior temporal lobe hematoma, in conjunction with subarachnoid hemorrhage, is typical of a ruptured middle cerebral artery aneurysm[98] (see Chapter 23).

Subarachnoid hemorrhage is visualized by MRI only when there are large focal blood collections. CT is more sensitive. The sensitivity of MRI was superior to the sensitivity of CT for detection of aneurysmal subarachnoid hemorrhage in only one study, which has been the subject of the "devil's advocate."[99, 100]

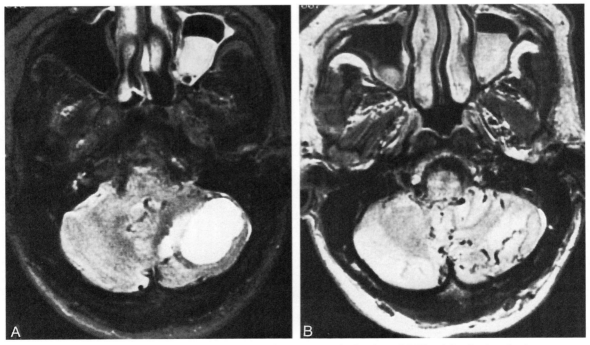

FIGURE 21–19. Cerebellar hemorrhage in the subacute stage. *A,* On the axial T2-weighted spin-echo image, the hemorrhage appears bright. *B,* The proton density–weighted spin-echo image of an adjacent slice shows multiple flow voids, consistent with an AVM.

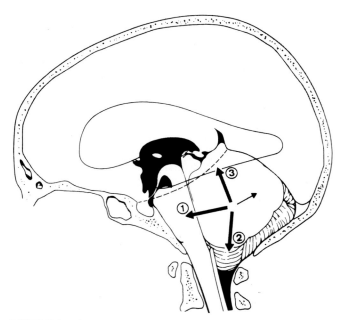

FIGURE 21–20. Possible mass effects from a posterior fossa hemorrhage. The hemorrhage may compress the brain stem (1), leading to necrosis of the tegmentum, and cause cerebellar tonsillar herniation (2) or superior cerebellar tentorial herniation (3) or both. Hydrocephalus may ensue due to compromise of CSF outflow. (Courtesy of U. Ebeling, MD, University of Bern, Switzerland.)

Using fluid-attenuated inversion recovery (FLAIR) sequences, Noguchi and coworkers[101] reliably visualized acute subarachnoid hemorrhage 2 hours to 4 days after the ictus. The hemorrhage was seen as an area of high signal intensity relative to normal CSF and brain parenchyma.[101]

Superficial siderosis of the central nervous system is a rare condition characterized by hemosiderin deposition in the leptomeninges and the outer layers of the brain, spinal cord, and cranial nerves in contact with the CSF, best seen as hypointensity on T2-weighted images.[102] Clinical signs are progressive hearing loss and ataxia. Common causes include chronic subarachnoid hemorrhage, long-term anticoagulation, vascular malformations, subdural hematomas, and hemorrhagic neoplasms.

Vascular Malformations

Vascular malformations of the brain are categorized as AVMs (Fig. 21–23), cavernous angiomas (Fig. 21–24), capillary telangiectasias, and venous malformations (Figs. 21–25 and 21–26; see also Figs. 21–16 and 21–19). AVMs are more commonly located in the cerebral hemispheres, whereas capillary telangiectasias are most often found in the diencephalon, brain stem, and cerebellum.[103] An AVM contains a tangle of congenitally malformed vascular channels buried in the brain, known as a nidus. Within the nidus there are direct arteriovenous communications that permit marked increase in regional blood flow through the lesion. The feeding arteries have lost the capability of autoregulation, and the draining veins are usually dilated because of increased blood flow. Because an AVM is often in continuity with the ventricles or cerebral surface, a rupture of the nidus can produce parenchymatous as well as subarachnoid and intraventricular hemorrhage. A cavernous angioma and a capillary telangiectasia are low-flow malformations of the arterioles and capillaries, respectively, without enlarged feeding arteries or draining veins; a venous angioma is a cluster

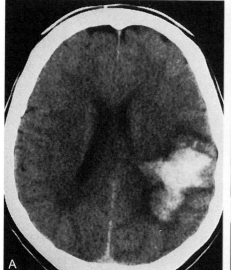
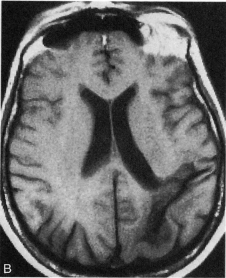
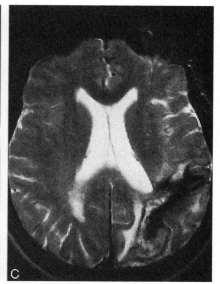

FIGURE 21–21. A 64-year-old woman presented with a left lobar parietal lobar hemorrhage. *A,* CT scan of the acute hemorrhage. *B,* High-field MR image obtained 10 months later. The axial T1-weighted spin-echo image demonstrates enlargement of the posterior horn of the left lateral ventricle and adjacent to it a long subcortical low intensity stripe. *C,* On the T2-weighted spin-echo image (TR/TE = 2800/90), the area of the previous hemorrhage is predominantly hypointense. The signal loss is due to old hemoglobin breakdown products such as ferritin and hemosiderin. These substances are superparamagnetic and produce T2 shortening.

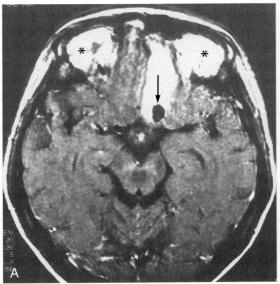

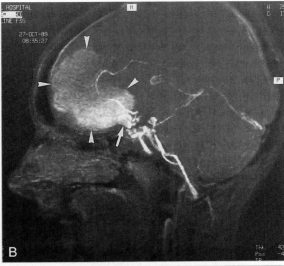

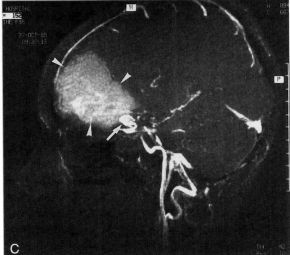

FIGURE 21–22. Left frontal lobe hemorrhage from an ophthalmic artery aneurysm. *A,* On a T1-weighted image the subacute hematoma is hyperintense and the aneurysm *(arrow)* is hypointense owing to flow void. Orbital fat is marked with an asterisk. *B,* On a three-dimensional time-of-flight MR angiogram, the hematoma remains visible owing to the bright methemoglobin *(arrowheads).* The aneurysm is not well seen *(arrow). C,* On a two-dimensional time-of-flight MR angiogram, slow flow is better visualized and the aneurysm *(arrow)* is conspicuous against the bright hematoma *(arrowheads). (A to C* from Mattle H, Edelman RR, Atkinson DJ: Zerebrale Angiographie mittels Kernspintomographie. Schweiz Med Wochenschr 122:323–333, 1992.)

of deep medullary veins draining abnormally, in a centripetal fashion, to a venous nidus.

MRI is an extremely sensitive imaging modality for the detection of a vascular malformation and is capable of demonstrating the precise anatomic relationship of its feeding arteries, nidus, and draining veins.[1, 104–107] On spin-echo sequences, signal loss in an AVM is due to hemorrhage, rapidly flowing blood, or calcification. On gradient-echo images, blood vessels with flowing blood have a bright signal pattern because of flow-related enhancement, whereas hemosiderin and calcification are seen as a signal void (see Fig. 21–16). However, so-called bright blood gradient-echo techniques (see Chapter 9) may underestimate the true extent of the vascularity of an AVM, because rapid and turbulent flow can result in nonrecoverable signal loss within the AVM. Calcification within an AVM is best evaluated by CT. The presence of hemosiderin in an AVM does not necessarily indicate previous clinical episodes of bleeding, because histologic study often shows hemosiderin-laden macrophages in the walls of an uncomplicated AVM (see Fig. 21–25). Gradient-

echo imaging may also be useful for demonstrating residual flow in an AVM after a recent hemorrhage, where the compressive effects of the hematoma on the AVM make contrast CT difficult to interpret.[104]

MRI is superior to CT in detecting so-called occult or cryptic vascular malformations in the brain, which are defined as vascular malformations not demonstrated by angiography[105, 108, 109] (see Fig. 21–25). Occult vascular malformations are usually low-flow vascular lesions that have a propensity to bleed. Histologically, they include capillary telangiectasia, cavernous angioma, venous angioma, and rarely some true AVMs. On CT scans, all of these vascular lesions may contain punctate calcification. Furthermore, they may all show mild or no enhancement and exhibit minimal or no mass effect on adjacent structures. There is seldom any associated surrounding edema. With CT the differential diagnosis of such a lesion includes a calcified glioma, granuloma, hamartoma, or old hemorrhage.

With MRI an occult vascular malformation has a characteristic appearance. It consists of a circumscribed region of low signal intensity, most prominent

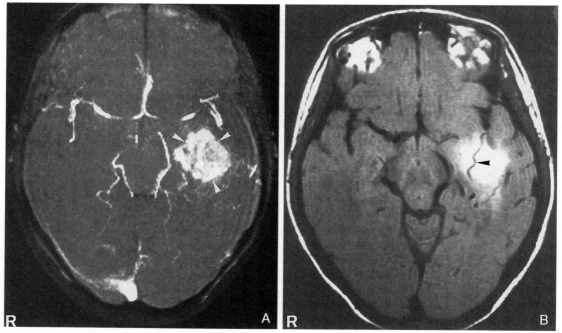

FIGURE 21–23. Left temporal hemorrhage from an arteriovenous malformation. *A,* On the gradient-echo image the hematoma appears bright due to methemoglobin *(arrowheads)* and no abnormal vessel is visualized. *B,* On the spin-echo image with flow presaturation below the section to be imaged, flow voids of abnormal vessels posterior to the hematoma and an abnormal vessel running through the hematoma *(arrowhead)* are visible. (*A* and *B* from Mattle H, Edelman RR, Atkinson DJ: Zerebrale Angiographie mittels Kernspintomographie. Schweiz Med Wochenschr 122:323–333, 1992.)

on T2-weighted images, representing hemosiderin deposition, which is on the periphery of the lesion (see Fig. 21–25). Within the hemosiderin rim are multiple areas of higher but different signal intensities that correspond to hematomas in various stages of evolution. Often scattered within the areas of hemorrhage are further foci of decreased signal intensity caused by calcification and more hemosiderin. Simple hematomas associated with trauma, surgery, hypertension, or tumors have a single cavity. Hemorrhagic contusions and infarctions may have multiple collections but are of the same age and have other associated parenchymal findings. The diagnostic feature of an occult vascular malformation with MRI is the recognition of a lesion-containing hemorrhage in various stages of evolution, indicative of recurrent bleeding. In a series of 63 vascular malformations of the brain stem, Abe and colleagues[67] found that clinical data, in conjunction with the MRI findings, were helpful in determining the true nature of such lesions.[67] However, a word of caution: although the MRI appearance was initially thought to be diagnostic for an occult vascular malformation, one report has shown a number of hemorrhagic neoplasms with similar MRI features.[110] Further details on MRI of vascular malformations are given in Chapter 23.

Amyloid Angiopathy

Amyloid angiopathy is estimated to account for 2% to 10% of all brain hemorrhages.[111, 112] Amyloid deposition in small and medium-sized cerebral vessels with-

out systemic amyloidosis has been found in 18% of men and 28% of women at autopsy.[113] Its frequency increases with age, and there is an association with Alzheimer-type changes such as neuritic plaques and neurofibrillary tangles, but there is no correlation with hypertension or atherosclerosis.[114] The frontal lobes are more frequently affected than the parietal, occipital, or temporal lobes.[86] Vessel walls, weakened and made brittle by amyloid deposition, may undergo spontaneous or traumatic rupture or develop miliary aneurysms with subsequent hemorrhage.[115] Lobar hemorrhages due to amyloid angiopathy commonly affect the elderly and are usually located in the cortex or subcortical white matter. Sometimes there is associated subarachnoid, subdural, or intraventricular hemorrhage.[115] An additional feature is a tendency to produce recurrent hemorrhages over months or years[112] (Fig. 21–27). A bilateral hemispheric leukoencephalopathy is a frequent radiologic and histologic concomitant of cerebral amyloid angiopathy.[116–119] In about one third of patients, a progressive dementia of the Alzheimer type is present. Although confirmation of the diagnosis of amyloid angiopathy needs a surgical or autopsy specimen, it is suggested by the MRI findings of two or more lobar hematomas of varying age in an elderly patient. Unfortunately, no therapeutic measure prevents progression of the disease.

Subcortical "Slit" Hemorrhage

Cole and Yates described cortical penetrators as an additional site for aneurysm formation in hypertensive

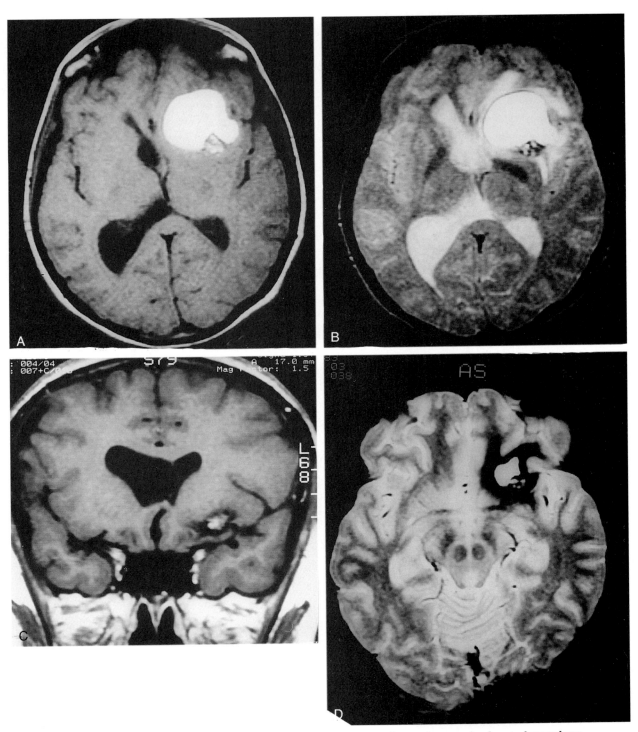

FIGURE 21–24. A 30-year-old woman presented with a cavernous hemangioma and subacute hemorrhage below and lateral to the anterior horn of the left lateral ventricle. T1-weighted *(A)* and T2-weighted *(B)* spin-echo images were obtained 2 weeks after the ictus. The angioma is visible at the posterior border of the hematoma. Nine months later most of the methemoglobin has been degraded to hemosiderin, causing a large border of signal loss on T1-weighted *(C)* and even more on T2-weighted *(D)* images.

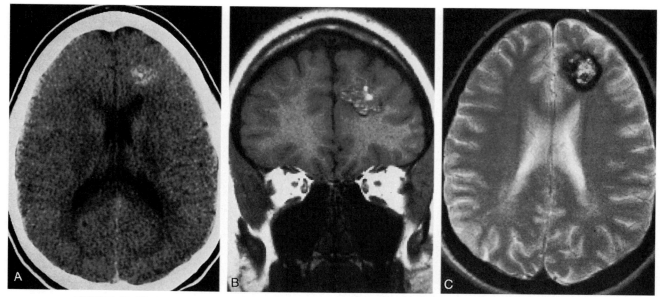

FIGURE 21–25. Occult vascular malformation in a 22-year-old woman who suffered from seizures for many years. *A,* CT scan shows irregular hyperdensity in the left frontal lobe most likely representing calcification within a vascular malformation but indistinguishable from a calcified low-grade glioma. *B,* On the coronal T1-weighted spin-echo image, small areas of bright signal are seen due to either flow-related enhancement within abnormal vessels or extracellular methemoglobin from small subclinical hemorrhages. *C,* T2-weighted spin-echo image shows a hypointense ring around the vascular malformation. The presence of this ring is considered to be the result of chronic hemosiderin deposition developing from previous subclinical hemorrhages and also the consequence of a magnetic susceptibility effect because of subtle differences in the local magnetic fields between vascular malformation and surrounding brain. A hypointense ring rarely occurs around low-grade gliomas.

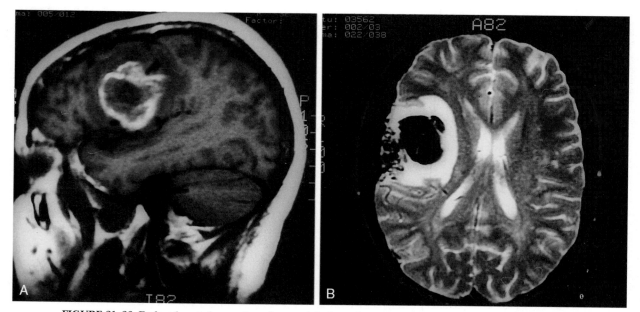

FIGURE 21–26. Early subacute hemorrhage from a right frontal vascular malformation in a 44-year-old woman. T1-weighted (1.5 T, TR/TE = 420/16) *(A)* and T2-weighted (TR/TE = 2500/90) *(B)* spin-echo images. The multiple abnormal vessels lateral to the hematoma are best seen on *B* as flow voids.

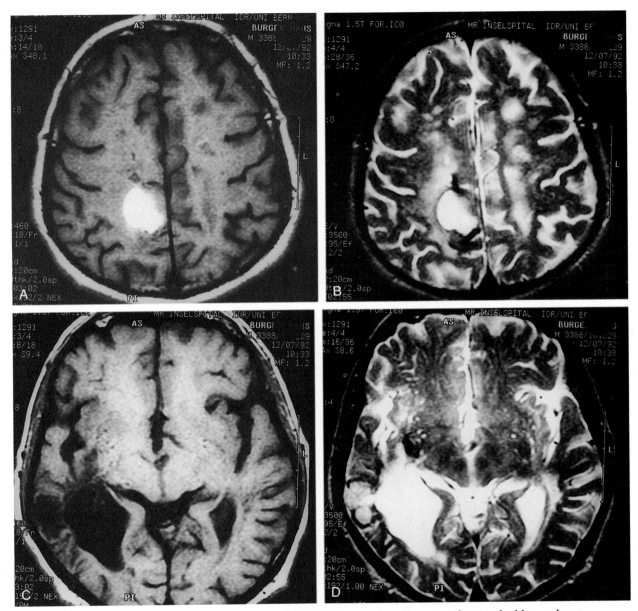

FIGURE 21–27. A 63-year-old farmer presented with left leg paresis and recurrent intracerebral hemorrhages presumably due to amyloid angiopathy. T1-weighted spin-echo (TR/TE = 460/18) and T2-weighted fast spin-echo (TR/TE = 3500/95, effective) images. *A* and *B* demonstrate a subacute subcortical hematoma close to the right motor strip. *C* and *D* show enlargement of the right posterior horn due to substance loss of the right parietal lobe. The right parietal lobe has been damaged from previous hemorrhages. The hemorrhages can still be recognized because of the hemosiderin-laden cyst margins. Note the extensive white matter changes in *B* and *D* that are present in most patients with amyloid angiopathy.

patients.[120] These can bleed and give rise to small hematomas at the junction between cortical gray matter and underlying white matter. The appearance of these hematomas is lens or slit shaped. When slit hemorrhages are seen but there is no evidence or history of hypertension, other causes of lobar hemorrhage must be sought.

Bleeding Diathesis

Hemorrhagic disorders that occur with anticoagulants (warfarin [Coumadin], heparin), thrombocyto-penia, leukemia, liver disease, hemophilia, fibrinolysis, disseminated intravascular coagulation associated with sepsis, and other rare diseases predispose to intracranial hemorrhage.[121–125] Antiplatelet agents such as aspirin or warfarin have also been associated with a moderate excess of hemorrhage and hemorrhagic stroke when compared with placebo.[126] Warfarin, widely used as an oral anticoagulant for the prevention of arterial and venous thrombosis and embolism, increases the risk of brain hemorrhage between 8- and 11-fold.[127] Anticoagulation-related brain hemorrhages represent the most serious side effect of anticoagulant treatment and generally have a dismal prognosis. Compared with hypertensive hemorrhage, an apparent difference in topographic distribution has been noted. Anticoagulation-related brain hemorrhages show a predilection for the cerebral lobes and the cerebellum (Figs. 21–28 and 21–29). The onset of clinical signs tends to be slower than with hypertensive hemorrhage.[128] Neither CT nor MRI shows any special features with this hemorrhage type. The diagnosis relies on history and laboratory findings.

Drug Use and Abuse

A number of "street drugs" such as heroin,[129] methamphetamine, amphetamine, pseudoephedrine,[130, 131] pentazocine and tripelenamine,[132] phenylpropanolamine,[133] and cocaine (especially in the form of "crack"[134]) have been implicated as a cause of brain hemorrhage. Transiently elevated blood pressure or angiographic changes suggestive of vasculitis have been implicated as etiologic factors.[130, 135] Generally, cerebrovascular complications of these drugs present as ischemic stroke, but occasionally they present as brain hemorrhage closely after use of the drugs. The majority of the hematomas are located in the subcortical hemispheric white matter, and occasionally multiple hemorrhages occur simultaneously. Except for antithrombotic and antiplatelet agents, medically used drugs hardly ever cause brain hemorrhage as an unwanted side effect. One rare example is brain hemorrhage associated with use of L-asparaginase.[136]

Hemorrhage Associated with Tumor

Bleeding into preexisting brain tumors accounts for 10% of all brain hemorrhages.[137] The clinical manifestation is either an acute new focal neurologic deficit or worsening of a preexisting deficit, often associated

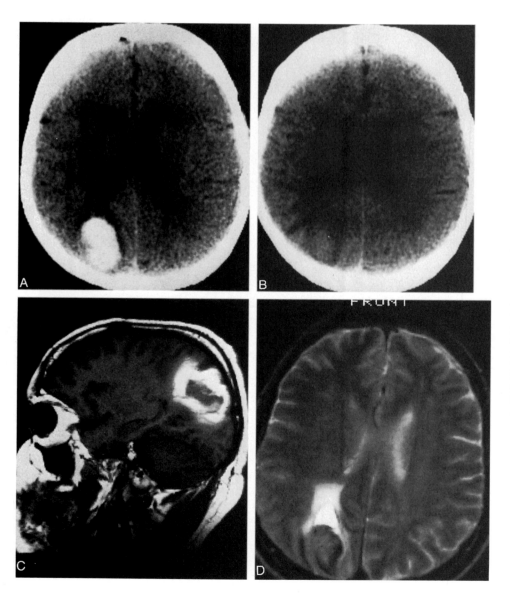

FIGURE 21–28. A 51-year-old normotensive man suffered a right parieto-occipital subcortical hemorrhage due to anticoagulation. *A,* Acute clot appears hyperdense on CT scan. *B,* A follow-up CT scan 6 weeks later shows the resolving hematoma demarcated by a hypodense rim. The center is isodense with normal brain parenchyma. *C,* High-field T1-weighted spin-echo image obtained 10 days after the first CT scan demonstrates T1 shortening in the periphery of the hematoma. *D,* The T2-weighted spin-echo image shows retracted blood clot and supernatant plasma. The fluid-rich plasma is bright, whereas the clot appears darker.

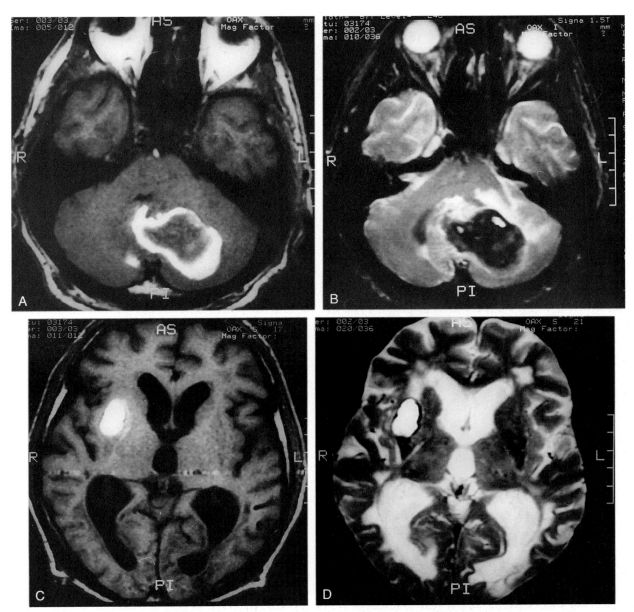

FIGURE 21–29. A 71-year-old man with arterial hypertension suffered both cerebellar and right basal ganglia hemorrhage while taking anticoagulant medication. T1-weighted *(A)* and T2-weighted *(B)* spin-echo images at 1.5 T show a cerebellar hematoma in the early subacute stage. T1-weighted *(C)* and T2-weighted *(D)* spin-echo images show a hematoma in the right basal ganglia in the late subacute stage. Note the areas with hyperintense signal in the white matter of both hemispheres, predominantly surrounding the anterior and posterior horns and typical for vascular changes *(D)*.

with a decreased level of consciousness. Only 1% to 2% of primary or metastatic tumors present as a hemorrhage.[137] Of primary brain tumors that bleed, glioblastoma multiforme, oligodendroglioma, and ependymoma are the most common types. Metastases most prone to bleeding are those of melanoma, choriocarcinoma, and bronchogenic, renal cell, and thyroid carcinoma.[138] Primary brain tumors are usually deeply seated and therefore produce deep hemorrhages, whereas metastases and their hemorrhages are more often subcortical or cortical.[139] The pathogenesis of tumoral hemorrhage is probably dependent on the

degree of malignancy as well as on the rate of growth and vascularity of the tumor. In cardiac myxoma, metastases to the brain cerebral aneurysms form, which may be responsible for bleeding.[140]

In general, the diagnosis of tumor as the underlying cause of a brain hemorrhage is difficult, because the hematoma may obliterate evidence of the neoplasm. However, Atlas and colleagues[16] and Destian and co-workers[3] have reported MRI findings on spin-echo images, that appear to be specific for tumoral hemorrhage (Fig. 21–30). They compared the signal intensity patterns of simple intracerebral hematomas with those

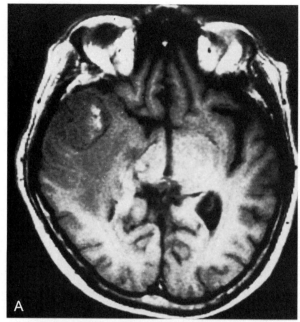

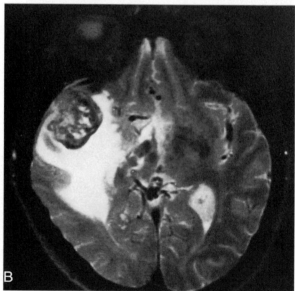

FIGURE 21–30. A 70-year-old man presented with lung carcinoma. The T1-weighted *(A)* and T2-weighted *(B)* spin-echo images demonstrate hemorrhage into a temporal lobe metastasis. The diagnosis is suggested by the more heterogeneous signal intensity pattern than is encountered in simple hematomas, the presence of marked edema, and an ill-defined hemosiderin ring around the lesion. Unlike in a simple hematoma, in which methemoglobin formation starts at the periphery, the bright signal pattern resulting from methemoglobin is seen centrally on the T1-weighted image *(A)*.

of hematomas due to an underlying neoplasm (Figs. 21–31 and 21–32). Their findings may be summarized as follows:

1. Signal intensity patterns are generally more heterogeneous with neoplasia than with simple hematomas. In contrast to the orderly evolution of signal intensity changes in simple hematomas, multiple stages of hematoma evolution are often present simultaneously in a tumor.

2. Evolution of a tumoral hemorrhage is slower than that of a simple hematoma.

3. Presence of a well-defined, complete hemosiderin rim found around simple hematomas is reduced or absent in tumoral hemorrhages. However, in later stages, tumoral hemorrhages may also demonstrate a hemosiderin ring, although usually incomplete or attenuated.

4. Areas of abnormal signal intensity typical of tumor tissue suggest underlying neoplasia. This abnormal signal pattern is usually hypointense or isointense relative to cortex on T1-weighted spin-echo images and hyperintense on T2-weighted images.

5. Tumoral hemorrhage is suggested by the presence of edema that persists in the subacute and chronic stages (see Fig. 21–30), unlike transient, perihematoma edema seen in acute simple hematomas.

6. Unlike simple hematomas, in which high signal intensity on T1-weighted images originates in the rim of the lesion, increased signal intensity (due to paramagnetic methemoglobin formation) may originate centrally within some tumoral hemorrhages. The reason for this discrepancy may relate to the oxygen tension.[141] In a simple hematoma, the oxygen tension may be so low centrally as to inhibit the oxidation of deoxyhemoglobin to methemoglobin. This delays the development of central high signal intensity on T1-weighted images. On the other hand, there is evidence that the oxygen tension in the central portions of neoplasms is greater than that in simple hematomas (although lower than in normal tissues). In tumoral hemorrhages, enough oxygen may be present in the central region to support methemoglobin formation.

Aside from these features, the simplest means to differentiate tumor from nontumor hemorrhages is to administer a contrast agent such as Gd-DTPA.

In many cases, it is possible to differentiate hemorrhagic neoplasm from hematoma on the basis of the appearance on MR images. However, in some instances the diagnosis is only suspected by the finding of systemic malignancy or by biopsy of the hematoma cavity at the time of surgical evacuation (see also Chapter 17).

Hemorrhagic Infarction

Hemorrhagic infarction occurs in about 20% of all infarcts, and the hemorrhage almost always originates in the cortex[34] (Fig. 21–33) or from deep perforators (Fig. 21–34). Four conditions predispose ischemic brain tissue to hemorrhage,[34, 142] and all are due to the phenomenon of reperfusion: 1) when an arterial embolus lyses and moves distally (Fig. 21–35); 2) when collateral vessels supply ischemic brain tissue; 3) when hypotension is followed by restoration of normal blood pressure; and 4) when temporal lobe herniation transiently occludes a posterior cerebral artery. The first two conditions predispose watershed zones to hemorrhagic infarction. Other causes of hemorrhagic infarction include hypertension, anticoagulation, fat embolism, and venous infarction.[143, 144] In fat embolism, multiple petechial hemorrhages in the cerebral white

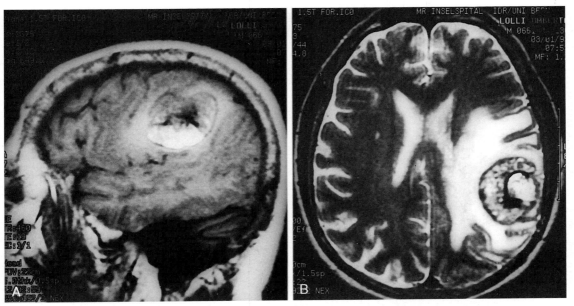

FIGURE 21–31. A 57-year-old man presented with a hemorrhage into a bronchial carcinoma metastasis. *A,* Parasagittal T1-weighted spin-echo image (1.5 T, TR/TE = 460/19). *B,* Axial T2-weighted turbo spin-echo image (TR/TE = 3900/85, effective). The hemorrhage seems to be less diffuse within the metastasis than in Figure 21–30 and in a later stage with hemosiderin in the center.

matter are a common finding, and occasionally larger hemorrhagic infarctions are seen in this entity.[145] Cerebral venous or sinus thrombosis may cause hemorrhagic infarction or frank hemorrhage[146] (Figs. 21–36 and 21–37). Enhanced CT can make the diagnosis of complete sagittal sinus thrombosis ("delta" sign) but is insensitive to partial sinus thrombosis as well as cortical venous occlusion.[147] MRI, particularly in conjunction with flow-imaging techniques, may prove superior to CT in this disorder.[148, 149]

In autopsy studies, some infarcts are devoid of blood and therefore pallid (pale infarction), others show mild congestion especially at their margins, and still others show extensive extravasation of blood from many small vessels in the infarcted tissue (red or hemorrhagic infarction). Although many infarcts are of the same type, either pale or hemorrhagic, others are mixed.

Hemorrhagic infarction remained an autopsy diagnosis until the advent of CT. Because of the paramagnetic properties of blood and its degradation products, MRI is even more sensitive than CT in the detection of hemorrhagic infarction. The MRI appearances are those of subcortical edema due to the ischemia, added to which are the various stages of a hemorrhage, as described earlier. However, there is one important

FIGURE 21–32. A 71-year-old man presented with hemorrhage into a glioma. The diagnosis was verified by stereotactic biopsy. *A,* Axial T1-weighted spin-echo image (1.0 T, TR/TE = 600/15). *B,* Axial T2-weighted spin-echo image (TR/TE = 3400/90). The signal pattern of the hematoma is more heterogeneous than in nontumoral bleedings; however, in this patient there is only little mass effect and edema surrounding the glioma.

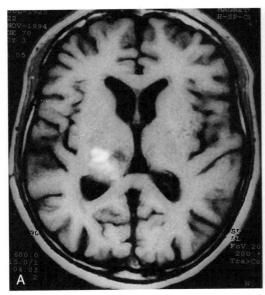
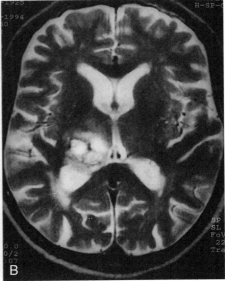

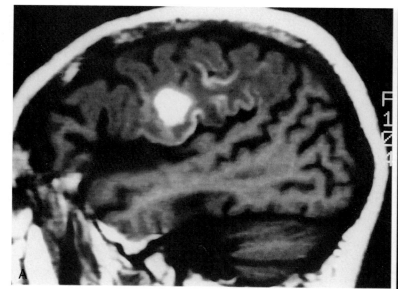

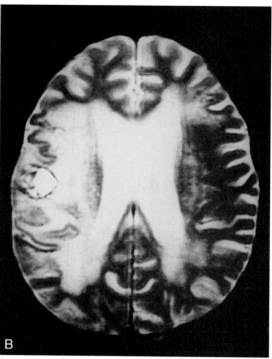

FIGURE 21–33. A 53-year-old man had a large right middle cerebral artery stroke of unknown cause. A subacute hematoma is in the infarcted area, and petechial hemorrhage in the cortex is visualized as cortical hyperintensity on the T1-weighted image (A) and as cortical hypointensity on the T2-weighted image (B).

difference. Hecht-Leavitt and coworkers[34] observed that in the acute stage of hemorrhagic infarction there was less low intensity on T2-weighted images than in intraparenchymal hemorrhage. They believe this to be the result of a higher local oxygen tension in hemorrhagic infarction because, of early vascular recanalization and luxury perfusion (see Fig. 21–35B). (See Chapter 24 for additional information on cerebral ischemia and infarction.)

Miscellaneous Rare Types of Hemorrhage

In addition to brain hemorrhages, miscellaneous rare types of hemorrhage have been reported, some of them associated with acute rise in arterial pressure: medical conditions with acute hypertension such as eclampsia, pheochromocytoma, and glomerulonephritis; after carotid endarterectomy[44]; after surgical correction of congenital heart defects[150]; on exertion and

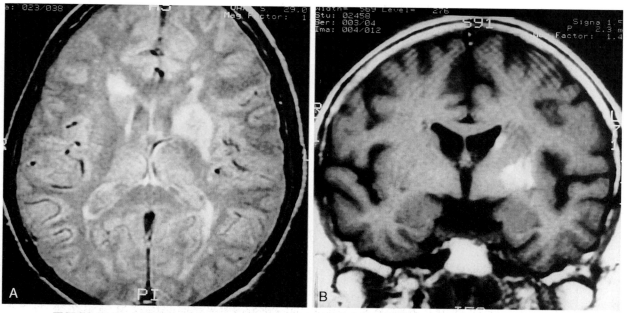

FIGURE 21–34. A 70-year-old woman presented with a lenticulostriate infarct. Note the infarct on the proton density–weighted spin-echo image performed on a 1.5-T scanner (A), which contains methemoglobin as seen on the T1-weighted image (B).

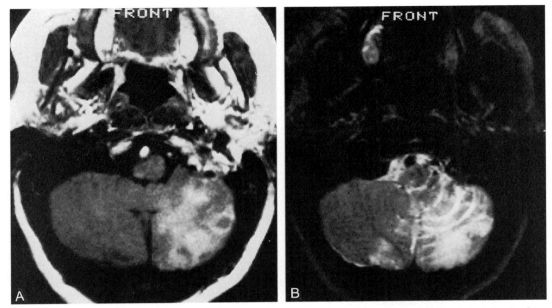

FIGURE 21–35. A 69-year-old woman presented with an embolic hemorrhagic cerebellar infarction in the region of the posterior inferior cerebellar artery. Inhomogeneous signal pattern involves the left and, to a lesser extent, the right cerebellar hemisphere. *A,* On the T1-weighted image, bright areas representing hemorrhage are interspersed with normal-appearing tissue. This appearance is atypical for most simple hematomas and occurs because of the inhomogeneous distribution of hemorrhage within the infarct. *B,* On the T2-weighted image the entire infarction appears bright and the hemorrhagic components are poorly distinguished. The cerebellar folia are well seen, indicating no mass effect of the infarct.

exposure to cold weather[151]; after administration of vasopressor drugs; and after sympathetic stimulation with severe dental pain[152] or painful urologic examination. Furthermore, supratentorial brain hemorrhage has complicated posterior fossa surgery.[153, 154] All these hemorrhages are preferentially located in the cerebral lobes. Brain stem and thalamic hemorrhages combined with subarachnoid hemorrhage have followed balloon occlusion of an extracranial vertebral arteriovenous fistula.[155]

PRIMARY INTRAVENTRICULAR HEMORRHAGE

Intraventricular hemorrhages can be separated into two groups: 1) those without clinical or neuroradiologic evidence of a lesion in the adjacent brain parenchyma and 2) those resulting from erosion of the ventricular wall by a juxtaventricular lesion or rupture of a hemorrhage into the ventricles as outlined earlier[156, 157] (for an example, see Fig. 21–18). The first group is commonly referred to as primary intraventric-

FIGURE 21–36. A 50-year-old woman had right hemiparesis due to superior sagittal sinus (SSS) and cortical venous thrombosis. T1-weighted (1.5 T, TR/TE = 400/15) *(A)* and T2-weighted (TR/TE = 3000/90) *(B)* images. On both images gross edema of the left hemisphere is visible, and there are multiple mainly cortical hemorrhages in the early subacute stage. On the T1-weighted image there is bright signal in the SSS. Normally the SSS shows as a flow void. However, a clot in the SSS is conformed only when there is bright signal also in the coronal or sagittal images or when gradient-echo images demonstrate absence of flow. SSS thrombosis often causes hemorrhage in both hemispheres.

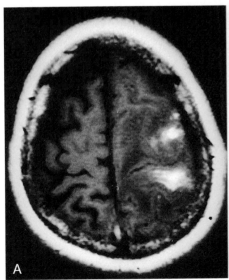
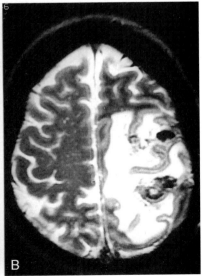

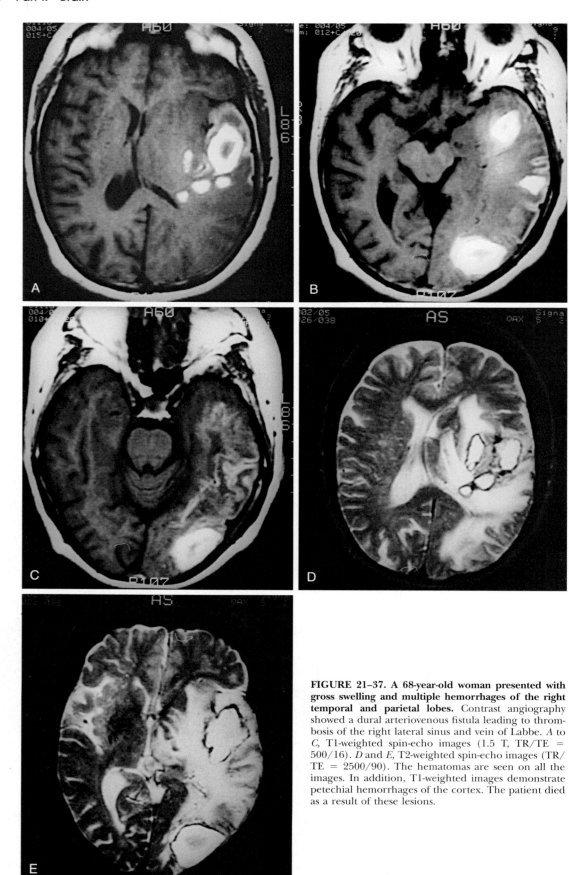

FIGURE 21–37. A 68-year-old woman presented with gross swelling and multiple hemorrhages of the right temporal and parietal lobes. Contrast angiography showed a dural arteriovenous fistula leading to thrombosis of the right lateral sinus and vein of Labbe. *A* to *C*, T1-weighted spin-echo images (1.5 T, TR/TE = 500/16). *D* and *E*, T2-weighted spin-echo images (TR/TE = 2500/90). The hematomas are seen on all the images. In addition, T1-weighted images demonstrate petechial hemorrhages of the cortex. The patient died as a result of these lesions.

ular hemorrhage and is rare. Primary intraventricular hemorrhage has been described with aneurysms, vascular malformations, and tumors within the choroid plexus or involving the anterior choroidal or lenticulostriate vessels,[156, 158] but in many cases the cause is never detected. Primary intraventricular hemorrhage and periventricular hemorrhage are also common complications in premature infants.[159] The presenting features include headache, confusion, altered sensorium to a variable extent, and minimal or absent focal neurologic signs. Clinical distinction between subarachnoid hemorrhage and primary intraventricular hemorrhage is impossible. The diagnosis is made by CT or MRI. Occasionally, with CT or MRI, a localized clot in the ventricles instead of diffusely spreading blood is seen simulating tumor. However, tumor can easily be ruled out on a follow-up scan. Altered sensorium as an initial presentation is associated with a grave prognosis, whereas in uncomplicated primary intraventricular hemorrhage the outcome is favorable.[157] When neurologic deterioration appears to be secondary to acute hydrocephalus, temporary ventriculostomy is indicated.

PITUITARY HEMORRHAGE

Degenerative changes such as small cysts or areas of hemorrhage occur as a gross or microscopic feature of nearly 28% of pituitary adenomas[160] (Fig. 21–38). They are far more frequent than the catastrophic entities of pituitary apoplexy (see Fig. 21–21) or hemorrhage into a normal pituitary gland (Sheehan's syndrome). The frequency of small intratumoral hemorrhages in pituitary adenomas has been attracting attention, because MRI has made hemorrhagic foci within the adenomas easier to detect. However, decreased signal intensity due to the paramagnetic field effects of hemosiderin is much less common in intratumoral hemorrhage in pituitary adenomas. This is probably because these extracerebral tumors lack a blood-brain barrier, so that there is less accumulation of hemosiderin-laden macrophages. There is evidence that pituitary adenomas treated with bromocriptine are at greater risk for intratumoral hemorrhage, which is often asymptomatic (see Chapter 18).[161]

INTRACEREBRAL HEMORRHAGE OF UNDETERMINED CAUSE

In a certain group of patients, the clinical and radiologic work-up will not be able to detect the reason for the hemorrhage. In patients in whom hypertension or amyloid angiopathy is not the likely cause of hemorrhage, angiography is needed to help decide whether there is an anatomic explanation such as a vascular malformation or tumor causing the hemorrhage. If the initial angiogram is normal, in many institutions the study is repeated in 2 to 3 months when pressure from the hematoma has subsided.[50] If no abnormality is seen at that time, CT or MRI 4 to 6 months later is suggested to be certain not to overlook an underlying pathologic process. Once the sensitivity of MRI is established for detecting these lesions in the acute and later stages, it should further reduce the need for angiography.

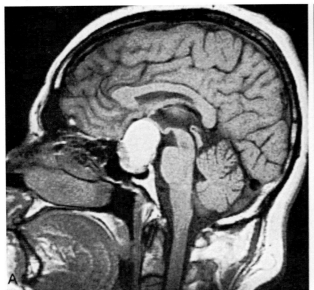
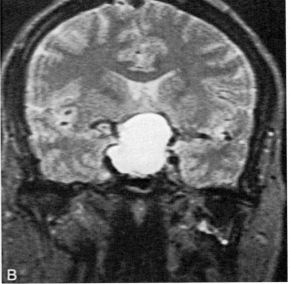

FIGURE 21–38. A 40-year-old man presented with surgically proven hemorrhage into chromophobe pituitary adenoma. The sagittal T1-weighted image *(A)* as well as the coronal T2-weighted image *(B)* show bright signal consistent with extracellular methemoglobin. Note the absence of a dark rim around the hematoma, which is usually present around intracerebral hematomas. This is considered a consequence of an absent blood-brain barrier in the pituitary, enabling iron-laden macrophages to mobilize away from the hematoma. A cholesterol-containing cyst without hemorrhage in this area can have the same signal characteristics.

FACTORS INFLUENCING OUTCOME OF INTRACEREBRAL HEMORRHAGE AND THERAPEUTIC IMPLICATIONS

Alertness is bound to integrity of the reticular activating system. A unilateral mass can jeopardize its function either by displacing the brain stem laterally[162] or by impaction of portions of the medial temporal lobe between the tentorial edge and the adjacent brain stem, causing compression and damage of the midbrain.[163] The oculomotor nerve is compressed as well. This process is called *transtentorial herniation*. Bilateral cerebral masses may compress the low diencephalon in the tentorial opening without shifting it horizontally. This is termed *central* or *central descending transtentorial herniation*. Pupillary enlargement and altered level of consciousness are considered the surest clinical signs of transtentorial herniation.

On CT scans, effacement of the tentorial cisterns, horizontal shift and depression of the pineal body, and contralateral hydrocephalus are the findings in tentorial herniations with a unilateral mass. In central herniation, obliteration of the basal subarachnoid cisterns is associated with downward shift of the pineal calcium.[164] In MRI the displacement and torquing of the brain stem can be appreciated directly.

Negative prognostic signs in patients with intracerebral hemorrhage include initial stupor or coma, significant midline shift on the angiogram[165] or CT scan,[166–168] large hemorrhage size,[169] and intraventricular extension of blood. Patients with large temporal or temporoparietal hematomas appear to be at greater risk for brain stem compression than those with hematomas in other locations.[170] Of patients who survive the hemorrhage, only one fourth show persistent severe neurologic deficits at 1 year.[171]

Medical treatment is of critical importance. Blood pressure must be maintained within acceptable limits. Hypertension should be corrected only if values are extremely high (systolic greater than 180 to 200 mm Hg). Increased intracranial pressure can rarely be managed by medical means alone (hyperventilation, hyperosmotic agents), and medical measures usually have to be followed by surgical evacuation of the hematoma. It is generally agreed that in patients with large lobar and putaminal hematomas and decreasing levels of consciousness, surgical evacuation of the hematoma can be lifesaving. In cerebellar hematomas a worsening sensorium is a distinct indication for surgery.[50] The clinical course of cerebellar hemorrhage is unpredictable.[83, 86] Rapid deterioration to coma and death can occur without warning. Hematomas with a diameter of 3 cm or less on CT scans usually have a favorable outcome with medical treatment.[172, 173] However, these patients need careful monitoring in the intensive care unit of an adequately equipped center for at least 48 hours. With larger lesions, immediate surgical removal should be considered, because the morbidity of surgical intervention is low and the chance of rapid and irreversible deterioration is considerable.[174] When a patient is in deep coma, removal of the hematoma can still result in good recovery,

especially if the interval between decrease of consciousness and surgery is short. Ventricular drainage may be necessary to treat persisting hydrocephalus after evacuation of the hematoma. Ventricular drainage alone does not relieve pressure on the brain stem and bears the danger of superior cerebellar tentorial herniation.[175]

If there is loss of pupillary reaction and brain stem function, surgery offers little chance for clinical improvement. There is also little to be gained by surgery in patients with thalamic and pontine hemorrhage. When hydrocephalus develops in thalamic hemorrhage, emergency ventricular drainage may be necessary as an isolated measure or in conjunction with surgical evacuation of the clot.

When amyloid angiopathy is suggested, surgery should be avoided and delayed as long as possible, because the vessels are fragile and surgical evacuation is often attended by uncontrollable hemorrhage and postoperative recurrent bleeding.[176] Hematomas due to aneurysms, arteriovenous malformations, and tumors are treated essentially in the same way as other forms of spontaneous brain hemorrhage. In patients who require surgical removal of the hematoma, efforts should be made to repair the aneurysm or AVM at the same operation to prevent postoperative bleeding.[50] When a tumor is suspected, the wall of the hematoma cavity should be sampled for microscopic examination. The role of stereotactic techniques to remove hematomas needs to be studied further, and also the place of surgery in the neurologically stable patient is not yet established. It has not been proved that evacuation of a hematoma in a neurologically stable patient would improve the outcome; therefore, it is usually not done. In a patient with a typical basal ganglia hematoma, surgery offers no benefit, and the patient should be treated conservatively.[177]

Other therapeutic measures are useful in certain conditions. In anticoagulant-related hemorrhage, administration of vitamin K and clotting factors or fresh frozen plasma may help stem bleeding.[178] Thrombocytopenic patients may benefit from platelet transfusion,[179] and hemophiliacs may experience improvement from infusion of appropriate clotting factors.[180]

CEREBRAL HEMORRHAGE IN NEONATES

The most frequent and severe complication in premature neonates is periventricular and intraventricular hemorrhage (Figs. 21–39 to 21–41). It occurs in 30% to 40% of all neonates born before 32 completed weeks of gestation.[159, 181, 182] The hemorrhage originates in the subependymal germinal matrix because of fragile vessels in this area. Most often it is located in the caudate nucleus. Germinal matrix hemorrhage has been divided into four grades depending on its extension: grade I hemorrhage is restricted to the germinal matrix; grade II hemorrhage breaks into the ventricles; grade III hemorrhage breaks into the ventricles and is associated with hydrocephalus; and grade IV hemorrhage extends into the cerebral hemispheres. The clin-

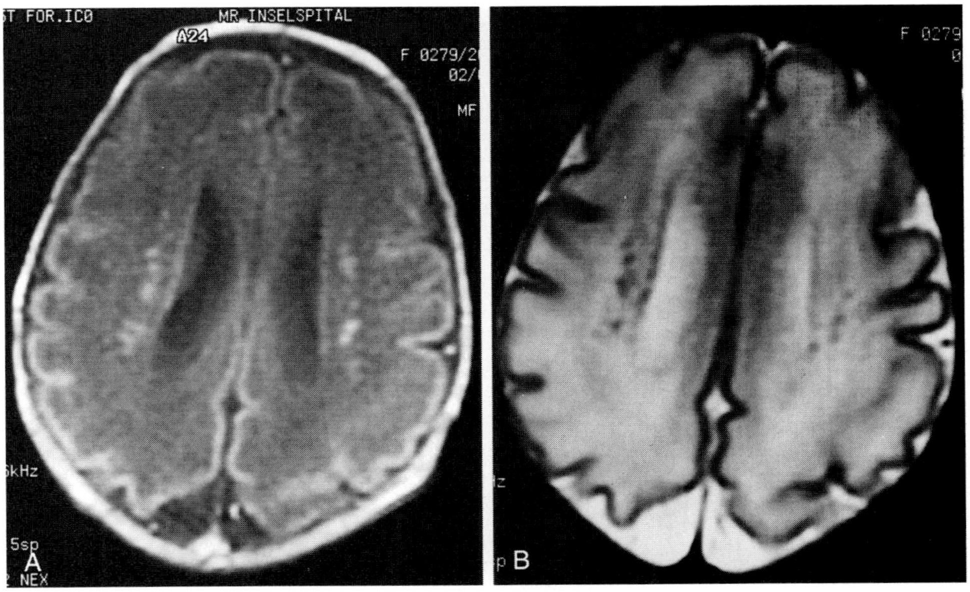

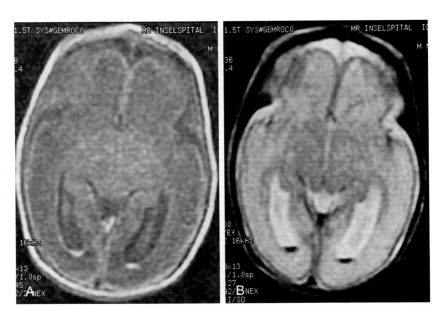

FIGURE 21–39. Grade I germinal matrix hemorrhage in a 31-week premature 4-day-old girl. There are small foci of abnormal signal bilaterally in the germinal matrix zone, bright on the axial T1-weighted spin-echo image (1.5 T, TR/TE = 360/19) *(A)* and dark on the T2-weighted turbo spin-echo image (TR/TE = 4000/119, effective) *(B)*.

ical manifestation ranges from no signs to neurologic devastation. More widespread intraparenchymal hematomas seem to be associated with leukomalacia, which may be preexisting or a consequence of the hemorrhage.[159, 182]

In the full-term neonate, periventricular and intraventricular hemorrhage is less frequent. The causes of bleeding in full-term neonates are more diverse than in preterm infants. They include peripartum asphyxia, mechanical birth trauma, coagulation abnormalities, and infection. The hemorrhage most often originates from the choroid plexus, the choroidal veins, or the residual germinal matrix.[183–185]

Ultrasonography is useful for detecting germinal matrix hemorrhages larger than 5 mm but is less sensitive for early diagnosis of periventricular leukomalacia. Ultrasonography and CT may detect acute germinal and

parenchymal hemorrhage in newborns better than MRI. However, a few days after birth, the conspicuity of hemorrhage on MR images rises over visualization by the other modalities.[186, 187]

HEAD TRAUMA AND RELATED HEMORRHAGES

Trauma constitutes the most frequent cause of death and disability in the early decades of life.[188] In most places, transportation accidents are most frequent, followed by falls, whereas in some cities injuries from guns outnumber those from traffic accidents.[189] Men are more often involved in accidents than women. The male-to-female ratio ranges from 2.2:1 to 4.5:1.

Clinicians separate head injuries into open and

FIGURE 21–40. Grade III germinal matrix hemorrhage in a 27-week premature 5-day-old boy. *A,* Axial T1-weighted spin-echo image (1.5 T, TR/TE = 380/15). *B,* Axial T2-weighted turbo spin-echo image (TR/TE = 3600/85, effective). The lateral ventricles are dilated, and there are blood-CSF levels in the posterior horns.

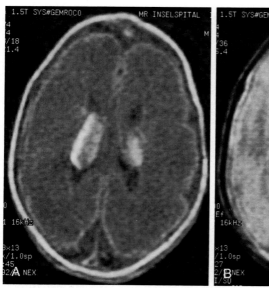
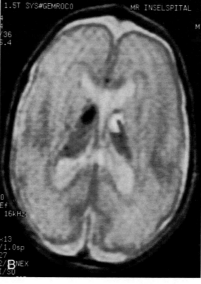

FIGURE 21–41. Five-day-old 29-week preterm boy with extensive bilateral hemorrhage of the choroid plexus. *A,* Axial T1-weighted image (1.5 T, TR/TE = 360/15). *B,* Axial T2-weighted turbo spin-echo image (TR/TE = 4000/85, effective).

closed trauma. Closed nonpenetrating head injuries are by far more common than open lesions due to direct lacerations or missiles. Clinical descriptions of different severities of head injuries have been given as early as in the Middle Ages. Clinicians differentiate cerebral concussion (commotio cerebri), contusion (contusio cerebri), and compression (compressio cerebri). Concussion is defined as a short traumatic loss of consciousness and reversible disturbance of autonomic functions resulting in nausea, dizziness, and headache. At times, concussion can cause transient amnesia without loss of consciousness. A concussion should leave no trace in the brain parenchyma. Unlike concussion, contusion represents bruising of brain tissue at the point of impact, and compression denotes hematomas or other space-occupying lesions such as edema. Both cause longer lasting or permanent neurologic deficits, such as loss of consciousness, vomiting, stiff neck, and seizures, and depending on the site of the lesion, there will be transient or permanent amnesia, cognitive defects, and motor and sensory deficits. Many injuries are unattended by witnesses, and amnesia, cognitive deficits, and clouding of consciousness often limit the patient's ability to give a history. In addition, noncerebral injuries such as chest, abdominal, or limb lacerations can cause blood loss, hypotension and shock, or hypoxia and dominate the clinical scenario.

Extensive knowledge of head trauma has been collected by Duret in France, Bollinger in Germany, and Cushing in the United States toward the end of the last century.[190] In their anatomic studies they observed most of today's known primary injuries and secondary injuries that lead to delayed deterioration of trauma patients. Holbourn studied mechanical injuries to the brain in a gelatin model and observed two major mechanisms: 1) direct injuries due to contact phenomena of the brain with the skull and 2) indirect injuries, which are rotationally induced shear-strain lesions that typically are bilateral and multiple and occur remote from the site of impact.[191, 192] At Holbourn's time, radiographic evaluation of trauma patients consisted of skull radiographs to rule out a fracture or displacement of the pineal gland from the midline. Extent and site of a potential intracranial hematoma were determined by angiography; however, intracerebral lesions were mostly missed. The advent of CT revolution-

TABLE 21–7. CLASSIFICATION OF TRAUMATIC CRANIOCEREBRAL LESIONS

PRIMARY TRAUMATIC LESIONS
Scalp hematoma/laceration, skull fracture
Primary neuronal injuries
  Cortical contusion
  Diffuse axonal injury
  Subcortical gray matter injury
  Primary brain stem injury (diffuse axonal injury, direct lacerations, pontomedullary tears)
Primary hemorrhages
  Subdural hematoma
  Epidural hematoma (arterial, venous)
  Intraventricular hemorrhage
Primary vascular injuries
  Carotid-cavernous fistula
  Arterial pseudoaneurysm
  Arterial dissection, laceration, or occlusion
  Dural sinus laceration or occlusion
Traumatic pia-arachnoid injuries
  Post-traumatic arachnoid cyst
  Subdural hygroma
Cranial nerve lesions

SECONDARY TRAUMATIC LESIONS
Major territorial infarction
Boundary and terminal zone infarction
Diffuse hypoxic injury
Diffuse brain swelling, edema
Pressure necrosis (due to brain displacement and herniation)
Secondary "delayed" hemorrhage
Secondary brain stem injury (mechanical compression, secondary hemorrhages, infarction, pressure necrosis)
Other (e.g., fatty embolism, infection)

Modified from Gentry LR: Imaging of closed head injuries. Radiology 191:1–17, 1994.

ized diagnostic evaluation of head injuries. CT accurately and rapidly localizes intracranial hematomas and permits expeditious surgical treatment. CT also visualizes nonhemorrhagic lesions, brain displacement and herniation, cerebral edema, hydrocephalus, traumatic infarcts, and skull fractures.[193] All this has made CT the study of choice for diagnosing neurotrauma. However, CT is limited because it does not show all shearing injuries and contusions. Missing shearing injuries and contusions usually does not have implications in the immediate management of neurotrauma patients, but it can have later clinical and important medicolegal implications. MRI has shown distinctive advantages over CT in demonstrating brain lesions, and therefore trauma patients constitute an increasing number of cases referred for MRI. Several studies[194–206] and an excellent review[207] on MRI of head trauma have been published.

A classification of traumatic intracranial lesions that can be diagnosed by modern imaging methods is given in Table 21–7.

PRIMARY NEURONAL INJURIES

Cortical Contusion

Contusions are the most common type of intracerebral traumatic lesions (Figs. 21–42 and 21–43). They result from bruising of the brain tissue and involve primarily the superficial gray matter. They tend to be larger than diffuse axonal injuries, are ill defined, and contain petechial hemorrhages or foci of small and large hematomas. They are often multiple and tend to involve the frontal and temporal lobes along the anterior, lateral, and inferior surfaces. The parietal and occipital lobes and the cerebellum are less frequently involved. On CT scans performed shortly after the trauma, only hemorrhage within a contusion may be seen. Nonhemorrhagic contusions may be missed on CT scans before edematous swelling of the contused areas develops. MRI is superior to CT for detection of contusion. In one series the sensitivity of CT was 68%, compared with 96% for MRI.[208] In addition, MRI is more likely to portray the true volume and extent of contused tissue, although it does not differentiate damaged tissue from traumatic edema unequivocally. The MRI signal in contusional hemorrhage evolves in the same way as in spontaneous intracerebral hemorrhage with time.

Diffuse Axonal Injury, Subcortical Gray Matter Injury, and Primary Brain Stem Injury

Rotational forces during head impact cause shear stress to the axons and may cause diffuse axonal injuries (Figs. 21–44 to 21–46). They tend to occur in three major anatomic sites: 1) the hemispheric white matter, 2) the corpus callosum, and 3) the dorsolateral and upper parts of the brain stem. In mild trauma,

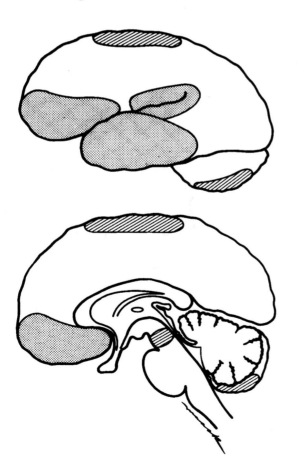

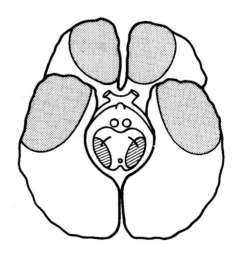

☐ Frequent

▨ Occasional

FIGURE 21–42. Anatomic diagrams depict typical locations of contusional traumatic brain injuries. (From Osborn AG: Diagnostic Neuroradiology—A Text-Atlas. St. Louis: Mosby–Year Book, 1994, p 217.)

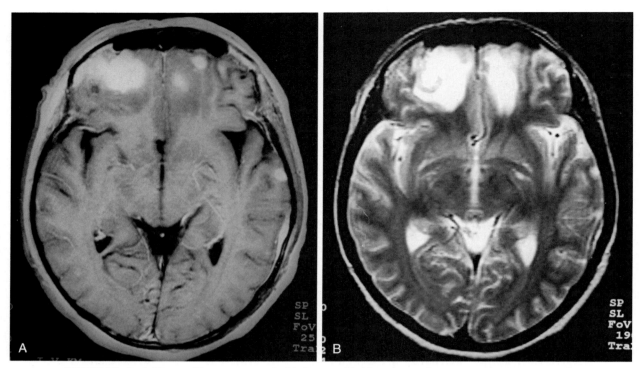

FIGURE 21–43. A 55-year-old man presented with fronto-orbital hematomas due to contusions as seen on the T1-weighted spin-echo image *(A)*. In addition, there is a small cortical hematoma in the left temporal lobe just anterior to a thin subdural hematoma. Note the marked edema surrounding the frontal hematomas that is hypointense on the T1-weighted image *(A)* and hyperintense on the T2-weighted spin-echo image *(B)*.

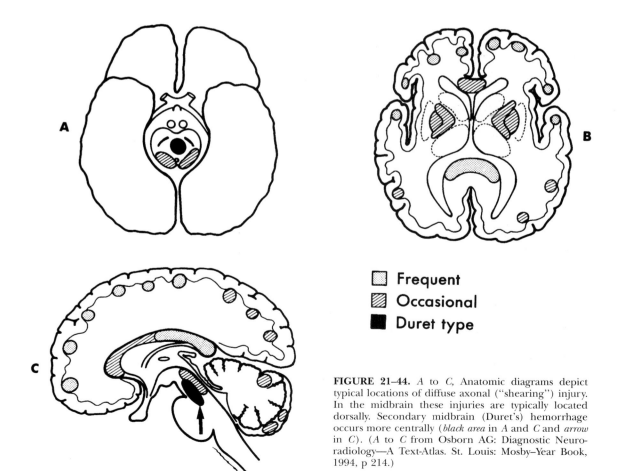

☐ Frequent
▨ Occasional
■ Duret type

FIGURE 21–44. *A* to *C,* Anatomic diagrams depict typical locations of diffuse axonal ("shearing") injury. In the midbrain these injuries are typically located dorsally. Secondary midbrain (Duret's) hemorrhage occurs more centrally (*black area* in *A* and *C* and *arrow* in *C*). (*A* to *C* from Osborn AG: Diagnostic Neuroradiology—A Text-Atlas. St. Louis: Mosby–Year Book, 1994, p 214.)

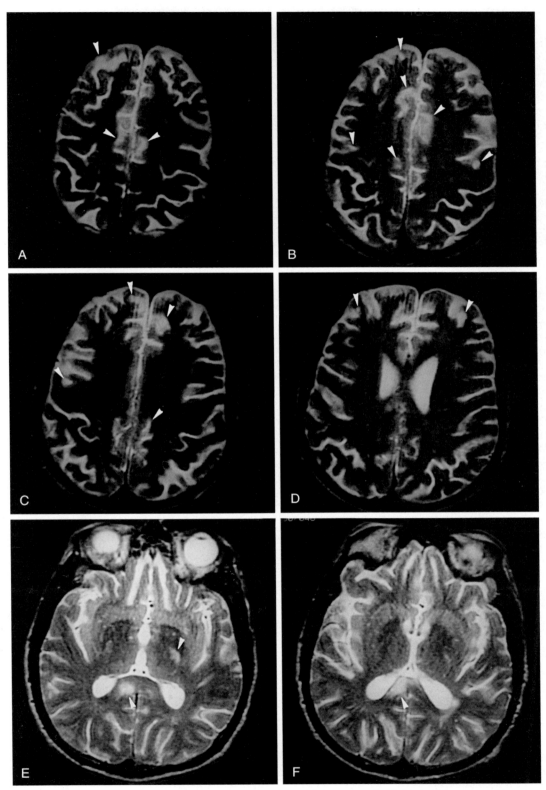

FIGURE 21–45. A 50-year-old cyclist suffered a closed head injury. *A* to *D,* Multiple diffuse axonal injuries occurred subcortically at the junction of the gray and white matter *(arrowheads). E* and *F,* Axonal injuries are also evident in the posterior part of the corpus callosum and in the left basal ganglia *(arrowheads).* All images are T2-weighted spin-echo images (1.5 T, TR/TE = 2500/90).

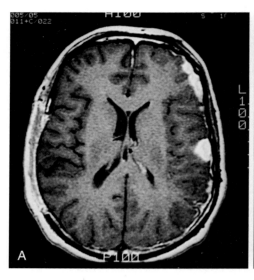 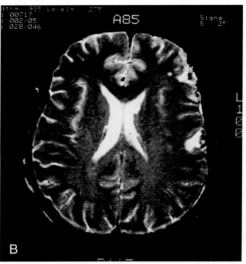

FIGURE 21–46. Hemorrhagic cortical contusions of the left frontal lobe. *A*, T1-weighted spin-echo image after gadolinium injection. *B*, T2-weighted spin-echo image.

diffuse axonal injuries may be limited to the frontal and temporal white matter. With more severe trauma, the corpus callosum, especially the posterior parts, may also be involved; in even greater trauma, lesions in the brain stem occur. With increasing severity of the trauma, involvement of the brain becomes sequentially deeper.[207, 209] Eighty percent of diffuse axonal injuries are nonhemorrhagic, and 20% contain petechial hemorrhage.[204, 205] The majority of these lesions are located at the junction of the gray and white matter. Lobar diffuse axonal injuries involve the parasagittal regions of the frontal lobes, the periventricular regions of the temporal lobes, and, less often, the parietal and occipital lobes, the internal and external capsules, and the cerebellum. Diffuse axonal injuries of the corpus callosum typically occur in conjunction with lobar white matter lesions and are mostly in the posterior parts of the callosal body and the splenium. They are frequently associated with intraventricular hemorrhage.[203] Brain stem lesions are small and usually nonhemorrhagic. They encompass the dorsolateral midbrain, upper pons, and superior cerebellar penduncles[206] (Fig. 21–47). The brain stem lesions may be mediated by tensile and shear-strain forces generated by rotational acceleration of the head or by direct contusion with the free edge of the tentorium.

Cortical contusions cause less impairment of consciousness than diffuse axonal injuries or primary brain stem lesions. Severe prolonged loss of consciousness occurs only when the contusions are quite large, multiple, bilateral, or associated with diffuse axonal injuries. Admission Glasgow Coma Scale scores for patients with primary brain stem diffuse axonal injuries are usually lower than for those with any other type of primary brain injury. Patients with brain stem lesions tend to regain consciousness slowly, and some degree of permanent neurologic impairment and disability is typical.[207, 210]

In some patients a type of subcortical gray matter injury occurs, characterized by multiple petechial hemorrhages in the upper brain stem, the thalamus, and around the third ventricle and by foci of larger hematomas in the basal ganglia. Disruption of multiple small perforating blood vessels causes this form of subcortical gray matter injury.[211] These patients mostly die shortly after the trauma.

The MRI signal changes of diffuse axonal injuries are loss of signal pattern on T1-weighted images and hyperintense signal pattern on T2-weighted images. When the lesions are hemorrhagic, the signal changes produced by the hemoglobin and its breakdown products dominate the appearance of the images.

PRIMARY HEMORRHAGES

According to anatomic location, extracerebral hemorrhages are classified as epidural or subdural hematomas.

Epidural Hematoma (Arterial, Venous)

Epidural hematomas occur between the dura and the inner table of the skull. They are mostly of arterial origin and are associated with skull fractures in approximately 90% of cases. They usually arise at the moment of impact and need more than 1 hour to become clinically symptomatic.[212] As early as 1 hour after the trauma they may be neurosurgically relevant, and the longer the diagnosis and treatment are delayed, the higher the mortality.

The most common bleeding artery is the middle meningeal artery, which is traumatized after linear fracture of the temporal bone. In children, stretching and tearing of this vessel can occur without a fracture. Therefore, most epidural hematomas are situated in the temporal or temporoparietal regions. Five percent of the epidural hematomas are bilateral, and 5% are in the compartment below the tentorium.[213, 214] The arterial force of the bleeding dissects the dura from the bone. Epidural hematomas may cross dural attachments but not sutures. Venous epidural hematomas are less common than those of arterial origin. They usually result from direct or indirect damage of a dural

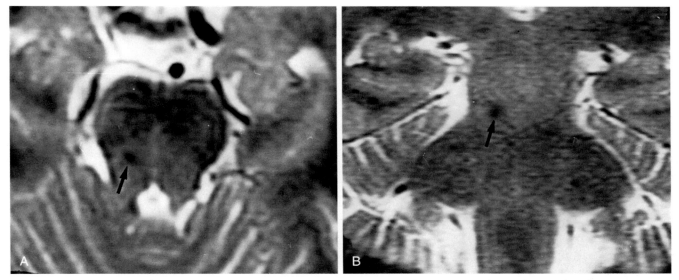

FIGURE 21–47. A 24-year-old man suffered a severe head trauma in a motor vehicle accident. When he regained consciousness several hours later he complained of persistent vertical diplopia. MRI 3 months later shows an old hemorrhage in the dorsolateral brain stem between the midbrain and pons *(arrows)*, which is compatible with a primary hemorrhagic contusion of the brain stem. Axial *(A)* and coronal *(B)* fast spin-echo images (1.5 T, TR/TE = 3800/80, effective).

sinus with frontal, parietal, occipital, or sphenoid bone fractures.[215, 216]

With CT and MRI the hematoma is biconvex or lenticular and compresses and displaces the brain away from the calvaria.[217] Venous hematomas are more variable in shape than arterial epidural hematomas. The dura can be seen stripped away from the inner table of the skull as a thin line of low signal intensity between the brain and the hematoma.[204] The cortical veins are also displaced and are sometimes visible at the inner side of the dural line. A fracture can be recognized because of the hemorrhage or fluid extending between the fracture margins. In venous epidural hematomas the fracture line crosses the corresponding dural sinus, which is generally occluded. Its patency or occlusion can be documented on spin-echo images by looking at flow voids and flow-related enhancement in conjunction with flow-sensitive gradient-echo images.[218] In general, an acute epidural hematoma is isointense or slightly hyperintense relative to gray matter on T1-weighted images and isointense on T2-weighted spin-echo images. They mostly contain oxyhemoglobin, but a small area of low signal intensity may be seen consistent with deoxyhemoglobin. With time, signal changes evolve as in intracerebral and subdural hematomas.

Subdural Hematoma

Subdural hematomas (Figs. 21–48 and 21–49) are located between the dura attached to the skull's inner table and the arachnoid covering the brain. The presumed pathogenetic mechanism is stretching and tearing of cortical bridging veins at the moment of trauma, and this rupture results in bleeding into the subdural space. When the arachnoid is also torn, the blood in the subdural space will mix with CSF. Arterial subdural hematomas or bleeding from a parenchymal brain hemorrhage into the subarachnoid and subdural space is less common.

The interval between trauma and onset of clinical symptoms ranges from less than 1 hour to several months. This interval is relied on for various temporal classifications of subdural hematomas. Hematomas with an interval of less than 1 to 4 days are classified as acute, those with an interval between 2 and 20 days as subacute, and those with an interval longer than 10 to 20 days as chronic.[219, 220] In longer standing hematomas, rebleeding can occur from vascularized neomembranes or because stretched cortical veins rupture as they pass the enlarged fluid-filled subdural space. Neurologic manifestations are highly variable. They depend on size, location, degree of bleeding, mass effect, and concomitant injuries and include headache, mental status alterations, and motor and sensory deficits. Mass effect is associated with deterioration of consciousness and can cause secondary injuries. It can occur rapidly and needs prompt neurosurgical intervention to reduce mortality and permanent morbidity.

CT and MRI show that subdural hematomas are crescent-like collections of blood between the inner table of the skull and the brain. They are usually more extensive than epidural hematomas. Unlike epidural hematomas they cross sutures but not dural attachments. Common locations are over the frontoparietal convexities and in the middle cranial fossa. They can spread diffusely over the affected hemisphere. Interhemispheric or supra-tentorial and infratentorial subdural hematomas also occur alone or in conjunction with hematomas over the convexities.

The MRI signal of subdural hematomas evolves in a

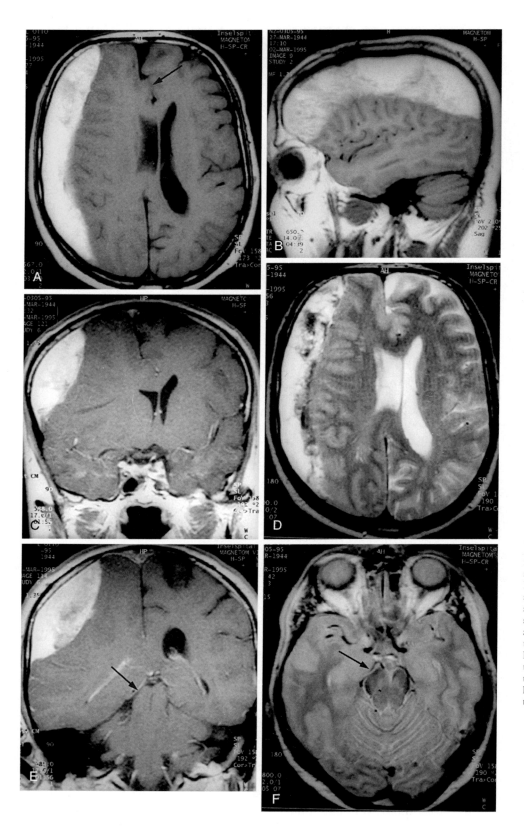

FIGURE 21–48. A 51-year-old farmer presented with headache and left hemiparesis and ataxia. He had been attacked by a boar and sustained a closed head injury 2 weeks before MRI. On MR images there is a subacute subdural hematoma with subfalcial and early transtentorial herniation. At surgery the hematoma was liquefied and there were multiple membranes. *A,* Axial T1-weighted spin-echo image (1.5 T, TR/TE = 567/12) demonstrates a midline shift of more than 1 cm and subfalcial herniation of the cingulate gyrus *(arrow).* *B,* Parasagittal T1-weighted spin-echo image (TR/TE = 650/14) shows the extension of the hematoma over the frontal and parietal lobes. Unlike an epidural hematoma it crosses the coronal suture of the skull. *C,* Coronal T1-weighted spin-echo image (TR/TE = 588/17 after gadolinium injection) shows also the midline shift, compression, and distortion of the right lateral ventricle and the subfalcial herniation. *D,* Axial T2-weighted turbo spin-echo image (TR/TE = 3800/90, effective) reveals more heterogeneous signal within the hematoma. The hypointense areas represent membranes within the hematoma or more recent hemorrhage. *E,* Coronal T1-weighted image (TR/TE = 588/17 after gadolinium injection) visualizes a mild shift and compression of the brain stem *(arrow).* *F,* Axial proton density–weighted turbo spin-echo image (TR/TE = 3800/18, effective) shows asymmetry of the hippocampal gyrus, which protrudes on the right *(arrow)* more toward the brain stem than on the left and is typical for early transtentorial herniation.

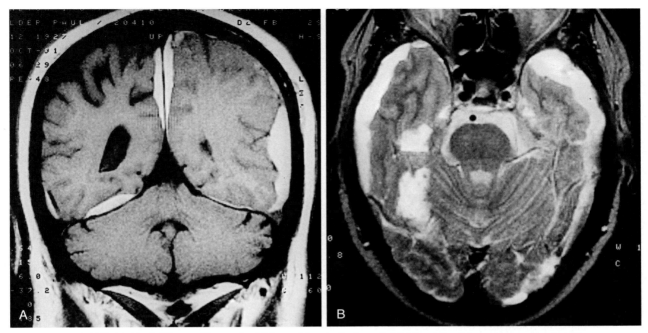

FIGURE 21–49. A 73-year-old man had bilateral hemispheric and falcial subdural hematomas. On the T1-weighted spin-echo image *(A)* a blood collection is recognized also on the right tentorium, which could be mistaken as an intracerebral hemorrhage *(B, T2-weighted spin-echo image)*.

similar way as does the signal of intraparenchymal hematomas.[13, 221–224] Acute hematomas with oxyhemoglobin have a signal intensity similar to that of brain parenchyma on both T1- and T2-weighted images. When hemoglobin converts to deoxyhemoglobin after the first hours, signal intensity on T2- and T2*-weighted images will be low. On T1-weighted images, signal intensity changes only little. In the subacute stage, 2 to 3 days after the trauma, deoxyhemoglobin will be converted to methemoglobin, which produces marked shortening of signal pattern on T1-weighted images. On T2- and T2*-weighted images, signal intensity remains low until lysis of red blood cells. After this occurs, the hematoma becomes hyperintense relative to brain parenchyma on T2- and T2*-weighted images. The lysis starts at the periphery of the hematoma. In the chronic stage, the appearance of subdural hematomas differs from that of intraparenchymal hematomas. On T1-weighted images the signal pattern ranges from slightly hypointense to isointense relative to gray matter, and on T2- or T2*-weighted images a hyperintense signal pattern persists. Hemosiderin and thus signal loss on T2- or T2*-weighted images occur infrequently; and when it is noted, it is usually associated with thickened membranes and rebleeding. Owing to the absence of a blood-brain barrier in the subdural space, hemosiderin is more readily reabsorbed into the bloodstream. In repeated hemorrhages the clearance mechanism may be poorly functional, resulting in greater hemosiderin deposition.[222] In chronic subdural hematomas, septa and adhesions often develop after repeated hemorrhages, giving rise to multiple compartments in dissimilar stages of evolution.[207] Each compartment may have a different signal intensity, and sedimentation of blood elements may cause layering of fluids with different signal intensities.

Intraventricular Hemorrhage

In most patients, rotationally induced tearing of subependymal veins causes intraventricular hemorrhage.[203] Therefore, intraventricular hemorrhage is often associated with diffuse axonal injuries of the corpus callosum. In patients without these injuries of the corpus callosum, intraventricular hemorrhage is due to dissection of large intracerebral hematomas into the ventricles. Intraventricular blood is, in general, hyperintense relative to CSF on T1-weighted images.

Subarachnoid Hemorrhage

Traumatic subarachnoid hemorrhage is frequently associated with other types of hemorrhage (mostly intracerebral hematomas from cortical contusions). The imaging characteristics do not differ from subarachnoid hemorrhage from other causes.

Subdural Hygromas

Fluid collections with similar shapes as chronic subdural hematomas and signal characteristics like CSF are called subdural hygromas (Fig. 21–50). Cortical veins in hygromas and chronic subdural hematomas are seen at the margin of the displaced cortex. Unlike in cerebral atrophy, cerebral veins are not seen traversing the widened CSF spaces.[222, 225] Presumably, subdural hygromas result from arachnoid tears.

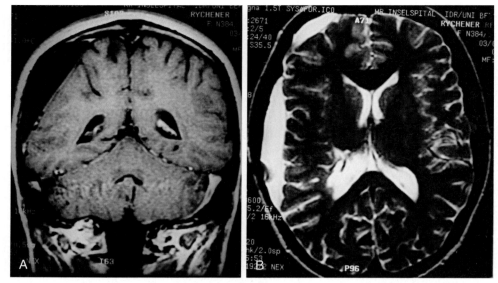

FIGURE 21–50. Subdural hygroma in a 25-year-old woman who has substantial substance loss of the right temporal lobe from surgical resection of a pilocystic grade I astrocytoma 8 years earlier. The hygroma shows the same signal as CSF, low on the T1-weighted spin-echo image (1.5 T, TR/TE = 600/19) *(A)* and bright on the T2-weighted fast spin-echo image (TR/TE = 3600/85Ef) *(B)*.

PRIMARY VASCULAR INJURIES

Primary traumatic vascular injuries comprise the following: carotid-cavernous fistulas; arterial pseudoaneurysm; arterial dissections, lacerations, or occlusions; and dural sinus lacerations or occlusions. Traumatic dissections of the carotid arteries, unlike spontaneous dissections, are more frequently bilateral. The imaging characteristics of these traumatic lesions do not differ significantly from those arising spontaneously.

In trauma patients with cerebrovascular ischemic lesions, dissections of the extracranial cerebral vessels causing emboli, and thus secondary vascular injuries to the brain, have to be considered. Typical clinical findings are unilateral hemispheric signs and ipsilateral Horner's syndrome. At our institution, these patients are evaluated with cerebrovascular ultrasonography.[226] When ultrasonography confirms a suspected dissection, MRI is performed to visualize the hematoma in the vessel wall. The MRI findings in traumatic dissections do not differ from those of spontaneous dissections.

TRAUMATIC PIA-ARACHNOID INJURIES

Arachnoid cysts are intra-arachnoid space-occupying lesions filled with clear CSF.[227] Their etiology is controversial; some may be traumatic. Occasionally, arachnoid cysts are complicated by intracystic or subdural hemorrhage, which may be spontaneous or occur after minor trauma.[228]

SECONDARY TRAUMATIC LESIONS

Secondary traumatic lesions include major territorial infarctions, boundary and terminal zone infarctions,

diffuse hypoxic injuries and diffuse brain swelling, fatty embolism, and infections. The brain stem can also be damaged indirectly by a variety of mechanisms, such as pressure necrosis due to displacement of the cerebral hemispheres and herniation, mechanical compression by infratentorial space-occupying lesions, or secondary "delayed" hemorrhage. Unlike primary brain stem injuries, which are located in the dorsolateral quadrants of the midbrain and upper pons, secondary brain stem hemorrhages and infarctions involve the ventromedial parts of the midbrain and pons.[229] Secondary hemorrhages consist of centrally located midline lesions. They are also called Duret's hemorrhages and may vary from numerous small focal collections of blood to massive central tegmental hemorrhages in the entire brain stem. They are usually associated with indirect signs such as large supratentorial hematomas, severe diffuse brain swelling, compression of the fourth ventricle and the basal cisterns, herniation of the parahippocampal gyrus into the tentorial incisura, infarcts in the vertebrobasilar distribution, and signs of compression and displacement of the upper brain stem.[206]

CT OR MRI EVALUATION OF HEAD TRAUMA?

CT is the modality of choice in the initial examination of patients with head trauma, especially when the patient is hemodynamically or neurologically unstable. All lesions relevant for the immediate treatment of the trauma patient can be detected by CT. In addition, CT is more sensitive for detection of fracture.[208] However, MRI is more helpful than CT in detecting, localizing, and characterizing diffuse axonal injuries in the cerebral white matter, corpus callosum, and brain stem. CT is insensitive in the detection of these lesions when they are nonhemorrhagic. We share Gentry's opinion[207] that all patients with moderate to severe head injuries should be evaluated with MRI at some time during the first 2 weeks using both T1- and T2-weighted sequences. Most parenchymal lesions are best visualized during the first 2 weeks and disappear in the ensuing weeks. The presence of contusions may have significant management and also medicolegal implications.

REFERENCES

1. Smith HJ, Strother CM, Kikuchi Y, et al: MR imaging in the management of supratentorial intracranial AVMs. AJNR 9:225–235, 1988.
2. Gomori JM, Grossman RI, Hackney DB, et al: Variable appearances of subacute intracranial hematomas on high-field spin-echo MR. AJNR 8:1019–1026, 1988.
3. Destian S, Sze G, Krol G, et al: MR imaging of hemorrhagic intracranial neoplasms. AJNR 9:1115–1122, 1988.
4. DiChiro G, Brooks RA, Girton ME, et al: Sequential MR studies of intracerebral hematomas in monkeys. AJNR 7:193–199, 1986.
5. Edelman RR, Johnson K, Buxton R, et al: MR of hemorrhage: a new approach. AJNR 7:751–756, 1986.
6. Grossman RI, Gomori JM, Goldberg HI, et al: MR of hemorrhagic conditions. Acta Radiol Suppl 369:56–58, 1986.
7. Tanaka T, Sakai T, Uemura K, et al: MR imaging as predictor of delayed posttraumatic cerebral hemorrhage. J Neurosurg 69:203–209, 1988.
8. Zimmerman RD, Heier LA, Snow RB, et al: Acute intracranial hemorrhage: intensity changes on sequential MR scans. AJNR 9:47–57, 1988.
9. Komiyama M, Baba M, Hakuba A, et al: MR imaging of brainstem hemorrhage. AJNR 9:261–268, 1988.
10. Jenkins A, Hadley DM, Teasdale GM, et al: Magnetic resonance imaging of acute subarachnoid hemorrhage. J Neurosurg 68:731–736, 1988.
11. Satoh S, Kadoya S: Magnetic resonance imaging of subarachnoid hemorrhage. Neuroradiology 30:361–366, 1988.
12. Nose T, Enomoto T, Hyodo A, et al: Intracerebral hematoma developing during MR examination. J Comput Assist Tomogr 11:184–185, 1987.
13. Hosoda K, Tamaki N, Masuruma M, et al: Magnetic resonance images of chronic subdural hematomas. J Neurosurg 67:677–683, 1987.
14. Grossman RI, Gomori JM, Goldberg HI, et al: MR imaging of hemorrhagic conditions of the head and neck. Radiographics 8:441–454, 1988.
15. Hackney DB, Atlas SW, Grossman RI, et al: Subacute intracranial hemorrhage: contribution of spin density to appearance on spin-echo images. Radiology 165:199–202, 1987.
16. Atlas SW, Grossman RI, Gomori JM, et al: Hemorrhagic intracranial malignant neoplasms: spin-echo MR imaging. Radiology 164:71–77, 1987.
17. Winkler ML, Olsen WL, Mills TC, Kaufman L: Hemorrhagic and nonhemorrhagic brain lesions: evaluation with 0.35-T fast MR imaging. Radiology 165:203–207, 1987.
18. Atlas SW, Mark AS, Grossman RI, Gomori JM: Intracranial hemorrhage: gradient-echo MR imaging at 1.5 T. Radiology 168:803–807, 1988.
19. Bradley WG Jr: MRI of hemorrhage and iron in the brain. In: Stark DD, Bradley WG Jr, eds. Magnetic Resonance Imaging. St. Louis: CV Mosby, 1988, pp 359–374.
20. Norman D: Vascular disease: hemorrhage. In: Brant-Zawadzki M, Norman D, eds. Magnetic Resonance Imaging of the Central Nervous System. New York: Raven Press, 1987, pp 209–220.
21. Gomori JM, Grossman RI: Mechanisms responsible for MR appearance and evolution of intracranial hemorrhage. Radiographics 8:427–440, 1988.
22. Barkovich AJ, Atlas SW: Magnetic resonance imaging of intracranial hemorrhage. Radiol Clin North Am 26:801–820, 1988.
23. Schlesinger SD: MRI of intracranial hematomas and closed head trauma. In: Pomeranz SJ, ed. Craniospinal Magnetic Resonance Imaging. Philadelphia: WB Saunders, 1989, pp 399–435.
24. Hayman LA, McArdle CB, Tabes KH, et al: MR imaging of hyperacute intracranial hemorrhage in the cat. AJNR 10:681–686, 1989.
25. Brooks RA, DiChiro G, Patronas N: MR imaging of cerebral hematomas at different field strengths: theory and applications. J Comput Assist Tomogr 13:194–206, 1989.
26. Bradley WG: MR appearance of hemorrhage in the brain. Radiology 189:15–26, 1993.
27. Fullerton GD: Physiologic basis of magnetic relaxation. In: Stark DD, Bradley WG, eds. Magnetic Resonance Imaging. 2nd ed. St. Louis: Mosby–Year Book, 1992, pp 88–108.
28. Hayman LA, Taber KH, Ford JJ, Bryan RN: Mechanisms of MR signal alteration by acute intraxcerebral blood: old concepts and new theories. AJNR 12:899–907, 1991.
29. Janick PA, Hackney DB, Grossman RI, Asakura T: MR imaging of various

30. Hayman LA, Ford JJ, Taber KH, et al: T2 effect of hemoglobin concentration: assessment with in vitro MR spectroscopy. Radiology 168:489–491, 1988.
31. Jones KM, Mulkern RV, Mantello MT, et al: Brain hemorrhage: evaluation with fast spin-echo and conventional dual spin-echo images. Radiology 182:53–58, 1992.
32. Weingarten K, Zimmerman RD, Cahill PT, Deck MDF: Detection of acute intracerebral hemorrhage on MR imaging: ineffectiveness of prolonged interecho interval pulse sequences. AJNR 12:475–479, 1991.
33. Edelman RR, Wielopolski P, Schmitt F: Echo-planar MR imaging. Radiology 192:600–612, 1994.
34. Hecht-Leavitt C, Gomori JM, Grossman RI, et al: High-field MRI of hemorrhagic cortical infarction. AJNR 7:581–585, 1986.
35. Maeder PP, Holtås SL, Basibüyük LN, et al: Colloid cysts of the third ventricle: correlation of MR and CT findings with histology and chemical analysis. AJNR 11:575–581, 1990.
36. Woodruff WW, Djang WT, McLendon RE, et al: Intracerebral malignant melanoma: high-field-strength MR imaging. Radiology 165:209–213, 1987.
37. Gomori JM, Grossman RI, Shields JA, et al: Choroidal melanomas: correlation of NMR spectroscopy and MR imaging. Radiology 158:443–445, 1986.
38. Atlas SW, Grossman RI, Hackney DB, et al: Calcified intracranial lesions: detection with gradient-echo-acquisition rapid MR imaging. AJR 150:1383–1389, 1988.
39. Dell LA, Brown MS, Orrison WW, et al: Physiologic intracranial calcification with hyperintensity on MR imaging: case report and experimental model. AJNR 9:1145–1148, 1988.
40. De Haan J, Grossman RI, Civitello L, et al: High-field magnetic resonance imaging of Wilson's disease. J Comput Tomogr 11:132–135, 1987.
41. Roh JK, Lee TG, Wie BA, et al: Initial and follow-up brain MRI findings and correlation with the clinical course in Wilson's disease. Neurology 44:1064–1068, 1994.
42. Caplan L: Intracerebral hemorrhage revisited. Neurology 38:624–627, 1988. Editorial.
43. Cole A, Aube M: Late-onset migraine with intracerebral hemorrhage: a recognizable syndrome. Neurology 37(suppl 1):238, 1987.
44. Pomposelli FB, Lamparello PJ, Riles TS, et al: Intracranial hemorrhage after carotid endarterectomy. J Vasc Surg 7:248–255, 1988.
45. Feldmann E: Intracerebral hemorrhage. Stroke 22:684–691, 1991.
46. Ojemann RG, Mohr JP: Hypertensive brain hemorrhage. Clin Neurosurg 23:220–244, 1976.
47. Caplan LR: General symptoms and signs. In: Kase CS, Caplan LR, eds. Intracerebral Hemorrhage. Boston: Butterworth-Heinemann, 1994, pp 31–44.
48. Bae HG, Lee KS, Yun IG, et al: Rapid expansion of hypertensive intracerebral hemorrhage. Neurosurgery 31:35–41, 1992.
49. Herbstein DS, Schaumburg HH: Hypertensive intracerebral hematoma. An investigation of the initial hemorrhage and rebleeding using chromium Cr[51]-labeled erythrocytes. Arch Neurol 30:412–414, 1974.
50. Ojemann RG, Heros RC: Spontaneous brain hemorrhage. Stroke 14:468–475, 1983.
51. Fulgham JR, Wijdicks EFM: Deterioration with hemorrhage. Neurology 45:602, 1995. Letter.
52. Mohr JP, Caplan LR, Melski JW, et al: The Harvard Cooperative Stroke Registry: a prospective registry. Neurology 28:754–762, 1978.
53. Bogousslavsky J, Van Melle G, Regli F: The Lausanne Stroke registry: analysis of 1,000 consecutive patients with first stroke. Stroke 19:1083–1092, 1988.
54. Foulkes MA, Wolf PA, Price TR, et al: The Stroke Data Bank: design, methods, and baseline characteristics. Stroke 19:547–554, 1988.
55. Toffel GJ, Biller J, Adams HP: Nontraumatic intracerebral hemorrhage in young adults. Arch Neurol 44:483–485, 1987.
56. Schuetz HJ, Dommer T, Boedeker RH, et al: Changing pattern of brain hemorrhage during 12 years of computed axial tomography. Stroke 23:653–656, 1992.
57. Gross CR, Kase CS, Mohr JP, et al: Stroke in south Alabama: incidence and diagnostic features—a population based study. Stroke 15:249–255, 1984.
58. Fisher CM: Pathological observations in hypertensive cerebral hemorrhage. J Neuropathol Exp Neurol 30:536–550, 1971.
59. Charcot JM, Bouchard C: Nouvelles recherches sur la pathogénie de l'hémorrhagie cérébrale. Arch Physiol Norm Pathol 1:110–127, 643–665, 725–734, 1868.
60. Kim JS, Lee JH, Lee MC: Small primary intracerebral hemorrhage. Clinical presentation of 28 cases. Stroke 25:1500–1506, 1994.
61. Loes DJ, Smoker WRK, Biller J, Cornell SH: Nontraumatic lobar intracerebral hemorrhage: CT/angiographic correlation. AJNR 8:1027–1030, 1987.
62. Huber P: Krayenbühl/Yasargil. Zerebrale Angiographie für Klinik und Praxis. Stuttgart, Germany: Thieme Publishers, 1979.
63. Stein RW, Kase CS, Hier DB, et al: Caudate hemorrhage. Neurology 34:1549–1554, 1984.

64. Kase CS, Mohr JP: Supratentorial intracerebral hemorrhage. In: Barnett HJM, Mohr JP, Stein BM, Yatsu FM, eds. Stroke: Pathophysiology, Diagnosis, and Management. New York: Churchill Livingstone, 1986, pp 525–547.

65. Weisberg LA: Thalamic hemorrhage: clinical-CT correlations. Neurology 36:1382–1386, 1986.

66. Huang C, Woo E, Yu YL, Chan FL: Lacunar syndromes due to brainstem infarct and haemorrhage. J Neurol Neurosurg Psychiatry 51:509–515, 1988.

67. Abe M, Kjellberg RN, Adams RD: Clinical presentations of vascular malformations of the brain stem: comparison of angiographically positive and negative types. J Neurol Neurosurg Psychiatry 52:167–175, 1989.

68. Kase CS, Maulsby GO, Mohr JP: Partial pontine hematomas. Neurology 30:652–655, 1980.

69. Silverstein A: Primary pontine hemorrhage. In: Vinken PJ, Bruyn GW, eds. Handbook of Clinical Neurology, Volume 12, Vascular Diseases of the Nervous System, Part II. Amsterdam: North Holland Publishing, 1972, pp 37–53.

70. Caplan LR, Goodwin JA: Lateral tegmental brainstem hemorrhages. Neurology 32:252–260, 1982.

71. Fisher CM: Some neuro-ophthalmological observations. J Neurol Neurosurg Psychiatry 30:383–392, 1967.

72. Henn V, Lang W, Hepp K, Reisine H: Experimental gaze palsies in monkeys and their relation to human pathology. Brain 107:619–636, 1984.

73. Sand JJ, Biller J, Corbett JJ, et al: Partial dorsal mesencephalic hemorrhages: report of three cases. Neurology 36:529–533, 1986.

74. Weisberg LA: Mesencephalic hemorrhages: clinical and computed tomographic correlations. Neurology 36:713–716, 1986.

75. Stern LZ, Bernick C: Spontaneous, isolated mesencephalic hemorrhage. Neurology 36:1627, 1986. Letter.

76. Mangiardi JR, Epstein FJ: Brainstem haematomas: review of the literature and presentation of five new cases. J Neurol Neurosurg Psychiatry 51:966–976, 1988.

77. Getenet JC, Vighetto A, Nighoghossian N, Trouillas P: Isolated bilateral third nerve palsy caused by a mesencephalic hematoma. Neurology 44:981–982, 1994.

78. Biller J, Gentry LR, Adams HP Jr, Morris DC: Spontaneous hemorrhage in the medulla oblongata: clinical MR correlations. J Comput Assist Tomogr 10:303–306, 1986.

79. Kase CS, Caplan LR: Hemorrhage affecting the brain stem and cerebellum. In: Barnett HJM, Mohr JP, Stein BM, Yatsu FM, eds. Stroke: Pathophysiology, Diagnosis, and Management. New York: Churchill Livingstone, 1986, pp 621–641.

80. Mumenthaler M: Neurologie. 9 Auflage. Stuttgart: Thieme Publishers, 1986.

81. Caplan LR, Stein RW: Stroke: A Clinical Approach. Boston: Butterworth, 1990.

82. Barinagarrementeria F, Cantú C: Primary medullary hemorrhage. Report of four cases and review of the literature. Stroke 25:1684–1687, 1994.

83. Ott KH, Kase CS, Ojemann RG, Mohr JP: Cerebellar hemorrhage: diagnosis and treatment. Arch Neurol 31:160–167, 1974.

84. Dunne JW, Chakera T, Kermode S: Cerebellar haemorrhage—diagnosis and treatment: a study of 75 consecutive cases. Q J Med 64:739–754, 1987.

85. McKissock W, Richardson A, Walsh L: Spontaneous cerebellar haemorrhage. Brain 83:1–9, 1960.

86. Fisher CM, Picard EH, Polak A, et al: Acute hypertensive cerebellar hemorrhage: diagnosis and surgical treatment. J Nerv Ment Dis 140:38–57, 1965.

87. Ebeling U, Huber P: Der akute raumfordernde Prozess in der hinteren Schädelgrube. Klinik und computertomographischer Befund. Schweiz Med Wochenschr 116:1394–1401, 1986.

88. Weingarten K, Barbut D, Filippi C, Zimmerman RD: Acute hypertensive encephalopathy: findings on spin-echo and gradient-echo MR imaging. AJR 162:665–670, 1994.

89. Kase CS, Williams PJ, Wyatt DA, Mohr JP: Lobar intracerebral hematomas: clinical and CT analysis of 22 cases. Neurology 32:1146–1450, 1982.

90. Hilt DC, Buchholz D, Krumholz A, et al: Herpes zoster ophthalmicus and delayed contralateral hemiparesis caused by cerebral angiitis. Diagnosis and management approaches. Ann Neurol 14:543–553, 1983.

91. Hart RG, Kagan-Hallet K, Joerns SE: Mechanisms of intracranial hemorrhage in infective endocarditis. Stroke 18:1048–1056, 1987.

92. Weisberg LA, Stazio A, Shamsnia M, et al: Nontraumatic parenchymal brain hemorrhages. Medicine 69:277–295, 1990.

93. Schütz H: Spontane intrazerebrale Hämatome: Pathophysiologie, Klinik und Therapie. Heidelberg, Germany: Springer-Verlag, 1988.

94. Ropper AH, Davis KR: Lobar cerebral hemorrhages: acute clinical syndromes in 26 cases. Ann Neurol 8:141–147, 1980.

95. Lipton RB, Berger AR, Lesser ML, et al: Lobar versus thalamic and basal ganglion hemorrhage: clinical and radiologic features. J Neurol 234:86–90, 1987.

96. Ausman JI, Diaz FG, Malik GM, et al: Current management of cerebral aneurysms: is it based on facts or myths? Surg Neurol 24:625–635, 1985.

97. Jellinger K: Pathology and aetiology of intracranial aneurysms. In: Pia HW, Langmaid C, Zierski J, eds. Cerebral Aneurysms. Advances in Diagnosis and Therapy. Berlin: Springer-Verlag, 1979, pp 5–41.

98. Hayvard RD, O'Reilly GV: Intracranial haemorrhage. Accuracy of computerized transverse axial scanning in predicting the underlying aetiology. Lancet 1:1–4, 1976.

99. Ogawa T, Inugami A, Shimosegawa E, et al: Subarachnoid hemorrhage: evaluation with MR imaging. Radiology 186:345–351, 1993.

100. Atlas SW: MR imaging is highly sensitive for acute subarachnoid hemorrhage . . . not! Radiology 186:319–322, 1993. Ogawa T, Uemura K: Reply. Radiology 186:323, 1993.

101. Noguchi K, Ogawa T, Inugami A, et al: MR imaging of acute subarachnoid hemorrhage with fluid-attenuated inversion recovery pulse sequences. Radiology 193:462S, 1994.

102. Daniele D, Bracchi M, Riva A, et al: Superficial siderosis of the central nervous system: neuroradiological evaluation of two cases. Eur Neurol 32:270–273, 1992.

103. Mohr JP, Nichols FC, Tatemichi TK, Stein BM: Vascular malformations of the brain: clinical considerations. In: Barnett HJM, Mohr JP, Stein BM, Yatsu FM, eds. Stroke: Pathophysiology, Diagnosis, and Management. New York: Churchill Livingstone, 1986, pp 679–705.

104. Needell WM, Maravilla KR: MR flow imaging in vascular malformations using gradient recalled acquisition. AJNR 9:637–642, 1988.

105. Rigamonti D, Drayer BP, Johnson PC, et al: The MRI appearance of cavernous malformations (angiomas). J Neurosurg 67:518–524, 1987.

106. Rigamonti D, Spetzler RF, Drayer BP, et al: Appearance of venous malformations on magnetic resonance imaging. J Neurosurg 69:535–539, 1988.

107. Farmer JP, Cosgrove GR, Villemure JG, et al: Intracerebral cavernous angiomas. Neurology 38:1699–1704, 1988.

108. Gomori JM, Grossman RI, Goldberg HI, et al: Occult cerebral vascular malformations: high-field MR imaging. Radiology 158:707–713, 1986.

109. Ogilvy CS, Heros RC, Ojeman RG, New PF: Angiographically occult arteriovenous malformations. J Neurosurg 69:350–355, 1988.

110. Sze G, Krol G, Olsen WL, et al: Hemorrhagic neoplasms: MR mimics of occult vascular malformations. AJNR 8:795–802, 1987.

111. Jellinger K: Cerebrovascular amyloidosis with cerebral haemorrhage. J Neurol 214:195–206, 1977.

112. Vinters HV: Cerebral amyloid angiopathy: a critical review. Stroke 18:311–324, 1987.

113. Masuda J, Tanaka K, Ueda K, Omae T: Autopsy study of incidence and distribution of cerebral amyloid angiopathy in Hisayama, Japan. Stroke 19:205–210, 1988.

114. Vonsattel JP, Myers RH, Hedley-Whyte ET, et al: Cerebral amyloid angiopathy without and with cerebral hemorrhages: a comparative histological study. Ann Neurol 30:637–649, 1991.

115. Cosgrove CR, Leblanc R, Meagher-Villemure K, Ethier R: Cerebral amyloid angiopathy. Neurology 35:625–631, 1985.

116. Gray F, Dubas F, Roullet E, et al: Leukoencephalopathy in diffuse hemorrhagic cerebral amyloid angiopathy. Ann Neurol 18:54–59, 1985.

117. Loes DJ, Biller J, Yuh WTC, et al: Leukoencephalopathy in cerebral amyloid angiopathy: MR imaging in four cases. Am J Neuroradiol 11:485–488, 1990.

118. Hendricks HT, Franke CL, Theunissen PHMH: Cerebral amyloid angiopathy: diagnosis by MRI and brain biopsy. Neurology 40:1308–1310, 1990.

119. Awasthi D, Voorhies RM, Eick J, Mitchell WT: Cerebral amyloid angiopathy presenting as multiple intracranial lesions on magnetic resonance imaging. J Neurosurg 75:458–460, 1991.

120. Cole FM, Yates P: Intracerebral microaneurysms and small cerebrovascular lesions. Brain 90:759–768, 1967.

121. Franke CL, de Jonge J, van Swieten JC, et al: Intracerebral hematomas during anticoagulant treatment. Stroke 21:726–730, 1990.

122. Forsting M, Mattle HP, Huber P. Anticoagulation-related intracerebral hemorrhage. Cerebrovasc Dis 1:97–102, 1991.

123. Carlson SE, Aldrich MS, Greenberg HS, Topol EJ: Intracerebral hemorrhage complicating intravenous tissue plasminogen activator treatment. Arch Neurol 45:1070–1073, 1988.

124. Wijdicks EFM, Jack CR: Intracerebral hemorrhage after fibrinolytic therapy for acute myocardial infarction. Stroke 24:554–557, 1993.

125. Wijdicks EFM, Silbert PL, Jack CR, Parisi JE: Subcortical hemorrhage in disseminated intravascular coagulation associated with sepsis. AJNR 15:763–765, 1994.

126. Kase CS: Bleeding disorders. In: Kase CS, Caplan LR, eds. Intracerebral Hemorrhage. Boston: Butterworth-Heinemann, 1994, pp 117–152.

127. Wintzen AR, de Jonge H, Loeliger EA, Bots GTAM: The risk of intracerebral hemorrhage during oral anticoagulant treatment: a population study. Ann Neurol 16:553–558, 1984.

128. Kase CS, Robinson RK, Stein RW, et al: Anticoagulant-related intracerebral hemorrhage. Neurology 35:943–948, 1985.

129. Brust JCM, Richter RW: Stroke associated with addiction to heroin. J Neurol Neurosurg Psychiatry 39:194–199, 1976.

130. Rumbaugh CL, Bergeron RT, Fang HC, McCormick R: Cerebral angiographic changes in the drug abuse patient. Radiology 101:335–344, 1971.

131. Delaney P, Estes M: Intracranial hemorrhage with amphetamine use. Neurology 30:1125–1130, 1980.

132. Caplan LR, Thomas C, Banks G: Central nervous system complications of addiction to "T's and Blues." Neurology 32:623–628, 1982.

133. Fallis RJ, Fisher M: Cerebral vasculitis and hemorrhage associated with phenylpropanolamine. Neurology 35:405–407, 1985.
134. Levine SR, Welch KMA: Cocaine and stroke. Stroke 19:779–783, 1987.
135. Kase CS: Intracerebral hemorrhage: non-hypertensive causes. Stroke 17:590–595, 1986.
136. Feinberg WM, Swenson MS: Cerebrovascular complications of L-asparaginase therapy. Neurology 38:127–133, 1988.
137. Scott M: Spontaneous intracerebral hematoma caused by cerebral neoplasms. Report of eight verified cases. J Neurosurg 42:338–342, 1975.
138. Mandybur TI: Intracranial hemorrhage caused by metastatic tumors. Neurology 27:650–655, 1977.
139. Zimmerman RA, Bilaniuk LT: Computed tomography of acute intratumoral hemorrhage. Radiology 135:355–359, 1980.
140. Mattle HP, Maurer D, Sturzenegger M, et al: Cardiac myxomas: a long term study. J Neurol, in press.
141. Gatenby RA, Coia LR, Richter MP, et al: Oxygen tension in human tumors: in vivo mapping using CT-guided probes. Radiology 156:211–214, 1985.
142. Fisher CM, Adams RD: Observations on brain metabolism with special reference to the mechanism of hemorrhagic infarction. J Neuropathol Exp Neurol 10:92–93, 1951.
143. Ott BR, Zamani A, Kleefield J, Funkenstein HH: The clinical spectrum of hemorrhagic infarction. Stroke 17:630–637, 1986.
144. Lodder J, Krijne-Kubat B, Broekman J: Cerebral hemorrhagic infarction at autopsy: cardiac embolic cause and the relationship to the cause of death. Stroke 17:626–629, 1986.
145. McCarthy M, Norenberg MD: Pontine hemorrhagic infarction in nontraumatic fat embolism. Neurology 38:1645–1647, 1988.
146. Bousser MG, Chiras J, Sauron B, et al: Cerebral venous thrombosis: a review of 38 cases. Stroke 16:199–213, 1985. Erratum in Stroke 16:738, 1985.
147. Buonanno FS, Moody DM, Ball MR, Laster DW: Computed cranial tomographic findings in cerebral sinovenous occlusion. J Comput Assist Tomogr 2:281–290, 1978.
148. Sze G, Simmons B, Krol G, et al: Dural sinus thrombosis: verification with spin-echo techniques. AJNR 9:679–686, 1988.
149. Edelman RR, Wentz KU, Mattle H, et al: Projection arteriography and venography in the body and head: initial clinical results using magnetic resonance. Radiology 172:351–357, 1989.
150. Humphreys RP, Hoffman HJ, Mustard WT, Trusler GA: Cerebral hemorrhage after heart surgery. J Neurosurg 43:671–675, 1975.
151. Caplan LR, Neely S, Gorelick PB: Cold-related intracerebral hemorrhage. Arch Neurol 41:227, 1984.
152. Barbas N, Caplan L, Baquis G, et al: Dental chair intracerebral hemorrhage. Neurology 37:511–512, 1987.
153. Seiler RW, Zurbrügg HR: Supratentorial intracerebral hemorrhage after posterior fossa operation. Neurosurgery 18:472–474, 1986.
154. Haines S, Maroon J, Janetta P: Supratentorial intracerebral hemorrhage following posterior fossa surgery. J Neurosurg 49:881–886, 1978.
155. Kondoh T, Tamaki N, Takeda N, et al: Fatal intracranial hemorrhage after balloon occlusion of an extracranial vertebral arteriovenous fistula. J Neurosurg 69:945–948, 1988.
156. Gates PC, Barnett HJM, Vinters HV, et al: Primary intraventricular hemorrhage in adults. Stroke 17:872–877, 1986.
157. Verma A, Maheshwari MC, Bhargava S: Spontaneous intraventricular haemorrhage. J Neurol 234:233–236, 1987.
158. Darby DG, Donnan GA, Saling MA, et al: Primary intraventricular hemorrhage: clinical and neuropsychological findings in a prospective stroke series. Neurology 38:68–75, 1988.
159. Volpe JJ: Neonatal intraventricular hemorrhage. N Engl J Med 304:886–891, 1981.
160. Kraus JF: Neoplastic diseases of the human hypophysis. Arch Pathol 39:343–349, 1945.
161. Yousem DM, Arrington JA, Zinreich SJ, et al: Pituitary adenomas: possible role of bromocriptine in intratumoral hemorrhage. Radiology 170:239–243, 1989.
162. Ropper AH: Lateral displacement of the brain and level of consciousness in patients with an acute hemispheral mass. N Engl J Med 314:953–958, 1986.
163. Plum F, Posner JB: The Diagnosis of Stupor and Coma. 3rd ed. Philadelphia: FA Davis, 1980.
164. Hahn F, Gurney J: CT signs of central descending transtentorial herniation. AJNR 6:844–845, 1985.
165. McKissock W, Richardson A, Tyler J: Primary intracerebral haemorrhage. A controlled trial of surgical and conservative treatment in 180 unselected cases. Lancet 2:221–226, 1961.
166. Portenoy RK, Lipton RB, Berger AR, et al: Intracerebral haemorrhage: a model for the prediction of outcome. J Neurol Neurosurg Psychiatry 50:976–979, 1987.
167. Tuhrim S, Dambrosia JM, Price TR, et al: Prediction of intracerebral hemorrhage survival. Ann Neurol 24:258–263, 1988.
168. Francke CL, van Swieten JC, Algra A, van Gijn J. Prognostic factors in patients with intracerebral hematoma. J Neurol Neurosurg Psychiatry 55:653–657, 1992.
169. Broderick JP, Brott TG, Duldner JE, et al: Volume of intracerebral hemorrhage. A powerful and easy-to-use predictor of 30-day mortality. Stroke 24:987–993, 1993.
170. Andrews BT, Chiles BW 3d, Olsen WL, Pitts LH: The effect of intracerebral hematoma location on the risk of brain-stem compression and on clinical outcome. J Neurosurg 69:518–522, 1988.
171. Fieschi C, Carolei A, Fiorelli M, et al: Changing prognosis of primary intracerebral hemorrhage: results of a clinical and computed tomographic follow-up study of 104 patients. Stroke 19:192–195, 1988.
172. Little JR, Tubman DE, Ethier R: Cerebellar hemorrhage in adults. J Neurosurg 48:575–579, 1978.
173. Heiman TD, Satya-Murti S: Benign cerebellar hemorrhages. Ann Neurol 3:366–368, 1978.
174. Crowell RG, Ojemann RG: Spontaneous brain hemorrhage: surgical considerations. In: Barnett HJM, Mohr JP, Stein BM, Yatsu FM, eds. Stroke: Pathophysiology, Diagnosis, and Management. New York: Churchill Livingstone, 1986, pp 1191–1206.
175. Cuneo RA, Caronna JJ, Pitts L, et al: Upward transtentorial herniation: seven cases and a literature review. Arch Neurol 36:618–623, 1979.
176. Tyler KL, Poletti CE, Heros RC: Cerebral amyloid angiopathy with multiple intracerebral hemorrhages. Neurosurgery 57:286–289, 1982.
177. Heiskanen O: Treatment of spontaneous intracerebral and intracerebellar hemorrhages. Stroke 24(suppl I):I94–I95, 1993.
178. Mattle H, Kohler S, Huber P, et al: Anticoagulation-related intracranial extracerebral haemorrhage. J Neurol Neurosurg Psychiatry 52:829–837, 1989.
179. Woerner FJ, Abildgaard CF, French BN: Intracranial hemorrhage in children with idiopathic thrombocytopenic purpura. Pediatrics 67:453–460, 1981.
180. Yoshida M, Hayashi T, Kuramoto S, et al: Traumatic intracranial hematomas in hemophiliac children. Surg Neurol 12:115–118, 1979.
181. Hutchinson AA, Barrett JM, Fleischer AC: Intraventricular hemorrhage in the premature infant. N Engl J Med 307:1272–1273, 1982.
182. Volpe JJ: Neurology of the Newborn. Philadelphia: WB Saunders, 1987.
183. Palma PA, Miner ME, Morriss FH: Intraventricular hemorrhage in the neonate born at term. Am J Dis Child 133:941–944, 1979.
184. Scher MS, Wright FS, Lockman LA, et al: Intraventricular hemorrhage in the term neonate. Arch Neurol 39:769–772, 1982.
185. Fenichel GM, Webster DL, Wong WK: Intracranial hemorrhage in the term newborn. Arch Neurol 41:30–34, 1984.
186. McArdle CB, Richardson CJ, Hayden CK, et al: Abnormalities of the neonatal brain: MR imaging. Part I. Intracranial hemorrhage. Radiology 163:387–394, 1987.
187. Zürrer M, Martin E, Boltshauser E: MR imaging of intracranial hemorrhage in neonates and infants at 2.35 tesla. Neuroradiology 33:223–229, 1991.
188. National Research Council, Committee on Trauma Research: Injury in America: A Continuing Public Health Problem. Washington, DC: National Academy Press, 1985.
189. Jennett B, Frankowski RF: The epidemiolgy of head injury. In: Vinken PJ, Bruyn GW, Klawans HL, Braakmann R, eds. Handbook of Clinical Neurology, Volume 57, Revised Series 13, Head Injury. Amsterdam: Elsevier Science Publishers, 1990, pp 1–16.
190. Caplan LR: Head trauma and related hemorrhage. In: Kase CS, Caplan LR, eds. Intracerebral Hemorrhage. Boston: Butterworth-Heinemann, 1994, pp 221–241.
191. Holbourn AHS: Mechanics of head injuries. Lancet 2:438–441, 1943.
192. Holbourn AHS: Mechanics of brain injuries. Br Med Bull 3:147–149, 1945.
193. Gentry LR: Head trauma. In: Atlas SW, ed. Magnetic Resonance Imaging of the Brain and Spine. New York: Raven Press, 1990, pp 439–466.
194. Han JS, Kaufman B, Alfidi RJ, et al: Head trauma evaluated by magnetic resonance and computed tomography: a comparison. Radiology 150:71–77, 1984.
195. Moon KL Jr, Brant-Zawadzki M, Pitts LH, Mills CM: Nuclear magnetic resonance imaging of CT-isodense subdural hematomas. AJNR 5:319–322, 1984.
196. Gandy SE, Snow RB, Zimmerman RD, Deck MDF: Cranial nuclear magnetic resonance imaging in head trauma. Ann Neurol 16:254–257, 1984.
197. Levin HS, Hadnel SF, Goldman AM, et al: Magnetic resonance imaging after "diffuse" nonmissile head injury. Arch Neurol 42:963–968, 1985.
198. Zimmerman RA, Bilaniuk LT, Hackney DB, et al: Head injury: early results comparing CT and high-field MR. AJNR 7:757–764, 1986.
199. Langfitt TW, Obrist WD, Alavi A, et al: Computerized tomography, magnetic resonance imaging, and positron emission tomography in the study of brain trauma: preliminary observations. J Neurosurg 64:760–767, 1986.
200. Snow RB, Zimmerman RD, Gandy SE, Deck MDF: Comparison of magnetic resonance imaging and computed tomography in the evaluation of head injury. Neurosurgery 18:45–52, 1986.
201. Jenkins A, Teasdale G, Hadley MDM, et al: Brain lesions detected by magnetic resonance imaging in mild and severe head injuries. Lancet 2:445–446, 1986.
202. Hesselink JR, Dowd CF, Healy ME, et al: MR imaging of brain contusions: a comparative study with CT. AJNR 9:269–278, 1988.
203. Gentry LR, Thompson B, Godersky JC: Trauma to the corpus callosum: MR features. AJNR 9:1129–1138, 1988.

204. Gentry LR, Godersky JC, Thompson BH, Dunn VD: Prospective comparative study of intermediate-field MR and CT in the evaluation of closed head trauma. AJNR 9:91–100, 1988.
205. Gentry LR, Godersky JC, Thompson BH: MR imaging of head trauma: review of the distribution and radiopathologic features of traumatic lesions. AJNR 9:101–110, 1988.
206. Gentry LR, Godersky JC, Thompson BH: Traumatic brain stem injury: MR imaging. Radiology 171:177–187, 1989.
207. Gentry LR. Imaging of closed head injury. Radiology 191:1–17, 1994.
208. Orrison WW, Gentry LR, Stimac GK, et al: Blinded comparison of cranial CT and MR in closed head injury evaluation. AJNR 15:351–356, 1994.
209. Adams JH, Doyle D, Ford I, et al: Diffuse axonal injury in head injury: definition, diagnosis, and grading. Histopathology 15:49–59, 1989.
210. Adams JH, Graham DI, Murray LS, Scott G: Diffuse axonal injury due to nonmissile head injury in humans: an analysis of 45 cases. Ann Neurol 12:557–563, 1982.
211. Adams JH, Graham DI, Scott G, et al: Brain damage in fatal non-missile head injury. J Clin Pathol 33:1132–1145, 1980.
212. Frowein RA, Schiltz F, Stammler U: Early posttraumatic intracranial hematomas. Neurosurg Rev 12(suppl 1):184–189, 1989.
213. Darker SR, Bhargava N: Bilateral epidural hematoma. Acta Neurchir 110:29–32, 1991.
214. Rivano C, Borzone M, Altomonte M, Capuzzo T: Traumatic posterior fossa extradural hematomas. Neurochirurgia 35:43–47, 1992.
215. Guillermain P: Traumatic extradural hematomas. In: Vigouroux RP, ed. Advances in Neurotraumatology, Volume I. Vienna: Springer-Verlag, 1986, pp 1–18.
216. Pozzati E, Tognetti F, Cavallo M, Acciarri N: Extradural hematomas of the posterior fossa: observations on a series of 32 consecutive cases treated after the introduction of computed tomography scanning. Surg Neurol 32:300–303, 1989.
217. Zimmerman RA, Bilaniuk LT: Computed tomography staging of traumatic epidural bleeding. Radiology 144:809–812, 1982.
218. Mattle HP, Wentz KU, Edelman RR, et al: Cerebral venography with magnetic resonance. Radiology 178:453–458, 1991.
219. Frowein RA, Firsching R: Classification of head injury. In: Vinken PJ, Bruyn GW, Klawans HL, Braakman R, eds. Handbook of Clinical Neurology, Volume 57, Revised Series 13, Head Injury. Amsterdam: Elsevier Science Publishers, 1990, pp 101–122.
220. Cooper PR: Post-traumatic intracranial mass lesions. In: Cooper PR, ed. Head Injury. 2nd ed. Baltimore: Williams & Wilkins, 1987, pp 238–284.
221. Sipponen JT, Sepponen RE, Sivula AS: Chronic subdural hematoma: demonstration by magnetic resonance. Radiology 150:79–85, 1984.
222. Fobben ES, Grossman RI, Atlas SW, et al: MR characteristics of subdural hematomas and hygromas at 1.5 T. AJNR 10:687–693, 1989.
223. Ebisu T, Naruse S, Horikawa Y, et al: Nonacute subdural hematoma: fundamental interpretation of MR images based on biochemical and in vitro MR analysis. Radiology 171:449–453, 1990.
224. Wilms G, Marchal G, Geusens E, et al: Isodense subdural haematomas on CT: MRI findings. Neuroradiology 34:497–499, 1992.
225. McCluney KW, Yeakley JW, Fenstermacher MJ, et al: Subdural hygroma versus atrophy on MR brain scans: "the cortical vein sign." AJNR 13:1335–1339, 1992.
226. Sturzenegger M, Mattle HP, Rivoir A, et al: Ultrasound findings in carotid artery dissection: analysis of 43 patients. Neurology 45:691–698, 1995.
227. Robertson SJ, Wolpert SM, Runge VM: MR imaging of middle cranial fossa arachnoid cysts: temporal lobe agenesis syndrome revisited. AJNR 10:1007–1010, 1989.
228. Eustace S, Toland J, Stack J: CT and MRI of arachnoid cyst with complicating intracystic and subdural hemorrhage. J Comput Assist Tomogr 16:995–997, 1992.
229. Adams H, Mitchell DE, Graham DI, Doyle D: Diffuse brain damage of immediate impact type. Its relationship to "primary brain-stem damage" in head injury. Brain 100:489–502, 1977.

22

Epilepsy

RICHARD J. FRIEDLAND ▪ RICHARD A. BRONEN

The word *epilepsy* is derived from the Greek word *epilepsia* meaning "to take hold of or to seize." Clinical descriptions of epileptic seizures were recorded more than 2000 years ago by Hippocrates.[1] A seizure is a distinct clinical episode characterized by a transient disturbance in mentation, abnormal movements of the body, or both that results from excess electrical brain activity. The terms *seizure* and *epilepsy* are not synonymous. Epilepsy is a condition in which an individual experiences recurrent unprovoked seizures; the term does not indicate or specify an underlying cause.

Epilepsy is a common neurologic disorder, affecting 0.5% to 1.0% of the U.S. population.[2, 3] In evaluating the patient with epilepsy, it is helpful to be familiar with causes commonly associated with this disease. The underlying cause of epilepsy depends on the characteristics of the population studied, such as seizure classification, age of the patient, and response to medical treatment[4, 5] (Table 22–1). Epidemologic studies of epilepsy identified a cause in only 25% of patients: trauma, 5%; vascular malformation, 6%; neoplasm, 2%; developmental malformation, 5%; infection, 4%; and other, 1%.[6] In more selected studies of patients undergoing surgical therapy for epilepsy, hippocampal sclerosis is the most common cause of epilepsy (50% to 70%), followed by perinatal hypoxia or injury (13% to 35%), tumors (15%), vascular malformations (3%), traumatic scarring (2%), and hamartomas (2%). Less common abnormalities include infections, migrational abnormalities, tuberous sclerosis, cortical dysplasias, cysts, and infarcts[7–12] (Table 22–2).

There are two recognized schemes for classifying epilepsy. One scheme groups patients into those with epilepsy syndromes, based on clinical characteristics. The epilepsy syndromes are defined by age at onset, type of seizure, and presence of an underlying lesion. By grouping patients into epileptic syndromes one can define therapy and assign prognosis.[13, 14] A discussion of each of the individual epilepsy syndromes is beyond the scope of this chapter.

The second classification scheme, devised by the International League Against Epilepsy in 1981, is based on the type of seizures. Seizures can be classified as either 1) generalized, with initial neuronal activation occurring simultaneously in both hemispheres or 2) partial, with initial activation of a limited set of neu-rons in a single region of cortex. Generalized seizures are subcategorized as either absence, tonic-clonic, clonic, tonic, myoclonic, or atonic. Absence seizures are characterized by a sudden cessation of ongoing conscious activity and a blank stare. The term *tonic* describes rigid extensor posturing, whereas clonic refers to a repeated jerking motion of the extremities. Myoclonic seizures are sudden, brief, and often violent muscular contractions. Atonic seizures are manifested by a sudden focal or generalized loss of muscle tone. Partial seizures, also known as focal seizures, can be subdivided into 1) simple, with no impairment of consciousness; 2) complex, with impaired consciousness; or 3) focal, with secondary generalization. A study of 1220 epileptic adults by Keränen and colleagues[13] found partial seizures in 56%, generalized seizures in 27%, and seizures that were not classifiable in the remaining 18%.

The distinction between generalized and focal seizures is a critical one because they have different therapeutic implications. Although generalized seizures are usually well controlled with medication, 15% to 30% of patients with partial epilepsy continue to have seizures despite maximal medical treatment.[15, 16] Most have an epileptogenic focus in the temporal lobe. Intractable epilepsy has important social, medical, and financial repercussions to both the individual and society.[17] Epilepsy causes social disabilities and carries an increased risk of injury or death compared with these risks in the general population.[18, 19] Surgery to control seizures can be considered in patients with at least 2 years of medically refractory epilepsy. There may be 150,000 to 200,000 surgical candidates in the United States.[15, 20, 21] Localization of the epileptogenic focus is most important in patients deemed surgical candidates.

Before we discuss the different techniques used to determine the seizure focus, we must review some terminology. The term *epileptogenic lesion* refers to a structural abnormality, found by imaging or pathologic studies, that causes the seizure disorder. The *epileptogenic zone* is an area of cortex that must be completely resected to eliminate the patient's seizures.[22] Although the epileptogenic lesion and the epileptogenic zone are often closely related to each other, they may not be synonymous.

Presently, no single technique can precisely identify

TABLE 22–1. ETIOLOGY OF EPILEPSY CATEGORIZED BY AGE AT ONSET OF SEIZURE

	CAUSE FOR AGE				
CAUSE	0–2 y	3–20 y	21–40 y	41–60 y	>60 y
Anoxia	X				
Metabolic abnormalities or inborn error of metabolism	X				
Congenital or developmental malformations	X	X			
Infection	X	X			
Phacomatosis (tuberous sclerosis, Sturge-Weber disease, neurofibromatosis)	X	X			
Primary generalized seizures		X			
Hippocampal sclerosis		X			
Trauma	X	X	X	X	
Vascular malformation			X		
Tumor			X	X	X
Cerebrovascular accident				X	X

From Bronen RA: Evaluation of the seizure patient. In: Huckman MS, ed. American Roentgen Ray Society Neuroradiology Categorical Course Syllabus. Orlando, FL: American Roentgen Ray Society, 1992, pp 147–158.

the epileptogenic zone. In the past, detection of the epileptogenic zone was based almost entirely on findings of electroencephalography (EEG). Scalp EEG is not as accurate as invasive EEG monitoring and often has difficulty localizing an abnormality within a lobe or sometimes a hemisphere. However, because of its ability to depict neuroanatomy, magnetic resonance imaging (MRI) is ideally suited for identifying a focal brain abnormality and can detect structural lesions with a high degree of sensitivity.[2, 4, 7, 11, 23–25] MRI and video monitoring EEG are widely available and are the most critical noninvasive studies in the evaluation of the epileptogenic zone (Fig. 22–1).

Other noninvasive tests include computed tomography (CT), single photon emission CT (SPECT), positron emission tomography (PET), magnetoencephalography, intracarotid sodium amobarbital testing, and neurologic and neuropsychologic testing. CT has limited value in the work-up of intractable epilepsy. In a study of 113 patients with resective surgery for epilepsy at Yale, the epileptic abnormality was localized by CT in 28% of patients compared with 86% of patients by MRI. The probability of a positive CT scan after a normal MR image was 0%. Functional tests such as PET and SPECT are commonly coregistered with MRI for better anatomic localization. A localized reduction in cerebral blood flow by SPECT or a decrease in cerebral metabolism by PET has a relatively high sensi-

tivity and a moderate specificity for localization of an epileptogenic focus, particularly when the temporal lobe is involved. SPECT is unique because it can be performed during ictus (a clinical seizure). PET has better spatial resolution and can use various tracer elements to measure functional disorders but is limited by high cost and lack of widespread availability. Because these imaging modalities identify different structural and functional properties of the epileptogenic zone, they often provide different and complementary information. Comparison of these modalities is nearly impossible, owing to the rapid pace of technologic refinements[26] (Table 22–3).

The algorithm for determining the seizure focus and resectability varies depending on institutional philosophy and available resources. Most centers use a combination of EEG and neuroimaging as their primary means of determining the epileptogenic zone. If these studies localize the seizure focus and all studies are concordant, invasive EEG testing may not be necessary. If these tests are discordant, EEG recordings from intraparenchymal depth electrodes or subdural electrodes are warranted.

ROLE OF MRI IN SURGERY FOR EPILEPSY

The primary role of MRI is to locate and define anatomic epileptogenic lesions. MRI findings may also influence whether the patient is a candidate for surgery, the type of surgery, the need for invasive EEG evaluation, and the prognosis of postoperative seizure control. Patients undergo a multitude of presurgical tests to determine the relationships of the MRI-identified lesion, the epileptogenic zone, and the functional (eloquent) cortex. As previously discussed, concordance of all noninvasive tests with the MRI findings may preclude the need for invasive testing, which is associated with an increased morbidity of 2% to 5%.[7, 27, 28] MRI is also useful in planning the placement of invasive electrodes, such as the surgical placement of subdural grids or depth electrodes.

Most abnormalities can be categorized into diagnos-

TABLE 22–2. ETIOLOGY OF MEDICALLY INTRACTABLE EPILEPSY

CAUSE	SURGICAL SERIES (%)	MRI SERIES* (%)
Hippocampal sclerosis	50–70	57
Tumor	10–20	14
Vascular	3–5	4
Developmental causes	2	11
Perinatal or miscellaneous causes	13–35	7
No lesion		9

*Data from Jackson GD: New techniques in magnetic resonance and epilepsy. Epilepsia 35(suppl 6):S2–S13, 1994.

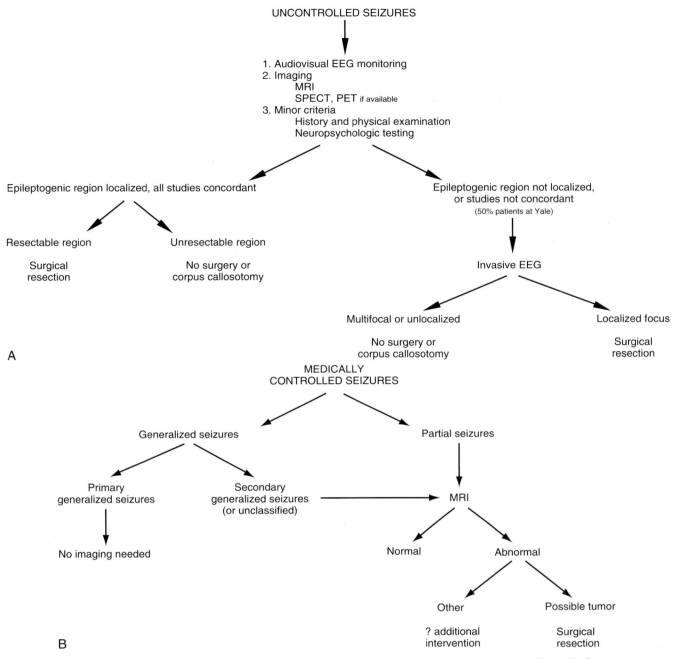

UNCONTROLLED SEIZURES

1. Audiovisual EEG monitoring
2. Imaging
    MRI
    SPECT, PET if available
3. Minor criteria
    History and physical examination
    Neuropsychologic testing

Epileptogenic region localized, all studies concordant

Epileptogenic region not localized, or studies not concordant
(50% patients at Yale)

Resectable region

Unresectable region

Surgical resection

No surgery or corpus callosotomy

Invasive EEG

Multifocal or unlocalized

Localized focus

No surgery or corpus callosotomy

Surgical resection

A

MEDICALLY CONTROLLED SEIZURES

Generalized seizures

Partial seizures

Primary generalized seizures

Secondary generalized seizures (or unclassified)

MRI

No imaging needed

Normal

Abnormal

Other

Possible tumor

? additional intervention

Surgical resection

B

FIGURE 22–1. *A*, Algorithm for medically *uncontrolled* seizures. The decision tree for patients with medically intractable epilepsy is based primarily on EEG and imaging. *B*, Decision tree for MRI of medically *controlled* seizures. It is often difficult to determine primary from secondary generalization of seizure activity, especially in the pediatric population. Some neurologists advocate the use of MRI as a screening tool in all patients with epilepsy except those with definite primary generalized seizures. (*A* and *B* from Bronen RA: Epilepsy: the role of MR imaging. AJR 159:1165–1174, 1992.)

tic groups by their MRI features. One can generally distinguish among neoplasms, arteriovenous malformations (AVMs), cavernous hemangiomas, certain infections, cicatricial processes, diffuse atrophic processes, migration anomalies, hippocampal sclerosis, and sometimes hamartomas and cortical dysplasias.[7, 29] Some lesions are subtle, such as in hippocampal sclerosis and migrational abnormalities, whereas others are

obvious but easily confused with other lesions, such as focal cortical dysplasia of Taylor and tumors. The correct categorization of a lesion has significant impact on treatment of patients and on surgical decisions. MRI has radically improved our recognition and understanding of three broad categories of epileptogenic abnormalities: 1) hippocampal sclerosis; 2) focal lesions, such as tumors; and 3) nonvascular develop-

TABLE 22–3. COMPARISON OF IMAGING
MODALITIES*

| MODALITY | PATHOLOGY STANDARD | | EEG STANDARD | |
	TLE Sensitivity	TLE Specificity	TLE† Sensitivity	ETLE‡ Sensitivity
PET	81	22	84	33
SPECT, interictal	70	36	66	60
SPECT, ictal	93	13	90	81
MRI	69§	68§	55§	42§

*Comparison of imaging modalities was from studies using either pathology or EEG as the standard. TLE = temporal lobe epilepsy; ETLE = extratemporal lobe epilepsy.

†Specificity of all techniques for TLE is 68%–86%.

‡Specificity of all techniques for ETLE is 93%–95%.

§This table is based on a review of the literature; it does not reflect current sensitivities, especially for MRI. More recent literature suggests that the sensitivity and specificity of MRI are at least 80%–90%.

From Spencer SS: The relative contributions of MRI, SPECT, and PET imaging in epilepsy. Epilepsia 35(suppl 6):S72–S89, 1994.

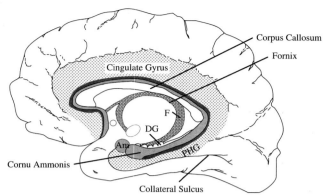

FIGURE 22–2. A diagram of the medial aspect of the brain with the brain stem removed. The hippocampus, which is composed of two gray matter layers, the cornu ammonis and the dentate gyrus (DG), is located on the medial aspect of the temporal lobe. The hippocampus is located superior to the parahippocampal gyrus (PHG) and posterior to the amygdala (AM). The major efferent fibers of the hippocampus eventually form the fimbria and fornix (F). The hippocampus is part of the limbic system that is composed of both gray matter and white matter tracts arcing along the medial aspect of the cerebrum. (Reprinted from Magn Reson Imaging, Volume 9, Bronen RA, Cheung G: Relationship of hippocampus and amygdala to coronal MRI landmarks. Pages 449–457, Copyright 1991, with kind permission from Elsevier Science Ltd, The Boulevard, Langford Lane, Kidlington OX5 1GB, UK.)

mental abnormalities, such as heterotopic gray matter. The remainder of the chapter is devoted to selected lesions associated with medically intractable epilepsy.

HIPPOCAMPAL SCLEROSIS

Hippocampal sclerosis is characterized by hippocampal neuronal loss and gliosis associated with medial temporal lobe epilepsy. It is also commonly known as mesial temporal sclerosis, Ammon's horn sclerosis, and end folium sclerosis. We prefer the term *hippocampal sclerosis* because our definition of this entity is based on changes found exclusively within the hippocampus.[30] The focus in this section is on the anatomy, pathology, and significance of hippocampal sclerosis as they relate to MRI.

ANATOMY AND PATHOLOGY

Familiarity with the normal anatomy, variations, and pathology of the hippocampus and temporal lobe is essential to evaluate this region adequately.[31] Hippocampal terminology is often confusing; we use the terms *hippocampal formation* and *hippocampus* synonymously.[32] The hippocampus is a curved structure located along the medial temporal lobe (Fig. 22–2). The hippocampus is divided into three segments based on its morphology and its relationship to the brain stem: the head, the body, and the tail (Fig. 22–3). The head is located at the anterior aspect of the brain stem. It can be recognized by digitations that resemble toes and, therefore, is also referred to as the pes hippocampus. The body is a cylindrical structure in the axial plane situated adjacent to the brain stem. The tail rapidly narrows as it sweeps upward behind the brain stem.[31, 33–36] In cross section, the hippocampus is a complex functional unit composed of two interlocking C-shaped gray matter structures: the cornu ammonis and the dentate gyrus (Fig. 22–4). The alveus, fornix,

and fimbria are the major white matter tracts that form the efferent pathways to the remainder of the brain. Structures surrounding the hippocampus include the parahippocampal gyrus inferiorly, connected to the hippocampus by the subiculum; the ambient (perimesencephalic) cistern medially, which separates the hippocampus from the brain stem; the choroidal fis-

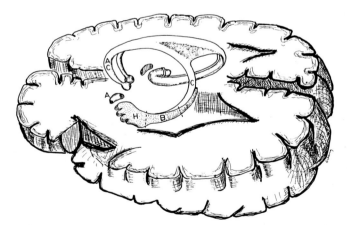

FIGURE 22–3. The hippocampus is an arc of gray matter along the medial aspect of the temporal lobe. It can be divided into the head (H), which is bulbous and has digitations; the body (B), which is relatively uniform and is located adjacent to the brain stem; and the tail (T), which narrows as it ascends behind the brain stem. The amygdala (A) is located anterior to the hippocampal head. Efferent fibers from the hippocampus eventually become the fornix. The crus of the fornix is labeled (C), and the column of the fornix is labeled (AC). (Reprinted from Magn Reson Imaging, Volume 9, Bronen RA, Cheung G: Relationship of hippocampus and amygdala to coronal MRI landmarks. Pages 449–457, Copyright 1991, with kind permission from Elsevier Science Ltd, The Boulevard, Langford Lane, Kidlington OX5 1GB, UK.)

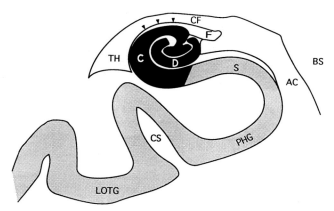

FIGURE 22–4. Coronal diagram of the right hippocampus. The hippocampus is made up of two U-shaped laminas of gray matter—the dentate gyrus (D) and cornu Ammonis (C). Efferent fibers from the hippocampus form the white matter track, the alveus *(arrowheads)*, which converge medially to become the fimbria (F). TH = temporal horn; CF = choroidal fissure; AC = ambient cistern; BS = brain stem; S = subiculum; PHG = parahippocampal gyrus; CS = collateral sulcus; LOTG = lateral occipital temporal gyrus. (From Bronen RA: Epilepsy: the role of MR imaging. AJR 159:1165–1174, 1992.)

sure and temporal horn superiorly; and the temporal horn laterally.[31, 33–36]

MRI of the amygdala and hippocampus is best performed in the coronal plane, perpendicular to the long axis of the hippocampus. The amygdala and hippocampus are isointense relative to gray matter on all pulse sequences (Figs. 22–5 and 22–6). The best landmark for separating amygdala from hippocampus is the anterior temporal horn, known as the uncal recess. The amygdala is always superior to the temporal horn. When there is a paucity of cerebrospinal fluid (CSF) within the uncal recess of the temporal horn, the alveus, which is the white matter of the hippocampal head, can be used to delineate the borders of these structures. The amygdala-hippocampal junction occurs at the level of the suprasellar cistern and basilar artery bifurcation. The hippocampal head can be recognized by its digitations and bulbous appearance. The hippocampal body appears as an oval gray matter structure, capped by the white matter of the alveus and fimbria. The internal architecture of the hippocampus may be visualized with high-resolution studies, using fast spin-echo (FSE) or inversion recovery techniques (see Figs. 22–6, 22–7B, and 22–13A and B). The temporal horn is situated lateral and superior to the body. The hippocampal tail narrows markedly as it ascends around the brain stem. Many centers use the crus of the fornix to delineate the posterior boundary of the hippocampus for quantitative studies.[35–40]

The initial gross anatomic description of hippocampal sclerosis was made by Bouchet and Cazauviel in 1825; Sommer was the first to report the microscopic changes within the hippocampus of epileptics in 1880.[20] Falconer and colleagues[41] coined the term *mesial temporal sclerosis* because they noted changes that affected not only the hippocampus but also the entorhinal cortex and the amygdala.

Histologically, hippocampal sclerosis is characterized by a pattern of neuronal cell loss principally involving the pyramidal cell layer in sectors CA1, CA3, and CA4 and the granular cell layer of the dentate gyrus[42] (Fig. 22–7). Hippocampal neuronal loss ranges from 30% to 60% compared with control subjects. Morphologic and cytochemical reorganization of the dentate gyrus is marked. This is characterized by selective loss of inhibitory interneurons, abnormal sprouting of axons, reorganization of neurotransmitter receptors, alterations in second-messenger systems, and hyperexcitability of granule cells. It is postulated that an insult to the developing brain during childhood, such as a complicated febrile seizure, damages hippocampal inhibitory interneurons. This initial damage leads to the reorganization of the dentate gyrus with the creation of an aberrant hyperexcitable synaptic system, which is clinically manifested as recurrent seizures.[42, 43]

Clinically, patients with hippocampal sclerosis present with intractable temporal lobe epilepsy and have an EEG focus arising from the hippocampus. There is often a history of a complicated febrile seizure in early childhood, occurring in 9% to 50% of cases.[44] However, only 2% to 7% of children with febrile convulsions develop epilepsy. Hippocampal sclerosis is seen in 65% of patients with intractable temporal lobe epilepsy in surgical and autopsy series.[8] Reports show that up to 50% of children with temporal lobe epilepsy have hippocampal sclerosis.[45, 46] Surgical resection of the hippocampus and anterior temporal lobe can cure epilepsy in up to 90% of patients with hippocampal sclerosis. Thus, preoperative identification of this disorder is imperative.[8, 47–49]

MRI FEATURES

The two most consistent MRI features for diagnosing hippocampal sclerosis are volume loss and signal changes in the ipsilateral hippocampus (Figs. 22–8 to 22–12). Most studies have reported hippocampal signal changes as hyperintense on T2-weighted sequences. Other hippocampal findings include hypointensity and disruption of the normal internal architecture on T1-weighted sequences (Fig. 22–13). Currently, many authors believe that visual analysis by a trained observer is 80% to 90% sensitive for the detection of hippocampal sclerosis under optimal conditions.[4, 7, 20, 50–56] In one series of 123 patients with histologically confirmed hippocampal sclerosis, MRI had a sensitivity of 98% with a specificity of 93%.[50] Volume loss and T2 signal changes can be assessed quantitatively as well as by visual inspection. Quantitative data may increase diagnostic accuracy and reliability and are especially important for research endeavors.

An atrophic or an asymmetrically small hippocampus is the most common MRI finding seen in hippocampal sclerosis (see Figs. 22–8 to 22–11). Compared with visual assesment, quantitative volume analysis of the hippocampus increases sensitivity to 80% to 100%, presumably by detecting subtle atrophic changes.[39, 54, 57–61] Most volumetric studies use either thin spoiled

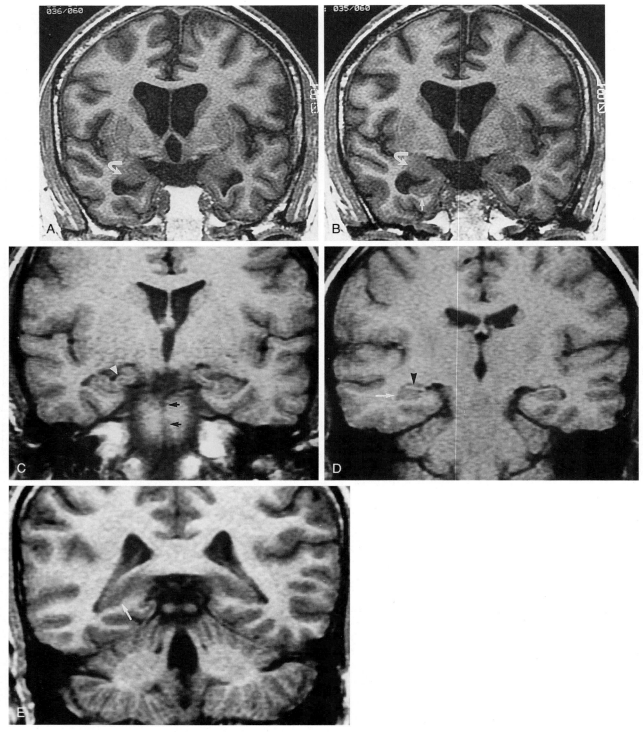

FIGURE 22–5. Coronal T1-weighted images of the normal amygdala and hippocampus proceeding from anterior *(A)* to posterior *(E)*. *A,* The temporal horn lies inferior to the amygdala *(curved white arrow)* at the level of the suprasellar cistern. *B,* The temporal horn is lateral and superior to the hippocampus *(straight arrow)*; the amygdala *(curved arrow)* is situated above the temporal horn. *C,* The digitations *(white arrowhead)* identify this as the hippocampal head located at the anterior aspect of the brain stem. Note the basilar artery *(short black arrows)*. *D,* The hippocampal body *(white arrow)* is oval and found adjacent to the brain stem. The white matter tracts of the alveus and fimbria *(black arrowhead)* are observed superior to the hippocampus. *E,* The hippocampal tail *(arrow)* is demonstrated as it ascends posterior to the brain stem. *(A to E reprinted from Magn Reson Imaging, Volume 9, Bronen RA, Cheung G: Relationship of hippocampus and amygdala to coronal MRI landmarks. Pages 449–457, Copyright 1991, with kind permission from Elsevier Science Ltd, The Boulevard, Langford Lane, Kidlington OX5 1GB, UK.)*

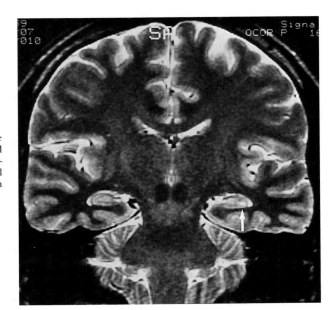

FIGURE 22–6. Coronal T2-weighted fast spin-echo (FSE) image at the level of the brain stem. The internal architecture of the hippocampal body is better demonstrated using the FSE technique than with T1-weighted conventional spin-echo sequences (seen in Fig. 22–5). A normal developmental variant, the hippocampal sulcus remnant, is seen within the left hippocampus *(arrow)*.

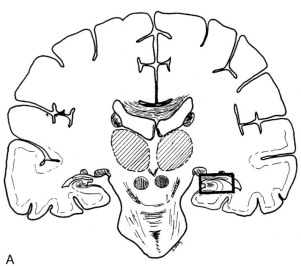

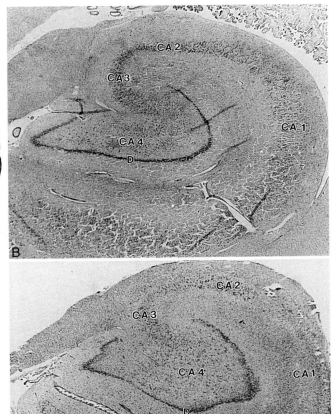

FIGURE 22–7. Hippocampal sclerosis. *A,* Coronal diagram with the rectangle showing the region of interest in *B* and *C. B,* Coronal histologic section of a normal hippocampus. Note the layer formed by neurons in the cornu Ammonis (CA1 to CA4) and the dentate gyrus (D), whose granules stain darkly in this micrograph. This contrasts to other regions, which are predominantly composed of white matter and do not stain. *C,* Coronal histologic section from a patient with hippocampal sclerosis. The dark-staining neurons are absent or markedly diminished, especially in CA1, CA3, CA4, and the dentate gyrus regions. (*A* to *C* from Bronen RA, Cheung G, Charles JT, et al: Imaging findings in hippocampal sclerosis: correlation with pathology. AJNR 12[5]:933–940, 1991. © by American Society of Neuroradiology.)

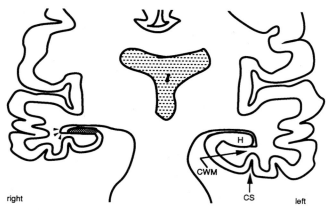

FIGURE 22–8. This diagram depicts the archetypical features of hippocampal sclerosis seen on coronal MR images. The right hippocampus is atrophic and hyperintense *(shaded)*. The temporal horn is expanded *(arrowheads)* but the temporal lobe and collateral white matter (CWM) are atrophic. H = hippocampus; CS = collateral sulcus. (From Bronen RA, Cheung G, Charles JT, et al: Imaging findings in hippocampal sclerosis: correlation with pathology. AJNR 12[5]:933–940, 1991. © by American Society of Neuroradiology.)

gradient-recalled (SPGR) or FSE images. Both techniques appear to be accurate, reproducible, and invaluable for expanding our understanding of hippocampal sclerosis. Volumetric measurements of the hippocampus have shown correlation with the amount of atrophy and the degree of neuronal cell loss, a history of childhood febrile seizures, age at onset of seizure, verbal memory performance, epileptiform EEG abnormalities, and postoperative seizure control.[39, 57–59, 61–65] Two studies have formally compared the sensitivities of simple visual inspection and quantitative volume analysis for the detection of this disorder, with disparate results. Jack and associates[53] found little difference

(71% versus 76%, respectively), whereas Cendes and coworkers[66] found volume measurements to be significantly better (56% versus 92%). We believe that quantitative analysis will increase sensitivity slightly compared with visual assessment by a well-trained observer.[67]

The other major imaging feature of hippocampal sclerosis is a hyperintense signal pattern within the hippocampus on long repetition time (TR) sequences (see Figs. 22–8 to 22–12). Early MRI studies underestimated the true incidence of signal abnormalities because of unrecognized subtle signal intensity changes, imaging artifacts that obscure pathologic processes, lack of coronal imaging, and failure to appreciate normal anatomic temporal lobe variations.[31, 34, 38, 40, 52, 55, 57] More recent studies have noted this finding in 70% to 100% of cases.[51, 54, 67, 68] The increased signal intensity is thought to reflect gliosis. Jackson and associates[51] have shown that quantitative evaluation of the signal is a sensitive (70%) and reliable method for lateralizing hippocampal sclerosis. T2 relaxometry also allows detection of hippocampal sclerosis in subjects without associated volume loss and detection of bilateral disease.[50, 51, 69]

Although most cases of hippocampal sclerosis are detected by assessing hippocampal volumes and T2 signal changes, other imaging findings may be beneficial in subtle cases and can increase sensitivity. Jackson and associates[40] noted that the normal hippocampal internal architecture was replaced by an abnormal hypointense signal pattern on T1-weighted images (see Fig. 22–13). Derangement of the normal cytoarchitecture within the hippocampus is seen best on inversion recovery sequences or FSE high-resolution images[40, 50, 52] (see Figs. 22–6, 22–12, and 22–13). Other imaging findings associated with hippocampal sclerosis include ipsilateral temporal lobe volume loss, dilatation of the

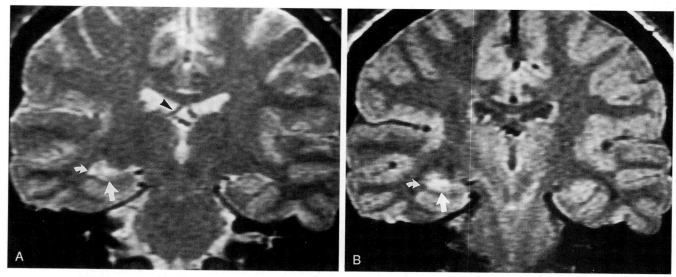

FIGURE 22–9. Right hippocampal sclerosis. T2-weighted *(A)* and proton density–weighted *(B)* coronal MR images show an atrophic, hyperintense right hippocampus *(straight arrow)* compared with the normal hippocampus on the left. The hyperintense signal is not due to the adjacent CSF within the temporal horn, which is seen laterally *(curved arrow)*. Note the decreased size of the ipsilateral fornix *(arrowhead)*. (*A* and *B* from Bronen RA, Cheung G, Charles JT, et al: Imaging findings in hippocampal sclerosis: correlation with pathology. AJNR 12[5]:933–940, 1991. © by American Society of Neuroradiology.)

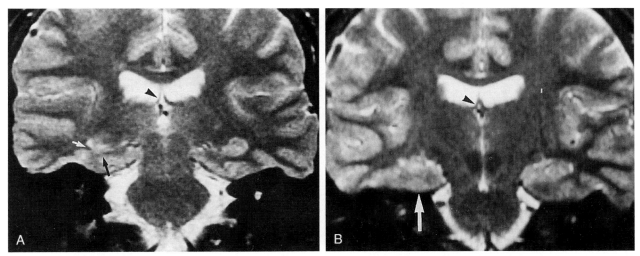

FIGURE 22–10. Right hippocampal sclerosis. Coronal T2-weighted images show an atrophic and hyperintense right hippocampus *(black arrow)* consistent with right hippocampal sclerosis. *A,* The white matter between the hippocampus and collateral sulcus, known as the collateral white matter, is markedly decreased on the ipsilateral side *(white arrow)*. *B,* On a more anterior slice, the collateral white matter on the ipsilateral side has vanished. In this case it is difficult to define the boundaries of the hippocampus. A reader might visually include the parahippocampal gyrus gray matter *(large white arrow)* as part of the hippocampus and thus miss the hippocampal atrophy signifying hippocampal sclerosis. Note other findings associated with hippocampal sclerosis, including ipsilateral temporal lobe atrophy and decrease in the diameter of the fornix *(arrowheads)*. (*A* and *B* from Bronen RA, Cheung G, Charles JT, et al: Imaging findings in hippocampal sclerosis: correlation with pathology. AJNR 12[5]:933–940, 1991. © by American Society of Neuroradiology.

ipsilateral temporal horn, and loss of the collateral white matter[7, 24, 56, 70] (see Fig. 22–8). One should interpret these findings with caution because normal asymmetries of these structures occur.[31, 34, 38, 71] Two findings associated with hippocampal sclerosis are thinning of the ipsilateral fornix and mammillary body atrophy[72–73a] (see Figs. 22–9A and 22–10A). Detection of multiple primary and secondary imaging criteria in-

crease diagnostic confidence.* There is no role for contrast-enhanced studies in the detection of hippocampal sclerosis.[74]

MRI has furthered our understanding of hippocampal sclerosis by permitting in vivo detection of this entity and by elucidating its regional and bilateral dis-

---

*References 4, 7, 20, 50, 51, 56, 67, 69.

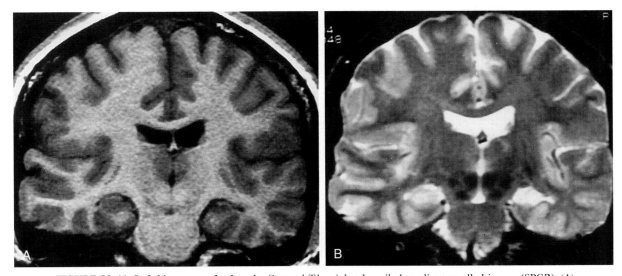

FIGURE 22–11. Left hippocampal sclerosis. Coronal T1-weighted spoiled gradient-recalled image (SPGR) *(A)* and coronal T2-weighted image *(B)*. Because atrophy occurs more frequently than signal changes in hippocampal sclerosis, sequences that optimize gray matter—white matter distinctions such as the SPGR sequence *(A)* are crucial for detecting hippocampal sclerosis. Inversion recovery sequences or FSE T2-weighted images also maximize gray matter–white matter contrast (see Figs. 22–4 and 22–12). The atrophy is best seen in *A*, whereas the signal changes are seen in *B*. (*A* and *B* from Bronen RA: Epilepsy: the role of MR imaging. AJR 159:1165–1174, 1992.)

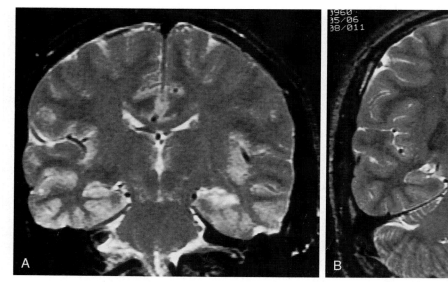

FIGURE 22–12. Left hippocampal sclerosis. Coronal T2-weighted conventional spin-echo *(A)* and FSE *(B)* sequences both demonstrate the hyperintense left hippocampus. Note how much more precisely the FSE sequence localizes the signal changes within the hippocampus. The subiculum is not involved.

tribution. MRI findings indicate that hippocampal sclerosis is not always associated with medically refractory epilepsy as commonly reported. It appears that the medical literature reflects a selection bias in favor of surgically treated cases of intractable epilepsy. Triulzi and associates[75] reported imaging characteristics consistent with hippocampal sclerosis in patients with medically controlled temporal lobe epilepsy; these patients are not surgical candidates and thus will not have histologic confirmation.

The distribution and bilaterality of abnormalities have important implications for surgery if the generator of the seizure is related to MRI findings. MRI abnormalities associated with hippocampal sclerosis affect the entire hippocampus in most patients, but regional involvement (of limited portions of the hippocampus or amygdala) occurs in a substantial number of patients. The most frequently affected region is the hippocampal body (95%), in contrast to the head in 63%, the tail in 75%, and the amygdala in 16%. Detection of regional MRI findings may alter the surgical procedure. For example, if MRI showed abnormalities localized predominantly to the hippocampal tail, the temporal lobectomy may be extended to include this region, although one study implied that good outcomes can be obtained without using this strategy.[7, 62, 76–78a] It is also important to identify bilateral hippocampal sclerosis because patients with symmetric bilateral hippocampal sclerosis may not have as favorable an outcome as those with unilateral hippocampal sclerosis after unilateral temporal lobectomy. Review of autopsy studies indicates that asymmetric bilateral damage (i.e., predominantly unilateral hippocampal sclerosis) occurs in about 80%, symmetric bilateral hippocampal sclerosis occurs in about 10%, and unilateral hippocampal sclerosis occurs in approximately 10%.[8] One MRI study found asymmetric bilateral hippocampal atrophy in 20% and symmetric atrophy in

4% of patients with hippocampal sclerosis. As expected, patients with asymmetric bilateral disease (with a predominant unilateral component of atrophy) all had good outcomes after temporal lobectomy, whereas those with symmetric bilateral atrophy did poorly.[79] However, other investigators found good outcomes after temporal lobectomy in patients with bilateral atrophy.[79a] Another study using T2 relaxometry found evidence for bilateral hippocampal sclerosis in 29% of patients.[51]

Presurgical identification of hippocampal sclerosis has important prognostic and therapeutic significance.[78a] Evidence at MRI of hippocampal sclerosis correlates with an EEG-defined abnormality in 70% to 100% of patients.[54, 63, 80] In patients with a concordant EEG and a lateralizing MR image, a satisfactory postoperative outcome occurs in 97% of cases.[63] When hippocampal atrophy alone is identified by MRI without an EEG-defined focus, there is an 86% positive predictive value for excellent postoperative seizure control.[80] If no MRI abnormality is observed in a surgical candidate, the postoperative success rate for seizure control drops to only 44%.[63, 80]

Although an atrophic hyperintense hippocampus is indicative of hippocampal sclerosis in the correct clinical context, hippocampal atrophy and signal changes can be seen in other disorders. Hippocampal atrophy, usually subtle and bilateral, has been reported in Alzheimer's disease, aging, amnestic syndromes, and schizophrenia.[79, 81, 82] It may be seen in conjunction with diffuse atrophic processes or cerebral hemiatrophy. Hippocampal signal changes may be due to tumors, inflammatory disorders (such as herpes encephalitis or the paraneoplastic syndrome of limbic encephalitis), or infarctions in addition to hippocampal sclerosis.[83] Most of these entities can be distinguished by their clinical presentation in conjunction with imaging findings. Epileptic patients with hippo-

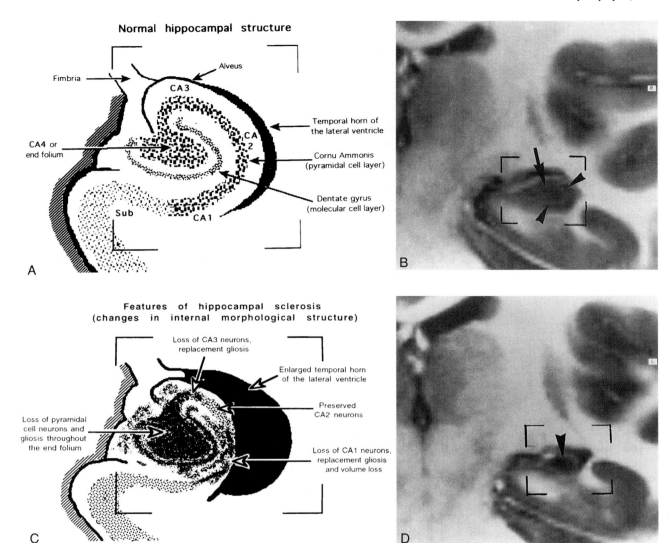

FIGURE 22–13. Coronal internal morphologic characteristics of a normal hippocampus shown diagrammatically *(A)* and with an inversion recovery MRI sequence *(B)*. Observe the alternating gray and white matter within the cornu ammonis and dentate gyrus. This architecture can also be recognized on FSE images (see Fig. 22–6) and in histologic sections (see Fig. 22–7*B*). *C* and *D* show the changes within the hippocampus in a patient with hippocampal sclerosis both diagrammatically and by inversion recovery coronal MRI sequences. The alternating layers of gray and white matter are replaced by a diffuse hypointensity throughout the hippocampus, which is thought to be due to neuronal cell loss and glial proliferation. (*A* to *D* from Jackson GD: New techniques in magnetic resonance and epilepsy. Epilepsia 35[suppl 6]:S2–S13, 1994.)

campal sclerosis or hippocampal tumors may have similar clinical presentations, but MRI can usually predict the correct diagnosis. Unlike the situation with tumors, the signal changes are confined entirely to the hippocampus in hippocampal sclerosis. Hippocampal atrophy is never seen with tumors unless there is concomitant hippocampal sclerosis.[7] Developmental anomalies, such as the hippocampal sulcus remnant, should not be mistaken for tumors or hippocampal sclerosis (Fig. 22–14; see Fig. 22–6). This normal variant is isointense relative to CSF on all pulse sequences, is usually 1 to 2 mm in diameter, is situated between the dentate gyrus and cornu ammonis, and occurs in 10% to 20% of persons. It develops when the hippocampal sulcus does not normally involute medially in utero, resulting in a residual cystic cavity within the hippocampus.[38, 84]

DUAL PATHOLOGY

Dual pathology, the coexistence of hippocampal sclerosis and another lesion, occurs in 8% to 22% of epileptic patients undergoing surgery.[8] This should not be confused with the mild decrease in hippocampal neuronal cell density associated with temporal lobe tumors.[49] These patients are not considered to have dual pathologic conditions because they do not exhibit the axonal reorganization and immunohistochemical abnormalities that are typically seen in hippocampal sclerosis.[85] Patients with dual pathologic conditions commonly have a long history of a seizure disorder beginning at an early age.[8, 86] The preoperative detection of dual pathologic conditions can have a significant impact on surgical planning and outcome, be-

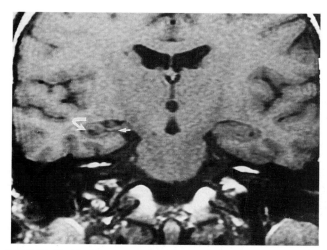

FIGURE 22–14. Hippocampal sulcus remnant. The hippocampal cyst *(curved arrow)* on this T1-weighted coronal image is a normal anatomic variant and should not be confused with a pathologic process. When the medial aspect of the hippocampal sulcus *(straight arrow)* does not obliterate in utero, a residual cavity may persist, as seen bilaterally in this subject. The hippocampal sulcus remnant is isointense relative to CSF on all pulse sequences and is contiguous with the hippocampal sulcus. (Reprinted by permission of the publisher from Bronen RA, Cheung G: MRI of the normal hippocampus. Magn Reson Imaging 9:497–500, 1991. Copyright 1991 by Elsevier Science Inc.)

cause these patients do not respond well to simple lesionectomy.[87]

Several issues must be considered when evaluating MR images. First, the relationship between the MRI abnormality and the epileptogenic zone must be investigated. During a 3-year period, we found multiple abnormalities at MRI in 17% of our epileptic patients treated surgically at Yale. Most additional lesions were incidental findings (such as cysts and nonspecific focal signal abnormalities); thus, the majority of patients did not have two epileptogenic abnormalities or dual pathology. Second, hippocampal sclerosis may not be discovered in patients with dual pathology because many physicians may concentrate on the lesion and not thoroughly assess the hippocampus (Fig. 22–15). For detection of dual pathology, one needs either a high index of suspicion when assessing scans visually or use of quantitative hippocampal data (such as volumetrics or T2 values). Finally, mass lesions arising in the medial temporal lobe may obscure visualization of the hippocampus, making detection of hippocampal sclerosis impossible with MRI.

FOCAL EPILEPTOGENIC LESIONS

The term *focal lesions* or *foreign tissue lesion* has been used in the epilepsy literature to describe a focus of abnormal tissue within brain parenchyma not due to disorders of nonvascular development or hippocampal sclerosis. This term includes neoplasms, vascular malformations, infections, and scarring processes (cicatrix or discrete atrophy).[29]

The incidence of focal lesions is estimated to be 15% to 25% in studies of the general epileptic population as

well as surgically treated epileptic patients.[4, 7, 88, 89] Because up to 90% of patients are seizure free after surgery, the preoperative detection of a focal lesion in a patient with intractable epilepsy is particularly important. However, the detection of lesions in patients without intractable epilepsy is equally important because surgical resection may decrease antiepileptic medications, reduce seizure frequency, alleviate the seizures, or remove a tumor that has the potential to evolve into a malignant neoplasm.[90]

Identification of a focal lesion is predictive of surgical success and an excellent long-term outcome.[89] When the location of a lesion is identical to that of the epileptogenic focus, complete removal of that lesion offers an 82% to 94% chance of a seizure-free outcome.[91, 92] Complete removal correlates with postoperative success based on seizure abatement, reduction of antiepileptic medication, and improvement in psychologic and cognitive performance. Even incomplete lesionectomy can result in a significant rate of seizure-free outcomes (73%).[91, 92] Incomplete resections may act by decreasing the critical epileptogenic mass required for seizure generation or by disrupting electrical pathways required for seizure propagation. If the patient's lesion was remote from the site of epileptogenesis, removal of either the lesion or the epileptogenic zone alone usually results in a less favorable outcome.[93]

Several points need to be emphasized regarding MRI of epileptogenic focal lesions. MRI is effective at detecting and localizing focal lesions with a sensitivity approaching 100%.[2, 20, 24, 94] The Yale experience has been similar, with MRI correctly detecting all 41 neoplastic and vascular lesions in surgically treated epileptic patients during a 3-year period.[29] Epileptogenic focal lesions have a number of features in common. Most lesions are found in the temporal lobe. Because epilepsy is usually a cortical process, these lesions are predominantly cortical or subcortical (Fig. 22–16). In one study, more than 85% of surgical epileptogenic lesions involved either the cortex or the junction of gray matter and white matter.[29] These lesions are usually chronic and benign, as evidenced by lengthy seizure histories. Imaging features supporting their benign nature include the lack of significant mass effect or edema. Because the majority of epileptogenic lesions are present for more than a decade and involve the brain periphery (i.e., cortex), it is not uncommon to discover associated calvarial remodeling[4, 29, 92] (see Fig. 22–16). This is an important caveat to remember because calvarial changes are traditionally thought to be due to lesions outside the brain parenchyma (i.e., extra-axial), yet these lesions are intra-axial.

NEOPLASMS

Brain tumors are responsible for seizures in 2% to 4% of the general epileptic population.[6, 88] In adults with medically intractable epilepsy, the prevalence of neoplasms rises to 10% to 20% and may be even higher in children.[8-10, 12, 24, 95-97] Conversely, 50% to

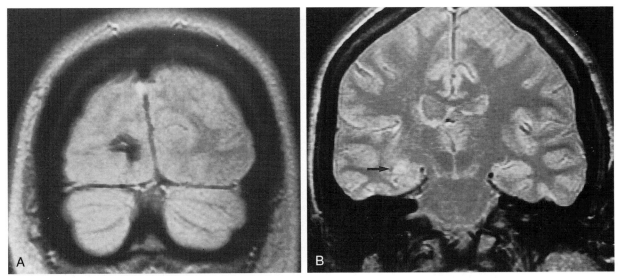

FIGURE 22–15. Dual pathology. *A,* Coronal proton density–weighted image shows a temporal-occipital vascular malformation characterized by signal void surrounding a central region of hyperintensity. *B,* A more anterior image through the temporal lobe reveals subtle hyperintensity in an atrophic right hippocampus *(arrow).* This second abnormality, hippocampal sclerosis, was missed by some observers. This patient underwent epilepsy surgery twice; final diagnosis was hippocampal sclerosis and a thrombosed AVM. The imaging appearance of this thrombosed AVM is identical to that of a cavernous malformation.

76% of patients with cerebral neoplasms present with seizures.[98, 99] In the Montreal series of 230 gliomas, seizures occurred in 92% of oligodendrogliomas, 70% of astrocytomas, and 35% of glioblastomas.[100] The spectrum of neoplastic lesions encountered in a series of patients with surgically treated epilepsy differs from that observed in a conventional neurosurgical tumor series. Epileptogenic lesions include astrocytomas, oligodendrogliomas, mixed tumors, pilocytic astrocytomas, pleomorphic xanthoastrocytomas, gangliogliomas, and dysembryoplastic neuroepithelial tumors. Extra-axial tumors rarely cause epilepsy.

Most patients with epilepsy due to neoplasms have normal neurologic examination results and have had stable epilepsy for at least a decade.[92, 95] The phenomenology and auras produced by neoplastic lesions are indistinguishable from those of other causes, such as hippocampal sclerosis. The seizure characteristics that the patient manifests are usually related to the location of the lesion. Most tumors causing epilepsy are located in the cortex or subcortical regions (91%) of the temporal lobe (70%) and present with partial complex seizures.[29, 92]

Because medically intractable epilepsy is a chronic illness, it is not surprising that most epileptogenic tumors are low-grade neoplasms, and long-term survival is excellent.[89] Slow-growing cortically based, low-grade gliomas causing chronic epilepsy appear to derive from

FIGURE 22–16. Low-grade glioma. T1-weighted *(A)* and T2-weighted *(B)* axial images demonstrate a cystic subcortical lesion. The mass has remodeled the overlying calvaria, a finding usually associated with an extra-axial lesion. Epileptogenic masses frequently cause calvarial remodeling because of their chronicity and peripheral location. *(A* and *B* from Bronen RA: Epilepsy: the role of MR imaging. AJR 159:1165–1174, 1992.)

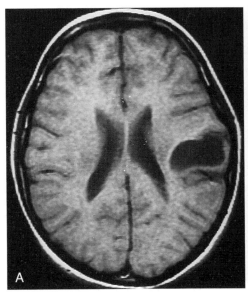
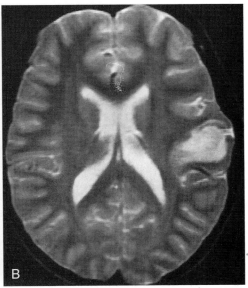

a different astrocytic lineage as compared with white matter–based low-grade gliomas, which have a short (<1 year) period of preoperative symptoms.[101] Patients with chronic epilepsy due to gliomas tend to have a good prognosis regardless of the tumor grade. In one report of 65 patients, the average seizure history was 15 years and only 1 of 65 patients died as a result of their tumor.[92]

Some of the general imaging characteristics of epileptogenic neoplasms have already been mentioned. These lesions are found predominantly within or adjacent to gray matter, have little mass effect or edema, and may produce calvarial remodeling.[4, 7, 92] In a Yale series of 33 epileptogenic tumors, one third demonstrated features of calvarial remodeling[29] (see Fig. 22–16). Although subgroups of tumors usually have characteristic imaging features, these traits may not be sufficiently unique to allow a preoperative histologic diagnosis in an individual case. Similar imaging features are found in many tumors causing epilepsy. A brief discussion of the more common epileptogenic tumors is presented next (see also Chapter 17).

Astrocytomas

Well-differentiated gliomas are the most common epileptogenic neoplasm.[92, 99, 100] The peak incidence of the supratentorial astrocytoma ranges from 20 to 50 years of age. Imaging of low-grade astrocytomas usually demonstrates a well-circumscribed lesion with little mass effect and no edema.[102] Various patterns of contrast enhancement can be observed. Calcification is detected in about 20% of astrocytomas by CT but can be missed by MRI.[103] Hemosiderin has been identified within macrophages adjacent to epileptogenic gliomas

in 25% and may play a role in epileptogenesis.[92, 104] The signal intensity of most low-grade astrocytomas is hypointense relative to gray matter on T1-weighted images and hyperintense on T2-weighted images (see Fig. 22–16).

Oligodendrogliomas

One half of the cases are pure oligodendrogliomas, whereas the other half are mixed tumors, containing an astrocytic component.[105] Imaging of oligodendrogliomas may suggest the diagnosis based on location, a cystic component (20%), patchy enhancement (50%), linear or nodular calcification (30% to 40%), hemorrhage (20%), absence of edema, or calvarial erosion (17%), although none of these findings are specific for this lesion.[106–108] MR signal characteristics of oligodendrogliomas are similar to those of other gliomas, isointense relative to gray matter on T1-weighted images and hyperintense on T2-weighted images. Calcification, hemorrhage, and cystic changes are responsible for the heterogeneous appearance (Fig. 22–17). Gradient-echo sequences are better than spin-echo sequences for the detection of calcification and hemorrhage.[107]

Gangliogliomas

Although gangliogliomas are rare in the general population, they frequently occur in patients with epilepsy.[25] These tumors occur most frequently in the first and second decades of life.[105, 109] Gangliogliomas are often cystic, well circumscribed, and calcified and may contain a mural nodule. The temporal lobes are the most frequent site of involvement, although these tu-

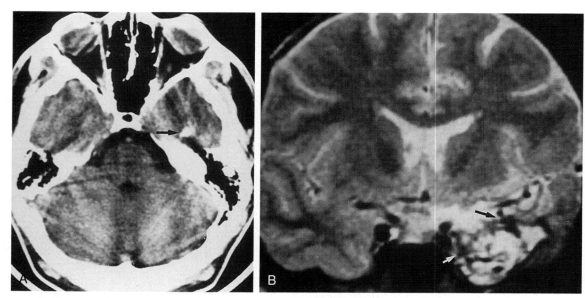

FIGURE 22–17. Mixed glioma. *A,* Beam hardening artifact obscures a large portion of the left temporal lobe mass on this axial CT scan. The region of high attenuation *(arrow)* is suggestive of a calcified lesion such as a glioma, but it could also be artifactual. *B,* Coronal T1-weighted MR image shows a heterogeneous mass much larger than that suspected on the basis of the CT scan. The heterogeneity is due to cystic changes (regions of increased signal intensity), calcification *(black arrow)*, and hemosiderin *(white arrow)*. These are typical findings associated with pure or mixed oligodendrogliomas. This epilepsy patient had a low-grade astrocytoma with oligodendrocytic features. (*A* and *B* from Bronen RA: Epilepsy: the role of MR imaging. AJR 159:1165–1174, 1992.)

mors are found throughout the brain.[105, 109, 110] MRI commonly demonstrates a heterogeneous mass that is predominantly hypointense on T1-weighted images and hyperintense on T2-weighted images[110] (Fig. 22–18). Cystic lesions may show a heterogeneous signal that is slightly hyperintense relative to CSF with all sequences. Most gangliogliomas show some contrast enhancement.[110] Resection of the lesion is considered curative. Postoperatively, most patients are free of seizures and have an excellent long-term survival.[92]

Dysembryoplastic Neuroepithelial Tumors

Dysembryoplastic neuroepithelial tumor is a rare entity described by Daumas and colleagues.[111] These pa-

tients usually present in childhood and have a long seizure history and no focal neurologic deficits. The histologic picture of these lesions is unique and shows astrocytes, oligodendrocytes, and neural elements in an intracortical location and sometimes associated with focal cortical dysplasias. These lesions can be confused histologically with gangliogliomas and oligodendrocytomas. CT often shows a well-circumscribed hypodense lesion without edema that may enhance after contrast medium administration (18%) or calcify (23%) but is normal in 10%.[111] Similar to the situation with other indolent lesions, remodeling of the overlying calvaria may occur. The MRI appearance consists of a focal lobulated cortical mass of low signal intensity on T1-weighted images, high signal intensity on T2-weighted

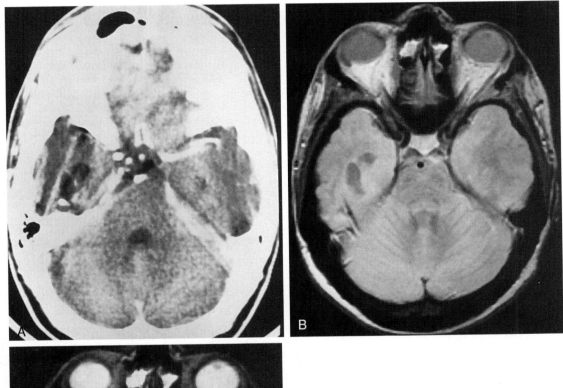

FIGURE 22–18. Ganglioglioma. *A,* Enhanced CT scan shows a hypodense mass with calcification in the right temporal lobe. Proton density–weighted *(B)* and T2-weighted *(C)* axial images reveal this to be a multilobulated lesion, isointense relative to CSF, without associated edema. Calcification and cyst formation are typical of gangliogliomas. Note that the calcification demonstrated by CT is not well seen with MRI. (Reprinted from Magn Reson Imaging, Volume 13, Bronen RA, Fulbright RK, Spencer SS, et al: MR characteristics of neoplasms and vascular malformations associated with epilepsy, Pages 1153–1162, Copyright 1995, with kind permission from Elsevier Science Ltd, The Boulevard, Langford Lane, Kidlington OX5 1GB, UK.)

images without adjacent edema, and a variable signal intensity on the proton density–weighted images[112] (Fig. 22–19). A nodular gyriform thickening has been reported as a feature unique to dysembryoplastic neuroepithelial tumors that may allow one to distinguish them from other glial tumors.[112, 113] Patients have an excellent prognosis after complete or even incomplete surgical excision of these tumors.[114]

VASCULAR MALFORMATIONS

Approximately 5% of epilepsy is caused by a vascular abnormality, usually a cavernous malformation or an AVM.* MRI detects almost all intracranial vascular lesions.[11, 12, 24, 70] We found CT to be less sensitive than MRI. During a 3-year period, CT predicted the correct pathology in only six of eight epileptogenic vascular malformations compared with eight of eight by MRI (see also Chapter 23).[29]

Cavernous Malformation (Cavernous Hemangioma)

Cavernous malformations are large vascular spaces without discrete arteries or veins.[105, 115] These lesions may contain calcification, hemorrhage, or thrombus. Cavernous malformations occur in about 0.5% of the population, affect all age groups, and may be multiple (10% to 40%) or familial.[116] Seizures are the most frequent clinical presentation, particularly in cases of multiple cavernous malformations.[117] Compared with AVMs, cavernous malformations are more likely to cause medically refractory seizures.[116]

Imaging is excellent for detecting vascular malformations, but it cannot reliably differentiate between

*References 6, 10, 24, 25, 70, 88, 95, 96.

cavernous malformations and small partially thrombosed AVMs (Fig. 22–20; see Fig. 22–15). These lesions have similar CT and MRI appearances. They are sometimes labeled as occult vascular malformations because their angiographic appearance is usually normal or "occult," but occasionally a faint blush is seen. CT findings consist of a focal hyperdense enhancing lesion without mass effect or edema that may calcify.[118] MRI is the best imaging modality for diagnosing occult vascular malformations, because CT cannot reliably distinguish these lesions from low-grade neoplasms. Occult vascular malformations have characteristic MRI features.[119] A reticulated hyperintense focus within the center of the lesion is demonstrated, indicative of subacute or chronic hemorrhage. This is surrounded by a rim of signal void, representing paramagnetic hemosiderin from prior hemorrhage. The hemosiderin ring is best seen on gradient-echo or T2-weighted sequences. Initially, this appearance was believed to be pathognomonic for occult vascular malformations, but experience has shown that any hemorrhagic lesion, such as a hemorrhagic metastasis, can have these features.[120] However, a lesion with these characteristics in a patient who has had a seizure will almost always be an occult vascular malformation.[29]

Most seizures caused by cavernous malformations can be controlled medically. Surgical resection is indicated in patients with medically intractable epilepsy and a surgically accessible causative cavernous hemangioma. Surgical excision may eliminate seizures, reduce the frequency and severity of the seizures, or allow tapering of antiepileptic medication.[121]

Arteriovenous Malformation

AVMs are the most common congenital vascular malformations. An AVM consists of a group of vessels that form direct arteriovenous shunts without an in-

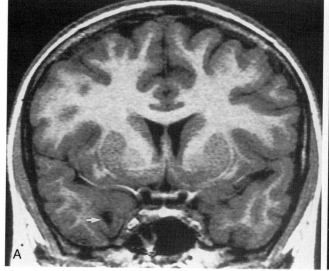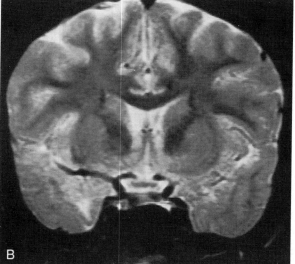

FIGURE 22–19. Dysembryoplastic neuroepithelial tumor. Coronal T1-weighted *(A)* and T2-weighted *(B)* images demonstrate a cystic lesion *(arrow)* in a subcortical location within the right temporal lobe. This lesion is associated with abnormally thickened gray matter medially and superiorly.

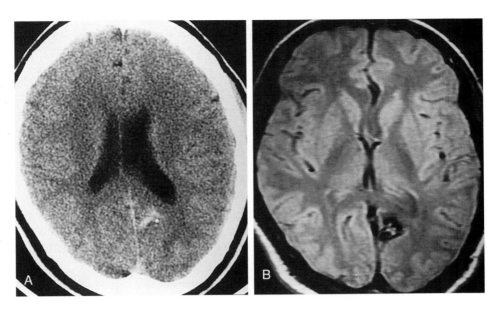

FIGURE 22–20. Cavernous hemangioma. *A,* CT scan shows a focus of calcification without adjacent edema or mass effect. Either a vascular malformation or a tumor could have this appearance. *B,* MR image is typical for an occult vascular malformation and not a tumor. The axial proton density–weighted image shows a central area containing a speckled pattern of high and low signal intensity surrounded by a hypointense rim from hemosiderin with minimal mass effect. (*A* and *B* from Bronen RA: Epilepsy: the role of MR imaging. AJR 159:1165–1174, 1992.)

tervening capillary network. The association of epilepsy with AVMs may be due to 1) focal cerebral ischemia from arteriovenous shunting and steal phenomenon or 2) adjacent hemosiderin deposition and secondary epileptogenesis.[116, 122] Epilepsy is the second most common clinical presentation of AVMs after hemorrhage. The risk of seizure disorder in patients with AVMs varies from 18% to 42%.[123, 124] The risk of developing seizures rises with the size of the lesion, proximity to the cortex, and involvement of the frontal or temporal lobes.[123–125] These malformations have a characteristic angiographic appearance with dilated tortuous arteries entering a nidus and early venous drainage (arteriovenous shunting). AVMs that are difficult to characterize by CT include small AVMs, thrombosed or partially thrombosed AVMs, and AVMs that have hemorrhaged. Although CT and MRI are nearly equal in their ability to detect AVMs, angioarchitectural features are better assessed with MRI. Both T1-weighted and T2-weighted sequences demonstrate a region of serpiginous flow voids that represents the AVM nidus, dilated arterial supply, and draining veins. Interspersed within the signal voids are areas of heterogeneous signal from calcification, hemorrhage, and gliosis.

Improvement in seizure control usually occurs with treatment of an epileptogenic AVM by embolization, radiosurgery, or surgical excision.[116] Although previous reports questioned the efficacy of surgical treatment of AVMs for seizure relief, more recent reports indicate that surgical excision is an effective method of seizure control.[99, 116, 123–126]

INFECTION

Infections are a frequent cause of seizures worldwide, although they are uncommon in the United States. The number of seizures caused by infections in the United States has increased because of the spread of human immunodeficiency virus and increased resistance of infections to antimicrobial therapy. In a study of 630 patients with human immunodeficiency virus infection, 50 of 70 patients with new-onset seizures had an infection as the cause of the seizures.[127] Most infections present as nonspecific ring-enhancing lesions associated with vasogenic edema. Neurocysticercosis and tuberculosis are common causes of epilepsy in Third World countries (see also Chapter 20).

Neurocysticercosis

Neurocysticercosis, caused by the pork parasite *Taenia solium,* is one of the most common causes of epilepsy worldwide, affecting 2% to 4% in endemic populations.[128] Epilepsy is the most frequent sign of neurocysticercosis, possibly because the parasites are found primarily in the gray matter.[129] CT and MRI findings reflect the various locations and stages of cysticercosis (Fig. 22–21). Lesions may occur in the brain parenchyma or meningeal spaces or within the ventricles. In the acute phase, when the parasite is alive and there is little host reaction, a cystic mass lacking significant enhancement or edema may be seen. At this stage MRI is more sensitive than CT and shows a cystic mass, isointense relative to CSF, which contains a hyperintense mural nodule best detected on long-TR, short-TE sequences.[130, 131] The death of the larvae leads to an exuberant host reaction and a fibrous capsule. At this stage, MRI demonstrates a ring-enhancing cystic mass associated with edema. As the host inflammatory response diminishes, lesion enhancement and surrounding edema also decrease. The lesion eventually involutes, leaving normal parenchyma or residual focal calcification best visualized with CT.[131] The cysticidal drugs albendazole and praziquantel are effective in the treatment of neurocysticercosis and improve the prognosis of patients with seizures by decreasing the frequency of seizures or eliminating them.[132]

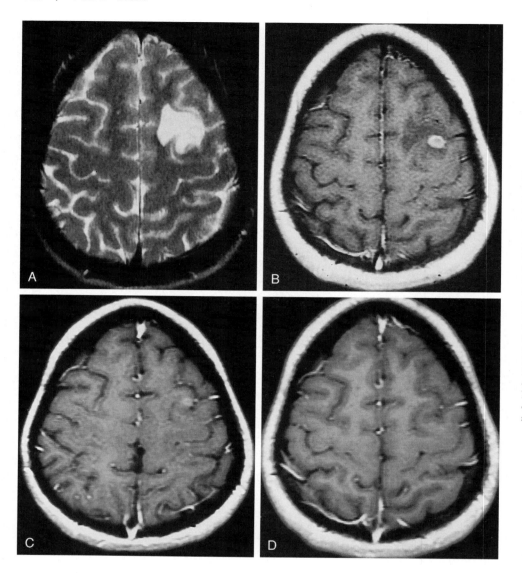

FIGURE 22–21. Cysticercosis. A 30-year-old woman who traveled extensively in Mexico as a teenager presented with seizures. T2-weighted *(A)* and enhanced T1-weighted *(B)* axial images show a ring-enhancing lesion in the left frontal lobe with considerable mass effect and edema. Although the differential diagnosis includes cysticercosis, abscess, primary neoplasm, and metastatic disease, the travel history suggests cysticercosis. *C,* Enhanced MR image after 1 month of treatment with praziquantel shows that the lesion is smaller and has less intense enhancement. The mass effect and edema have also diminished. *D,* Nine months after treatment, the enhanced MR image shows no residual abnormalities.

Tuberculomas

Tuberculomas, although uncommon in the United States, constitute between 10% and 40% of intracranial mass lesions in developing nations.[133–136] Patients with intracranial tuberculomas may present with focal seizures or elevated intracranial pressure but are often otherwise neurologically intact. The CT appearance of parenchymal tuberculomas is nonspecific. They may be solid or ring enhancing and solitary or multiple (10% to 34%).[137] The thickness of ring enhancement and associated edema varies considerably. Calcification is rare, occurring in only 1% to 6% of tuberculomas.[138] The MRI appearance of tuberculomas is also variable, depending on the host's reaction and the amount of macrophages, fibrosis, and gliosis.[139] As these components increase, there is a tendency for granulomas to become more hypointense on T2-weighted sequences.[140] Tuberculomas and adjacent edema are usually hypointense on T1-weighted images. After the intravenous administration of gadolinium, a nodular or ring-like enhancement of the lesion is observed.

Transient Signal Abnormalities

Transient signal abnormalities have been reported in patients with seizures. These may be due to a number of diverse causes, including infections, focal status epilepticus, and Rasmussen's encephalitis. Reports from India and Mexico suggest cysticercosis or tuberculosis as causes. Other reports have found that imaging abnormalities parallel clinical seizure activity. Transient imaging abnormalities may appear in the patient with frequent seizures and thus caution should be exercised when invasive studies are recommended. In these cases, signal changes may reflect focal cerebral edema, although attempts to correlate seizure with MRI changes have not usually been successful.[7, 141–143]

ATROPHIC PROCESSES

Tissue loss, which may be focal or diffuse, is the final common pathway for many processes affecting the central nervous system, including trauma, infarctions, and infections. Most focal atrophic processes associated with epilepsy are the result of trauma. Infarction is the most common cause of seizures in the elderly. Seizures caused by infarction are often self-limited and only rarely progress to a chronic epileptic disorder. Hippocampal sclerosis is a specialized atrophic process that has been discussed. Diffuse atrophic processes, involving large sections of the brain or the entire hemisphere, are usually due to perinatal insults but can be due to entities such as Sturge-Weber syndrome, Rasmussen's encephalitis, or infantile spasms.[144, 145] Diffuse atrophic entities associated with medically refractory epilepsy may be amenable to surgery for palliation, usually in the form of functional hemispherectomy or corpus callosotomy.[144]

TRAUMA

Head trauma has been recognized as a cause of epilepsy for thousands of years.[100] The prevalence of post-traumatic epilepsy is significant because of the large number of head injuries.[146] Fortunately, only a small proportion of patients with head injuries develop post-traumatic epilepsy. Accepted risk factors for the development of late-onset seizures include severe head trauma, especially injuries that pierce the dura; early post-traumatic seizures (seizures occurring within the first week of the event); intracranial hemorrhage; and depressed skull fractures.[147, 148] CT can document post-traumatic hemorrhages such as intracerebral hemorrhages and identify extra-axial collections. Months after the injury, cortical and subcortical atrophy may be detected by CT or MRI.[149]

PERINATAL INSULTS

Perinatal and neonatal causes of epilepsy represent a diverse group of insults rather than a single disease entity and include birth hypoxia, metabolic disorders, infections, and intracranial hemorrhage. Focal, hemispheric, or global injury to the brain may result. Seizure foci arise from viable tissue at the penumbra of the injury site, regions that are hyperintense on long-TR, short-TE images (Fig. 22–22). Areas isointense relative to CSF on all pulse sequences usually represent areas of complete tissue loss or macrocystic changes. The role of MRI is to accurately assess the location and extent of tissue damage in those patients deemed surgical candidates.[150]

STURGE-WEBER SYNDROME

The Sturge-Weber syndrome (encephalotrigeminal angiomatosis) is a neurocutaneous syndrome characterized by the association of a facial capillary angioma with ipsilateral leptoangiomatosis. This disease is believed to be due to persistence of embryonic vasculature.[151] The clinical hallmarks of the disease are unilateral cutaneous facial nevus, epilepsy, retardation, hemiplegia, and ocular abnormalities. Like other neurocutaneous syndromes, there is wide variability in the clinical manifestations of the disease. Epilepsy is the most common and usually the first neurologic manifestation of this disorder.

CT and MRI findings in Sturge-Weber syndrome usually include hemiatrophy, cortical calcification, choroid plexus calcification, and enhancement of the pial angioma (Fig. 22–23). Unilateral cerebral atrophy is

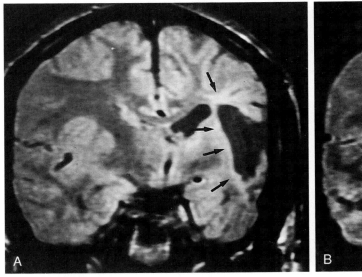
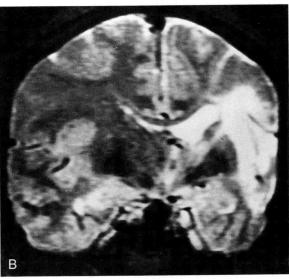

FIGURE 22–22. Diffuse atrophic process. Coronal proton density–weighted *(A)* and T2-weighted *(B)* images demonstrate a small left cerebral hemisphere with focal tissue loss adjacent to the sylvian fissure. The findings are consistent with a perinatal middle cerebral artery infarction. The vague hyperintense rim *(arrows)* surrounding the complete tissue loss represents gliosis in the penumbra. It is in this partially viable tissue of the penumbra that multifocal seizure generation occurs. (*A* and *B* from Bronen RA: Epilepsy: the role of MR imaging. AJR 159:1165–1174, 1992.)

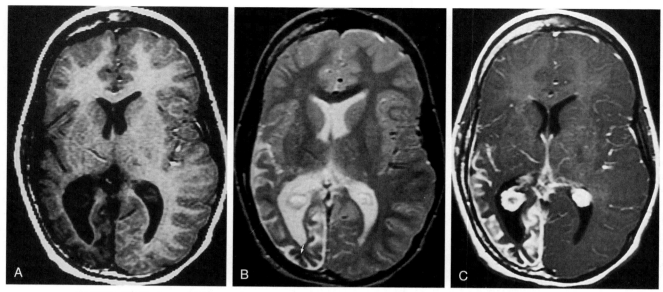

FIGURE 22–23. Sturge-Weber syndrome. *A,* T1-weighted axial image demonstrates right hemiatrophy with focal parieto-occipital volume loss and enlargement of the adjacent lateral ventricle. *B,* Gyriform hypointensity *(arrow)* is seen on the T2-weighted image, indicative of dystrophic calcification or hemosiderin. *C,* Enhanced T1-weighted image shows the classic pial-meningeal enhancement and ipsilateral enlargement of the ipsilateral choroid plexus.

frequently accompanied by secondary changes, such as thickening of the ipsilateral hemicranium, frontal sinus enlargement, and petrous bone enlargement. The cortical calcification has been described as serpiginous, gyriform, or "tram track"–like and is commonly found in the parietal and occipital lobes. Although these findings are all part of the spectrum of Sturge-Weber syndrome, prominent enhancement of the pial angioma (adjacent to cerebral atrophy) and the ipsilateral choroid plexus on contrast MRI is often crucial in making the diagnosis (see also Chapter 16).[152–154]

RASMUSSEN'S ENCEPHALITIS

The hallmark of Rasmussen's (chronic) encephalitis (epilepsia partialis continua) is intractable epilepsy beginning in childhood and leading to severe neurologic and mental impairment. Antecedent history of an infectious or inflammatory episode involving the patient or a family member is present in two thirds of cases.[155] Patients commonly develop medically refractory epilepsy, hemiparesis, dysphasia, and hemianopsia. Although the disease is self-limited and rarely fatal, only 10% of patients are left with no permanent neurologic sequelae.[156] Rasmussen's encephalitis tends to localize in one hemisphere but can present with bilateral involvement.[156] Although the cause of this disorder is unknown, early microscopic changes parallel those identified in viral infections. Other research raises the possibility that autoantibodies to a glutamate receptor, which is an excitatory neurotransmitter, may increase neuronal excitation and lead to seizures.[157]

At the onset of symptoms, CT and MRI findings are often normal.[156] CT scans obtained later in the course of the disease show marked unihemispheric

atrophy with ipsilateral ventriculomegaly. Some atrophic changes may be seen in the contralateral hemisphere, although these may be on the basis of the chronic anoxia and the trauma of the seizures.[16] MRI experience with Rasmussen's encephalitis is limited. During the acute stage, we have seen hyperintense signal foci on long-TR images that change in size and location over time. In the chronic stage, T2-weighted images demonstrate significant unilateral atrophic changes and signal hyperintensity in the periventricular region and basal ganglia that may represent edema[156, 158] (Fig. 22–24). Rasmussen's encephalitis is often refractory to medical treatment. Hemispherectomy may be necessary to gain control over the seizures.

NONVASCULAR DEVELOPMENTAL ABNORMALITIES

Nonvascular developmental abnormalities are often associated with seizure disorders but were frequently unrecognized before the MRI era.[159–163] These anomalies can be classified into three categories based on their MRI appearance, although there is some overlap: 1) focal lesions, 2) unilateral disorders, and 3) generalized or bilateral abnormalities (Table 22–4). The recognition, localization, and classification of these anomalies have important prognostic and therapeutic implications.[159, 160] The type of developmental anomaly may influence surgical treatment. For example, patients with epilepsy with the congenital bilateral perisylvian syndrome appear to derive benefit from corpus callosotomy rather than resective surgery.[160]

Focal developmental disorders are sometimes described as "cortical dysplasia" in the literature. One

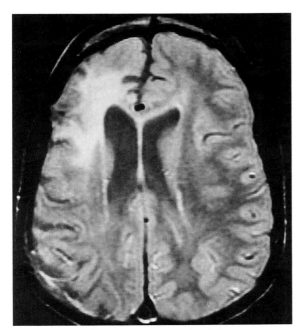

FIGURE 22–24. Rasmussen's encephalitis. This child had chronic persistent seizures for many years. A proton density–weighted axial image shows hyperintensity throughout the white matter of the right frontal lobe. In patients with long-standing Rasmussen's encephalitis, there is often hemispheric volume loss, as seen in this case.

should be careful not to mistake the cortical developmental disorder or MRI cortical dysplasia for the pathologic entity known as focal cortical dysplasia described by Taylor and coworkers.[164] Focal cortical dysplasia of Taylor is part of the spectrum of disorders found within the MRI category of cortical dysplasia. A better general term for the cortical abnormalities found by MRI is *cortical developmental disorder*. Other focal developmental disorders include polymicrogyria,

TABLE 22–4. DEVELOPMENTAL DISORDERS CAUSING SEIZURES

FOCAL*

Focal cortical dysplasia of Taylor
Tuberous sclerosis
Polymicrogyria (congenital bilateral perisylvian fissure syndrome)
Schizencephaly
Focal subcortical heterotopia
Temporal lobe encephalocele

GENERALIZED

Lissencephaly (agyria)
Pachygyria
Band heterotopia (double cortex syndrome)
Subependymal heterotopia

UNILATERAL

Hemimegalencephaly
Sturge-Weber syndrome

*Although these disorders may be solitary, they frequently present as bilateral or multiple focal anomalies. Focal developmental disorders or cortical migration disorders are sometimes termed *cortical dysplasia*. This includes the pathologic entity focal cortical dysplasia of Taylor, but these terms are not synonymous.

schizencephaly, focal subcortical heterotopia, and tuberous sclerosis. These lesions may also be bilateral or multiple (see also Chapter 16).

FOCAL CORTICAL DYSPLASIA OF TAYLOR

Focal cortical dysplasia of Taylor and its variants encompass a wide spectrum of abnormalities that range from mild cortical disruption without abnormal cellular elements to severe abnormalities with marked cortical dyslamination and many bizarre cellular elements.[164] These lesions are thought to be among the most epileptogenic lesions associated with epilepsy.[165] They can be unifocal or multifocal. Focal cortical dysplasias often occur in the precentral, central, and insular regions.[165] Severe multifocal cortical dysplasia can be difficult to differentiate from hemimegalencephaly and from cortical tubers in tuberous sclerosis. Clinical symptoms relate to the location of the lesion or the associated medically refractory epilepsy.[166]

MRI findings include increased cortical thickness, poor gray matter–white matter differentiation, and a shallow abnormal gyral-sulcal pattern[163, 167] (Fig. 22–25). Some lesions, particularly those with more severe architectural distortion, demonstrate increased signal intensity in the adjacent subcortical white matter on long-TR pulse sequences.[165] The imaging-defined abnormality may underestimate the extent of the histologic abnormality. Mild or microscopic cortical disorganization may be undetectable by MRI using current techniques.[165]

TUBEROUS SCLEROSIS AND HAMARTOMAS

Tuberous sclerosis (Bourneville's disease) is an autosomal dominant multisystem disorder with high pen-

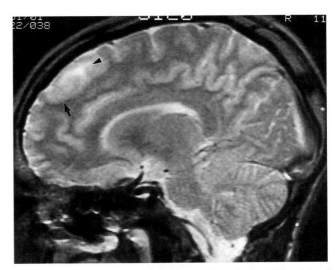

FIGURE 22–25. Cortical dysplasia of Taylor. Sagittal T2-weighted image demonstrates a focal abnormality in the frontal lobe. There is a hyperintense signal *(arrowhead)* in the subcortical white matter associated with cortical thickening *(arrow)*. On an adjacent slice (not shown), a linear signal abnormality was seen extending medially from the lesion toward the ventricle (similar to findings occurring in tuberous sclerosis). The cortex medial to the signal abnormality is thinned, and the remainder of the adjacent cortex demonstrates architectural distortion.

etrance, variable expression, and a prevalence of up to 1 in 10,000.[168, 169] The primary abnormality is a disorder of cell migration, proliferation, and differentiation that leads to the formation of hamartomas. The classic clinical triad of papular facial nevus (adenoma sebaceum), seizures, and mental retardation is found in less than half of patients, although myoclonic seizures and mental retardation are common.[169, 170] Because of the protean clinical manifestations of tuberous sclerosis, MRI can be invaluable in establishing the diagnosis.[171] Some authors believe that the number and location of imaging-defined brain abnormalities correlate with the frequency of seizure activity and the patient's intelligence.[172]

The cortical tuber or hamartoma is the hallmark of tuberous sclerosis. A hamartoma is a mass of disorganized but mature cells indigenous to that part of the brain. The term designates a tumor-like but non-neoplastic formation or an error in tissue development.[105] Hamartomas that cause epilepsy can be seen in isolation, not associated with tuberous sclerosis. The cortical hamartoma of tuberous sclerosis is similar to focal cortical dysplasia of Taylor both histologically and by MRI characteristics (Fig. 22–26). In fact, the pathologic description for cortical dysplasia of Taylor has been forme fruste tuberous sclerosis. Other intracranial abnormalities observed with tuberous sclerosis include white matter abnormalities and subependymal giant cell astrocytomas.

POLYMICROGYRYIA

Polymicrogyria is a term used to describe abnormal secondary gyri. The clinical manifestations depend on

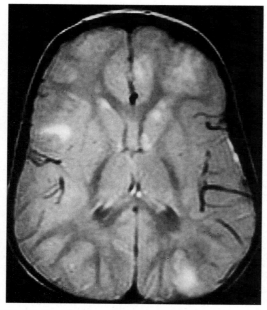

FIGURE 22–26. Tuberous sclerosis. An axial proton density–weighted image demonstrates multiple subcortical and periventricular subependymal foci of high signal intensity without significant mass effect. The multiplicity of the lesions suggests the correct diagnosis—multiple hamartomas in a patient with tuberous sclerosis. However, if there is a single lesion, differentiation from a glioma or cortical dysplasia of Taylor may be impossible. (From Bronen RA: Epilepsy: the role of MR imaging. AJR 159:1165–1174, 1992.)

the amount and location of involved brain. Patients commonly present with developmental delay and seizures. Patients with severe cases may have hypotonia and microcephaly.[163, 170]

MRI of polymicrogyria may demonstrate paradoxical smoothing of the brain surface. The cortex may be slightly thickened, although usually less so than with pachygyria. The inner surface of the cortex adjacent to the white matter is smooth, lacking the normal interdigitations. Long-TR images occasionally demonstrate increased signal intensity in the subcortical white matter adjacent to the polymicrogyral cortex.

Kuzniecky and colleagues have described a constellation of clinical and imaging findings due to polymicrogyria—the congenital bilateral perisylvian syndrome.[159, 167, 170] These patients have congenital pseudobulbar palsy, intellectual delay, and epilepsy that is intractable in 50%. The characteristic feature of this syndrome is abnormal development of the sylvian fissures and adjacent opercular regions bilaterally (Fig. 22–27). The sylvian fissures are abnormally long, extending to the vertex of the brain. The gray matter of the opercula lining the sylvian fissure is abnormally thick. Patients with congenital bilateral perisylvian syndrome and epilepsy may obtain significant seizure relief from corpus callosotomy.

SCHIZENCEPHALY

Schizencephaly describes a gray matter–lined cleft extending from the lateral ventricle through the cortex to the pia.[173] Two subtypes of schizencephaly are recognized. The closed lip or type I cleft occurs when the walls of the cleft are in apposition, whereas the open lip or type II cleft occurs when the walls are separated. The gray matter lining the cleft is usually polymicrogyric; the adjacent cortex may be normal or polymicrogyric. These lesions are believed to be due to in utero vascular injuries and thus are usually unilateral, involving the frontoparietal distribution of the middle cerebral artery. The clinical condition of the patient is dictated by the severity, location, and presence or absence of bilaterality.[174] Patients with bilateral schizencephaly often have severe developmental delay, severe motor dysfunction, and intractable seizures presenting in childhood. Patients with unilateral schizencephaly usually have a better prognosis and present with mild developmental delay, intellectual impairment, and focal motor seizures (see Figs. 16–41 and 16–42).[175]

HETEROTOPIA

Heterotopia is ectopic gray matter or gray matter in an abnormal location (Fig. 22–28). It is caused by an arrest or problem in the migration of primitive neuroblasts en route to the cortex from their periventricular origin. Heterotopias may occur focally or diffusely and may be subependymal or subcortical.[162, 175a]

Subependymal heterotopias can range from small nodular collections of neurons to a continuous layer of neurons lining the ependyma. Barkovich and Kjos[176]

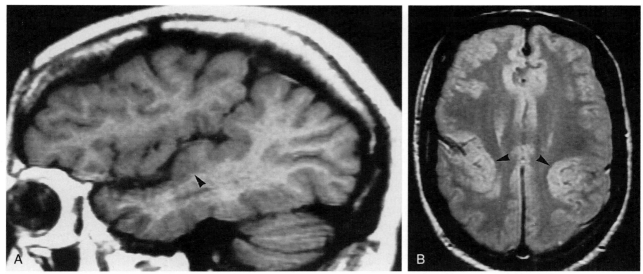

FIGURE 22–27. Congenital bilateral perisylvian syndrome. *A,* Sagittal T1-weighted images show the sylvian fissure extending to the vertex *(arrowhead).* This abnormality is characteristic of the congenital bilateral perisylvian syndrome. *B,* Axial proton density–weighted image shows a markedly thickened opercular cortex *(arrowheads)* around the sylvian fissure due to polymicrogyria.

have reported that 90% of patients with this form of heterotopia have diffuse involvement of the subependyma. These patients often have mild developmental delay and normal neurologic examinations and do not present with seizures until the second decade of life.[176] The seizures in these patients are often amenable to medical therapy.[170]

Subcortical heterotopias have a range of clinical, pathologic, and imaging presentations, depending on the location and severity of the underlying lesion and concomitant abnormalities in the cerebral cortex.[170] Patients may be normal or may present with developmental delay accompanied by focal or generalized seizures. Heterotopias are always isointense relative to gray matter on all MRI pulse sequences and demonstrate no contrast enhancement.[163, 177]

Band heterotopia, or double cortex syndrome, is an

anomaly of the central nervous system associated with mild to moderate mental retardation, epilepsy, and behavioral problems; it has been reported only in females. MRI reveals a bilateral band of gray matter between the lateral ventricle and cortex, separated by white matter. This laminar form of heterotopia is distinctive, and its recognition has important therapeutic implications. These patients often have medically intractable epilepsy that several authors believe is ameliorated by corpus callosotomy.[178, 179]

LISSENCEPHALY AND PACHYGYRIA

Lissencephaly, or complete lack of gyral formation, is an uncommon severe migrational disorder. Medically refractory seizures often develop within the first

FIGURE 22–28. Heterotopia. Axial T1-weighted *(A)* and T2-weighted *(B)* images demonstrate gray matter lining the ventricular surface *(arrowheads),* giving it a nodular appearance. The signal intensity is isointense relative to gray matter on all pulse sequences and it does not enhance with administration of contrast medium (not shown), confirming the diagnosis. Note the cortical migrational disorder (probably representing polymicrogyria) in the overlying cortex *(arrow).*

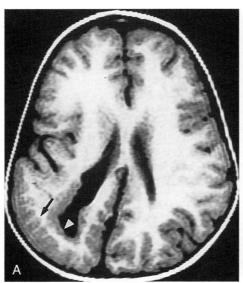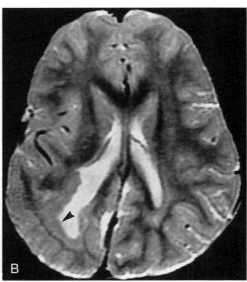

year of life in these severely retarded and hypotonic patients.[180] MRI in children with type I lissencephaly reveals a thickened smooth cortex with shallow, smooth open vertical sylvian fissures resulting in a characteristic figure-eight appearance of the brain. A second form of lissencephaly, type II or Walker's lissencephaly, has a different MRI appearance consisting of hydrocephalus, hypomyelination of the white matter, and thickening of the cortex. Medical and surgical management of seizures in patients with these disorders is often ineffective.

Pachygyria is considered a less severe form of lissencephaly. Instead of agyria there is a paucity of gyri, which are thickened.[181] Compared with lissencephaly, patients with pachygyria have less severe clinical neurologic dysfunction, although developmental delay, microcephaly, and seizures are common. The MRI hallmark of pachygyria is a broad, thick cerebral cortex with shallow sulci, usually regionalized without the global dysmorphism as seen in lissencephaly (see Figs. 16–37 and 16–38).

HEMIMEGALENCEPHALY

Hemimegalencephaly, or unilateral megalencephaly, describes an uncommon entity of hamartomatous overgrowth of all or a portion of a cerebral hemisphere.[182] This disorder is often associated with abnormalities of neuronal migration and cortical sulcation, including heterotopias, pachygyria, polymicrogyria, and agyria.[170]

Clinically, these patients often present in the first 6 months of life with medically refractory seizures.[183] The seizures are often unilateral but may have secondary generalization. Most patients have severe developmental delay or mental retardation, although cases of near-normal intellectual development and neurologic function exist.[183] Unilateral hemiparesis and hemianopsia are common; less frequent findings include macrocephaly and unilateral somatic hemihypertrophy.

MR images are virtually pathognomonic for this disorder, typified by unilateral enlargement of all or part of a hemisphere associated with ipsilateral ventriculomegaly (Fig. 22–29). There is a paucity of normal-appearing white matter, and much of the identified white matter has abnormal signal characteristics. Cortical abnormalities such as pachygyria and polymicrogyria are frequently present. Imaging recognition of this syndrome in conjunction with the patient's clinical condition often directs therapy. Hemispherectomy may be performed in patients with severe motor deficits. Focal cortical resection of an MRI- and EEG-defined abnormality area can be performed in patients with mild neurologic symptoms.[165]

IMAGING PARAMETERS AND THE APPROACH

Although MRI protocols for epilepsy vary widely, they must be able to detect hippocampal sclerosis as

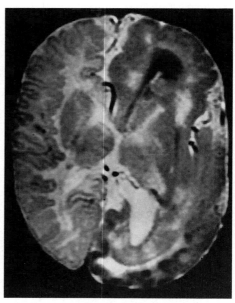

FIGURE 22–29. Hemimegalencephaly. T2-weighted image shows unilateral enlargement of the left cerebral hemisphere with heterotopic gray matter and abnormal sulcation of the cortex in this 4-month-old infant. The ipsilateral lateral ventricle appears enlarged and there is a paucity of normal white matter. These features are characteristic of hemimegalencephaly.

well as focal epileptogenic lesions and developmental disorders.[7, 20, 40, 54, 184, 185] For optimal evaluation of hippocampal sclerosis, imaging is best obtained orthogonal to the long axis of the hippocampus in the coronal oblique plane. MRI of hippocampal sclerosis requires evaluation of both morphologic and signal abnormalities. T1-weighted sequences, such as inversion recovery or three-dimensional SPGR, best depict structural abnormalities and focal volume loss, although some advocate FSE T2-weighted sequences.[54, 186] Coronal SPGR sequences provide not only excellent gray matter–white matter differentiation but also thin slices (1.0 to 3.0 mm thick), which may improve the detection of subtle asymmetries of hippocampal size and help account for head rotation. This sequence is also invaluable for recognizing subtle migrational abnormalities.[186a] Coronal inversion recovery sequences are touted for superior contrast resolution, which allows direct inspection of the internal architecture within the hippocampus.[40] T2-weighted images assess for signal abnormalities. Some authors advocate conventional spin-echo T2-weighted imaging as more sensitive to hippocampal signal changes, whereas other authors rely on FSE T2-weighted imaging[54, 186] (see Fig. 22–12). We find long-TR imaging sequences in the axial and coronal planes to be the most useful for detecting focal epileptogenic lesions. Fluid-attenuated inversion recovery (FLAIR) imaging has been reported to increase the yield for detecting abnormalities missed by conventional spin-echo sequences.[185, 187] MRI with contrast enhancement has little value in the routine imaging of patients with epilepsy but is useful in selected cases.[23, 154, 188] Once a lesion is detected by MRI, contrast enhancement may increase diagnostic confidence, improve delineation of a lesion, assist in differentiating between aggressive and nonaggressive lesions, and help direct lesion biopsy. Contrast enhancement is also helpful in Sturge-Weber syndrome because it can distinguish this entity from other forms of epilepsy-associated hemiatrophy (see Fig. 22–23). In patients who have undergone surgery for resection of an enhancing lesion, enhanced imaging is important during follow-up studies to monitor for residual or recurrent disease.

Although the correct imaging sequences are vital for successful interpretation, it is essential that a systematic approach is used to review scans because of the subtle nature of many epileptogenic lesions. At our institution we routinely assess the images for the following: 1) symmetry of hippocampal size and signal intensity in the coronal plane for hippocampal sclerosis (we account for head rotation by evaluating symmetry of the internal auditory canals and the atria of the lateral ventricles[35]); 2) the periventricular regions of the lateral ventricles for heterotopia (there is never gray matter superior to the caudate nucleus or inferior or lateral to the temporal horn); 3) cortex for thickening due to cortical migration anomalies; 4) subtle cortical signal changes indicative of peripheral tumors, vascular malformations, or developmental disorders; 5) the inferior aspect of the temporal poles for encephaloceles[189]; 6) focal or diffuse areas of volume loss to detect the atrophic disorders; and 7) the obvious lesion or mass, because the obvious lesion may not be the only source of the seizures or it may be incidental (we do not want to miss dual pathology cases with concurrent hippocampal sclerosis). Every epilepsy patient study is reviewed using this seven-step approach, which can increase observer sensitivity (Bronen R, unpublished data).

FUTURE TRENDS

Advances in MRI will continue to enhance our understanding and evaluation of epilepsy. Current research includes improving imaging resolution (by use of phased-array surface coils or high-field [4.0 T] magnets), MR spectroscopy, functional MRI (FMRI) for ictal imaging or mapping brain function adjacent to an epileptogenic focus, and diffusion-weighted imaging. Studies of MR spectroscopy in patients with temporal lobe epilepsy have shown a reduction in N-acetyl aspartate, which is a marker for neuronal cell mass, and an increase in compounds containing creatine plus phosphocreatine and choline (which may be markers for gliosis) on the ipsilateral side. Other compounds important in epilepsy that can be detected by spectroscopy include intracellular pH, lactate, free fatty acids, γ-aminobutyric acid, and glutamate.[50, 190, 191] Diffusion-weighted imaging has detected changes in the path length of water diffusion in the rat during status epilepticus. This technology may prove useful for mapping recent intense seizure activity in humans as well.[192]

FMRI uses fast MRI techniques to detect brain activity, which can be coregistered to conventional MR images for exquisite anatomic localization. This technique exploits the differences in the magnetic susceptibility of oxyhemoglobin and deoxyhemoglobin for measurement of regional blood flow, which is related to brain activity. The most promising use of FMRI for epilepsy involves mapping the function of the brain adjacent to an epileptogenic focus for surgical planning.[193] Investigations of motor, sensory, and cognitive testing are already under way.[194] Another potential use of FMRI is in the dynamic detection of seizure foci. Jackson and associates[195] have shown that FMRI can detect cortical activation occurring during partial motor seizures before clinical seizure activity. The spread of the seizure was imaged dynamically from its focal origin to the remainder of the brain.[195] FMRI has the potential to replace other forms of functional testing, such as intracarotid artery amobarbital (Amytal) testing for memory and speech and perhaps interictal SPECT imaging.

REFERENCES

1. Glaser G: Historical perspectives and future directions. In: Wyllie E, ed. The Treatment of Epilepsy: Principles and Practice. Philadelphia: Lea & Febiger, 1993, pp 3–9.
2. Sperling MR, Wilson G, Engel JJ, et al: Magnetic resonance imaging in intractable partial epilepsy: correlative studies. Ann Neurol 20:57–62, 1986.
3. Hauser W, Annegers J, Kurland L: Prevalence of epilepsy in Rochester, 73Minnesota 1940–1980. Epilepsia 32:429–445, 1990.
4. Bronen RA: Evaluation of the seizure patient. In: Huckman MS, ed. American Roentgen Ray Society Neuroradiology Categorical Course Syllabus. Orlando, FL: American Roentgen Ray Society, 1992, pp 147–158.
5. Niedermeyer E: The Epilepsies. Diagnosis and Management. Baltimore: Urban & Schwarzenberg, 1990, pp 85–108.
6. Hauser WA, Annegers JF: Risk factors for epilepsy. Epilepsy Res Suppl 4:45–52, 1991.
7. Bronen RA: Epilepsy: the role of MR imaging. AJR 159:1165–1174, 1992.
8. Babb TL, Brown WJ: Pathological findings in epilepsy. In: Engel JJ, ed. Surgical Treatment of the Epilepsies. New York: Raven Press, 1987, pp 511–540.
9. Currie S, Heathfield KWG, Henson RA, Scott DF: Clinical course and prognosis of temporal lobe epilepsy. Survey of 666 patients. Brain 94:173–190, 1971.
10. Bruton CJ: The Neuropathology of Temporal Lobe Epilepsy. Oxford, Oxford University Press, 1988.
11. Dowd CF, Dillon WP, Barbaro NM, Laxer KD: Magnetic resonance imaging of intractable complex partial seizures: pathologic and electroencephalographic correlation. Epilepsia 32:454–459, 1991.
12. Duncan JS, Sagar HJ: Seizure characteristics, pathology, and outcome after temporal lobectomy. Neurology 37:405–409, 1987.
13. Keränen T, Sillanpää M, Riekkinen PJ: Distribution of seizure types in an epileptic population. Epilepsia 29:1–7, 1988.
14. Wyllie E, Lüders H: Classification of seizures. In: Wyllie E, ed. The Treatment of Epilepsy: Principles and Practice. Philadelphia: Lea & Febiger, 1993, pp 359–368.
15. Spencer SS: Surgical options for uncontrolled epilepsy. Neurol Clin 4:669–695, 1986.
16. Engell JJ, Shewon D: Who should be considered a surgical candidate? In: Engel JJ, ed. Surgical Treatment of the Epilepsies. New York: Raven Press, 1993, pp 23–34.
17. Taylor D: Epilepsy as a chronic sickness: remediating its impact. In: Engle JJ, ed. Surgical Treatment of the Epilepsies. New York: Raven Press, 1993, pp 11–22.
18. Hauser W: The natural history of temporal lobe epilepsy. In: Lüders HO, ed. Epilepsy Surgery. New York: Raven Press, 1992, pp 133–141.
19. Klennerman P, Sander J, Shorvon S: Mortality in patients with epilepsy. J Neurol Neurosurg Psychiatry 56:149–152, 1993.
20. Jack CR: Epilepsy: surgery and imaging. Radiology 189:635–646, 1993.
21. Spencer SS, Katz A: Arriving at the surgical options for intractable seizures. Semin Neurol 10:422–430, 1990.
22. Lüders H, Awad I: Conceptual considerations. In: Lüders HO, ed. Epilepsy Surgery. New York: Raven Press, 1992, pp 52–62.
23. Cascino GD, Jack CJ, Hirschorn KA, Sharbrough FW: Identification of

the epileptic focus: magnetic resonance imaging. Epilepsy Res Suppl 5:95–100, 1992. Review.

24. Kuznicky R, de la Sayette V, Ethier R, et al: Magnetic resonance imaging in temporal lobe epilepsy: pathological correlations. Ann Neurol 22:341–347, 1987.

25. Wolf HK, Campos MG, Zentner J, et al: Surgical pathology of temporal lobe epilepsy. Experience with 216 cases. J Neuropathol Exp Neurol 52:499–506, 1993.

26. Spencer SS: The relative contributions of MRI, SPECT, and PET imaging in epilepsy. Epilepsia 35(suppl 6):S72–S89, 1994.

27. Spencer SS, Spencer DD, Schwartz SS: The treatment of epilepsy with surgery. Merritt-Putnam Q 5:3–17, 1988.

28. Van Buren JM: Complications of surgical procedures in the diagnosis and treatment of epilepsy. In: Engel JJ, ed. Surgical Treatment of the Epilepsies. New York: Raven Press, 1987, pp 465–475.

29. Bronen R, Fulbright R, Spencer D, et al: MR characteristics of neoplasms and vascular malformations associated with epilepsy. Magn Reson Imaging, in press.

30. Kim J, Kraemer D, Spencer D: The neuropathology of epilepsy. In: Hopkins A, Shorvon S, Cascino G, eds. Epilepsy. London: Chapman & Hall, 1995, pp 243–267.

31. Bronen R, Cheung G: MRI of the temporal lobe: normal variations with special reference toward epilepsy. Magn Reson Imaging 9:501–507, 1991.

32. Bronen RA: Hippocampal and limbic terminology. AJNR 13:943–945, 1992.

33. Duvernoy HM: The Human Hippocampus. An Atlas of Applied Anatomy. Munich: JF Bergmann, 1988.

34. Bronen RA: Anatomy of the temporal lobe. In: Spencer SS, Spencer DD, eds. Surgery for Epilepsy. Boston: Blackwell Scientific Publications, 1991, pp 103–118.

35. Bronen RA, Cheung G: Relationship of hippocampal and amygdala to coronal MRI landmarks. Magn Reson Imaging 9:449–457, 1991.

36. Naidich TP, Daniels DL, Haughton VM, et al: Hippocampal formation and related structures of the limbic lobe: anatomic-MR correlation. Part I. Surface features and coronal sections. Radiology 162:747–754, 1987.

37. Naidich TP, Daniels DL, Haughton VM, et al: Hippocampal formation and related structures of the limbic lobe: anatomic-MR correlation. Part II. Sagittal sections. Radiology 162:755–761, 1987.

38. Bronen RA, Cheung G: MRI of the normal hippocampus. Magn Reson Imaging 9:497–500, 1991.

39. Watson C, Andermann F, Gloor P, et al: Anatomic basis of amygdaloid and hippocampal volume measurement by magnetic resonance imaging. Neurology 42:1743–1750, 1992.

40. Jackson GD, Berkovic SF, Duncan JS, Connelly A: Optimizing the diagnosis of hippocampal sclerosis using MR imaging. AJNR 14:753–762, 1993.

41. Falconer MA, Serafetinides EA, Corsellis JAN: Etiology and pathogenesis of temporal lobe epilepsy. Arch Neurol 10:233–248, 1964.

42. Babb TL, Lieb JP, Brown WJ, et al: Distribution of pyramidal cell density and hyperexcitability in the epileptic human hippocampal formation. Epilepsia 25:721–728, 1984.

43. De Lanerolle NC, Brines ML, Kim JH, et al: Neurochemical remodelling of the hippocampus in human temporal lobe epilepsy. Epilepsy Res Suppl 9:205–219, 1992.

44. Weiser H, Engel JJ, Williamson P, et al: Surgically remediable temporal lobe syndromes. In: Engel JJ, ed. Surgical Treatment of the Epilepsies. New York: Raven Press, 1993, pp 49–63.

45. Grattan SJ, Harvey AS, Desmond PM, Chow CW: Hippocampal sclerosis in children with intractable temporal lobe epilepsy: detection with MR imaging. AJR 161:1045–1048, 1993.

46. Kuznicky R, Murro A, King D, et al: Magnetic resonance imaging in childhood intractable partial epilepsies: pathologic correlations. Neurology 43:681–687, 1993.

47. Kuks JB, Cook MJ, Fish DR, et al: Hippocampal sclerosis in epilepsy and childhood febrile seizures. Lancet 342:1391–1394, 1993.

48. Lévesque MF, Nakasato N, Vinters HV, Babb TL: Surgical treatment of limbic epilepsy associated with extrahippocampal lesions: the problem of dual pathology. J Neurosurg 75:364–370, 1991.

49. Kim JH, Guimaraes PO, Shen MY, et al: Hippocampal neuronal density in temporal lobe epilepsy with and without gliomas. Acta Neuropathol 80:41–45, 1990.

50. Jackson GD: New techniques in magnetic resonance and epilepsy. Epilepsia 35(suppl 6): S2–S13, 1994.

51. Jackson GD, Connelly A, Duncan JS, et al: Detection of hippocampal pathology in intractable partial epilepsy: increased sensitivity with quantitative magnetic resonance T2 relaxometry. Neurology 43:1793–1799, 1993.

52. Jackson GD, Berkovic SF, Tress BM, et al: Hippocampal sclerosis can be reliably detected by magnetic resonance imaging. Neurology 40:1869–1875, 1990.

53. Jack CJ, Sharbrough FW, Twomey CK, et al: Temporal lobe seizures: lateralization with MR volume measurements of the hippocampal formation [see comments]. Radiology 175:423–429, 1990.

54. Tien RD, Felsberg GJ, Castro C, et al: Complex partial seizures and mesial temporal sclerosis: evaluation with fast spin-echo MR imaging. Radiology 189:835–842, 1993.

55. Berkovic SF, Andermann F, Olivier A, et al: Hippocampal sclerosis in temporal lobe epilepsy demonstrated by magnetic resonance imaging. Ann Neurol 29:175–182, 1991.

56. Bronen RA, Cheung G, Charles JT, et al: Imaging findings in hippocampal sclerosis: correlation with pathology. AJNR 12:933–940, 1991.

57. Ashtari M, Barr WB, Schaul N, Bogerts B: Three-dimensional fast low-angle shot imaging and computerized volume measurement of the hippocampus in patients with chronic epilepsy of the temporal lobe. AJNR 12:941–947, 1991.

58. Cascino GD, Jack CJ, Parisi JE, et al: Magnetic resonance imaging–based volume studies in temporal lobe epilepsy: pathological correlations. Ann Neurol 30:31–36, 1991.

59. Cendes F, Andermann F, Gloor P, et al: MRI volumetric measurement of amygdala and hippocampus in temporal lobe epilepsy. Neurology 43:719–725, 1993.

60. Cook MJ: Mesial temporal sclerosis and volumetric investigations. Acta Neurol Scand Suppl 152:109–114, 1994.

61. Lencz T, McCarthy G, Bronen RA, et al: Quantitative magnetic resonance imaging in temporal lobe epilepsy: relationship to neuropathology and neuropsychological function. Ann Neurol 31:629–637, 1992.

62. Cook MJ, Fish DR, Shorvon SD, et al: Hippocampal volumetric and morphometric studies in frontal and temporal lobe epilepsy. Brain 115:1001–1015, 1992.

63. Jack CJ, Sharbrough FW, Cascino GD, et al: Magnetic resonance image-based hippocampal volumetry: correlation with outcome after temporal lobectomy. Ann Neurol 31:138–146, 1992.

64. Trenerry MR, Jack CJ, Sharbrough FW, et al: Quantitative MRI hippocampal volumes: association with onset and duration of epilepsy, and febrile convulsions in temporal lobectomy patients. Epilepsy Res 15:247–252, 1993.

65. Trenerry MR, Jack CJ, Ivnik RJ, et al: MRI hippocampal volumes and memory function before and after temporal lobectomy. Neurology 43:1800–1805, 1993.

66. Cendes F, Leproux F, Melanson D, et al: MRI of amygdala and hippocampus in temporal lobe epilepsy. J Comput Assist Tomogr 17:206–210, 1993.

67. Bronen R, Anderson A, Spenser D: Quantitative MR for epilepsy: a clinical and research tool? AJNR 15:1157–1160, 1994.

68. Meiners L, van Gils A, Jansen G, et al: Temporal lobe epilepsy: the various MR appearances of histologically proven mesial temporal sclerosis. AJNR 15:1547–1555, 1994.

69. Jackson GD, Kuznicky RI, Cascino GD: Hippocampal sclerosis without detectable hippocampal atrophy. Neurology 44:42–46, 1994.

70. Brooks BS, King DW, El Gammal T, et al: MR imaging in patients with intractable complex partial epileptic seizures. AJNR 11:93–99, 1990.

71. Jack CR, Twomey CK, Zinsmeister AR, et al: Anterior temporal lobes and hippocampal formations: normative volumetric measurements from MR images in young adults. Radiology 172:549–554, 1989.

72. Baldwin GN, Tsuruda JS, Maravilla KR, et al: The fornix in patients with seizures caused by unilateral hippocampal sclerosis: detection of unilateral volume loss on MR images. AJR 162:1185–1189, 1994.

73. Mamourian AC, Rodichok L, Towfight J: The asymmetric mamillary body: association with medial temporal lobe disease demonstrated with MR. AJNR 16:517–522, 1995.

73a. Kim JH, Tien RD, Felsberg GJ, et al: Clinical significance of asymmetry of the fornix and mammillary body on MR in hippocampal sclerosis. AJNR 16:509–515, 1995.

74. Bronen R: Is there any role for gadopentetate dimeglumine administration when searching for mesial temporal sclerosis in patients with seizures? AJR 164:503, 1995.

75. Triulzi F, Franceschi M, Fazio F, Del Maschio A: Nonrefractory temporal lobe epilepsy: 1.5-T MR imaging. Radiology 166:181–185, 1988.

76. Spencer DD, Spencer SS, Mattson RH, et al: Access to the posterior medial temporal lobe structures in the surgical treatment of temporal lobe epilepsy. Neurosurgery 15:667–671, 1984.

77. Kim J, Tien R, Felsberg GJ, et al: MR measurements of the hippocampus for lateralization of temporal lobe epilepsy: value of measurements of the body versus the whole structure. AJR 163:1453–1457, 1994.

78. Bronen R, Fulbright R, Kim J, et al: Regional distribution of MR findings in hippocampal sclerosis. AJNR 16:1193–1200, 1995.

78a. Kim JK, Tien RD, Felsberg GJ, et al: Fast spin-echo MR in hippocampal sclerosis: correlation with pathology and surgery. AJNR 16:627–636, 1995.

79. Jack CRJ, Petersen RC, O'Brien PC, Tangalos EG: MR-based hippocampal volumetry in the diagnosis of Alzheimer's disease. Neurology 42:183–188, 1992.

79a. King D, Spencer SS, McCarthy G, et al: Bilateral hippocampal atrophy in medial temporal lobe epilepsy. Epilepsia 36:905–910, 1995.

80. Kuznicky R, Burgard S, Faught E, et al: Predictive value of magnetic resonance imaging in temporal lobe epilepsy surgery. Arch Neurol 50:65–69, 1993.

81. Suddath RL, Christison GW, Torrey EF, et al: Anatomic abnormalities in the brains of monozygotic twins discordant for schizophrenia. N Engl J Med 322:789–794, 1990.

82. Squire L, Amaral D, Press G: Magnetic resonance imaging of the hippocampal formation and mammillary nuclei distinguish medial temporal lobe epilepsy and diencephalic amnesia. J Neurosci 10:3106–3107, 1990.

83. Tien R, Felsberg G, Krishnan R, Heinz E: MR imaging of diseases of the limbic system. AJR 163:657–665, 1994.

84. Sasaki O, Tanaka R, Koike T, et al: Excision of cavernous angioma with preservation of coexisting venous angioma. Case report. J Neurosurg 75:461–464, 1991.

85. De Lanerolle NC, Kim JH, Robbins RJ, Spencer DD: Hippocampal interneuron loss and plasticity in human temporal lobe epilepsy. Brain Res 495:387–395, 1989.

86. Jay V, Becker LE, Otsubo H, et al: Pathology of temporal lobectomy for refractory seizures in children. Review of 20 cases including some unique malformative lesions. J Neurosurg 79:53–61, 1993.

87. Cascino GD, Jack CJ, Parisi JE, et al: Operative strategy in patients with MRI-identified dual pathology and temporal lobe epilepsy. Epilepsy Res 14:175–182, 1993.

88. Hauser WA, Kurland LT: The epidemiology of epilepsy in Rochester, Minnesota, 1935 through 1967. Epilepsia 16:1–66, 1975.

89. Kuzniecky R, Cascino G, Palmini A, et al: Structural neuroimaging. In: Engel JJ, ed. Surgical Treatment of the Epilepsies. New York: Raven Press, 1993, pp 197–209.

90. Cascino G, Boon P, Fish D: Surgically remediable lesional syndromes. In: Engel JJ, ed. Surgical Treatment of the Epilepsies. New York: Raven Press, 1993, pp 77–86.

91. Awad IA Rosenfield J, Ahl J, et al: Intractable epilepsy and structural lesions of the brain: mapping, resection strategies and siezure outcome. Epilepsia 32:179–186, 1991.

92. Fried I, Kim J, Spencer D: Limbic and neocortical gliomas associated with intractable seizures: a distinct clinicopathological group. Neurosurgery 34:815–823, 1994.

93. Fish D, Andermann F, Olivieri A: Complex partial seizures and posterior temporal or extratemporal lesions: surgical strategies. Neurology 41:1781–1784, 1991.

94. Bergen D, Bleck T, Ramsey R, et al: Magnetic resonance imaging as a sensitive and specific predictor of neoplasms removed for intractable epilepsy. Epilepsia 30:318–321, 1989.

95. Boon PA, Williamson PD, Fried I, et al: Intracranial, intraaxial, space-occupying lesions in patients with intractable partial seizures: an anatomoclinical, neuropsychological, and surgical correlation. Epilepsia 32:467–476, 1991.

96. Heinz ER, Crain BJ, Radtke RA, et al: MR imaging in patients with temporal lobe seizures: correlation of results with pathologic findings. AJNR 11:827–832, 1990.

97. Drake J, Hoffman H, Kobayashi J, et al: Surgical management of children with temporal lobe epilepsy and mass lesions. Neurosurgery 21:792–797, 1987.

98. Hirsch JF: Epilepsy and brain tumours in children. J Neuroradiol 16:292–300, 1989.

99. Rasmussen T: Surgery of epilepsy associated with brain tumors. Adv Neurol 8:227–239, 1975.

100. Le Blanc F, Rasmussen T: Cerebral Seizures and Brain Tumors. Amsterdam: North Holland, 1974.

101. Piepmeier JM, Fried I, Makuch R: Low-grade astrocytomas may arise from different astrocyte lineages. Neurosurgery 33:627–632, 1993.

102. Atlas SW: Intraaxial brain tumors. In: Atlas SW, ed. Magnetic Resonance Imaging of the Brain and Spine. New York: Raven Press, 1991, pp 223–326.

103. Holland B, Kucharcyk W, Brant-Zawadski M, et al: MR imaging of calcified intracranial lesions. Radiology 125:119–125, 1985.

104. Spencer SS, Spencer DD, Kim J, et al: Gliomas in chronic epilepsy. In: Wolf P, Janz D, Dreifuss FE, eds. Advances in Epileptology: XVIth Epilepsy International Symposium. New York: Raven Press, 1987, pp 39–41.

105. Russell D, Rubenstein L: Pathology of Tumors of the Nervous System. Baltimore: Williams & Wilkins, 1989.

106. Lee YY, Van TP: Intracranial oligodendrogliomas: imaging findings in 35 untreated cases. AJR 152:361–369, 1989.

107. Masters L, Zimmerman R: Imaging of supratentorial brain tumors in adults. Neuroimaging Clin North Am 3:649–669, 1993.

108. Mork S, Lindegaard K, Halvorsen T: Oligodendroglioma: incidence and biological behavior in a defined population. J Neurosurg 63:881–889, 1985.

109. Dorne H, O'Gorman A, Melanson D: Computed tomography of intracranial ganglioglioma. AJNR 7:281–285, 1986.

110. Castillo M, Davis P, Takei Y, Hoffman J: Intracranial ganglioglioma: MR, CT and clinical findings in 18 patients. AJNR 11:109–114, 1990.

111. Daumas-Duport C, Scheithauer BW, Chodkiewicz JP, et al: Dysembryoplastic neuroepithelial tumor: a surgically curable tumor of young patients with intractable partial seizures. Report of thirty-nine cases. Neurosurgery 23:545–556, 1988.

112. Kuroiwa T, Bergey GK, Rothman MI, et al: Radiologic appearance of the dysembryoplastic neuroepithelial tumor. Radiology 197:233–238, 1995.

113. Kuroiwa T, Kishikawa T, Kato A, et al: Dysembryoplastic neuroepithelial tumors: MR findings. J Comput Assist Tomogr 18:352–356, 1994.

114. Kirkpatrick PJ, Honavar M, Janota I, Polkey CE: Control of temporal lobe epilepsy following en bloc resection of low-grade tumors. J Neurosurg 78:19–25, 1993.

115. Okazaki H: Fundamentals of Neuropathology. New York: Igaku-Shoin, 1983.

116. Kraemer D, Awad I: Vascular malformations and epilepsy: clinical considerations and basic mechanisms. Epilepsia 35(suppl 6):S30–S43, 1994.

117. Fortuna A, Ferrante L, Mastronardi L, et al: Cerebral cavernous angioma in children. Childs Nerv Syst 5:201–207, 1989.

118. Kucharczyk W, Lemme-Pleghos L, Uske A, et al: Intracranial vascular malformations: MR and CT imaging. Radiology 156:383–389, 1985.

119. Gomori JM, Grossman RI, Goldberg HI, et al: Occult cerebral vascular malformations: high-field MR imaging. Radiology 158:707–713, 1986.

120. Sze G, Krol G, Olsen W, et al: Hemorrhagic neoplasms: MR mimics of occult vascular malformations. Am J Neuroradiol 8:795–802, 1987.

121. Robinson JR, Awad IA, Little JR: Natural history of the cavernous angioma. J Neurosurg 75:709–714, 1991.

122. Yeh H, Tew J: Management of arteriovenous malformations of the brain. Contemp Neurosurg 9:1–8, 1988.

123. Crawford P, West C, Shaw M, et al: Cerebral arteriovenous malformations and epilepsy: factors in the development of epilepsy. Epilepsia 27:270–275, 1986.

124. Piepgras DG, Sundt TJ, Ragoowansi AT, Stevens L: Seizure outcome in patients with surgically treated cerebral arteriovenous malformations. J Neurosurg 78:5–11, 1993.

125. Crawford P, West C, Chadwich D, et al: Arteriovenous malformations of the brain: natural history in unoperated patients. J Neurol Neurosurg Psychiatry 49:1–10, 1986.

126. Yeh HS, Tew JJ, Gartner M: Seizure control after surgery on cerebral arteriovenous malformations. J Neurosurg 78:12–18, 1993.

127. Wong M, Suite N, Labar D: Seizures in human immunodeficiency virus infection. Arch Neurol 47:640–642, 1990.

128. Del Brutto O, Sotelo J: Neurocysticercosis: an update. Rev Infect Dis 10:1075–1087, 1988.

129. Sotelo J, Guerrero V, Rubio F: Neurocysticercosis: a new classification based on active and inactive forms: a study of 753 cases. Arch Intern Med 145:442–445, 1985.

130. Suss R, Maravilla K, Thompson J: MR imaging of cysticercosis: comparison with CT and anatomicopathologic features. AJNR 7:235–242, 1986.

131. Teitelbaum G, Otto R, Lin M, et al: MR imaging of neurocysticercosis. AJR 153:857–866, 1989.

132. Vazquez V, Sotelo J: The course of seizures after treatment for cerebral cysticercosis [see comments]. N Engl J Med 327:696–701, 1992.

133. Olivier A, Gloor P, Andermann F: Occipitotemporal epilepsy studied with stereotactically implanted depth electrodes and successfully treated by temporal resection. Ann Neurol 11:428–432, 1982.

134. Bhargava S, Tandon P: Intracranial tuberculomas: a CT study. Br J Radiol 53:935–945, 1980.

135. Rhamamurthi B, Rhamamurthi R, Vasudevan M: Changing concepts in the treatment of tuberculomas of the brain. Childs Nerv Syst 2:242–243, 1986.

136. Salgado P, Del BO, Talamas O, et al: Intracranial tuberculoma: MR imaging. Neuroradiology 31:299–302, 1989.

137. Jinkins JR: Computed tomography of intracranial tuberculosis. Neuroradiology 33:126–135, 1991.

138. Whelan M, Stern J: Intracranial tuberculoma. Radiology 138:75–81, 1981.

139. Bowen B, Post MJD: Intracranial infection. In: Atlas SW, ed. Magnetic Resonance Imaging of the Brain and Spine. New York: Raven Press, 1991, pp 501–538.

140. Gupta RK, Pandey R, Khan EM, et al: Intracranial tuberculomas: MRI signal intensity correlation with histopathology and localised proton spectroscopy. Magn Reson Imaging 11:443–449, 1993.

141. Kennedy A, Schon F: Epilepsy: disappearing lesions appearing in the United Kingdom. BMJ 302:933–935, 1991.

142. Cox JE, Matthews VP, Santos CC, Elster AD: Seizure-induced transient hippocampal abnormalities on MR: correlation with positron emission tomography and electroencephalography. AJNR 16:1736–1738, 1995.

143. Riela AR, Sires BP, Penry JK: Transient magnetic resonance imaging abnormalities during partial status epilepticus. J Child Neurol 6:143–145, 1991.

144. Andermann F, Freeman J, Vigevano F, Pals H: Surgically remediable diffuse hemispheric syndromes. In: Engel JJ, ed. Surgical Treatment of the Epilepsies. 2nd ed. New York: Raven Press, 1993, pp 87–101.

145. Cusmai R, Ricci S, Pinard JM, et al: West syndrome due to perinatal insults. Epilepsia 34:738–742, 1993.

146. Dinner D: Posttraumatic Epilepsy. In: Wyllie E, ed. The Treatment of Epilepsy: Principles and Practice. Philadelphia: Lea & Febiger, 1993, pp 654–658.

147. Jennett W, Lewin W: Traumatic epilepsy after closed head injuries. J Neurol Neurosurg Psychiatry 23:295–301, 1960.

148. Caveness W: Onset and cessation of fits following craniocerebral trauma. J Neurosurg 20:570–583, 1963.

149. Heikkinen ER, Ronty HS, Tolonen U, Pyhtinen J: Development of post-traumatic epilepsy. Stereotact Funct Neurosurg 55:25–33, 1990.

150. Dietrich RB, el Saden S, Chugani HT, et al: Resective surgery for intractable epilepsy in children: radiologic evaluation. AJNR 12:1149–1158, 1991.

151. Roizin L, Gold G, Berman H: Congenital vascular anomalies and their histopathology in Sturge-Weber syndrome. J Neuropathol Exp Neurol 18:75–97, 1959.

152. Wasenko J, Rosenbloom S, Duchesneau P, et al: The Sturge-Weber syndrome: comparison of MR and CT characteristics. AJNR 11:131–134, 1990.
153. Benedikt R, Brown D, Ghaed V, et al: Sturge-Weber syndrome: cranial MR imaging with Gd-DTPA. AJNR 14:409–415, 1993.
154. Elster AD, Mirza W: MR imaging in chronic partial epilepsy: role of contrast enhancement. AJNR 12:165–170, 1991.
155. Rasmussen T, Andermann F: Update on the syndrome of "chronic encephalitis" and epilepsy. Cleve Clin J Med 56(suppl Part 2):S181–S184, 1989.
156. Zupanc ML, Handler EG, Levine RL, et al: Rasmussen encephalitis: epilepsia partialis continua secondary to chronic encephalitis. Pediatr Neurol 6:397–401, 1990.
157. Rogers SW, Andrews PI, Gahring LC, et al: Autoantibodies to glutamate receptor GluR3 in Rasmussen's encephalitis. Science 265:648–651, 1994.
158. Tien RD, Ashdown BC, Lewis DJ, et al: Rasmussen's encephalitis: neuroimaging findings in four patients. AJR 158:1329–1332, 1992.
159. Kuzniecky R, Andermann F, Tampieri D, et al: Bilateral central microgyria: epilepsy, pseudobulbar palsy, clarification by MRI. Ann Neurol 25:547–554, 1989.
160. Kuzniecky R, Andermann F: The congenital bilateral perisylvian syndrome: imaging findings in a multicenter study. CBPS Study Group. AJNR 15:139–144, 1994.
161. Palmini A, Andermann F, Olivier A, et al: Neuronal migration disorders: a contribution of modern neuroimaging to the etiologic diagnosis of epilepsy. Can J Neurol Sci 18:580–587, 1991.
162. Barkovich AJ, Gressens P, Evrard P: Formation, maturation, and disorders of brain neocortex. AJNR 13:423–446, 1992.
163. Barkovich A, Chuang S: MR of neuronal migrational anomalies. AJNR 8:1009–1017, 1987.
164. Taylor D, Falconer M, Bruton C, Corsellis J: Focal cortical dysplasia of the cerebral cortex in epilepsy. J Neurol Neurosurg Psychiatry 34:369–387, 1971.
165. Palmini A, Gambardella A, Andermann F, et al: Operative strategies for patients with cortical dysplastic lesions and intractable epilepsy. Epilepsia 35(suppl 6):S57–S71, 1994.
166. Kuzniecky R, Berkovic S, Andermann F, et al: Focal cortical myoclonus and rolandic cortical dysplasia: clarification with MRI. Ann Neurol 23:317–325, 1988.
167. Kuzniecky R, Andermann F, Guerrini R: Congenital bilateral perisylvian syndrome: study of 31 patients. The CBPS Multicenter Collaborative Study. Lancet 341:608–612, 1993.
168. Braffman BH, Bilaniuk LT, Naidich TP, et al: MR imaging of tuberous sclerosis: pathogenesis of this phakomatosis and literature review. Radiology 183:227–238, 1992.
169. Curatolo P, Cusmai R, Cortesi F, et al: Neuropsychiatric aspects of tuberous sclerosis. Ann N Y Acad Sci 615:8–16, 1991.
170. Kuzniecky RI: Magnetic resonance imaging in developmental disorders of the cerebral cortex. Epilepsia 35(suppl 6):S44–S56, 1994.
171. Roach ES, Kerr J, Mendelsohn D, et al: Detection of tuberous sclerosis in parents by magnetic resonance imaging. Neurology 41:262–265, 1991.
172. Jambaque I, Cusmai R, Curatolo P, et al: Neuropsychological aspects of tuberous sclerosis in relation to epilepsy and MRI findings. Dev Med Child Neurol 33:698–705, 1991.
173. Yakovalev P, Wadsworth R: Schizencephalies: a study of the congenital clefts in the cerebral mantle. I. Clefts with fused lips. J Neuropathol Exp Neurol 5:116–130, 1946.
174. Aniskiewicz AS, Frumkin NL, Brady DE, et al: Magnetic resonance imaging and neurobehavioral correlates in schizencephaly. Arch Neurol 47:911–916, 1990.
175. Barkovich AJ, Kjos BO: Schizencephaly: correlation of clinical findings with MR characteristics [see comments]. AJNR 13:85–94, 1992. Review.
175a. Lehericy S, Dormant D, Semah F, et al: Developmental abnormalities of the medial temporal lobe in patients with temporal lobe epilepsy. AJNR 16:617–626, 1995.
176. Barkovich AJ, Kjos BO: Gray matter heterotopias: MR characteristics and correlation with developmental and neurologic manifestations. Radiology 182:493–499, 1992.
177. Smith AS, Weinstein MA, Quencer RM, et al: Association of heterotopic gray matter with seizures: MR imaging. Radiology 168:195–198, 1988.
178. Landy HJ, Curless RG, Ramsay RE, et al: Corpus callosotomy for seizures associated with band heterotopia. Epilepsia 34:79–83, 1993.
179. Palmini A, Andermann F, Aicardi J, et al: Diffuse cortical dysplasia, or the "double cortex" syndrome: the clinical and epileptic spectrum in 10 patients. Neurology 41:1656–1662, 1991.
180. Pavone L, Rizzo R, Dobyns WB: Clinical manifestations and evaluation of isolated lissencephaly. Childs Nerv Syst 9:387–390, 1993.
181. Crome L: Pachygyria. J Pathol Bacteriol 71:335–352, 1956.
182. Babyn P, Chuang S, Daneman A, Withers C: Sonographic recognition of unilateral megalencephaly. J Ultrasound Med 11:563–566, 1992.
183. Fusco L, Ferracuti S, Fariello G, et al: Hemimegalencephaly and normal intellectual development. J Neurol Neurosurg Psychiatry 55:720–722, 1992.
184. Chan S, Silver A, Hilal S, et al: STIR MR imaging of the normal and abnormal temporal lobe. Presented at the American Society of Neuroradiology Conference, Vancouver, 1993.
185. Bergin P, Fish D, Shorvon S, et al: FLAIR imaging in partial epilepsy: improving the yield of MRI. Epilepsia 34:121, 1993. Abstract.
186. Jack CJ, Krecke K, Luetmer P, et al: Diagnosis of mesial temporal sclerosis with conventional versus fast spin-echo MR imaging. Radiology 192:123–127, 1994.
186a. Barkovitch AJ, Rowley HA, Andermann F: MR in partial epilepsy: value of high-resolution volumetric techniques. AJNR 16:339–344, 1995.
187. Ryberg JN, Hammond CA, Grimm RC, et al: Initial clinical experience in MR imaging of the brain with a fast fluid-attenuated inversion-recovery pulse sequence. Radiology 193:173–180, 1994.
188. Cascino GD, Hirschorn KA, Jack CR, Sharbrough FW: Gadolinium-DTPA–enhanced magnetic resonance imaging in intractable partial epilepsy. Neurology 39:1115–1118, 1989.
189. Leblanc R, Tampieri D, Robitaille Y, et al: Developmental anterobasal temporal encephalocele and temporal lobe epilepsy. J Neurosurg 74:933–939, 1991.
190. Prichard JW, Rosen BR: Functional study of the brain by NMR. J Cereb Blood Flow Metabol 14:365–372, 1994. Review.
191. Ng T, Comair Y, Xue M, et al: Temporal lobe epilepsy: Presurgical localization with proton chemical shift imaging. Radiology 193:465–472, 1994.
192. Zhong J, Petroff O, Prichard J, Gore J: Changes in water diffusion and relaxation properties of rat cerebrum during status epilepticus. Magn Reson Med 30:241–246, 1993.
193. Jack CJ, Thompson RM, Butts RK, et al: Sensory motor cortex: correlation of presurgical mapping with functional MR imaging and invasive cortical mapping. Radiology 190:85–92, 1994.
194. McCarthy G, Blamire AM, Rothman DL, et al: Echo-planar magnetic resonance imaging studies of frontal cortex activation during word generation in humans. Proc Natl Acad Sci USA 90:4952–4956, 1993.
195. Jackson GD, Connelly A, Cross JH, et al: Functional magnetic resonance imaging of focal seizures. Neurology 44:850–856, 1994.

Aneurysms and Vascular Malformations

JOHN PERL, II ■ THOMAS J. MASARYK
PATRICK A. TURSKI

Magnetic resonance imaging (MRI), computed tomography (CT), and catheter angiography are all at the forefront of the diagnostic evaluation of intracranial vascular disease. The specific modality employed for the diagnostic evaluation of arteriovenous malformations (AVMs) and intracranial aneurysms is based on the urgency of clinical presentation. Nevertheless, these modalities are frequently complementary in establishing the diagnosis, in characterizing the lesion, in planning therapy, and in evaluating results after therapy.

The advances in MRI and MR angiography have produced powerful tools to reveal detailed architectural features of intracranial vascular disease noninvasively, supplanting CT in the evaluation of most intracranial vascular disease in the nonemergent clinical scenario. With the exception of the detection of calcification and acute subarachnoid blood, it is generally accepted that MRI is the most sensitive and specific in detecting occult or symptomatic structural vascular lesions of the central nervous system.[1] With advances in MRI flow techniques, not only can morphologic information about a vascular abnormality be detected but physiologic information such as cerebral blood rheology and flow quantification can also be obtained. Although continued improvement in MRI hardware and additional innovation in pulse sequence design should improve the abilities of MRI to completely evaluate vascular lesions, it is important to recognize that catheter angiography remains an integral technique in the presurgical evaluation of most central nervous system aneurysms, parenchymal AVMs, and dural arteriovenous fistulas (AVFs).

INTRACRANIAL ANEURYSMS

It is estimated that 28,000 intracranial aneurysms rupture annually in North America, with nearly half of the initial survivors succumbing within the first month after rupture.[2] Although the exact prevalence of unruptured aneurysms is unknown, autopsy series estimate the prevalence of incidental unruptured aneurysms at 1.3% to 7.9%.[3, 4] In an angiographic study, Atkinson and associates[5] revealed a 1% prevalence of anterior circulation aneurysms. The significant morbidity and mortality associated with ruptured aneurysms combined with the low but real prevalence of incidental aneurysms emphasize the need to evaluate symptomatic and high-risk asymptomatic patients.[6–11]

CLASSIFICATION AND LOCATION

Classification of aneurysms is based on either the histology (true in pseudoaneurysm), gross morphologic architecture, or cause of the aneurysm. The morphologic appearance is described as saccular or fusiform, with the most common type being the congenital saccular (berry) aneurysm, constituting 90% of all intracranial aneurysms. Fusiform aneurysms account for only about 7% of cases.[3] The types of aneurysms other than berry aneurysm include atherosclerotic, dissecting (Fig. 23–1), flow related, mycotic, neoplastic, and traumatic (Fig. 23–2).

Aneurysms can be located intradurally or extradurally. Generally, extradural aneurysms arise below the origin of the ophthalmic artery from the internal carotid artery (C-3 segment). Intradural aneurysms most often involve the bifurcation of vessels at the base of the brain, specifically the middle cerebral artery, the distal internal carotid artery, and the vertebrobasilar trunk.[12] Aneurysms located at branch points of peripheral cerebral vessels are uncommon and if present should suggest infectious, traumatic, myxomatous, or neoplastic causes.[13–15] Anterior circulation aneurysms constitute about 85% of cases.[3, 16] Multiplicity occurs in 12% to 31% with a propensity for mirror occurrence.[17]

Giant saccular aneurysms are defined as aneurysms with a greatest diameter exceeding 2.5 cm.[18] These lesions constitute 5% to 7% of intracranial aneurysms, although a prevalence as high as 13% has been published.[19–22] In two early reports, giant aneurysms were noted to arise more commonly from the anterior circu-

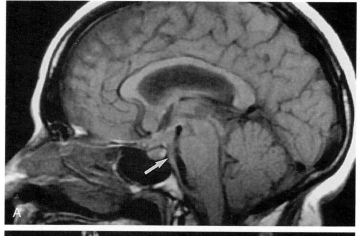

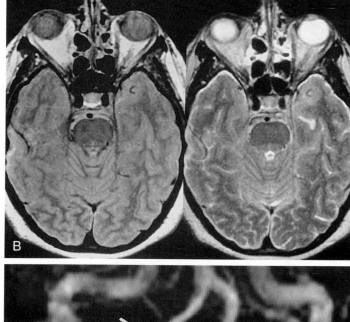

FIGURE 23–1. Subarachnoid hemorrhage due to a dissecting vertebral artery aneurysm. *A,* Sagittal T1-weighted image demonstrates relatively high signal intensity in the subarachnoid space in the prepontine and suprasellar cistern *(arrow)* compared with normal low signal intensity of cerebrospinal fluid. *B,* Short–echo time (TE), long–repetition time (TR) and long-TE, long-TR axial images show a relatively high heterogeneous signal pattern in the prepontine cistern on the T2-weighted image compared with cerebrospinal fluid. *C,* A three-dimensional time-of-flight (3D TOF) MR angiogram shows a triangular dissecting vertebral artery aneurysm *(arrow)* arising off the right vertebral artery distal to the origin of the posterior inferior cerebellar artery. *D,* The catheter angiogram demonstrates the same lesion.

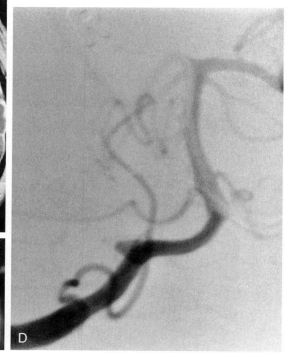

lation; however, the exact locations of these aneurysms differ from smaller saccular aneurysms.[4, 23] The most frequent locations of giant aneurysms are the intradural (Fig. 23–3) and cavernous segments of the internal carotid artery, followed by the vertebrobasilar arterial system, the middle cerebral artery, and the anterior communicating/anterior cerebral artery junction. A review of the literature by Nukui and coworkers[24] documented the distribution of giant aneurysms as follows: intradural internal carotid artery–ophthalmic artery, 21%; middle cerebral artery, 16%; anterior communicating/anterior cerebral artery junction, 12%; internal carotid artery bifurcation, 9%; basilar artery/superior cerebellar artery, 8%; basilar artery tip, 7%; cavernous internal carotid artery, 6%; vertebral artery, 4%; vertebrobasilar artery junction, 3%; posterior cerebral artery, 3%; intradural internal carotid artery/posterior communicating artery, 3%; posterior communicating artery, 1%; posterior inferior cerebellar artery, 1%.

A small but unique subset of giant intracerebral aneurysms is seen in children and constitutes less than 5% of lesions, occurring with greatest frequency at the middle cerebral arteries, the carotid terminus, and the posterior circulation. These aneurysms are frequently associated with other congenital anomalies (e.g., connective tissue disorders), and this coexistence is cited in support of an underlying genetic etiology or cofactor in the development of intracranial aneurysms.[25, 26] Giant fusiform aneurysms also occur in the intracranial circulation, albeit less commonly, and they tend to involve the vertebrobasilar artery.[20, 27] These vascular dilatations are often related to atherosclerotic deterioration of the

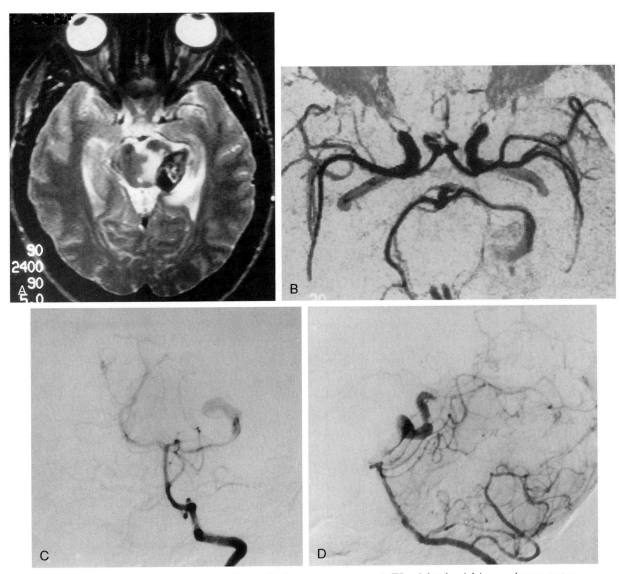

FIGURE 23–2. Traumatic left posterior cerebral artery aneurysm. *A*, T2-weighted axial image demonstrates the extra-axial hemorrhagic mass. Note the high signal intensity in the adjacent midbrain and mesial temporal lobe. Some of the low signal intensity within the mass represents flow void. *B*, A 3D TOF MR angiogram demonstrates a fusiform aneurysm arising off the left posterior cerebral artery. The high signal intensity adjacent to the flowing spins is due to small amounts of methemoglobin within thrombus, which is artifactually included in the maximal intensity projection (MIP) MR angiogram. There is anterior and lateral displacement of the posterior cerebral artery due to the mass of the aneurysm. *C* and *D*, Catheter angiograms demonstrate similar findings of a fusiform posterior cerebral artery aneurysm with displacement of the posterior cerebral artery.

vessel wall or, less commonly, collagen-vascular disease: Marfan's syndrome, Ehlers-Danlos disease, and pseudoxanthoma elasticum.[28, 29]

Patients with giant aneurysms present in one of two ways: 1) acute headaches and meningismus from subarachnoid hemorrhage (SAH), and 2) symptoms due to mass effect. Giant aneurysms are more likely than smaller saccular aneurysms to present with symptoms secondary to mass effect, such as headache, focal deficit, and seizures. Aneurysm rupture and the accompanying intracranial hemorrhage occur in 13% to 76% (average 35%) of patients with giant aneurysms.[22]

MORPHOLOGY AND RHEOLOGY

Aneurysm morphology results in different flow characteristics, which have implications related to the clinical stability and growth of the lesion and are reflected in the appearance on MR flow images.[30] Turbulent flow is not commonly present in any aneurysm. Flow within the aneurysm, although not always laminar, is seldom chaotic. Using mathematic models and computer simulations, Perktold[31] predicted flow in an axisymmetric aneurysm model, revealing complex consistent intra-aneurysm flow fields, with varying shear

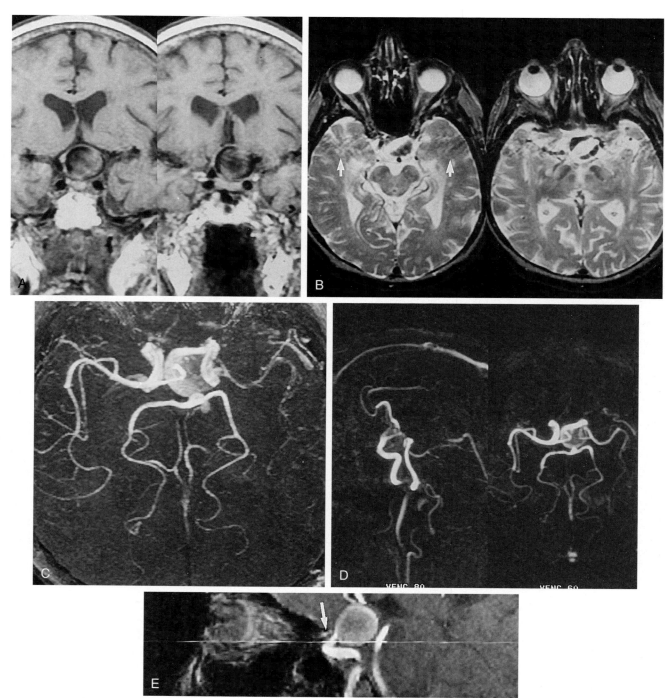

FIGURE 23–3. Giant paraophthalmic unruptured aneurysm. *A,* T1-weighted spin-echo images show a round lesion of heterogeneous signal intensity with a hypointense periphery and a higher signal intensity center located predominantly in the suprasellar cistern. The low signal intensity on the periphery is most likely related to spin dephasing from rapidly moving blood, and the higher signal pattern in the central area is probably due to flow-related enhancement, with slower flow being higher in signal intensity. *B,* Long-TE, long-TR axial images display the same phenomena. Note the thicker hypointense rim of the aneurysm because of the longer TE. In addition, note the ghost artifact arising from the intra-aneurysmal flow, a spin-phase phenomenon *(arrows).* *C,* On a 3D TOF axial MR angiogram the aneurysm projects medially. The inflow stream (highest signal intensity) is along the periphery of the aneurysm. *D,* Two-dimensional (2D) phase-contrast (PC) images with two different velocity encodings. Note the image with the velocity encoding of 80 cm/s demonstrates little vascular signal intensity within the aneurysm, with the exception of the inflow stream. The axial 2D PC image with a velocity encoding of 60 cm/s shows a much higher intra-aneurysmal signal pattern. *E,* Multiplanar reconstruction from the 3D TOF data set allows localization of the aneurysm above the origin of the ophthalmic artery *(arrow).*

stresses in different locations within the aneurysm. Strother and coworkers[32] demonstrated that the geometric relationship between an aneurysm and its parent artery is the primary factor determining the intra-aneurysm flow pattern. Flow patterns are highly predictable. Flow transitions represent intermediate stages between true laminar flow and turbulence and were observed in all aneurysm geometries.

Lateral saccular aneurysms project nearly perpendicularly from the side of the parent artery and are frequently encountered in the region of the cavernous internal carotid (C-4 segment) artery. The characteristic blood flow is a discrete inflow path along the distal edge of the aneurysm ostium, continuing in a circular fashion along the lateral margin of the aneurysm and exiting adjacent to the proximal edge of the aneurysm ostium. Centrally, there is recirculation of the blood (see Fig. 23–3). This flow pattern has been described in experimental and human lateral saccular aneurysms.[32] Both phase-contrast (PC) and time-of-flight (TOF) MR angiograms demonstrate the central flow as low signal intensity (see Fig. 23–3). The low signal intensity is thought to be due to saturation effects rather than intravoxel dephasing. Optimal visualization of the slow central flow is best performed with a PC technique with low velocity encoding[33, 34] (see Fig. 23–3 and Chapter 25).

The two main flow features of lateral aneurysms that determine the MR angiographic appearance are 1) the greatest flow velocity is within the inflow stream along the periphery of the aneurysm lumen and 2) the maximal flow velocity and therefore shear stress are at the neck not the dome of the aneurysm. The work of Strother and associates[32] suggests that these stresses are maximal at the trailing edge of the aneurysm neck, the presumed site of continued enlargement. Factors predisposing to such lesions include congenital or acquired defects in the arterial wall at points of hemodynamic stress, a condition that may be precipitated or aggravated by hypertension and atherosclerosis. Giant saccular aneurysms are thought to arise from enlarging, smaller berry aneurysms.[35, 36] Additional studies suggest that disturbed flow within the sac contributes to the disruption of the endothelial surface, with secondary clot formation.[37] Sutherland and colleagues[38] demonstrated that giant aneurysms are physiologically dynamic lesions, accumulating and dissipating platelets and fibrin thrombus debris in an irregular fashion.

Partial thrombosis of giant aneurysms is common because the volume of the aneurysm sac is disproportionately large relative to the size of the aneurysm orifice to the parent artery (Fig. 23–4), resulting in intra-aneurysmal slow flow and stasis, which enhances platelet aggregation at the inner wall.[22] Mural thrombus within a giant aneurysm usually begins peripherally and progresses centripetally in a laminated pattern, with the majority of thrombus accumulating on the wall opposite the aneurysm ostium. Therefore, giant aneurysms may appear substantially different on sequential MRI and MR angiographic examinations, even in the absence of intervening therapy.

Bifurcation aneurysms are most often located at the middle cerebral artery or internal carotid artery bifurcation. The flow characteristics of bifurcation aneurysms have been well documented in experimental models.[32] Inflow is at the edge of the aneurysm ostium nearest the long axis of the parent artery. Rapid helical flow is the most common flow pattern in these aneurysms, with rotation of flow in the direction of the outflow branch. Because outflow is predominantly into one of the two branch vessels, the conspicuity of small branch vessels adjacent to the aneurysm may be reduced on imaging studies (MR angiography more than catheter angiography). With MR angiography, signal loss may occur from intravoxel dephasing but the relatively high inflow allows adequate demonstration of the contour of the aneurysm.

The most common terminal aneurysm occurs at the basilar tip. The flow into terminal aneurysms is determined by the part of the aneurysm ostium closest to a straight line drawn through the center of the parent artery. Outflow is at the opposite edge of the aneurysm ostium and typically extends almost exclusively into the branch vessel closest to the outflow stream. As with bifurcation aneurysms, flow within terminal aneurysms is rapid and rotary.[39]

In light of the complex flow conditions, occasional difficulties may be encountered in adequately visualizing the flow within intracranial aneurysms using MRI and MR angiographic techniques.

Anatomic Imaging

The imaging evaluation of aneurysms includes demonstration of the location, size, number, and morphologic appearance in addition to the architecture of the neck in cases of saccular aneurysms. Moreover, evaluation for the presence of associated vascular variants or anomalies (e.g., hypoplastic/aplastic segments of the circle of Willis, carotid/basilar artery anastomosis, and supply or absence of vertebral or carotid arteries) is imperative. The imaging appearance is influenced by the size and location of the aneurysm; the presence of subarachnoid, intraventricular, or intraparenchymal blood; intra-aneurysmal blood flow; and the composition of the aneurysm wall. Besides the clinical grade, the presence of subarachnoid or parenchymal clot, vasospasm, cerebral edema, infarction, and hydrocephalus is important for prognosis and also for medical and surgical management.[13]

MRI and MR angiographic techniques are substantially robust to permit reliable diagnosis of an intracranial aneurysm and whether the aneurysm is solitary or multiple. These techniques provide morphologic characteristics such as the size, shape, location, relationship of the aneurysm to the parent artery, adjacent vessels and dural reflections, presence of larger branches (not perforating arteries) that arise off the aneurysm wall, and demonstration of the neck of the aneurysm. All of these factors influence the surgical or endovascular approach to the treatment of these lesions.

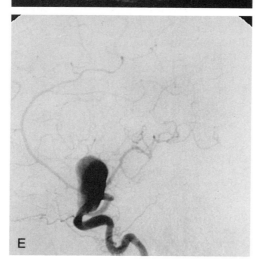

FIGURE 23–4. Giant partially thrombosed paraophthalmic artery aneurysm. *A,* Sagittal T1-weighted image reveals a large laminated region along the margins of the aneurysm wall and dome with an inferior flow void. Note the rim of low signal intensity and the high signal intensity within the periphery of the thrombus from the presence of methemoglobin. *B,* Short-TE, long-TR images demonstrate the laminated mural thrombus with the high signal intensity centrally, a flow-related phenomenon. *C,* On the long-TE, long-TR images, note the varying hypointensity due to blood byproducts in different stages of breakdown within the thrombosed portion of the aneurysm. A ghost artifact is identified arising off only the patent portion of the aneurysm. There is also high signal intensity in the adjacent brain parenchyma due to the edema. *D* and *E,* Anteroposterior and lateral catheter angiograms demonstrate only the patent portion of the aneurysm lumen. MR angiography depicts the true size of the aneurysm more accurately than catheter or MR angiography.

SCREENING ASYMPTOMATIC PATIENTS AT RISK

At this time the evaluation of asymptomatic cerebral aneurysms is evolving. Certain populations are at high risk for harboring cerebral aneurysms. These include patients with polycystic kidney disease (PKD), cerebral AVMs, fibromuscular dysplasia, coarctation of the aorta, a family history of SAH or aneurysms, and some connective tissue disorders.[7, 11, 28, 29, 40–46] Because of the low but potentially serious morbidity, invasive studies are not typically performed in the asymptomatic patient unless an aneurysm is suggested by another imaging modality. CT, which requires enhancement with an intravenously administered iodinated contrast agent, has significant limitations in its ability to detect small or asymptomatic aneurysms.[47, 48] This may change with the advent and refinement of spiral (helical) CT angiographic techniques.[48a] Alternatively, MR angiography exhibits promise as a screening procedure for asymptomatic aneurysms, especially in high-risk populations (Fig. 23–5). The noninvasive nature and the short acquisition time of three-dimensional Fourier transform TOF (3DFT TOF) MR angiography make the widespread screening for aneurysms possible but also raise many questions related to outcome for the patient (see Chapter 25).

Despite the high morbidity and mortality due to SAH associated with intracranial aneurysms, there is no consensus regarding the true natural history and risk of rupture of intact asymptomatic intracranial aneurysms. Calculating the risk of rupture, regardless of size, is complicated by the lack of clear discrimination between symptomatic and asymptomatic aneurysms in most studies. The annual risk of rupture of an asymptomatic aneurysm has been estimated as less than 0.5% to 2%. Symptomatic intact aneurysms are associated with a significantly higher risk of hemorrhage, and these aneurysms rupture at a rate of at least 4% per year.[49–52] Although the natural history of incidental aneurysms and of those discovered during the investigation of SAH from another source was shown to be similar in one study,[51] this point has never been properly investigated and, in fact, the risk of rupture for these two groups of aneurysms may be dissimilar.[52] The most important predictor of the cost and benefit of screening is the prevalence of aneurysms, and studies of the prevalence of aneurysms in asymptomatic subjects have as yet been small or biased.

A screening study using 3D TOF MR angiography in the detection of intracranial aneurysms in patients with familial intracranial aneurysms has been performed.[43] The prevalence of intracranial aneurysms among this Finnish cohort was 10%, estimated to be 10 times higher than the general population. All patients with MR angiography–detected aneurysms were studied by digital subtraction catheter angiography. Ten aneurysms were less than 6 mm in diameter, and six were between 7 and 14 mm. Catheter angiography demonstrated one more aneurysm than MR angiography (the size of this aneurysm was not revealed).

Three studies have estimated the prevalence of aneurysms in asymptomatic individuals with a history of autosomal dominant PKD.[6, 10, 44] The prevalence was estimated to range from 4% to 11.7%. It was also noted that a subset of patients with PKD with a familial history of aneurysm had a prevalence that is much higher. Chapman and colleagues[44] identified two patients with aneurysms among 29 subjects with a family history of ruptured intracranial aneurysms employing high-resolution CT; the point estimate (best guess) for the prevalence of aneurysm based on this study is 7% (95% confidence interval is 0.02 to 0.23). Huston and coworkers[6] used MR angiography to identify 6 patients with aneurysms among 27 patients with a family history of aneurysm or SAH; the point estimate for the prevalence of aneurysm based on this study is 22% (95%

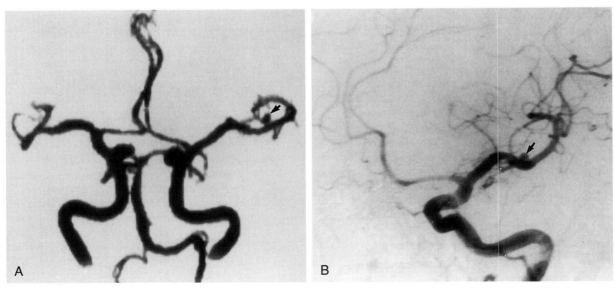

FIGURE 23–5. Berry aneurysm in a patient with autosomal dominant polycystic kidney disease. *A,* A 3D TOF MR angiogram with vessel tracking postprocessing algorithm discloses a left middle cerebral artery bifurcation aneurysm *(arrow). B,* Catheter angiogram shows the same lesion *(arrow).*

confidence interval is 0.08 to 0.42). Ruggieri and associates[10, 53] likewise used MR angiography to identify 5 patients with a saccular intracranial aneurysm among 27 patients with a family history or suspected family history of aneurysm; the point estimate for the prevalence of aneurysm based on this study is 19% (95% confidence interval is 0.09 to 0.42 [adjusted for the estimated false-negative rate of MR angiography]). In a fourth study of patients without PKD, Nakagawa and coworkers[8] used a combination of catheter angiography and MR angiography to screen 400 Japanese patients with a family or clinical history of cerebrovascular disease; 26 patients (6.5%) had aneurysms. Volunteers with a family history of SAH within the second degree of consanguinity revealed a higher prevalence of aneurysms (17.9%).

It was concluded by Levey and associates,[40] in a rigorous decision analysis of patients with PKD, that catheter angiography should not be performed on a routine basis in this population because its benefit becomes significant if the prevalence of aneurysms exceeds 30%, the treatment complication rate is less than 1%, and the patient is younger than 25 years of age. Some investigators indicate that MR angiography may be the optimal noninvasive study for detection of asymptomatic intracranial aneurysms.[6, 10, 45] The current data suggest that MRI with MR angiography is a noninvasive test that has the sensitivity and specificity to have a significant impact on screening high-risk asymptomatic populations.[9]

Black,[46] in an editorial, reviewed the issues concerning screening patients with adult PKD. Although it is clear that MR angiography has the ability to detect aneurysms, the real issue is whether detection actually increases life expectancy of patients with high risk of aneurysms. The arguments favoring screening include the likelihood of serious complication from an aneurysm rupture as being approximately 70%,[54] instead of Levey's initial estimate of 37%.[40] However, the probability of a serious complication resulting from surgery is also believed to be slightly higher than the initial 1% to 3%.[40, 45] With these modifications the screening examination is expected to increase the life expectancy of a typical 48-year-old patient with PKD by only 2 weeks.[46] In addition, it is important to recognize that the size of many of the aneurysms detected in these studies was less than 4 mm. Some authors suggest the risk of rupture of these aneurysms is lower.[49] Black,[46] therefore, concluded that screening asymptomatic patients with MR angiography may not be indicated because of the uncertainty about the natural history and the subsequent risk/benefit ratio of surgical repair if an intracranial aneurysm is detected. In institutions where the surgical complication rate is extremely low and the expected risks and benefits of aneurysm surgery are well understood by patients, however, screening may be an appropriate clinical plan in asymptomatic patients.[46] Clearly, this is vastly different from screening symptomatic patients.

ACUTE SYMPTOMATIC EVALUATION

An important limitation to the use of MRI and MR angiography in the detection of aneurysms is the insensitivity to SAH.[55, 56] This may change because newer hardware and pulse sequences are promising for increasing the sensitivity of MRI to SAH. One study utilizing a fluid-attenuated inversion recovery (FLAIR) pulse sequence revealed equal sensitivity of MRI and CT for detecting SAH.[56a] Patients presenting with signs and symptoms of acute SAH should be studied by CT as part of the initial evaluation. Alternatively, those presenting clinically with intracranial mass lesions may initially be evaluated with MRI followed by conventional intra-arterial angiography.

Computed Tomography

SAH from aneurysm rupture is most commonly an acute event accompanied by severe headache and often followed by altered consciousness or focal neurologic deficit. CT allows sensitive assessment of the subarachnoid and ventricular spaces and is equally crucial to the detection of acute hemorrhage into brain parenchyma and in distinguishing acute hemorrhage from bland infarction or cerebral edema.[57]

Nonenhanced CT is approximately 90% sensitive in detecting SAH within the first 24 hours after the initial event and approximately 50% sensitive if examination is performed within a week after the initial event.[58, 59] Subarachnoid blood is metabolized between 6 and 10 days after the hemorrhage[57]; therefore, CT should be performed as early as possible after the ictus to optimize the chance of demonstrating SAH. As blood is progressively broken down it becomes more isodense relative to cerebrospinal fluid. Therefore, the longer the interval between the time of the CT examination and the onset of SAH, the higher the rate of failure in detecting the presence of SAH. In the acute period, nonenhanced CT does not exclude a small amount of SAH. If there is no contraindication, a lumbar puncture should be performed for patients suspected of having an SAH if the nonenhanced CT scan is unrevealing.

The location of the SAH is often predictive of the location of the aneurysm rupture. However, because of overlap of different hemorrhage patterns the distribution of subarachnoid blood is not always pathognomonic for a specific site of a ruptured aneurysm.[57, 59, 60] Of note is the report by Davis and associates,[61] which did not correlate any relationship between the ruptured aneurysm site and CT findings; some patterns of SAH may imply nonaneurysmal or cryptogenic etiology.[62, 63]

Nevertheless, the following patterns, described by Silver and coworkers[64] in 81 consecutive patients with SAH, may focus attention to a particular aneurysm site. Hemorrhage in the suprasellar cistern and the interhemispheric fissure is most suggestive of an anterior communicating artery aneurysm. Blood in a sylvian fissure is common for an ipsilateral middle cerebral artery aneurysm. Both suprasellar cistern SAH and sylvian fissure SAH suggest an aneurysm located at the internal carotid terminus or at the origin of the posterior communicating artery. Prepontine and ambient cistern hemorrhages favor a basilar tip aneurysm. Prepontine blood should also raise the possibility of a ruptured posterior inferior cerebellar artery aneurysm.

Spin-Echo MRI

The size of a nonthrombosed aneurysm at MRI correlates well with the catheter angiographic size. Both catheter angiography and MR angiography underestimate the size of partially thrombosed aneurysms. Compared with CT, MRI certainly provides superior delineation of the exact location and the relationship to the adjacent neural structures.[65–68] The artery from which the aneurysm arises is frequently identified, but demonstration of the aneurysm neck is often not possible.[9]

SAH is the most common imaging finding of acute aneurysm rupture. Intraparenchymal hemorrhage, intraventricular hemorrhage, or subdural blood collection may accompany aneurysm rupture as well. The location of an intracerebral hematoma is a more accurate predictor than the pattern of SAH in determining the site of a ruptured aneurysm.[57–59, 69] An anterior septum pellucidum (septal) or inferior frontal hematoma is highly predictive of an anterior communicating artery aneurysmal rupture. Posterior communicating artery or terminal internal carotid artery aneurysms may present with anterior temporal lobe or temporal horn hematomas. Middle cerebral artery aneurysms are associated with hematomas in the anterior temporal lobe or insular regions or both. Although MRI is insensitive to acute small SAH, the tissue contrast in smaller parenchymal hematomas adjacent to an aneurysm and larger SAH allows detection. This is important in a patient with multiple cerebral aneurysms in which one has ruptured,[13, 43, 70, 71] especially in patients with no angiographic or CT findings to suggest the location of the rupture.

After hypertensive hemorrhage, ruptured saccular aneurysms are the second most common cause for intraventricular hemorrhage.[72] Anterior communicating artery aneurysm ruptures are most often associated with intraventricular extension of SAH, followed by rupture of posterior inferior cerebellar artery or basilar artery tip aneurysms.[60] Intraventricular hemorrhage may accompany intraparenchymal hematomas adjacent to the site of aneurysm rupture.

Subdural hematomas occasionally occur as complications of ruptured intracranial aneurysms. Aneurysms of the anterior communicating artery or anterior cerebral artery may rupture into the interhemispheric subdural space.[73] Peripheral middle cerebral artery aneurysms have reportedly ruptured into the frontoparietal subdural space.[74] Posterior communicating artery and middle cerebral artery bifurcation aneurysms have notably ruptured into the subtemporal subdural space.

A less common mode of acute presentation of intracranial aneurysm is that of nonhemorrhagic cerebral infarction. This is most frequently seen with giant aneurysms. Flow through the patent lumen of giant aneurysms containing poorly organized thrombus can dislodge clot, producing a transient ischemic attack or thromboembolic infarction.

The major reason why conventional MRI is not the initial examination of choice for suspected aneurysm rupture is that it is notoriously insensitive for detecting acute SAH.[75, 76] With newer pulse sequences, such as FLAIR, the sensitivity of MRI for SAH may equal or exceed that of CT.[56a] The specificity of MRI for detecting extravasated blood products is dependent on the progressive breakdown of hemoglobin.[77–79] The diminished sensitivity of MRI in the acute stages of SAH is thought to relate to the higher partial pressure of oxygen within the cerebrospinal fluid compared with brain parenchyma.[75] The higher oxygen partial pressure delays conversion of oxyhemoglobin to deoxyhemoglobin and methemoglobin. This conversion is responsible for altering the relaxation rates of neighboring protons (i.e., changing the local cerebrospinal fluid signal) and increasing the conspicuity of hemorrhage on MR images. When present, blood can be recognized as areas of relative high signal intensity in the normally low-signal-intensity subarachnoid cisterns and sulci on T1-weighted images (see Fig. 23–1). The pathophysiology of blood breakdown products in the subarachnoid space is far more variable and less predictable than brain parenchyma. The variability is attributed to delayed conversion of diamagnetic oxyhemoglobin to paramagnetic deoxyhemoglobin and the presence of methemoglobin in the subarachnoid space. The metabolism of subarachnoid paramagnetic blood breakdown products is sufficiently unreliable as to preclude the use of MRI for suspected life-threatening SAH.[80, 81]

The signal changes on routine MR images produced by intraparenchymal hemorrhage and thrombus are variable, although often dramatic and quite specific. The recognition and characterization of the MRI findings in intracranial hemorrhage are understandable after considering the context of the findings, which depend on 1) the location, specifically subarachnoid versus intraparenchymal; 2) the oxidative state of hemoglobin and the subsequent breakdown products; 3) the type of imaging pulse sequence used (T1 versus T2, spin-echo versus gradient-echo, conventional spin-echo versus rapid acquisition with relaxation enhancement [RARE] sequences); and 4) the field strength of the machine used to acquire the images.[66, 77, 82]

The explanation for the predictable evolutionary MRI appearance of parenchymal hemorrhage at high magnetic fields in conventional spin-echo imaging is outlined by Gomori and colleagues.[77] Signal intensity patterns of blood breakdown products on T1- and T2-weighted images evolve in three general time frames: 1) the acute stage (<7 days old), 2) the subacute stage (<1 month, >1 week), and 3) the chronic stage (>1 month). In the acute stage, intraparenchymal hematomas are isointense or slightly hypointense relative to normal gray matter on T1-weighted images, with an area of marked hypointensity on the T2-weighted scans. This appearance is attributable to the presence of intracellular deoxyhemoglobin. Although paramagnetic, deoxyhemoglobin demonstrates minimal proton-electron dipolar-dipolar interaction because of limited access to water protons and thus has low signal intensity on T1-weighted images. However, ferrous deoxyhemoglobin also produces significant heterogeneity of magnetic susceptibility and thus low signal intensity on T2-weighted images.[83] With intraparenchymal hematomas, after the first few days the T2-weighted images also demonstrate a peripheral area of high signal intensity within the surrounding brain related to reactive edema. In the subacute stage, thrombus begins to acquire a ring of high signal intensity on T1-weighted images that gradually fills from the periphery; somewhat later a similar effect is observed on the T2-weighted images. This high signal intensity is believed to be due to the oxidation of deoxyhemoglobin to ferric methemoglobin, which is not only paramagnetic but also accessible to water protons. The methemoglobin is initially intracellular and also produces significant local susceptibility changes on the T2-weighted images, which is responsible for its low signal intensity initially. With red blood cell lysis this effect dissipates, ultimately resulting in high signal intensity on the T2-weighted scans as well. The paramagnetic effects of methemoglobin have been reported to persist for up to 1 year. After approximately 3 weeks an outer ring of low signal intensity gradually appears at the site of hemorrhage, which is most prominent on the T2-weighted images. This corresponds to the appearance of macrophages at the margins of the thrombus that digest the red blood cells, leaving hemosiderin and ferritin (Fig. 23–6). These materials produce significant magnetic susceptibility changes, which result in low signal intensity on both T1- and T2-weighted images. This effect is accentuated on more T2-weighted images and can persist indefinitely. This phenomenon increases with the square of the magnetic field and is directly proportional to the echo time (TE).[77, 84–87]

This description of evolving hemorrhage pertains primarily to "conventional," dual-echo, spin-echo im-

aging. Because of the inferior signal refocusing of gradient-echo techniques, the T2* signal loss observed secondary to magnetic susceptibility phenomena is much more pronounced on these types of images.[66, 88] Alternatively, with the newer RARE spin-echo techniques now popular in clinical practice, this phenomenon is less dramatic, owing to the inherent signal refocusing of successive 180° refocusing pulses or possibly to the T2-filtering effects of variable k-space sampling[82, 89, 90] (see also Chapters 7 and 21).

MR Angiography

Catheter angiography as the exclusive vascular imaging modality for evaluation of patients with acute SAH is being challenged. In one case report of a patient with SAH, MR angiography demonstrated the ruptured anterior communicating artery aneurysm that was undetected by catheter angiography.[91] A second study comparing MR angiography with catheter angiography in the setting of SAH is encouraging.[92] Fourteen patients presenting with acute SAH were evaluated with both modalities. In 3 of the 14 patients no abnormalities were detected on either diagnostic test, and 2 patients had two aneurysms. MR angiography detected all the aneurysms with the exception of one, a 2-mm middle cerebral artery aneurysm. Catheter angiography failed to detect a 5-mm middle cerebral artery aneurysm. These preliminary data suggest that MRI and MR angiography may have a role in the setting of SAH, especially if the catheter angiogram is unrevealing.

SYMPTOMATIC, UNRUPTURED ANEURYSMS

Spin-Echo MRI

Pathologically, giant intracranial aneurysms are characterized as mass lesions composed of variable

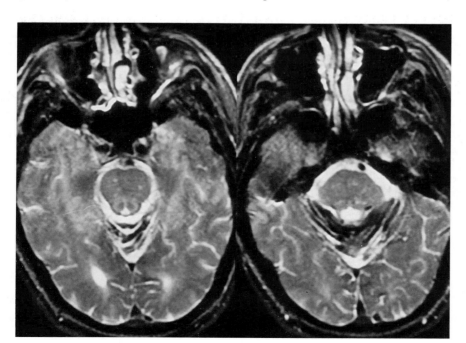

FIGURE 23–6. Superficial siderosis. Axial T2-weighted images demonstrate marked hypointensity of the cerebellar vermis due to deposition of hemosiderin and ferritin on the brain parenchyma from a remote SAH.

amounts of differing age thrombus or flowing blood within a patent lumen. There may also be variable degrees of calcification within the wall and edema involving the adjacent brain parenchyma. Due to its high contrast, multiplanar imaging capability, sensitivity to edema, ischemia and blood breakdown products, and responsiveness to motion, MRI is ideal for evaluating giant aneurysms.[77, 93–96] MRI has exquisite sensitivity to parenchymal edema in the presence of ischemia or inflammation.[97] When seen on spin-echo images, intracranial giant aneurysms typically exhibit a peripheral area of low signal intensity on T1-weighted studies, with an associated larger irregular area of high signal intensity on T2-weighted studies in the brain adjacent to the aneurysm (see Fig. 23–4). The dominant effect responsible for these signal changes is the presence of additional free water protons within edematous tissue relative to adjacent normal brain. Several reports describe in detail the collective findings of edema and thrombus about the focal areas of blood flow anticipated with giant intracranial aneurysms at MRI.[68, 93, 98] When present, the thrombus is typically laminated along the confines of the aneurysm wall and dome. The physiologically dynamic nature of these lesions results in the clot often demonstrating alternating layers of high and low signal intensity on both T1- and T2-weighted studies, reflecting the varying stages of blood breakdown products (see Fig. 23–4). The characteristic curvilinear calcification often noted within mural thrombus on a CT scan is not readily discernible from chronic clot with MRI. The constellation of MRI signal derangements provides a characteristic appearance for giant aneurysms, as well as the opportunity to demonstrate and quantify the local vasculature noninvasively with a variety of flow-sensitive techniques.[68, 93]

The MRI depiction of flow is complex; however, recognition of the telltale signs of motion often confirms the diagnosis of aneurysm amid an otherwise long differential diagnosis of mass lesions.[68] Blood flow (motion) during either excitation or sampling results in two types of corresponding effects on the MRI signal intensity of moving spins: 1) the wash-in/wash-out or "flight" of spins relative to the timing and placement of a radiofrequency pulse produces so-called TOF effects, and 2) spins moving during the application, and in the direction of an imaging gradient, produce a shift in signal phase dependent on the type of flow (e.g., constant velocity, turbulent) and gradient in the flow direction (i.e., spin-phase phenomena).[37, 96] These flow-induced changes in MRI signal form the basis of identifying and quantifying flow; in effect, motion itself is an agent of contrast. Depending on the imaging technique, TOF and spin-phase phenomena may produce high or low signal intensity at an area of flow.

Often all or part of the aneurysm has a patent lumen. On T2-weighted spin-echo scans this is almost always recognized as a dark area secondary to the TOF effect known as *flow void*, as well as concomitant signal loss due to spin dephasing (see Fig. 23–4). Although due to different mechanisms, both phenomena are dependent on the long TE values used for such sequences; therefore, the longer the TE, the more reliable is the signal loss due to blood flow. With T1-weighted or short-TE, long–repetition time (TR) scans, a second TOF effect known as *flow-related enhancement* may be present that can produce high signal intensity within the patent aneurysm lumen, especially if the aneurysm is near the first image slice encountered along the direction of flow (so-called entry slice phenomenon, a form of flow-related enhancement) (see Fig. 23–4). Spin-phase phenomena secondary to motion along imaging gradients may still be present, but they are reduced at shorter TE values. In addition to simply loss of signal, these spin-phase effects are also responsible for the ghost artifact seen in the phase-encoding direction on these scans, which is highly characteristic of pulsatile flow arising from the lumen of the aneurysm[99] (see Fig. 23–3).

Other nonvascular flow phenomena may potentially result in a false-positive diagnosis of aneurysm. Cerebrospinal fluid motion from adjacent transmitted vascular pulsations may give rise to areas of cerebrospinal fluid hypointensity surrounding a vessel, simulating the flow void of an aneurysm. This is usually noted on long-TR, short-TE and long-TR, long-TE images as hypodensities adjacent to vessels such as the basilar artery.[100] These phenomena are accentuated in pulse sequence techniques without flow compensation schemes (Fig. 23–7). Another manifestation of the same phenomenon with both large and small vessels are phase shift artifacts, which are recognized as a series of alternating dark and light bands arising from the pulsating vessels due to spatial signal misregistration in the phase-encoding direction. These artifacts are particularly troublesome mimics of fusiform aneurysms of the posterior circulation. Usually, they can be distinguished as large areas of flow void that do not have the same association with layered thrombus commonly seen with saccular giant aneurysms.[101]

Another pitfall in MRI evaluation of aneurysms is the apparent flow void that can be seen in the paraclinoid region and may be confused with a pneumatized anterior clinoid process or other bony structures of the skull base[23] (Fig. 23–8). Such relationships are also important, because the proximity of a given lesion to the skull base and sinuses may hinder satisfactory clip placement. This pitfall may be avoided if a gradient-echo flow-imaging protocol is used. Small nonthrombotic aneurysms usually demonstrate the signal characteristics of the supplying vessel, specifically the fast-flow–related enhancement or bright signal, not flow void.

MR Angiography

Manipulation of the radiofrequency excitation pulse sequence to maximize the TOF effect known as flow-related enhancement has led to a variety of TOF MR angiography techniques. With this method, vascular contrast is maximized by the rapid flow of blood through the region of interest. This has been exploited to best advantage for the detection of small berry aneurysms[9, 10, 44] (see Fig. 23–5). In addition to radiofrequency pulse manipulations used to produce TOF angiograms, gradient-modified images that produce vas-

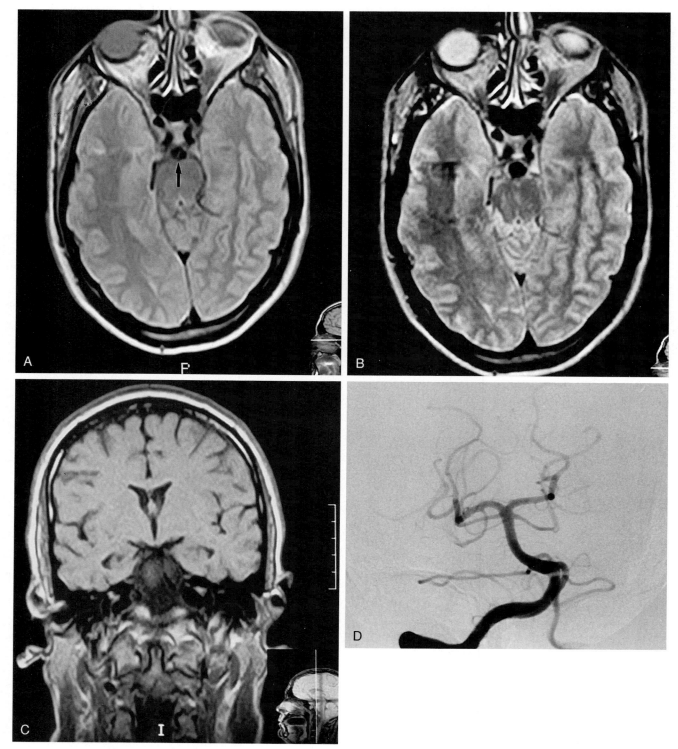

FIGURE 23–7. "Basilar tip" aneurysm. Short-TE, long-TR *(A)* and long-TE, long-TR *(B)* images demonstrate enlargement of the basilar artery tip, suggestive of basilar tip aneurysm *(arrow)*. Also note the alternating dark and light bands (ghost artifact) arising off the pulsatile vessel. *C,* T1-weighted coronal image shows subtle but possible enlargement of the basilar tip. All of these images were obtained without a flow compensation scheme, resulting in the inaccurate diagnosis of a basilar tip aneurysm. *D,* Catheter angiogram of the same patient demonstrates a normal basilar bifurcation.

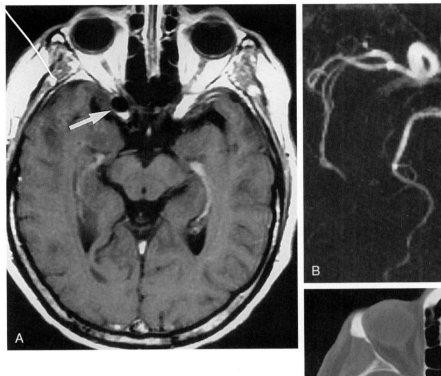

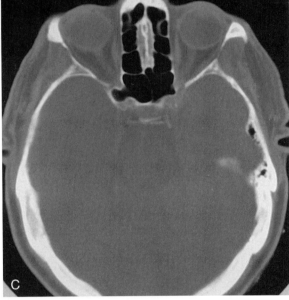

FIGURE 23–8. Pneumatized anterior clinoid. *A,* T1-weighted image reveals an area of low signal intensity *(arrow)* that could represent a flow void and inappropriately be diagnosed as an aneurysm. *B,* A 3D TOF MR angiogram shows no aneurysm in this region. *C,* Axial CT scan discloses the pneumatized anterior clinoid.

cular contrast on the basis of spin-phase phenomena can be obtained and are known as PC MR angiography. Acquisition times for comparable resolution of 3D studies are typically longer for PC than the analogous TOF angiograms. Additional cine MR angiographic techniques exist that can demonstrate flow and flow disturbances within aneurysms; with some, it is possible to quantify blood flow and flow velocities[102–104] (see also Chapter 25). Giant intracranial aneurysms, which are conspicuous on spin-echo images, may not demonstrate the same level of vascular contrast with MR angiography, owing to slower, disturbed flow within the aneurysm lumen.[105–107] In addition, most clinical TOF techniques employ a maximal intensity projection (MIP) algorithm to create the angiographic image from the original image data set. Although expeditious, it does not completely exclude the angiogram signal from stationary tissue, which can become problematic with tissue with high signal intensity such as fat and paramagnetic blood breakdown products. The inclusion of stationary signal into the flow image may result in image degradation, or in a misleading diagnosis or imply flow in stationary tissue[106–108] (see Fig. 23–2). Currently, the spatial resolution of 3DFT TOF MR angiography is approximately 0.8 mm, still less than catheter angiography but adequate to detect 2- to 3-mm aneurysms. This may be of practical importance because both Locksley[49] and McCormick and coworkers[109] reported no SAHs from aneurysms smaller than 3 mm. Therefore, the aneurysms of most clinical concern are detected by current MR angiographic techniques (see Fig. 23–5).

In a retrospective study by Ross and associates,[9] 3DFT TOF MR angiography combined with MRI resulted in a combined sensitivity of 95% and a specificity of 100% compared with catheter digital subtraction angiography. These results are encouraging, but several limitations of the study and 3DFT technique were illuminated. First, the incidence of aneurysms within the study group was much higher than in the population as a whole, introducing bias into the sensitivity value. Second, vascular contrast depends on the presence of adequate inflow; slow-flow lesions, such as giant or fusiform intracranial aneurysms were poorly visualized or underestimated in size, although these were easily detected on the spin-echo images. Although the anterior communicating artery, middle cerebral artery, and basilar tip aneurysms were typically well defined, the carotid siphon proved problematic to characterize fully because of signal dropout from the uncompensated turbulent flow. Solutions to these limitations include targeted MIPs, better flow compensation, shorter TE, and reduced slice thickness.[9] Another important conclusion to be drawn from this investigation is the importance of examination of the individual partitions from the 3DFT MR angiography data set, which revealed aneurysms not visualized on the MIP postprocessed angiogram. Although tedious, this is particularly important for adequate evaluation of the carotid siphon.

In a blind prospective study, the sensitivity of spin-echo MRI, 3D PC MR angiography, and 3D TOF MR angiography for the detection of known intracranial aneurysms was evaluated.[110] All 16 patients harboring 27 intracranial aneurysms were previously studied with catheter angiography. Sensitivities of the MRI sequences were calculated as follows: axial T1-weighted images, 26%; axial T2-weighted images, 48%; 3D PC MR angiography (256 × 128 matrix), 44.1%; and 3D TOF MR angiography (512 × 256 matrix), 55.6%. If the analysis was restricted to aneurysms 5 mm or larger, the sensitivity was increased to T1-weighted images, 37.5%; T2-weighted images, 62.5%; 3D PC MR angiography, 75%; and 3D TOF MR angiography, 87.5%. Interestingly, two aneurysms identified on the T2-weighted images were not seen on the TOF MR angiogram because of adjacent blood products. Moreover, in a limited retrospective analysis of several patients with smaller aneurysms, all aneurysms 3 mm or larger could be identified. However, the authors concluded that in prospective evaluation, 5-mm aneurysms appear to be the critical size for reliable detection.[110] A second study by Korogi and colleagues[111] evaluated intracranial aneurysms in 61 patients with a total of 78 aneurysms. Sensitivity in detecting aneurysms for the five observers for small aneurysms (less than 5 mm) was 56%, and it was 86% for medium-sized aneurysms (greater than 5 mm but less than 12 mm). Detection of aneurysms arising off the carotid artery was more difficult than that of aneurysms of the anterior or middle cerebral arteries. Prospectively, 13 aneurysms were missed by all five observers; all were 4 mm or less in diameter, but 8 of the 13 aneurysms were identified retrospectively. The results of these studies should be interpreted with caution because analysis was performed without the spin-echo images and individual MR angiographic partitions. Moreover, targeted MIPs were not performed. A reasonable conclusion from the presentation of these data suggests

that both MRI and MR angiography are valuable techniques in screening patients suspected of harboring aneurysms.[112] Moreover, it is imperative that evaluation of a patient suspected of having an aneurysm include routine MRI in combination with an MR angiographic technique. MR angiographic evaluation includes both evaluation of individual partitions as well as MIPs. Reliance on several MIP images from a 3D TOF MR angiogram or a single image from a two-dimensional (2D) PC acquisition represents an incomplete evaluation.[112] Small aneurysms, specifically aneurysms less than 5 mm, are not detected as reliably as large aneurysms.

Early work by Huston and colleagues[105] suggested that 3D PC techniques yielded better results than TOF techniques. The same authors' more recent work in a prospective comparison concludes that 3D TOF techniques are more appropriate for screening of intracranial aneurysms.[110] It is also important to recognize that both PC and TOF techniques have individual strengths and weaknesses as well as pitfalls. The merits of each technique should be optimized and applied appropriately to render the most useful information.

The predominant rheologic feature of fusiform and giant aneurysms is slow flow along the wall, often resulting in laminated mural thrombus. These lesions are typically conspicuous on spin-echo images, but, as discussed previously, they may not demonstrate the same level of vascular contrast, owing to slow, disturbed flow within the aneurysm lumen.[105–107] As a result, the aneurysm size and associated thrombus can best be evaluated with spin-echo MRI. Because PC MR angiography is not dependent on rapid flow and uses a true subtraction scheme to generate the images, it avoids misregistration of clot into the final image and is often better suited in the evaluation of giant aneurysms.[34, 105] If an aneurysm is partially thrombosed, MR angiography may underestimate the true size or not detect an aneurysm in a fashion analogous to catheter angiography.

There have been significant advances in acquisition and postprocessing techniques that will no doubt continue to improve image quality and enhance its role in the diagnostic armamentarium (see Fig. 23–5). Occasionally, the flexibility of postprocessing with the 3D data set of MR angiographic images may allow visualization of certain aneurysms, as well as delineate the morphology of the aneurysm such as branch vessels better than catheter angiography[107] (Fig. 23–9). A variety of preprocessing and postprocessing innovations have also been attempted to minimize the pitfalls of MIP-rendered images. These include magnetization transfer and fat saturation pulses to minimize signal from nonvascular stationary tissue, macromolecular paramagnetic contrast agents, and multiple overlapping thin-slab 3D acquisition schemes.[113–116]

Finally, beyond simple static angiographic display of vascular anatomy, MR flow-sensitive techniques have also been used to create multiplanar reconstructions of aneurysms, which are useful in defining the aneurysm neck or determining intradural or extradural location (see Fig. 23–3).

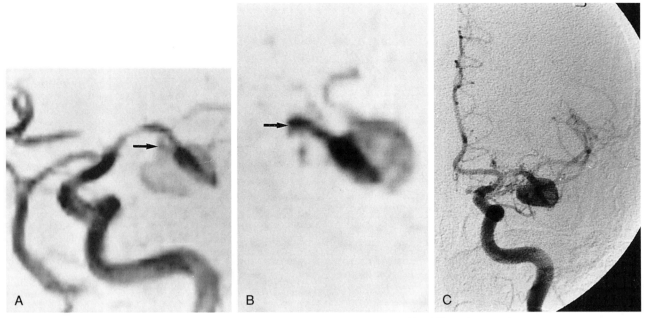

FIGURE 23–9. Middle cerebral artery bifurcation aneurysm. *A,* A 3D TOF MR angiogram demonstrates an aneurysm arising off the middle cerebral artery bifurcation. The distal branch of the middle cerebral artery arises off the superior medial aspect of the aneurysm *(arrow)*. *B,* Targeted MIP image displays the aneurysm again, with the efferent limb *(arrow)* and the afferent vessel arising off the aneurysm. In both MR angiograms, the relative high signal intensity represents the inflow stream within the aneurysm. *C,* The saccular middle cerebral aneurysm is clearly demonstrated, but the relationships of the parent and branch vessels to the neck of the aneurysm are not revealed on the angiogram and were not demonstrated in spite of multiple oblique images.

COMPLICATIONS OF ANEURYSM RUPTURE

Hydrocephalus

The development of hydrocephalus after rupture of an aneurysm is a common occurrence. Blood in the subarachnoid space increases cerebrospinal fluid protein levels, producing adhesions or inflammatory changes in the subarachnoid spaces that may ultimately result in communicating hydrocephalus. In addition, obstructive hydrocephalus may occur if intraventricular hemorrhage is present, especially if blood is present in the third or fourth ventricles. Distention of the ventricles may damage the ventricle-brain barrier, thereby allowing cerebrospinal fluid to spread through the extracellular space within the periventricular white matter, so-called noncytotoxic nonvasogenic cerebral edema.[117–119]

MRI and CT are accurate modalities for detecting the presence and degree of hydrocephalus. Hydrocephalus-related cerebral edema is visualized as periventricular decreased signal intensity on T1-weighted images and a hyperintense signal pattern on T2-weighted images compared with gray matter. The signal abnormalities are frequently seen extending from the frontal horns toward the frontal poles in patients with obstructive hydrocephalus. The mechanism of these signal changes has been attributed to transventricular passage of cerebrospinal fluid due to a change in ependymal permeability secondary to increased intraventricular pressure.[118] Periventricular signal abnormalities are seen most often in patients with acute or subacute obstructive hydrocephalus due to tumors and also in the presence of papilledema or a decreased level of consciousness.[119] After ventricular shunt placement, the ventricular enlargement and abnormal signal changes resolve.

Aneurysm Rebleeding

For untreated aneurysms one cause of clinical deterioration that occurs after SAH is rebleeding with its significant morbidity and mortality. The rates of rebleeding after aneurysm rupture vary among different series and are as high as 15% to 20% within the first 2 weeks and 50% by 6 months.[24, 101, 120] However, it is agreed that the risk is significant and greatest within the first 2 weeks after the initial rupture. By 6 months the annualized rebleeding rate is estimated to be 2% to 3%. Rebleeding in the first few days may be difficult to determine because the blood in the subarachnoid space from the initial SAH may mask further bleeding into the subarachnoid space. Increased volume of SAH or intraventricular hemorrhage in addition to new or expanding intraparenchymal hemorrhage are signs that indicate rebleeding. At 1 week after the initial SAH, blood in the subarachnoid space should be almost isodense relative to parenchymal gray matter on CT scans. If at this point there is new hyperdense SAH, rebleeding has probably occurred.

Cerebral Vasospasm

Vasospasm is one of the main causes of morbidity and mortality after acute aneurysm rupture. Arterial spasm may be local or diffuse and symptomatic or asymptomatic. Approximately 40% of patients develop vasospasm after aneurysmal SAH. Fifty percent of patients with angiographic evidence of vasospasm develop delayed ischemic deficits, and the mortality of patients who develop delayed ischemic deficits is approximately 50%. These deficits typically develop between day 3 and day 13 after SAH.[121]

The size and location of the subarachnoid hematoma in the basal cisterns are reliable findings to predict subsequent vasospasm.[61, 62, 122] Vasospasm occurred in 20 of 22 patients with large thick hematomas and in 5 of 19 patients with no blood or diffuse SAH on CT scans. Black[123] described a high association of both vasospasm (74%) and hydrocephalus (67%) with large SAHs. Decreased attenuation on CT scans indicative of ischemia or infarction also has a strong correlation with vasospasm. Ischemic findings at MRI would also be expected to have a strong correlation with vasospasm. Infarction secondary to vasospasm occurs mainly in the peripheral cortex and adjacent white matter.[124]

POST-TREATMENT EVALUATION AND ANEURYSM THROMBOSIS

Because MRI's sensitivity to the motion of blood flow permits the preoperative recognition of aneurysms on the basis of flow phenomena such as ghost artifact and MR angiography, the post-treatment scans can also reveal the effect of treatment on vascular occlusion or aneurysm thrombosis.[125]

Although open clipping of such lesions usually calls for intraoperative or postoperative catheter angiography to assess these lesions and reliably exclude a small aneurysm rest, several studies suggest that postoperative MRI of patients with a successfully clipped aneurysm is safe and provides more useful information than does CT.[126, 127] Regardless of the chemical composition of the aneurysm clip, most CT images are markedly degraded by beam-hardening artifacts arising from the aneurysm clip. Often with MRI the artifacts are produced due to the magnetic properties of the alloys within the surgical clips, resulting in local image distortion due to inhomogeneities produced in the magnetic field. The amount of artifact created on both imaging modalities relates to both the clip size and the alloy used in production of the clip.[127] The difficulty arises in distinguishing the ferromagnetic from the nonferromagnetic clip once it has been placed in the patient. The safety of a magnetic clip for imaging does not imply that there will be no artifact, rather that there will be no deflection and thus no risk of dislodging of the aneurysm clip.[127–129] Skepticism regarding the routine use of MRI for postoperative evaluation of surgically clipped aneurysms relates to the potential for ferromagnetic interaction between the imager and

clip, leading to vascular disruption with possible catastrophic consequences.[130, 131] Although there are numerous published reports testing MRI-compatible aneurysm clips, news of a fatal complication has led to renewed caution and recommendations for tighter quality assurance programs by both manufacturers and treating physicians.[132] Aneurysms wrapped with muslin gauze at surgery may be successfully evaluated with MR angiographic techniques, as long as no other sources of artifact are nearby.

Aneurysms not amenable to surgical treatment may be approached by endovascular techniques. These techniques primarily consist of parent artery occlusion (hunterian) or direct aneurysm occlusion. Fox and colleagues[133] successfully treated 65 of 67 patients by proximal parent artery occlusion with a detachable balloon. Complete obliteration of the aneurysm in 65 of 84 patients by direct balloon placement into the lumen of the aneurysm was achieved by Higashida and associates[134] (this method of treating aneurysms has for the most part been abandoned). More recently, direct occlusion of aneurysms with preservation of the parent artery is being performed with Guglielmi detachable coils with good success.[135] Hunterian closure of the parent artery may be assessed by MRI. With regard to aneurysms treated by proximal balloon occlusion or a Drake tourniquet, several small series of patients with giant aneurysms thrombosed by parent artery embolization were followed with MRI.[65, 126, 136–139] In Strother's series of the aneurysms that were 100% occluded, all demonstrated a decrease in physical size on follow-up MRI.[65] The one patient who had a 90% obliteration of the lumen demonstrated no change in the size of giant aneurysm during a 2-year follow-up. Thrombus formation in an incompletely thrombosed giant aneurysm differs from organizing thrombus in a completely thrombosed aneurysm (Fig. 23–10). The thrombosis after occlusion is due to stasis, a mechanism analogous to venous (red) thrombosis rather than arterial (white) thrombosis. This is reflected in the appearance on MR images. Iatrogenically induced thrombosis demonstrates an area of hyperintensity at 5 to 10 days on short-TR, short-TE and long-TR, short-TE images. The long-TR, long-TE images demonstrate hypointensity. At 4 to 6 weeks, induced thrombus was hyperintense on all spin-echo sequences where native, spontaneous mural thrombus still had areas of hypointensity, but these had increased in signal intensity from the subacute stage (5 to 10 days).[65, 137]

There have been reports of persistent or increasing mass effect after treatment by proximal artery occlusion.[65] MRI is useful in the detection of mass effect or ischemia secondary to vascular compression. Vasogenic or ischemic edema is typically perceived by prolongation of T1 (low signal) and T2 (high signal) relaxation times of brain parenchyma on nonenhanced scans. The sensitivity of MRI in detecting infarcts in the first 24 hours is approximately 80% compared with a sensitivity of approximately 50% for CT.[140] The earliest changes of infarction visualized on MR images are enlargement and distortion of cortical gyri due to tissue swelling. These morphologic changes are best visu-

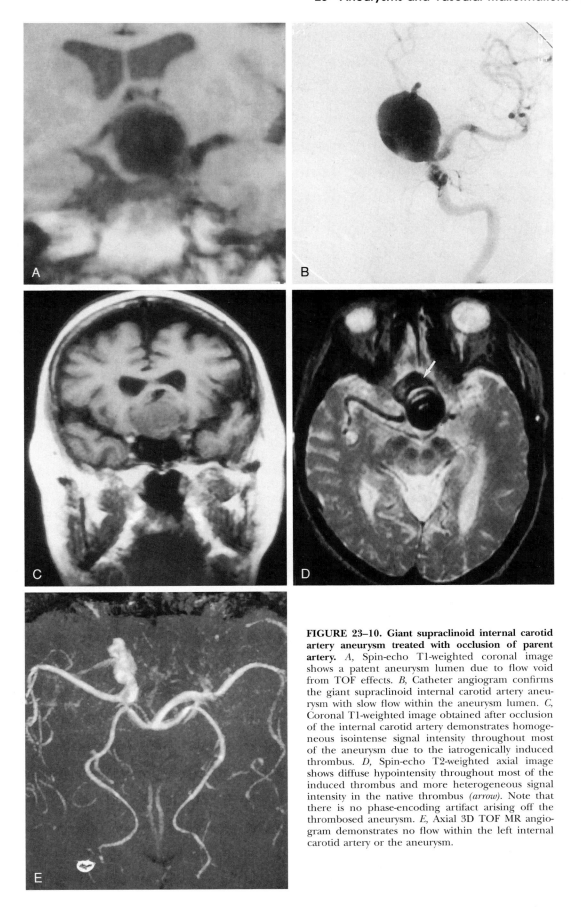

FIGURE 23–10. Giant supraclinoid internal carotid artery aneurysm treated with occlusion of parent artery. *A,* Spin-echo T1-weighted coronal image shows a patent aneurysm lumen due to flow void from TOF effects. *B,* Catheter angiogram confirms the giant supraclinoid internal carotid artery aneurysm with slow flow within the aneurysm lumen. *C,* Coronal T1-weighted image obtained after occlusion of the internal carotid artery demonstrates homogeneous isointense signal intensity throughout most of the aneurysm due to the iatrogenically induced thrombus. *D,* Spin-echo T2-weighted axial image shows diffuse hypointensity throughout most of the induced thrombus and more heterogeneous signal intensity in the native thrombus *(arrow).* Note that there is no phase-encoding artifact arising off the thrombosed aneurysm. *E,* Axial 3D TOF MR angiogram demonstrates no flow within the left internal carotid artery or the aneurysm.

alized with short-TE, short-TR sequences and can be seen within 2 to 6 hours after infarction.[141] Slightly later, increased T2 signal intensity is visualized in the involved tissue as the result of developing cytotoxic edema. Reports of use of paramagnetic contrast agents suggest even earlier detection of ischemia.[142]

The post-therapeutic assessment of patients treated by direct aneurysmal closure with endovascular placement of balloons includes identifying the location of the occluding balloon or coils, assessing the presence of thrombus, and determining residual flow in the parent artery or aneurysm. Tsuruda and associates[143] evaluated five patients treated with detachable balloons. Three of these patients had residual flow within the treated aneurysms. 3D TOF MR angiography identified the residual aneurysm lumen in two of these patients. Methemoglobin within the thrombus obscured the flow in the third patient. A second potential pitfall is slow flow within the aneurysm rest. Evaluation of patients treated with Guglielmi detachable coils with MR angiography has not been published. A canine study with both PC and TOF techniques was compared with catheter angiography and revealed detection of only two of eight aneurysm rests.[144] Both MR angiographic techniques were degraded by the susceptibility artifact from the coils. Clinical implementation of both techniques has occasionally been successful (Fig. 23–11).

VASCULAR MALFORMATIONS

Pial vascular malformations of the brain have been traditionally categorized as AVMs, cavernous malformations (CMs), capillary telangiectasia, and venous angiomas.[145, 146] An additional category of vascular malformation should be recognized, that is, the dural AVM, which is more appropriately categorized as the dural AVF.

From a clinical standpoint it is important to recognize the natural history of each of these malformations and to identify characteristics that can be predictors of behavior of a lesion over time.

ARTERIOVENOUS MALFORMATIONS

Clinical Features

Central nervous system pial AVMs are less common than are intracranial aneurysms, occurring in approximately 0.15% of the U.S. population.[147] AVMs are congenital vascular abnormalities resulting from direct connections between the arteries and veins from the failure of regression of the primitive direct communications between the arterial and venous systems.[146] The actual arteriovenous connection is through a nest of abnormal vessels supplanting the normal capillary bed. The clinical presentation of AVMs is predominantly through intracranial hemorrhage, incapacitating headaches, seizures, and progressive neurologic deficits related to adjacent brain ischemia.[148, 149] Larger AVMs

are more likely to present with seizures, ischemia, or both,[150] whereas smaller AVMs more often hemorrhage.[151]

The natural history of untreated AVMs is an annual rate of hemorrhage of 2% to 4%, with subsequent morbidity and mortality related to hemorrhage of 2% to 3% and 1% annually, respectively.[148–151] In addition, the mortality from an unruptured AVM is approximately 1% per year and the mortality associated with the first hemorrhage is approximately 10%. Graf and colleagues[152] concluded that the incidence of rebleeding after an initial hemorrhage from a brain AVM is approximately 6% per year and then returns to the normal annualized rate of 2% to 4% per year thereafter.

Morphologic evaluation of AVMs has been performed to attempt to predict aggressive or a more benign course. Marks and coworkers[149] performed a detailed angiographic analysis in 65 patients with intracranial AVMs and identified features that correlated positively with hemorrhage. Specifically, these consisted of central venous drainage, periventricular or intraventricular location, and the presence of an intranidal aneurysm. Negatively correlated findings were AVMs with any peripheral venous drainage and AVMs with arteries providing collateral flow (so-called angiomatous change) to ischemic brain about the AVM. Another morphologic feature that reportedly increases the risk of hemorrhage is a small AVM with a nidus diameter of 3 cm or less.[151]

Definitive treatment for AVMs may involve surgery, endovascular therapy, or radiation therapy. A subset of these AVMs (specifically, those that are large and in deep or eloquent parts of the brain) are particularly problematic and require a coordinated, multimodality approach to their management.[153]

Because of the multimodality approach of treating AVMs, it is important to establish not only the diagnosis but also the morphologic and physiologic features of the lesion, which facilitate appropriate therapeutic decisions. To arrive at an appropriate therapeutic plan, specific features of the AVM need to be demonstrated. The afferent arterial feeding pedicles should be characterized as 1) direct terminal feeders supplying only the AVM (Fig. 23–12) or 2) indirect arterial pedicles supplying both the AVM and normal brain distal to the malformation, so-called passage vessels. A second variety of indirect supply angiomatous change is important, because this supply to the malformation may enlarge after incomplete treatment of the direct arterial supply.[154, 155] Angiomatous change (collateral flow) may appear similar to the AVM nidus; however, distinguishing features include absence of the arteriovenous shunting and slower circulation.[155] Other architectural aspects of the arterial supply that are important include the presence of AVFs and flow-related saccular aneurysms (21% of cases) seen on the supplying pedicle to the AVM.[156]

In addition to the afferent supply, determination of the nidus size is important. The nidus is a pathologic network of abnormal vascular channels replacing the normal arteriolar and capillary network and resulting

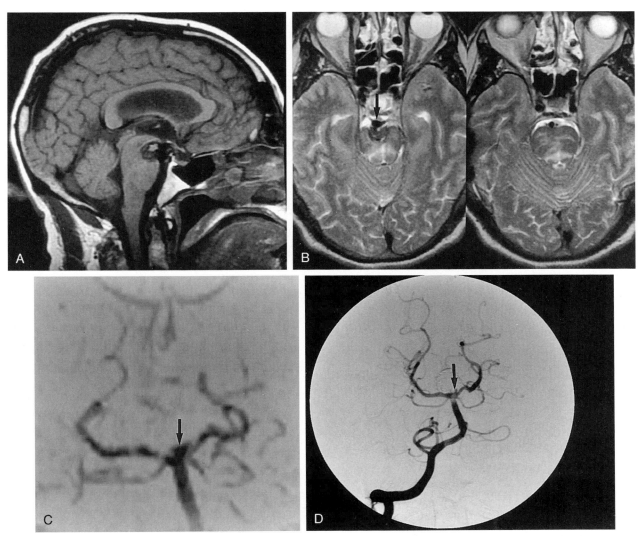

FIGURE 23–11. Basilar tip aneurysm after treatment with Guglielmi detachable coils. *A,* Spin-echo T1-weighted sagittal image reveals heterogeneous signal intensity in the interpeduncular cistern due to a combination of local field inhomogeneity from the intra-aneurysm location of the coils and thrombus. *B,* Axial T2-weighted images reveal decreased signal intensity from a combination of the intra-aneurysmal coils and thrombus. The distal tip of the basilar artery is still somewhat enlarged *(arrow).* Note the high signal intensity within the pons. *C,* Frontal view from a 3D TOF MR angiogram shows residual flow in the base of the aneurysm *(arrow). D,* Corresponding angiogram demonstrating the small aneurysm rest *(arrow),* which was subsequently treated with additional coils.

in a low resistance, arteriovenous connection. Nidus size varies, as does its configuration; it may be compact, diffuse, and occasionally multicompartmental.[154] Often, 3D TOF MR angiography allows the most accurate determination of the nidus size (see Fig. 23–12).

The efferent side of the AVM is also variable. Several large draining veins that coalesce to a single larger vein or represent several independent large veins are the most common pattern. Venous drainage is categorized as 1) superficial drainage into the sagittal, cavernous, transverse, sigmoid, and sphenoparietal sinuses (Fig. 23–13) or 2) deep draining pattern that empties into the internal cerebral veins, basal vein of Rosenthal, vein of Galen, and straight sinus (see Fig. 23–12).

Besides the AVM itself, its location in the brain parenchyma is also an important consideration for management and potential treatment options. Specifically, if it is located in a region controlling a readily identifiable, focal neurologic function, this area is termed *eloquent.*[157]

Several proposed grading schemes for intracranial AVMs have been formulated to predict the surgical risk of excision.[157, 158] Most of these systems revolve around the issues of nidus size, of location, and of the pattern of venous drainage. The grading systems of Spetzler and Martin[157] and of Shi and Chen[158] both provide a framework for the MRI and MR angiographic evaluation of AVMs. The more commonly used Spetzler and Martin classification assigns a cumulative, numeric score for the nidus size, the eloquence of adjacent brain, and the venous pattern to arrive at a designation in ascending severity from I to VI.[157] Sur-

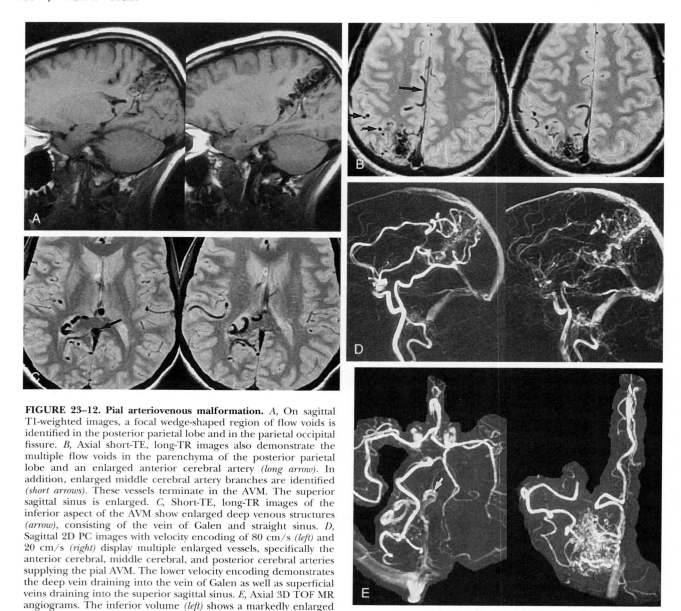

FIGURE 23–12. Pial arteriovenous malformation. *A,* On sagittal T1-weighted images, a focal wedge-shaped region of flow voids is identified in the posterior parietal lobe and in the parietal occipital fissure. *B,* Axial short-TE, long-TR images also demonstrate the multiple flow voids in the parenchyma of the posterior parietal lobe and an enlarged anterior cerebral artery *(long arrow).* In addition, enlarged middle cerebral artery branches are identified *(short arrows).* These vessels terminate in the AVM. The superior sagittal sinus is enlarged. *C,* Short-TE, long-TR images of the inferior aspect of the AVM show enlarged deep venous structures *(arrow),* consisting of the vein of Galen and straight sinus. *D,* Sagittal 2D PC images with velocity encoding of 80 cm/s *(left)* and 20 cm/s *(right)* display multiple enlarged vessels, specifically the anterior cerebral, middle cerebral, and posterior cerebral arteries supplying the pial AVM. The lower velocity encoding demonstrates the deep vein draining into the vein of Galen as well as superficial veins draining into the superior sagittal sinus. *E,* Axial 3D TOF MR angiograms. The inferior volume *(left)* shows a markedly enlarged posterior cerebral artery as well as the deep draining vein *(arrow).* The more cephalad volume depicts the AVM nidus more accurately than does the PC image and also reveals the enlarged anterior and middle cerebral arteries terminating into the AVM.

gery is the current treatment modality of choice for removal of lower grade AVMs. Endovascular therapy is often recommended in patients with larger AVMs to obliterate a portion, either to ease the surgical excision or to convert a large AVM into a lesion that can be treated with radiation. Incomplete embolization often provides palliation of the symptoms and can arrest the neurologic decline in patients harboring large AVMs, but it does not reduce the risk of hemorrhage.[157, 159] Stereotactic radiosurgery tends to be reserved for AVMs that are approximately 3 cm in size or less and are located in or near eloquent brain, such that other therapy would pose a high risk to the patient. The ultimate cure rate with stereotactic radiosurgery for small AVMs without AVFs is approaching 90%[160] (see Fig. 23–13). Because of the success of treating patients with AVMs with stereotactic radiosurgery and the increasing availability of radiosurgery centers, the assessment of nidal flow as a method of evaluation of AVM obliteration is important.[161, 162]

Anatomic Imaging

The complete diagnostic evaluation of AVMs requires a multimodality approach. Catheter angiography clearly remains the diagnostic technique that accurately depicts the arterial vascular supply, the angioarchitecture of the AVM, and the venous drainage. In addition, it most accurately identifies whether the AVM is supplied exclusively from pial vessels or a mixed supply from both dural and pial vessels.

Several articles[163–166] agree that MRI provides most

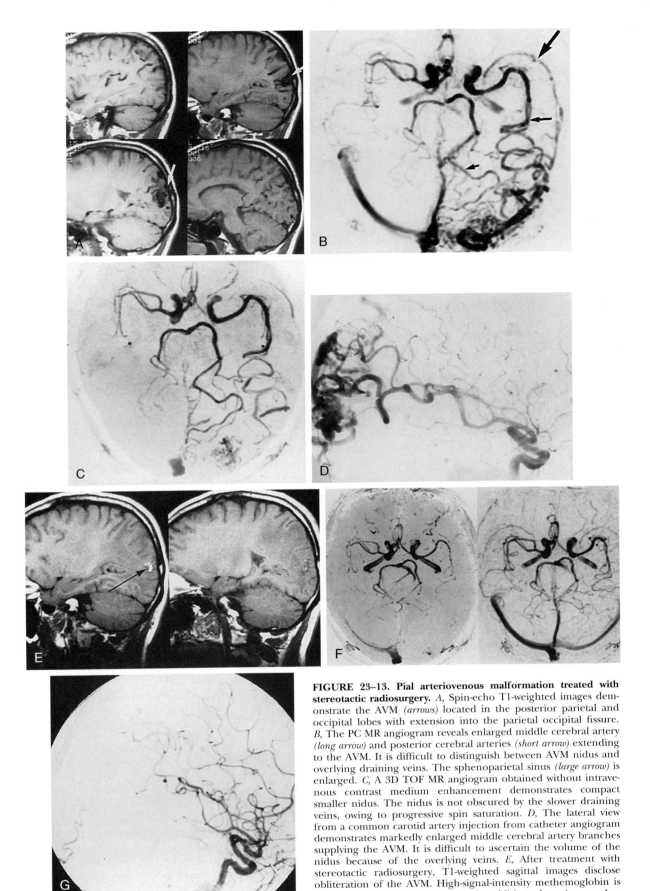

FIGURE 23–13. Pial arteriovenous malformation treated with stereotactic radiosurgery. *A,* Spin-echo T1-weighted images demonstrate the AVM *(arrows)* located in the posterior parietal and occipital lobes with extension into the parietal occipital fissure. *B,* The PC MR angiogram reveals enlarged middle cerebral artery *(long arrow)* and posterior cerebral arteries *(short arrow)* extending to the AVM. It is difficult to distinguish between AVM nidus and overlying draining veins. The sphenoparietal sinus *(large arrow)* is enlarged. *C,* A 3D TOF MR angiogram obtained without intravenous contrast medium enhancement demonstrates compact smaller nidus. The nidus is not obscured by the slower draining veins, owing to progressive spin saturation. *D,* The lateral view from a common carotid artery injection from catheter angiogram demonstrates markedly enlarged middle cerebral artery branches supplying the AVM. It is difficult to ascertain the volume of the nidus because of the overlying veins. *E,* After treatment with stereotactic radiosurgery, T1-weighted sagittal images disclose obliteration of the AVM. High-signal-intensity methemoglobin is present within the nidus *(arrow).* In addition, there is some low signal intensity within the adjacent brain, most likely due to edema. *F,* The 3D TOF MR angiogram *(left)* and a 2D PC MR angiogram *(right)* of the same patient 18 months after radiosurgery show no residual AVM on either study. *G,* A catheter angiogram performed after the MR angiogram confirms obliteration of the AVM.

accurate architectural detail of the relationship of the AVM nidus to the adjacent cerebral anatomy and the best 3D representation (see Fig. 23–12). This information has substantially enhanced optimizing the surgical, endovascular, and stereotactic radiosurgery approaches to AVMs. The imaging characteristics of AVMs with MRI consist of focal round, serpentine, and linear flow voids that represent the enlarged vessels with shunting blood. The signal intensity at times is heterogeneous, owing to a combination of flow-related enhancement and even echo rephasing in areas of slower flow.[96] Although the diagnosis is usually obvious in larger AVMs, occasionally the only clue to the presence of a small vascular malformation with MRI or MR angiography may be that of an enlarged deep venous structure.[167] In a review by LeBlanc and coworkers[164] of 15 patients, the imaging findings of vascular signal voids were found in all patients and in approximately one third of patients there was focal perilesional high signal intensity on T2-weighted images that was thought to represent gliosis or edema. Because of the pivotal role of the nidus size on therapy, Smith and associates[166] in a retrospective fashion compared MRI with both CT and conventional angiography in 15 consecutive patients with AVMs. The authors determined that MRI was superior to both CT and catheter angiography and demonstrated the exact anatomic relationship of the nidus, the afferent arteries, and the draining veins, as well as determined the extent of AVM nidus obliteration after embolization. MRI was more sensitive than CT in demonstrating associated parenchymal abnormalities and subacute hemorrhage. However, MRI still had a low sensitivity for detecting remote hemorrhage within the AVM. In a study by Noorbehesht and colleagues[165] of supratentorial AVM size, CT, MRI, and catheter angiography were compared. In general, the size of the malformation with MRI was found to be smaller than that of conventional angiographic studies. Discrepancy in size increased as the AVM size increased. Interestingly, the AVM size with CT and catheter angiography was essentially equivalent. They concluded the discrepancy between the actual nidus size on the different modalities was due to the inherent ability of MRI to distinguish AVM nidus from the draining veins. In addition, the multiplanar capability of MRI revealed a more accurate 3D representation of the AVM nidus. The detection of any flow through the nidus becomes especially important subsequent to therapy with endovascular techniques or stereotactic radiosurgery (see Fig. 23–13). Both the pretreatment and post-treatment MRI and MR angiography must provide detailed information, including the afferent and efferent AVM blood supply, precise location, and size of the AVM nidus and evaluation of the flow through the nidus itself.[161]

It is known that MRI is extremely helpful in detecting parenchymal hemorrhage. Gomori and colleagues[77, 87] described the characteristic signal intensities on the T1- and T2-weighted spin-echo sequences in the evolution of cerebral parenchymal hematomas, allowing the differentiation between blood products in different oxidative states. Detecting these abnormalities in patients with cerebral AVMs is more difficult because of the adjacent mixed signal intensities from both blood vessels and dystrophic calcifications. In addition, in patients who have been treated with endovascular therapy, embolic agents containing metal fragments (tantalum or tungsten powder) or oily contrast material (Lipiodol, iophendylate [Pantopaque], or Ethiodol) can be difficult to differentiate from blood byproducts. The signal intensity from the metallic fragments is close to that of hemosiderin. The oily contrast media have high signal intensity on the T1-weighted images but can be differentiated from methemoglobin by the marked signal loss of Lipiodol on T2-weighted images.[168]

Several authors have investigated the MRI characteristics of hemorrhage in patients with AVMs. Prayer and associates[168] studied 51 patients with 59 angiographically proven AVMs in high-field MRI instruments. Evidence of previous hemorrhage was identified in 83% of patients with hemorrhages and 44% of patients with symptoms that suggested hemorrhage and, interestingly, in 20% of patients with no clinical history of previous hemorrhage. Chappell and colleagues[169] studied the ability to determine remote hemorrhage using both spin-echo and gradient-echo imaging in 50 patients with high-flow AVMs. Forty-eight percent of the patients had had a prior clinical hemorrhage documented by CT or MRI at the time of the ictus. Decreased signal intensity indicating the presence of hemosiderin and ferritin was seen in 14 of 19 T2-weighted spin-echo images and 18 of 19 gradient-echo images for a sensitivity of 74% and 95%, respectively. No patient without a prior episode of clinical bleeding demonstrated evidence of iron deposition at MRI, in contrast to Prayer and associates' results. They evaluated architectural features of the lesion that would correlate positively with a prior hemorrhage. As with a catheter angiographic study by Marks and coworkers,[149] central venous drainage in periventricular or intraventricular AVM locations correlated positively with prior clinical hemorrhage.[169] The presence of an intranidal aneurysm or collateral flow (angiomatous change) could not be detected with MRI.

MR Angiography and Post-therapy Evaluation

The feasibility and utility of the 3D TOF MR angiographic techniques in the evaluation of pial AVMs have been demonstrated in preliminary studies in which diagnostically useful information concerning the feeding arteries, draining veins, and nidus location were obtained. However, current MR angiographic techniques have problems, including areas of signal void within tortuous feeding arteries (from complex flow), inability to differentiate flow from methemoglobin within an associated subacute hematoma, and lack of visualization of slower distal venous spins due to progressive spin saturation.[106]

There have been two attempts to minimize this problem of spin saturation. In one approach, MR angiograms were obtained in 26 patients with congenital intracranial vascular lesions, with a single thick 3DFT volume in 15 cases and a technique using multiple sequentially acquired thin volumes in 11 subjects.[170] The authors observed a significant improvement in visualization of the slowly flowing venous spins with the multiple thin-volume method as compared with the single-volume technique. A less significant improvement was noted with the single thick-volume method when intravenous gadolinium diethylenetriaminepentaacetic acid (Gd-DTPA) was administered. Edelman and colleagues[171] compared a single thick-volume 3DFT TOF technique and a sequential 2DFT TOF technique in 10 patients with AVMs. Similar to the findings with multiple thin 3DFT volumes, the reduction of spin saturation obtained with the sequential 2DFT technique allowed significantly improved visualization of draining veins. The single thick-volume 3DFT technique, however, was better for the delineation of small arteries, owing to its higher spatial resolution and lower sensitivity to spin dephasing (smaller voxel size and shorter TE). An additional feature of this investigation was the application of selective spatial presaturation pulses to determine the territories supplied by a particular vessel. By selectively saturating inflowing blood from the anterior, middle, and posterior cerebral arteries while acquiring flow-compensated 2DFT images of the nidus, the authors were able to correctly define which of these arteries contributed feeding vessels to the AVM in all 10 cases, as confirmed by conventional contrast angiography.

Kauczor and colleagues[162] evaluated the role of 3DFT TOF MR angiography after stereotactic radiosurgery in 18 patients prospectively. MR angiography demonstrated reduction of nidus flow in 9 patients after 6 months and 15 patients after 1 year status post treatment (see Fig. 23–13). The MR angiographic technique was more sensitive than spin-echo imaging and revealed a reduction of the nidus size in two patients after 6 months and in eight patients at 1 year of follow-up. The MR angiographic signal intensity of the feeding arteries was reduced in nine patients and diminished veins were seen in six patients, implying reduced flow through the AVM (see Fig. 23–13). Correlation with conventional angiography was performed in all patients. Other authors have reported excellent success using tandem 2D gradient-echo images with and without gradient moment nulling to evaluate AVM after stereotactic radiosurgery. In a subset of patients in whom conventional angiograms were performed, there were no false-positive or false-negative results using this MRI diagnostic algorithm.[161]

In addition to follow-up of radiosurgery, the use of 3DFT TOF MR angiographic techniques as a database for treatment planning for stereotactic radiosurgery has been reported. An advantage of using 3D TOF MRA data sets is that they permit more accurate delineation of the stereotactic target and the adjacent brain parenchyma more reliably than does CT.[172–174] Concern over the geometric distortion inherent to the magnet as well as magnetic field heterogeneities induced by the patient and gradient nonlinearities is currently less of a problem because of improved MRI hardware and correction algorithms, resulting in distortions of approximately 1 mm.[173]

3D PC MR angiography has not enjoyed the same enthusiasm in evaluating the architecture of AVMs as TOF techniques. In a small study by Nussel and colleagues,[163] 10 patients with AVMs were examined by PC MR angiography and catheter angiography. In seven of these patients, data about vascular supply were obtained using this 3D PC (velocity-encoding values were not presented) technique, complementing the MR images. In three patients with small AVMs, the lesion could not be definitely detected.

PC MR angiographic flow analysis techniques provide opportunities for evaluation of blood flow in the vascular supply to an AVM. Marks and colleagues[175] evaluated 16 patients with intracerebral AVMs. In this study, velocity and volume flow rates in both carotid arteries and the basilar artery were calculated by using a PC cine MR angiographic technique. As expected, flow and velocity measurements were significantly elevated in all three arteries in patients with AVMs. The flow in the carotid artery ipsilateral to the AVM was significantly greater than the flow in the contralateral carotid artery. In four patients who underwent partial embolization, a corresponding decrease in flow was observed. Turski and coworkers,[104] reporting preliminary data using cardiac gated PC MR angiography, demonstrated flow rates in the arterial supply in the AVMs at 200 cm/s and venous flow rates at 20 cm/s. As work in this area continues to develop, flow quantification of AVMs may allow assessment of responses to therapy (see also Chapter 25).

CAVERNOUS MALFORMATIONS

Epidemiology and Pathophysiology

CMs have frequently been included in a group of vascular malformations with different pathologic characteristics, which collectively are called *angiographically occult vascular malformations*. This is a nonspecific term whose only common feature is the absence of abnormal vascularity by catheter angiography. Physiologically, the common feature to all of these lesions is extremely slow blood flow. They are composed pathologically of thrombosed AVMs, capillary telangiectasias, CMs, and venous angiomas.[145, 146] The CT and MRI findings are becoming better established as more rigorous evaluations of angiographically occult malformations have been performed. MRI has provided dramatic improvement in identifying and localizing angiographically occult cerebrovascular malformations.[84, 94, 95, 176–180]

Pathologic studies have demonstrated that multiple lesions occur in approximately 25% of cases.[146] Rigamonti and coworkers,[177] in an MRI-based series, demonstrated multiple lesions in approximately 50% of the patients. Studies by both Robinson and colleagues[178] and Requena and colleagues,[176] based on the MRI diagnosis of CM, revealed that 11% to 13% of patients harbored multiple malformations. Although many

CMs are often sporadic, familial occurrences have been described by several authors.[181-183] Familial populations have a much higher incidence of multiple lesions (73%) compared with the sporadic expression (10% to 15%).[146] As a result, the natural history has become more clearly elucidated and therefore the clinical management of CM is evolving.[176, 178, 180]

CMs are hamartomatous lesions composed of enlarged sinusoidal vascular spaces with a single layer of attenuated endothelium devoid of elastin or smooth muscle. The sinusoids are separated from each other by connective tissue with no intervening neural tissue. The brain parenchyma immediately surrounding the lesion is gliotic and may contain small slow-flowing arteries and veins.[184] In addition, a rim of parenchyma surrounding the lesion is hemosiderin stained.[147, 177]

The true prevalence and incidence of CMs are not precisely known. In McCormick's prospective autopsy study of 4069 consecutive brains, 165 patients were found to have one or more vascular malformations of the brain. The number of venous malformations was 105 (2.6%); capillary telangiectasia, 28 (0.69%); AVMs, 24 (0.59%); CMs, 16 (0.39%); and varix malformations of the brain, 4 (0.1%).[145] The prevalence of CMs in McCormick's series closely parallels that of a retrospective study performed by Robinson and colleagues.[178] This consisted of 14,035 MRI examinations that were evaluated in a 5-year period. In those studies, there were 76 lesions identified in 66 patients, constituting a prevalence of 0.47%.

Intra-axial Cavernous Malformations

Clinical Presentation

The most frequently associated clinical presentation with CMs is seizures, described in the range of 40% to 70%. Focal neurologic deficits, including sensory disturbances, hemiparesis, diplopia, and ataxia, are the next most common presentations. These symptoms relate to both the size and the location of the lesion and account for 35% to 50% of presentations. In addition, some patients present with headaches; however, because of the nonspecific and nonlocalizing nature of this presentation, it has only been reported in 25% to 30% of patients.[178, 185, 186]

Robinson and colleagues[178] reviewed the MR images of 76 lesions in 66 patients and demonstrated that most intracranial CMs occur within the frontal and temporal lobes. Approximately 70% of these lesions were in the cerebral hemispheres, and approximately 5% of the lesions were considered deep lesions affecting the diencephalon and septal region. The infratentorial lesions were almost equally split between the cerebellar hemisphere and brain stem locations. The pons is the most common site for brain stem CMs.[187] In another study of 56 CMs in 47 patients,[176] 59% were supratentorial, the most common location being in the temporal and parietal regions, and 39% of the lesions were infratentorial, the most common locations being the pons and the cerebellum. Of significant clinical and therapeutic importance is the association of ve-

nous angiomas with CMs in 5% to 16% of cases.[178, 180, 188] The size of CMs varies widely, ranging from several millimeters to 4 cm or greater.

In the pre-MRI era "angiographically occult malformations" were grouped without using strict histologic features of CMs. With more recent rigorous studies using primarily MRI with histologic confirmation, imaging characteristics of CMs have become more firmly established. Although the MRI appearance of CMs is relatively specific, other vascular malformations and some neoplasms may demonstrate similar morphologic appearance.[176, 177, 189, 190]

Intracranial extracerebral CMs have also been described but are considerably rarer than intracerebral lesions, most commonly involving the cavernous sinus. They have also been described arising from cranial nerves.[191-193]

Anatomic Imaging

The sensitivity of CT in the detection of CMs is less than that of MRI. However, CT is frequently the first imaging study obtained in patients with acute clinical presentations. On nonenhanced CT scans, CMs appear as focal nodular heterogeneous hyperdensities relative to adjacent brain. A minority of lesions are hypodense compared with brain. After intravenous contrast medium administration, there is variable but commonly faint enhancement.[95, 176, 179] Punctate areas of increased attenuation coefficient (probably related to calcifications) are seen in approximately 14% of cases. Transient increased attenuation is also seen with acute hemorrhage that frequently has associated surrounding edema and mass effect.[177, 179] In six episodes of acute brain stem hemorrhages into pathologically proven CMs observed on CT scans by Zimmerman and associates,[180] none had evidence of SAH or fourth ventricular hemorrhage. This is not the case for cryptic AVMs. This observation is postulated to be a result of a lack of a capsule in the true AVMs, and thus hemorrhage follows the path of least resistance.

The high sensitivity of MRI to subacute and chronic hemorrhage makes it the examination of choice in the evaluation of CMs. The signal changes associated with parenchymal hemorrhage have been described previously; however, some issues are worth noting. The preferential T2 relaxation enhancement in acute hematomas and with hemosiderin is field dependent, increasing as the square of the magnetic field.[77, 84, 87] For this reason it is advantageous to image patients with suspected or known CMs on high-field MRI units. This has been supported clinically in the detection of occult CMs.[84, 177] In addition, the susceptibility effect due to the hemosiderin is directly related to the length of the TE. Therefore, the hypointense rim thickens with longer TE-weighted images[77] (Fig. 23–14). Gradient-echo MRI can detect both acute and chronic hemorrhage not seen on conventional spin-echo techniques. This is attributed to the inferior signal refocusing of gradient-echo techniques. The T2* signal loss observed secondary to magnetic susceptibility phenomena is much more pronounced on these types of

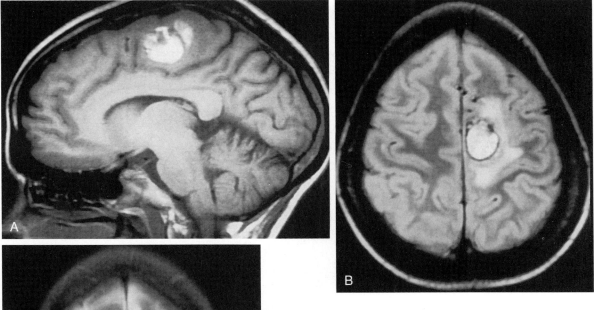

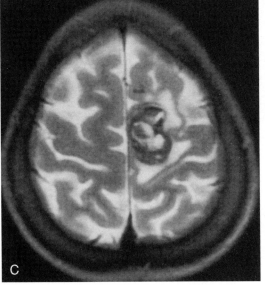

FIGURE 23–14. Cavernous malformation with recent hemorrhage. *A,* Spin-echo sagittal image demonstrates a predominantly high-signal-intensity area consistent with methemoglobin in the posterior frontal lobe in the supplementary motor area in a patient who presented with seizures. Note the hypointensity surrounding the posterior aspect of the malformation. *B,* Short-TE, long-TR image shows the lesion with a hypointense rim and edema in the adjacent white matter. *C,* Long-TE, long-TR image shows thickening of the hypointense rim due to the longer TE.

images.[66, 88] Thus, with patients with suspected CMs, a gradient-echo sequence could be illuminating, especially if a low-field MRI unit or if newer RARE spin-echo techniques are used. Because of the inherent signal refocusing of successive 180° refocusing pulses and possibly T2 filtering effects of variable k-space sampling, the RARE or fast spin-echo sequences are less sensitive to magnetic susceptibility effects.[82, 89, 90]

CMs have well-defined rounded or multilobulated margins. The typical appearance of the CMs on MR images consists of a reticulated central core, a result of blood byproducts in various states of evolution and of mixed low and high signal intensity with the surrounding hemosiderin ring[176, 177, 189, 194] (see Fig. 23–14). In addition, some of the mixed signal intensity may be due to calcifications. Occasionally, small regions of high signal intensity surrounding the hemosiderin rim may be seen due to edema, brain parenchymal gliosis, or both (see Fig. 23–14). No vessels are identified, although a small vessel adjacent to the CM may be due to a coexistent venous angioma (Fig. 23–15). Distinguishing a CM from a mixed malformation

becomes important before surgical extirpation of the CM. The surgery is directed at removing the CM and sparing the venous malformation. The sparing of the venous malformation is important because this frequently drains normal brain and removing these veins may result in a venous infarction. Small CMs may appear as petechial areas of decreased signal intensity.[176, 188, 189, 194]

Because the appearance of CMs is merely due to hemorrhage in evolution, it is not surprising that the appearance can be nonspecific. Other diagnostic considerations include a thrombosed AVM and hemorrhagic neoplasms. Differentiation from neoplasm may be possible, because most metastases greater than 5 mm have moderate to extensive vasogenic edema, whereas CMs have little or no vasogenic edema. Two caveats must be considered: 1) a recent hemorrhage into a CM will have edema but often with evidence of a hemosiderin rim within the lesion (see Fig. 23–14), and 2) corticosteroids often reduce the amount of edema. Multiplicity of lesions, especially if not all are hemorrhagic, would favor metastatic disease. CT may

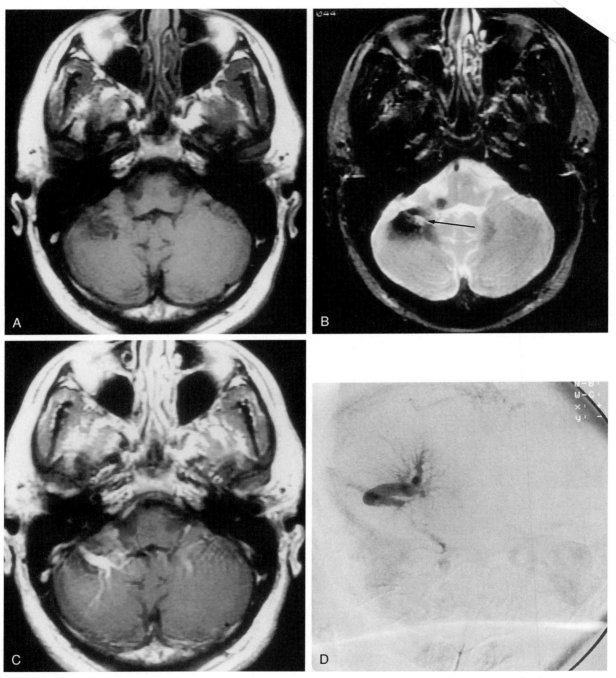

FIGURE 23–15. Mixed vascular malformation. *A,* Spin-echo T1-weighted axial image demonstrates a focal area of decreased signal intensity within the right cerebellar hemisphere. *B,* T2-weighted axial image reveals marked hypointensity within the cerebellar hemisphere in the same location. Note the central area of higher signal intensity *(arrow)* corresponding to flow within the venous malformation. In addition, focal hypointensity is identified in the left inferior cerebellar peduncle. The hypointense lesions are consistent with a CM. *C,* T1-weighted image after the administration of Gd-DTPA demonstrates the classic caput medusae appearance of the venous angioma. *D,* Venous phase of a catheter angiogram also exhibits the classic appearance of a venous angioma. At surgery, the CM was removed, sparing the venous malformation.

be helpful in some situations because metastases are frequently hypodense and do not commonly contain calcifications.[176, 189, 190] CMs, on the other hand, are most often hyperdense and often contain calcifications.[179]

MR Angiography

MR angiography is of limited value in imaging CMs. CMs are frequently identified with MRI due to the associated blood and blood byproducts. The lesions are angiographically occult due to the extremely slow flow through the malformation. The role of MR angiography lies in imaging of mixed malformations. The angiographic features of the venous malformation, consisting of the typical caput medusae of veins converging on a central venous structure, can be identified. Imaging algorithms should include a 2D TOF sequence due to its superior sensitivity slow flow. In addition, use of contrast medium, which results in preferential T1 relaxation, may be helpful to increase the signal intensity of the flowing blood (see Fig. 23-15).

Extra-axial Cavernous Malformations

Extracerebral intracranial CMs are rare. Approximately 40 of these malformations have been reported in the literature. These malformations are most commonly located in the middle cranial fossa in close association with the cavernous sinus. They tend to affect women with a higher frequency than do intracerebral CMs. The clinical presentation is usually of an acute or subacute onset of diplopia, impaired visual acuity, and visual field defects. Other findings include exophthalmos and facial weakness.[191–193]

Anatomic Imaging

CT demonstrates secondary changes of bony erosion of the adjacent structures, specifically the orbital fissure, middle cranial fossa floor, dorsum sella, and posterior clinoid. In addition, usually a discrete hyperdense mass with homogeneous enhancement is present after contrast medium administration. Calcifications are not a frequent finding. The amount of enhancement and the rarity of calcifications are in contrast to the intracerebral CMs. Of significant clinical importance is that although the extracerebral CMs may appear relatively hypovascular on imaging studies, they bleed profusely at surgery, causing life-threatening hemorrhages.[191]

Extracerebral intracranial CMs at MRI also do not share the same features of the intraparenchymal CMs. Extracerebral CMs tend to be isointense with gray matter on short-TR, short-TE images and hyperintense on the long-TR, long-TE images. They vividly enhance after the administration of contrast agent.[191] The most common differential diagnosis is that of a meningioma, which is commonly isointense relative to brain on T1- and T2-weighted images. Another feature that may allow differentiation between meningiomas is a

frequent association of hyperostosis with meningiomas, which has not been described with extracerebral CMs. In contrast to the intracerebral CMs, there is a lack of the markedly hypointense rim, owing to the absence of the hemosiderin-laden macrophages around the malformation.

VENOUS MALFORMATIONS

Venous malformations (angiomas) were once thought to be quite rare, but, with the advent of CT and MRI, they are now known to be common vascular malformations that are usually discovered incidentally. Morphologically, they are characterized by mildly dilated, radially oriented medullated veins that converge into a linear subcortical transcerebral vein, which drains into a superficial or ependymal vein. Drainage can occur centrally toward the subependymal veins. Arteriovenous shunting is not identified. Approximately 50% of these lesions are identified in the frontal lobe and 25% in the cerebellar white matter. Pure venous malformations drain normal brain, and therefore as an isolated malformation they are rarely associated with hemorrhage.[195–197] A retrospective analysis by Garner and colleagues[198] evaluated the natural history of venous angiomas in 100 patients diagnosed with imaging techniques. Contrary to earlier works, they found a predominantly benign natural history with only 1 of 14 patients with a pure venous angioma presenting with hemorrhage. This was estimated to represent a 0.22% per year risk of hemorrhage. Transient focal deficits, seizures, and headaches were the most common presenting symptoms.[198] Up to one third of these malformations can be associated with a CM[199] (see Fig. 23-15).

Anatomic Imaging

In a study by Ostertun and associates,[196] evaluation of 20 patients with 21 developmental venous malformations was done with a 2DFT TOF technique. MR angiography was diagnostic in 17 of the 21 developmental venous abnormalities when both the 2DFT slices (number not specified) and the MIPs were interpreted. MRI alone frequently identified the draining of veins, but after Gd-DTPA administration MRI was diagnostic in 17 of 18 cases.

Occasionally, the radially oriented medullary veins can be visualized on 3DFT TOF angiograms, but they are frequently identified only after the intravenous administration of contrast medium. The 2DFT TOF technique, because of its sensitivity to slow flow, is ideal for imaging venous malformations. The typical MR angiographic findings are similar to the catheter angiographic findings with the curvilinear venous channel coursing toward a subependymal, cortical, or dural sinus (Fig. 23-16). In addition, PC MR angiography can be helpful if an extremely low velocity encoding (5 cm/s) is selected to take advantage of a slow flow seen in these lesions. Intravenous contrast medium enhancement may also increase the detectability of the

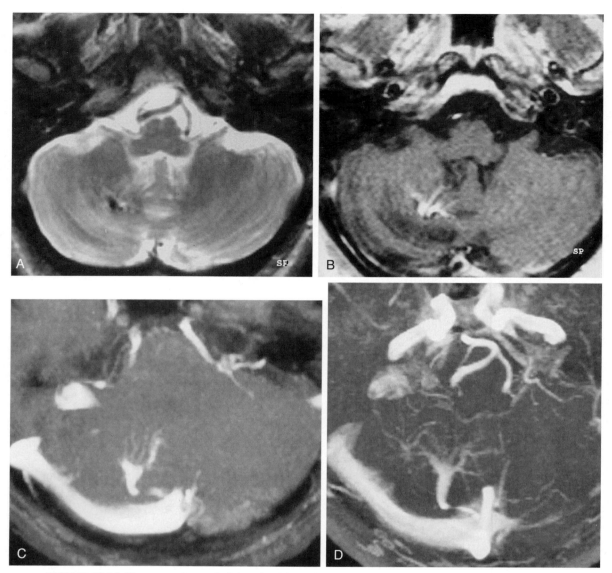

FIGURE 23–16. Venous angioma. *A,* Spin-echo T2-weighted axial image discloses a focal area of decreased signal intensity in the mesial right cerebellar hemisphere. *B,* T1-weighted axial image after the administration of Gd-DTPA reveals multiple radiating vascular structures projecting toward the larger draining vein corresponding to the hypodensity on the T2-weighted image. The malformation drains normal brain parenchyma. *C,* A 2D TOF MR angiogram (which is sensitive to slow flow) demonstrates the typical appearance of a venous angioma with a focal stenosis at its connection with the torcular. *D,* A 3D TOF MR angiogram after the administration of Gd-DTPA to increase vascular signal demonstrates the venous angioma to best advantage because of it superior resolution.

lesions with all MR angiographic techniques (see Fig. 23–16). If hemorrhage is identified on the accompanied MRI examination, a coexisting CM should be strongly suspected.[196]

DURAL ARTERIOVENOUS FISTULAS

Dural AVFs are thought to represent an acquired or developmental anomaly responsible for 15% of intracranial vascular malformations[200, 201] (Figs. 23–17 and 23–18). The most common locations involve the dural sinuses along the skull base, usually the cavernous, transverse, and sigmoid sinus. Dural AVMs have a vari-

ety of clinical presentations depending on the location and the venous drainage pattern. Signs and symptoms may include headaches, pulsatile tinnitus, otalgia, bruit, exophthalmos, chemosis, and cranial nerve palsies.[202–204] The neurologic deficit relates to the severity of the induced venous hypertension resulting from the arterial-to-venous shunt.[205] Cortical venous involvement is often associated with venous hypertension and parenchymal hemorrhage (see Fig. 23–18).

Anatomic Imaging

DeMarco and colleagues[202] evaluated 12 patients with angiographically proven dural AVFs. The spin-

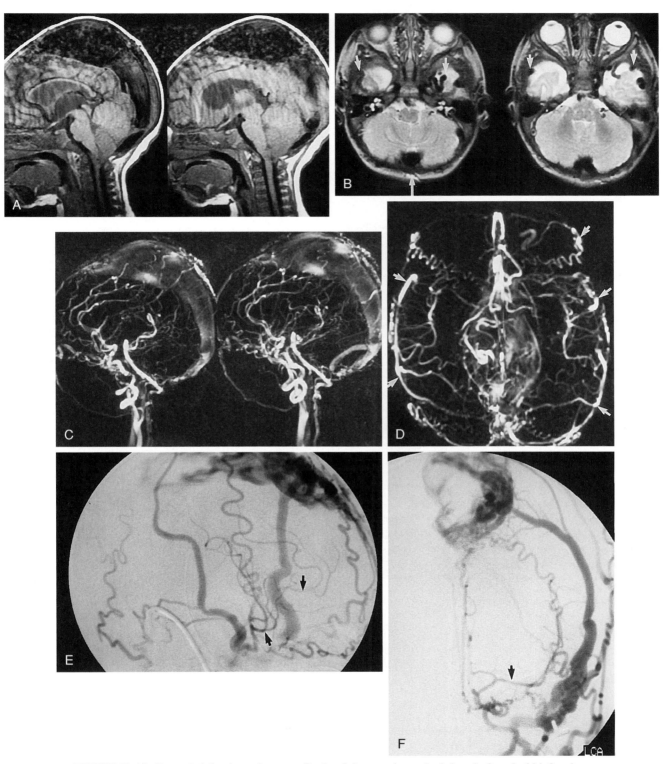

FIGURE 23–17. Congenital dural arteriovenous fistula of the superior sagittal sinus in 2-week-old infant born with congestive heart failure. *A*, Sagittal T1-weighted images demonstrate the markedly enlarged superior sagittal sinus with extensive ghost artifact degrading the images. *B*, Axial T2-weighted images show the markedly enlarged torcular *(long arrow)*. In addition, note the markedly enlarged external carotid artery branches, specifically the middle meningeal arteries *(short arrows)*. *C*, Sagittal 2D PC MR angiogram with velocity encodings of 60 cm/s *(left)* and 30 cm/s *(right)*. Note the markedly enlarged superior sagittal sinus, with most of the arteriovenous connections not identified on the 60 cm/s image. On the lower velocity encoding, more of the dural sinuses are visualized. *D*, Axial 3D TOF MR angiogram demonstrates markedly enlarged dural and scalp arteries *(arrows)*. Note that the superior sagittal sinus is only faintly seen, most likely due to the complex and rapid flow. Lateral *(E)* and anteroposterior *(F)* projections from a catheter angiogram show markedly enlarged external carotid artery branches supplying the superior sagittal sinus. Note that the intracranial vessels are normal in size *(arrows)*.

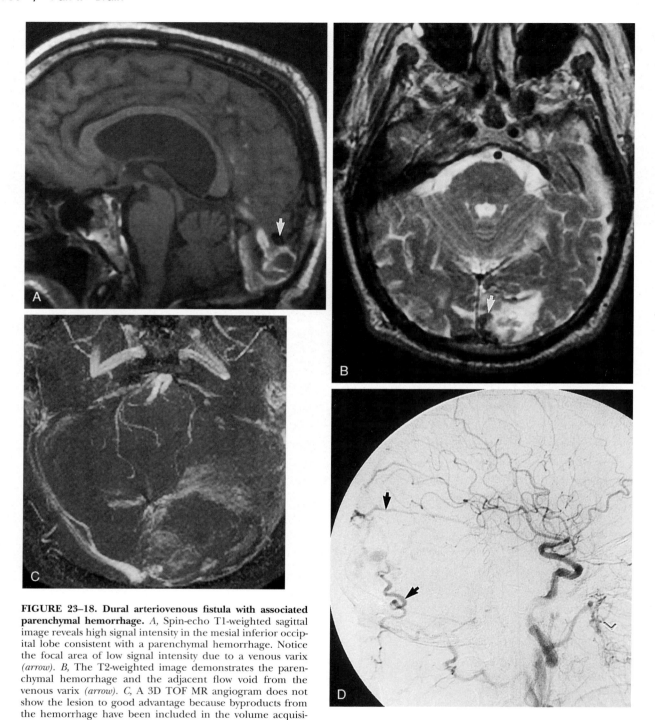

FIGURE 23–18. Dural arteriovenous fistula with associated parenchymal hemorrhage. *A,* Spin-echo T1-weighted sagittal image reveals high signal intensity in the mesial inferior occipital lobe consistent with a parenchymal hemorrhage. Notice the focal area of low signal intensity due to a venous varix *(arrow)*. *B,* The T2-weighted image demonstrates the parenchymal hemorrhage and the adjacent flow void from the venous varix *(arrow)*. *C,* A 3D TOF MR angiogram does not show the lesion to good advantage because byproducts from the hemorrhage have been included in the volume acquisition. *D,* Lateral conventional angiogram shows the fistula with a venous varix. Note supply to the malformation through the posterior branch of the middle meningeal artery *(top arrow)* and the occipital artery *(bottom arrow)*.

echo images revealed abnormal dilated draining veins in 8 of the 12 patients (see Fig. 23–18). The site of the dural AVF was never identified with MRI. Primary complications of dural AVMs include infarction, intraparenchymal hematoma, and subdural hematoma. Willinsky and colleagues[206] evaluated 13 patients with dural AVFs with associated cortical venous drainage. The predominant finding was dilated pial vessels in 10 of

13 patients, hydrocephalus in 2 patients, and parenchymal hemorrhage as well. A venous occlusion was identified in two patients, a finding seen only in one patient in DeMarco and colleagues' series. An associated finding in four patients with known neurologic deficits was high signal intensity on the long-TR images in the brain parenchyma, which is thought to reflect venous hypertension with resultant passive congestion of the

brain. Supratentorially, this was predominantly bihemispheric, but infratentorially it predominantly involved an isolated cerebellar hemisphere. Both studies suggested that in patients with parenchymal or subdural hemorrhage or secondary signs of venous occlusive disease with prominent pial vessels, a conventional angiogram should be performed for further evaluation. In a study by Chen and associates,[205] identification of dural AVF proved difficult with spin-echo MRI, confirming an earlier study by DeMarco and colleagues.[202] In six of the seven patients in this study, nine dural AVFs were identified by MR angiography. There was good correlation between MR angiography and conventional angiography. There is a well-established association of dural sinus thrombosis with dural AVM. In this MR angiographic study, occlusion of the dural sinus was not identified on any spin-echo images, but MR angiography also failed to diagnose the dural sinus thrombosis in two of the three cases. This particular issue may be addressed better using techniques sensitive to slow flow, specifically PC or 2D TOF MR angiographic techniques.

It is important to note a study by Chen and associates[205] in which Gd-DTPA was used in all cases except one case of cavernous sinus involvement. There was no attempt to perform 3D TOF MR angiography before and after the administration of the contrast agent. Although contrast was believed to improve the identification of the dural AVFs, caution was expressed when imaging cavernous sinus dural AVFs because flow-related enhancement may not be well differentiated from the normal contrast enhancement of the cavernous sinus, a difficulty not experienced by Chen and associates (Fig. 23–19).

In addition to the dural AVFs that consist of numerous tiny anastomoses between the dural arteries and veins or the cavernous sinus, there can occasionally be a direct fistula from the carotid artery into the cavernous sinus. This finding is usually associated with trauma or is secondary to a ruptured cavernous carotid aneurysm. With MR angiography, the appearance is slightly different because this is an extremely high flow fistula directly into the cavernous sinus without multiple tiny dural connections.

VASCULAR COMPRESSION OF THE FACIAL OR TRIGEMINAL NERVE

CLINICAL BACKGROUND

Trigeminal neuralgia and many cases of hemifacial spasm are believed to be due to vascular compression of the nerve root as it exits from the pons, often called the nerve root exit zone[207] (Fig. 23–20). Other causes associated with trigeminal neuralgia and hemifacial spasm include extra-axial mass lesions in the cerebellopontine angle and intraparenchymal lesions, including multiple sclerosis.[208] Although some consider vascular compression of the fifth and seventh cranial nerves as controversial, there is support for neurovascular compression by neuropathologic and electrophysiologic studies.[209] Several studies with MRI and MR angiography have supported the notion of compression of the exiting nerve with demonstration of the compressing vascular structures preoperatively, with clinical improvement occurring after microvascular decompression.[208, 210–217]

ANATOMIC IMAGING

In an early study using MRI alone, all 13 patients with clinically documented hemifacial spasm had identification of a vascular structure at the root exit zone; however, a similar finding was also found in 21% of the asymptomatic patients. In addition, identifying the vessel involved was not possible in this MRI-based study.[214] Bernardi and coworkers[216] described 37 patients with hemifacial spasm with 16 age-matched control subjects in whom MRI, MR angiography, and MR tomographic angiography were applied in the study of hemifacial spasm. Sixty-five percent of patients with hemifacial spasm had ipsilateral vascular compression of the facial nerve or the pons, whereas only 6.3% of control patients had similar patterns of vascular compression. The MR tomographic angiography technique was found to be more sensitive and more specific in vascular decompression.

Marked elongation and widening of the basilar artery may result in compression of the adjacent brain stem and exiting nerve roots as well as physiologic changes that are associated with slow flow due to the enlarged vessel, commonly called basilar dolichoectasia. This can result in cranial nerve palsies in up to 60% of patients, and symptoms of vertebrobasilar insufficiency or vertebrobasilar ischemic infarctions can be identified in approximately 55% of these patients. Trigeminal neuralgia is most often caused by arterial branches arising off the distal vertebral or the basilar arteries or veins. Occasionally, it is caused by the vertebral or basilar artery itself. In one surgical series, 31 of 1404 consecutive patients treated by microvascular decompression for typical trigeminal neuralgia were found to have vascular compression by either the basilar or vertebral arteries.[217] As with vascular compression in hemifacial spasm and trigeminal neuralgia, 3D TOF MR angiography can be useful in identifying the cranial nerve compression or compression of the midbrain itself (see Fig. 23–20). In patients with extremely slow flow, PC employing low-velocity encoding or 2D TOF MR angiographic techniques are useful. In patients with vertebrobasilar insufficiency or ischemic symptoms, these findings can direct therapy, which may include antiplatelet aggregating drugs.

MR tomographic angiography consists of using a conventional 3DFT TOF MR angiographic technique and reformatting the original data in submillimeter coronal, sagittal, and oblique sections with the window and level adjusted to allow visualization of both vascular structures and the adjacent brain stem parenchyma in nerve root exit zones.[208, 217] The coronal re-forma-

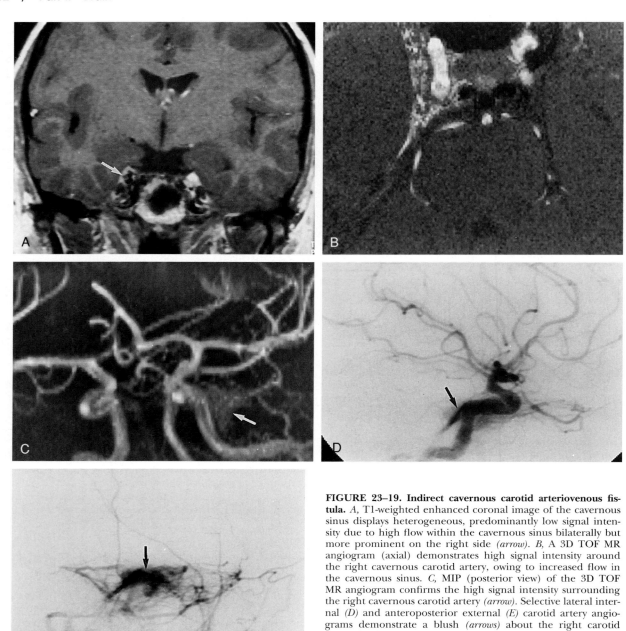

FIGURE 23–19. Indirect cavernous carotid arteriovenous fistula. *A,* T1-weighted enhanced coronal image of the cavernous sinus displays heterogeneous, predominantly low signal intensity due to high flow within the cavernous sinus bilaterally but more prominent on the right side *(arrow)*. *B,* A 3D TOF MR angiogram (axial) demonstrates high signal intensity around the right cavernous carotid artery, owing to increased flow in the cavernous sinus. *C,* MIP (posterior view) of the 3D TOF MR angiogram confirms the high signal intensity surrounding the right cavernous carotid artery *(arrow)*. Selective lateral internal *(D)* and anteroposterior external *(E)* carotid artery angiograms demonstrate a blush *(arrows)* about the right carotid artery in the cavernous sinus and the multiple tiny vessels supplying the dural fistula.

tions appear to be the most reliable for graphically demonstrating the route exit zone of the seventh cranial nerve in 65%, with axial MR angiography in 51%, compared with MRI in 27%, of patients.[217] Gadolinium-enhanced MRI was found to be of no additional value. Similar findings were published by Felber and associates[210] in 14 patients with unilateral hemifacial spasm. MRI in combination with MR angiography demonstrated the neurovascular contact in 12 of 14 patients and only 4 of 20 control subjects. The vessels that can contribute to neurovascular compression include the vertebral artery, posterior cerebellar artery, anterior inferior cerebellar artery, and, less commonly, cochlear or basilar arteries. Occasionally, venous structures have been implicated in the cause of hemifacial spasm. In these particular cases, the 3DFT TOF technique will not demonstrate the slower venous flow, owing to saturation effects as well as the presence of the venous presaturation pulse. Because of the multiple vascular structures that may be causing the vascular decompression, identifying the offending vessel has been helpful in directing the surgical approach.[208, 210, 212, 213, 217]

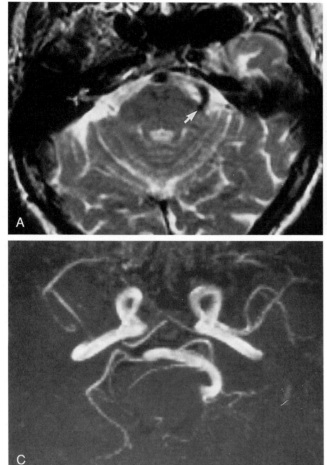

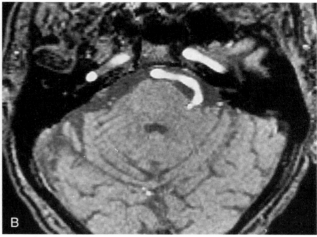

FIGURE 23–20. Hemifacial spasm and vascular compression. *A*, Long-TE, long-TR image revealing severe tortuousity of the distal vertebral artery, which impacts the pons at the nerve root exit zone *(arrow)*. *B*, A 3D TOF MR angiogram (axial partition) shows the tortuous vertebral artery impacting the right side of the pons at the nerve root exit zone. *C*, The collapsed view demonstrates the vascular anatomy without the benefit of the adjacent parenchyma, making this image less useful in the diagnosis of vascular compression.

REFERENCES

1. Atlas SW: Intracranial vascular malformations and aneurysms. In: Atlas SW, ed. Magnetic Resonance Imaging of the Brain and Spine. New York: Raven Press, 1991, pp 379–409.
2. Drake CG: Management of cerebral aneurysm. Stroke 12:273–283, 1981.
3. Housepian EM, Pool JL: A systematic analysis of intracranial aneurysms from the autopsy file of Presbyterian Hospital. J Neuropathol Exp Neurol 17:409–423, 1958.
4. McCormick WF: Problems and pathogenesis of intracranial arterial aneurysms. In: Toole JF, Moosey J, Janeway R, eds. Cerebrovascular Disorders. 2nd ed. New York: Grune & Stratton, 1971, pp 219–231.
5. Atkinson JLD, Sundt TM, Houser OW, Whisnant JP: Angiographic frequency of anterior circulation intracranial aneurysms. J Neurosurg 70:551–555, 1989.
6. Huston J III, Torres VE, Sulivan PP, et al: Value of magnetic resonance angiography for the detection of intracranial aneurysms in autosomal dominant polycystic kidney disease. J Am Soc Nephrol 3:1871–1877, 1993.
7. Leblanc R, Worsley KJ, Melanson D, Tampieri D: Angiographic screening and elective surgery of familial cerebral aneurysms: a decision analysis. Neurosurgery 35:9–18, 1994.
8. Nakagawa T, Hashi K: The incidence and treatment of asymptomatic unruptured cerebral aneurysms. J Neurosurg 80:217–223, 1994.
9. Ross JS, Masaryk TJ, Modic MT, et al: Intracranial aneurysms: evaluation by MR angiography. AJNR 11:449–456, 1990.
10. Ruggieri PM, Poulas N, Obuchowski N, et al: Occult intracranial aneurysms in polycystic kidney disease: screening with MR angiography. Radiology 191:33–39, 1994.
11. ter Berg HWM, Dippel DWJ, Limburg M, et al: Familial intracranial aneurysms. Stroke 23:1024–1030, 1992.
12. Hacker RS, Krall SM, Fox JL. Data I. In: Fox JL, ed. Intracranial Aneurysms, Volume 1. New York: Springer-Verlag, 1983, pp 19–117.
13. Fox JL: Management of aneurysms of anterior circulation of intracranial procedures. In: Youmans JR, ed. Neurological Surgery. 3rd ed. Philadelphia: WB Saunders, 1990, pp 1689–1732.
14. Hove B, Andersen BB, Christiansen TM: Intracranial oncotic aneurysms from choriocarcinoma. Case report and review of the literature. Neuroradiology 32:526–528, 1990.
15. Nakstad P, Nornes H, Hauge HN: Traumatic aneurysms of the pericallosal arteries. Neuroradiology 28:335–338, 1986.
16. Ojemann RG, Crowell RM: Intracranial aneurysms and subarachnoid hemorrhage: incidence, pathology, clinical features and medical management. In: Ojermann RG, Crowell RM, eds. Surgical Management of Cerebrovascular Disease. Baltimore: Williams & Wilkins, 1983, p 128.
17. Wilkins RH: Update: subarachnoid hemorrhage and saccular intracranial aneurysm. Surg Neurol 15:92–101, 1981.
18. Sahs AL, Perret GE, Locksley HB, Nishioka H: Intracranial Aneurysms and Subarachnoid Hemorrhage: A Cooperative Study. Philadelphia: JB Lippincott, 1969.
19. Bull J: Massive aneurysms at the base of the brain. Brain 92:535–570, 1969.
20. Locksley HB: Report of the cooperative study of intracranial aneurysms and subarachnoid hemorrhage. Section V, Part II. Natural history of subarachnoid hemorrhage, intracranial aneurysms and arteriovenous malformations based on 6,368 cases in the cooperative study. J Neurosurg 23:321–368, 1966.
21. Morely TP, Barr HWK: Giant intracranial aneurysms: diagnosis, course and management. Clin Neurosurg 16:73–94, 1969.
22. Pia HW, Zierski J: Giant cerebral aneurysms. Neurosurg Rev 5:117–148, 1982.
23. Gean AD, Pile-Spellman J, Heros RC: A pneumatized anterior clinoid mimicking an aneurysm on MR imaging. Report of two cases. J Neurosurg 71:128–132, 1989.
24. Nukui H, Imai S, Fukamachi A, et al: Bilaterally symmetrical giant aneurysms of the internal carotid artery within the cavernous sinus, associated with an aneurysm of the basilar artery. Neurol Surg 5:479–484, 1977.
25. Herman JM, Rekate HL, Spetzler RF: Pediatric intracranial aneurysms: simple and complex cases. Pediatr Neurosurg 17:66–73, 1991.
26. Scholten FG, ter Berg HWM, Hofstee N, Vellenga CJRL: Giant aneurysm of the posterior cerebral artery in a one-year-old child. Eur J Radiol 15:56–58, 1992.

27. Segal HD, McLaurin RL: Giant serpentine aneurysm: report of two cases. J Neurosurg 46:115–120, 1977.
28. Matsuda M, Matsuda I, Handa H, Okamoto K: Intracavernous giant aneurysm associated with Marfan's syndrome. Surg Neurol 12:119–121, 1979.
29. Rubinstein MK, Cohen NH: Ehlers-Danlos syndrome with multiple intracranial aneurysms. Neurology 14:125–132, 1964.
30. Steiger HJ, Poll A, Liepsch DW, Reuler HJ: Basic flow structures in saccular aneurysms: a flow visualization study. Heart Vessels 3:55–65, 1987.
31. Perktold K: On the path of fluid particles in an axisymmetrical aneurysm. J Biomech 20:311–317, 1987.
32. Strother CM, Graves VB, Rappe A: Aneurysm hemodynamics: an experimental study. AJNR 13:1089–1095, 1992.
33. Turjman F, Tournut P, Baldy-Porcher C, et al: Demonstration of subclavian steal by MR angiography. J Comput Assist Tomogr 16:756–759, 1992.
34. Turski PA, Korosec F: Technical features and emerging clinical applications of phase contrast MRA. Neuroimaging Clin North Am 2:785–800, 1992.
35. Allcock JM, Canham PB: Angiographic study of the growth of intracranial aneurysms. J Neurosurg 45:617–621, 1976.
36. Artmann H, Vonofakos D, Meuller H, Gran H: Neuroradiologic and neuropathologic findings with growing giant intracranial aneurysms. Surg Neurol 21:391–401, 1984.
37. Ferguson GG: Physical factors in the initiation, growth and rupture of intracranial saccular aneurysms. J Neurosurg 37:666–667, 1972.
38. Sutherland GR, King ME, Peerless SJ, et al: Platelet interaction within giant intracranial aneurysms. J Neurosurg 56:53–61, 1982.
39. Steiger HJ, Liepsch DW, Poll A, Reulen JH: Hemodynamic stress in terminal saccular aneurysms—a laser Doppler study. Heart Vessels 4:162–169, 1988.
40. Levey AS, Pauker SG, Kassirer JP: Occult intracranial aneurysm in polycystic kidney disease. When is cerebral arteriography indicated? N Engl J Med 308:986–994, 1983.
41. Perret G, Nishioka H: Report on the cooperative study of intracranial aneurysms and subarachnoid hemorrhage. Section VI. Arteriovenous malformations. An analysis of 545 cases of cranio-cerebral arteriovenous malformations and fistulae reported to the cooperative study. J Neurosurg 25:467–490, 1966.
42. Belber CJ, Hoffman RB: The syndrome of intracranial aneurysm associated with fibromuscular hyperplasia of the renal arteries. J Neurosurg 28:556–559, 1969.
43. Ronkainen A, Hernesniemi J, Ryynanen M, et al: A ten percent prevalence of asymptomatic familial intracranial aneurysms: preliminary report on 110 magnetic resonance angiography studies in members of 21 Finnish familial intracranial aneurysm families. Neurosurgery 35:208–212, 1994.
44. Chapman AB, Rubinstein D, Hughes R, et al: Intracranial aneurysms in autosomal dominant polycystic kidney disease. N Engl J Med 327:916–920, 1992.
45. Weibers DO, Torres VE: Screening for unruptured intracranial aneurysms in autosomal dominant polycystic kidney disease. N Engl J Med 327:953–955, 1992.
46. Black WC: Intracranial aneurysm in adult polycystic kidney disease: is screening with MR angiography indicated? Radiology 191:18–20, 1994.
47. Asari S, Satoh T, Sakurai M, et al: Delineation of unruptured cerebral aneurysms by CT angiotomography. J Neurosurg 57:527–534, 1982.
48. Aoki S, Sasaki Y, Machida T, et al: Cerebral aneurysms: detection and delineation using 3-D-CT angiography. AJNR 13:1115–1120, 1992.
48a. Vieco PT, Shuman WP, Alsofrom GF, Gross CE: Detection of circle of Willis aneurysms in patients with subarachnoid hemorrhage: a comparison of CT angiography and digital subtraction angiography. AJR 165:425–430, 1995.
49. Locksley HB: Natural history of subarachnoid hemorrhage, intracranial aneurysms and arteriovenous malformations. Based on 6368 cases in the cooperative study. J Neurosurg 25:219–239, 1966.
50. Wiebers DO, Whisnant JP, O'Fallon WM: The natural history of unruptured intracranial aneurysms. N Engl J Med 304:696–698, 1981.
51. Winn HR, Almaani WS, Berga SL, et al: The long-term outcome in patients with multiple aneurysms. Incidence of late hemorrhage and implications for treatment of incidental aneurysms. J Neurosurg 59:642–651, 1983.
52. Wiebers DO, Whisnant JP, Sundt TM Jr, et al: Intracranial aneurysm size and potential for rupture. J Neurosurg 67:476, 1987. Letter.
53. Obuchowski NA, Modic MT, Magdinec M: Current implications for the efficacy of noninvasive screening for occult intracranial aneurysms in patients with a family history of aneurysms. J Neurosurg 83:42–49, 1995.
54. Harbaugh RE: Unruptured intracranial aneurysms: decision making and management. Contemp Neurosurg 13(12):1–6, 1991.
55. De La Paz RL, New PFJ, Buonanno FS, et al: NMR imaging of intracranial hemorrhage. J Comput Assist Tomogr 8:599, 1984.
56. Atlas SW: MR imaging is highly sensitive for acute subarachnoid hemorrhage . . . not! Radiology 186:319–322, 1993.
56a. Noguchi K, Toshihide O, Inugami A, et al: Acute subarachnoid hemorrhage: MR imaging with fluid-attenuated inversion recovery pulse sequences. Radiology 196:773–777, 1995.

57. Scotti G, Ethier R, Melancon D, et al: Computed tomography in the evaluation of intracranial aneurysms and subarachnoid hemorrhage. Radiology 123:85–90, 1977.
58. Ghoshhjra K, Scotti L, Marasco J, et al: CT detection of intracranial aneurysm in subarachnoid hemorrhage. AJR 132:613–616, 1979.
59. Liliequist B, Lindquist M, Valdimarsson E: Computed tomography and subarachnoid hemorrhage. Neuroradiology 14:21–26, 1977.
60. Laissy J-P, Normand G, Monroc M, et al: Spontaneous intracerebral hematomas from vascular causes. Predictive value of CT compared with angiography. Neuroradiology 33:291–295, 1991.
61. Davis JM, Davis KR, Crowell RM: Subarachnoid hemorrhage secondary to ruptured intracranial aneurysm: prognostic significance of cranial CT. AJNR 1:17–21, 1980.
62. Alexander MSM, Dias PS, Uttley D: Spontaneous subarachnoid hemorrhage and negative cerebral panangiography. J Neurosurg 64:537–542, 1986.
63. van Gijn J, van Dongen KJ, Vermeulen M, Hijdra A: Permesencephalic hemorrhage: a nonaneurysmal and benign form of subarachnoid hemorrhage. Neurology 35:493–497, 1985.
64. Silver AJ, Pederson ME, Ganti SR, et al: CT of subarachnoid hemorrhage due to ruptured aneurysm. AJNR 2:549–552, 1981.
65. Strother CM, Eldevik P, Kikuchi Y, et al: Thrombus formation and structure and the evolution of mass effect in intracranial aneurysms treated by balloon embolization: emphasis on MR findings. AJNR 10:787–796, 1989.
66. Atlas SW, Mark AS, Grossman RI, Gomori JM: Intracranial hemorrhage: gradient-echo imaging at 1.5T. Radiology 168:803–807, 1988.
67. Biondi A, Scialfa G, Scotti G: Intracranial aneurysms: MR imaging. Neuroradiology 30:214–218, 1988.
68. Olsen WL, Brant-Zawadzki M, Hodes J, et al: Giant intracranial aneurysms: MR imaging. Radiology 163:431–435, 1987.
69. Almaani WS, Richardson AE: Multiple intracranial aneurysms: identifying the ruptured lesion. Surg Neurol 9:303–305, 1978.
70. Stone JL, Crowell RM, Gandhi YN, Jafar JJ: Multiple intracranial aneurysms: magnetic resonance imaging for determination of the site of rupture. Report of a case. Neurosurgery 23:97–100, 1988.
71. Zimmerman RA, Atlas S, Bilaniuk LT, et al: Magnetic resonance imaging of cerebral aneurysm. Acta Radiol 369:107–109, 1986.
72. Little JR, Blomquist GA Jr, Ethier F: Intraventricular hemorrhage in adults. Surg Neurol 8:143–149, 1977.
73. Fein JM, Rovit RL: Interhemispheric subdural hematoma secondary to hemorrhage from a callosal-marginal artery aneurysm. Neuroradiology 1:183–186, 1970.
74. Sadik AR, Adachi M, Ransohoff J: Rupture of intracranial aneurysm. Neurosurgery 20:609–612, 1963.
75. Grossman RI, Kemp SS, Yulp C, et al: The importance of oxygenation in the appearance of subarachnoid hemorrhage on high field magnetic resonance imaging. Acta Radiol, in press.
76. Neill JM, Hasting AB: The influence of the tension of molecular oxygen upon certain oxidations of hemoglobin. J Biol Chem 63:479–484, 1925.
77. Gomori JM, Grossman RI, Goldberg HI, et al: Intracranial hematomas: imaging by high field MR. Radiology 157:87–93, 1985.
78. Zimmerman RD, Hein LA, Snow RB, et al: Acute intracranial hemorrhage: intensity changes on sequential MR scans at 0.5 T. AJNR 9:47–53, 1988.
79. Zimmerman RD, Deck MF: Intracranial hematomas: imaging by high field MR. Radiology 159:565–569, 1986.
80. Ogawa T, Inugami A, Shimosegawa E, et al: Subarachnoid hemorrhage: evaluation with MR imaging. Radiology 186:345–351, 1993.
81. Bradley WG Jr, Schmidt PG: Effect of methemoglobin formation on the MR appearance of subarachnoid hemorrhage. Radiology 156:99–103, 1985.
82. Norbash AM, Glover GH, Enzmann DR: Intracerebral lesion contrast with spin-echo and fast spin-echo pulse sequence. Radiology 185:661–665, 1992.
83. Thulborn KR, Waterton JC, Matthews PM, Radda GK: Oxygenation dependence of the transverse relaxation time of water protons in whole blood at high field. Biochim Biophys Acta 714:265–270, 1982.
84. Gomori JM, Grossman RI, Goldberg HI, et al: Occult cerebral vascular malformations: high-field MR imaging. Radiology 158:707–713, 1986.
85. Hardy PA, Kucharczyk W, Henkelman RM: The cause of signal loss in MR images of old hemorrhagic lesions. Radiology 174:549–555, 1990.
86. Thulborn KR, Sorensen AG, Kowal NW, et al: The role of ferritin and hemosiderin in the MR appearance of intracerebral hemorrhage: a histopathological study in rats. AJNR 11:291–297, 1990.
87. Gomori JM, Grossman RI, Hackney DB, et al: Variable appearances of subacute intracranial hematomas on high-field spin-echo MR. AJNR 8:1019–1026, 1987.
88. Edelman RR, Johnson K, Buxton R, et al: MR of hemorrhage: a new approach. AJNR 7:751–756, 1986.
89. Henning J, Nauerth A, Friedburg H: RARE imaging: a fast imaging method for clinical MR. J Magn Reson Med 3:823–833, 1986.
90. Jones KM, Mulkern RV, Mantello MT, et al: Brain hemorrhage: evaluation with fast spin-echo and conventional dual spin-echo images. Radiology 182:53–58, 1992.

91. Curnes JT, Shogry MEC, Clark DC, Elsner HJ: MR angiographic demonstration of an intracranial aneurysm not seen on conventional angiography. AJNR 14:971–973, 1992.
92. Gouliamos A, Gotsis E, Vlahos L, et al: Magnetic resonance angiography compared to intra-arterial digital subtraction angiography in patients with subarachnoid haemorrhage. Neuroradiology 35:46–49, 1992.
93. Atlas SW, Grossman RI, Goldberg HI, et al: Partially thrombosed giant intracranial aneurysms: correlation of MR and pathologic findings. Radiology 162:111–114, 1987.
94. Lemme-Plaghos L, Kucharczyk W, Brant-Zawadzki M, et al: MRI of angiographically occult vascular malformations. AJR 146:1223–1228, 1986.
95. New PFJ, Ojemann RG, Davis KR, et al: MR and CT of occult vascular malformations of the brain. AJR 147:985–993, 1986.
96. Bradley WG Jr, Waluch V, Lai K-S, et al: The appearance of rapidly flowing blood on magnetic resonance images. AJR 143:1167–1174, 1984.
97. Unger E, Gado M, Fulling K, et al: Acute cerebral infarction in monkeys: an experimental study using MR imaging. Radiology 162:789–795, 1987.
98. Vorkapic P, Czech T, Pendl G, et al: Clinico-radiological spectrum of giant intracranial aneurysms. Neurosurg Rev 14:271–274, 1991.
99. Nadel L, Braun IF, Kraft KA, et al: Intracranial vascular abnormalities: value of MR phase imaging to distinguish thrombus from flowing blood. AJNR 11:1133–1140, 1990.
100. Burt TB: MR of CSF flow phenomenon mimicking basilar artery aneurysm. AJNR 8:55–58, 1987.
101. Iwama T, Andoh T, Sakai N, et al: Dissecting and fusiform aneurysms of vertebro-basilar systems: MR imaging. Neuroradiology 32:272–279, 1990.
102. Hennig J, Muri M, Brunner P, Friedburg H: Quantitative flow measurement with the fast Fourier flow technique. Radiology 166:237–240, 1988.
103. Dixon WT, Du LN, Gado M, Rossnick S: Projection angiograms of blood labeled by adiabatic fast passage. Magn Reson Med 3:454–462, 1986.
104. Turski PA, Korsec FR, Partington CR, et al: Cardiac-gated and variable-velocity-phase MR angiography for evaluation of intracranial aneurysms and arteriovenous malformations. Radiology 177(P):281, 1990. Abstract.
105. Huston J III, Rufenacht DA, Ehman RL, Wiebers DO: Intracranial aneurysms and vascular malformations: comparison of time-of-flight and phase-contrast MR angiography. Radiology 181:721–730, 1991.
106. Masaryk TJ, Modic MT, Ross JS, et al: Intracranial circulation: preliminary clinical results with three-dimensional (volume) MR angiography. Radiology 171:793–799, 1989.
107. Sevick RJ, Tsuruda JS, Schmalbrock P: Three-dimensional time-of-flight MR angiography in the evaluation of cerebral aneurysms. J Comput Assist Tomogr 14:874–881, 1990.
108. Anderson CM, Saloner D, Tsuruda J, et al: Artifacts in maximum-intensity-projection display of MR. AJR 154:623–629, 1990.
109. McCormick WF, Acosta-Rua GJ: The size of intracranial saccular aneurysms. An autopsy study. J Neurosurg 33:422–427, 1970.
110. Huston J III, Nichols DA, Luetner PH, et al: Blinded prospective evaluation of sensitivity of MR angiography to known intracranial aneurysms: importance of aneurysm size. AJNR 15:1607–1614, 1994.
111. Korogi Y, Takahashi M, Mabuchi N, et al: Intracranial aneurysms: diagnostic accuracy of three-dimensional, Fourier transform, time-of-flight MR angiography. Radiology 193:181–186, 1994.
112. Litt AW: MR angiography of intracranial aneurysms: proceed, but with caution. AJNR 15:1615–1616, 1994.
113. Edelman RR, Ahn SS, Chien D, et al: Improved time-of-flight MR angiography of the brain with magnetization transfer contrast. Radiology 184:295–299, 1992.
114. Blatter DD, Parker DL, Robison RO: Cerebral MR angiography with multiple overlapping thin slab acquisition. Part I. Quantitative analysis of vessel visibility. Radiology 179:805–811, 1991.
115. Runge VM, Kirsch JE, Lee C: Contrast-enhanced MR angiography. J Magn Reson Imaging 3:233–239, 1993.
116. Bogdanov AA Jr, Weissleder R, Frank HW, et al: A new macromolecule as a contrast agent for MR angiography: preparation, properties, and animal studies. Radiology 187:701–706, 1993.
117. Graeb DA, Robertson WD, Lapointe JS, et al: Computed tomographic diagnosis of intraventricular hemorrhage: etiology and prognosis. Radiology 43:91–96, 1982.
118. Mori K, Murata T, Nakano Y, Handa H: Periventricular lucency in hydrocephalus on computerized tomography. Surg Neurol 8:337–340, 1977.
119. Moseley IF, Radii EW: Factors influencing the development of periventricular lucencies in patients with raised intracranial pressure. Neuroradiology 17:65–69, 1979.
120. Juul R, Fredriksen TA, Ringkjob R: Prognosis in subarachnoid hemorrhage of unknown etiology. J Neurosurg 64:359–362, 1986.
121. Weir BKA: The effect of vasospasm on morbidity and mortality after subarachnoid hemorrhage from ruptured aneurysm. In: Wilkins RH, ed. Cerebral Arterial Spasm. Baltimore: Williams & Wilkins, 1980, pp 385–393.
122. Kistler JP, Crowell RM, Davis KR, et al: The relation of cerebral vasospasm to the extent and location of subarachnoid blood visualized by CT scan: a prospective study. Neurology 33:424–436, 1983.
123. Black PM: Hydrocephalus and vasospasm after subarachnoid hemorrhage from ruptured intracranial aneurysms. Neurosurgery 18:12–16, 1986.
124. Ohta H, Ito Z: Cerebral infarction due to vasospasm, revealed by computed tomography. Neurol Med Chir 21:365–372, 1981.
125. Pagni CA, Valentini C, Cento A, Forni C: Giant aneurysm of the internal carotid bifurcation successfully clipped. Case report and description of postoperative CT scan and MRI modifications. J Neurosurg Sci 35:147–152, 1991.
126. Brothers MF, Fox AJ, Lee DH, et al: MR imaging after surgery for vertebrobasilar aneurysm. AJNR 11:149–161, 1990.
127. Holtas S, Olsson M, Romner B, et al: Comparison of MR imaging and CT in patients with intracranial aneurysm clips. AJNR 9:891–897, 1988.
128. Becker RL, Norfray JF, Teitelbaum GP, et al: MR imaging in patients with intracranial aneurysm clips. AJNR 9:885–889, 1988.
129. Shellock FG, Morisoli S, Kanal E: MR procedures and biomedical implants, materials, and devices: 1993 update. Radiology 189:587–599, 1993.
130. Kanal E, Shellock FG: MR imaging of patients with intracranial aneurysm clips. Radiology 187:612–614, 1993.
131. Romner B, Olsson M, Ljunggren B, et al: Magnetic resonance imaging and aneurysm clips: magnetic properties and image artifacts. J Neurosurg 70:426–431, 1989.
132. Food and Drug Administration: Caution needed when performing MRI scans on patients with aneurysm clips. FDA Med Bull 23(2):2–3, 1993.
133. Fox AJ, Vinuela F, Pelz DM: Use of detachable balloons for proximal artery occlusion in the treatment of unclippable cerebral aneurysms. J Neurosurg 66:40–46, 1987.
134. Higashida RT, Halbach VV, Barnwell SL: Treatment of intracranial aneurysms with preservation of the parent vessel: results of percutaneous balloon embolization in 84 patients. AJNR 11:633–640, 1990.
135. Guglielmi G, Vinuela F, Duckwiler G, et al: Endovascular treatment of posterior circulation aneurysms by electrothrombosis using electrically detachable coils. J Neurosurg 77:515–524, 1992.
136. Hecht ST, Horton JA, Yonas H: Growth of a thrombosed giant vertebral artery aneurysm after parent artery occlusion. AJNR 12:449–451, 1991.
137. Kwan ESK, Wolpert SM, Scott RM, Runge V: MR evaluation of neurovascular lesions after endovascular occlusion with detachable balloons. AJNR 9:523–531, 1988.
138. Kwan ESK, Heilman CB, Shucart WA, Klucznik RP: Enlargement of basilar artery aneurysms following balloon occlusion—"water-hammer effect." J Neurosurg 75:963–968, 1991.
139. Kondoh T, Fujita K, Yamashita H, et al: Giant intracranial aneurysms: magnetic resonance imaging follow-up and clinical symptoms. Neurol Med Chir (Tokyo) 31:330–335, 1991.
140. Yuh WTC, Crain MR, Loes DJ, et al: MR imaging of cerebral ischemia: findings in the first 24 hours. AJNR 12:621–629, 1991.
141. Bryan RN, Levy LM, Whitlow WD, et al: Diagnosis of acute cerebral infarction: comparison of CT and MR imaging. AJNR 12:611–620, 1991.
142. Sato A, Takahashi S, Soma Y, et al: Cerebral infarction: early detection by means of contrast enhanced cerebral arteries at MR imaging. Radiology 178:443–449, 1991.
143. Tsuruda JS, Sevick RJ, Halbach VV: Three-dimensional time-of-flight MR angiography in the evaluation of intracranial aneurysms treated by endovascular balloon occlusion. AJNR 13:1129–1136, 1992.
144. Perl J II, Turski PA, Strother CM, Graves VB: Flow dynamics in experimental lateral, terminal and bifurcation aneurysms assessed by phase contrast speed MRA imaging: confirmation of MRA flow features by conventional angiography. In: Proceedings of the 32nd Annual Meeting of the American Society of Neuroradiology, Nashville, Tennessee, May 3–7, 1994, p 219.
145. McCormick WF: The pathology of vascular ("arteriovenous") malformations. J Neurosurg 24:807–816, 1966.
146. Russel DS, Rubenstein LJ: Pathology of Tumours of the Nervous System. Baltimore: Williams & Wilkins, 1989, pp 727–746.
147. Jellinger K: Vascular malformation of the central nervous system: a morphological overview. Neurosurg Rev 9:177–216, 1986.
148. Brown RD Jr, Wiebers DO, Forbes G, et al: The natural history of unruptured intracranial arteriovenous malformations. J Neurosurg 68:352–357, 1988.
149. Marks MP, Lane B, Steinberg GK, Chang PJ: Hemorrhage in intracerebral arteriovenous malformations: angiographic determinants. Radiology 176:807–813, 1990.
150. Waltimo O: The relationship of size, density and localization of intracranial arteriovenous malformations to the type of initial symptom. J Neurol Sci 19:13–19, 1973.
151. Spetzler RF, Hargraves RW, McCormick PW, et al: Relationship of perfusion pressure and size to risk of hemorrhage from arteriovenous malformations. J Neurosurg 76:913–923, 1992.
152. Graf CJ, Perret GE, Torner JC: Bleeding from cerebral arteriovenous malformations as part of their natural history. J Neurosurg 58:331–337, 1983.
153. Spetzler RF, Martin NA, Carter LP, et al: Surgical management of large AVM's by staged embolization and operative excision. J Neurosurg 67:17–28, 1987.
154. Berenstein A, Lasjaunias P: Classification of brain arteriovenous malformations In: Berenstein A, Lasjaunias P, eds. Surgical Neuroangiography. Berlin: Springer-Verlag, 1992, pp 1–86.
155. Marks MP, Lane B, Steinberg G, Chang P: Vascular characteristics of

intracerebral arteriovenous malformations in patients with clinical steal. AJNR 12:489–496, 1991.

156. Willinsky R, Lasjaunias P, Terburgge K, et al: Brain arteriovenous malformations: analysis of the angioarchitecture in relationship to hemorrhage. J Neuroradiol 15:225–237, 1988.

157. Spetzler RF, Martin NA: A proposed grading system for arteriovenous malformations. J Neurosurg 65:476–483, 1986.

158. Shi YQ, Chen XC: A proposed scheme for grading intracranial arteriovenous malformations. J Neurosurg 65:484–489, 1986.

159. Dawson RC III, Tarr RW, Hect ST, et al: Treatment of arteriovenous malformations of the brain with combined embolization and stereotactic radiosurgery: results after one and two years. AJNR 11:857–864, 1990.

160. Betti OO, Munari C, Rosler R: Stereotactic radiosurgery with the linear accelerator: treatment of arteriovenous malformations. Neurosurgery 24:311–321, 1989.

161. Quisling RG, Peters KR, Friedman WA, Tart RP: Persistent nidus blood flow in cerebral arteriovenous malformation after stereotactic radiosurgery: MR imaging assessment. Radiology 180:785–791, 1991.

162. Kauczor HU, Engenhart R, Layer G, et al: 3D TOF MR angiography of cerebral arteriovenous malformations after radiosurgery. J Comput Assist Tomogr 17:184–190, 1993.

163. Nussel F, Wegmuller H, Huber P: Comparison of magnetic resonance angiography, magnetic resonance imaging and conventional angiography in cerebral arteriovenous malformation. Neuroradiology 33:56–61, 1991.

164. Leblanc R, Levesque M, Comair Y, Ethier R: Magnetic resonance imaging of cerebral arteriovenous malformations. Neurosurgery 21:15–20, 1987.

165. Noorbehesht B, Fabrikant JI, Enzmann DR: Size determination of supratentorial arteriovenous malformations by MR, CT and angio. Neuroradiology 29:512–518, 1987.

166. Smith HJ, Strother CM, Kikuchi Y, et al: MR imaging in the management of supratentorial intracranial AVMs. AJNR 9:225–235, 1988.

167. Pernicone JR, Siebert JE, Potchen EJ: Demonstration of an early draining vein by MR angiography. J Comput Assist Tomogr 15:829–831, 1991.

168. Prayer L, Wimberger D, Stiglbauer R, et al: Haemorrhage in intracerebral arteriovenous malformations: detection with MRI and comparison with clinical history. Neuroradiology 35:424–427, 1993.

169. Chappell PM, Steinberg GK, Marks MP: Clinically documented hemorrhage in cerebral arteriovenous malformations: MR characteristics. Radiology 183:719–724, 1992.

170. Marchal G, Bosmans H, Van Fraeyenhoven L, et al: Intracranial vascular lesions: optimization and clinical evaluation of the three-dimensional time-of-flight MR angiography. Radiology 175:443–448, 1990.

171. Edelman RR, Wentz KU, Mattle HP, et al: Intracerebral arteriovenous malformations: evaluation with selective MR angiography and venography. Radiology 173:831–837, 1989.

172. Ehricke HH, Schad LR, Gademann G, et al: Use of MR angiography for stereotactic planning. J Comput Assist Tomogr 16:35–40, 1992.

173. Mehta MP, Petereit D, Turski P, et al: Magnetic resonance angiography: a three-dimensional database for assessing arteriovenous malformations. J Neurosurg 79:289–293, 1993.

174. Petereit D, Mehta M, Turski P, et al: Treatment of arteriovenous malformations with stereotactic radiosurgery employing both magnetic resonance angiography and standard angiography as a database. Int J Radiat Oncol Biol Phys 25:309–313, 1993.

175. Marks M, Pelc N, Ross MR, Enzmann DR: Determination of cerebral blood flow with phase-contrast cine MR imaging technique evaluation of normal subjects and patients with arteriovenous malformations. Radiology 182:467–476, 1992.

176. Requena I, Arias M, Lopez-Ibor L, et al: Cavernomas of the central nervous system: clinical and neuroimaging manifestations in 47 patients. J Neurol Neurosurg Psychiatry 54:590–594, 1991.

177. Rigamonti D, Drayer BP, Johnson PC, et al: The MRI appearance of cavernous malformations (angiomas). J Neurosurg 67:518–524, 1987.

178. Robinson JR, Awad IA, Little JR: Natural history of the cavernous angioma. J Neurosurg 75:709–714, 1991.

179. Savoiardo M, Strada L, Passerini A: Intracranial cavernous hemangiomas: neuroradiologic review of 36 operated cases. AJNR 4:945–950, 1983.

180. Zimmerman RS, Spetzler RF, Lee KS, et al: Cavernous malformations of the brain stem. J Neurosurg 75:32–39, 1991.

181. Allard JC, Hochberg FH, Frankin PD, et al: Magnetic resonance imaging in a family with hereditary cerebral arteriovenous malformations. Arch Neurol 46:184–187, 1989.

182. Rigamonti D, Hadley MN, Drayer BP, et al: Cerebral cavernous malformations. Incidence and familial occurrence. N Engl J Med 319:343–347, 1988.

183. Rutka ST, Brant-Zawadzki M, Wilson CT, et al: Familial cavernous malformations: diagnostic potentials of magnetic resonance imaging. Surg Neurol 29:467–474, 1988.

184. McCormick WF: Pathology of vascular malformations of the brain. In: Wilson CB, Stein BM, eds. Intracranial Vascular Malformations. Baltimore: Williams & Wilkins, 1984, pp 44–63.

185. Simard JM, Garcia-Bengochea F, Ballinger WE Jr, et al: Cavernous angioma: a review of 126 collected and 12 new clinical cases. Neurosurgery 18:162–172, 1986.

186. Tagle P, Huete I, Mendez J, et al: Intracranial cavernous angioma: presentation and management. J Neurosurg 64:720–723, 1986.

187. McCormick WF, Hardman JM, Boulter TR: Vascular malformations ("angiomas") of the brain, with special reference to those occurring in the posterior fossa. J Neurosurg 28:241–251, 1968.

188. Rigamonti D, Spetzler RF: The association of venous and cavernous malformations. Report of four cases and discussion of the pathophysiological, diagnostic, and therapeutic implications. Acta Neurochir (Wien) 92:100–105, 1988.

189. Rapacki TFX, Brantley MJ, Furlow TW Jr, et al: Heterogeneity of cerebral cavernous hemangiomas diagnosed by MR imaging. J Comput Assist Tomogr 14:18–25, 1990.

190. Sze G, Krol G, Olsen WL, et al: Hemorrhagic neoplasms: MR mimics of occult vascular malformations. AJR 149:1223–1230, 1987.

191. Momoshima S, Shiga H, Yuasa Y, et al: MR findings in extracerebral cavernous angiomas of the middle cranial fossa: report of two cases and review of the literature. AJNR 12:756–760, 1991.

192. Sepehrnia A, Tatagiba M, Brandis A, et al: Cavernous angioma of the cavernous sinus: case report. Neurosurgery 27:151–155, 1990.

193. Steinberg GK, Marks MP, Shuer LM, et al: Occult vascular malformations of the optic chiasm: magnetic resonance imaging diagnosis and surgical laser resection. Neurosurgery 27:466–470, 1990.

194. Awad IA, Robinson JR Jr, Mohanty S, Estes M: Mixed vascular malformations of the brain: clinical and pathogenetic considerations. Neurosurgery 33:179–188, 1993.

195. Valavanis A, Wellauer J, Yasargil MG: The radiological diagnosis of cerebral venous angioma: cerebral angiography and CT. Neuroradiology 24:193–199, 1983.

196. Ostertun B, Solymosi L: Magnetic resonance angiography of cerebral developmental venous anomalies: its role in differential diagnosis. Neuroradiology 35:97–104, 1993.

197. Augustyn GT, Scott JA, Olson E, et al: Cerebral venous angiomas: MR imaging. Radiology 156:391–395, 1985.

198. Garner TB, Del Curling O Jr, Kelly DL Jr, Laster DW: The natural history of intracranial venous angiomas. J Neurosurg 75:715–722, 1991.

199. Wilms G, Bleus E, Demaerel P, et al: Simultaneous occurrence of developmental venous anomalies and cavernous angiomas. AJNR 15:1247–1254, 1994.

200. Barnwell SL, Halbach VV, Dowd CF, et al: Multiple dural arteriovenous fistulas of the cranium and spine. AJNR 12:441–445, 1991.

201. Houser WO, Campbell KJ, Campbell JR, Sundt TM: Arteriovenous malformation affecting the transverse dural venous sinus: an acquired lesion. Mayo Clin Proc 54:651–661, 1979.

202. DeMarco K, Dillon WP, Halbach VV, Tsuruda JS: Dural arteriovenous fistula: evaluation with MR imaging. Radiology 175:193–199, 1990.

203. Halbach VV, Higashida RT, Hieshima GB, et al: Dural fistulas involving the cavernous sinus: results of treatment in 30 patients. Radiology 63:437–442, 1987.

204. Halbach VV, Higashida RT, Hieshima GB, et al: Dural fistulas involving the transverse and sigmoid sinuses: results in 28 patients. Radiology 163:443–447, 1987.

205. Chen JC, Tsuruda JS, Halbach VV: Suspected dural arteriovenous fistula: results with screening MR angiography in seven patients. Radiology 183:265–271, 1992.

206. Willinsky R, Terbrugge K, Montanera W, et al: Venous congestion: an MR finding in dural arteriovenous malformations with cortical venous drainage. AJNR 15:1501–1507, 1994.

207. Jannetta PJ, Abbasy M, Maroon JC, et al: Etiology and definitive microsurgical treatment of hemifacial spasm: operative techniques and results in 47 patients. J Neurosurg 47:321–328, 1977.

208. Adler CH, Zimmerman RA, Savino PJ, et al: Hemifacial spasm: evaluation by magnetic resonance imaging and magnetic resonance tomographic angiography. Ann Neurol 32:502–506, 1992.

209. Neilsen VK, Janetta PJ: Pathophysiology of hemifacial spasm: III. Effects of facial nerve decompression. Neurology 34:891–897, 1984.

210. Felber S, Birbamer G, Aichner F, et al: Magnetic resonance imaging and angiography in hemifacial spasm. Neuroradiology 34:413–416, 1992.

211. Furuya Y, Ryu H, Uemura K, et al: MRI of intracranial neurovascular compression. J Comput Assist Tomogr 16:503–505, 1992.

212. Harsh GR, Wilson CB, Hieshima GB, Dillon WP: Magnetic resonance imaging of vertebrobasilar ectasia in tic convulsif. J Neurosurg 74:999–1003, 1991.

213. Nagaseki Y, Horikoshi T, Omata T, et al: Oblique sagittal magnetic resonance imaging visualizing vascular compression of the trigeminal or facial nerve. J Neurosurg 77:379–386, 1992.

214. Tash R, DeMerritt J, Sze G, Leslie D: Hemifacial spasm: MR imaging features. AJNR 12:839–842, 1991.

215. Tien RD, Wilkins RH: MRA delineation of the vertebral-basilar system in patients with hemifacial spasm and trigeminal neuralgia. AJNR 14:34–36, 1993.

216. Bernardi B, Zimmerman RA, Savino PJ, Adler C: Magnetic resonance tomographic angiography in the investigation of hemifacial spasm. Neuroradiology 35:606–611, 1993.

217. Linskey ME, Jho HD, Jannetta PJ: Microvascular decompression for trigeminal neuralgia caused by vertebrobasilar compression. J Neurosurg 81:1–9, 1994.

Stroke and Cerebral Ischemia

TEREASA M. SIMONSON ▪ WILLIAM T. C. YUH

Stroke affects 400,000 people annually in the United States and is the third leading cause of death.[1] However, only a small percentage of patients die as a result of stroke, making this the leading cause of disability and the third most costly disease affecting adults.[2] The word *stroke* is a clinical term referring to the sudden onset of neurologic symptoms such as loss of or decreased consciousness, sensation, or voluntary motion. Usually this is due to ischemia. If ischemia is prolonged, cell death or infarction occurs. Infarction can be classified by the overall cause of ischemia, such as arterial vascular occlusion (secondary to embolism or thrombosis), venous occlusion, anoxia, hypoxemia, or hypotension. Hypoglycemia may also be contributory in some cases.

Acute, subacute, or chronic infarction refers to the time from symptom onset. The location of the infarction depends on the vessels involved: lobar infarctions, which occur in the cerebrum or cerebellum; lacunar infarctions, which tend to occur as small foci in the basal ganglia, internal capsule, thalamus, or brain stem; and watershed infarctions. The age of the patient can also affect the location of the injury. Periventricular leukomalacia, for example, is typical in hypoxic premature infants but does not occur in adults.

The clinical role of neuroimaging in acute stroke has been primarily threefold: 1) to assess the cause of neurologic dysfunction, which may be a process mimicking ischemia such as tumor or infection; 2) to provide radiologic evidence of tissue ischemia and define the vascular territories involved; and 3) to rule out the presence of hemorrhage or hematoma in anticipation of treatment (usually systemic anticoagulation).

This chapter is a review of the current, readily available applications of magnetic resonance imaging (MRI) in the detection and characterization of cerebral ischemia.

MRI AND PATHOPHYSIOLOGY

The detection of brain ischemia by MRI depends on the evaluation of four features: 1) vascular flow abnormalities, 2) mass effect, 3) parenchymal signal characteristics, and 4) parenchymal enhancement by contrast material (Table 24–1).

TABLE 24–1. MRI FINDINGS IN ACUTE CEREBRAL ISCHEMIA

MECHANISM	MRI FINDINGS	POSSIBLE CAUSES	ESTIMATED TIME* (h)
Flow kinetics	Absent flow	Slow flow; occlusion	Early
	Arterial enhancement	Accentuation of flow derangement	Early
Biophysiologic	T1 morphologic change	Cytotoxic edema (free water)	2–4
	T2 signal change	Blood-brain barrier breakdown; vasogenic edema; macromolecular binding	8
	T1 signal change	Blood-brain barrier breakdown; vasogenic edema; macromolecular binding	16–24
Combination	Delayed parenchymal enhancement†	Impaired delivery of significant contrast agent	>24‡
	Early exaggerated enhancement§	Intact delivery of contrast agent; blood-brain barrier leakage; focal hyperemia	2–4§

*Time at which findings generally could first be detected by available MRI; this does not necessarily imply the exact time of onset.
†Typical findings in completed cortical infarctions.
‡Usually not detected before 5–7 d.
§Found in cases with transient or partial occlusions and in watershed infarctions.
From Yuh WTC, Crain MR, Loes DJ, et al: MRI of cerebral ischemia: findings in the first 24 hours. AJNR 12(4):621–629, 1991, © by American Society of Neuroradiology.

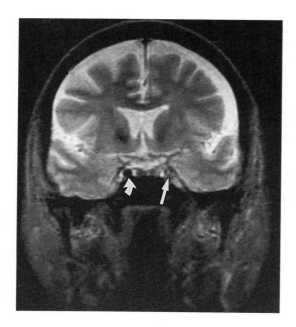

FIGURE 24–1. Arterial occlusion. A 63-year-old man presented with acute onset of diminished vision in the left eye. Coronal T2-weighted image (repetition time/echo time = 2000/100) obtained 18 hours after symptom onset shows absence of flow void phenomenon in the left internal carotid artery *(straight arrow)*. Note normal right internal carotid artery flow void *(curved arrow)*. (From Yuh WTC, Crain MR, Loes DJ, et al: MR imaging of cerebral ischemia: findings in the first 24 hours. AJNR 12[4]:621–629, 1991, © by American Society of Neuroradiology.)

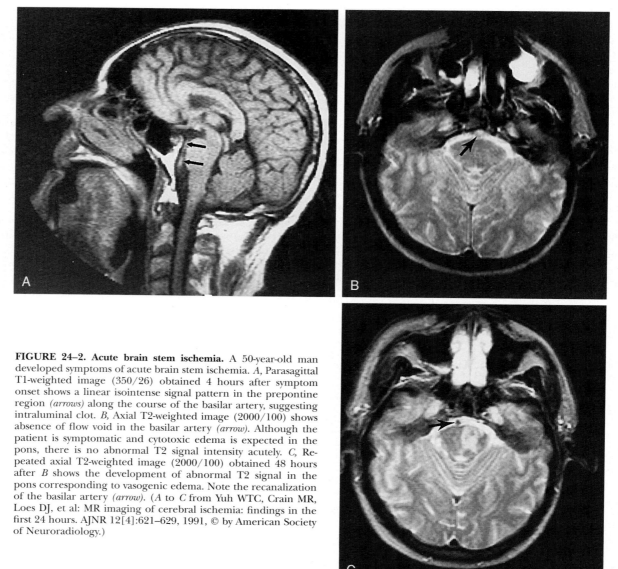

FIGURE 24–2. Acute brain stem ischemia. A 50-year-old man developed symptoms of acute brain stem ischemia. *A,* Parasagittal T1-weighted image (350/26) obtained 4 hours after symptom onset shows a linear isointense signal pattern in the prepontine region *(arrows)* along the course of the basilar artery, suggesting intraluminal clot. *B,* Axial T2-weighted image (2000/100) shows absence of flow void in the basilar artery *(arrow)*. Although the patient is symptomatic and cytotoxic edema is expected in the pons, there is no abnormal T2 signal intensity acutely. *C,* Repeated axial T2-weighted image (2000/100) obtained 48 hours after *B* shows the development of abnormal T2 signal in the pons corresponding to vasogenic edema. Note the recanalization of the basilar artery *(arrow)*. (*A* to *C* from Yuh WTC, Crain MR, Loes DJ, et al: MR imaging of cerebral ischemia: findings in the first 24 hours. AJNR 12[4]:621–629, 1991, © by American Society of Neuroradiology.)

Normal cerebral blood flow is 50 to 55 mL/100 g/ min.[3] Brain injury due to inadequate oxygen delivery occurs as cerebral blood flow drops below 22 mL/100 g/min.[4] This mechanical blood flow alteration during acute ischemia is a phenomenon that can be detected by MRI immediately after the event. In normal arteries, high-velocity or turbulent blood flow is seen on MR images as an absence of signal intensity (flow void phenomenon). Loss of flow void phenomenon, especially in a symptomatic patient, therefore indicates significant compromise of arterial blood flow by either low-velocity flow or occlusion. On the T1-weighted image, a signal abnormality will be seen within the occluded vessel, which tends to be isointense or hyperintense compared with brain parenchyma. Flow void phenomena are usually best evaluated on T2-weighted images, however, because of the longer echo time and distinct contrast between the low signal intensity of the blood vessel and the high signal intensity of cerebrospinal fluid (CSF) (Fig. 24–1).

In the evaluation of flow abnormalities in the distal internal carotid and middle cerebral arteries, the axial imaging plane is preferred because the entire course of these vessels can be demonstrated in a few images with little interference from flow-related enhancement (entrance phenomenon). Optimal evaluation of the basilar artery frequently requires both sagittal T1-weighted images to detect intraluminal clot and axial T2-weighted images to detect the absence of flow void phenomenon (Fig. 24–2). Flow-related enhancement in the basilar artery is frequently seen on axial views and on images enhanced with contrast medium. This should not be mistaken for a flow abnormality.

Vascular flow abnormalities in acute ischemia can be further accentuated by contrast material. Abnormal arterial enhancement is readily detected on T1-weighted images because of excellent contrast with the relatively dark CSF background. Arterial enhancement most likely represents low-velocity flow associated with stenosis, occlusion, or mass effect from brain swelling in the presence of poor collateral circulation[5] (Fig. 24–3).

Vascular stenosis and occlusion of larger vessels can also be evaluated with MR angiography using either phase-contrast or time-of-flight effects (see Chapter 25). Flow enhancement can be augmented by the gradient-echo technique using a short repetition time. This technique can be used with MR scanners that do not have the MR angiographic option.

The remaining three factors affecting the MRI appearance of brain ischemia are biologic processes that may occur early but require some time to develop changes detectable on MR images. These biologic tissue responses to acute ischemia include changes in tissue water content, mass effect, breakdown of the blood-brain barrier, and loss of autoregulation. The change in tissue water content probably represents a complex interplay between the somewhat arbitrary distinctions of cytotoxic and vasogenic edema (see Table 24–1). In chronic infarction, however, the increased tissue water content is a result of encephalomalacia and gliosis after ischemic necrosis. Infarcted

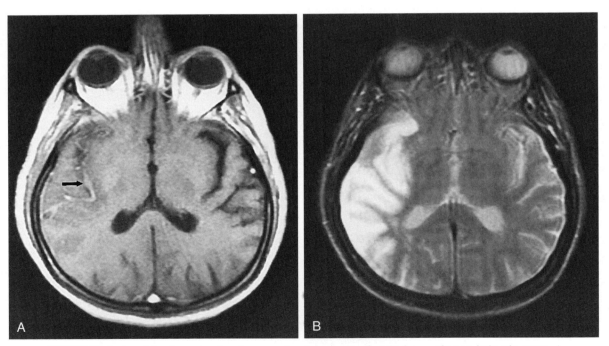

FIGURE 24–3. Arterial enhancement and vasogenic edema in the first 24 hours after an ischemic event. *A,* Postcontrast axial T1-weighted image (583/20) demonstrates abnormal arterial enhancement *(arrow)* in the distribution of the right middle cerebral artery. *B,* Corresponding T2-weighted image (2000/100) shows abnormal parenchymal signal intensity in a gyriform pattern in the distribution of the right middle cerebral artery corresponding to vasogenic edema. These findings are typical of complete ischemia. (*A* and *B* from Crain MR, Yuh WTC, Greene GM, et al: Cerebral ischemia: evaluation with contrast-enhanced MR imaging. AJNR 12[4]:631–639, 1991, © by American Society of Neuroradiology.)

tissue, due to its increased water content, typically appears hyperintense on T2-weighted images and isointense to hypointense on T1-weighted images.

Cytotoxic edema, the first factor, is characterized by intracellular water accumulation secondary to metabolic and cell membrane dysfunction early after the onset of the ischemic insult (within the first 6 hours). The degree of water shift during this phase has been reported to be 3% to 5% of total tissue water content.[6, 7] Cytotoxic edema is predominantly a result of a free water and electrolyte shift without associated protein shift and is probably responsible for the brain swelling that occurs within the first few hours. Intracellular levels of sodium, lactate, calcium, and free fatty acids increase as extracellular potassium increases. Restoration of blood flow will reverse these changes. Despite

marked local accumulation of intracellular free water, cytotoxic edema occurring early in ischemia does not show increased T2 signal intensity (Fig. 24–4). This is probably due to a lack of binding of this free water to macromolecules, which facilitates proton relaxation.[8]

Vasogenic edema, the second factor, has been described as a predominantly extracellular accumulation of water associated with the breakdown of the blood-brain barrier. Both water and protein macromolecules shift into the interstitium when blood-brain barrier breakdown occurs approximately 6 hours after blood flow is interrupted.[6, 7, 9, 10] Signal change depends not only on the amount of water shift but also on the binding of free water to macromolecules. However, increased T2 signal intensity is not reliably seen until 8 hours after the ischemic insult[8, 11] (Table 24–2; see Table 24–1).

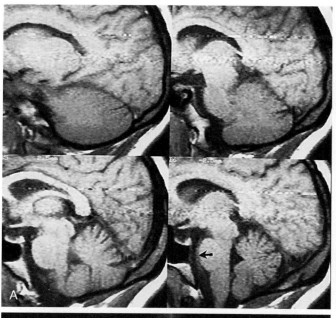

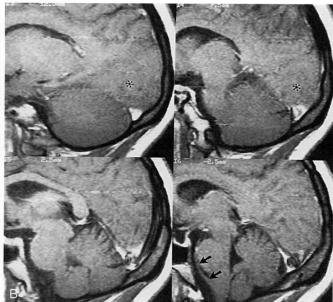

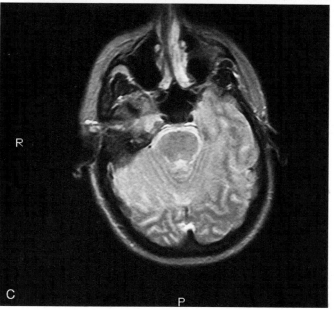

FIGURE 24–4. **Basilar artery occlusion.** A 35-year-old woman developed stroke-like symptoms that rapidly progressed from cerebellar dysfunction to unresponsiveness. *A,* Precontrast parasagittal T1-weighted images (450/20) obtained 2.5 hours after symptom onset show an isointense signal pattern in the prepontine cistern consistent with basilar artery thrombosis *(arrow). B,* Corresponding postcontrast parasagittal images obtained 40 minutes after *A* show development of massive brain swelling in the occipital lobes *(asterisk)* and cerebellum. The thrombosis of the basilar artery is even more prominent *(arrows). C,* Axial T2-weighted image (2000/100) obtained just before administration of contrast medium shows no parenchymal signal abnormality. Mass effect from cytotoxic edema without T2 signal abnormalities can be seen in the first 6 to 8 hours of acute ischemia. (*A* to *C* from Yuh WTC, Crain MR, Loes DJ, et al: MR imaging of cerebral ischemia: findings in the first 24 hours. AJNR 12[4]:621–629, 1991, © by American Society of Neuroradiology.)

TABLE 24–2. TYPICAL MRI FINDINGS IN THREE ISCHEMIC STROKE MODELS*

MODEL	VASCULAR		MASS EFFECT (POSITIVE OR NEGATIVE)	SIGNAL CHANGE†	PE	SIZE OF LESION DEMONSTRATED BY Gd AND T2-WEIGHTED IMAGE	COMMENTS
	Flow Void	AE					
Complete ischemia							
Acute (<7 d)							
Cortical	+	++	+++	+++	−	T2 > Gd	Usually severe symptoms
Noncortical	−	−	±	++	−		Usually infarction
Subacute (7 d–3 mo)							
Cortical	±	−	+	++	+++	T2 > Gd	AE usually disappears after day 7, when PE starts
Noncortical	−	−	±	++	+		
Chronic (>3 mo)							
Cortical	±	−	+‡	+	−	T2 > Gd	Usually infarction
Noncortical	−	−	+‡	+	−		
Incomplete ischemia							
Acute	−	−	+	±	+++	Gd ≥ T2	Usually minimal symptoms
Subacute or chronic	−	−	−	±	−		
Watershed ischemia							
Acute	−	−	++	++	++	Gd ≥ T2	Usually severe symptoms with infarction
Subacute or chronic	−	−	+	++	−	T2 > Gd	

*AE = arterial enhancement; PE = parenchymal enhancement; Gd = gadolinium.
†Changes usually after 8 h.
‡Negative mass effect.
From Yuh WTC, Crain MR: Magnetic resonance imaging of acute cerebral ischemia. Neuroimaging Clin North Am 2:428, 1992.

Signal change due to vasogenic edema or gliosis is better demonstrated on the first echo of the multiecho sequence (proton density–weighted image) when the infarcted or ischemic tissue is located in the cortex or periventricular region. This is because the signal contrast between these lesions and CSF is more apparent than on T2-weighted images. When located deep within the white matter, subcortical gray matter, or brain stem, an infarct or ischemia is often better seen on T2-weighted images. Signal change on T1-weighted images is less apparent because of the limited signal contrast between the ischemic tissue and surrounding normal tissue.

During acute ischemia, mass effect may be detected as a morphologic change associated with sulcal obliteration, effacement of ventricles, or structural enlargement (see Fig. 24–4). Mass effect probably results from the abnormal accumulation of water predominantly by cytotoxic edema in the early phase (first 6 hours) of brain ischemia and by vasogenic edema in the later phase (after 6 hours). In the chronic phase of infarction, "negative mass effect" caused by loss of brain parenchyma can be observed. Associated focal enlargement of sulci and ventricles as well as focal atrophy will be seen. Mass effect is best seen on T1-weighted images, which provide better anatomic detail as well as contrast with adjacent CSF signal intensity. Mass effect is more readily demonstrated in cortical infarct than in small noncortical lesions.

Parenchymal enhancement, the last factor, is caused by the abnormal accumulation of contrast agent in the ischemic or infarcted tissue (Fig. 24–5). The currently available chelated gadolinum contrast agents are normally confined to the intravascular space by a tight capillary junction (i.e., intact blood-brain barrier). When the blood-brain barrier breaks down, which occurs experimentally 6 hours after the onset of ischemia, contrast material leaks from the capillary bed into the ischemic or infarcted tissue. However, insufficient or absent blood supply to the infarcted tissue can hinder the delivery of contrast material. Thus, despite the breakdown of the blood-brain barrier, parenchymal enhancement is usually not demonstrated in early complete occlusive ischemia (see Fig. 24–4). Parenchymal enhancement does not occur until the reestablishment of a sufficient blood supply by collateral neovascularity or vessel recanalization 5 to 7 days after the acute event (Table 24–3). When delivery of contrast material is reestablished to the ischemic or infarcted tissue, the immature blood-brain barrier and lack of normal autoregulation in the proliferating vessels allow leakage and pooling of contrast agent in the affected tissue (see Fig. 24–5). Parenchymal enhancement, therefore, usually does not occur until 5 to 7 days after the acute event and may persist until the completion of the reparative process (maturation of the neovasculature), usually several months after the acute event.

Parenchymal enhancement before 7 days and even before 6 hours has been reported in clinical and experimental studies[8, 12, 13] (Fig. 24–6). This early enhancement suggests intact delivery of contrast material to the ischemic tissue in incomplete occlusion or nonocclusive ischemia. The cause of the abnormal accumulation of contrast material within the brain parenchyma before blood-brain barrier breakdown is expected (i.e.,

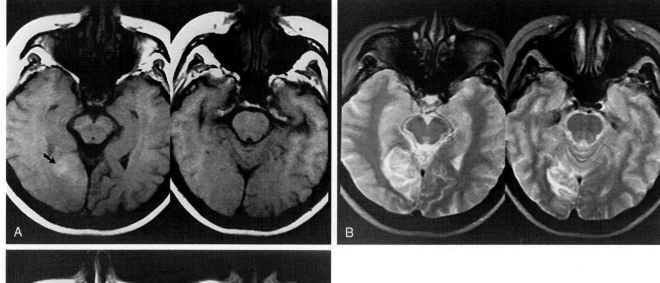

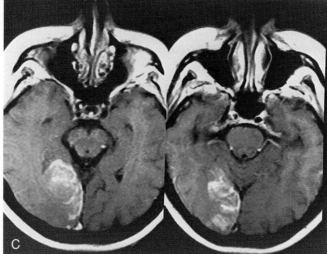

FIGURE 24–5. Posterior cerebral artery infarction. Infarction of right posterior cerebral artery occurred 10 days after symptom onset. *A*, Axial T1-weighted images (583/20) show mass effect in the distribution of the right posterior cerebral artery along with a well-defined increased signal intensity representing reperfusion petechial hemorrhage *(arrow)*. *B*, Axial T2-weighted images (2000/100) show abnormal parenchymal signal in the region demonstrating mass effect on the T1-weighted image. *C*, Axial contrast-enhanced T1-weighted images (583/20) demonstrate gyriform enhancement in the right posterior cerebral artery distribution. This is the typical enhancement appearance seen in the subacute to chronic stages of cortical infarction.

TABLE 24–3. SUMMARY OF TYPICAL PATTERNS OF ENHANCEMENT

MRI FINDINGS AND OUTCOME	COMPLETE ISCHEMIA (PROGRESSIVE ENHANCEMENT)		INCOMPLETE ISCHEMIA (EARLY OR INTENSE ENHANCEMENT) (n=15)*
	Cortical (n=36)	Noncortical (n=31)	
Parenchymal enhancement Pattern			
Acute (≤7 d)	Usually absent† (1/27)‡	Infrequent§ (9/30)	Early (10)
Subacute (≥7 d)	Progressive gyriform	Peripheral → central	Intense (5)
Extent (area involved)			
Acute	Contrast material < T2 signal (34/36)	Contrast material < T2 signal (26/31)	Contrast material ≥ T2 signal (13/15)
Arterial enhancement			
Acute	Frequent (30/36)	Infrequent‖ (5/31)	Infrequent (2/15)
Clinical outcome	Infarction	Infarction	Reversible/minimal neurologic dysfunction versus irreversible/infarction¶

*Five cases of transient ischemia and 10 cases limited to a watershed zone.
†Single case with faint enhancement at 6 d.
‡Number of positive cases/number of cases imaged.
§All enhancing lesions were small and had faint peripheral enhancement.
‖When positive, usually involved basilar artery.
¶Infarction in many cases of watershed zone ischemia.
From Crain MR, Yuh WTC, Greene GM, et al: Cerebral ischemia: evaluation with contrast-enhanced MR imaging. AJNR 12(4):631–639, 1991, © by American Society of Neuroradiology.

within 6 hours) is unclear and requires further study. Because absence of vasogenic edema is also frequently associated with this early parenchymal enhancement within the first 6 hours of symptoms, local dysautoregulation and hyperemia resulting in abnormal intravascular pooling of blood and contrast material in the ischemic area seem the most likely explanation.

NEW MRI TECHNIQUES

New developments in MRI have been applied to evaluating ischemia, including MR spectroscopy, diffusion imaging, and perfusion imaging.[14]

Spectral changes caused by ischemia are detectable within minutes after the insult due to altered cellular metabolism. Proton MR spectroscopy is used to evaluate acid-base balance (e.g., the presence of lactate in ischemic tissue).[15, 16] Phosphorus spectroscopy can evaluate the decrease in cellular energy substrates and the increase in their breakdown products.[17, 18] Although intense research interest centers around spectroscopy, clinical application has been limited because of long acquisition times (see Chapter 30).

Diffusion imaging is another method of detecting hyperacute changes associated with ischemia before morphologic abnormalities develop on conventional spin-echo images.[19–23] Diffusion maps of the brain can be calculated and displayed, showing regions of signal hyperintensity representing slower water proton diffusion correlating with acute cerebral ischemia. This decrease in the calculated apparent diffusion coefficient is seen in the acute cytotoxic edema stage of ischemia in which more water is restricted to the intracellular compartment. The apparent diffusion coefficient increases in the vasogenic edema stage, probably due to the increase in extracellular bulk water[19] (see Chapter 26).

Perfusion mapping can be done using fast MRI techniques (e.g., echo planar) to acquire rapid sequential images tracking an intravenously administered bolus of contrast material through the brain.[24–26] The contrast material causes T2 shortening or loss of signal intensity, which can be graphed over time. These data can then be used to calculate relative cerebral blood flow, blood volume, and mean tissue transit time, which can be displayed as gray-scale brain maps (Fig. 24–7).

These new experimental techniques may serve to increase our understanding of the pathophysiology of ischemia. Whether these techniques will prove practical in acute stroke evaluation remains to be seen. An acute stroke evaluation strategy needs to be extremely rapid, reliable, and convenient to facilitate therapeutic intervention.

CLINICAL ASPECTS AND TREATMENT

As treatment modalities evolve for stroke, emergent clinical assessment is expected to become standard. Effective treatment requires intervention as early as possible after the event. Therefore, initial management should include a thorough history to establish the time and features of symptom onset. Symptoms suggesting stroke include abrupt onset of one or more of the following: hemiparesis or monoparesis, decreased consciousness, headache, dysphasia or dysarthria, visual field deficit or diplopia, vertigo, ataxia, vomiting, or sensory loss. A neurologic and cardiovascular assessment must be done immediately to assess the extent of neurologic deficit and to determine possible contributory factors, such as hypertension or carotid bruit (stenosis). Other causes of neurologic decline such as infection and trauma should be considered during the physical examination. The neurologic assessment must be repeated at regular intervals to determine whether

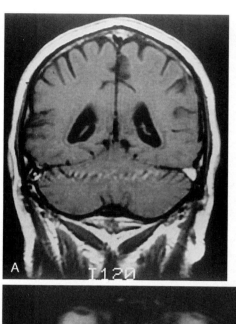
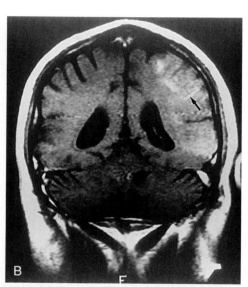
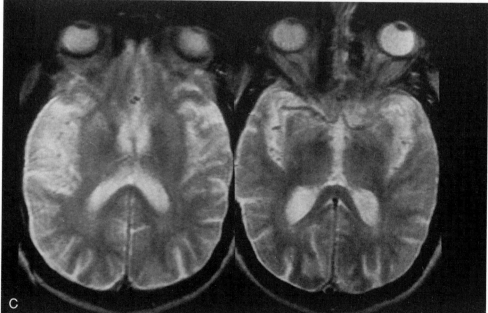

FIGURE 24–6. Abnormal parenchymal enhancement 2 hours after transient acute neurologic symptoms. Coronal noncontrast *(A)* and corresponding postcontrast *(B)* T1-weighted images (350/20) show prominent parenchymal enhancement on the left along with enhancement of a few cortical vessels *(B, arrow).* This enhancement markedly decreased on a follow-up study performed 24 hours later (not shown). *C,* Axial T2-weighted images (2000/90) show no abnormal signal pattern.

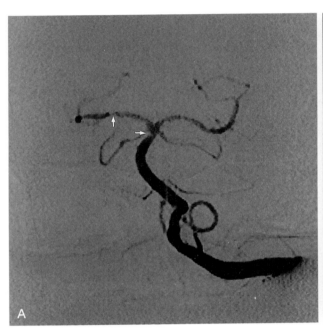

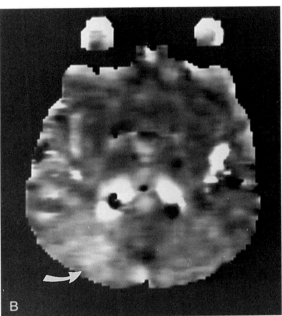

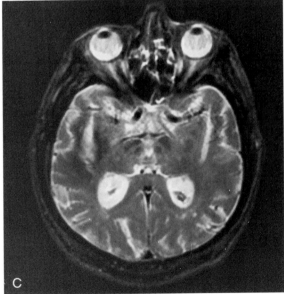

FIGURE 24–7. Perfusion mapping. A 78-year-old man presented with transient ischemic attacks. *A,* Conventional angiogram demonstrates atherosclerotic irregularities along the distal basilar and proximal right posterior cerebral artery *(arrows).* *B,* The mean tissue transit time map done to evaluate cerebral perfusion using the dynamic echo-planar contrast T2*-weighted technique of following a contrast bolus shows relative hypoperfusion in the right posterior and middle cerebral artery watershed region *(arrow).* Areas with a prolonged tissue transit time appear relatively hyperintense. Note the bright ventricles that have no vascular flow. *C,* T2-weighted image (2000/100) shows no definite abnormal signal pattern. Perfusion imaging can detect subclinical regions of hypoperfusion.

the disease process is progressing, stabilized, or regressing.

Noncontrast computed tomography (CT) to determine whether the stroke is hemorrhagic has become the standard because all treatment options depend on this initial information. CT detects nearly all intracerebral hematomas larger than 1 cm.[27] However, it cannot assess vascular disease directly.

Controversy has developed in regard to the role of MRI in stroke. Some advocate emergent MRI with MR angiography to evaluate both the brain parenchyma and the vascular system. This "one-stop shopping" concept has a certain appeal. However, issues of MRI compatibility with monitoring equipment, length of scan time, and round-the-clock availability need to be resolved. Protocols for rapid assessment and treatment of patients must be developed.

When compared with the aggressive therapies used in myocardial ischemia, the treatment of acute cerebral ischemia appears tentative. However, new developments in drug treatment have shown potential benefits. These include neuroprotective agents to reduce the extent of tissue injury[28] and selective endovascular thrombolytic therapy to reverse the underlying thromboembolic pathology.[29] Thrombolytic therapy is limited by a narrow, 6-hour time window after symptom onset to avoid revascularization injury and hemorrhage into ischemic tissue.[30-32] These treatment modalities have not yet gained widespread use. Nevertheless, in the future, early intervention will be the key to optimal treatment of acute ischemic stroke.

NONOCCLUSIVE INFARCTS

ANOXIA OR HYPOXIA

The word *stroke* is often presumed to mean brain ischemia caused by arterial occlusive disease. Although arterial occlusion is the most common mechanism, stroke may be caused by nonocclusive processes that result in decreased oxygen delivery to the brain parenchyma, in brain ischemia, and ultimately in infarction.

Nonocclusive causes of ischemia tend to have a more global impact on the brain with MRI characteristic patterns. Impaired circulation caused by hypovolemia or poor cardiac output, frequently in combination with anemia, hypoxemia, or anoxia, can have a severe impact on the brain, resulting in multiple watershed infarcts, diffuse cerebral edema, or ischemia of basal ganglia, depending on the severity of the insult (Fig. 24–8). Cortical and basal ganglia enhancement with gadolinium reflects the sensitivity of gray matter to hypoxia.[33] Poor oxygenation can also occur in carbon monoxide poisoning, causing abnormal increased signal intensity in the basal ganglia (see Fig. 24–8). Hypoglycemia, usually superimposed on low flow states or hypoxia, can also contribute to similar brain injury from lack of substrate for glycolysis. Generally, hypoglycemia in and of itself does not cause permanent brain damage.

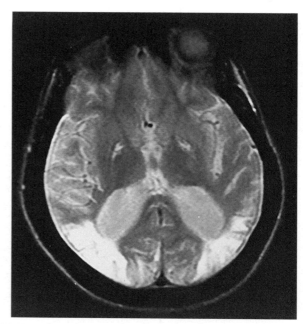

FIGURE 24–8. Carbon monoxide poisoning resulting in cardiac arrest. T2-weighted image (2000/100) after resuscitation shows symmetric abnormal signal pattern in the basal ganglia and posterior watershed areas. The abnormal globus pallidus signal pattern is classically associated with carbon monoxide poisoning. Symmetric watershed ischemia can be seen after systemic hypotension.

PERIVENTRICULAR LEUKOMALACIA

Premature infants are especially vulnerable to hypoxic brain injury. The periventricular region in these infants contains end-arteries and is therefore a vascular watershed. In addition, premature infants have immature cerebral autoregulation such that systemic blood pressure is directly proportional to cerebral blood flow. Thus, the periventricular region is especially vulnerable to systemic hypotension and hypoxia, resulting in a characteristic appearance called *periventricular leukomalacia.*

MRI is most often performed in patients with chronic periventricular leukomalacia, whereas neurosonography at the bedside is preferred in the acute unstable infant. The MRI appearance of end-stage periventricular leukomalacia exhibits a characteristic triad of findings:

1. Abnormally increased periventricular white matter signal intensity on the proton density– and T2-weighted sequences, most commonly in the peritrigonal white matter and the periventricular white matter dorsal to the internal capsule at the level of the foramen of Monro
2. Marked loss of periventricular white matter, especially in the peritrigonal region
3. Compensatory focal ventricular enlargement adjacent to regions of abnormal white matter signal intensity[34] (see Fig. 27–25)

In addition, on inversion recovery images, decreased signal intensity is observed in the periventricular white matter. The coronal plane best demonstrates these abnormalities. Early in the disease, a delay in myelination of the remaining white matter is observed; however, this is transient.

ARTERIAL OCCLUSION

ATHEROSCLEROSIS

Atherosclerosis is the most common arterial occlusive disease and tends to occur in the elderly. Although atherosclerosis causes stenosis in larger arteries and may be associated with significant reduction in flow, most strokes caused by atherosclerosis are secondary to thromboemboli rather than hypoperfusion. Less frequently, associated hypoperfusion or inadequate collateral circulation may cause stroke, often in a watershed distribution (see Fig. 24–7).

WATERSHED INFARCT

Watershed infarct, occurring in the end-arterial zones between two major vascular distributions, is frequently associated with severe carotid disease. In a study of 51 patients with watershed infarcts, 45% had ipsilateral occlusion of the internal carotid artery.[35] Eighty-eight percent of those patients had either severe stenosis (greater than 75%) or occlusion of that artery. The cerebral blood flow associated with severe internal carotid artery disease may be adequate in the absence of systemic stressors. However, concomitant factors such as hypertension, hypovolemia, elevated hematocrit, hypotension, and hypoxia related to chronic lung disease may acutely exceed cerebral blood flow reserves, resulting in watershed infarction (see Fig. 24–8). These concomitant factors are frequently associated with watershed infarction. For example, 86% of patients with watershed infarct suffer from chronic obstructed airway disease from heavy cigarette use.[35] When watershed infarcts are observed with MRI, the lowest axial cut should always be checked for abnormal signal in the internal carotid artery lumen, indicating obstruction or slow flow. Embolic watershed infarcts are also possible and have been produced experimentally.[36]

EMBOLI

Ninety-five percent of thromboembolic phenomena are secondary to atherosclerosis. Other sources of embolic infarct include cardiac emboli (in patients with valvular disease), intracardiac thrombi, and atrial myxomas. In patients with cardiac shunts, venous thrombi from the peripheral circulation may reach the brain. Septic emboli, fat emboli from major long bone fractures, air emboli from surgical procedures or hyperbaric accidents, and microemboli associated with open heart surgery and aortography are other possible sources.[37] Emboli are usually multiple and lodge in small distal arterial branches, producing peripheral infarcts. Many of these will be in the watershed zones. Frequently, the thromboemboli are quickly lysed with reestablishment of cerebral circulation and resolution of the neurologic deficits. However, if restoration of circulation occurs after tissue infarction, hemorrhagic transformation may occur. This is usually seen in the cortical gray matter, which is more sensitive to hypoxia than white matter. MRI is sensitive to the T1 shortening of methemoglobin associated with hemorrhage and is consequently more sensitive than CT in detecting hemorrhagic transformation of infarction.

Multiple peripheral infarctions in more than one vascular distribution suggest emboli. If the infarction is unilateral, internal carotid artery disease should be suspected. If the infarction is bilateral, a systemic source of emboli should be considered.

WALLENBERG'S SYNDROME

Numerous syndromes have been described associated with cerebellar and brain stem ischemia. The most frequent and well known is Wallenberg's (lateral medullary) syndrome caused by the occlusion of the posterior inferior cerebellar artery (Fig. 24–9). Ipsilateral symptoms include paralysis of the soft palate, pharynx, and larynx with dysphagia and dysphonia, facial anesthesia to pain and temperature, corneal reflex loss, and Horner's syndrome. Contralateral loss of pain and temperature sensation in the limbs and trunk is also present. This syndrome can also result from vertebral artery occlusion.

STROKE IN CHILDREN OR YOUNG ADULTS

In a young adult or child, stroke should prompt suspicion of one of the less common causes of ischemia, such as sickle cell disease, moyamoya disease, venous occlusive disease, or vasculitis.

Stroke occurs in 6% to 16% of children with sickle cell disease,[38] and 25% of these children will die of a subsequent stroke.[39] Vascular occlusion or stenosis tends to occur in the large vessels, such as the proximal anterior cerebral artery, the middle cerebral artery, and the internal carotid artery. The posterior circulation is rarely affected.[40, 41] MRI will show ischemia or infarction in major vascular distributions (41%), watershed regions (31%), or small subcortical or cortical regions (28%).[42] The appearance is identical with the pattern of stroke evolution seen in adults.

Another rare cause of cerebral infarction is moyamoya disease. The cause of this occlusive disease of large vessels is not known. The supraclinoid internal carotid artery is stenotic, and numerous collaterals are present characteristically through the thalamoperforate, thalamogeniculate, and lenticulostriate vessels. These vessels produce the pathognomonic "puff of smoke" seen on conventional angiography. The associated cerebral infarcts and parenchymal hemorrhages seen with MRI are nonspecific. However, this diagnosis can frequently be made on conventional T1- and T2-

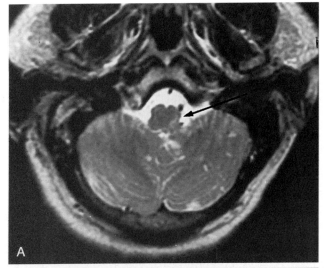

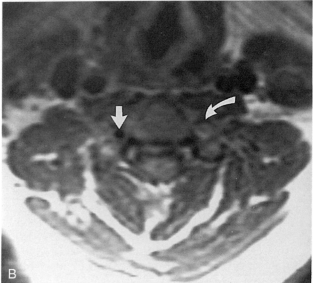

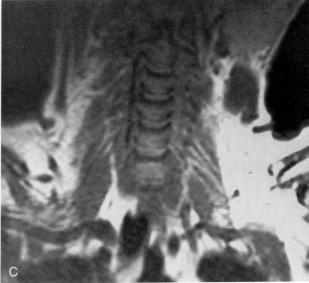

FIGURE 24–9. Wallenberg's (lateral medullary) syndrome. *A,* Axial T2-weighted image (2000/100) shows a hyperintense signal pattern in the left lateral aspect of the medulla *(arrow). B,* Axial T1-weighted image (500/20) of the cervical spine shows absence of flow void in the left vertebral artery *(curved arrow).* Note the normal flow void in the right vertebral artery *(straight arrow). C,* Coronal T1-weighted image (550/20) again shows normal flow void in the right vertebral artery with no evidence of flow void in the expected region of the left vertebral artery. Although Wallenberg's syndrome is associated with occlusion of the posterior inferior cerebellar artery, it can also occur due to vertebral artery occlusion.

weighted images because numerous small flow voids representing the moyamoya vessels are seen in both thalami and basal gangla (Fig. 24–10). MR angiography can also demonstrate these vessels[43] (see Fig. 25–33). A moyamoya disease–like appearance can result from acquired distal internal carotid artery stenosis resulting from conditions such as sickle cell disease, neurofibromatosis, or tuberculous meningitis.

ARTERIAL DISSECTION

Another cause of arterial occlusion or stenosis is dissection of a major vessel. Hyperextension or rotational injuries to the neck may damage the carotid or vertebral arteries. Vertebral fractures tend to injure the vertebral artery, whereas basilar skull fractures may injure the petrous or clinoid portion of the internal carotid artery. Symptoms from these injuries are frequently delayed, possibly for days, and are secondary to thrombosis, embolism, and infarction. Spontaneous

dissections may also occur. Thus, the vascular injury may be unsuspected.

MRI can be used to screen for vascular injury. Lack of flow void on conventional spin-echo images suggests thrombosis or slow flow. A characteristic ring of abnormal signal around a vessel on the axial view is diagnostic of dissection.[44] Usually, the abnormal signal is hyperintense in comparison with that of fat due to the presence of methemoglobin (Fig. 24–11; also see Figs. 25–29 and 25–30).

VENOUS OCCLUSION

Venous sinus occlusive disease (VSOD) is a serious, potentially lethal (20% to 78%)[45] problem that often presents a confusing, nonspecific clinical picture. Stroke-like symptoms with a relatively slow onset, especially in the presence of predisposing factors, may suggest the diagnosis. Precipitating factors include otitis media and mastoiditis, pregnancy and the puerpe-

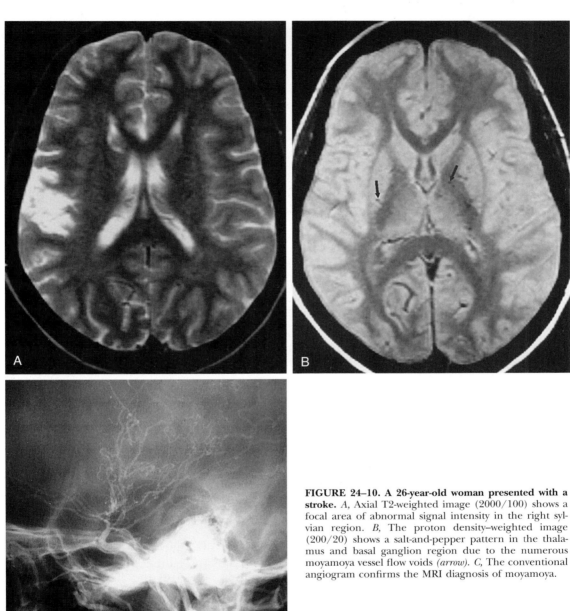

FIGURE 24–10. A 26-year-old woman presented with a stroke. *A,* Axial T2-weighted image (2000/100) shows a focal area of abnormal signal intensity in the right sylvian region. *B,* The proton density–weighted image (200/20) shows a salt-and-pepper pattern in the thalamus and basal ganglion region due to the numerous moyamoya vessel flow voids *(arrow). C,* The conventional angiogram confirms the MRI diagnosis of moyamoya.

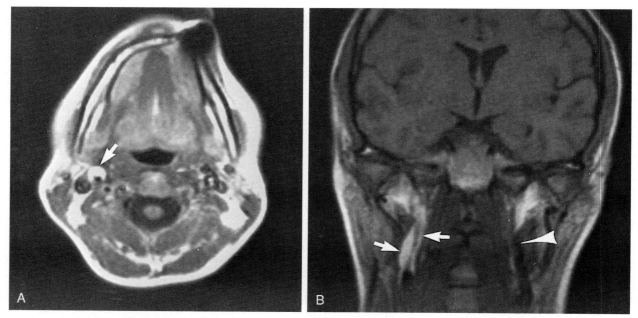

FIGURE 24–11. Carotid dissection. *A,* Axial T1-weighted image (500/20) shows a hyperintense ring or collar around the right internal carotid artery flow void *(arrow),* corresponding to methemoglobin within the wall of the artery. *B,* The corresponding coronal T1-weighted image (550/20) shows a tubular encasement of abnormal hyperintense signal pattern surrounding the barely visible right internal carotid artery flow void *(arrows).* Note the normal contralateral internal carotid artery flow void *(arrowhead).*

rium, oral contraceptives, hypercoagulable states, sickle cell anemia, severe dehydration, trauma, and Behçet's syndrome. Often, however, the diagnosis is unsuspected before radiologic evaluation.

MRI will demonstrate abnormal signal intensity and lack of flow in the venous sinus. This needs to be distinguished from an intraluminal signal pattern resulting from slow venous flow. MR venography can be helpful. Two-dimensional phase-contrast MR venography with relatively low-velocity encoding will demonstrate the patent venous sinuses. This is a convenient, noninvasive way to make the diagnosis and follow therapeutic response (Fig. 24–12A and B) (see Chapter 25).

Three brain parenchymal patterns associated with VSOD may be observed.[46] In the first state, brain swelling is observed as cortical sulci effacement and mass effect without abnormal T2 signal intensity. This may be caused by increased intravascular volume due to venous congestion and early edema. The second stage occurs as venous pressure increases, causing a transudate of fluid into the brain interstitium. Increased T2 signal intensity is seen, especially in the periventricular region. Abnormal signal intensity in the bilateral thalamus at this stage suggests deep venous obstruction. The ventricles may also be enlarged, owing to increased CSF production secondary to transependymal flow of interstitial fluid into the ventricle as well as to decreased CSF absorption secondary to venous hypertension (see Fig. 24–12). There is no abnormal enhancement because the blood-brain barrier is intact. Up to this point, parenchymal changes associated with VSOD are reversible and should *not* be called venous infarction, which implies irreversible cell death. Selec-

tive endovascular thrombolysis with urokinase at this stage may cause a dramatic clinical recovery and complete resolution of MRI abnormalities.[47]

In the third stage, hemorrhage occurs when venous hypertension causes vascular rupture. This intraparenchymal hematoma is the main source of tissue damage associated with VSOD. Only at this hemorrhagic stage should the process be called venous infarction.

BEHÇET'S DISEASE

Behçet's disease is a rare multisystem disease that can cause VSOD. It is prevalent in Japan, the Mediterranean, and the Middle East. Behçet's disease presents with the clinical triad of oral ulcers, genital ulcers, and uveitis. Neurologic symptoms occur in 10% to 25% of these patients, are often nonspecific, and include headache, confusion, cranial nerve palsies, and cerebellar signs.[48] In addition to VSOD, focal white matter lesions may be present in the brain stem, basal ganglia, or cerebral white matter. Lesions do not necessarily correlate with clinical symptoms[49] and are often larger on T2-weighted images than on T1-weighted images, presumably because of edema. Areas of active inflammation enhance with gadolinium (Fig. 24–13). After treatment with corticosteroids, abnormal signal pattern may persist on T1- and T2-weighted images, but abnormal enhancement will resolve.[50, 51] This may indicate residual demyelination and gliosis after the active inflammation has resolved.

ANTIPHOSPHOLIPID ANTIBODY

Antiphospholipid antibody is also associated with systemic and cerebral vascular occlusive disease,[52] usu-

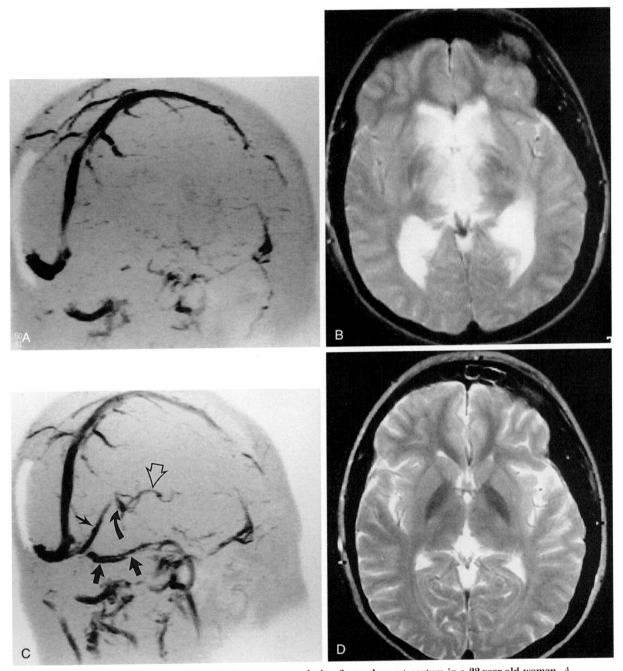

FIGURE 24–12. Left transverse and deep venous occlusion 3 months post partum in a 22-year-old woman. *A,* A two-dimensional sequential oblique parasagittal gradient-echo MR angiogram (31/10/1 NEX [number of excitations]) with a flip angle of 50° shows lack of flow in the left transverse and deep veins. *B,* T2-weighted image (2500/100) shows periventricular and thalamic edema, mild hydrocephalus, and sulcal effacement. Deep venous thrombosis tends to be associated with symmetric thalamic edema. *C,* Gradient-echo MR angiogram (32/8/1 NEX) with a flip angle of 40° performed 2 weeks after successful thrombolytic therapy with endovascular urokinase shows flow in previously absent deep veins. Large straight arrows indicate transverse sinus; the small straight arrow, the straight sinus; the curved arrow, the vein of Galen; the open arrow, the internal cerebral vein. *D,* Corresponding axial T2-weighted image (2500/100) shows complete resolution of the paraventricular and thalamic edema. The hydrocephalus has also resolved. The patient recovered completely. (*A* and *C* from Yuh WTC, Simonson TM, Wang AM, et al: Venous sinus occlusive disease: MR findings. AJNR 15[2]:309–316, 1994, © by American Society of Neuroradiology.)

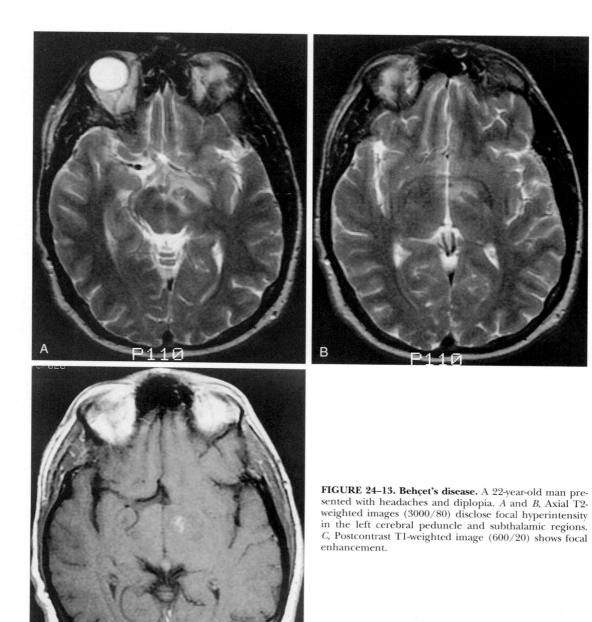

FIGURE 24–13. Behçet's disease. A 22-year-old man presented with headaches and diplopia. *A* and *B*, Axial T2-weighted images (3000/80) disclose focal hyperintensity in the left cerebral peduncle and subthalamic regions. *C*, Postcontrast T1-weighted image (600/20) shows focal enhancement.

ally with venous thrombosis, but arterial occlusion in multiple sites has also been observed. The exact interaction between the antiphospholipid immunoglobulin and the coagulation cascade is unknown. This diagnosis should be considered when evaluating VSOD or arterial ischemia in a patient with no risk factors for thrombo-occlusive disease. Antiphospholipid antibody has been reported as a cause of VSOD in pregnancy.[53] If antiphospholipid antibodies are found, the patient should be treated with long-term anticoagulation.

CEREBRAL ARTERITIS

INFECTIOUS ARTERITIS

Small vessel occlusive disease caused by vasculitis can produce a pattern of infarction similar to that of multiple emboli. Vasculitis or arteritis may be either septic or nonseptic. Cerebral infarctions resulting from vasculitis develop in up to one fourth of children with complicated bacterial meningitis, usually caused by *Haemophilus influenzae*.[54] Tuberculosis vasculitis tends to involve the basilar vessels including the supraclinoid internal carotid arteries and the M1 segments of the middle cerebral arteries. Syphilis typically affects both cortical arteries and veins. A variety of fungi can cause mycotic arteritis. Some fungi such as *Aspergillus* and *Actinomyces* may invade vascular walls and produce multiple hemorrhagic infarctions.

NECROTIZING ANGIITIS

Noninfectious arteritides include collagen-vascular diseases (systemic lupus erythematosus, scleroderma,

and rheumatoid arthritis), granulomatous diseases such as sarcoidosis, reaction to drug abuse (methamphetamine, heroin, and cocaine), Wegener's granulomatosis, polyarteritis nodosa, and giant cell arteritis.

Common MRI findings associated with vasculitis include numerous, bilateral supratentorial infarctions involving both gray and white matter. Infarctions in the deep white matter including the corpus callosum and capsular tracts may also be present[55] (see Fig. 27–24). Hemorrhagic infarctions or hemorrhagic transformation may be seen in one third to one half of patients with MRI[55, 56] (Fig. 24–14). When there is a clinical suspicion of vasculitis, MRI is the imaging modality of choice. When an MRI study is negative, there is little likelihood of finding vasculitis with cerebral angiography.[56]

FIBROMUSCULAR DYSPLASIA

Fibromuscular dysplasia (FMD), unlike vasculitis, usually does not involve the small intracranial vessels. The larger cervical internal carotid artery and vertebral arteries are more likely to demonstrate the alternating focal narrowing and dilatation ("string of beads") appearance characteristic of this disease. Although FMD may be found incidentally at angiography, some patients present with stroke-like symptoms.

In an evaluation of two-dimensional time-of-flight MR angiography, Heiserman and associates[57] suggested that artifacts, including skull base susceptibility, motion of the patient, and swallowing, may mimic the appearance of FMD.[57] On the other hand, the multiple focal changes in lumen diameter associated with FMD

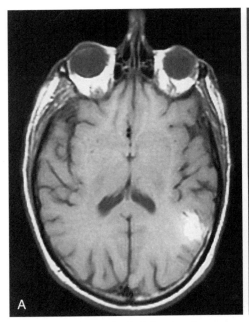
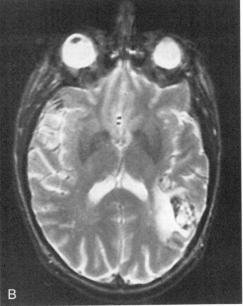

FIGURE 24–14. Hemorrhagic infarction in a young woman. *A,* Axial T1-weighted image (583/20) shows abnormal hyperintense signal pattern in the left temporal cortex corresponding to a hematoma. *B,* Axial T2-weighted image (2000/100) shows mixed signal intensity in the same region. Edema is seen surrounding the hemorrhage. This type of cortical hemorrhagic infarction is common with vasculitis. In an older person, hemorrhagic transformation of a thromboembolic infarct or amyloid angiopathy would be more likely causes.

will result in intravoxel dephasing due to nonlaminar flow. Thus, FMD will appear as areas of stenosis as well as decreased signal intensity with MR angiography (see Fig. 25–31).

MIGRAINE

Migraine headache is a common disease, occurring in 8.7 million females and 3.4 million males in the United States.[58] Although the cause of migraines is unknown, it definitely involves the cerebral vasculature. Whether the vasomotor changes are the cause or the effect of the disease is less clear. Transient regional cerebral blood flow reductions can be measured during migraine headache by a variety of techniques, including xenon 133 CT, positron emission tomography, and MR perfusion imaging.[59]

On conventional MR images, as many as 44% of migraineurs have nonspecific white matter hyperintensities on T2-weighted images.[60] Fazekas and colleagues[61] found the number of patients with white matter lesions varies with migraine type: 53% of "classic" migraine patients with prodrome and 18% of "common" migraine patients without prodrome.[61] Histologically, these white matter lesions consist of perivascular edema, demyelination, and gliosis without evidence of infarction (Fig. 24–15). Thus, transient cerebral hypoperfusion is probably not the cause of these lesions.

Migraine-related stroke is rare and occurs in 4% of migraineurs.[62] Migraine appears to increase the relative risk of known stroke risk factors such as hypertension, oral contraceptives, and pregnancy. However, nearly one third of migraine patients who suffer a stroke have no other risk factors, and these are presumed migraine-induced strokes.[62] The appearance of these strokes is indistinguishable from that of strokes due to other causes.

HYPERTENSIVE ENCEPHALOPATHY AND ECLAMPSIA

Hypertensive encephalopathy is caused by an abrupt, dramatic elevation in blood pressure resulting in progressive neurologic symptoms. Headache, nausea, vomiting, and altered mentation may progress to stupor, coma, and death if the diagnosis is not promptly made and treatment instituted. Severe hypertension of this type may develop as a complication of late pregnancy known as eclampsia.

The MRI appearance is the same whether or not the hypertension is related to pregnancy.[63] Punctate or confluent areas of increased signal intensity on T2-weighted images may be found in the subcortical white matter, centrum semiovale, deep white matter, or basal ganglia or in a gyriform pattern in the gray matter[64] (Fig. 24–16). Focal swelling and abnormal signal intensity in the occipital lobes can be associated with blindness. Many of these abnormalities resolve with control of the blood pressure.[65] Petechial hemorrhages are another common finding, and detection is improved with the use of gradient-echo MRI because this technique has increased sensitivity to blood products. Larger parenchymal hemorrhages may also be present. Hemorrhage suggests irreversible damage.[66]

Small (<15 mm) lacunar infarcts in the basal ganglia and capsular area are frequently attributed to chronic hypertension, although diabetes atherosclerosis and microaneurysms are alternative hypotheses. Small hemorrhages in the brain stem, basal ganglia, and capsular regions are also more frequent in patients with chronic hypertension. Small infarcts or hemor-

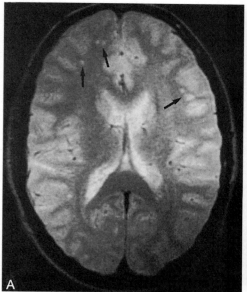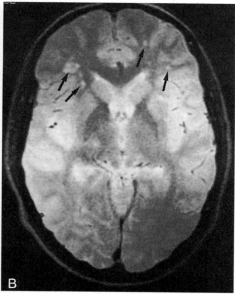

FIGURE 24–15. Migraine headaches with associated white matter lesions. *A* and *B*, Axial T2-weighted images reveal multiple small lesions *(arrows)* in the subcortical white matter, primarily involving the frontal lobes.

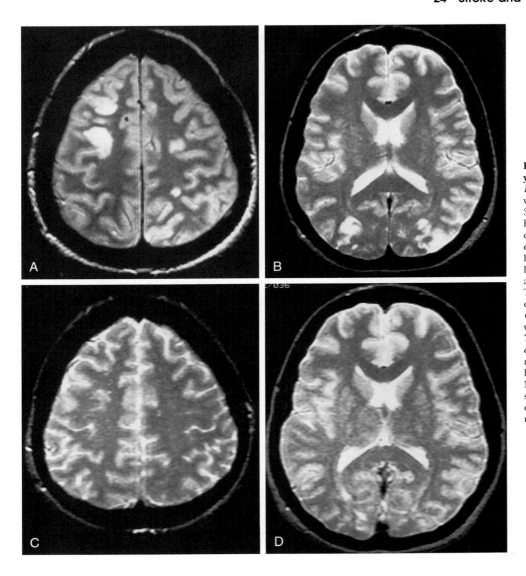

FIGURE 24–16. Eclampsia in a 24-year-old pregnant woman. *A* and *B*, Axial proton density– and T2-weighted images (spin echo 2800/30, 70) show multiple areas of high signal intensity within both cerebral hemispheres. The bilateral involvement of the occipital lobes is typical for eclampsia. The lesions involve the cortex and adjacent subcortical white matter. T1-weighted images (not shown) did not reveal any hemorrhage. *C* and *D*, Follow-up axial T2-weighted images (spin echo 2800/70) obtained 6 days later disclose complete resolution of the abnormalities. (*A* to *D* from Schwaighofer BW, Hesselink JR, Healy ME: MR demonstration of reversible brain abnormalities in eclampsia. J Comput Assist Tomogr 13:310–312, 1989.)

rhages in these regions should prompt a blood pressure evaluation.

DIFFERENTIAL DIAGNOSIS

The two primary mechanisms of ischemic stroke are thrombo-occlusive disease and emboli. It is often difficult to distinguish the two. However, the presence of multiple vascular territory involvement is highly suggestive of emboli, as is coexistent embolic disease in other organs such as the retina. Another feature distinguishing the two is presentation: thrombotic stroke is associated with a stepwise clinical progression, whereas embolic stroke has a maximal neurologic deficit at symptom onset.

Usually, the precipitating factors in nonocclusive infarct are known (e.g., carbon monoxide poisoning, cardiac arrest), and MRI is performed to evaluate the extent of brain damage.

Stroke in young adults or children, or stroke with unusual or slow progression, should suggest some of the less common causes of ischemia. Sickle cell disease, moyamoya disease, VSOD, and vasculitis are all possible causes of ischemia in young patients. It is important to discover the cause of ischemia in these cases to begin effective and appropriate treatment. MRI and MR angiography can often suggest the correct diagnosis by defining the pattern of parenchymal and vascular involvement.

REFERENCES

1. Monthly Vital Stat Rep 40(suppl 2):1–20, 1992.
2. Imakita S, Nishimura T, Naito H, et al: Magnetic resonance imaging of human cerebral infarction: enhancement with Gd-DTPA. Neuroradiology 29:422–429, 1987.
3. Yonas H, Gur D, Good BC, et al: Stable xenon CT blood flow mapping for evaluation of patients with extracranial-intracranial bypass surgery. J Neurosurg 62:324–333, 1985.
4. deVries EJ, Seckhar LN, Horton JA, et al: A new method to predict safe resection of the internal carotid artery. Laryngoscope 100:85–88, 1990.
5. Mueller DP, Yuh WTC, Fisher DJ, et al: Arterial enhancement in acute ischemia: clinical and angiographic correlation. AJNR 14:661–668, 1993.
6. Schuier FJ, Hosmann KA: Experimental brain infarcts in cats. II. Ischemic brain edema. Stroke 11:593–601, 1980.
7. Gotoh O, Asano T, Koide T, Takakura K: Ischemic brain edema following

occlusion of the middle cerebral artery in the rat. I. The time courses of the brain, water, sodium, and potassium contents and blood-brain barrier permeability to ^{125}I-albumin. Stroke 16:101–109, 1985.

8. Yuh WTC, Crain MR, Loes DJ, et al: MR imaging of cerebral ischemia: findings in the first 24 hours. AJNR 12:621–629, 1991.

9. Hossman KA, Schuier FJ: Experimental brain infarcts in cats. I. Pathophysiologic observations. Stroke 11:583–591, 1988.

10. Bell BA, Symon L, Branston MN: CBF and time thresholds for the formation of ischemic cerebral edema, and effect of reperfusion in baboons. J Neurosurg 62:31–41, 1985.

11. Simonson T, Ryals TJ, Yuh WTC, et al: MR imaging and HMPAO scintigraphy in conjunction with balloon test occlusion: value in predicting sequelae after permanent carotid occlusion. AJNR 13:1063–1068, 1992.

12. Crain MR, Yuh WTC, Greene GM, et al: Cerebral ischemia: evaluation with contrast-enhanced MR imaging. AJNR 12:631–639, 1991.

13. McNamara MT, Brant-Zawadzki M, Berry I: Acute experimental cerebral ischemia: MR enhancement using Gd-DTPA. Radiology 158:701–705, 1986.

14. Moonen CTW, van Zijl PCM, Frank JA, et al: Functional magnetic resonance imaging in medicine and physiology. Science 250:53–61, 1990.

15. Duijn JH, Matson GB, Maudsley AA, et al: Human brain infarction: proton MR spectroscopy. Radiology 183:711–718, 1992.

16. Baker LL, Kucharczyk J, Sevick RJ, et al: Recent advances in MR imaging/spectroscopy of cerebral ischemia. AJR 156:1133–1143, 1991.

17. Sappey-Marinier D, Hubesch B, Matson GB, Weiner MW: Decreased phosphorus metabolite concentrations and alkalosis in chronic cerebral infarction. Radiology 182:29–34, 1992.

18. Crockard HA, Gadian DG, Frackowiak RSJ, et al: Acute cerebral ischaemia: concurrent changes in cerebral blood flow, energy metabolites, pH, and lactate measured with hydrogen clearance and ^{31}P and ^{1}H nuclear magnetic resonance spectroscopy. II. Changes during ischaemia. J Cereb Blood Flow Metab 7:394–402, 1987.

19. Le Bihan D, Turner R, Douek P, Patronas N: Diffusion MR imaging: clinical applications. AJR 159:591–599, 1992.

20. Moseley ME, Kucharczyk J, Mintorovitch J, et al: Diffusion-weighted MR imaging of acute stroke: correlation with T2-weighted and magnetic susceptibility–enhanced MR imaging in cats. AJNR 11:423–429, 1989.

21. Sevick RJ, Kanda F, Mintorovitch J, et al: Cytotoxic brain edema: assessment with diffusion-weighted MR imaging. Radiology 185:687–690, 1992.

22. Pierpaoli C, Righini A, Linfante I, et al: Histopathologic correlates of abnormal water diffusion in cerebral ischemia: diffusion-weighted MR imaging and light and electron microscopic study. Radiology 189:439–448, 1993.

23. Kucharczyk J, Mintorovitch J, Asgari HS, Moseley M: Diffusion/perfusion MR imaging of acute cerebral ischemia. Magn Reson Med 19:311–315, 1991.

24. Tzika AA, Massoth RJ, Ball WS Jr, et al: Cerebral perfusion in children: detection with dynamic contrast-enhanced T2*-weighted MR images. Radiology 187:449–458, 1993.

25. Kucharczyk J, Roberts T, Moseley ME, Watson A: Contrast-enhanced perfusion-sensitive MR imaging in the diagnosis of cerebrovascular disorders. J Magn Reson Imaging 3:241–245, 1993.

26. Edelman RR, Mattle HP, Atkinson DJ, et al: Cerebral blood flow: assessment with dynamic contrast-enhanced T2*-weighted MR imaging at 1.5 T. Radiology 176:211–220, 1990.

27. Tarr RW, Hecht ST, Horton JA: Nontraumatic intracranial hemorrhage. In: Latchaw RE, ed. MR and CT Imaging of the Head, Neck, and Spine. 2nd ed. St. Louis: CV Mosby, 1991, pp 267–299.

28. Kucharczyk J, Chew W, Derugin N, et al: Nicardipine reduces ischemic brain injury: magnetic resonance imaging/spectroscopy study in cats. Stroke 20:268–273, 1989.

29. Del Zoppo GJ, Zeumer H, Harker LA: Thrombolytic therapy in acute stroke: possibilities and hazards. Stroke 17:595–607, 1986.

30. Miller CL, Lampard DG, Alexander K, Brown WA: Local cerebral blood flow following transient cerebral ischemia. I. Onset of impaired reperfusion within the first hour following global ischemia. Stroke 11:534–541, 1980.

31. Ginsberg MD, Budd WW, Welsh FA: Diffuse cerebral ischemia in the cat. I. Local blood flow during severe ischemia and recirculation. Ann Neurol 3:482–492, 1978.

32. Kagstrom E, Smith M-L, Siesjo BK: Recirculation in the rat brain following incomplete ischemia. J Cereb Blood Flow Metab 3:183–192, 1983.

33. Takahashi S, Higano S, Ishii K, et al: Hypoxic brain damage: cortical laminar necrosis and delayed changes in white matter at sequential MR imaging. Radiology 189:449–456, 1993.

34. Baker LL, Stevenson DK, Enzmann DR: End-stage periventricular leukomalacia: MR evaluation. Radiology 168:809–815, 1988.

35. Bogousslavsky J, Regli F: Unilateral watershed cerebral infarcts. Neurology 36:373–377, 1986.

36. Pollanen MS, Deck JHN: The mechanism of embolic watershed infarction: experimental studies. Can J Neurol Sci 17:395–398, 1990.

37. Moody DM, Bell MA, Challa VR, et al: Brain microemboli during cardiac surgery or aortography. Ann Neurol 28:477–486, 1990.

38. Wiznitzer M, Ruggieri PM, Masaryk TJ, et al: Diagnosis of cerebrovascular disease in sickle cell anemia by magnetic resonance angiography. J Pediatr 117:551–555, 1990.

39. Rao VM, Sebes JI, Steiner RM, Ballas SK: Noninvasive diagnostic imaging in hemoglobinopathies. Hematol Oncol Clin North Am 5:517–533, 1991.

40. El Gammal TE, Adams RJ, Nichols FT, et al: MR and CT investigation of cerebrovascular disease in sickle cell patients. AJNR 7:1043, 1986.

41. Goldberg HI, Zimmerman RA: Sickle cell anemia: central nervous system. Semin Roentgenol 22:205–212, 1987.

42. Adams RJ, Nichols FT, McKie V, et al: Cerebral infarction in sickle cell anemia: mechanism based on CT and MRI. Neurology 38:1012–1017, 1988.

43. Yamada I, Matsushima Y, Suzuki S: Moyamoya disease: diagnosis with three-dimensional time-of-flight MR angiography. Radiology 184:773–778, 1992.

44. Goldberg HI, Grossman RI, Gomori JM, et al: Cervical internal carotid artery dissecting hemorrhage: diagnosis using MR. Radiology 158:157–161, 1986.

45. Wilkins RH, Rengachary SS, eds: Neurosurgery Update II: Vascular, Spinal, Pediatric, and Functional Neurosurgery. New York: McGraw-Hill, 1991, p 442.

46. Yuh WTC, Simonson TM, Wang AM, et al: Venous sinus occlusive disease: MR findings. AJNR 15:309–316, 1994.

47. Tsai FY, Higashida RT, Matovich V, Alfieri K: Acute thrombosis of the intracranial dural sinus: direct thrombolytic treatment. AJNR 13:1137–1141, 1991.

48. Banna M, El-Ramahi K: Neurologic involvement in Behçet disease: imaging findings in 16 patients. AJNR 12:791–796, 1991.

49. Erdem E, Carlier R, Idir ABC, et al: Gadolinium-enhanced MRI in central nervous system Behçet's disease. Neuroradiology 35:142–144, 1993.

50. Nüssel F, Wegmüller H, Laseyras F, et al: Neuro-Behçet: acute and sequential aspects by MRI and MRS. Eur Neurol 31:399–402, 1991.

51. Kazui S, Naritomi H, Imakita S, et al: Sequential gadolinium-DTPA enhanced MRI studies in neuro-Behçet's disease. Neuroradiology 33:136–139, 1991.

52. Bacharach JM, Stanson AW, Lie JT, Nichols DA: Imaging spectrum of thrombo-occlusive vascular disease associated with antiphospholid antibodies. Radiographics 13:417–423, 1993.

53. McClean BN, Whitehead PJ, Campbell MJ: Antiphospholipid syndrome in pregnancy. Br J Hosp Med 48:504–506, 1992.

54. Kerr L, Filloux FM: Cerebral infarction as a remote complication of childhood *Haemophilus influenzae* meningitis. West J Med 157:179–182, 1992.

55. Greenan TJ, Grossman RI, Goldberg HI: Cerebral vasculitis: MR imaging and angiographic correlation. Radiology 182:65–72, 1992.

56. Harris KG, Tran DD, Sickels WJ, et al: Diagnosing intracranial vasculitis: the roles of MR and angiography. AJNR 15:317–330, 1994.

57. Heiserman JE, Drayer BP, Fram EK, Keller PJ: MR angiography of cervical fibromuscular dysplasia. AJNR 13:1454–1457, 1992.

58. Stewart WF, Lipton RB, Celentano DD, Reed ML: Prevalence of migraine headache in the United States: relation to age, income, race, and other sociodemographic factors. JAMA 267:64–69, 1992.

59. Lauritzen M, Olesen J: Regional cerebral blood flow during migraine attacks by xenon-133 inhalation and emission tomography. Brain 107:447–461, 1984.

60. Jacome DE, LeBorgne JL: MRI studies in basilar artery migraine. Headache 30:88–90, 1990.

61. Fazekas F, Koch M, Schmidt R, et al: The prevalence of cerebral damage varies with migraine type: an MRI study. Headache 32:287–291, 1992.

62. Welch KMA, Levine SR: Migraine-related stroke in the context of the International Headache Society classification of head pain. Arch Neurol 47:458–462, 1990.

63. Schwartz RB, Jones KM, Kalina P, et al: Hypertensive encephalopathy: findings on CT, MR imaging and SPECT imaging in 14 cases. AJR 159:379–383, 1992.

64. Sanders TG, Clayman DA, Sanchez-Ramos L, et al: Brain in eclampsia: MR imaging with clinical correlation. Radiology 180:475–478, 1991.

65. Schwaighofer BW, Hesselink JR, Healy ME: MR demonstration of reversible brain abnormalities in eclampsia. J Comput Assist Tomogr 13:310–312, 1989.

66. Weingarten K, Barbut D, Filippi C, Zimmerman RD: Acute hypertensive encephalopathy: findings on spin-echo and gradient-echo MR imaging. AJR 162:665–670, 1993.

Basic Principles of MR Angiography and Flow Analysis: Cerebrovascular Applications

PATRICK A. TURSKI

Sometime early in the 21st century magnetic resonance (MR) angiography will replace conventional catheter angiography as the primary method of imaging the cerebrovascular system. This evolution of neurovascular imaging will be the direct result of innovations in MR hardware, data acquisition, and display techniques. Extraordinary leaps in computational speed will enable the radiologist to rapidly generate detailed integrated three-dimensional (3D) images of the brain parenchyma and vascular structures complete with re-creations of the endovascular surface. A large body of information on flow physiology will also be applied to MR data sets. Flow features will be quantified by their spin phase characteristics, thus creating an entire new field of in vivo cerebrovascular MR rheology.[1] Unfortunately, before we enter this "brave new world" of cerebrovascular imaging we must pass through a transition period in which the exact role of MR angiography in our current everyday practice of radiology is incompletely defined. Consequently, in this chapter a practical introduction is provided that will enable those interested in clinical MR angiography to begin to apply these techniques to their daily practice of radiology. This summary is only a starting point, and new information will undoubtably become available that will supersede these recommendations. In addition, several books also cover the topic of MR angiography in considerably more detail.[2, 3] However, most of the concepts presented here can be generally applied, even to advanced MR systems with powerful gradient subsystems.

Early in the development of clinical MR imaging (MRI) it became apparent that flowing blood had MR properties different from those of stationary tissue.

Initially, these properties were considered artifacts and attempts were made to reduce these flow-related artifacts. While trying to eliminate flow artifacts, it was recognized that important new information was contained within the physical events that propagated flow artifacts. Two distinct types of flow-related processes were recognized. The first was the observation that under certain conditions spins moving into a slice would have bright signal intensity compared with the surrounding stationary tissue.[4, 5] This observation eventually gave rise to the family of MR angiographic techniques based on inflow enhancement and called *time-of-flight (TOF) MR angiography*. Other investigators[6, 7] discovered a definable relationship between the velocity of blood flow and the phase of a moving spin as it passed through a magnetic field gradient. This discovery led to the development of a second family of MR angiographic techniques based on spin phase and later termed *phase-contrast MR angiography* (see also Chapter 9).

TIME-OF-FLIGHT MR ANGIOGRAPHIC TECHNIQUES

To better understand TOF MR angiography, imagine the spin conditions for an axial T1-weighted gradient-echo MR image through the neck. During the gradient-echo acquisition, the stationary spins experience a rapid series of radiofrequency (RF) pulses—one every repetition time (TR). After several RF pulses, an equilibrium magnetization is established in the stationary spins. The magnitude of the equilibrium magnetization is less than the fully relaxed state. This reduced

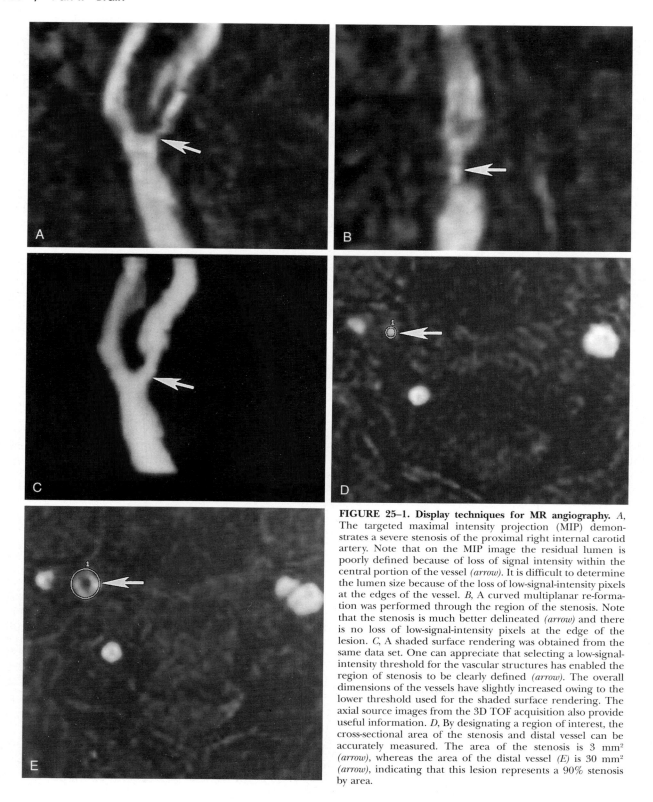

FIGURE 25–1. Display techniques for MR angiography. *A,* The targeted maximal intensity projection (MIP) demonstrates a severe stenosis of the proximal right internal carotid artery. Note that on the MIP image the residual lumen is poorly defined because of loss of signal intensity within the central portion of the vessel *(arrow)*. It is difficult to determine the lumen size because of the loss of low-signal-intensity pixels at the edges of the vessel. *B,* A curved multiplanar re-formation was performed through the region of the stenosis. Note that the stenosis is much better delineated *(arrow)* and there is no loss of low-signal-intensity pixels at the edge of the lesion. *C,* A shaded surface rendering was obtained from the same data set. One can appreciate that selecting a low-signal-intensity threshold for the vascular structures has enabled the region of stenosis to be clearly defined *(arrow)*. The overall dimensions of the vessels have slightly increased owing to the lower threshold used for the shaded surface rendering. The axial source images from the 3D TOF acquisition also provide useful information. *D,* By designating a region of interest, the cross-sectional area of the stenosis and distal vessel can be accurately measured. The area of the stenosis is 3 mm² *(arrow)*, whereas the area of the distal vessel *(E)* is 30 mm² *(arrow)*, indicating that this lesion represents a 90% stenosis by area.

equilibrium magnetization is responsible for the partial saturation of the stationary spins that occurs in TOF imaging. When the signal from the stationary tissue is read out, a relatively reduced signal intensity is detected. Now consider the spins in the blood flowing into the partially saturated imaging slice. These spins have been outside the imaging slice and have not seen the prior RF pulses. These flowing spins have not undergone saturation and are fully magnetized. If these spins remain within the slice during readout they will generate a relatively large signal intensity compared with the saturated stationary tissues. This phenomenon is the basic contrast mechanism in TOF MR angiography. Vascular structures are visible because inflow enhances their signal intensity compared with the saturated stationary tissues. TOF effects can be used to visualize flow in a series of two-dimensional (2D) slices; a 3D gradient-echo volume; or multiple, overlapping, thin 3D slabs (called MOTSA or multislab TOF). Each method is discussed here in relation to its common clinical application.

2D Time-of-Flight Examination and Image Display

The 2D TOF studies are generated from a stack of 1.5- to 2-mm-thick T1-weighted gradient-echo slices. The slices can overlap or be contiguous. If necessary, a large number of slices can be obtained to cover the vascular structure of interest. At the end of the examination the slices are combined, creating a volume of MR data. To visualize the vascular structure within this volume of tissue, special display methods must be applied. The most direct method is to project the brightest pixel along a ray into a plane. This projection image is a collapse of the bright vascular structures into a predetermined plane. By using the maximal intensity projection (MIP) ray tracing technique the vessels can be displayed with reduced detection of the overlying soft tissues. Specific vascular structures are projected into the desired plane by selecting a subvolume of the original data set and generating a targeted MIP image.[8]

One serious limitation of the MIP process is that low-signal-intensity pixels at the edge of the vessel are lost owing to the automated thresholding that selects only bright pixels to display. This results in an overall reduction in the apparent lumen size and elimination of low-signal-intensity regions adjacent to or within a region of stenosis. The loss of the low-signal-intensity pixels contributes to MR angiographic overestimation of vascular stenosis.[9, 10] (Fig. 25–1).

A simple method for overcoming the limitations of the MIP process is to display the vessels in cross section using a multiplanar re-formation program. Unlike the MIP method, multiplanar re-formations do not apply a threshold to the re-formatted image and the low-signal-intensity pixels at the edge of the vessel can easily be identified. More recent versions of the multiplanar software allow curved re-formations to be generated that conform to the geometry of the vessel. Careful review of the re-formatted images can provide a more accurate assessment of vascular stenosis than can the MIP projections.[11]

An alternative display technique termed *shaded surface rendering* is more flexible. In this technique, the user selects the desired pixel signal intensity threshold. Low-signal-intensity pixels can be included in the surface-rendered image. Additional postprocessing is required, but shaded surface rendering provides an aesthetically pleasing display of the vascular structures[12] (Fig. 25–2).

The main advantage of the 2D TOF acquisition is that it is quite sensitive to slow blood flow. Inflow enhancement is best detected when thin 1.5- to 2.0-mm slices are obtained and the flow is perpendicular to the image plane. The 2D TOF technique has proved useful for identifying nearly occluded vessels with severely reduced flow or slow flow within venous structures (Fig. 25–3).

Detecting intravascular signal requires that the spins are in coherent phase relationships at the time of readout. One can imagine that within flowing blood this can be difficult to achieve, particularly in the case of pathologic flow conditions. One method of increasing vascular signal intensity is by using balanced gradients during the acquisitions to compensate for

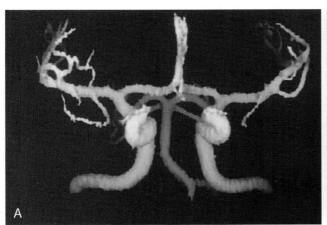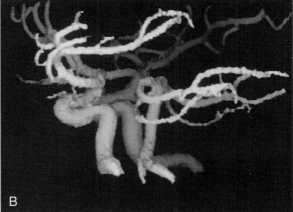

FIGURE 25–2. Shaded surface rendering of the intracranial vasculature. The surface-rendered vascular images are projected from an anterior view *(A)* and a right posterior oblique view *(B)*. In both instances, vascular shading has resulted in depth cueing of the arterial structures. The complex geometries of the carotid siphons and distal basilar artery are easily appreciated.

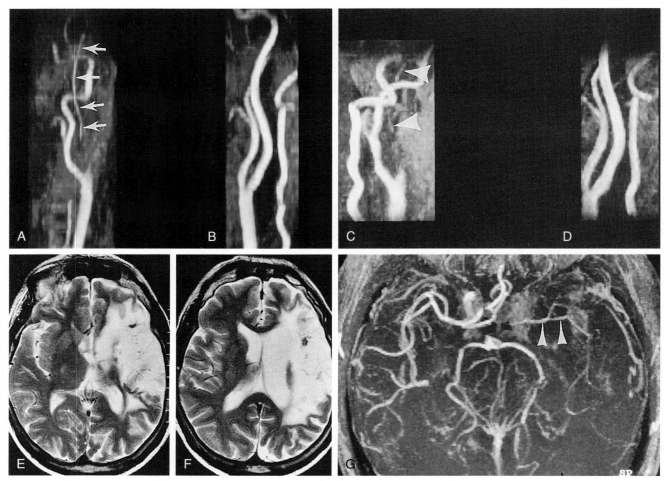

FIGURE 25–3. Detection of slow flow by 2D TOF MR angiography. Lateral views of the left *(A)* and right *(B)* carotid bifurcation from a 2D TOF acquisition. There is a small residual lumen of the left internal carotid artery that is easily identified on the 2D TOF acquisition *(arrows)*. The 3D TOF examination of the left *(C)* and right *(D)* bifurcation poorly demonstrates the residual lumen of the left internal carotid artery owing to saturation of the slow flow within this vessel *(arrowheads, C)*. There is minimal disease at the origin of the right internal carotid artery. *E* and *F,* Axial T2-weighted images identify an extensive region of infarction corresponding to the entire left middle cerebral artery distribution. *G,* The 3D TOF MR angiogram was obtained with intravenous contrast medium enhancement to sensitize the technique to slow flow. Venous structures such as the internal cerebral veins can be visualized. In addition, the extremely slow flow within the small left middle cerebral artery *(arrowheads)* is also appreciated. The reduced flow within the middle cerebral artery is due to its isolated nature with no evidence of collateral flow from the anterior communicating artery or posterior communicating artery. There is also reduced demand for flow owing to the large area of infarction. *(A to G* from Turski P: Magnetic resonance angiography. In: Forbes G [ed]: Syllabus: Special Course in Neuroradiology. Oak Brook, IL: RSNA Publications, 1994.)

constant-velocity flow. By balancing the gradients, the signal from spins with constant velocity can be recovered. In most instances only "first-order flow compensation" is practical because compensating for higher orders of motions such as acceleration and jerk prolong the echo time (TE).[13]

Echo Time

A complementary method for increasing flow signal (by reducing dephasing) is to substantially shorten the TE. The loss of signal from dephasing effects is approximately proportional to the TE squared. For example, reducing the TE from 4 to 2 ms will decrease the signal loss due to dephasing effects from approxi-

mately 16 to 4. In the past, short TE values were difficult to achieve owing to limitations in the strength of the gradient amplifiers. New gradient coils and amplifiers are now available that provide rapid rise times and high gradient amplitudes. The rise time and gradient amplitude are used to describe a quantity called the *slew rate.* The slew rate is expressed in tesla per meter per second and is defined as the maximal gradient amplitude divided by the rise time to the maximal amplitude of the gradients. For example, a slew rate of 76.6 T/m/s is equal to a maximal gradient amplitude of 0.0230 T/m divided by rise time to maximal amplitude of 0.0003 second (Fig. 25–4). Gradient performance is now commonly described in terms of the gradient system slew rate. The greater the slew rate,

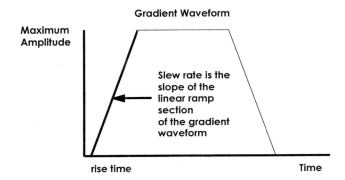

FIGURE 25–4. Gradient slew rate. To accurately describe gradient performance, a quantity called the slew rate is commonly used. The slew rate is defined as the maximal gradient amplitude divided by the time to reach the maximal gradient strength. A rapid gradient slew rate allows imaging systems to provide MR angiographic pulse sequences with short TE values.

the faster the gradients can achieve maximal amplitude. Less time is needed to complete the gradient pulse, allowing the TE to be shortened. MRI systems with slew rates of 77 T/m/s are now commercially available, providing MR angiographic 2D sequences with TE values of less than 5 ms and 3D MR angiographic sequences with TE values of less than 2.4 ms. Even more powerful gradient systems are on the hori-

zon that will shorten the TE to less than 2 ms, substantially improving the ability to detect signal from complex flow conditions (Fig. 25–5).

Spatial Saturation Pulses

Occasionally, it is desirable to eliminate the signal pattern from vascular structures that overlap the re-

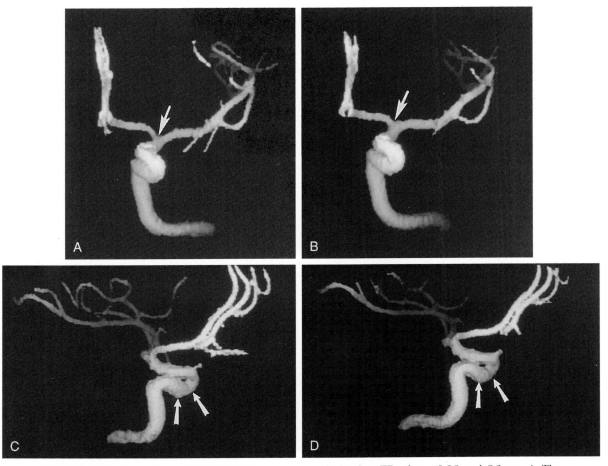

FIGURE 25–5. Comparison of 3D TOF MR angiograms obtained at TE values of 6.9 and 2.3 ms. *A,* The anterior view of the left internal carotid artery bifurcation reveals signal loss at a TE of 6.9 ms *(arrow). B,* The same region when studied using a gradient-echo technique and TE of 2.3 ms reveals an increase in the vascular signal of the proximal A1 segment *(arrow).* Similarly, *(C)* the lateral projections through the carotid siphon reveal that there is artifactual vascular irregularity of the carotid siphon at a TE of 6.9 ms *(arrows),* whereas the same region studied with TE of 2.3 ms *(D)* shows a smooth vascular lumen with no evidence of irregularity *(arrows).*

gion of interest. This is commonly encountered in MR angiography of the carotid bifurcation where the internal jugular veins can obscure the proximal internal carotid artery. Vascular signal can be eliminated by the placement of spatial saturation (SAT) bands through the vessel to be nulled. A superior SAT band is routinely used in 2D TOF MR angiography of the neck to eliminate the flow signal from the internal jugular veins that are entering the slice from above.[14] Ordinarily, the SAT band is close to the slice and moves (or walks) with the slice as the slice position changes (Fig. 25–6). When there is to-and-fro motion of the blood, spins may move in and out of the SAT band, resulting in reduced signal intensity. In this instance, the gap between the SAT band and the slice should be increased to move the SAT band away from the flow region.

It is also desirable to reduce the signal from fat by selecting a TE that places fat and water out of phase. This is a periodic event that occurs at 6.9 ms at 1.5 T. By selecting a TE that places fat and water out of phase, orbital and subcutaneous fat signal can be significantly reduced, improving the detection of small vascular structures.

The most common problems encountered with 2D TOF angiography include misregistration of the axial slices due to motion of the patient, saturation of in-plane blood flow, and loss of vascular signal owing to long TE values necessary for thin-slice 2D imaging.

3D TIME-OF-FLIGHT MR ANGIOGRAPHY

Rather than acquiring a single slice, it is also possible to perform a T1-weighted 3D gradient-echo acquisition with a small flip angle (e.g., 20° to 30°), short TE, and short TR that also demonstrates inflow enhancement. These studies are called 3D TOF angiograms. The 3D volumes can be acquired as one large single volume or as a series of overlapping 3D slabs. The major strengths of 3D TOF angiography are high spatial resolution, relatively short scan times, short TE values, and high signal-to-noise ratio. The most significant weaknesses of 3D TOF are reduced sensitivity to slow

flow and the tendency of short-T1 materials such as methemoglobin (or fat) to appear bright in the image and thus simulate flow.[15]

Several modifications of 3D TOF MR angiography have been introduced to increase the detection of flow signal intensity. The most significant advance is the ramped RF pulse (also called a tone pulse) that substantially reduces the saturation of blood as it flows through the imaging volume.[16] The ramped RF excitation linearly varies the flip angle across the 3D slab. If an inferior to superior ramp factor of 2 is used, then the flip angle will double from the entry slice to the exit slice. Flow from above will be suppressed, and saturation of inferior to superior flow will be reduced. Unfortunately, background signal intensity will also vary owing to the ramped RF pulse[17] (Fig. 25–7).

Magnetization transfer (MT) uses an off-resonance RF pulse to further suppress background signal.[18] This is accomplished by applying an RF pulse at a frequency separate from the unbound water frequency. The MT pulse saturates the spins that are bound to proteins. These saturated bound spins rapidly exchange with the free unbound spins in the surrounding tissue. The result is partial saturation of the unbound spins. MT suppresses brain signal approximately 50%, whereas blood signal is suppressed only 15%. Fat signal is not suppressed and appears increased in intensity relative to other stationary tissues when an MT pulse is applied.

The reduced background signal allows smaller vessels to be identified. MT is used primarily for intracranial MR angiographic examinations. The prominent fat signal makes MT less useful in examinations of the carotid bifurcations. Probably the most desirable approach is to combine the ramped RF pulse and the MT pulse (Fig. 25–8).

MULTIPLE OVERLAPPING THIN-SLAB TIME OF FLIGHT

The multislab technique improves flow sensitivity by decreasing the dwell time of flowing spins within the thin imaging volume. The spins pass through the thin slab much more quickly than a thick 3D volume acquisition. The flowing spins are less saturated in the thin

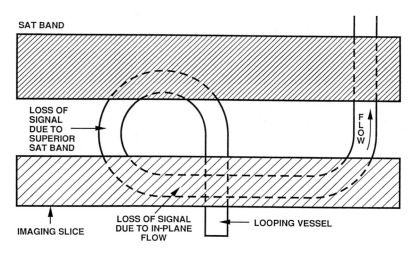

FIGURE 25–6. Elimination of unwanted vascular signal by saturation pulses. In this diagram an axial 2D TOF slice is depicted. A superior SAT band is applied to eliminate any signal from venous flow originating from above the slice plane. Note that this configuration of imaging slice and SAT band can lead to artifactual signal loss if the vessel geometry results in adverse interaction with the SAT band. (From Turski P, ed: Vascular Magnetic Resonance Imaging. 2nd ed. Volume 3 of General Electric Applications Guide. Waukesha, WI: GE Medical Systems, 1994.)

SAT BAND

LOSS OF SIGNAL DUE TO SUPERIOR SAT BAND

FLOW

IMAGING SLICE

LOSS OF SIGNAL DUE TO IN-PLANE FLOW

LOOPING VESSEL

ramp slope = 2

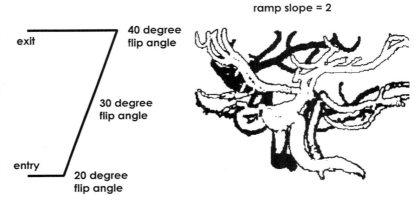

FIGURE 25–7. To reduce the saturation of blood as it flows through the imaging volume, the flip angle can be varied. A small flip angle is used at the entry site to reduce saturation, and a large flip angle is used near the exit site of the slab to increase the detection of signal from vascular structures. The ramp slope can be varied to match the velocity of flow and the slab thickness. For most intracranial applications a ramp slope of 2, in which the entry slice has a 20° flip angle, the midvolume a 30° flip angle, and the exit slice a 40° flip angle, is commonly used. (From Turski P, ed: Vascular Magnetic Resonance Imaging. 2nd ed. Volume 3 of General Electric Applications Guide. Waukesha, WI: GE Medical Systems, 1994.)

exit — 40 degree flip angle

30 degree flip angle

entry — 20 degree flip angle

slab because they are in the imaging slab only for a short time and experience only a few RF pulses. Many slabs can be obtained sequentially, similar to a 2D TOF examination, allowing a larger region to be covered. Inflow can also be increased by stacking the slabs from superior to inferior to avoid saturation of slow flow as the spins move from inferior to superior through the carotid artery. Although multislab TOF MR angiography generates excellent flow signal, each slab requires

several minutes to acquire, making the technique rather time intensive.

Unfortunately, it is necessary to overlap the 3D slabs approximately 25% to reduce the variation in vascular and background signal intensity (i.e., the "venetian blind" artifact) that occurs at the junction points of the slabs. The amount of overlap can be minimized by applying a slightly ramped RF excitation. Approximately one fourth of the slope used for intracranial imaging is used to reduce the flow saturations. A small ramp slope has a minor effect on background signal intensity, yet further reduces the saturation of spins as they move through the imaging slab. The advantage of using a slightly ramped RF pulse is that the flow signal is more evenly distributed within the slab and the number of overlap slices can be reduced, increasing coverage per unit of imaging time while minimizing saturation of slow flow[19] (Fig. 25–9; see Fig. 25–1).

PHASE-BASED MR ANGIOGRAPHY: MEASURING VELOCITY AND FLOW RATE

BASIC CONCEPTS OF BLOOD FLOW

In most instances, blood flows fastest near the center of the vessel and slowest adjacent to the wall. This

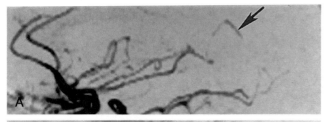

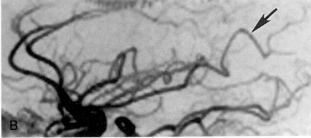

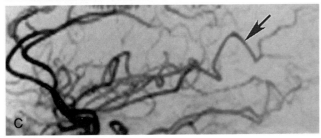

FIGURE 25–8. Comparison of 3D TOF imaging with magnetization transfer (MT) and ramped RF pulse. *A,* 3D TOF MR angiogram. Note that the angular artery is poorly visualized *(arrow). B,* After the application of MT the angular artery *(arrow)* is better delineated. *C,* With the application of a ramped RF pulse, the saturation of the flowing spins has been decreased and the angular artery is now optimally visualized *(arrow).* (Courtesy of Matt Bernstein, PhD, GE Medical Systems, Waukesha, WI.)

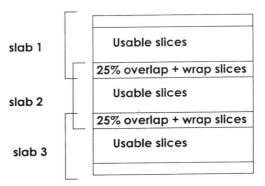

slab 1	Usable slices
	25% overlap + wrap slices
slab 2	Usable slices
	25% overlap + wrap slices
slab 3	Usable slices

FIGURE 25–9. Multislab TOF imaging. To provide greater coverage, multiple overlapping 3D TOF slabs are typically used to examine the carotid bifurcation. It is necessary to overlap the slabs to reduce artifacts at the junction points. A small ramp slope can be used to reduce the number of overlap slices. MT is not applied to multislab imaging of the carotid bifurcations owing to the resulting high signal intensity of the adjacent fat. (From Turski P, ed: Vascular Magnetic Resonance Imaging. 2nd ed. Volume 3 of General Electric Applications Guide. Waukesha, WI: GE Medical Systems, 1994.)

pattern of flow is the result of viscosity leading to friction within blood components and between blood and the vessel wall. This friction is called shear stress. The velocity gradient that is created perpendicular to the vessel wall is called the shear rate. It defines the rate of the change in flow velocity as one moves from the center of the vessel toward the wall. The shear rate or velocity gradient is greatest near the vessel wall and decreases as one approaches the center of the vessel. Laminar flow predominates in most larger arterial structures. Flow is laminar when the velocities are distributed along regular lines or layers. In the ideal situation of constant flow in a straight vessel, the velocities would be distributed as concentric shells. If viewed in cross section, these layers of flow would assume a parabolic profile[20] (Fig. 25–10).

Peak velocity is the maximal velocity encountered in the vessel lumen. For nonpulsatile vessels the average velocity is one-half peak velocity. Flow (Q) is defined as the average velocity (V) in centimeters per second times the cross-sectional area (A) of the vessel in square centimeters, or $Q = V \cdot A$. In pulsatile vessels, flow may be expressed as the average over the cardiac cycle. Typically, for clinical applications flow rate is described in milliliters per minute rather than cubic centimeters per second. In MRI, velocity and flow measurements are spatially averaged over the size of the imaging voxel (1 to 3 mm³). Unlike Doppler ultrasonography, MR flow measurements are not instantaneous and are temporally averaged over 16 or 32 intervals during the TR.[21, 22]

2D PHASE-CONTRAST PROJECTION SLAB COMPLEX DIFFERENCE IMAGING

The most basic phase-contrast technique acquires the image data as a 2D projection slab ranging from 20 to 100 mm in thickness. A bipolar flow-encoding gradient is added to the scan sequence to make the phase-contrast scans sensitive to velocity-dependent phase shifts. Stationary spins will refocus at the end of the bipolar gradient pulse, whereas spins with constant velocity will acquire a phase shift that is directly proportional to the velocity of blood flow. For most neurovascular applications, the flow-encoding gradients are applied along all three orthogonal directions: anterior to posterior, right to left, and superior to inferior.[23]

Elimination of the stationary tissue from the angiographic image is accomplished by using a four-point technique in which a flow-compensated gradient-echo acquisition of the stationary spins is interleaved with the three flow-encoded acquisitions.[24] The stationary spins are subtracted from the data set to remove the background signal intensity. The flow images are then combined to generate the angiographic or "speed" image. The subtraction of the stationary tissue also eliminates any high-signal-intensity material such as methemoglobin or fat from the phase-contrast angiogram.

The amplitude of the bipolar gradient determines the velocity encoding (V_{enc}) and defines the velocity that will produce maximal signal intensity. By varying the amplitude of the bipolar gradients one can generate phase-contrast angiograms that emphasize fast, intermediate, or slow flow. A larger amplitude of the bipolar flow encoding gradient will sensitize the technique to slow flow, and a small bipolar flow-encoding gradient will sensitize the scan to fast flow.[25]

Two methods are currently used to process the phase-contrast scan data. The first is called complex difference processing in which a difference signal proportional to the sine of the phase angle is displayed. Complex difference processing is used for imaging thick slabs (20 to 100 mm) containing large amounts of soft tissues and vascular structures. Unfortunately, a spoiler gradient used in the complex difference technique to reduce the signal from stationary tissue destroys the quantitative velocity-phase relationships needed to measure velocity and flow.

VELOCITY AND FLOW FROM 2D PHASE-CONTRAST PHASE DIFFERENCE THIN SLICES

An alternative method of processing the 2D phase-contrast scan data that maintains the quantitative phase-velocity relationship is called phase difference processing. Two interleaved acquisitions are obtained with opposite polarities of the bipolar gradient, and the difference in the phase shift between these two acquisitions is then calculated. The resulting phase difference is directly proportional to velocity, the gyromagnetic ratio, and the change in the first gradient moment with respect to time (or, more simply, the

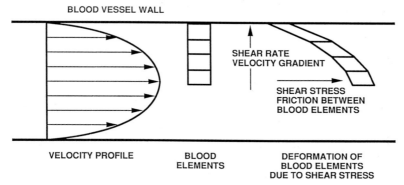

BLOOD VESSEL WALL

SHEAR RATE
VELOCITY GRADIENT

SHEAR STRESS
FRICTION BETWEEN
BLOOD ELEMENTS

VELOCITY PROFILE   BLOOD ELEMENTS   DEFORMATION OF BLOOD ELEMENTS DUE TO SHEAR STRESS

FIGURE 25–10. In this diagram, laminar flow has resulted in a parabolic flow profile within the vessel. The highest velocities typically occur near the center of the vessel. Note that because of the friction between blood elements there is resulting shear stress that produces a velocity gradient. This velocity gradient can be quantitated and is a measure of shear rate. These physiologic principles are important because they produce spin dephasing and saturation that alters the appearance of MR angiograms. Shear rate also plays a role in activation of the coagulation system and generates stress on the vascular wall. (From Turski P, ed: Vascular Magnetic Resonance Imaging. 2nd ed. Volume 3 of General Electric Applications Guide. Waukesha, WI: GE Medical Systems, 1994.)

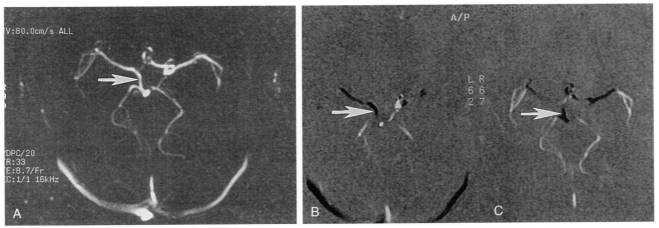

FIGURE 25–11. Velocity imaging using a 2D phase-contrast phase difference technique. To determine the direction of blood flow, axial phase-contrast images were obtained through the circle of Willis. *A,* The speed image reveals complete occlusion of the right internal carotid artery. A prominent right posterior communicating artery is identified *(arrow). B* and *C,* The corresponding velocity image encoded for flow in the anterior to posterior direction indicates that flow is reversed in the posterior communicating artery *(arrows).* Flow in the direction of the flow-encoded gradient is represented as bright pixels, whereas flow in the opposite direction (posterior to anterior) is represented by dark pixels. (*A* to *C* from Turski P, ed: Flow Analysis. Volume 6 of General Electric Applications Guide. Waukesha, WI: GE Medical Systems, 1994.)

area of the flow-encoding gradient). Thus, for a specific pixel the phase difference between the two acquisitions is directly proportional to the velocity of flow along the applied axis of the bipolar flow-encoding gradient. Unfortunately, unwanted phase shifts may occur due to eddy currents, a patient's motion, and other factors. The subtraction of two sets of data that differ only by their first gradient moment minimizes the adverse effects of eddy currents and magnetic field inhomogeneities. Thus, the phase difference is calculated on a pixel-by-pixel basis, yielding an image in which the signal intensity can be made proportional to the velocity of blood flow.[26]

Each flow direction can be individually displayed. Flow along the direction of the flow-encoding axis is displayed as bright signal pixels, and flow in the opposite direction is displayed as dark (or black) pixels.

The ability to determine the direction of blood flow can be helpful for identifying collateral blood flow pathways (Fig. 25–11). A useful feature of phase-contrast flow analysis is the ability to measure average blood flow from a nongated 2D phase-contrast slice.[27] This is accomplished by obtaining a thin 2D phase-contrast slice perpendicular to the vessel of interest with flow encoding along the axis of the vessel. The intravascular signal intensity is summed, allowing measurement of the total flow across the slice. The velocity and flow rate represented by the intravascular signal intensity are average values because the 2D phase-contrast scans are obtained throughout the cardiac cycle and over many cardiac cycles (Fig. 25–12). Measuring flow volume from a single nongated 2D phase-contrast slice is most applicable to arteries that do not have excessive pulsatility or triphasic flow pat-

FIGURE 25–12. Flow analysis based on a 2D phase-contrast slice. Flow encoding was in the superior to inferior direction; thus, the inferior to superior flow velocities are displayed as negative values. Regions of interest have been drawn around the basilar arteries. A background phase correction was also performed. The volume flow rate was also measured from a nongated 2D phase-contrast slice through the same location. The average flow rate measured 79.7 mL/min. (From Turski P, ed: Flow Analysis. Volume 6 of General Electric Applications Guide. Waukesha, WI: GE Medical Systems, 1994.)

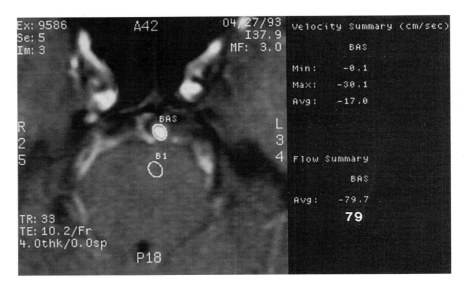

TABLE 25–1. PHASE-CONTRAST FLOW ANALYSIS PROTOCOLS*

PHASE-CONTRAST TECHNIQUE	TE (ms)	TR (ms)	FLIP ANGLE	FC	THK (mm)	NEX	MTX	FOV (cm)	V_enc (cm/s)
Cine phase contrast	8.6	30–40	30°–45°	+	4	2	128 × 256	12–18	125
2D phase contrast	8.7	30–40	30°	+	4	4	192 × 256	12–18	125
									40 (veins)
3D phase contrast 60 slices	8.2	24	20°	+	1	1	128 × 256	16	80

*TE = echo time; TR = repetition time; FC = flow compensation; THK = slice thickness; NEX = number of excitations; MTX = matrix; FOV = field of view; V_{enc} = velocity encoding.

terns. The 2D phase-contrast slice method is particularly useful for measuring nonpulsatile venous flow within the superior sagittal sinus. The 2D phase-contrast scans can be obtained in 1 to 2 minutes depending on the desired resolution and number of excitations. Higher resolution images (512 × 256, ¾ field of view [FOV]) can be obtained, reducing the partial-volume effects that occur at the edges of small intracranial arteries. Typical scanning parameters are summarized in Table 25–1.

2D Cine Phase-Contrast Complex Difference Slab Imaging

Cine phase-contrast angiograms can be obtained by applying bipolar flow-encoding gradients to conventional cine gradient-echo scans. In this approach, electrocardiographic or peripheral gating is used to trigger the examination. The scan data are collected continuously during the cardiac cycle. The image data are reconstructed so that information obtained during various portions of the cardiac cycle is displayed in a time-resolved fashion. In the situation in which a thick volume is imaged, the complex difference technique is used. Cine phase-contrast complex difference imaging provides images in which the vascular structures can be visualized with time resolution, overcoming the problems associated with flow pulsatility.[28, 29]

Cine Phase-Contrast Phase Difference Method for Quantifying Blood Flow

A single cine phase-contrast slice is oriented perpendicular to the vessel of interest. Flow is detected as it passes through the slice by using a bipolar flow-encoding gradient applied along the axis of flow.[30] In the cine phase-contrast sequence, the bipolar flow-encoding gradient generates a phase shift for moving spins proportional to their velocity.[31, 32] Typically, 16 or 32 velocity and flow measurements are calculated at sequential points in the cardiac cycle, providing time-resolved flow information[33] (Fig. 25–13). The resulting velocity waveform allows assessment of pulsatility and variations in flow dynamics during the cardiac cycle.

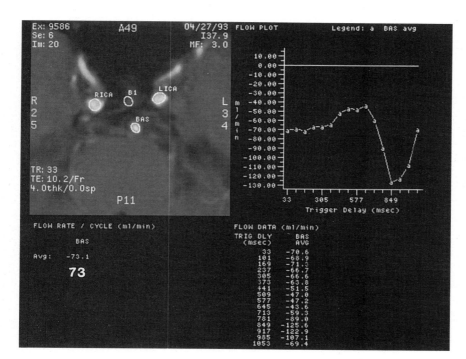

FIGURE 25–13. Flow analysis based on a 2D cine phase-contrast slice. The cine phase-contrast acquisition was obtained using peripheral gating through the same region as in Figure 25–12. The pulse delay results in the systolic peak velocities occurring at a trigger delay of 849 ms. Peak velocities are displayed for 16 points in the cardiac cycle for each vessel. In addition, the average velocity for each vessel is calculated. The basilar artery volume flow data are displayed in this plot. Note that the systolic peak flow occurs at a trigger delay of 849 ms. The average flow rate is 73.1 mL/min. (From Turski P, ed: Flow Analysis. Volume 6 of General Electric Applications Guide. Waukesha, WI: GE Medical Systems, 1994.)

The cine examination can be triggered by cardiac or peripheral gating. Cardiac gating typically results in the systolic flow information being displayed early in the flow waveform (i.e., systole followed by diastole). Peripheral gating is easier to set up and is generally more reliable than cardiac gating. Because of the pulse delay in peripheral gating, the systolic portion of the flow waveform may be displaced in time. In normal vessels this is not a problem because the systolic portion of the waveform is usually obvious. However, pulsatility may be reduced in pathologic conditions and precise identification of systole may be difficult in these instances.

The small size of the intracranial vessels requires that thin slices (3 mm) be used to reduce partial-volume effects at the vessel edge. The slice should be oriented as perpendicular to the vessel as possible. Oblique orientations of the scan plane can introduce errors in flow measurements due to overestimation of the vessel's cross-sectional area. A flip angle of 30° to 45° is suggested to minimize saturation of the flowing spins as they move through the slice. Although high-resolution images improve vessel edge detection, the longer data acquisition results in unacceptable scan times. A practical approach is to obtain images with 256×256 resolution using an FOV of 16 to 18 cm. The minimal TE available (with flow compensation) is routinely used along with TR 40 to 50 ms. The flow-encoding direction is selected to sensitize the acquisition to flow through the slice (e.g., superior to inferior flow encoding for an axial section through the internal carotid arteries).

3D PHASE-CONTRAST IMAGING

The phase-contrast angiographic data can be acquired as a 3D volume acquisition analogous to 3D TOF MR angiography. By using the four-point technique, a flow-compensated 3D gradient-echo acquisition is interleaved with three additional flow-encoded 3D volume acquisitions.[34] For 3D phase-contrast angiography, phase difference processing is used to generate magnitude-weighted phase images demonstrating flow direction.[35] The scan data are also reconstructed, providing magnitude images and speed images (angiogram).

VELOCITY AND FLOW FROM 3D PHASE-CONTRAST ACQUISITIONS

Average velocity data can also be obtained from a 3D phase-contrast to volume acquisition. The advantages of using the 3D phase-contrast technique are that thin 1- to 1.5-mm slices can be obtained, reducing partial-volume averaging of the vessel wall; and voxel sizes are small compared with 2D phase-contrast imaging, decreasing intravoxel dephasing. Flow measurements are improved when the vessel edge is well resolved, and the vessel is oriented exactly perpendicular to the imaging plane. By reviewing the entire 3D volume, several slices can be identified that display the vascular structures in direct cross section. These slices are then used for the velocity and flow calculations. The 3D phase-contrast angiograms are also obtained

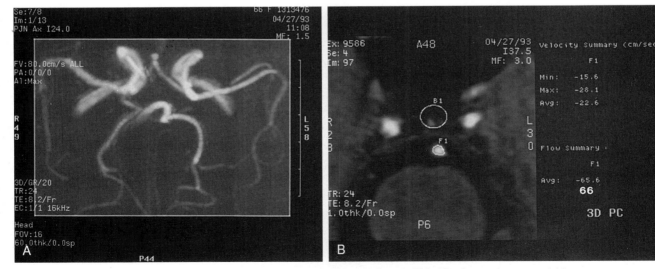

FIGURE 25–14. Flow analysis based on a 3D phase-contrast slice. *A*, This 3D phase-contrast acquisition was obtained in the axial plane (V_{enc} of 80 cm/s) through the same region as Figure 25–12. The 3D phase-contrast examination reveals that the posterior cerebral artery has a fetal origin and originates from the right internal carotid artery. Thus, the basilar artery supplies only the posterior fossa and left posterior cerebral artery. This anatomic variation results in a lower flow rate for the basilar artery than would ordinarily be encountered if both posterior cerebral arteries were supplied by the basilar artery. *B*, A single axial 1-mm-thick section from the 3D phase-contrast examination was used for flow analysis. The average flow rate measures 66 mL/min using the 3D phase-contrast data. (*A* and *B* from Turski P, ed: Flow Analysis. Volume 6 of General Electric Applications Guide. Waukesha, WI: GE Medical Systems, 1994.)

TABLE 25–2. COMPARISON OF PHASE-CONTRAST TECHNIQUES

TECHNIQUE	ADVANTAGES	DISADVANTAGES
Cine phase contrast	Time-resolved flow dynamics Waveform analysis Assessment of pulsatile flow	Requires gating Longer scan times More difficult to process flow data
2D phase contrast	Short scan times Provides average velocity and flow	Pulsatility can degrade accuracy No time-resolved information
3D phase contrast, 12 or 28 slices	Thin sections Reduced partial-volume effects	Pulsatility can degrade accuracy No time-resolved information
3D phase contrast, 60 slices	Thin sections Reduced partial-volume effects Potential to reformat images perpendicular to vessel	Longer scan times More difficult to process Pulsatility can degrade accuracy No time-resolved information

throughout the cardiac cycle and over many cardiac cycles so the velocities and flow rates, represented by intravascular signal intensity, are average values (Fig. 25–14). The problem with 3D phase-contrast flow analysis is the relatively long scan time associated with the acquisition. A typical 60-slice 3D phase-contrast examination with a 128 × 256 matrix, ¾ FOV of 22 ×

16, V_{enc} of 80, flip angle of 20°, TR of 26 ms, TE of 8.3 ms, and 1-mm partitions requires approximately 12 minutes to perform. Image reconstruction would also require additional time and would generate 60 anterior to posterior flow images, 60 superior to inferior flow images, 60 right-to-left flow images, 60 magnitude images, and 20 reprojections, for a total of 260 images

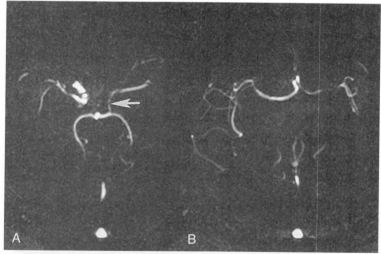

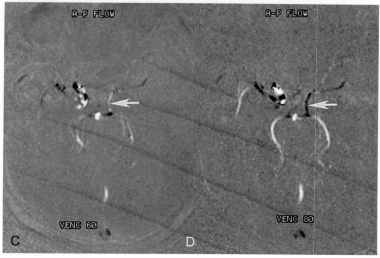

FIGURE 25–15. Phase wrap or aliasing due to incorrect selection of the velocity encoding. *A* and *B,* In this patient, the left internal carotid artery is occluded *(arrow)* and there is collateral flow through the posterior communicating artery. *C,* Velocity images were initially obtained at a V_{enc} of 60 cm/s. This resulted in an incorrect display of the flow direction due to aliasing or phase wrap *(arrow). D,* The examination was repeated with a V_{enc} of 80 cm/s. The posterior to anterior flow within the left posterior communicating artery *(arrow)* is now properly displayed. To accurately represent velocity and flow rate, aliasing (or phase wrap) can be avoided by selecting a V_{enc} that exceeds the maximal velocity within the vessel of interest.

from one examination. Shorter, more practical scans can be obtained using a 12- or 28-slice acquisition. The 12-slice 3D phase-contrast studies can also be obtained with thicker partitions (e.g., 2 to 4 mm) to cover a large volume in less time (Table 2–2).

PHASE WRAP OR ALIASING

A potential problem in flow and velocity imaging is phase wrap or aliasing. Phase wrap occurs when a V_{enc} is selected that does not equal or exceed the maximal velocity present within the vessel of interest. For flow analysis, the V_{enc} is selected so that all velocities within the vessel of interest fall within a range that produces a phase difference between $+180°$ and $-180°$. For example, if a V_{enc} of 100 cm/s is selected, velocities between -100 and $+100$ cm/s will have linearly varying signal intensity corresponding to the appropriate phase difference. Spins that are moving in the direction of the flow-encoding gradient will be represented by bright pixels and flow in the opposite direction by dark pixels.

If there are spins that have velocities greater than 100 cm/s, however, they will phase wrap or alias and the incorrect signal intensity will be displayed. Phase wrap compromises the ability to calculate flow measurements. A V_{enc} of 80 to 150 cm/s is generally used for intracranial flow analysis studies to avoid this problem. Therefore, when one wants to maintain the flow and velocity information in a phase-contrast MR angiogram using phase difference technique, it is important to select a V_{enc} that equals or exceeds the highest velocity spins within the vessel of interest. However, selecting a V_{enc} that is excessively high will prevent aliasing but will also result in a degradation of the signal-to-noise ratio for that acquisition[36, 37] (Fig. 25–15).

LIMITATIONS OF PHASE-CONTRAST FLOW ANALYSIS

The causes of inaccurate flow measurements can be divided into 1) incorrect selection of the V_{enc} resulting in flow aliasing (V_{enc} too low) or poor detection of slow flow (V_{enc} too high); 2) partial loss of intravascular signal due to intravoxel dephasing due to turbulent flow; 3) saturation of in-plane flow; 4) incorrect selection of the vessel region of interest; 5) excessive obliquity of the slice plane; and 6) eddy currents. Saturation effect can be reduced by increasing the TR or by decreasing the flip angle. Eddy currents adversely affect the phase-contrast flow measurements by inducing a larger or smaller phase shift than desired. The result is degradation of the quantitative phase-velocity relationships and increased background signal intensity. These adverse effects are reduced by the use of shielded gradient coils and eddy compensation corrections. Unfortunately, some eddy current artifacts persist and, in general, a background phase correction is performed by sampling stationary tissue adjacent to the vessel of interest.[38]

One method of improving reproducibility of the flow measurement uses manual thresholding to create a vessel edge corresponding to a defined pixel signal intensity. This can be accomplished by careful selection of the window width and level. Selecting a window width of 1 on the phase-velocity image creates a flow map of bright and dark pixels. A cursor can be placed on the vessel of interest to determine the maximal intensity (e.g., 1000). By readjusting the window level to 500 (one half of the maximum) many of the partial-volume pixels at the vessel edge are excluded and the vessel edge becomes rigorously defined by its signal intensity. The calculated flow rates may be lower than reported values owing to the smaller vessel area that results from low-signal-intensity pixels at the vessel edge.

Validation studies by Tang and colleagues[39] showed that poor resolution of the vessel edge and partial-volume effects were the major obstacles to accurate flow measurements. These researchers also noted that at least 16 voxels must cover the cross-sectional area of the vessel lumen to obtain a measurement accuracy within 10% (Fig. 25–16).

PHYSIOLOGIC PROCESSES THAT AFFECT FLOW MEASUREMENTS

Immediately after birth, middle cerebral artery flow velocities are low but increase rapidly in the first week of life. Velocities reach their maximum at age 6 years, with peak velocities of approximately 100 cm/s. Middle

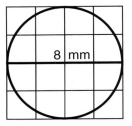
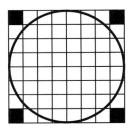

FIGURE 25–16. Partial-volume effects for velocity and flow measurements. The accuracy of velocity and flow measurements depends greatly on the resolution of the vessel wall. Typically it is necessary to have 16 pixels within the vessel to clearly delineate the wall. Note in the diagram that the accuracy of the flow measurement improves as the resolution of the vessel wall increases. PC MRA = phase-contrast MR angiography.

True area of vessel = 50.2 mm². By partial-volume averaging at the corners of the vessel, PC MRA calculates an area of 0.64 mm².

By doubling the resolution, partial-volume averaging is decreased by excluding the dark pixels from the measurement — the area of the vessel now measures 0.60 mm².

cerebral artery velocities decline throughout life, falling to approximately 40 cm/s by the seventh decade.[40]

Hematocrit has a marked effect on cerebral flow velocities. Middle cerebral artery flow velocities measured by transcranial Doppler exceed age-adjusted norms for hematocrits less than 35%. Velocities decrease in patients with polycythemia owing to the elevated hematocrit.

The main metabolic factors that alter cerebral blood flow are PO_2, PCO_2, and cerebral metabolic demand. The PO_2 must fall to 50 mm Hg before cerebral blood flow is increased due to hypoxia. Blood flow is unaffected by elevated PO_2 levels. The effects of PCO_2 are much more dramatic. By increasing PCO_2 levels from 20 to 60 mm Hg (e.g., by breathing 5% carbon dioxide), middle cerebral artery flow velocities increase an average of 52.5%. Brain activation also affects the intracranial flow. For example, middle cerebral artery flow velocities have been noted to increase approximately 11% after activation of the motor cortex by hand movements.

Autoregulation is the process by which the flow to the brain is maintained at relatively constant levels despite variations in perfusion pressure. Cerebral autoregulation may depend on an inherent capacity of vascular smooth muscle to contract when it is stretched or on the washing away of carbon dioxide and other vasodilating metabolites when the perfusion pressure and blood flow are increased. Autoregulation is disturbed after head trauma or stroke and in patients with severe hypertension or arteriovenous malformations (AVMs) (Fig. 25–17).

Minor changes in cardiac output do not dramatically alter intracranial flow velocities if autoregulation is intact. Transient changes in middle cerebral artery velocities are observed owing to increased cardiac output, but autoregulation rapidly returns flow to normal

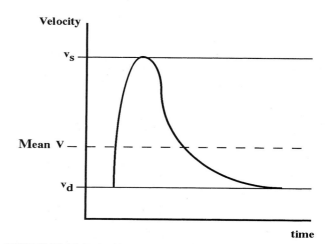

FIGURE 25–18. Pulsatility index (Gosling): PI = $(v_s - v_d)/V$. The pulsatility index has been defined as the systolic peak velocity (v_s) minus the diastolic velocity (v_d) divided by the mean velocity (V). This index allows accurate description of flow pulsatility.

levels. Patients with hypertension, head injury, vascular malformations, or stroke may have disturbed autoregulation, and cerebral blood flow may be more closely coupled to cardiac output in these instances.

Pulsatility analysis is the investigation of the excursions of the blood velocity waveform during one cardiac cycle. It has been used extensively for transcranial Doppler evaluations of intracranial flow. The most commonly used pulsatility index was described by Gosling and associates[41] and is defined as the maximal vertical excursion of the velocity waveform divided by its mean height (Fig. 25–18). This measurement reflects the amplitude of the first harmonic of the velocity waveform. A low pulsatility index, as measured by transcranial Doppler, has been associated with low peripheral resistance. For example, arterial feeders to AVMs have high flow velocities and volume flow rates, yet the pulsatility is usually lower than normal intracranial arteries. Pulsatility increases in the feeder arteries after embolization or surgery.[42] Similarly, reduced pulsatility is often observed distal to a severe stenosis or in vessels supplied by collateral pathways.[43] Lindegaard and coworkers[44] also identified reduced pulsatility in the middle cerebral artery distal to a 75% stenosis of the proximal internal carotid artery.

A significant limitation of cine phase-contrast imaging for providing pulsatility data is the relatively poor temporal resolution of this technique when compared with transcranial Doppler evaluation. The peak velocities are more accurately measured by transcranial Doppler because the sampling is virtually instantaneous throughout the cardiac cycle. The current temporal resolution of cine phase-contrast flow analysis is 16 or 32 measurements during the cardiac cycle. Thus, the highest flow velocity could fall between the 16 (or 32) phases of the cardiac cycle, resulting in imprecise measurements of the peak velocities.[45]

NORMAL FLOW RATES

Measuring flow rates for intracranial arteries is technically difficult, and there are few established normal

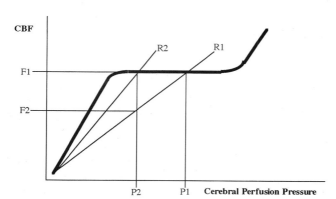

FIGURE 25–17. The relationship of pressure, flow, and resistance during autoregulation. Assuming flow F1 and perfusion pressure P1, the resistance is indicated by R1. If the pressure suddenly drops to P2, flow would drop an equal percentage to F2. Within seconds, autoregulation becomes effective in the brain, changing the resistance to R2, whereby flow is restored to the original value. The thick line indicates that autoregulation is effective only within a range of perfusion pressures. When the reserve capacity for vasodilatation has been exhausted, cerebral perfusion pressure is fixed to cardiac output and varies with blood pressure. (Modified from Aaslid R: Cerebral hemodynamics. In: Newell DW, Aaslid R, eds. Transcranial Doppler. New York: Raven Press, 1992, p 50.)

TABLE 25–3. MEAN ± SE OF THE BLOOD FLOW MEASUREMENTS DETERMINED BY CINE MR ANGIOGRAPHY AND PEAK BLOOD FLOW AS DETERMINED FROM 16 IMAGES*

VESSEL	RIGHT BLOOD FLOW (mL/min) Mean	Peak	Right Vessel Area (cm²)	LEFT BLOOD FLOW (mL/min) Mean	Peak	Left Vessel Area (cm²)
Carotid	302 ± 21	389 ± 28	0.22 ± 0.06	337 ± 19	440 ± 31	0.22 ± 0.06
A1-ACA	88 ± 11	105 ± 13	0.10 ± 0.04	75 ± 10	91 ± 11	0.09 ± 0.04
PCALL	44 ± 5	52 ± 6	0.06 ± 0.02	42 ± 5	48 ± 6	0.06 ± 0.02
MCA	127 ± 7	152 ± 10	0.15 ± 0.04	108 ± 7	126 ± 8	0.13 ± 0.04
PCA	51 ± 4	64 ± 5	0.09 ± 0.3	53 ± 4	68 ± 5	0.09 ± 0.04
Basilar	161 ± 11	203 ± 13	0.14 ± 0.03			

*A1-ACA = A1 segment of anterior cerebral artery; PCALL = pericallosal artery; MCA = middle cerebral artery; PCA = posterior cerebral arteries.
From Enzmann DR, Ross MR, Marks MP, Pelc NJ: Blood flow in major cerebral arteries measured by phase-contrast cine MR. AJNR 15(1):123–129, 1994, © by American Society of Neuroradiology.

flow values. It is therefore important not to place too much emphasis on an absolute flow number. The best results are obtained by comparing flow values to internal standards such as an analogous contralateral vessel (e.g., the opposite middle cerebral artery). Nonetheless, cine phase-contrast velocity and volume flow measurements for normal carotid and basilar arteries have been reported by several authors.

In an early study, Marks and associates[46] noted in normal adult subjects (mean age, 44 years) the following velocity and flow values: right internal carotid artery peak velocity 63 cm/s and volume flow rate 352 ± 21 mL/min, left internal carotid artery peak velocity 60 cm/s and volume flow rate of 342 ± 15 mL/min, and basilar artery peak velocity 51 cm/s and volume flow rate 164 ± 12 mL/min. Mattle and colleagues[47] described volume flow rates (normal subjects) for the middle cerebral artery using a bolus tracking technique. The middle cerebral artery peak velocity was 69.8 cm/s and the volume flow rate was 150 mL/min (range, 138 to 161 mL/min). Velocities for the middle cerebral artery decreased with increasing age.

Enzmann and coworkers[48] have extensively studied intracranial flow rates and flow velocities in normal volunteer subjects (Tables 25–3 and 25–4). Note that the peak flow velocities range from 29 cm/s for the posterior cerebral artery to 62 cm/s for the middle

TABLE 25–4. MEAN (± 1 STANDARD DEVIATION) OF THE BLOOD VELOCITY IN EACH OF THE MAJOR CEREBRAL VESSELS AS DETERMINED BY CINE MR ANGIOGRAPHY*

VESSEL	MR PEAK BLOOD VELOCITY (mL/min) Right	Left
Carotid	51 ± 3	43 ± 4
A1-ACA	52 ± 11	44 ± 6
PCALL	30 ± 2	31 ± 2
MCA	62 ± 5	47 ± 5
PCA	29 ± 2	27 ± 1
Basilar	56 ± 5	

*Abbreviations are as in Table 25–3.
From Enzmann DR, Ross MR, Marks MP, Pelc NJ: Blood flow in major cerebral arteries measured by phase-contrast cine MR. AJNR 15(1):123–129, 1994, © by American Society of Neuroradiology.

cerebral artery. These values should be taken into consideration when selecting the V_{enc} for phase-contrast flow studies.

CONTRAST ENHANCEMENT AND MR ANGIOGRAPHY

For both TOF and phase-contrast techniques, when the TR is shorter than the longitudinal relaxation time (T1) the longitudinal magnetization of the spin ensemble reaches a steady state that is much less than the fully relaxed value. As mentioned earlier, this is the basis for the vessel to static tissue contrast in TOF imaging. The static tissue is more saturated and has a lower steady-state magnetization (and lower signal intensity) compared with the inflowing blood, which is initially much higher in signal intensity. As blood flows through the imaging volume, it will experience multiple RF pulses and will become partially saturated. For slowly flowing blood the equilibrium magnetization is similar to the equilibrium magnetization of the stationary tissues and the vessels are not easily detected. Therefore, slowly flowing blood would be easier to detect on MR angiography (both TOF and complex difference phase-contrast techniques) if the equilibrium magnetization and intravascular signal intensity are increased relative to stationary tissue. This is accomplished by catalytically shortening the T1 of blood by administering a gadolinium chelate[49] (Fig. 25–19).

Runge and coworkers[50] have documented the improved detection of slow flow in pathologic conditions after the administration of gadolinium chelates. Fortunately, the blood-brain barrier restricts gadolinium to the intravascular space under normal conditions. After the administration of the contrast material, flowing blood establishes a new steady-state magnetization at a higher signal intensity level. The T1 shortening and resulting signal increase are proportional to the concentration of the gadolinium chelate. This relationship is nearly linear for concentration of gadolinium up to 0.5 mmol/kg. At higher doses, the nonlinear relationship between gadolinium concentration and vessel signal intensity is probably due to the loss of signal intensity that occurs at high concentrations of paramagnetic agents owing to the shortening of T2 relaxation time.[51] In the clinical setting, the intravascular concentration

SIGNAL VS RF NUMBER VS T1 AND TIP ANGLE

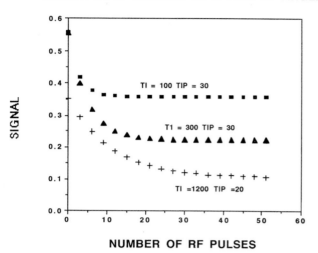

FIGURE 25–19. Effect of contrast enhancement on blood signal intensity. The equilibrium magnetization plots for three blood T1 values are displayed. The lowest equilibrium magnetization corresponds to unenhanced blood (T1 = 1200 ms) moving through a 3D TOF imaging volume. After saturation, the spins have a relatively low signal intensity. The next plot indicates the equilibrium magnetization of blood after contrast enhancement (T1 = 300 ms). Note that the overall signal intensity of the moving spins has dramatically increased. The final plot represents the equilibrium magnetization of blood after a triple dose of a gadolinium chelate (T1 = 100 ms).

drops rapidly owing to renal excretion reducing the overall effect of the contrast agent.

One problem associated with contrast-enhanced TOF MR angiography is that the extracellular gadolinium chelates are nonspecific MR contrast agents. Many normal and pathologic tissues will enhance because of absence or increased permeability of the blood-brain barrier. The high-signal-intensity enhanced stationary tissue will obscure vessels in the MIP images and may simulate flow signal pattern or degrade vessel detail.

A serious limitation for both contrast-enhanced TOF and phase-contrast angiography is that SAT bands become ineffective when the T1 of blood is significantly reduced. Venous structures such as the internal jugular vein cannot be eliminated from the MR angiogram by the selective placement of SAT bands and may obscure the carotid bifurcation. Similarly, arterial structures cannot be selectively eliminated by saturation techniques when contrast material is administered. Clinical trials have shown that the effects of enhancement with a contrast agent on phase-contrast angiographic vascular signal are complicated by the V_{enc} dependence of the sequence.[52] At a V_{enc} of 40 to 80 cm/s, slow spins have relatively low signal intensity and are poorly visualized. In this instance, contrast material will improve the detection of slow flow by increasing the magnitude of the steady-state magnetization above background noise levels.

The real clinical importance of enhanced MR angiography is that a larger spectrum of velocities and vessels can be detected after enhancement. This is particularly advantageous when one wants to detect slow flow within a nearly occluded artery or venous flow in pathologic conditions. The increased signal from small vessels also allows images to be obtained with higher resolution and better delineation of the small vessels. When an MT pulse is applied to a 3D TOF examination, there is even greater detection of the small contrast-enhanced vessels because of the suppression of the background signal[53] (Fig. 25–20).

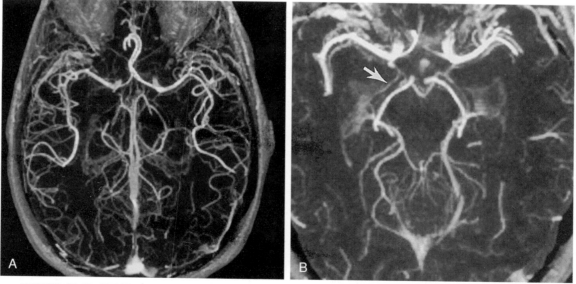

FIGURE 25–20. MT 3D TOF imaging with intravenous contrast enhancement. There is a synergistic effect of contrast enhancement with MT enabling enhanced structures to be more easily appreciated. This is particularly noticeable in contrast-enhanced MT 3D TOF MR angiograms. *A,* In this axial collapse image after administration of intravenous contrast material, the 3D TOF MR angiogram with MT shows an extensive vascular enhancement. *B,* A subvolume of the imaging data set has been projected into the axial plane. In the subvolume the anterior choroidal artery *(arrow)* can be appreciated.

ALTERED FLOW IN CEREBRAL ISCHEMIA

The MR angiographic examination focuses on the larger extracranial and intracranial vessels and attempts to identify compromised blood flow and to determine the severity and cause of the flow reduction. Usually, reduced or absent flow within the internal carotid, vertebral, basilar, anterior, middle, and posterior cerebral arteries can be identified with confidence.

FLOW RESTRICTIVE EXTRACRANIAL LESIONS

MR angiography of the proximal internal carotid artery begins with a 2D TOF examination to locate the site of the bifurcations and identify nearly occluded vessels.[54] The region of the proximal internal carotid artery is then further defined by obtaining a multislab 3D TOF MR angiogram.[55, 56] There is a tendency for MR angiography to overestimate the degree of stenosis when displayed only as a series of MIP images. Signal loss in the stenotic segment from spin dephasing can be reduced but not completely eliminated by using a short TE and small voxels. In general, the accuracy of MR angiography for defining the percentage of carotid artery stenosis using the North American Symptomatic Carotid Endarterectomy Trial (NASCET) index [1 − (stenosis diameter ÷ distal lumen diameter) × 100 = % stenosis] has been acceptable only when measurements are made from 3D re-formations rather than the MIP images. By using 3D re-formations, the low-signal-intensity pixels that define the true edge of the vessel can be better identified[57] (Fig. 25–21).

Regional hypoperfusion may occur distal to a severely stenotic internal carotid artery if there is inadequate collateral circulation. In this situation, the vessel remains patent but flow is so severely reduced that the cerebral hemisphere ipsilateral to the stenosis experiences chronic hypoperfusion and ischemia. When the cross-sectional area of an arterial lumen is reduced by more than 50%, the flow velocity at the stenosis begins to increase above normal values. This velocity increase is necessary to maintain the normal flow rate across the arterial obstruction. As the stenosis approaches 80%, the velocity increase does not completely compensate for the compromised lumen, resulting in a reduction in the flow rate. If the stenosis is greater than 95%, the flow rate distal to the stenosis may drop to a such a low level that collateral flow by means of the circle of Willis is necessary to maintain ipsilateral hemispheric perfusion. If the collateral circulation is inadequate, regional hypoperfusion may occur distal to the flow restrictive stenosis. Regional hypoperfusion can be detected by the identification of reduced vessel diameter, decreased intravascular signal intensity, decreased visualization of distal vessels secondary to saturation of the slower flow, altered flow in the circle of Willis or ophthalmic collateral arteries, and reduced arterial flow rates.[58] There may also be intermittent reduction in vascular flow related to variations in cardiac output or other factors resulting in transient epi-sodes of ischemia. In these patients there may be a role for MR perfusion or cerebral blood volume imaging.[59, 60]

Embolic infarcts are characterized by the sudden onset of focal neurologic signs. Infarction occurs when an artery supplying the brain is suddenly occluded by atherosclerotic plaque or thrombus that has embolized from a more proximal source. Emboli most commonly originate from sites of stenosis or ulceration in the proximal internal carotid artery and flow distally into the distribution of the middle cerebral artery. Approximately 25% of embolic infarcts are thought to be caused by emboli originating in the cardiac chambers or from diseased heart valves. The middle cerebral artery and the posterior cerebral artery are the most common vessels occluded by embolic disease. Frequently, the emboli rapidly lyse, resulting in reperfusion and potentially hemorrhagic areas of infarction. Hypoperfusion of the cerebral hemisphere during transient occlusion may result in watershed infarction occurring at the anastomotic border zones between the major vascular territories. MR angiography can also be used to exclude the carotid bifurcation as a source of emboli in patients with underlying cardiac disease[61] (Fig. 25–22) (see also Chapter 24).

INTERNAL CAROTID ARTERY OCCLUSION

Vascular thrombosis occurs as clot forms in situ in an artery that has reduced blood flow caused by a constricting atherosclerotic plaque. Thrombosis usually results in decreased or absent perfusion in the vascular distribution normally supplied by the thrombosed vessel. It is essential that the MR angiographic technique selected is capable of excluding the possibility of slow flow in a nearly occluded carotid artery. This can be accomplished by obtaining a 2D TOF axial acquisition through the cervical internal carotid artery or a high-resolution complex difference phase-contrast slab examination encoded for low flow velocities (i.e., 10 to 20 cm/s). Intravenous contrast material may also be helpful for increasing intravascular signal in slow flow vessels. If contrast enhancement is used, one must be careful not to confuse enhancing soft tissue with collateral flow.

Another consideration in the evaluation of internal carotid artery occlusion is the presence of collateral flow through the circle of Willis. The potential for collateral flow probably explains the variable clinical presentation of patients with internal carotid artery occlusion.[62] Collateral flow may occur through intact portions of the circle of Willis or through extracranial to intracranial pathways (i.e., the ophthalmic artery). Unfortunately, a complete circle of Willis is present in only 21% of patients.[63] When a complete circle of Willis is present, collateral flow occurs through the anterior communicating artery and the posterior communicating arteries. Ordinarily, after internal carotid artery occlusion the anterior communicating artery provides adequate collateral flow to the anterior cerebral artery ipsilateral to the occluded internal carotid

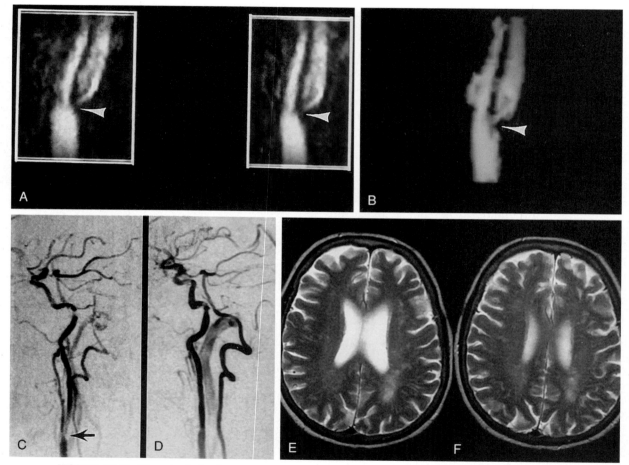

FIGURE 25–21. Flow restrictive internal carotid artery stenosis. In this patient the 3D TOF examination through the proximal internal carotid artery is displayed as an MIP image *(A)* and lateral shaded surface rendering *(B)*. Note the severe proximal internal carotid artery stenosis *(arrowheads)*. *C* and *D*, Sagittal 2D phase-contrast images through the cervical internal carotid arteries reveal reduced signal intensity *(arrow)* of the left internal carotid artery when compared with the right. Flow measurements through the internal carotid arteries indicated a slightly elevated flow volume of 386 mL/min on the right and a reduced flow volume of 142 mL/min on the left. *E* and *F,* Axial T2-weighted images also demonstrate evidence of ischemic changes involving the deep white matter of the left hemisphere.

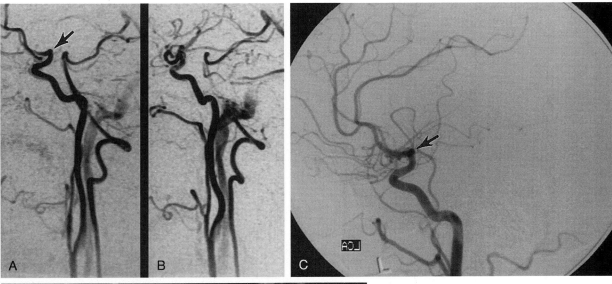

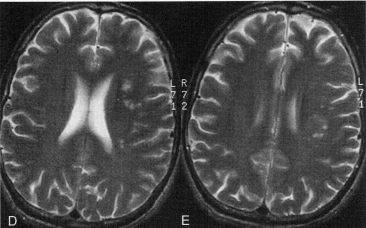

FIGURE 25–22. Middle cerebral artery embolus demonstrated by phase-contrast MR angiography. Sagittal 2D phase-contrast images were obtained through the left *(A)* and right *(B)* cervical internal carotid arteries. There is absence of flow within the left middle cerebral artery *(arrow)* when compared with the right. *C,* This finding was confirmed by conventional angiography where there was proximal occlusion of the left middle cerebral artery *(arrow).* Note that on the T2-weighted images *(D* and *E)* the patient has suffered a relatively minor ischemic injury.

artery. Thus, the middle cerebral artery territory is the most prone to infarction from carotid occlusion (Fig. 25–23).

With the TOF techniques, flow direction in the circle of Willis can be determined by the careful placement of presaturation bands over the carotid or basilar arteries during the acquisition of a 3D TOF MR angiogram. When the presaturation band is placed over the carotid artery, flow through this vessel will become saturated and distal flow will not be visible on the MR angiogram. Any collateral flow originating from this vessel will also "drop out" of the MR angiogram (Fig. 25–24).

An alternative approach uses phase-contrast flow imaging. 2D or 3D phase-contrast angiograms are obtained using phase difference processing. When the 2D phase-contrast phase difference method is used, slices up to 20 mm in thickness can be generated without loss of the phase-velocity relationships. If a 3D phase-contrast acquisition is chosen, 12, 28, or 60 slices can be obtained through the region of interest. In both acquisitions, phase maps are generated that display flow in the directions anterior to posterior, right to left, and superior to inferior.[64] A V_{enc} of 80 cm/s or higher is suggested to prevent aliasing of flow in collateral vessels with high-velocity flow (see Fig. 25–11).

CEREBRAL VASOMOTOR RESERVE

An important concept in the application of phase-contrast MR flow information is that the cerebral vaso-

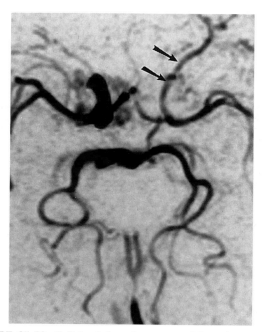

FIGURE 25–23. Collateral flow demonstrated by axial 2D phase-contrast angiography. In this patient there is complete occlusion of the proximal left internal carotid artery. Note that collateral flow has been established to the left hemisphere through a markedly hypertrophied left ophthalmic artery *(arrows)*. Only a relatively low-flow signal is identified related to the left posterior communicating artery and A2 segment of the anterior cerebral artery, suggesting that the ophthalmic artery is the dominant collateral pathway in this patient.

motor reserve will become exhausted as soon as the resistance arteries of the brain are maximally dilated. In this instance, the vessels are refractory to any further vasodilator stimulus, such as hypercapnia. This condition is important to recognize because any further reduction in perfusion pressure will result in cerebral ischemia. Therefore, intermittent reduction in vascular flow related to variations in cardiac output or other factors can produce transient episodes of ischemia.[65]

Vasomotor reactivity can be tested by measuring volume flow rates in the resting state and after induced vasodilatation. Transcranial Doppler studies have demonstrated that during 5% carbon dioxide inhalation, middle cerebral artery flow velocities increase by up to 52.5% in normal subjects. In patients with symptomatic carotid occlusions, middle cerebral artery velocities remain stable or increase only modestly, indicating that the middle cerebral artery vascular territory is already maximally vasodilated. Similar findings have been observed after the intravenous administration of acetazolamide,[66] providing a practical alternative to 5% carbon dioxide inhalation for measuring vasomotor reserve using cine phase-contrast techniques (Fig. 25–25).

SUBCLAVIAN STEAL SYNDROME

After proximal subclavian artery occlusion, blood flow is reversed in the ipsilateral vertebral artery and redirected away from the basilar artery into the arm. Occasionally, after exercise, the increased demand for blood flow in the arm may result in inadequate blood flow to the posterior circulation. This syndrome is characterized on MR angiograms by reversed flow in the vertebral artery ipsilateral to the subclavian occlusion. The degree of subclavian steal can be quantitatively measured by obtaining an axial cine phase-contrast study and measuring flow in both vertebral arteries throughout the cardiac cycle. Basilar artery steal during exercise can also be quantified. In addition, flow analysis techniques have the ability to assess the results of percutaneous transluminal angioplasty or vascular reconstructive surgery[67, 68] (Fig. 25–26).

POSTERIOR CIRCULATION

The majority of lateral medullary and proximal internal carotid artery infarcts are in fact due to vertebral artery occlusion.[69] Occasionally, embolic proximal internal carotid artery infarcts are identified. Lateral medullary infarcts have a characteristic feature of crossed sensory disturbance; that is, there is loss of pain and temperature sensation on the same side of the face and the opposite side of the body. MR angiography can be definitive in identifying vertebral artery thrombosis by using a phase-contrast technique with a low V_{enc} (10 to 20 cm/s) or 3D TOF (ramped RF and MT) acquisition[70] (Fig. 25–27).

The clinical syndrome of basilar artery occlusion due to thrombosis may arise in several ways: 1) occlusion in the basilar artery, usually in the lower third at the

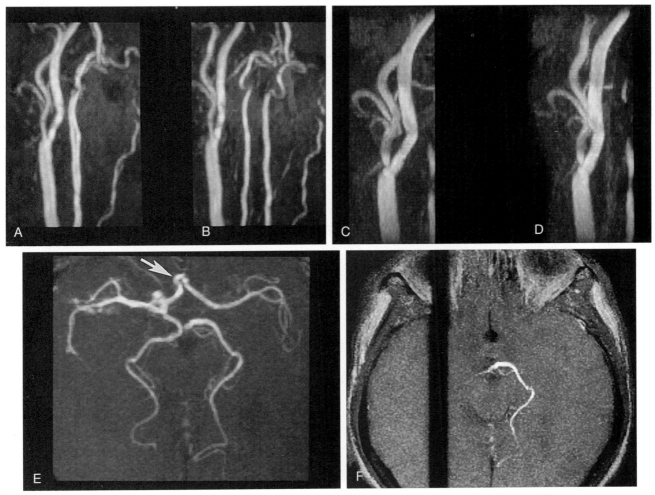

FIGURE 25–24. Collateral blood flow defined by the selective use of saturation pulses. *A* and *B*, MIP images through the cervical region from the 2D TOF acquisition indicate complete occlusion of the proximal left common carotid artery. *C* and *D*, MIP images from the multislab 3D TOF examination reveal minimal atherosclerotic plaque at the origin of the right internal carotid artery. *E*, The 3D TOF multislab intracranial examination identifies brisk flow into the left middle cerebral artery across the anterior communicating artery *(arrow)*. It is unclear as to the direction of blood flow in the posterior communicating artery because there is a fetal origin of the posterior cerebral artery and a hypoplastic P1 segment. To better define these flow relationships, a SAT band was placed over the right internal carotid artery, eliminating the flow signal from this vessel. *F*, The resulting 3D TOF image indicates that only the left posterior cerebral artery receives flow from the basilar artery and that in fact the P1 segment is quite hypoplastic. This implies that the right internal carotid artery supplies not only both middle cerebral arteries but also the right posterior cerebral artery.

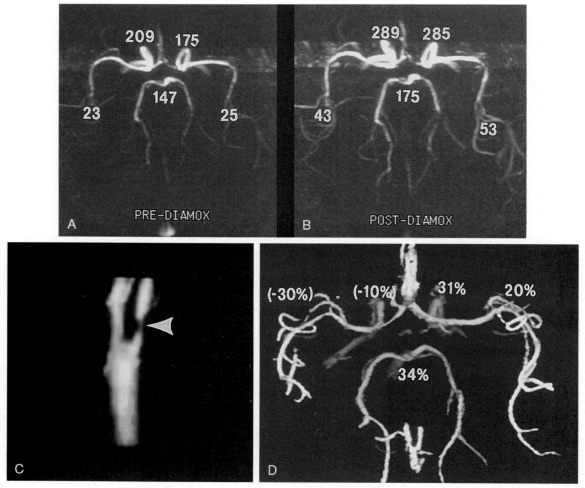

FIGURE 25–25. 3D phase-contrast flow analysis obtained before and after the administration of acetazolamide: normal and pathologic conditions. *A,* Flow measurements were made from individual superior to inferior flow-encoded axial slices of the 3D phase-contrast data set. *B,* After the administration of acetazolamide (17 mg/kg), the 3D phase-contrast acquisition was repeated. Identical axial sections were used to measure flow in the carotid basilar and branches of the middle cerebral artery. Typically, there is approximately a 25% increase in flow within the intracranial vessels after acetazolamide. A lack of response to this agent indicates loss of autoregulation. *C,* In a different patient a severe stenosis of the proximal right internal carotid artery *(arrowhead)* was identified. *D,* Flow measurements before and after acetazolamide are displayed on the surface-rendered images through the circle of Willis region. Note that there is a normal response to acetazolamide on the left, whereas ipsilateral to the carotid stenosis there is, in fact, a decrease in middle cerebral artery flow. This suggests that this patient has less autoregulation on the right and is unable to respond to variations in carotid output.

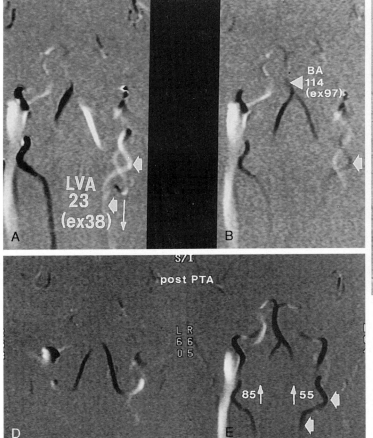

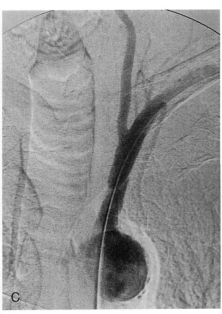

FIGURE 25–26. Left subclavian steal syndrome: quantitation of the vertebral and basilar artery steal during exercise. *A,* The superior to inferior flow image obtained during systole indicates reversed (superior to inferior) flow in the left vertebral artery *(arrows). B,* Note that the image obtained during diastole reveals inferior to superior flow in the left vertebral artery *(arrow).* This biphasic flow is due to the high peripheral resistance of the left brachial artery. The resting level of the left vertebral artery steal was 23 mL/min. After exercise, the left vertebral artery steal increased to 38 mL/min. Basilar artery *(arrowhead)* flow rates were also measured at rest (114 mL/min) and during exercise (97 mL/min), indicating the blood being diverted from the posterior circulation during exercise. *C,* The left subclavian artery stenosis was treated with percutaneous transluminal angioplasty. *D* and *E,* The follow-up flow analysis demonstrated inferior to superior flow in the left (55 mL/min) and right (85 mL/min) vertebral arteries *(arrows).* (*A* to *D* from Turski P: Magnetic resonance angiography. In: Forbes G [ed]: Syllabus: Special Course in Neuroradiology. Oak Brook, IL: RSNA Publications, 1994.)

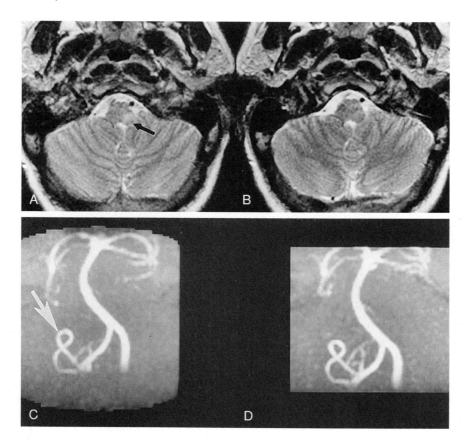

FIGURE 25–27. Lateral medullary infarct. *A* and *B*, Axial fast spin-echo T2-weighted images reveal an area of high signal intensity involving the dorsolateral aspect of the left medulla *(arrow)*. *C* and *D*, The 3D TOF coronal MIP images demonstrate occlusion of the left posterior inferior cerebellar artery. The right posterior inferior cerebellar artery *(arrow)* is well seen. (*A* to *D* from Turski P: Magnetic resonance angiography. In: Forbes G [ed]: Syllabus: Special Course in Neuroradiology. Oak Brook, IL: RSNA Publications, 1994.)

site of an atherosclerotic lesion; 2) occlusion of both vertebral arteries due to proximal stenoses; or 3) occlusion of a single dominant vertebral artery. Thrombosis frequently involves only a branch of the basilar artery rather than the trunk. When the obstruction is embolic, the embolus usually lodges at the upper bifurcation of the basilar artery or in one of the posterior cerebral arteries. If emboli are small enough to pass through the vertebral artery, they can traverse the basilar artery and ultimately lodge in the posterior cerebral artery. The majority of cerebellar emboli arise from atherosclerotic debris or thrombus generated on the surface of irregular or ulcerative atherosclerotic plaque or distal to a severe stenosis[71] (Fig. 25–28).

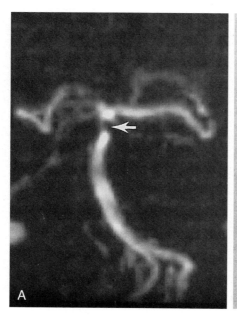

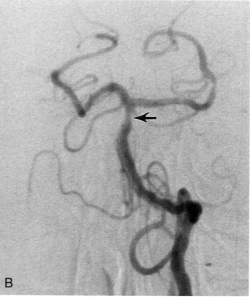

FIGURE 25–28. Basilar artery stenosis. *A*, In this patient, the distal basilar artery is involved by atherosclerotic disease. Distal flow appears to be compromised *(arrow)*. *B*, The subsequent conventional intra-arterial digital subtraction angiogram confirms the presence of the stenosis *(arrow)*, although it does not appear to be restricting flow.

DISSECTING HEMATOMA AND ALTERED FLOW

Dissection of the carotid or vertebral artery is usually the result of trauma. The traumatic insult may be quite minor. Complaints of headache and neck pain are common. Horner's syndrome may occur from damage to the sympathetic nerves. The MR angiographic diagnosis relies on the identification of high-signal-intensity hematoma in the wall of the vessel. Usually, 3D TOF axial source images are able to separate the residual lumen from the hematoma[72] (Figs. 25–29 and 25–30). Thin axial T1-weighted, spin density, and T2-weighted images are also useful for defining the extent of the hematoma. These should be obtained with superior and inferior saturation pulses to eliminate any confusing flow signal. Occasionally, pseudoaneurysms may form as the hematoma resolves; therefore, follow-up examinations are usually required.[73, 74]

FIBROMUSCULAR DYSPLASIA

Fibromuscular dysplasia is caused by idiopathic cellular proliferation in the vascular intima and media. The disease may involve the cervical internal carotid or vertebral arteries. Alterations in the size of the vessel lumen occur in a periodic fashion and creates a "string of beads" configuration on angiographic studies. Progression of this morphologic change may result in long segments of stenosis or saccular dilatations of the affected vessel. The internal carotid artery is involved three times more commonly than the vertebral artery. The diseased vessels are more prone to dissection and aneurysm formation. The cause of fibromuscular dysplasia remains obscure; therapy for symptomatic patients includes anticoagulants and percutaneous transluminal angioplasty.

The diagnosis of fibromuscular dysplasia may be problematic using MR angiographic techniques. Misregistration artifacts on 2D TOF images may occasionally mimic the findings of fibromuscular dysplasia. The use of multiple overlapping thin slabs improves detection, and 2D phase-contrast techniques may also help confirm the diagnosis[75] (Fig. 25–31).

INTRACRANIAL STENOSIS AND MOYAMOYA DISEASE

The most commonly used method for imaging the intracranial circulation is a 60-slice, ramped RF, 3D TOF acquisition with MT using a 512 × 192 matrix, FOV of 22 × 16, and 1-mm partitions. This approach enables evaluation of the circle of Willis, the proximal middle cerebral arteries, and the distal basilar artery. Unfortunately, because the 3D TOF technique is not particularly sensitive to slow flow, there may be instances in which vessel patency is overlooked, owing to saturation of the slow flow distal to an area of severe stenosis.[76–78] Some authors[79] have recommended using a multislab approach to increase the sensitivity of the examination to slow flow (Fig. 25–32).

Moyamoya disease is an idiopathic process that re-

sults in occlusion of the large vessels at the base of the brain with secondary neovascularization. Extensive small anastomotic channels develop by means of the perforating and leptomeningeal vessels, which allows continued brain perfusion. The disease is limited to the intracranial circulation and is almost always associated with symptoms of cerebral ischemia. Progressive vascular occlusion occurs owing to intimal proliferation. The cause of the disease is unknown. Percutaneous angioplasty, surgical revascularization procedures, and antiplatelet drugs may offer some benefit. The main clinical presentation is transient ischemic attacks, infarction, or hemorrhage. Ischemic changes predominate in the pediatric age group, in which mental retardation is a common clinical finding (Fig. 25–33).

Yamada and coworkers[80] imaged 26 patients with moyamoya disease and compared conventional catheter angiography with 3D TOF MR angiography. In this study, MR angiography accurately depicted 217 of 264 arteries (82%). In 37 vessels the vascular signal could not be detected on the MIP images or the degree of stenosis was overestimated. Conventional angiography demonstrated collateral moyamoya vessels in all 52 hemispheres, whereas 3D TOF demonstrated moyamoya vessels in only 53 hemispheres (80%). In addition, 3D TOF MR angiography demonstrated only 18 of 28 large leptomeningeal and transdural collaterals. The authors noted that the small moyamoya and collateral vessels can frequently be visualized on the source images from 3D TOF studies but are nearly eliminated from the MIP images. The loss of small vessels from the MIP images is due to the low intravascular signal intensity and small vessel size, so it is difficult to separate these vessels from the background tissue.

VASCULITIS

Inflammation and necrosis of the cerebral arteries may occur as a result of infectious or immune-related processes. Bacterial, tubercular, fungal, syphilitic, and viral infections have been implicated in cerebrovasculitis. Immune-related disorders include polyarteritis nodosa, systemic lupus erythematosus, sarcoidosis, and Wegener's granulomatosis. Vasculitis may also occur secondary to amphetamine abuse or as a primary central nervous system angiitis. The MR angiographic findings parallel those appreciated in larger vessels with conventional angiography. These include segmental narrowing and dilatation in the proximal intracranial arteries. Occasionally, peripheral aneurysms may also be encountered (Fig. 25–34) (see also Chapter 24).

FLOW FEATURES OF VASCULAR MALFORMATIONS

Most AVMs are supratentorial with a large component of the AVM located superficially in the pia. Malformations completely restricted to the dura are termed *dural AVMs*. Spinal vascular malformations are

Text continued on page 816

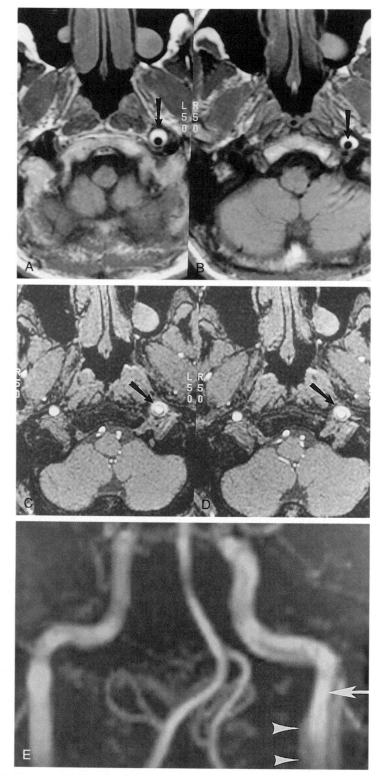

FIGURE 25–29. Spontaneous dissection of the internal carotid artery. The axial T1-weighted *(A and B)* and source 3D TOF *(C and D)* images demonstrate a high-signal-intensity hematoma within the wall of the left internal carotid artery *(arrows)*. *E,* The coronal MIP image from the 3D TOF angiogram also displays the high-signal-intensity hematoma within the wall of the internal carotid artery *(arrowhead)* as well as the residual lumen *(arrows)*. *(A to E* from Turski P: Magnetic resonance angiography. In: Forbes G [ed]: Syllabus: Special Course in Neuroradiology. Oak Brook, IL: RSNA Publications, 1994.)

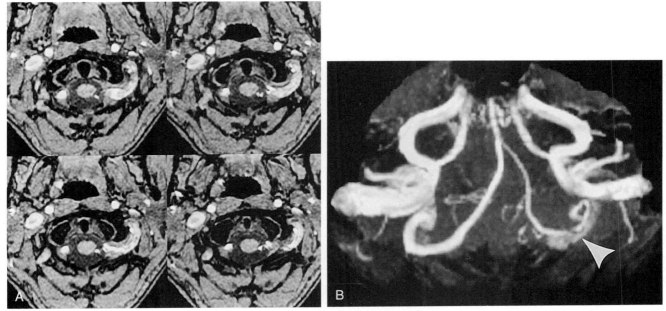

FIGURE 25–30. Traumatic dissection of the left vertebral artery. *A*, Axial source images from the 3D TOF acquisition reveal a high-signal-intensity hematoma within the wall of the left vertebral artery. *B*, The MIP images confirm the presence of the hematoma *(arrowhead)* within the wall of the vertebral artery. Although the lumen is somewhat compromised, normal flow signal is maintained within the left vertebral artery.

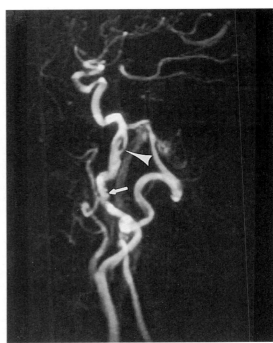

FIGURE 25–31. Fibromuscular dysplasia. The sagittal 2D phase-contrast image demonstrates a beaded appearance *(arrow)* of the proximal internal carotid artery with a subsequent slight dilatation of the vessel. Note that in the region of the dilatation there is a central low-signal-intensity region indicating complex flow *(arrowhead)*.

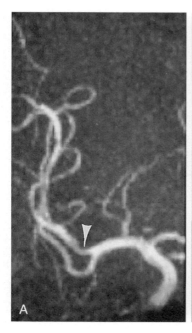

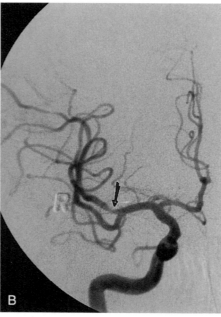

FIGURE 25–32. **Stenosis of the middle cerebral artery.** *A*, The 3D multislab image through the proximal middle cerebral artery reveals a moderate stenosis of this vessel *(arrowhead)*. *B*, The stenosis *(arrow)* was confirmed by conventional angiography. Flow measurements through the middle cerebral artery indicated a normal flow volume of 132 mL/min and a normal pulsatility index.

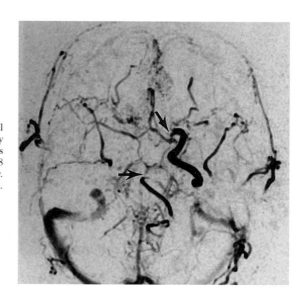

FIGURE 25–33. **Moyamoya disease.** In this patient, a 2D phase-contrast axial projection image reveals severe stenosis of the distal left internal carotid artery *(upper arrow)*, occlusion of the right internal carotid artery, and severe stenosis of the distal basilar artery *(lower arrow)*. Flow analysis indicated a flow rate of 98 mL/min in the basilar artery and 138 mL/min in the left internal carotid artery. The diminished cerebral blood flow accounts for the patient's cognitive decline.

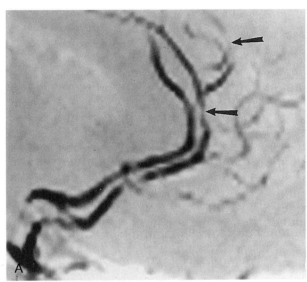

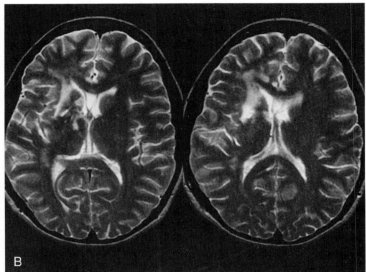

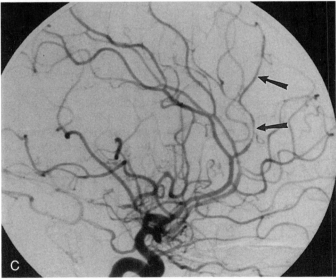

FIGURE 25–34. Intracranial vasculitis associated with systemic lupus erythematosus. *A,* In this patient, a 3D TOF image revealed several segments of reduced signal intensity *(arrows). B,* The T2-weighted images also demonstrated multiple areas of infarction. *C,* The findings of central nervous system vasculitis were confirmed by conventional angiography: distal branches of the anterior cerebral artery demonstrated variations in vessel diameter *(arrows).*

most often dural in location and frequently contain direct arteriovenous fistulas.[81] The arterial supply to the malformation may be derived from a terminal feeding artery, an artery that supplies normal brain tissue and the AVM, or an artery that has undergone angiomatous change and vasodilatation in response to intracranial steal. Arteries that terminate in the AVM can be embolized or clipped at surgery without injury to adjacent normal brain tissue.[82]

The nidus of the AVM represents the area of arteriovenous shunting within the malformation. It is, therefore, the low-resistance portion of the malformation and is thus responsible for the hemodynamic changes related to the malformation.[83] Two types of arteriovenous communications have been observed within the nidus. The first is a tangle of small vascular loops that have a few interconnections and simulate small veins or capillaries. The second type of connection is the direct arteriovenous fistula in which there is a relatively large direct communication between the arterial and venous components of the AVM, as is frequently encountered in vein of Galen malformations. AVMs may contain a single compact nidus with all the vascular channels related to one geographic region, or they can be multicentric with more than one nidus. There may also be several hemodynamic compartments within the nidus. Vascular pedicles that are small before surgical intervention may rapidly enlarge once they become the hemodynamically dominant vascular system[84, 85] (Fig. 25–35).

The draining veins are usually divided into superficial groups that drain into the sagittal, sphenoparietal, cavernous, transverse, and sigmoid sinuses and deep groups that drain into the subependymal veins, internal cerebral veins, the basal vein of Rosenthal, the vein of Galen, and straight sinus.

By combining 3D TOF and phase-contrast methods, MR angiography can identify the arterial supply to the AVM, determine the size and location of the AVM nidus, define the location and morphology of the venous drainage, identify high-flow aneurysms, and attempt to detect the presence of fistulas within the AVM. Sagittal 2D phase-contrast angiograms are acquired at V_{enc} values of approximately 80 and 20 cm/s. By generating images that emphasize different velocities it is possible to qualitatively assess the flow within the AVM (Fig. 25–36). The additional advantages of this approach are that the arterial supply is well defined at the higher V_{enc} and the venous drainage is delineated at the lower V_{enc}. The high spatial resolution that can be achieved with 3D TOF angiography provides information regarding the size and morphology of the AVM nidus. Mukherji and colleagues[86] compared 2D and 3D TOF MR angiographic techniques for delineation of nidus size and concluded that an AVM nidus greater than 0.36 cm could be reliably identified by 2D TOF MR angiography. High-flow aneurysms and fistulas may also be visible on the 3D TOF angiograms. The ability to define the size and location of the AVM nidus is essential for the proper selection of patients for surgery, endovascular therapy,[87] or focused radiation therapy[88, 89] (Fig. 25–37).

Dural AVMs have a natural history somewhat different from that of pial AVMs. Frequently, patients complain of pulsatile tinnitus,[90] bruit, headache, hemifacial spasm, or other symptoms related to vascular enlargement and compression of adjacent neural structures. Dural arteriovenous fistulas may be difficult to detect on spin-echo images but are usually identifiable on thin-slab 3D TOF examinations or on phase-contrast slab images obtained at a low V_{enc} (Fig. 25–38).

There is a well-established association of dural AVMs with dural sinus thrombosis. In most instances, the dural sinus thrombosis precedes the formation of the AVM and, in fact, may contribute to the formation of the AVM by encouraging the formation of collateral venous drainage. The combination of dural sinus occlusion and increased flow through the malformation may produce venous hypertension. Nonhemorrhagic neurologic deficit, venous aneurysms (varices), or hemorrhage may occur secondary to local increases in venous pressure.[91]

Transcranial Doppler has demonstrated the following flow conditions in association with AVMs.[92] Minimal velocity changes are associated with small AVMs that are located a long distance form the proximal basal cerebral arteries and have small shunts. Prominent velocity changes are related to larger AVMs located more centrally with high shunt volumes and few feeding arteries. Transcranial Doppler flow characteristics suggest that arteries exclusively supplying the AVM have a low resistance and pulsatility index. Elevated systolic and diastolic flow velocities are also encountered in these vessels. Peak velocities greater than 180 cm/s may occasionally be encountered in high-flow AVMs. The AVM feeders have low resistance with high flow rates and steal blood flow away from adjacent brain structures. The AVM feeders do not respond to hypercapnia (i.e., no carbon dioxide reactivity). Neighboring arteries supplying normal brain parenchyma show diminished carbon dioxide reactivity with no cerebrovascular reserve capacity and reduced flow velocities.

Flow analysis has also proved useful for quantitating the results of endovascular therapy of AVMs.[93] Marks and colleagues[14] noted an increase in flow rates in both ipsilateral and contralateral internal carotid arteries in 16 patients with large AVMs. For the internal carotid arteries ipsilateral to the AVM, volume flow rates were 563 ± 48 mL/min, mean velocities were 90.0 ± 7.8 cm/s, and peak systolic velocities were 117.2 ± 9.2 cm/s. In these patients, volume flow rates were also elevated in the contralateral internal carotid artery (422 ± 29 mL/min) and the basilar artery (385 ± 42 mL/min). After embolization of the AVMs, repeated flow analysis revealed a reduction in the total cerebral blood flow.

Phase-contrast flow analysis has also demonstrated that AVMs containing large direct arteriovenous fistulas have markedly elevated flow rates and little variation in flow velocity from systole to diastole, resulting in a low pulsatility index.[94] In large AVMs the arterial feeders have low resistance and divert blood flow away form adjacent brain structures. The AVM feeders do

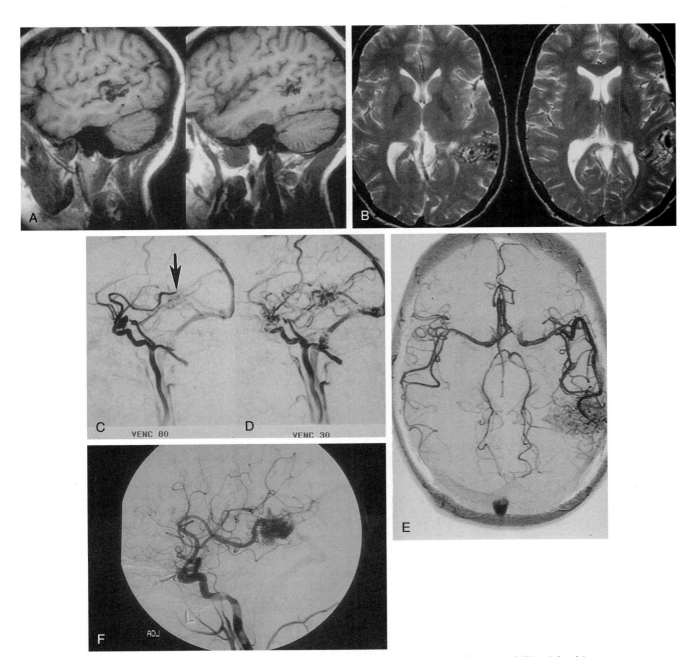

FIGURE 25–35. Temporal lobe AVM combining MRI and MR angiography. *A,* The sagittal T1-weighted image indicates an AVM involving the superior and middle temporal lobe gyri. The lesion is close to Wernicke's area. *B,* The T2-weighted images show a deep component of the AVM that has a triangle configuration. *C,* 2D phase-contrast images were also obtained at a V_{enc} of 80 cm/s, demonstrating the arterial supply to the AVM *(arrow).* *D,* At a lower V_{enc} of 20 cm/s, the slower flow components of the AVM nidus can be appreciated. *E,* The 3D TOF angiogram obtained through the AVM nidus clearly defines the margin of the nidus and reveals dilatation of the arterial feeders. *F,* A conventional angiogram confirms the "en passant" nature of the feeding artery that not only supplies the AVM but also flows distally to supply normal brain tissue.

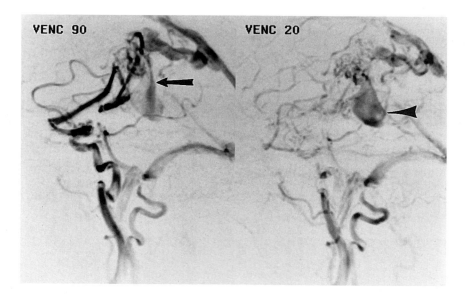

FIGURE 25–36. Arteriovenous fistula demonstrated by MR angiography. This patient has a right parietal AVM with a direct arteriovenous fistula and a large varix associated with the venous drainage. *Left,* On the phase-contrast angiogram obtained at a V_{enc} of 90 cm/s, the flow jet arising from the arteriovenous fistula can be identified *(arrow). Right,* At a V_{enc} of 20 cm/s, the varix associated with the venous drainage is better visualized *(arrowhead). (Left* and *right* from Turski P: Magnetic resonance angiography. In: Forbes G [ed]: Syllabus: Special Course in Neuroradiology. Oak Brook, IL: RSNA Publications, 1994.)

FIGURE 25–37. Occipital lobe AVM treated by focused radiosurgery. The initial 3D TOF MR angiograms were obtained without *(A)* and with *(B)* intravenous contrast material. There is a small well-defined AVM involving the parietal occipital region *(arrows),* supplied by branches of the posterior cerebral artery and middle cerebral artery. *C* and *D,* One year after focused radiation therapy, the MR angiograms were repeated. There is complete obliteration of the vascular malformation, which was confirmed by conventional angiography. *(A* to *D* from Turski P: Magnetic resonance angiography. In: Forbes G [ed]: Syllabus: Special Course in Neuroradiology. Oak Brook, IL: RSNA Publications, 1994.)

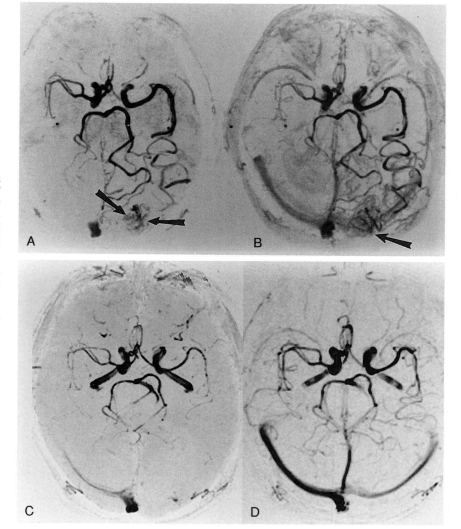

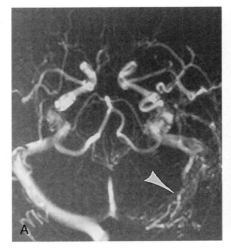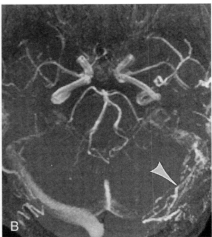

FIGURE 25–38. Dural AVM of the transverse sinus after lateral sinus thrombosis. *A*, The axial phase-contrast angiogram reveals increased vascularity in the region of the left transverse sinus *(arrowhead)*. The jugular bulb is visualized and fills through collateral venous pathways. *B*, The 3D TOF angiogram obtained through the same region also demonstrates the increased vascularity of the left transverse sinus *(arrowhead)* but is less sensitive to the slow flow in the jugular bulb. (*A* and *B* from Turski P: Magnetic resonance angiography. In: Forbes G [ed]: Syllabus: Special Course in Neuroradiology. Oak Brook, IL: RSNA Publications, 1994.)

not respond to acetazolamide or hypercapnia (i.e., no carbon dioxide reactivity) (Fig. 25–39) (see also Chapter 23).

INTRACRANIAL ANEURYSMS AND FLOW CHARACTERISTICS

Despite the potential of MR angiography as a noninvasive method for identifying intracranial aneurysms,[95] the limitation in spatial resolution of this technique requires that it be used cautiously in this population of patients.[96] Failure to detect an intracranial aneurysm may result in inappropriate therapy and subsequent devastating subarachnoid hemorrhage. The identification of intracranial aneurysms before hemorrhage is of critical importance because nearly 50% of patients presenting with acute subarachnoid hemorrhage die within the first 30 days after rupture.[97, 98] Thus, using MR angiography to identify intracranial aneurysms places a tremendous responsibility on the radiologist. During MR angiography, particular care must be taken to obtain the highest spatial resolution possible and to perform a thorough review of the imaging data. Targeted MIP subvolumes and multiplanar re-formations must be obtained to reduce vessel overlap and enable the aneurysms to be profiled in relation to the parent artery. In most instances, 3D TOF MR angiography has been most successful in identifying small intracranial aneurysms (3 to 5 mm in diameter or larger) in the region of the circle of Willis.[99, 100] In addition, 3D TOF techniques, using multiple, thin overlapping slabs[101] or ramped RF and MT, have improved the detection of aneurysms by improving visualization of slow flow.[102, 103]

An important factor in the detection of intracranial aneurysms by 3D TOF MR angiography is the TE. The complex flow patterns and shear stress encountered within intracranial aneurysms may lead to signal loss from intravoxel dephasing. The degree of signal loss from intravoxel dephasing can be reduced by shortening the TE and decreasing the voxel size.

Additional information regarding the flow dynamics of the aneurysm can be obtained by using phase-contrast techniques.[104] A useful approach is to obtain a 2D phase-contrast angiogram in a plane that profiles the aneurysm and parent vessel. This requires review of the the 3D TOF angiogram before the prescription of the phase-contrast slice. The V_{enc} of the phase-contrast angiogram can be selected to emphasize the inflow jet, the impact zone, or the slow vortex flow. Another advantage of the phase-contrast slab angiogram is that high-signal-intensity thrombus will not appear in the angiographic image, thus better delineating the residual lumen. In addition, time-resolved cine phase-contrast angiograms can be acquired to define variations in the size and configuration of the aneurysm during the cardiac cycle.[105] Occasionally, a portion of the aneurysm wall will bulge during systole, suggesting that this portion of the aneurysm wall may be more likely to rupture. Thus, phase-contrast angiography plays an important adjunctive role to 3D TOF MR angiography for the presurgical work-up of patients with intracranial aneurysms.

Vortex flow and stasis within lateral saccular aneurysms (Fig. 25–40) can be identified by concentric circles of variable signal intensity on 2D or cine phase-contrast images. The slow vortex flow results in the accumulation of platelets and leukocytes along the intimal surface, leading to thrombus formation, thickening of the aneurysm wall, and aneurysm growth rather than rupture.[106] Two main features of these aneurysms affect their appearance on phase-contrast MR angiographic flow studies. The first is that the flow velocity is greatest within the inflow jet and adjacent to the wall of the aneurysm. The maximal flow velocity and shear stress are not found at the dome of the aneurysm but at the neck. The second is that vortex flow and thrombus tend to occur in concentric layers. Terminal and bifurcation aneurysms have a more variable flow appearance with a distinct inflow jet and a high-stress impact zone. The impact zone experiences significant pulsatile force, and these lesions are more prone to rupture. Strother and coworkers[107] have also shown that the geometric relationship between an aneurysm and its parent artery is the principal factor that determines the intra-aneurysm flow pattern (Fig. 25–41).

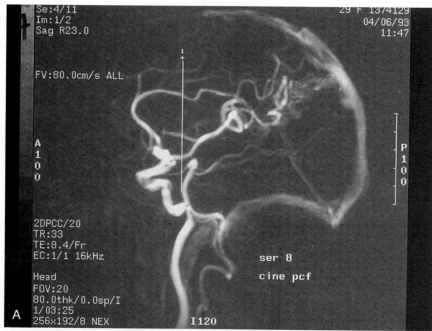

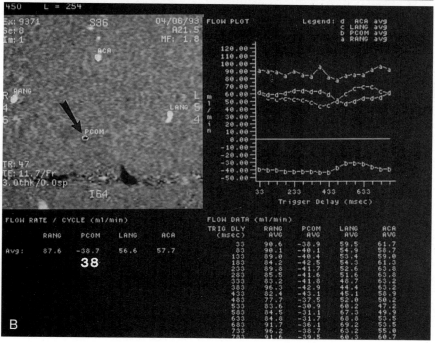

FIGURE 25–39. Right parietal AVM with flow analysis. *A,* A sagittal 2D phase-contrast slab image was obtained as a localizer before a cine phase-contrast examination. The vertical line indicates the location of the coronal cine phase-contrast slice. *B,* Velocity measurements were made through the right angular artery, the right posterior communicating artery, the left angular artery, and the anterior cerebral artery on the right. Note that there is reversed flow in the right posterior communicating artery *(arrow).* Volume flow rates were calculated for the same vessels. Note that the volume flow rate of the right angular artery of 87.6 mL/min was only modestly increased when compared with the left angular artery, which measured 56.6 mL/min. The reversed flow in the right posterior communicating artery measured 38.7 mL/min, indicating a shunt from the posterior to the anterior circulation.

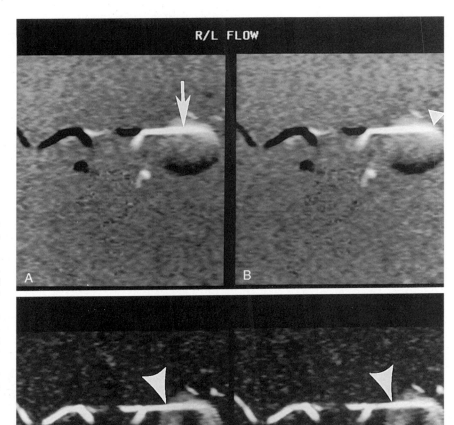

FIGURE 25–40. Giant middle cerebral artery aneurysm flow dynamics. *A* and *B,* Two systolic speed images are displayed from a coronal cine phase-contrast phase difference acquisition. Note the inflow jet *(arrow)* and vortex flow *(arrowhead)* associated with the giant aneurysm. *C* and *D,* The images for right to left flow display velocity as a function of pixel signal intensity. One can appreciate the high shear rate that occurs in the region of the inflow jet as a rapid change in pixel signal intensity. Note the impact zone along the superior lateral aspect of the aneurysm *(arrowhead).* (*A* to *D* from Turski P: Magnetic resonance angiography. In: Forbes G [ed]: Syllabus: Special Course in Neuroradiology. Oak Brook, IL: RSNA Publications, 1994.)

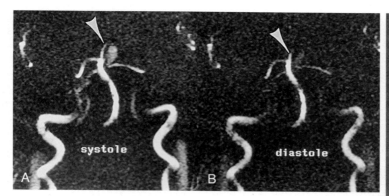

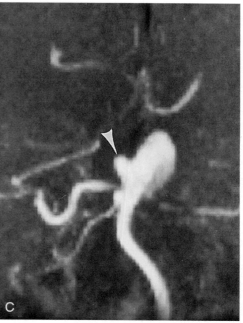

FIGURE 25–41. Basilar tip aneurysm. *A* and *B*, Coronal cine phase-contrast images obtained through the basilar tip aneurysm indicate that the impact zone of the inflow jet is maximal along the inferior right lateral aspect of the aneurysm *(arrowhead)*. Note that the flow continues to be prominent even during diastole. *C*, A subsequent 3D TOF MR angiogram obtained with MT shows the development of a daughter aneurysm at the site of the impact zone *(arrowhead)*. (*A* to *C* from Turski P: Magnetic resonance angiography. In: Forbes G [ed]: Syllabus: Special Course in Neuroradiology. Oak Brook, IL: RSNA Publications, 1994.)

VASOSPASM

Cerebral vasospasm is a severe complication of subarachnoid hemorrhage. Vasospasm may also be encountered in patients suffering from preeclampsia or eclampsia. Imaging of the intracranial circulation with 3D TOF MR angiography can be helpful in patients who are able to tolerate the MR examination. High-quality images and high-resolution techniques are capable of resolving vasospasm involving the M1, A1, and P1 segments of the anterior cerebral vessels. Particular care should be taken in the assessment of the supraclinoid internal carotid arteries where flow effects may result in artifactual loss of signal intensity. MR angiography also provides the opportunity to evaluate vessels serially with a noninvasive examination[108] (see also Chapter 23).

VENOUS DISEASES AND FLOW

VENOUS MALFORMATIONS

Venous malformations are common lesions characterized by small, radially oriented medullary veins that drain into a linear, subcortical venous trunk that courses to the cortex and empties into an enlarged, cortical vein on the brain surface. Venous malformations are interposed with normal brain tissue and, as isolated malformations, are rarely associated with hemorrhage unless there is thrombosis of the main draining venous trunk. Occasionally, mixed venous-cavernous malformations are encountered. In these instances, hemorrhage may be observed related predominantly to the cavernous component of the malformation.

The radially oriented medullary tributaries can be visualized on 3D TOF angiograms after intravenous injection of contrast material. Enhanced axial source images from the 3D TOF acquisition provide detailed images of the dilated medullary veins, adjacent brain structures, and venous drainage pathways (Fig. 25–42) (see Chapter 23).

VENOUS THROMBOSIS

Venous thrombosis may be difficult to clinically recognize due to the nonspecific nature of the symptoms

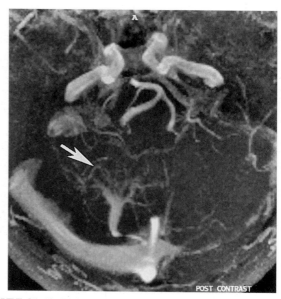

FIGURE 25–42. Right cerebellar venous angioma. The 3D TOF MR angiogram obtained after intravenous contrast enhancement reveals multiple, small, deep venous structures *(arrow)* coalescing into one large venous channel that drains into the torcular Herophili. (From Turski P: Magnetic resonance angiography. In: Forbes G [ed]: Syllabus: Special Course in Neuroradiology. Oak Brook, IL: RSNA Publications, 1994.)

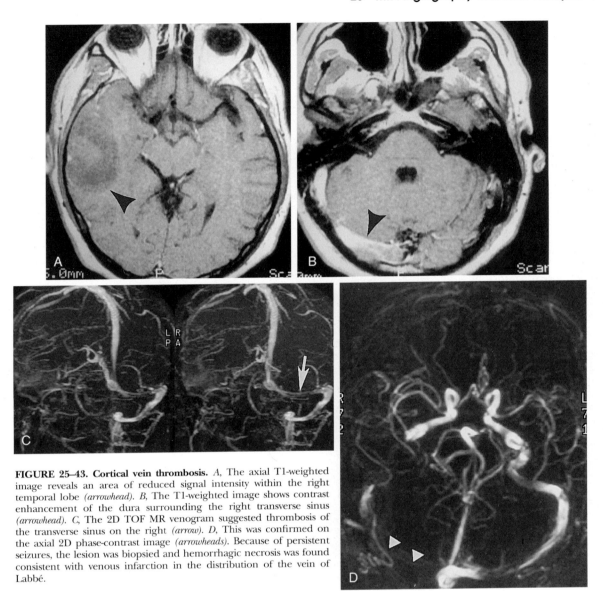

FIGURE 25–43. Cortical vein thrombosis. *A,* The axial T1-weighted image reveals an area of reduced signal intensity within the right temporal lobe *(arrowhead). B,* The T1-weighted image shows contrast enhancement of the dura surrounding the right transverse sinus *(arrowhead). C,* The 2D TOF MR venogram suggested thrombosis of the transverse sinus on the right *(arrow). D,* This was confirmed on the axial 2D phase-contrast image *(arrowheads).* Because of persistent seizures, the lesion was biopsied and hemorrhagic necrosis was found consistent with venous infarction in the distribution of the vein of Labbé.

and the variable severity of the patient's complaints.[109] Acute thrombosis of the cerebral venous system may give rise to a sudden increase in intracranial pressure, producing violent headache, convulsions, paralysis, and death. Patients with slowly developing or incomplete thrombosis frequently present only with the symptom of persistent severe headache. Occasionally, transverse sinus and internal jugular vein thromboses are incidentally identified on MR images with minimal clinical symptoms.[110] Cerebral venous thrombosis may occur from primary aseptic causes,[111] such as dehydration and hypercoagulable states, or secondary to a prior infectious process involving the soft tissues of the face, vascular structures, or meninges.[112] Because of the variable pattern of signal intensity that may be encountered within the normal and pathologic dural sinuses on spin-echo images, it is desirable to use an additional acquisition to further evaluate the venous structures. MR venographic techniques have gained rapid acceptance as fast and effective to confirm the diagnosis of venous thrombosis[113] (Fig. 25–43).

The most commonly used method is to create a 2D TOF venogram by acquiring 1.5- to 2.0-mm-thick slices in the oblique coronal plane. Approximately 110 slices are required to cover the entire intracranial venous system. A presaturation pulse is placed inferiorly to reduce the signal from arterial structures.[114]

A fast and perhaps more effective method for imaging blood flow within the dural sinuses is to obtain complex difference 2D phase-contrast slab images. The phase-contrast angiograms are made sensitive to venous flow rates by selecting a V_{enc} of 20 cm/s. A 4-cm-thick midline sagittal phase-contrast angiogram is obtained through the sagittal and straight sinuses. Clinically useful images that clearly demonstrate the dural sinuses can be obtained in approximately 3 minutes. The midline sagittal phase-contrast angiogram displays flow in the sagittal sinus as well as the internal cerebral veins, vein of Galen, and straight sinus.[115] After the sagittal acquisition, a second phase-contrast slab angiogram is acquired in the axial plane through the lateral sinuses and jugular veins. In this projection, the con-

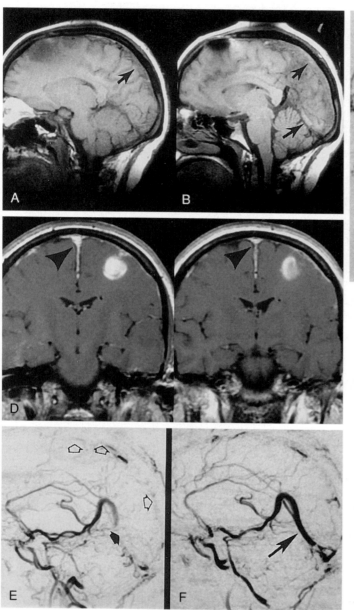

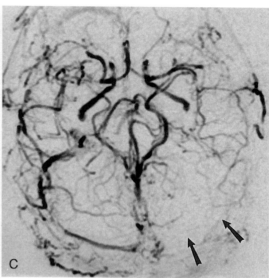

FIGURE 25–44. Sagittal sinus thrombosis. *A* and *B*, Sagittal T1-weighted images obtained during the acute phase reveal isointense thrombus *(arrows)* within the sagittal sinus. *C*, Complete thrombosis of the sagittal sinus and nearly complete thrombosis of the transverse sinus *(arrows)* are confirmed on the 2D phase-contrast image. *D*, Follow-up examination reveals marked enhancement of the dura surrounding the sagittal sinus and persistent thrombus within the sagittal sinus *(arrowheads)*. *E* and *F*, The initial and follow-up sagittal 2D phase-contrast images indicate partial recanalization of the straight sinus, *(short arrow* compared with *long arrow)*, but persistent thrombosis of the sagittal sinus *(open arrows)*.

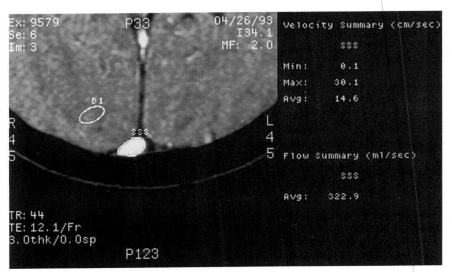

FIGURE 25–45. Superior sagittal flow analysis.
The 2D phase-contrast technique is nearly ideal for measuring flow in nonpul- satile vessels such as the cerebral venous system. In this example an axial 2D phase-contrast slice is obtained through the posterior aspect of the superior sagittal sinus. Flow at this location measured 322.9 mL/min.

fluence of the dural sinuses is well visualized, as are the transverse and sigmoid segments of the lateral sinus (Fig. 25–44).

Phase-contrast angiography has several desirable features that favor successful imaging of the dural sinuses. The phase-contrast angiograms are sensitive to flow in all directions, facilitating imaging of complex geometries such as the sigmoidal sinus. There is also better visualization of in-plane flow due to the subtraction of background tissue. Most importantly, high-signal-intensity thrombus is subtracted from the flow image along with the other stationary soft tissues. The result is an MR venogram that is sensitive to slow flow and displays only moving spins[116–118] (see also Chapter 24).

VENOUS FLOW MEASUREMENTS

Cine phase-contrast studies by Jordan and associates[119] have shown that the average flow in the dural sinuses can also be measured by obtaining a single nongated phase-contrast slice (Fig. 25–45). However, the flow values obtained with the cine phase-contrast and single-slice phase-contrast methods are lower than the previously reported mean flow value of approximately 420 mL/min measured by using bolus tracking techniques.[120] Peak velocities for the sagittal sinus ranged from 24 to 44.5 cm/s in this study. By using a combination of MR angiography and phase-contrast flow analysis techniques, it may be possible not only to determine the degree of venous compromise but also to quantitate the flow rate through the affected venous channel.

CONCLUSION

Through the application of noninvasive vascular imaging techniques, such as MR angiography, the care of patients with a variety of vascular lesions can be significantly enhanced. The safety of MR angiography will aid in its acceptance as the primary method to image the vascular system. The MR angiographic 3D data sets and ability to measure flow may one day give rise to multidimensional integrated examinations that display "form and function" of the vascular system.

REFERENCES

1. Napel S, Lee DH, Frayne R, Rutt BK: Visualizing three-dimensional flow with simulated streamlines and three-dimensional phase-contrast MR imaging. J Magn Reson Imaging 2:143–153, 1992.
2. Anderson CM, Edelman RR, Turski, PA: Clinical Magnetic Resonance Angiography. New York: Raven Press, 1993.
3. Potchen EJ, Siebert JE, Haacke EM, Gottschalk A: Magnetic Resonance Angiography. St. Louis: CV Mosby, 1993.
4. Mills C, Brant-Zawadzki M, Crooks L, et al: Nuclear magnetic resonance: principles of blood flow imaging. AJNR 4:1161–1166, 1983.
5. Wehrli F, MacFall J, Axel L, et al: Approaches to in-plane and out-of-plane flow imaging. Noninvasive Med Imaging 1:127–136, 1984.
6. Moran R: A flow velocity zeugmatographic interlace for NMR imaging in humans. Magn Reson Imaging 1:197–203, 1982.
7. Perman WH, Moran PR, Moran RA, Bernstein MA: Artifacts from pulsatile flow in MR imaging. J Comput Assist Tomogr 10:473–483, 1986.
8. Keller PJ, Drayer DP, Fram EK, et al: MR angiography with two dimensional acquisition and three dimensional display. Radiology 173:527–532, 1989.
9. Anderson CM, Saloner D, Tsuruda JS, et al: Artifacts in maximum-intensity-projection display of MR angiograms. AJR 154:623–629, 1990.
10. Patel MR, Klufas RA, Kim D, et al: MR angiography of the carotid bifurcation: artifacts and limitations. AJR 162:1431–1437, 1994.
11. De Marco JK, Nesbit GM, Wesbey GE, Richardson D: Prospective evaluation of extracranial carotid stenosis: MR angiography with maximum-intensity projections and multiplanar reformation compared with conventional angiography. AJR 163:1205–1212, 1994.
12. Atlas SW: MR angiography in neurologic disease. Radiology 193:1–16, 1994.
13. Urchuk S, Plewes D: Mechanisms of flow-induced signal loss in MR angiography. J Magn Reson Imaging 2:453–462, 1992.
14. Bowen, Quencer RM, Margosian P, Pattany PM: MR angiography of occlusive disease of the arteries in the head and neck: current concepts. AJR 162:9–18, 1994.
15. Tkach JA, Ruggieri PM, Ross JS, et al: Pulse sequence strategies for vascular contrast in time-of-flight carotid MR angiography. J Magn Reson Imaging 3:811–820, 1993.
16. Atkinson D, Brant-Zawadzki M, Gillan G, et al: Improved MR angiography: magnetization transfer suppression with variable flip angle excitation and increased resolution. Radiology 190:890–894, 1994.
17. Turski P, ed: Vascular Magnetic Resonance Imaging. 2nd ed. Volume 3 of General Electric Applications Guide. Waukesha, WI: GE Medical Systems, 1994.
18. Edelman RR, Ahn SS, Chien D, et al: Improved time of flight angiography of the brain with magnetization transfer contrast. Radiology 184:395–399, 1992.
19. Ding X, Tkach JA, Ruggieri PR, Masaryk TJ: Sequential three-dimen-

sional time-of-flight MR angiography of the carotid arteries: value of variable excitation and postprocessing in reducing venetian blind artifact. AJR 163:683–688, 1994.

20. Kerber CW, Liepsch D: Flow dynamics for radiologist. Practical considerations in the live human. AJNR 15:1076–1086, 1994.

21. Turski PA: Phase contrast angiography. In: Anderson CM, ed. Clinical Magnetic Resonance Angiography. New York: Raven Press, 1993, pp 43–71.

22. Haake EM, Smith AS, Lin W: Velocity quantitation in magnetic resonance imaging. Top Magn Reson Imaging 3:34–49, 1991.

23. Turski PA, Korosec F: Technical features and emerging clinical applications of phase contrast magnetic resonance angiography. Neuroimaging Clin North Am 2:785–800, 1992.

24. Pelc NJ, Bernstein MA, Shimakawa A, Glover GH: Encoding strategies for three-direction phase-contrast MR imaging of flow. J Magn Reson Imaging 1:405–413, 1991.

25. Wagle WA, Dumoulin CL, Souza SP, et al: 3DFT MR angiography of the carotid and basilar arteries. AJNR 10:911–919, 1989.

26. Bernstein MA, Ikezaki Y: Comparison of phase-difference and complex-difference processing in phase-contrast MR angiography. Magn Reson Imaging 10:725–729, 1991.

27. Enzmann DR, Marks MP, Pelc NJ: Comparison of cerebral artery blood flow measurements with gated cine and ungated phase-contrast techniques. J Magn Reson Imaging 3:705–712, 1993.

28. Dumoulin CL, Souza SP, Walker MF, et al: Time resolved magnetic resonance angiography. Magn Reson Med 6:275–286, 1988.

29. Spitzer CE, Pelc NJ, Lee JN, et al: Rapid MR imaging of blood flow with a phase-sensitive, limited-flip-angle, gradient recalled pulse sequence: preliminary experience. Radiology 176:255–262, 1990.

30. Spritzer CE, Pelc NJ, Lee NJ, et al: Preliminary experience with rapid MR flow imaging using a phase sensitive limited flip angle gradient refocused pulse sequence. Radiology 176:256–261, 1990.

31. Firmin DN, Nayler GL, Klipstein RH et al: In vivo validation of MR velocity imaging. J Comput Assist Tomogr 11:751–756, 1987.

32. Sommer G, Noorbehesht B, Pelc N, et al: Normal renal blood flow measurement using phase-contrast cine magnetic resonance imaging. Invest Radiol 27:465–470, 1992.

33. Evans AJ, Fumiharu I, Grist TA, et al: Magnetic resonance imaging of blood flow with a phase subtraction technique. Invest Radiol 28:109–115, 1993.

34. Dumoulin CL, Souza SP, Walker MF, et al: Three-dimensional phase-contrast angiography. Magn Reson Med 9:139–149, 1989.

35. Pernicone JR, Siebert JE, Potchen EJ, et al: Three-dimensional phase-contrast MR angiography in the head and neck: preliminary report. AJNR 11:457–466, 1990.

36. Bogren HG, Buonocore MH: Blood flow measurements in the aorta and major arteries with MR velocity mapping. J Magn Reson Imaging 4:119–130, 1994.

37. Sondergaard L, Ståhlberg F, Thomsen C, et al: Accuracy and precision of MR velocity mapping in measurement of stenotic cross-sectional area, flow rate, and pressure gradient. J Magn Reson Imaging 3:433–437, 1993.

38. Hamilton CA, Moran PR, Santago P II, Rajala SA: Effects of intravoxel velocity distributions on the accuracy of the phase-mapping method in phase-contrast MR angiography. J Magn Reson Imaging 4:752–755, 1994.

39. Tang CT, Blatter DD, Parker DL: Accuracy of phase contrast flow measurements in the presence of partial volume effects. J Magn Reson Imaging 3:377–385, 1993.

40. Adams RJ, Nichols FT, Hess DC: Normal values and physiologic variables. In: Newell DW, Aaslid R, eds. Transcranial Doppler. New York: Raven Press, 1992, pp 41–49.

41. Gosling RG, King DH: Arterial assessment by Doppler shift ultrasound. Proc R Soc Med 67:447–449, 1974.

42. Batjer HH, Purdy PD, Giller CA, et al: Evidence of redistribution of cerebral blood flow during treatment for an intracranial arteriovenous malformation. Neurosurgery 25:599–605, 1989.

43. Grolimund P, Seiler RW, Aaslid R, et al: Evaluation of cerebrovascular disease by combined extracranial and transcranial Doppler sonography. Experience in 1039 patients. Stroke 18:1018–1024, 1987.

44. Lindegaard KF, Bakke SJ, Grolimund P, et al: Assessment of intracranial hemodynamics in carotid artery disease by transcranial Doppler ultrasound. J Neurosurg 63:890–898, 1985.

45. Hangiadreou N, Rossman P, Riederer SJ: Analysis of MR phase contrast measurements of pulsatile velocity waveforms. J Magn Reson Imaging 12:387–394, 1993.

46. Marks MP, Pelc NJ, Ross MR, Enzmann DR: Determination of cerebral blood flow with a phase-contrast cine MR imaging technique: evaluation of normal subjects and patients with arteriovenous malformations. Radiology 182:467–476, 1992.

47. Mattle H, Edelman RR, Wentz KU, et al: Middle cerebral artery: determination of flow velocities with MR angiography. Radiology 181:527–530, 1991.

48. Enzmann DR, Ross MR, Marks MP, Pelc NJ: Blood flow in major cerebral arteries measured by phase-contrast cine MR. AJNR 15:123–129, 1994.

49. Marchal G, Bosmans H, McLachlan SJ: Magnetopharmaceuticals as contrast agents. In: Potchen EJ, Haacke EM, eds. Magnetic Resonance Angiography, Concepts and Applications. St. Louis: CV Mosby, 1993, pp 305–343.

50. Runge VM, Kirsch JE, Lee C: Contrast-enhanced MR angiography. J Magn Reson Imaging 3:233–239, 1993.

51. Haustein J, Laniado M, Niendorf HP, et al: Triple-dose versus standard-dose gadopentetate dimeglumine: a randomized study in 199 patients. Radiology 186:855–860, 1993.

52. Tu R, Kennell T, Turski P, et al: Preliminary assessment of gadodiamide-enhanced, complex-difference phase-contrast magnetic resonance angiography. Acad Radiol 1:S47–S55, 1994.

53. Lin W, Haacke EM, Smith AS, Clampitt ME: Gadolinium-enhanced high-resolution MR angiography with adaptive vessel tracking: preliminary results in the intracranial circulation. J Magn Reson Imaging 2:277–284, 1992.

54. Heiserman J, Drayer B, Fram E, et al: Carotid artery stenosis: clinical efficacy of two-dimensional time-of-flight angiography. Radiology 182:761–768, 1992.

55. Masaryk T, Obuchowski N: Noninvasive carotid imaging: caveat emptor. Radiology 186:325–331, 1993.

56. Polak JF, Bajakian RL, Oleary DH, et al: Detection of internal carotid artery stenosis: comparison of MR angiography, color Doppler sonography, and arteriography. Radiology 182:35–40, 1992.

57. Anderson C, Saloner D, Lee R, et al: Assessment of carotid artery stenosis by MR angiography: comparison with x-ray angiography and color-coded Doppler ultrasound. AJNR 13:989–1003, 1992.

58. Davis WL, Turski PA, Gorbatenko KG, Weber D: Correlation of cine MR velocity measurements in the internal carotid artery with collateral flow in the circle of Willis: preliminary study. J Magn Reson Imaging 3:603–609, 1993.

59. Rosen BR, Belliveau JW, Vevea JM, Brady TJ: Perfusion imaging with NMR contrast agents. Magn Reson Med 14:249–265, 1990.

60. Vanninen RL, Manninen HI, Partanen PLK, et al: Carotid artery stenosis: clinical efficacy of MR phase-contrast flow quantification as an adjunct to MR angiography. Radiology 194:459–467, 1995.

61. Ringelstein EB, Zeumer H, Angelou D: The pathogenesis of strokes from internal carotid occlusion. Diagnostic and therapeutic implications. Stroke 14:867–875, 1983.

62. Fisher M: Occlusion of the internal carotid artery. Arch Neurol Psychiatry 65:346–377, 1951.

63. Riggs HE, Rupp C: Variation in form of circle of Willis. Arch Neurol 8:24–30, 1963.

64. Pernicone JR, Siebert JE, Laird TA, et al: Determination of blood flow direction using velocity-phase image display with 3D phase-contrast MR angiography. AJNR 13:1435–1438, 1992.

65. Ringelstein EB, Otis SM: Physiologic testing of vasomotor reserve and collateral flow via the circle of Willis. In: Newell DN, Aasbid R, eds. Transcranial Doppler. New York: Raven Press, 1992, pp 83–100.

66. Mandai K, Sueyoshi K, Fukunaga R, et al: Acetazolamide challenge for three-dimensional time-of-flight MR angiography of the brain. AJNR 15:659–665, 1994.

67. Chong BW, Kerber CW, Buxton RB, Frank LR: Blood flow dynamics in the vertebrobasilar system: correlation of a transparent elastic model and MR angiography. AJNR 15:733–745, 1994.

68. Klingelhöfer J, Conrad B, Benecke R, Frank B: Transcranial Doppler ultrasonography of carotido-basilar collateral circulation in subclavian steal. Stroke 19:1036–1042, 1988.

69. Mohn JP, Caplan LR, Melski JW, et al: The Harvard cooperative stroke registry: a prospective registry of cases hospitalized with stroke. Neurology 28:754–762, 1978.

70. Wentz KU, Röther J, Schwartz A, Mattle HP: Intracranial veretebrobasilar system: MR angiography. Radiology 190:105–110, 1994.

71. Knepper L, Biller J, Adams, HP Jr, et al: MR imaging of basilar artery occlusion. J Comput Assist Tomogr 14:32–35, 1990.

72. Lévy C, Laissy JP, Raveau V, et al: Carotid and vertebral artery dissections: three-dimensional time-of-flight MR angiography and MR imaging versus conventional angiography. Radiology 190:97–103, 1994.

73. Bui LN, Brant-Zawadzki M, Verghese P, Gillan G: Magnetic resonance angiography of cerviocranial dissection. Stroke 24:126–131, 1993.

74. Turski P: Intracranial magnetic resonance angiography and stroke. In: Anderson C, ed. Clinical Magnetic Resonance Angiography. New York: Raven Press, 1993, pp 309–340.

75. Heiserman JE, Drayer BP, Fram EK: MR angiography of cervical fibromuscular dysplasia. AJNR 13:1454–1456, 1992.

76. Crosby D, Turski P, Davis W: Magnetic resonance angiography and stroke. Neuroimaging Clin North Am 2: 509–531, 1992.

77. Fugita N, Hirabuki N, Fujii K, et al: MR imaging of middle cerebral artery stenosis and occlusion: value of MR angiography. AJNR 15:335–341, 1994.

78. Johnson BA, Heiserman JE, Drayer BP, Keller PJ: Intracranial MR angiography: its role in the integrated approach to brain infarction. AJNR 15:901–908, 1994.

79. Davis WL, Blatter DD, Harnsberger HR, Parker DL: Intracranial MR angiography: comparison of single-volume three-dimensional time-of-flight and multiple overlapping thin slab acquisition techniques. AJR 163:915–920, 1994.

80. Yamada I, Suzuki S, Matsushima Y: Moyamoya disease: comparison of assessment with MR angiography and MR imaging versus conventional angiography. Radiology 196:211–218, 1995.

81. McCormick WF: Pathology of vascular malformations of the brain. In: Wilson CB, Stein BM, eds. Intracranial Arteriovenous Malformations. Baltimore: Williams & Wilkins, 1984, pp 44–63.

82. Yasargil MG: AVM of the Brain, History, Embryology, Pathology, Hemodynamics, Diagnostic Studies, Microsurgical Anatomy. New York: Georg Thieme, 1986.

83. Atlas SW: Intracranial vascular malformations and aneurysms. In: Atlas SW, ed. Magnetic Resonance Imaging of the Brain and Spine. New York: Raven Press, 1991, pp 379–409.

84. Martin N, Vinters H: Pathology and grading of intracranial vascular malformations. In: Barrow DL, ed. Neurosurgical Topics: Intracranial Vascular Malformations. Park Ridge, IL: American Association of Neurological Surgeons Publications, 1990, pp 2–31.

85. Marks MP, Lane B, Steinberg GK, Chang PJ: Hemorrhage in intracerebral arteriovenous malformations: angiographic determinants. Radiology 176:807–813, 1990.

86. Mukherji SK, Quisling RG, Kubilis PS, Finn JP: Intracranial arteriovenous malformations: quantitative analysis of magnitude contrast MR angiography versus gradient-echo MR imaging versus conventional angiography. Radiology 196:187–193, 1995.

87. Dawson RC III, Tarr RW, Hecht ST, et al: Treatment of arteriovenous malformations of the brain with combined embolization and stereotactic radiosurgery: results after one and two years. AJNR 11:857–864, 1990.

88. Betti OO, Munari C, Rosler R: Stereotactic radiosurgery with the linear accelerator: treatment of arteriovenous malformations. Neurosurgery 24:311–321, 1989.

89. Winston KR, Lutz W: Linear accelerator as a neurosurgical tool for stereotactic radiosurgery. Neurosurgery 22:454–464, 1988.

90. Dietz RR, Davis WL, Harnsberger HR, et al: MR imaging and MR angiography in the evaluation of pulsatile tinnitus. AJNR 15:879–889, 1994.

91. Turski P: MRA of vascular malformations. In: Anderson C, ed. Clinical Magnetic Resonance Angiography. New York: Raven Press, 1993, pp 247–288.

92. Hassler W, Burger R: Arteriovenous malformations. In: Newell DW, Aaslid R, eds. Transcranial Doppler. New York: Raven Press, 1992.

93. Wasserman BA, Lin W, Tarr RW, et al: Cerebral arteriovenous malformations: flow quantitation by means of two-dimensional cardiac-gated phase-contrast MR imaging. Radiology 194:681–686, 1995.

94. Kesava P, Baker E, Mehta M, Turski P: Preradiosurgery classification of AVM's using MRI, 3D TOF MRA, anatomic surface rendering and phase contrast flow analysis. In: Book of Abstracts. Annual Meeting of the American Roentgen Ray Society, Washington, DC, 1995.

95. Ruggieri PM, Poulos N, Masaryk TJ, et al: Occult intracranial aneurysms in polycystic kidney disease: screening with MR angiography. Radiology 191:33–39, 1994.

96. Teresi LM, Davis SJ: Cerebrovascular malformations. In: Stark DD, Bradley WG, eds. Magnetic Resonance Imaging. 2nd ed. St. Louis: Mosby–Year Book, 1992, pp 963–987.

97. Sundt TM Jr, Whisnant JP: Subarachnoid hemorrhage from intracranial aneurysms. Surgical management and natural history of disease. N Engl J Med 299:116–122, 1978.

98. Drake CG: Management of cerebral aneurysm. Stroke 12:273–280, 1981.

99. Huston J III, Nichols DA, Luetmer PH, et al: Blinded prospective evaluation of sensitivity of MR angiography to known intracranial aneurysms: importance of aneurysm size. AJNR 15:1607–1614, 1994.

100. Ronkainen A, Puranen MI, Hernesniemi JA, et al: Intracranial aneurysms: MR angiographic screening in 400 asymptomatic individuals with increased familial risk. Radiology 195:35–40, 1995.

101. Bladder DD, Parker DL, Sunskee A, et al: Cerebral MR angiography with multiple overlapping thin slab acquisition. Part II. Early clinical experience. Radiology 183:379–389, 1992.

102. Sevick RJ, Tsuruda JS, Schmalbrock P: Three dimensional time of flight MR angiography in the evaluation of cerebral aneurysms. J Comput Assist Tomogr 14:874–881, 1990.

103. Ross JS, Masaryk TJ, Modic MT, et al: Intracranial aneurysms: evaluation by MR angiography. AJNR 11:449–456, 1990.

104. Huston J, Rufenacht DA, Ehman RL, Wiebers DD: Intracranial aneurysms and vascular malformations: comparison of time of flight and phase contrast MR angiography. Radiology 181:721–730, 1991.

105. Tsuruda JS, Halbach VV, Higashida RT, et al: MR evaluation of large intracranial aneurysms using cine low flip angle gradient refocused imaging. AJNR 9:415–424, 1988.

106. Artman H, Vonofakos D, Muller H, Grau H: Neuroradiologic and neuropathologic findings with growing giant intracranial aneurysm: review of the literature. Surg Neurol 21:391–401, 1984.

107. Strother CM, Graves VB, Rappe A: Aneurysm hemodynamics: an experimental study. AJNR 13:1089–1095, 1992.

108. Ito T, Sakai T, Inagawa S, et al: MR angiography of cerebral vasospasm in preeclampsia. AJNR 16:1344–1346, 1995.

109. Schutta H: Cerebral venous thrombosis. In: Joynt R ed. Clinical Neurology, Volume 1. Philadelphia: JB Lippincott, 1991, pp 1–67.

110. Hullcelle PJ, Dooms GC, Mathurin P, et al: MRI assessment of unsuspected dural sinus thrombosis. Neuroradiology 31:217–221, 1989.

111. Kalbag RM, Woolf AL: Cerebral Venous Thrombosis. New York: Oxford University Press, 1967.

112. Southwick FS, Richardson EP, Swartz MN: Septic thrombosis of the dural venous sinuses. Medicine 65:82–106, 1986.

113. Vogl TJ, Bergman C, Villringer A, et al: Dural sinus thrombosis: value of venous MR angiography for diagnosis and follow-up. AJR 162:1191–1998, 1994.

114. Mattle HP, Wentz KN, Edelman RR, et al: Cerebral venography with MR. Radiology 178:453–458, 1991.

115. Rippe DJ, Boyko OB, Spritzer CE, et al: Demonstration of dural sinus occlusion by the use of MR angiography. AJNR 11:199–201, 1990.

116. Tsuruda JS, Shimakawa A, Pelc NJ, Saloner D: Dural sinus occlusions: evaluation with phase-sensitive gradient-echo MR imaging. AJNR 12:481–488, 1991.

117. Nadel L, Braun IF, Kraft KA, et al: Intracranial vascular abnormalities: value of MR phase imaging to distinguish thrombus from flowing blood. AJR 156:373–380, 1991.

118. Shulthess GK, Augustiny N: Calculation of T2 values versus phase imaging for the distinction between flow and thrombus in MR imaging. Radiology 164:549–554, 1987.

119. Jordan JE, Pelc NJ, Enzman DR: Velocity imaging and flow quantitation in the superior sagittal sinus and dural venous sinuses with ungated and cine gated 2D phase contrast MR. Presented at the 30th Annual Meeting of the American Society of Neuroradiology, St. Louis, 1992, p 58.

120. Mattle H, Edelman RR, Reis MA, Atkinson DJ: Flow quantification in the superior sagittal sinus using magnetic resonance. Neurology 40:813–815, 1990.

26

Diffusion and Perfusion MRI: Functional Brain Imaging

STEVEN WARACH

Magnetic resonance imaging (MRI) is well recognized as a diagnostic modality for identifying structural pathology of the brain. Development of methods for imaging aspects of brain physiology has generated much excitement because of the potential of providing diagnostic information about altered brain function in disease states as well as opening up the possibility of studying brain pathophysiology and higher cortical functions. MRI methods can measure various aspects of cerebral perfusion, the self-diffusion of water in the brain, and relative concentrations of brain metabolites. The latter is included in the discussions of MR spectroscopy and spectroscopic imaging in Chapter 30. The lack of ionizing radiation, greater spatial and temporal resolution, and more certain anatomic cross-registration are distinct advantages of functional MRI methods over older functional neuroimaging methods.

The possibility of obtaining functional information along with structural imaging has generated a great deal of interest and enthusiasm for the potential to improve diagnosis and guide therapies more objectively. This is especially true for ischemic stroke, the third leading of cause of death in the United States and the leading cause of long-term disability in the elderly, with an approximate cost to society of $30 billion per year.[1] Initial diagnosis in acute stroke may be in error in up to 30% of cases, even with the aid of computed tomography and conventional MRI.[2]

Accurate and early diagnosis is essential for the optimal design of clinical trials and, therefore, for the development and implementation of rational therapies to minimize the size of the infarction and reverse the vascular pathology. However, the accuracy of the initial bedside diagnosis of cerebral ischemia has been estimated to be 70% to 75% when compared with the final diagnosis, as determined by the progression of the illness and follow-up laboratory and radiologic studies.[3-5] The clinical course of stroke is highly variable, and large numbers of patients are needed for assessment of new forms of therapies if only clinical end points are used. Using the size of tissue damage as an end point has been impractical because there has been no method of identifying the extent of ischemic injury early in stroke, before initiation of therapy, to which the final infarct size can be compared. Furthermore, on clinical grounds alone, it is frequently impossible in the first hours after a patient presents to the physician to distinguish between an ischemic insult that will leave no fixed deficit and one that will cause permanent disability or death.

If only clinical end points are used, it is possible that true therapeutic effects of drugs may be overwhelmed by the variability in clinical outcome and lost in the statistical error. Pharmacologic therapies are aimed at protecting the brain from infarction; an effective therapy would therefore lead to smaller infarcts. Because severity of clinical deficit does not necessarily correlate with infarct size, clinical outcome is not the optimal method of evaluating the neuroprotective effect of a therapy. A better end point for the evaluation of therapeutic efficacy would be a quantitative measure of tissue injury. Until now, such a measure has not been practical because there has been no method of visualizing and thereby quantifying the volume of early ischemic injury before therapeutic intervention in humans. Drugs directed against various steps in the pathophysiologic development of ischemic neuronal injury have been shown to limit infarct size due to ischemic stroke in animal models, and these drugs are undergoing clinical trials. One of the rationales underlying the development of these drugs is the concept of the existence of an ischemic penumbra. The ischemic penumbra is an area of abnormal perfusion hypothesized to surround the central core of complete ischemia and infarction. This area is postulated to be at high risk for imminent infarction. The ischemic penumbra has never been conclusively demonstrated in patients with stroke, and therefore little is known about its relationship to the evolution of human stroke. A better understanding of the ischemic penumbra of human stroke may permit more accurate diagnosis and prognosis early in the course of the illness and may provide a more objective basis for deciding which patients are most likely to benefit from intervention. The central principle of the ischemic penumbra hypothesis is that within the region of ischemia (or oligemia) there are two distinct populations of neurons: 1) those in which energy failure has occurred, the first step in the cascade of molecular events leading to ischemic neuronal death; and 2) those in which energy-dependent ionic homeostasis is preserved. The potential of diffusion-weighted imaging (DWI) and perfusion imaging is that these techniques may provide more accurate early diagnosis, permit quantification of lesion volume, help define the ischemic penumbra, and identify thresholds of potentially reversible ischemic injury.

Other neurologic diseases such as Alzheimer's disease and epilepsy have associated perfusion abnormalities as seen with positron emission tomography (PET) and single photon emission computed tomography. MRI methods for diagnosis of perfusion abnormalities in these diseases would have the advantages of being obtained during the same session of routine diagnostic imaging, lack of ionizing radiation, superior spatial resolution, and easier cross-registration between anatomic and functional studies.

DIFFUSION-WEIGHTED IMAGING

BACKGROUND

In its most familiar usage, diffusion refers to the dispersion of molecules from a region of high concentration to one of low concentration by random molecular motion. DWI measures the self-diffusion of water, or the movement of water among other water molecules. This is due to the random molecular movement, or brownian motion, of the molecules. The rate of diffusion is determined by the kinetic energy of the particles and is therefore temperature dependent. In biologic tissue, diffusion is not truly random because structural constituents of the tissue (e.g., membranes) and chemical interactions of water with macromolecules present barriers to diffusion. Therefore, we refer to the self-diffusion of water in tissue as apparent diffusion. A detailed discussion of the physics of diffusion and its measurement by MRI is presented in Chapter 8. The general principle of measuring diffusion with MRI is the addition of a pair of strong gradient pulses to an otherwise standard pulse sequence, such that the first dephases the spins and the second completely rephases the spins if they have not moved in position. Where there is a net translation of protons in the time between the application of the two diffusion-sensitizing gradient pulses, their spins are not perfectly in phase and signal attenuation results. The degree of signal attenuation is related not only to the magnitude of the molecular translation but also to the strength of the diffusion weighting, described by the so-called b value. The b value is specific for the particular pulse se-

quence and is a function of the diffusion gradient strength (G), the duration of the diffusion gradient pulse (δ), and the time of the diffusion measurement (Δ), that is, the time between the leading edge of the two diffusion gradients. For most clinical applications the contribution to the b value of the other imaging gradients is considered negligible. For the example of measuring diffusion by a pair of bipolar diffusion gradients, the b value due to the diffusion gradients is equal to $\gamma^2 G^2 \delta^2 (\Delta - \delta/3)$, where γ is the gyromagnetic ratio of hydrogen. Calculation of the diffusion coefficient, or in tissue more accurately termed the *apparent diffusion coefficient* (ADC), requires a minimum of two acquisitions of different b values. The ADC is the negative slope of the regression line fitting b versus the natural log of the signal intensity (Fig. 26–1). The accuracy of the ADC measurement is therefore related to both the range and the number of b values used for measurement. For two b values, ADC $= \ln(SI_2/SI_1)/(b_1 - b_2)$. The two limiting factors in DWI are the maximal gradient strength of the imaging system and the ability to avoid or correct for artifacts due to brain and head motion.

The contrast on strongly diffusion-weighted images is determined primarily by the differential signal attenuation from various tissue types. This depends to some extent on the signal intensity without attenuation from the strong diffusion gradients, but in general, at high b values, regions of lower ADC appear hyperintense relative to regions of higher ADC. Normal brain parenchyma therefore appears more intense than fluid-filled spaces (ventricles, watery cysts), but less intense than acute ischemic infarctions, which have reduced diffusion. Synthetic images of ADC may also be created by calculating the ADC on a pixel-by-pixel basis. In the ADC maps, regions of higher ADC appear hyperintense relative to regions of lower ADC. Contrast in

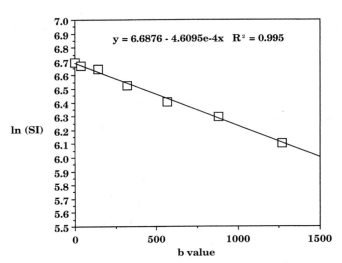

FIGURE 26–1. The apparent diffusion coefficient (ADC) of brain is the negative slope of the regression line best fitting the points of b value versus the natural log of the signal intensity ln(SI). In this example taken from a patient with a 2-hour-old ischemic stroke, the ADC = 4.6095×10^{-4} mm²/s. The goodness of fit of this curve has an R² of 0.995.

DWI and ADC maps may also depend on the direction along which the diffusion gradient is applied. ADC is lower in the direction of the applied diffusion gradient in which fewer barriers are encountered (e.g., parallel to the long axis on axonal bundles) and is higher where more barriers are encountered.[5a] This diffusion anisotropy may be exploited to study the normal anatomy as well as white matter disease. Anisotropy can be minimized by imaging the trace of the diffusion tensor.[6–8] In practice, diffusion trace imaging may be accomplished by averaging images obtained with diffusion gradient directions applied in three orthogonal planes.

CLINICAL DIFFUSION IMAGING

The first report of DWI in animals was in 1984.[9] This was soon followed by early results showing changes in diffusion contrast and ADC in various neurologic diseases.[10–12] A number of reports of case series followed, indicating the potential diagnostic utility of DWI in a variety of neurologic conditions.

Arachnoid cysts can be differentiated from epidermoid tumors because the former have high ADC, characteristic of cerebrospinal fluid, whereas the latter have lower ADC, characteristic of solid tissue.[13] Components of brain tumors may be distinguishable with DWI.[14] Cystic and necrotic portions of the tumors have the highest ADC, and tumor in areas that enhance with gadolinium on T1-weighted images has the lowest ADC.

In one report of 10 patients with pseudotumor cerebri, the diffusion coefficient of brain was increased both globally and periventricularly, suggestive of increased extracellular water edema due to transependymal flow of water from the ventricles into the parenchyma.[15]

In multiple sclerosis, a higher ADC has been observed in acute and chronic plaques than in the patients' normal-appearing white matter, which was observed to have higher ADC than normal white matter in control subjects.[16] The authors of this study suggested that the latter result is evidence that even normal-appearing white matter of patients is abnormal. The higher ADC in plaques was attributed to tissue loss from demyelination and edema.

Because diffusion is temperature dependent, mapping regional differences in brain temperature with DWI has been proposed[17–19] and demonstrated to be sensitive to detecting differences as little as 0.2°C in phantoms. ADC measurements in rat brain vary directly with body temperature,[20] and ADC is decreased with hypothermia.[21]

Anisotropic DWI has been used to study the development of myelination[22–24] and the orientation of white matter tracts in the human brain.[25–30]

ISCHEMIC STROKE (see Chapter 24)

The greatest interest in the clinical use of DWI has been in its application to cerebral ischemia. The dis-

covery by Moseley and coworkers[31–33] that experimental ischemia causes a drop in ADC within minutes and a distinct region of hyperintensity in diffusion-weighted images that closely correlated the localization of infarcts seen on postmortem histopathologic studies[34] has generated a great deal of excitement. It was obvious that DWI had enormous potential for improving understanding of ischemic pathophysiology, improving the accuracy of clinical diagnosis in ischemic stroke, and aiding the development of effective therapies in stroke. This observation of hyperacute DWI intensity of experimental ischemic lesions and decreased ADC has been replicated in numerous laboratories, using different types of animal models and various imaging techniques.[8, 35–48]

Studies of patients with acute stroke have been difficult for several practical reasons. The technique is sensitive to net translational movements due to causes other than diffusion. Small brain movements due to cardiac and respiratory pulsations[49] or involuntary head movements degrade image quality and affect ADC calculations. These artifacts may be reduced with cardiac and respiratory gating as well as with the use of navigator echoes,[50, 51, 51a] but larger, voluntary head movements are not well compensated for by these strategies, and navigator echoes are most effective when the diffusion gradient is applied along the phase-encoding direction. It is essential that the patient voluntarily remain still for the duration of the data acquisition. The nature of the acute illness in this elderly population renders many patients unable to cooperate because of cognitive deficits, emotional agitation, or comorbid medical conditions. Head restraints and pharmacologic sedation are of limited usefulness in this population because of ineffectiveness in controlling voluntary movements or medical contraindication. On the basis of our experience, my colleagues and I estimate that approximately one third of patients with acute stroke with moderate or severe acute deficits are unable to cooperate adequately for diffusion measurements if the acquisition times are greater than 5 to 10 minutes. Fast imaging methods are needed for the DWI to be widely applicable for these patients. The patient with subacute or chronic stroke is generally more cooperative, and measurements have been achieved using acquisition methods that take longer.[11, 12, 52] The results for ADC in these subacute and chronic cases were variable but tended to increase over time and were clearly elevated chronically.[52]

Warach and colleagues reported the first successful DWI of patients with hyperacute stroke[53] using a turbo stimulated-echo acquisition mode (turboSTEAM) method[54] on a conventional clinical imager at 1.5 T with gradient strengths of 9 mT/m applied in all three directions. Using a b value of 357 s/mm² relative to no diffusion weighting, acute lesions were identified as early as 105 minutes after onset. DWI demonstrated cerebral infarcts in 32 patients at various times after the onset of ischemic symptoms and revealed the regions of ischemic injury sooner than conventional T2-weighted spin-echo imaging; four hyperacute infarcts were shown only by DWI. Acute infarcts had significantly lower ADC than noninfarcted regions by 34% in the first 12 hours, 49% from 12 to 24 hours, and 42% from 24 to 48 hours. This relative difference rose progressively thereafter. Two cases are illustrated in Figures 26–2 and 26–3. Chronic infarcts showed a relative increase in ADC and were readily distinguishable from acute infarcts (Fig. 26–4). Although the results were promising, several technical limitations were apparent. The moderate b value seemed to underestimate the apparent size of the hyperacute lesion in DWI. Patients' head motions were frequent, even on this sample preselected for cooperativity, and degraded the images. A single-slice acquisition time (a prepulse succeeded by four averaged turboSTEAM acquisitions) for each b value was 27 seconds. A complete multislice survey of the brain was impractically long, given the need for standard imaging, patients' uncooperativeness, and the demands of acute stroke management. These problems were since overcome by the use of stronger gradients and echo-planar imaging (EPI).

DWI using EPI has been accomplished and is well suited to the study of ischemic stroke.[35, 55] Single-shot EPI permits whole-brain multislice imaging to be completed in several seconds, and the stronger gradients required by EPI allow for higher b values. This has now been accomplished for acute human stroke.[56] DWI of the entire brain could be completed in 3 seconds, or using seven different b values (maximal b = 1271 s/mm^2) in 48 seconds. Early ischemic lesions were identified with DWI as hyperintense regions of decreased ADC in all patients who subsequently developed infarction, before changes were evident with conventional MRI in cases studied earlier than 6 hours after onset of ischemic symptoms (Figs. 26–5 to 26–7). Lesions as small as 4 mm in diameter were identified. Acute lesions were seen in white matter as well as gray matter and in the brain stem and cerebellum as well as in the cerebral hemispheres. The extent of lesions within white matter was best defined by controlling for the anisotropic effect of axonal orientation (Fig. 26–8). The mean ADC ($\pm$ standard deviation) for control regions in the 36 patients was 0.92 ($\pm$ 0.29) $\times$ 10^{-3} mm^2/s. The mean ADC of ischemic regions was 56% of control values at 6 hours or less and stayed significantly reduced for 3 to 4 days after onset of ischemia. The relative ADC increased progressively over time to be pseudonormalized at 5 to 10 days and elevated in the chronic state, making the distinction of acute infarcts adjacent to chronic infarcts readily apparent (Figs. 26–9 and 26–10). Thus, in two different samples of stroke patients and using two different techniques, the

hyperacute lesions had a 40% to 50% decrease in ADC and a similar evolution to chronic elevation over time.

In patients with severe clinical deficits, a lesion in DWI has been associated with little clinical recovery, whereas no lesion is associated with spontaneous recovery.[56] In several cases spontaneous regression of the lesion on DWI was observed along with clinical improvement. This has been found for small lesions of presumed cardioembolic source in which, it is presumed, spontaneous reperfusion has occurred. For large lesions seen only in DWI within the first 6 hours, inevitable evolution into fixed lesions occurred on T2-weighted and T1-weighted imaging.

Except for the relatively unusual circumstance in which a lesion regresses and clinical deficits resolve, the rise in ADC toward control values over the first several weeks does not represent a true normalization of tissue diffusion but the combination of several pathologic processes. As can be readily appreciated by the increased signal intensity in proton density–weighted and T2-weighted imaging at these times, the brain is abnormal and an infarct is present and evolving. This early approach toward control ADC values may be termed a *pseudonormalization*, an inevitable point in the transition of decreased ADC acutely to increased ADC chronically. This observation points out that one cannot interpret the direction of diffusion change by using only a diffusion-weighted image without knowledge of the T2-weighted imaging (b = 0) or calculation of the ADC. The presence of increased T2-weighted signal intensity with normal ADC, subacutely, indicates that the tissue is not normal. Increased signal intensity (hyperintensity) may be seen in DWI in areas of increased diffusion if the T2-weighted image is sufficiently hyperintense. Signal characteristics and ADC values typical at each stroke stage are listed in Table 26–1.

Although all lesions displayed decreased diffusion acutely, there was variability within and between lesions, especially at later times. Within lesions there was heterogeneity of ADC, contributing to variability in the measurements.

The biophysical basis of the reduced ADC in acute ischemia is a matter of considerable debate. The emerging consensus is that it is directly related to a reduction in extracellular volume and an increase in intracellular volume. Cells swell early after ischemia, presumably reflecting intracellular accumulation of sodium and water, and the ADC of water measured with MRI is decreased.[32, 57, 58] The hyperacute decrease in diffusion does not reflect change in water content of

TABLE 26–1. SIGNAL CHARACTERISTICS AND APPARENT DIFFUSION COEFFICIENT TYPICAL AT EACH STROKE STAGE

STAGE	T2-WEIGHTED IMAGE	DIFFUSION-WEIGHTED IMAGE	APPARENT DIFFUSION COEFFICIENT
Hyperacute (0–6 h)	Normal	Increased	Decreased
Acute (6–48 h)	Normal to increased	Increased	Decreased
Subacute (3–10 d)	Increased	Increased	Decreased to normal
Chronic	Increased	Decreased to increased	Increased

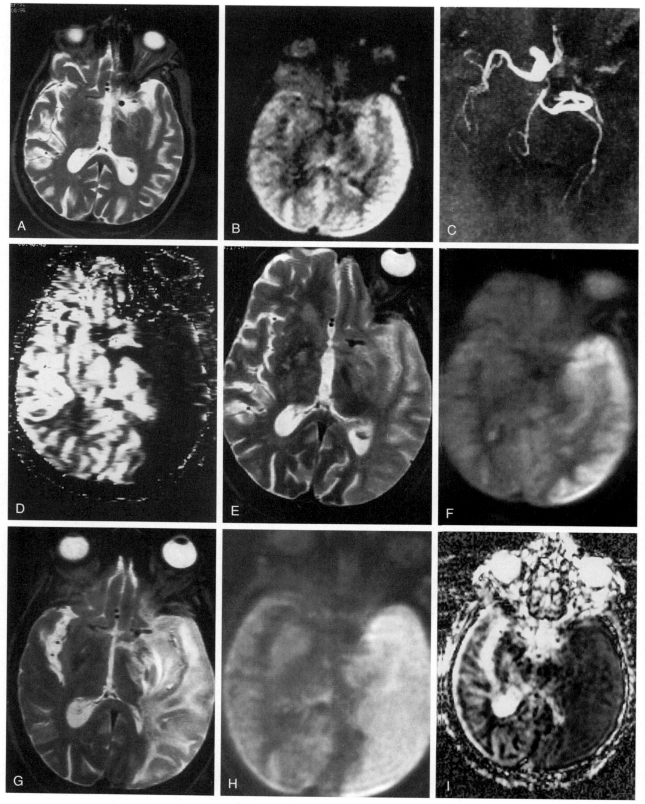

FIGURE 26–2 *See legend on opposite page*

the lesion in the first few hours because there is no increase in signal intensity on proton density–weighted or T2-weighted imaging,[44, 56, 59] and, therefore, because there is a change in the relative size of the intracellular and extracellular compartments of water, there must be associated a change in the distribution of water: from extracellular to intracellular. In animal models of stroke, there is an evolution in the onset and volume of lowered diffusion over time, with the diffusion hyperintensity exceeding the lesion on T2-weighted images for as much as 12 hours,[32, 34, 60] and anisotropy of diffusion even within acute ischemic lesions is preserved.[60] The size of the diffusion lesion has been reported to increase in the first 48 hours after experimental stroke,[38] and we have observed in stroke in humans that many lesions continue to evolve in size even beyond 2 days. Whether the hyperacute drop in ADC in this region is due to an increased intracellular fraction of water, decreased fraction of a relatively less restricted extracellular space, increased tortuosity of the extracellular space leading to greater restriction to diffusion, reduced membrane permeability to water, or some combination of these factors remains to be determined. Many studies of DWI in experimental stroke in animal models have provided insights into ischemic pathophysiology and the development of drugs to block or reverse ischemic neuronal injury and reveal the potential of DWI for applications to stroke patients.

The hypothesis originally put forward by Moseley that the hyperacute decrease in ADC is associated with cytotoxic edema[32] has been supported by a number of lines of evidence, and it is generally accepted that the hyperacute diffusion changes occur, along with a reduction in extracellular volume and an increase in intracellular volume. Electrical impedance is increased in acute stroke, consistent with decreased extracellular space.[61] Simultaneous ADC measurements and electrical impedance measurements of ischemic tissue have confirmed that the ADC drop is associated with a decrease in extracellular space.[62] There is evidence that restricted diffusion occurs in both normal and ischemic brain and that the drop in ADC in ischemic

tissue may be explained by more restricted diffusion, because the diffusion coefficient in ischemic and normal tissue does not increase as diffusion time increases beyond 50 ms[60]; if unrestricted, diffusion would increase with increasing diffusion times. In determining the true extent of an acute ischemic lesion into the white matter, images representing the trace of the diffusion tensor (the average of three diffusion images with orthogonal diffusion directions) provide a much more accurate delineation of affected area than images representing the diffusion in only one direction by minimizing anisotropic effects.[8, 56]

Within minutes after the onset of ischemia in experimental models, there is a decrease in diffusion by 40% to 50%.[33, 36, 57] Theoretically, this could be due to a drop in brain temperature or to a direct effect of decreased perfusion by a contribution to the diffusion measurement or by a reduction in brain pulsations, respectively. These other effects have been proved not to significantly contribute to the ADC drop by the elegant experiments of Davis and coworkers,[57] who measured ADC every 10 seconds after the induction of focal or global cerebral ischemia and found a 1- to 2-minute lag between the onset of ischemia and the diffusion decrease and also that the magnitude of the ADC decline exceeds that which could be accounted for by the associated drop in temperature. During these first minutes of ischemia-induced diffusion decrease there is an associated decrease (approximately 40%) in the activity of the energy-requiring Na^+,K^+-ATPase that maintains ionic gradients.[58] ADC does not decrease until tissue perfusion falls below levels known to be critical for maintenance of Na^+,K^+-ATPase activity.[36] After 60 minutes of ischemia not only was Na^+,K^+-ATPase activity decreased, but water content and sodium concentration were increased, and potassium concentration was decreased in the ischemic hemisphere.[58] A topographic coincidence was demonstrated between changes on diffusion images, the pattern of histologic damage, adenosine triphosphate (ATP)–depleted areas, and local tissue acidosis.[47] A decrease in diffusion comparable to that induced by ischemia may also be reproduced by intraparenchymal

FIGURE 26–2. T2-weighted, turboSTEAM diffusion-weighted (b = 357 s/mm²), and dynamic blood volume images from a 68-year-old woman 105 minutes, 13 hours, and 9 days after she suffered a sudden onset of global aphasia, right-sided hemiplegia, and right homonymous hemianopsia from which she never recovered. *A*, T2-weighted image at 105 minutes shows no parenchymal lesion in the left hemisphere. *B*, Diffusion-weighted image at 105 minutes demonstrates hyperintensity in the cerebral cortex of the left hemisphere relative to the right. Relative ADC was 0.60. *C*, A single-slab three-dimensional time-of-flight MR angiogram demonstrated absence of flow throughout the intracranial portion of the left internal carotid artery. *D*, Relative blood volume map using dynamic contrast enhancement and susceptibility-weighted imaging with a fast low-angle shot (FLASH) sequence demonstrates hypoperfusion throughout the left middle cerebral artery territory. *E*, T2-weighted image at 13 hours shows early changes (increased signal intensity) of evolving parenchymal lesion in the left hemisphere. *F*, Diffusion-weighted image at 13 hours demonstrates greater degree of hyperintensity in the area of evolving infarct. Relative ADC was 0.40. *G*, T2-weighted image at 9 days shows the fully evolved infarct. *H*, Diffusion-weighted image at 9 days demonstrates a matching area of hyperintensity. *I*, ADC map at 9 days shows decreased ADC, with relative ADC 0.60. (*A, B*, and *E* to *H* from Warach S, Chien D, Li W, et al: Fast magnetic resonance diffusion-weighted imaging of acute human stroke. Neurology 42:1717–1723, 1992.)

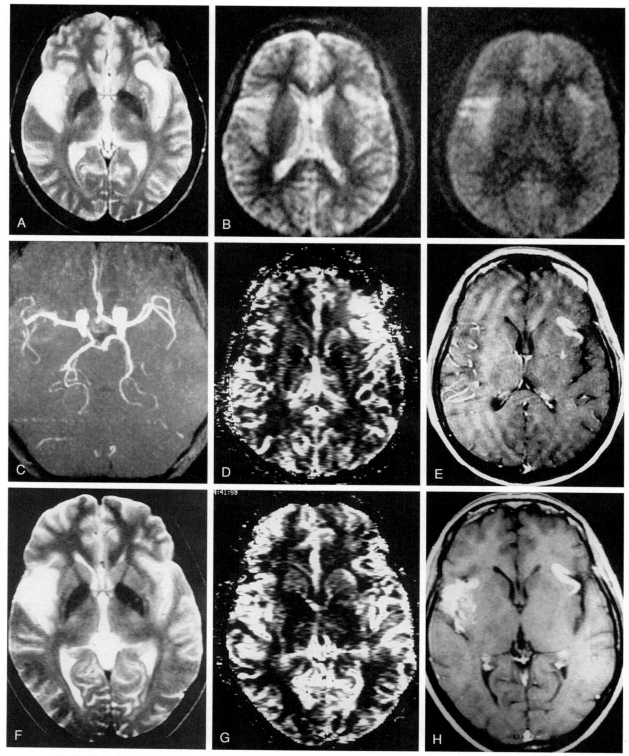

FIGURE 26–3. *A,* T2-weighted image from a patient with acute (12 hours) and subacute (1 week) infarcts in the right (acute) and left (subacute) peri-insular regions. *B,* TurboSTEAM images with no diffusion weighting or diffusion weighting (b = 357 s/mm²) showing hyperintensities greater in acute than subacute lesions. *C,* A three-dimensional time-of-flight MR angiogram suggests reduced flow through the insular branches of the right middle cerebral artery. *D,* Relative blood volume map using dynamic contrast enhancement and susceptibility-weighted imaging with a FLASH sequence demonstrates hypoperfusion in the acute (right) infarct and hyperperfusion of the subacute (left) infarct. *E,* Postcontrast T1-weighted image showing gyriform enhancement in the subacute infarct. Intravascular enhancement is seen in the arterial supply to the acute infarct. *F,* T2-weighted image 1 week later. *G,* Relative blood volume map demonstrates normalization of perfusion in both infarcts. *H,* Postcontrast T1-weighted image showing gyriform enhancement in both subacute infarcts.

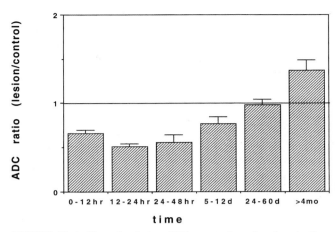

FIGURE 26–4. Plot of relative ADC versus time for the six time groups of 32 patients using turboSTEAM. Error bars represent the standard error of the mean of the group means. The unity line signifies no difference between lesion and control. Note that the relative ADC is decreased in the earliest four groups, lowest at 12 to 24 hours, and increased for the chronic group. (From Warach S, Chien D, Li W, et al: Fast magnetic resonance diffusion-weighted imaging of acute human stroke. Neurology 42:1717–1723, 1992.)

infusions of oubain, an inhibitor of Na+,K+-ATPase, and by infusions into the brain of glutamate or *N*-methyl-D-aspartate, mediators of ischemic neurotoxicity.[63] The hyperacute decrease in ADC is therefore considered to be a marker of failure of Na+,K+-ATPase activity in response to cerebral ischemia. The significance of the decreased ADC as a marker of energy failure is that it may permit the definition of the ischemic penumbra: an area of reduced perfusion sufficient to cause potentially reversible clinical deficits but insufficient to cause disrupted ionic homeostasis due to Na+,K+-ATPase failure[64, 65] or ADC decrease.[36] In other words, combined perfusion and diffusion imaging may identify the penumbra as a region of symptomatic hypoperfusion that has normal diffusion. Transient decreases in ADC have been seen during depolarizations associated with acute ischemic injury,[66] which may also be a marker for spreading depression.[67] The number of these peri-infarct depolarizations has been associated with evolution of infarction. Observations in animal models support the idea that combined DWI and perfusion imaging can delineate the core and penumbra of stroke. There is delayed evolution of infarction in territories where the perfusion defect is less severe.[68] In a model of stenosis, ADC decrease and infarction were associated with the greatest reductions in perfusion, whereas surrounding areas of variable degrees of hypoperfusion were associated with variable and lesser degrees of ADC decrease.[45] The study of Busza and colleagues[36] most convincingly demonstrates the relationship of perfusion thresholds to ADC decrease: diffusion-weighted images remained unchanged until cerebral blood flow was reduced to 15 to 20 mL/100 g/min and below, after which hyperintensity increased in DWI as cerebral blood flow was lowered further.

In general, there is a correspondence of the area of acute ADC decrease and postmortem histopathology.[31,]

[34, 40, 41, 44, 47, 69] Histologically, the increase in ADC as the infarct evolves to the chronic state progresses from edema to gliosis to cyst formation.[70] In the core of the infarct, the ADC becomes elevated when electron microscopy reveals cellular lysis.[71]

There is variability of ADC decrease with an infarct, and evolution to infarction is predicted by more severe decreases in ADC or an increase in proton density.[41, 44] Much work has been directed toward demonstrating the reversibility of ischemic lesions on DWI, with reperfusion or pharmacologic manipulations, and in identifying thresholds of irreversibility. Substantial resolution of DWI lesions without evolution of infarction has been demonstrated with early (1 hour or less) reperfusion.[34, 69] Areas of reversibility appear less intense on DWI,[69] and thresholds of reversibility in the rat have been estimated to be either less than 0.55×10^{-5} cm^2/s[72] or a reduction of greater than 0.25×10^{-5} cm^2/s relative to the contralateral hemisphere.[73] In studies of global ischemia, animals without recovery of ADC exhibited global depletion of ATP and glucose and severe lactic acidosis, whereas animals with recovery of ADC showed replenishment of ATP and glucose to near control and a substantial reversal of lactic acidosis.[48]

Reversal of ischemia in animal models sufficiently early causes reversal of the diffusion decrease that is not greater than a threshold value and prevents infarction.[34, 73] Hypothermia during reperfusion causes a more rapid normalization of ADC.[21] Antagonists of *N*-methyl-D-aspartate receptors[62, 74] or calcium influx,[75–78] mediators of ischemic neurotoxicity, and early reperfusion[34, 73, 79] in animal models may cause reversal of some diffusion-weighted abnormalities, often in excess of 50% of lesion size if therapy begins sufficiently early.

Experimentally induced conditions other than acute ischemia have been demonstrated to cause decreases in ADC. These include experimental status epilepticus (14% to 18% reduction)[80] and hyponatremia.[81] DWI has been reported to distinguish traumatic from ischemic brain lesions; the former displayed increased ADC.[82] Cerebral ischemia is the only condition in humans in which reduced ADC has been observed.

PERFUSION IMAGING

In the broadest sense, brain perfusion refers to one or more of various aspects of cerebral blood flow. Parenchymal blood flow is the ratio of cerebral blood volume to the transit time of blood through the tissue. The different techniques of perfusion MRI typically deal with blood volume, transit times, and blood flow as *relative* measures. The theoretic basis and methodologic details of MRI perfusion techniques are described in Chapter 8. In brief, the two perfusion strategies that have found applicability to clinical conditions and scientific questions are based either on induced changes in intravascular magnetic susceptibility or on tagging inflowing arterial spins.

The susceptibility-based techniques use either injected paramagnetic contrast agents or endogenous

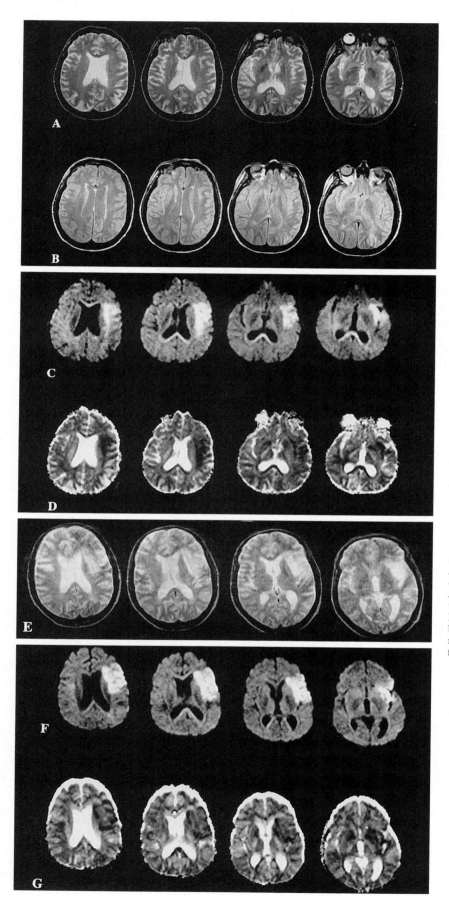

FIGURE 26–5. Three-hour infarct shown by EPI multislice DWI. *A,* T2-weighted images 3 hours after stroke onset show no acute infarct (four slices); a small chronic hemorrhagic infarct is present at the left parieto-occipital junction. *B,* Proton density–weighted images 3 hours after stroke onset show no acute infarct. *C,* Diffusion-weighted images 3 hours after stroke onset show extensive DWI hyperintensity indicative of acute ischemic injury and reduced ADC. *D,* ADC map at 3 hours shows reduced ADC in acute lesion as darker areas. The ADC at the core of the lesion was 4.45×10^{-4} mm²/s, and in the control contralateral region it was 8.17×10^{-4} mm²/s; the ADC ratio is therefore 0.54. Darker areas distant from the stroke reflect in part anisotropic diffusion in white matter. Eight days after onset T2-weighted images *(E),* diffusion-weighted images *(F),* and ADC map *(G)* show the extent of the lesion. The conventional T2-weighted images at 8 days are compromised by motion artifact, which did not affect the diffusion-weighted images. Note that on the ADC map at 8 days a darker rim of low ADC surrounds the infarct, which displays the pseudonormalization of the ADC that occurs at this time (ADC in the core is 0.96 of control). At any given time the state of the brain must be evaluated by T2-weighted imaging, DWI, and ADC measurements to adequately characterize the disease. (*A* to *G* from Warach S, Gaa J, Siewert B, et al: Acute human stroke studied by whole brain echo planar diffusion-weighted magnetic resonance imaging. Reprinted with permission from Ann Neurol 37:231–241, 1995.)

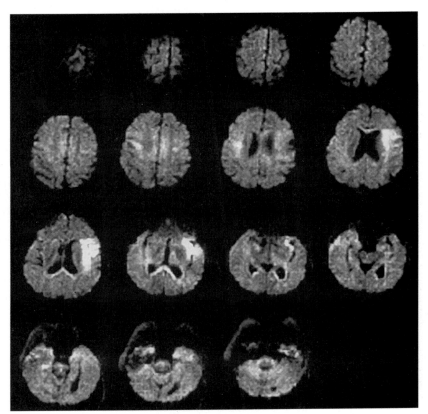

FIGURE 26–6. Multislice imaging permits definition of full extent of lesion volume. Heavily diffusion-weighted image 3 hours after stroke (same patient as in Fig. 26–2) shows the diffusion abnormality as hyperintensity in 15 contiguous 7-mm-thick slices. The total time for acquisition was approximately 3 seconds.

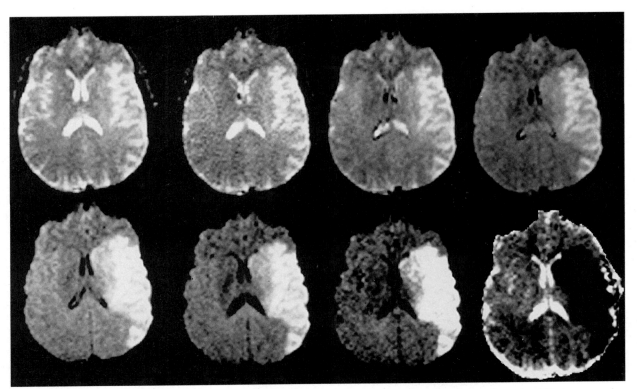

FIGURE 26–7. EPI DWI 12 hours after stroke from a left internal carotid artery occlusion shows the diffusion abnormality as hyperintensity in 10 contiguous 7-mm-thick slices. Diffusion sensitivity at one transverse slice position (b values 0, 35, 141, 318, 565, 883, and 1271 s/mm²) increases from upper left to right. In the lower right is a synthetic ADC map. Note that with no diffusion weighting (T2-weighted echo-planar image) little abnormality is seen, but as diffusion sensitivity increases, the lesion stands out from the surrounding tissue as relatively hyperintense. The ADC map shows the acute infarct as the dark area representing decreased diffusion (ADC = 4.77×10^{-4} mm²/s; ADC is 62% of contralateral control region). (From Warach S, Gaa J, Siewert B, et al: Acute human stroke studied by whole brain echo planar diffusion-weighted magnetic resonance imaging. Reprinted with permission from Ann Neurol 37:231–241, 1995.)

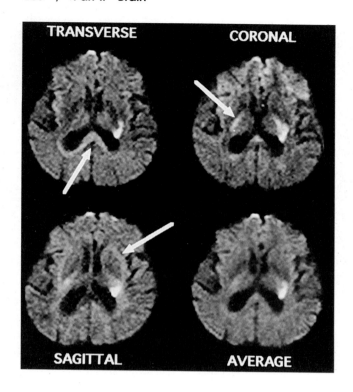

FIGURE 26–8. Anisotropic diffusion-weighted image defines boundary of white matter lesions. Seven-hour lesion is evident in the left internal capsule with diffusion gradients applied in transverse, coronal, and sagittal directions. White matter tracts oriented perpendicularly to the orientation of the diffusion gradient appear relatively hyperintense *(arrows)*, whereas those parallel to the diffusion gradient appear isointense or hypointense. The hyperintensity of the ischemic lesion is present regardless of direction of diffusion gradient, but its boundary blends in with the hyperintensity due to axonal anisotropy. The average of the DWI from the three diffusion directions produces a diffusion image relatively free of anisotropy. Hyperintensity at the inferior frontal poles at the top of this image is caused by susceptibility artifact. (From Warach S, Gaa J, Siewert B, et al: Acute human stroke studied by whole brain echo planar diffusion-weighted magnetic resonance imaging. Reprinted with permission from Ann Neurol 37:231–241, 1995.)

changes in the concentration in an intrinsic paramagnetic molecule—deoxyhemoglobin—to induce intravascular susceptibility changes related to brain perfusion. Deoxygenation increases magnetic susceptibility within the erythrocytes and thus creates local field gradients around these cells. Diffusion of water through these field gradients with increasing blood deoxygenation causes dephasing and loss of signal intensity.[83, 84] The latter technique, the so-called blood oxygen level–dependent (BOLD) technique, depends not only on flow changes but also on a mismatch between flow changes and changes in oxygen extraction ratio. The applications of BOLD are discussed later in the context of functional localization.

Dynamic contrast-enhanced susceptibility-weighted perfusion imaging, also referred to as contrast agent bolus tracking,[33, 85, 86] may be used to image signal changes due to relative differences in cerebral blood volume. The susceptibility differences induced by paramagnetic agents set up local magnetic field gradients in the tissue, and diffusion of water through these gradients leads to a loss of phase coherence and thus a decrease in signal intensity in the tissue surrounding the vessels. The amount of signal loss can be quantified and is directly proportional to cerebral blood volume in normal brain. The quantifiable variable of interest is $\Delta R2^*$, which is equal to $-\ln(S_i/S_o)/TE$, where $\Delta R2^*$ is defined as $\Delta(1/T2^*)$ as a result of contrast infusion. S_o is the precontrast signal intensity and S_i is the signal intensity at time t_i. The sum of $\Delta R2^*$, $\Sigma \Delta R2^* \; \Delta t$, for

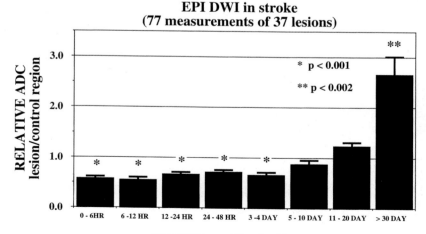

FIGURE 26–9. Mean ADC ratio (ADCR; lesion/control) at time from onset after stroke. The ADC is reduced by 56% early in the course and rises progressively over time, approaching symmetry at 5 to 10 days and elevated chronically. Analysis of variance with time as the between group factor was significant at $P < .001$ $F(7,68) = 25.80$. In the earliest five time groups up to and including 3 to 4 days the ADCR is significantly reduced (comparison of mean versus 1.0 by one-tailed Student's t-test gives $P < .001$, symbolized by * in the graph). In the chronic group the ADCR is elevated (one-tailed t-test, $t_{(df = 7)} = 7.11$, $P < .002$, symbolized by ** in the graph). (From Warach S, Gaa J, Siewert B, et al: Acute human stroke studied by whole brain echo planar diffusion-weighted magnetic resonance imaging. Reprinted with permission from Ann Neurol 37:231–241, 1995.)

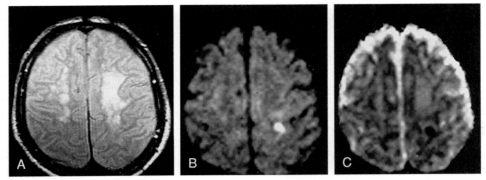

FIGURE 26–10. Diffusion-weighted image distinguishes acute from chronic lesions. *A,* Proton density–weighted image 22 hours after onset of weakness of the right hand demonstrates extensive areas of hyperintensity throughout the left hemisphere. *B,* DWI readily distinguishes the small lesion near the left central sulcus from surrounding areas of chronic changes. *C,* ADC map confirms that the acute lesion has reduced ADC (dark) and that chronic vascular changes in white matter have elevated ADC relative to contralateral tissue. (*A* to *C* from Warach S, Gaa J, Siewert B, et al: Acute human stroke studied by whole brain echo planar diffusion-weighted magnetic resonance imaging. Reprinted with permission from Ann Neurol 37:231–241, 1995.)

all of the images in the series (assuming the time between images, Δt, is sufficiently short) is a value known to be proportional to cerebral blood volume in healthy brain tissue.[87] Analysis of images may be done qualitatively or quantitatively. Qualitatively, the images can be viewed as a cine loop to observe the relative drops in signal intensity or are postprocessed, subtracting or dividing the enhanced images from the precontrast images such that signal intensity is directly related to blood volume (hyperintense). Using a spin-echo sequence and R2 calculations may preferentially measure changes associated with small and medium-sized arteries.[87a] By estimating the arterial input function from signal changes in proximal arteries, tissue blood volume and blood flow may potentially be quantified.[87b]

Blood flow imaging with MRI by spin labeling of the arterial input to a slice has the appeal that it is completely noninvasive, is a more direct assessment of cerebral blood flow, and potentially may generate absolute quantification. Cerebral blood flow quantification has been accomplished by continuous adiabatic inversion of arterial spins.[88, 89] The theoretic basis of this technique has been detailed in Chapter 8. Qualitative mapping of cerebral blood flow has also been described using EPI, a single inversion pulse to inflowing arterial spins, and subtraction of tagged and untagged EPI images.[90] This technique, termed EPI signal targeting with alternating radiofrequency (EPISTAR) has been used for both clinical applications and functional localization (Fig. 26–11).

Dynamic contrast-enhanced susceptibility weighting has been used to define and study the regions of ischemia in animal models of stroke, wherein, compared with normally perfused brain, the degree of signal reduction is markedly less within minutes of ischemia due to reduced blood volumes, before changes in T2-weighted images.[31, 33, 69, 91, 92] As discussed earlier, complete to near-complete ischemia corresponds to an acute hyperintensity on DWI, but partial decreases in perfusion are associated with normal diffusion. Early reperfusion is associated with reversal of

a large proportion of the lesion in DWI. Oxygenation changes in the brain during apnea can be characterized using BOLD imaging.[93]

CLINICAL PERFUSION IMAGING

Clinical perfusion imaging has been described in various neurologic conditions,[94, 95] including cerebral infarctions, arteriovenous malformations, and brain tumors using a fast low-angle shot (FLASH) sequence on a conventional 1.5-T imager. The method is used to particular advantage with EPI,[96, 97] which has superior temporal resolution, allowing for more accurate concentration-time curves, and multislice imaging capabilities. Three-dimensional bolus tracking using a frequency-

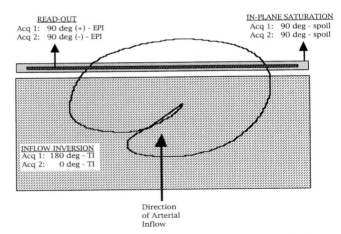

FIGURE 26–11. EPISTAR technique. The 180° tagging pulse is applied during alternate acquisitions. The presaturation pulse is applied to the plane of section during each EPI acquisition. The untagged acquisition is subtracted from the tagged acquisition to produce relative maps of cerebral blood flow. Details of the pulse sequence are described in the text. (From Edelman RR, Siewert B, Darby DG, et al: Qualitative mapping of cerebral blood flow and functional localization with echo-planar MR imaging and signal targeting with alternating radiofrequency. Radiology 192:513–520, 1994.)

shifted BURST sequence on a conventional 1.5-T scanner has also been described.[98]

Several promising clinical applications of perfusion imaging have been described. In ischemic infarction, dynamic relative cerebral blood volume mapping reveals well-demarcated decreases in perfusion and $\Delta R2*$ in areas of infarction.[59, 94, 95, 99] In one study of acute infarcts, dynamic contrast-enhanced T2*-weighted MRI and MR angiography were used to evaluate cerebral blood volume and the intracranial arterial system in 34 patients within 48 hours after the onset of cerebral ischemia.[59] A single-slice FLASH technique was used on a 1.5-T clinical imager. In 24 of the cases an abnormality on T2-weighted spin-echo images was identified that corresponded to the acute clinical deficit. Intracranial MR angiography demonstrated occlusions or severe stenoses of major vessels supplying the area of infarction in 16 of these 24 cases. MR angiography showed acute arterial occlusions or stenoses of the internal carotid, middle cerebral stem and branches, basilar, and posterior cerebral arteries but could not show small branch vessel occlusions. Decreased blood volume (observed on dynamic scans as less signal reduction relative to normal tissue after bolus injection of gadolinium diethylenetriaminepentaacetic acid [Gd-DTPA]) correlated well with MR angiographic abnormalities. In 15 of the 16 cases with MR angiographic lesions, decreased blood volume was observed by qualitative examination of the images. In these 16 cases, the mean rate ($\pm$ SEM) of the area under the curve for T2* change, $\Sigma\Delta R2*$ dt, previously shown to be proportional to cerebral blood volume in healthy brain tissue, was 0.018 ± 0.004 less ($P < .001$) in the area of infarction than in normal control regions of the same brain. The mean transit time to peak signal reduction after bolus injection was 4.03 ± 1.45 seconds delayed in the area distal to the arterial occlusion ($P = .014$). Areas of decreased blood volume were more apparent and more extensive than the lesion on T2-weighted spin-echo images in two cases of internal carotid occlusion (5 hours, 16 hours) and two cases of middle cerebral artery occlusion (6 hours, 11 hours). In two cases of large infarction more than 40 hours old, an area of blood volume abnormality could be seen to match the T2-weighted lesion, although the MR angiogram was normal. Infarcts less than 2 cm in diameter were not reliably shown by MR angiography or blood volume studies. In conclusion, there was good correlation between lesions with MR angiography and decreased blood volume in acute infarcts, and both techniques demonstrated lesions early in the clinical course. More recently, multislice EPI has been used to study acute infarcts with dynamic contrast-enhanced T2*-weighted imaging. The greater sensitivity of EPI permits investigation of the entire ischemic area and an evaluation of the ischemic penumbra[100] (Fig. 26–12).

Dynamic blood volume imaging of patients with brain tumors has been accomplished and may provide unique information about tumor grade and vascularity that is not appreciated from conventional T2-weighted or gadolinium-enhanced T1-weighted imaging[94, 95,] [97, 101–103] (Figs. 26–13 to 26–15). The relationship between relative cerebral blood volume and tumor type and grade has been shown most convincing by Aronen and associates[101] in 19 cases of histologically examined gliomas. Relative cerebral blood volume was directly related to tumor grade, with the highest relative cerebral blood volume values associated with mitotic activity and vascularity, but not with cellular atypia, endothelial proliferation, necrosis, or cellularity.

It is known from radionuclide imaging that active epileptic foci cause increased cerebral blood flow at the site of the foci. MRI using a FLASH sequence and dynamic contrast enhancement with gadolinium demonstrated relative hyperperfusion of the right temporoparietal cortex in a patient in focal status epilepticus. A single photon emission computed tomography scan also demonstrated hyperperfusion of the right temporoparietal cortex. Perfusion MRI, single photon emission computed tomography, and the electroencephalogram (EEG) normalized when the seizures ended.[104] Focal increases in BOLD signal intensity using FLASH were observed during partial motor seizures in a 4-year-old boy. MRI revealed activation associated in the contralateral hemisphere with each of five consecutive clinical seizures, and also during a period that was not associated with a detectable clinical seizure. The activity was associated with abnormal cortical structures.[104]

FUNCTIONAL LOCALIZATION OF BRAIN ACTIVITY

The first functional localization of normal brain activity with MRI was described by Belliveau and coworkers[105] in 1991 using dynamic contrast-enhanced T2*-weighted imaging with EPI and simple visual stimulation. They showed increases in blood volume in calcarine cortex during visual stimulation. This was soon followed by reports of noninvasive functional localization of primary sensory and motor tasks[106–108] using EPI at 1.5 T[106, 107] with BOLD imaging[106, 107] and cerebral blood flow imaging using inversion tagging of arterial inflow[106] or gradient-echo imaging at 4.0 T without EPI.[108]

This relatively new field has generated an enormous amount of excitement because localization with functional MRI offers better spatial and temporal resolution, more straightforward anatomic registration of results, less expense, and greater availability than PET functional neuroimaging and without radiation exposure. The activity has focused on technical developments as well as using the techniques to localize brain functions.

The initial study by Belliveau and coworkers[105] accomplished the functional localization using gadolinium injections and EPI at 1.5 T. Functional localization has also been demonstrated using bolus tracking of gadolinium with FLASH imaging.[109, 110] In addition to BOLD imaging with EPI at 1.5 T and gradient-echo imaging at 4.0 T, BOLD functional MRI has been accomplished without EPI, using gradient-echo sequences,[111, 112] spin-echo or fast spin-echo sequences[113]

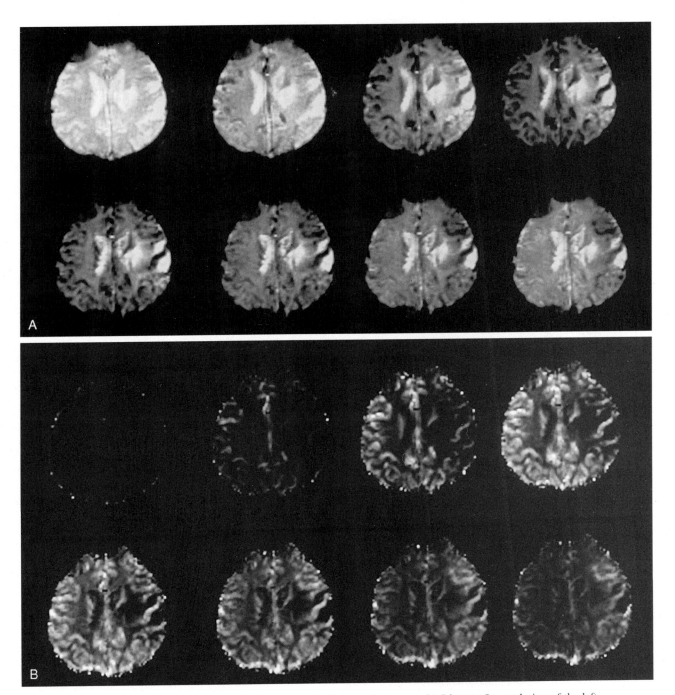

FIGURE 26–12. EPI dynamic blood volume mapping in acute human stroke 2 hours after occlusion of the left middle cerebral artery. *A*, Eight gradient-echo EPI images (echo time of 60 ms) after an intravenous bolus injection of a gadolinium-containing contrast agent (Gd-DTPA). Each image is acquired in approximately 100 ms, and they are 2 seconds apart from upper left to right. Darkened images show reduced signal intensity due to the passage of gadolinium and are related to blood volume. *B*, Images as in *A* but processed into relative blood volume ($\Delta R2^*$) maps. Brighter areas display increased blood volume. Note core of complete absence of blood volume in region of left hemisphere (right side of image) and delayed flow surrounding the core, suggestive of an ischemic penumbra.

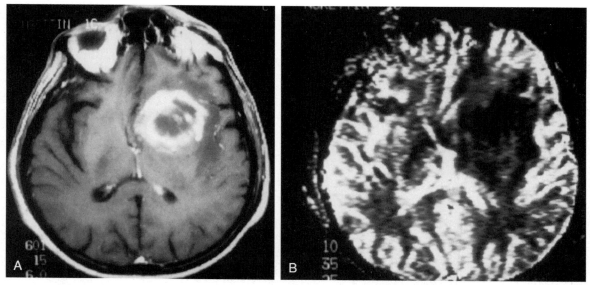

FIGURE 26–13. Glioma shown on postcontrast T1-weighted image *(A)* with hypoperfusion of mass and surrounding edema *(B)* using dynamic contrast enhancement and susceptibility-weighted imaging with a FLASH sequence for relative blood volume mapping.

on conventional 1.5 T scanners, and EPI at 4 T.[114] A three-dimensional BOLD acquisition using an echo-shifted FLASH sequence has also been described, in which a three-dimensional data set may be collected in 20 seconds.[98] The arterial spin tagging technique EPISTAR has been used for functional localization by detecting local increases in relative cerebral blood flow.[90]

BOLD signal changes increase with field strength.[115] Although much variability exists among subjects and studies, the percent BOLD signal intensity increase is typically 2% to 5% at 1.5 T and up to 20% to 30% increase at 4.0 T.

As previously discussed, the BOLD effect is attributed to increased venous oxyhemoglobin that results from a functional increase in cerebral blood flow that exceeds tissue oxygen extraction. There is a well-recognized latency of several seconds between the onset of a stimulus and a functional increase in signal intensity in BOLD images. A rapid small decrease in BOLD signal intensity has been discovered to occur within the first 500 ms after stimulus onset.[116] This fast negative

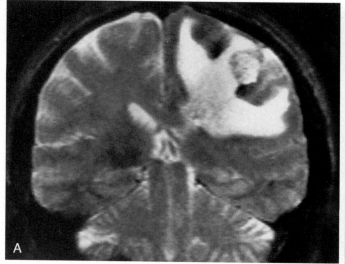

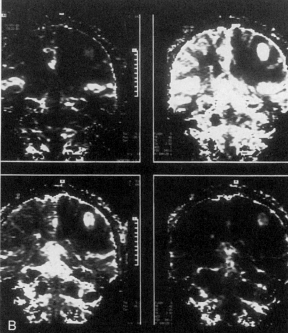

FIGURE 26–14. *A,* Metastatic brain tumor shows mass with surrounding edema on T2-weighted image. *B,* With dynamic contrast-enhanced susceptibility-weighted imaging with FLASH, the mass is hyperperfused and a surrounding region of hypoperfusion is seen in the area of edema.

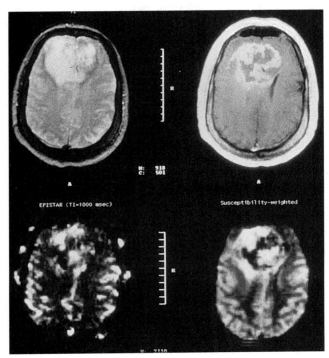

FIGURE 26–15. Glioblastoma multiforme on T2-weighted image *(upper left)*, postcontrast T1-weighted image *(upper right)*, EPISTAR relative blood flow map *(lower left)*, and relative blood volume map by dynamic contrast-enhanced susceptibility-weighted imaging with EPI *(lower right)*.

response has been attributed to increased oxygen consumption, followed by a slower vascular response with overcompensation in blood oxygenation to give the familiar increased signal intensity on BOLD images after several seconds. This hypothesized basis for the functional BOLD response is supported by optical imaging data, which indicate that 200 to 400 ms after neuronal activity local oxygen utilization increases, followed 200 to 400 ms later by an increase in blood volume, and then less than 1000 ms after that by an increase in oxyhemoglobin.[117]

High-resolution BOLD imaging correlated with high-resolution MR angiography has demonstrated that the source of the signal change at 1.5 T is almost always from susceptibility changes in surface cortical veins.[118] These observations are the central issue in the so-called brain versus vein debate: Does the functional change in BOLD localize to cortex or to draining veins on the surface of the brain and in sulci? This question is important only to the extent that precise anatomic localization is necessary. For many questions gross localization seems sufficient, especially given the tradition of approximate localization that is the norm in literature on PET. Ultimately, the potential of MRI for high spatial resolution will attract scientific questions in need of precise localization.

In addition to the brain versus vein debate, there is controversy as to what extent signal changes in BOLD images are due to oxygenation changes versus inflow effects.[119, 120] Although there may be both inflow and oxygenation changes detectable with BOLD imaging,

the changes due to T2* relaxation are probably dominant.[118, 121, 122] Parenchymal signal changes, as opposed to large surface veins, may be favored by spin-echo or asymmetric spin-echo methods at 1.5 T, but with a reduction in the magnitude of the functional response,[123, 124] or by longer echo times of gradient-echo sequences at higher fields.[125]

In principle, inflow techniques are theoretically more appealing because they depend only on a functional increase in cerebral blood flow, whereas the BOLD effect depends on both a cerebral blood flow increase and a mismatch in the relationship of cerebral blood flow increase with oxygen extraction ratio. This relationship has not been well established for subcortical regions or for different developmental stages. In other words, techniques that look at flow directly are one step closer to neuronal activity and avoid the brain versus vein dilemma. Kwong[125a] used selective and nonselective inversion pulses to demonstrate functional increases in flow. Edelman and associates[90] found this as well with EPISTAR, generating functional cerebral blood flow maps, analogous to PET (Fig. 26–16). The latter technique has been used to study functional principles of the human motor cortices, and the results have closely matched results from cerebral blood flow imaging by PET.[125b] Differences in BOLD and EPISTAR activation are under investigation, but preliminary evidence suggests that the former is more sensitive to changes, both from movement artifact and stimulus related, whereas the latter displays more task-specific signal changes and better contrast.

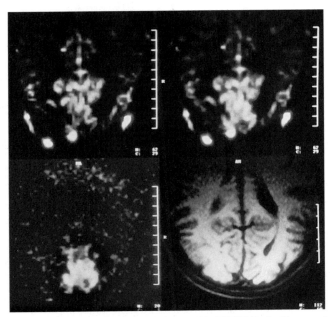

FIGURE 26–16. Functional activation with EPISTAR. As illustrated in the turboFLASH image in the lower right, the images were acquired in a plane parallel to the calcarine sulcus. In the upper left is the EPISTAR image without stimulation. In the upper right is the EPISTAR image during full-field flashing (8 Hz) lights. Note the increase in signal intensity in the occipital cortex. In the lower left is the difference of stimulation minus rest, illustrating the region of increased cerebral blood flow with this visual activation.

Methods of statistical analysis of functional localization experiments were discussed in detail in Chapter 8. The most appropriate analyses for EPI time series experiments are techniques that cross-correlate the presence or absence of stimulus with signal change. These techniques are done with either parametric or nonparametric statistics.[126, 127]

Initial validations of functional MRI techniques for functional localization involved simple sensory or motor tasks. Replications of experiments similar to those reported in the literature on functional neuroimaging by PET have been reported. Motor cortex has been investigated with regard to distribution of contralateral versus ipsilateral activation and the interaction with handedness[128, 129] and the involvement of primary and nonprimary motor cortex in actual and imagined movements.[130, 131] Language functions have also been investigated using a word activation task,[132] silent word generation,[133, 134] or auditory stimuli.[135] Changes have also been localized in association with visual imagery.[136] New insights into brain function and localization have begun to emerge from functional MRI literature. Response to a simple visual stimulation was greater in a group of schizophrenic patients than in control subjects.[137]

Simultaneous recording of an EEG during EPI and triggering a BOLD acquisition to an EEG event have been accomplished.[138] By careful selection and arrangement of analog multiplexed cable-telemetry equipment to eliminate both ferrous materials and radiofrequency interference, a stable, readable EEG can be obtained without interfering with the image quality of the MRI. In some subjects, an exaggerated ballistocardiogram artifact is seen on the EEG recording, but this rarely renders the tracing unreadable. We use gold or silver surface electrodes connected to a preamplifier-multiplexor unit that rests just outside the head coil. The unit connects to a cable that plugs into a box attached to the magnet room and by fiberoptics conducts the signal to a demultiplexor and EEG recorder that sits next to the scanning console. In this way, EEG events can be manually or potentially automatically used to trigger an EPI sequence, thereby time locking the EEG event to a functional response in the brain. This technical capability permits more accurate neurophysiologic control during the acquisition of echo-planar functional MRI studies. This combination of modalities will aid functional localization in epilepsy and sleep and may permit functional localization of cognition-related EEG potentials. BOLD imaging has been used for functional localization as part of neurosurgical planning and agreed with subsequent intraoperative recordings.[139]

BOLD signal increase has also been observed after injection of acetazolamide, presumably because of increased cerebral blood flow without an increase in oxygen utilization.[140] It is well established that cerebral blood flow increases directly with the partial pressure of carbon dioxide in arterial blood ($Paco_2$). This effect has also been observed in BOLD signal intensity.[141] Thus, studies of functional localization with BOLD must optimally control for the variability in signal intensity due to $Paco_2$, either by measuring and corrected for $Paco_2$ on an image-by-image basis or by covarying global signal intensity in the overall analysis.

SODIUM IMAGING

Sodium has been suggested to be an alternative nucleus to protons for obtaining different information about biologic systems. The reduced sensitivity of sodium imaging, relative to that of protons, is due to the lower biologic concentration and its intrinsic nuclear properties of lower gyromagnetic ratio and quadripolar character. These characteristics have meant long acquisition times to obtain images of limited spatial resolution. Important biologic information is potentially available from the sodium image. Because the ability of a cell to maintain ion homeostasis is a measure of its viability, the sodium MRI signal can be used to monitor quantitative changes in cell density and cell viability.[142–144] Such interpretations have applications in following therapy in oncology, in which the goal is to selectively kill tumor cells, and for monitoring interventions in cerebrovascular disease and stroke, in which the goal is to preserve brain tissue.

To realize such applications, a method that can produce high-quality sodium images at 1.5 T in 20 minutes was developed by Thulborn and colleagues at the University of Pittsburgh Medical Center.[144–146] This method combines a custom-designed, quadrature detection mode, volume radiofrequency coil with a special three-dimensional acquisition scheme that allows efficient coverage of k-space with minimal T2* signal loss and an efficient reconstruction algorithm. An example of the images obtained with a human volunteer is shown in Figure 26–17. With the development of high-field systems, imaging times can be expected to be less than 10 minutes.

CONCLUSIONS

In summary, functional MRI, and particularly localization studies, have generated an enormous amount of enthusiasm, fueled greatly by the relative ease of performing a functional MRI experiment. This enthusiasm must be tempered by the knowledge that the applications, results, and interpretations are not as straightforward as they may seem to the uninitiated. Several fundamental issues are unresolved: the basis of the signal change, sources of and solutions for artifact, the problem of precise localization, and the appropriate statistical analyses. As this technology is handed over from physicists and radiologists to basic and clinical neuroscientists, there is a welcome move afoot to establish a consensus across laboratories regarding experimental design and analysis. Such consensus not only will improve communication and reliability across laboratories but also will serve as a foundation for the inevitable technical innovations that are always right around the corner.

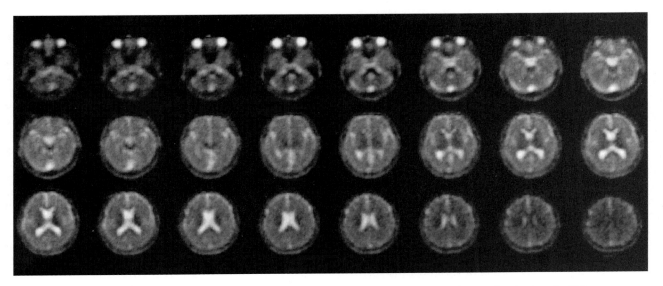

FIGURE 26–17. Multiple axial partitions of a three-dimensional acquisition of a human head using the ^{23}Na signal. The acquisition parameters are echo time = 0.4 ms, repetition time = 100 ms, number of projections = 506, number of signal averages = 12, total acquisition time = 20 minutes, and isotropic voxel size = 0.7 × 0.7 × 0.7 cm³. (Courtesy of the research team at the MR Research Center at the University of Pittsburgh Medical Center: Fernando E. Boada, Sam Chang, Joseph S. Gillen, Gary Shen, Lalith Talagala, Xiaohong Zhou, and Keith R. Thulborn.)

Acknowledgment

I thank Dr. Keith R. Thulborn and his colleagues at the MR Research Center at the University of Pittsburgh Medical Center for providing discussion.

Appendix

METHODS

DIFFUSION-WEIGHTED IMAGING

The limiting factor in DWI is the maximal gradient strength and speed of the MRI system. Our recommendation for clinical DWI is EPI or comparable single-shot technique to achieve multislice imaging with multiple b values and orthogonal diffusion gradient directions to control for anisotropic effects. EPI permits these to be acquired in a practical amount of time for acutely ill clinical patients. We have found that measurement of lesion volume for acute stroke requires the highest b value used to be at least 880 s/mm² with an echo time of 100 ms to see the full extent of the lesion. The greater the range of b values and the greater the number, the more accurate will be the ADC calculation. Ideally, one could acquire all images in a single measurement, although for less cooperative or unstable patients a quicker study at the highest and lowest b values is more appropriate.

In my colleagues' and my study of acute stroke patients,[56] the pulse sequence used for DWI was a single-shot spin-echo EPI sequence with an echo time of 100 ms, 128 × 128 acquisition matrix, and readout time of 64 ms. We used a field of view of 30 cm, a 7-mm slice thickness, acquired with no gap, transverse slice orientation, and the diffusion gradient applied in the transverse (x) direction. Diffusion anisotropy, the directional dependence of the diffusion measurement, can be investigated by applying the diffusion gradient in sagittal and coronal directions separately. Diffusion gradient strength (G) was varied between 0 and 30 mT/m by increments of 5 mT/m. The duration of the diffusion gradient (δ) was 20 ms, and the diffusion time (Δ) was 56.01 ms for the majority of studies. The diffusion sensitivities (b values), neglecting the small contribution of the other imaging gradients, were 0, 35, 141, 318, 565, 883, and 1271 s/mm². In selected cases, higher b values could be used by increasing gradient strength or timing factors, depending on the limitations of the MRI system. Diffusion-weighted images generated by one single-shot EPI acquisition yield enough signal-to-noise ratio and contrast to be diagnostic. Although averaging multiple acquisitions would improve the signal-to-noise ratio, it would also prolong the study and reintroduce the problem of motion artifact. We used an implementation in which all seven diffusion sensitivities are acquired in a single measurement with a total acquisition time of 48 seconds. With the use of a preparation radiofrequency pulse and a 6-second delay between sequential radiofrequency stimulation at each slice position, all images are acquired sequentially for each diffusion sensitivity. For extremely uncooperative patients, a single diffusion-weighted sequence with a high b value is adequate for lesion detection and can be acquired in approximately 3 seconds for 20 images.

PERFUSION IMAGING: DYNAMIC BLOOD VOLUME IMAGING

Dynamic maps of cerebral blood volume can be acquired with gradient-echo techniques using long echo times during the dynamic bolus injection of a paramagnetic contrast agent. By using long echo times, the image becomes T2* weighted and thus strongly susceptibility weighted, enhancing the signal loss when the contrast agent reaches the blood vessels and capillary bed. The magnitude of the signal loss and thus the sensitivity of the technique depend directly on field strength and the concentration of the gadolinium-based contrast material, which determine the strength of the susceptibility effect. Most experience has been at 1.5 T, but adequate studies can be done at 1.0 T. On conventional hardware we have performed these studies using a FLASH sequence with the repetition time/echo time/flip angle/number of excitations = 35/25/10°/1, slice thickness = 8 mm, acquisition matrix = 256 × 80, and rectangular field of view = 23 × 17 cm. A single slice was repeatedly scanned. The dynamic MR images were acquired at a single slice location corresponding to the level of most clinical relevance. Scan time per image was approximately 2.8 seconds with no interscan delay; 25 images were acquired. After approximately four images were obtained, 0.1 mmol/kg of Gd-DTPA was administered intravenously by manual injection over approximately 5 seconds followed by a saline flush. If available, an MRI-compatible power injector may be used to yield consistency of injection speed. Otherwise, one can layer the denser gadolinium beneath 10 to 15 mL of normal saline in a large syringe and manually inject the contrast medium immediately followed by the saline. Doses up to 0.2 mmol/kg are permissible with other approved agents (gadodiamide or gadoteridol). Ideally, one needs as compact a bolus injection as possible to maximize the intravascular concentration during the first pass through the brain. Injection with the use of an 18-gauge intravenous catheter in an antecubital vein is the preferred technique to minimize resistance to the injection.

There are several advantages to using EPI with dynamic contrast imaging. The speed of EPI acquisitions renders each slice insensitive to motion and permits improved time resolution (more frequent sampling to improve quantification) and multislice acquisitions. Single-shot EPI is also inherently susceptibility weighted, even more so with a gradient-echo EPI sequence. Spin-echo EPI is sufficiently susceptibility weighted for dynamic contrast bolus tracking to be successful. An interesting and important difference in the results using gradient-echo versus spin-echo EPI is that the latter preferentially detects signal changes associated with smaller vessels, minimizing the signal changes around larger vessels, which can sometimes overwhelm parenchymal changes associated with arteriolar and capillary flow.[147] The relative disadvantage of using spin-echo EPI is that the magnitude of the signal change is less and the contrast-to-noise ratio between different tissues is reduced. This can be compensated for by using reduced spatial resolution (more susceptibility weighting) or injecting a greater quantity of contrast medium. The echo times used are 60 ms for gradient-echo EPI and 100 ms for spin-echo EPI. Slice parameters and positioning are identical to those for the DWI-EPI sequence. For combined diffusion and perfusion imaging, the results of the DWI are used to select the minimal number of perfusion slices that will cover the area of abnormality. Typically, 12 slice levels can be selected. At the start of the acquisition an intravenous bolus of contrast agent is injected as described earlier. At each slice position an image is acquired every 2 seconds. Twenty-five measurements of each slice are acquired, for a total acquisition time of 50 seconds.

PERFUSION IMAGING: EPISTAR

The basic idea of EPISTAR is to tag blood using a selective inversion pulse in a feeding vessel and then image it after it has flowed into a target vessel. The tagging pulse is applied on alternate acquisitions, and the images are then subtracted. The image subtraction eliminates background tissue while maintaining a large intravascular signal. There are 128 phase-encoding steps collected over 64 ms with a bandwidth of 2 kHz/pixel; the echo is markedly asymmetric along the phase-encoding direction to shorten the echo time to 16 ms. The field of view my colleagues and I typically use is 32 cm, with a section thickness of 8 mm. In the first image, blood is tagged by a 23-ms duration hyperbolic secant inversion pulse with a section-selection gradient of 1.3 mT/m and a nominal slab thickness of 90 mm. The center of the inverted slab is positioned 60 mm caudal to the plane of section; thus, the superior edge of the inverted region is 15 mm from the center of the plane of section. A 90° radiofrequency saturation pulse with twice the thickness of the plane of section is applied to the section immediately before the inversion pulse, followed by a spoiler gradient 7 ms in duration with an amplitude of 9 mT/m. This saturation pulse eliminates potential contamination from the side lobes of the inversion pulse that might leave spurious residual signal intensity after image subtraction. The inversion time corresponds to the time between the tag and the first radiofrequency applied during the readout. A complex subtraction between tagged and untagged acquisitions provides only signal from blood that moved into the section of interest during inversion time. Gradient timing and amplitudes are kept identical during the sequence execution to reduce eddy currents that may introduce inhomogeneous subtraction of stationary material. In the second image, no inversion pulse is applied. Magnetization transfer effects can be minimized by applying 180° radiofrequency tagging pulses that are positioned equidistant from the slice during both odd and even acquisitions, one proximal to the slice (arterial tag) and one distal (control tag). The inversion time may be varied to see more proximal or more distal parts of the arterial circulation. To improve the signal-to-noise ratio, each image is acquired multiple times and averaged. At short inflow times of a few hundred milliseconds, the proximal arterial branches are depicted. As the inversion time is lengthened, progressively more distal portions of the middle cerebral vascular system are shown until the blood reaches the brain cortex (inversion time ~1000 ms for the parameters used). Typically, from 16 acquisitions (scan time = 32 seconds for an inflow time of 1 second) to 96 acquisitions (scan time = 192 seconds for an inflow time of 1 second) are used. The images can be reconstructed individually to be used for functional localization and task activation as described next for BOLD.

PERFUSION IMAGING: BOLD

Because BOLD contrast depends on susceptibility changes, the sequence strategies are the same as those for dynamic contrast studies. Without EPI, susceptibility-weighted sequences, such as FLASH, with long echo times are used (typically echo times of 30 to 60 ms, with repetition times of 60 to 90 ms). The advantages of EPI are the same as mentioned previously: more susceptibility weighting, greater multislice capability, and better time resolution. With EPI, images are typically repeated every 2 to 4 seconds at each slice position and a prolonged time series of alternating tasks is acquired. Echo times for gradient-echo EPI are typically 50 to 60 ms. BOLD, with spin-echo or asymmetric spin-echo sequences, may be used to minimize the signal coming from larger veins, but with an overall loss of sensitivity. Repeated acquisitions of the same slice are performed during performance of various tasks or during rest. For cross-correlational statistical analyses, several rounds of each task, ideally randomly ordered or counterbalanced, are repeated. Typically, a task condition is maintained for 20 to 60 seconds before the next task is introduced; four to eight rounds of tasks are repeated during a single measurement. Because there is a 2- to 5-second latency for the BOLD signal intensity to change with stimulation, shorter task durations may not be as reliable. The two biggest challenges of BOLD experiments have to do with 1) the props and paraphernalia needed for presentation of stimuli and recording of behavioral response while the·subject lies inside the magnet bore and 2) the necessity to keep the head motionless. The latter is a problem even in highly motivated, cooperative subjects. Solutions range from padding the subject's neck and head to requiring the subject to bite on a bite-bar that has been individually molded; the former seeks to minimize the urge to move from discomfort, whereas the latter, although it more actively inhibits movement, introduces a cognitive-motor task that may interact with the question of interest and may not simply subtract out during analysis. No solution is perfect, and corrections for motion are applied to data analysis either by attempts to realign images before statistical analysis or by the cross-correlational statistical analysis itself. As mentioned earlier, if precise spatial localization of response is not needed, larger fields of view and thicker slices improve BOLD sensitivity by increasing the susceptibility weighting.

REFERENCES

1. Wolf PA, Cobb JL, D'Agostino RB: Epidemiology of stroke. In: Barnett HJM, Mohr JP, Stein BM, Yatsu FM, eds. Stroke: Pathophysiology, Diagnosis, and Management. 2nd ed. New York: Churchill Livingstone, 1992, pp 3–27.
2. Special report from the National Institute of Neurological Disorders and Stroke. Classification of cerebrovascular diseases III. Stroke 21:637–676, 1990.
3. Chimowitz MI, Logigian EL, Caplan LR: The accuracy of bedside neurological diagnoses. Ann Neurol 28:78–85, 1990.
4. Calanchini PR, Swanson PD, Gotshall RA, et al: Cooperative study of hospital frequency and character of transient ischemic attacks. IV. The reliability of diagnosis. JAMA 238:2029–2033, 1977.
5. von Arbin M, Britton M, de Faire U, et al: Accuracy of bedside diagnosis in stroke. Stroke 12:288–293, 1981.
5a. Moseley ME, Cohen Y, Kucharczyk J, et al: Diffusion-weighted MR imaging of anisotropic water diffusion in cat central nervous system. Radiology 176:439–445, 1990.
6. Basser PJ, Mattiello J, LeBihan D: MR diffusion tensor spectroscopy and imaging. Biophys J 66:259–267, 1994.
7. Basser PJ, Mattiello J, LeBihan D: Estimation of the effective self-diffusion tensor from the NMR spin echo. J Magn Reson B 103:247–254, 1994.
8. van Gelderen P, de Vleeschouwer MH, DesPres D, et al: Water diffusion and acute stroke. Magn Reson Med 31:154–163, 1994.
9. Wesbey GE, Moseley ME, Ehman RL: Translational molecular self-diffusion in magnetic resonance imaging. II. Measurement of the self-diffusion coefficient. Invest Radiol 19:491–498, 1984.
10. Le Bihan D, Breton E, Lallemand D, et al: MR imaging of intravoxel incoherent motions: application to diffusion and perfusion in neurologic disorders. Radiology 161:401–407, 1986.
11. Le Bihan D, Breton E, Lallemand D, et al: Separation of diffusion and perfusion in intravoxel incoherent motion MR imaging. Radiology 168:497–505, 1988.
12. Ebisu T, Naruse S, Horikawa Y, et al: The application of in vivo diffusion weighted magnetic resonance imaging to intracranial disorders. No To Shinkei 43:677–684, 1991.
13. Tsuruda JS, Chew WM, Moseley ME, Norman D: Diffusion-weighted MR imaging of the brain: value of differentiating between extraaxial cysts and epidermoid tumors. AJNR 11:925–931; discussion 932–934, 1990.
14. Tien RD, Felsberg GJ, Friedman H, et al: MR imaging of high-grade cerebral gliomas: value of diffusion-weighted echoplanar pulse sequences. AJR 162:671–677, 1994.
15. Sorensen PS, Thomsen C, Gjerris F, Henriksen O: Brain water accumulation in pseudotumour cerebri demonstrated by MR-imaging of brain water self-diffusion. Acta Neurochir Suppl 51:363–365, 1990.
16. Christiansen P, Gideon P, Thomsen C, et al: Increased water self-diffusion in chronic plaques and in apparently normal white matter in patients with multiple sclerosis. Acta Neurol Scand 87:195–199, 1993.
17. Le Bihan D, Delannoy J, Levin RL: Temperature mapping with MR imaging of molecular diffusion: application to hyperthermia. Radiology 171:853–857, 1989.
18. Delannoy J, Chen CN, Turner R, et al: Noninvasive temperature imaging using diffusion MRI. Magn Reson Med 19:333–339, 1991.
19. Samulski TV, MacFall J, Zhang Y, et al: Non-invasive thermometry using magnetic resonance diffusion imaging: potential for application in hyperthermic oncology. Int J Hyperthermia 8:819–829, 1992.
20. Hasegawa Y, Latour LL, Sotak CH, et al: Temperature dependent change of apparent diffusion coefficient of water in normal and ischemic brain of rats. J Cereb Blood Flow Metab 14:383–390, 1994.
21. Jiang Q, Chopp M, Zhang ZG, et al: The effect of hypothermia on transient focal ischemia in rat brain evaluated by diffusion- and perfusion-weighted NMR imaging. J Cereb Blood Flow Metab 14:732–741, 1994.
22. Nomura Y, Sakuma H, Takeda K, et al: Diffusional anisotropy of the human brain assessed with diffusion-weighted MR: relation with normal brain development and aging. AJNR 15:231–238, 1994.
23. Rutherford MA, Cowan FM, Manzur AY, et al: MR imaging of anisotropically restricted diffusion in the brain of neonates and infants. J Comput Assist Tomogr 15:188–198, 1991.
24. Sakuma H, Nomura Y, Takeda K, et al: Adult and neonatal human brain: diffusional anisotropy and myelination with diffusion-weighted MR imaging. Radiology 180:229–233, 1991.
25. Chenevert TL, Brunberg JA, Pipe JG: Anisotropic diffusion in human white matter: demonstration with MR techniques in vivo [see comments]. Radiology 177:401–405, 1990.
26. Doran M, Hajnal JV, Van Bruggen N, et al: Normal and abnormal white matter tracts shown by MR imaging using directional diffusion weighted sequences. J Comput Assist Tomogr 14:865–873, 1990.

27. Hajnal JV, Doran M, Hall AS, et al: MR imaging of anisotropically restricted diffusion of water in the nervous system: technical, anatomic, and pathologic considerations. J Comput Assist Tomogr 15:1–18, 1991.

28. Douek P, Turner R, Pekar J, et al: MR color mapping of myelin fiber orientation. J Comput Assist Tomogr 15:923–929, 1991.

29. Coremans J, Luypaert R, Verhelle F, et al: A method for myelin fiber orientation mapping using diffusion-weighted MR images. Magn Reson Imaging 12:443–454, 1994.

30. Kinosada Y, Ono M, Okuda Y, et al: MR tractography—visualization of structure of nerve fiber system from diffusion weighted images with maximum intensity projection method. Nippon Igaku Hoshasen Gakkai Zasshi 53:171–179, 1993.

31. Moseley ME, Kucharczyk J, Mintorovitch J, et al: Diffusion-weighted MR imaging of acute stroke: correlation with T2-weighted and magnetic susceptibility-enhanced MR imaging in cats. AJNR 11:423–429, 1990.

32. Moseley ME, Cohen Y, Mintorovitch J, et al: Early detection of regional cerebral ischemia in cats: comparison of diffusion- and T2-weighted MRI and spectroscopy. Magn Reson Med 14:330–346, 1990.

33. Moseley ME, Mintorovitch J, Cohen Y, et al: Early detection of ischemic injury: comparison of spectroscopy, diffusion-, T2-, and magnetic susceptibility–weighted MRI in cats. Acta Neurochir Suppl 51:207–209, 1990.

34. Mintorovitch J, Moseley ME, Chileuitt L, et al: Comparison of diffusion- and T2-weighted MRI for the early detection of cerebral ischemia and reperfusion in rats. Magn Reson Med 18:39–50, 1991.

35. Moseley ME, Sevick R, Wendland MF, et al: Ultrafast magnetic resonance imaging: diffusion and perfusion. Can Assoc Radiol J 42:31–38, 1991.

36. Busza AL, Allen KL, King MD, et al: Diffusion-weighted imaging studies of cerebral ischemia in gerbils. Potential relevance to energy failure. Stroke 23:1602–1612, 1992.

37. Berry I, Gigaud M, Manelfe C: Experimental focal cerebral ischaemia assessed with IVIM*-MRI in the acute phase at 0.5 tesla. Neuroradiology 34:135–140, 1992.

38. Verheul HB, Berkelbach van der Sprenkel JW, Tulleken CA, et al: Temporal evolution of focal cerebral ischemia in the rat assessed by T2-weighted and diffusion-weighted magnetic resonance imaging. Brain Topogr 5:171–176, 1992.

39. van Bruggen N, Cullen BM, King MD, et al: T2- and diffusion-weighted magnetic resonance imaging of a focal ischemic lesion in rat brain. Stroke 23:576–582, 1992.

40. Minematsu K, Li L, Fisher M, et al: Diffusion-weighted magnetic resonance imaging: rapid and quantitative detection of focal brain ischemia. Neurology 42:235–240, 1992.

41. Helpern JA, Dereski MO, Knight RA, et al: Histopathological correlations of nuclear magnetic resonance imaging parameters in experimental cerebral ischemia. Magn Reson Imaging 11:241–246, 1993.

42. Moseley ME, de Crespigny AJ, Roberts TP, et al: Early detection of regional cerebral ischemia using high-speed MRI. Stroke 24(suppl):I60–I65, 1993.

43. Bizzi A, Righini A, Turner R, et al: MR of diffusion slowing in global cerebral ischemia. AJNR 14:1347–1354, 1993.

44. Knight RA, Dereski MO, Helpern JA, et al: Magnetic resonance imaging assessment of evolving focal cerebral ischemia: comparison with histopathology in rats. Stroke 25:1252–1261; discussion 1261–1262, 1994. Erratum in Stroke 25:1887, 1994.

45. Roberts TP, Vexler Z, Derugin N, et al: High-speed MR imaging of ischemic brain injury following stenosis of the middle cerebral artery. J Cereb Blood Flow Metab 13:940–946, 1993.

46. Roussel SA, van Bruggen N, King MD, et al: Monitoring the initial expansion of focal ischaemic changes by diffusion-weighted MRI using a remote controlled method of occlusion. NMR Biomed 7:21–28, 1994.

47. Back T, Hoehn-Berlage M, Kohno K, Hossmann KA: Diffusion nuclear magnetic resonance imaging in experimental stroke. Correlation with cerebral metabolites. Stroke 25:494–500, 1994.

48. Hossmann KA, Fischer M, Bockhorst K, Hoehn-Berlage M: NMR imaging of the apparent diffusion coefficient (ADC) for the evaluation of metabolic suppression and recovery after prolonged cerebral ischemia. J Cereb Blood Flow Metab 14:723–731, 1994.

49. Poncelet BP, Wedeen VJ, Weisskoff RM, Cohen MS: Brain parenchyma motion: measurement with cine echo-planar MR imaging [see comments]. Radiology 185:645–651, 1992.

50. Ordidge RJ, Helpern JA, Qing ZX, et al: Correction of motional artifacts in diffusion-weighted MR images using navigator echoes. Magn Reson Imaging 12:455–460, 1994.

51. Anderson AW, Gore JC: Analysis and correction of motion artifacts in diffusion weighted imaging. Magn Reson Med 32:379–387, 1994.

51a. de Crespigny AJ, Marks MP, Enzmann DR, Moseley ME: Navigated diffusion imaging of normal and ischemic human brain. Magn Reson Med 33:720–728, 1995.

52. Chien D, Kwong KK, Gress DR, et al: MR diffusion imaging of cerebral infarction in humans. AJNR 13:1097–1102; discussion 1103–1105, 1992.

53. Warach S, Chien D, Li W, et al: Fast magnetic resonance diffusion-weighted imaging of acute human stroke. Neurology 42:1717–1723, 1992. Erratum in Neurology 42:2192, 1992.

54. Merboldt KD, Hanicke W, Bruhn H, et al: Diffusion imaging of the human brain in vivo using high-speed STEAM MRI. Magn Reson Med 23:179–192, 1992.

55. Turner R, Le Bihan D, Maier J, et al: Echo-planar imaging of intravoxel incoherent motion. Radiology 177:407–414, 1990.

56. Warach S, Gaa J, Siewert B, et al: Acute human stroke studied by whole brain echo planar diffusion-weighted magnetic resonance imaging. Ann Neurol 37:231–241, 1995.

57. Davis D, Ulatowski J, Eleff S, et al: Rapid monitoring of changes in water diffusion coefficients during reversible ischemia in cat and rat brain. Magn Reson Med 31:454–460, 1994.

58. Mintorovitch J, Yang GY, Shimizu H, et al: Diffusion-weighted magnetic resonance imaging of acute focal cerebral ischemia: comparison of signal intensity with changes in brain water and Na$^+$,K$^+$-ATPase activity. J Cereb Blood Flow Metab 14:332–336, 1994.

59. Warach S, Li W, Ronthal M, Edelman RR: Acute cerebral ischemia: evaluation with dynamic contrast-enhanced MR imaging and MR angiography. Radiology 182:41–47, 1992.

60. Moonen CT, Pekar J, de Vleeschouwer MH, et al: Restricted and anisotropic displacement of water in healthy cat brain and in stroke studied by NMR diffusion imaging. Magn Reson Med 19:327–332, 1991.

61. Hossmann KA: Cortical steady potential, impedance and excitability changes during and after total ischemia of cat brain. Exp Neurol 32:163–175, 1971.

62. Verheul HB, Balazs R, Berkelbach van der Sprenkel JW, et al: Comparison of diffusion-weighted MRI with changes in cell volume in a rat model of brain injury. NMR Biomed 7:96–100, 1994.

63. Benveniste H, Hedlund LW, Johnson GA: Mechanism of detection of acute cerebral ischemia in rats by diffusion-weighted magnetic resonance microscopy. Stroke 23:746–754, 1992.

64. Hakim AM: The cerebral ischemic penumbra. Can J Neurol Sci 14:557–559, 1987.

65. Astrup J, Siesjo BK, Symon L: Thresholds in cerebral ischemia—the ischemic penumbra. Stroke 12:723–725, 1981.

66. Gyngell ML, Back T, Hoehn-Berlage M, et al: Transient cell depolarization after permanent middle cerebral artery occlusion: an observation by diffusion-weighted MRI and localized ^{1}H-MRS. Magn Reson Med 31:337–341, 1994.

67. Latour LL, Hasegawa Y, Formato JE, et al: Spreading waves of decreased diffusion coefficient after cortical stimulation in the rat brain. Magn Reson Med 32:189–198, 1994.

68. Quast MJ, Huang NC, Hillman GR, Kent TA: The evolution of acute stroke recorded by multimodal magnetic resonance imaging. Magn Reson Imaging 11:465–471, 1993.

69. Minematsu K, Li L, Sotak CH, et al: Reversible focal ischemic injury demonstrated by diffusion-weighted magnetic resonance imaging in rats. Stroke 23:1304–1310; discussion 1310–1311, 1992.

70. Takahashi M, Fritz-Zieroth B, Chikugo T, Ogawa H: Differentiation of chronic lesions after stroke in stroke-prone spontaneously hypertensive rats using diffusion-weighted MRI. Magn Reson Med 30:485–488, 1993.

71. Pierpaoli C, Righini A, Linfante I, et al: Histopathologic correlates of abnormal water diffusion in cerebral ischemia: diffusion-weighted MR imaging and light and electron microscopic study. Radiology 189:439–448, 1993.

72. Dardzinski BJ, Sotak CH, Fisher M, et al: Apparent diffusion coefficient mapping of experimental focal cerebral ischemia using diffusion-weighted echo-planar imaging. Magn Reson Med 30:318–325, 1993.

73. Hasegawa Y, Fisher M, Latour LL, et al: MRI diffusion mapping of reversible and irreversible ischemic injury in focal brain ischemia. Neurology 44:1484–1490, 1994.

74. Lo EH, Matsumoto K, Pierce AR, et al: Pharmacologic reversal of acute changes in diffusion-weighted magnetic resonance imaging in focal cerebral ischemia. J Cereb Blood Flow Metab 14:597–603, 1994.

75. Kucharczyk J, Mintorovitch J, Sevick R, et al: MR evaluation of calcium entry blockers with putative cerebroprotective effects in acute cerebral ischaemia. Acta Neurochir Suppl 51:254–255, 1990.

76. Kucharczyk J, Mintorovitch J, Moseley ME, et al: Ischemic brain damage: reduction by sodium-calcium ion channel modulator RS-87476. Radiology 179:221–227, 1991.

77. Seega J, Elger B: Diffusion- and T2-weighted imaging: evaluation of oedema reduction in focal cerebral ischaemia by the calcium and serotonin antagonist levemopamil. Magn Reson Imaging 11:401–409, 1993.

78. Minematsu K, Fisher M, Li L, et al: Effects of a novel NMDA antagonist on experimental stroke rapidly and quantitatively assessed by diffusion-weighted MRI. Neurology 43:397–403, 1993.

79. Minematsu K, Fisher M, Li L, Sotak CH: Diffusion and perfusion magnetic resonance imaging studies to evaluate a noncompetitive N-methyl-D-aspartate antagonist and reperfusion in experimental stroke in rats. Stroke 24:2074–2081, 1993.

80. Zhong J, Petroff OA, Prichard JW, Gore JC: Changes in water diffusion and relaxation properties of rat cerebrum during status epilepticus. Magn Reson Med 30:241–246, 1993.

81. Sevick RJ, Kanda F, Mintorovitch J, Arieff AI, et al: Cytotoxic brain edema: assessment with diffusion-weighted MR imaging. Radiology 185:687–690, 1992.

82. Hanstock CC, Faden AI, Bendall MR, Vink R: Diffusion-weighted imaging differentiates ischemic tissue from traumatized tissue. Stroke 25:843–848, 1994.

83. Thulborn KR, Waterton JC, Matthews PM, Radda GK: Oxygenation dependence of the transverse relaxation time of water protons in whole blood at high field. Biochim Biophys Acta 714:265–270, 1982.

84. Ogawa S, Lee TM, Kay AR, Tank DW: Brain magnetic resonance imaging with contrast dependent on blood oxygenation. Proc Natl Acad Sci USA 87:9868–9872, 1990.

85. Villringer A, Rosen BR, Belliveau JW, et al: Dynamic imaging with lanthanide chelates in normal brain: contrast due to magnetic susceptibility effects. Magn Reson Med 6:164–174, 1988.

86. Rosen BR, Belliveau JW, Chien D: Perfusion imaging by nuclear magnetic resonance. Magn Reson Q 5:263–281, 1989.

87. Belliveau JW, Rosen BR, Kantor HL, et al: Functional cerebral imaging by susceptibility-contrast NMR. Magn Reson Med 14:538–546, 1990.

87a. Weisskoff RM, Zuo CS, Boxerman JL, Rosen BR: Microscopic susceptibility variation and transverse relaxation: theory and experiment. Magn Reson Med 31:601–610, 1994.

87b. Rempp KA, Brix G, Wenz F, et al: Quantification of regional cerebral blood flow and volume with dynamic susceptibility contrast-enhanced MR imaging. Radiology 193:637–641, 1994.

88. Roberts DA, Detre JA, Bolinger L, et al: Quantitative magnetic resonance imaging of human brain perfusion at 1.5 T using steady-state inversion of arterial water. Proc Natl Acad Sci USA 91:33–37, 1994.

89. Williams DS, Detre JA, Leigh JS, Koretsky AP: Magnetic resonance imaging of perfusion using spin inversion of arterial water. Proc Natl Acad Sci USA 89:212–216, 1992. Erratum in Proc Natl Acad Sci USA 89:4220, 1992.

90. Edelman RR, Siewert B, Darby DG, et al: Qualitative mapping of cerebral blood flow and functional localization with echo-planar MR imaging and signal targeting with alternating radio frequency. Radiology 192:513–520, 1994.

91. Finelli DA, Hopkins AL, Selman WR, et al: Evaluation of experimental early acute cerebral ischemia before the development of edema: use of dynamic, contrast-enhanced and diffusion-weighted MR scanning. Magn Reson Med 27:189–197, 1992. Erratum in Magn Reson Med 28:339, 1992.

92. Wendland MF, White DL, Aicher KP, et al: Detection with echo-planar MR imaging of transit of susceptibility contrast medium in a rat model of regional brain ischemia. J Magn Reson Imaging 1:285–292, 1991.

93. de Crespigny AJ, Wendland MF, Derugin N, et al: Rapid MR imaging of a vascular challenge to focal ischemia in cat brain. J Magn Reson Imaging 3:475–481, 1993.

94. Edelman RR, Mattle HP, Atkinson DJ, et al: Cerebral blood flow: assessment with dynamic contrast-enhanced T2*-weighted MR imaging at 1.5 T. Radiology 176:211–220, 1990.

95. Guckel F, Brix G, Rempp K, et al: Assessment of cerebral blood volume with dynamic susceptibility contrast enhanced gradient-echo imaging. J Comput Assist Tomogr 18:344–351, 1994.

96. Worthington BS, Bullock P, Stehling M, et al: Clinical experience with contrast enhanced echo-planar imaging of the brain. Magn Reson Med 22:255–258; discussion 265–267, 1991.

97. Rosen BR, Belliveau JW, Aronen HJ, et al: Susceptibility contrast imaging of cerebral blood volume: human experience. Magn Reson Med 22:293–299; discussion 300–303, 1991.

98. Duyn JH, Mattay VS, Sexton RH, et al: Three-dimensional functional imaging of human brain using echo-shifted FLASH MRI. Magn Reson Med 32:150–155, 1994.

99. Bock JC, Sander B, Hierholzer J, et al: The regional cerebral circulation in infarct patients. Rapid dynamic T2*-weighted MRT after a bolus injection of gadolinium-DTPA. Rofo Fortschr Geb Rontgenstr Neuen Bildgeb Verfahr 156:382–387, 1992.

100. Warach S, Wielopolski P, Edelman RR: Identification and characterization of the ischemic penumbra of acute human stroke using echo planar diffusion and perfusion imaging. In: Proceedings of the 12th Annual Meeting of the Society of Magnetic Resonance in Medicine, New York, 1993, p 263.

101. Aronen HJ, Gazit IE, Louis DN, et al: Cerebral blood volume maps of gliomas: comparison with tumor grade and histologic findings. Radiology 191:41–51, 1994.

102. Bock JC, Sander B, Hierholzer J, et al: The regional blood flow in intracranial tumors: a comparison of HMPAO-SPECT with a newer magnetic resonance tomographic procedure. Rofo Fortschr Geb Rontgenstr Neuen Bildgeb Verfahr 157:378–383, 1992.

103. Rogowska J, Preston K Jr, Aronen HJ, Wolf GL: A comparative analysis of similarity mapping and eigenimaging as applied to dynamic MR imaging of a low grade astrocytoma. Acta Radiol 35:371–377, 1994.

104. Jackson GD, Connelly A, Cross JH, et al: Functional magnetic resonance imaging of focal seizures. Neurology 44:850–856, 1994.

105. Belliveau JW, Kennedy DN Jr, McKinstry RC, et al: Functional mapping of the human visual cortex by magnetic resonance imaging. Science 254:716–719, 1991.

106. Kwong KK, Belliveau JW, Chesler DA, et al: Dynamic magnetic resonance imaging of human brain activity during primary sensory stimulation. Proc Natl Acad Sci USA 89:5675–5679, 1992.

107. Bandettini PA, Wong EC, Hinks RS, et al: Time course EPI of human brain function during task activation. Magn Reson Med 25:390–397, 1992.

108. Ogawa S, Tank DW, Menon R, et al: Intrinsic signal changes accompanying sensory stimulation: functional brain mapping with magnetic resonance imaging. Proc Natl Acad Sci USA 89:5951–5955, 1992.

109. Moonen CT, Barrios FA, Zigun JR, et al: Functional brain MR imaging based on bolus tracking with a fast T2*-sensitized gradient-echo method. Magn Reson Imaging 12:379–385, 1994.

110. Zigun JR, Frank JA, Barrios FA, et al: Measurement of brain activity with bolus administration of contrast agent and gradient-echo MR imaging. Radiology 186:353–356, 1993.

111. Connelly A, Jackson GD, Frackowiak RS, et al: Functional mapping of activated human primary cortex with a clinical MR imaging system. Radiology 188:125–130, 1993.

112. Cao Y, Towle VL, Levin DN, Balter JM: Functional mapping of human motor cortical activation with conventional MR imaging at 1.5 T. J Magn Reson Imaging 3:869–875, 1993.

113. Constable RT, Kennan RP, Puce A, et al: Functional NMR imaging using fast spin echo at 1.5 T. Magn Reson Med 31:686–690, 1994.

114. Turner R, Jezzard P, Wen H, et al: Functional mapping of the human visual cortex at 4 and 1.5 tesla using deoxygenation contrast EPI. Magn Reson Med 29:277–279, 1993.

115. Ugurbil K, Garwood M, Ellermann J, et al: Imaging at high magnetic fields: initial experiences at 4 T. Magn Reson Q 9:259–277, 1993.

116. Ernst T, Hennig J: Observation of a fast response in functional MR. Magn Reson Med 32:146–149, 1994.

117. Frostig RD, Lieke EE, Ts'o DY, Grinvald A: Cortical functional architecture and local coupling between neuronal activity and the microcirculation revealed by in vivo high-resolution optical imaging of intrinsic signals. Proc Natl Acad Sci USA 87:6082–6086, 1990.

118. Lai S, Hopkins AL, Haacke EM, et al: Identification of vascular structures as a major source of signal contrast in high resolution 2D and 3D functional activation imaging of the motor cortex at 1.5T: preliminary results. Magn Reson Med 30:387–392, 1993.

119. Frahm J, Merboldt KD, Hanicke W, et al: Brain or vein—oxygenation or flow? On signal physiology in functional MRI of human brain activation. NMR Biomed 7:45–53, 1994.

120. Duyn JH, Moonen CT, van Yperen GH, et al: Inflow versus deoxyhemoglobin effects in BOLD functional MRI using gradient echoes at 1.5 T. NMR Biomed 7:83–88, 1994.

121. Menon RS, Ogawa S, Tank DW, Ugurbil K: Tesla gradient recalled echo characteristics of photic stimulation-induced signal changes in the human primary visual cortex. Magn Reson Med 30:380–386, 1993.

122. Ogawa S, Menon RS, Tank DW, et al: Functional brain mapping by blood oxygenation level–dependent contrast magnetic resonance imaging. A comparison of signal characteristics with a biophysical model. Biophys J 64:803–812, 1993.

123. Hoppel BE, Weisskoff RM, Thulborn KR, et al: Measurement of regional blood oxygenation and cerebral hemodynamics. Magn Reson Med 30:715–723, 1993.

124. Bandettini PA, Wong EC, Jesmanowicz A, et al: Spin-echo and gradient-echo EPI of human brain activation using BOLD contrast: a comparative study at 1.5 T. NMR Biomed 7:12–20, 1994.

125. Kim SG, Hendrich K, Hu X, et al: Potential pitfalls of functional MRI using conventional gradient-recalled echo techniques. NMR Biomed 7:69–74, 1994.

125a. Kwong KK: Functional magnetic resonance imaging with echo planar imaging. Magn Reson Q 11:1–20, 1995.

125b. Schlaug G, Sanes JN, Seitz RJ, et al: Movement rate determines cerebral blood flow changes as assessed by PET and functional MRI. In: Proceedings of the 24th Annual Meeting of the Society for Neuroscience, Miami, FL, 1994, p 147.

126. Bandettini PA, Jesmanowicz A, Wong EC, Hyde JS: Processing strategies for time-course data sets in functional MRI of the human brain. Magn Reson Med 30:161–173, 1993.

127. Friston KJ, Jezzard P, Turner R: Analysis of functional MRI time series. Hum Brain Mapping 1:153–171, 1994.

128. Kim SG, Ashe J, Georgopoulos AP, et al: Functional imaging of human motor cortex at high magnetic field. J Neurophysiol 69:297–302, 1993.

129. Kim SG, Ashe J, Hendrich K, et al: Functional magnetic resonance imaging of motor cortex: hemispheric asymmetry and handedness. Science 261:615–617, 1993.

130. Tyszka JM, Grafton ST, Chew W, et al: Parceling of mesial frontal motor areas during ideation and movement using functional magnetic resonance imaging at 1.5 tesla [see comments]. Ann Neurol 35:746–749, 1994.

131. Rao SM, Binder JR, Bandettini PA, et al: Functional magnetic resonance imaging of complex human movements. Neurology 43:2311–2318, 1993.

132. McCarthy G, Blamire AM, Rothman DL, et al: Echo-planar magnetic resonance imaging studies of frontal cortex activation during word generation in humans. Proc Natl Acad Sci USA 90:4952–4956, 1993.

133. Hinke RM, Hu X, Stillman AE, et al: Functional magnetic resonance imaging of Broca's area during internal speech. Neuroreport 4:675–678, 1993.

134. Rueckert L, Appollonio I, Grafman J, et al: Magnetic resonance imaging functional activation of left frontal cortex during covert word production. J Neuroimaging 4:67–70, 1994.

135. Binder JR, Rao SM, Hammeke TA, et al: Functional magnetic resonance imaging of human auditory cortex [see comments]. Ann Neurol 35:662–672, 1994.

136. Le Bihan D, Turner R, Zeffiro TA, et al: Activation of human primary visual cortex during visual recall: a magnetic resonance imaging study. Proc Natl Acad Sci USA 90:11802–11805, 1993.

137. Renshaw PF, Yurgelun-Todd DA, Cohen BM: Greater hemodynamic response to photic stimulation in schizophrenic patients: an echo planar MRI study. Am J Psychiatry 151:1493–1495, 1994.

138. Ives JR, Warach S, Schmitt F, et al: Monitoring the patient's EEG during echo planar MRI. Electroencephalogr Clin Neurophysiol 87:417–420, 1993.

139. Jack CR Jr, Thompson RM, Butts RK, et al: Sensory motor cortex: correlation of presurgical mapping with functional MR imaging and invasive cortical mapping. Radiology 190:85–92, 1994.

140. Bruhn H, Kleinschmidt A, Boecker H, et al: The effect of acetazolamide on regional cerebral blood oxygenation at rest and under stimulation as assessed by MRI. J Cereb Blood Flow Metab 14:742–748, 1994.

141. Rostrup E, Larsson HB, Toft PB, et al: Functional MRI of CO_2 induced increase in cerebral perfusion. NMR Biomed 7:29–34, 1994.

142. Christensen JD, Barrere BJ, Boada FE, et al: Quantitative sodium tissue concentration mapping of rat brain tumors. In: Proceedings of the 12th Annual Meeting of the Society of Magnetic Resonance in Medicine, New York, 1993, p 978.

143. Barrere BJ, Christensen JD, Boada FE, et al: Absolute tissue sodium concentration maps of rat brain by $^{23}Na/^{1}H$ MR projection imaging. In: Proceedings of the 12th Annual Meeting of the Society of Magnetic Resonance in Medicine, New York, 1993, p 400.

144. Boada FE, Christensen JD, Huang-Hellinger FR, et al: Quantitative in vivo tissue sodium concentration maps: the effects of biexponential relaxation. Magn Reson Med 32:219–223, 1994.

145. Boada FE, Gillen J, Thulborn KR: Constant sampling density transversals for faster three dimensional sodium imaging: a theoretical study. In: Proceedings of the Second Annual Meeting of the Society of Magnetic Resonance, San Francisco, 1994, p 417.

146. Boada FE, Gillen J, Thulborn KR: Optimized data acquisition, reconstruction and post-processing techniques for quantitative sodium imaging. In: Proceedings of the 1st IEEE International Conference on Image Processing, Austin, 1994, vol 3, pp 20–24.

147. Weisskoff RM, Zuo CS, Boxerman JL, Rosen BR: Microscopic susceptibility variation and transverse relaxation: theory and experiment. Magn Reson Med 31:601–610, 1994.

White Matter Disease

JOHN R. HESSELINK

Magnetic resonance imaging (MRI) is exquisitely sensitive for detecting brain abnormalities. Particularly in the evaluation of white matter diseases, MRI far outperforms any other imaging technique. Lesions that may be quite subtle or even invisible by computed tomography (CT) are often clearly seen on the MR image. The MR signal characteristics of white matter lesions are similar and relatively nonspecific, but other distinguishing features are often present to assist in diagnosis, such as the pattern of the abnormality, location, and enhancement features.

The white matter is affected by many disease processes. Neoplastic and infectious diseases readily invade both the gray matter and the white matter. Cerebral infarction destroys the cortex and the underlying white matter, but chronic ischemia predominantly affects the white matter. The primary demyelinating disease is multiple sclerosis (MS), but many other metabolic and inflammatory disorders result in deficient or abnormal myelination.

Histologically, myelin abnormalities are either demyelinating or dysmyelinating. Demyelination implies destruction of myelin. Dysmyelination refers to defective formation or maintenance of myelin resulting from dysfunction of the oligodendrocytes. Most of the dysmyelinating disorders are caused by metabolic defects that present in infancy. White matter diseases in older children and adults are generally demyelinating disorders or a combination of the two processes.

The terminology used to describe abnormal white matter includes leukodystrophy, leukoencephalopathy, leukomalacia, and leukoencephalitis. They are Latin or Greek derivations of words that describe their appearance on pathologic examination. *Leukodystrophy* refers to "bad or disordered white matter." *Leukoencephalopathy* means "diseased white matter within the head." *Leukomalacia* translates as "white matter softening." Finally, *leukoencephalitis* implies "infection or inflammation of white matter." Because in most cases these diseases were named before their causes were known, the names describe the effect of the disease on brain tissue and not the cause. It would be confusing and misleading to use these words in a classification scheme because the causes of many white matter diseases have been determined. For example, the virus causing progressive multifocal leukoencephalopathy has been identified, so it would be more accurate to call it a leukoencephalitis.

As an aside, the name *multiple sclerosis* defies all logic and is entirely nonspecific. Based on its name, it could just as well be a multifocal sclerotic bone disease. It probably got its name from the pathologic appearance of old inactive plaques. Nonetheless, the name will stay with us, and despite its nonspecificity everyone knows what it means.

Valk and van der Knaap[1] proposed a new classification scheme for myelin disorders based on etiology. The two major categories are hereditary and acquired. Hereditary disorders encompass primarily the metabolic diseases. The acquired disorders are subdivided into 1) noninfectious-inflammatory, 2) infectious-inflammatory, 3) toxic-metabolic, 4) hypoxic-ischemic, and 5) traumatic disorders. No classification system is perfect, but for the most part this one follows a logical pattern. In this scheme, the category of trauma includes radiation and hydrocephalus. I have elected to discuss radiation injury separately; hydrocephalus is covered in Chapter 29. Also, because deep white matter ischemia and MS are so important in MR image interpretation, they are discussed first under separate categories.

NORMAL WHITE MATTER

The white matter of the brain includes the major commissural tracts, the cortical association fibers, and all the cortical afferent and efferent fibers. Histologically, the white matter contains nerve fibers, supporting cells, interstitial space, and vascular structures. White matter consists mostly of axons with their envelope of myelin, along with two types of neuroglial cells: oligodendrocytes and astrocytes. Axons are extensions of neurons that reside within the gray matter of the brain, spinal cord, and ganglia. The myelin is produced and maintained by oligodendrocytes. The oligodendrocyte extends its cell membrane and wraps around the axon cylinder multiple times. Although the axon may be several feet long, the oligodendrocyte has more regional duty. The myelin of one axon represents contributions from many oligodendrocytes. At the same time, one oligodendrocyte myelinates segments of up to 50 axons.[2]

The myelin sheath has a lamellar structure with alternating layers of lipid and protein. The ratio of lipid to protein is quite high, ranging from 70% to 80% lipid (phospholipid, cholesterol, galactolipid) and 20% to 30% protein.[3] As a result of its high lipid content, myelin is relatively dehydrated. Overall, white matter has a water content of 72%, compared with 82% for gray matter.

Myelin functions as an insulator of the axons, and its structure facilitates rapid transmission of impulses. Segmental interruptions of the myelin sheath, called nodes of Ranvier, expose the axonal membrane to the extracellular environment. When the nerve fiber depolarizes, the electrical impulse jumps from node to node, markedly increasing the rate of propagation.

Development and maturation of white matter in the developing fetus and young child are discussed in Chapter 16. Adult myelin is stable, and it is metabolized and replenished rather slowly. Any disease process that disrupts the axon or myelin interferes with function. In the case of a demyelinating injury, as long as the oligodendrocytes are preserved the brain has the capacity to remyelinate regions of destroyed myelin. However, except for extremely small lesions the remyelination is frequently incomplete, and the new myelin is thinner than the original.

Myelin has relatively short T2 and T1 relaxation times, primarily owing to its lipid content. As a result, normal myelin is hypointense relative to gray matter on T2-weighted MR images and hyperintense on T1-weighted images. If a disease process reduces the myelin content, the white matter becomes less hydrophobic and takes on more water. Less myelin and more water protons prolong both T1 and T2, resulting in more signal intensity on T2-weighted images and less signal intensity on T1-weighted images.

Regions of the forceps major posterior and superior to the ventricular trigones are the last to myelinate during development. Moreover, the axons are less compact, and more interstitial space is present. As a result, the white matter of the forceps major has relatively longer T1 and T2 relaxation times, especially in children but also in adults.[4]

AGING EFFECTS ON THE WHITE MATTER

As a result of the high sensitivity of T2-weighted spin-echo pulse sequences, MR images frequently reveal high-signal-intensity foci within the subcortical white matter. Estimates of the incidence of these hyperintensities in the brains of healthy, elderly persons have ranged from 30% to 90%.[5–8] Gerard and Weisberg[5] found subcortical lesions in only 10% of patients older than 60 years of age unless cerebrovascular symptoms or risk factors were present; if both were present, the frequency increased to 84%. To a certain extent, the presence of these hyperintensities limits the sensitivity of MRI for white matter disease. They are often normal variants or related to deep white matter ische-

mia, but they can be mistaken for, or can obscure, more serious pathologic conditions.

VIRCHOW-ROBIN PERIVASCULAR SPACES

When nutrient vessels penetrate the brain substance, the pia mater is carried along with the vessel down to the capillary level. The small subarachnoid space that follows the pia is called the Virchow-Robin (VR) space. These perivascular cerebrospinal fluid (CSF) spaces appear as punctate areas of high signal intensity on T2-weighted images. They become essentially isointense relative to white matter on proton density–weighted images and as a result of their fluid contents are distinctly hypointense on T1-weighted images. The signal intensity on the proton density–weighted image will vary depending on the specific pulse sequence used. For example, with fast spin-echo sequences the proton density–weighted image has more T2 weighting, and the VR spaces have often slightly higher signal intensity than the white matter.

The VR spaces are commonly seen within the superficial white matter on higher axial sections through the cerebral hemispheres, where nutrient arteries for the deep white matter enter the brain (Fig. 27–1A and B). Another common location is the lower basal ganglia at the level of the anterior commissure, where the lenticulostriate arteries enter the anterior perforated substance (Fig. 27–1C and D). They are often clustered around the lateral aspects of the anterior commissure.[9] The VR spaces are usually no more than 1 or 2 mm; however, in the basal ganglia they can reach 5 mm. If small high-signal-intensity foci are observed in these areas on T2-weighted images, they should be dismissed as normal structures, unless corroborative evidence of disease is found on other brain sections. On the other hand, normal VR spaces are generally not visible in the middle or upper thirds of the basal ganglia. Occasionally, extremely large (1 cm or more) VR spaces are observed in the basal ganglia region (Fig. 27–2). If the patient is young and has no risk factors for vascular or degenerative disease, these large VR spaces are probably normal variants, representing a confluence of penetrating arteries and veins.

Not infrequently, VR spaces in the brain stem are sufficiently large to be seen on MR images. On T2-weighted axial images they are sectioned longitudinally and appear as hyperintense linear structures coursing in a ventrolateral direction. Their linear character generally distinguishes them from small brain stem infarcts.[10]

If the brain becomes atrophic and loses volume, it retracts away from the vessels and extracellular fluid fills the space. On postmortem studies, these perivascular fluid spaces appear like a network of tunnels within the brain substance. These changes have been termed *état criblé* (sieve-like) by Durand-Fardel.[11] These fluid spaces simply represent dilated VR spaces. Brain atrophy results in dilated VR spaces in the same manner that the cortical sulci become enlarged. As expected, in older patients with atrophic brains the VR spaces are larger and appear more numerous.[12] On T2-weighted

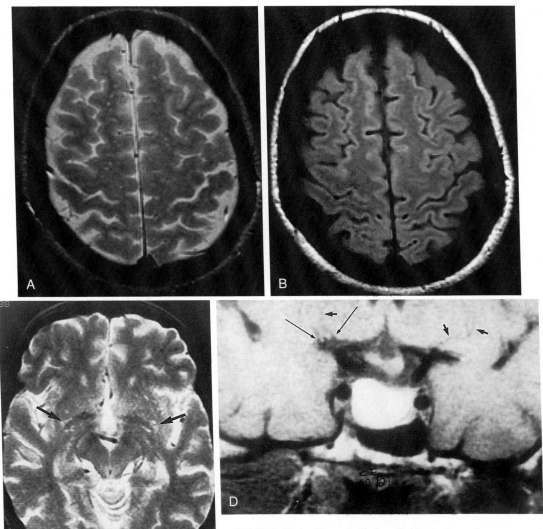

FIGURE 27–1. Normal Virchow-Robin perivascular spaces. *A,* Axial T2-weighted image (spin echo [SE], repetition time/echo time = 3000/80) through the vertex of the brain shows multiple punctate hyperintensities within the white matter. *B,* On a corresponding proton density–weighted image (SE, 3000/20), the hyperintensities disappear or become isointense relative to the white matter, characteristic of normal perivascular CSF spaces. *C,* Axial scan (SE, 3000/80) at the level of the anterior commissure reveals small high-signal-intensity foci *(arrows)* clustered about the lateral aspects of the commissure, all representing VR spaces surrounding penetrating lenticulostriate arteries. *D,* Coronal T1-weighted image (SE, 600/20) at the level of the optic chiasm shows small CSF projections *(long arrows)* representing VR spaces following the lenticulostriate arteries as they enter the base of the brain. These VR spaces are in similar position to those in *C.* The thin-caliber lentriculostriate arteries, along with their accompanying VR spaces *(short arrows),* can be followed deeper into the brain substance. The patient also had an incidental pituitary hemorrhage.

images, the dilated perivascular spaces appear as punctate hyperintense foci if cut in cross section or may have a linear, vessel-like configuration if sectioned longitudinally (Fig. 27–3). On proton density–weighted and T1-weighted images, the fluid spaces should follow the signal characteristics of CSF or water.[13]

Deep White Matter Ischemia

Pathophysiology

As the brain ages, structural, chemical, and metabolic changes occur that are reflected on the MR images. Most important for interpretation of MRI are the changes related to deep white matter ischemia. The deep white matter of the cerebral hemispheres receives its blood supply from long, small-caliber arteries and arterioles that penetrate the cerebral cortex and traverse the superficial white matter fiber tracts. The white matter does not have as generous a blood supply as the gray matter and is more susceptible to ischemia. As the nutrient arteries become narrowed by arteriosclerosis and lipohyalin deposits within the vessel walls, the white matter becomes ischemic on a chronic basis.

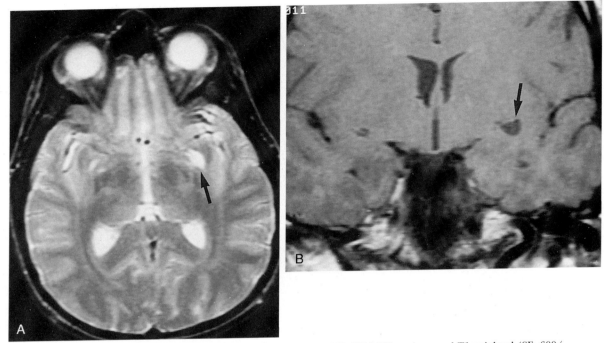

FIGURE 27–2. Large VR space. *A* and *B,* Axial T2-weighted (SE, 3000/80) and coronal T1-weighted (SE, 600/20) images show a 1-cm cyst-like lesion *(arrows)* in the left cerebral hemisphere. It has sharp, smooth margins, follows CSF signal, has no surrounding gliosis, and is positioned along the lateral aspect of the anterior commissure near other smaller VR spaces; therefore, it likely represents a large VR space.

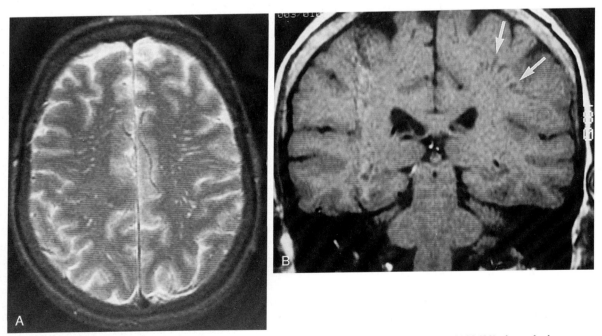

FIGURE 27–3. Abnormally dilated perivascular spaces *(état criblé). A,* Axial scan (SE, 3000/80) through the centrum semiovale shows many hyperintensities within the white matter that are more prominent than normally seen. Some are round, and others have a more linear character, as if following the course of vessels. *B,* On a T1-weighted image (SE, 600/20) the dilated VR spaces are distinctly hypointense *(arrows)* and exhibit a radial pattern in the left cerebral hemisphere.

Pathologically, one of the first changes in the aging brain is an increase in the perivascular interstitial fluid, predominantly at the arteriolar level of the vascular tree. With continued progressive ischemia of the white matter, additional histologic changes are observed, including atrophy of axons and myelin and tortuous, sclerotic, and thickened vessels. Maintenance of the myelin becomes deficient, resulting in "myelin pallor" on microscopic sections. Mild gliosis and increased interstitial fluid accompany the changes in the myelin.[14, 15]

Necrosis is not seen until severe ischemia leads to frank infarction of brain tissue. In the larger white matter lesions, Marshall and colleagues[16] demonstrated central areas of necrosis, axonal loss, and demyelination characteristic of true infarction. The central infarcts were surrounded by large peripheral zones of astrocytic reaction. The peripheral zones of "isomorphic gliosis" also exhibited high signal intensity on T2-weighted images and made the lesions appear much larger than the actual size of the infarcts. Their findings give support to the idea that the white matter hyperintensities represent a spectrum of pathologic changes associated with the vascular abnormalities.

As mentioned previously, the observed changes are secondary to chronic ischemia of the deep white matter and are found more often in patients with ischemic cerebrovascular disease, hypertension, and aging. A combination of arteriolar disease and episodic brain hypoperfusion probably leads to the histopathologic changes. Hypoperfusion can be caused by episodes of hypotension, hypoxia secondary to cardiac or carotid artery disease, hypertension, or aging.[17]

The white matter changes have been called atrophic perivascular demyelination, perivascular atrophy,[18] incomplete infarction, deep white matter infarction,[16] microangiopathic leukoencephalopathy,[7] Binswanger's disease, and subcortical arteriosclerotic encephalopa-

thy.[19] None of these terms are satisfying because they do not accurately reflect all the observed histologic changes, and they seem to overstate their clinical significance. There is no general agreement about what terminology most correctly describes the subcortical hyperintensities seen on T2-weighted MR images. It seems clear that the varied histologic changes are depicted on MR images as nonspecific foci of high signal intensity that, at present, cannot be distinguished. Therefore, more nonspecific terms might be appropriate, such as *deep white matter ischemia* or *white matter hyperintensities of aging*. In our MRI interpretations we also give a qualitative rating of the observed changes, such as "normal for age," "slightly advanced for age," and so on. A popular term used in the neurology literature is *leukoaraiosis*.[20]

Imaging Features

The most common locations for the hyperintensities are the subcortical and periventricular white matter, optic radiations, basal ganglia, and brain stem, in decreasing order of frequency.[14] The lesions are of high signal intensity on T2-weighted and proton density–weighted images and have well-defined but irregular margins (Fig. 27–4). They are mildly hypointense on T1-weighted images, but the contrast between the lesions and the normal brain is much less than that on T2-weighted images (Fig. 27–5). The white matter changes are not associated with breakdown of the blood-brain barrier and do not enhance. The process tends to be multifocal, but as the lesions enlarge, a more confluent pattern may develop.[21] As mentioned, lesions are often found in the internal capsule and putamen, common locations for lacunar infarcts (see section on differential diagnosis), and the brain stem can be involved. In fact, if patchy foci are seen within the brain stem without symptoms and with associated

FIGURE 27–4. Deep white matter ischemia: subcortical pattern. *A* and *B,* Axial proton density–weighted and T2-weighted scans (SE, 3000/20,80) demonstrate multiple focal hyperintensities within the subcortical white matter. The lesions are variable in size and shape. Some are discrete and well defined; others are irregular with indistinct margins. The borders of some in the left hemisphere are merging and becoming confluent.

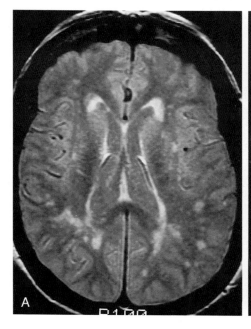
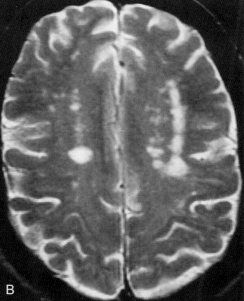

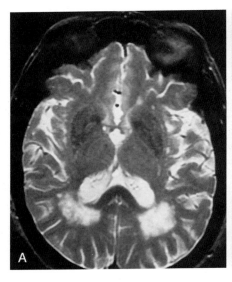

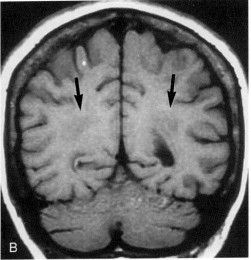

FIGURE 27–5. Deep white matter ischemia: signal intensity. A, Axial T2-weighted image (SE, 3000/80) shows large patchy areas of hyperintensity in the forceps major, bilaterally. Note that the lesions are separated from the atria of the lateral ventricles by a band of uninvolved white matter, to distinguish them from the characteristic ependymal-based plaques of MS. B, On a coronal T1-weighted image (SE, 600/20), the lesions are barely perceptible as mildly hypointense areas within the white matter (arrows).

changes of subcortical white matter ischemia, the brain stem foci probably represent changes of chronic ischemia as well. The subcortical U fibers receive their blood supply from shorter cortical arteries and are generally not involved by the process. Similarly, the corpus callosum is usually spared because it is supplied by the nearby pericallosal arteries.

Another pattern of white matter abnormality associated with deep white matter ischemia is a more or less continuous band of abnormal signal bordering the lateral ventricles (Fig. 27–6). This phenomenon should not be confused with the "periventricular halo" associated with obstructive hydrocephalus, which has a different mechanism (see Chapter 29). The brain has no lymphatics, and the bulk flow of interstitial water is centripetal toward the dorsolateral angles of the lateral ventricles. The fluid is removed by the ependymal cells and excreted into the ventricles by an active transport mechanism. Normally, this mechanism is efficient and water does not accumulate around the ventricles ex-

cept for small "CSF caps" around the frontal and occipital horns (Fig. 27–7). If the transport system is disrupted by an ependymitis or increased intraventricular pressure, periventricular fluid is observed on imaging studies.

In the case of white matter ischemia the transport mechanism remains intact, but the ischemia results in mild interstitial edema that exceeds the capacity of the ependymal transport system. The chronic accumulation of water around the ventricles adversely affects myelin maintenance and over time induces partial but irreversible loss of myelin that is reflected as myelin pallor of the periventricular white matter on pathologic examination. On T2-weighted MR images this white matter abnormality appears as a hyperintense band of variable thickness located along the dorsolateral angles of the ventricles, closely apposed to the ependymal surface.[21] A slightly heterogeneous texture and irregular outer margins distinguish it from the phenomenon of transependymal CSF flow or periven-

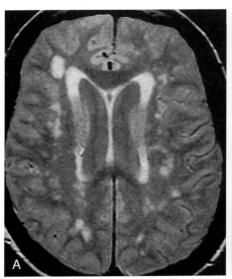

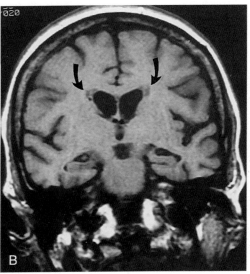

FIGURE 27–6. Deep white matter ischemia: periventricular pattern. A, Proton density–weighted image (SE, 3000/20) reveals a band of hyperintensity bordering the lateral ventricles. Multiple subcortical white matter lesions are also present. B, On a coronal T1-weighted scan (SE, 600/20), the periventricular bands are seen as discrete low-density areas (arrows) at the dorsolateral angles of the ventricles.

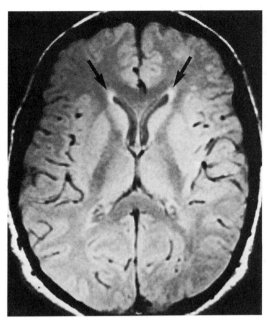

FIGURE 27–7. Normal frontal CSF caps. On a proton density–weighted image (SE, 3000/20), hyperintensity *(arrows)* surrounds the tips of the frontal horns of both lateral ventricles, representing normal accumulation of fluid in the area.

tricular halo of obstructive hydrocephalus (see section on differential diagnosis). On T1-weighted images the periventricular lesions are of lower signal intensity than the subcortical white matter lesions, probably due to increased water content (compare Fig. 27–6 with Fig. 27–5).

Functional Significance

Considerable debate reigns about the significance of the periventricular and subcortical white matter hyperintensities. In general, correlation between these findings and neurologic function is poor. A patient may have many high-signal-intensity foci within the white matter and be functioning perfectly normally for age. Nonetheless, these foci are not necessarily a normal part of aging because many elderly patients do not have them. Careful neuropsychologic studies have revealed that patients who have more of these lesions perform less well on neuropsychologic tests and are more likely to have cognitive deficits.[22] Steingart and colleagues[23] also noted a correlation with abnormalities of gait, limb power, plantar response, and the rooting and palmomental reflexes. They concluded that the observed white matter abnormalities may play a role in the development of intellectual impairment in the elderly. Drayer[7] suggested calling the process *normal aging* when a patient has the hyperintensities and *successful aging* when no lesions are present.

T2-weighted images, having high sensitivity for increased water content of the brain, detect the changes of deep white matter ischemia much earlier than does CT. A few small lesions may be found as early as the middle or late 40s, and then it becomes a clinical

problem to decide what further tests, if any, are necessary to rule out, beyond a reasonable doubt, other significant pathology. An additional problem is how to relate the scan findings to the patient without causing undue alarm. Perhaps we must accept that the brain degenerates with aging just like other organ systems. Everyone develops degenerative changes in the joints with aging, some more than others. Probably, a similar phenomenon occurs in the brain. Fortunately, the brain has a large reserve, so that minor structural changes do not significantly alter function.

MULTIPLE SCLEROSIS

CLINICAL FEATURES

MS is a chronic inflammatory disease of myelin that features a relapsing and remitting course with evidence of disseminated lesions in the white matter of the central nervous system. It is found predominantly in the northern climates of Canada, the United States, and Europe. The incidence of MS is 30 to 80 individuals per 100,000 population, and it is more prevalent in women than men (1.7:1.0). More than 250,000 Americans are afflicted, and MS is the most common disabling neurologic disease of young adults. More than two thirds of patients are between 20 and 40 years old.[24] The female-to-male ratio is even higher in children, and the disease tends to be more severe.[25]

The clinical course is characterized by acute, transient attacks of focal neurologic dysfunction. The presenting symptom is usually weakness or numbness in one or more extremities or visual loss secondary to optic neuritis. In general, patients recover function from these acute episodes, but some residual neurologic deficit is common. Over time, the initial relapsing and remitting course may advance to a more chronic progressive phase. Repeated attacks result in permanent white matter damage and chronic disability.[26]

A number of variants of MS have been described, including neuromyelitis optica (Devic's disease), concentric sclerosis (Baló's disease), and Schilder's diffuse sclerosis. Neuromyelitis optica is a severe form of optic neuritis that is often bilateral and leads to blindness. It is frequently associated with transverse myelitis and accompanied by lower extremity motor and sensory deficits. Concentric sclerosis is fortunately a relatively rare variant of MS. It has a monophasic course but is rapidly progressive and often fatal within a few years. A concentric or lamellar pattern of demyelination is characteristic of this disease.[27] Schilder's disease is a demyelinating disease of children. It shares many of the same symptoms with MS, but its course is more progressive, and intellectual and psychiatric problems are more common.

The diagnosis of MS is usually established by a combination of history, physical examination, laboratory tests, and imaging findings. The classification system most commonly used by neurologists was developed by Poser and colleagues,[28] which sets criteria to make the diagnosis of clinically definite or clinically probable

MS. The most definitive laboratory evidence is oligoclonal bands in the CSF demonstrated by protein electrophoresis. The MR findings are discussed further on.

The cause of MS is uncertain, but the most popular view is that an initial viral infection is followed sometime later by an autoimmune reaction that attacks the myelin. On histologic examination, acute MS plaques show partial or complete destruction and loss of myelin with sparing of axon cylinders. They occur in a perivenular distribution and are associated with a neuroglial reaction and infiltration of mononuclear cells and lymphocytes. The perivascular demyelination gives the appearance of a finger pointing along the axis of the vessel. In the pathologic literature, these elongated lesions have been named *Dawson's fingers*. Active demyelination is accompanied by transient breakdown of the blood-brain barrier. Chronic lesions show predominantly gliosis. MS plaques are distributed throughout the white matter of the optic nerves, chiasm and tracts, cerebrum, brain stem, cerebellum, and spinal cord.[24]

IMAGING FEATURES

The sensitivity of MRI has been reported as 67% in definite and probable MS combined[29] and as 76%[30] to 85%[31] in definite MS alone. These rates compare with published sensitivity figures for CT, ranging from 25% (routine enhanced CT)[31] to 60% (double-dose enhanced CT).[30] In general, CT enhanced with contrast medium performs as well as plain MRI in detecting acute plaques that are associated with breakdown of the blood-brain barrier and enhance, but MRI is far superior for evaluating patients with chronic progressive MS. Reports indicate that MRI is more helpful than evoked potentials or CSF findings for diagnosing MS[32]; and in patients with isolated cord symptoms, MRI of the brain was more sensitive than the laboratory tests.[33] Detection of spinal cord plaques remains problematic because the images are often degraded by swallowing artifacts and by respiratory and cardiac motion.

MS plaques are seen best with T2-weighted spin-echo pulse sequences (long repetition time, long echo time), except for lesions closely apposed to an ependymal surface, where they may be obscured by the high-signal-intensity CSF. These lesions are depicted better by proton density–weighted scans (long repetition time, short echo time) or with fluid-attenuated inversion recovery (FLAIR) pulse sequences,[33a] because the high-signal-intensity plaques are contrasted against the lower signal intensity CSF (Fig. 27–8). In general, T1-weighted images are less sensitive. MS plaques are hyperintense on T2-weighted and proton density–weighted images and hypointense on T1-weighted scans (Fig. 27–9). Specific signal intensities of MS lesions vary depending on the magnetic field strength, the pulse sequence parameters, and partial-volume effects. Occasionally, acute plaques may have a thin rim of relative T2 hypointensity or T1 hyperintensity (see Fig. 27–9B). The T1 hyperintensity has been attributed to free radicals, lipid-laden macrophages, and protein accumulations.[34]

MS plaques are usually discrete foci with well-defined margins. Most are small and irregular, but larger lesions can coalesce to form a confluent pattern. Multiple focal periventricular lesions can give a "lumpy-bumpy" appearance to the ventricular margins.[35] As a result of their perivenular distribution, many periventricular plaques have an ovoid configuration, with their long axis oriented transversely on an axial scan.[36] The ovoid lesion is the imaging correlate of Dawson's finger (see Figs. 27–8A and 27–9A). In general, MS plaques have a homogeneous texture without evidence of cystic or necrotic components. Hemorrhage is not a feature of MS lesions. Edema and mass effect are also uncommon.

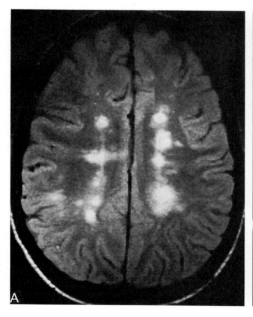
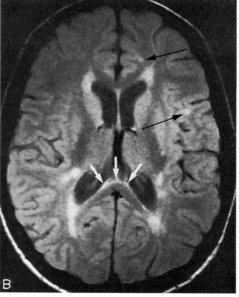

FIGURE 27–8. MS in a 22-year-old woman. *A,* Axial scan (SE, 3000/20) shows multiple plaques within the centrum semiovale bilaterally. *B,* On a proton density–weighted image (SE, 3000/20), MS plaques are clustered about the lateral atria. Two additional plaques *(black arrows)* are present in the subcortical U fibers. A long, arcing plaque *(white arrows)* involves the inner fibers of the splenium of the corpus callosum.

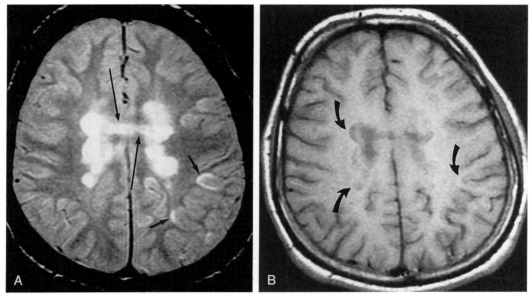

FIGURE 27–9. MS: Dawson's fingers, subcortical U fiber plaques. *A*, Proton density–weighted image (SE, 3000/30) demonstrates multiple plaques in the centrum semiovale. Note the finger-like bands of hyperintensity representing Dawson's fingers *(long arrows)*, extending medially from the plaques. Also, distinctive curvilinear plaques *(short arrows)* involve the subcortical U fibers. *B*, On a corresponding T1-weighted image (SE, 600/20) the plaques are hypointense. Note a thin rim of hyperintensity bordering some of the plaques *(arrows)*.

The periventricular white matter is a favorite site for MS plaques, particularly along the lateral aspects of the atria (see Fig. 27–8*B*) and occipital horns. The corpus callosum, corona radiata, internal capsule, visual pathways, and centrum semiovale are also commonly involved. When more than a few lesions are present, symmetric involvement of the cerebral hemispheres seems to be the rule. Any structures that contain myelin can harbor MS plaques, including the brain stem (Fig. 27–10), spinal cord, subcortical U fibers (see Fig. 27–9*A*) and even within the gray matter of the cerebral cortex and basal ganglia. A distinctive site in the brain stem is the ventrolateral aspect of the pons at the fifth nerve root entry zone[37] (see Fig. 27–10*B*). Brain stem and cerebellar plaques are more prevalent in the adolescent age group.[38]

Lesions of the corpus callosum have been a special focus of study. On axial sections, plaques in the corpus callosum above the lateral ventricles have a transverse orientation along the course of the nerve fiber tracts and vessels. Sagittal proton density–weighted images are especially helpful for depicting the small callosal lesions closely apposed to the superior ependymal surface of the lateral ventricles[39] (Fig. 27–11). Sagittal thin-section fast FLAIR appears to be even more sensitive for detecting MS plaques in the corpus collosum. Early edema and demyelination along subependymal veins produce a striated appearance.[39a] In a review of 40 patients by Simon and colleagues,[40] 30% had focal plaques in the corpus callosum. More than half also had long, inner callosal-subcallosal lesions that the authors described as "arcing" transversely through the corpus callosum and crossing the midline. The lesions were between 1 and 8 mm thick and were most often

seen on axial sections through the genu and splenium (see Figs. 27–8*B* and 27–11*A*).

Brain atrophy can be a prominent part of long-standing, chronic MS. Ventricular dilatation and sulcal enlargement are the most obvious changes. Atrophy of the corpus callosum is also present in 40% of patients (see Fig. 27–11*C*) and is seen best on T1-weighted sagittal images. The atrophy progresses from the ependymal surface toward the outer fibers of the corpus callosum. When Simon and associates[40] compared their 40 patients with MS with a control group, the corpus callosum measured 6.0 mm (range, 5.0 to 7.2 mm) in the normal group and only 4.3 mm (range, 3.0 to 5.4 mm) in the patients with MS.

In patients with advanced disease, Drayer and associates[41] noted decreased signal intensity (T2 shortening) in the putamen and thalamus on T2-weighted images. They postulated that the effect is likely due to abnormal accumulation of iron or other trace metals.

Involvement of the visual pathways, particularly the optic nerves, frequently occurs sometime during the course of disease. Patients may present with optic neuritis, although in about half of those cases, MRI will unveil other silent lesions in the brain.[42] Imaging plaques in the optic nerves is a challenge even for MRI. Nonenhanced spin-echo sequences are not sensitive, and generally some type of fat suppression is required. This can be achieved with short-tau inversion recovery (STIR) sequences or with chemical-shift methods.[43] Probably the most sensitive method for detecting acute MS of the optic nerves is the combination of gadolinium (Gd) enhancement and chemical-shift imaging[44] (Fig. 27–12). Most MRI systems now incorporate some type of frequency-selective method for fat

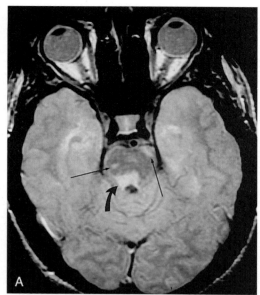

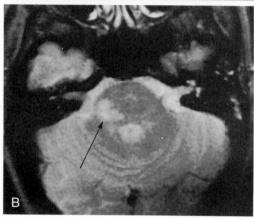

FIGURE 27–10. Brain stem plaques. *A,* Axial proton density–weighted scan (SE, 3000/30) through the upper pons reveals a large plaque *(curved arrow)* in the tegmentum of the pons and two smaller lesions *(thin arrows)* in the basis pontis. *B,* T2-weighted scan (SE, 3000/70) through the pons shows a plaque *(arrow)* in the ventrolateral pons at the fifth nerve root entry zone.

suppression. Although multiplanar imaging is usually performed to evaluate the optic nerves, partial-volume effects are minimized in the coronal plane.

The spinal cord is commonly involved by MS, and patients may present with a transverse myelitis. All levels of the cord can be affected, but most plaques are found in the cervical region. Because the white matter fiber tracts are positioned along the outer aspects of the cord, MS plaques are often based along a pial surface and have an elongated configuration. Signal characteristics are similar to those of lesions in the brain. Edema associated with acute plaques may lead to cord swelling, simulating an intramedullary tumor (Fig. 27–13). In chronic MS, cord atrophy can result from focal lesions or axonal degeneration from distal disease.[45]

Nonenhanced MRI cannot judge lesion activity, because plaques almost always remain evident after they disappear on CT scans.[29] Although the water content of acute plaques decreases over time, the T1 and T2 relaxation times of acute and chronic plaques have sufficient overlap that quantitative MRI cannot distinguish between old and new lesions.[46] Quantitative brain analyses of patients with MS have shown that the T1 and T2 relaxation times are prolonged not only in acute and chronic plaques but also in normal-appearing white matter.[47] The latter finding is noteworthy because it suggests that the white matter involvement in MS is a diffuse process, rather than the focal nature portrayed on the imaging studies and on clinical examination. Diffuse white matter involvement has been confirmed further with magnetization transfer (MT) measurements.[47a]

The clinical correlation of signs and symptoms with supratentorial disease is poor because most of the lesions seen by MRI are old and inactive. Because up to 83% of patients with brain stem and cerebellar plaques exhibit acute neurologic deficits, the correlation is better with lesions of the posterior fossa. In patients with MS with internuclear ophthalmoplegia, MRI has detected corresponding midbrain plaques even though CT findings were normal.[48] A system of grading overall disease severity by MRI has been found to correlate with clinical rating scales.[49] On the other hand, although half of patients with MS have evidence of psychologic morbidity, the type and severity of dysfunction do not correlate well with the MRI abnormalities. The lesion load on MRI tends to correlate better with cognitive dysfunction than with working memory deficits.[50]

Gadolinium Enhancement

Because acute MS plaques are associated with transient breakdown of the blood-brain barrier, Gd contrast agents produce enhancement of these lesions on T1-weighted images (Fig. 27–14). Enhancement is observed for 8 to 12 weeks after acute demyelination. Thus, Gd-enhanced MRI can be used to assess lesion activity just like CT enhanced with contrast medium. Either nodular or ring-like enhancement may be seen early after contrast medium injection (see Figs. 27–13*B* and 27–14*C*), but the central areas tend to fill in and become more homogeneous on delayed scans. Immediate postcontrast scans are most sensitive for detecting MS, and delayed scanning is not necessary. In a study by Grossman and associates,[51] Gd-enhanced MRI detected more enhancing lesions than "high-iodine" CT, and the lesions found correlated better with clinically active disease and recent deficits. Gd-enhanced MRI can be used to follow the progression of disease and to assess the response to therapy.[52]

Nesbit and colleagues[34] reviewed the histologic changes in MS lesions that had varying degrees of blood-brain barrier breakdown. They noted that the level of contrast enhancement correlated with the degree of macrophage infiltration but did not correlate with perivascular lymphocyte infiltration. Their data support the hypothesis that breakdown of the blood-brain barrier is related to macrophage migration and

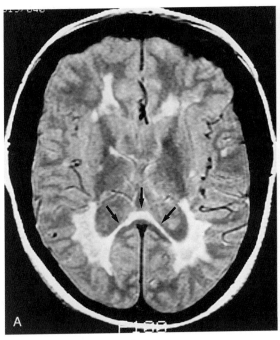

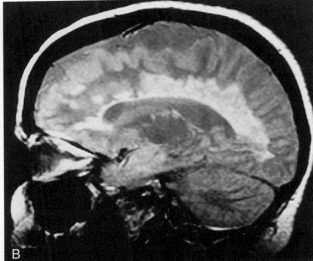

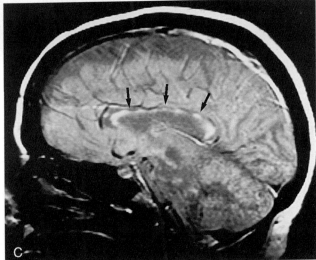

FIGURE 27–11. MS: corpus callosum. *A,* Axial proton density–weighted scan (SE, 3000/30) shows confluent plaques around the atria of the lateral ventricles and involvement of the inner fibers of the splenium of the corpus callosum *(arrows). B* and *C,* Proton density–weighted images (SE, 3000/30). The parasagittal section *(B)* shows extensive confluent involvement extending from the ependymal surface of the lateral ventricle into the white matter of the cerebral hemisphere. A midline sagittal section *(C)* demonstrates the typical lumpy-bumpy pattern *(arrows)* in the corpus callosum. Also noted is atrophy of the corpus callosum.

infiltration. It has also been noted that the enhancement peak for MS lesions may be delayed to 45 or 60 minutes after injection. This may be related to partial or incomplete breakdown of the blood-brain barrier in MS plaques, as opposed to a complete disruption of the blood-brain barrier in neoplastic or infectious lesions.[53]

Leptomeningeal enhancement has been reported with acute relapsing MS.[54] This is not a common phenomenon, but its occurrence is explained by pathologic reports of lymphoplasmocytic infiltration of the leptomeninges in 41% of cases at autopsy, mostly associated with active demyelination in brain plaques.[55]

Occasionally, large MS plaques, also called tumefactive MS, may produce mass effect and simulate other mass lesions. However, compared with neoplastic or inflammatory processes, MS plaques have minimal surrounding edema and relatively less mass effect for the overall size of the white matter lesion (Fig. 27–15). Lack of enhancement or the enhancement pattern may assist further characterization of these unusual

plaques. In most cases, additional periventricular plaques help solidify the diagnosis of MS.[56]

ADVANCED MR TECHNIQUES

Three advanced MR techniques that are still investigational include MR spectroscopy, MT contrast, and anisotropic diffusion imaging.

MR Spectroscopy

Localized proton spectroscopy has shown significantly lower *N*-acetylaspartate/cholesterol and *N*-acetyl-aspartate/phosphocreatine ratios in MS plaques compared with normal control subjects.[57] The ratios were reduced by the same amount, indicating that the changes were due to a decrease in the *N*-acetylaspartate peak density. Elevation of mobile lipids have also been reported in acute plaques, probably as a result of myelin breakdown[58] (see Chapter 30).

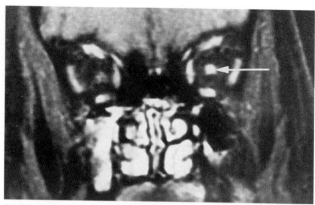

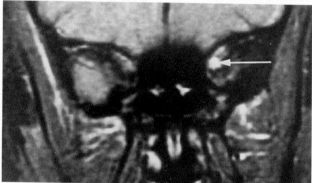

FIGURE 27–12. Optic neuritis. Gadolinium-enhanced T1-weighted images (SE, 600/20, fat suppressed) obtained in the coronal plane through the retrobulbar region of the orbits reveals enhancement of the left optic nerve *(arrows)*. The right optic nerve does not enhance because of an intact blood-brain barrier.

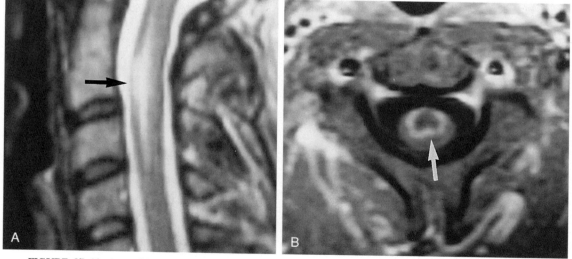

FIGURE 27–13. Acute MS of the spinal cord. The patient had recent onset of bilateral leg weakness and paresthesias. *A,* Sagittal T2-weighted image (fast SE, 3600/102, effective) shows an elongated plaque in the upper cervical cord *(arrow)*, associated with fusiform swelling of the cord. *B,* An axial Gd-enhanced image (SE, 800/12) reveals ring enhancement of the plaque *(arrow)* and confirms the cord swelling.

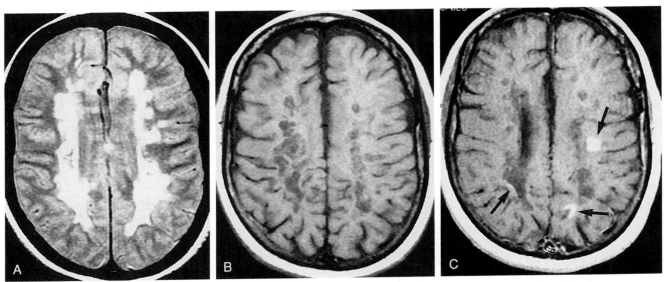

FIGURE 27–14. Enhancing MS plaques in a patient with acute presentation. *A* and *B*, Proton density–weighted (SE, 3000/30) and T1-weighted (SE, 600/20) images disclose multiple plaques in the periventricular white matter. The plaques are discrete, well defined, and variable in shape and size. Some of the plaques have merged to form a more confluent pattern. *C*, On a contrast-enhanced scan (SE, 600/20), some of the plaques enhance *(arrows)*, indicating that they are active lesions. The chronic plaques do not enhance.

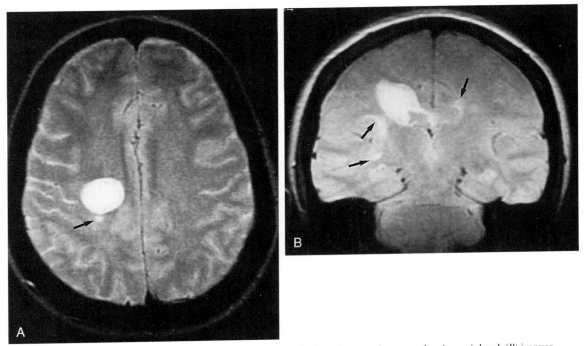

FIGURE 27–15. MS: mass-like plaque. Axial T2-weighted *(A)* and coronal proton density–weighted *(B)* images (SE, 3000/30,80) show a 2-cm mass in the right centrum semiovale. The diagnosis of MS is suggested by a number of features, including well-defined margins without surrounding edema, close apposition to an ependymal surface (coronal view), relatively little mass effect for lesion size, and the presence of additional plaques *(arrows)*.

Magnetization Transfer Imaging

MT makes use of the property that relatively immobile protons of myelin have broad resonances compared with free water protons. Off-resonance radiofrequency pulses can be applied to selectively saturate portions of the immobile proton pool, and subsequent exchange with mobile protons results in partial saturation of the mobile pool and decreased signal intensity from free water. The MT effect is most prominent in normally myelinated white matter, and the effect is less in areas of demyelination[59] (see Chapter 1).

In patients with MS, the MT ratios become progressively lower with increasing hypointensity of lesions on T1-weighted images, reflecting progressive demyelination and breakdown of macromolecular structure. MT imaging has higher sensitivity for MS abnormalities and may improve the ability of MRI to characterize MS plaques and to separate edema from demyelination.[59a]

Diffusion-Weighted Imaging

Diffusion-weighted imaging uses strong magnetic field gradient pulses to amplify the dephasing effects of normal molecular motions, resulting in attenuation of the MR signal. Diffusion is maximal in fluids such as CSF and less in solid tissues that have structure and restrict molecular motions. In white matter, molecular motion is further restricted by the axonal walls and myelin sheaths, so that diffusion is anisotropic, occurring mainly along the long axis of the fiber tracts.[60] Diffusion studies of myelination in infants suggest that the myelin sheath is primarily responsible for the diffusion anisotropy in white matter. In normal white matter the reduction of MR signal depends heavily on the orientation of the fiber tracts and the gradient direction. Maximal signal loss occurs when the gradient pulses are parallel to the fiber tracts. With demyelination and vasogenic edema, the diffusional effects would be greater and less dependent on gradient direction, so contrast could be achieved between normal and diseased white matter with diffusion imaging[61] (see Chapter 8). In a study of experimental allergic encephalomyelitis, diffusion-weighted imaging was more sensitive to white matter disease than T2-weighted images.[62]

SUMMARY

In summary, MRI is without question the diagnostic imaging procedure of choice in patients with clinically suspected MS. Moreover, it can be conclusively stated that CT is inadequate. MRI is so exquisitely sensitive for detecting MS that the absence of plaques at MRI makes the diagnosis of active MS involving the brain extremely unlikely. Finally, the interpretation of MRI studies is aided by the usual occurrence of MS in a younger group of patients than that associated with the more benign periventricular hyperintensities of aging. When an atypical presentation of MS is being considered in an older patient, the nonspecificity of white matter lesions becomes quite troublesome. This problem is discussed later in the section on differential diagnosis.

INFECTIOUS AND INFLAMMATORY DISORDERS

PROGRESSIVE MULTIFOCAL LEUKOENCEPHALOPATHY
(see also Chapter 20)

Progressive multifocal leukoencephalopathy (PML) is a demyelinating disease that results from reactivation of a latent DNA papovavirus in an immunocompromised host. The JC virus, named after the initials of the patient from whom it was first isolated, primarily infects oligodendrocytes, resulting in failure of these cells to maintain myelin. In the past, most cases occurred in patients with Hodgkin's disease, in patients with chronic lymphocytic leukemia, or in those treated with corticosteriods or immunosuppressive drugs. Today, PML is more often associated with acquired immunodeficiency syndrome (AIDS) and has been reported in 5.3% of AIDS patients.[63] The opportunistic infection causes progressive neurologic deterioration, including motor and sensory dysfunction, visual deficits, personality change, memory loss, and disturbances of speech and cognition. There is no effective therapy, and death usually ensues within 6 to 9 months.

The predominant pathologic abnormality is focal demyelination and myelin pallor on cut sections of the involved brain. Histologic examination reveals large, swollen oligodendrocytes with multiple intranuclear inclusions laden with virus particles. The deformed oligodendrocytes are most numerous at the peripheral margins of demyelination. An associated astrocytosis features mostly large multinucleate astrocytes.[64] Perivascular inflammation is not seen in PML, to distinguish it from the immune-mediated demyelinating disorders.

PML has an affinity for subcortical white matter, and the classic distribution is in the parieto-occipital lobes. It is not primarily a periventricular process, but as the disease progresses the deeper white matter is also affected. Any white matter structures can be involved, but lesions of the corpus callosum are much less common than in MS, for example. Brain stem and cerebellar lesions are found in about one third of patients; occasionally, they can be the solitary presenting lesion. Basal ganglia and thalamic sites generally represent extension from lesions in the internal capsule or damage to white matter fibers coursing through the gray matter structures.[65]

The white matter lesions of PML are patchy and round or oval at first but then become confluent and large. The process is often distinctly asymmetric and initially involves the peripheral white matter, following the contours of the gray matter–white matter interface to give outer scalloped margins (Fig. 27–16). Lesions tend to be homogeneous with well-defined margins. The prolonged T1 and T2 relaxation times reflect the loss of myelin and increased water (see Fig. 20–25).

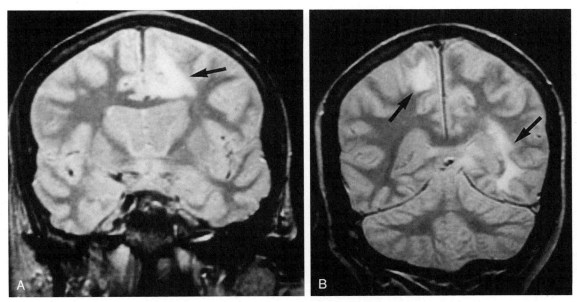

FIGURE 27–16. PML. *A* and *B*, Coronal proton density–weighted images (SE, 3000/30) show patchy hyperintense foci *(arrows)* within both cerebral hemispheres. The lesions involve the more peripheral subcortical white matter, giving them scalloped outer margins.

Mass effect and contrast enhancement are rarely seen.[66]

Mark and Atlas[67] reported that atypical features are common on MR images. A little hemorrhage or peripheral enhancement should not eliminate PML from diagnostic consideration. The gray matter was affected in 50% of their cases. When subcortical lesions extend outward to involve the adjacent cortex, the gray matter–white matter margins become indistinct and the disease process may simulate a cortical encephalitis, cerebritis, or even cerebral infarction. Occasionally, PML may extend across the corpus callosum like a lymphoma or glioma. These atypical features suggest a more aggressive form of PML in the AIDS population.

ACUTE DISSEMINATED ENCEPHALOMYELITIS

Acute disseminated encephalomyelitis is a demyelinating disease that is thought to be of autoimmune origin. It usually occurs within 2 weeks after one of the childhood viral infections, such as measles or chickenpox, or after vaccination against rabies or smallpox. It has also been reported in association with chronic Epstein-Barr virus infection.[68] The clinical picture is one of abrupt onset with a monophasic course, to distinguish it from MS and most other white matter diseases. Initial headache, seizures, and drowsiness may progress to profound lethargy and even coma. Brain stem involvement can produce nystagmus, diplopia, and dysarthria. Because it is a myelinoclastic process, lesions usually correlate with discrete clinical symptoms.[69] Although variable, recovery is often surprisingly good. Acute hemorrhagic leukoencephalitis is a more fulminant variant of acute disseminated encephalomyelitis.

Lesions are found in the white matter of the brain stem, cerebrum, and cerebellum, and as a rule are asymmetric and few (Fig. 27–17). There is no predilection for the periventricular white matter. The lesions are typically hyperintense on T2-weighted images and hypointense on T1-weighted images and without hemorrhage or calcification. Despite the acute demyelinating picture, enhancement with contrast medium has been reported in only a few cases.[70] Involvement of the deep gray matter has also been reported[71] (see Fig. 20–10).

SUBACUTE SCLEROSING PANENCEPHALITIS

Subacute sclerosing panencephalitis is another autoimmune disease that presents a few years after measles infection. It is characterized by a progressive relentless course, often leading to death within 2 years. Fortunately, the incidence of this disease has markedly decreased with the introduction of measles vaccine. Diagnosis is established by clinical features and the presence of measles antibody in the CSF and serum. Histologic examination shows severe myelin and axonal loss, inflammation, gliosis, and nuclear inclusions in the oligodendrocytes and neurons. The white matter changes are patchy and nonspecific but tend to involve the parietal lobes.[72]

SUBACUTE ENCEPHALITIS CAUSED BY HUMAN IMMUNODEFICIENCY VIRUS

A subacute encephalitis involving the white matter is seen in up to 30% of patients with AIDS. Levy and colleagues[73] reported that 54 (17%) of 315 patients in their clinical series had subacute encephalitis. In another series, 31.4% had microglial nodular encephali-

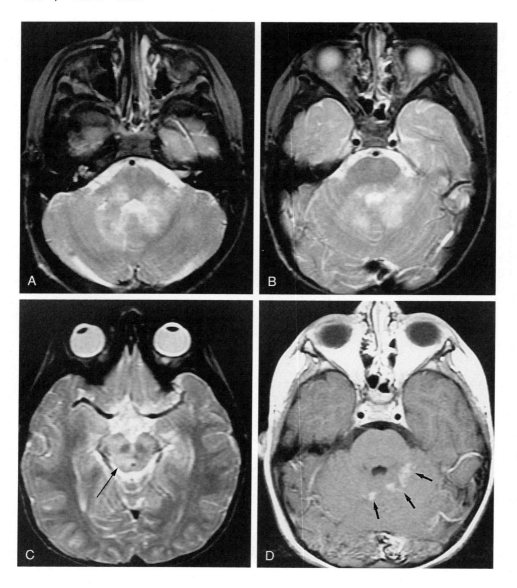

FIGURE 27–17. Acute disseminated encephalomyelitis. A 10-year-old child developed progressive brain stem dysfunction 2 weeks after an influenza-like syndrome. *A* and *B*, Contiguous axial T2-weighted images (SE, 3000/80) through the brain stem demonstrate patchy hyperintensities with indiscrete margins within the tegmentum of the pons, middle cerebellar peduncles, and the deep white matter of both cerebellar hemispheres. *C*, A higher section discloses abnormal high signal intensity *(arrow)* within the right midbrain as well. *D*, On a Gd-enhanced scan (SE, 600/20), some of the lesions in the cerebellum enhance *(arrows)*.

tis suggesting human immunodeficiency virus (HIV), and cytomegalovirus was found in only 14.4% of those cases.[74] The two viruses often coexist in brain specimens taken from patients with AIDS.[75] Additional studies have confirmed a predominant HIV etiology for the microglial nodules and the subacute white matter encephalitis.[76]

The MRI picture is one of bilateral, diffuse, patchy to confluent areas of increased signal intensity on T2-weighted images with poorly defined margins involving the white matter of the cerebrum, cerebellum, and brain stem[77] (see Fig. 20–23). The white matter changes are not as striking as in many other demyelinating diseases. Initially, the images may show only a hazy mottled pattern of hyperintensity within the centrum semiovale. HIV encephalitis does not enhance with Gd. The MR appearance is distinct from that of PML, and the clinical setting readily separates it from other white matter abnormalities.

In a study of 21 patients with HIV encephalitis,[78] both CT and MRI were found to be relatively insensi-

tive to the early stages of involvement, manifested pathologically by widespread microscopic microglial nodules with multinucleate giant cells. The secondary changes of atrophy were well seen by both modalities in the majority of patients, whereas parenchymal lesions consistent with demyelination were noted in three of seven patients studied by MRI.

A study by Chrysikopoulos and colleagues[79] of 24 patients with biopsy-proven HIV encephalitis revealed similar results. Neither MRI nor CT could detect the microglial nodules or multinucleate giant cells, the hallmark of HIV encephalitis. Atrophy, the most common finding, was found in 18. White matter abnormality was imaged only in four patients. The white matter changes seen by MRI and CT correlated pathologically with demyelination and vacuolation associated with severe HIV infection.

HEREDITARY METABOLIC DISORDERS

The group of hereditary metabolic disorders includes a long list of diseases that affect the gray and white matter to varying degrees. This section discusses briefly the major diseases that affect primarily the white matter, including the classic leukodystrophies. The names and terminologies of these disorders are confusing because they were derived from the pathologic literature before their metabolic defects were discovered. As the specific biochemical and enzyme defects are being elucidated, these diseases are being classified more appropriately. The ones with "cause unknown" are listed under the general category of primary white matter disorders.

The classic leukodystrophies include adrenoleukodystrophy, Krabbe's globoid cell, and metachromatic leukodystrophy and a few other less well-known entities. They have in common a genetic origin and involve the peripheral nerves as well as the central nervous system. Each is caused by a specific inherited biochemical defect in the metabolism of myelin proteolipids that results in abnormal accumulation of a metabolite in brain tissue. Progressive visual failure, mental deterioration, and spastic paralysis develop early in life; however, variants of these diseases have a more delayed onset and a less progressive course.[24] The other primary white matter disorders include Alexander's disease, Canavan's disease, Cockayne's syndrome, and Pelizaeus-Merzbacher disease.[80]

All of the previously mentioned white matter diseases are characterized by symmetric massive involvement of the white matter (Fig. 27–18). MRI is quite sensitive for detecting the white matter damage, but it is not specific. Van der Knaap and coworkers[81] developed a computer-based pattern recognition program in an attempt to enhance the specificity of image interpretation. Their program uses information about brain structures involved, lesion characteristics, and special features, such as calcification, ventricular size, and enhancement with Gd.

Two metabolic disorders, Hurler's disease and Lowe's syndrome, are associated with cystic changes in the cerebral white matter. Hurler's disease is one of the mucopolysaccharidoses, caused by an enzymatic defect in the degradation of heparan, dermatan, or keratan sulfate. The cystic lacunar lesions in the white matter are dilated perineuronal spaces filled with mucopolysaccharide gargoyle cells.[82] Lowe's syndrome, one of the aminoacidurias also known as the oculocerebrorenal syndrome, results from defects in the amino acid transport mechanism. In addition to the renal deficiencies, these patients develop ocular problems and patchy white matter lesions with cystic components.[83] (For a more in-depth discussion of metabolic disorders, see Chapter 28.)

ACQUIRED TOXIC-METABOLIC DISORDERS

EFFECTS OF CHEMOTHERAPEUTIC AGENTS

Many of the cancer chemotherapeutic drugs are neurotoxic. The blood-brain barrier limits the direct entry of these substances into the brain, but the barrier may be damaged by the disease process or by the therapeutic agent itself. Also, in the case of central nervous system disease, agents may be given to open the blood-brain barrier to allow greater access of the anticancer drug to the tumor. Lipid solubility and intrathecal administration are other factors that increase delivery to the brain. The chemotherapeutic agents commonly associated with leukoencephalopathy include methotrexate, cisplatin, cytarabine, carmustine, and thiotepa. The combination of chemotherapy and radiation has a synergistic effect, resulting in greater damage to the white matter than either therapy alone.[84] Combinations of chemotherapeutic agents are also commonly used.[85]

Both acute and delayed effects are observed with chemotherapy. The acute changes develop during

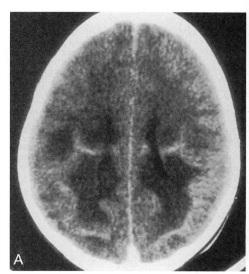
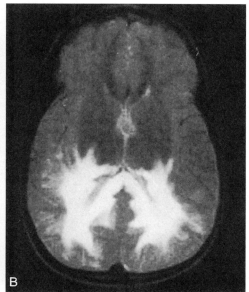

FIGURE 27–18. Adrenoleukodystrophy. *A*, CT scan of a young child demonstrates bilateral hypodense areas within the white matter of the occipital and posterior parietal lobes. The involvement is relatively symmetric and confluent. *B*, A T2-weighted MR image in the same child shows hyperintensity in the same areas of the posterior cerebral white matter. The posterior temporal lobe is also involved, and the abnormality extends into the splenium of the corpus callosum.

therapy, often within the first few days of initiating treatment. High-dose intravenous methotrexate is the most common cause, but acute neurotoxicity has also been reported with cytarabine.[86] The bilateral diffuse white matter hyperintensity is transient, and patients may be entirely asymptomatic.

The delayed effects of chemotherapy range from asymptomatic white matter hyperintensities to a severe necrotizing leukoencephalopathy. The onset of clinical and imaging findings is earlier than that observed with radiation, usually a few weeks or months after therapy. The reported incidence of necrotizing leukoencephalopathy varies widely, but it is much higher with central nervous system leukemia or when combinations of intravenous and intrathecal chemotherapy and radiation are employed.

Early in the course of disease, histologic examination shows widespread white matter edema with mild gliosis, which can advance to loss of oligodendroglia and multifocal demyelination, axonal swelling, astrocytic hypertrophy, and coagulation necrosis. Petechial hemorrhage and increased macrophage activity have also been reported. Unlike radiation changes, hyalinization and fibrinoid necrosis of arterioles are not seen with chemotherapy alone.[87]

MRI initially reveals patchy involvement of the periventricular white matter and centrum semiovale, which evolves to a confluent pattern. The process tends to spare the deep white matter tracts, brain stem, and cerebellum. Enhancement or mass effect is seen only in the most severe cases. Long-term follow-up often shows some brain atrophy, and in children treated for cancer, cerebral calcification is commonly found.[88, 89]

Compared with radiation change, the leukoencephalopathy associated with chemotherapy is detected earlier but is not as permanent. Wilson and colleagues[90] conducted a longitudinal study of 25 children with acute lymphocytic leukemia, performing serial MRI from baseline to 3 years after initiation of therapy. Bilateral symmetric white matter abnormalities were noted in 17 patients, but the changes observed with MRI were largely reversible, showing marked improvement at follow-up imaging. Clinical symptoms were relatively mild. Although 12 children showed neuropsychologic deficits, no correlation was found between MRI findings and neuropsychologic deficits (see also Chapter 28).

IMMUNOSUPPRESSANT THERAPY

Leukoencephalopathy is also associated with immunosuppressant therapy. The cyclosporines are the most widely immunosuppressants used, and neurologic complications occur in about 20% of transplant patients receiving cyclosporine. The cause of neurotoxicity is not known, but the proposed mechanisms range from a demyelinating process, ischemia from vasospasm, to hypertensive encephalopathy. MRI reveals lesions with high signal intensity on T2-weighted nonenhanced images. There is a predilection for the posterior cerebral white matter, and in severe cases the adjacent gray matter can be involved. The white matter injury appears to be reversible. At least, the MRI findings resolve in few weeks and follow clinical recovery.[91]

White matter damage has also been reported with FK 506, a newer immunosuppressant drug. MRI features include multifocal hyperintensities on T2-weighted images, a diffuse confluent involvement of the white matter with focal hemorrhage, and brain atrophy.[92, 93]

CENTRAL PONTINE MYELINOLYSIS

Central pontine myelinolysis is a disorder characterized pathologically by dissolution of the myelin sheaths of fibers within the central aspect of the basis pontis. In extreme cases there may be extension to the pontine tegmentum, midbrain, thalamus, internal capsule, and cerebral cortex.[94] The myelinolysis occurs with relative sparing of the nerve cells and axon cylinders. Many patients are asymptomatic, and at the other extreme are patients whose symptoms are masked by coma. Most clinically diagnosed cases present with spastic quadriparesis, pseudobulbar palsy, and acute changes in mental status, with progression possible to altered levels of consciousness and death. Survival is possible with varying residual neurologic deficits. Although initial reports were largely confined to chronic alcoholics, central pontine myelinolysis has also been seen in patients with electrolyte disturbances, particularly hyponatremia that has been rapidly corrected.

The use of MRI has increased the number of positive imaging studies in patients with central pontine myelinolysis. In a study by Miller and colleagues[95] of 13 patients with central pontine myelinolysis (5 diagnosed clinically, 8 diagnosed at autopsy), only one of nine CT examinations was positive, whereas 10 of 11 patients had positive MRI studies. The lesions with MRI were seen best as areas of hypointensity on inversion recovery images and hyperintensity on T2-weighted images in the central pons with sparing of the pontine tegmentum and ventrolateral pons. All lesions had an oval shape on sagittal images, a bat-wing configuration on coronal images, and various shapes on the axial images (Fig. 27–19; also see Fig. 28–26). Associated lesions were noted in three patients in the periventricular white matter, basal ganglia, and corticomedullary junction (see Fig. 28–27). Follow-up imaging at 6 months and 1 year revealed little or no change despite clinical recovery.

The clinical symptoms can be quite mild despite obvious pontine hyperintensity on MR images.[96] The extrapontine lesions often resolve completely, leaving some residual pontine abnormality. Enhancement is not a feature of this disease, but severe cases may show peripheral enhancement of the pontine lesions.[97]

CARBON MONOXIDE

Carbon monoxide poisoning causes distinctive bilaterally symmetric lesions within the globus pallidus (see Fig. 28–28). Associated low signal intensity in the thalamus and putamen is probably due to iron deposition.

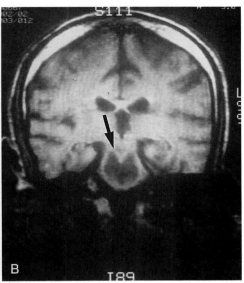

FIGURE 27–19. Central pontine myelinolysis. Axial T2-weighted *(A)* and coronal T1-weighted *(B)* images disclose a prominent abnormality *(arrows)* in the basis pontis. The lesion has well-defined margins, has a homogeneous texture, and exhibits prolongation of both T1 and T2 relaxation times.

Also, Chang and colleagues[98] reported a delayed encephalopathy occurring 1 to 2 months after carbon monoxide intoxication. A bilateral confluent pattern of hyperintensity was seen in the cerebral white matter on T2-weighted images. Improvement on follow-up clinical and MRI examinations suggests a reversible demyelinating process.

RADIATION INJURY

Radiation to the brain produces acute, early delayed, and late changes. The acute changes occur during the course of irradiation and represent mild vasogenic edema secondary to an acute inflammatory response of the capillary endothelium. The endothelium is the most radiosensitive tissue in the brain. These changes resolve after therapy and are not observed on imaging studies.

Early delayed changes develop during the second month after irradiation, are responsive to corticosteroid therapy, and generally resolve within 6 weeks. It is a multifocal demyelinating process similar to MS. Enhancing lesions can be found in the brain stem, basal ganglia, and deep cerebral white matter.[99]

Late radiation injury starts later but has a progressive and insidious course. The effects on the brain can be focal or diffuse, depending on whether whole brain or more focused radiation was given. The clinical picture is variable. Many patients are entirely asymptomatic; as a rule, severe imaging abnormalities are required for patients to have symptoms. Impairment of mental function is the most common problem and may include personality change, memory deficiencies, confusion, learning difficulties, and, in severe cases, dementia.[100]

A few months after irradiation, demyelination is seen histologically, associated with proliferation of the glial elements and mononuclear cells. This condition can progress to irreversible damage to the capillary endothelium, perivascular inflammation, breakdown of the blood-brain barrier, diffuse vasogenic edema of the cerebral white matter, necrotic foci, vacuolation, and petechial hemorrhage. Endothelial hyperplasia also occurs, resulting in reduced cerebral blood flow. The pathologic changes of radiation necrosis continue to evolve for a number of years after the initial irradiation. The location and amount of brain injury are related to the radiation dose, fractionation methods, and the portals used.[101]

The effects of late radiation injury to the brain are first detected on imaging studies about 6 to 8 months after the initial therapy. MRI detects more lesions than CT, and the abnormalities appear more extensive with MRI than with CT.[102] The characteristic pattern of diffuse radiation injury is symmetric, high-signal-intensity foci on T2-weighted images in the periventricular white matter (Fig. 27–20; see also Fig. 28–35). There is initial sparing of the corpus callosum and the subcortical arcuate fibers. The changes parallel those seen in ischemia, but the lesions are more prevalent and a confluent pattern usually develops.[103] As the process extends outward to involve the peripheral arcuate fibers of the white matter, the margins become scalloped (Fig. 27–21), a helpful feature in the differential diagnosis.[104] With time, atrophy becomes a part of the picture, as shown by enlargement of the ventricles and cortical sulci. There is relative sparing of the posterior fossa, basal ganglia, and internal capsules, but in more severe cases these structures are also involved. Deposition of hemosiderin in the basal ganglia has been reported. As observed histologically, imaging findings may continue to progress for 2 or more years after radiation therapy.[105]

With focal high-dose therapy, radiation necrosis may lead to profound edema, mass effect, and enhancement with Gd. Especially in these cases, distinguishing radiation change from recurrent tumor can be extremely difficult, if not impossible. Frequently, biopsy is required to clarify the issue.[103]

Enhancement of radiation lesions depends on the

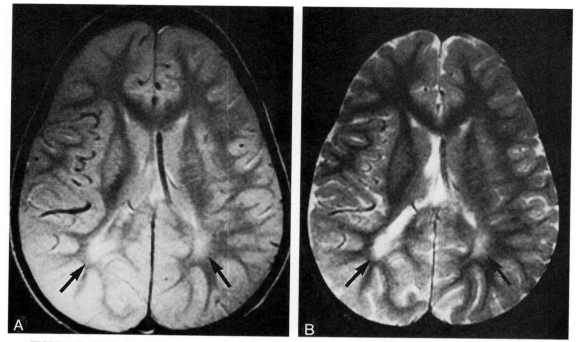

FIGURE 27–20. Early radiation injury 8 months after irradiation for a posterior fossa tumor. *A* and *B,* Axial scans (SE, 3000/30,80) show focal areas of high signal intensity *(arrows)* within the forceps major bilaterally. A shunt catheter is present in the left lateral ventricle.

degree of blood-brain barrier breakdown. With mild injury to the blood-brain barrier, only vasogenic edema may be observed. More severe injuries result in leakage of the macromolecules of contrast agents across the blood-brain barrier into the interstitial space to produce enhancement of the area. In an experimental study of radiation injury, Hecht-Leavitt and colleagues[105] noted that the nonenhancing lesions showed only edema and demyelination, whereas the enhancing lesions demonstrated histologic changes of necrosis with inflammatory infiltrates (see also Chapter 28).

TRAUMATIC SHEAR INJURIES

Patients with head trauma constitute a large percentage of the cases referred for neuroimaging. Initially, the role of MRI in these patients was considered limited due to the time required for the examination, difficulty in using life-support and monitoring equipment within the scanning room, and problems in imaging acute hemorrhage. Although some of these problems remain, MRI has come to be used more frequently in these patients, particularly in the subacute period.

The most common head injuries result from blunt or nonpenetrating trauma. These frequently induce a temporary or longer loss of consciousness, and the brain may suffer gross damage despite the lack of a skull fracture or penetrating injury. The spectrum of intracranial injury from head trauma includes extracerebral hemorrhage, brain contusion, intracerebral hemorrhage, and diffuse axonal injuries or white matter shear injuries. Traumatic intracranial hemorrhage is

discussed in Chapter 21. This section discusses the effect of trauma on the white matter.

Severe head injuries are often associated with rotational forces that produce shear stresses on the brain parenchyma. The brain itself has little rigidity and is extremely incompressible. Brain volume can be decreased only by exerting great pressure. On the other hand, the brain is soft and malleable. Relatively little effort is required to distort the shape of the brain. The parenchyma is of relatively uniform density, except for differences between the CSF of the ventricles and surrounding brain tissue. Slight differences in density also exist between gray matter and white matter.[106]

When the skull is rapidly rotated, it carries along the superficial brain parenchyma but the deeper structures lag behind, causing axial stretching, separation, and disruption of nerve fiber tracts. Shear stresses are most marked at junctions between tissues of differing densities.[107] As a result, shear injuries commonly occur at gray matter–white matter junctions (see Fig. 21–45), but they are also found in the deep white matter of the corpus callosum, centrum semiovale, brain stem (mostly the midbrain and rostral pons), and cerebellum.[108] Lesions in the basal ganglionic regions are usually found along the borders between the ganglia and the internal or external capsules, in other words, the deep gray matter–white matter junctions of the cerebral hemispheres. The thalamic and basal ganglia injuries are hemorrhagic in slightly more than 50% of cases[109] (Fig. 27–22). On the other hand, shear injuries of the corpus callosum and centrum semiovale are more often nonhemorrhagic[110] (Fig. 27–23).

Attempts to correlate CT findings with acute and chronic sequelae of closed head trauma have been

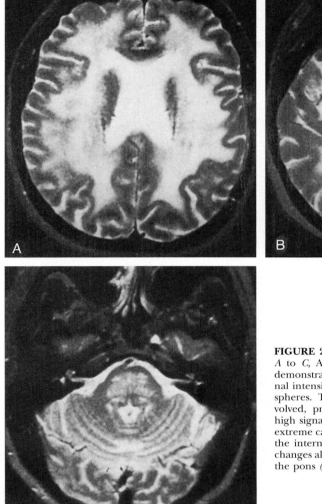

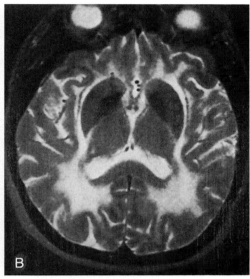

FIGURE 27-21. Severe advanced radiation injury. *A to C,* Axial T2-weighted images (SE, 3000/80) demonstrate extensive confluent areas of high signal intensity within the white matter of both hemispheres. The peripheral white matter is also involved, producing scalloped outer margins. The high signal intensity extends into the external and extreme capsules *(B),* but there is relative sparing of the internal capsules and basal ganglia. Radiation changes also affect the fiber tracts coursing through the pons *(C).*

discouraging, largely related to the insensitivity of CT to many cerebral injuries. Chiefly among these, poorly seen by CT and well seen by MRI, are the diffuse axonal injuries or white matter shear injuries. These injuries constitute the most frequent MRI findings in head trauma, constituting 40% of all lesions in one study of 40 patients.[111] Shear injuries are most often multiple, ovoid, and parallel to white matter fiber bundles. They are hyperintense on T2-weighted and hypointense on T1-weighted scans, unless hemorrhagic components are present, in which case more complex patterns are observed. During transition phases of hematoma evolution, combinations of methemoglobin, hemosiderin rings, and peripheral edema can result in layers of different signal intensity and a target-like appearance.[112]

The axial plane is the primary plane of imaging for shear injuries, but supplemental coronal views are helpful for assessing injuries to the body of the corpus callosum. Fast scanning techniques or gradient-echo images have lower resolution but are useful in uncoop-

erative patients. Contrast enhancement has little role in the evaluation of traumatic brain injuries.

Studies indicate that the added information provided by MRI in many traumatic conditions is clinically useful. MRI defines the exact extent of large extracerebral fluid collections and the presence of small collections better than CT, but rarely has the surgical management of the patient been altered by this information. However, the medical management and prognosis of the patient were often altered significantly by the additional information provided by MRI.[113] Diffuse axonal injuries have been associated with impaired consciousness and poor prognosis. Exact correlation of MRI with clinical status has been variable. In a study of 20 patients with mild and moderate closed head injuries, lesions documented by MRI correlated more closely with deficits on neuropsychologic testing than did lesions noted by CT.[114] Kelly and colleagues[115] studied 100 patients with head trauma, and in the 24 patients with post-traumatic syndrome (a constellation of complaints including headache, vertigo, memory

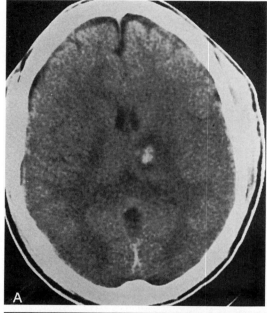

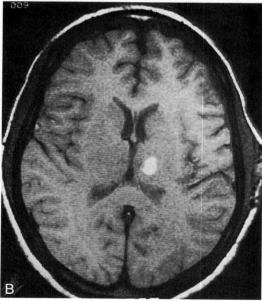

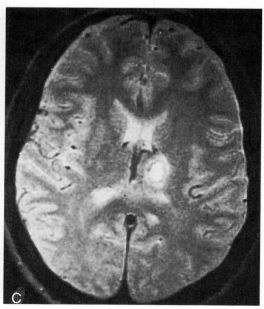

FIGURE 27–22. Hemorrhagic thalamic contusion. *A*, CT scan 2 days after injury reveals hemorrhage in the left thalamus. *B*, T2-weighted image 13 days after injury shows high-signal-intensity subacute hemorrhage. *C*, T2-weighted image reveals high signal intensity centrally with a low-signal-intensity rim from hemosiderin deposition, surrounded by higher signal intensity edema. (*A* to *C* from Hesselink JR, Dowd CF, Healy ME, et al: MR imaging of brain contusions: a comparative study with CT. AJNR 9:269–278, 1988. © by American Society of Neuroradiology.)

FIGURE 27–23. Shear injury of the corpus callosum, bilateral subdural hygromas, and small subdural hematoma. *A*, CT scan illustrates blood along the posterior falx *(arrow)*. No abnormality of the corpus callosum is identifiable. *B*, Proton density–weighted image demonstrates high-signal-intensity contusion in the splenium of the corpus callosum *(arrow)* and small right occipital subdural hematoma. Isointense subdural collections are present over the frontal lobes bilaterally, consistent with subdural hygromas *(arrowheads)*. *C*, T2-weighted image demonstrates similar findings. (*A* to *C* from Hesselink JR, Dowd CF, Healy ME, et al: MR imaging of brain contusions: a comparative study with CT. AJNR 9:269–278, 1988. © by American Society of Neuroradiology.)

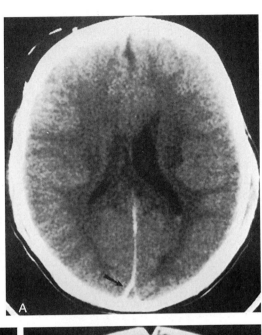

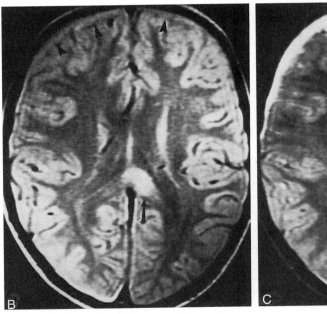

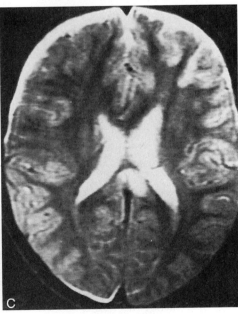

loss, attention deficits, and emotional instability), all had a normal CT and MRI study.

Overall, most investigators believe that MRI is superior to CT for imaging head trauma except in cases of acute (less than 48 to 72 hours) moderate to severe head trauma. In these cases the ease and rapidity of obtaining CT and its high sensitivity for acute hemorrhage make it the preferred imaging modality. The role of MRI in symptomatic patients after minimal head trauma remains uncertain, given the high percentage of normal studies in these cases. MRI is especially indicated in patients whose signs and symptoms are disproportionately greater than expected on the basis of CT findings.[116]

DIFFERENTIAL DIAGNOSIS

Because the periventricular hyperintensities have common histologic features, such as increased interstitial water, demyelination, and gliosis, it should not be surprising that their MRI appearance can be quite similar. Nevertheless, differential clues are often present on the images. The normal VR spaces should not be a problem. They are round, are no more than 1 or 2 mm, and are seen on the higher axial sections through the cerebral hemispheres and on lower sections through the basal ganglia at the level of the anterior commissure.

The major problem is distinguishing MS from the chronic changes of deep white matter ischemia and aging. MS is a disease of young adults, whereas the changes of ischemia are seen predominantly in patients older than 60 years old, but overlap of the age groups does occur. MS plaques tend to be closely apposed to the atria and occipital horns of the lateral ventricles. The corpus callosum is frequently involved, and plaques can be found in the subcortical U fibers

and even the cortical gray matter. The plaques in the corpus callosum often have a characteristic horizontal orientation. Lesions at the fifth nerve root entry zone and in the spinal cord are further evidence of MS. In a study by Yetkin and his group[117] of a series of patients with MS, hypertension, dementia, and normal control subjects, the specificity of the MRI diagnosis of MS was 95% to 99%.

White matter ischemia usually spares the corpus callosum and the subcortical U fibers. There is often a history of hypertension, stroke, and cardiovascular disease. A multifocal process with little or no neurologic dysfunction also suggests the diagnosis.

Many of the other white matter diseases have special features. PML occurs in an immunocompromised host and involves the peripheral white matter in a patchy and asymmetric fashion. The hereditary metabolic disorders occur in children and exhibit a symmetric, diffuse, and confluent pattern of involvement. Other infectious and inflammatory disorders have an acute clinical course and a history of a recent viral infection, vaccination, or AIDS.

Cerebral arteritis, secondary to collagen-vascular disease or granulomatous disease, can also result in multifocal periventricular hyperintensities (Fig. 27–24). Moreover, these diseases occur in young adults and can produce a neurologic picture similar to that of MS. Associated systemic features are important diagnostic clues for vasculitis, and the brain images usually reveal cortical infarcts in addition to the periventricular lesions[118, 119] (see Chapter 24).

Migraine is another neurologic problem associated with periventricular abnormalities. In a study by Soges and colleagues,[120] periventricular hyperintensities were found in 41% of patients with classic or common migraine and in 57% of patients with complicated migraine. The white matter lesions resemble deep white matter ischemia or vasculitis more than MS (see Fig.

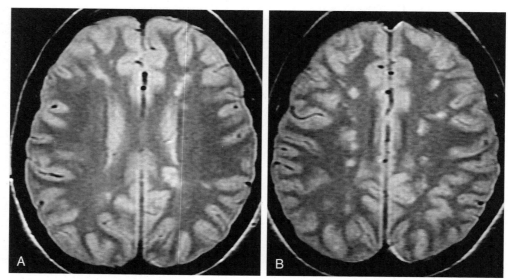

FIGURE 27–24. Cerebral arteritis in a 21-year-old woman with systemic lupus erythematosus. *A* and *B*, Axial proton density–weighted images (SE, 3000/30) disclose multiple discrete hyperintensities within the subcortical white matter. A lower section (not shown) also revealed a right occipital cortical infarct.

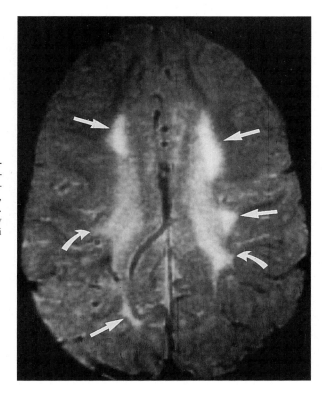

FIGURE 27–25. A 2-year-old child with cerebral palsy secondary to periventricular leukomalacia. A T2-weighted image demonstrates multiple high-signal-intensity lesions *(straight arrows)* within the periventricular white matter. Some lesions have coalesced with the lateral ventricles *(curved arrows)*, resulting in a wavy appearance to the lateral borders of the ventricles. Overall, the volume of white matter is markedly reduced, particularly posteriorly. Relatively little white matter separates the cortical gyri and sulci from the ventricles.

24–15), and the classic pattern of headaches usually identifies these patients (see Chapter 24).

Periventricular leukomalacia is caused by neonatal hypoxia or ischemia, but it may be imaged during adulthood when these patients are being reevaluated or seen for other neurologic problems. It affects predominantly the periventricular white matter along the posterior bodies and atria of the lateral ventricles. The involvement tends to be symmetric and is often associated with regional loss of white matter volume and ventricular dilatation. The lesions have scalloped outer margins, and the ventricular surface may also be irregular due to coalescence of cystic components with the adjacent ventricles[121] (Fig. 27–25) (see Chapter 24).

A number of processes can cause a more or less continuous band of abnormal signal intensity within the white matter bordering the ventricles. Because the abnormal signal pattern is due to fluid accumulation and some loss of myelin, it is hyperintense on T2-weighted scans and hypointense on T1-weighted scans. Transependymal CSF flow from hydrocephalus usually appears as a smooth halo of relatively even thickness (Fig. 27–26). It also has the associated findings of

lateral ventricles enlarged out of proportion to the cortical sulci, dilated inferior recesses of the third ventricle, and smooth elevation and thinning of the corpus callosum (see Chapter 29). As mentioned earlier, deep white matter ischemia can result in myelin pallor of the periventricular white matter, but it is more heterogeneous, the margins are less sharply defined, and it involves predominantly the white matter along the upper outer margins of the lateral ventricles. Cytomegalovirus ventriculitis or ependymitis results from reactivation of a latent herpesvirus in an immunocompromised host, usually in the setting of HIV infection. T2 hyperintensity often outlines the entire lateral and third ventricles (see Fig. 20–24), and in severe cases the fourth ventricle as well. The associated inflammatory reaction results in Gd enhancement of the ependyma and subependymal white matter. The enhancement is linear, continuous, and of variable thickness[122, 123] (see Chapter 20).

Signal intensity on T1-weighted, proton density–weighted, and T2-weighted images is important information for characterizing lesions (Table 27–1). The proton density–weighted image is often helpful for

TABLE 27–1. SIGNAL INTENSITIES OF WHITE MATTER LESIONS

LESION	T2-WEIGHTED IMAGING	PROTON DENSITY–WEIGHTED IMAGING	T1-WEIGHTED IMAGING
VR spaces	High	Isointense	Low
Deep white matter ischemia	High	High	Slightly low
Cerebral infarct	High	High	Low
Infarct with cavitation	High	Isointense (center) High (perimeter)	Low
MS	High	High	Low

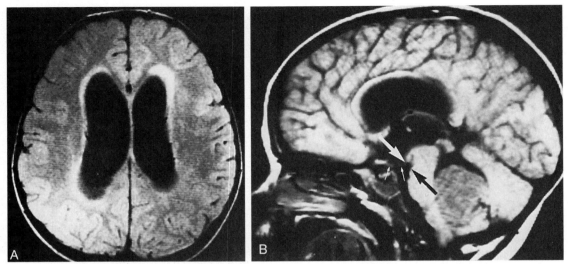

FIGURE 27–26. Acute obstructive hydrocephalus in an 8-year-old child with a medulloblastoma. *A*, Proton density–weighted scan (SE, 2000/25) shows dilated lateral ventricles with a periventricular halo of high signal. The halo is closely apposed to the ventricular surface and has smooth outer margins. *B*, A midline sagittal scan (SE, 600/25) discloses the large tumor that has grown into the fourth ventricle, obstructing CSF pathways. The corpus callosum is elevated and thinned. The mamillopontine distance is markedly reduced *(large arrows)*, and the hypothalamus is bowed inferiorly *(small arrows)*.

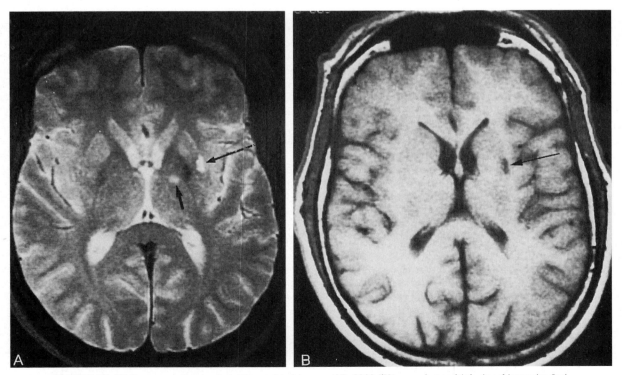

FIGURE 27–27. Lacunar infarcts. *A*, A T2-weighted image (SE, 2000/70) reveals two high-signal-intensity foci, one in the putamen *(long arrow)* and another in the region of the internal capsule *(short arrow)*. (From Brown JJ, Hesselink JR, Rothrock JF: MR and CT imaging of lacunar infarcts. AJNR 9:477–482, 1988. © by American Society of Neuroradiology.) *B*, On a T1-weighted scan (SE, 600/20), the putaminal infarct *(arrow)* is hypointense, owing to cystic necrosis. The other lesion is isointense, with signal characteristics identical with those of deep white matter ischemia. The clinical picture suggested a second infarct.

differentiating significant disease from the more benign processes. VR spaces, *état criblé*, brain cysts, and ventricular diverticula are all isointense relative to brain on the proton density–weighted image. The other entities show increased signal intensity. Unfortunately, the changes of deep white matter ischemia are also of higher signal intensity than the brain and CSF. Cystic or necrotic components of lacunar infarcts may be isointense on proton density–weighted images, but they often have an associated peripheral zone of increased signal intensity due to gliosis, and they are distinctly hypointense on T1-weighted images[124] (Fig. 27–27).

Enhancement is a helpful feature. Acute MS plaques, subacute infarcts, radiation necrosis, and adrenoleukodystrophy are associated with breakdown of the blood-brain barrier and enhance with use of Gd. Enhancement patterns provide additional diagnostic clues. The CSF spaces and chronic changes of white matter ischemia and aging will not enhance. Most of the hereditary metabolic disorders and the immune mediated inflammatory disorders do not enhance.

Hyperintense foci are commonly seen in the posterior limb of the internal capsule on T2-weighted images. The foci are of low signal intensity on T1-weighted images and are round or oval, homogeneous, well-defined, and symmetric. Correlative anatomic studies showed these hyperintense foci to represent fibers of the corticospinal tract. The signal characteristics are likely due to prominent clear spaces wedged between large axons with thick myelin sheaths.[125]

All of the features just discussed are helpful for evaluating periventricular white matter abnormalities. Sometimes, a definitive diagnosis cannot be made from the images alone, and a list of differential diagnoses must be considered and correlated with clinical information. Occasionally, one or two punctate subcortical hyperintensities may be found in a young healthy patient with no focal symptoms, no risk factors for vascular diseases, no history of trauma or neurologic disease, and imaging features that do not fit with any of the aforementioned entities. Correlative pathology is not available in these cases, but the lesions most likely represent focal gliosis related to a prior subclinical infection (prenatal or postnatal) or some indeterminant developmental event. None of these punctate lesions have ever been reported to evolve into something significant, such as tumor, or to be a seizure focus; therefore, in all probability they are of no clinical significance.

REFERENCES

1. Valk J, van der Knaap MS: Classification of myelin disorders. In: Valk J, van der Knaap MS. Magnetic Resonance of Myelin, Myelination and Myelin Disorders. Berlin: Springer-Verlag, 1989, pp 4–8.
2. Valk J, van der Knaap MS: White matter and myelin. In: Valk J, van der Knaap MS. Magnetic Resonance of Myelin, Myelination and Myelin Disorders. Berlin: Springer-Verlag, 1989, pp 4–21.
3. Byrd SE, Darling CF, Wilczynski MA: White matter of the brain: maturation and myelination on magnetic resonance in infants and children. Neuroimaging Clin North Am 3:247–266, 1993.
4. Staudt M, Schropp C, Staudt F, et al: Myelination of the brain in MRI: staging system. Pediatr Radiol 23:169–176, 1993.
5. Gerard G, Weisberg LA: Magnetic resonance imaging in adult white matter disorders and hydrocephalus. Semin Neurol 6:17–23, 1986.
6. Kirkpatrick JB, Hayman LA: White-matter lesions in MR imaging of clinically healthy brains of elderly subjects: possible pathologic basis. Radiology 162:509–511, 1987.
7. Drayer BP: Imaging of the aging brain. Part I. Normal findings. Radiology 166:785–796, 1988.
8. George AE, de Leon MJ, Kalnin A, et al: Leukoencephalopathy in normal and pathologic aging: 2. MRI of brain lucencies. AJNR 7:567–570, 1986.
9. Jungreis CA, Kanal E, Hirsch WL, et al: Normal perivascular spaces mimicking lacunar infarction: MR imaging. Radiology 169:101–104, 1988.
10. Elster AD, Richardson DN: Focal high signal on MR scans of the midbrain caused by enlarged perivascular spaces: MR-pathologic correlation. AJNR 11:1119–1122, 1990.
11. Durand-Fardel M: Traité du Ramollissement du Cerveau. Paris: Bailliere, 1843.
12. Heier LA, Bauer CJ, Schwartz L, et al: Large Virchow-Robin spaces: MR-clinical correlation. AJNR 10:929–936, 1989.
13. Braffman BH, Zimmerman RA, Trojanowski JQ, et al: Brain MR: pathologic correlation with gross and histopathology. 1. Lacunar infarction and Virchow-Robin spaces. AJNR 9:621–628, 1988.
14. Awad IA, Johnson PC, Spetzler RF, et al: Incidental subcortical lesions identified on magnetic resonance imaging in the elderly. II. Postmortem pathological correlations. Stroke 17:1090–1097, 1986.
15. Fazekas F, Kleinert R, Offenbacher H, et al: Morphologic correlate of incidental punctate white matter hyperintensities on MR images. AJNR 12:915–921, 1991.
16. Marshall VG, Bradley WG, Marshall CE, et al: Deep white matter infarction: correlation of MR imaging and histopathologic findings. Radiology 167:517–522, 1988.
17. Kobari M, Meyer JS, Ichijo M, Oravez WT: Leukoaraiosis: correlation of MR and CT findings with blood flow, atrophy, and cognition. AJNR 11:173–281, 1990.
18. Challa VR, Moody DM: White-matter lesions in MR imaging of elderly subjects. Radiology 164:874–878, 1987.
19. Burger PC, Burch JG, Kunze U: Subcortical arteriosclerotic encephalopathy (Binswanger's disease): a vascular etiology of dementia. Stroke 7:626–631, 1976.
20. Hachinski VC, Potter P, Merskey H, et al: Leuko-araiosis. Arch Neurol 44:21–23, 1987.
21. Zimmerman RD, Fleming CA, Lee BCP, et al: Periventricular hyperintensity as seen by magnetic resonance: prevalence and significance. AJNR 7:13–20, 1986.
22. Brant-Zawadzki M, Fein G, VanDyke C, et al: MR imaging of the aging brain: patchy white-matter lesions and dementia. AJNR 6:675–682, 1985.
23. Steingart A, Hachinski VC, Lau C, et al: Cognitive and neurologic findings in subjects with diffuse white matter lucencies on computed tomographic scan (leuko-araiosis): Arch Neurol 44:32–35, 1987.
24. Adams RD, Victor M: Principles of Neurology. 2nd ed. New York: McGraw-Hill Book Company, 1981, pp 524–702.
25. Ebner F, Millner MM, Justich E: Multiple sclerosis in children: value of serial MR studies to monitor patients. AJNR 11:1023, 1990.
26. Swanson JW: Multiple sclerosis: update in diagnosis and review of prognostic factors. Mayo Clin Proc 64:577–586, 1989.
27. Korte JH, Bom EP, Vos LD, et al: Baló concentric sclerosis: MR diagnosis. AJNR 15:1284–1285, 1994.
28. Poser CM, Paty DW, Scheinberg L, et al: New diagnostic criteria for multiple sclerosis: guidelines for research protocols. Ann Neurol 13:227–231, 1983.
29. Jacobs L, Kinkel PR, Kinkel WR: Impact of nuclear magnetic resonance imaging on the assessment of multiple sclerosis patients. Semin Neurol 6:24–32, 1986.
30. Jackson JA, Leake DR, Schneiders NJ, et al: Magnetic resonance imaging in multiple sclerosis: results in 32 cases. AJNR 6:171–176, 1985.
31. Sheldon JJ, Siddharthan R, Tobias J, et al: MR imaging of multiple sclerosis: comparison with clinical and CT examinations in 74 patients. AJNR 6:683–690, 1985.
32. Gebarski SS, Gabrielsen TO, Gilman S, et al: The initial diagnosis of multiple sclerosis: clinical impact of magnetic resonance imaging. Ann Neurol 17:469–474, 1985.
33. Edwards MK, Farlow MR, Stevens JC: Cranial MR in spinal cord MS: diagnosing patients with isolated cord symptoms. AJNR 7:1003–1006, 1986.
33a. Rydberg JN, Hammond CA, Grimm RC, et al: Initial clinical experience in MR imaging of the brain with a fast fluid-attenuated inversion-recovery pulse sequence. Radiology 296:173–180, 1994.
34. Nesbit GM, Forbes GS, Scheithauer BW, et al: Multiple sclerosis: histopathologic and MR and/or CT correlation in 37 cases at biopsy and three cases at autopsy. Radiology 180:467–474, 1991.
35. Runge VM, Price AC, Kirshner HS, et al: The evaluation of multiple sclerosis by magnetic resonance imaging. Radiographics 6:203–212, 1986.
36. Horowitz AL, Kaplan RD, Grewe G, et al: Ovoid lesion: a new MR observation in patients with multiple sclerosis. AJNR 10:303–305, 1989.
37. Simon JH: Neuroimaging of multiple sclerosis. Neuroimaging Clin North Am 3:229–246, 1993.

38. Osborn AG, Harnsberger HR, Smoker WRK, et al: Multiple sclerosis in adolescents: CT and MR findings. AJNR 11:489–494, 1990.
39. Gean-Marton AD, Vezina LG, Marton KI, et al: Abnormal corpus callosum: a sensitive and specific indicator of multiple sclerosis. Radiology 180:215–221, 1991.
39a. Hashemi RH, Bradley WG, Chen DY, et al: Suspected multiple sclerosis: MR imaging with a thin-section fast FLAIR pulse sequence. Radiology 196:505–510, 1995.
40. Simon JH, Holtas SL, Schiffer RB, et al: Corpus callosum and subcallosal-periventricular lesions in multiple sclerosis: detection with MR. Radiology 160:363–367, 1986.
41. Drayer B, Burger P, Hurwitz B, et al: Reduced signal intensity on MR images of thalamus and putamen in multiple sclerosis: increased iron content? AJNR 8:413–419, 1987.
42. Jacobs L, Munschauer FE, Kaba SE: Clinical and magnetic resonance imaging in optic neuritis. Neurology 41:14–19, 1991.
43. Lee DH, Simon JH, Szumowski J, et al: Optic neuritis and orbital lesions: lipid-suppressed chemical shift MR imaging. Radiology 179:543–546, 1991.
44. Tien RD, Hesselink JR, Szumowski J: MR fat suppression combined with Gd-DTPA enhancement in optic neuritis and perineuritis. J Comput Assist Tomogr 15:223–227, 1991.
45. Larsson E-M, Holtas S, Nilsson O: Gd-DTPA–enhanced MR of suspected spinal multiple sclerosis. AJNR 10:1071–1076, 1989.
46. Larsson HBW, Frederiksen J, Kjaer L, et al: In vivo determination of T_1 and T_2 in the brain of patients with severe but stable multiple sclerosis. Magn Reson Med 7:43–55, 1988.
47. Miller DH, Johnson G, Tofts PS, et al: Precise relaxation time measurements of normal-appearing white matter in inflammatory central nervous system disease. Magn Reson Med 11:331–336, 1989.
47a. Loevner LA, Grossman RI, Cohen JA, et al: Microscopic disease in normal-appearing white matter on conventional MR images in patients with multiple sclerosis: assessment with magnetization-transfer measurements. Radiology 196:511–515, 1995.
48. Atlas SW, Grossman RI, Savino PJ, et al: Internuclear ophthalmoplegia: MR-anatomic correlation. AJNR 8:243–247, 1987.
49. Edwards MK, Farlow MR, Stevens JC: Multiple sclerosis: MRI and clinical correlation. AJNR 7:595–598, 1986.
50. Wallace CJ, Seland TP, Fong TC: Multiple sclerosis: the impact of MR imaging. AJR 158:849–857, 1992.
51. Grossman RI, Gonzalez-Scarano F, Atlas SW, et al: Multiple sclerosis: gadolinium enhancement in MR imaging. Radiology 161:721–725, 1986.
52. Grossman RI, Braffman BH, Brorson JR, et al: Multiple sclerosis: serial study of gadolinium-enhanced MR imaging. Radiology 169:117–122, 1988.
53. Kermode AG, Tofts PS, Thompson AJ, et al: Heterogeneity of blood-brain barrier changes in multiple sclerosis: an MRI study with gadolinium-DTPA enhancement. Neurology 40:229–235, 1990.
54. Barkhof F, Valk J, Hommes OR, et al: Meningeal Gd-DTPA enhancement in multiple sclerosis. AJNR 13:397–400, 1992.
55. Guseo A, Jellinger K: The significance of perivascular infiltrations in multiple sclerosis. J Neurol 211:51–60, 1975.
56. Giang DW, Poduri KR, Eskin TA: Multiple sclerosis masquerading as a mass lesion. Neuroradiology 34:150–154, 1992.
57. Van Hecke P, Marchal G, Johannik K, et al: Human brain proton localized NMR spectroscopy in multiple sclerosis. Magn Reson Med 18:199–206, 1991.
58. Wolinsky JS, Narayana PA, Fenstermacher MJ: Proton magnetic resonance spectroscopy in multiple sclerosis. Neurology 40:1764–1769, 1990.
59. Wolff SD, Balaban RS: Magnetization transfer contrast (MTC) and tissue water proton relaxation in vivo. Magn Reson Med 10:135–144, 1989.
59a. Loevner LA, Grossman RI, McGowan JC, et al: Characterization of multiple sclerosis plaques with T1-weighted MR and quantitative magnetization transfer. AJNR 16:1473–1479, 1995.
60. Chenevert TL, Brunberg JA, Pipe JG: Anisotropic diffusion within human white matter: demonstration with NMR techniques in vivo. Radiology 177:401–405, 1990.
61. Le Bihan D, Turner R, Douek P, Patronas N: Diffusion MR imaging: clinical applications. AJR 159:591–599, 1992.
62. Heide AC, Richards TL, Alvord EC, et al: Diffusion imaging of experimental allergic encephalomyelitis. Magn Reson Med 29:478–484, 1993.
63. Stoner GL, Ruschkwetisch CF, Walker DL, Webster HD: JC papovavirus large tumor (T)-antigen expression in brain tissue of acquired immune deficiency syndrome (AIDS) and non-AIDS patients with progressive multifocal leukoencephalopathy. Proc Natl Acad Sci USA 23:2271–2275, 1986.
64. Greenfield JG: Greenfield's Neuropathology. 4th ed. New York: John Wiley & Sons, 1984, pp 261–288.
65. Whiteman JLH, Post MJD, Berger JR, et al: Progressive multifocal leukoencephalopathy in 47 HIV-seropositive patients: neuroimaging with clinical and pathologic correlation. Radiology 187:233–240, 1993.
66. Guilleux MH, Steiner RE, Young IR: MR imaging in progressive multifocal leukoencephalopathy. AJNR 7:1033–1035, 1986.
67. Mark AS, Atlas SW: Progressive multifocal leukoencephalopathy in patients with AIDS: appearance on MR images. Radiology 173:517–520, 1989.
68. Shoji H, Kusuhara T, Honda Y, et al: Relapsing acute disseminated encephalomyelitis associated with chronic Epstein-Barr virus infection: MRI findings. Neuroradiology 34:340–342, 1992.
69. Atlas SW, Grossman RI, Goldberg HI, et al: MR diagnosis of acute disseminated encephalomyelitis. J Comput Assist Tomogr 10:798–801, 1986.
70. Caldemeyer KS, Harris TM, Smith RR, et al: Gadolinium enhancement in acute disseminated encephalomyelitis. J Comput Assist Tomogr 15:673–675, 1991.
71. Baum PA, Barkovich AJ, Koch TK, Berg BO: Deep gray matter involvement in children with acute disseminated encephalomyelitis. AJNR 15:1275–1283, 1994.
72. Winer JB, Pires M, Kermode A, et al: Resolving MRI abnormalities with progression of subacute sclerosing panencephalitis. Neuroradiology 33:178–180, 1991.
73. Levy RM, Bredesen DE, Rosenbloom ML: Neurologic manifestations of the acquired immunodeficiency syndrome (AIDS): experience at UCSF and review of the literature. J Neurosurg 62:475–495, 1985.
74. Anders KH, Guerra WF, Tomiyasu U, et al: The neuropathology of AIDS: UCLA experience and review. Am J Pathol 124:537–557, 1986.
75. Wiley CA, Nelson JA: Role of human immunodeficiency virus and cytomegalovirus in AIDS encephalitis. Am J Pathol 133:73–81, 1988.
76. Shaw GM, Harper ME, Hahn BH, et al: HTLV-III infection in brains of children and adults with AIDS encephalopathy. Science 227:177–182, 1985.
77. Post MJD, Tate LG, Quencer RM, et al: CT, MR and pathology in HIV encephalitis and meningitis. AJNR 9:469–476, 1988.
78. Post MJD, Berger JR, Quencer RM: Asymptomatic and neurologically symptomatic HIV-seropositive individuals: prospective evaluation with cranial MR imaging. Radiology 178:131–139, 1991.
79. Chrysikopoulos HS, Press GA, Grafe MR, et al: Encephalitis caused by human immunodeficiency virus: CT and MR imaging manifestations with clinical and pathologic correlation. Radiology 175:185–191, 1990.
80. Lee BCP: Magnetic resonance imaging of metabolic and primary white matter disorders in children. Radiol Clin North Am 3:267–289, 1993.
81. van der Knaap MS, Valk J, de Neeling N, et al: Pattern recognition in magnetic resonance imaging of white matter disorders in children and young adults. Neuroradiology 33:478–493, 1991.
82. Murata R, Nakajima S, Tanaka A, et al: MR imaging of the brain in patients with mucopolysaccharidosis. AJNR 10:1165–1170, 1989.
83. O'Tuama L, Laster DW: Oculocerebrorenal syndrome: case report with CT and MR correlates. AJNR 8:555–557, 1987.
84. Rowley HA, Dillon WP: Iatrogenic white matter diseases. Neuroimaging Clin North Am 3:379–404, 1993.
85. Stemmer SM, Stears JC, Burton BS, et al: White matter changes in patients with breast cancer treated with high-dose chemotherapy and autologous bone marrow support. AJNR 15:1267–1273, 1994.
86. Vaughn DJ, Jarvik JG, Hackney D, et al: High-dose cytarabine neurotoxicity: MR findings during the acute phase. AJNR 14:1014–1016, 1993.
87. Lee YY, Nauert C, Glass JP: Treatment-related white matter changes in cancer patients. Cancer 57:1473–1482, 1986.
88. Ebner F, Ranner G, Slavc I, et al: MR findings in methotrexate-induced CNS abnormalities. AJNR 10:959–964, 1989.
89. Lien HH, Blomlie V, Saeter G, et al: Osteogenic sarcoma: MR signal abnormalities of the brain in asymptomatic patients treated with high-dose methotrexate. Radiology 179:547–550, 1991.
90. Wilson DA, Nitschke R, Bowman ME, et al: Transient white matter changes on MR images in children undergoing chemotherapy for acute lymphocytic leukemia: correlation with neuropsychologic deficiencies. Radiology 180:205–209, 1991.
91. Truwit CL, Denaro CP, Lake JR, et al: MR imaging of reversible cyclosporin A–induced neurotoxicity. AJNR 12:651–659, 1991.
92. Eidelman BH, Abu-Elmagd K, Wilson J, et al: Neurologic complications of FK 506. Transplant Proc 23:3175–3178, 1991.
93. Friese CE, Rowley H, Lake J, et al: Similar clinical presentation of neurotoxicity following FK 506 and cyclosporine in a liver transplant patient. Transplant Proc 23:3173–3174, 1991.
94. Adams RD, Victor M, Mancall EL: Central pontine myelinolysis. A hitherto undescribed disease occurring in alcoholic and malnourished patients. Arch Neurol Psychiatry 81:154–172, 1959.
95. Miller GM, Baker HC Jr, Okazaki H, Whisnant JP: Central pontine myelinolysis and its imitators: MR findings. Radiology 168:795–802, 1988.
96. Korogi Y, Takahashi M, Shinzato J, et al: MR findings in two presumed cases of mild central pontine myelinolysis. AJNR 14:651–654, 1993.
97. Ho VB, Fitz CR, Yoder CC, et al: Resolving MR features in osmotic myelinolysis (central pontine and extrapontine myelinolysis). AJNR 14:163–167, 1993.
98. Chang KH, Han MH, Kim HS, et al: Delayed encephalopathy after acute carbon monoxide intoxication: MR imaging features and distribution of cerebral white matter lesion. Radiology 184:117–122, 1992.
99. Yamashita J, Handa H, Yumitori K, Mitsuyuki A: Reversible delayed radiation effects on the brain after radiotherapy of malignant astrocytoma. Surg Neurol 13:413–417, 1980.
100. Valk PE, Dillon WP: Radiation injury of the brain. AJNR 12:45–62, 1991.
101. Lampert PW, Davis RL: Delayed effects of radiation on the human CNS: "early" and "late" delayed reactions. Neurology 14:912–917, 1964.

102. Dooms GC, Hecht S, Brant-Zawadzki M, et al: Brain radiation lesions—MR imaging. Radiology 158:149–155, 1986.
103. Tsuruda JS, Kortman KE, Bradley WG, et al: Radiation effects on cerebral white matter: MR evaluation. AJNR 8:431–437, 1987.
104. Curnes JT, Laster DW, Ball MR, et al: Magnetic resonance imaging of radiation injury to the brain. AJNR 7:389–394, 1986.
105. Hecht-Leavitt C, Grossman RI, Curran WJ, et al: MR of brain radiation injury: experimental studies in cats. AJNR 8:427–430, 1987.
106. Holbourn AHS: Mechanisms of head injuries. Lancet 2:438–441, 1943.
107. Adams JH, Mitchell DE, Graham DI, Doyle D: Diffuse brain damage of immediate impact type: its relationship to primary brainstem damage in head injury. Brain 100:489–502, 1977.
108. Peerless SJ, Rewcastle NB: Shear injuries of the brain. Can Med Assoc J 96:577–582, 1966.
109. Hesselink JR, Dowd CF, Healy ME, et al: MR imaging of brain contusions: a comparative study with CT. AJNR 9:269–278, 1988.
110. Gentry LR, Godersky JC, Thompson B, Dunn VD: Prospective comparative study of intermediate-field MR and CT in the evaluation of closed head trauma. AJNR 9:91–100, 1988.
111. Gentry LR, Godersky JC, Thompson B: MR imaging of head trauma: review of the distribution and radiopathologic features of traumatic lesions. AJNR 9:101–110, 1988.
112. Sklar EML, Quencer RM, Bowen BC, et al: Magnetic resonance applications in cerebral injury. Radiol Clin North Am 30:353–366, 1992.
113. Zimmerman RA, Bilaniuk LT, Hackney DB, et al: Head injury: early results of comparing CT and high-field MR. AJNR 7:757–764, 1986.
114. Levin HS, Amparo E, Eisenberg HM, et al: Magnetic resonance imaging and computerized tomography in relation to the neurobehavioral sequelae of mild and moderate head injuries. J Neurosurg 66:706–713, 1987.
115. Kelly AB, Zimmerman RD, Snow RB, et al: Head trauma: comparison of MR and CT—experience in 100 patients. AJNR 9:699–708, 1988.
116. Gentry LR: Primary neuronal injuries. Neuroimaging Clin North Am 1:411–432, 1991.
117. Yetkin FZ, Haughton VM, Papke RA, et al: Multiple sclerosis: specificity of MR for diagnosis. Radiology 178:447–451, 1991.
118. Aisen AM, Gabrielsen TO, McCune WJ: MR imaging of systemic lupus erythematosus involving the brain. AJNR 6:197–201, 1985.
119. Greenan UJ, Grossman RI, Goldberg HI: Cerebral vasculitis: MR imaging and angiographic correlation. Radiology 182:65–72, 1992.
120. Soges LJ, Cacayorin ED, Petro GR, Ramachandran TS: Migraine: evaluation by MR. AJNR 9:425–429, 1988.
121. Flodmark O, Lupton B, Li D, et al: MR imaging of periventricular leukomalacia in childhood. AJNR 10:111–118, 1989.
122. Post MJD, Hensley GT, Moskowitz LB, Fischl M: Cytomegalic inclusion virus encephalitis in patients with AIDS: CT, clinical, and pathologic correlation. AJNR 7:275–280, 1986.
123. Kalayjian RC, Cohen ML, Bonomo BA, Flanigan TP: Cytomegalovirus ventriculoencephalitis in AIDS—a syndrome with distinct clinical and pathologic features. Medicine 72:67–76, 1993.
124. Brown JJ, Hesselink JR, Rothrock JF: MR and CT imaging of lacunar infarcts. AJNR 9:477–482, 1988.
125. Yagishita A, Nakano I, Oda M, Hirano A: Location of the corticospinal tract in the internal capsule at MR imaging. Radiology 191:455–460, 1994.

28

Metabolic, Congenital Neurodegenerative, and Toxic Disorders

WILLIAM S. BALL, JR. ■ ANTONIUS DEGRAUW

Development of the brain is not only the product of careful morphologic evolution but also the result of a well-orchestrated process of balanced cellular metabolism that is most responsible for its maturation and function. Congenital malformations are most commonly thought of as alterations in morphology and structure, thus generally overlooking those ultrastructural alterations in cellular metabolism that may be equally devastating to the normal development of the child. A number of degenerative pathologic processes may involve the central nervous system (CNS) in children and adults and are increasingly being recognized owing to advances in neuroimaging. These disorders are often referred to as metabolic, congenital neurodegenerative, or toxic disorders and are classified on the basis of recognized gross anatomic or cellular morphologic changes, recognized metabolic abnormalities, or the known agents that lead to recognizable patterns of neurotoxicity. Common to all of these conditions in childhood are their injurious effects on normal maturation of the CNS at a time of maximal growth and development. In adults, loss of motor, sensory, and neurocognitive function may result.

Metabolic and congenital neurodegenerative disorders, which are often grouped together, are responsible for abnormal growth and development manifesting in infancy, later in childhood, and even into adulthood. Classifications may vary, but the cellular organelle designation scheme described by Valk and van der Knaap,[1] which is based on abnormal cellular morphology and/or function of the lysosome, peroxisome, or mitochondria, is most pertinent. Not all metabolic or congenital neurodegenerative disorders fall under this classification. Some are recognized as falling outside the categories based on the cellular morphology of the lysosome, peroxisome, or mitochondria, whereas others are yet to be classified as to their origin or are poorly understood. We have, for the purpose of discussion, grouped these disorders into the primary leukodystrophies, into disorders of known amino acid metabolism, or into a group of miscellaneous disorders for lack of any unifying features. Although most of these conditions are considered congenital, clinical manifestations may not begin until the adult years. Delayed recognition is most commonly the result of slow progression, borderline enzyme deficiencies, changing hormonal influences with increasing age, or clinical interaction of the enzymatic deficiency with the normal cellular process of aging.

In addition, the delicate balance of the developing CNS, as well as the more mature CNS, may be influenced by a variety of external agents that lead to gross morphologic injury, cellular dysfunction, or both. Although some of these conditions are considered toxic (e.g., carbon monoxide poisoning, drug abuse), others are the result of complications of legitimate medical therapy or are secondary to other disease states affecting the human body.

Differentiation of toxic conditions from metabolic and congenital neurodegenerative disorders based on imaging alone may, at times, prove difficult. In addition, separating the various types of metabolic from congenital neurodegenerative disorders by imaging may prove difficult. This difficulty is related to the fact that different conditions may have similar pathophysiologic pathways of CNS involvement and, therefore, may look similar. In addition, within the same process, there may be variable morphologic expression depending on severity or the stage of involvement. Despite such problems, imaging still plays an essential role in the diagnosis, evaluation, and follow-up of this group of CNS disorders.

IMAGING

For imaging to play a role in these disorders, it must be sensitive to anatomic changes within both gray and white matter, not only according to gross morphology but also according to tissue ultrastructure. For this purpose, magnetic resonance imaging (MRI) is clearly superior to computed tomography (CT) or ultrasonography. Advantages of MRI include superb anatomic resolution with excellent delineation of both gray and white matter, the ability to image in multiple projections with equal ability, and the capability to differentiate normal from pathologic conditions based on the tissue-related characteristics known as T1- and T2-weighted relaxation.

In this application, the complete MRI examination must consist of sequences that optimally represent both brain morphologic picture and relaxation characteristics. For this purpose, the "complete" examination must combine both T1- and T2-weighted imaging. Routinely, we begin each examination with a T1-weighted spin-echo (SE) sagittal sequence (repetition time [TR] = 500 to 600 ms, echo time [TE] = 10 to 15 ms), which not only serves as a localizer but also allows evaluation of both structure and myelination of the central commissures (e.g., corpus callosum) and deep white matter tracts, which may go undeveloped in many of these conditions. This is then followed by T1- and T2-weighted imaging in the axial projection from the base of the brain to the vertex. T1-weighted imaging may consist of any one of the available T1-weighted sequences, including SE (TR = 400 to 600 ms, TE = 8 to 15 ms), inversion recovery (IR) (TR = 2000 to 3000 ms, TE = 10 to 15 ms, inversion time [TI] = 600 to 800 ms), or gradient acquisition with a spoiled gradient (TR = 30 to 60 ms, TE = 13 to 15 ms, flip angle = 45° to 65°). Although all three produce satisfactory results, subtle variations among the techniques require that consistency in their selection be an important prerequisite to consistency in interpretation.

For T2-weighted imaging, either SE (TR = 2500 to 3000 ms, TE = 35 to 45 and 90 to 120 ms) or fast SE (TR = 2500 ms, TE = 17/119 effective) sequences are used. Gradient acquisition imaging has less T2-weighted signal intensity and, therefore, is less sensitive to early changes in demyelination. For this reason, it is seldom used in the work-up of metabolic, neurodegenerative, or toxic conditions.

METABOLIC AND CONGENITAL DISORDERS

LYSOSOMAL DISORDERS

Disorders centered on a cellular organelle known as the lysosome encompass a wide variety of cellular enzyme deficiencies, primarily involving hydrolases, that lead to an abnormal accumulation of undigested material (lipid, carbohydrates, or mucopolysaccharides) within the lysosome, their subsequent rupture into the cytoplasm of the cell, and, as a result, eventual cellular disruption.[2, 3] The lysosome is both a source of intracellular hydrolytic enzyme and a storage organelle that plays an important function in the autophagocytosis of unwanted cellular particulates. Lysosomal abnormalities are generally subdivided based on the specific pathway that is affected; however, such abnormalities

can be further divided pathologically based on whether there is predominant involvement of white matter, gray matter, or both. Conditions primarily affecting the white matter are the *sphingolipidoses,* such as metachromatic leukodystrophy and globoid cell leukodystrophy (Krabbe's disease), whereas the *mucolipidoses* (I cell disease), *lipidoses* (Niemann-Pick disease), *gangliosidoses,* and *mucopolysaccharidoses* involve predominantly gray matter initially with secondary changes in the white matter.

Metachromatic Leukodystrophy

Metachromatic leukodystrophy is an autosomal recessive disorder secondary to a deficiency in the enzyme arylsulfatase A, an important constituent in the breakdown and reutilization of myelin.[4] Absence of this enzyme, based on enzyme assay in white blood cells and urine, leads to the abnormal accumulation of sulfatides in the cell, imparting the typical metachromatic reaction seen by light microscopy.[4] The clinical presentation of this condition is divided into four groups based on the age at presentation as connatal (from birth), late infantile (6 to 25 months), early juvenile (4 to 6 years), and juvenile (6 to 10 years).[5] The late infantile form is the most common type and typically presents with a gait disorder (pyramidal and cerebellar syndrome).[6, 7] The other types are associated with behavior problems as well as disturbances in gait.[8] Additional clinical findings of diagnostic importance include evidence of a demyelinating polyneuropathy and an increased total protein content in the cerebrospinal fluid (CSF). It is now understood that manifestations and onset may be related to the percentage of arylsulfatase A activity that is present. Decreased activity can often be demonstrated in the parents or siblings of clinically affected children or both. Progressive neurologic dysfunction leads to paralysis, mental deterioration, blindness, and a persistent vegetative state within several years.

Pathologic changes consist of metachromatic granules representing engorged lysosomes in white matter, neurons, and peripheral nerve biopsy specimens. Oligodendrocytes are reduced in number, and areas of demyelination predominate throughout the deep white matter region. Oddly enough, there is early sparing of the white matter subcortical arcuate fibers or U fibers until late in the disease process. An inflammatory response is typically absent, which accounts for a lack of enhancement in this disorder, but, eventually, myelinated white matter is replaced by astrogliosis and scarring.

On CT scans, there is diffuse low attenuation of white matter compared with gray matter, with no early evidence of atrophy. The findings of MRI, although not pathognomonic, may be suggestive, based on the appearance of diffuse deep white matter involvement with relative sparing of subcortical white matter (Fig. 28–1). The MRI findings consist of an initially focal patchy, but later diffuse, hyperintense T2-weighted signal pattern within the white matter of the centrum semiovale. The deep central white matter is involved

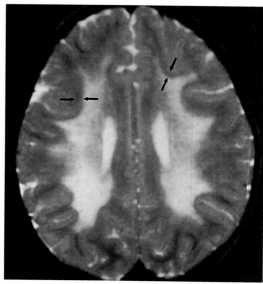

FIGURE 28–1. Metachromatic leukodystrophy. TR/TE = 2500/100. A diffuse hyperintense signal pattern is evident throughout the deep white matter, with relative sparing of the subcortical region (U fibers) *(arrows)*. White or gray matter volume loss is absent in the early stage of this disorder.

initially, with late recruitment of the peripheral subcortical fibers (U fibers). Contrast enhancement is generally absent. Eventually, white matter volume decreases over time as does the gray matter volume, leading to the appearance of diffuse atrophy of all regions with marked enlargement of the ventricles and extra-axial fluid spaces. At this end stage, differentiation of this condition from even diffuse hypoxic or ischemic injury may not be possible based on imaging alone.

Globoid Cell Leukodystrophy (Krabbe's Disease)

Globoid cell leukodystrophy (Krabbe's disease) arises from a deficiency in the enzyme galactocerebroside β-galactosidase (galactosylceramidase I), leading to the accumulation of cerebroside, galactosylsphingosine (toxic to the oligodendrocyte), and abnormal myelin (dysmyelination).[9] This disorder is thought to be an autosomal recessive one, and an abnormality localized to chromosome 14 has been described.[10] Accumulation of abnormal metabolites in the lysosomes of white matter histiocytes gives them a globoid appearance and is responsible for this entity's commonly referred to name. The clinical onset is generally earlier than that of metachromatic leukodystrophy, typically between 3 and 5 months of age. Early clinical signs include pyramidal tract syndrome with depressed deep tendon reflexes because of a demyelinating polyneuropathy. The CSF total protein level is also increased. Progressive neurologic deterioration starts with irritability that evolves into a vegetative state and death by 2 to 3 years of age.[11]

Pathologic changes include a marked reduction in the number of oligodendrocytes. Multinucleate globoid-appearing cells as well as reactive macrophages

are scattered throughout the white matter region. Demyelination may be extensive and eventually leads to gliosis and scarring in the white matter region. Gray matter involvement in the basal ganglia region is not uncommon.

On CT scans, diffuse stippled calcifications in the basal ganglia have been described and should be considered in the differential diagnosis of any cause of calcification of the basal ganglia in the first 2 years of life (Table 28–1). Additional early changes include increased density in the distribution of the thalami, cerebellum, caudate head, and brain stem that may precede the abnormal low attenuation of white matter in the centrum semiovale.[12] The appearance of Krabbe's disease at MRI is described as being one of two patterns. A patchy hyperintense periventricular signal pattern on T2-weighted images, consistent with dysmyelination, may eventually coalesce into a more diffuse pattern in the white matter, and in this form there is often involvement of the thalami with a hyperintense signal pattern as well (Fig. 28–2). This pattern may eventually develop into one of diffuse atrophy similar to that described for metachromatic leukodystrophy. A second pattern is that of patchy low signal intensity on T2-weighted images in a similar distribution to the hyperdense regions seen on CT scans and is thought to represent a paramagnetic effect from calcium deposition in the region.[13] Finelli and coworkers[14] described two infants with early CT changes, one of whom had a normal MRI examination, suggesting that the CT findings may precede the MRI findings in selected cases.[14] Delayed myelination may be the first finding seen with MRI in infants with this disorder;

TABLE 28–1. CAUSES OF BASAL GANGLIA CALCIFICATIONS IN CHILDHOOD

METABOLIC AND NEURODEGENERATIVE DISEASES

Lysosomal disorders
  Globoid cell leukodystrophy (Krabbe's disease)
Mitochondrial leukodystrophies
Primary disorders of white matter
  Cockayne's syndrome
Disorders in amino acid metabolism
  Glutaricacidemia Types I and II
  Methylmalonicacidemia
  Propionicacidemia
  Maple syrup urine disease
  Homocystinuria
Miscellaneous disorders
  Hallervorden-Spatz disease
  Wilson's disease
  Mannosidosis
Hypoparathyroidism, hyperparathyroidism
Pseudohyperparathyroidism

DESTRUCTIVE AND INFLAMMATORY CONDITIONS

Osmotic myelinolysis
Carbon monoxide poisoning
Radiation injury
Chemotherapy-induced injury
Human immunodeficiency virus infection
TORCH (toxoplasmosis, other infections, rubella, cytomegalovirus, and herpes simplex) infections
Hemolytic-uremic syndrome
Hypoxic-ischemic encephalopathy

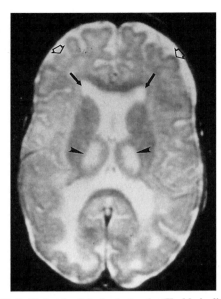

FIGURE 28–2. Globoid cell leukodystrophy (Krabbe's disease). TR/ TE = 2500/90. Hyperintense signal pattern can be seen throughout the white matter but is greatest in the posterior parieto-occipital region and adjacent to the anterior horns of the lateral ventricles *(solid arrows)*. There is also a symmetric hyperintense signal pattern in the thalami *(arrowheads)*. Changes of early gray matter volume loss occur over the cerebral convexities *(open arrows)*.

therefore, any child with a delay in myelination based on imaging without a previous history for insult should be evaluated for early changes of a metabolic or neurodegenerative process such as Krabbe's disease (Fig. 28–3). Demaerel and colleagues[13] reported their MRI findings in a single adult patient with this disorder. Findings consisted of bilateral symmetric hyperintense signal pattern on T2-weighted images in the periventricular parieto-occipital white matter and along the corticospinal tracts.[13]

Gangliosidoses

Gangliosidoses are divided into two primary groups referred to as the GM_1 and GM_2 gangliosidoses. In GM_1 gangliosidosis, the primary enzyme deficiency is that of β-galactosidase, whereas an abnormal accumulation of gangliosides is the result of a hexosaminidase deficiency in GM_2 gangliosidosis. The clinical presentation of GM_1 gangliosidosis is typically in infancy with features that are often confused with Hurler's disease, such as pitting edema of the face, hypotonia, developmental delay, hepatosplenomegaly, macrocephaly, and cherry-red spots involving the macula of the retina (50%). The course is progressive, with death within 2 years. A juvenile form presents later with progressive ataxia but without many of the course features of the infantile variety.[15]

Tay-Sachs disease is a form that falls under the category of GM_2 gangliosidosis (type I).[16, 17] It occurs predominantly in Jewish children of eastern European origin as an autosomal disorder, but it may be seen in other ethnic groups as well. The enzyme deficiency is that of hexosaminidase A isoenzyme. The initial

presentation is shortly after birth and consists of progressive psychomotor deterioration, hypotonia, seizures, blindness, and progressive macrocephaly. Cherry-red macular spots are found in 90% of affected children. This condition is generally progressive, resulting in death by 2 or 3 years of age. Sandhoff's disease (type II) is a second condition in this group with a clinical course similar to Tay-Sachs disease and is the result of a deficiency of both the A and B isoenzymes of hexosaminidase.[18]

Pathologically, white and gray matter is affected in both conditions, but the latter is affected to a greater degree. Demyelination does, however, form an important part of this group of disorders and is primarily responsible for the initial MRI findings.[17] Accumulation of the abnormal lysosomal metabolite can be found in neurons of the cerebrum, cerebellum, basal ganglia, brain stem, and spinal cord. With MRI, Yoshikawa and associates[17] demonstrated involvement of the caudate heads, putamina, and thalami in this disorder. All areas appeared hyperintense on T2-weighted images. The brain is enlarged secondary to the abnormal accumulation of gangliosides. Fukumizu and coworkers[16] related the changing appearance at MRI to the three primary clinical stages of the disease. Initially in the first phase (0 to 14 months), high signal intensity was found on T2-weighted images in the basal ganglia and white matter. The caudate heads appeared swollen. This appearance gradually progresses to diffuse atrophy, coinciding with the second and third clinical phases (15 to 24 months and after 24 months, respectively) (Fig. 28–4). With the loss of neurons, generalized cortical atrophy is identified. Cystic degeneration may occur in white matter regions, followed by astrogliosis and volume loss.

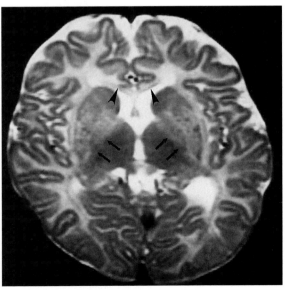

FIGURE 28–3. Globoid cell leukodystrophy (Krabbe's disease). TR/ TE = 3000/100. In this early stage of infantile Krabbe's disease, the most prominent feature is the hypomyelination for age in a 14-month-old infant. This is especially evident as absence of myelin in the internal capsule *(arrows)* and the corpus callosum *(arrowheads)*.

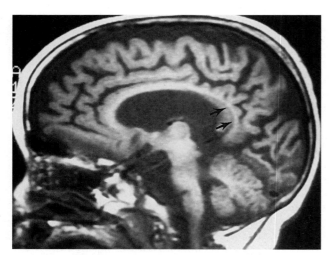

FIGURE 28–4. Tay-Sachs disease. TR/TE = 500/15. At this late stage in the disease process, the most prominent feature is that of diffuse atrophy of both supratentorial and infratentorial structures. Note thinning of the posterior corpus callosum *(arrows)*, indicating significant white matter volume loss centrally.

On CT scans, the white matter appears hypodense. The basal ganglia may also appear hypodense in GM_2 gangliosidosis. Hyperdense thalami have been reported in Sandhoff's disease.[19] On T2-weighted images, the white matter and basal ganglia are often hyperintense without any special characteristics to separate this disorder from similar or other demyelinating conditions (Table 28–2). Vertebral changes with beaking and wedging on plain radiographs may actually provide more of a clue to this group of disorders than does MRI of the brain.

Mucopolysaccharidoses

Of the lysosomal abnormalities affecting predominately gray matter, the mucopolysaccharidoses are the best known.[3] The primary defect is a failure to break down sulfates (dermatan, heparan, and keratan), leading to overladen mucopolysaccharide-filled histiocytes within brain, bone, skin, and other organs. There are six distinct types within this general group: Hurler's, Hunter's, Sanfilippo's, Morquio's, Maroteaux-Lamy, and Sly's; the classic prototype is that of Hurler's disease. Coarse facial and bony features as well as complex skeletal manifestations are well-known clinical characteristics. Death usually comes within the first decade of life.

The MRI findings reflect the pathologic changes of perivascular histiocytic infiltration and the accumulation of mucopolysaccharide within astrocytes and the centrum semiovale, leading to marked overexaggerated prominence of the perivascular spaces.[20–22] Demyelination is most commonly secondary to neuronal degeneration and loss but may also reflect the direct deposition of glycosaminoglycans in the white matter region. Eventually, these processes lead to volume loss of both the gray and white matter regions.

Diffuse patchy low density on CT scans and high

signal intensity in the white matter on T2-weighted images, however, are found more often in Hurler's disease and Hunter's disease than in the other mucopolysaccharidoses[21] (Fig. 28–5). The prominent perivascular spaces extend as fluid spaces with CSF signal intensity on T1- and T2-weighted images from the surface of the cortex to the corpus callosum.[23, 24] Prominent spaces within the corpus callosum may also be seen. Neuronal injury and degeneration lead to diffuse cerebral and cerebellar cortical atrophy with ventricular dilatation and widening of the extra-axial fluid spaces over the cerebral convexities. White matter demyelination secondary to neuronal degeneration appears as a patchy hyperintense signal pattern without a characteristic pattern of involvement scattered throughout the cerebrum on T2-weighted images (see Fig. 28–5). Skull base changes seen best on CT scans include a J-shaped sella, thickening of the bony calvaria, and stenosis at the craniocervical junction (Fig. 28–6).

PEROXISOMAL DISORDERS

The peroxisome is another of the cellular organelles that is home to a host of enzyme activities critical to proper cellular function.[25] It consists of a single-layered membrane that is generally round and forms an internal matrix to which various enzyme foci appear to be attached. The principal function for each peroxisomal

TABLE 28–2. CAUSES OF ABNORMAL MRI SIGNAL IN BASAL GANGLIA

DESTRUCTIVE PROCESSES
Hypoxic-ischemic encephalopathy
Carbon monoxide poisoning
Osmotic myelinolysis
Hemolytic-uremic syndrome
Hepatic encephalopathy
Radiation injury
Chemotherapy-induced injury

INFLAMMATORY CONDITIONS
Acute and chronic encephalomyelitis
Human immunodeficiency virus infection and acquired immunodeficiency syndrome
Cytomegalovirus infection (microvascular angiopathy)

METABOLIC AND NEURODEGENERATIVE DISORDERS
Lysosomal disorders
   Globoid cell leukodystrophy (Krabbe's disease)
Mitochondrial leukodystrophies
Primary disorders of white matter
   Cockayne's syndrome
Disorders in amino acid metabolism
   Glutaricacidemia
   Methylmalonicacidemia
   Propionicacidemia
   Maple syrup urine disease
   Homocystinuria
Miscellaneous disorders
   Hallervorden-Spatz disease
   Wilson's disease
   Mannosidosis
Neurofibromatosis type 1
Juvenile Huntington's disease

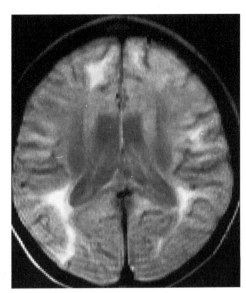

FIGURE 28–5. Hurler's disease (mucopolysaccaridosis). TR/TE = 2500/35. Multiple patchy areas of increased signal intensity are scattered throughout the white matter of both hemispheres, representing demyelination as a result of abnormal metabolite deposition and secondary axonal degeneration from primary neuronal injury. Despite the pathologic involvement of the gray matter, the cortical mantle appears grossly normal.

enzyme is still in the process of discovery. Known functions include oxidation of very-long-chain fatty acids, synthesis of bile acids, formation of plasmalogens, glycerol ether lipid synthesis, and phytanic and pipecolic acid metabolism. Morphologic abnormalities (absence, decreased size, or deficient numbers) or specific single or multiple enzyme defects lead to a variety of clinical

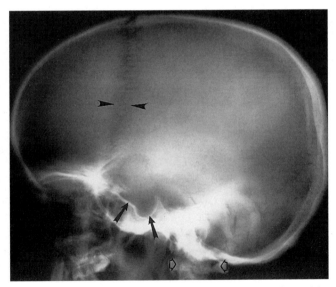

FIGURE 28–6. Hurler's disease (mucopolysaccaridosis). Many of the diagnostic features of this group of disorders can be identified by a skeletal survey. Characteristic involvement of the calvaria includes a J-shaped sella (*solid arrows*), macrocrania, splitting of the sutures due to leptomeningeal infiltration by metabolites (*arrowheads*), and stenosis of C-1 at the craniocervical junction (*open arrows*).

syndromes classified in a generalized group known as the peroxisomal disorders.[26]

Zellweger's and Related Infantile Syndromes (Group I)

Zellweger's syndrome is the prototypical abnormality in peroxisome morphology in which there is a complete or near-complete absence of the peroxisome unit on electron micrographs (Table 28–3). Manifestations begin in utero with the development of cortical dysplasias, which are a hallmark of this disorder. The cortical dysplasias have been previously described as taking the form of "migrational defects."[27] Our observations in six infants with this disorder indicate that the cortical morphology is most consistent with pachygyria, ulegyria, polymicrogyria, and thickening of the cortical mantle, all of which suggest more "encephaloclastic" features with disorganization in the later stages of migration rather than a true lissencephaly (Fig. 28–7). Other organ systems such as the liver may be involved.

Clinical features include cataracts, optic atrophy, peculiar facies (high prominent forehead), large fontanelle, malshaped ears, and stippling of the epiphyses as seen on conventional radiographs.[27] Severe hypotonia is often the first manifestation to call attention to this disorder. Clinical severity is directly related to the amount of enzyme deficiency that is present. Variants of Zellweger's syndrome have also been described that do not quite fit into the typical prototype but still have many features in common with Zellweger's syndrome.[28] Related clinical conditions include neonatal adrenoleukodystrophy (ALD), infantile Refsum's disease, and hyperpipecolic acidemia. Death usually results from many of these conditions within the first 2 years of life. Clinical and morphologic features of Zellweger's syndrome may be similar in neonatal ALD, which is characterized by the presence of multiple recognizable enzyme deficiencies with grossly normal, but deficient numbers of, peroxisomes. Specific conditions include pipecolic and phytanic acidemia and a deficiency of plasmalogen synthetase. This condition also presents with hypotonia in the first months of life, but without many of the facial features of Zellweger's syndrome.

TABLE 28–3. DISORDERS INVOLVING THE PEROXISOME

GROUP I: PEROXISOMES EITHER ABSENT OR REDUCED IN NUMBER
Zellweger's syndrome
Zellweger's variants
Neonatal adrenoleukodystrophy
Infantile Refsum's disease
Hyperpipecolic acidemia
GROUP II: SINGLE ENZYME DEFECT IN PEROXISOME
X-linked adrenoleukodystrophy
Pseudo-Zellweger's syndrome
Others
GROUP III: ABNORMAL STRUCTURE PEROXISOME
Rhizomelic chondrodysplasia punctata

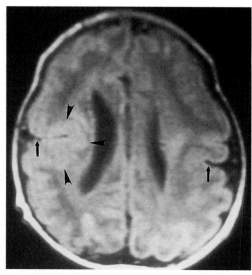

FIGURE 28–7. Zellweger's disease. TR/TE = 500/15. The cortical mantle appears immature with diffuse pachygyria, prominence of the sylvian fissues *(arrows)*, and multiple areas of thickening on the cortical gray matter *(arrowheads)* consistent with diffuse cortical dysplasia. This appearance is typical of this and other infantile forms of peroxisomal dysfunction.

Abnormalities in the form of cortical dysplasias are also found in these conditions as well.

The diagnosis of this group of infantile forms in peroxisomal function and morphology is highly suggestive in infants with severe unexplained hypotonia and findings on MR images of cortical dysplasia.[25] Other findings seen by MRI are those of subependymal cysts and marked delay in myelination with diffuse increased white matter signal intensity on T2-weighted images. Myelination is typically delayed at the time of birth and fails to progress in a normal fashion within the first year of life. Unfortunately, little is known about any delayed sequelae as seen by imaging because of the brief life span of affected infants. Enhancement can be seen in neonatal ALD as a result of an inflammatory response to the demyelination seen with this condition.

Adrenoleukodystrophy (Group II)

Within this group are included X-linked ALD,[29] adrenomyeloneuropathy,[30] Refsum's disease,[31] and pseudo-Zellweger's syndrome (see Table 28–3). X-linked ALD is also a peroxisomal disorder in which the morphology of the organelle is found to be normal by electron microscopy but a single enzyme defect leads to the accumulation of very-long-chain fatty acids and progressive CNS deterioration in the form of a chronic progressive encephalopathy.[32–35] Acyl CoA synthetase is the enzyme that is absent in this disorder. It is an enzyme required for the breakdown of long-chain fatty acids and their incorporation into cholesterol esters for myelin synthesis. This "classic" form of ALD is an X-linked disorder (males) with a clinical onset at age 5 to 7 years with behavioral problems, followed by a rapidly progressive decline in neurologic function

and death within the ensuing 5 to 8 years. The first indication of this condition may include mental status changes or a decline in school performance. Varying degrees of adrenal insufficiency are also present but may require laboratory evaluation for detection. Insufficiency to the point of Addison's disease is uncommon. Rarely, the adrenal insufficiency may actually precede the neurologic symptoms. Clinical symptoms may begin with subtle alterations in neurocognitive function but eventually progress to severe spasticity and visual deficits, leading finally to a vegetative state and death.[36] A milder autosomal recessive form is also recognized in adults known as adrenomyeloneuropathy and is covered in the subsequent section.

X-linked ALD has been described as having a typical appearance at CT and MRI with predominant posterior involvement that with time progresses from posterior to anterior into the frontal lobes and from the deep white matter to the peripheral subcortical white matter.[32, 34] On CT scans, the involvement appears as generally symmetric low attenuation in a butterfly distribution across the splenium of the corpus callosum, surrounded on its periphery by an enhancing zone (inflammatory intermediate zone).[33] Three zones are readily distinguished on MR images: 1) an inner zone of astrogliosis and scarring corresponds to the low-density zone seen on CT scans that appears hypointense on T1-weighted images and hyperintense on T2-weighted sequences; 2) an intermediate zone of active inflammation that appears isointense on T1-weighted images and isointense or hypointense on T2-weighted images; and 3) an outer zone of active demyelination that appears minimally hypointense on T1-weighted images and hyperintense on T2-weighted scans (Fig. 28–8). Enhancement that follows gadolinium administration can often be found within the intermediate zone of active inflammation and may disappear as the first change after bone marrow transplantation[32] (Fig. 28–9). Rarely, involvement can be entirely anterior in a similar butterfly distribution; unilateral and asymmetric involvement has also been described.

Treatment centers on the use of bone marrow transplantation to prevent or attenuate progression of the disease. Unfortunately, such treatment is generally not instituted until late in the course of the disease when irreversible injury to the brain has already occurred. After a bone marrow transplant, the first finding is often the disappearance of enhancement within the intermediate zone of inflammation. The progression of disease from posterior to anterior and from deep white matter to the periphery of the brain may slow compared with its previous course, but hyperintense signal changes are not significantly reversed.

Pseudo-Zellweger's syndrome represents a variant of the true form in which several enzyme functions also appear to be absent but there are normal concentrations of phytanic acid.

Refsum's Disease

In this rare single-enzyme defect of peroxisomal function, a deficiency in phytanic acid 2-hydroxylase

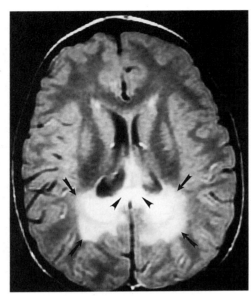

FIGURE 28–8. X-linked adrenoleukodystrophy. TR/TE = 2500/35. In this disorder there is a characteristic pattern of increased signal intensity involving both posterior trigones (*arrows*) of the centrum semiovale and the splenium of the corpus callosum (*arrowheads*), representing diffuse astrogliosis, inflammatory reaction, and demyelination.

prevents the metabolic breakdown of phytanic acid to form part of the myelin structure.[31, 37] This condition may affect myelination both in the CNS and in the peripheral nerves and thus presents with both central encephalopathy and a peripheral neuropathy. Skeletal manifestations are common in this disorder and include an epiphyseal dysplasia and a peculiar shortening or elongation of the second metatarsal.

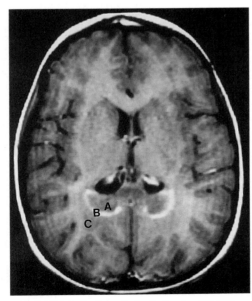

FIGURE 28–9. X-linked adrenoleukodystrophy. TR/TE = 500/15, plus gadolinium. The gadolinium enhancement defines three zones: an inner zone of astrogliosis (A), an enhancing zone of inflammatory reaction (B), and an outer zone of active demyelination (C).

CT may reveal diffuse low density throughout the white matter of the cerebrum and cerebellum. Enhancement is generally absent. Similar regions appear hyperintense on T2-weighted images. Cranial nerves occasionally appear enlarged. With only mild demyelination, the MR image is often normal or may not show evidence of demyelination until the fourth or fifth decade of life.

Adrenomyeloneuropathy

Adrenomyeloneuropathy is believed by many to represent a recessive form of ALD that does not manifest until later in life, typically in adulthood.[30, 38] It is believed to be secondary to a similar single-enzyme defect; however, its precise etiology is unclear. It may arise in families with a previous history of X-linked ALD among males in the family. Oddly enough, this condition more commonly affects females than males. Clinical manifestations include the slow onset of neuromuscular weakness, yet overt CNS manifestations secondary to demyelination are less common and may not manifest until late in the disease process. Clinical progression does not necessarily correspond with the severity of imaging findings at the time of initial diagnosis.

Imaging is best accomplished with MRI. In about half of cases, the MR image is within normal limits for age. High signal intensity on T2-weighted imaging representing demyelination can be identified in the corticospinal and spinocerebellar tracts of the brain stem. Abnormal signal intensity may eventually extend into the midbrain and posterior limb of the internal capsule; however, the typical deep white matter involvement as seen in ALD is less common. When present, it is less extensive than in ALD and is generally seen only late in the disease process. Demyelination of cerebellar deep white matter can be found, primarily centered on pontocerebellar tracts of the middle cerebellar peduncles, pontocerebral tracts, and medial lemniscus.

MITOCHONDRIAL DISORDERS

The mitochondria of the cell is an important organelle involved in the respiratory chain vital for the production of adenosine triphosphate (ATP), the fuel for most of the energy needs of the cell. This function is primarily accomplished by the DNA-encoded production of various polypeptide enzymes required in the respiratory cycle. Abnormalities in the structure of the mitochondrial DNA (Table 28–4) and alterations in respiratory oxidation with various enzyme deficiencies may involve the Krebs cycle and cytochrome-electron transfer system, leading to an inability to provide sufficient quantities of ATP.[39] Abnormal accumulation of lactate, pyruvate, and alanine in blood, serum, CSF, brain, and muscle may be found in many of these disorders as a result of dysfunction in pyruvate metabolism through the respiratory cycle.

Although many new conditions are being discovered

TABLE 28–4. GENETIC BASIS OF THE MITOCHONDRIAL DISORDERS

POINT MUTATIONS IN MITOCHONDRIAL DNA

Myoclonic epilepsy with ragged red fibers (MERRF syndrome)
Mitochondrial encephalomyopathy, lactic acidosis, stroke-like episodes (MELAS syndrome)
Maternally inherited myopathy or cardiomyopathy
Multiple inherited subcutaneous lipomatosis
Leber's hereditary optic neuropathy
ATP mutation diseases

DELETIONS IN MITOCHONDRIAL DNA

Kearns-Sayre syndrome
Pearson's marrow/pancreas syndrome

NUCLEAR DNA ABNORMALITIES

Myoneurogastrointestinal disorder and encephalopathy syndrome
Infantile cytochrome oxidase deficiency
Leigh's disease

as being related to mitochondrial dysfunction (see Table 28–4), foremost among them are the disorders classified as Leigh's disease; mitochondrial encephalomyopathy, lactic acidosis, and stroke-like episodes (MELAS); and myoclonic epilepsy with ragged red fibers (MERRF). Clinical features may vary considerably among these disorders and include muscle weakness, easy fatigability, seizures, headaches, and mental status changes. Considerable overlap may exist between conditions such as MERRF and other mitochondrial disorders such as Kearns-Sayre syndrome. Often a frequent overlap in signs and symptoms within this group of disorders leaves the biochemical, pathologic, and neuroimaging abnormalities as the best means for diagnosis.

Leigh's Disease

The classification of disorders in mitochondrial dysfunction is evolving. Leigh's disease actually represents a group of enzyme deficiencies related to the respiratory chain, but often with similar clinical manifestations and findings by neuroimaging.[40, 41] This disorder is also known as subacute necrotizing encephalomyopathy, reflecting pertinent histologic changes. It generally presents clinically within the first 2 years of life but may begin with symptoms of hypotonia in the newborn period or as late as adulthood.[42] Clinical signs that are slowly progressive include ophthalmoplegia, cerebellar signs, and spasticity. Other features include psychomotor regression, extrapyramidal signs, blindness, nystagmus, respiratory compromise, and cranial nerve palsies. Early onset of symptoms within the first years of life is generally fatal, whereas a later onset is generally associated with a more slowly progressive course.

Pathologically, this disorder involves both gray and white matter of the brain and spinal cord.[42] Common sites of anatomic involvement include the basal ganglia (specifically the globus pallidus and putamen), the thalami, the midbrain, the pons, the cerebellum, and the medulla. Pathologic changes include spongiform degeneration, demyelination, and vascular compromise and proliferation.

Abnormal low signal intensity on T1-weighted images (Fig. 28–10) or high signal intensity on T2-weighted images in the basal ganglia, periaqueductal gray matter, and brain stem and cerebellum is characteristic of Leigh's disease.[43–46] Involvement within the medulla characteristically appears to follow tracts that may encompass the entire length of the brain stem. Such a distribution is helpful in differentiating this condition from vascular or inflammatory conditions that may involve the brain stem as well. Bilateral symmetric involvement of the basal ganglia (globus pallidus and putamen) with decreased signal intensity on T1-weighted images and increased signal intensity on T2-weighted images is highly suggestive of this condition.[42] Rarely, late involvement may include the deep white matter of the centrum semiovale as areas of increased signal intensity on T2-weighted images consistent with demyelination. Lactate accumulation within these regions may be recognized on proton MR spectroscopy.[47]

MELAS Syndrome

The combination of myopathy, encephalopathy, lactic acidosis, and stroke-like episodes is recognized as MELAS syndrome as first described by Pavlakis and associates.[48] The stroke-like episodes may involve both infratentorial and supratentorial structures and have been described by Rosen and colleagues[49] as "migrating." The initial presentation is, therefore, not uncommonly that of an acute cerebrovascular occlusion. Genetic point mutations within mitochondria have been discovered and may eventually provide information as to the origin of the dysfunction.[50] Such

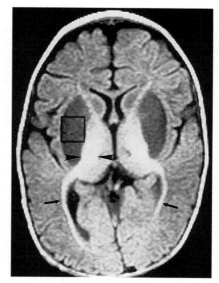

FIGURE 28–10. Leigh's disease. TR/TE/TI, 2500/15/600 IR. The lentiform nuclei appear low in signal intensity (box) bilaterally. This would appear hyperintense on an SE T2-weighted image. Note the normal myelination of the optic radiations (arrows) but an increase in signal intensity in the region of the posterior limb of the internal capsule and the lateral thalami (arrowheads). This may represent myelin clumping secondary to the ongoing metabolic insult.

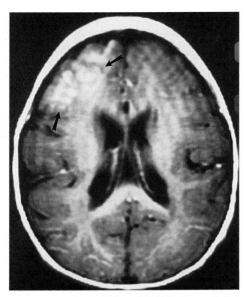

FIGURE 28–11. MELAS. TR/TE = 500/15, plus gadolinium. Gyral swelling and enhancement are identified in the right frontal region *(arrows)* consistent with the stroke-like episode. Such episodes are characteristic of this and other mitochondrial disorders.

mutations also provide the means for a more specific means to diagnose this and other mitochondrial disorders. Early clinical development is usually normal; however, rapid deterioration may follow the first clinical signs and symptoms. A specific enzyme defect is unknown at this time in MELAS. Likewise, the etiology and pathophysiology of the stroke-like episodes are unclear. Abnormal mitochondrial function within cerebrovascular smooth muscle and alterations in cerebral metabolism have been linked to the abnormal pathophysiology of this disorder.[51]

On MR images, stroke-like manifestations may involve both the infratentorial and the supratentorial structures (Fig. 28–11). Both white matter and cortical gray matter are involved as with stroke.[52] Areas of involvement appear hypointense on T1-weighted images and hyperintense on T2-weighted scans and are indistinguishable from cerebrovascular occlusion in children. In our experience, hemorrhage within the area is uncommon. Unlike in Leigh's disease, there is no propensity to involve the basal ganglia region. Stroke-like regions appear avascular on T2*-weighted MR perfusion imaging, single photon emission CT or positron emission tomography, supporting their ischemic nature. Proton spectroscopy in several of our cases is consistent with acute or subacute injury with a decrease in *N*-acetylaspartate and creatine/phosphocreatine ratio, and minimal to moderate lactate accumulation in involved tissue. Lesions may appear to come and go over time. The end result is typically that of maturation of the region to an area of encephalomalacia.

MERRF Syndrome

MERRF syndrome refers to a heterogeneous group of conditions that have in common the clinical presentation of myoclonus, epilepsy, and pathologic changes on muscle biopsy specimens of ragged red fibers.[42] Ragged red fibers on muscle biopsy specimens are not solely related to this group but can be seen occasionally in other mitochondrial disorders. The clinical course is often referred to as episodic, consisting of nausea and vomiting, intermittent blindness and hemiparesis, weakness, and mental deterioration. Elevated lactate levels are found in serum and CSF and can be detected in brain as well by proton MR spectroscopy.[53, 54] Other disorders with myoclonus as a prominent feature such as Baltic myoclonus and Lafora's disease must be excluded clinically.

The relationship between MERRF and the conditions known as Kearns-Sayre syndrome and ophthalmoplegia plus is poorly defined. All have similar clinical presentations, except in Kearns-Sayre syndrome sources report the presence of external ophthalmoplegia, retinitis pigmentosa, and heart block that are not a characteristic of MERRF.[55–57] Many signs and symptoms are similar, however, as well as the presence of elevated lactate levels in blood and serum and the findings of ragged red fibers on muscle biopsy specimens. Hypoparathyroidism or pseudohypoparathyroidism may account for the calcifications found within the basal ganglia in this disorder (Fig. 28–12). The genetic basis for these inherited disorders is supported by the findings of point mutations on mitochondrial DNA that result in abnormal function of the respiratory cycle in both MERRF and Kearns-Sayre syndrome, but sporadic occurrence is also found with Kearns-Sayre syndrome.[39]

The CT findings are similar to those of other disorders in mitochondrial dysfunction. Low density can be found scattered throughout the white matter region; however, unlike in MELAS and Leigh's disease, as

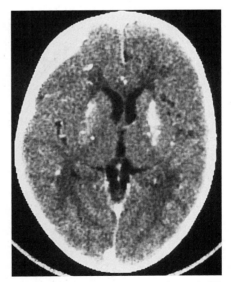

FIGURE 28–12. Kearns-Sayre syndrome. Enhanced CT scan. Calcifications are identified within the lateral lobe of the globus pallidus bilaterally. The white matter is slightly low in density compared with the adjacent gray matter (especially in the frontal region) owing to some hypomyelination.

reported by Seigel and colleagues,[58] calcification can be found within the basal ganglia and dentate nuclei in Kearns-Sayre syndrome as well as in MERRF (see Fig. 28–12). Diffuse atrophy eventually involves the cerebrum as well as the cerebellum, and enhancement is not a feature of either of these disorders.

At MRI, a diffuse patchy hyperintense signal pattern on T2-weighted images can be identified scattered throughout the white matter but may appear most prominent in the posterior trigonal regions (Fig. 28–13). A hyperintense signal pattern on T2-weighted images can also be found within the gray matter regions of the basal ganglia and dentate nuclei of the cerebellum. In the presence of calcification, both the basal ganglia and dentate regions may actually have increased signal intensity on T1-weighted images. Barkovich and coworkers[42] reported that in their experience early involvement is within the peripheral white matter (subcortical white matter) and posterior trigones, which are both regions that tend to myelinate late.

Other less common disorders of mitochondrial function include Alpers' disease, Menkes' disease, and carnitine deficiency. In Alpers' disease, both the brain and the liver are predominantly involved.[59] Clinical presentation includes myoclonic epilepsy, dementia, spasticity, and developmental delay that begins within the first several years of life and tends to be rapidly progressive. Several enzyme deficiencies have been reported in this condition that involve the electron transport chain within the mitochondria.[60] Gray matter involvement may be a prominent feature at imaging, especially involving the occipital and posterior temporal regions; otherwise, the findings are similar to those reported with other mitochondrial disorders. Menkes' disease does, however, have a characteristic clinical presentation with features that are well known to this

disorder.[61, 62] The classic presentation is that of hypotonia, seizures, and sparse fragile hair that is easily broken, which gives this condition its name of Menkes' kinky-hair syndrome. Also characteristic are the findings at cerebral angiography of dilated tortuous vessels within the region of the circle of Willis. This disorder is actually one of secondary dysfunction of the mitochondria due to a deficiency of copper, which is required for the proper development of cytochrome c. At imaging, Menkes' syndrome appears as diffuse atrophy with prominence of the extra-axial fluid spaces through which run the tortuous and dilated cerebral arteries. Hyperintense signal pattern within white matter on T2-weighted images indicates a lack of myelination with this disorder but may be related to a relative lack of blood flow secondary to the vascular involvement. These changes may progress despite adequate replacement of serum copper. Finally, carnitine deficiency may also lead to mitochondrial dysfunction. Imaging changes are most often related to delayed myelination or patchy demyelination.

PRIMARY DISORDERS OF WHITE MATTER (LEUKODYSTROPHIES)

Within this general classification we have elected to include those conditions in which there is suspected a primary defect in the formation of normal myelination. This includes conditions in which there is a failure to form normal myelin (hypomyelination) or in which abnormal myelin is produced. The terms *demyelination* and *dysmyelination* both refer to pathologic processes that are indistinguishable by MRI except, on occasion, by their pattern of involvement. For this reason, separation on imaging based on these terms is inappropriate except for this discussion.

Hypomyelination

Pelizaeus-Merzbacher Disease

Pelizaeus-Merzbacher disease represents a primary defect in myelin formation.[63] Several different subtypes have been described. The most common presentation is that of the slowly progressive classic form (type I) that presents in infancy and is believed to represent an X-linked recessive inheritance pattern. A second pattern (type II or Seitelberger type) begins in the neonatal period (connatal), is believed to be either X linked or autosomal recessive, and is more rapidly progressive. The common clinical features of the classic form include early nystagmus ("dancing eyes"), poor head control, spasticity, ataxia or extrapyramidal movement disorders, and severe developmental delay. These findings become slowly progressive within the first decade of life, eventually leading to death in late adolescence or young adulthood. In the connatal form, symptoms are similar but tend to become more rapidly progressive, with death within the first decade of life.

Although no specific enzyme defect has been iso-

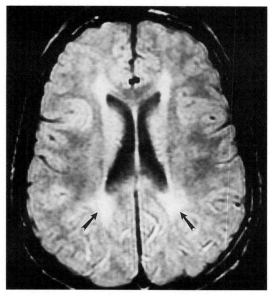

FIGURE 28–13. MERRF syndrome. TR/TE = 2500/35. Abnormal increased signal appears in a periventricular distribution but is especially prominent in the region of the posterior trigones (*arrows*).

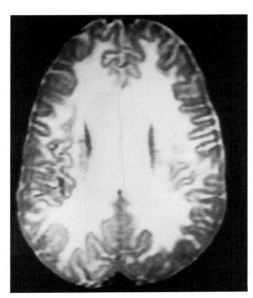

FIGURE 28–14. Pelizaeus-Merzbacher disease. TR/TE = 2500/100. Diffuse abnormal hyperintense signal pattern involves the deep and superficial white matter, virtually obscuring the lateral ventricles. Note the secondary thinning of the overlying gray matter as a result of neuroaxonal degeneration.

lated, a primary defect in the formation of normal myelin is suspected.[63] Pathologic changes, therefore, consist primarily of hypomyelination without early neurodegeneration. Evidence for breakdown of myelin is typically lacking.

As expected, the imaging findings are consistent with a marked delay in myelination from the onset.[64, 65] On CT scans, the appearance is that of diffuse low attenuation of white matter. On MR images, there is a pattern of marked delay in the normal temporal pattern of myelination; therefore, the white matter appears diffusely hypointense on T1-weighted images and diffusely hyperintense on T2-weighted sections[64, 65] (Fig. 28–14). Eventually, myelin that is present tends to be patchy without any particular distribution within the white matter region. In the end stage of the disease, white matter volume actually appears to be decreased, with thinning of the corpus callosum. Excess iron deposition in the later stages of the disease may be found within the basal ganglial region and appears markedly hypointense on the T2-weighted images.

Cockayne's Disease

Cockayne's disease is believed most likely to represent a similar process to Pelizaeus-Merzbacher disease. It differs predominantly by greater involvement of peripheral nerves, with resultant peripheral neuropathy. It is divided into two types, both of which are autosomal recessive disorders. A congenital form (type II) begins in the neonatal period; however, the most common or classic form (type I) presents near the end of the first year of life. Both conditions present clinically with wasting of subcutaneous tissue, microcephaly, mental retardation, deafness, intracranial calcifica-

tions, and peripheral neuropathy. Additional features include renal disease with hypertension, flexion contractures and disproportionate elongation of the limbs, photosensitive dermatitis, and cataracts. The two forms differ primarily in the age at onset and the progression of the disease. A diagnosis can be made after the demonstration of photosensitivity of cultured skin fibroblasts to the lethal effects of ultraviolet light.

The diagnosis is made primarily on the basis of the clinical presentation and on the CT finding of intracranial calcifications within the basal ganglia and subcortical white matter[66, 67] (Fig. 28–15). Cerebellar atrophy may be a prominent feature, followed by loss of white matter volume. On MR images, the features are similar to those of Pelizaeus-Merzbacher disease and represent diffuse hypomyelination seen best with T2-weighted imaging. Subcortical white matter is also involved early in this disorder.

Other Leukodystrophies

Two additional disorders that deserve some mention under metabolic and neurodegenerative conditions are Alexander's disease and Canavan's disease. Both are characterized by macrocrania, progressive neurologic deterioration, and psychomotor retardation.

Alexander's Disease

The exact cause of Alexander's disease has not been discovered.[68] It generally presents in males within the first year of life, with a progressive course ending in death in the first decade. As with most leukodystrophies, Alexander's disease is a rapidly progressive disorder with a clinical propensity toward increasing meg-

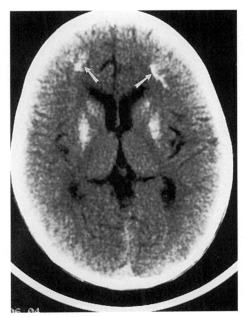

FIGURE 28–15. Cockayne's disease. Noncontrast CT scan. Calcifications are identified in the globus pallidus and caudate head bilaterally, as well as in the subcortical white matter *(arrows)*. Subcortical involvement is often noted early in this disorder.

alencephaly, spastic quadriparesis, seizures, and psychomotor retardation. The early presentation is generally between 7 and 14 years of age, but this disorder may not present until adulthood, in which case it may mimic multiple sclerosis.

Involvement is predominantly of frontal lobes early in the course of the disease in the majority of cases[68, 69] (Fig. 28–16). Diffuse involvement is common late in the course of the disease. Brain weight may actually be increased; pathologically, the cytoplasm of degenerating astrocytes, perivascular spaces, and subependymal zones appears to be packed with Rosenthal fibers. Early in the course of the disease, the white matter is most affected; soon, however, gray matter involvement becomes evident.

At CT and MRI, there is often bilaterally symmetric involvement of the frontal lobes.[68, 69] On CT scans, the appearance is that of low attenuation in the white matter in which deep gray matter and subependymal tissue appears isodense or even hyperdense. A similar distribution is found at MRI. On the T1-weighted images, the areas have low signal intensity, with gray matter being isointense and the anterior limb of the internal capsule hyperintense. These same areas appear markedly hyperintense on the T2-weighted images. Enhancement with gadolinium is the result of breakdown in the blood-brain barrier from the infiltrative process. Progression of the disease is from anterior to posterior, quite unlike that found in Canavan's disease and ALD.[70] The body and splenium of the corpus callosum; the posterior parietal, occipital, and temporal lobes; the cerebellum; and the brain stem are all relatively spared by the process until late in the disease. Eventually those areas involved become significantly atrophic.

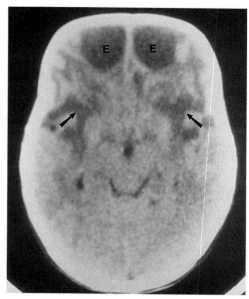

FIGURE 28–16. Alexander's disease. Noncontrast CT scan. Anterior involvement is characteristic of this disorder when combined with macrocrania. In addition to cystic encephalomalacia of the anterior frontal lobes (E), diffuse white matter edema is progressing posterior to involve the adjacent frontotemporal lobes as well (*arrows*).

Canavan's Disease

As in Alexander's disease, the hallmark of Canavan's disease is that of progressive macrocrania.[71] This disorder is one of autosomal dominant inheritance occurring primarily in children with lineage from the Jewish sect of Ashkenazi and arises from a deficiency in the enzyme N-acetylaspartoacylase.[72] The clinical presentation early within the first year of life consists of macrocrania, hypotonia, and seizures, progressing to psychomotor retardation, developmental delay, spasticity, and unrelenting seizures. Choreoathetoid movement and myoclonus may be prevalent features of this disorder. The onset of symptoms may be as early as in the first 3 months of life. Progressive neurologic deterioration eventually produces a vegetative state and death by 3 to 4 years of age. Prognosis, therefore, is uniformly poor. Rarely, a juvenile form with later onset and a more protracted clinical course has been described.

Pathologic changes primarily center on the findings of spongiform degeneration of the brain parenchyma. Brain weight may significantly increase within the first 20 months of life by as much as one half. Eventually, atrophy results in the brain weight returning to normal for age, and, finally, the brain actually decreases in weight in the late stages of the disease. The process of cavitation first begins in the cortical gray and subcortical white matter but rapidly progresses to involve the entire brain. No specific regions are typically affected first, although there may be a slight tendency for this condition to involve the posterior half of the brain early on. There is also relative early sparing of the basal ganglia, external and internal capsules, and corpus callosum. Optic nerve atrophy is often present. Cerebellar involvement is common and displays similar pathologic features. The most prominent pathologic feature is the diffuse vacuolar degeneration that occurs in the white matter, giving rise to the term *spongy degeneration*.

The underlying metabolic defect brought on by the N-acetylaspartoacylase deficiency results in the accumulation of high levels of N-acetylaspartate in serum and urine.[72] Assay of this metabolite in urine has been the principal method of diagnosis in the past.

At imaging, although early involvement of the occipital lobes has been reported, eventually all parts of the brain may be involved.[73, 74] More characteristic is the pattern of diffuse involvement of white matter, with relative early sparing of subcortical white matter tracts (U fibers) (Fig. 28–17). Also characteristic is the early relative sparing of the basal ganglia; of the internal, external, and extreme capsules; and of the corpus callosum. Eventually the condition becomes more permeative and involves all parts of the brain, both infratentorial and supratentorial. The involvement appears as low signal intensity on T1-weighted images and as high signal intensity on T2-weighted images. On CT scans, the same regions have low density without enhancement.[75] With basal ganglia involvement, the medial portion of the globus pallidus is affected before there is involvement of the putamen.

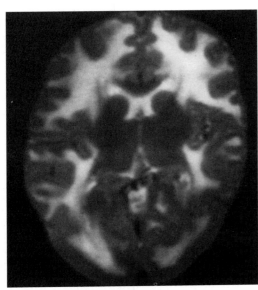

FIGURE 28–17. Canavan's disease. TR/TE = 2500/100. Diffuse abnormal hyperintense signal pattern is identified throughout the white matter but is actually greatest in the frontal regions in this early stage of involvement. Diffuse involvement is more typical, however, of this disorder. Both deep and subcortical white matter appears to be equally affected.

MRI not only allows for anatomic characterization of the lesions in this disorder but also may provide a specific diagnosis. Proton spectroscopy has been used to demonstrate a marked increase in *N*-acetylaspartate with respect to age.[47] There may be, at the same time, other metabolic evidence of neurodegeneration such as elevation of levels of choline compounds and depression of total creatine level with respect to *N*-acetylaspartate.

DISORDERS OF AMINO ACID METABOLISM

Disorders affecting amino acid metabolism comprise a heterogeneous group of disorders with respect to brain metabolism, with a characteristic clinical expression and not so characteristic imaging. Unlike disorders affecting the lysosome, peroxisome, or mitochondria, these conditions are not necessarily associated with any particular cellular organelle. Those deficiencies in amino acid metabolism that do reside within a particular organelle structure may have a similar clinical presentation to more specific disorders involving the organelle directly. Although the amino acid disorders are a rare group, when left untreated, they may result in significant irreversible, yet preventable, brain injury with mental retardation. Foremost among this group are the disorders of phenylketonuria, methylmalonicacidemia and propionicacidemia, tyrosinemia, nonketotic hyperglycinemia, maple syrup urine disease, and homocystinemia. They are subdivided mainly according to whether there is a specific enzyme deficiency or whether the defect is predominantly in the transport of a specific amino acid.

All of these conditions are inherited as an autosomal recessive pattern. The onset of CNS injury may actually precede significant clinical problems; therefore, it is imperative that the diagnosis be made early to correct the metabolic effect of the condition through dietary manipulation. We first discuss phenylketonuria as the classic example of an amino acid disorder. The imaging findings in this condition serve as an example of many of the other conditions within this diagnostic classification.

Phenylketonuria

Probably the most well known of the amino acid disorders is phenylketonuria. Familiarity with this condition by most physicians has primarily been through the efforts of congressional legislation. All newborns by law must be evaluated for this condition before discharge from the nursery. It is an autosomal recessive disorder resulting from enzyme deficiencies impairing the ability to convert phenylalanine to tyrosine (phenylalanine hydroxylase, dihydropteridine reductase, 6-pyruvoyltetrahydropterin synthase). Its frequency is on the order of 1 in 14,000 live births.[76]

If phenylketonuria is left untreated, injury to the CNS by the elevation of phenylalanine leads to irritability, mental deterioration, seizures, psychotic behavior, developmental delay, hypertonia and hyperreflexia, and movement disorders. Other physical evidence for this condition includes eczema, fair skin and hair, chronic vomiting, and a peculiar musty odor. The child is normal at birth but soon is noted to fail to meet developmental milestones within the first year of life. By this time, despite minimal clinical signs, brain injury may be irreversible. The clinical deterioration is progressive and may prove fatal if left untreated.

The severity of the clinical condition is in part dependent on the degree of enzyme defect. A more malignant course may be encountered that is rapidly progressive despite appropriate dietary restriction and may prove fatal in as many as 20% of cases.[77]

As a result in the enzyme deficiencies, accumulation of phenylalanine leads to the overproduction of phenylpyruvic and phenylacetic acids, as well as phenylacetylglutamine, which are all toxic to the developing nervous system. Pathologically, the white matter of the cerebrum, the cerebellum, and the optic tracts is most often affected. Diffuse demyelination with the absence of myelin degradation products is evident. This is followed by spongy degeneration and vacuolation of the white matter with glial scarring. Neuronal loss may be evident in the gray matter as well.[78]

At imaging, the CT scan is generally normal until late in the disease process, when there may be diffuse low density to the white matter region without enhancement. At MRI, the first evidence for this condition may be that of delayed myelination of structures for age.[79, 80] The earliest finding is that of increased T2 signal in the posterior trigonal regions and around the optic radiations, which correlate well with similar changes of demyelination found on histopathologic studies.[79] This pattern may then progress to involve both the deep and then superficial white matter of the anterior and posterior parietal and frontal lobes (Fig. 28–18). The cerebellar white matter shows a similar increase in signal intensity on the T2-weighted images; however, the brain stem is usually spared.[81] With progression, white matter volume is lost, resulting in diffuse dilatation of the lateral ventricles. Finally, secondary gray matter volume loss is evident late in the course of the untreated disease. Many of these findings may be attenuated or absent in the presence of early and adequate dietary phenylalanine restriction,[79] but generally there is poor correlation of treatment or neurologic impairment with the presence of atrophic and signal changes as seen at MRI.[80]

Organic Acidurias

Included within this group of disorders are organic acidurias related to certain deficiencies in mitochondrial protein synthesis and degradation. Thus, these conditions may have in common many clinical features found in the disorders of mitochondrial dysfunction previously described. The three most common include glutaricacidemia types I and II,[82] methylmalonicacidemia,[83] and propionicacidemia. In glutaricacidemia types I and II, a deficiency exists in the oxidation of glutaryl CoA by glutaryl-CoA dehydrogenase. Symptoms consist primarily of hypotonia, developmental delay, and choreoathetosis. Occasionally, the clinical onset is more acute, simulating an acute encephalitis.

In methylmalonicacidemia, there is a deficiency in the coenzyme B_{12}–mediated conversion of methylmalonic CoA to succinyl CoA or in the methylmalonyl-CoA mutase. The result is the inhibition of oxidative metabolism, resulting in ketoacidosis, increased sensitivity to excitatory neurotransmitter toxicity, hyperammonemia, or a direct toxic effect of methylmalonic

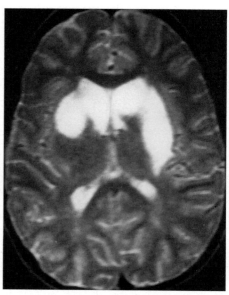

FIGURE 28–19. Organic aciduria (methylmalonicacidemia). TR/TE = 2500/100. This patient presented with an acute encephalopathy. MRI demonstrates a marked hyperintense signal pattern in the caudate heads and anterior lentiform nuclei bilaterally and in the posterior lentiform nucleus on the left. An organic aciduria was found after an exhaustive work-up for infection proved negative.

acid on the CNS. In both conditions, the diagnosis is generally confirmed by the increased excretion of either glutaric acid or methylmalonic acid in the urine. Propionicacidemia is secondary to a deficiency in propionyl-CoA carboxylase and presents in a similar fashion to methylmalonicacidemia.

Each of these conditions affects oxidative metabolism in the mitochondria, so it is not surprising that they have clinical, pathologic, and imaging features similar to those of the primary mitochondrial disorders. They often present clinically with the secondary effects of severe ketoacidosis. Pathologically, the neostriatum is involved with the globus pallidus more often in methylmalonicacidemia, and the caudate head and putamen in glutaricacidemia type I. Involvement includes volume loss and bilateral striatal necrosis. The entire neuronal population may be lost. Central pontine myelinolysis can occur simultaneously.

Imaging findings in the organic acidurias include changes in the basal ganglia that appear of low density on CT scans and hyperintense on T2-weighted MR images similar to findings in Leigh's disease.[84] Diffuse low density on CT scans or hyperintense signal on T2-weighted sequences may be found in the encephalitic form of the disease, as well as enhancement in the basal ganglia in the acute form[83] (Fig. 28–19). A diffuse hyperintense signal pattern on T2-weighted images develops within the white matter, followed by diffuse atrophy involving both white and gray matter. Stroke-like episodes similar to those of MELAS may occasionally be found as a clinical presentation of the organic acidurias.

Nonketotic Hyperglycinemia

Nonketotic hyperglycinemia is inherited in an autosomal recessive fashion and involves a defect in the

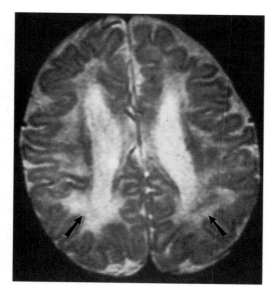

FIGURE 28–18. Phenylketonuria. TR/TE = 2500/100. Diffuse increased signal intensity is seen throughout the white matter but is especially prominent in the region of the posterior trigones (*arrows*). Note that in this poorly compliant patient there is diffuse gray matter volume loss despite some dietary restrictions.

cleavage of glycine to serine. As a result, there is an accumulation of glycine within the CNS. The clinical presentation may be as early as the first 72 hours of life and be life threatening.[85, 86] Early symptoms include lethargy, hypotonia, myoclonus, and seizures, which may lead to an unresponsive state and apnea. The electroencephalogram typically demonstrates a burst suppression type of background. This condition eventually leads to a vegetative state or severe mental retardation, or both. Many infants die within the first year of life.

The enzyme defect leads to the excessive accumulation of glycine in serum and brain, which has an inhibitory neurotransmitter effect on synaptic function. Elevated glycine levels further disrupt brain development by the effect of glycine on embryologic development and on myelin production. Glycine in high concentrations may affect normal development of the corpus callosum in utero or postnatally, leading to dysgenesis. Oddly enough, there is poor correlation between the degree of volume loss and the CSF or plasma levels of glycine.[87] Glycine may also disrupt myelin production by the oligodendrocytes. Pathologic changes include spongiform degeneration of the white matter, demyelination, gliosis, neuronal loss, and diffuse atrophy.

MRI reveals a normal pattern of delayed myelination in brain stem and cerebellum in infants younger than 4 months of age.[87] At the same time, myelination of supratentorial regions is usually lacking (Fig. 28–20). Progressive delay in myelination follows and remains markedly delayed by 1 to 2 years of age. The corpus callosum is typically dysplastic and thin and is also markedly delayed in its myelination.[88, 89] Hypodensities on CT scans and hyperintense foci on T2-weighted MR images in the periventricular regions are the result of the spongiform degeneration in this condition.[90–92] Atrophy may be an early finding. Press and associates[87] found parenchymal loss as early as 4 days of age that steadily progressed until age 27 months. Atrophy is generally accompanied by compensatory enlargement of the ventricles, which should not be confused with hydrocephalus.

Maple Syrup Urine Disease

Most often recognized because of its unusual name, maple syrup urine disease is a branched chain ketonuria that results from the deficiency of α-keto acid decarboxylase complex. This results in the accumulation of leucine, isoleucine, valine, and α-keto acids in the urine, which gives the urine a maple syrup or burnt odor. The incidence is 5 to 10 per 1 million live births. Its clinical presentation is quite early within the first weeks of life (75%) as hypotonia, lethargy and vomiting, failure to thrive, and seizures, with episodes of hypoglycemia in more than half the patients. Death follows within weeks if the disease is not treated.[90, 93] Early treatment can prevent the consequences of brain injury through dietary restriction of the branched chain amino acids and dialysis to remove glycine. Despite these efforts, the process in utero often leads to impairment to a variable extent.[94]

Imaging studies in the newborn period are often normal, but they soon show evidence of diffuse edema. The pattern of edema affects the deep cerebellar white matter, dorsal brain stem, cerebral peduncles, and posterior limb of the internal capsule in an ascending pattern that corresponds to patterns of early myelination.[95] Eventually the edema may spread to involve the basal ganglia (globus pallidus) and cerebral hemispheres. The edema resolves within the first 2 months, however, leaving a pattern of diffuse atrophy.

In the edema phase, the white matter tracts appear diffusely hypodense on CT scans, hypointense on T1-weighted MR images, and hyperintense on T2-weighted MR images. Cystic changes may correspond to the spongiform changes seen pathologically in the cerebellar white matter, dorsal brain stem, cerebral peduncles, and posterior limbs of the internal cap-

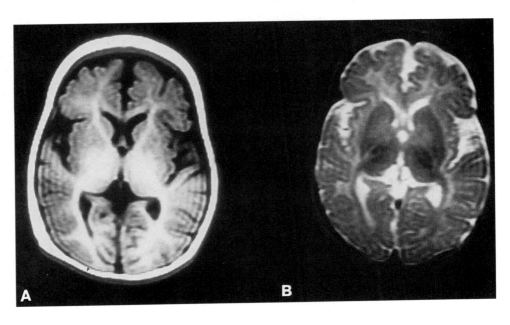

FIGURE 28–20. Nonketotic hyperglycinemia. *A:* TR/TE = 500/15; *B:* TR/TE = 2500/100. *A,* The brain appears immature with prominent sylvian fissures. Despite some myelination seen in *A,* the thalami appear too hyperintense. *B,* This section confirms there is indeed some delay in overall myelination for a 20-month-old child.

sules. With early treatment, these findings may resolve. Residual foci of hyperintensity on T2-weighted images in the lateral lemnisci may persist.[94] A low-density zone around the lateral ventricles or low attenuation foci in the brain stem have also been reported on CT scans.[95]

Homocystinuria

Homocystinuria is a rare hereditary deficiency in the enzyme cystathionine β-synthase. It is characterized clinically by mental retardation, seizures, dislocation of the lens of the eye, and neurologic deficits from cerebrovascular ischemia. Cerebrovascular occlusion can involve both the arteries and veins. Endothelial injury results from abnormal metabolite accumulation in the blood, intimal fibrosis, and discontinuity of the elastic membrane, predisposing to thrombosis and thromboembolism. In short, the vessels suffer from premature aging in which atherosclerosis and increased platelet adhesiveness are said to contribute to the risk for vascular occlusion.

Multiple infarcts are common throughout the brain. Rarely, stroke is responsible for the initial presentation of this disorder.[96–98] Cochran and Packman[97] described an acute presentation of stroke and venous sinus thrombosis in an otherwise healthy teenager with homocystinuria. Therapy consists of methionine restriction to improve blood flow and reduce the risk for stroke.

The MRI findings are predominantly related to the cerebrovascular occlusive disease that accompanies this disorder (Fig. 28–21). Multifocal lacunar infarctions or areas of ischemia are scattered throughout the white matter region. Prominence of perivascular spaces in the basal ganglia region suggests the complication of

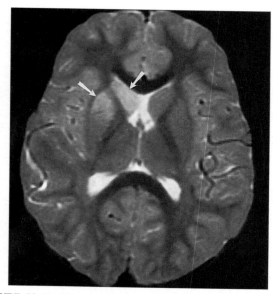

FIGURE 28–21. Homocystinuria. TR/TE = 2500/90. High signal intensity in the caudate head and anterior lentiform nucleus on the right (arrows) reflects changes secondary to developing infarction in this young adult with known homocystinuria and premature atherosclerosis.

moyamoya disease with collateral circulation through lenticulostriate vessels.

MISCELLANEOUS DISORDERS

Hallervorden-Spatz Disease

Hallervorden-Spatz disease overlaps considerably with neuroaxonal dystrophy, and many researchers believe these are related disorders. This condition and neuroaxonal dystrophy are both characterized by dystrophic axons and abnormal pigmentation within the basal ganglia. Neuroaxonal dystrophies are generally classified into infantile, late infantile, juvenile, Hallervorden-Spatz, and presenile and senile forms.

The classic type occurring in childhood is that of the infantile or juvenile forms. Onset for the infantile form begins early in the first year of life and progresses to death at the end of the first decade. Symptoms include tremors, gait disturbances, increasing rigidity of the extremities, choreoathetoid movement disorders, language delay, and mental deterioration. Dystonia is a prominent feature of this disorder. The juvenile form overlaps with the presenile form and may not begin until the second decade of life.

The pathologic changes are similar to those of the adult form of the disease. The substantia nigra appears enlarged owing to abnormal pigmentation. A similar process is identified in the globus pallidus bilaterally. Iron deposition corresponds to these same regions, but in a premature fashion.[99, 100] Spheroids (axonal swellings) are present in both Hallervorden-Spatz disease and neuroaxonal dystrophy within the CNS and in peripheral nerves.

CT demonstrates both abnormal low density and high density within the midbrain and globus pallidus bilaterally. The abnormal increased density likely reflects abnormal calcification within the region. Enhancement is typically lacking. At MRI, the classic findings are the premature deposition of paramagnetic iron in a distribution corresponding to that found on pathologic studies[99–103] (Fig. 28–22). Marked abnormal T2 shortening in the pallidum with an anteromedial area of high signal intensity has been described as the "eye of the tiger" sign.[100] This area of increased signal intensity on T2-weighted images corresponds well to areas of loose tissue with vacuolization found at histopathologic examination.[100] Similar changes have been identified in other forms of neuroaxonal dystrophy.

Wilson's Disease

Hepatolenticular degeneration, or Wilson's disease, is inherited in an autosomal recessive fashion and is a result of an inborn error in copper metabolism. It typically presents in young adults with chronic hepatic insufficiency and neurologic deterioration. Copper fails to be excreted in the bile; thus, it accumulates in the body, especially in liver, brain, kidney, and red blood cells. This then results in a CNS copper toxicosis with accumulation of copper in the basal ganglia. The

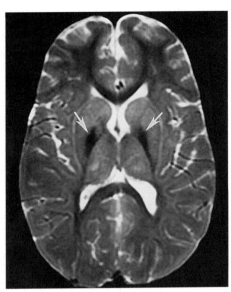

FIGURE 28–22. Hallervorden-Spatz disease. TR/TE = 2500/100. Premature symmetric low signal intensity is identified in the medial lobe of globi pallidi in this 5-year-old girl *(arrows)*. These changes represent the premature deposition of iron that may be seen in Hallervorden-Spatz disease or other forms of neuroaxonal dystrophy. Other causes include hypoxic-ischemic injury, which is obviously not present in this child.

clinical presentation is primarily that of extrapyramidal signs, hepatic insufficiency, and Kayser-Fleischer corneal rings. Either the hepatic toxicity or the neurologic findings may predominate. Neurologic dysfunction begins with changes in mentation, abnormalities in speech or language, and difficulty in swallowing. They progress slowly and may eventually lead to death.

On CT scans, the basal ganglia are typically low in attenuation, especially the globus pallidus and putamen[104] (Fig. 28–23). Atrophy of these structures eventually follows. The white matter may also have low density. Eventually, white matter volume loss leads to compensatory dilatation of the lateral ventricles. On MR images, the basal ganglia, corresponding to changes seen on CT scans, are hyperintense on T1-weighted images and the first echo of the T2-weighted sequence similar to other causes of hepatic dysfunction. The same areas are typically hyperintense on T2-weighted images early in the course of the disease, but the hyperintensity may actually decrease late in the process, corresponding to an increased signal intensity on the T1-weighted images.[104–108] The corresponding surrounding white matter demonstrates progressive increase in T2 signal intensity from demyelination and gliosis.

Galactosemia

Galactosemia is the result of a deficiency in galactose 1-phosphate uridyltransferase, which is an essential enzyme in the metabolism of galactose. The disorder, therefore, presents in infants soon after the institution of milk in the diet. Clinical features include failure to thrive, hepatomegaly with jaundice, vomiting and diarrhea, cataracts, increased intracranial pressure, and mental deterioration. It can be identified by the presence of increased amounts of reducing substances in the stool. Neurologic dysfunction is the result of the accumulation of galactose, galactose 1-phosphate, and galactitol in the brain and eye, as well as of severe hypoglycemia.[109, 110]

On CT scans, there is commonly diffuse low attenuation of white matter in a pattern similar to that of diffuse edema. This pattern may go unnoticed on MR images early on. The most consistent early finding at MRI is that of a delay in myelination as seen on T1- or T2-weighted images. This may appear as an absence of the normal dropoff in peripheral white matter signal intensity on the T2-weighted images.[111] Hyperintense signal intensity throughout the white matter may be seen on T2-weighted images in the older child as a result of demyelination. Patchy areas of focal increased signal intensity on T2-weighted images have also been reported and are thought to represent damaged areas of white matter.[111] Eventually a pattern of mild cerebral or cerebellar atrophy is found.

Mannosidosis

Both mannosidosis and fucosidosis are believed to represent disorders in the development of glycoproteins and glycolipid by defects in lysosomal hydrolases. In this regard, they are closely linked to the mucopolysaccharidoses. They are of autosomal recessive inheritance. Typical clinical features include coarse clinical appearances and mental deterioration. The course varies from chronic and mild to rapidly progressive and severe. Two groups emerge: a more severe infantile form (type I) and a less severe adult form (type II). The defect is in the mannosidase activity, leading to a

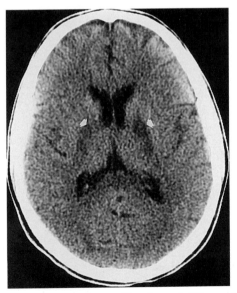

FIGURE 28–23. Wilson's disease. Unenhanced CT scan. The globi pallidi appear low in density without calcification *(arrows)*. Although nonspecific, such findings are consistent with, and when seen should suggest, Wilson's disease in the differential diagnosis.

deficiency in the isoenzymes A and B. Pathologically, there is an increase in brain weight. Vacuolization of cells occurs with an increase in storage elements in neuroglial cells, astrocytes, and endothelial cells. Neuronal degeneration is also the result of this process.

Findings at CT may include cerebellar and cerebral atrophy, shown as patchy low density in the white matter region perhaps due to demyelination. Dietemann and associates[112] described seven modifications on MR images in eight children with this disorder. Included were brachycephaly, a thickened calvaria, a vertically oriented chiasmatic sulcus, poor pneumatization of the sphenoid body, a partially empty sella, cerebellar atrophy, and signal alterations in the white matter. The signal alterations consisted of a hyperintense signal pattern on T2-weighted images in the posterior trigonal regions that was symmetric and consistent with demyelination.

TOXIC AND SYSTEMIC DISORDERS WITH CENTRAL NERVOUS SYSTEM INVOLVEMENT

A variety of toxins may affect the developing and mature CNS. Many of the toxic agents are more of historical interest (e.g., milk of bismuth; mercury), whereas current lifestyles and risks still provide ample exposure of the brain to a wide variety of toxins (e.g., carbon monoxide, illicit drugs, alcohol, pharmaceuticals). In addition, a variety of disorders related to dysfunction in other organ systems may have secondary CNS involvement that leads to morbidity or mortality. Renal disease and hepatic disease are two of the most common to secondarily involve the CNS, but there are many others.

CENTRAL PONTINE MYELINOLYSIS

Central pontine myelinolysis refers to a toxic form of demyelination that primarily involves the central pons but may be extrapontine as well. It occurs predominantly in chronic alcoholics and debilitated or malnourished adults as a result of an osmotic myelinolysis, but it has rarely been reported associated with liver disease, Addison's disease, or diuretic use[113] (Table 28–5). We have more recently encountered this condition as a complication of liver transplantation in

TABLE 28–5. CAUSES OF OSMOTIC MYELINOLYSIS

Chronic alcohol abuse
Debilitation or malnutrition
Chronic hyperalimentation
Liver disease
Addison's disease
Chronic diuretic use
Liver transplantation
Radiation or chemotherapy
Hyponatremia (correction of)
Hypernatremia (correction of)

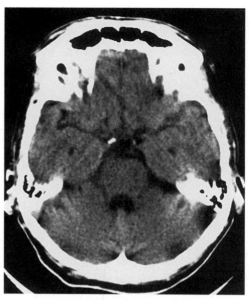

FIGURE 28–24. Central pontine myelinolysis. Noncontrast CT scan. Despite progressive symptoms related to pontine necrosis in this known male alcoholic, the noncontrast CT scan remains grossly normal.

both adults and children. It rarely affects the pediatric age group, but it is being increasingly recognized in patients younger than 18 years of age. In adults, more than 75% of cases can be found in chronic alcoholics. Many cases have been linked to the too rapid correction of hyponatremia by hyperosmotic loading. Symptoms include acute changes in mental status or coma, spastic quadriparesis, and pseudobulbar palsy with difficulty in swallowing. Death is the end result in the majority of cases, but, with survival, permanent neurologic deficits are common.

At autopsy, symmetric demyelination is found at the base of the pons. There is sparing of the ventrolateral longitudinal fiber tracts. The neurons and their axons are generally spared. Demyelination is accompanied by a decrease in the number of oligodendrocytes. In severe cases, demyelination gives way to white matter necrosis and cavitation. Demyelination may be found in extrapontine sites, including the basal ganglia, thalami, midbrain, corticomedullary junction of the cerebrum, and cerebellum.

On CT scans, the regions involved may appear normal or myelinolysis appears as low density of involved areas, most prominent in the central pons (Fig. 28–24). Enhancement is generally lacking, but it can occur as a result of breakdown in the blood-brain barrier. The corresponding histopathologic areas appear as decreased signal intensity on T1-weighted images and as increased signal intensity on the T2-weighted examination[113–116] (Fig. 28–25). Involvement, except in severe cases, is isolated to the basilar pons, with relative sparing of the tegmental region (Fig. 28–26). Extrapontine involvement has similar signal characteristics on both T1- and T2-weighted images (Fig. 28–27). Changes in both the pontine and the extrapontine regions typically persist despite recovery; however, they may com-

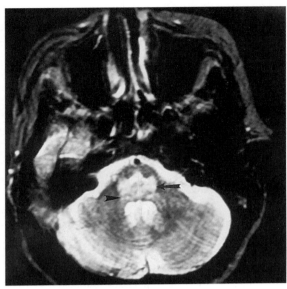

FIGURE 28–25. Central pontine myelinolysis. TR/TE = 2500/90. MRI in same patient as in Figure 28–24 reveals hyperintense signal pattern bilaterally in the pons consistent with a central pontine myelinolysis. Note that there is equal involvement of both the basilar *(arrow)* and the tegmentum pons *(arrowhead)*, which is somewhat atypical for this disorder.

pletely resolve after clinical improvement. Ho and coworkers[114] reported a transient increase in T1 signal in the basal ganglia in an adolescent recovering from myelinolysis. They thought that this was likely the result of either a regional release of myelin breakdown products or the mixing of free (axonal) and bound (myelin) waters to produce the T1 shortening (see also Chapter 27).

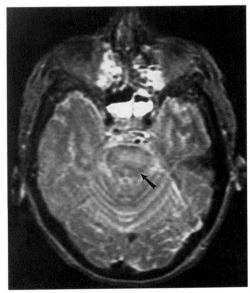

FIGURE 28–26. Central pontine myelinolysis. TR/TE = 2500/90. In a more typical pattern of involvement, a hyperintense signal pattern predominantly involves the basilar portion of the pons with relative sparing of the tegmentum *(arrow)*.

CARBON MONOXIDE POISONING

Unfortunately, the incidence of carbon monoxide poisoning either accidentally or as a means of suicide remains high within the United States. Acute poisoning produces a severe anoxic episode that leads to coma and death if proper steps for recovery are not undertaken. With appropriate management, recovery is generally quick within several days unless severe neurologic impairment has resulted from the anoxic insult. After a brief recovery, progressive neurologic deterioration may occur in a small percentage of cases (1% to 12%) and is known as postanoxic delayed encephalopathy.[117] Symptoms of this delayed process include mental status changes, gait disturbances, extrapyramidal signs, and mutism.

Pathologic changes consist of neurodegeneration of the basal ganglia (specifically the globus pallidus), neuronal injury, necrosis of Sommer's sector of the hippocampus, and demyelination of the periventricular white matter. Obvious necrosis of the pallidum may occur in severe cases. Other manifestations are directly related to the length of the anoxic episode.[118]

Imaging findings correlate well with neuropathologic data.[117, 119] On CT scans, evidence of infarction of the caudate head and putamen with low density is typically bilateral and symmetric[120] (Fig. 28–28). Lesions are best identified at MRI, however, as areas of low signal intensity on T1-weighted images and as a hyperintense signal pattern on T2-weighted images (Fig. 28–29). Bilateral lesions of the thalami were reported with carbon monoxide poisoning in a child by Tuchman and colleagues[119] at MRI examination. The lesions involved the anterior thalami and were accompanied by symmetric changes of hyperintense T2 signal pattern in the centrum semiovale.

Delayed encephalopathy leads to white matter lesions that can also be identified at MRI. In a report by Chang and associates,[117] 15 patients had a clinical course after the acute event consistent with a delayed encephalopathy from carbon monoxide. A symmetric hyperintense T2 signal pattern was identified within the centrum semiovale, including the subcortical white matter, the corpus callosum, and both the external and internal capsules. In 10 of the patients, the putamina and thalami had low signal intensity on the T2-weighted images, suggesting iron deposition within these structures. With time, and clinical improvement, the signal changes decrease toward normal, but they may never return to a normal baseline appearance. Focal areas of necrosis may develop in the globus pallidus and centrum semiovale (see also Chapter 27).

DRUG ABUSE

A variety of substances have become sources of abuse in today's society. Many of them have a direct detrimental effect on both the developing and the mature brain in children and adults. Most prevalent are the toxic effects secondary to the use and chronic abuse of alcohol, cocaine, amphetamines, and heroin.

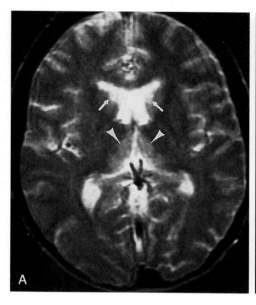
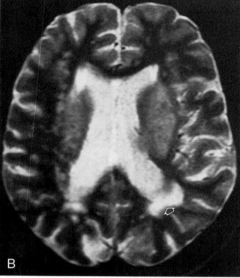

FIGURE 28–27. Central extrapontine myelinolysis. *A* and *B:* TR/TE = 2500/90. Hyperintense signal pattern involves the caudate heads *(arrows)* and medial thalami *(arrowheads)* in *A* and the periventricular region *(open arrow)* and centrum semiovale in *B.*

Ethanol

In addition to central pontine myelinolysis, chronic alcohol abuse may involve the CNS in two other ways. The most common is that of a degenerative encephalopathy known as Wernicke's (Wernicke-Korsakoff) encephalopathy, followed by a far less common manifestation known by the exotic name of Marchiafava-Bignami disease.[121]

Wernicke's Encephalopathy

Wernicke's encephalopathy is the result of a nutritional deficiency of thiamine.[121] Although it most com-

monly occurs in chronic alcoholism, it has also been reported as a complication in additional situations of nutritional deprivation, including patients undergoing dialysis or hyperalimentation or after gastric plication or stapling, carcinomas, chronic small bowel obstruction, anorexia nervosa, and intentional prolonged starvation.[122] The clinical presentation may be acute or intermittent and consists of nystagmus, cranial nerve palsies, mental status changes such as amnesia, abnormalities in gait, and, eventually, coma and death if the disorder is untreated. The classic triad of ophthalmoplegia, ataxia, and apathy was first described by Wernicke, but it is generally present in only one fourth to one third of patients. The term *Korsakoff's syndrome*

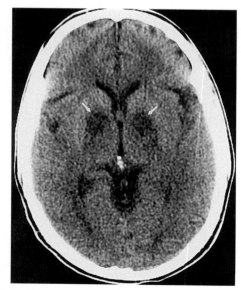

FIGURE 28–28. Carbon monoxide poisoning. Noncontrast CT scan. Several days after carbon monoxide asphyxiation there are symmetric low densities of the globi pallidi *(arrows)*. These changes are more likely due to anoxic-ischemic injury rather than the direct result of the carbon monoxide intoxication.

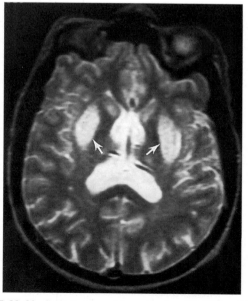

FIGURE 28–29. Carbon monoxide poisoning. TR/TE = 2500/90. Two weeks after carbon monoxide asphyxiation, a symmetric hyperintense signal pattern can be identified in the caudate heads and lentiform nuclei *(arrows)* bilaterally.

refers to a chronic dementia in which the severity involving learning and memory tends to be proportionately greater compared with other neurocognitive function.[121] Confabulation is also a prominent feature.

Pathologically, acute changes involve both white and gray matter of the hypothalamus, mamillary bodies, thalami, periventricular region, floor of the fourth ventricle, midline cerebellum, and periaqueductal and tectal regions.[123] Blood vessels within the involved areas appear prominent as a result of dilatation, thickening of the adventitia, an increase in the size of the endothelial cells, and capillary proliferation. As a result, there are alterations acutely in the blood-brain barrier.[124] Additional changes consist of necrosis and a proliferation of astrocytic and microglial cells. Hemorrhage may occur within the involved regions in 20% to 25% of cases and may cause sudden death.

CT grossly underestimates the disease process. Not uncommonly, the CT scan is normal in the presence of a severe symptom complex.[125] Changes, when present, consist of low attenuation with or without enhancement in the involved regions, especially with symmetric low density in the thalami. MRI has considerably improved our ability to make this diagnosis.[122, 125–129] Areas of involvement may appear as low signal intensity on T1-weighted images but are best identified as areas of increased signal intensity on T2-weighted images corresponding to the areas that appear abnormal on histologic study (Fig. 28–30). In the late stage of the disease, focal volume loss with gliosis results in dilatation of the third ventricle and aqueduct.

Schroth and associates[124] related enhancement in the third ventricular region and around the aqueduct or fourth ventricle in the acute phase to disruption of the blood-brain barrier due to involvement of the capillaries. Enhancement was also identified within the mamillary bodies and quadrigeminal plate by D'Aprile and coworkers[126] during the acute phase of the disorder, and mamillary enhancement alone has been reported as the only acute sign by Shogry and Curnes.[127] Enhancement may disappear altogether, as well as signal changes, with appropriate dietary therapy; however, the signal changes on T2-weighted images may persist. If the disease is left untreated or when treatment is late in the course of the disease process, atrophic changes may be identified at follow-up CT or MRI as mamillary atrophy and dilatation of the third ventricle and aqueduct.[125]

Marchiafava-Bignami Disease

Sounding more like an Italian opera than a disease state, Marchiafava-Bignami disease is a rare complication of chronic alcohol use first described in malnourished men of Italian decent from the consumption of locally made red wine.[121] It is now recognized as a complication of any chronic alcohol consumption. It consists primarily of a toxic leukomalacia that typically involves the corpus callosum, anterior commissure, and centrum semiovale with demyelination and white matter necrosis. Involvement of the centrum semiovale has also been reported.

MRI findings consist of early prominence of the perivascular spaces in the corpus callosum best seen on sagittal midline sections. These areas soon develop into areas of necrosis that have low signal intensity on T1-weighted images and high signal intensity on T2-weighted images. The centrum semiovale also appears increased in signal intensity predominantly involving the deep white matter regions.

Gallucci and colleagues[130] reported in a series of 35 asymptomatic patients with chronic alcoholism that 14 patients demonstrated multifocal white matter hyperintensities compared with a group of 35 control subjects in whom no similar findings were evident at MRI. These authors suggested that when ethanol is ingested in sufficient quantities for a prolonged time white matter injury may result even in currently asymptomatic individuals.

Maternal Alcohol Abuse

Maternal abuse of alcohol is also a well-known cause of CNS and extraneural injury to the developing fetus. The fetal alcohol syndrome consists of microcephaly, developmental delay, facial anomalies, cardiac defects, and ear abnormalities. The incidence is reported at 1.1 in 1000 live births in the United States. It is considered to be the most common single cause of mental retardation. Microcephaly, which is a prominent feature of this disorder, is the result of deficient brain growth. Mental retardation is variable. Features of minimal brain dysfunction, hyperactivity, and attention deficit disorders are common even in children with apparent normal intellect. Defects involving the CNS commonly include migrational anomalies best identi-

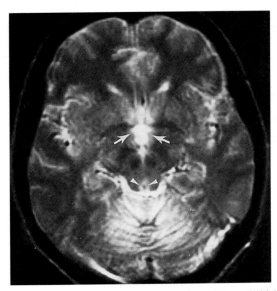

FIGURE 28–30. Wernicke's encephalopathy. TR/TE = 2500/90. A subacute onset of symptoms with hypothalamic dysfunction and mental status changes suggested a diagnosis of Wernicke's encephalopathy in this patient with chronic alcoholism. MRI revealed a hyperintense signal pattern in the basal ganglia, the hypothalamus (*arrows*), the periaqueductal gray matter (*arrowheads*), and the posterior fossa.

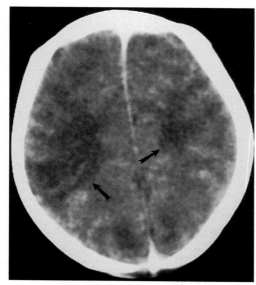

FIGURE 28–31. Cerebral infarction secondary to maternal cocaine use. Enhanced CT scan. Bilateral abnormal low density involves both gray and white matter but does not enhance *(arrows).* These findings, along with focal neurologic deficits, confirmed the diagnosis of infarction developing soon after birth in this term infant. By history, the infant's mother used cocaine throughout her pregnancy.

fied by MRI; however, any defect in organogenesis, neurulation, histogenesis, or maturation may be identified. Jacobson and coworkers[131] found that the greatest effect on the developing fetus may be when alcohol use and smoking are combined during pregnancy with illicit drug use.

Methanol

Accidental or intentional ingestion of methanol may produce CNS toxicity. Most common have been reports describing bilateral putaminal necrosis from in-farction. Less common manifestations include atrophy, symmetric neocerebellar infarctions, intracerebral hemorrhage (most often involving the basal ganglia), and diffuse edema.[132] The pattern of putaminal involvement is similar to that described in carbon monoxide poisoning.

Illicit Drugs

Narcotic addiction in pregnant women is one example of toxic exposure to the developing brain that is increasing in our civilized society. Both cocaine and heroin may cause CNS injury in the developing fetus and newborn.[133] Heier and colleagues[134] reported a 17% incidence of cerebral infarction in infants whose mothers met criteria for maternal cocaine abuse, as compared with a control group (2%) (Fig. 28–31). The incidence of midline and other congenital malformations was 12% in the abuse group, compared with none in the control group (Fig. 28–32). Most CNS malformations consisted of neural tube defects and are best identified either on physical examination or by MRI in the case of suspected cephaloceles. The authors indicated that the high incidence of stroke and CNS malformations was related to vasospasm caused by the cocaine abuse. Singer and colleagues[133] further demonstrated an increased incidence for intraventricular hemorrhage in extremely low birth weight infants exposed to cocaine in utero (Fig. 28–33). In our study population we have found, in addition to lacunar and arterial infarctions, a number of term cases with the appearance of periventricular leukomalacia, suggesting injury in utero of small vessels (Fig. 28–34). Lacunar infarctions appear on CT scans as focal areas of low density, typically within the white matter region, which follow CSF on all pulse sequences with MRI. The appearance of a pattern reminiscent of periventricular leukomalacia is an interesting finding. At CT or MRI, the appearance is that of decreased white matter vol-

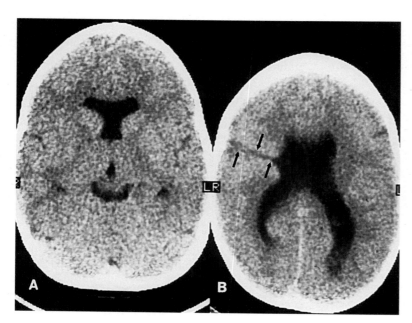

FIGURE 28–32. Congenital malformation secondary to cocaine exposure. *A* and *B*, Noncontrast CT scans. There is absence of the septum pellucidum, ventricular dysplasia, and a closed-lip schizencephaly on the right *(arrows).* By history, this mother used cocaine throughout her pregnancy but with a far greater frequency in the first trimester.

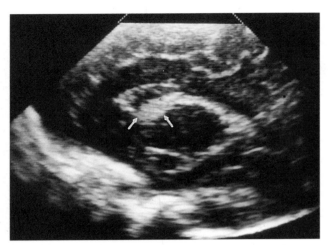

FIGURE 28–33. Intracranial hemorrhage secondary to cocaine exposure. Ultrasound scan. A grade I germinal matrix hemorrhage is evident in the region of the caudothalamic groove as seen on this sagittal ultrasound section *(arrows)*.

ume loss, where gray matter approaches the ventricular surface. The overlying gray matter of the cortex is relatively spared anatomically but not necessarily functionally. These findings support the presence of the insult in utero before a period of 34 weeks' gestational age, at a time before complete vascular maturity of the developing telencephalic vasculature. There may be persistent increased signal intensity on the remaining white matter on T2-weighted images owing to gliosis and scarring from the ischemic insult.

CENTRAL NERVOUS SYSTEM EFFECTS OF RADIATION AND CHEMOTHERAPY

Radiation therapy and intrathecal and systemic chemotherapy can generate a cascade of events leading to cerebral toxicity.[135] The mechanism of injury is complex. Mechanisms include vascular injury, cell-mediated glial injury, and an immune-mediated response. Vascular injury consists primarily of proliferative obstruction of small and medium-sized vessels, endothelial cell injury, alterations in the local fibrinolytic pathway, and eventual thrombosis, infarction, and parenchymal necrosis. Withers and coworkers[136] postulated that direct injury to the parenchyma, especially to the microglial cells, oligodendrocytes, and axons, was primarily responsible for the CNS injury. Proton spectroscopic findings of neurodegeneration in several of our patients would support evidence of neuronal injury but cannot differentiate primary from vascular-mediated cell death. Whether parenchymal injury is in fact primary or secondary to a vascular-mediated event remains controversial.

Actual patterns of injury found at MRI reflect both a loss of parenchymal and cellular elements and the vascular mechanism of injury.[135] Vascular injury from ischemia, infarction, and necrosis appears on MR images as focal or regional zones of high signal intensity within white matter on T2-weighted images (Fig. 28–35). Focal hemorrhage appears as punctate areas of low signal intensity on the same T2-weighted images. White matter necrosis rarely simulates a mass lesion; however, this presentation is far more common in adults, a higher percentage of whom are administered megadoses of radiation or more intense chemotherapy

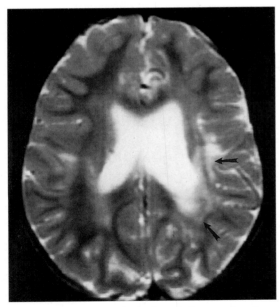

FIGURE 28–34. Periventricular leukomalacia secondary to cocaine exposure. TR/TE = 3000/100. There is evidence of central white matter volume loss, greater on the left than on the right, and hyperintense signal pattern representing gliosis *(arrows)*. Minimal gray matter volume loss is present on the left as well. Because there were no known problems at the time of this term birth, these findings strongly suggest that the injury occurred in utero during the last trimester. The mother used cocaine throughout the pregnancy.

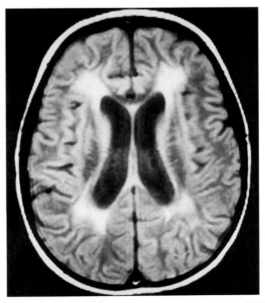

FIGURE 28–35. Leukomalacia secondary to irradiation. TR/TE = 2500/35. Radiation-induced leukomalacia appears as diffuse increased signal intensity in the white matter in a periventricular distribution. Despite this ominous appearance, the child remained asymptomatic. On a follow-up examination in 6 months, the leukomalacia had all but disappeared.

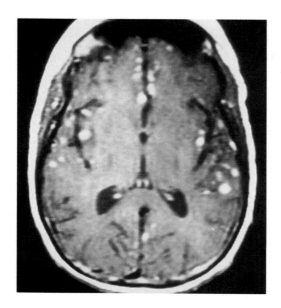

FIGURE 28–36. Radiation-induced vasculitis. TR/TE = 500/15, plus gadolinium. Diffuse punctate areas of enhancement appear along Virchow-Robin spaces 6 weeks after craniospinal irradiation. Biopsy failed to identify recurrent tumor or infection and was consistent with radiation vasculitis, which responded to systemic corticosteroids. The MR image reverted to normal during the next 4 weeks with corticosteroid therapy.

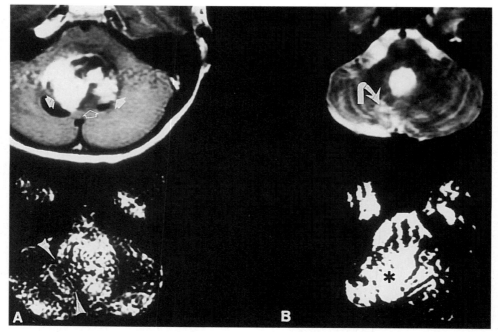

FIGURE 28–37. Use of perfusion imaging to separate recurrent tumor from radiation injury. *A, top:* TR/TE = 500/15, plus gadolinium; *A, bottom:* T2*-weighted perfusion image; *B, top:* TR/TE = 2500/100; *B, bottom:* T2*-weighted perfusion image. *A,* An intraventricular tumor is identified within the fourth ventricle *(top).* Enhancement appears within the solid portion of the tumor *(arrows)* 5 minutes after the administration of gadolinium. Note that not all of the solid tumor enhances *(open arrow).* In the same section *(bottom),* this first-pass T2*-weighted perfusion image reveals flow to the solid tumor that is seen as low signal intensity *(arrowheads).* This indicated adequate perfusion of the tumor, which corresponds to the areas of breakdown in blood-brain barrier seen on more delayed T1-weighted images as enhancement. *B,* One year postoperatively and after irradiation to the area, abnormal signal intensity posterior to the fourth ventricle developed *(top)* and was suggestive of tumor *(curved arrow);* there was, however, no T1 enhancement. On the first-pass T2*-weighted perfusion image of the same area *(bottom)* there is decreased perfusion, as one might expect in radiation injury. Therefore, this area remains hyperintense (*). Biopsy revealed radiation-induced and postsurgical changes but no residual tumor.

for inoperable brain tumors. Diffuse high signal intensity throughout the white matter is common and represents both vascular compromise and ischemia as well as white matter demyelination and cellular injury[137-140] (see Fig. 28–35). Multifocal enhancement occurring after gadolinium administration appears within the deep and superficial white matter as a result of vascular endothelial compromise with breakdown of the blood-brain barrier (Fig. 28–36). The enhancement often correlates well with the onset of clinical symptoms, but it may persist, despite clinical improvement, and develop into a pattern that appears to wax and wane and eventually disappears over time.

More severe white matter involvement, known as necrotizing leukoencephalopathy, results in extensive areas of white matter necrosis and demyelination. This can eventually lead to central white matter volume loss and scarring in a distribution similar to that found in periventricular leukomalacia. We have found T2*-weighted perfusion imaging can be of some help in differentiating changes caused by chemotherapeutically induced injury due to ischemia and decreased blood flow from recurrent tumor with normal to increased blood flow in a similar fashion to that found with positron emission tomography or single photon emission CT (Fig. 28–37). Differentiating the hypometabolism of chemotherapy injury from the hypermetabolism of recurrent tumor by positron emission tomography, however, remains the most sensitive method for separating the radiation injury from recurrent tumor (see also Chapter 27).

CEREBRAL EFFECTS FROM RENAL AND LIVER DISEASES

Disorders arising within other organ systems are well known to produce systemic effects that may involve the CNS in both adults and children. Foremost among these have been secondary CNS involvement associated with either hepatic or renal disease. Uremia in end-stage renal disease leads to significant metabolic and nutritional imbalances that can result in CNS involvement. As we have seen, Wernicke's encephalopathy is one manifestation that can result from end-stage renal disease or its management. Complications of end-stage renal toxicity may result in neurologic manifestations from hypertension, hypocalcemia, hypercalcemia, hyperparathyroidism, or aluminum toxicity. Anlar and associates[141] described additional CNS manifestations of end-stage renal disease in two children who developed patchy cerebral white matter edema either from uremia or as a result of hypertension and hyponatremia (Fig. 28–38). On CT scans, the appearance was that of multifocal patchy low attenuation in white matter that generally held to a symmetric pattern of involvement. Diffuse cortical atrophy may be an additional manifestation of chronic renal disease secondary to therapy or chronic nutritional deprivation (Fig. 28–39).

Uremic encephalopathy refers specifically to the effect of uremic toxins on the CNS. The clinical presen-

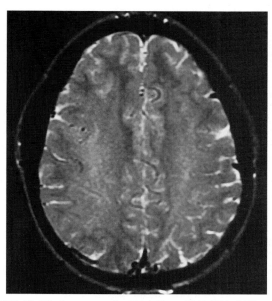

FIGURE 28–38. Acute uremia. TR/TE = 2500/100. Diffuse high signal intensity permeates the centrum semiovale bilaterally on this T2-weighted image. These findings are consistent with diffuse edema coinciding with mental status changes and decreased sensorium in this patient with acute renal failure and a creatinine value of 4.0 mg/dL.

tation includes mental status changes, difficulty with speech, gait abnormalities, tremors clonus, and a confusional state. The exact pathophysiology of this condition is unclear but may include manifestations secondary to neurotransmitter toxicity, parathyroid hormone, calcium abnormalities, brain osmolality, or alterations in cerebral blood flow. Okada and colleagues[142] described CT and MRI findings in one such patient with

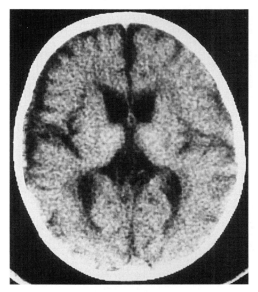

FIGURE 28–39. Chronic uremic encephalopathy. Noncontrast CT scan. Diffuse volume loss involves both gray and white matter. This patient has undergone chronic dialysis but was noncompliant in frequency for more than a year. One year earlier the CT scan was normal.

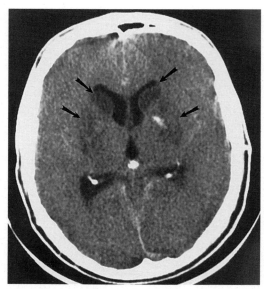

FIGURE 28–40. Subacute uremic encephalopathy. Enhanced CT scan. There is low density involving the caudate heads and lentiform nuclei bilaterally *(arrows)*. A focal area of hemorrhage is seen in the left globus pallidus. Note the poor gray matter–white matter differentiation of both cerebral hemispheres.

uremic encephalopathy. These authors found low density in the basal ganglia, internal capsule, and centrum semiovale on CT scans, which corresponded to areas of hyperintense signal pattern on T2-weighted MR images (Fig. 28–40). Oddly enough, these findings returned to normal after renal hemodialysis, and the patient was left without any neurologic deficit.

CNS involvement may also complicate the hemolytic-uremic syndrome in children caused by gram-negative infections,[143, 144] such as with *Escherichia coli*. Manifestations include acute renal failure, hemolytic anemia, thrombocytopenia, neurologic involvement from infarctions secondary to disseminated intravascular coag-

ulation, and a microvascular angiopathy with thrombosis. Infarctions may involve any portion of the CNS and have imaging characteristics of a typical infarction. Patterns of hemorrhagic or nonhemorrhagic infarction involving the basal ganglia are common. Ischemic infarction involving the basal ganglia appears hypointense on T1-weighted images and hyperintense on T2-weighted SE images. If hemorrhage develops, the signal characteristics will change to reflect the presence of either acute or subacute blood. Transient signal changes (hyperintensity) may also be identified in a paramedian watershed distribution on MR images in children or adults with malignant hypertension secondary to hemolytic-uremic syndrome or other causes of hypertension, but they resolve after control and a return of the blood pressure to normal levels.

Likewise, chronic hepatic failure from a variety of causes may lead to CNS manifestations similar to those described earlier for Wilson's disease. In children, the CNS manifestations in Reye's syndrome are well known and include diffuse brain swelling and injury to the basal ganglia or cortex (Fig. 28–41). The result may leave the child with a diffusely atrophic brain and neurologic deficit. There is a predilection for involvement of type II Alzheimer's astrocytes in both the cortex and the basal ganglia, neuronal injury, and laminar necrosis of the cortex in chronic hepatic toxicity. Demyelination and subcortical microcavitation may also occur. Imaging findings reflect this histologic distribution of injury as well. CT is less sensitive to these changes compared with MRI. Findings include diffuse edema, low density of the basal ganglia, and a pattern of diffuse cortical atrophy. At MRI, involved areas appear hyperintense on T1-weighted images and hyperintense on the first echo of the T2-weighted images but may actually decrease in signal intensity on the second echo of the T2-weighted sequence[145] (Fig. 28–42).

The clinical presentation of chronic hepatic encephalopathy is often subtle and underestimated on routine

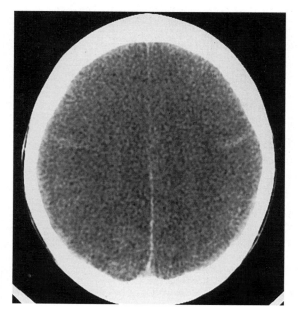

FIGURE 28–41. Reye's syndrome. Noncontrast CT scan. This child presented with a Glasgow Coma Scale score of 6, hepatomegaly, and elevated serum ammonia levels. CT revealed diffuse low density and loss of the gray matter–white matter interface consistent with acute cerebral edema. A diagnosis of Reye's syndrome was made clinically and confirmed at autopsy.

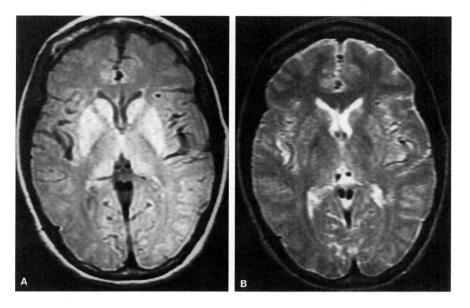

FIGURE 28–42. Hepatic encephalopathy. *A* and *B:* TR/TE = 2500/35, 100. Bilateral symmetric hyperintense signal pattern on the first *(A)* and second *(B)* echos of this T2-weighted sequence involves the basal ganglia and thalami. Note a decrease in signal intensity on the second echo compared with the first, suggesting that it may be a predominant T1 effect that accounts for the signal changes on the first echo.

neurologic examination. Manifestations may be evident only after an extensive neurocognitive evaluation. Ross and colleagues[146] demonstrated the utility of not only conventional MRI but also proton spectroscopy in the early diagnosis of hepatic encephalopathy before overt clinical manifestations were obvious. In their study, agreement was 94% between the neurocognitive evaluation and evidence of neurodegeneration by proton spectroscopy. Most pronounced was a reduction in the myoinositol component, which had an 84% correlation with evidence of hepatic encephalopathy on neuropsychiatric examination.

Overt clinical manifestations of hepatic encephalopathy include tremors, incoordination, gait abnormali- ties, spasticity, asterixis, and seizures. When these findings are present, the conventional MR image is more likely to show changes of CNS involvement (Fig. 28–43). These changes may remain, however, quite subtle and predominantly involve the basal ganglia region. The basal ganglia may appear hypointense on T1-weighted images, but a hyperintense signal pattern on the same sequence is most often seen.[145] A hyperintense signal pattern on T2-weighted images is best observed on the first echo of the T2-weighted sequence (see Fig. 28–42). Typically, the signal intensity then drops on the second echo, such that the basal ganglia appear isointense or hypointense on the long echo. These changes may or may not be accompanied by

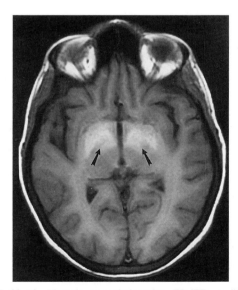

FIGURE 28–43. Hepatic encephalopathy. TR/TE = 500/13. A change in the sensorium in this patient with acute hepatic necrosis prompted the MRI. Hyperintense signal pattern consistent with hepatic encephalopathy is identified on the T1-weighted image, involving predominantly the basal ganglia and hypothalamus *(arrows)*.

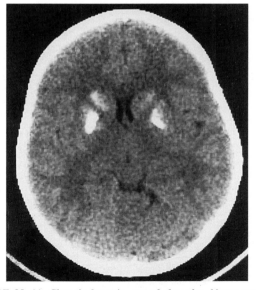

FIGURE 28–44. Chronic hepatic encephalopathy. Noncontrast CT scan. Bilaterally symmetric calcifications involve both caudate heads and lentiform nuclei in this young patient with chronic liver failure. Despite these findings, she remained neurologically intact except for a mild tremor.

calcification as seen by CT and may reflect a microvascular angiopathy, deposition of paramagnetic substances, or protein binding as a result of the toxicity of the hepatic failure (Fig. 28–44).

REFERENCES

1. Valk J, van der Knaap MS: Magnetic Resonance of Myelin, Myelination, and Myelin Disorders. Berlin: Springer-Verlag, 1989, p 82.
2. Kendall BE: Disorders of lysosomes, peroxisomes, and mitochondria. AJNR 13:621, 1992.
3. McKusick VA, Neifeld EF: The mucopolysaccharide storage diseases. In: Stanbury JB, Wyngaarden JB, Frederickson DS, et al, eds. The Metabolic Basis of Inherited Disease. New York: McGraw-Hill, 1983, p 751.
4. Suzuki K, Suzuki H, Chen C: Metachromatic leukodystrophy: isolation and chemical analysis of metachromatic granules. Science 151:1231, 1966.
5. Alves D, Pires MM, Guimaraes A, et al: Four cases of late onset metachromatic leukodystrophy in a family: clinical, biochemical and neuropathologic studies. J Neurol Neurosurg Psychiatry 49:1417, 1986.
6. Norman R: Diffuse progressive metachromatic leukoencephalopathy. Brain 70:234, 1947.
7. Hagberg B: Clinical symptoms, signs, and tests in metachromatic leukodystrophies. In: Folch-Pi J, Bauer H, eds. Brain Lipids and Lipoproteins and the Leukodystrophies. Amsterdam: Elsevier Science Publishing, 1963, p 134.
8. Finelli PF: Metachromatic leukodystrophy manifesting as a schizophrenic disorder: computed tomographic correlation. Ann Neurol 18:94, 1985.
9. Hagberg B: Krabbe's disease: clinical presentation of neurological variants. Neuropediatrics 15(suppl):11, 1984.
10. Zlotogora J, Chakraborty S, Knowlton R, et al: Krabbe's disease locus mapped to chromosome 14 by genetic linkage. Am J Hum Genet 47:37, 1990.
11. D'Agostino AM, Sayre GP, Hagles AB: Krabbe's disease. Arch Neurol 8:82, 1963.
12. Kwan E, Drace J, Enzmann D: Specific CT findings in Krabbe's disease. AJNR 5:453, 1984.
13. Demaerel P, Wilms G, Verdu P, et al: MR findings in globoid cell leukodystrophy. Neuroradiology 32:520, 1990.
14. Finelli DA, Sawyer RN, Horwitz SJ: Deceptively normal MR in early infantile Krabbe disease. AJNR 15:167–171, 1994.
15. O'Brien JS: Generalized gangliosidosis. J Pediatr 75:167, 1969.
16. Fukumizu M, Yoshikawa H, Takashima S, et al: Tay-Sachs disease: progression of changes on neuroimaging in four cases. Neuroradiology 34:483, 1992.
17. Yoshikawa H, Yamada K, Sakuragawa N: MRI in the early stage of Tay-Sachs disease. Neuroradiology 34:394, 1992.
18. Okada S, McCrea M, O'Brien JS: Sandhoff's disease (GM$_2$-gangliosidosis type 2): clinical, chemical and enzyme studies in five patients. Pediatr Res 6:606, 1972.
19. Stalker HP, Han BK: Thalamic hyperdensity: a previously unreported sign of Sandhoff's disease. AJNR 10:S82, 1989.
20. Ishimoda-Matsubayashi S, Kuru Y, Sumie H, et al: MRI findings in the mild type of mucopolysaccaridosis II (Hunter's syndrome). Neuroradiology 32:328, 1990.
21. Murata R, Nakajima S, Tanaka A, et al: MR imaging of the brain in patients with mucopolysaccharidosis. AJNR 10:1165, 1989.
22. Gabrielli O, Salvolini U, Maricotti M, et al: Cerebral MRI in two brothers with mucopolysaccharidosis type I and different clinical phenotypes. Neuroradiology 34:313, 1992.
23. Lee C, Dineen TE, Brack M, et al: Mucopolysaccharidoses: characterization by cranial MR imaging. AJNR 14:1285, 1993.
24. Watts RWE, Spellacy E, Kendall BE, et al: CT studies on patients with mucopolysaccharidoses. Neuroradiology 21:9, 1981.
25. van der Knapp MS, Valk J: MR spectrum of peroxisomal disorders. Neuroradiology 33:30, 1991.
26. Monnens LA, Heymans HSA: Peroxisomal disorders: clinical characterization. J Inherit Metab Dis 10(suppl):23, 1987.
27. Volpe JJ, Adams RD: Cerebro-hepato-renal syndrome of Zellweger: an inherited disorder of neuronal migration. Acta Neuropathol 20:175, 1972.
28. Kelly RI, Datta NS, Dobryns WB, et al: Neonatal adrenoleukodystrophy: new cases, biochemical studies and differentiation from Zellweger's and related peroxisomal polydystrophy syndromes. Am J Med Genet 23:869, 1986.
29. Moser HW, Naidu S, Kumar AJ, et al: The adrenoleukodystrophies. Crit Rev Neurobiol 5:29, 1987.
30. Schaumburg HH, Powers JM, Raine CS, et al: Adrenomyeloneuropathy: a probable variant of adrenoleukodystrophy. II. General pathologic, neuropathologic and biochemical aspects. Neurology 27:1114, 1977.
31. Valk J, van der Knaap MS: Refsum's disease. In: Valk J, van der Knaap MS, eds. Magnetic Resonance of Myelin, Myelination, and Myelin Disorders. Berlin: Springer-Verlag, 1989, p 113.
32. Tzika AA, Ball WS Jr, Vigneron DB, et al: Childhood adrenoleukodystrophy: assessment with proton MR spectroscopy. Radiology 189:467, 1993.
33. Kumar AJ, Rosenbaum AE, Naidu S, et al: Adrenoleukodystrophy: correlating MR imaging with CT. Radiology 165:497, 1987.
34. Jenson ME, Sawyer RW, Braun IF, et al: MR imaging appearance of childhood adrenoleukodystrophy with auditory, visual and motor pathway involvement. Radiographics 10:53, 1990.
35. Pasco A, Kalifa G, Sarrazin JL, et al: Contribution of MRI to the diagnosis of cerebral lesions of adrenoleukodystrophy. Pediatr Radiol 21:161, 1991.
36. Valk J, van der Knaap MS: Adrenoleukodystrophy. In: Valk J, van der Knaap MS: Magnetic Resonance of Myelin, Myelination, and Myelin Disorders. Berlin: Springer-Verlag, 1989, p 104.
37. Dubois J, Sebag G, Argyropoulou M, et al: MR findings in infantile Refsum's disease: case report of two family members. AJNR 12:1159, 1991.
38. Moser H, Moser A, Naidu S, et al: Clinical aspects of adrenoleukodystrophy and adrenomyeloneuropathy. Dev Neurosci 13:254, 1991.
39. Karpati G, Shoubridge EA: Mitochondrial encephalomyopathies due to electron transport chain defects. Curr Neurol 13:133, 1993.
40. Tulinius MH, Holme E, Kristiansson B, et al: Mitochondrial encephalomyopathies in childhood. I. Biochemical and morphologic investigations. J Pediatr 199:242, 1191.
41. Tulinius MH, Holme E, Kristiansson B, et al: Mitochondrial encephalomyopathies in childhood. II. Clinical manifestations and syndromes. J Pediatr 119:242, 1991.
42. Barkovich AJ, Good WV, Koch TK, et al: Mitochondrial disorders: analysis of their clinical and imaging characteristics. AJNR 14:1119, 1993.
43. Geyer CA, Sartor KJ, Preasky AJ, et al: Leigh disease (subacute necrotizing encephalomyelopathy): CT and MR findings in five cases. J Comput Assist Tomogr 12:40, 1988.
44. Davis PC, Hoffman JC, Braun IF, et al: MR of Leigh's disease. AJNR 8:71, 1987.
45. Medina L, Chi TL, DeVivo DC, et al: MR findings in patients with subacute necrotizing encephalomyelopathy (Leigh syndrome): correlation with biochemical defect. AJNR 11:379, 1990.
46. Manzi SV, Hager KH, Murtagh FR, et al: MR imaging in a patient with Leigh's disease (subacute necrotizing encephalomyelopathy). Pediatr Radiol 21:62, 1990.
47. Tzika AA, Ball WS Jr, Vigneron DB, et al: Clinical proton spectroscopy of neurodegenerative disease in childhood. AJNR 14:1267, 1993.
48. Pavlakis SG, Phillips PC, DiMauro S, et al: Mitochondrial myopathy, encephalopathy, lactic acidosis, and stroke-like episodes: a distinctive clinical syndrome. Ann Neurol 16:481, 1984.
49. Rosen L, Phillips S, Enzmann D, et al: Magnetic resonance imaging in MELAS syndrome. Neuroradiology 32:168, 1990.
50. King MP, Koga Y, Davidson M, et al: Defects in mitochondrial protein synthesis and respiratory chain activity segregate with the tRNA^{Leu}(UUR) mutation associated with mitochondrial encephalopathy, lactic acidosis, and stroke-like episodes. Mol Cell Biol 12:480, 1992.
51. Ciafaloni E, Ricci E, Shanske S, et al: MELAS: clinical features, biochemistry, and molecular genetics. Ann Neurol 31:391, 1992.
52. Abe K, Inui T, Hirono N, et al: Fluctuating MR images with mitochondrial encephalopathy, lactic acidosis, stroke-like syndrome (MELAS). Neuroradiology 32:77, 1990.
53. Wallace DC, Zheng X, Lott MT, et al: Familial mitochondrial encephalopathy (MERRF): genetic, pathophysiological, and biochemical characterization of a mitochondrial DNA disease. Cell 55:601, 1988.
54. Fukuhara N: MERRF: a clinicopathological study. Relationship between myoclonic epilepsies amd mitochondrial myopathies. Rev Neurol 147:476, 1991.
55. Demange P, Pham-Gia H, Kalifa G, et al: MR of Kearns-Sayre syndrome. AJNR 12:375, 1989.
56. Leutner C, Layer G, Zierz S, et al: Cerebral MR in ophthalmoplegia PLUS. AJNR 15:681, 1994.
57. Kearns T, Sayre G: Retinitis pigmentosa, external ophthalmoplegia, and complete heart block. Arch Ophthalmol 60:280, 1958.
58. Seigel RS, Seeger JF, Gabrielson TO, et al: Computed tomography in oculocraniosomatic disease. Neuroradiology 130:159, 1979.
59. Harding BN: Progressive neuronal degeneration of childhood with liver disease (Alpers-Huttenlocher syndrome): a personal review. J Child Neurol 5:273, 1990.
60. Boyd SG, Harden A, Egger J, et al: Progressive neuronal degeneration of childhood with liver disease (Alpers disease): characteristic neurophysiological features. Neuropediatrics 17:75, 1986.
61. Johnson DE, Coleman L, Poe L: MR of progressive neurodegenerative change in treated Menkes' kinky hair disease. Neuroradiology 33:181, 1991.
62. Ichihashi K, Yano S, Kobayashi S, et al: Serial imaging of Menkes disease. Neuroradiology 32:56, 1990.
63. Gencic S, Abuelo D, Ambler M, et al: Pelizaeus-Merzbacher disease: an X-linked neurologic disorder of myelin metabolism with a novel mutation in the gene encoding proteolipid protein. Am J Hum Genet 45:435, 1989.

64. Silverstein AM, Hirsch DK, Trobe JD, et al: MR imaging of the brain in five members of a family with Pelizaeus-Merzbacher disease. AJNR 11:495, 1990.
65. Andre M, Monin P, Moret C, et al: Pelizaeus-Metzbacher disease: contribution of magnetic resonance imaging to an early diagnosis. Neuroradiology 17:216, 1990.
66. Damaerel P, Wilms G, Verdu P, et al: MRI in the diagnosis of Cockayne's syndrome: one case. J Neuroradiol 17:157, 1990.
67. Boltshauser E, Yalcinyaka C, Wichmann W, et al: MRI in Cockayne syndrome type I. Neuroradiology 31:276, 1989.
68. Schuster V, Horwitz AE, Kreth HW, et al: Alexander's disease: cranial MRI and ultrasound findings. Pediatr Radiol 21:133, 1991.
69. Farrell K, Chaung S, Becker LE: Computed tomography in Alexander's disease. Ann Neurol 15:605, 1984.
70. Trommer BL, Naidich TP, Del Cento MC, et al: Noninvasive CT diagnosis of infantile Alexander disease: pathologic correlation. J Comput Assist Tomogr 7:509, 1983.
71. Buchanan DS, Davis RL: Spongy degeneration of the central nervous system: a report of four cases and a review of the literature. Neurology 15:207, 1965.
72. Matalon R, Kaul R, Casanova J, et al: Aspartocyclase deficiency: the enzyme defect in Canavan's disease. J Inherit Metab Dis 12(suppl 2):329, 1989.
73. Brismar J, Brismar G, Gascon G, et al: Canavan disease: CT and MR imaging of the brain. AJNR 11:805, 1990.
74. Austin SJ, Connelly A, Gadian DG, et al: Localized 1H NMR spectroscopy in Canavan's disease: a report of two cases. Magn Reson Med 19:439, 1991.
75. McAdams HP, Geyer CA, Done SL, et al: CT and MR imaging of Canavan's disease. AJNR 11:3397, 1990.
76. Crome L, Pare CMB: Phenylketonuria: a review and a report of the pathological findings in four cases. J Ment Sci 106:862, 1960.
77. Gudinchet F, Maeder P, Meuli RA, et al: Cranial CT and MRI in malignant phenylketonuria. Pediatr Radiol 22:223, 1992.
78. Malamud N: Neuropathology of phenylketonuria. J Neuropathol Exp Neurol 25:254, 1966.
79. Shaw DWW, Weinberger E, Maravilla KR: Cranial MR in phenylketonuria. J Comput Assist Tomogr 14:458, 1990.
80. Pearsen KD, Gean-Marton AD, Levy HL, et al: Phenylketonuria: MR imaging of the brain with clinical correlation. Radiology 177:437, 1990.
81. Shaw DWW, Maravilla KR, Weinberger E, et al: MR imaging of phenylketonuria. AJNR 12:403, 1991.
82. Goodman SI, Kohlhoff JG: Glutaric aciduria: inherited deficiency of glutaryl-CoA dehydrogenase activity. Biochem Med 13:138, 1975.
83. Andreula CF, De Blasi R, Carella A: CT and MR studies in methylmalonic acidemia. AJNR 12:410, 1991.
84. Gebarski SS, Gabrielson TO, Knake JE, et al: Cerebral CT findings in methylmalonic and propionic acidurias. AJNR 4:955, 1983.
85. Sisson MC: Amniotic fluid embolism. Crit Care Nurs Clin North Am 4:667, 1992.
86. Roessmann U, Miller RT: Thrombosis of the middle cerebral artery associated with birth trauma. Neurology 30:889, 1980.
87. Press GA, Barshop BA, Haas RH, et al: Abnormalities of the brain in nonketotic hyperglycinemia: MR manifestations. AJNR 10:315, 1989.
88. Bisset GS III, Schwartz DC, Meyer RA, et al: Clinical spectrum and long-term follow-up of isolated mitral valve prolapse in 119 children. Circulation 62:423, 1980.
89. Kouvaras G, Bacoulas G: Association of mitral valve leaflet prolapse with cerebral ischaemic events in the young and middle-aged patient. Q J Med 55:387, 1985.
90. Tada H, Morooka K, Arimoto K, et al: [N-Isopropyl-p-[I¹²³] iodoamphetamine single photon emission computed tomography (I¹²³-IMP SPECT) and child neurology]. No To Hattatsu 24:462, 1992.
91. Rice GPA, Ebers GC, Bondar RL, et al: Mitral valve prolapse: a cause of stroke in children? Dev Med Child Neurol 23:352, 1981.
92. Woodhurst WB, Robertson WD, Thompson GB: Carotid injury due to intraoral trauma: case report and review of the literature. Neurosurgery 6:559, 1980.
93. Dusser A, Goutieres F, Aicardi J: Ischemic strokes in children. J Child Neurol 1:131, 1986.
94. Mintz M, Epstein LG, Koenigsberger MR: Idiopathic childhood stroke is associated with human leukocyte antigen (HLA)-B51. Ann Neurol 31:675, 1992.
95. Brismar J, Aqeel A, Brismar G, et al: Maple syrup urine disease: findings on CT and MR scans of the brains in 10 infants. AJNR 11:1219, 1990.
96. Newman M, Mitchell JRA: Homocystinuria presenting as multiple arterial occlusions. Q J Med 53:251, 1984.
97. Cochran FB, Packman S: Homocystinuria presenting as sagittal sinus thrombosis. Eur Neurol 32:1, 1991.
98. Favre JP, Becker F, Lorcerie B, et al: Vascular manifestations in homocystinuria. Ann Vasc Surg 6:294, 1992.
99. Schaffert DA, Johnson SD, Johnson PC, et al: Magnetic resonance imaging in pathologically proven Hallervorden-Spatz disease. Neurology 39:440, 1989.
100. Savoiardo M, Halliday WC, Nardocci N, et al: Hallervorden-Spatz disease: MR and pathologic findings. AJNR 14:155, 1992.
101. Littrup PJ, Gebarski SS: MR imaging of Hallervorden-Spatz disease. J Comput Assist Tomogr 9:491, 1985.
102. Ambrosetto P, Nonni R, Bacci A, et al: Late onset familial Hallervorden-Spatz disease: MR findings in two sisters. AJNR 13:394, 1992.
103. Tanfani G, Mascalchi M, Dal Pozzo GC, et al: MR imaging in a case of Hallervorden-Spatz disease. J Comput Assist Tomogr 11:1057, 1987.
104. Abdollah A, Tampieri D, Melanson D: Wilson's disease: computed tomography and magnetic resonance imaging findings. J Can Assoc Radiol 42:130, 1991.
105. Aisen AM, Martel W, Gabielson TO, et al: Wilson disease of the brain: MR imaging. Radiology 157:137, 1985.
106. Brugieres P, Combes C, Ricolfi F, et al: Atypical MR presentation of Wilson disease: a possible consequence of paramagnetic effect of copper. Neuroradiology 34:222, 1992.
107. Wimberger DM, Kramer J, et al: Cranial MRI in Wilson's disease. Neuroradiology 32:211, 1990.
108. Starosta-Rubinstein S, Young AB, Kluin K, et al: Clinical assessment of 31 patients with Wilson's disease. Correlation with structural changes on magnetic resonance imaging. Arch Neurol 44:365, 1987.
109. Donnell GN, Collado M, Koch R: Growth and development of children with galactosemia. J Pediatr 58:836, 1961.
110. Lo W, Packman S, Nash S, et al: Curious neurologic sequela in galactosemia. Pediatics 73:309, 1964.
111. Nelson MD, Wolff JA, Cross CA, et al: Galactosemia: evaluation with MR imaging. Radiology 184:255, 1992.
112. Dietemann JL, Filippi de la Palavesa MM, Tranchant C, et al: MR findings in mannosidosis. Neuroradiology 32:485, 1990.
113. Miller GM, Baker HC Jr, Okazaki H, et al: Central pontine myelinolysis and its imitators: MR findings. Radiology 168:795, 1988.
114. Ho VB, Fitz CR, Yoder CC, et al: Resolving features in osmotic myelinolysis (central pontine and extrapontine myelinolysis). AJNR 14:163, 1992.
115. Korogi Y, Takahashi M, Shinzato J, et al: MR findings in two presumed cases of mild central pontine myelinolysis. AJNR 14:651, 1993.
116. Thompson AJ, Brown MM, Swash M, et al: Autopsy validation of MRI in central pontine myelinolysis. Neuroradiology 30:175, 1988.
117. Chang KH, Han MH, Kim HS, et al: Delayed encephalopathy after acute carbon monoxide intoxication: MR imaging features and distribution of cerebral white matter lesions. Radiology 184:117, 1992.
118. Lapresle J, Fardeau M: The central nervous system and carbon monoxide poisoning, II. Anatomical study of brain lesions following intoxication with carbon monoxide (22 cases). Prog Brain Res 24:31, 1967.
119. Tuchman RF, Moser FG, Moshe SL: Carbon monoxide poisoning: bilateral lesions in the thalamus on MR imaging of the brain. Pediatr Radiol 20:478, 1990.
120. Nardizzi LR: Computerized tomographic correlate of carbon monoxide poisoning. Arch Neurol 36:38, 1979.
121. Victor M, Adams RD, Collins GH: The Wernicke-Korsakoff Syndrome and Related Neurologic Disorders due to Alcoholism and Malnutrition. 2nd ed. Philadelphia: FA Davis, 1989, pp 1–117.
122. Victor M: MR in the diagnosis of Wernicke-Korsakoff syndrome. AJNR 11:895, 1990.
123. Thompson AD, Ryle PR, Shaw GK: Ethanol, thiamine, and brain damage. Alcohol Alcohol 1:27, 1983.
124. Schroth G, Wichmann W, Valavanis A: Blood-brain-barrier disruption in acute Wernicke encephalopathy: MR findings. J Comput Assist Tomogr 15:1059, 1991.
125. Yokote K, Miyagi K, Kuzuhara S, et al: Wernicke encephalopathy: follow-up study by CT and MR. J Comput Assist Tomogr 15:853, 1991.
126. D'Aprile P, Gentile MA, Carella A: Enhanced MR in the acute phase of Wernicke encephalopathy. AJNR 15:591, 1994.
127. Shogry MEC, Curnes JT: Mamillary body enhancement on MR as the only sign of acute Wernicke encephalopathy. AJNR 15:172, 1994.
128. Dorai-swamy PM, Massey EW, Enright K, et al: Wernicke-Korsakoff syndrome caused by psychogenic food refusal: MR findings. AJNR 15:594, 1994.
129. Gallucci M, Bozzao A, Splendiani A, et al: Wernicke encephalopathy: MR findings in five patients. AJNR 11:887, 1990.
130. Gallucci M, Amicarelli I, Rossi A, et al: MR imaging of white matter lesions in uncomplicated chronic alcoholism. J Comput Assist Tomogr 13:395, 1989.
131. Jacobson JL, Jacobson SW, Sokol RJ, et al: Effects of alcohol use, smoking, and illicit drug use on fetal growth in black infants. J Pediatr 124:757, 1994.
132. Chen JC, Schneiderman JF, Wortzman G: Methanol poisoning: bilateral putaminal and cerebellar cortical lesions on CT and MR. J Comput Assist Tomogr 15:522, 1991.
133. Singer LT, Yamashita TS, Hawkins S, et al: Increased incidence of intraventricular hemorrhage and developmental delay in cocaine-exposed, very low birth weight infants. J Pediatr 124:765, 1994.
134. Heier LA, Carpanzano CR, Mast J, et al: Maternal cocaine abuse: the spectrum of radiologic abnormalities in the neonatal CNS. AJNR 12:951, 1991.
135. Ball WS, Prenger EC, Ballard ET: Neurotoxicity of radio/chemotherapy in children: pathologic and MR correlation. AJNR 13:761, 1992.
136. Withers HR, Peters LJ, Kogelnik HS: The pathology of late effects of

radiation. In: Meyn RE, Withers HR, eds. Radiation Biology in Cancer Research. New York: Raven Press, 1980, p 439.

137. Wilson DA, Nitschke R, Bowman ME, et al: Transient white matter changes on MR images in children undergoing chemotherapy for acute lymphocytic leukemia: correlation with neuropsychologic deficiencies. Radiology 180:205, 1991.

138. Ebner F, Ranner G, Slavc I, et al: MR findings in methotrexate-induced CNS abnormalities. AJNR 10:959, 1989.

139. Vaughn DJ, Jarvik JG, Hackney D, et al: High-dose cytarabine neurotoxicity: MR findings during the acute phase. AJNR 14:1014, 1993.

140. Truwit CL, Denaro CP, Lake JR, et al: MR imaging of reversible cyclosporin A induced neurotoxicity. AJR 157:851, 1991.

141. Anlar B, Erzen C, Saarci U: Patchy cerebral white matter edema in chronic renal failure. Pediatr Radiol 19:444, 1989.

142. Okada J, Yoshikawa K, Matsuo H, et al: Reversible MRI and CT findings in uremic encephalopathy. Neuroradiology 33:524, 1991.

143. Hahn JS, Havens PL, Higgns JJ, et al: Neurological complications of hemolytic-uremic syndrome. J Child Neurol 4:108, 1989.

144. Sherwood JW, Wagle WA: Hemolytic uremic syndrome: MR findings of CNS complications. AJNR 12:703, 1991.

145. Brunberg JA, Kanal E, Hirsch W, et al: Chronic acquired hepatic failure: MR imaging of the brain at 1.5T. AJNR 12:909, 1991.

146. Ross BD, Jacobson S, Villamil F, et al: Subclinical hepatic encephalopathy: proton spectroscopic abnormalities. Radiology 193:457, 1994.

Neurodegenerative Disorders

ANDREI I. HOLODNY ■ AJAX E. GEORGE
JAMES GOLOMB ■ MONY J. DE LEON

The development of magnetic resonance imaging (MRI) has greatly enhanced the radiologic assessment of neurodegenerative disorders, including the dementias, movement disorders, hydrocephalus, and temporal lobe epilepsy. MRI and computer postprocessing of the images can discern structural as well as functional changes in the human brain that may be sensitive as well as specific for the neurodegenerative disorder.

DEMENTIA

ALZHEIMER'S DISEASE

Alzheimer's disease (AD)[1, 2] is now recognized as one of the most significant health problems of our century.[3] AD is estimated to afflict 10% of people older than 65 years of age and 50% of individuals older than the age of 85 years.[4] It is the most common dementing disorder of the elderly.[5] Despite the high prevalence of AD, the diagnosis in vivo is often a problem. According to the Diagnostic and Statistical Manual of Mental Disorders (DSM-III-R),[6] patients with AD usually present with "a multifaceted loss of intellectual abilities, such as memory, judgment, abstract thought, and other higher cortical functions, and changes in personality and behavior." However, these clinical signs are far from specific for AD and often overlap signs of other clinical entities.

Early reports of the gross pathologic examination of the postmortem brain in AD also failed to determine specific diagnostic criteria. They revealed a pattern of generalized atrophy of the cerebral cortex. However, the degree of cerebral atrophy was not constant and in certain cases atrophy was even absent.[7] In addition, cerebral atrophy is not specific for AD, as there is a large overlap with other dementing processes as well as with the normal process of aging.

The only definitive way to make a diagnosis of AD is by histopathologic examination.[8] The histopathologic changes consist of neurofibrillary tangles and senile plaques that are accentuated in the medial temporal lobe and the temporal-parietal association cortices.[9–11]

Clinical-pathologic correlation studies have found an overall accuracy rate of 60% to 90%.[12–16] Therefore, the clinical diagnosis of AD is often unclear, especially in the mild and early cases of dementia. Because brain biopsy is not a viable option for the vast majority of suspected AD cases, the neuroradiologic findings are becoming increasingly important.

It was not until the early 1980s that a specific part of the brain—the hippocampal formation—was implicated in the pathogenesis of AD. Hyman and colleagues[17] described the specific histopathologic changes that occur in the degenerated hippocampal formation of patients with AD. In 1991, Price and coworkers[18] reported that in early cases of AD, the histopathologic markers are restricted to the hippocampus and parahippocampal gyrus. From these reports, it followed that the earliest anatomic and histologic changes in AD occurred in the hippocampal formation and that the other changes observed in postmortem studies described previously were secondary in both importance and temporal development to the changes in the hippocampal formation.

In terms of what is known about the neural pathways, the implication of hippocampal formation involvement in AD also seems correct. The affected neurons in the hippocampus are those that have reciprocal connections with the association cortices, basal forebrain, thalamus, and hypothalamus—in other words, structures that are crucial to memory and cognition. Damage to these hippocampal neurons therefore correlates well with the neuropsychologic impairment observed in patients with AD. The observed pattern of degeneration results in "isolation" of the hippocampal formation from the neocortical association areas.[17] In 1985, Ball and colleagues,[19] acknowledging the central role of the hippocampal formation in the development of AD, proposed a new definition for AD—that of a hippocampal dementia. Therefore, the research efforts of a number of groups, including our own, to establish radiologic criteria for the diagnosis of AD have been centered on the hippocampal formation.

Before the recognition of the importance of temporal lobe disease in AD, several early computed tomography studies in the 1970s and early 1980s were able to show weak correlations among ventricular enlargement, cortical atrophy, and dementia related to presumed AD.[20, 21]

As the spatial resolution of computed tomography improved and attention was directed to the temporal lobes, enlargement of the cerebrospinal fluid (CSF) spaces in the perihippocampal region was identified as indicative of volume loss in the hippocampus and parahippocampal gyrus. A number of studies, including work by LeMay and Kido and their associates, demonstrated that evaluation of the structures of the medial temporal lobe can differentiate patients with AD from normal age-matched control subjects.[22–24] George and coworkers,[25] using a "reverse angle" scanning plane paralleling the long axis of the temporal lobes, found a sensitivity of 82%, a specificity of 75%, and an overall accuracy of 80% in the ability to discriminate patients with AD from normal age-matched control subjects by subjectively evaluating atrophy of the temporal lobes and dilatation of the parahippocampal fissures. De Leon and colleagues[26] suggested that this measure had value in the prediction of future dementia in mildly impaired adults.

The advent of high-resolution MRI greatly facilitated visualization of the medial aspect of the temporal lobes and the hippocampus (Figs. 29–1 to 29–4). In addition, by obtaining images in the coronal plane, the hippocampus and the perihippocampal fissures are visualized directly. A number of studies have demonstrated a significant decrease in the size of the hippocampal formation in patients with AD compared with normal control subjects.

In 1988, Seab and associates[27] reported that volumetric measures of coronal MRI scans of the hippocam-

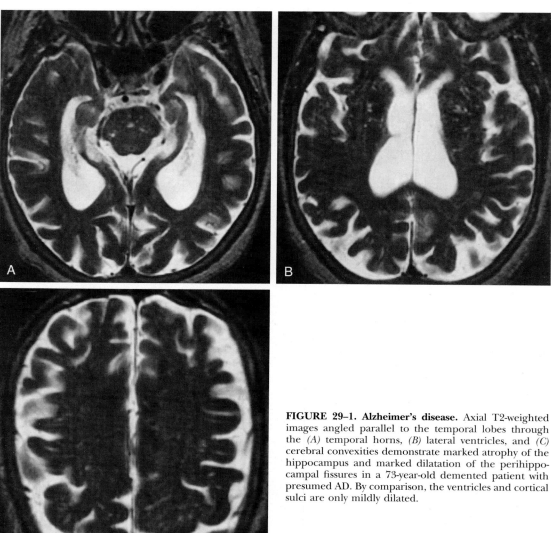

FIGURE 29–1. Alzheimer's disease. Axial T2-weighted images angled parallel to the temporal lobes through the (A) temporal horns, (B) lateral ventricles, and (C) cerebral convexities demonstrate marked atrophy of the hippocampus and marked dilatation of the perihippocampal fissures in a 73-year-old demented patient with presumed AD. By comparison, the ventricles and cortical sulci are only mildly dilated.

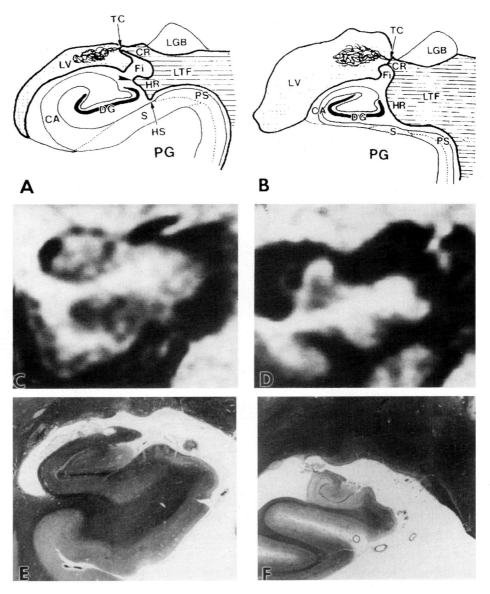

FIGURE 29–2. Alzheimer's disease. Coronal sections at the level of the lateral geniculate bodies of the control (*A, C,* and *E*) and AD (*B, D,* and *F*) brains. *A* and *B,* Drawings; *C* and *D,* T1-weighted MR images; *E* and *F,* histologic slices stained with the Loyez method. In the AD brain, the lateral part of the transverse fissure (LTF) is dilated and the choroidal recess (CR) and hippocampal recess (HR) are enlarged. Atrophy of the parahippocampal gyrus (PG) including the subiculum (S) is apparent. Hippocampal atrophy encompasses the cornu Ammonis (CA), sparing the dentate gyrus (DG). Structures: Fi = fimbria; HS = hippocampal sulcus; LGB = lateral geniculate body; LV = lateral ventricle; PS = presubiculum; TC = tela choroidea; arrowhead = fimbrio-dentate sulcus. (*A* to *F* from Narkiewicz O, de Leon MJ, Convit A, et al: Dilatation of the lateral part of the transverse fissure of the brain in Alzheimer's disease. Acta Neurobiol Exp [Warsz] 53: 457–465, 1993.)

pus, ventricles, subarachnoid spaces, and brain parenchyma demonstrated a reduction of 40% in the hippocampal volume of the AD group compared with the control subjects, with no overlap. The measures of brain atrophy and ventricular and sulcal enlargement also showed a difference between the two group means; however, there was a significant overlap. This paper suggested that diminished hippocampal size as seen with MRI may be able to differentiate between AD and normal aging.

In 1991, Kesslak and coworkers[28] showed that the hippocampus and parahippocampal gyrus showed significant atrophy with a reduction in size of more than 40% in AD patients "in the mild to moderate stages of the disease" compared with normal control subjects. In addition, there was no overlap between the two groups. Of the volumetric measures taken by these investigators, the size of the hippocampus showed the greatest difference. Hippocampal and parahippocam-

pal gyrus volumes also had the highest correlation with scores in the Mini-Mental State Examination.

In 1992, Jack and colleagues[29] obtained volumetric measures of temporal lobe structures from MR images. They found that the volume of the hippocampal formation effectively differentiated between a group of patients suffering from dementia of the Alzheimer type (with a Global Deterioration Scale score of 3 or 4) and normal age-matched control subjects ($P < .001$). These investigators noted an overlap of only 3 of the 42 patients in the two groups.

Milder degrees of hippocampal atrophy occur in approximately one third of cognitively normal older adults. In such persons, hippocampal atrophy is associated with diminished recent memory performance.[30, 31]

In 1991, Rusinek and associates[32] described an MRI method that permitted accurate determination of regional volumes of gray matter, white matter, and CSF. This technique utilized dual inversion recovery pulse

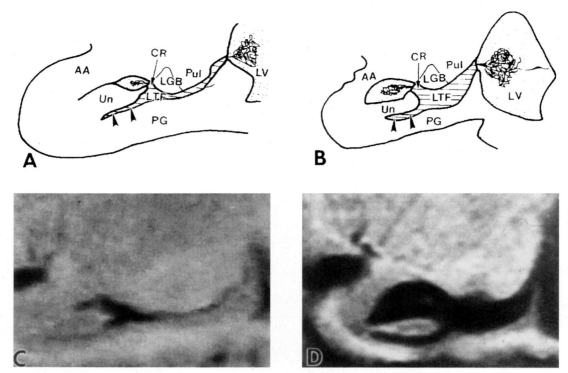

FIGURE 29–3. Alzheimer's disease. Sagittal section of the lateral part of the transverse fissure (LTF) in control (*A* and *C*) and AD (*B* and *D*) brains. *A* and *B,* Drawings; *C* and *D,* T1-weighted MR images. In AD, the LTF is enlarged in dorsoventral dimension; atrophy of the parahippocampal gyrus (PG) occurs, as does severe atrophy of the uncus (Un). Structures: AA = amygdaloid body; CR = choroidal recess; LGB = lateral geniculate body; LV = lateral ventricle; Pul = pulvinar; arrowheads = uncal sulcus. (*A* to *D* from Narkiewicz O, de Leon MJ, Convit A, et al: Dilatation of the lateral part of the transverse fissure of the brain in Alzheimer's disease. Acta Neurobiol Exp [Warsz] 53:457–465, 1993.)

sequences that were designed to compensate for partial-volume effects. In the first sequence the gray matter–white matter contrast is maximized. The second sequence is designed to maximize the CSF signal and suppress the brain signal as originally described by Condon and colleagues.[33] By algebraically manipulating the signal of these two pulse sequences in the same brain region, the volumes of gray matter, white matter, and CSF are determined. In a study of 14 AD patients and 14 age-matched control subjects, the percentage of gray matter in brains of the AD patients was significantly lower than in the control subjects (44.9% ± 4.4% versus 50.2% ± 3.2%). The greatest loss in neocortical gray matter (13.8%, $P < .001$) and the greatest increase in surrounding CSF ($P < .01$) occurred in the temporal lobes of the AD patients. Reduction in gray matter volume was also observed in the AD group in the frontal and occipital lobes but to a lesser extent. No significant regional white matter changes were detected. These findings are in agreement with postmortem studies of brains of patients with AD.[34, 35]

Another study by Lehericy and coworkers[36] used detailed volumetric analysis based on MRI to show that patients with clinically mild AD (Mini-Mental status ≥ 21) showed significant atrophy not only of the hippocampal formation but also of the amygdala when compared with normal age-matched control subjects. There was no difference in the size of the caudate nucleus and the ventricles between these two groups.

It has been suggested that measurement of the interuncal distance on axial MR images may be reflective of hippocampal formation atrophy and may be able to distinguish patients with AD.[37] However, other reports have not confirmed this observation. A report by Early and colleagues[38] has shown that interuncal distance does not show significant correlation with the amygdala and hippocampal volume and does not serve to discriminate between AD patients and control subjects. A commentary by de Leon and associates[39] concluded that at present the interuncal distance is not a useful tool in the diagnosis of AD.

Work by de Leon and associates[40] has shown that dilatation of the perihippocampal CSF spaces and associated hippocampal atrophy can be used as a predictor of the development of AD. In a group of 86 nondemented elderly adults who were either normal or had mild memory impairment, who were studied at two points in time 4 years apart, dilatation of the perihippocampal CSF spaces was 91% sensitive and 89% specific in predicting the development of AD.

In the past, the value of neuroimaging in the evaluation of AD was limited to the exclusion of other pathologic conditions such as multiple infarcts, subdural hematoma, and metastatic disease. The work just outlined defines radiographic characteristics that appear to be both sensitive and specific for AD. Thus, the radiologic diagnosis of AD is becoming increasingly a diagnosis of inclusion.[41]

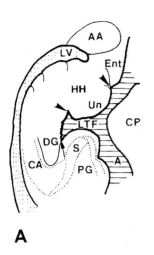

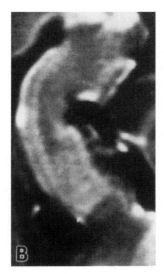

A

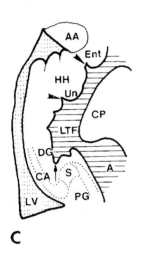

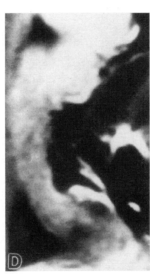

C

FIGURE 29–4. Alzheimer's disease. Axial section of the lateral part of the transverse fissure (LTF) in control *(A and C)* and AD *(B and D)* brains. *A* and *C,* Drawings; *B* and *D,* postmortem axial MR images. *D,* Severe dilatation of the LTF is seen in the AD brain. Atrophy of the cornu Ammonis (CA) and parahippocampal gyrus (PG) is apparent. Structures: A = ambient cistern; AA = amygdaloid body; CP = cerebral peduncle; DG = dentate gyrus; Ent = entorhinal cortex; HH = head of hippocampus; LV = lateral ventricle; S = subiculum; Un = uncus; arrowheads = hippocampal sulcus; arrow = uncal sulcus. *(A to D from Narkiewicz O, de Leon MJ, Convit A, et al: Dilatation of the lateral part of the transverse fissure of the brain in Alzheimer's disease. Acta Neurobiol Exp [Warsz] 53:457–465, 1993.)*

PICK'S DISEASE

Pick's disease is another cause of dementia in the elderly population. Pick's disease is much less prevalent than AD. The clinical onset in most patients is suggestive of frontal lobe damage. It is characterized by an insidious deterioration of intellectual capacity, difficulty in concentration and memory, and a slow but steady progression to marked dementia. Pathologic studies have demonstrated atrophy of the brain, particularly of the frontal lobes and the anterior aspects of

the temporal lobes. The parietal and occipital lobes are usually spared. Histologically, intense loss and misalignment of neurons and subcortical gliosis in the affected areas of the brain are observed. Many of the remaining neurons are small and contain a characteristic Pick body. Pick's body is a well-defined or poorly defined lesion in the neuron that is seen with Bielschowsky's silver stain and antibody immunostaining.[7]

Radiographically, Pick's disease presents as marked atrophy of the anterior temporal and frontal lobes. The sulci of these lobes become so atrophic that they have been described as icicle-like. The posterior aspect of the superior frontal gyrus and the brain posterior to it are usually spared.[42]

MULTIPLE-INFARCT DEMENTIA

Multiple-infarct dementia is the second most common type of dementia in the elderly, representing 10% to 20% of cases in patients older than 65 years old.[43] Clinically, these patients present with a sudden onset of dementia, day-to-day fluctuation, and spontaneous improvement early in the disease. There is also evidence of arteriosclerosis such as strokes, coronary artery disease, and hypertension.

These patients present radiographically with focally dilated fissures and multiple areas of focal cortical volume loss. Multiple subcortical infarcts and infarcts involving certain strategic structures (e.g., parts of the thalamus, caudate, or the genu of the internal capsule) can also result in dementia. Multiple-infarct dementia should be differentiated from periventricular white matter disease, which appears as focal areas of decreased attenuation on computed tomographic scans and increased signal intensity on balanced and T2-weighted images and which has been shown not to be dementing in itself.[44] These white matter lesions, which are referred to as unidentified bright objects or leukoaraiosis, are due to hypertensive-type microvascular disease and associated demyelination (Fig. 29–5).

CREUTZFELDT-JAKOB DISEASE

Creutzfeldt-Jakob disease is a rare cause of rapidly progressive dementia that has an incidence of approximately 1 case per million each year. Although most cases occur sporadically, approximately 10% to 15% are inherited in an autosomal dominant fashion with variable penetrance. The disease is one of several associated neurodegenerative illnesses whose pathogenesis is related to a small, nonviral, 30- to 35-kd proteinaceous infectious particle known as a prion. The loci of disease involve the cerebral and cerebellar cortices as well as the basal ganglia, where neuronal loss, reactive astrocytosis, and the formation of cytoplasmic vacuoles within the glia and neurons give the tissue a characteristic spongiform appearance with light microscopy. These changes all occur in the absence of an inflammatory response. The clinical syndrome is

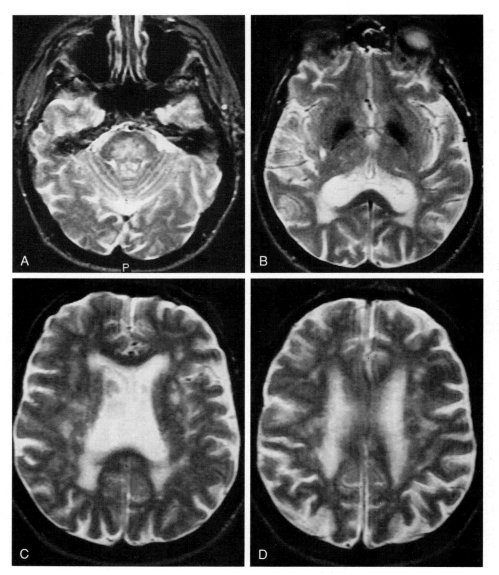

FIGURE 29–5. Microvascular disease. *A* to *D,* Axial T2-weighted images demonstrate multiple foci of white matter abnormalities including the brain stem. The U fibers and the corpus callosum are spared.

typically one of rapid cognitive decline, often with psychosis and delirium. Motor abnormalities of cerebellar dysfunction can appear and almost all patients evidence pronounced myoclonus before the final phase of deepening unresponsiveness and coma. The time course of the disease from presentation until death is usually less than 1 year. Diagnosis can be established by brain biopsy.

In the early stages of the disease, the computed tomographic scan and even the MR image may be normal.[45] The earliest reported changes are symmetric increased signal intensities in the basal ganglia[46–49] (Fig. 29–6) and occasionally in the white matter.[50] Occasionally, the changes in the basal ganglia occur before the typical clinical and neurophysiologic signs of Creutzfeldt-Jakob disease develop.[51]

During the late stages of the disease, patients develop significant atrophy. Serial MR images reveal that this atrophy is rapidly progressive.[45] Symmetric increased T2 signal abnormality with a mass effect in the occipital cortex, predominantly in a gray matter

distribution, has been reported.[52] A study using MR spectroscopy detected a decrease in *N*-acetylaspartate and other metabolites in late disease.[53] It should be stressed that an initial normal MR image does not exclude Creutzfeldt-Jakob disease in a middle-aged or elderly patient with rapid-onset dementia.[45]

DISORDERS WITH PROMINENT MOTOR DISABILITY

HUNTINGTON'S DISEASE

Huntington's disease (HD) (Fig. 29–7) is a degenerative neurologic disease that is inherited in an autosomal dominant fashion with complete penetrance and is determined by a gene localized to the short arm of chromosome 4. Patients usually become symptomatic before the age of 50 years and tend to present with abnormalities of affect and personality. In time, dementia becomes evident, accompanied by gradual disin-

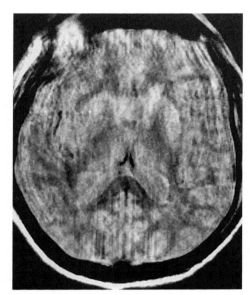

FIGURE 29–6. Creutzfeldt-Jakob disease. Axial balanced image of a 72-year-old patient with rapid-onset dementia and biopsy-proven Creutzfeldt-Jakob disease demonstrates abnormally increased signal intensity in the basal ganglia.

transmitters acetylcholine and γ-aminobutyric acid. In early cases, neuronal loss is generally first appreciated in the head of the caudate.[54] This has been confirmed by a number of MRI studies that show atrophy of the basal ganglia in patients with HD, which is most prominent in the head of the caudate. However, one study found that in mild HD, atrophy of the putamen was more prominent than atrophy of the caudate and that the size of the putamen was a better discriminator between patients with HD and normal subjects.[56]

A number of investigators have reported that in addition to atrophic changes in the basal ganglia, patients with HD present with areas of abnormal T2-weighted signal hyperintensity in the basal ganglia. Two groups have reported that such changes are present in all patients with the rigid form of HD but only occasionally in the classic hyperkinetic form.[57, 58]

More advanced cases of HD present with atrophy of other parts of the central nervous system including the olives, pons, and cerebellum[59]; the thalamus, mesial temporal lobe, and white matter tracts[60]; and the cerebral cortex.[61] Cortical atrophy, as seen with MRI, has been shown to correlate well with specific neuropsychologic deficits.[61]

tegration of motor control and the emergence of choreoathetoid movements. Occasionally, rigidity rather than chorea is the most salient motor abnormality (the Westphal variant).

Neuropathologically, the most conspicuous finding in patients with HD is atrophy of the basal ganglia, which generally proceeds medial to lateral and dorsal to ventral.[54–56] Degenerative changes can also affect the frontal and temporal cortices. The small ganglion cells of the caudate and putamen undergo progressive depletion, which is preceded by simplification of their dendritic structure. The degenerative process is accompanied by diminished concentrations of the neuro-

PARKINSON'S DISEASE

Parkinson's disease (PD) affects approximately 1% of the population older than 50 years of age and is perhaps the most common neurologic explanation for progressive motor impairment in elderly adults. The disease is caused by an acceleration of the normal age-dependent depletion of dopamine-synthesizing pigmented cells in the pars compacta of the substantia nigra. The loss of dopaminergic input to the striatum caused by this cell loss produces a characteristic syndrome of which the most salient features are progressive bradykinesis, rigidity, masked facies, hypophonia,

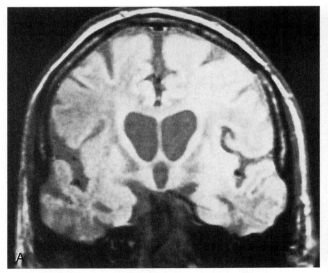
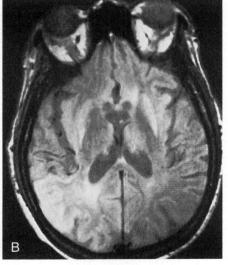

FIGURE 29–7. Huntington's disease. A, Coronal proton density–weighted image demonstrates atrophy of the caudate nuclei, associated with dilatation of the frontal horns of the lateral ventricles. B, On the axial image, the putamen is also small and atrophic.

festinating gait with stooped posture, and a coarse resting tremor. Dementia may occur in up to 30% of patients, which may reflect the concomitant presence of AD. In addition to loss of cells in the substantia nigra, autopsy reveals a loss of pigmented cells in the locus caeruleus and the dorsal motor nucleus of the vagus. These regions exhibit reactive astrocytosis and some of the remaining neurons contain eosinophilic cytoplasmic inclusions called Lewy's bodies.

Radiographically, PD patients present with a significant narrowing of the pars compacta of the substantia nigra, best visualized with T2-weighted sequences (Fig. 29–8). Multiple studies have demonstrated that there is little overlap between PD patients and normal age-matched control subjects.[62–65] Early PD has been reported to present with asymmetry of the pars compacta.[66]

MULTIPLE-SYSTEM ATROPHY

In contrast to PD, in which extrapyramidal clinical manifestations result from a loss of dopaminergic input to the striatum, other diseases produce progressive motor dysfunction by means of primary degenerative processes that simultaneously affect groups of several subcortical anatomic structures. This group of disorders has been referred to by the clinical term *Parkinson-plus syndrome* or by the anatomic term *multiple-system atrophy* (MSA). Various forms of MSA can present with a clinical picture similar to that of PD. These two disorders can be especially difficult to differentiate clinically early in the presentation. Neurologically, MSA is suspected when presumed parkinsonian patients fail to respond to L-dopa administration. Anatomically, the patient's disease is due to the involutional change undergone by various combinations of striatal, cerebellar, pontine, brain stem, and spinal cord nuclei. With the growing ability of MRI to show

detailed anatomy, a number of investigators have demonstrated the atrophic and signal abnormality changes in patients with the various forms of MSA, which allows differentiation from PD.

One neuropathologic pattern of MSA is termed striatonigral degeneration (SND). In this condition, a PD-like syndrome results from progressive atrophy and neuronal depletion of the putamen and caudate accompanied by cell loss in the zona compacta of the substantia nigra without Lewy's body deposition. Radiographically, patients with SND also exhibit thinning of the pars compacta of the substantia nigra similar to that seen in PD.[64, 65] This is expected from the histopathology of the disease. However, a number of specific findings in SND allow one to differentiate it from PD radiographically. The most prominent distinguishing feature of SND is hypointensity in the putamen.[65, 67–71] This is thought to be due to increased iron deposition.[72, 73] Focal atrophy in the quadrigeminal plate[74] and the putamen[67] has also been reported. These findings are not seen in PD. For MSA patients who present with hemiparkinsonism, MRI findings have consistently demonstrated abnormalities including T2 hypointensity of the posterior lateral putamen and atrophy of the putamen, caudate nucleus, and pars compacta of the substantia nigra on the contralateral side.[69, 75]

Another form of MSA is olivopontocerebellar atrophy (OPCA), in which degeneration involves the pontine nuclei, transverse pontine fibers, middle cerebellar peduncles, cerebellar cortex, and inferior olives. Clinically, the syndrome results in progressive ataxia and bulbar dysfunction. OPCA is typically a disorder of adult onset and can be both familial (usually autosomal dominant) and sporadic. Radiographically, patients present with atrophy of the transverse fibers of the pons and the cerebellum,[71, 76] as well as the middle cerebellar peduncles[77] (Fig. 29–9). There is a mild

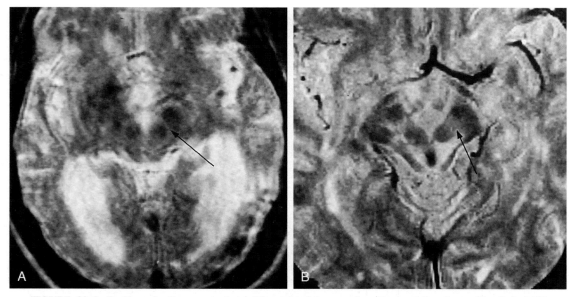

FIGURE 29–8. Parkinson's disease. *A*, Axial T2-weighted image of a 71-year-old patient with clinical PD demonstrates narrowing of the pars compacta of the substantia nigra *(arrow)*, which measures 2 mm. *B*, An axial balanced image from a normal patient for comparison. The pars compacta measures 5 to 6 mm *(arrow)*.

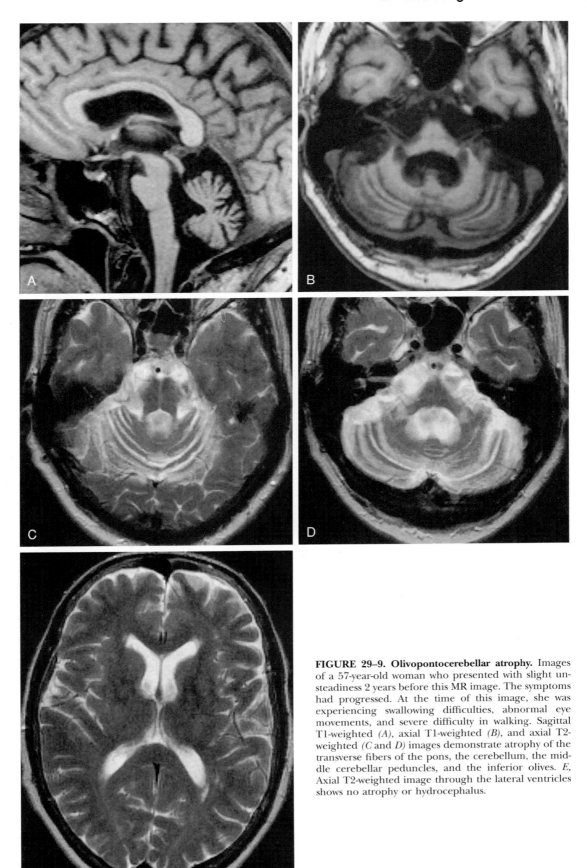

FIGURE 29–9. Olivopontocerebellar atrophy. Images of a 57-year-old woman who presented with slight unsteadiness 2 years before this MR image. The symptoms had progressed. At the time of this image, she was experiencing swallowing difficulties, abnormal eye movements, and severe difficulty in walking. Sagittal T1-weighted *(A)*, axial T1-weighted *(B)*, and axial T2-weighted *(C* and *D)* images demonstrate atrophy of the transverse fibers of the pons, the cerebellum, the middle cerebellar peduncles, and the inferior olives. *E,* Axial T2-weighted image through the lateral ventricles shows no atrophy or hydrocephalus.

decrease in the width of the pars compacta of the substantia nigra.[64] The T2 hypointensity seen in SND is not seen in OPCA.[68] These radiographic findings are in concert with the histopathologic picture. They appear to be specific for the disease and should be identified before the diagnosis of OPCA is made.

Other cases have been identified in which the anatomic loci of degenerative change are even more widespread and involve brain stem motor nuclei, corticospinal pathways, and such spinal cord structures as the dorsal columns, anterior horns, and spinocerebeller tracts. OPCA can occur independently or in tandem with SND.

Many patients with MSA undergo cell loss in the autonomic intermediolateral nuclei of the spinal cord that produces symptoms of orthostatic hypotension, incontinence, and sexual dysfunction in addition to the symptoms of MSA. This is known as Shy-Drager syndrome. MRI findings in Shy-Drager syndrome reflect the atrophic changes and T2 abnormalities seen in MSA.[74, 78]

PROGRESSIVE SUPRANUCLEAR PALSY

Progressive supranuclear palsy (Fig. 29–10) is a neurodegenerative disorder without known familial predilection that affects middle-aged and older adults. The pathologic changes involve neuronal loss and astrocytosis in the globus pallidus, dentate nucleus, and several diencephalic structures including the subthalamic nucleus, periaqueductal gray matter, and pretectal regions. Single-stranded neurofibrillary disease is a distinctive histopathologic feature of this condition. The clinical presentation is characterized by pseudobulbar signs, supranuclear oculomotor disturbances, axial dystonia, gait dysfunction, and dementia.

Radiographically, patients with progressive supranu-

clear palsy present with atrophy of the pretectum and of the dorsal pons.[79] In addition, decreased T2 relaxation times were reported in the superior colliculi, the globus pallidus, and the putamen, which were more pronounced than in patients with MSA.[80] These radiographic findings are confirmed by the histopathology of the disease and are useful in separating progressive supranuclear palsy from clinically similar entities such as PD.[80]

FRIEDREICH'S ATAXIA

Friedreich's ataxia is a progressive spinocerebellar degeneration transmitted by both autosomal dominant and recessive modes of inheritance that affects both children and young adults. The pathologic manifestation consists of spinal cord degeneration involving the dorsal columns, lateral corticospinal tracts, Clarke's column, and spinocerebellar tracts. Degeneration also occurs in the dorsal root ganglia, dentate nucleus, cerebellar vermis, and inferior olive. Children typically present with ataxia and are often incapable of walking by 5 years. Later, bilateral Babinski's signs with areflexia, tremor, slurred speech, and nystagmus appear. Other associated abnormalities include pes cavus deformity, kyphoscoliosis, and cardiomyopathy.

Radiographically, Friedreich's ataxia spinal cord atrophy is often severe[81] and is seen even in early cases.[82] Moderate cerebellar or bulbar atrophy is occasionally seen.[81] In advanced cases, atrophy of the cerebellar vermis and medulla has been reported[83] (Fig. 29–11).

AMYOTROPHIC LATERAL SCLEROSIS

Amyotrophic lateral sclerosis (ALS) is the most common form of a broader class of motor system diseases characterized by primary degeneration of the motor neurons in the brain, brain stem, and spinal cord. In ALS, both anterior horn neurons and pyramidal Betz's cells in the primary motor cortex (precentral gyrus) undergo progressive involutional change. Histopathologic features include astrocytosis, lipofuscin deposition, and occasionally the accumulation of intracytoplasmic inclusion bodies. Secondary degeneration of the descending corticospinal fibers occurs with variable demyelination and lipid-filled macrophage buildup. The corticospinal tract involvement is most evident in the lateral and anterior columns of the lower spinal cord but can also affect the cerebral white matter of the internal capsule, corona radiata, and centrum semiovale. These changes result in a clinical presentation of progressive appendicular weakness and atrophy combined with signs of spasticity.

A number of abnormalities were identified in the cortices of patients with ALS. T2 hypointensities in the precentral gyrus, the location of the perikarya of the motor neurons that are affected by ALS, have been reported. These areas of signal abnormality are thought to represent increased deposition of iron.[84, 85]

The subcortical white matter tracts of patients with

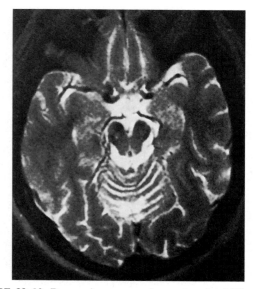

FIGURE 29–10. Progressive supranuclear palsy. Axial T2-weighted image discloses atrophy of the midbrain, with prominence of the perimesencephalic cisterns.

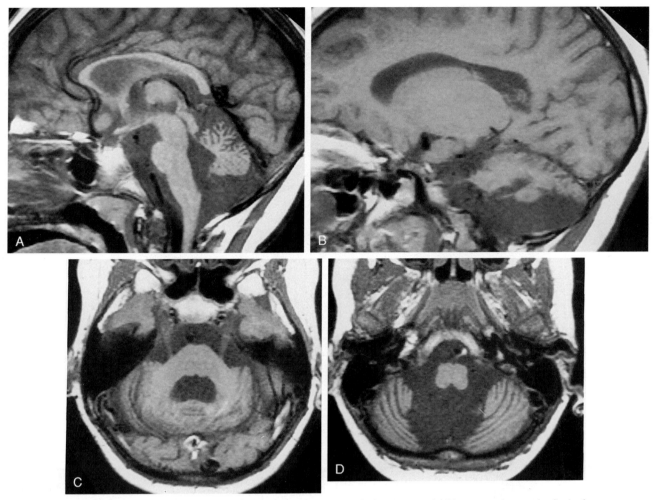

FIGURE 29–11. Freidreich's ataxia. Images of a 4-year-old girl who presented with progressive ataxia. Sagittal *(A and B)* and axial *(C and D)* T1-weighted images demonstrate severe atrophy of the cerebellum.

ALS occasionally demonstrate abnormal hyperintensity on T2-weighted images. These areas of signal abnormality have been reported to extend from the motor cortex to the centrum semiovale, the corona radiata, and the pons.[86–90] Histopathologic studies have shown that this is the location of the corticospinal tract that is composed of the upper motor neurons that originate in the precentral gyrus, descend to the spinal cord, and govern volitional movement, that is, the neurons that are affected in ALS. In addition, patients with ALS occasionally demonstrate areas of hypointensity on T1-weighted images as well as hyperintensity on balanced and T2-weighted images in the third quarter of the posterior limb of the internal capsule.[86] Radiologic-pathologic studies have shown that these signal abnormalities represent degeneration of the corticospinal tract and myelin pallor.[86] The signal abnormalities were found predominantly in patients with hyperreflexia indicating upper motor neuron disease. They have been shown to be distinctly different from normally appearing areas of hypointensity on T1-weighted images and hyperintensity on T2-weighted images, which represent normal fibers of the corticospinal tract traversing the internal capsule. The abnormal signal seen in ALS was distinctly hyperintense relative to gray matter on T2- and hypointense on T1-weighted images, and the normally appearing corticospinal tract was isointense relative to gray matter on T1- and T2-weighted images.[86]

Similar areas of T2 hyperintensity were identified in the corticospinal tracts in the spinal cord.[91]

HYDROCEPHALUS

Hydrocephalus is defined as an increase in the amount of CSF in the cranial cavity, associated with dilatation of the ventricular system. Hydrocephalus, derived from the Greek, literally means water on the brain. It is due to structural (e.g., tumor, aqueductal stenosis, incisural block) or functional (e.g., overproduction of CSF associated with choroid plexus papilloma, increased CSF protein, pacchionian absorption deficits, superior sagittal sinus hypertension, or thrombosis) obstruction of the CSF pathways. Thus, hydrocephalus is always obstructive. For this reason the term

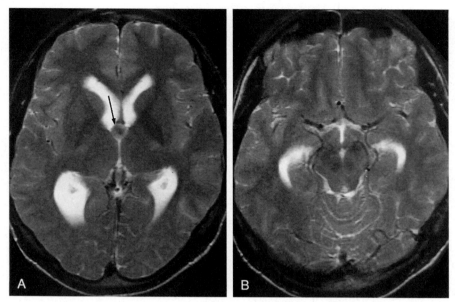

FIGURE 29–12. Colloid cyst. Images of a 24-year-old patient with postural headaches. *A*, Axial T2-weighted image through the foramen of Monro demonstrates the colloid cyst *(arrow)* that is causing the dilatation of the lateral ventricles. *B*, Axial T2-weighted image through the temporal lobes demonstrates enlargement of the temporal horns of the lateral ventricles.

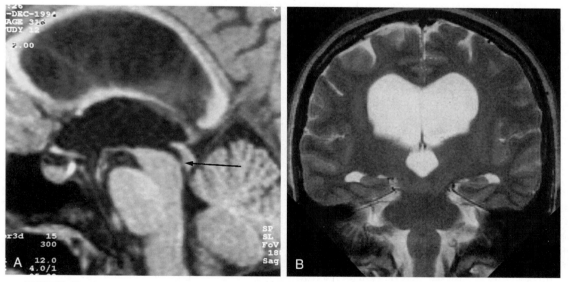

FIGURE 29–13. Aqueductal stenosis. Images of a 47-year-old woman who presented with a seizure. *A*, Sagittal T1-weighted image shows markedly enlarged lateral and third ventricles and a small fourth ventricle. The arrow points to the area of stenosis. *B*, Coronal T2-weighted image again demonstrates marked enlargement of the third and lateral ventricles, including the temporal horns. There is no dilatation of the perihippocamal fissures. The hippocampi are also well preserved.

hydrocephalus ex vacuo to denote cerebral atrophy is best avoided.

Hydrocephalus is traditionally divided into communicating, in which the ventricular system communicates with the rest of the subarachnoid spaces, and obstructive or noncommunicating. It should be noted that complete CSF obstruction is incompatible with life. Although the terms communicating and obstructive hydrocephalus have prevailed and are in common use, it would be more accurate to think of hydrocephalus as either obstructive intraventricular or obstructive extraventricular.

In obstructive hydrocephalus, an area of stenosis is identified along the normal ventricular CSF pathways that causes dilatation of the proximal ventricular system. The distal segments of the ventricular system are normal or smaller than normal. Obstructive hydrocephalus can be caused by several types of lesions, both malignant and benign. These include colloid cyst (Fig. 29–12), aqueductal stenosis (Fig. 29–13), and tumors along the pathway of CSF drainage.

Communicating hydrocephalus is diagnosed radiographically when an area of stenosis or obstruction is not seen. This is often associated with trauma, surgery, or inflammatory or carcinomatous meningitis or may occur after subarachnoid hemorrhage. The site of obstruction may be the incisura of the tentorium (incisural block). Less commonly, the obstruction is due to a structural or functional CSF resorption deficit at the level of the pacchionian granulations.

NORMAL-PRESSURE HYDROCEPHALUS

The condition known as normal-pressure hydrocephalus (NPH) was originally described by Adams and colleagues[92] and Hakim and Adams[93] in 1965. NPH is one of the few potentially treatable causes of gait impairment, motor deficits, and dementia in the elderly. NPH is characterized by gait disturbance that is often severe (magnetic or apractic gait), dementia that is often mild, and urinary incontinence that is of variable occurrence.[92–97] However, these clinical signs can be present in a number of disorders of the elderly that can be difficult to differentiate on clinical grounds.

In appropriate candidates, marked improvement can be accomplished by ventricular shunting.[98] After shunting, motor improvement may be dramatic whereas cognitive improvement is generally modest.[98, 99] Severe dementia is generally a limiting factor, suggesting that irreparable damage has set in or that there is coexisting AD.[100] The patient's preoperative memory deficits may improve after shunt placement. Severely demented patients may not improve sufficiently to justify a surgical procedure. Thus, the identification of other coexisting conditions, especially AD, becomes an important objective preoperatively.[100, 101]

A number of radiographic criteria have been described for NPH (Figs. 29–14 to 29–16). Patients with NPH often have large ventricles whose size is out of proportion to the degree of cortical atrophy and to the cognitive deficit, which is typically mild. This discrepancy between ventricular size and expected severity of sulcal enlargement is one of the earliest and most reliable radiologic signs that has been used to select shunt candidates. Ventricular enlargement associated with hydrocephalus is typically severe, whereas ventricular enlargement associated with atrophy related to AD is of mild to moderate degree even in patients with advanced AD.

Relatively mild cognitive deficits are also characteristic of this condition. NPH can be an incidental finding in normal volunteers who test in the normal range. Motor deficits, however, are often severe and the patient may be confined to a wheelchair or bed.

Ventricular enlargement in hydrocephalus is characterized by stretching and bowing of the pericallosal

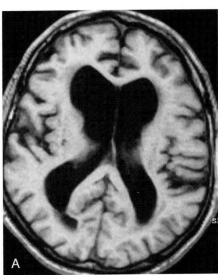 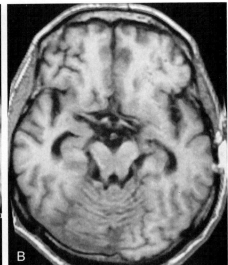

FIGURE 29–14. Normal-pressure hydrocephalus. Images of a 75-year-old patient. Axial T1-weighted images through the *(A)* lateral ventricles and *(B)* temporal horns demonstrate dilatation of the lateral ventricles out of proportion to the sulci. The temporal horns are also dilated. There is no evidence for atrophy of the hippocampus or prominence of the perihippocampal fissures.

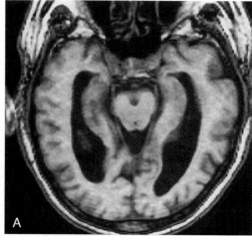

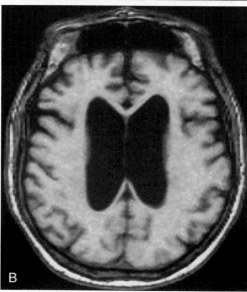

FIGURE 29–15. Normal-pressure hydrocephalus. Images of an 82-year-old patient. Axial T1-weighted images angled parallel to the temporal lobes through the (A) temporal horns and (B) lateral ventricles demonstrate dilatation of the lateral ventricles including the temporal horns. The hippocampi are intact and the perihippocampal fissures are not dilated.

arteries and of the corpus callosum, which can be of marked degree. These findings are shown to good advantage by the sagittal projection,[102] which represents a major contribution of MRI to the diagnosis of hydrocephalus. Even in advanced cases of atrophy typically caused by AD, the corpus callosum tends to undulate and the pericallosal arteries are not severely stretched and bowed.

In addition, in hydrocephalus, the temporal horns and the third ventricle tend to become rounded or ballooned as they enlarge. Enlargement of the temporal horns even in severe atrophy does not involve the lateral convex bowing seen in hydrocephalus. Similarly, as the third ventricle is enlarged with atrophy, the lateral walls tend to remain parallel to each other.

Decreased height of the intrapeduncular cistern (a mamillopontine distance less than 1 cm) caused by downward pressure by the distended third ventricle has been described as an important sign strongly favoring hydrocephalus over atrophy.[102]

A number of studies have been aimed specifically at differentiating NPH from other disorders, most notably AD. As atrophy of the hippocampal formation appears to characterize AD, it has been proposed that this criterion can be used to differentiate been AD and NPH. Golomb and colleagues[100] reported that hippocampal volume is preserved in nondemented NPH patients and suggested that the presence of hippocampal atrophy might indicate the coexistence of AD.

Holodny and associates[103] compared the MR images of a group of mildly impaired (Global Deterioration Scale ≤ 5) AD patients with preshunt MR images of a group of aged-matched NPH patients. The patients in the AD group showed no evidence of gait disorder. This criterion tended to eliminate patients with concurrent NPH. The patients in the NPH group showed at least an initial positive response to ventricular shunting. The scans were evaluated both subjectively and objectively. The objective measurements of the perihippocampal fissures and the lateral ventricles were performed using a computer-assisted technique designed to eliminate partial-volume artifacts. The greatest difference between the two groups was shown for the degree of atrophy of the hippocampal formation and resultant dilatation of the perihippocampal fissures. There was no overlap between the two groups. In the NPH group that responded to shunting, there was either no atrophy or mild atrophy of the hippocampal formation. This finding suggests that patients with preserved hippocampal formations, that is, those who presumably have not undergone irreversible cell destruction in this area, may be considered for ventricular shunting. An excellent correlation was also found between the subjective assessments and the objective measurements generated by computer analysis. This finding suggests that atrophy of the hippocampal formation can be evaluated on routine MR images and that this evaluation often provides salient clinical information.

The presence of a signal void in the aqueduct has been proposed as a sign of NPH.[104] However, CSF signal void as an isolated finding indicates patency of the aqueduct and is present in patients with atrophy as well as those with hydrocephalus.[105–107] Quantification of CSF velocities[108] and flow patterns could prove to be useful in differentiating atrophy and hydrocephalus.

Similarly, current and future MRI studies will address the question of whether brain motion as reflected in strain patterns is different in patients with hydrocephalus. Will functional MRI brain studies, such as diffusion scans, replicate the results of positron emission tomographic metabolic measures of brain or single photon emission computed tomography of brain perfusion? The latter types of studies show characteristically diffuse metabolic and blood flow deficits in hydrocephalus[109] and characteristic focal temporal and parietal lobe deficits in AD.[110–112]

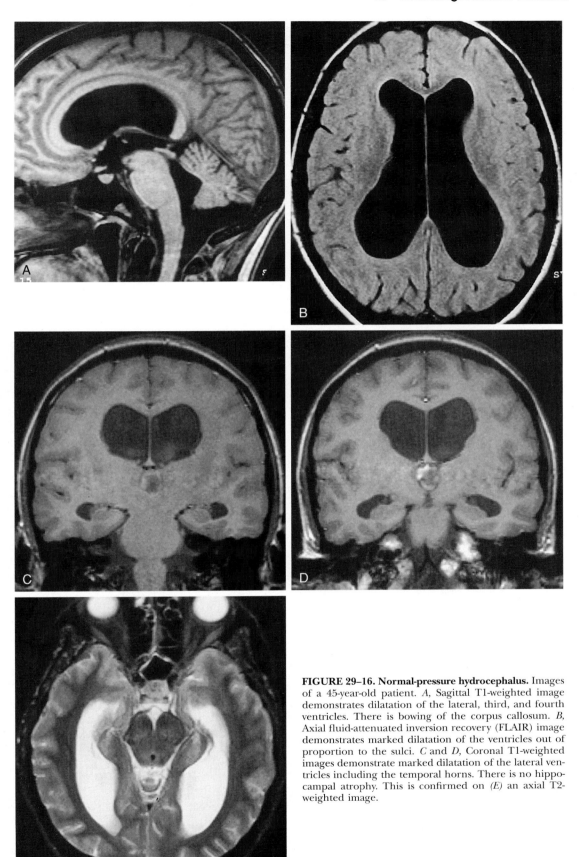

FIGURE 29–16. Normal-pressure hydrocephalus. Images of a 45-year-old patient. *A*, Sagittal T1-weighted image demonstrates dilatation of the lateral, third, and fourth ventricles. There is bowing of the corpus callosum. *B*, Axial fluid-attenuated inversion recovery (FLAIR) image demonstrates marked dilatation of the ventricles out of proportion to the sulci. *C* and *D*, Coronal T1-weighted images demonstrate marked dilatation of the lateral ventricles including the temporal horns. There is no hippocampal atrophy. This is confirmed on *(E)* an axial T2-weighted image.

REFERENCES

1. Alzheimer A: Über eine eigenartige Erkrankung der Hirninde. Allg Z Psychiatr 64:146–148, 1907.
2. Alzheimer A. Über eine eigenartige Erkrankung der Hinrinde. Zentralbl Gesamte Neurol Psychiatr 18:177–179, 1907.
3. Katzman R: Alzheimer's disease. N Engl J Med 314:964–973, 1986.
4. Evans DA, Funkenstein HH, Albert MS, et al: Prevalence of Alzheimer's disease in a community population of older persons: higher than previously reported. JAMA 262:2551–2556, 1990.
5. Terry RD: Senile dementia of the Alzheimer type. Ann Neurol 14:497–506, 1983.
6. American Psychiatric Association: Diagnostic and Statistical Manual of Mental Disorders. 3rd ed, revised. Washington, DC: American Psychiatric Association, 1987.
7. Adams JH, Duchen LW: Greenfield's Neuropathology. New York: Oxford University Press, 1992.
8. McKhann G: Clinical diagnosis of Alzheimer's disease. Neurology 34:939–944, 1984.
9. Ball M: Neuronal loss, neurofibrillary tangles, and granulovacuolar degeneration in the hippocampus with aging and dementia. Acta Neuropathol (Berl) 37:111–118, 1977.
10. Wilcock G, Esiri M: Plaques, tangles, and dementia. J Neurol Sci 56:343–356, 1982.
11. Mann D: The neuropathology of Alzheimer's disease: a review with pathogenetic, aetiological and therapeutic consideration. Mech Ageing Dev 31:213–255, 1985.
12. Terry RD: Senile dementia of the Alzheimer type. Ann Neurol 14:497–506, 1983.
13. Katzman R: Alzheimer's disease. N Engl J Med 314:964–973, 1986.
14. Wade J, Mirsen T, Hachinski V, et al: The clinical diagnosis of Alzheimer's disease. Arch Neurol 44:24–29, 1987.
15. Joachim CL, Morris JH, Selkoe D: Clinically diagnosed Alzheimer's disease: autopsy neuropathological results in 150 cases. Ann Neurol 24:50–56, 1988.
16. Morris JC, McKeel DW Jr, Fulling K, et al: Validation of clinical diagnostic criteria for Alzheimer's disease. Ann Neurol 24:17–22, 1988.
17. Hyman BT, Van Horsen GW, Damasio AR, Barnes CL: Alzheimer's disease: cell-specific pathology isolated the hippocampus. Science 225:1168–1170, 1984.
18. Price JL, Davis PB, Morris LC, White DL: The distribution of tangles, plaques and related immunohistochemical markers in healthy aging and Alzheimer's disease. Neurobiol Aging 12:295–312, 1991.
19. Ball MJ, Fisman M, Hachinski V, et al: A new definition of Alzheimer's disease: a hippocampal dementia. Lancet 1:14–16, 1985.
20. de Leon MJ, Ferris SH, Blau I, et al: Correlations between computerised tomographic changes and behavioural deficits in senile dementia. Lancet 2:859–860, 1979. Letter.
21. George AE, de Leon MJ, Rosenbloom S, et al: Ventricular volume and cognitive deficit: a computed tomographic study. Radiology 149:493–498, 1983.
22. LeMay M, Stafford JL, Sandor T, et al: Statistical assessment of perceptual CT scan ratings in patients with Alzheimer's type dementia. J Comput Assist Tomogr 10:802–809, 1986.
23. Sandor T, Albert M, Stafford J, Harpley S: Use of computerized CT analysis to discriminate between Alzheimer patients and normal control subjects. AJNR 9:1181–1187, 1988.
24. Kido DK, Caine ED, LeMay M, et al: Temporal lobe atrophy in patients with Alzheimer disease: a CT study. AJNR 10:551–555, 1989.
25. George AE, de Leon MJ, Stylopoulos LA, et al: CT diagnostic features of Alzheimer disease: importance of the choroidal/hippocampal fissure complex. AJNR 11:101–107, 1990.
26. de Leon MJ, George AE, Stylopoulos LA, et al: Early marker for Alzheimer's disease: the atrophic hippocampus. Lancet 2:672–673, 1989. Letter.
27. Seab JP, Jagust WJ, Wong STS, et al: Quantitative NMR measurements of hippocampal atrophy in Alzheimer's disease. Magn Reson Med 8:200–208, 1988.
28. Kesslak JP, Nalcioglu O, Cotman CW: Quantification of magnetic resonance scans for hippocampal and parahippocampal atrophy in Alzheimer's disease. Neurology 41:51–55, 1991.
29. Jack CR, Petersen RC, O'Brien PC, Tangalos EG: MR based hippocampal volumetry in the diagnosis of Alzheimer's disease. Neurology 42:183–188, 1992.
30. Golomb J, de Leon MJ, Kluger A, et al: Hippocampal atrophy in normal aging: an association with recent memory impairment. Arch Neurol 50:967–976, 1993.
31. Golomb J, Kluger A, de Leon MJ, et al: Hippocampal formation size in normal human aging: a correlate of delayed secondary memory performance. Learning Memory 1:45–54, 1994.
32. Rusinek H, de Leon MJ, George AE, et al: Alzheimer disease: measuring loss of cerebral gray matter with MR imaging. Radiology 178:109–114, 1991.
33. Condon BR, Patterson J, Wyper D, et al: A quantitative index of ventricular and extraventricular CSF volumes using MR imaging. J Comput Assist Tomogr 10:784–792, 1986.
34. De la Monte, SM: Quantification of cerebral atrophy in pre-clinical and end-stage Alzheimer's disease. Ann Neurol 25:450–459, 1989.
35. Terry RD, Peck A, DeTheresa R, et al: Some morphometric aspects of the brain in senile dementia of the Alzheimer type. Ann Neurol 10:184–192, 1981.
36. Lehericy S, Baulac M, Chiras J, et al: Amygdalohippocampal MR volume measurements in the early stages of Alzheimer disease. AJNR 15:929–937, 1994.
37. Dahlbeck JW, McCluney KW, Yeakley JW, et al: The interuncal distance: a new MR measurement for the hippocampal atrophy of Alzheimer disease. AJNR 12:931–932, 1991.
38. Early B, Escalona PR, Boyko OB, et al: Interuncal distance measurements in healthy volunteers and in patients with Alzheimer disease. AJNR 14:907–910, 1993.
39. de Leon MJ, George AE, Golomb J: The case for interuncal distance. AJNR 15:1286–1290, 1994.
40. de Leon MJ, Golomb J, George AE, et al: The radiologic prediction of Alzheimer disease: the atrophic hippocampal formation. AJNR 14:897–906, 1993.
41. Narkiewicz O, de Leon MJ, Convit A, et al: Dilatation of the lateral part of the transverse fissure of the brain in Alzheimer's disease. Acta Neurobiol Exp (Warsz) 53:457–465, 1993.
42. Drayer BP: Imaging of the aging brain: II. Pathological conditions. Radiology 166:797–806, 1988.
43. Tomlinson BE, Blessed G, Roth M: Observations on the brains of demented old people. J Neurol Sci 11:205–242, 1970.
44. George AE, de Leon MJ, Kalnin A: Leukoencephalopathy in normal and pathologic aging: 2. MRI of brain lucencies. AJNR 7:567–570, 1986.
45. Urchino A, Yoshinaga M, Shiokawa O, et al: Serial MR imaging in Creutzfeldt-Jakob disease. Neuroradiology 33:364–367, 1991.
46. Milton WJ, Atkas SW, Lavi E, Mollman JE: Magnetic resonance imaging of Creutzfeldt-Jakob disease. Ann Neurol 29:438–440, 1991.
47. Di Rocco A, Molinari S, Stollman AL, et al: MRI abnormalities in Creutzfeldt-Jakob disease. Neuroradiology 35:584–585, 1993.
48. Barboriak DP, Provenzale JM, Boyko OB: MR diagnosis of Creutzfeldt-Jakob disease: significance of high signal intensity in the basal ganglia. AJR 162:137–140, 1994.
49. Tartaro A, Fulgente T, Delli Pizzi C, et al: MRI alterations as an early finding in Creutzfeldt-Jakob disease. Eur J Radiol 17:155–158, 1993.
50. Yamamoto K, Morimatsu M: Increased signal in the basal ganglia and white matter on magnetic resonance imaging in Creutzfeldt-Jakob disease. Ann Neurol 32:114, 1992. Letter.
51. Rother J, Schwartz A, Harle M, et al: Magnetic resonance imaging follow-up in Creutzfeldt-Jakob disease. J Neurol 239:404–406, 1992.
52. Falcone S, Quencer RM, Bowen B, et al: Creutzfeldt-Jakob disease: focal symmetrical cortical involvement demonstrated by MR imaging. AJNR 13:403–406, 1992.
53. Graham GD, Petroff OA, Blamire AM, et al: Proton magnetic resonance spectroscopy in Creutzfeldt-Jakob disease. Neurology 43:2065–2068, 1993.
54. Vonsattel JP, Meyers RH, Stevers TJ: Neuropathologic classification of Huntington's disease. J Neuropathol Exp Neurol 44:559–577, 1985.
55. Roos RAC, Pruyt JFM, de Vries J, Bots GTA: Neuronal distribution in the putamen in Huntington's disease. J Neurol Neurosurg Psychiatry 48:422–425, 1985.
56. Harris GJ, Pearlson GD, Peyser CE, et al: Putamen volume reduction on magnetic resonance imaging exceeds caudate changes in mild Huntington's disease. Ann Neurol 31:69–75, 1992.
57. Oliva D, Carella F, Savoiardo M, et al: Clinical and magnetic resonance features of the classical and akinetic-rigid variants of Huntington's disease. Arch Neurol 50:17–19, 1993.
58. Savoiardo M, Strada L, Oliva D, et al: Abnormal MRI signal in the rigid form of Huntington's disease. J Neurol Neurosurg Psychiatry 54:888–891, 1991.
59. Sax DS, Bird ED, Gusella JF, Myers RH: Phenotypic variation in 2 Huntington's disease families with linkage to chromosome 4. Neurology 39:1332–1336, 1989.
60. Jernigan TL, Salmon DP, Butters N, Hesselink JR: Cerebral structure on MRI, Part II: Specific changes in Alzheimer's and Huntington's diseases. Biol Psychiatry 29:68–81, 1991.
61. Starkstein SE, Brandt J, Bylsma F, et al: Neuropsychological correlates of brain atrophy in Huntington's disease: a magnetic resonance imaging study. Neuroradiology 34:487–489, 1992.
62. Duguid JR, De La Paz R, DeGroot J: Magnetic resonance imaging of the midbrain in Parkinson's disease. Ann Neurol 20:744–747, 1986.
63. Braffman BH, Grossman RI, Goldberg HI, et al: MR imaging of Parkinson's disease with spin-echo and gradient-echo sequences. AJR 152:159–195, 1989.
64. Aotsuka A, Shinotoh H, Hirayama K, et al: Magnetic resonance imaging in multiple system atrophy. Rinsho Shinkeigaku 32:815–821, 1992.
65. Stern MB, Braffman BH, Skolnick BE, et al: Magnetic resonance imaging in Parkinson's disease and parkinsonian syndromes. Neurology 39:1524–1526, 1989.

66. Huber SJ, Chakeres DW, Paulson GW, Khanna R: Magnetic resonance imaging in Parkinson's disease. Arch Neurol 47:735–737, 1990.

67. O'Brien C, Sung JH, McGeachie RE, Lee MC: Striatonigral degeneration: clinical, MRI and pathological correlation. Neurology 40:710–711, 1990.

68. Tsuchiya K: High-field MR findings of multiple system atrophy. Nippon Igaku Hoshasen Gakkai Zasshi 50:772–779, 1990.

69. Kume A, Shiratori M, Takahashi A, et al: Hemi-parkinsonism in multiple system atrophy: a PET and MRI study. J Neurol Neurosurg Psychiatry 52:1221–1227, 1989.

70. Sullivan EV, De La Paz R, Zipursky RB, Pfefferbaum A: Neuropsychological deficits accompanying striatonigral degeneration. J Clin Exp Neuropsychol 13:773–778, 1991.

71. Testa D, Savoiardo M, Fetoni V, et al: Multiple system atrophy. Clinical and MR observations on 42 cases. Ital J Neurol Sci 14:211–216, 1993.

72. De Volder AG, Francart J, Laterre C, et al: Decreased glucose utilization in the striatum and frontal lobe in probable striatonigral degeneration. Ann Neurol 26:239–247, 1989.

73. Rutledge JN, Hilal SK, Silver AJ, et al: Study of movement disorders and brain iron by MR. AJNR 8:397–411, 1987.

74. Savoiardo M, Strada L, Girotti F, et al: MR imaging in progressive supranuclear palsy and Shy-Drager syndrome. J Comput Assist Tomogr 13:555–560, 1989.

75. Kato T, Kume A, Ito K, et al: Asymmetrical FDG-PET amd MRI findings of striatonigral system in multiple system atrophy with hemiparkinsonism. Radiat Med 10:87–93, 1992.

76. Mukai E, Makino N, Fujishiro K: Magnetic resonance imaging of parkinsonism. Rinsho Shinkeigaku 29:720–725, 1989.

77. Savoiardo M, Strada L, Girotti F, et al: Olivopontocerebellar atrophy: MR diagnosis and relationship to multisystem atrophy. Radiology 174:693–696, 1990.

78. Pastakia B, Polinsky R, Di Chiro G, et al: Multiple system atrophy (Shy-Drager syndrome): MR imaging. Radiology 159:499–502, 1986.

79. Taniwaki T, Hosokawa S, Goto I, et al: Positron emission tomography (PET) in "pure akinesia." J Neurol Sci 107:34–39, 1992.

80. Drayer BP, Olanow W, Burger P, et al: Parkinson plus syndrome: diagnosis using high field MR imaging of brain iron. Radiology 159:493–498, 1986.

81. Nicolau A, Diard F, Fontan D, et al: Magnetic resonance imaging in spinocerebellar degenerative diseases. Pediatrie 42:359–365, 1987.

82. Wessel K, Schroth G, Diener HC, et al: Significance of MRI-confirmed atrophy of the cranial spinal cord in Friedreich's ataxia. Eur Arch Psychiatry Neurol Sci 238:225–230, 1989.

83. Ormerud IE, Harding AE, Miller DH, et al: Neuropsychological deficits accompanying striatonigral degeneration. J Clin Exp Neuropsychol 13:773–788, 1991.

84. Oba H, Araki T, Ohtomo K, et al: Amyotrophic lateral sclerosis: T2 shortening in motor cortex at MR imaging. Radiology 189:843–846, 1993.

85. Ishikawa K, Nagura H, Yokota T, Yamanouchi H: Signal loss in the motor cortex on magnetic resonance images in amyotrophic lateral sclerosis. Ann Neurol 33:218–222, 1993.

86. Yagashita A, Nakano I, Oda M, Hirano A: Location of the corticospinal tract in the internal capsule at MR imaging. Radiology 191:455–460, 1994.

87. Abe K, Yorifuji S, Nishikawa Y: Reduced isotope uptake restricted to the motor area in patients with amyotrophic lateral sclerosis. Neuroradiology 35:410–411, 1993.

88. Udaka F, Sawada H, Seriu N, et al: MRI and SPECT findings in amyotrophic lateral sclerosis. Neuroradiology 34:389–393, 1992.

89. Iwasaki Y, Kinoshita M, Ikeda K, et al: MRI in patients with amyotrophic lateral sclerosis: correlation with clinical features. Int J Neurosci 59:253–258, 1991.

90. Goodin DS, Rowley HA, Olney RK: Magnetic resonance imaging in amyotrophic lateral sclerosis. Ann Neurol 23:418–420, 1988.

91. Freidman DP, Tartaglino LM: Amyotrophic lateral sclerosis: hyperintensity of the corticospinal tracts on MR images of the spinal cord. AJR 160:604–606, 1993.

92. Adams RD, Fisher CM, Hakim S: Symptomatic occult hydrocephalus with "normal" cerebrospinal fluid pressure: a treatable syndrome. N Engl J Med 273:117–126, 1965.

93. Hakim S, Adams RD: The special clinical problem of symptomatic hydrocephalus with normal cerebrospinal fluid pressure. J Neurol Sci 2:307–327, 1965.

94. Pickard JD: Adult communicating hydrocephalus. Br J Hosp Med 27:35–40, 1982.

95. Messert B, Wannamaker B: Reappraisal of the adult occult hydrocephalus syndrome. Neurology 24:224–230, 1974.

96. Tomlinson BE, Corsellis JAN: Ageing and dementias. In: Adams JH, Corsellis JAN, Duchen LW, eds. Greenfield's Neuropathology. 4th ed. New York: John Wiley & Sons, 1984, pp 951–1025.

97. Vassilouthis J: The syndrome of normal pressure hydrocephalus. J Neurosurg 61:501–509, 1984.

98. Fischer CM: Hydrocephalus as a cause of disturbance of gait in the elderly. Neurology 32:1358–1363, 1982.

99. Huckman M: Normal pressure hydrocephalus: evaluation of diagnostic and prognostic tests. AJNR 2:385–395, 1981.

100. Golomb J, de Leon MJ, George AE, et al: Hippocampal atrophy correlates with severe cognitive impairment in elderly patients with suspected normal pressure hydrocephalus. J Neurol Neurosurg Psychiatry 57:590–593, 1994.

101. Golomb J, de Leon MJ, Kluger A, et al: Hippocampal atrophy in normal aging. An association with recent memory impairment. Arch Neurol 50:967–973, 1993.

102. El Gammal T, Allen MB Jr, Brooks BS, Mark EK: MR evaluation of hydrocephalus. Am J Neuroradiol 8:591–597, 1987.

103. Holodny AI, Waxman R, George AE, et al: The MRI differential diagnosis of normal pressure hydrocephalus and cerebral atrophy: significance of the medial temporal fissure. Presented at the Annual Meeting of the American Society of Neuroradiology, Vancouver, BC, May 1993.

104. Bradley WG Jr, Kortman KE, Burgoyne B: Flowing cerebrospinal fluid in normal and hydrocephalic states: appearance on MR images. Radiology 159:611–616, 1986.

105. Citrin C, Sherman JL, Gangarosa RE, Scanlon D: Physiology of the CSF flow-void sign: modification by cardiac gating. AJNR 7:1021–1024, 1986.

106. Sherman JL, Citrin CM, Gangarosa RE, Bowen BJ: The MR appearance of CSF flow in patients with ventriculomegaly. AJR 148:193–199, 1987.

107. Stollman AL, George AE, Pinto RS, de Leon MJ: Diagnostic and prognostic significance of MRI periventricular T2 high signal lesions and signal void in hydrocephalus. Acta Radiol Suppl 369:388–391, 1986.

108. Bradley WG Jr, Whittemore AR, Kortman KE, et al: Marked cerebrospinal fluid void: indicator of successful shunt in patients with suspected normal-pressure hydrocephalus. Radiology 178:459–466, 1991.

109. George AE, de Leon MJ, Miller J, et al: Positron emission tomography of hydrocephalus: metabolic effects of shunt procedures. Acta Radiol Suppl 369:435–439, 1986.

110. Ferris SH, de Leon MJ, Wolf AP, et al: Positron emission tomography in the study of aging and senile dementia. Neurobiol Aging 1:127–131, 1980.

111. de Leon MJ, Ferris SH, George AE, et al: Positron emission tomographic studies of aging and Alzheimer disease. AJNR 4:568–571, 1983.

112. Holman BL: Perfusion and receptor SPECT in the dementias. J Nucl Med 27:855–860, 1986.

MR Spectroscopy of the Brain: Neurospectroscopy

BRIAN ROSS ■ THOMAS MICHAELIS

STRUCTURE OF THE PRESENT CHAPTER

The changes in clinical spectroscopy since the first edition of this book dictated a division of the chapter into two. Theoretic and technical aspects of nuclear magnetic resonance (NMR) spectroscopy, describing the methods necessary to perform reliable clinical examinations, are now discussed in Chapter 11. Only human applications in neurodiagnosis and clinical management are discussed here.

^{31}P magnetic resonance spectroscopy (MRS) dominated in earlier years and is still paramount in clinical applications to regions outside the brain, but ^{31}P has been almost completely displaced by ^{1}H MRS for studies of the brain. The ease of ^{1}H MRS and the sheer volume of clinical studies of the brain warrant a chapter dealing solely with neurospectroscopy. Because it would require unnecessary duplication to discuss pathogenesis and clinical features of each disease studied with MRS, we recommend that each section be read in conjunction with the appropriate magnetic resonance imaging (MRI) chapter, where such details are given. To facilitate this, the subheadings of the section on current clinical uses include cross-references to the appropriate MRI chapters.

NEUROSPECTROSCOPY: A DEFINITION

We define neurospectroscopy as the field of study resulting from MRS examination of the human brain. Diseases and pathologies of the brain are commonly classified as 1) structural (including degenerative, tumor, and embryogenic defects), 2) physiologic (essentially interruption of blood supply), and 3) biochemical or genetic. Of the last, some are receptor and neurotransmitter related (e.g., dopamine in Parkinson's disease) but many are directly or indirectly related to distur-

bances of the pathways of oxidative, anabolic, and catabolic intermediary metabolism; the tricarboxylic acid (TCA) cycle; glutamine and glutamate turnover; glycolysis; ketogenesis; or fatty acid metabolism. Genetic diseases involve mutations of nuclear or mitochondrial DNA. Positron emission tomography and to a lesser extent single photon emission computed tomography (SPECT), MR angiography, functional MRI (FMRI), and diffusion imaging address blood flow, glucose turnover, and oxygen consumption, and positron emission tomography and SPECT are uniquely able to "image" targeted receptor ligands. However, until the advent of NMR, no direct noninvasive assay of the products of gene expression, the cerebral metabolites, was available. No neuronal marker, no astrocyte marker, and no technique for directly determining energy metabolism existed. These gaps are now filled by neurospectroscopy and, with increased clinical experience, a diagnostic need for MRS of the brain emerges (Table 30–1).

TABLE 30–1. TWELVE MOST PREVALENT USES OF NEUROSPECTROSCOPY, 1984 TO 1994

1. Differential diagnosis of coma
   Neurodiagnosis of symptomatic patients
2. Subclinical hepatic encephalopathy and pretransplantation evaluation
3. Differential diagnosis of dementia (rule out Alzheimer's disease)
4. Therapeutic monitoring in cancer ± radiation
5. Neonatal hypoxia
6. "Work-up" of inborn errors of metabolism
7. "Added value" in routine MRI
8. Differential diagnosis of white matter disease, especially multiple sclerosis, adrenoleukodystrophy, and human immunodeficiency virus infection
9. Prognosis with acute cerebrovascular accident and stroke
10. Prognosis in head injury
11. Surgical planning in temporal lobe epilepsy
12. Muscle disorders

TABLE 30–2. METHODS OF MR SPECTROSCOPY APPLICABLE TO THE BRAIN*

CLINICAL METHOD	RADIO-FREQUENCY COIL AVAILABLE	CLINICAL IMPLEMENTATION AT 1.5 T
Localized ¹H MRS		
Long echo	+	+
Short echo	+	+
Quantitation	+	+
Phase-encoded imaging of metabolites	+	+
Fast metabolite imaging	+	+
Automation	+	+
Osmolality	+	+
Functional MRS	+	+
Localized ³¹P MRS		
Pulse-acquired spectroscopy	+	+
Decoupled ¹H-³¹P		+
Phase-encoded imaging	+	+
Fast phosphocreatine imaging	+	+
Magnetization transfer (flux)		+
Localized ¹³C MRS		
Natural abundance		
¹³C enriched-flux measures	+	+
¹H-¹³C heteronuclear method	+	+
(Localized) ¹⁵N MRS		
¹⁵N enriched-flux measures		
¹H-¹⁵N heteronuclear methods		
Localized ¹⁹F MRS		
¹⁹F, drug detection	+	+
¹⁹F, imaging and blood flow methods	+	+
(¹⁹F probes for Ca²⁺ and Mg²⁺ determination)†		+
²³Na MRS		

*The great variety of available localization techniques has been described in detail (Chapter 11). The first application of MRS with surface coil demonstrated the potential of MRS for noninvasive insights into metabolism.[152] The lack of proper localization with this easy and straightforward technique has been partly overcome by improvements.[153] However, in the clinical setting of neurospectroscopy, more advanced localization techniques are used. Currently, ISIS,[154] STEAM,[155, 156] or PRESS[157, 158] sequences are most frequently used as single-voxel or chemical-shift imaging (CSI) techniques for localized MRS. ¹H MRS performed with long or (better) short echo times allows the quantitation of important metabolites.[14, 64, 99, 159-165] Automation of the measurement (shimming, water suppression, acquisition[166] and of the data processing (phasing, fitting)[167] should lead to a fully automated examination in the near future. Additional metabolic information is obtained by using spectral editing techniques, which are currently used for the identification of low-concentration metabolites or overlapping resonance.

†Toxic in vivo.

METHODS FOR CLINICAL NEUROSPECTROSCOPY

"Methodik ist Alles," said Otto Warburg,[1] and at least 20 methods are available for neurospectroscopy. Table 30–2 outlines the currently available methods of MRS as applied to the brain. Details are given in Chapter 11. Localized ¹H MRS methods include long echo, short echo, stimulated-echo acquisition mode (STEAM), point-resolved spectroscopy (PRESS), and quantitative, phase-encoded metabolite, "fast" metabolite, automated, and functional imaging. Localized ³¹P MRS methods include pulse-acquired imaging, depth-resolved surface coil spectroscopy (DRESS), image-selected in vivo spectroscopy (ISIS), decoupled ¹H-³¹P, phase-encoded metabolite imaging, fast phosphocreatine (PCr) imaging, and magnetization transfer (flux). Each method has contributed to some aspect of neurophysiologic research or has found clinical application. All of the methods offer useful and specific

information, and older methods re-emerge from time to time. An example is the renewed interest in ³¹P MRS with proton decoupling, to identify separately the components of the choline (Cho) peak seen in routine ¹H MRS (Fig. 30–1). However, with this wealth of methods the uninitiated would be forgiven if they found the different spectral appearances confusing or even unhelpful. For this reason we have been selective in the use of figures in this chapter, employing only a limited number of formats for ease of interpretation.

SHORT HISTORY OF NEUROSPECTROSCOPY: MILESTONES IN THE BRAIN (Table 30–3)

MRS of the brain began with ³¹P spectroscopic studies of anesthetized rats and other small animals. Noninvasive assays of adenosine triphosphate (ATP) and PCr (expressed as metabolite ratios) and of intracellular pH gave exciting new insights. Direct metabolic rate determination in vivo, using ³¹P magnetization transfer, was among the first biologic applications of this now widespread technique.

Global ischemia provided a simple means of testing the methods of MRS and confirming the dependence of cerebral energetics on oxidative metabolism and glycolysis. A practical future for MRS was demonstrated

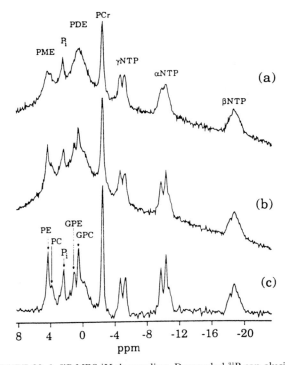

FIGURE 30–1. ³¹P MRS ¹H decoupling. Decoupled ³¹P can elucidate the phosphorylcholine (PC) versus the glycerophosphorylcholine (GPC) contribution to differentiate between systemic and local neuroregulation. PME = phosphomonoester; P_i = inorganic phosphate; PDE = phosphodiester; PCr = phosphocreatine; γ-NTP = nucleoside triphosphates; PE = phosphoethanolamine; GPE = glycerophosphorylethanolamine. (Courtesy of Truman Brown, PhD, Fox Chase Cancer Center, Philadelphia, PA.)

TABLE 30–3. NINE MILESTONES OF NEUROSPECTROSCOPY

EXPERIMENT	CLINICAL INSIGHT
1. ^{31}P NMR brain of anesthetized rats and small animals ATP + Cr → ADP + PCr ADP + Pi → ATP (pH)	Gerbil "stroke."
2. ^{31}P NMR of human newborns	Prognosis in hypoxic-ischemic disease.
3. Localized ^{31}P NMR of adult human brain	Human (brain) tumors are alkaline.
4. Phosphomonoesters and phosphodiesters	Beginnings of the new neurochemistry.
5. N-Acetylaspartate	A neuronal marker reflecting multiple disease states.
6. Integration of imaging and spectroscopy	Image guidance of MRS and metabolite imaging; anatomic dissociation from neurochemistry.
7. Single-voxel MRS (e.g., ^{1}H, ^{13}C, ^{15}N)	Neurochemical disorder is independent of anatomic changes; a role for accurate single measurements.
8. Functional MRS	Reversible neurochemical change precedes other changes.
9. Automation and quantitation	The gross disturbance in neurochemical homeostasis occurs only in severe disease, in which speed and precision of MRS analysis permit access to unique and transient biochemical events.

with the gerbil stroke model, when carotid ligation was clearly shown to produce ipsilateral changes of anerobic metabolism: loss of PCr and ATP, increase of inorganic phosphate (P$_i$), and acidification of the affected hemisphere.[2] It is hard now to realize that before those studies rapid freezing of whole animals, brain blowing, and surgical biopsy were the only effective sources of knowledge of such events.

MRS of the human brain, which began with newborns, quickly verified the predictions based on animal studies that hypoxic-ischemic disease of the brain could be monitored by the changes in high-energy phosphates, P$_i$ and pH.[3–5] The predictive value of MRS has been demonstrated in several hundred newborn infants. The outcome after severe hypoxic-ischemic encephalopathy in newborn humans is determined by the intracerebral pH and P$_i$/ATP ratio.

Wide-bore high-field magnets (from Oxford Magnet Technology) permitted extension to adults and infants older than a few weeks of age.[6] As a result, three areas of human neuropathology have been extensively illuminated by ^{31}P MRS. Using brain tumor as a target of newly evolving localization techniques (the early studies of infants employed no localization beyond that conferred by the surface coil), Oberhaensli and colleagues[7] began the slow process of overturning three decades of thought about brain tumors in particular, showing their intracellular pH to be generally

alkaline, not acidic. A new generation of drugs in oncology will be designed to enter alkaline intracellular environments rather than the acidic environment measured in the interstitial fluid.

^{31}P MRS findings in adult stroke exactly mirrored the findings in hypoxic-ischemic disease of newborns and even appear to offer predictive value through intracellular pH and the P$_i$/ATP ratio.[8] This work in turn has led to a large body of research on experimental models of stroke, which now guides the application of MRS to humans.

The third area of work stimulated by the advent of ^{31}P MRS was that on degenerative disease of the brain, including Alzheimer's disease (AD).[9] Commencing with in vitro studies of tissue extracts, two hitherto unrecognized groups of compounds, seen in the ^{31}P spectrum as phosphomonoesters (PMEs) and phosphodiesters (PDEs), were empirically shown to be altered. Much of the work was unsatisfying because the identity and metabolic significance of these "peaks," unlike those of ATP, PCr, and P$_i$, were incompletely understood. Nevertheless, a promising new area of neurochemistry was opened by ^{31}P MRS and then extended to in vivo brain analysis in patients. Modern neurospectroscopy is much more like this than was anticipated by the earlier investigators. What MRS has done in neurochemistry is what virtually all spectroscopic techniques have done in their time. By providing noninvasive assays of less well known metabolites and pathways, MRS has identified a "new" neurochemistry. A perfect example of this new knowledge emerged with the advent of water-suppressed ^{1}H MRS of the brain in vivo.

N-Acetylaspartate (NAA), a neuronal marker,[10] was rediscovered in 1983.[11] Of the many expected and new resonances now identified in clinical practice of neuro-MRS, none has led to more diagnostic information than NAA. Its identity, concentration, and distribution are now well established. Early experiments with animals showed loss of NAA in stroke. Large numbers of studies of humans show NAA absent or reduced in brain tumor (glioma), ischemia, degenerative disease, inborn errors of metabolism, and trauma, so that to a first approximation the histochemical identification of NAA (and N-acetylaspartylglutamate) with neurons and axons and its absence from mature glial cells are confirmed. The clinical use of ^{1}H MRS as an assay of neuron "number" is justified. In the 10 years since its introduction, 50 to 100 clinical applications of this assay have emerged and placed neurospectroscopy far ahead in the introduction of MRS into routine clinical practice.

The first generation of MRS studies was performed without image guidance. Although MRI is not essential to our understanding of neurochemistry, the combined use of these two powerful tools permitted the direct demonstration that there is often a dissociation in space between anatomically obvious events in the brain and biochemical changes. Metabolite imaging (see Table 30–2) has confirmed this important principle in stroke, tumors, multiple sclerosis (MS), and degenerative diseases.

Dissociation in Time

The other side of the same coin is the realization that abnormalities in the anatomy, as revealed by MRI, are not essential to the detection of biochemical disorders by MRS. A simplified method of localization permitted the routine use of MRS to assay neurochemistry in a single place, albeit rather large, in the cerebral cortex, cerebellum, or midbrain. This method, now generally known as single-voxel MRS, was pioneered by Frahm and by Shulman and is largely responsible for showing that biochemical disorders commonly underlie neurologic disease.[12–19] MRS is therefore well poised for "early" diagnosis.

Reversible biochemical changes accompany several physiologic events, providing a biochemical basis for functional imaging. In addition to inborn errors of metabolism and hereditary diseases, which are relatively rare, several of the major neurologic scourges of our time reveal functional biochemical disturbance: neonatal hypoxia, cerebral palsy, neurologic aspects of acquired immunodeficiency syndrome (AIDS), dementias, stroke, epilepsies, neuroinfections, and many encephalopathies are now seen to have a biochemical component. Often this can be diagnosed only with MRS.

Automation and Quantitation

Even when MRI identifies disease accurately and early, there is a strong possibility that MRS could do so earlier and therefore increase the window of therapeutic opportunity so much needed in neurology. Automation permits universal access, including urgent MRS in acute, reversible neurologic diseases and large-scale clinical trials. Quantitation (see Table 30–2), a long-overlooked area, gives the precision of measurement required to demonstrate conclusively incremental metabolic responses to intervention and therapy.

INTRODUCTORY NEUROCHEMISTRY

BIOCHEMICAL COMPOSITION OF THE BRAIN

Just as an atlas of neuroanatomy is provided in order to understand better the neuropathologic derangements indicated by MRI appearances, for MRS it is useful to describe the basic building blocks of the brain in terms of neurochemistry. For MRS this consists not only of an understanding of the major anatomic structures used for image guidance but also of some commentary on the chemical composition of neurons and astrocytes, myelin and cerebrospinal fluid (CSF), and the surrounding meninges, skull, and scalp.

Although it is obviously an oversimplification, brain may be defined biochemically as water plus dry matter.

WATER. As in other tissues, the water is divided into intracellular and extracellular (about 85% and 15%, respectively). Intracellular water, which is further divided into cytoplasmic and mitochondrial compartments, about 75% and 25%, respectively, contains all of the important neurochemicals. These are either unique to intracellular water, such as lipids, proteins, amino acids, neurotransmitters, and low-molecular-weight substances, or at least are quite different in concentration in the intracellular compared with the extracellular and CSF compartments. Glucose is an exception, being found in proportions 5:3:1 in blood, CSF, and brain water, respectively. Amino acids are generally distributed 20:1 in brain water versus CSF or blood. Brain water and extracellular fluid are distinct from the large CSF compartment, whose volume depends greatly on the location selected for study, and from the intravascular blood, which constitutes up to 6% of brain water.

DRY MATTER. Seen through the MR image and the MRS assays of water, the 20% or so of brain that really matters is largely invisible—hence, the occasional use of the terms "missing" or "invisible" in the literature. Covered by these terms are all macromolecules (DNA, RNA, and most proteins and phospholipids), as well as cell membranes, organelles (including the dry matter of the mitochondria, the cristae), and myelin. The term dry matter is almost equivalent to the biochemist's term dry weight and can be used as a more constant unit with which to determine the concentration of key neurochemicals. This is particularly relevant in pathologies in which brain water (or the wet weight/dry weight ratio) may be altered, such as edema, tumors, inflammation, or infarction. Metabolite concentrations may be more accurately compared in terms of millimoles per gram dry weight than by the more usual millimoles per gram wet weight or per milliliter of brain water.

MYELIN AND MYELINATION. As mentioned earlier, for the most part myelin is inaccessible to in vivo NMR spectroscopy (whereas myelin contributes to the ready differentiation of white matter from gray matter in MRI). This is the result of its macromolecular structure. The nature of myelin water is discussed elsewhere (see Chapters 1, 8, and 27). The composition of myelin is nevertheless of some interest to the in vivo spectroscopist because of the changes that may occur in demyelinating and many other diseases. Whereas the major components phosphatidylcholine, phosphatidylethanolamine, phosphatidylserine, and phosphatidylinositol are probably immobile and NMR invisible, their putative breakdown products, phosphorylcholine, glycerophosphorylcholine, Cho, and *myo*-inositol (mI) are a normal feature of the ^{1}H or ^{31}P brain spectrum. These molecules are frequently encountered in discussions of clinical spectroscopy, even though their precise relationship to myelin is far from clear. This is nowhere more important than in the detection of developmental changes in the brain. The MRI appearances, on which we depend heavily for "dating" infants, are accompanied by no less dramatic changes in the MR spectrum. These are presumed to be related in some as yet ill-defined way to myelination.

EDEMA. This important concept in neurophysiology and in clinical diagnosis by MRI has not yet been clearly defined in MRS assays of brain water. One possibility is that edema, as seen in MRI, represents less than 1% of total brain water and falls within the limits of error of present methods of NMR water assay. These methods rely heavily on differences in T2 relaxation between water in various states. Although it is T2 relaxation that distinguishes edema in MRI, the differences are either too small or too local to be measured directly.

METABOLISM. Intermediary metabolism of the brain is not much different from that of other less specialized tissues. Amino acids, carbohydrates, fatty acids, and lipids, including triglycerides, form a complex network of biosynthetic and degradative pathways, as found in almost all other mammalian cells. The network is maintained by the thermodynamic equilibrium of hundreds of identified enzymes, and relative rates of flux through the various pathways are equally closely controlled. Hence, the concentrations of all but a few key molecules (messengers and, in the special case of the brain, neurotransmitters) are kept remarkably constant. For this reason, a thoroughly reproducible brain "spectrum" can be obtained with MRS. Conversely, predictable and reversible changes, such as increased lactate and glutamate, reduced ATP, and increased adenosine diphosphate (ADP), accompany limitation of oxygen supply, resulting from altered redox state of the pyridine nucleotide coenzymes of electron transport, making MRS the tool for acute conditions and short-term therapeutic monitoring.

COMPARTMENTATION. Mitochondrial energetics, the enzymes of which are controlled by nonmendelian genetics, consist of the electron transport chain and of oxidative phosphorylation, which provides virtually all of the high-energy phosphate bonds to maintain ion pumps, neurotransmission, cell volume, and active transport of nutrients. ATP, the essential "currency" of this process, is buffered in brain, skeletal muscle, and the heart (but not in most other tissues) by another high-energy system, that of creatine kinase, creatine (Cr), and PCr. These molecules are readily observed in MR spectra. Cytoplasmic enzymes control aerobic glycolysis and the formation of lactate, which supplements ATP synthesis. Glycolysis is massively activated by the Pasteur effect under hypoxic conditions, which obviously limit mitochondrial energy production. Lactate and glutamate are both formed in excess when the mitochondrial redox state changes. It is possible that a similar activation of glycolysis accompanies functional changes (as in FMRI) and electrical activation (as in seizures).

FUELS OF OXIDATIVE PHOSPHORYLATION. Glucose dominates the fuel supply of the brain, and its supply via blood flow is strongly protected. Vascular occlusion, because it results in glucose deprivation, oxygen lack, and CO_2 and H^+ accumulation, results in rather different neurochemical insults from those of pure hypoxia such as is seen in respiratory failure or near-drowning (ND). Thus, hypoxia and ischemia are different to the spectroscopist, whereas the terms might not have to be distinguished for the purposes of MRI.

In severe conditions of starvation, when glucose is not available, fatty acids and ketone bodies can sustain

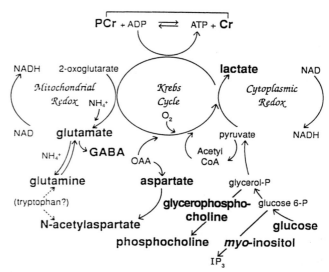

FIGURE 30–2. Major metabolic pathways important in ¹H MRS. GABA = γ-aminobutyric acid; OAA = oxaloacetic acid; CoA = coenzyme A; P = phosphate; IP_i = inositol trisphosphate; NAD(H) = nicotinamide adenine dinucleotide (reduced).

cerebral energy metabolism, and this may be the normal state of affairs for the milk-fed newborn. Unlike other tissues, the brain does not apparently require insulin to utilize glucose, so in diabetic patients the marked alterations in cerebral metabolism (and in the MR spectrum) are secondary to the systemic metabolic disorder.

SUMMARY: THE NEW NEUROCHEMISTRY

Figure 30–2 depicts some of the neurochemical pathways that have become more relevant since the advent of neuro-MRS. The energetic interconversion of ATP, PCr, and P_i, together with intracellular pH, which is readily monitored by ³¹P MRS, is central in thinking about stroke. The major peaks of the ¹H MR spectrum, corresponding to NAA, total Cr (Cr + PCr), total Cho (including phosphorylcholine and glycerophosphorylcholine), mI, and glutamate plus glutamine (Glx), were only infrequently encountered in neurochemical discussion of physiology or disease before the advent of MRS. They now join glucose uptake and oxygen consumption as the most easily measured neurochemical events and must become increasingly important in neurologic discussion.

Because of the concentration limit (of protons) of about 0.5 to 1.0 mM for NMR detection, virtually all true neurotransmitters, including acetylcholine, norepinephrine, dopamine, and serotonin (the exceptions are glutamate, glutamine, and α-aminobutyric acid), are currently beyond detection by conventional neuro-MRS. Similarly, the hormone messenger inositol polyphosphates and cyclic adenosine monophosphate (AMP) are not detected. This leaves important gaps in the new neurochemistry.

Another evident shortcoming of NMR is the inaccessibility of most macromolecules because of their limited mobility. Accordingly, phospholipids, myelin, proteins, nucleosides, and nucleotides, as well as RNA and DNA, are effectively invisible to this family of methods. Exceptions may be glycogen, a macromolecule in heart, skeletal muscle, and liver, which is readily detectable in ^{13}C spectra, and the broad signals from phospholipids in the ^{31}P spectrum and from low-molecular-weight proteins in ^1H spectra of the brain.

How to "Read" a Proton Spectrum

Conventional maps of neurochemistry are of somewhat limited use in understanding MR spectra, because the limits of detectability, about 0.5 to 1.0 mM, rather inconveniently deprive us of "seeing" almost all amino acids, carbohydrates, and fatty acids that make up the network, as well as all neurotransmitters with the exception of glutamate and α-aminobutyric acid. This rather simplifies the MR spectrum of normal human brain. Conversely, and conveniently, levels of these common neural metabolites, which are elevated in response to single-enzyme defects, site-specific gene mutations, or other inborn errors, can often be readily detected for diagnostic purposes, as can iatrogenic (drug) or toxicologically ingested (ethanol) molecules. Together, these provide a rich diagnostic pattern of cerebral metabolites for the neurospectroscopist.

The ^1H spectrum of the normal human brain is most readily understood by referring to Figure 30–3. Each metabolite has a "signature,"[15] which, when added to those of the other major metabolites, results in a complex spectrum of overlapping peaks. For all practical purposes, because of its ease and universal access, ^1H spectroscopy in clinical practice is synony-mous with neurospectroscopy. Although such spectra are familiar to all, it is crucial to adopt a rigorous approach to acquiring and interpreting spectra, so that they can form the basis of a clinical report.

Figure 30–4 is composed of four spectra from "gray matter" acquired by an automated procedure (PROBE [proton brain exam]), using a 1.5-T scanner, STEAM, and a short echo (echo time [TE] = 30 ms). The equivalent spectra acquired with a long echo (TE = 135 or 270 ms) would look substantially different but could be similarly interpreted by referring to a "normal" spectrum acquired under identical conditions.

The top spectrum is for a healthy volunteer. Reading from right to left, there are two broad resonances that are believed to be due to intrinsic cerebral proteins or lipids. The first and tallest sharp peak, resonating at 2.0 ppm, is assigned to the neuronal marker NAA. The next cluster of small peaks consists of the coupled resonances of β- and γ-glutamine plus glutamate (Glx). However, the tallest peak of this cluster, at approximately 2.6 ppm, actually represents NAA, which has three peaks, one of which overlaps the glutamine resonance. The second tallest resonance, labeled Cr (at about 3.0 ppm), represents Cr plus PCr, and adjacent to this is another prominent but smaller peak assigned to Cho. A small peak to the left of the Cho peak is that of *scyllo*-inositol (sI). A prominent peak at 3.6 ppm is assigned to mI. To the left of the mI peak, two small peaks of the α-Glx triplet are clearly seen, and to the left is the second Cr peak. Variations in the degree of water suppression affect the intensities of the metabolite peaks closest to the water frequency at 4.7 ppm, that is, the second Cr peak and its immediate neighbors. However, this effect of water suppression has no

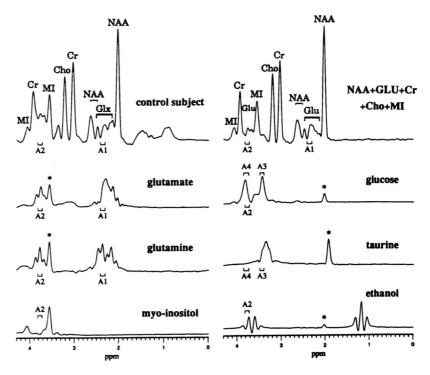

FIGURE 30–3. Localized in vivo and in vitro ^1H MR spectra, obtained with a stimulated-echo sequence at 1.5 T, illustrate the identification of the cerebral metabolites. At the top left is a normal brain spectrum (the sum of results for 10 age-matched control subjects). At the top right is a reference spectrum for an aqueous solution composed of 36.7 mmol/L NAA, 25.0 mmol/L Cr, 6.3 mmol/L choline chloride, 30.0 mmol/L glutamine, and 22.5 mmol/L mI (adjusted to pH 7.15 in a phosphate buffer). The remaining spectra were recorded from solutions of individual biochemicals. To simulate in vivo conditions, all spectra were subjected to a line shape transformation yielding gaussian peaks of approximately 4-Hz line width. The integration ranges used to detect changes in the cerebral levels of Glx (glutamine or glutamate) (A1 + A2) and glucose (A3 + A4) are indicated. The peaks labeled with an asterisk originated from glycine, NAA, or acetate, which were added to the various solutions as chemical shift references (the methyl peak of NAA was set to 2.02 ppm). All spectra were scaled individually and cannot be used for direct quantitation. (From Kreis R, Ross BD, Farrow NA, Ackerman Z: Metabolic disorders of the brain in chronic hepatic encephalopathy detected with ^1H MRS. Radiology 182:19–27, 1992.)

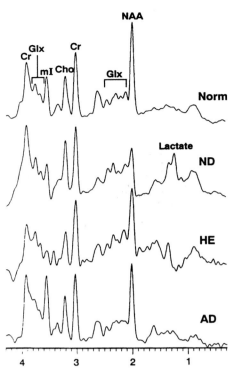

FIGURE 30–4. ¹H MR spectra of "gray matter" acquired with PROBE. Spectra, from top to bottom, are for a healthy volunteer and patients with ND, hepatic encephalopathy (HE), and probable AD. All spectra were acquired with a 1.5-T scanner, using STEAM and a short echo (repetition time [TR]/echo time [TE] = 1.5/30).

influence on the diagnostic value of spectra. The three major resonances (NAA, Cr, and mI) provide a steep angle up from left to right in normal spectra acquired at short TE.

In the spectrum for ND, a lipid peak and overlying lactate doublet peak (at 1.3 ppm) replace the normally nearly flat baseline. NAA is almost completely depleted, and there is a characteristic pattern of increased glutamine resonances (2.2 to 2.4 ppm). The Cho/Cr peak ratio is apparently increased, compared with the normal ratio, but in this case the impression is created by a reduction in Cr intensity (which can be ascertained only from a quantitative spectrum).

The spectrum for a patient with acute hepatic encephalopathy (HE) shows peaks in the lipid-lactate region that cannot be reliably interpreted. The NAA/Cr ratio is clearly reduced, and the cluster of peaks designated Glx is increased. The Cho/Cr ratio is if anything slightly less than normal, but the most striking change is the almost complete absence of mI. This also makes the increased α-Glx peaks to the left of mI more easily visible.

The spectrum for probable AD also has a characteristic appearance, with NAA much reduced (NAA/Cr ratio close to 1); Glx is if anything reduced, and the Cho/Cr ratio is in this case slightly higher than normal. The prominent mI peak is almost equal to the Cr and NAA peaks, giving the spectrum its characteristic flat appearance. In each case (not shown) MRI was essentially normal and gave little or no diagnostic in-

formation, whereas the spectrum is now well established as characteristic for the disease state described.

CURRENT CLINICAL USES OF MR SPECTROSCOPY

DEVELOPMENTAL DISORDERS
(see Chapters 16 and 28)

For normal development, the evolution of MRS changes in the newborn brain, from in utero (in a single near-term fetus)[20] to 300+ weeks of gestational age, is now well described[21] (Fig. 30–5). The findings add significantly to the information routinely obtained in MRI. Van der Knaap and colleagues[22] have correlated the evolution of changes in the ³¹P and ¹H MR spectra with the development of myelination, but without short-TE spectra with which to define changes in mI and with no quantitative data. Normative curves for normal development now established for two cerebral locations (Fig. 30–6) confirm earlier published long-TE and ³¹P findings and unpublished data.[21, 23] mI dominates the spectrum at birth (12 mmol/kg), and Cho is responsible for the strongest peak in older

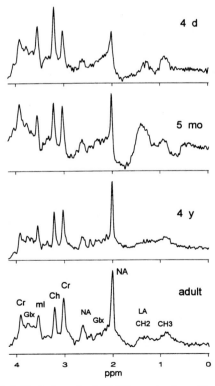

FIGURE 30–5. Typical cerebral ¹H MR spectra for subjects of different age. The relative amplitudes of the main peaks in short-TE STEAM spectra vary drastically with age. The spectra were obtained from a periventricular area in the parietal cortex. Acquisition parameters: 30-ms TE, 1500-ms TR, 128 to 256 averages, voxel sizes 8 to 10 cm³ for children and 12 to 16 cm³ for adults. (Modified from Kreis R, Ernst T, Ross BD: Development of the human brain: in vivo quantification of metabolite and water content with proton magnetic resonance spectroscopy. Magn Reson Med 30:1–14, 1993.)

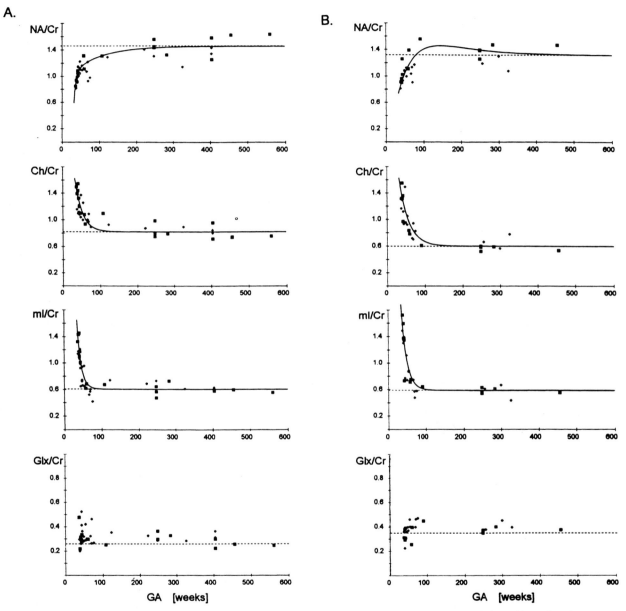

FIGURE 30–6. Time courses of metabolite peak amplitude ratios versus gestational age of the subject. *A* and *B*, Normative curves for the parietal (mostly white matter) and occipital (predominantly gray matter) locations, respectively. The curves are well defined for the first year of life, in which the most dramatic changes take place. The normative curves are specific for the acquisition parameters used. (*A* and *B* modified from Kreis R, Ernst T, Ross BD: Development of the human brain: in vivo quantification of metabolite and water content with proton magnetic resonance spectroscopy. Magn Reson Med 30:1–14, 1993.)

TABLE 30–4. ABSOLUTE CONCENTRATIONS FOR DIFFERENT AGE GROUPS (MMOL/KG BRAIN TISSUE, MEAN ± 1 SEM) AND SIGNIFICANCE TESTS FOR THE DIFFERENCES FOUND*

GROUP	n (ROIs)	GESTATIONAL AGE (GA) (WK)	POSTNATAL AGE (WK)	NA	Cr	Ch	mI
<42 GA	11	38.7 ± 0.7	3.9 ± 1.6	4.82 ± 0.54	6.33 ± 0.32	2.41 ± 0.11	10.1 ± 1.1
42–60 GA	8	50.2 ± 1.8	9.3 ± 1.9	7.03 ± 0.41	7.28 ± 0.28	2.23 ± 0.06	8.52 ± 0.92
<2 postnatal	6	40.0 ± 1.0	0.8 ± 0.2	5.52 ± 0.64	6.74 ± 0.43	2.53 ± 0.12	12.4 ± 1.4
2–10 postnatal	7	41.9 ± 1.5	3.8 ± 0.9	5.89 ± 0.21	6.56 ± 0.44	2.16 ± 0.09	7.69 ± 0.62
Adult	10		1440 ± 68	8.89 ± 0.17	7.49 ± 0.12	1.32 ± 0.07	6.56 ± 0.43
P value: <42 GA versus adult				<.0001	<.0001	<.0001	.001
P value: <42 GA versus 42–60 GA				.0007	.02	.07	.10
P value: 42–60 GA versus adult				<.0001	.16	<.0001	.0003
P value: <2 postnatal versus adult				<.0001	.005	<.0001	<.0001
P value: < postnatal versus 2–10 postnatal				.7	.8	.02	.004
P value: 2–10 postnatal versus adult				<.0001	.001	<.0001	.007

*NA (NAA) and Ch (Cho) are used interchangeably.

Modified from Kreis R, Ernst T, Ross BD: Development of the human brain: in vivo quantification of metabolite and water content with proton magnetic resonance spectroscopy. Magn Reson Med 30:1–14, 1993.

infants (2.5 mmol/kg). Cr (plus PCr) and *N*-acetyl (NA) groups (of which the major component is NAA) are at significantly lower concentrations in the neonate than in the adult (6 and 5 mmol/kg, respectively). NAA and Cr increase while Cho and particularly mI decrease during the first few weeks of life[21] (Table 30–4). Increased NAA and Cr are determined by gestational age, whereas the falling concentration of mI correlates best with postnatal age (Fig. 30–7). Absolute metabolite concentrations depend on metabolite T1 and T2 relaxation. Whereas T1 values change significantly with age for the metabolites NA, Cr, and mI, that for Cho is not altered. The T2 value for NAA appears to show important changes between newborns and adults, whereas those for Cr, Cho, and mI seem to be unimportant.

Quantitative ¹H MRS is expected to be of particular value in diagnosis and monitoring of disease in infants[21] (see Fig. 30–7), because metabolite ratios are often misleading. This may be particularly useful in the period before myelination is apparent in the developing brain.

MR Spectroscopy of Inborn Errors of Metabolism

Inborn errors of metabolism, although relatively rare, make up a large proportion of pediatric clinical practice. Extensive reviews of MRI discuss "pattern recognition" in differential diagnosis. Something similar can be done for MRS. Figures 30–8 and 30–9 attempt to draw together examples of common inborn errors. Despite profound methodologic differences, in each case the MR spectrum is diagnostic.

MRS may fill in part of the gap in the diagnostic work-up of inborn errors of metabolism. MRS data for lysosomal and peroxisomal disorders are limited, and generally nonspecific abnormalities related to loss of myelin or to neuronal damage have been described. Nevertheless, even these preliminary data may convey important information and reveal distinct patterns of metabolic disturbances, involving the neuronal marker

NAA (see Fig. 30–8), lactate, and separate abnormalities of Cho, Cr plus PCr, mI, and sI, which may point to a significant new role for MRS in the critical area of early diagnosis of inborn errors. The fact that results are, at present, available for rather small numbers of patients limits our ability to define these disorders more precisely. The early reports suggest, however, that these are just the additional pieces of information that are needed to fill the gap that exists between the subtle enzyme defect and the gross disturbances of neuroanatomy and pathology that constitute the MR image. Until now, the strength of MRS has been in defining mitochondrial disorders, disorders of amino acid and organic acid metabolism, and urea cycle disorders. Especially in the case of atypical and nondiagnostic MRI findings, the demonstration of elevation of cerebral lactate or other substances may be a lead in the diagnostic work-up.

Three types of spectroscopic abnormalities are seen in inborn metabolic errors:

1. Nonspecific spectroscopic abnormalities related to MRI-visible brain damage, including demyelination or atrophy
2. Generic (nonspecific) spectroscopic changes that are largely unassociated with particular changes in MRI, for instance, loss of neuronal marker NAA, loss of high-energy metabolites, or changes in glutamine or glutamate
3. Specific spectroscopic abnormalities directly related to the chemistry of the inborn error under investigation, such as phenylalanine in phenylketonuria and glycine in hyperglycinemia (these changes may be associated with MRI abnormalities)

Nonspecific cerebral damage associated with inborn errors of metabolism may consist of disturbance of brain maturation, demyelination, or neuronal degeneration. In demyelinating disorders, it is primarily the myelin sheath that is lost; secondarily, axonal damage and loss occur.

In demyelinating disorders, the rarefaction of white matter implies that the total amount of membrane

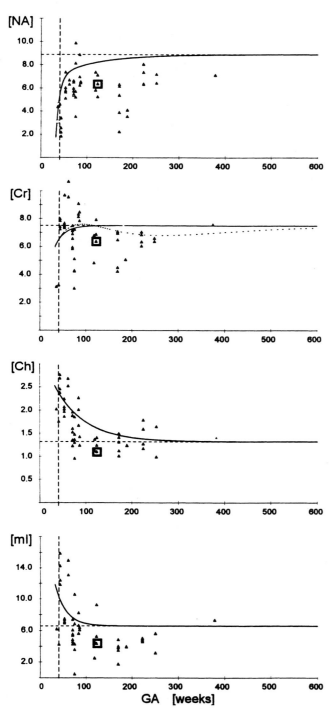

FIGURE 30–7. Alterations of semiquantitatively determined concentrations with pathology. The data represented as normative curves are contrasted with data (▲) for children with a range of nonlocalized cerebral disease. Because relaxation and background changes cannot be ruled out for each particular patient, the data can be read as concentrations only with caution. This semiquantitative approach is still clinically useful in finding out which features in a spectrum remain normal and which are subject to change.

phospholipids per volume of brain tissue decreases. Myelin sheaths consist of condensed membranes with a high lipid content. Gliotic scar tissue contains far fewer membranes and, therefore, far fewer phospholipids per volume. In view of this loss of membrane

phospholipids, a decrease in PDEs in the ^{31}P spectrum is expected. The PDE peak in brain spectra has been shown to contain signals from mobile phospholipids present in membranes[24] and also from intermediary products in the turnover of membrane phospholipids.[25] A decrease in the PDE/β-ATP ratio has been found and is proportional to the extent of the demyelination.[26] The PME peak contains signals from mainly phosphocholine and phosphoethanolamine, both intermediary products in the metabolism of membrane phospholipids.[25] The size of the PME peak has been shown to be proportional to the rate of membrane phospholipid synthesis.[27] A variable decrease in PME/β-ATP ratio has been observed only in severe demyelination.[26] There are two possible explanations for the PME/β-ATP ratio being normal unless demyelination is severe: either the processes of phospholipid synthesis are relatively insensitive to the disappearance of a considerable quantity of membranes or losses of PME and β-ATP occur in parallel. The neuronal damage and loss accompanying demyelination are reflected in a decrease in NAA in the ^{1}H spectra. In active demyelination, an elevation of Cho and lactate has been reported repeatedly, in addition to elevation of fatty acids, presumably representing the breakdown products of myelin.

In neuronal degenerative disorders, no white matter rarefaction occurs. As expected, the PDE/β-ATP ratio has been found to remain in the normal range.[26] The neuronal damage is reflected in a decrease in NAA, which is present in the cytosol of neurons and is probably lost early in neuronal dysfunction. In infarction, a decrease in NAA occurs within hours, whereas the removal of dead neurons starts only after days.

MRS provides a sensitive and valuable extension of the diagnostic information offered by MRI. As a quantitative method it is more sensitive than MRI to subtle changes in disease. Because metabolic abnormalities precede many of the MRI changes discussed in this chapter, such MRS findings may be of value as early diagnostic indicators in siblings screened for a disease.

Several specific spectroscopic changes that are characteristic of a particular inborn error or a subclass of inborn errors are now recognized. Examples (see Figs. 30–8 and 30–9) include elevated glutamine in hyperammonemias, elevation of a peak at 3.35 ppm assigned to sI in some peroxisomal disorders[28] and highly elevated NAA in Canavan's disease.[29] Others, assigned with less certainty at present, include a peak at 0.9 to 1 ppm assigned to branched chain amino acids and oxo acids in maple syrup urine disease,[30, 31] a peak at 3.55 ppm assigned to glycine in nonketotic hyperglycinemia,[31] and a peak of unknown origin at 1.1 ppm in propionicacidemia.[30] Lactate is typically elevated in many mitochondrial disorders[29] but is elevated as well in several other conditions, such as hypoxia-ischemia and inflammation.

Both MRI and MRS may be of help in screening children with a suspected inborn error of metabolism to provide clues for the diagnosis and give direction to the biochemical investigations. The value of MRS, as of any new test, lies as much in the unexpected findings as in those carefully planned. Hence, there is

Text continued on page 942

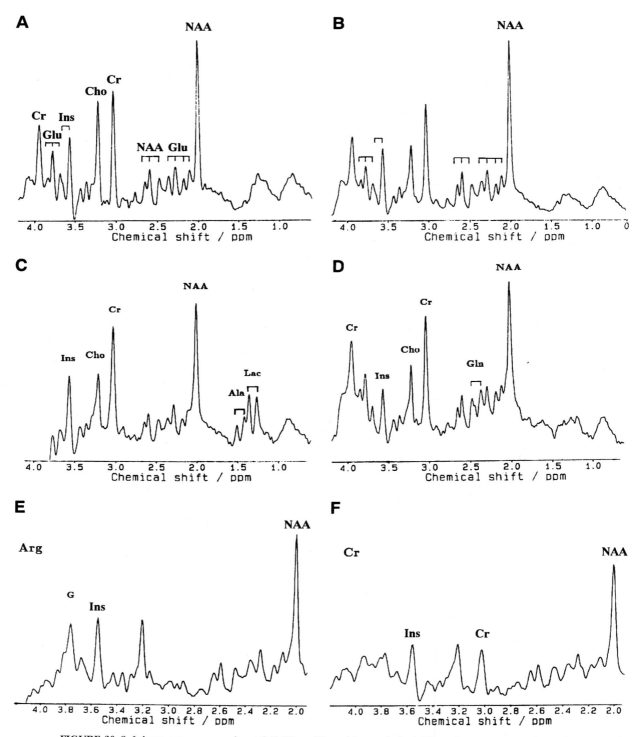

FIGURE 30–8. Inborn errors: examples at 2 T, TE = 20 ms (short echo). *A,* Normal gray matter at 4 months. *B,* Normal gray matter at 2 years (for normal white matter see Fig. 30–6). Ins = mI. *C,* Leigh's disease: white matter at 11 months. *D,* Zellweger's syndrome variant: gray matter at 15 months. *E,* Guanidinoacetate methyltransferase deficiency (Frahm-Hanefeld syndrome) with total Cr deficiency, *(F)* partially restored after treatment.

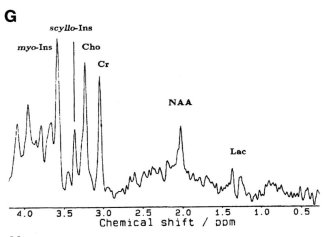

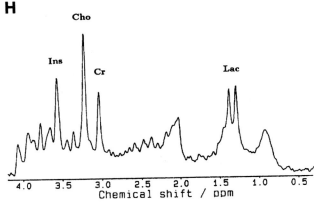

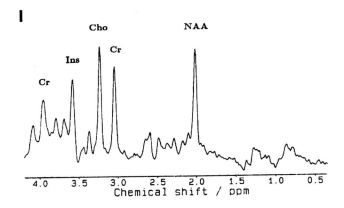

FIGURE 30–8 *Continued G,* Metachromatic leukodystrophy. *H,* Severe adrenoleukodystrophy (ALD). *I,* Adrenal insufficiency only (ALD variant). (*A, B,* and *D* from Bruhn H, Kruse B, Korenke GC, et al: Proton NMR spectroscopy of cerebral metabolic alterations in infantile peroxisomal disorders. J Comput Assist Tomogr 16:335–344, 1992. *C, E,* and *F* from Michaelis T, Helms G, Merboldt KD, et al: First observation of *scyllo*-inositol in proton NMR spectra of human brain in vitro and in vivo. In: Proceedings of the 11th Annual Meeting of the Society of Magnetic Resonance in Medicine, Berlin, 1992, p 541. *H* and *I* from Kruse B, Hanefeld F, Merboldt K-D, et al: Localized proton MR spectroscopy in hemimegalencephaly. In: Proceedings of the 12th Annual Meeting of the Society of Magnetic Resonance in Medicine, New York, 1993, p 1570. *G* from Kruse B, Hanefeld F, Christen HJ, et al: Alterations of brain metabolites in metachromatic leukodystrophy as detected by localized proton magnetic resonance spectroscopy in vivo. J Neurol 241:68–74, 1993.)

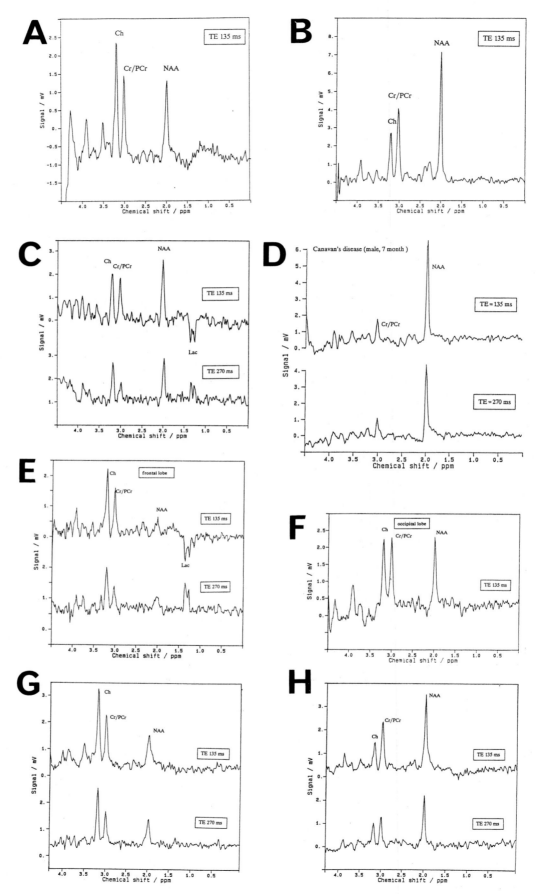

FIGURE 30–9. *See legend on opposite page*

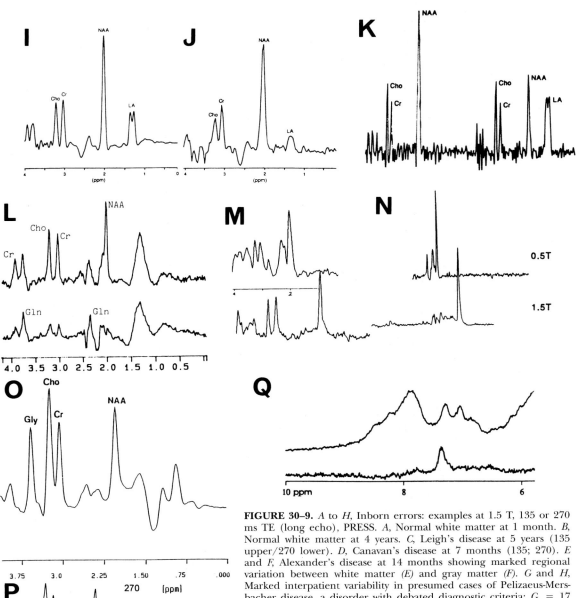

FIGURE 30–9. *A* to *H*, Inborn errors: examples at 1.5 T, 135 or 270 ms TE (long echo), PRESS. *A*, Normal white matter at 1 month. *B*, Normal white matter at 4 years. *C*, Leigh's disease at 5 years (135 upper/270 lower). *D*, Canavan's disease at 7 months (135; 270). *E* and *F*, Alexander's disease at 14 months showing marked regional variation between white matter *(E)* and gray matter *(F)*. *G* and *H*, Marked interpatient variability in presumed cases of Pelizaeus-Mersbacher disease, a disorder with debated diagnostic criteria: *G*, = 17 months, early onset; *H*, 6 years, late onset. *I* to *Q*, Mitochondrial encephalopathies: Significant effects of field strength, sequence, and TE. *I*, Kern-Sayer syndrome (PRESS 272). *J*, Mitochondrial encephalopathy with ragged red fibers (MERRF) (PRESS 272). *K*, Region variations in MELAS syndrome (chemical-shift imaging). *L*, Ornithine transcarbamylase deficiency (PRESS 135). *M*, Normal (PRESS 41 ms) dramatically refocused at 0.5 T, barely present at 1.5 T. *N*, Glx phantom used to ensure accurate assignment. *O*, Nonketotic hyperglycinemia (PRESS 135), glycine or mI? *P*, Age-matched normal STEAM, 30 to 270 ms. The progressive disappearance of mI increases certainty of glycine rather than mI. *Q*, Phenylketonuria (PRESS 20). Difference spectroscopy ensures identity of resonance at 7.37 ppm. (*A* to *H* courtesy of Wolfgang Grodd, MD, University of Tübingen, Germany. *I* to *K* courtesy of Douglas Arnold, MD, University of Montreal, Canada. *L* courtesy of David Gadian, PhD, Royal College of Surgeons, London, UK. *M* and *N* courtesy of Robert Prost, PhD, University of Wisconsin, Milwaukee. *O* courtesy of W. Heindel, MD, University of Cologne, Germany. *P* from Kreis R, Ernst T, Ross BD: Development of the human brain: in vivo quantification of metabolite and water content with proton magnetic resonance spectroscopy. Magn Reson Med 30:424–437, 1993. *Q* from Kreis R, Pietz J, Penzien J, et al: Unequivocal identification and quantitation of phenylalanine in the brain of patients with phenylketonuria by means of localized in vivo ¹H MRS. In: Proceedings of the Second Annual Meeting of the Society of Magnetic Resonance, San Francisco, 1994, p 308.)

a need for good quality control, so that artifacts are not treated as novel chemical aberrations. The ease with which ¹H MRS of the brain can now be performed makes this area of study most likely to expand. Until now, little work has been done in the area of carrier detection with the help of MRS. As carriers often have minor metabolic abnormalities, which do not lead to structural damage, MRS may prove of greater use than MRI.

Abnormal Development

In inborn errors there are two broad categories of central nervous system involvement[22]: primarily structural and primarily functional abnormalities. Inborn errors of metabolism are presumably present from the beginning of embryogenesis and so a number of them lead to disturbances of normal brain development. Zellweger's syndrome, Pelizaeus-Merzbacher disease, glutaricaciduria type I, aminoacidopathies, phenylketonuria, metachromatic leukodystrophy, globoid cell leukodystrophy (Krabbe's disease), and gangliosidoses are just some of the inborn errors of metabolism in which (it is presumed) the anatomic abnormality by which they are recognized in MRI results primarily from metabolic interference with normal brain development. In one example,[32] an infant with an abnormal thirst control mechanism presented with hypernatremia and a markedly ''hyperosmolar'' brain chemistry on MRS examination (see later) and was discovered at the same time to have a minor and incomplete holoprosencephaly on MRI. Presumably, the anatomic defect underlay the complex biochemical disorder uncovered by MRS.[33]

However, many of the primary defects are in pathways involving macromolecules or membrane lipids, invisible to NMR. Unless the inborn error of metabo-

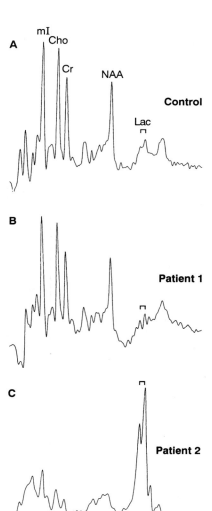

FIGURE 30–11. Good and bad outcomes after hypoxic encephalopathy. Localized, short-TE ¹H MR spectra of the gray matter of a control subject *(A)*, patient 1 *(B)*, and patient 2 *(C)*. The metabolite resonances of NAA, total creatine (Cr), Cho, mI, and lactate (Lac) are indicated. In *A* and *B* a possible trace of lactate is detectable, but the spectra are otherwise identical. Patient 1 presented with an Apgar score of 0-0-2 after birth, and hypoxic encephalopathy was prevented by the standard resuscitation measures applied. This contrasts with severe abnormalities in patient 2. In *C*, major abnormalities are lack of NAA, excess lactate, excess mI at 3.58 ppm, and the unknown doublet resonance at 1.15 ppm assigned to 1,3-propanediol (see also Fig. 30–45). *(A to C from Michaelis T, Cooper K, Kreis R, Ross BD, unpublished; see also Cady EB, Lorek A, Penrice J, et al: Detection of propan-1,2-diol in neonatal brain by in vivo proton magnetic resonance spectroscopy. Magn Reson Med 32:764–767, 1994.)*

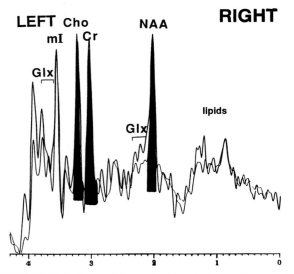

FIGURE 30–10. Left and right parietal hemispheres after arteriovenous extracorporeal membrane oxygenation in a patient of 26 days postnatal age. ¹H MRS showed a normal spectrum for both parietal hemispheres despite total ligation of the left carotic artery. No significant differences in principal metabolites are seen.

lism results in accumulation of a low-molecular-weight species detectable in conventional or edited versions of MRS, the underlying biochemical disorder is not apparent. Thus, it is to the primarily functional abnormalities that we turn for examples in which MRS assists diagnosis. Here, because it can offer greater specificity than can MRI, MRS may be of value in the work-up of difficult cases.

Neonatal Hypoxia

Extracorporeal membrane oxygenation, an extracorporeal life support technique that is used to maintain cerebral oxygenation in sick, hypoxemic infants and that usually necessitates ligation of one carotid artery, is without dramatic effect on the MR spectrum of the newborn brain (Fig. 30–10). Not only is the spectrum essentially normal but also, as there is no distinguishable difference between left and right parietal cortex, we can presume carotid ligation to be relatively benign. Another example of an essentially normal brain spectrum after what was presumed to be severe perinatal hypoxic encephalopathy is shown in Figure 30–11. This example is in contrast to the dramatic abnormalities that are regularly detected by means of ¹H MRS in newborns with true hypoxic encephalopathy (Fig. 30–12); NAA is depleted and Cho, lactate, and lipid accumulate in both cerebral hemispheres despite rather normal MRI. Anatomic heterogeneity of hypoxic damage and the progression of the biochemical damage over time are illustrated in Figure 30–13. Progressive loss of NAA, Cr, and mI with time reflects the evolution of hypoxic damage between days 5, 12, and 42 after birth. The occipital (gray) region is most severely affected and the frontal least; the effect on the parietal cortex is intermediate. This patient clearly demonstrates a further general point: that lipid is one of the metabolic markers of cerebral hypoxia in the neonate.

The severity of changes in MRS appears to correlate

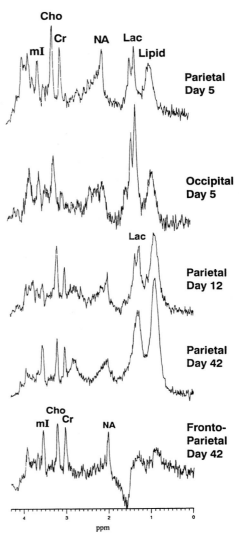

FIGURE 30–13. Anatomic heterogeneity of hypoxic damage and progression of the biochemical damage over time. On day 5, MRS is dramatically abnormal and MRI is equivocal, showing normal or modest edema (not shown). The occipital cortex is marked by overall low signal intensity with virtually absent NA and great excesses of lactate and lipid. Even in the parietal cortex, lactate and lipid are prominent; mI is considerably below normal for age in both locations. (Note: no line broadening was applied to spectra for day 5 and day 42.) Changes in parietal cortex on day 12 are reflected by progressive loss of NA and Cr and apparent increasing lactate and lipid intensities, which by day 42 dominate the spectrum as the total signal intensity falls. There is some increase in the mI/Cr ratio at this late stage of hypoxia. Even at this late stage, MRS of the frontoparietal cortex is virtually normal (the inverted lipid peak is from without the region of interest and probably outside the brain). MRI of the frontoparietal cortex was also normal. MRI on day 12 showed encephalomalacia in the occipital lobe, and by day 42 there was complete occipital lobe atrophy.

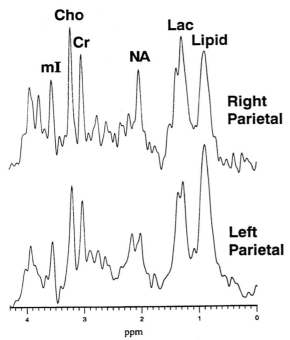

FIGURE 30–12. Newborn hypoxic encephalopathy. Two-week-old infant, hypoxic episode at birth. The ¹H MR spectra show severe hypoxic changes, including a reduced NA/Cr ratio, excess lactate and intravoxel lipid. Ischemic damage is considerably more severe on the left, but lactate and lipid are prominent on both left and right parietal spectra. MRI was reported to demonstrate left posteroparietal and occipital ischemic infarction and right occipital ischemia, with changes more marked on the left.

with the clinical outcome. Paradoxically, recovery of cerebral metabolites after severe hypoxic encephalopathy might be best explained by cortical atrophy (Figs. 30–14 and 30–15). Despite the obvious lack of NAA at delivery, the spectrum acquired several weeks later shows NAA and an almost normal spectrum. However, the marked ventricular dilatation at MRI (see Fig. 30–

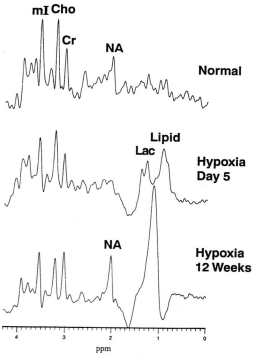

FIGURE 30–14. Hypoxic encephalopathy in prematurity. ^{1}H MR spectra illustrating the paradoxical recovery of cerebral metabolites after severe hypoxic encephalopathy (see Fig. 30–15 for images) in an infant at 31 weeks of gestational age (control age = 34 to 35 weeks). (Modified from Ross B, Ernst T, Kreis R: Magnetic resonance spectroscopy in pediatric hypoxic-ischemic disorders. In: Faerber EN, ed. CNS Magnetic Resonance Imaging in Infants and Children. Cambridge, UK: Cambridge University Press, 1995, pp 279–328.)

15*B*) confirms that this is most probably the result of consolidation of surviving neurons within a smaller volume of brain. Delayed neuronal development and delayed NAA synthesis are a more speculative but possible alternative in the extremely premature infant.

For completeness, also illustrated are the spectra and images (Fig. 30–16*A* and *B*) of an infant with middle cerebral artery occlusion, indistinguishable from the neurochemical profile of adult stroke, and another with multiple intracerebral hemorrhage (Fig. 30–17*A* and *B*).

MR Spectroscopy in Children

Although undoubtedly we will eventually recognize special features, at present ^{1}H MRS findings in children appear to be representative of the changes seen in adults with the same disease and for that reason are dealt with under the appropriate disease headings. Published case reports on Reye's syndrome,[34, 35] hypernatremia,[32] head injury,[36] and diabetes mellitus[37] illustrate this general point. MS in children 7 to 16 years of age has a similar appearance on ^{1}H MRS to that in adults.[38]

Seizure and Epilepsies

Seizures have so many different causes that it is not surprising that systematic studies with MRS are lacking.

Nevertheless, we can identify several specific spectra (see Figs. 30–8 and 30–9), associated with inborn errors of metabolism, which present as seizures, and to a considerable body of work on older children with temporal lobe epilepsy. Using either symmetrically placed pairs of voxels or entire data sets of chemical-shift imaging (CSI), most authors can point to a significant reduction in NAA/Cr ratio in one temporal lobe compared with the other. Even "blinded" studies appear to select the affected lobe with clinically useful reproducibility and precision.

One word of caution concerns the difficulty of obtaining spectra of the required excellent quality from both temporal lobes. Nevertheless, this approach is in clinical use in a number of centers.[39–47]

Seizures in infants and children certainly appear to warrant an MRS examination, even though we cannot discern one specific pattern of changes.

CEREBRAL NEOPLASMS (see Chapter 17)

MRI has proved a boon to the neuroradiologist examining the brain for evidence of neoplasms, and in the purely diagnostic sense there are few remaining questions that MRI cannot answer. Nonenhancing lesions still present diagnostic problems, as does the differentiation between the acute edematous lesion of MS and glioma. Peritumoral edema is poorly understood based on MRI alone, and because the extent of tumors visualized by computed tomography (CT) and that visualized by MRI can be different, the surgeon or radiotherapist may not have concise advice about an optimal biopsy site or the extent of desired therapy. Finally, the most often asked question concerns the appearance of recurrent tumor after radiation therapy, that is, the distinction between tumor and radiation necrosis.

MRS has addressed some of these questions and achieved a measure of success. Thorough reviews are available.[48–51] Specifically, CSI performed in several different ways and in several centers readily documents the heterogeneity of brain tumors and the great regional differences in individual subjects[51–59] (Fig. 30–18). The loss of spectral resolution and quantitative information is more than compensated for. Metabolic heterogeneity in human brain tumors is now detectable with three-dimensional, high-spatial-resolution (0.2 to 0.4 mL) ^{1}H MR spectroscopic imaging.[60] Differences among solid tumor, necrosis, and viable brain tissue can be shown in single cases. The method uses phased-array surface coils, which are difficult to use but may be needed if real clinical progress in brain tumor management is to be achieved. More effort has been expended on the areas in which MRS has special advantages. These include the following:

1. The attempt to provide better differential diagnosis than is achievable with MRI alone
2. Definition of tumor grade, aggressivity, and relevant biochemistry, in particular the importance of measuring tumor lactate and possibly also of Cho

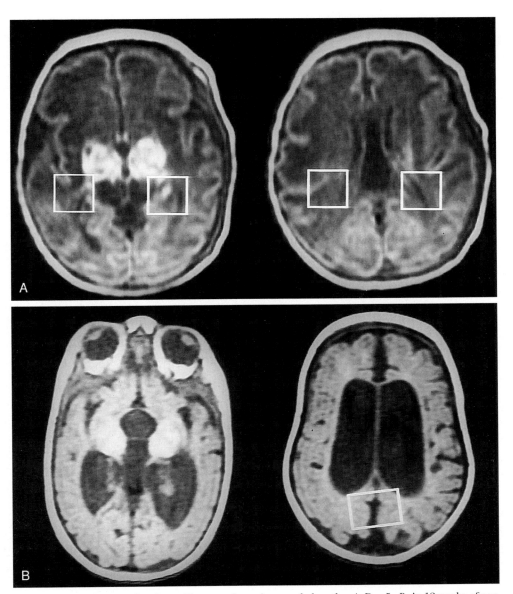

FIGURE 30–15. Images of patient with severe hypoxic encephalopathy. *A,* Day 5. *B,* At 12 weeks of age.

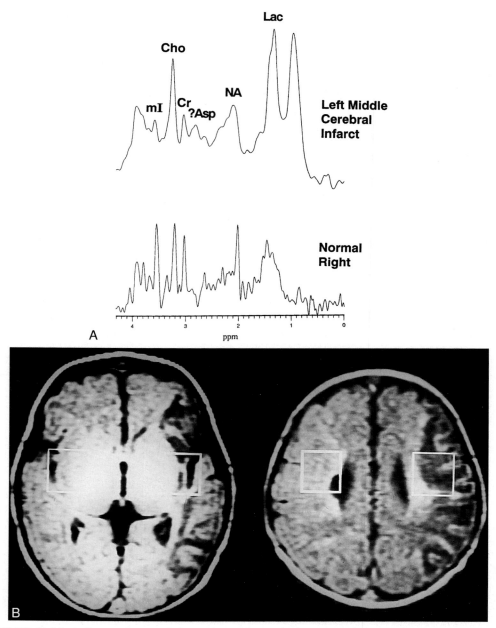

FIGURE 30–16. *A,* Spectra from an infant with middle cerebral artery occlusion. Differences in line width account for some of the apparent differences in spectral appearance of the focal lesion. However, dramatically lower NAA, Cr, and mI, together with increased lactate and lipid, distinguish the hemisphere with "stroke" from the presumed normal hemisphere. *B,* Images indicating location of volumes of interest and of infarcted hemispheres in the distribution of the left middle cerebral artery.

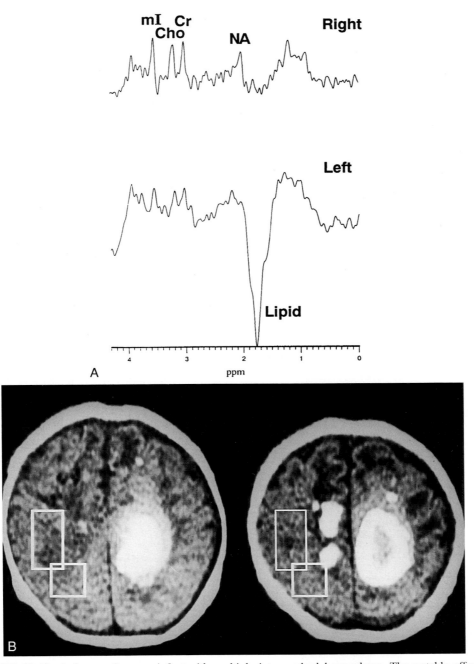

FIGURE 30–17. *A*, Spectra from an infant with multiple intracerebral hemorrhage. The notable effect of hemorrhage is to produce line broadening and lipid artifacts that distort the ¹H spectrum. In the contralateral hemisphere, NAA is lower than expected, indicating damage beyond the obvious local regions of hemorrhage noted by MRI *(B)*.

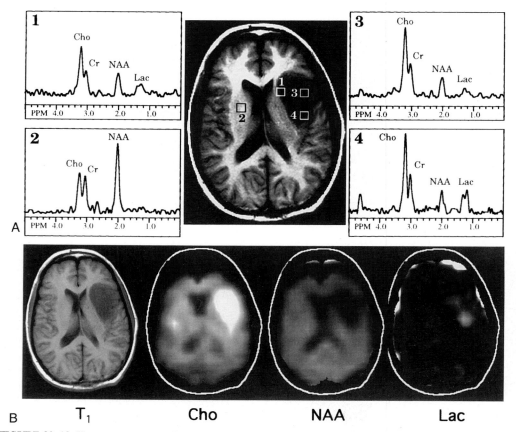

FIGURE 30–18. Heterogeneous metabolism of brain tumor. CSI permits multiple metabolite distribution maps of tumor and surrounding tissue to be prepared in a little more than 30 minutes. *A,* Shows four individual spectra extracted from the CSI data set in the locations indicated on the axial water images. Loss of NAA is uniform throughout the tumor region, but excess of lactate is most marked in location number 4. Excess Cho fills the tumor region of the MR image. *B,* Images reconstructed from CSI data to show the precise anatomic distribution of those metabolic changes that correspond to tumor on T1-weighted MR images. (*A* and *B* courtesy of Peter Barker, PhD, Johns Hopkins University, Baltimore, MD.)

3. Monitoring of a successful tumor response before tumor regression during nonsurgical treatments and, conversely, the early definition of tumor recurrence

Basic Neurochemistry of Tumors

Five biochemical defects are common to the majority of brain tumors, as measured by MRS (Fig. 30–19): NAA is decreased, lactate is increased, lipid is increased (see inset in Fig. 30–19), Cr plus PCr is decreased (as is PCr determined alone), and Cho is increased. This increase in Cho is readily recognized in ^1H spectra as an increase in the Cho/Cr ratio and in ^{31}P spectra as an increase in PME. Further information in the ^{31}P spectrum indicates an alkaline (not acid) intratumor pH and often increased P_i relative to ATP.[7] However, it should be remembered that in ^1H and ^{31}P spectra all metabolite concentrations are often reduced, so these peak ratios correctly reflect relative changes rather than absolute increments or decrements.[61] This aspect of tumor diagnosis and analysis becomes clearer when quantitative MRS is applied.

Quantitative MRS, performed either systematically in absolute terms or by inference, comparing voxels representing tumors with those representing surrounding normal brain, takes account of heterogeneous anatomy of tumors, including regions of necrosis or cysts. The most thorough studies have used metabolite imaging (CSI or other techniques) to throw new light on the metabolic heterogeneity of brain tumors. These results, when combined with the insights from MRI, significantly alter management.

Significance of Changes in Tumor Spectra

Reduction or absence of NAA expresses the absence of neurons and axons in most tumors, which are histologically derived from astrocytes (which entirely lack NAA [gliomas], connective tissue [meningiomas], ectoderm [craniopharyngioma]) or from remote tissues of non-neuronal origin (virtually all secondary tumors). Lactate, normally undetectable in brain, accumulates in cysts, necrotic tissues, or active tumors because of the high rate of glycolysis (of glucose to lactate) in even aerobic tumors of all types. Heterogeneous distribution of lactate reflects its accumulation in cysts, regions of high tumor activity or, conversely, areas of tumor necrosis. Alanine, an alternative reduced partner of pyruvate derived from glycolysis, has been systematically reported in meningiomas, an observation that at present is interesting rather than helpful.

Lipid signals commonly associated with tumor spectra have usually been ascribed to necrotic regions in untreated tumors or to treatment-responsive necrosis in treated tumors, and this is probably correct for in vivo tumor spectra.[62] On the other hand, in high-resolution spectra of brain tumor biopsy specimens more specific lipids are identifiable[63] (Fig. 30–20). These are probably contributors to the unresolved lipid peaks of the in vivo tumor itself.

Decreased Cr plus PCr or decreased PCr itself is an inconstant finding in tumors. When found, it has usually been ascribed to the low-energy status of glycolytic tumors in general. In the case of secondary tumors the explanation is more straightforward, as most tissues that commonly metastasize to brain (kidney, lung, breast, lymphoma, prostate) lack both PCr and creatine kinase. On the other hand, elevated Cho (or PME) is nearly always observed and has been substantiated by in vitro chemical assays on tumor biopsy specimens. Proliferation of cell membranes, the explanation usually offered, is too vague; breakdown of NMR-invisible phosphatidylcholine, to release NMR-visible phosphorylcholine and glycerophosphorylcholine, is another possibility without experimental support at present. More likely, brain tumors share with other tumors the property of increased synthesis of phosphorylcholine and glycerophosphorylcholine.

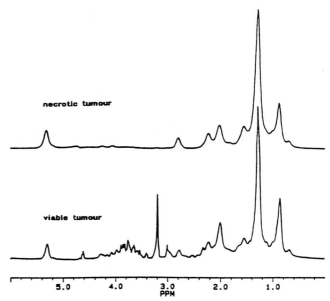

FIGURE 30–20. Absolute intensity ex vivo ^{1}H MR spectra (scale × ½) at 37°C of samples from two biopsies of a subependymal giant cell tumor in a patient with tuberous sclerosis, representing histologically 99% necrotic tumor and histologically 99% viable tumor. The free induction decay for the upper spectrum was acquired with half the receiver gain used for that of the lower spectrum. (From Kuesel AC, Donnelly SM, Halliday W, et al: Mobile lipids and metabolic heterogeneity of brain tumours as detectable by ex vivo ^{1}H MR spectroscopy. NMR Biomed 7:172–180, 1994. Reprinted by permission of John Wiley & Sons Ltd.)

Alkaline pH in brain tumors, conflicting as it does with accepted dogma and with the accumulation of (presumably) acidic lactate, has been slow to gain acceptance. It is now readily resolved: ^{31}P MRS determines intracellular pH (which is alkaline), whereas other methods have measured extracellular pH (which is acidic).

In summary, there is a good theoretic basis for all of the neurochemical information concerning brain tumors now available with MRS. Attempts have been made to refine this information into a better tool for differential diagnosis, grading, and staging, as discussed in the following.

Differential Diagnosis of Tumors with MR Spectroscopy: Grading and Therapeutic Monitoring

Several papers provide a basis on which MR spectra, particularly ^{1}H spectra, might contribute to the differentiation of tumors. One group[49, 50] arrived at the distinctions shown in Table 30–5, which may prove generally useful in clinical practice.

In summary, we must say that not only is differentiation extremely problematic when based on the spectrum alone but also there is an alarming overlap with the spectral appearance of focal lesions such as MS, AIDS masses, or even infarcts, which are not neoplastic (see subsequent sections). That is not to dismiss MRS for the differentiation of tumors from one another.

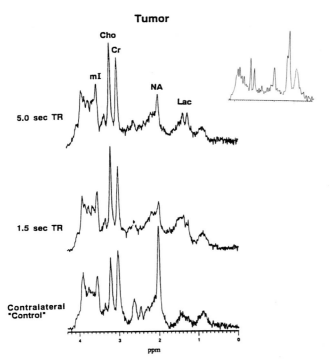

FIGURE 30–19. An obvious primary tumor showing absent NA, increased Cho/Cr ratio, and, particularly at longer TR values, increased lactate (in all cases. TE = 30 ms). *Inset,* Spectrum from a second patient showing the now classic profile of lipid plus lactate, probably representing recurrence after therapy.

TABLE 30–5. ¹H MRS DISTINCTION OF HIGH- AND LOW-GRADE GLIAL BRAIN TUMORS*

TUMOR CHARACTERISTIC	P VALUE
Increased lactate/Cr in high (8) versus low (3) grades	<.002
Increased Cho/NAA in malignant (9) versus benign (14) versus brain (5)	.05
Decreased NAA/(Cr + PCr) in malignant (9) versus benign (14) versus brain (5)	.05

*Number of patients in parentheses.
From Negendank W, Sauter R, Brown T, et al: Intratumoral lipids and lactate in ¹H MRS in vivo in astrocytic tumors. In: Proceedings of the Second Annual Meeting of the Society of Magnetic Resonance, San Francisco, 1994, p 1296.

When MRS results are taken in conjunction with careful analysis of the available imaging sequences, SPECT or positron emission tomography, some statements appear to be justified (Table 30–6).

The clinical impact of MRS in this area has been explored by Norfray and colleagues (Norfray JF, Tomita T, Strauss L, et al, unpublished manuscript, 1994). They undertook the task of translating this application into clinical management and reported "changes in therapeutic decision" based on sequential, automated MRS in 6 of 11 pediatric patients with brain tumors.

SPONTANEOUS HEMORRHAGE
(see Chapter 21)

Appearances at MRI

Differences in MR image intensity, which permit definitive diagnosis and dating of recent or older intracerebral hemorrhage, are due in large part to magnetic field inhomogeneities induced by deposition of iron and accumulation of hemoglobin and its breakdown products. These conditions are extremely unfavorable for MRS, resulting in signal loss, poor water shim, and broad metabolite resonances. It is a reasonable generalization to say that regions of obvious hemorrhage in the brain should be strenuously avoided by the clinical neurospectroscopist. In rare cases, when the radiologist is still confused by high-intensity signals that might represent fat, MRS is definitive, because the

TABLE 30–6. POSSIBLE DISCRIMINATORS IN ¹H MRS OF MALIGNANT BRAIN TUMORS

DISCRIMINATOR	AUTHOR
Lipid A grade	Ott et al.[58]
Low NAA, low Cr, normal Cho (no specificity)	Peeling (cited in Negendank[49])
Low NAA, low Cr, high Cho, high lactate, tumor type	Negendank[49]
Glioma versus meningioma versus neurolemmoma versus cyst versus breast secondary	Bruhn[52]
Peritumoral edema—T2	Lowry (cited in Negendank[49])

*Number of cases in parentheses.

chemical shift of lipid (0.9 to 1.2 ppm) is pathognomonic.

The pathogenesis of intracranial hemorrhage differs with age, being closely correlated with prior hypoxic-ischemic injury in the neonatal brain and with arteriolar damage related to amyloid angiopathy in the older population (see Chapter 7).

Predictive Value of MR Spectroscopy in Neonatal Cerebral Hemorrhage

Finding hemorrhage in one location should lead to MRS examination of the contralateral hemisphere or another apparently innocent region to look for evidence of hypoxic encephalopathy. This is widespread, according to the studies of Volpe[63a] and reports of positron emission tomography studies. In the next section, we deal with hemorrhage in an infant, illustrating the deleterious effect of hemorrhage on spectral detail, rendering it effectively uninterpretable. But it also demonstrates the severe hypoxic damage in apparently normal areas of the brain on MRI images. The same argument might be applied to cerebral hemorrhage detected by CT or MRI in adults. MRS probably has an important contribution to make in defining the severity of hypoxic damage to surrounding brain and dating the hypoxic insult. (This should be differentiated from the task of dating the hemorrhage, for which MRI is well suited.)

Surgical Intervention in Older Adults with Cerebral Hemorrhage

Surgical correction is often a high priority in therapy for recent intracranial bleeding. Patients with amyloid angiopathy are poor candidates for surgery and should be excluded if possible. The knowledge that 30% of patients with amyloid angiopathy also have AD (Chapter 29) gives an opportunity for MRS that has not yet been tested. Because ¹H MRS has 90% sensitivity for AD versus normal findings and negative predictive value, excluding AD in about 80% of patients with other dementias (see later section on AD), this single examination should be considered in the presurgical evaluation of patients with hemorrhage.

TRAUMATIC HEMORRHAGE: MR SPECTROSCOPY IN CLOSED HEAD TRAUMA (DIAGNOSIS, PROGNOSIS, AND NEUROPATHOLOGY)
(see Chapters 21 and 27)

MRI is superior to CT in detection of intracerebral hemorrhage after trauma, so that once the difficulties of life support and monitoring of patients have been overcome, MRI provides several opportunities for improving the management of patients with severe closed head injury. Although the major sites of hemorrhagic injury are the inferior temporal and frontal lobes (because of the local bony structures), shear injuries that are considered much more damaging occur in cortical white matter.

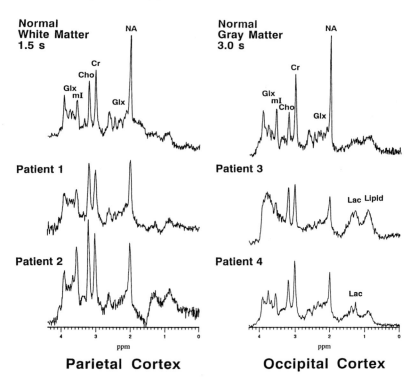

FIGURE 30–21. Quantitative ¹H MRS to monitor progression after closed head injury. The location of voxels was selected to represent tissue that is apparently normal at MRI. The exception is patient 3, who had suffered extensive and obvious tissue damage. Patient 1: elevated cerebral Cho and reduced NA levels in a 32-year-old male, unconscious 7 days after head injury. Patient 2: elevated cerebral Cho, Cr, and mI levels with nearly normal NA in a female unconscious for 2.5 months. Patient 3: reduced Cr, NA, and mI levels with intracerebral lactate and lipid accumulation in a 2.5-year-old child unconscious 5 weeks after closed head injury. Patient 4: reduced Cr and NA levels with lactate (~2.5 mM) in an 8-year-old child maintained with a ventilator 5 days after closed head injury. The top spectrum on each side is for the appropriate age-related control subject.

Shear injuries in the thalamus and basal ganglia are seen with MRI (but not CT) because of the hemorrhage that is present in 50% of cases. For this and many other reasons, outcome correlated much more closely with MRI than with CT findings. But in this series (Chapters 21 and 27), 24 of 100 patients did not have MRI changes, and for these patients correlation of MRI results with outcome was poor. In trauma, MRS can fill this diagnostic void by identifying subtle neurochemical defects in the absence of abnormality in any imaging study.

MRS appears to show three patterns of disease[37] (Fig. 30–21) (diffuse axonal injury, patient 1; hyperosmolar state, patient 2; and hypoxic injury, patients 3 and 4).

Outcome, which is so difficult to predict from clinical or imaging evidence, appears to be well correlated with the NAA/Cr ratio and NAA level (Ross BD, Arcinue E, Caron W, et al, unpublished results), and more subtle aspects of outcome are often illuminated with follow-up MRS[64] (Fig. 30–22; three spectra for patient 2).

For patients with head injury, MRI is informative in most cases, but MRS shows an even wider range of abnormalities, some of which are apparent in normal-looking brains. MRS might reflect diffuse axonal injury. In severe cases, hypoxic encephalopathy (see ND example later) or reduction of the NAA level may be used to predict poor outcome.[36, 65]

MR SPECTROSCOPY OF EPILEPSY
(see Chapter 22)

There is little doubt that MRS, carefully performed, can distinguish between the two temporal lobes in patients with intractable epilepsy. The NAA/Cr ratio is significantly reduced in the affected lobe. This information is being used both to avoid surface electroencephalographic electrodes and ultimately to guide sur-

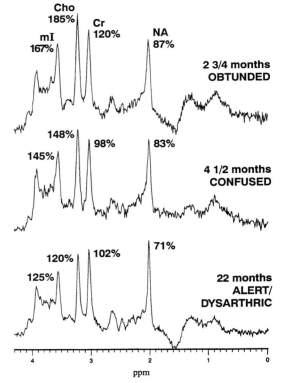

FIGURE 30–22. MRS progression after trauma. Spectra for the parietal white matter of a 28-year-old woman in a hyperosmolar state after head injury.

TABLE 30–7. PRINCIPAL NEUROCHEMICAL CHANGES OF STROKE*

	HYPOXIA (ND)	ISCHEMIA	HEMORRHAGE
Instant	pH ↓, lactate ↑, PCr ↓, ATP ↓	?	?
Early	NAA ↓, lactate ↑ or normal (determines outcome)	NAA ↓, lactate ↑ (lipid ?) Reversible ?	Poor spectral quality
Late	NAA ↓ ↓, lactate ↑ ↑, Cr ↓, lipid ↑	Lactate ↓	Diffuse axonal injury ± lactate ± lipid common
Chronic	NAA ↓, Cho ↑, mI ↑, lipid ↑ ↑	Lactate ↑ or ↓	? elevated Cho

*? signifies insufficient clinical studies. ↑ ↓ indicate metabolite increased or decreased; ↑ ↑ or ↓ ↓ indicate dominating increase or decrease in metabolite concentration.

gery. Relevant references were given in the section on seizure and epilepsies.

STROKE AND CEREBRAL ISCHEMIA
(see Chapter 24)

In general, it can be stated with confidence that MRS is more sensitive than MRI in detecting hypoxic damage (related to vascular or other disease) and is also diagnostic at a much earlier stage in the disease. Thus, whereas the exquisite sensitivity of MRI to developing cerebral edema gives warnings as early as 2 to 4 hours after vascular occlusion, MRS is affected within seconds and would certainly give positive results at the earliest moment at which a clinician condoned the risks of moving the patient to the MRS suite. Indeed, several studies in the past 8 years confirm in humans

what was well established in experimental animals, that a characteristic metabolite profile occurs in strokes. MRS of stroke is reviewed extensively by Howe and colleagues.[66]

The nature, chronology, and severity of biochemical insults that can be anticipated both early and later after a major stroke are detailed in Table 30–7 and illustrated by Figures 30–23 to 30–25.

Stroke is a complex disorder, with three major pathogenetic components: hypoxia, ischemia, and hemorrhage. Each has a characteristic pathologic biochemistry. Next, the type of pathologic injury has its own impact on the biochemical evolution of the stroke. This component is reflected in the complex events that characterize MRS changes observed in stroke over time. Finally, and probably of the greatest clinical significance, graded injuries are apparent depending on the distance from the nearest fully oxygenated loca-

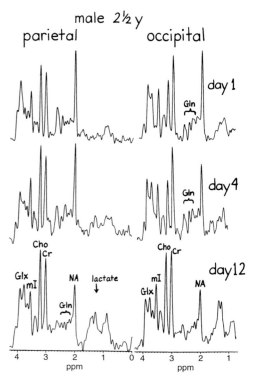

FIGURE 30–23. MRS progression in hypoxia after ND. More severe regional changes are considered to be due to a "watershed" effect. Thus, NA falls earlier and more severely in the occipital than in the parietal location, where excess Glx and lactate are also more marked.

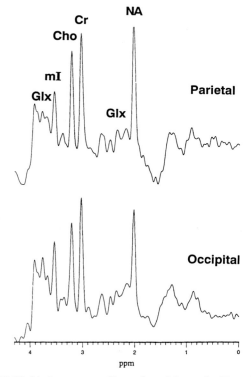

FIGURE 30–24. Long-term effect of partial anoxia. Note that the NAA/Cr ratio is reduced, with the effect being most marked in the gray matter of occipital cortex (watershed area?). The Cho/Cr ratio is inappropriately elevated in the occipital region of interest, possibly another consequence of hypoxia. Spectra from a 3-month-old child.

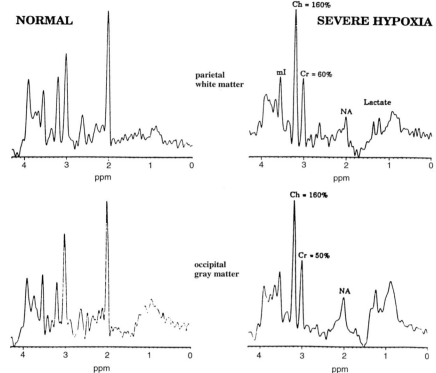

FIGURE 30–25. Spectra from a 17-year-old asthmatic patient with cardiac arrest. The spectra from parietal white matter and occipital gray matter show identical dramatic loss of NA and a small quantity of lactate. The values for Cho and Cr refer to quantitative elevation and loss of each metabolite, indicative of severe long-standing hypoxic damage.

tion. This is the concept of watershed injuries in global ischemia and of the "penumbra" of salvageable brain tissue as distance from the stroke center increases.[67]

Chemical-Shift Imaging of Stroke

Single-voxel MRS has been used to define all of the biochemical changes in stroke: loss of NAA and Cr and accumulation of lactate and Cho. The all-important features, including the extent and severity of ischemia and the peripheral penumbra, can best be defined by CSI[57, 68] (Fig. 30–26). Figure 30–26A demonstrates the presence of both lipid and lactate in typical single-voxel ^{1}H spectrum after stroke.[69]

Clinical Implications

It has not yet become clear how and when to apply this wealth of metabolic information in stroke management. Welch[8] emphasized the need for early assessment of stroke to determine salvageable volumes within a 6-hour therapeutic "window." Few MRS studies have actually been performed in this time; several (including that illustrated) are achieved within 24 hours. This may be called "acute," and the value of MRS may be in diagnosis of ischemic damage. Late changes, including further loss of NAA, accumulation of lactate and lipid,[69] and the late "reappearance" of lactate first noted by Petroff and colleagues,[70] may also be of clinical interest if methods for dealing with the secondary repair after stroke become available.[71]

Newer results from Prichard and colleagues[72] summarize their experience with 32 patients examined at approximately day 5. Lactate intensity in the "worst" CSI voxel correlated with: 1) lesion size, 2) SPECT score, 3) Toronto stroke scale, and 4) outcome index. NAA, by contrast, correlated with outcome index but not with items 1 to 3. Lipid and Cho or Cr changes were not considered. Barker and coworkers[73] concurred with others that these additional biochemical markers also convey clinical information, possibly even with prognostic value.

The ultimate role of MRS is therefore still unclear, but to the present observers it is apparent that Welch is correct—the earlier MRS is performed, the more likely we are to see potentially salvageable tissues conserved by therapy. Conversely, new precision in prognosis after stroke—a notoriously difficult area of medical management—can already be offered by MRS performed as early as 5 days and as late as several weeks after stroke.

All of these considerations provide strong evidence that MRS is beneficial for stroke patients.

FUNCTIONAL MR SPECTROSCOPY
(see Chapter 26)

FMRI has opened new areas of brain research and diagnosis and has brought MRI one step closer to MRS. Whereas single MRS determinations are static and only remotely linked to brain function, rapidly sequential MRS acquisitions can be truly regarded as functional MRS and can be used to define further the physiologic responses to activation.

Functional MRS currently involves two concepts: 1)

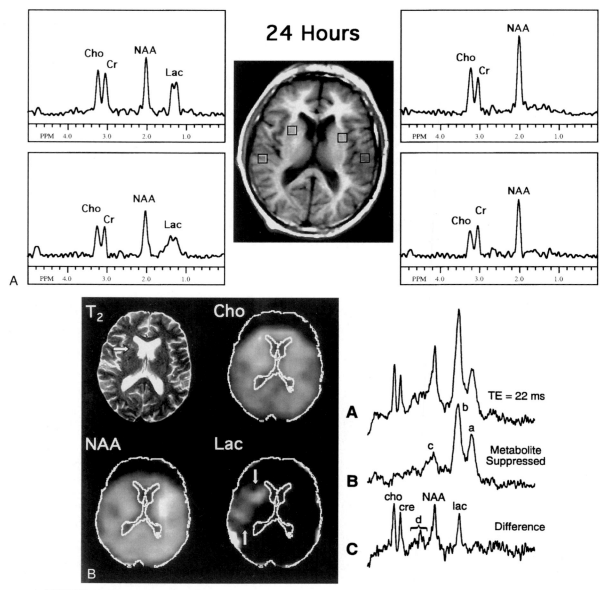

FIGURE 30–26. Spectra obtained 23 days after subcortical stroke. Heterogeneity of metabolism is readily identified, with the potential advantage of identifying salvageable neuronal tissue in the stroke "penumbra." Compare with Figure 30–18. *A,* Individual spectra abstracted from a CSI data set numbered on the MR image. *B,* Lactate excess and loss of NAA from the stroke are confirmed in metabolite images. (*A* and *B* courtesy of Peter Barker, PhD, Johns Hopkins University, Baltimore, MD.) *Inset: A,* Definition of lipid and lactate in an infarct single-voxel difference technique *(C)* based on the ability of an inversion recovery pulse *(B)* to remove low-molecular-weight metabolites from the spectrum. (*Inset* spectra *A, B,* and *C,* courtesy of J. W. Prichard, MD, Yale University, New Haven, CT.)

localized water proton spectroscopy (hemoglobin/oxy-hemoglobin = T2* of water) and 2) metabolic flux (glucose → lactate; glucose → glutamate [TCA cycle]; PCr ⇌ ATP → ADP; NAA → ?).

Localized Water Proton Spectroscopy

This method[74, 75] can detect changes in hemoglobin oxygenation in larger brain volumes with a time resolution of 0.025 to 5 seconds. This lower limit is so superior to that achieved by FMRI that new, fast response of the occipital cortex to visual stimulation becomes apparent. It remains to be seen whether this is sufficient to monitor all-important communication pathways within the brain, which are currently beyond the reach of FMRI.

Metabolic Flux

The more familiar aspects of this topic are dealt with later in the section on metabolic disease. Here we deal exclusively with the modern use—functional brain activation in response to sensory, motor, or even cognitive tasks.

Glucose consumption in the occipital cortex increases with visual stimulation. This is inferred from the demonstration by Merboldt and colleagues[76] that the steady-state cerebral glucose concentration (0.8 mM) falls to about 0.4 mM during 16-Hz photic stimulation and confirmed by the calculation of cerebral metabolic rate in similar ^{1}H MRS studies.[77] Glucose flux in the occipital cortex increases 22% in response to 8-Hz photic stimulation.

Enhanced lactate production from glucose (the direct result of falling glucose concentration) in response to photic stimulation is less certain. Sappey-Marinier[78] and Prichard[79] and their colleagues observed the expected increase in steady-state concentration of lactate, but Merboldt and coworkers[76] reported no change. Finally, flux into [^{13}C]glutamate increased with photic stimulation, confirming that TCA cycle activity (and presumably oxygen consumption) also increases.

Together, this information is consistent and vital to the understanding of FMRI, because slow metabolic adaptation must occur to support the detectable blood flow and oxygenation responses if there is a physiologic basis for these phenomena. Applications of these and other largely ^{1}H-based MRS examinations to the analysis of function in other brain areas are probably premature. Changes in NAA concentration are not to be expected, but changes in PCr (as a reflection of increased ADP concentration) and possibly even total Cr, as well as pH[78, 80] (Lee JH, Ernst T, Farrow N, unpublished observations), have a theoretic basis.

WHITE MATTER DISEASES
(see Chapters 27 and 28)

Aging Brain

The checkered history of deep white matter changes at MRI—they have been considered in turn MS, deep white matter infarcts, and signs of normal aging—is somewhat clearer since the advent of MRS. P. B. Barker (personal communication) and Weiner and colleagues[81, 82] have demonstrated that even quite sizable deep white matter infarct areas in the centrum ovale have normal metabolite ratios on long-TE MRS. No evidence of lactate or of an elevated Cho/Cr ratio in deep white matter infarcts has been obtained. This removes any suggestion that these brain regions are

actually ischemic. However, the fact remains that 84% of patients with cerebrovascular risk factors have deep white matter infarcts and only 10% of control subjects have them. MRS shows definite but small changes in the "normal" ^{1}H MRS profile of the aging brain. The NAA/Cr ratio and NAA level fall in (occipital) gray matter. The Cho/Cr ratio is higher on average than in younger normal subjects, and the mI/Cr ratio is somewhat lower. None of these changes exceed 10%, even up to the age of 90+ years (Table 30–8).

Multiple Sclerosis

Because it is the pattern of distribution rather than specific appearance that aids the detection of MS, MRI is greatly superior to MRS in diagnosis. However, despite useful studies with gadolinium enhancement, dating of MS plaques and, in particular, correlating acute activity in the plaque with neurologic activity in the patient have been only partially successful. This task becomes increasingly urgent as effective therapies are introduced in clinical trials. When the plaque is large enough to be analyzed with a single MRS voxel, the following changes are characteristic[66]: a low NAA/Cr ratio is universally recorded, the Cho/Cr ratio is generally elevated,[83] and the mI/Cr ratio is increased in short-TE spectra[38, 84] (Moats RA, Mandigo JC, Watson L, et al, submitted).

Progression of MS is more clearly documented by reduction in the NAA/Cr ratio than by MRI.[83, 85] Activity in the MS plaque is also well defined by MRS. Surveys in Canada[84] and the United Kingdom[86] indicate that large, extremely active, acute MS lesions have a characteristic ^{1}H MR spectrum (Fig. 30–27). Lipid, lactate, high Cho/Cr ratio, and elevated mI have been interpreted as evidence of myelin breakdown and acute activity in seven of eight cases[84] and 10 of 24 lesions.[86] In some instances, reversal of these changes has been reported, and there are indications that this is accompanied by regression of the acute neurologic symptoms.[87] In single-voxel MRS studies of brain regions containing chronic MS plaques, an increased mI/Cr ratio may be the only residual change (Koopmans R, Michaelis T, Wycoff R, Ross B, unpublished work, 1993). It seems probable, therefore, that the addition of MRS to routine MRI for patients with established MS would improve activity assessment. This could translate into improved quality of clinical trials

TABLE 30–8. FINDINGS FOR NORMAL AGING*

AGE RANGE (y)	N	NAA/CR	CHO/CR	mI/CR
Gray matter				
16–25	10	1.41 ± 0.08	0.56 ± 0.05	0.60 ± 0.04
26–37	10	1.38 ± 0.08	0.61 ± 0.08	0.60 ± 0.04
40–78	12	1.26 ± 0.09	0.60 ± 0.05	0.59 ± 0.06
White matter				
16–25	10	1.54 ± 0.09	0.77 ± 0.05	0.59 ± 0.05
26–37	10	1.49 ± 0.07	0.78 ± 0.06	0.60 ± 0.04
40–78	12	1.41 ± 0.12	0.82 ± 0.08	0.63 ± 0.05

*Valid for TE of 30 ms, TR of 1500, 3000, and 5000 ms.

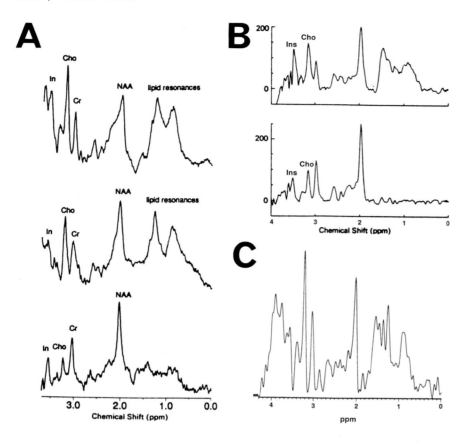

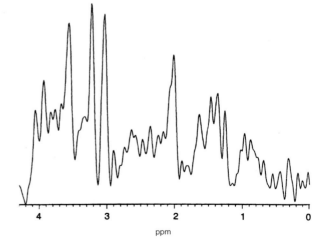

FIGURE 30–27. Active MS plaque. Comparable MRS appearances were reported from London *(A)*, Edmonton *(B)*, and Pasadena *(C)* in large enhancing lesions. The spectrum in *C* is quantitative, indicating percentages of control values for NAA (66%), Cr (50%), and Cho (170%), with lipid, lactate, and possibly alanine present.

of newer therapeutic agents, that is, management of patients.

Leukodystrophies

In the past, the term leukodystrophy was used to describe both adult and infantile white matter diseases. Childhood diseases, which are increasingly recognized from specific patterns of change in MRI,[22] are dealt with in the earlier section on inborn errors. Undifferentiated white matter disease appears to be rare. The MRS patterns have not been described in any large series of patients. In children, adrenoleukodystrophy (ALD), metachromatic leukodystrophy, Canavan's disease, Alexander's disease, and a leukodystrophy with universally low ^{1}H metabolite levels[88] have been to some extent characterized by ^{1}H MRS. Because these disorders have all been considered as disorders of myelination (a view that is no longer accurate), they are considered in detail in the earlier section (see Figs. 30–8 and 30–9). All result in rather impressive changes in the ^{1}H spectrum, varying from a minor change in sI in a preclinical case of ALD, through NAA depletion and increased Cho/Cr ratio in ALD with normal MRI but biochemical evidence of ALD, to major disturbances of the MR spectrum for the regions of the brain shown by MRI to be most affected.

Leukoencephalitides

Diseases that clearly involve an infectious agent, such as herpes encephalitis and Rasmussen's disease, not surprisingly result in major abnormalities of the MR spectrum. The specificity of these changes to one disease has not been established, and although the neurochemical disturbance is striking in newborns, children, and adults (Fig. 30–28), it is not known whether any or all of these changes are reversible. Hence, the possible role of MRS in prognosis remains to be explored.

The anatomic extent of the disease might be determined with MRS, as the focal form of Rasmussen's disease, for example, appears to be associated with

FIGURE 30–28. Herpes encephalitis. PROBE spectrum from parietal cortex. Low signal-to-noise ratio implies loss of brain mass. Cho, mI, and lactate are increased relative to Cr, and NAA is reduced.

normal spectroscopic findings for brain areas that are normal at MRI and grossly abnormal spectra of the focal lesion(s).

Radiation Effects

The MRI appearance of the brain after widespread x-irradiation is characteristic, but the differentiation of this from edema of unknown cause is not straightforward. MRS patterns for a brain exposed to x-rays can be strikingly abnormal, even when the MRI finding is unimpressive, with loss of NAA and an increase in Cho. Radiation necrosis in the presence or absence of recurrent brain tumor has already been discussed; studies using the Cho/Cr ratio to differentiate between the two entities appear promising.

The first effects of radiation are on the endothelium, but this does not result in any observable change at MRI. Demyelination, which appears about 6 to 8 months after radiation and continues to develop for up to 2 years, as judged by MRI, must surely be preceded by some of these changes in MRS. If so, then MRS offers predictive value for the extent and severity of postirradiation necrosis.

INFLAMMATION

Human Immunodeficiency Virus and Acquired Immunodeficiency Syndrome
(see Chapter 20)

The case of human immunodeficiency virus (HIV) infection is instructive and may apply to other, better understood inflammatory diseases of the brain. Several authorities reported a steady decline of the NAA/Cr ratio in patients who are HIV positive but do not yet have proven AIDS. More striking is the reporting of positive MRS findings in patients with HIV serologic results but normal MRI findings at the time of the MRS examination.[89–97] Although better sequences, more careful reading, or more rigorous evaluations of immunologic status could explain such a discrepancy, the most likely answer is that MRS, by detecting the unsuspected underlying neurochemical changes of HIV infection, gives an early warning of MRI changes to come. The therapeutic consequences of this conclusion are striking, particularly for such a generally serious disease. If treatment of HIV can prevent neurologic deterioration,[97] then MRS must become an indispensable tool in this area.

Other infections of the central nervous system might behave similarly, but we do not have the results of clinical studies in hand. If herpes encephalitis can be defined before overt changes are seen with MRI, it is to be hoped that outcomes of treatment would be significantly improved by performing and interpreting ^{1}H MRS.

Several studies define abnormal MRS in association with abnormalities of MRI in encephalitis, HIV, and AIDS-related masses. There is persuasive evidence that MRS changes precede those in MRI, so there is a debate about what to do when a patient manifests such MRS changes (in particular, reduced NAA and increased Cho). We lack reports of systematic MRS studies of abscess, meningitis, and encephalitis.

Several neurologic complications of AIDS are recognized, and MRI is the method of choice for their detection and differentiation. In cases in which focal lesions still prove difficult to diagnose, yet therapeutic choices demand an accurate answer, preliminary studies with MRS look promising. Figure 30–29 shows such a study, in which it was concluded that MRS could displace unpopular and hazardous brain biopsy in this clinical arena (Miller BL, personal communication, 1995).

Hydrocephalus (see Chapter 29)

From the MR radiologist's perspective, the major goal for MR is to distinguish hydrocephalus from brain atrophy (what used to be known as hydrocephalus ex vacuo) with sufficient certainty to guide therapy. As the universal choice for treatment of other forms of hydrocephalus is invasive surgery, with installation of a shunt in both infants and adults, this is not a trivial issue. Initally, it was believed that transependymal flow, with periventricular hyperintensity on MR images, characterized true hydrocephalus and could be used to indicate an increase in intraventricular pressure with confidence. The work of Zimmerman and coworkers[98] appears to refute this. Detection of a flow void is now taken as the hallmark. In case of remaining diagnostic confusion, there is a strong suggestion that MRS does, or will, differentiate these disease entities with a high degree of certainty.

Atrophy is characterized by enlarged ventricles and widened sulci; if this differentiator is applicable in adults with dilated ventricles, then the CSF and brain water assay of Ernst and colleagues[99] can be applied. In a series of patients presenting with dementia, the atrophy index was always increased. The effect was significantly greater in patients with probable AD than other forms of dementia, but it cannot be used alone to diagnose AD (see section on degenerative diseases). The MRS brain water assay is performed as follows. On an axial image, a voxel 20 mm thick and 27 mm anteroposterior by 21 mm wide, bridging the calcarine sulcus of the left and right occipital lobes, is prescribed. Water T2-weighted signal is determined from seven different TE acquisitions, plotted as a double exponential. Three (rather than two) compartments are defined: brain water, CSF (7% to 25% or even 30%), and dry matter. As described by Ernst and colleagues, the CSF compartment in this location is an atrophy index. Indeed, it is increased as expected, from 10% in normal elderly people to 15% in those with general dementias and 18% in those with AD. In three patients with normal-pressure hydrocephalus, however, the atrophy index was increased also (Blüml S, Ross B, unpublished observations, 1995). Furthermore, for patients with severe ventricular dilatation and for infants, the inclusion of ventricular CSF in the

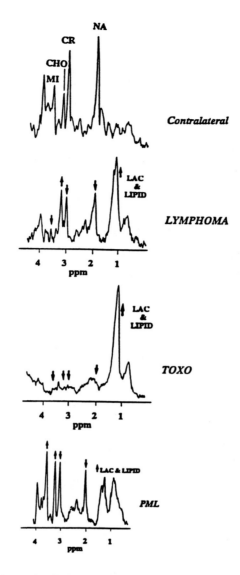

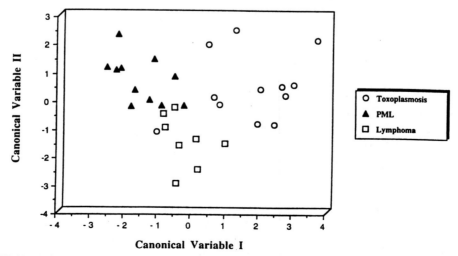

Stepwise Discriminant Analysis of Brain Masses in AIDS

○ Toxoplasmosis
▲ PML
□ Lymphoma

FIGURE 30–29. ¹H MRS readily distinguishes the different metabolite profiles of commonly occurring AIDS brain masses. (Modified from Chang L, Miller BL: Proton magnetic resonance spectroscopy of brain lesions in AIDS. Radiology 197:525–531, 1995.)

prescribed voxel is inevitable, with considerable loss of sensitivity for this atrophy assay.

Cortical atrophy implies relative loss of gray matter. The MR spectrum should reflect the increased proportion of white matter in the standard occipital gray matter location. The most obvious difference between white matter and gray matter spectra is the relative increase in Cho (Cho/Cr = 0.83 versus 0.59). Proportional increases in the Cho/Cr ratio of gray matter are sometimes but not always noted in patients with atrophy related to dementia. In patients with normal-pressure hydrocephalus, the Cho/Cr ratio is significantly increased, but the number of patients is still too small for diagnostic certainty. For infants younger than 1 year of age, this assay is of limited value, because the Cho/Cr ratio is higher anyway than in older children and exceeds the normal white matter value of adults.

Atrophy ex vacuo implies loss of brain substance and destruction of nervous tissue with quantitative loss of key neurochemicals. NAA, the neuronal marker, is exquisitely sensitive to nutritional deprivation, whether because of oxygen lack or vascular occlusion. It is not surprising, therefore, that a reduced NAA/Cr ratio is a frequent finding in pediatric neurospectroscopy. In one case investigated, a shunt had been placed several months earlier after the detection of marked ventricular dilatation at 6 months of age. However, pressure was not elevated, and the child's condition continued to deteriorate. MRS showed a significant reduction in the NAA/Cr ratio of the remnant rim of cerebral cortex. It seems most likely, therefore, that cortical atrophy and loss of brain substance were consequences of prior metabolic disease. Although no neuropathologic diagnosis is yet available for this child, hydrocephalus was probably ruled out by the use of MRS.

The increased pressure of true hydrocephalus impairs nutrient supply and particularly limits energy supply to the developing brain. In the absence of the ependymal brightness sign of increased and persistent high intraventricular pressure, how are we to determine that this is the case and accordingly develop a higher index of suspicion of the need for emergency shunting? If the mechanism suggested is correct, then cerebral PCr and ATP should fall. Although ^{31}P MRS, the logical method for finding this, has not been performed, we have reported one case[100] in which combined PCr imaging and ^{1}H MRS were used to demonstrate a reduction in the putative energy markers of cerebral function. Apart from hydrocephalus in the presence of a shunt and nebulous neurologic symptoms, this 26-year-old patient had normal imaging studies. A significantly reduced Cr level was determined in quantitative ^{1}H MRS. The PCr image of the surviving cortex had somewhat low intensity, indicating possible loss of PCr throughout the compressed brain.

In summary, MRS has a potentially valuable role in examination of hydrocephalus, in which conventional MRI leaves some important unanswered questions. MR CSF flow methods are more sensitive than conventional MRI but are surprisingly little used. No comparative study of MRS versus CSF flow methods has been performed to date.

DEGENERATIVE DISEASES (see Chapter 29)

Parkinson's Disease

Parkinson's disease is a disorder of the dopa and dopamine system, particularly in the basal ganglia. It is perhaps not surprising, therefore, that despite a carefully conducted multicenter trial, no reproducible abnormalities have been defined by ^{1}H MRS at long TE values. There may be some differences in the spectra for the basal ganglia in treated versus untreated Parkinson's disease, but we must be cautious because of the virtually diagnostic excess of iron in this region and the resulting susceptibility changes in Parkinson's disease as shown by MRI.

Alzheimer's Disease

CT and MRI performed in a routine way make little direct contribution to the diagnosis of dementia or of AD in particular. Their role is to eliminate other, usually space-occupying disorders. With special measurements, the temporal lobe atrophy can become a rather specific and sensitive tool for the diagnosis of late AD. On the other hand, MRS is showing genuine promise of defining dementia (based on the reduction in NAA/Cr ratio and of NAA level). In more than one series, the addition of even nonquantitative MRS improved the precision of diagnosis of AD when added to MRI.[101] Elevation of the Cho/Cr ratio (although predicted by postmortem studies) is neither reproducible nor specific to AD, because the Cho/Cr ratio increases with age and in several other conditions, including stroke and possibly multiple-infarct dementia. More specificity and a possible alternative view of pathogenesis are accorded by the measurement of the mI/Cr ratio in short-TE MRS. The mI/Cr ratio and mI level are increased (Figs. 30–30 and 30–31). Other dementias share the feature of a low NAA/Cr ratio, but the mI/Cr ratio distinguishes AD from normal older age and from other dementias (Figs. 30–32 and 30–33).

Dementia in Down's syndrome, which is pathogenetically similar to AD, is also marked by an increased mI/Cr ratio (Fig. 30–34). It is possible, therefore, that both in ruling out AD in the elderly and in making an early diagnosis of dementia in Down's syndrome, MRS will be superior to imaging with either SPECT or MRI. At present, clinical diagnosis of AD has a sensitivity of 80% to 90%. Based on the same clinical criteria (i.e., assuming the sensitivity of this flawed "gold standard" to be 100%), MRS can be equally precise in distinguishing AD from normal with specificity greater than 80%. AD is distinguished from other proven dementias with a specificity of 65%, but AD is excluded with 80% efficiency by the MRS examination.[102]

Pick's Disease

In life, the definition of Pick's disease and its distinction from AD rest on the peculiarly "frontal lobe" clinical symptoms and the obvious frontal lobe atrophy

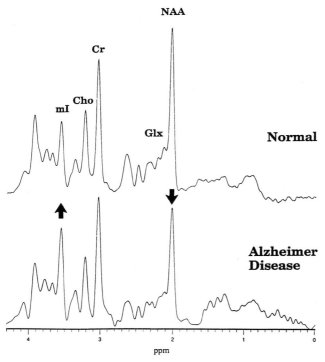

FIGURE 30–30. ¹H MR spectra of the occipital cortex (gray matter) of a patient with probable AD compared with an age-matched normal subject. Peaks are scaled to Cr and provide a measure of concentration of individual metabolites.

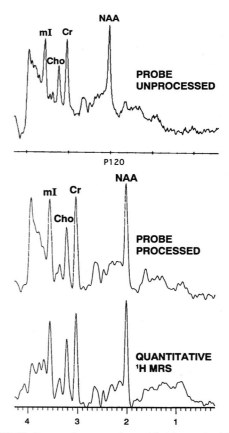

FIGURE 30–31. Spectra from a patient with AD acquired by PROBE *(top)* compared with a quantitative spectrum *(bottom)* of the same patient. Note the increased precision conferred by routine postprocessing of the spectrum *(middle).* (Modified from Shonk TK, Moats RA, Gifford P, et al: Probable Alzheimer disease: diagnosis with proton MR spectroscopy [see comments]. Radiology 195:65–72, 1995.)

revealed by CT or MRI. Neuropathologically, Pick's disease and AD are quite distinct from each other. However, in a limited series, MRS has not been successful in distinguishing frontal lobe dementias (including Pick's) from AD when the single voxel is acquired from the occipital region (see Fig. 30–33). The obvious strategy of examining the frontal lobe has not yet been successful, principally because of the poor magnetic field homogeneity in this brain region. This uncertainty has been resolved by Chang and colleagues,[102a] who found that marked loss of NAA from frontal cortex, excess mI/Cr, and possibly also excess lactate offered a clear distinction between frontal lobe dementia and AD.

Huntington's Disease

Huntington's disease correctly belongs under metabolic diseases, now that MRS has been successful in demonstrating excess lactate in these patients.[103] Furthermore, this disease offers one of the relatively few instances in which MRS has both guided the choice of treatment (coenzyme Q) and monitored its successful implementation.[104]

Creutzfeldt-Jakob Disease

This rare disorder gives few if any clues at MRI. MRS findings, on the other hand, are markedly abnormal in the single case report from Bruhn and colleagues[105]

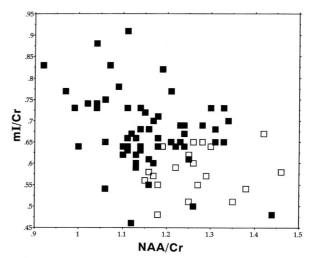

FIGURE 30–32. Distribution of mI/Cr and NAA/Cr ratios in patients with clinically verified probable AD (■) compared with age-matched normal subjects (□). (Modified from Shonk TK, Moats RA, Gifford P, et al: Probable Alzheimer disease: diagnosis with proton MR spectroscopy [see comments]. Radiology 195:65–72, 1995.)

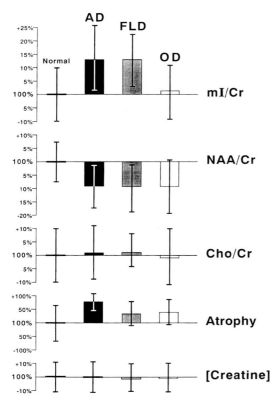

FIGURE 30–33. MRS and CSF volumes (atrophy index) in differentiation of AD from other clinical dementias (OD). Note the marked overlap between frontal lobe dementia (FLD) and AD. (Modified from Shonk TK, Moats RA, Gifford P, et al: Probable Alzheimer disease: diagnosis with proton MR spectroscopy [see comments]. Radiology 195:65–72, 1995.)

(Fig. 30–35) and readily distinguished from findings of AD.

METABOLIC DISEASE (see Chapter 28)

Surprisingly, this area has been remarkably rewarding for MRI. Many reports of pattern recognition related to inborn errors of metabolism serve to make MRI a necessary part of the diagnosis.[22] But the neuroradiologist's contact with metabolic diseases in adults is extremely limited. Central pontine myelinolysis, Leigh's disease, Wilson's disease, and Hallervorden-Spatz disease were the four general areas discussed in the first edition of this book. Although there are several more in the present edition, the impact of MRS is now considerably greater than that of MRI. In general, in the presence of normal or nondiagnostic MRI appearances, carefully selected MRS studies can specifically identify dozens of different neurologic diseases and modify a large area of neurodiagnosis.

Metabolic disturbances of liver, kidney, endocrine, or other systems have remote effects; those of the brain result in a variety of well-defined encephalopathies. When severe, these disorders present as coma. Plum and Posner[106] published a comprehensive account of human coma. Many cases were the result of presumed metabolic events with normal brain anatomy, setting the stage for noninvasive elucidation by means of biochemically based techniques. Among these techniques are MR angiography, diffusion imaging, positron emission tomography, SPECT, and multinuclear NMR spectroscopy (MRS). MRS has increasingly been used to identify specific biochemical changes in the brain, from which information on diagnosis and pathogenesis of these poorly understood disorders is beginning to emerge.

As a model for this group of disorders, we discuss HE, with additional remarks about diabetic, hyperosmolar, and hypoxia-induced encephalopathies.

Hepatic Encephalopathy

A triad of changes (loss of mI, increased Glx, and reduced Cho) characterizes patients with chronic HE, and, more usefully, defines subclinical HE. Patients with transjugular intrahepatic portal-systemic shunt (TIPS) develop these characteristic metabolite changes as evidence of HE after shunting. Transplant recipients undergo complete reversal of these biochemical abnormalities within weeks after successful transplantation. Exaggerated MRS changes are seen in acute fulminant HE and the rare Reye's syndrome even when the MRI results are normal.

Neurochemical Pathology of HE

HE is an excellent example of metabolic encephalopathy,[107] with identifiable neurotoxins originating in

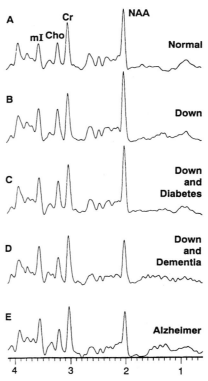

FIGURE 30–34. Dementia of Down's syndrome. The marked similarity of the MR spectrum to that in AD is noted, as is the presumably much earlier onset of one of the two biochemical changes, the increase in the mI/Cr ratio.

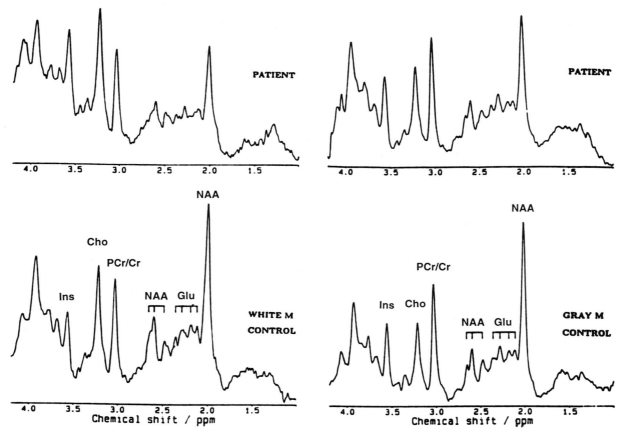

FIGURE 30–35. MR spectra from a patient with Creutzfeldt-Jakob disease at 2 T. Note the excellent definition of glutamate resonances at higher field. The principal change is in white matter (in contrast to AD), with reduction of the NAA/Cr ratio and an apparent increase in mI/Cr and Cho/Cr ratios. The latter is also a distinction from AD.

a systemic disease. In animal studies, several distinct neurotoxins have been identified. The earliest of these was ammonia,[108, 109] which is normally fully removed from portal blood by hepatic urea synthesis.[110, 111] The combination of the loss of biosynthetic liver function and the diversion of nondetoxified blood to the brain by so-called portal-systemic shunts accounts for the frequently demonstrated excess of cerebral and CSF glutamine[112] (Equation 1):

$$NH_4^+ + glutamate \underset{glutaminase}{\overset{GS}{\rightleftharpoons}} glutamine \quad (1)$$

The enzyme glutamine synthetase (GS) responsible for this reaction is located exclusively in astrocytes.[113] Resynthesis of glutamate and of α-aminobutyric acid from glutamine (both vital neurotransmitter amino acids) occurs principally in neurons.[114]

Lest it be thought that ammonia toxicity accounts for all of the clinical syndromes covered by the term HE, the interested reader is referred to Butterworth and Layrargues[115] for an extensive review of several other well-documented alternatives. Metabolic theories abound; failure of oxidative energy metabolism (a corollary of glutamate and 2-oxoglutarate depletion from the Krebs cycle), tryptophan and serotonin (5-hydroxy-

tryptamine) accumulation, branched chain amino acid deficits, endogenous benzodiazepine agonists that modify access of α-aminobutyric acid to its inhibitory receptors, and neurotoxic fatty acids, octanoate in particular, have all been proposed.

An attractive unifying theory proposed by Zieve[116] is that multiple neurotoxins derived from liver, blood, or the diet gain access via portal-systemic shunts to a previously "sensitized" brain. No mechanism of sensitization is known, but with the advent of MRS a candidate has been proposed in the form of cerebral mI depletion.[18]

Animal Studies in HE Using Multinuclear Nuclear Magnetic Resonance Spectroscopy

Three groups[117–119] independently perfected methods for the noninvasive determination of cerebral glutamine (including a variable contribution from glutamate in each assay) with ^{1}H NMR spectroscopy (now referred to as MRS) and confirmed the elevation of this metabolite in a variety of animal models of acute liver failure with HE. One of these groups[117] also demonstrated a hitherto unrecognized abnormality, the significant reduction of cerebral Cho-containing compounds in the ^{1}H spectra of rats with acute HE.

Subsequently, ^{15}N NMR[120, 121] and [1]H-^{15}N hetero-nuclear multiple-quantum coherence identified cerebral glutamine unequivocally in vivo in HE produced by ammonia infusion in the normal and portacaval-shunted rat, respectively.

Finally, in extracts of brain from portacaval-shunted rats, high-performance liquid chromatography confirmed the accumulation of glutamine and the depletion of glycerophosphorylcholine (which is the explanation for the reduced Cho in the prior ^{1}H NMR study), as well as demonstrating the expected depletion by 50% or more of the cerebral mI and sI contents.[122] This result confirmed the observations that first emerged from human studies with short-TE ^{1}H MRS[18, 123, 124] and established the validity of the portacaval-shunted rat for future experimental studies.

Pathogenesis, Diagnosis, and Therapeutic Management of HE in Humans: Emerging Role of Proton MR Spectroscopy

Studies using STEAM-localized, short-TE ^{1}H MRS defined the changes in 10 patients with clinically confirmed chronic HE. The average increase in cerebral glutamine was estimated as 50%, Cho decreased 14%, and mI decreased by 45%[125] (Fig. 30–36). Similar findings have been obtained at 2 T by Bruhn and colleagues[123, 126] and at 1.5 T by McConnell and coworkers[127] using PRESS at short or long TE values.

An early study that used long-TE PRESS-localized ^{1}H MRS failed to identify the depletion of mI but was the first to show clearly Cho depletion in human brain.[128]

Energetics of the Human Brain in HE

The predicted cerebral energy deficit (reduction in ATP concentration) has been shown convincingly only in mice and tree shrews.[129] ^{31}P MRS should be the easiest tool with which to establish any energy deficit in HE (as predicted). Ross,[130] Tropp,[131] Luyten,[132] Barbara,[133] and Morgan[134] and their colleagues have obtained conflicting and hence unconvincing data with ^{31}P MRS on such effects in humans. Using quantitative ^{1}H MRS, however, Geissler and colleagues[135] showed a small and significant increase in cerebral Cr level after liver transplantation in humans. Because total Cr is the sum of PCr and Cr, this may indicate that patients with HE have an energy deficit. The difficulty confronted by ^{31}P MRS in demonstrating such an effect, with a sensitivity 10% that of ^{1}H MRS, becomes obvious. As reduced cerebral oxygen consumption and reduced blood flow are recognized abnormalities in HE, the ^{13}C NMR techniques pioneered by Shulman and associates[136] may be best suited to demonstrate the anticipated reduction in the overall rate of the TCA cycle.

From these clinical studies, it appears that ^{1}H MRS, particularly if applied with effective water suppression to reveal mI, is currently most efficient for the elucidation of pathogenesis of HE and also, as shown later, for its early clinical diagnosis. Direct measurement of mI by ^{13}C NMR may become a valuable adjunct.[137]

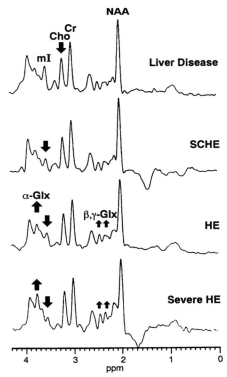

FIGURE 30–36. Development of HE in human subjects (1.5-T spectra). A series of spectra of parietal cortex (white matter) acquired under closely similar conditions (GE Signa, 1.5 T MR scanner, STEAM localization, TR = 1500 ms, TE = 30 ms, number of excitations = 128) from different patients is presented. A normal spectrum for comparison is that in Figure 30–25. The spectrum for liver disease is relatively normal, with a slight decrease in Cho. In subclinical HE (SCHE), there is a definite decrease in mI with a minor increase in the glutamine regions (glutamine plus glutamate = Glx). In HE (grade 1), there is a significant increase in the Glx regions and mI is further depleted. The spectrum in severe (grade 3) HE shows more severe changes in the biochemical markers of this disease, notably glutamine.

Subclinical HE

As indicated, HE is a group of diseases presumed to have identical etiology but presenting a great variety of distinct clinical pictures. Underlying all of them is believed to be the entity of subclinical HE, although it is by no means clear that the HE and coma of fulminant (extremely acute) liver failure goes through any truly subclinical phase.

^{1}H MRS accurately reflects the entity of subclinical HE,[138, 139] and in preliminary studies it also appears to mirror the progressive and increasingly severe syndromes of overt HE defined by Parsons-Smith grades 1 to 4 (see Fig. 30–36). Elevation of glutamine is rather more obvious at 2 T (Fig. 30–37) but presents little difficulty at 1.5 T.

Figure 30–36 should not be taken as proof, however, that in the individual patient such an orderly progression of neurochemical dysfunction occurs. Longitudinal studies have not been performed in sufficient numbers to be certain of this. Nevertheless, it is tempting to suggest, as Figure 30–36 appears to indicate, that in the brain exposed to liver toxins, depletion of Cho

CONTROL

HEPATIC ENCEPHALOPATHY

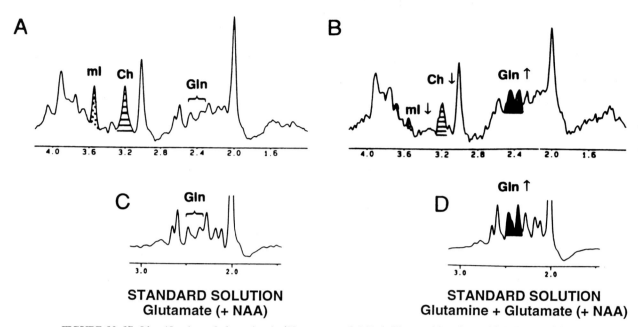

STANDARD SOLUTION
Glutamate (+ NAA)

STANDARD SOLUTION
Glutamine + Glutamate (+ NAA)

FIGURE 30–37. Identification of glutamine in ¹H spectra at 2.0 T. A 51-year-old patient with HE caused by a surgical portacaval shunt is compared with a normal control subject. Spectra were obtained from an occipital gray matter location and show the expected changes of HE: increased glutamine and decreased Cho/Cr and mI/Cr. With the improved resolution at 2 T, separate analysis of glutamine and glutamate is possible. Spectra from model solutions of *(C)* 5 mM glutamate + 5 mM NAA and *(D)* 5 mM glutamine + 5 mM glutamate + 5 mM NAA indicate that in this patient the increase in glutamine occurs without obvious depletion of cerebral glutamate. Spectra were acquired on Siemens 2.0-T clinical spectrometer with STEAM localization; TR/TE = 3000/20. (*A* to *D* modified from Bruhn H, Merboldt K-D, Michaelis T, et al: Proton MRS of metabolic disturbances in the brain of patients with liver cirrhosis and subclinical hepatic encephalopathy. Soc Magn Reson Med 10:400, 1991. Abstract.)

(possibly glycerophosphorylcholine) precedes the loss of mI and sI, with later accumulation of glutamine. If this sequence is correct, perhaps sensitization of the brain is the result of depletion of mI or Cho or both. In keeping with a theory of many years standing, increasing cerebral glutamine underlies the neurologic syndromes of severe, overt, chronic HE of grades 1 to 4, as well as perhaps, that of acute, fulminant HE and coma. Figure 30–38 shows the similar but more severe neurochemical changes of Reye's syndrome, giving an effective indication of what may be seen in acute HE. Unfortunately, published spectra for patients with fulminant HE are limited and difficult to interpret.[140]

myo-Inositol Depletion and the Induction of HE

A human "experiment" that goes some way toward verifying this sequence is the interventional procedure known as TIPS, which is a lifesaving procedure in cirrhosis-induced hematemesis. Not surprisingly, TIPS induces clinical HE in up to 90% of survivors.[138, 141] ¹H MRS performed both before and after TIPS in 10 patients showed a universal increase in mean intracerebral glutamine after the procedure. More important,

in a small number of individuals in whom mI was normal before to TIPS, a progressive reduction in mI/Cr ratio and development of subclinical and clinical HE follow the introduction of the shunt (Fig. 30–39).

Restoration of Cerebral myo-Inositol and Choline Accompanies Reversal of HE

Yet another common human "experiment," that of orthotopic liver transplantation, allows the reverse process to be unequivocally demonstrated, thereby establishing a firm, albeit circumstantial, link between mI depletion and the syndromes of subclinical and overt HE (Fig. 30–40). Glx and Cho also recovered. Indeed, an overshoot of cerebral Cho is consistently observed, perhaps linking the earlier Cho depletion with deficient hepatic biosynthesis of some relevant precursor of glycerophosphorylcholine.

Ornithine Transcarbamylase Deficiency

A description of MRS in HE would be incomplete without consideration of a rare but informative inborn error of hepatic urea synthesis, ornithine transcarbamylase deficiency. The single known biochemical consequence is hyperammonemia. Gadian and colleagues[142] demonstrated the inevitable elevation of cerebral glutamine in two such patients (see Fig. 30–9), and Ross and coworkers[19] showed the extraordinary parallel with HE in depletion of cerebral mI.

Contribution of Nuclear Magnetic Resonance in Clinical HE

PATHOGENESIS OF HE. Both experimentally and clinically, NMR (particularly ^{1}H MRS) supports the classic concept of HE as a disorder of cerebral ammonia metabolism, whether it involves ammonia toxicity or glutamine synthesis (as a newer variant of the theory would have it).[143] The concept of an underlying brain

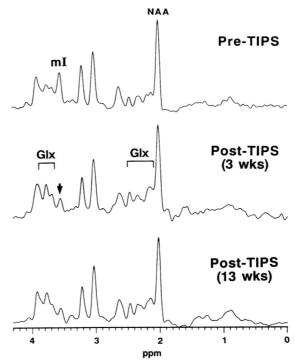

FIGURE 30–39. Effect of TIPS on the ^{1}H MR spectrum. Spectra are for a 30-year-old woman, 5 days after a hematemesis caused by esophageal varices and chronic alcoholic liver disease. Spectra acquired from a parietal white matter location (GE Signa, 1.5 T, volume = 12.5 cm³, STEAM TR = 1500 ms, TE = 30 ms, number of excitations = 128) before the TIPS procedure show no abnormalities apart from a small but significant reduction in Cho/Cr ratio, attributable to liver disease (top). Three weeks after TIPS, changes are seen in the Glx and mI regions and there is a further reduction of the Cho/Cr ratio (middle). The bottom spectrum shows the progression of changes seen 13 weeks after TIPS; Glx is markedly increased and mI is significantly reduced. (From Shonk T, Moats R, Lee JH, et al: Increased incidence of sub-clinical hepatic encephalopathy associated with TIPS procedure. Gastroenterology 104:A-449, 1993. Abstract.)

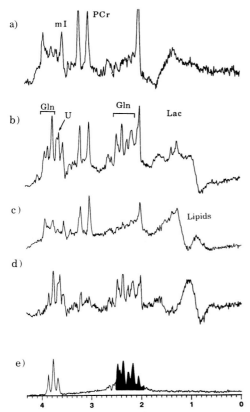

FIGURE 30–38. ^{1}H MRS in acute HE associated with Reye's syndrome. In vivo ^{1}H MR spectra were acquired from a parietal white matter region in infant brain from (a) a 10-month-old normal subject and a patient on (b) day 2 after admission and (c) day 8 after admission. d, Difference (b − c) between day 2 and day 8. e, Solution with 15 mM glutamine. All spectra are scaled. Spectral assignments: Lac = lactate (1.3 ppm); NAA (2.02 ppm); Gln = glutamine (2.10 to 2.50 ppm and 3.65 to 3.90 ppm); Cr + PCr (3.03 ppm); Cho = choline-containing compounds (3.23 ppm); mI (3.56 ppm); X = unassigned (3.62 ppm). Notable abnormalities are a huge accumulation of cerebral glutamine, reduced Cho, and later reduced mI, all of which reflect liver failure. In addition, there are decreases in NAA and Cr and appearance of the unassigned peak. Reye's syndrome, a toxic viral disease associated with aspirin intake, produces severe neuronal damage and may not therefore completely correspond to the picture of acute liver failure. An occipital gray matter region gave almost identical results. (a to e from Ernst T, Ross BD, Flores R: Cerebral MRS in infant with suspected Reye's syndrome. Lancet 340 [8817]:486, 1992. Letter. © by The Lancet Ltd 1992.)

sensitization receives substantial new impetus and deserves further research in animal models. Either "Cho" (glycerophosphorylcholine) depletion, perhaps resulting from failure of hepatic synthesis of a necessary precursor, or cerebral mI depletion could fulfill the role of sensitizer. In neither case is there a precedent, so basic research is urgently required. NMR is likely to play a crucial role in such investigations, and the portacaval-shunted rat is a convenient model. ^{13}C NMR and ^{31}P NMR are the only methods for unequivocally determining mI as distinct from the lower concentrations of inositol 1-phosphate and glycine with which mI coresonates in the ^{1}H MR spectrum.

PROTON MR SPECTROSCOPY FOR DIAGNOSIS. Early in these investigations, it became apparent that mI depletion and Glx accumulation occurred when clinical HE was absent. Other systemic or metabolic diseases (apart from ornithine transcarbamylase deficiency, already discussed) did not result in mI depletion, so ^{1}H MRS offers a unique opportunity for early, specific diagnosis of this still perplexing condition. Paradoxically, there is at present little enthusiasm

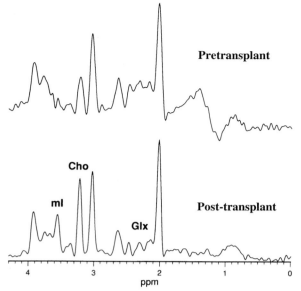

FIGURE 30–40. Restoration of biochemical abnormalities after liver transplantation. The patient was a 30-year-old man with chronic HE secondary to hepatitis, subsequently successfully treated by liver transplantation. Spectra were acquired 6 months apart from the same parietal white matter location (15.0 cm³, STEAM, TR = 1500 ms, TE = 30 ms, 128 excitations) and scaled to the same Cr intensity for comparison. The abnormalities before liver transplantation, increased α-, β-, and γ-glutamine and reduced the Cho/Cr and mI/Cr ratios *(upper spectrum)*, were completely reversed 3 months after transplantation and the Cho/Cr ratio exceeded normal *(lower spectrum)*.

for this, probably because prevention (with lactulose or neomycin) and treatment (by liver transplantation) of overt or severe HE is relatively straightforward (albeit rather costly in the case of orthotopic liver transplantation. If a ready medical means of restoring cerebral mI were to be discovered, the value of ¹H MRS in diagnosis might increase.

UNANSWERED QUESTIONS IN NEUROLOGY OF HE. Wilson's disease, caused by excess copper deposition, is believed to result in an encephalopathy analogous to HE. Not surprisingly, the ¹H MRS findings in Wilson's disease are rather different, lacking either mI depletion or glutamine accumulation (Ross B, Weiner L, unpublished observations, 1992).

Myelopathy can be a rare presenting feature of chronic HE. It presents with paraplegia. Although neurologic considerations suggest cord involvement, the ¹H MRS findings in the parietal cortex are typical of those for other patients with the more classic clinical presentation (see figure 4 in Ross and coworkers[19]).

Often noted in MRI, the basal ganglia may be "bright" in inversion recovery images of patients with known HE. There is no consistent relationship to ¹H MRS findings (mI depletion, reduced Cho/Cr ratio, and excess Glx are observed in this location), and increasingly this MRI finding is recognized as nonspecific. Nevertheless, the extrapyramidal signs, the changes on postmortem examination, and these inconsistent MRI findings continue to suggest that there

may be as yet unrecognized underlying neurochemical changes in the basal ganglia in HE.

Other Systemic Encephalopathies

Diabetes Mellitus

Like HE, diabetic encephalopathy is common and obviously metabolic in origin. Three principal syndromes are recognized: diabetic ketoacidosis, lactic acidosis, and nonketotic hyperosmolar coma.

Elevated cerebral glucose,[144] significant excess of mI, a reversible accumulation of Cho, and the presence of ketone bodies have been detected in various patients with varying severity of diabetic encephalopathy.[37]

The most surprising finding of ¹H MRS, which requires further study, is the identification of acetone (rather than the more widely anticipated β-hydroxybutyric acid and acetoacetate) as the ketone of human diabetic ketoacidotic encephalopathy[37] (Fig. 30–41).

Long-term neurologic and cerebral complications of

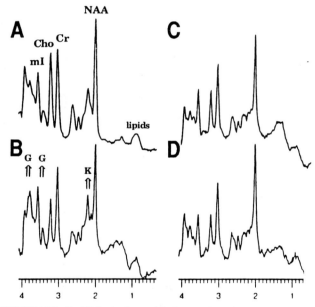

FIGURE 30–41. Diabetic ketoacidosis: cerebral ¹H spectra during two episodes and recovery. *A*, Episode 1, spectrum acquired 3 days after admission to hospital, at a time when the patient had supposedly totally recovered and was ready to be discharged. A peak characteristic of the presence of ketone (K) bodies was noted at 2.22 ppm, obtained from an 18-cm³ volume in the left parietal lobe. The patient relapsed into diabetic ketoacidosis 2 days later. *B*, Episode 2, spectrum acquired 5 months later from an occipital gray matter location (10.3 cm³) during a second episode. In addition to the ketone peak, peaks for glucose (G) were seen. *C*, Recovery, 6 days after episode 2 (from the same occipital location), when no more ketone bodies were detected in the urine. *D*, Occipital cortex of an age- and sex-matched healthy subject. Acquisition conditions: GE Signa, 1.5 T, 4X software; STEAM, TR = 1500 ms, TE = 30 ms, 128 excitations. More detailed analysis of peak K indicates the resonance frequency to be that of acetone rather than acetoacetate, the ketone body more commonly identified in blood and urine of diabetics in coma. (*A* to *D* from Kreis R, Ross BD: Cerebral metabolic disturbances in patients with sub-acute and chronic diabetes mellitus by proton magnetic resonance spectroscopy. Radiology 184:123–130, 1992.)

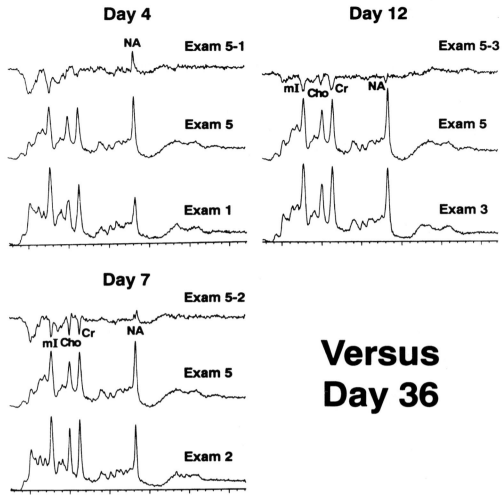

Day 4

Exam 5-1

NA

Exam 5

Exam 1

Day 12

Exam 5-3

mI Cho Cr NA

Exam 5

Exam 3

Day 7

Exam 5-2

mI Cho Cr NA

Exam 5

Exam 2

Versus Day 36

FIGURE 30–42. Time course of changes in principal cerebral organic osmolytes during correction of severe dehydration. A series of spectra were obtained from the same (occipital gray matter) brain location in a 14-month-old child recovering from severe dehydration and hypernatremia (plasma sodium 195 mEq/L, normal range 135 to 142 mEq/L) using identical acquisition conditions. Spectra were processed and scaled identically to permit subtraction of sequential spectra (difference spectroscopy). The day of examination refers to the interval since admission to the hospital. Examinations are numbered sequentially, from first (exam 1) to last (exam 5) on day 36. Compared with a relevant normal spectrum (spectrum *D* in Fig. 30–41), the principal abnormality appears to be reversal of the intensities of NAA (reduced) and mI (increased), so that mI dominates the spectrum. These changes slowly reverse and are nearly normal on day 36. The resultant difference spectra more clearly identify the progressively falling concentrations of several metabolites, with a possible elevation in the resonance peak assigned to the neuronal marker NAA. Quantitative MRS defines the principal abnormality as a threefold increase in the concentration of the cerebral osmolyte, mI. (From Lee JH, Arcinue E, Ross BD: Organic osmolytes in the brain of an infant with hypernatremia. N Engl J Med, 1994, 331:439–442. Copyright 1994. Massachusetts Medical Society. All rights reserved.)

diabetes contribute to the much increased mortality. The biochemical basis of these conditions may lie in the changes in Cho, NAA, mI, ketones, and glucose that are now recognized by ^{13}C and ^{1}H MRS to be present in the acutely and chronically diabetic brain.

Hyperosmolar State: Identification of Idiogenic Organic Osmolytes by Proton MR Spectroscopy

Lien and colleagues[145] first used ^{1}H MRS to investigate a "new" family of cerebral metabolites, collec-

tively known as organic osmolytes because of their postulated role in the maintenance of cerebral osmotic equilibrium. Such molecules were also first thoroughly researched in the papilla of the kidney with the help of in vitro NMR.[146]

First in sporadic cases of diabetic hyperosmolar coma[37] and in a patient after closed head injury[64] and then most convincingly in a single infant with holoprosencephaly and deficient thirst mechanisms, these concepts were confirmed as contributing to human encephalopathy by the use of ^{1}H MRS (Fig. 30–42). mI was three times normal, and other resonances, also markedly affected, returned toward normal with treatment. Difference spectroscopy is particularly helpful in identifying these changes.[100, 147]

Hyponatremia

The pathogenesis of morbidity associated with hyponatremia is postulated to be determined by the state of intracellular cerebral osmolytes. Previously inaccessible, these metabolites can now be quantitated by ^{1}H MRS. An in vivo quantitative assay of osmolytes in 12 patients with chronic hyponatremia (mean serum sodium level of 120 mEq/L) and 10 normal control subjects was performed. Short-TE ^{1}H MRS of occipital gray and parietal white matter locations revealed dramatic reductions in the concentrations of several metabolites (Fig. 30–43). In gray matter, mI was most profoundly reduced, at 49% of the control value. Cho-containing compounds were reduced 36%; Cr, 19%; and NAA 11% from control values. Similar changes were found in white matter. Recovery of osmolyte concentrations was demonstrated in four patients studied 8 to 14 weeks later. These results are consistent with a reversible osmolyte reduction under hypo-osmolar stress in the intact human brain, and they lead to

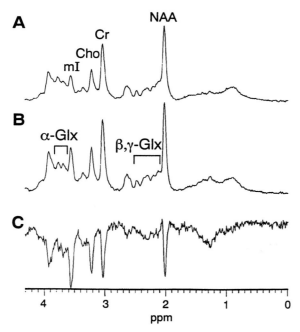

FIGURE 30–43. Summed and difference spectra of gray matter in hyponatremia. Individual spectra were processed on an absolute scale. Spectra of 11 hyponatremic patients *(A)* and 10 control subjects *(B)* were summed and then subtracted (patients minus controls) to yield the difference spectrum *(C)*, which is enlarged threefold. The negative peaks of the four major metabolites represent a decline in concentration. The fifth peak at 3.95 ppm represents the methylene protons of Cr and is proportional to the methyl-creatine peak at 3.05 ppm. *(A to C* from Videen JS, Michaelis T, Pinto P, Ross BD: Human cerebral osmolytes during chronic hyponatremia. A proton magnetic resonance spectroscopy study [see comments]. Reproduced from The Journal of Clinical Investigation, 1995, vol 95, pp 788–793 by copyright permission of The American Society for Clinical Investigation.)

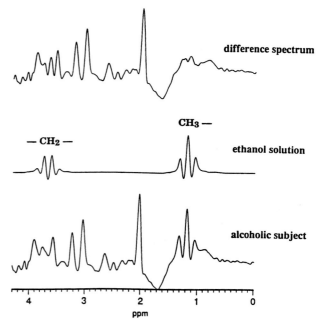

FIGURE 30–44. Difference spectroscopy to identify intracerebral ethanol in a patient with liver disease. *Bottom,* ^{1}H MR spectrum from parietal cortex in a 30-year-old woman with proven alcoholic liver disease shows no chronic HE but demonstrates an additional triplet. *Middle,* Spectrum recorded from an aqueous solution of ethanol has a triplet similar to that seen in the patient's spectrum and a quartet that is not apparent in the patient's spectrum. The chemical-shift scale was determined with other solution spectra containing known internal standards. *Top,* The difference spectrum shows coincidence of the resonances at 1.0 to 1.35 ppm seen in the patient with the triplet of ethanol, whereas negative peaks between 3.5 and 3.8 ppm indicate absence of the expected quartet resonances.

novel suggestions for treatment and monitoring of this common clinical event.

Diffuse metabolic changes in brain biochemistry are the result of complex interactions of disordered biochemistry in many other organs and tissues. HE, diabetic coma and hyperosmolar states, and hypoxic encephalopathy are examples of conditions in which accurate application of quantitative NMR spectroscopy sheds new light. Diagnostic utility of MRS in metabolic encephalopathies should increase as new therapeutic options are developed.

Detection of Xenobiotics in Brain

Relatively few drugs accumulate in the millimolar range in brain because of the effective blood-brain barrier. Three exceptions, readily demonstrable in ^{1}H spectra, are mannitol (Blüml S, Norfray J, Hungerford D, Ross B, unpublished assignment of resonance in Figure 2c of Moats and coworkers[150]; not shown), ethanol (Fig. 30–44), and the ubiquitous drug solvent propylene glycol (or 1,2-propanediol; Fig. 30–45). These findings can, however, be of utmost clinical importance in diagnosis, determining, for example, that a prospective liver transplant recipient is still drinking or that a pediatric case of lactic acidosis may be drug related.[148, 149]

PRACTICAL CONSIDERATIONS: CHEMICAL-SHIFT IMAGING VERSUS SINGLE VOXEL

FOCAL DISEASE AND CURRENT USES FOR METABOLITE MAPPING

Tumors, white matter disease, MS, stroke, and epilepsies have been the subject of exhaustive studies with localized MRS, and all result in defined patterns of abnormality. As expected with largely focal disease, there has been a considerable discrepancy between the spectrum and the MRI appearance and difficulty in defining the role of MRS. Robust metabolite imaging methods have made it useful to perform CSI for patients with tumor, to indicate sites preferred for biopsy, for example. Regional differences in stroke, lateraliz-

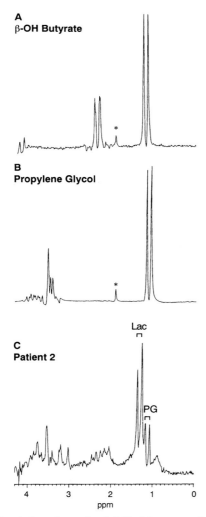

FIGURE 30–45. Propylene glycol (PG; 1,2-propanediol) is clearly identified as the source of the resonances in the infant brain *(C)* at 1.14 and 3.52 ppm; compare with standards in *A* and *B*. Lactate is possibly D-lactate, a toxic metabolite of *dl*-propylene glycol. Propylene glycol is a commonly used solvent of pediatric drugs. (*A* to *C* from Michaelis T, Cooper K, Kreis R, Ross B: Proton MRS reveals two unusual cases of neonatal hypoxic encephalopathy. In: Proceedings of the Third Annual Meeting of the Society of Magnetic Resonance, Nice, France, 1995.)

ing changes in temporal lobe epilepsy, regional and temporal changes in MS, which may indicate progression of disease, and dramatically different spectra from affected and unaffected regions of the cortex in developing leukodystrophies make these techniques more informative than single spectra obtained for arbitrarily selected regions of the MR image.

SINGLE-VOXEL MR SPECTROSCOPY: CHARACTERISTIC DIFFERENCES AND UNIFYING CONCEPTS

With 3 or 4 peaks in the long-TE spectrum (used generally in CSI) and 8 to 10 peaks in the short-TE spectrum, several distinct patterns of disease emerge that can be summarized in the form of a differential diagnosis (Table 30–9). With care, these patterns assume diagnostic importance and make a serious contribution to clinical discussions. Whether this translates into medical management is entirely a function of the confidence with which the results can be presented.

QUALITY CONTROL, AUTOMATION, CLINICAL TRIALS, AND ADDED VALUE OF MR SPECTROSCOPY

It is a weakness of MRS research that individual centers select their own acquisition conditions. This has certainly been a major handicap in preparing this chapter. As used to be the case with MRI, the expert can usually interpret abnormalities, given a relevant normal study and information about the sequence. However, this is not always so. Even small changes can have pathologic and prognostic significance when expressed in numeric form as ratios or absolute quantities, and therefore a system of quality assurance for MRS is necessary. There should be a greater effort to standardize and thereby accelerate the pooling of data for such important issues as outcome and cost-benefit analysis. Large-scale trials have been successfully completed for 1) automated single-voxel, short-TE examinations, showing less than 10% variations between 10 different MR sites, and 2) long-TE examinations of normal individuals and patients with different pathologic conditions (tumor, Parkinson's disease, HIV, dementia, stroke, MS), showing sufficient reproducibility between more than 20 international MRS centers, for clinical utility.

OUTCOME ANALYSES FOR CLINICAL MR SPECTROSCOPY

Several studies are available with which to define the clinical need for an MRS examination of the brain.

1. HIV: About 20% of MRI-negative patients have significant abnormalities at MRS (Marseilles).
2. ALD: 25% of MRI-negative boys, with an affected sibling, show significant abnormality at MRS (Göttingen).

TABLE 30–9. DIFFERENTIAL DIAGNOSTIC USES OF MR SPECTROSCOPY

METABOLITE (NORMAL CEREBRAL CONCENTRATION)	INCREASED	DECREASED
Lactate (~1 mM, not "visible")	Often Hypoxia, anoxia, ND, intracranial hemorrhage, stroke, hypoventilation (e.g., inborn errors of TCA), Canavan's disease, Alexander's disease, hydrocephalus	Unknown
NAA (5, 10, or 15 mM)	Rarely Canavan's disease	Often Developmental delay, infancy, hypoxia, anoxia, ischemia, intracranial hemorrhage, herpes II encephalitis, ND, hydrocephalus, Alexander's disease, epilepsy, neoplasm, MS, stroke, normal-pressure hydrocephalus, diabetes mellitus, closed head trauma
Glutamate and/or glutamine (? 10 mM; ? 5 mM)	Chronic HE, acute HE, hypoxia, ND, ornithine transcarbamylase deficiency	Unknown Possibly AD
mI (5 mM)	Neonate, AD, diabetes mellitus, recovered hypoxia, hyperosmolar states	Chronic HE, hypoxic encephalopathy, stroke, tumor
Cr + PCr (8 mM)	Trauma, hyperosmolar states, increasing with age	Hypoxia, stroke, tumor, infant
Glucose (~1 mM)	Diabetes mellitus, parenteral feeding, ? hypoxic encephalopathy	Not detectable
Cho (1.5 mM)	Trauma, diabetes, white versus gray matter, neonates, after liver transplantation, tumor, chronic hypoxia, hyperosmolar states, elderly, normal, AD	Asymptomatic liver disease, HE, stroke, nonspecific dementias, hyponatremia, syndrome of inappropriate antidiuretic hormone secretion (SIADH)
Acetoacetate, acetone, ethanol, aromatic amino acids, xenobiotics (propanediol, mannitol)	Detectable in specific settings	

3. ND: 5 of 5 good-outcome and 12 of 12 poor-outcome cases were defined by MRS performed between days 2 and 4 after rescue (Pasadena).

4. Temporal lobe epilepsy: 55 of 60 patients had successful determination by MRS of unilateral disease before surgery or open electroencephalography (London).

ADDED VALUE OR COSTS AND BENEFITS OF NEUROSPECTROSCOPY

Another approach to viewing MRI as a beneficial examination and to computing the added (diagnostic) value of neurospectroscopy was undertaken by Moats and colleagues.[150] If MRS is positive when MRI is negative, or if MRS shows definitive abnormalities in diseases for which MRI or other neuroimaging techniques are not currently indicated, it should be possible to calculate a crude figure for the added value of MRS. Figure 30–46 shows the preliminary results of a three-center trial in which MRI and automated MRS were performed "blind." Results for each were reported independently, and then the results were coordinated to define MRI positive (black column), MRS positive (gray column), and MRI positive plus MRI negative but MRS positive (black and gray column) for each center. Added value varied from 21% in an inpatient center, with relatively high success for MRI alone, to 28% in an outpatient center, where MRI was characteristically less successful alone. Not unexpectedly, when cases were selected based on MRS criteria alone, diagnoses were positive for MRS in 93% to 97% of cases.

HAS NEUROSPECTROSCOPY A FUTURE?

All high-technology innovative methods are under attack to prove their cost-effectiveness before being more widely implemented. MRS has several of the necessary attributes: methods are relatively uniform, robust, and widely available; a pattern of diagnostic uses is emerging; and a group of indications with unique diagnostic information has been found and translated into rather simplistic added value. The real cost/benefit ratio of neurospectroscopy has yet to be established. However, as pointed out 14 years ago by Epstein[151]:

The clinical applications of NMR and even its availability are sure to have a byproduct. Disorders formerly regarded as routine will invite new speculation about their pathophysiology. The introduction of a new technique to the bedside always stimulates intellectual reverberations that go beyond the narrow range of the instrument. Perhaps the most important contribution of NMR to clinical medicine will be that it will make us start thinking about familiar diseases in a new way.

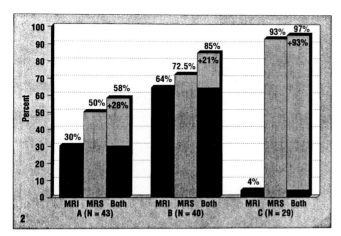

FIGURE 30–46. Results of a clinical trial to determine added value of neurospectroscopy. PROBE was performed in addition to MRI in three different clinical settings: outpatient private practice (A), inpatient county hospital (B), and MRS research unit (C). Black bars represent MRI-positive cases; gray bars, MRS-positive cases; and black and gray bars, MRI-positive cases + MRI-negative but MRS-positive cases. Added value was 28% in the outpatient center, where MRI was less successful alone, and 21% in the inpatient center, which had relatively high success for MRI alone. When cases were selected for MRS indications, added value was 93%.

Physicians using MRS to look at diseases "in a new way" will undoubtedly find ways to modify time-honored, but wrong, medical practice to benefit their patients.

WHAT HAVE WE LEARNED FROM NEUROSPECTROSCOPY?

N-ACETYLASPARTATE

Most observations with ¹H MRS strongly support the original formulation of NAA as a neuronal marker (Fig. 30–47). However, this simple conclusion must be modified in some particulars. There is evidence that NAA is also found in a precursor cell of the oligodendrocyte. The time course of appearance of NAA in human embryology is still unknown, but the best estimate is that NAA biosynthesis may begin in the middle trimester; that is, it is not dependent on the existence of MRI-visible myelin, which is only slowly added to the brain in the months after birth. Furthermore, the finding of approximately equal concentrations of NAA in white matter and gray matter of the human brain makes it inescapably obvious that NAA is also a component of the axon or the axonal sheath in humans. In addition to NAA, there is good evidence now for the existence of N-acetylaspartylglutamate in human (as well as animal) brain, with the preponderance in white matter and posterior and inferior regions of adult brain, especially the cerebellum.

Human pathobiology supports the idea of NAA as a neuronal marker, loss of NAA being generally an accompaniment of diseases in which neuronal loss is documented. Glioma, stroke, the majority of dementias, and hypoxic encephalopathy all show loss of NAA. It should be pointed out, however, that persuasive as

such conclusions may be, they remain circumstantial until a postmortem analysis with neuronal quantification is performed.

But NAA is obviously an axonal marker too, as supported by the loss of NAA in many white matter diseases (leukodystrophies of many kinds have been studied) and in MS plaques. Perhaps most convincing, loss of NAA occurs earlier in gray matter than in white matter in hypoxic encephalopathy after recovery from ND. We might hypothesize that the loss of neurons is followed by degeneration of axons in this setting.

If NAA is a neuronal marker, can we ever expect to see recovery of NAA in clinical practice? This has often been proposed but is perhaps best understood now not as evidence of neuronal recovery (still to be viewed as unlikely) but in terms of one of four possible alternatives:

1. Axonal recovery, after a less than lethal insult to the neuron, such as in MS plaques or in the rare syndrome of mitochondrial encephalopathy, lactic acidosis, and stroke-like episodes (MELAS syndrome).

NAA

Biosynthesis (slow) precedes myelination

Oligodendroglia/neurons

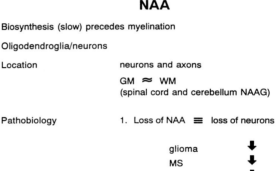

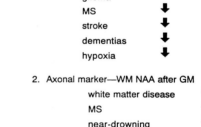

FIGURE 30–47. NAA. Little was known of this important neurochemical before the advent of clinical MRS. Studies of disease answer many questions about the pathobiology of NAA. GM = gray matter; WM = white matter.

2. An artifact of cortical atrophy. As neuronal death occurs, the consolidation of surviving brain tissue is well documented by neuropathologic studies and by the finding of ventricular dilatation and cortical atrophy at MRI. MRS, which determines local ratios or even concentrations of NAA, would record a real increase in the local concentration of this metabolite. This must not be interpreted as recovery but corrected for tissue volume and weight in some way and carefully distinguished from what seem to be the rather rarer examples described earlier.

3. Survival (or recovery) of a peak at 2.01 ppm in the ^{1}H spectrum is due not to NAA but to *N*-acetylaspartylglutamate and several other metabolites that contribute to this spectral region, so a metabolic explanation other than neuronal recovery must be sought. For this reason, "NAA" may respond to metabolic events other than those usually attributed to neurons and axons. A small decrease in the NAA peak in diabetes mellitus may be explained better in terms of another metabolite in this location.

4. NAA might also be a reversible cerebral osmolyte, increasing or decreasing in response to hyperosmolar states and decreasing noticeably in hypo-osmolar states, such as sodium depletion. These electrolyte disturbances, it must be recalled, are extremely common in hospitalized patients.

CREATINE AND PHOSPHOCREATINE

We know that in human brain at least these two compounds, which are in rapid chemical enzymatic exchange, represent a single-T2 species, likely to be in rapid exchange despite evidence of compartmentation. The idea that there might be a metabolically distinct pool of total Cr, which arose from the discrepancy between earlier biochemical and MRS quantitation in human subjects, is now considered less likely. When the same units are used, MRS gives an estimate of 8 mM Cr + PCr in human gray matter, compared with the published value of 8.6 mM for rapidly frozen rat brain. On the other hand, the Cr concentration in human gray matter significantly exceeds that measured in white matter, so there is some support for the results of tissue culture studies, in which Cr appears to be more related to neurons than to astrocytes.

As with NAA, MRS studies have thrown interesting light on the factors that might control Cr + PCr in human brain. In addition to the well-known regulation by enzymatic equilibrium, which permits a presumably crucial role of PCr in energetics of ATP synthesis, two new concepts have emerged. One is that cerebral Cr is controlled by distant events, because of the complex biosynthetic pathway through liver and kidney enzymes. Before Cr can be available for transport to the brain, it must be synthesized (Fig. 30–48). The absolute cerebral Cr concentration falls in chronic liver disease and recovers after liver transplantation. Even more striking is the discovery of a new human inborn error of Cr biosynthesis that is manifested as absence of cerebral Cr from the ^{1}H spectrum.

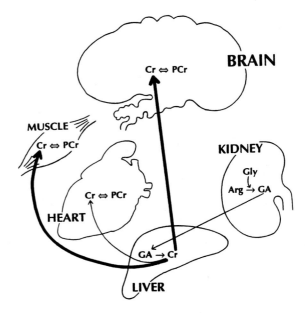

creatine (Cr); phosphocreatine (PCr); arginine (Arg); glycine (Gly); guanidinoacetate (GA)

FIGURE 30–48. The Cr pool. Cr synthesis requires participation of kidney and liver. Tissues may express creatine kinase, in which case PCr is present. Other tissues lack PCr. Cancers both with and without PCr are recognized.

The third method of regulation of cerebral Cr content is surprising, in view of the crucial nature of cerebral energy conservation. This is the marked modification of cerebral Cr by osmotic (Donnan's) forces, increased in hyperosmolar states and decreased in the common setting of hypo-osmolar states related to sodium depletion. The explanation for this apparent overriding of the all-important enzyme equilibrium (Gibbs') forces is probably that discovered for the mammalian heart and for cancer cells. That is, the Gibbs equilibrium and the Donnan equilibrium are closely linked. When all equilibria are interdependent, the total Cr + PCr may rise or fall to maintain the osmotic equilibrium. We presume, but cannot tell from ^{1}H MRS alone, that even under these circumstances, the PCr/Cr ratio continues to comply with the overriding requirements of the thermodynamic equilibrium between PCr and ATP, described in the equation in Figure 30–49.

In summary, therefore, the simple approach of assuming that Cr is constant and can be used as an internal reference for the other metabolite peaks of the ^{1}H spectrum is not valid. Cr intensity can actually increase. Second, the idea that a reduction in the total Cr peak must reflect failure of energy metabolism is also not correct, without supporting evidence. These ideas are summarized in Figure 30–49 as the three forces that control cerebral creatine.

CHOLINES

A number of new ideas concerning the Cho resonance and its component cerebral metabolites have emerged from clinical studies (Fig. 30–50). Although theoretically associated with myelin, the Cho concentration in cerebral white matter is not much higher than that in gray matter, even though this is the impression one gains from constantly seeing ^{1}H spectra, in which the Cho/Cr ratio is much higher and closer to 1.0 in short-TE spectra of white matter. The explanation lies in the difference in Cr concentration between the two locations, approximately 20% higher in gray matter. Thus, the Cho concentrations are virtually identical: 1.6 mM in white matter and 1.4 mM in gray matter. These values also appear to answer the question of whether the Cho head groups of phosphatidylcholine contribute to the ^{1}H spectrum of human brain in vivo. The answer is almost certainly no, because the total of free Cho plus phosphorylcholine plus glycerophosphorylcholine, determined by chemical means in human brain biopsy specimens and postmortem samples, is close to 1.5 mM, leaving little room for any other major Cho metabolite to be visible in the resonance.

1. Single-T2 species
2. Rapid exchange
3. Invisible pool?—not likely (8.0 vs 8.6 mM)
4. Neuron vs glial marker—(8.0 vs 6.3 mM; GM vs WM; unlikely)

3rd "force" controls [Cr]

(a) Enzyme equilibrium: early hypoxia, no change in [Cr + PCr]; Cr/PCr ↑

(b) Biosynthesis in liver and kidney: liver disease ↓ [Cr]

(c) Gibbs-Donnan equilibrium [Cr] ↑ or ↓

**Gibbs-Donnan Equilibrium
Control Cell Volume and Biochemistry in Brain**

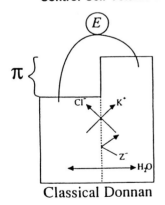 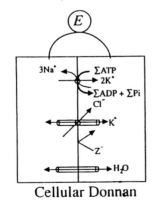

$$[\Sigma P_i] = \frac{[\Sigma 3PG]\,[\Sigma LACT]\,[\Sigma P\text{-}Cr]\,[H^+]}{[\Sigma DHAP]\,[\Sigma PYR]\,[\Sigma Creatine]} \times \frac{K_{LDH} \times K_{CK} \times K_{TPI}}{K_{G \cdot G}}$$

1. Electrolytes, metabolites **and** osmolytes "interact."

2. Metabolites (even PCr) might be osmolytes.

ERGO: We will observe reversible changes in [Cr] **and** [NAA]

FIGURE 30–49. Creatine. From studies of diseases, and a development in the theory of regulation of cell volume and metabolism, at least three major events may alter brain Cr concentration. (Based on Masuda T, Dobson VP, Veech RL: Gibbs-Donnan near-equilibrium of heart. J Biol Chem 265:20321–20334, 1990.)

1. A myth dispelled by QMRS
   Cho WM **NOT** > Cho GM
       1.6   vs   1.4
   (impression due to GM Cr > WM Cr)

2. No visible head groups of Pt Cho

3. Local and systemic; regulated by development; aging

Local	Systemic
Tumor	Diabetes
MS	Liver
(AD)	Renal failure
(depression)	Dialysis
Head Injury	Osmotic events
Stroke	Post-transplant (liver)
Hypoxia; brain death	
WM disease	
(ALD etc)	
Radiation	
HIV infection/inflammation	

4. PC vs GPC decoupled ^{31}P

FIGURE 30–50. What have we learned: cholines. Local, systemic, and biosynthetic events modifying MRS-visible choline(s).

Some light is thrown on the meaning of the Cho resonance from consideration of the many local and systemic events that alter the Cho concentration in brain (see Table 30–9). As with Cr, osmotic events are among these. The finding that many focal, inflammatory, and hereditary diseases result in increased Cho concentration has led to the speculation that these metabolites represent breakdown products of myelin. This is almost certainly an oversimplification. Conversely, the finding that several systemic disease processes also modify cerebral Cho indicates that biosynthesis and hormonal influences outside the brain, possibly in the liver, can markedly alter the composition and concentration of the Cho peak. These remain to be elucidated. Although ^{1}H spectroscopy offers little hope of distinguishing the different components, decoupled ^{31}P spectroscopy undoubtedly can do so, giving the opportunity to use disease processes to further understand these interesting metabolites.

MYO-INOSITOL (SCYLLO-INOSITOL)

Figure 30–51 illustrates some remarkable facts that have emerged concerning this simple sugar alcohol, which was rediscovered with the advent of short-TE in vivo human brain spectroscopy.[18] Its concentration fluctuates more than that of any of the other major compounds detected in the ^{1}H spectrum—more than 10-fold, from three times adult normal values in newborn infants and hypernatremic states to almost zero in HE. Although mI has been recognized as a cerebral osmolyte since 1990 and because of its cellular specificity is believed to be an astrocyte marker, evidence is incomplete. Like Cho, mI has been considered a breakdown product of myelin because it is seen at an apparently increased concentration in MS plaques,

Myo-inositol (*scyllo*-inositol)

10-fold Fluctuations

1. Astrocyte marker; little evidence
2. Osmolyte; hyper (x3)+ hyponatremia (x 1/2); newborn x2 post-natal
3. Myelin "product" in MS and HIV
4. Metabolic "marker" (IPP$_3$)
   AD—Down syndrome
   Diabetes
   Hepatic Encephalopathy:
   (a) SCHE?
   (b) Neuropsych. marker?

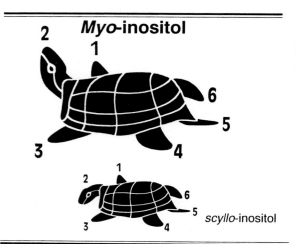

FIGURE 30–51. What have we learned: mI. Although little is known with certainity, cerebral mI is a significant metabolite, with several functions beyond that of an osmolyte (see Fig. 30–52). The "turtle" ideogram is provided to explain why an extremely low tissue concentration of *scyllo*-inositol (sI) is visible. sI resonates as a singlet (all protons symmetric) in contrast to the multiplet of mI (one asymmetric proton—the turtle's "head"). SCHE = subclinical hepatic encephalopathy.

FIGURE 30–52. Reactions involving mI. Enzymes of biosynthesis (labeled a, b, h) and degradation (labeled c, d, e) and those intermediate in the inositol polyphosphate signaling pathways (labeled f, g) are identified.

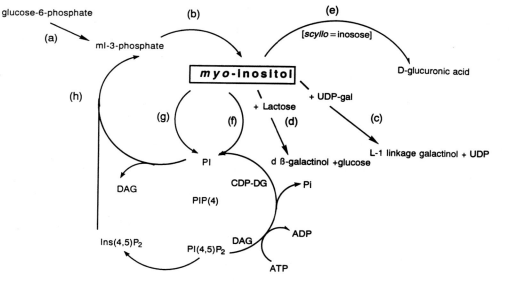

HIV infection, and metachromatic leukodystrophy. But the evidence is particularly indirect and rather weak on this point. Despite attempts to confine the role of mI to that of a chemically inert osmolyte or cell marker, it is important to remember that mI is at the center of a complex metabolic pathway that contains among other products the inositol polyphosphate messengers, inositol 1-phosphate, phosphatidylinositol, glucose 6-phosphate, and glucuronic acid (Fig. 30–52). Any or all of these products may be involved in the diseases listed in Table 30–9 as resulting in marked alterations in mI or sI concentration.

GLUTAMINE AND GLUTAMATE

Provided care is taken and the appropriate sequences are applied, even at 1.5 T the two amino acids that contribute to the spectral regions 2.2 to 2.4 ppm and 3.6 to 3.8 ppm can be readily separated. Glutamine, particularly when present at elevated concentrations, can be determined with some precision. Even

1. **Glutamine (5 mM) and glutamate (10 mM) ARE distinguishable at 1.5 T, 2 T, and 4 T**

2. ΔGlutamine: common   ΔGlutamate: rare

⬆	⬇	⬇
HE	AD	AD
Reyes	hyponatremia	
OTC def	(post-transplant)	
hypoxic-ischemic	liver	
hyperosmolar		
valproate (NH$_3$ ↑)		

3. GABA
     ↑ "vigibatrine"

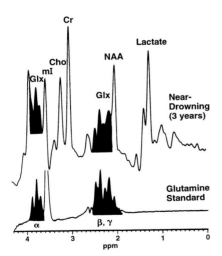

FIGURE 30–53. What have we learned: glutamine and glutamate (Glx). The spectra show massive elevation of cerebral glutamine in "pure" hypoxia. This is one example of several neuropathologies in which glutamine, rather than glutamate, accumulates.

better separation is achieved at 2.0 T, at which glutamate can be unequivocally identified and quantified. It is glutamine concentration, rather than that of glutamate, that appears to respond to disease (Fig. 30–53). Glutamate concentration decreases in AD and has not been shown convincingly to increase under any circumstance to date. On the other hand, increased cerebral glutamine concentration occurs in many settings, from Reye's syndrome and HE to hypoxic encephalopathy. The latter case appears contrary to popular neurochemical theory.

A much closer look at glutamate turnover is achieved through the use of either ^{13}C or ^{15}N MRS (the former in human brain). Mason and Gruetter (Shulman RG, personal communication, 1994) determined the rates of the TCA cycle, glucose consumption, glutamate formation from 2-oxoglutarate, and finally the rate of glutamine synthesis in vivo. Their data are consistent with the long-held view of two glutamate compartments. Although no explanation is yet available for the accumulation of glutamine rather than glutamate in hypoxic brain, the work of Kanamori and colleagues[120, 121] with ^{15}N MRS offers some clues. Thus, the rate of phosphate-activated glutaminase, the sole pathway of glutamine breakdown to glutamate, is under tight metabolic control in the (rat) brain. Because there is a cycle converting glutamate to glutamine and back (Fig. 30–54), it may be that phosphate-activated glutaminase holds the answer to the regulation of cerebral glutamate concentration in hypoxia. This apparent paradox (Fig. 30–55) is important, because so much neurochemical theory tends to the view of glutamate accumulation as a neurotoxin, explaining a number of pathologies. On the clinical horizon are new insights with ^{13}C and ^{15}N.

SUMMARY: WHAT HAVE WE LEARNED?

Rather than the simple enzymatic equilibria employed in most neurochemical descriptions of the brain, there are four kinds of metabolic regulation in the brain, at the macroscopic level, shown in Figure 30–56. This model should lead to some new interpretations of pathology in disease and widen the already extensive clinical value of neurospectroscopy.

When observing neuropathologic events through MRS, there seems to be a rather limited range of metabolic changes in response to disease. Tumor, MS, stroke, inflammation, and infections, as well as indirect trauma (closed head injury), produce similar patterns of change. This is not surprising and should not be condemned as lack of specificity when viewed from the perspective of making a clinical diagnosis via MRS. Rather, it should teach us more about the brain's response to injury and prevention and repair of injury.

The new neurochemistry described by MRS, using ^{1}H, ^{31}P, ^{13}C, and now ^{15}N, will in time result in new definitions of diseases, which may then be differently grouped according to their neurochemical pattern. Neurotherapeutic innovations will follow.

What we have not learned (Fig. 30–57), of course,

Mason/Gruetter
^{13}C

TCA cycle	0.7 ± 0.2 μmol/min
Glucose consumption	0.57 ±0.08 μmol/min
O_2 consumption	2.14 ± 0.48
α-KG ⇔ glutamate	57 ± 26 μmol/min

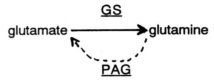

GS

glutamate ⟶ glutamine

PAG

0.47 μmol/min/g
(0.14 - 3.1 range)

Data consistent with two TCA compartments

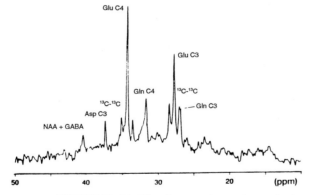

	Glu	Gln	GABA	Asp
^{13}C conc.	2.4±0.1	1.1±0.1	0.4±0.1	0.27±0.03
Min. total brain pool	9.1±0.7	4.3±0.7	1.2±0.3	1.0±0.2

FIGURE 30–54. What have we learned: γ-aminobutyric acid–glutamine–glutamate cycle. Although little has been learned from ¹H MRS, ¹³C studies permit critical reaction rates to be established in vivo, using spectra such as that illustrated. (Data from work of Mason[136] and Gruetter.[137])

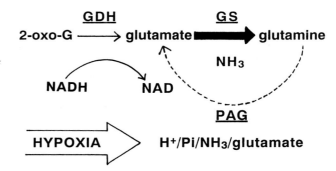

ANOMALY: Near-drowning and stroke

FIGURE 30–55. Anomaly of glutamate. Factors regulating glutamate conversion to glutamine.

1. There are 4 kinds of metabolic regulation in the brain:

   (a) Enzyme equilibria
   (b) Cell-cell interactions; inflammation, neoplasia, cell death, (de)myelination

   (c) Many systemic events

   (d) Gibbs-Donnan equilibria; cell-volume regulation

2. A LIMITED variety of pathological responses to disease: tumor ~ MS ~ stroke ~ inflammation ~ trauma

3. Neuro-diagnostic and therapeutic innovations follow the "NEW NEUROCHEMISTRY"

FIGURE 30–56. What have we learned: 1979 to 1994: 15 years of MRS of the brain.

1. Mechanism of **ANY** neurological disease or psychiatric disease.

2. Biosynthesis, turnover and function of NAA!

3. Role of neurochemistry in normal brain (e.g., in "functional" vs electrical reactions).

WHY NOT?
1. Wrong models: too microscopic
                     too micromolar
                     too "molecular"

2. Too **few** studies: MRI outnumbers MRS 1,000,000 to 1

FUTURE?
1. More diseases will fit current neurochemical models.

2. New MRS methods (diffusion/functional/interventional) will continue to shrink the unexplained areas.

FIGURE 30–57. What have we *not* learned?

will keep neurospectroscopists, neurologists, neuroradiologists, and neurochemists busy for the next 15 years. Undoubtedly, clinical studies will provide new insights that could not have been foreseen or planned for in the laboratory. The solutions will not all come from MRS, but neurospectroscopy has become a crucial diagnostic tool.

Acknowledgments

Ms. J. C. Mandigo-Bellinger typed the manuscript and prepared many of the figures. We are grateful to our colleagues Drs. Roland Kreis, Thomas Ernst, Else Rubæk Danielsen, Truda Shonk, John Videen, Rex Moats, Peter Barker, Bruce Miller, Linda Chang, Leslee Watson, and Joseph Norfray and Mr. Kenneth Cooper for permission to cite recent or unpublished work. The Clinical MRS Unit at Huntington Medical Research Institutes (HMRI) receives financial support from the L. K. Whittier Foundation, Jameson Foundation, Richard M. Lucas Foundation, and Norris Foundation and from the boards of HMRI and the Altadena Guild, without whom this chapter would not have been possible. The authors are visiting associates in the Department of Chemistry and Chemical Engineering at the California Institute of Technology. B. D. R. is professor of clinical medicine at the University of Southern California.

REFERENCES

1. Warburg O: Versuche an Überlebendem Carcinomgewebe: Methoden II. Die Herstellung der Gewebeschnitte. Biochem Z 142:317–333, 1923.
2. Thulborn KR, du Boulay GH, Radda GK: ^{31}P MRS of Stroke. In: Proceedings of the Xth International Symposium on Cerebral Blood Flow and Metabolism, Montreal, 1981, p 114.
3. Cady EB, Dawson MJ, Hope PL, et al: Non-invasive investigation of cerebral metabolism in newborn infants by phosphorus nuclear magnetic resonance spectroscopy. Lancet 1:1059–1062, 1983.
4. Hope PL, Costello AM, Cady EB, et al: Cerebral energy metabolism studied with phosphorus NMR spectroscopy in normal and birth-asphyxiated infants. Lancet 2:366–370, 1984.
5. Hamilton PA, Hope PL, Cady EB, et al: Impaired energy metabolism in brains of newborn infants with increased cerebral echodensities. Lancet 1:1242–1246, 1986.
6. Bottomley PA, Hart HR, Edelstein WA, et al: NMR imaging/spectroscopy system to study both anatomy and metabolism. Lancet 1:273–274, 1983.
7. Oberhaensli RD, Hilton Jones D, Bore PJ, et al: Biochemical investigation of human tumours in vivo with phosphorus-31 magnetic resonance spectroscopy. Lancet 2:8–11, 1986.
8. Welch KMA: The imperatives of magnetic resonance for the acute stroke clinician (plenary lecture). In: Proceedings of the 11th Annual Meeting of the Society of Magnetic Resonance in Medicine, Berlin, 1992, p 901.
9. Pettegrew JW, Minstew NJ, Cohen MM, et al: P-31 NMR changes in Alzheimer and Huntington diseased brain. Neurology 34:281–286, 1984.
10. Tallan HH: Studies on the distribution of N-acetyl-L-aspartic acid in brain. J Biol Chem 224:41–45, 1957.
11. Behar KL, den Hollander JA, Stromski ME, et al: High resolution ^{1}H NMR study of cerebral hypoxia in vivo. Proc Natl Acad Sci USA 80:4945–4948, 1983.
12. Frahm J, Michaelis T, Merboldt K-D, et al: Localized NMR spectroscopy in vivo: progress and problems. NMR Biomed 2:188–195, 1988.
13. Prichard JW, Alger JR, Behar KL, et al: Cerebral metabolic studies in vivo by ^{31}P NMR. Proc Natl Acad Sci USA 80:2748–2751, 1983.
14. Frahm J, Bruhn H, Gyngell ML, et al: Localized proton NMR spectroscopy in different regions of the human brain in vivo. Relaxation times and concentrations of cerebral metabolites. Magn Reson Med 11:47–63, 1989.
15. Michaelis T, Merboldt K-D, Hänicke W, et al: On the identification of cerebral metabolites in localized ^{1}H NMR spectra of human brain in vivo. NMR Biomed 4:90–98, 1991.
16. Hanstock CC, Rothman DL, Prichard JW, et al: Spatially localized ^{1}H NMR spectra of metabolites in the human brain. Proc Natl Acad Sci USA 85:1821–1825, 1988.
17. Frahm J, Michaelis T, Merboldt K-D, et al: Improvements in localized proton NMR spectroscopy of human brain. Water suppression, short echo times, and 1 ml resolution. J Magn Reson 90:464–473, 1990.
18. Kreis R, Farrow NA, Ross BD: Diagnosis of hepatic encephalopathy by proton magnetic resonance spectroscopy. Lancet 336:635–636, 1990.
19. Ross BD, Kreis R, Ernst T: Clinical tools for the 90's: magnetic resonance spectroscopy and metabolite imaging. Eur J Radiol 14:128–140, 1992.
20. Heerschap A, van den Berg P: Proton MR spectroscopy of the human fetus in utero. In: Proceedings of the 12th Annual Meeting of the Society of Magnetic Resonance in Medicine, New York, 1993, p 318.
21. Kreis R, Ernst T, Ross BD: Development of the human brain: in vivo quantification of metabolite and water content with proton magnetic resonance spectroscopy. Magn Reson Med 30:1–14, 1993.
22. van der Knaap MS, Ross BD, Valk J: Inborn errors of metabolism. In: Kucharcyzk J, Barkovich AJ, Moseley M, eds. Magnetic Resonance Neuroimaging. Boca Raton, FL: CRC Press, 1993.
23. Boesch C, Gruetter R, Martin E, et al: Variations in the in vivo ^{31}P MR spectra of the developing human brain during postnatal life. Radiology 172:197–199, 1989.
24. Murphy EJ, Rajagoplan B, Brindle KM, Radda GK: Phospholipid bilayer contribution to ^{31}P NMR spectra in vivo. Magn Reson Med 12:282–289, 1989.
25. Pettegrew JW, Kopp SJ, Minshew NJ, et al: ^{31}P nuclear magnetic resonance studies of phosphoglyceride metabolism in developing and degenerating brain: preliminary observations. J Neuropathol Exp Neurol 46:419–430, 1987.
26. van der Knaap MS, van der Grond J, Luyten PR, et al: ^{1}H and ^{31}P MRS of the brain in degenerative cerebral disorders. Ann Neurol 31:202–211, 1992.
27. van der Grond J, Dijkstra G, Roelofsen B, Mali WPTM: ^{31}P NMR determination of phosphomonoesters in relation to phospholipid biosynthesis in testis of the rat at different ages. Biochim Biophys Acta 1074:189–194, 1991.
28. Michaelis T, Helms G, Merboldt KD, et al: First observation of scyllo-inositol in proton NMR spectra of human brain in vitro and in vivo. In: Proceedings of the 11th Annual Meeting of the Society of Magnetic Resonance in Medicine, Berlin, 1992, p 541.
29. Grodd W, Kragelah-Mann I, Klose U, Sauter R: Metabolic and destructive brain disorders in children: findings with localized proton MR spectroscopy. Radiology 181:173, 1991.
30. Zimmerman RA, Wang Z: Proton spectroscopy of the pediatric brain. Riv Neuroradiol 5:5, 1992.
31. Kugel H, Heindel W, Roth B: Localized ^{1}H MR in the pediatric brain: a useful tool for the evaluation of metabolic diseases? In: Proceedings of the 11th Annual Meeting of the Society of Magnetic Resonance in Medicine, Berlin, 1992, p 2012.
32. Lee JH, Arcinue E, Ross BD: Organic osmolytes in the brain of an infant with hypernatremia. N Engl J Med 331:439–442, 1994.
33. Kreis R, Pfenninger J, Herschkowitz J, Boesch C: In vivo proton magnetic resonance spectroscopy in a case of Reye's syndrome. Intensive Care Med 21:1–3, 1995.
34. Kruse B, Hanefeld F, Merboldt K-D, et al: Localized proton MR spectroscopy in hemimegalencephaly. In: Proceedings of the 12th Annual Meeting of the Society of Magnetic Resonance in Medicine, New York, 1993, p 1570.
35. Ernst T, Ross BD, Flores R: Cerebral MRS in infant with suspected Reye's syndrome. Lancet 340:1296, 1992. Letter.
36. Ernst T, Ross BD, Shonk T, et al: Quantitative proton MRS for prognosis after closed head injury. In: Proceedings of the 12th Annual Meeting of the Society of Magnetic Resonance in Medicine, New York, 1993, 1, p 323.
37. Kreis R, Ross BD: Cerebral metabolic disturbances in patients with subacute and chronic diabetes mellitus by proton magnetic resonance spectroscopy. Radiology 184:123–130, 1992.
38. Bruhn H, Frahm J, Merboldt KD, et al: Multiple sclerosis in children: cerebral metabolic alterations monitored by localized proton magnetic resonance spectroscopy in vivo. Ann Neurol 32:140–150, 1992.
39. Matthews PM, Andermann F, Arnold DL: A proton magnetic resonance spectroscopy study of focal epilepsy in humans. Neurology 40:985–989, 1990.
40. Cendes F, Andermann F, Preul MC, Arnold DL: Proton MR spectroscopic imaging in the investigation of temporal lobe epilepsy. In: Proceedings of the 12th Annual Meeting of the Society of Magnetic Resonance in Medicine, New York, 1993, p 431.
41. Constantinidis I, Epstein CM, Peterman S, et al: Can ^{1}H MR spectroscopic imaging lateralize temporal lobe seizure foci? In: Proceedings of the 12th Annual Meeting of the Society of Magnetic Resonance in Medicine, New York, 1993, p 429.
42. Gadian DG, Connelly A, Cross JH, et al: Relationship of cognitive dysfunction to ^{1}H MRS assessment of temporal lobe pathology. In: Proceedings of the 12th Annual Meeting of the Society of Magnetic Resonance in Medicine, New York, 1993, p 430.
43. Hugg JW, Laxer KD, Matson GB, et al: Neuron loss localizes human temporal lobe epilepsy by in vivo proton magnetic resonance spectroscopic imaging. Ann Neurol 34:788–794, 1993.

44. Ng TC, Comair Y, Xue M, et al: Proton chemical shift imaging for the presurgical localization of temporal lobe epilepsy. In: Proceedings of the 12th Annual Meeting of the Society of Magnetic Resonance in Medicine, New York, 1993, p 428.

45. Breiter SN, Arroyo S, Mathews VP, et al: Proton MR spectroscopy in patients with seizure disorders. Am J Neuroradiol 15:373–384, 1994.

46. Cendes F, Andermann F, Preul MC, Arnold DL: Lateralization of temporal lobe epilepsy based on regional metabolic abnormalities in proton magnetic resonance spectroscopic images. Ann Neurol 35:211–216, 1994.

47. Gadian DG, Cross JH, Gordon I, et al: 1H MRS and interictal SPECT in children with intractable temporal lobe epilepsy. In: Proceedings of the Second Annual Meeting of the Society of Magnetic Resonance, San Francisco, 1994, p 344.

48. Negendank WG, Brown TR, Evelhoch JL, et al: Proceedings of a National Cancer Institute workshop: MR spectroscopy and tumor cell biology. Radiology 185:875–883, 1992.

49. Negendank W: Studies of human tumors by MRS: a review. NMR Biomed 5:303–324, 1992.

50. Negendank W, Zimmerman R, Gotsis E, et al: A cooperative group study of 1H MRS of primary brain tumors. In: Proceedings of the 12th Annual Meeting of the Society of Magnetic Resonance in Medicine, New York, 1993, p 1521.

51. Grad J, Stillman AE, Hall WA, et al: Serial study of brain tumors by MRS following radiation therapy. In: Proceedings of the 12th Annual Meeting of the Society of Magnetic Resonance in Medicine, New York, 1993, p 1522.

52. Bruhn H, Frahm J, Gyngell ML, et al: Noninvasive differentiation of tumors with use of localized H-1 MR spectroscopy in vivo. Initial experience in patients with cerebral tumors. Radiology 172:541–548, 1989.

53. Luyten PR, Marien AJH, Heindel W, et al: Metabolic imaging of patients with intracranial tumors: H-1 MR spectroscopic imaging and PET. Radiology 176:791–799, 1990.

54. Frahm J, Bruhn H, Hanicke W, et al: Localized proton NMR spectroscopy of brain tumors using short-echo time STEAM sequences. J Comput Assist Tomogr 15:915–922, 1991.

55. Segebarth CM, Baleriaux DF, Luyten PR, den Hollander JA: Detection of metabolic heterogeneity of human intracranial tumors in vivo by 1H NMR spectroscopic imaging. Magn Reson Med 13:62–76, 1990.

56. Calabrese G, Falini A, Santino P, et al: Clinical H-1 magnetic resonance spectroscopy in brain tumors. In: Proceedings of the 12th Annual Meeting of the Society of Magnetic Resonance in Medicine, New York, 1993, p 1526.

57. Kugel H, Heindel W, Lanfermann H, Lackner K: 1H NMR spectroscopic imaging—differentiation of human brain tumors and infarcts. In: Proceedings of the 12th Annual Meeting of the Society of Magnetic Resonance in Medicine, New York, 1993, p 1525.

58. Ott D, Hennig J, Ernst T: Human brain tumors: assessment with in vivo proton MR spectroscopy. Radiology 186:745–752, 1993.

59. de Certaines JD, Larsen VA, Podo F, et al: In vivo 31P MRS of experimental tumours. NMR Biomed 6:345–365, 1993.

60. Vigneron DB, Wald LL, Day M, et al: Detection of metabolic heterogeneity in human brain tumors by 3-dimensional high spatial resolution (0.2–0.4 cc) 1H MR spectroscopic imaging. In: Proceedings of the Second Annual Meeting of the Society of Magnetic Resonance, San Francisco, 1994, p 1170.

61. Ross BD, Narasimhan PT, Tropp J, Derby K: Amplification or obfuscation: is localization improving our clinical understanding of phosphorus metabolism? NMR Biomed 2:340–345, 1989.

62. Negendank W, Sauter R, Brown T, et al: Intratumoral lipids and lactate in 1H MRS in vivo in astrocytic tumors. In: Proceedings of the Second Annual Meeting of the Society of Magnetic Resonance, San Francisco, 1994, p 1296.

63. Kuesel AC, Donnelly SM, Halliday W, et al: Mobile lipids and metabolic heterogeneity of brain tumours as detectable by ex vivo 1H MR spectroscopy. NMR Biomed 7:172–180, 1994.

63a. Volpe JJ: Neurology of the Newborn. Philadelphia: WB Saunders, 1987.

64. Kreis R, Ernst T, Ross BD: Absolute quantitation of water and metabolites in the human brain. Part II. Metabolite concentrations. J Magn Reson 102:9–19, 1993.

65. Ernst T, Ross BD, Shonk T, Kreis R: Neurochemistry of coma: 1H MRS post traumatic encephalopathy. Advances in Proton MRS of the Brain, Oxford, December 16–18, 1992, p 11. Abstract.

66. Howe FA, Maxwell RJ, Saunders DE, et al: Proton spectroscopy in vivo. Magn Reson Q 9:31–59, 1993.

67. Truwit C, Kucharczyk J: Reversible cerebral ischemia. Neuroimaging Clin North Am 2:577–600, 1992.

68. van der Grond J, Balm R, Eikelboom BC, Mali WPTM: 1H MRSI of the hypoperfused brain. In: Proceedings of the Second Annual Meeting of the Society of Magnetic Resonance, San Francisco, 1994, p 611.

69. Graham GD, Rothman DL, Hwang J-H, et al: Spectroscopic assessment of alterations in lipids and small molecule metabolites in human brain after stroke. In: Proceedings of the Second Annual Meeting of the Society of Magnetic Resonance, San Francisco, 1994, p 187.

70. Petroff OAC, Graham GD, Blamire AM, et al: 1H spectroscopic imaging of stroke in man: histopathology correlates of spectral changes. In:

71. Graham GD, Blamire AM, Rothman DL, et al: Early temporal variation of cerebral metabolites after human stroke monitored by in vivo proton magnetic resonance spectroscopy. In: Proceedings of the 11th Annual Meeting of the Society of Magnetic Resonance in Medicine, Berlin, 1992, p 642.

72. Graham GD, Kalvach P, Blamire AM, et al: Clinical correlates of proton magnetic resonance spectroscopy findings after acute cerebral infarction. In: Proceedings of the 12th Annual Meeting of the Society of Magnetic Resonance in Medicine, New York, 1993, p 1483.

73. Barker PB, Gillard JH, van Zijl PCM, et al: Proton magnetic resonance spectroscopic imaging in acute stroke: identification of the ischemic penumbra. In: Proceedings of the Second Annual Meeting of the Society of Magnetic Resonance, San Francisco, 1994, p 186.

74. Hennig J, Ernst T, Speck O, et al: Detection of brain activation using oxygenation sensitive functional spectroscopy. Magn Reson Med 31:85–90, 1994.

75. Ernst T, Hennig J: Observation of a fast response in functional MR. Magn Reson Med 32:146–149, 1994.

76. Merboldt K-D, Bruhn H, Hanicke W, et al: Decrease of glucose in the human visual cortex during photic stimulation. Magn Reson Med 25:187–194, 1992.

77. Chen W, Novotny EJ, Zhu X-H, et al: Localized 1H NMR measurement of glucose consumption in the human brain during visual stimulation. In: Proceedings of the Second Annual Meeting of the Society of Magnetic Resonance, San Francisco, 1993, p 1528.

78. Sappey-Marinier D, Calabrese G, Hugg J, et al: Increased lactate in human visual cortex during photic stimulation. In: Proceedings of the Ninth Annual Meeting of the Society of Magnetic Resonance in Medicine, New York, 1990, p 106.

79. Prichard JW, Rothman DL, Novotny E, et al: Lactate rise detected by 1H NMR in human visual cortex during physiologic stimulation. Proc Natl Acad Sci USA 88:5829–5833, 1991.

80. Mora BN, Narasimhan PT, Ross BD, et al: 31P saturation transfer and phosphocreatine imaging in the monkey brain. Proc Natl Acad Sci USA 88:8372–8376, 1991.

81. Sappey-Marinier D, Deicken R, Fein G, et al: Alterations in brain phosphorus metabolite concentrations associated with areas of high signal intensity in white matter at MR imaging. Radiology 183:247–256, 1992.

82. Sappey-Marinier D, Calabrese G, Hetherington HP, et al: Proton magnetic resonance spectroscopy of human brain: applications to normal white matter, chronic infarction, and MRI white matter signal hyperintensities. Magn Reson Med 26:313–327, 1992.

83. Larsson HBW, Christiansen P, Jensen M, et al: Localized in vivo proton spectroscopy in the brain of patients with multiple sclerosis. Magn Reson Med 22:23–31, 1991.

84. Koopmans RA, Li DKB, Zhu G, et al: Magnetic resonance spectroscopy of multiple sclerosis: in-vivo detection of myelin breakdown products. Lancet 341:631–632, 1993.

85. Arnold DL, Riess GT, Matthews PM, et al: Use of proton magnetic resonance spectroscopy for monitoring disease progression in multiple sclerosis. Ann Neurol 36:76–82, 1994.

86. Davie CA, Barker GJ, Tofts PS, et al: Detection of myelin breakdown products by proton magnetic resonance spectroscopy. Lancet 341:630–631, 1993.

87. Arnold DL, Matthews PM, Francis GS, et al: Proton magnetic resonance spectroscopic imaging for metabolic characterization of demyelinating plaques. Ann Neurol 31:235–241, 1992.

88. Schiffman R, Moller JR, Trapp BD, et al: Childhood ataxia with diffuse central nervous system hypomyelination. Ann Neurol 35:331–340, 1994.

89. Menon DK, Baudouin CJ, Tomlinson D, Hoyle C: Proton MR spectroscopy and imaging of the brain in AIDS: evidence of neuronal loss in regions that appear normal with imaging. J Comput Assist Tomogr 14:882–885, 1990.

90. Jarvik JG, Lenkinski RE, Grossman RI, et al: Proton MR spectroscopy of HIV-infected patients: characterization of abnormalities with imaging and clinical correlation. Radiology 186:739–744, 1993.

91. Tracey I, Guimares AR, Carr CA, et al: The AIDS dementia complex: localized 1H MRS on human brain detects abnormal brain metabolism following HIV infection. In: Proceedings of the Second Annual Meeting of the Society of Magnetic Resonance, San Francisco, 1994, p 584.

92. Vion-Dury J, Confort-Gouny S, Nicoli F, et al: Localized brain proton MRS might identify different metabolic profiles in AIDS-related encephalopathies. In: Proceedings of the Second Annual Meeting of the Society of Magnetic Resonance, San Francisco, 1994, p 585.

93. Lu D, Pavlakis S, Frank Y, et al: Localized proton MR spectroscopy of the basal ganglia in normal children and children with AIDS. In: Proceedings of the Second Annual Meeting of the Society of Magnetic Resonance, San Francisco, 1994, p 583.

94. Wilkinson ID, Chinn RJS, Paley M, et al: Serial proton spectroscopy of brain parenchyma in HIV infection. In: Proceedings of the Second Annual Meeting of the Society of Magnetic Resonance, San Francisco, 1994, p 582.

95. Cousins JP, Tomalski W, Peters T, Wagle WA: NAA/choline and NAA/

Cr as markers of metabolic changes in HIV⁺ patients. In: Proceedings of the Second Annual Meeting of the Society of Magnetic Resonance, San Francisco, 1994, p 581.

96. Meyerhoff DJ, Poole N, Weiner MW, Fein G: Are proton metabolites affected in brain areas of heaviest HIV load? In: Proceedings of the Second Annual Meeting of the Society of Magnetic Resonance, San Francisco, 1994, p 580.

97. Hall-Craggs MA, Williams I, Wilkinson ID, et al: Proton spectroscopy in a cross-section of HIV positive asymptomatic patients receiving immediate compared with deferred zidovudine. In: Proceedings of the Second Annual Meeting of the Society of Magnetic Resonance, San Francisco, 1994, p 303.

98. Zimmerman RD, Fleming CA, Lee BCP: Periventricular hyperintensity as seen by magnetic resonance: prevalence and significance. Am J Neuroradiol 7:13–20, 1986.

99. Ernst T, Kreis R, Ross BD: Absolute quantitation of water and metabolites in the human brain. Part I. Compartments and water. J Magn Reson 102:1–8, 1993.

100. Lee JH, Ernst T, Ross BD: Phosphocreatine imaging of the brain: improved interpretation through quantitative ¹H MRS. In: Proceedings of the 12th Annual Meeting of the Society of Magnetic Resonance in Medicine, New York, 1993, p 1535.

101. Carr CA, Guimaraes AR, Growdon JH, Gonzalez RG: Combining proton MRS and MRI morphometry increases accuracy in the diagnosis of Alzheimer's disease. In: Proceedings of the 12th Annual Meeting of the Society of Magnetic Resonance in Medicine, New York, 1993, p 233.

102. Shonk TK, Moats RA, Gifford P, et al: Probable Alzheimer disease: diagnosis with proton MR spectroscopy [see comments]. Radiology 195:65–72, 1995.

102a. Chang L, Ernst T, Miller B, Melchor R: ¹H magnetic resonance spectroscopy in Alzheimer's disease and frontotemporal dementia. In: Proceedings of the Third Annual Meeting of the Society of Magnetic Resonance, Nice, France, 1995, p 387.

103. Jenkins BG, Koroshetz WJ, Beal MF, Rosen BR: Evidence for impairment of energy metabolism in vivo in Huntington's disease using localized ¹H NMR spectroscopy. Neurology 43:2689–2695, 1993.

104. Jenkins BG, Koroshetz WJ, Chen YI, et al: Lowering cerebral lactate levels in Huntington's disease by energy repletion: assessment using MRS. In: Proceedings of the Second Annual Meeting of the Society of Magnetic Resonance, San Francisco, 1994, p 576.

105. Bruhn H, Weber T, Thorwirth V, Frahm J: In vivo monitoring of neuronal loss in Creutzfeldt-Jakob disease by proton magnetic resonance spectroscopy. Lancet 337:1610, 1991.

106. Plum F, Posner JB: The Diagnosis of Stupor and Coma. 3rd ed. Philadelphia: FA Davis, 1986.

107. Sherlock S, Summerskill WHJ, White LP, Phear EA: Portal-systemic encephalopathy: neurological complications of liver disease. Lancet 2:453–457, 1954.

108. Bessman S, Bessman A: The cerebral and peripheral uptake of ammonia in liver disease with an hypothesis for the mechanism of hepatic coma. J Clin Invest 34:622–628, 1955.

109. Bessman S, Pal N: The Krebs cycle depletion theory of hepatic coma. In: Grisolia S, Baguena R, Mayor F, eds. The Urea Cycle. New York: John Wiley & Sons, 1976, pp 83–89.

110. Krebs HA, Henseleit K: Untersuchungen uber die Harnstoffbildung im Tierkorper. Hoppe-Seyler's Z Physiol Chem 210:33–66, 1932.

111. Geissler A, Kanamori K, Ross BD: Real time study of the urea cycle using ¹⁵N NMR in the isolated perfused rat liver. Biochem J 287:813–820, 1992.

112. Hourani B, Hamlin E, Reynolds T: Cerebrospinal fluid glutamine as a measure of hepatic encephalopathy. Arch Intern Med 127:1033–1036, 1971.

113. Norenberg MD, Martinez-Hernandez A: Fine structural localization of glutamine synthetase in astrocytes of rat brain. Brain Res 161:303–310, 1979.

114. Reubi J-C, van den Berg C, Cuenod M: Glutamine as precursor for the GABA and glutamate transmitter pools. Neurosci Lett 10:171–174, 1978.

115. Butterworth RF, Layrargues GP: Hepatic Encephalopathy: Pathophysiology and Treatment. Clifton, NJ: Humana Press, 1989.

116. Zieve L: Hepatic encephalopathy. In: Schiff L, Schiff ER, eds. Diseases of the Liver. 6th ed. Philadelphia: JB Lippincott, 1987, pp 925–948.

117. Deutz NEP, de Graaf AA, de Haan JB, et al: In vivo brain proton NMR spectroscopy (¹H NMRS) during acute hepatic encephalopathy (HE). J Hepatol [suppl]4:S13–S17, 1987.

118. Bates TE, Williams SR, Kauppinen RA, Gadian DG: Observation of cerebral metabolites in an animal model of acute liver failure in vivo: ¹H and ³¹P nuclear magnetic resonance study. J Neurochem 53:102–110, 1989.

119. Fitzpatrick SM, Hetherington HP, Behar KL, Shulman RG: The flux from glucose to glutamate in the rat brain in vivo as determined by ¹H-observed, ¹³C-edited NMR spectroscopy. J Cereb Blood Flow Metab 10:170–179, 1990.

120. Kanamori K, Ross BD: ¹⁵N NMR measurement of the in vivo rate of glutamine synthesis and utilization at steady state in the brain of hyperammonaemic rat. Biochem J 293:461–468, 1993.

121. Kanamori K, Parivar F, Ross BD: A ¹⁵N NMR study of in vivo cerebral glutamine synthesis in hyperammonemic rats. NMR Biomed 6:21–26, 1993.

122. Moats RA, Lien Y-HH, Filippi D, Ross BD: Decrease in cerebral inositols in rats and humans. Biochem J 295:15–18, 1993.

123. Bruhn H, Frahm J, Michaelis T, et al: Metabolic disturbances of the brain in patients with liver cirrhosis detected by proton magnetic resonance spectroscopy. Hepatology 14:121, 1991. Abstract.

124. Kreis R, Farrow NA, Ross BD: Localized ¹H NMR spectroscopy in patients with chronic hepatic encephalopathy. Analysis of changes in cerebral glutamine, choline and inositols. NMR Biomed 4:109–116, 1991.

125. Kreis R, Ross BD, Farrow NA, Ackerman Z: Metabolic disorders of the brain in chronic hepatic encephalopathy detected with ¹H MRS. Radiology 182:19–27, 1992.

126. Bruhn H, Merboldt K-D, Michaelis T, et al: Proton MRS of metabolic disturbances in the brain of patients with liver cirrhosis and subclinical hepatic encephalopathy. In: Proceedings of the 10th Annual Meeting of the Society of Magnetic Resonance in Medicine, San Francisco, 1991, p 400.

127. McConnell JR, Ong CS, Chu WK, et al: ¹H MRS of the brain in patients with liver failure. In: Proceedings of the 11th Annual Meeting of the Society of Magnetic Resonance in Medicine, Berlin, 1992, p 1957.

128. Chamuleau RAFM, Bosman DK, Bovee WMMJ, et al: What the clinician can learn from MR glutamine/glutamate assays. NMR Biomed 4:103–108, 1991.

129. Schenker S, Breen KJ, Hoyumpa AM: Hepatic encephalopathy: current status. Gastroenterology 66:121–151, 1974.

130. Ross BD, Morgan MR, Cox IJ, et al: Cerebral energy deficit in patients with chronic hepatic encephalopathy monitored with ³¹P MRS. J Cereb Blood Flow Metab 7:S396, 1987.

131. Ross BD, Roberts JP, Tropp J, et al: Phosphorus imaging of brain in HE. Magn Reson Imaging 7:82, 1989. Abstract.

132. Luyten PR, den Hollander JA, Bovée WMMJ, et al: ³¹P and ¹H NMR spectroscopy of the human brain in chronic hepatic encephalopathy. In: Proceedings of the Eighth Annual Meeting of the Society of Magnetic Resonance in Medicine, Amsterdam, 1989, p 375.

133. Barbara L, Barbiroli B, Gaiani S, et al: Abnormal brain energy metabolism assessed by ³¹P MRS in liver cirrhosis. Eur J Hepatol 2:2, 1993.

134. Taylor-Robinson S, Mallalieu RJ, Sargentoni J, et al: Cerebral ³¹P MRS in patients with chronic hepatic encephalopathy. In: Proceedings of the 12th Annual Meeting of the Society of Magnetic Resonance in Medicine, New York, 1993, p 89.

135. Geissler A, Farrow N, Villamil F, et al: Is hepatic encephalopathy reversed by liver transplantation? In: Proceedings of the 11th Annual Meeting of Society of Magnetic Resonance in Medicine, Berlin, 1992, p 647.

136. Mason GF, Gruetter R, Rothman DL, et al: Simultaneous determination of the rates of the TCA cycle, glucose utilization, alpha-ketoglutarate/glutamate exchange, and glutamine synthesis in human brain by NMR. J Cereb Blood Flow Metab 15:12–25, 1995.

137. Gruetter R, Novotny EJ, Boulware SD, et al: Localized ¹³C NMR spectroscopy in the human brain of amino acid labeling from D-[1-¹³C] glucose. J Neurochem 63:1377–1385, 1994.

138. Ross BD, Shonk T, Moats RA, et al: Proton MRS for the diagnosis of subclinical hepatic encephalopathy. In: Proceedings of the 12th Annual Meeting of the Society of Magnetic Resonance in Medicine, New York, 1993, p 131.

139. Ross BD, Jacobson S, Villamil FG, et al: Cerebral myo-inositol depletion defines sub-clinical hepatic encephalopathy. Hepatology 18:105A, 1993. Abstract.

140. Gupta RK, Saraswat VA, Poptani H, et al: Magnetic resonance imaging and localized in vivo proton spectroscopy in patients with fulminant hepatic failure. Am J Gastroenterol 88:670–674, 1993.

141. Shonk T, Moats R, Lee JH, et al: Increased incidence of sub-clinical hepatic encephalopathy associated with TIPS procedure. Gastroenterology 104:A-449, 1993. Abstract.

142. Gadian DG, Connelly A, Cross JH, et al: ¹H spectroscopy in two children with ornithine transcarbamylase deficiency. In: Proceedings of the 10th Annual Meeting of the Society of Magnetic Resonance in Medicine, San Francisco, 1991, p 193.

143. Hawkins RA, Jessy J, Mans AM, De Joseph MR: Effect of reducing brain glutamine synthesis on metabolic symptoms of hepatic encephalopathy. J Neurochem 60:1000–1006, 1993.

144. Bruhn H, Michaelis T, Merboldt K-D, et al: Monitoring cerebral glucose in diabetics by proton MRS. Lancet 337:745–746, 1991.

145. Lien Y-HH, Shapiro JI, Chan L: Effects of hypernatremia on organic brain osmoles. J Clin Invest 85:1427–1435, 1990.

146. Wong GG: Studies with in Vivo NMR. Ph.D. thesis, University of Oxford, 1981.

147. Lee JH, Ross BD: Quantitation of idiogenic osmoles in human brain. In: Proceedings of the 12th Annual Meeting of the Society of Magnetic Resonance in Medicine, New York, 1993, p 1553.

148. Michaelis T, Cooper K, Kreis R, Ross BD: Proton MRS reveals two unusual cases of neonatal hypoxic encephalopathy. Pediatrics, in press.

149. Cady EB, Lorek A, Penrice J, et al: Detection of propan-1,2-diol in neonatal brain by in vivo proton magnetic resonance spectroscopy. Magn Reson Med 32:764–767, 1994.

150. Moats RA, Watson L, Shonk T, et al: The "added value" of automated clinical proton MR spectroscopy of the brain. J Comput Assist Tomogr 19:480–491, 1995.

151. Epstein FH: Nuclear magnetic resonance: a new tool in clinical medicine. N Engl J Med 304:1360–1361, 1981.
152. Ackerman JJH, Bore PJ, Wong GG, et al: Mapping of metabolites in whole animals by 31P NMR using surface coils. Nature 283:167–170, 1980.
153. Bottomley PA, Roster TB, Darrow RD: Depth-resolved surface spectroscopy (DRESS) for in vivo 1H, 31P and 13C NMR. J Magn Reson 59:338–342, 1984.
154. Ordidge RJ, Connelly A, Lohman JAB: Image-selected in vivo spectroscopy (ISIS). A new technique for spatially selective NMR spectroscopy. J Magn Reson 66:283–294, 1986.
155. Frahm J, Merboldt K-D, Hänicke W: Localized proton spectroscopy using stimulated echoes. J Magn Reson 72:502–508, 1987.
156. Merboldt KD, Chien D, Hanicke W, et al: Localized 31P NMR spectroscopy of the adult human brain in vivo using stimulated-echo (STEAM) sequences. J Magn Reson 89:343–361, 1990.
157. Ordidge RJ, Bendall MR, Gordon RE, Connelly A: Volume selection for in vivo biological spectroscopy. In: Govil G, Khetrapal CL, Saran A, eds. Magnetic Resonance in Biology and Medicine. New Delhi: Tata McGraw-Hill, 1985, pp 387–397.
158. Bottomley PA. Spatial localization in NMR spectroscopy in vivo. Ann N Y Acad Sci 508:333–348, 1987.
159. Thulborn KR, Ackerman JJH: Absolute molar concentrations by NMR in inhomogeneous B1 fields. A scheme for analysis of in vivo metabolites. J Magn Reson 55:357–371, 1983.
160. Narayana PA, Johnston D, Flamig DP: In vivo proton magnetic resonance spectroscopy studies of human brain. Magn Reson Imaging 9:303–308, 1991.
161. Hennig J, Pfister H, Ernst T, Ott D: Direct absolute quantification of metabolites in the human brain with in vivo localized proton spectroscopy. NMR Biomed 5:193–199, 1992.
162. Michaelis T, Merboldt K-D, Bruhn H, et al: Absolute concentrations of metabolites in the adult human brain in vivo: quantification of localized proton MR spectra. Radiology 187:219–227, 1993.
163. Barker PB, Soher BJ, Blackband SJ, et al: Quantitation of proton NMR spectra of the human brain using tissue water as an internal concentration reference. NMR Biomed 6:89–94, 1993.
164. Christiansen P, Henriksen O, Stubgaard M, et al: In vivo quantification of brain metabolites by means of 1H MRS using water as an internal standard. Magn Reson Imaging 11:107–118, 1993.
165. Danielsen ER, Henriksen O: Quantitative proton NMR spectroscopy based on the amplitude of the local water suppression pulse. Quantification of brain water and metabolites. NMR Biomed 7:311–318, 1994.
166. Webb PG, Sailasuta N, Kohler S, et al: Automated single-voxel proton MRS: technical development and multisite verification. Magn Reson Med 31:365–373, 1994.
167. Provencher SW: Estimation of metabolite concentrations from localized in vivo proton NMR spectra. Magn Reson Med 30:672–679, 1993.

PART III

HEAD AND NECK

31

Orbital and Intraocular Lesions

MAHMOOD F. MAFEE

ORBIT

ANATOMY AND DEVELOPMENT

The orbits are two recesses that contain the globes, muscles, blood vessels, lymphatics, cranial nerves (II, III, IV, V, and VI), adipose and connective tissues, and most of the lacrimal apparatus. They are bordered by the periosteum and separated from the globe by Tenon's capsule. Anterior are the orbital septum and the lids.[1] The orbital cavity is pyramidal; its apex is directed posteriorly and medially and its base anteriorly and laterally at the orbital opening. Its bony walls separate it from the anterior cranial fossa superiorly, the ethmoid air cells and nasal cavity medially, the maxillary sinus inferiorly, and the lateral surface of the face and temporal fossa laterally and posteriorly[2] (Fig. 31–1).

Bony Orbit

Each orbit presents a roof, a floor, medial and lateral walls, a base or orbital opening, and an apex. At the posterior end of the junction of the roof with the medial wall, the optic canal and optic foramen establish communication between the orbit and the middle cranial fossa. The optic canal contains the optic nerve, ophthalmic artery, and sympathetic fibers (Fig. 31–2).

Superior Orbital Fissure

Just lateral and inferolateral to the optic canal, and separated from it by the optic strut, is the superior orbital fissure. It communicates with the middle cranial fossa and transmits the oculomotor, trochlear, and abducens nerves and the terminal branches of the ophthalmic nerve and the superior ophthalmic vein.

Inferior Orbital Fissure

At the posterior aspect of the orbit, the inferior and lateral walls of the orbit are separated by the inferior orbital fissure (see Fig. 31–2A). The fissure is bounded above by the greater wing of the sphenoid, below by the maxilla and the orbital process of palatine bone, and laterally by the zygomatic bone and the zygomaticomaxillary suture. In fact, the inferior orbital fissure extends obliquely as a gently curving continuation of the more medial pterygopalatine (sphenopalatine) fossa. The maxillary nerve is the most important structure traversing the inferior orbital fissure. In addition to the maxillary nerve, the inferior orbital fissure transmits the infraorbital vessels, the zygomatic nerve, and a few minute twigs from the pterygopalatine ganglion. Through the anterior part of the inferior orbital fissure, a vein passes to connect the inferior ophthalmic vein with the pterygoid venous plexus.[3]

TECHNICAL CONSIDERATIONS

High-quality orbital images have been produced at fields of 0.5 to 1.5 T. Most images in this section were obtained on a 1.5-T magnetic resonance (MR) imager. The spin-echo pulse sequence is the essential pulse sequence used for orbital imaging. Other useful pulse sequences include inversion recovery, short-tau inversion recovery (STIR), and gradient echo. The gradient-echo pulse sequences have limited application to the orbit because of signal loss resulting from magnetic susceptibility effects. STIR sequences provide high-contrast images but poor spatial resolution. We use STIR as an additional pulse sequence in cases of inflammatory and metastatic diseases. The use of gadolinium-based contrast agents has increased the sensitivity of MR imaging (MRI).[2-6] Postcontrast T1-weighted fat-suppressed pulse sequences in most cases appear to be most informative. One has to be careful with the technique of frequency-selective T1-weighted fat-suppressed pulse sequences. In these pulse sequences, extraocular muscles and lacrimal glands appear quite hyperintense. One should not misinterpret abnormal enhancement of these structures on fat-suppressed T1-weighted images after gadolinium diethylenetriamine-pentaacetic acid (Gd-DTPA) enhancement. The use of Gd-DTPA for intraocular tumors has proved valuable.

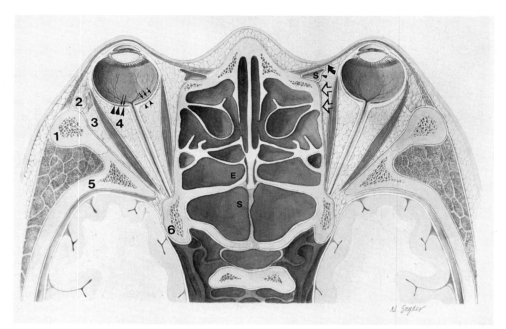

FIGURE 31–1. Diagram of an axial section of the orbits at the level of the optic nerve. Notice the periorbita or periosteum *(open arrows)*. The periorbita splits at the level of lacrimal sac (S), giving off lacrimal sac fascia *(arrowhead)*, and then forms the orbital septum *(curved arrow)*. Notice Tenon's capsule *(double arrowheads)*, sclera *(triple arrowheads)*, choroid *(double arrows)*, retina *(triple arrows)*, zygomatic bone (1), lacrimal gland (2), peripheral orbital fat (3), central orbital fat (4), greater wing of sphenoid bone (5), anterior clinoid (6), ethmoid (E), and sphenoid (s) sinuses.

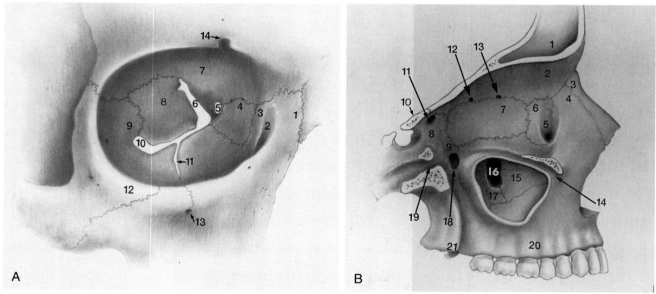

FIGURE 31–2. *A,* Schematic drawing of bony orbit. 1 = Frontal process of maxilla; 2 = lacrimal groove; 3 = lacrimal bone; 4 = lamina papyracea; 5 = optic canal (foramen); 6 = superior orbital fissure; 7 = frontal bone; 8 = greater wing of sphenoid; 9 = orbital plate of zygomatic bone; 10 = inferior orbital fissure; 11 = infraorbital groove; 12 = zygoma (malar bone); 13 = infraorbital foramen; 14 = supraorbital foramen; *B,* Schematic drawing of the orbital maxillary region. 1 = Frontal bone; 2 = orbital plate of frontal bone; 3 = nasal bone; 4 = frontal process of maxilla; 5 = lacrimal groove; 6 = lacrimal bone; 7 = lamina papyracea; 8 = sphenoid bone; 9 = palatine bone (orbital plate); 10 = lesser wing of sphenoid; 11 = optic canal; 12 = posterior ethmoid foramen; 13 = anterior ethmoid foramen; 14 = infraorbital canal (foramen); 15 = inferior concha; 16 = maxillary hiatus; 17 = palatine bone; 18 = sphenopalatine foramen opening into the pterygopalatine fossa; 19 = vidian canal, opening into the pterygopalatine fossa; 20 = alveolar process of maxilla; 21 = pterygoid palate.

TABLE 31–1. INTRACONAL (CENTRAL ORBITAL) LESIONS

MORE COMMON	LESS COMMON
Cavernous hemangioma	Capillary hemangioma
Optic nerve meningioma	Sclerosing hemangioma
Optic nerve glioma	Peripheral nerve tumors
Optic nerve granulomatous disease (sarcoid)	Neurofibroma
	Schwannoma
Optic neuritis (multiple sclerosis)	Leukemia
	Hematocele
Lymphoma	Optic nerve sheath cyst
Pseudotumor	Colobomatous cyst
Lymphangioma	Hemangioblastoma (optic nerve)
Venous angioma	
Varix	Chemodectoma (ciliary ganglion)
Arteriovenous malformation	
Carotid cavernous fistula	Necrobiotic xanthogranuloma
Hemangiopericytoma	Lipoma
Rhabdomyosarcoma	Amyloidosis
Metastasis	
Orbital cellulitis and abscess	

We use contrast to better differentiate tumors from subretinal fluid and to distinguish choroidal melanomas from choroidal hemangiomas. Optic nerve involvement and extraocular extension of intraocular tumors are best diagnosed on postcontrast fat-suppressed T1-weighted pulse sequences.

Computed Tomography Versus MRI

Because of its high-contrast resolution and ability to define hard and soft tissues, computed tomography (CT) had become the imaging method of choice for many orbital disorders. MRI, on the other hand, is a noninvasive technique that has remarkable sensitivity

TABLE 31–2. CAUSES OF ENLARGED EXTRAOCULAR MUSCLE AND COMMON ORBITAL PERIOSTEAL LESIONS

COMMON CAUSES OF ENLARGED EXTRAOCULAR MUSCLE	COMMON ORBITAL SUBPERIOSTEAL LESIONS
Graves' myositis	Subperiosteal cellulitis
Inflammatory myositis, including cysticercosis	Subperiosteal abscess
	Infiltration of neoplastic lesions of paranasal sinuses
Granulomatous myositis (less common), sarcoidosis	Infiltration of meningiomas (en plaque meningiomas)
Pseudotumor (myositic type)	Lymphomas
Lymphoma	Leukemia
Vascular lesions (hemangioma, arteriovenous malformation)	Plasmacytomas
	Extension of
Acromegaly	Lacrimal gland tumors
Pseudorheumatoid nodule	Dermoid and epidermoid cysts
Metastasis (breast, lung)	Hematoma and hematic cyst
	Cholesterol granuloma
	Fibrous histiocytoma (rare)
	Primary osseous or cartilaginous tumors (rare)
	Langerhans' histiocytosis (rare)
	Metastasis (neuroblastoma)

in differentiating various normal (Fig. 31–3A to L) and abnormal soft tissues. MRI is the imaging modality of choice for evaluation of neuro-ophthalmologic disorders. Except for foreign bodies, retinoblastomas (calcification), and osseous lesions, MRI has proved superior to CT for many orbital and intraocular applications.

ORBITAL PATHOLOGY

ORBITAL COMPARTMENTS

In descriptive terms, the orbit has been divided into the extraperiosteal, subperiosteal, extraconal, conal, and intraconal spaces. The intraconal space is separated from the other spaces by the rectus muscles and their intermuscular septa, which are denser in the anterior orbit and best seen on coronal MRI images (see Fig. 31–3H). Certain lesions have a predilection to present in specific or various orbital spaces (Tables 31–1 to 31–3). Some orbital and ocular disease may show dystrophic calcifications. The concept of various orbital spaces is useful for surgical planning for surgeons and differential diagnosis for radiologists.[2, 3, 7]

DEVELOPMENTAL ORBITAL CYSTS

The most frequent developmental cysts involving the orbit and periorbital structures are dermoid and epidermoid cysts.[1, 7] Both result from the inclusion of ectodermal elements during closure of the neural tube. The dermal elements that are pinched off along the cranio-orbitofacial suture lines, diploë, or within the meninges or scalp in the course of embryonic development give rise to these cysts. Both have a fibrous capsule of varying degrees of thickness. The epidermoid has a lining of keratinizing, stratified epithelium. The dermoid contains one or more dermal adnexal structures such as sebaceous glands and hair follicles. Teratomas are choristomatous tumors that contain tissue representing two or more germ layers. Endodermal derivatives such as gut or respiratory epi-

TABLE 31–3. EXTRACONAL PERIPHERAL ORBITAL LESIONS

MORE COMMON	LESS COMMON
Capillary hemangioma	Amyloidosis
Cholesterol granuloma	Fibrous histiocytoma
Dermoid and epidermoid cysts	Hemangiosarcoma
	Hemangiopericytoma
Lacrimal gland lesions	Hematic cyst
Inflammation	Lipoma
Lymphoma	Orbital encephalocele
Pseudotumor	Wegener's granulomatosis
Sarcoidosis	Aggressive fibromatosis
Epithelial tumors	
Lymphangioma	
Peripheral nerve tumors	
Plasmacytoma	
Rhabdomyocarcoma	
Sarcoidosis	

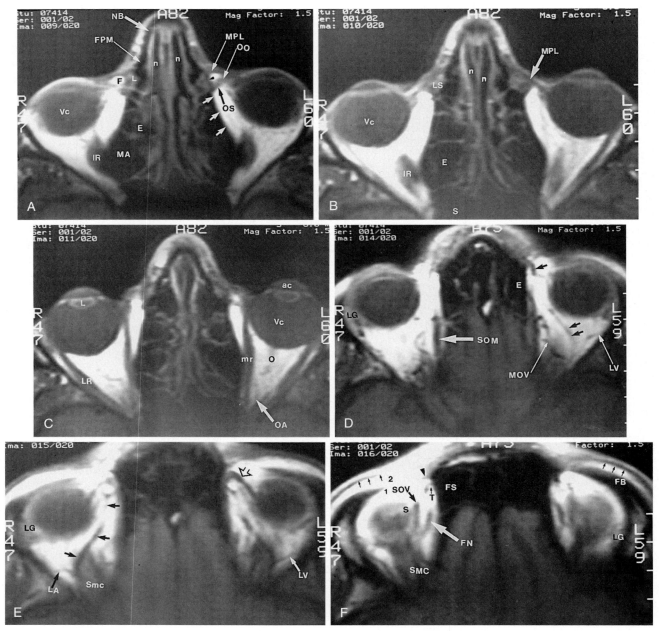

FIGURE 31–3. Normal MRI anatomy. *A,* Axial T1-weighted image obtained with surface coil shows nasal bone (NB), frontal process of maxilla (FPM), lacrimal sac (L), fat pad (F), nasal cavities (n), medial palpebral ligament (MPL), lacrimal portion of orbicularis oculi (OO), orbital septum (OS), ethmoid air cells (E), maxillary antrum (MA), inferior rectus (IR), and vitreous chamber (Vc). Notice the periorbita *(arrows)* and lacrimal fascia *(arrowhead).* The lacrimal sac is located in the lacrimal fossa and is enclosed by lacrimal fascia. The fascia is formed from the periorbita. *B,* Axial T1-weighted image obtained 3 mm cephalad to *A.* Notice medial palpebral ligament (MPL), nasal cavities (n), lacrimal sac (LS), ethmoid (E) and sphenoid (S) sinuses, inferior rectus muscle (IR), and vitreous chamber (Vc). *C,* Axial T1-weighted image obtained 3 mm cephalad to *B.* Notice anterior chamber (ac), vitreous chamber (Vc), medial rectus muscle (mr), optic nerve (O), ophthalmic artery (OA), lateral rectus (LR), and lens (L). *D,* Axial T1-weighted image obtained 9 mm cephalad to *C.* Notice superior ophthalmic vein *(solid arrows),* lacrimal vein (LV), medial ophthalmic vein (MOV), ethmoid sinus (E), and superior oblique muscle (SOM). *E,* Axial T1-weighted image obtained 3 mm cephalad to *D.* Notice lacrimal gland (LG), presumed lacrimal artery (LA), superior rectus levator palpebrae complex (Smc), superior ophthalmic vein *(solid arrows),* presumed lacrimal vein (LV), and reflected portion of the tendon of the superior oblique muscle *(open arrow).* *F,* Axial T1-weighted image obtained 3 mm cephalad to *E.* The orbital septum *(arrowhead)* separates the preaponeurotic fat pad (1) from the fat pad (2) underlying the orbicularis oculi *(triple arrows).* Notice frontal sinus (FS), trochlea (T), superior ophthalmic vein (SOV), sclera (S), presumed frontal nerve (FN), superior rectus levator palpebrae complex (SMC), lacrimal gland (LG), and frontal bone (FB).

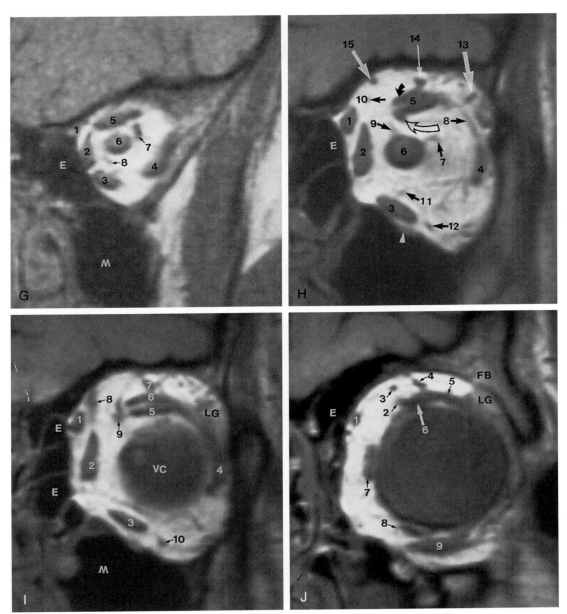

FIGURE 31–3. *Continued G,* Coronal T1-weighted image obtained with the surface coil. Notice superior oblique muscle (1), medial rectus muscle (2), inferior rectus muscle (3), lateral rectus muscle (4), superior rectus muscle (5), optic nerve (6), presumed ophthalmic artery (7), presumed oculomotor nerve (8), and ethmoid (E) and maxillary (M) sinuses. *H,* Coronal T1-weighted image obtained 3 mm anterior to G. Notice superior oblique muscle (1), medial rectus muscle (2), inferior rectus muscle (3), lateral rectus muscle (4), superior rectus muscle (5), levator palpebrae superioris *(solid curved arrow),* superior ophthalmic vein *(open curved arrow),* optic nerve (6), presumed posterior ciliary artery (7), intermuscular septum (8), presumed ciliary ganglion (9), nasociliary nerve (10), medial orbital vein or inferior muscular artery (11), inferior ramus of oculomotor nerve (12), lacrimal nerve artery and vein (13), frontal nerve (14), supratrochlear nerve (15), ethmoid sinus (E), and infraorbital nerve *(arrowhead).* *I,* Coronal T1-weighted image obtained 3 mm anterior to *H.* Notice superior oblique muscle (1), medial rectus muscle (2), inferior rectus (3), lateral rectus (4), superior rectus muscle (5), levator palpebrae superioris (6), frontal nerve (7), medial ophthalmic vein (8), ophthalmic artery (9), presumed inferior branch of oculomotor nerve (10), maxillary (M) and ethmoid (E) sinuses, and lacrimal gland (LG). VC = vitreous chamber. *J,* Coronal T1-weighted image obtained 3 mm anterior to *I.* Notice tendon of superior oblique muscle (1), reflected tendon of superior oblique muscle (2), under the tendon of superior rectus muscle (6), presumed superior ophthalmic vein (3), frontal nerve (4), tendon of levator palpebrae superioris (5), tendon of superior rectus muscle (6), tendon of medial rectus muscle (7), tendon of inferior rectus muscle (8), inferior oblique muscle (9), lacrimal gland (LG), frontal bone (FB), and ethmoid sinus (E).

Illustration continued on following page

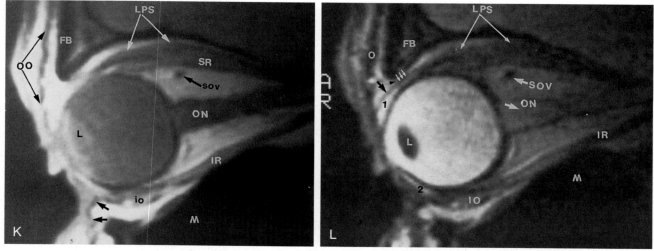

FIGURE 31–3. *Continued K,* Sagittal proton density–weighted image. Notice fibers of orbicularis oculi (OO), frontal bone (FB), lens (L), levator palpebrae superioris (LPS), superior rectus muscle (SR), superior ophthalmic vein (sov), optic nerve (ON), inferior rectus muscle (IR), maxillary antrum (M), inferior oblique muscle (io), and orbital septum *(double arrows)*. *L,* Sagittal T2-weighted image. Notice orbicularis oculi (O), frontal bone (FB), levator palpebrae superioris (LPS), superior ophthalmic vein (SOV), optic nerve (ON), inferior rectus muscle (IR), maxillary antrum (M), inferior oblique muscle (IO), lens (L), superior (1) and inferior (2) fornices, superior tarsal plate *(black arrow)*. Notice the tendon of insertion of levator palpebrae superioris *(three white arrows)*. This tendon is an aponeurosis that descends posterior to the orbital septum *(arrowhead)*. The tendinous fibers then pierce the orbital septum and become attached to the anterior surface of the superior tarsal plate.

thelium; ectodermal tissues such as skin and its appendages; and neural and mesodermal tissues such as connective tissues, smooth muscles, cartilage, bone, fat, and vessels may be present. Teratomas are evident at birth as grossly visible cystic orbital masses. The dermoid and epidermoid cysts favor the upper portion rather than the lower quadrants of the orbit for their growth.[7–10] They grow slowly, but at times these cysts can grow significantly, particularly in adults.[11] Epidermoids are seen on CT scans as nonenhancing masses (hypo- or isodense relative to adjacent soft tissues). There may be compression atrophy or significant scalloping of the adjacent bony orbital wall. Dermoids have similar CT findings. At times, fat density, fluid-fluid level, and calcification may be present in dermoids. The MRI characteristics of epidermoid include hypointensity in regard to brain in T1-weighted images and hyperintensity in T2-weighted images (Fig. 31–4). The fat components of dermoids show short-T1 and short-T2 signal characteristics (Fig. 31–5).

INFLAMMATORY DISEASES OF THE ORBIT

Orbital infections account for about 60% of primary orbital disease processes. The processes may be acute, subacute, or chronic. The majority of acute inflammatory disorders are of sinus origin. However, they may develop from an infectious process of the face or pharynx, trauma, or foreign bodies or may be secondary to septicemia. The bacteria most commonly involved are *Staphylococcus, Streptococcus,* pneumococcus, *Pseudomonas,* Neisseriaceae, *Haemophilus,* and mycobacteria. Herpes simplex and herpes zoster are the major viral

infections of the orbit. In immune-suppressed patients and poorly controlled diabetic patients, opportunistic infections such as infections with fungal and parasitic pathogens may be responsible for severe sinonaso-orbital infections.

Orbital Cellulitis and Sinusitis

Sinusitis is the most common cause of orbital cellulitis. Pathophysiologically, infection originating within the sinuses can spread readily to the orbit via the thin and often dehiscent bony wall and its many foramina or by means of the interconnecting valveless venous system of the face, sinus, and orbit. The classification of orbital cellulitis includes five categories or stages of orbital involvement from sinusitis: 1) inflammatory edema, 2) subperiosteal phlegmon and abscess, 3) orbital cellulitis, 4) orbital abscess, and 5) ophthalmic vein and cavernous sinus thrombosis. Limiting a particular inflammatory lesion to one of these categories is difficult, because they tend to overlap.

Preseptal cellulitis is the first stage of infection. It is often misdiagnosed as orbital or periorbital cellulitis. In this early stage the infection is actually still confined to the sinus. It is characterized by swelling of the eyelids. A slightly more advanced stage includes chemosis. CT or MRI at this stage demonstrates edema of the eyelids and inflammatory changes of the infected sinus or sinuses.

As the reaction of the orbital periosteum begins and gradually advances, the edema of the eyelids and conjunctivae becomes more generalized and the eye begins to protrude. Inflammatory tissue and edema collect beneath the periosteum to form a subperiosteal

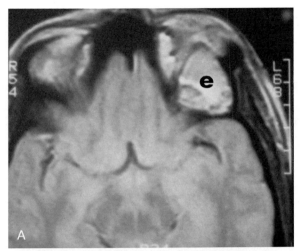

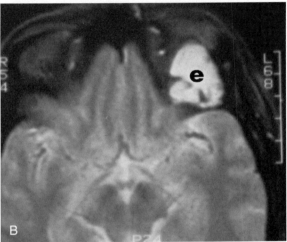

FIGURE 31–4. Epidermoid cyst. *(A)* Axial proton density–weighted (repetition time/echo time = 3500/30) and *(B)* T2-weighted (3500/80) images show a hyperintense mass in the superior portion of the left orbit, compatible with an epidermoid cyst (e).

phlegmon. Subsequently, pus may form and represent a subperiosteal abscess (Fig. 31–6). As the disease progresses, the inflammatory process may infiltrate the periorbital and retro-orbital fat to give rise to a true orbital cellulitis.[10, 12, 13]

Ophthalmic vein thrombosis and cavernous sinus thrombosis are serious complications of orbital and

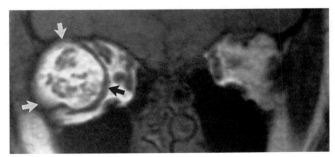

FIGURE 31–5. Dermoid cyst. Coronal T1-weighted image shows a large mass *(arrows)* compatible with a dermoid cyst.

sinonasal infections. Cavernous sinus thrombosis is heralded by profound central nervous system deficit and orbital functional impairment.[12]

Orbital Pseudotumor

Idiopathic inflammatory syndromes are usually referred to as orbital "pseudotumors," a clinically and histologically confusing category of lesions. In general, orbital pseudotumor comprises a broad category of orbital inflammatory diseases. It is defined as a nonspecific, idiopathic inflammatory condition for which no local identifiable cause or systemic disease can be found.[2, 3, 7, 14]

Pseudotumors may be classified as 1) acute or subacute idiopathic anterior orbital inflammation, 2) acute or subacute idiopathic diffuse orbital inflammation, 3) acute or subacute idiopathic myositic orbital inflammation, 4) acute or subacute idiopathic apical orbital inflammation, 5) idiopathic dacryoadenitis, and 6) perineuritis (optic nerve).

Computed Tomography and MRI

Of the various CT and MRI characteristics associated with different features of pseudotumors, the most common findings include enhancement with use of intravenous contrast medium (95%) (Fig. 31–7), infiltration of the retrobulbar fat (76%) (Fig. 31–8), proptosis (71%), extraocular muscle enlargement (57%), apical fat infiltration and edema (48%), muscle tendon sheath enlargement (Fig. 31–9) (43%), and optic nerve thickening (38%). Infiltration of the lacrimal gland is also common.

We have found no specific imaging findings, nor are there any specific clinical signs to establish the diagnosis of pseudotumors with absolute certainty. Classically, the rapid development of unilateral, painful ophthalmoplegia, proptosis, and chemosis with a rapid and lasting response to steroid therapy in an otherwise healthy patient is highly suggestive of pseudotumor. In the absence of a characteristic clinical presentation of pseudotumor or poor responsiveness to steroids, biopsy is necessary.

Thyroid Orbitopathy

Thyroid orbitopathy occurs most commonly in middle-aged women. It is characterized ophthalmologically by exophthalmos and in some patients by the gradual onset of diplopia, usually the vertical type. Initially, in the acute congestive phase, the retrobulbar orbital contents are markedly swollen and congested. Later, a more chronic, noncongestive phase follows, in which a restrictive type of limited eye movement often develops, secondary to infiltration of the extraocular muscles and to subsequent loss of elasticity. The involvement can be unilateral or bilateral. When bilateral, it is often fairly symmetric. The inferior rectus muscle is most commonly involved, leading to a limitation of elevation of the involved eye. The medial and superior rectus muscles are also frequently involved. The lateral

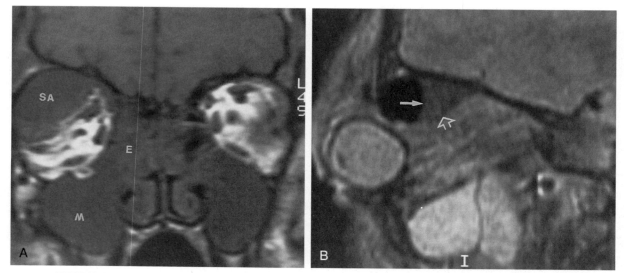

FIGURE 31–6. Sinogenic subperiosteal abscess. *A,* Coronal T1-weighted (800/20) image shows bilateral maxillary (M) and right ethmoid (E) sinusitis. Notice a well-defined mass in the superior portion of the right orbit compatible with a subperiosteal abscess (SA). *B,* Sagittal T2-weighted (2000/80) image shows an air-fluid level *(solid arrow)* within the subperiosteal abscess. Notice displaced periorbita *(open arrow).*

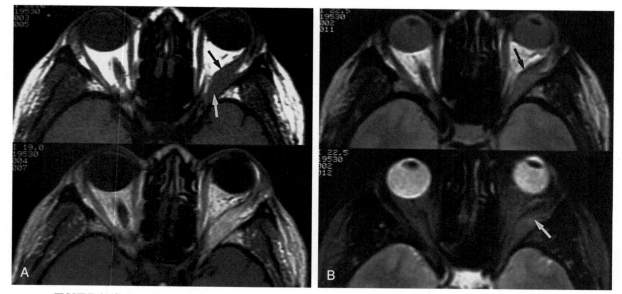

FIGURE 31–7. Pseudotumor. *A,* Axial precontrast T1-weighted *(top)* and post–Gd-DTPA T1-weighted *(bottom)* images show an infiltrative process involving the left lateral rectus muscle and adjacent peripheral orbital fat *(arrows).* *B,* Axial proton density–weighted *(top)* and T2-weighted *(bottom)* images show that the pseudotumor *(arrows)* appears isointense relative to fat on the T2-weighted image.

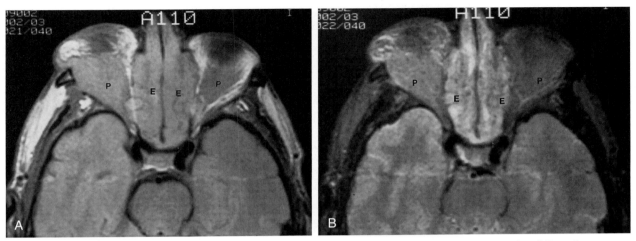

FIGURE 31–8. Pseudotumor. *(A)* Axial proton density–weighted and *(B)* axial T2-weighted images show bilateral infiltrative process in the retrobulbar spaces compatible with pseudotumor (P). Notice inflammatory polypoid changes in the ethmoids (E).

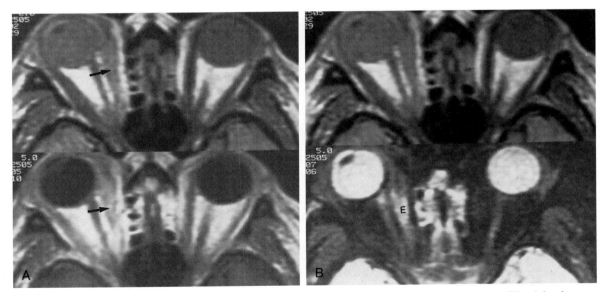

FIGURE 31–9. Myositic pseudotumor. *A,* Precontrast axial T1-weighted *(top)* and postcontrast T1-weighted *(bottom)* images showing thickening of right medial rectus muscle *(arrow)* including its tendinous part. Notice moderate degree of contrast enhancement. There is also involvement of right lateral rectus muscle. *B,* Axial proton density–weighted *(top)* and T2-weighted *(bottom)* images. Notice edema (E) of the right medial rectus muscle.

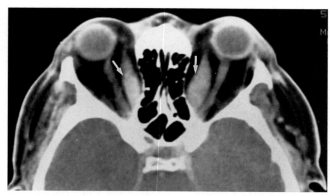

FIGURE 31–10. Thyroid ophthalmopathy. Axial CT scan shows marked bilateral enlarged medial rectus muscles *(arrows)*. Notice that their tendinous portions are spared.

rectus and superior oblique muscles are less commonly affected. The forced duction test result is almost always abnormal. Myopathy may occur at any time in the course of Graves' disease; laboratory evaluation may reveal hyperthyroidism, hypothyroidism, or euthyroidism.

Extraocular muscle enlargement in Graves' disease and associated compressive neuropathy, if any, can be visualized by CT and MRI (Figs. 31–10 and 31–11). Typically, enlargement involves the muscle belly, sparing its tendinous portion.[15] However, rare patients show thickening of the tendinous portion. Another helpful finding in thyroid myopathy is the presence of low-density areas within the muscle bellies on CT scans. These are probably the result of focal accumulation of lymphocytes, mucopolysaccharide deposition, and fatty degeneration. Other CT and MRI findings in thyroid orbitopathy are increased orbital fat, enlargement (engorgement) of the lacrimal glands, edema (fullness) of the eyelids, proptosis, and stretching of the optic nerve with or without associated "tenting" of the posterior globe.

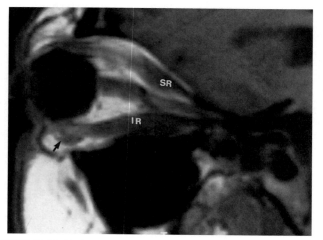

FIGURE 31–11. Thyroid ophthalmopathy. Sagittal T1-weighted image shows enlargement of superior (SR) and inferior (IR) rectus muscles. Notice also enlargement of inferior oblique muscle *(arrow)*.

Painful External Ophthalmoplegia (Tolosa-Hunt Syndrome)

Painful external ophthalmoplegia, or Tolosa-Hunt syndrome, is now considered an idiopathic inflammatory process and a regional variant of idiopathic orbital pseudotumors that, because of its anatomic location, produces typical clinical manifestations (Fig. 31–12). Pathologically, there is infiltration of lymphocytes and plasma cells along with thickening of the dura matter. The condition generally responds to systemic corticosteroid therapy. It is important to exclude the possibility of a neoplastic, inflammatory (particularly mycotic), or vasculogenic lesion. Carotid angiography and MRI are most useful in excluding aneurysm as a cause of the clinical signs and symptoms. Certain sellar, suprasellar, and parasellar lesions such as pituitary adenomas, meningiomas, craniopharyngiomas, neurogenic tumors, dermoid cysts, lymphoma, leukemic infiltration, extension of sinonasal and nasopharyngeal carcinomas, and metastatic lesions (e.g., melanoma, lung, breast, kidney, thyroid, prostate) may produce similar symptoms.

ORBITAL LYMPHOMA

Lymphomas are solid tumors of the immune system. Most are composed of monoclonal B cells. The extranodal presentation of non-Hodgkin's lymphomas is common, with an incidence ranging from 21% to 64%. Roughly 10% of non-Hodgkin's lymphomas present in the head and neck region. Lymphoid tumors account for 10% to 15% of orbital masses.[16]

Lymphoid neoplasms of the orbit span a large continuum of classifications from malignant lymphomas to benign pseudolymphomas or pseudotumors to the reactive and atypical lymphoid hyperplasias. There are no absolute imaging, clinical, or even laboratory tests that distinguish all types of benign orbital lymphoid lesions from orbital lymphomas or lesions that can simulate them.[16] A pleomorphic cellular infiltrate is correlated with more benign biologic activity. The more uniform the cellular appearance, the greater the likelihood that malignancy is present. Of all patients with orbital lymphoma, 75% have or will have systemic lymphoma. There is extensive overlap histologically from one type to another, and some forms of the benign process can transform over time into a more aggressive variety of lymphoma. True lymphoid tissue in the eye is found in the subconjunctiva and lacrimal gland. These two areas account for most orbital lymphoreticuloses.

Diagnostic Imaging

Ultrasonography, CT, and MRI can be used to evaluate orbital lymphomas. CT and MRI have made it possible to make a strong presumptive diagnosis of orbital lymphoma, especially when CT and MRI features are examined in conjunction with the clinical characteristics. The CT and MRI findings are usually

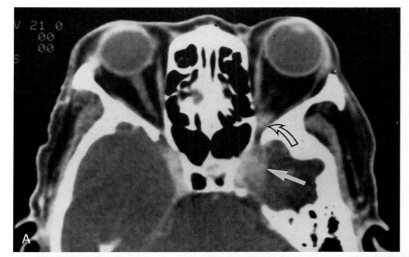

FIGURE 31–12. Tolosa-Hunt syndrome. The syndrome is due to tuberculosis of the orbital apex and superior orbital fissure region. *A,* Axial postcontrast CT scan shows infiltrative process involving the left cavernous sinus *(solid arrow)* and adjacent superior orbital fissure and orbital apex *(open arrow). B,* Axial proton density–weighted image shows increased soft tissue in the left cavernous sinus *(arrows)* and adjacent superior orbital fissure. Notice postoperative changes in the left temporal lobe and temporal fossa related to old surgical procedure. *C,* Axial proton density–weighted image after treatment for tuberculosis. Notice normal appearance of left cavernous sinus and superior orbital fissure and orbital apex.

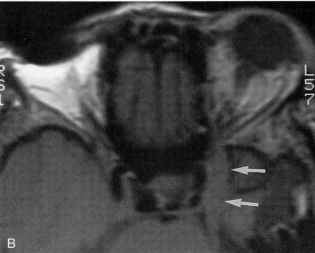
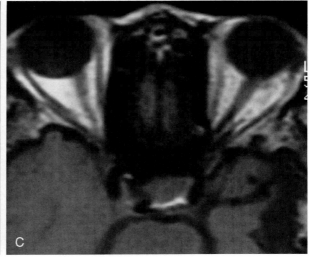

nonspecific and at times it can be impossible to differentiate orbital lymphomas from orbital pseudotumors, lacrimal gland tumors (Fig. 31–13), optic nerve tumors (Fig. 31–14), Graves' orbitopathy, primary orbital tumors, or orbital cellulitis. Orbital lymphomas are often

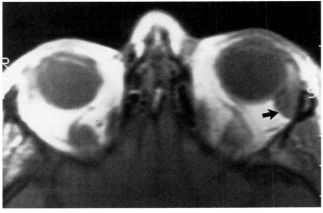

FIGURE 31–13. Lymphoma. Axial proton density–weighted image shows lymphomatous involvement of left lacrimal gland *(arrow).*

seen on CT scans as homogeneous masses of relatively high density[1] and sharp margins, which are more often seen in the anterior portion of the orbit, retrobulbar areas (see Fig. 31–14*A*), or the superior orbital compartment. Generally, the lesions mold themselves to preexisting structures without eroding the bone or enlarging the orbit. Mild to moderate enhancement is present.

A bulky lesion in the region of the lacrimal fossa that does not produce any bone erosion is most likely to be inflammatory or lymphoid in character. However, aggressive malignant lymphomas can produce frank destruction of bone, particularly in patients with myeloma.

MRI has proved to be as sensitive as CT for the diagnosis of orbital lymphoma and pseudotumors. Both pseudotumor and lymphoma may have an intermediate or hypointense signal on T1-weighted and proton density–weighted images and appear isointense relative to fat on T2-weighted images. Lymphomas may be more hypointense on T1-weighted images than pseudotumors (see Fig. 31–14*B*). Lymphomatous lesions may be hyperintense on T2-weighted images. Leukemic infiltration has MR appearances similar to

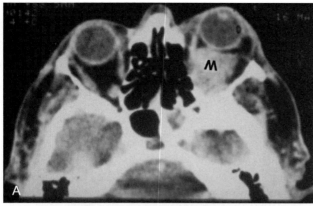

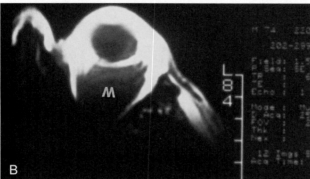

FIGURE 31-14. Lymphoma. *(A)* Axial CT scan and *(B)* axial T1-weighted image show a large retrobulbar mass (M) compatible with lymphoma.

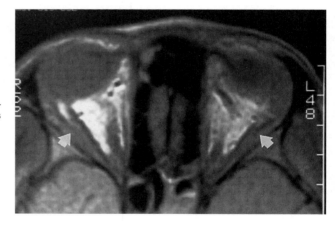

FIGURE 31-15. Leukemic infiltration of the orbits. Axial proton density–weighted image shows bilateral subperiosteal leukemic infiltrations *(arrows).*

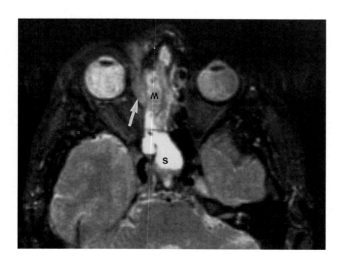

FIGURE 31-16. Lymphoma of sinonasal cavities with orbital involvement. Axial T2-weighted image shows a large mass (M) in the right nasal cavity and ethmoid air cells, extending into the orbit *(arrow).* Notice retained secretion in the right sphenoid (S).

those of lymphomatous lesions (Fig. 31–15). All criteria used for CT in the diagnosis of orbital pseudotumors and lymphoma in terms of morphology, location, homogeneity, contouring, and contrast enhancement (Gd-DTPA) can be used for MRI in the diagnosis of these conditions. Orbital lymphoma may at times be due to extension of lymphoma from a sinonasal cavity (Fig. 31–16).

VASCULAR CONDITIONS OF THE ORBIT

Capillary Hemangioma (Benign Hemangioendothelioma)

Capillary hemangiomas are tumors that occur primarily in infants during the first year of life. The tumor often increases in size for 6 to 10 months and then gradually involutes. The tumor most commonly occurs in the superior nasal quadrant. Involution generally commences by the 10th month of life. Microscopically, the tumor is composed of endothelial and capillary vessel proliferation with benign endothelial cells sur-

rounding small, capillary-sized vascular spaces. Capillary hemangiomas in and around the orbit usually have an arterial supply from the external and, to a lesser extent, the internal carotid arteries, and they are capable of bleeding profusely. These angiomas may extend intracranially through the superior orbital fissure, optic canal, and orbital roof. On CT scans, these lesions are seen as fairly well-marginated to poorly marginated, irregular, enhancing lesions. In our series, most of them were extraconal, although some of these lesions may be seen in the intraconal space. On dynamic CT study, these capillary hemangiomas characteristically show an intense, homogeneous enhancement.[17] MRI features of capillary hemangiomas are characteristic of long-T1 and long-T2 lesions. Prominent vascular structures may be present, seen as signal voids on MR images (Fig. 31–17). There is marked contrast enhancement after intravenous administration of Gd-DTPA.

Cavernous Hemangiomas

Cavernous hemangioma of the orbit, the most common orbital vascular tumor in adults, has distinctive

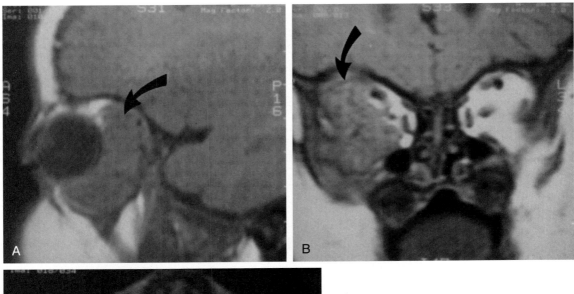

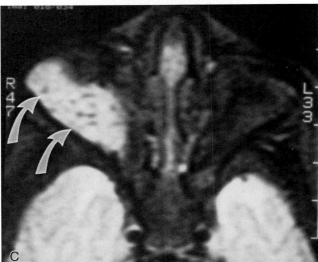

FIGURE 31–17. Capillary hemangioma. *(A)* Sagittal and *(B)* coronal T1-weighted (600/20) and *(C)* axial T2-weighted (2000/100) images show a large orbital mass *(arrows)* compatible with capillary hemangioma in this 5-month-old girl.

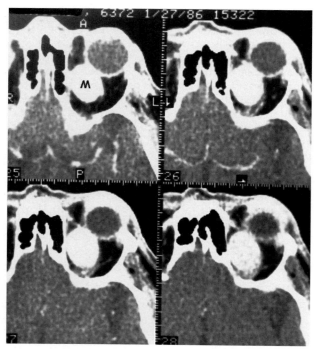

FIGURE 31–18. Cavernous hemangioma. Serial postcontrast CT scans show a markedly enhancing mass (M) compatible with a cavernous hemangioma.

clinical and histopathologic features. These tumors tend to occur in the second to fourth decades of life. They show a slowly progressive enlargement, whereas capillary hemangiomas gradually diminish in size. In contrast to the case with capillary hemangiomas, a prominent arterial supply is usually absent. Cavernous hemangiomas possess a distinct fibrous pseudocapsule and therefore appear as well-defined masses.[2, 7] Histologically, cavernous hemangiomas are composed of large dilated vascular channels (sinusoid-like spaces)

lined by thin, attenuated endothelial cells. These hemangiomas may be located anywhere in the orbit but frequently (83%) occur within the retrobulbar muscle cone. On CT scans, cavernous hemangiomas appear as well-defined, smoothly marginated, homogeneous, rounded, ovoid, or lobulated soft tissue of increased density with variable degrees of contrast enhancement (Fig. 31–18). The MRI features of cavernous hemangiomas are indicative of a lesion with long-T1 and long-T2 signal characteristics (Fig. 31–19). There is marked enhancement after intravenous administration of Gd-DTPA[17a] (Fig. 31–20).

Lymphangiomas

Orbital lymphangiomas occur in children and young adults. In contrast to the rapid, self-limited growth of infantile capillary hemangiomas, lymphangiomas gradually and progressively enlarge during the growing years. Cavernous lymphangiomas are composed of delicate, endothelium-lined, lymph-filled sinuses (filled with clear fluid or chocolate-colored unclotted fluid), which invade the surrounding connective tissue stroma. The interstitial tissue often shows lymphoid follicles and lymphocytic infiltration. Spontaneous hemorrhage within the lesion is common. Lymphangiomas may have distinct borders but are typically diffuse and not well capsulated, with portions of the lesion infiltrated within normal tissues of the lid and orbit (Fig. 31–21). They are usually multilobular, and complete surgical excision is seldom accomplished. Recurrence is common. They are more common in the extraconal space. On CT scans, these lymphangiomas appear as poorly circumscribed, often heterogeneous masses of increased density in the extraconal or intraconal space. Bone expansion may be present. Calcification is rare, and minimal to marked contrast enhancement may be present. With MRI, lymphangiomas are relatively hypointense or hyperintense on T1-

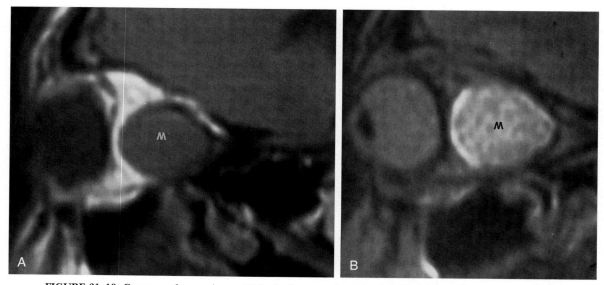

FIGURE 31–19. Cavernous hemangioma. *(A)* Sagittal proton density–weighted (2000/20) and *(B)* T2-weighted (2000/80) images show a well-defined intraconal mass (M) compatible with cavernous hemangioma.

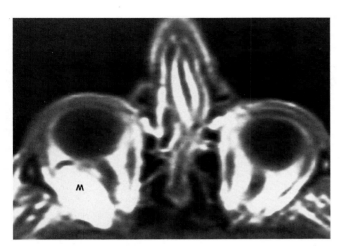

FIGURE 31–20. Cavernous hemangioma. Postcontrast axial T1-weighted (450/20) image shows an enhancing mass (M) compatible with cavernous hemangioma.

weighted images and usually quite hyperintense on T2-weighted images. Hemorrhage and fluid-fluid levels may be present. Their MRI characteristics should help to differentiate them from pseudotumors, hemangiomas, and many other lesions[2, 7] (see Fig. 31–21).

Hemangiopericytomas

Hemangiopericytomas are rare, slow-growing vascular neoplasms that arise from the pericytes of Zimmermann that normally envelop capillaries and postcapillary venules of practically all types of tissues. Histologically, these tumors are composed of scattered, capillary-like spaces surrounded by proliferating pericytes. Hemangiopericytomas may be divided into lobules by fibrovascular septa. About 50% of the cases are malignant and distant metastases, although uncommon, occur via the vascular and lymphatic routes.[2, 7, 18] The lungs are the most common sites for them. These lesions tend to recur if not excised completely. Wide surgical excision is the treatment of choice.

On CT scans, the margins of orbital hemangiopericytoma (particularly when the tumor is large), in contrast to cavernous hemangioma, may be slightly less distinct owing to their tendency to invade the adjacent tissues. Erosion of the underlying bone may be present. Marked contrast enhancement is often seen. Calcifications may be seen in hemangiopericytoma. Their MRI features are indicative of long-T1 and long-T2 lesions (Fig. 31–22). Hemangiopericytomas show intense enhancement on gadolinium-enhanced MR images (Fig. 31–23). MRI may not differentiate them from cavernous hemangioma, neurogenic tumor (Fig. 31–24), fibrous histiocytoma, meningioma, and other lesions. Angiography may be helpful in differentiating the tumors from cavernous hemangioma, meningiomas, and schwannomas. Hemangiopericytomas usually have an early florid blush, and cavernous hemangiomas show late minor pooling of the contrast agent or often behave as avascular masses. Meningiomas may show multiple tumor vessels and a late blush, and schwannomas may show no tumor blush. Hemangiopericytomas may be difficult to differentiate from other vasculogenic

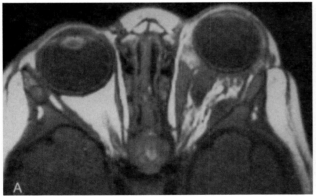

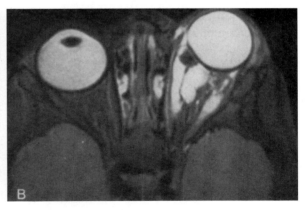

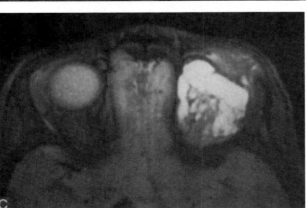

FIGURE 31–21. Lymphangioma. Proton density–weighted (A) and T2-weighted (B and C) axial scans show a heterogeneous mass within the left orbit of a 9-month-old child. The mass involves both the intraconal and the extraconal compartments. Multiple cystic components are hypointense relative to fat on proton density–weighted images and hyperintense relative to fat on T2-weighted images. The globe is markedly proptotic.

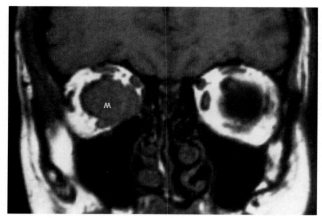

FIGURE 31–22. Hemangiopericytoma. Coronal T1-weighted (600/15) image shows an intraconal mass (M). Notice invasion of inferior and medial rectus muscles.

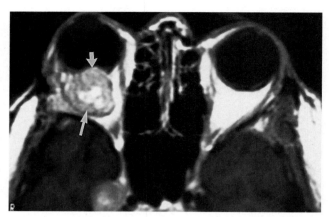

FIGURE 31–23. Recurrent hemangiopericytoma. Axial postcontrast T1-weighted image shows a recurrent hemangiopericytoma *(arrows)*. (Courtesy of Michael Rothman, MD, University of Maryland, Baltimore, MD.)

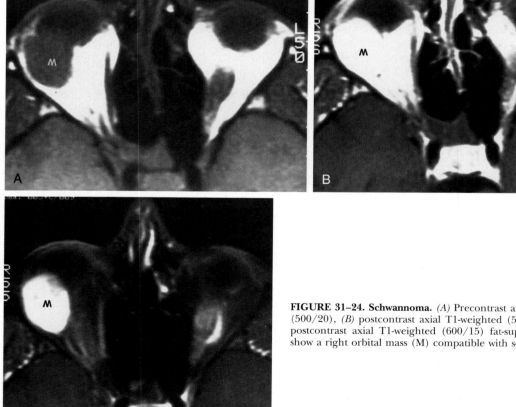

FIGURE 31–24. Schwannoma. *(A)* Precontrast axial T1-weighted (500/20), *(B)* postcontrast axial T1-weighted (500/20), and *(C)* postcontrast axial T1-weighted (600/15) fat-suppressed images show a right orbital mass (M) compatible with schwannoma.

tumors such as angioleiomyomas, malignant hemangioendothelioma (angiosarcoma), and fibrous histiocytoma.[19]

Orbital Varix

Primary orbital varices are congenital venous malformations characterized by proliferation of venous elements and massive dilation of one or more orbital veins presumably associated with congenital weakness in the venous wall.[2, 7] Orbital varices are the most common cause of spontaneous orbital hemorrhage. The CT appearance of orbital varix may be normal in axial sections but quite abnormal in coronal sections, particularly those obtained with the patient in a prone position, because of increased venous pressure. Any time an orbital varix is suspected, additional CT sections during the Valsalva maneuver are recommended. In suspected cases, MRI should also be done with the patient in the prone position. MRI of orbital varix in one of our patients with bilateral varices showed hyperintense lesions in T1-, proton density–, and T2-weighted images. Orbital varix may appear single or as several round or tubular images (Fig. 31–25) with or without associated calcifications.

Carotid Cavernous Fistulas

Carotid cavernous fistulas produce proptosis, chemosis, venous engorgement, pulsating exophthalmos, and auscultable bruit. Ischemic ocular necrosis resulting from carotid cavernous fistula has been reported. A carotid cavernous fistula may result from trauma or surgery or may occur spontaneously. Spontaneous carotid cavernous fistula has been reported in patients with osteogenesis imperfecta, Ehlers-Danlos syndrome, and pseudoxanthoma elasticum, probably caused by weakness of the vessel walls related to connective tissue disease. CT and MRI demonstrate proptosis with engorgement of the superior ophthalmic vein and frequently enlargement of the ipsilateral extraocular muscles (Fig. 31–26). There may be CT or MRI evidence of venous thrombosis in the lumen of the superior ophthalmic vein or cavernous sinus. Angiographic demonstration of the exact location of the carotid cavernous fistula is essential and aids in planning definitive therapy. At times, patients with anomalous intracranial venous drainage or dural vascular malformation may present with eye swelling and bluish discoloration over the periorbital region, mimicking carotid cavernous fistula[20] (Fig. 31–27).

OPTIC NERVE AND SHEATH LESIONS

Optic Nerve Sheath Meningioma

Optic nerve meningioma arises from either the arachnoid cells covering the optic nerve or extension into the orbit of an intracranial meningioma. Meningiomas are usually seen in middle-aged women.[21] Childhood optic nerve meningioma is much more aggressive than the adult form. Bilateral optic nerve meningiomas may occur in patients with or without neurofibromatosis. Bilateral optic nerve gliomas, however, always occur in patients with type 1 neurofibromatosis.

CT is an informative radiologic study for evaluating optic nerve meningioma. CT is best done with and without infusion of iodinated contrast medium. Thin sections (1.5 to 3 mm) are essential for visualizing the actual extent of small tumors. Because optic nerve meningioma is confined to the dura mater, it appears as a well-defined tubular thickening in 64% of cases. Optic nerve sheath meningiomas are commonly seen as localized eccentric expansion, often at the orbital apex. After injection of contrast medium, meningiomas often show homogeneous and well-defined enhancement. The "tram track" sign originally described with optic nerve meningioma, for which enhanced CT shows lucency in the center of an enlarged optic nerve–sheath complex with peripheral enhancement, is not a specific finding of optic nerve meningioma. This pattern of enhancement may be seen in pseudotu-

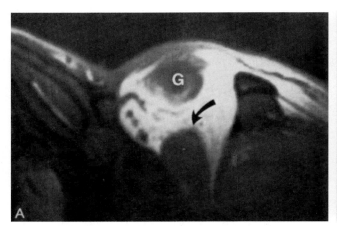
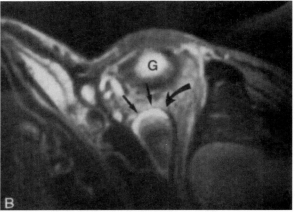

FIGURE 31–25. Orbital varix. T1-weighted *(A)* and T2-weighted *(B)* images show a mass *(curved arrow)* within the orbital apex. A small portion of the globe (G) is sectioned anteriorly. The mass has low signal intensity on the T1-weighted image but exhibits heterogeneous signal intensity on the T2-weighted image related to turbulent flow within the patent lumen of the varix. Some flow enhancement *(small arrows)* is present in the dome of the mass.

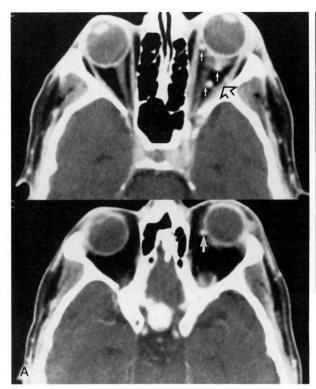

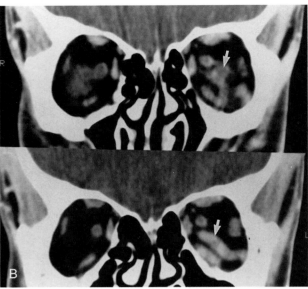

FIGURE 31–26. Carotid cavernous fistula. *A,* Postcontrast axial CT scans show several engorged veins *(small white arrows).* Notice enlargement of left lateral rectus muscle *(open arrow)* and prominent size of left cavernous sinus. *B,* Postcontrast coronal CT scans show enlarged left orbital veins *(arrows)* and moderate enlargement of rectus muscles on the involved side.

mors, lymphoma, leukemia, and optic neuritis. On CT scans, linear or granular calcifications within an optic nerve mass are almost always an indication of optic nerve meningioma. A large optic glioma, however, may rarely show focal calcification.

MRI can make multiple contributions to the imaging evaluation of optic nerve meningiomas and in my opinion is superior to CT. On MR images, meningioma can be seen as a uniform (Fig. 31–28) or round (globular) enlargement of the optic nerve (Fig. 31–29). Meningiomas may be hypointense relative to brain on T1- and proton density–weighted images and hyperintense on T2-weighted images. Intravenous injection of paramagnetic gadolinium usually results in moderate to marked enhancement of meningiomas. When intravenous gadolinium is used, an additional T1-weighted fat

suppression pulse sequence may prove valuable for enhancing meningioma (Fig. 31–30).

Optic Nerve Glioma (Juvenile Pilocytic Astrocytoma)

Optic nerve glioma is a tumor arising from the neuroglia. Although it is usually a tumor of childhood (2 to 6 years), it can be seen at birth and rarely in the adult years. Nine of 10 cases are symptomatic in the first two decades. Optic nerve glioma in children is a benign, well-differentiated, and slow-growing tumor.[22, 23] Bilateral optic nerve gliomas are characteristic of type 1 neurofibromatosis. The natural history of childhood optic glioma does not involve malignant transformation or systemic metastasis. Local invasion

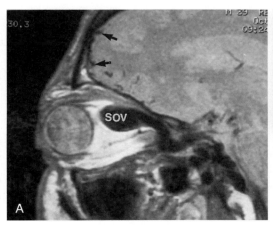

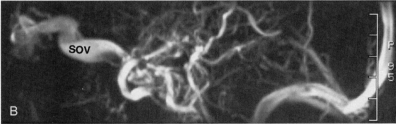

FIGURE 31–27. Intracranial vascular malformation. *A,* Sagittal proton density–weighted (3000/23) image shows marked engorgement of the superior ophthalmic vein (SOV) and cavernous sinus. Note engorged intracranial vessels *(arrows).* *B,* Three-dimensional phase-contrast MR angiogram shows the enlarged superior ophthalmic vein (SOV).

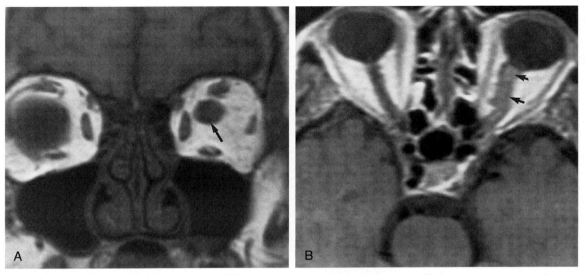

FIGURE 31–28. Meningioma. *A,* Coronal T1-weighted image shows enlargement of left optic nerve *(arrow). B,* Axial postcontrast MR image shows diffuse enhancement of optic nerve meningioma *(arrows).*

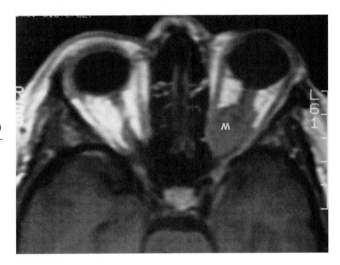

FIGURE 31–29. Meningioma. Postcontrast axial T1-weighted (600/20) image shows an infiltrative mass (M) around the left optic nerve compatible with meningioma.

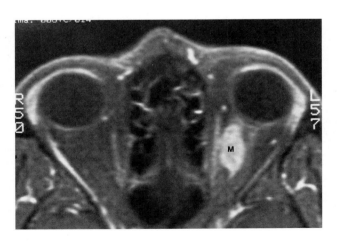

FIGURE 31–30. Meningioma. Postcontrast axial fat-suppressed T1-weighted image shows a meningioma (M) in this 36-year-old man. Note the eccentric growth pattern of this surgically proven meningioma.

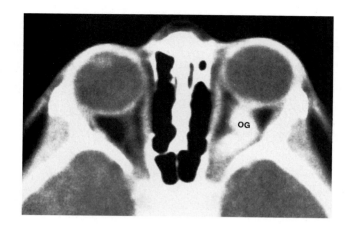

FIGURE 31–31. Juvenile optic nerve glioma. Postcontrast axial CT scan shows a markedly enhancing left optic glioma (OG). Note tortuousity and kinking of the optic glioma.

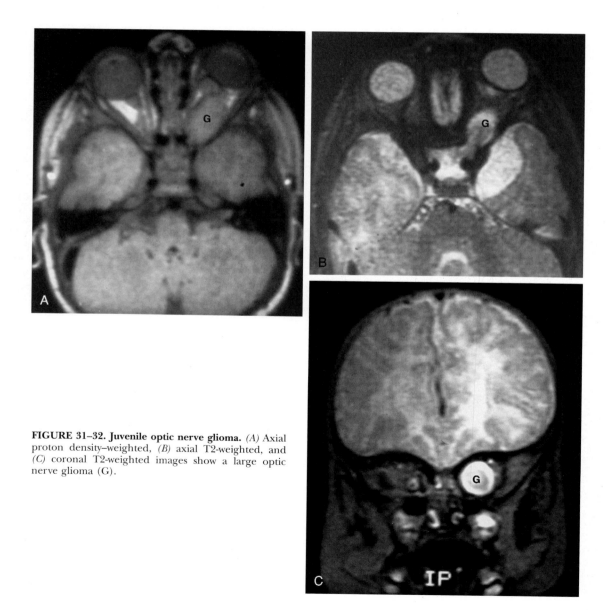

FIGURE 31–32. Juvenile optic nerve glioma. (A) Axial proton density–weighted, (B) axial T2-weighted, and (C) coronal T2-weighted images show a large optic nerve glioma (G).

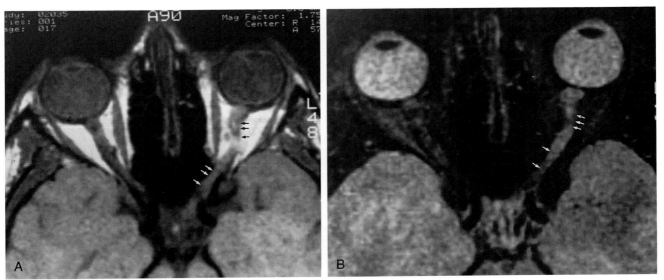

FIGURE 31–33. Optic neuritis. (A) Axial proton density–weighted and (B) axial T2-weighted images show moderate thickening of left optic nerve (arrows).

into the extraocular muscles rarely occurs. Thickening of perineural tissue seems to be responsible for the fusiform shape of optic nerve glioma. The primary sequela of this tumor is atrophy that results from damage to the optic nerve fibers and the optic nerve nutrient arteries. Malignant optic glioma is seen primarily in adults. It is a rare, fatal disease (glioblastoma multiforme) that usually extends from intracranial glioma.

Unenhanced axial CT shows well-defined fusiform enlargement of the optic nerve. Diffuse, tortuous enlargement of the optic nerve with a kinking and buckling (sinusoid) appearance is a characteristic feature of the childhood form of optic glioma. Calcification is rare in optic nerve gliomas. After intravenous administration of a contrast agent, they may show homogeneous or nonhomogeneous enhancement (Fig. 31–31). The inhomogeneity is the result of tumor infarction secondary to obliteration of the small nutrient arteries of the optic nerve.

MRI also readily demonstrates an enlarged fusiform and kinked optic nerve (Fig. 31–32). On T1-weighted images, the optic glioma appears isointense or slightly hyperintense relative to the white matter. On T2-weighted images, the lesion may show greater variability in intensity; however, it may appear hyperintense relative to the white matter. Intracranial extension of optic nerve gliomas can be better appreciated with MRI. Use of a paramagnetic contrast medium results in moderate to marked enhancement of gliomas, although usually less than that of meningiomas. At times, optic nerve gliomas may show significant arachnoid proliferation around the tumor (see also Chapter 18).

Nontumoral and Lymphomatous Enlargement of the Optic Nerve or Sheath

Primary or secondary involvement of optic nerve in cases of lymphoma, leukemia, sarcoid, tuberculosis, toxoplasmosis, syphilis, and optic neuritis has been reported.

Optic Neuritis

This condition is an acute inflammatory process involving the optic nerve and may present as optic nerve enlargement. Optic neuritis may be an early manifestation of multiple sclerosis. In optic neuritis, CT scans may occasionally show an enlarged optic nerve with some degree of contrast enhancement. On MR images, the optic neuritis may appear as a hyperintense lesion on proton density– and T2-weighted images (Fig. 31–33). MRI visualization of optic neuritis may be accentuated by a T1-weighted fat suppression technique after Gd-DTPA administration (Fig. 31–34).

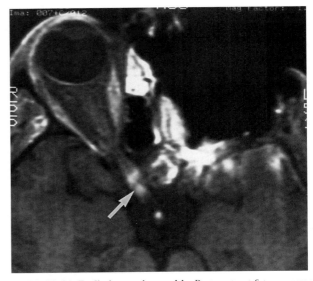

FIGURE 31–34. Radiation optic neuritis. Postcontrast fat-suppressed axial MR image shows enhancement of intracanalicular segment of the right optic nerve (arrow). Notice changes after left orbital exenteration.

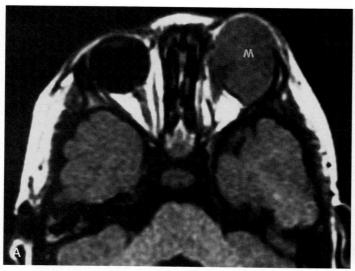
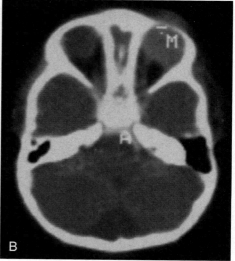

FIGURE 31–35. Rhabdomyosarcoma. *A,* Axial T1-weighted image shows a left orbital mass (M). *B,* Dynamic CT scan shows less enhancement of the mass (M), compared with the basilar (A) artery.

ORBITAL RHABDOMYOSARCOMA

Rhabdomyosarcoma is the most common primary orbital malignancy in children.[4] Clinically, its occurrence involves the differential diagnosis of acute and subacute proptosis of childhood. Changes in chemotherapy in the past decade have markedly improved the prognosis, particularly in orbital cases. Rhabdomyosarcoma arises in the orbit from extraocular muscles or from pluripotential mesenchymal elements.[3, 7] On the basis of their histopathologic features, most can be classified into one of three histologic types: embryonal, differentiated, or alveolar rhabdomyosarcoma. The embryonal type is the most common and the differentiated type the least frequent.[24]

Clinical Diagnosis

Rapidly progressing unilateral proptosis is the hallmark of orbital rhabdomyosarcoma. Congenital proptosis in infants is most likely to be caused by a rhabdomyosarcoma, hemangioma, or optic glioma, if primary, or by a neuroblastoma or leukemic deposit if secondary.

Differential Diagnosis

Clinically, the differential diagnosis of orbital rhabdomyosarcoma includes progressive, rapidly developing tumors and inflammatory conditions of childhood. These include neuroblastoma, chloroma, Langerhans' histiocytosis,[24a] lymphangioma, infantile hemangioma, teratoma, dermoid cysts, and orbital cellulitis.

Diagnostic Imaging

CT and MRI provide information about the orbital soft tissue structures and the relationship between them and adjacent bone, cranial fossae, and paranasal sinuses. Rhabdomyosarcoma is an aggressive malignant tumor capable of bone expansion and destruction. On CT scans, these tumors are seen as enhancing masses within the orbit. There may be associated bone destruction. The MRI features of orbital rhabdomyosarcoma are characteristic of long-T1 and long-T2 lesions (Fig. 31–35A). There is moderate to marked enhancement after intravenous injection of Gd-DTPA. CT and MRI can accurately define the anatomic location of the orbital mass, the involvement of various intraorbital structures, and the extension of tumor into the surrounding structures (Fig. 31–36). Dynamic CT is useful in differentiating rhabdomyosarcoma from highly vascular lesions such as capillary hemangioma (Fig. 31–35B). Although rare, at times rhabdomyosarcoma may be seen in adults (see Fig. 31–36). Biopsy should be obtained to establish the diagnosis. Rhabdomyosarcoma is sensitive to radiation therapy and chemotherapy.

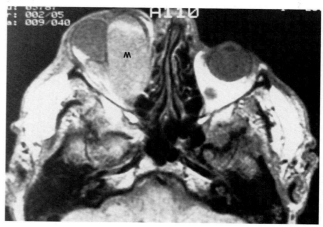

FIGURE 31–36. Rhabdomyosarcoma. Axial proton density–weighted image shows a large right orbital mass (M) compatible with rhabdomyosarcoma in this elderly man.

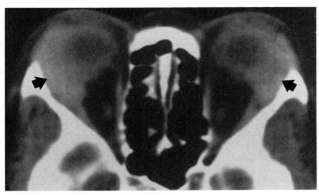

FIGURE 31–37. Sarcoidosis of lacrimal glands. Axial postcontrast CT scan shows marked bilateral diffuse enlargement of lacrimal glands *(arrows)*.

LACRIMAL GLAND AND FOSSA LESIONS

Lesions of the lacrimal gland and fossa present special problems in diagnosis and management. Because of the excellent prognosis for benign mixed tumor, provided it is completely excised at first surgery, these lesions should not undergo incisional biopsy but require en bloc excision along with adjacent tissues.[25–27] Because of the importance of preoperative diagnosis, all clinical ancillary findings should be integrated into the assessment of individual cases. In general, epithelial tumors represent approximately 50% of masses involving the lacrimal gland. The remaining 50% of lacrimal gland masses are the lymphoid or inflammatory type.[28, 29] Metastases to the parenchyma of the lacrimal gland are rare. Dermoid cysts are not true lacrimal gland tumors but rather arise from epithelial rests located in the orbit, particularly in the superolateral quadrant. Epithelial cysts, on the other hand, are intrinsic lesions that result from dilation of the lacrimal ducts.

Lymphomatous lesions of lacrimal gland include a broad spectrum from reactive lymphoid hyperplasia to malignant lymphomas of various types.[29] Inflammatory or lymphoid lesions of the lacrimal gland show diffuse enlargement of the gland (see Fig. 31–13). Contrast enhancement at CT or MRI may be marked, and there may be associated acute lateral rectus muscle myositis. In chronic dacryoadenitis, the gland also shows diffuse oblong enlargement. The glands may be massively enlarged in case of sarcoidosis (Fig. 31–37) or other conditions such as Mikulicz's syndrome, pseudotumors, and Wegener's granulomatosis.

Benign and malignant lymphoid tumors situated in the lacrimal gland also display diffuse enlargement with oblong contouring of the gland; however, these lesions are bulkier and frequently show more evidence of anterior and posterior extension and molding and draping on the globe. In general, inflammatory processes and lymphomas tend to involve all aspects of the lacrimal gland, often including its palpebral lobe (Fig. 31–38). However, neoplastic lesions of the gland rarely originate in the palpebral lobe of the gland, and there-fore there is often a tendency for posterior rather than anterior extension beyond the orbital rim (Fig. 31–39).

Because the lacrimal gland is histologically similar to the salivary gland, it is affected by similar disease processes. Epithelial tumors represent 50% of masses involving the lacrimal gland.[3, 7, 28] Half of these are pleomorphic (benign mixed) adenomas; the other half are malignant. Of the malignant tumors, adenoid cystic (adenocystic) is the most common, followed by pleomorphic (malignant mixed), mucoepidermoid, adenocarcinoma, squamous cell carcinoma, and undifferentiated (anaplastic) carcinoma. A significant number of these tumors arise within pleomorphic adenomas.

Jakobiec and colleagues[30] reviewed by CT 39 patients with solid masses in the lacrimal gland. Sixteen had parenchymal benign and malignant tumors: six benign mixed, one schwannoma, and nine malignant epithelial tumors that had rounded or globular soft tissue outlines and were frequently associated with continuous bone changes. Benign tumors had smooth encapsulated outlines, whereas the malignant tumors displayed microserrations indicative of infiltration (see Fig. 31–39). Calcifications are more common in malignant tumors of lacrimal gland. Inflammatory conditions in their series demonstrated diffuse, compressed, and molded enlargement of lacrimal gland in an oblong fashion, and there were no associated bone defects. They concluded that well-capsulated, rounded masses of long duration are likely to be benign mixed tumors. In contrast, inflammatory and lymphoid lesions of lacrimal gland were seen as a diffuse expansion of the lacrimal gland and the lesions molded themselves to preexisting orbital structures without eroding bone or enlarging the orbit.

Bone changes in the lacrimal gland fossa may be produced by benign or malignant epithelial tumors, parenchymal lacrimal gland tumors (such as schwannomas), and lesions originating within the subperiosteal space or bone, including benign orbital cyst, hematic cyst, eosinophilic granulomas, dermoid cysts, and metastatic carcinoma. Lymphoid and inflammatory processes rarely produce bone change.

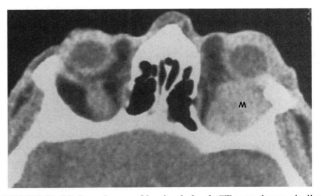

FIGURE 31–38. Lymphoma of lacrimal gland. CT scan shows a bulky mass (M) involving the left lacrimal gland and lacrimal fossa region. Notice deformity of the lateral orbital wall. Bone destruction is uncommon in lymphoma except in multiple myeloma and the malignant histiocytic type.

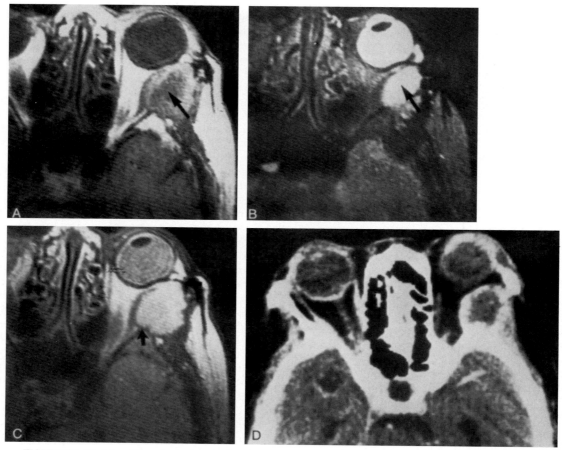

FIGURE 31–39. Adenoid cystic carcinoma. An ill-defined mass *(arrow)* invading the lateral rectus and breaking through the lateral wall of the orbit is shown on the T1-weighted *(A)*, T2-weighted *(B)*, and proton density–weighted *(C)* images. The central necrosis is most evident on the T2-weighted image. The orbital anatomy is much better demonstrated on the MR image than on the contrast-enhanced CT scan *(D)*. (*A* to *D* from Sullivan JA, Harms SE: Surface-coil MR imaging of orbital neoplasms. AJNR 7[1]:29–34, 1986.© by American Society of Neuroradiology.)

The MRI features of benign and malignant epithelial tumors of lacrimal gland are characteristic of long-T1 and long-T2 lesions. These tumors demonstrate moderate to marked enhancement after intravenous injection of Gd-DTPA (see Fig. 31–30).

HEMORRHAGIC LESIONS

Subperiosteal Orbital Hematomas

Acute subperiosteal orbital hematomas are a rare but serious complication of trauma, usually presenting as a painful unilateral proptosis. They may develop so insidiously as to defy explanation, especially when there is no definite history of injury. Spontaneous hemorrhage may occur as a complication of systemic disease such as leukemia, thrombocytopenia, blood dyscrasia, hemophilia, and other hemorrhagic systemic diseases.[2, 9] Subperiosteal hematomas develop as a result of rupture of subperiosteal blood vessels. The orbital roof is the most common place, and subperiosteal hematomas of the orbital roof occur almost exclusively in children and young adults, because the periorbita is not firmly adhered to the bone. They are less likely to occur later, because the periosteal bony connection may become firmer with age.[7]

Chronic Hematic Orbital Granulomatous Cysts

Most of the orbital hematomas, like other localized collections of blood, disappear within days. *Hematic cyst* is a term often used for deeply placed, incompletely resorbed hematoma (hemorrhagic cyst), which may remain unchanged and unidentified for long periods. Hematic cysts may develop as a complication of head trauma or prolonged retention of an orbital foreign body. These hematic cysts develop because orbital hemorrhage is too great to be absorbed quickly. Subclinical hemorrhage in the subperiosteal space or within the diploic space may also be incompletely resorbed, silently remaining as a cystic accumulation of hematogenous debris (chocolate-colored fluid), surrounded by a chronic granulomatous reaction and a wall of fibrous tissue (pseudocapsule) without any epithelial or endothelial lining.[7, 10] On histopathologic examination, a granulomatous reaction to blood debris including cholesterol clefts (cholesterol granuloma), hemosiderin, foreign body cells, pigment-collecting macrophages, and foam cells (lipid-laden macrophages) surrounded by a fibrous tissue is present.[7, 9]

The term *chronic orbital cyst* or cholesterol granuloma should be used only for cysts that have no epithelial or endothelial lining. Hemorrhage in an epidermoid (cholesteatoma) or dermoid cysts can produce changes similar to those of chronic orbital cysts, with cholesterol granuloma, giant cell foreign body reaction, and chocolate-colored fluid representing old hematoma.

Clinically, these patients usually present with diplopia and painless unilateral globe displacement. There may be a history of remote orbital trauma or of prior surgery. The radiographic features of chronic hematic cyst in the proper clinical setting can lead to a correct diagnosis. Confusion occurs when a history of trauma or orbital surgery is absent; hemorrhagic systemic disease, which might otherwise furnish a clue in the differential diagnosis, may also be absent. Hematic cysts are seldom reported along the floor of the orbit. The CT appearance of chronic hematic cyst includes a well-defined extraconal homogeneous or nonhomogeneous, nonenhancing mass in the subperiosteal, medullary, or diploic space (Fig. 31–40). The lesion often has a high CT attenuation value, which is related to the protein-rich fluid and hemosiderin deposition. Erosion and expansion of the surrounding bones are always observed, and at times flecks of calcium may be present (see Fig. 31–40A).

These cysts are infrequent but occasionally pose a challenge in the differential diagnosis of unilateral proptosis. The differential diagnosis includes lacrimal gland tumor or cyst, epidermoid cyst (see Fig. 31–4),

dermoid cyst, hemorrhagic extravasations within a dermoid or epidermoid cyst, teratomas, cholesterol granuloma, giant cell reparative granuloma, eosinophilic granuloma,[24a] encephalocele, and extension of inflammatory sinus disease into the orbit such as mucoceles and inflammatory polyps. Cholesterol granuloma cyst appears hyperintense on T1-, proton density–, and T2-weighted images. The lesion may be homogeneous or heterogeneous in appearance.

GLOBE

NORMAL ANATOMY

The eye consists of three primary layers: 1) the sclera, or outer layer, is composed primarily of collagen-elastic tissue; 2) the uvea, or middle layer of the eye, is richly vascular and contains pigmented tissue consisting of three components: iris, ciliary body, and choroid; and 3) the retina, or inner layer, which is the neural, sensory stratum of the eye. The sclera is covered by the Tenon capsule. The Tenon capsule (bulbar fascia) is a fibroelastic membrane that envelops the eyeball from the optic nerve to the level of ciliary muscle (Fig. 31–41).

IMAGING TECHNIQUES

CT of the globe should be performed using 1.5-mm collimation. Contiguous slices should be obtained. The major applications of CT for lesions of the globe include detecting foreign bodies and intraocular calcifi-

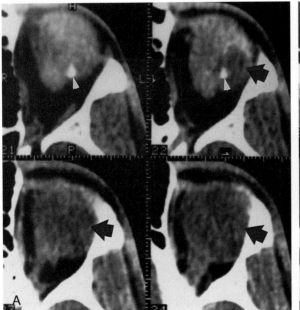
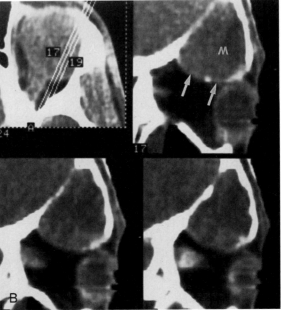

FIGURE 31–40. Cholesterol granuloma. *A,* Serial postcontrast axial CT scans show a low-density nonenhancing mass *(arrows)* in the region of left lacrimal fossa. Notice a focus of calcification *(arrowheads)*. *B,* Sagittal reformatted CT images show that the mass (M) is in the subperiosteal space and with the periosteum displaced inferiorly *(arrows)*.

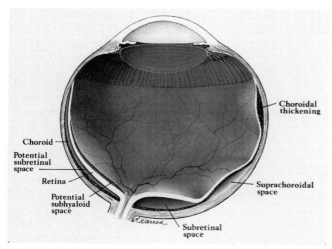

FIGURE 31–41. Diagram of a horizontal section of the globe at the level of the optic nerve, depicting coverings of the globe and various potential spaces. (From Mafee MF, Peyman GA: Retinal and choroidal detachments: role of magnetic resonance imaging and computed tomography. Radiol Clin North Am 25:487–507, 1987.)

cation. For intraocular tumors and other intraocular pathologic conditions, we prefer MRI as the initial study of choice.

MRI of the globe requires focused imaging techniques. Use of thin 3-mm sections with 0- to 0.6-mm interslice gap is recommended. Single-echo spin-echo pulse sequences, using a surface or head coil as the

receiving coil, are needed with a repetition time (TR) of 400 to 800 ms and an echo time (TE) of 20 to 25 ms (TR/TE = 400 to 800/20 to 25). Multiecho spin-echo pulse sequences are recommended with a TR of 1500 to 2500 ms and a TE of 20 to 100 ms. In our institution, the studies are most often performed with one excitation, a 256 × 256 matrix, and a 12- to 16-cm field of view. For shorter TR values (400 to 800 ms), the studies are often performed with two excitations. We use Gd-DTPA (0.1 mmol/kg body weight) for all suspected intraocular masses and infectious and infiltrative processes. We have found postcontrast fat-suppressed T1-weighted images useful for the detection of extraocular and optic nerve involvement of intraocular tumors.[3]

OCULAR PATHOLOGY

CONGENITAL LESIONS

Anophthalmia

Bilateral anophthalmia is a rare condition. Rudimentary tissue or no globe may be found by CT or MRI. The extraocular muscles, lacrimal glands, and eyelids are present (Fig. 31–42).

Microphthalmia

Microphthalmia can occur as an isolated disorder or may be associated with other craniofacial anomalies.

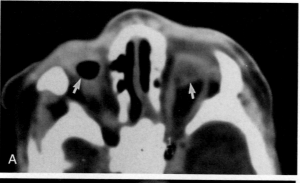

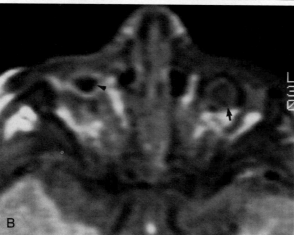

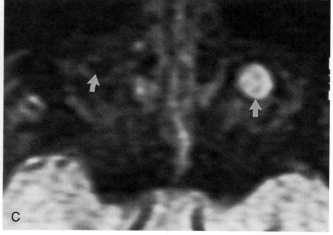

FIGURE 31–42. Bilateral anophthalmia. (A) CT scan, (B) proton density–weighted image, and (C) T2-weighted image show rudimentary globes (arrows and arrowhead). Some air is seen within the right rudimentary globe.

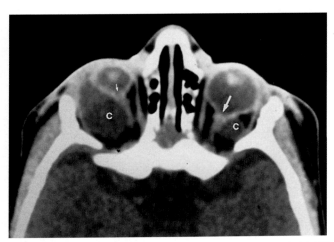

FIGURE 31–43. Microphthalmia with colobomatous cysts. Axial CT scan shows colobomas of the optic nerve head *(arrows)*. Notice bilateral colobomatous cysts (c).

Congenital rubella syndrome, persistent hyperplastic primary vitreous (PHPV), and retinopathy of prematurity are other causes of microphthalmia.

Macrophthalmia

Macrophthalmia is seen in patients with axial myopia, in patients with juvenile glaucoma who may have Sturge-Weber syndrome, and at times in patients with neurofibromatosis.

Coloboma and Morning Glory Anomaly

A coloboma is a notch, gap, hole, or fissure that is congenital or acquired and in which a tissue or portion of a tissue is lacking.[31, 32] A variety of ocular and systemic abnormalities may be seen with an optic nerve coloboma. Microphthalmos with cyst is an anomaly in which an eye with a retinochoroidal coloboma also has a cyst, which is usually attached to the inferior aspect of the globe (Fig. 31–43).

Morning glory disk anomaly was first characterized by Kindler in 1970.[32a] He described a unilateral congenital anomaly of the optic nerve head in 10 patients. Because of the similarity in appearance between the nerve head and a morning glory flower, he referred to the anomaly as the morning glory syndrome. Ophthalmoscopically, the abnormal nerve head has several characteristic findings. The disk is enlarged and excavated and has a central core of white tissue.

Diagnostic Imaging

The CT and MRI appearance of optic nerve head coloboma and the morning glory anomaly characteristically corresponds to its clinical appearance as a large funnel-shaped disk. The colobomatous cyst associated with coloboma of the optic nerve can easily be identified on CT and MR images. Any retroglobal cyst associated with a microphthalmic eye should raise suspicion of a colobomatous cyst (see Figs. 31–42 and 31–43).

OCULAR DETACHMENTS

Retinal Detachment

Retinal detachment occurs when the sensory retina is separated from the retinal pigment epithelium (see Fig. 31–41). Retinal detachment resulting from a hole (or tear) in the retina is referred to as rhegmatogenous retinal detachment. Fluid in the subretinal space can be detected by both CT and MRI. Retinal detachment is usually the result of retraction caused by a mass or a fibroproliferative disease in the vitreous such as vitreoretinopathy of prematurity or vitreoretinopathy of diabetes. Retinal detachment may be due to a choroidal mass or to an acute (viral) or chronic inflammatory process such as larval granuloma of *Toxocara* endophthalmitis. Retinal detachment may also occur because of retinal vascular leakage, which is seen in patients with Coats' disease, a primary vascular anomaly of the retina characterized by telangiectasis.[31, 33]

Computed Tomographic and MRI Evaluation

When a retinal detachment is identified, the principal question that must be answered is that of its cause. Retinal detachment and primary underlying disease can often be differentiated from each other by CT but MRI is even better.

On an axial CT or MR image taken below or above the lens, the retinal detachment appears as homogeneous increased density or increased intensity of the globe. The retina is thin and is therefore beyond the limits of resolution of CT and MRI scanners. However, it may be shown when outlined by significant contrast difference between the density or intensity of the subretinal effusion and the vitreous cavity[31, 33] (Fig. 31–44).

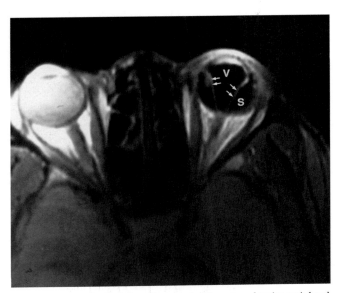

FIGURE 31–44. Retinal detachment. Axial proton density–weighted (2000/20) image shows the leaves *(arrows)* of the detached retina. The hypointensity of the vitreous (V) and subretinal space (S) is due to intravitreal injection of silicon.

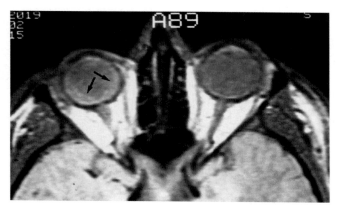

FIGURE 31–45. Serous retinal detachment. Axial proton density–weighted (2000/20) image shows the leaves of detached retina *(arrows)*. Notice subretinal effusion.

The appearance of retinal detachment varies with the amount of exudation and organization of subretinal materials (Fig. 31–45). In a section taken at the level of the optic disk, retinal detachment is seen with a characteristic indentation at the optic disk (see Fig. 31–45). When total retinal detachment is present and the entire vitreous cavity ablated, the leaves of the detached retina may or may not be clearly detected (Fig. 31–46). Retinal detachment is seen on coronal MR images as a characteristic folding membrane. The subretinal fluid in the exudative retinal detachment is rich in protein, giving higher CT numbers and stronger MRI signals than subretinal fluid (transudate) seen in rhegmatogenous detachment.

Retinal detachment is characteristically seen on CT or MR images as a V-shaped image, with its apex at the optic disk and its extremities toward the ciliary body (see Figs. 31–44 and 31–45). This appearance of retinal detachment may be confused with the appearance of

posterior choroidal detachment; however, posterior choroidal detachment in the region of the optic disk and macula involves detachment of the choroid that is restricted by the anchoring effect of the short posterior ciliary arteries and nerves as well as the vortex veins. This restriction usually results in a characteristic appearance where the leaves of the detached choroid, unlike the detached retina, do not extend to the region of the optic disk (Fig. 31–47).

Choroidal Detachment, Choroidal Effusion, and Ocular Hypotony

Choroidal detachment is caused by the accumulation of fluid (serous choroidal detachment) or blood (hemorrhagic choroidal detachment) in the potential suprachoroidal space between the choroid and the sclera. Serous choroidal detachment frequently occurs after intraocular surgery, penetrating ocular trauma, or inflammatory choroidal disorders. Hemorrhagic choroidal detachment occurs after a contusion, after a penetrating injury, or as a complication of intraocular surgery (ocular hypotony). Such detachment significantly influences the prognosis for the involved eye.[34]

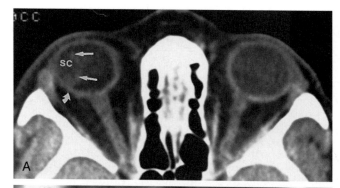

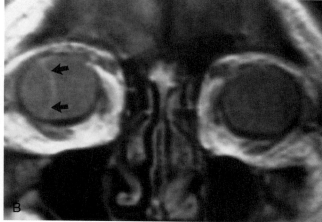

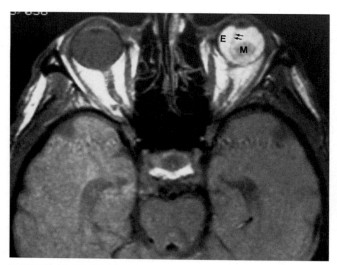

FIGURE 31–46. Total retinal detachment. Axial proton density–weighted (2000/20) image shows a large choroidal melanoma (M), resulting in total exudative retinal detachment. The leaves of the detached retina are seen abutting each other *(arrows)*. The exudate (E) in subretinal space appears hyperintense.

FIGURE 31–47. Serous choroidal detachment. *A,* Axial CT scan shows detached choroid *(straight arrows)*. Notice hypodense transudate in the suprachoroidal space (SC). Note that detached choroid is restricted at the expected location of vorticose vein *(curved arrow)*. *B,* Coronal proton density–weighted (2000/20) image shows the detached choroid *(arrows)*. The apparent increased intensity of right globe is probably due to leaking protein within the vitreous chamber.

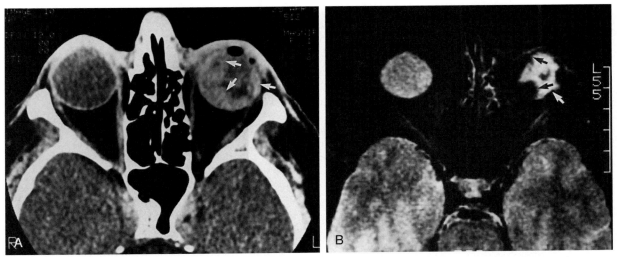

FIGURE 31–48. Hemorrhagic choroidal detachment. *A,* Axial CT scan shows several round images *(arrows)* of increased density, compatible with acute choroidal hemorrhage. *B,* Axial T2-weighted (200/80) image shows hypointense choroidal hemorrhages *(arrows).*

Computed Tomographic and MRI Evaluation

Serous choroidal detachment appears on CT scans as a semilunar or ring-shaped area of variable attenuation (see Fig. 31–47), and with MRI as variable-intensity images (see Fig. 31–46). The degree of attenuation depends on the cause but is generally greater with inflammatory disorders of the eyeball. Hemorrhagic choroidal detachment appears as a high or low mound-like image of high intensity on CT scans (Fig. 31–48A). It can be quite large and irregular.

MRI shows choroidal hematoma as a focal, well-demarcated, lenticular mass in the wall of the eyeball. The signal intensity of the choroidal hematoma depends on its age. In the first 48 hours, the hematoma is isointense to slightly hypointense relative to the normal vitreous body on T1- and proton density–weighted images but is markedly hypointense on T2-weighted images (Fig. 31–48B). After about 5 days, its signal intensity characteristics are different; it is relatively hyperintense on T1- and proton density–weighted images but rather hypointense on T2-weighted images. At this stage the choroidal hematoma may be confused with choroidal melanoma. The hematoma usually continues to increase in signal intensity on T1-, proton density–, and T2-weighted images and usually becomes markedly hyperintense with all MRI pulse sequences by 2 to 3 weeks.

Serous choroidal detachment and choroidal effusion have an appearance on CT and MRI different from that of choroidal hematoma. A choroidal effusion is usually seen as a crescentic or ring-shaped lesion on both CT scans and MR images. It does not resemble the lenticular appearance of a hematoma.

Posterior Hyaloid Detachment

Posterior hyaloid detachment usually occurs in adults older than the age of 50 years but may occur in children with PHPV. Posterior hyaloid detachment in adults is usually caused by liquefaction of the vitreous and may be associated with macular degeneration[33, 35] (Fig. 31–49).

LEUKOKORIA

Leukokoria is a white, pink-white, or yellow-white pupillary reflex (cat's eye). It is a sign that results from any intraocular abnormality that reflects the incident light back through the pupil toward the observer. This reflection of light is the result of a white or light-colored intraocular mass, membrane, retinal detach-

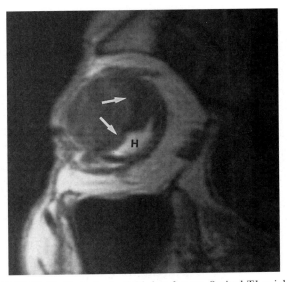

FIGURE 31–49. Posterior hyaloid detachment. Sagittal T1-weighted (1000/25) image shows a chronic hemorrhage (H) in the subretinal space. Notice a detached membrane *(arrow)* in front of the retina, compatible with surgically proven detached posterior hyaloid membrane.

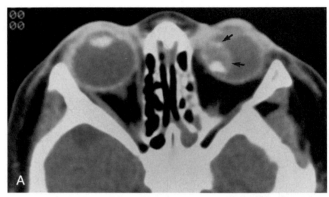

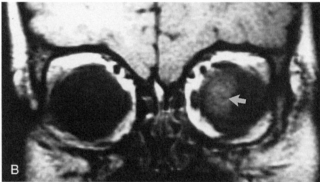

FIGURE 31–50. Retinoblastoma. *A,* Axial CT scan shows a partially calcified mass in the left globe *(arrows). B,* Coronal proton density–weighted (2000/20) image shows that the retinoblastoma *(arrow)* is hyperintense relative to vitreous.

ment, or retinal storage disease. When examining a child with leukokoria, the major diagnostic considerations are retinoblastoma, PHPV, retinopathy of prematurity, congenital cataract, Coats' disease, toxocariasis, total retinal detachment, and a variety of other nonspecific causes of leukokoria.[36, 37]

RETINOBLASTOMA

Retinoblastoma, the most common intraocular tumor of childhood, is a highly malignant, primary retinal tumor that arises from neuroectodermal cells (nuclear layer of the retina) that are destined to become retinal photoreceptors. The manner of intraocular and extraocular extension, patterns of metastasis and recurrence, ocular complications, and associated malignancies make the diagnosis of retinoblastoma one of the most challenging problems of pediatric ophthalmology and radiology. Retinoblastoma accounts for about 1% of all deaths from childhood cancer in the United States.

The diagnosis of retinoblastoma can usually be made by an ophthalmoscopic examination; however, the detection and clinical differentiation of retinoblastoma from a host of benign simulating lesions may be difficult. Bilateral retinoblastoma with coexistent pinealoblastoma (trilateral retinoblastoma)[37a] or coexistent pinealoblastoma and suprasellar tumor (primitive neu-

roectodermal tumor), so-called tetralateral retinoblastoma,[32] has a poor prognosis.

Diagnostic Imaging

Although ophthalmoscopic recognition of retinoblastoma is often reliable, imaging modalities should be used for all patients suspected of having a retinoblastoma to determine the presence of gross retrobulbar spread, intracranial metastasis, and a second tumor. Imaging techniques may allow differentiation of retinoblastoma from lesions such as 1) PHPV, 2) Coats' disease, 3) retinopathy of prematurity, 4) toxocariasis, 5) retinal detachment, 6) organized subretinal hemorrhage, 7) organized vitreous, 8) endophthalmitis, 9) retinal dysplasia, 10) retinal astrocytoma (hamartoma), 11) retinal gliosis, 12) myelinated nerve fibers, 13) choroidal hemangioma, 14) coloboma, 15) morning glory anomaly, 16) congenital cataract, 17) choroidal osteoma, 18) drusen of optic nerve head, and 19) other so-called pseudogliomas and leukokorias. These lesions may have a clinical appearance similar to that of retinoblastoma.

Ultrasonography, CT, and MRI are the most useful imaging techniques in the evaluation of these lesions. The tumor and calcification can be diagnosed by ultrasonography. However, the accuracy of ultrasonography for this condition is only 80%.

Histologically, 95% of retinoblastomas show calcifi-

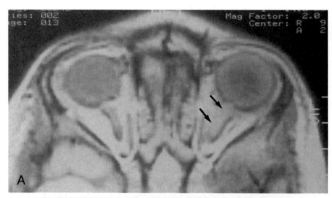

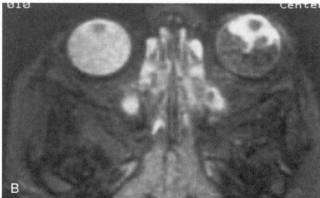

FIGURE 31–51. Retinoblastoma. *(A)* Axial proton density–weighted (2000/20) and *(B)* axial T2-weighted (2000/80) images show a large mass in the left globe that appears hypointense. Notice involvement of left optic nerve *(arrows).*

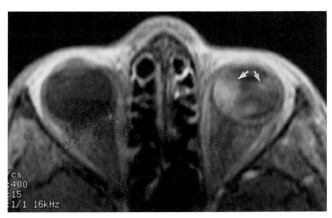

FIGURE 31–52. Retinoblastoma. Axial postcontrast fat-suppressed T1-weighted image shows enhancement of a diffuse retinoblastoma of the left globe *(arrows)*. There is no involvement of the optic nerve.

cations. More than 90% of retinoblastomas show evidence of calcification on a CT scan. The DNA released from necrotic cells in retinoblastoma has a propensity to form a DNA-calcium complex. The presence of intraocular calcification in children younger than 3 years of age is highly suggestive of retinoblastoma. In children older than 3 years of age, some of the simulating lesions, including retinal astrocytoma, retinopathy of prematurity, toxocariasis, and optic nerve head drusen can produce calcification.

In the diagnosis of retinoblastoma, MRI is not as specific as CT because of its lack of sensitivity in detecting calcification (Fig. 31–50A). However, the MRI appearance of retinoblastoma may be specific enough to differentiate retinoblastoma from simulating lesions. Retinoblastomas appear slightly or moderately hyperintense in relation to normal vitreous on T1- and proton density–weighted images (Fig. 31–50B). On T2-weighted images and at times on proton density–

weighted images, they appear as areas of markedly to moderately low signal intensity (Fig. 31–51). Tumors elevated 3 to 4 mm in height may not be definitely identified on MR images. Lesions less than 2 mm in height are not recognized by present MRI technology.[37] The use of Gd-DTPA has significantly improved the MRI sensitivity for the detection of retinoblastoma and (Fig. 31–52) in particular for the detection of optic nerve, subarachnoid, and intracranial spread of the tumor. Postcontrast fat suppression T1-weighted images are extremely sensitive in detecting optic nerve involvement.

In the diagnosis of retinoblastoma, CT is the study of choice because of its superior sensitivity for detecting calcification. Calcification as small as 2 mm can be reliably detected by CT. MRI, however, has superior contrast resolution and provides more information for differentiation of leukokoric eyes, as well as for optic nerve involvement and subarachnoid seeding.

Trilateral Retinoblastoma

Trilateral retinoblastoma is a clinical presentation in which a solitary, midline intracranial neoplasm occurs in association with bilateral retinoblastoma. The intracranial tumor is most commonly an undifferentiated, primitive neuroectodermal tumor in the pineal region (pinealoblastoma).[37–41] A case of tetralateral retinoblastoma has been reported in which bilateral retinoblastoma coexisted with a suprasellar mass[32] (Fig. 31–53). Both CT and MRI can demonstrate trilateral or tetralateral retinoblastoma as well as the occurrence of a second primary cancer[32, 37, 38] (Fig. 31–54).

PERSISTENT HYPERPLASTIC PRIMARY VITREOUS

PHPV is caused by failure of the embryonic hyaloid vascular system to regress normally. The basic lesion is

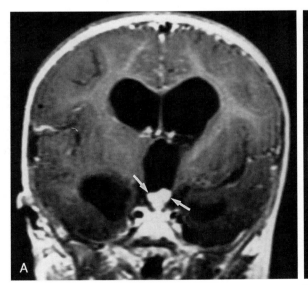
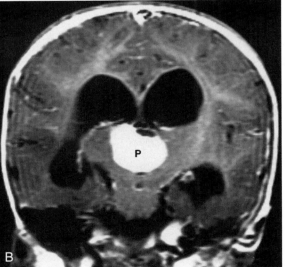

FIGURE 31–53. Retinoblastoma. Coronal postcontrast T1-weighted images *(A and B)* show a suprasellar mass *(arrows)* and a pinealoblastoma (P) in this child with bilateral retinoblastomas. Notice marked hydrocephalus.

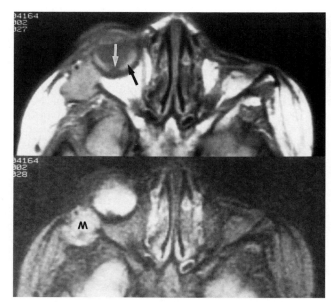

FIGURE 31–54. Second primary in a patient with bilateral retinoblastoma. Axial proton density–weighted *(top)* and T2-weighted *(bottom)* images show a postradiation regressed retinoblastoma *(white arrow)*, subretinal exudate *(black arrow)*, postenucleation changes of the left globe, and a destructive mass (M), presumed to be a sarcoma.

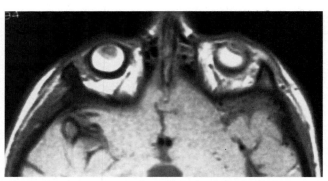

FIGURE 31–56. Persistent hyperplastic primary vitreous. Axial proton density–weighted (2000/20) image shows bilateral microphthalmia. The increased intensity of the globes is due to chronic hemorrhage in either the subretinal or subhyaloid space.

caused by persistence of various portions of the primary vitreous and tunica vasculosa lentis with hyperplasia and extensive proliferation of the associated embryonic connective tissue. Diagnosis of PHPV is often made difficult by its extremely broad array of clinical manifestations, etiologic heterogeneity, and frequently opaque ocular media.

The CT findings of PHPV include the following: 1) microphthalmos is usually detectable; 2) calcification is absent within or around the globe; 3) generalized increased density of the entire vitreous chamber may be visible; 4) enhancement on the CT image of abnormal intravitreal tissue may be seen after intravenous administration of contrast medium; 5) tubular, cylin-

drical, triangular, or other discrete intravitreal densities suggest the persistence of fetal tissue in Cloquet's canal or congenital nonattachment of the retina.[35]

The MRI appearance of PHPV of different causes may be different. MRI in patients with PHPV may reveal marked hyperintensity of the vitreous chamber on T1-weighted images (Fig. 31–55), proton density–weighted images (Fig. 31–56), and T2-weighted images. The MRI appearance of retinopathy of prematurity may be difficult to differentiate from that of PHPV (Fig. 31–57).

COATS' DISEASE

Coats' disease is a primary vascular anomaly of the retina characterized by idiopathic retinal telangiectasia and exudative retinal detachment (exudative retinopathy). The condition occurs more frequently in juvenile males than in females. The condition is also seen in adults and is almost always unilateral.

The CT and MRI findings in Coats' disease vary with the stages of progression of the disease. At early stages,

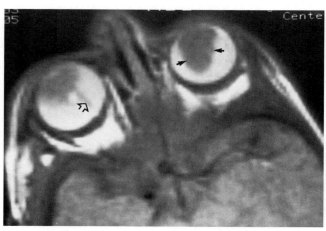

FIGURE 31–55. Persistent hyperplastic primary vitreous. Axial proton density–weighted image shows bilateral retinal detachments *(arrows)*. The increased subretinal intensity is due to chronic hemorrhage.

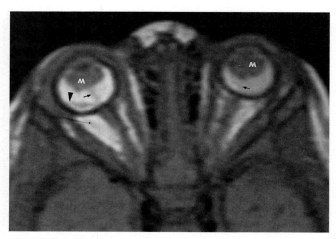

FIGURE 31–57. Retinopathy of prematurity. Axial proton density–weighted (2000/20) image shows bilateral detached retina *(arrows)*, fluid-fluid level *(arrowhead)* related to hemorrhage, and retrolental masses (m) resulting from scar and reactive tissues.

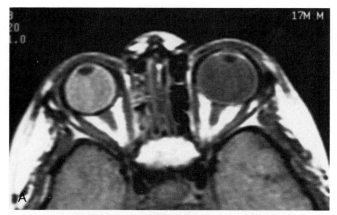

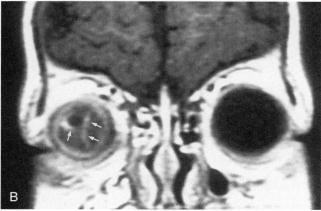

FIGURE 31–58. Coats' disease. A 17-month-old boy with leukokoric right eye. *A,* Axial proton density–weighted (2000/16) image shows increased intensity of the right globe. This is related to total retinal detachment. The detached leaves of the retina cannot be recognized; however, they are seen after gadolinium contrast study as seen in a coronal scan. *B,* Postcontrast coronal T1-weighted (400/17) image shows enhancing leaves of the detached retina *(arrows).* The leaves of the retina are thickened as well as enhanced. This is due to intraretinal telangiectasia and intraretinal exudate, which are characteristic of Coats' disease. Findings were confirmed after enucleation.

both techniques may yield little information. In the later stages of the disease, retinal detachment accounts for all of the pathologic findings with CT and MRI[31, 37, 42] (Fig. 31–58*A*). Enhancement of the detached leaves of the retina on enhanced MR images is highly suggestive, if not pathognomonic, of Coats' disease (Fig. 31–58*B*).

OCULAR TOXOCARIASIS (SCLEROSING ENDOPHTHALMITIS)

The granuloma of *Toxocara canis* is actually an eosinophilic abscess with the second-stage larvae of *Toxocara* within the abscess. The infection results from ingestion of eggs of the nematode *T. canis.* In these patients, death of the larvae results in a wide spectrum of intraocular inflammatory reactions.[4]

CT findings consist of a nonhomogeneous intravitreal density that corresponds to detached retina, organized vitreous, and inflammatory subretinal exudate.

In general, the proteinaceous subretinal exudate produced by inflammatory response to larval infiltration is seen as variable hyperintensity on T1-, proton density–, and T2-weighted images. Gd-DTPA MRI may delineate one or more foci (abscesses) of enhancement (Fig. 31–59).

MALIGNANT UVEAL MELANOMA

The uvea (iris, ciliary body, and choroid) is derived from the mesoderm and neuroectoderm and may harbor tumors of both origins. As it is the most highly vascular portion of the eyeball, it provides a suitable substrate for tumor cells. Most primary and metastatic ocular neoplasms involve the choroid, with the most common being malignant melanoma. Malignant melanomas of the uvea are unusual in black persons; the white/black ratio is about 15:1. Those involving the ciliary body and choroid are thought to originate from preexisting nevi.[31, 43]

Diagnostic Imaging

Although uveal melanomas can be accurately diagnosed by ophthalmoscopy, fluorescein angiography, or ultrasonography, misdiagnosis continues to occur, particularly when opaque media preclude direct visual-

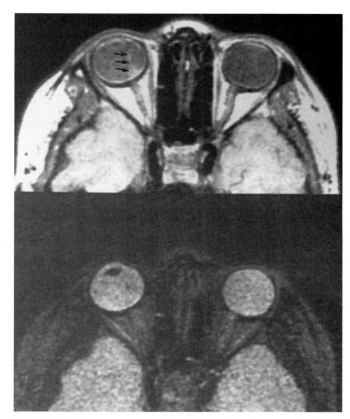

FIGURE 31–59. *Toxocara canis* granuloma. Axial proton density–weighted *(top)* and T2-weighted *(bottom)* images show an irregular mass *(arrows),* compatible with *Toxocara* granuloma. The lesion appears hyperintense on the T2-weighted image.

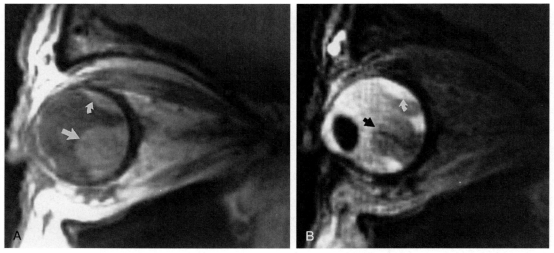

FIGURE 31–60. Choroidal melanoma. *(A)* Sagittal proton density–weighted (2000/20) and *(B)* T2-weighted (2000/80) images show a large melanoma *(straight arrows)* and associated subretinal exudate *(curved arrows)*.

ization.[43] CT has proved useful for demonstrating uveal melanoma and a wide variety of pathologic conditions. Most uveal melanomas are seen on CT scans as elevated, hyperdense, sharply marginated lesions.

MRI has been used to diagnose various intraocular lesions. On T1- and proton density–weighted images, uveal melanomas are seen as areas of moderately high signal intensity (greater signal intensity than vitreous)[43] (Fig. 31–60A). On T2-weighted images, melanomas are seen as areas of moderate to marked low signal intensity (lower intensity than vitreous) (Fig. 31–60B). These MRI characteristics of uveal melanomas are similar to those of retinoblastomas. Some of the ocular melanomas may be hyperintense on T2-weighted images. Discoid melanomas or ring melanomas may not be detected if they are not elevated more than 2 mm.

Associated retinal detachment is better visualized by MRI than by CT particularly after intravenous administration of Gd-DTPA (Fig. 31–61). Exudative retinal detachment is usually depicted on MR images as a dependent area of moderate to high signal intensity on T1-, proton density–, and T2-weighted images. Total retinal detachment may be present. Chronic retinal detachment and hemorrhagic subretinal fluid have varied MRI appearances, and at times the signal intensity of subretinal fluid may be identical to that of ocular melanoma.

Most uveal melanomas appear as a well-defined solid mass. At times, atypical features of ocular melanoma may be present. When necrotic or hemorrhagic foci are present within the uveal melanoma, the inhomogeneity within the tumor can be a problem. Some melanomas may be seen better on T2-weighted images. Other uveal melanomas may show no significant hypointensity on T2-weighted images.

The MRI diagnosis of uveal melanomas is greatly enhanced by the use of gadolinium contrast material. Uveal melanomas show moderate enhancement. Invasion of the sclera, extension of tumor in the optic disk and the Tenon capsule, and extraocular invasion can be easily detected by MRI particularly on postcontrast fat-suppressed T1-weighted images (Fig. 31–62).

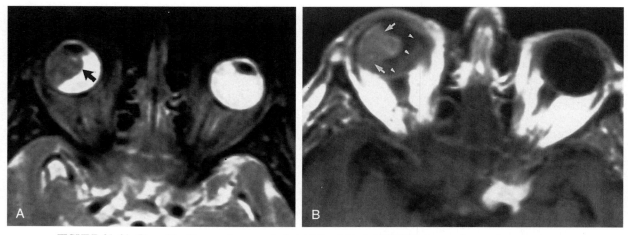

FIGURE 31–61. Choroidociliary melanoma. *A,* Axial T2-weighted (2800/80) image shows a large melanoma *(arrow)*. *B,* Postcontrast axial T1-weighted (500/20) image shows the melanoma *(arrows)* as well as associated subretinal exudate *(arrowheads)*. Notice enhancement of tumor and its distinction from subretinal exudate.

Differential Diagnosis

A number of benign and malignant lesions of the eye may be confused with malignant uveal melanoma. The main ocular conditions that may be mistaken for a malignant uveal melanoma include[44, 45]

1. Metastatic tumors
2. Choroidal detachment
3. Choroidal nevi
4. Choroidal hemangioma
5. Choroidal cyst
6. Neurofibroma
7. Schwannoma of the uvea
8. Leiomyoma
9. Adenoma
10. Medulloepithelioma
11. Retinal detachment
12. Diskiform degeneration of the macula
13. Others

CHOROIDAL AND RETINAL HEMANGIOMAS

Choroidal hemangiomas are seen usually in association with Sturge-Weber disease. Retinal angiomas, on the other hand, are seen in patients with von Hippel–Lindau disease. Sturge-Weber disease consists of capillary or cavernous hemangiomas with the cutaneous distribution of the trigeminal nerve and of a predominantly venous hemangioma of the leptomeninges.

Diagnostic Imaging

Although choroidal hemangioma can be diagnosed by ophthalmoscopy, fluorescein angiography, or ultrasonography, this is a lesion whose diagnosis on clinical grounds presents some difficulty. Choroidal hemangiomas are seen on plain CT scans as ill-defined images. They demonstrate intense enhancement on contrast infusion and dynamic CT scans.

With MRI, choroidal hemangioma may be seen as a hypointense or slightly hyperintense area on T1-

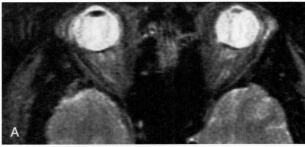
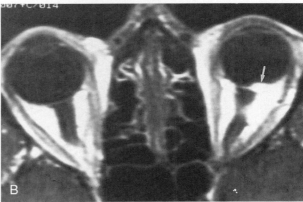

FIGURE 31–63. Choroidal hemangioma. *A,* Axial T2-weighted (2200/80) image shows no distinct lesion in either globe. *B,* Postcontrast T1-weighted (400/20) image shows an intense enhancement involving the presumed choroidal hemangioma *(arrow)* of the left globe.

weighted images and as a hyperintense area on T2-weighted images (Fig. 31–63A). Some choroidal hemangiomas are seen as a moderately intense area in T1-, proton density–, and T2-weighted images.[45] Choroidal hemangiomas show intense enhancement after intravenous administration of Gd-DTPA (Fig. 31–63B). Retinal angiomas, unlike choroidal angiomas, are often flat and difficult to image by CT and MRI.

UVEAL METASTASIS

Uveal metastasis can be confused with uveal melanoma both clinically and by imaging studies. Metastatic lesion of the uvea extends chiefly in the plane of the choroid with relatively little increase in thickness. Unlike uveal melanomas, which tend to form a protuberant mass, the metastatic lesions often have a mottled appearance and diffuse outline. The malignant cells (emboli) gain access to the eye via the blood stream by means of the short posterior ciliary arteries. This may be the reason why the site of the majority of the metastases is in the posterior half of the eye. The most common source of secondary carcinoma within the eye is breast or lung. Tumor metastasis may occur in both retina and choroid, both eyes being affected in about one third of the cases.

Uveal metastasis and lymphoreticular involvement of the choroid may have similar MRI characteristics. A mucin-producing metastatic lesion (adenocarcinoma)

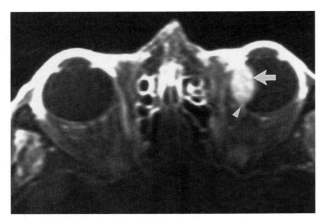

FIGURE 31–62. Choroidal melanoma. Postcontrast fat suppression axial T1-weighted (500/20) image shows a melanoma *(arrow).* Notice focal invasion of the eye wall *(arrowhead).*

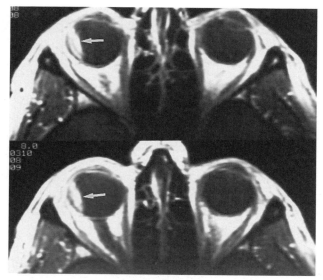

FIGURE 31–64. Choroidal metastasis. Postcontrast axial T1-weighted (400/25) images show an enhancing mass *(arrows)* compatible with metastasis from breast carcinoma.

may simulate uveal melanoma as well because the proteinaceous fluid tends to decrease T1 and T2 relaxation times of the lesion. Metastatic lesions from primary carcinoid tumor or other primary neoplasms may also simulate uveal melanomas. Metastatic lesions demonstrate moderate to marked enhancement after intravenous injection of Gd-DTPA. The MRI contrast study improves the detection of metastatic foci (Fig. 31–64).

REFERENCES

1. Rootman J, ed: Diseases of the Orbit. Philadelphia: JB Lippincott, 1988.
2. Mafee MF: The orbit. In: Som PM, Bergeron RT, eds. Head and Neck Imaging. St. Louis: Mosby–Year Book, 1991, pp 693–813.
3. Mafee MF: Imaging of the orbit. In: Valvassori GE, Mafee MF, Carter BL, eds. Imaging of the Head and Neck. New York: Thieme Medical Publishers, 1995, pp. 158–247.
4. Barakow JA, Dillon WP, Chew WM: Orbit, skull base and pharynx: contrast-enhanced fat suppression MR imaging. Radiology 179:191–198, 1991.
5. Tien RD, Hesselink JR, Szumowski J: MR fat suppression combined with Gd-DTPA enhancement in optic neuritis and perineuritis. J Comput Assist Tomogr 15:223–227, 1991.
6. Tien RD, Chu PK, Hesselink JR, Szumowski J: Intra- and paraorbital lesions: value of fat-suppression MR imaging with paramagnetic contrast enhancement. AJNR 12:245–253, 1991.
7. Mafee MF, Putterman A, Valvassori GE, et al: Orbital space-occupying lesions: role of CT and MRI; an analysis of 145 cases. Radiol Clin North Am 25:529–559, 1987.
8. Shields JA, ed: Diagnosis and Management of Orbital Tumors. Philadelphia: WB Saunders, 1989.
9. Henderson JW: Orbital Tumors. Philadelphia: WB Saunders, 1973, pp 116–123.
10. Mafee MF, Dobben GD, Valvassori GE: Computed tomography assessment of paraorbital pathology. In: Gonzalez CA, Becker MH, Flanagan JC, eds. Diagnostic Imaging in Ophthalmology. New York: Springer-Verlag, 1985, pp 281–302.
11. Grove AS: Giant dermoid cysts of the orbit. Ophthalmology 86:1513–1520, 1979.
12. Weber AL, Mikulis DK: Inflammatory disorders of the paraorbital sinuses and their complications. Radiol Clin North Am 25:615–630, 1987.
13. Hawkins DD, Clark RW: Orbital involvement in acute sinusitis. Clin Pediatr 16:464–471, 1977.
14. Flanders AE, Mafee MF, Rao VM, et al: CT characteristics of orbital pseudotumors and other orbital inflammatory processes. J Comput Assist Tomogr 13:40–47, 1989.
15. Trokel SL, Hilal SK: Recognition and differential diagnosis of enlarged extraocular muscles in computed tomography. Am J Ophthalmol 87:503–512, 1979.
16. Flanders AE, Espinosa GA, Markiewicz DA, et al: Orbital lymphoma. Radiol Clin North Am 25:601–612, 1987.
17. Mafee MF, Miller MT, Tan WS, et al: Dynamic computed tomography and its application to ophthalmology. Radiol Clin North Am 25:715–731, 1987.
17a. Wilms G, Taat H, Dom R, Thywissen C, et al: Orbital cavernous hemangioma: findings on sequential Gd-enhanced MRI. J Comput Assist Tomogr 19:548–551, 1995.
18. Bockwinkel KD, Diddams JA: Haemangiopericytoma: report of case and comprehensive review of literature. Cancer 25:896–901, 1970.
19. Jacomb-Hood J, Moseley IF: Orbital fibrous histiocytoma: computed tomography in 10 cases and a review of radiological findings. Clin Radiol 43:117–120, 1991.
20. Tech KE, Becker CJ, Lazo A, et al: Anomalous intracranial venous drainage mimicking orbital or cavernous arteriovenous fistula. AJNR 16:171–174, 1995.
21. Azar-Kia B, Naheedy MF, Elias DA, et al: Optic nerve tumors: role of MRI and CT. Radiol Clin North Am 25:561–581, 1987.
22. Hoyt WF, Baghdassarian SA: Optic glioma of childhood. Natural history and rationale for conservative management. Br J Ophthalmol 53:793–798, 1969.
23. Lewis A, Gerson P, Axelson K, et al: Von Recklinghausen neurofibromatosis II. Incidence of optic glioma. Ophthalmology 91:929–935, 1984.
24. Vade A, Armstrong D: Orbital rhabdomyosarcoma in childhood. Radiol Clin North Am 25:701–714, 1987.
24a. Erly WK, Carmody RF, Dryden RM: Orbital histiocytosis X. AJNR 16:1258–1261, 1995.
25. Stewart WB, Krohel GB, Wright JE: Lacrimal gland and fossa lesions: an approach to diagnosis and management. Ophthalmology 86:886–895, 1979.
26. Wright JE: Factors affecting the survival of patients with lacrimal gland tumors. Can J Ophthalmol 17:3–9, 1982.
27. Zimmerman LE, Sanders LE, Ackerman IV: Epithelial tumors of the lacrimal gland: prognostic and therapeutic significance of histologic types. Int Ophthalmol Clin 2:337–367, 1962.
28. Mafee MF, Haik BG: Lacrimal gland and fossa lesions: role of computed tomography. Radiol Clin North Am 25:767–779, 1987.
29. Yeo JH, Jakobiec FA, Abbott GF, et al: Combined clinical and computed tomographic diagnosis of orbital lymphoid tumors. Am J Ophthalmol 94:235–245, 1982.
30. Jakobiec FA, Yeo JH, Trokel SL, et al: Combined clinical and computed tomographic diagnosis of primary lacrimal fossa lesions. Am J Ophthalmol 94:785–807, 1982.
31. Mafee MF: Magnetic resonance imaging: ocular pathology. In: Newton TH, Bilaniuk LT, eds. Modern Neuroradiology, Volume 4. Radiology of the Eye and Orbit. New York: Clavadel Press/Raven Press, 1990, pp 1–35.
32. Mafee MF: Case 5: Calcifications of the eye. In: Som PM, ed. Head and Neck Disorders (Fourth Series) Test and Syllabus. Reston, VA: American College of Radiology, 1992, pp 71–116.
32a. Kindler P: Morning glory syndrome. Unusual congenital optic disc anomaly. Am J Ophthalmol 69:376–384, 1970.
33. Mafee MF, Peyman GA: Retinal and choroidal detachments: role of MRI and CT. Radiol Clin North Am 25:487–507, 1987.
34. Mafee MF, Peyman GA: Choroidal detachment and ocular hypotony: CT evaluation. Radiology 153:697–703, 1984.
35. Mafee MF, Goldberg MF, Valvassori GE, Capek V: Computed tomography in the evaluation of patients with persistent hyperplastic primary vitreous (PHPV). Radiology 145:713–714, 1982.
36. Haik BG, Saint Louis L, Smith ME, et al: Magnetic resonance imaging in the evaluation of leukocoria. Ophthalmology 92:1143–1152, 1985.
37. Mafee MF, Goldberg MF, Cohen SB, et al: Magnetic resonance imaging versus computed tomography of leukocoric eyes and use of in vitro proton magnetic resonance spectroscopy of retinoblastoma. Ophthalmology 96:965–975, 1989.
38. Provenzale J, Weber AL, Klintworth GK, McLendon RE: Radiologic-pathologic correlation: bilateral retinoblastoma with coexistent pineoblastoma (trilateral retinoblastoma). AJNR 16:157–165, 1995.
39. Jakobiec FA, Tso MO, Zimmerman LE, Danis P: Retinoblastoma and intracranial malignancy. Cancer 39:2048–2058, 1977.
40. Bader JL, Meadows AT, Zimmerman LE, et al: Bilateral retinoblastoma with ectopic intracranial retinoblastoma. Cancer Genet Cytogenet 5:203–213, 1982.
41. Finelli DA, Shurin SB, Bardenstein DS: Trilateral retinoblastoma: Two variations. AJNR 16:166–170, 1995.
42. Sherman JL, McLean IW, Brallier DR: Coats' disease. CT-pathologic correlation in two cases. Radiology 146:77–78, 1983.
43. Mafee MF, Peyman GA, Peace JH, et al: Magnetic resonance imaging in the evaluation and differentiation of uveal melanoma. Ophthalmology 94:341–348, 1987.
44. Mafee MF, Linder B, Peyman GA, et al: Choroidal hematoma and effusion: evaluation with MR imaging. Radiology 168:781–786, 1988.
45. Shields JA, Zimmerman LE: Lesions simulating malignant melanoma of the posterior uvea. Arch Ophthalmol 89:466–471, 1973.

Skull Base and Temporal Bone

KENT B. REMLEY

The skull base represents a unique and complex transition zone, separating the intracranial contents from the face and suprahyoid neck. The undulating surface and minimal craniocaudal dimensions of the cranial base require multiplanar imaging for accurate assessment. Disease processes can arise within the skull base primarily or can affect this region secondarily, from the intracranial compartment above or the spaces of the suprahyoid neck (deep face) below. In addition, numerous bony foramina and canals create many potential pathways for transcranial disease spread.

Newer cranial base surgical techniques have placed a greater demand on the radiologist to precisely define the location and extent of lesions involving the skull base. Although magnetic resonance imaging (MRI) is well established as the modality of choice for evaluating the internal auditory canal and the cerebellopontine angle, it is only in more recent years that MRI has also become the primary tool for imaging the skull base, and in many instances it serves as the definitive imaging study.

This chapter focuses on the anterior, central, and posterolateral skull base. It begins with a discussion of imaging techniques and technical considerations. Anatomy with emphasis on the skull base foramina and associated transcranial pathways of potential disease spread is then presented, followed by a discussion of congenital abnormalities and neoplasms of the anterior and central skull base. These two areas are discussed together because many of the same processes affect both regions. Discussion of pertinent anatomy and pathology involving the temporal bone follows. Skull base involvement from regional neoplasms, metastatic disease, and inflammatory and infectious diseases is presented in separate sections.

The chapter concludes with a section on the differential diagnosis of skull base processes. The terms *posterolateral skull base* and *temporal bone* are used interchangeably throughout the chapter, although technically the posterolateral skull base also includes the occipital bone contribution to the jugular foramen and the occipital condyle. Discussion of the anterior skull base is limited here primarily to congenital and neoplastic processes because this area is also discussed in Chapter 33.

IMAGING TECHNIQUES

GENERAL CONCEPTS

In many ways, MRI is ideally suited for evaluation of the complex anatomy of the cranial base. Multiplanar imaging capabilities, noninvasive vascular assessment, and superb ability to assess relationships between lesions of the skull base and the intracranial structures offer a significant advantage over computed tomography (CT). However, the insensitivity of MRI to calcification and cortical bone is an important drawback with this technique. CT is often used as an adjunct to MRI when knowledge of precise bone anatomy is required by the surgeon. Analysis of tumor calcification and the pattern of bone destruction can provide additional information regarding lesion diagnosis. When complex lesions are present, both techniques are required. If complete soft tissue information of the lesion is provided by the MR study, only a noncontrast CT examination need be performed using a high-resolution bone algorithm program.

In contrast to MRI of the brain or spine, protocols for imaging the skull base are less well defined and agreed on. Although imaging of the cerebellopontine angle and internal auditory canal has been fairly standardized, the addition of fast spin-echo (FSE) techniques to the repertoire of available pulse sequences has modified the imaging protocol for the base of the skull at many institutions. The complex geometry of the skull base and wide variety of different diseases therefore require a tailored examination in many instances. Because pathologic processes such as perineural tumor spread are often subtle, knowledge of the patient's history and clinical examination, particularly regarding the status of the cranial nerves, assumes paramount importance in directing the MR study. The following recommendations are intended to guide the physician with imaging of the cranial base and temporal bone. Individual imaging protocols I have used, based on the site of disease and skull base location, are provided in Table 32–1.

A standard head coil is used for imaging the skull base. The routine examination consists of imaging in sagittal, axial, and coronal planes. After a T1-weighted sagittal series, which serves as a localizing sequence, T2-weighted axial and T1-weighted coronal series are performed. A T1-weighted axial series may be performed in place of the coronal sequence, depending on the area of interest. The T1-weighted images are obtained for anatomic definition. Therefore, section thickness is kept to a minimum and is usually 3 mm. In general, coronal images are obtained from the posterior ethmoidal sinuses to the middle of the foramen magnum, but the sequence profile may be modified depending on the precise localization of the lesion on the T1 sagittal localizer. The T1-weighted sagittal sequence should be reviewed before setting up subsequent sequences, if possible, because it will often define the area of interest. Intravenous administration of MR contrast agent is used in all routine cases, given at standard dosage (0.1 mmol/kg). The coronal sequence is then repeated, and an axial sequence is performed from the hard palate to the suprasellar cistern.

Proton density– and T2-weighted images have been reported in the past to be of lesser value in evaluating the skull base, in part due to the significant increase in imaging time.[1] Often, however, the enhancement characteristics of histologically distinct neoplasms appear similar. Because the T2 relaxation times of tumors involving the skull base may vary significantly, T2-weighted images can yield important additional information regarding the correct diagnosis. Furthermore,

T2-weighted images can be of critical importance in differentiating inflammatory disease from tumor when the anterior skull base and sphenoidal sinuses are involved.[2] The T1- and T2-weighted appearances, including enhancement features, of specific skull base neoplasms are presented later in this chapter.

FSE imaging has been an important advancement in MRI of the extracranial head and neck.[3] This technique is discussed in depth elsewhere in this text and is not detailed here. Briefly, FSE imaging, by filling multiple lines of k-space with a single excitation pulse, allows for more rapid acquisition of T2-weighted images, thereby replacing the need for conventional spin-echo (SE) sequences in the head and neck. In addition, FSE imaging is less affected by the magnetic susceptibility artifacts encountered in the skull base and temporal bone. The time savings afforded by FSE imaging can be exchanged for thinner slices, greater resolution, and improved signal-to-noise ratio, as needed. In most cases, a single-echo long repetition time (TR), long echo time (TE) sequence is adequate when this technique is used.

The addition of fat suppression techniques to the MRI pulse sequence repertoire has also become a useful adjunct to standard T1- and T2-weighted SE imaging of the deep face and skull base.[4, 5] The idea behind employment of fat saturation is to improve lesion conspicuity when the suspected disease is located in an area containing fat (e.g., bone marrow, parapharyngeal space). In-depth discussion of methods of fat suppression in MRI is provided in Chapter 1. Chemical-shift fat suppression is the only commonly used technique to suppress fat signal with contrast-enhanced T1-weighted sequences. When an enhancing lesion is surrounded by fat, the margins of the lesion

TABLE 32–1. IMAGING PROTOCOLS FOR THE SKULL BASE*

LOCATION	AREA OF COVERAGE	PULSE SEQUENCES	COMMENTS
Anterior skull base	AP—frontal sinus to sella SI—frontal sinus to oral cavity	T1 sagittal localizer T2 axial (FSE or SE) T2 coronal Post-Gd T1 coronal Post-Gd T1 axial + FS	Post-Gd T1 sagittal optional FSE with FS recommended
Central skull base	AP—posterior orbits to middle pons SI—suprasellar cistern to oral cavity	T1 sagittal localizer T2 axial (FSE or SE) T1 coronal Post-Gd T1 coronal Post-Gd T1 axial + FS	Post-Gd T1 sagittal optional FSE with FS recommended MRA if arterial lesion suspected or vascular encasement or displacement present
Posterolateral skull base Jugular foramen Petrous apex	AP—posterior foramen magnum to nasopharynx or sphenoidal sinus SI—internal auditory canal to tongue base (jugular foramen); sella to foramen magnum (petrous apex)	T1 sagittal (side of interest) T1 axial T2 axial Post-Gd T1 coronal Post-Gd T1 axial + FS	MRA if arterial lesion suspected or vascular encasement or displacement present FSE with FS recommended MRV for all studies of the jugular foramen (single-slice gradient-echo sequence may be substituted or added)
Posterolateral skull base Internal auditory canal Middle ear/mastoid	AP—petrous apex through semicircular canals SI—sella to posterior mastoid (coverage for acoustic work-up); extend coverage posterior as needed for mastoid work-up	T1 axial T2 axial (whole brain) FSE T2 coronal of internal auditory canals (3-mm slices) Post-Gd T1 axial Post-Gd T1 coronal	Expand coverage posteriorly for mastoid disease MRV of signoidal sinus for mastoiditis or posterior temporal bone tumor

*AP = anterior-posterior; SI = superior-inferior; FS = fat saturation; SE = spin echo; FSE = fast spin echo; MRA = MR angiography; MRV = MR venography; post-Gd = after gadolinium enhancement.

or the lesion itself may become inapparent. By suppressing the surrounding fat signal pattern, any enhancement of the lesion is much more easily detected. Furthermore, suppression of the fat signal pattern can be helpful if there are no precontrast images for comparison. Fat suppression techniques can also be employed when there is a question of fat versus subacute hemorrhage (methemoglobin) or proteinaceous content within a mass. In contrast to standard T2-weighted SE imaging, the fat signal pattern is not significantly suppressed with FSE imaging. Therefore, fat suppression techniques should be used, if possible, to improve the conspicuity of lesions with moderately long T2 relaxation times.

It is important to realize the potential drawbacks and artifacts associated with fat suppression techniques. A slice penalty results from the additional time required to apply the fat-selective presaturation radiofrequency pulse. As a result, the TR may need to be lengthened, increasing imaging time. Magnetic susceptibility artifacts are commonly encountered with fat suppression techniques. Interface susceptibility artifacts ("blooming" artifact), resulting in signal loss at air-tissue interfaces, are a frequent problem in skull base imaging because of the paranasal sinuses and temporal bones. The coronal imaging plane is affected to a greater degree than is the axial plane. Therefore, if the radiologist elects to use fat suppression after gadolinium administration, the axial plane should be used if possible and a standard T1-weighted sequence should also be obtained in a different imaging plane. Bulk susceptibility artifact occurs in areas where tissue volumes change, such as the junction of the suprahyoid and infrahyoid neck.[5] This artifact can result in incomplete or asymmetric fat signal suppression or cause water signal suppression along one end of the frequency encoding gradient. Fat suppression failure artifacts are observed as focal areas of high signal intensity without geometric distortion at air-fat interfaces.[6] Metallic artifacts tend to be more prominent with fat suppression techniques, an important consideration when dental amalgam or surgical clips are near the area of interest. It is important to be aware of these artifacts when imaging the skull base so that scan techniques can be adjusted to minimize their impact. Short-tau inversion recovery (STIR) pulse sequences offer another method of fat suppression with T2-weighted–type image contrast enhancement. The details of these techniques are covered elsewhere, but they are used less commonly in the skull base and suprahyoid neck because of coverage limitations and increased sensitivity to motion.

TEMPORAL BONE AND INTERNAL AUDITORY CANAL

MRI of the temporal bone in clinical practice is done most commonly to evaluate the patient with signs and symptoms suggesting vestibulocochlear nerve disease. Patients referred to "rule out acoustic schwannoma" are evaluated with the standard head coil. T2-weighted axial images of the brain are obtained to evaluate for central causes of auditory pathway dysfunction. T1-weighted images of the internal auditory canals are obtained before and after gadolinium administration. I prefer to obtain the T1-weighted images in the axial plane, with an additional postcontrast T1-weighted coronal sequence as needed. Other authors prefer the coronal plane for their precontrast T1-weighted sequence. High-resolution, thin-section single-echo FSE images, obtained with either a head coil or a surface coil, enable the imager to visualize the facial and vestibulocochlear nerves within the internal auditory canal. Superb images of the internal auditory canal and membranous labyrinth can be obtained by using a dual 3-inch temporomandibular joint surface coil. Although some resolution is sacrificed when the head coil is substituted for the temporomandibular joint coil, there is no dropoff of signal intensity over the brain stem. As these latter techniques become refined, the need for routine contrast enhancement with MRI of the internal auditory canal may be significantly decreased. In addition to FSE techniques, several three-dimensional (3D) Fourier transformation MRI techniques have been advocated for evaluating the otic capsule and internal auditory canal.[7, 8]

MAGNETIC RESONANCE ANGIOGRAPHY

MR angiography is being used with increasing frequency for noninvasive evaluation of the major arterial and venous structures of the intracranial circulation and neck.[9] Arterial displacement, stenosis, and occlusion can be assessed without the need for catheter angiography. MR venography is a useful adjunct to standard T1- and T2-weighted sequences in evaluating the jugular foramen.[10] Both arterial and venous MR angiographic techniques may be needed for assessment of patients with suspected dural arteriovenous fistulas or jugular foramen tumors.[11]

Time-of-flight (TOF) and phase-contrast MR angiography techniques can both be used for vascular assessment of the skull base. I prefer to use two-dimensional (2D) TOF MR angiography for the initial assessment of the arterial structures of the neck and skull base and venous anatomy of the jugular foramen region. Phase-contrast MR angiography is useful if there is a question of vascular thrombosis. Hybrid TOF techniques such as multiple overlapping thin-slab acquisition (MOTSA) and 3D phase-contrast imaging are particularly valuable in evaluating vascular lesions that may have flow in multiple planes with variable velocities, such as dural arteriovenous fistulas.[12, 13] 3D T1-weighted sequences such as magnetization-prepared rapid gradient echo (MP-RAGE) and spoiled gradient-recalled acquisition in the steady state (GRASS) can be useful for evaluating smaller arterial structures around the skull base. The latter two techniques have the additional advantage of multiplanar reconstruction with exquisite anatomic definition of adjacent nonvascular structures. Finally, reference to source images is critical when evaluating anatomy and pathology with MR angiography. Proteinaceous cystic masses or hemorrhagic lesions containing methemoglobin produce

T1 shortening and are visible on the 3D TOF images. These lesions can simulate the vascular "blush" of a hypervascular tumor with conventional angiography.

NORMAL ANATOMY

A detailed discussion of the complex embryology and normal anatomy of the skull base is beyond the scope of this chapter, and the reader is referred to several excellent in-depth sources for this information.[14-17] The first portion of this section highlights the developmental anatomy of the anterior and central skull base because it pertains to the more common congenital abnormalities and tumors of the cranial base. The second half highlights normal anatomy including the skull base foramina as potential transcranial pathways for disease spread.

EMBRYOLOGY AND DEVELOPMENTAL ANATOMY

According to developmental anatomy, the skull is divided into two parts, the neurocranium and the viscerocranium. Each component can be further subdivided into membranous (formed directly from mesenchymal connective tissue) and cartilaginous (formed from endochondral ossification of cartilage) portions. The membranous neurocranium comprises the calvaria, whereas the cartilaginous neurocranium, or chondrocranium, forms the major portion of the cranial base. The facial bones arise from membranous viscerocranium, although several structures, including the middle ear ossicles, arise from cartilaginous viscerocranium. The chondrocranium ultimately forms the base of the occipital bone, the body and lesser wing of the sphenoid bone, the body and nasal portions of the ethmoid bone, and the petrous and mastoid segments of the temporal bone. The paired frontal bones, forming the majority of the anterior cranial fossa, the greater sphenoid wings, and lateral pterygoid plates, arise from membranous neurocranium.

Development of the chondrocranium begins at about the 40th day of gestation with the conversion of mesenchyme into cartilage.[1] The central mesenchyme envelops the rostral notochord, incorporating it into the eventual basiocciput and basisphenoid. The central, posterior, and midline anterior skull base is formed from the fusion of multiple cartilaginous precursors with subsequent endochondral ossification. The growth of the endochondral bones of the skull base occurs at multiple synchondroses: the intersphenoidal, spheno-occipital, basiexoccipital, and innominant synchondroses. The intersphenoidal synchondrosis, located between the presphenoid and postsphenoid segments, fuses shortly before birth. Closure of the innominant and basiexoccipital synchondroses occurs by 4 years of age.[18] The spheno-occipital synchondrosis, an easily recognized clival landmark on midline sagittal MR images, usually fuses by age 16 to 20 years, but it may remain visible until 25 years of age[18] (Fig. 32–1). Because growth of the skull base primarily depends on endochondral bone development, maturation parallels skeletal growth in general. As a result, congenital maldevelopment or delays in maturation of the appendicular skeleton may also be manifest in the base of the skull.

The anterior skull base is formed by the fusion of the orbital plates of the paired frontal bones and the ethmoid bone. In the early embryo, the paired frontal bones are separated from the developing nasal bones by a small fontanelle, the fonticulus nasofrontalis. A diverticulum of dura normally passes through the fonticulus into the developing nose.[16] This diverticulum

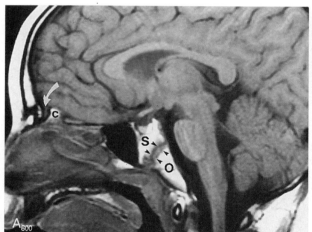
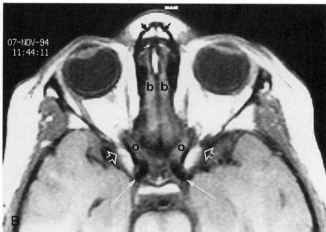

FIGURE 32–1. Normal anterior and central skull base anatomy. *A,* Midline sagittal T1-weighted image of the anterior and central skull base in a child shows the spheno-occipital synchondrosis *(arrowheads)* separating the basisphenoid (S) from the basiocciput (O) with fatty conversion of the marrow space. This synchondrosis may remain visible until age 25 years. The foramen cecum *(arrow)* is well visualized anterior to the crista galli (c). *B,* Axial T1-weighted image in the same patient demonstrates the optic nerves (o) within the optic canals, the superior orbital fissures *(open arrows),* and signal void within the internal carotid arteries *(long white arrows).* The olfactory tracts and olfactory bulbs (b) extend to the crista galli. The foramen cecum *(small white arrows)* is anterior to the crista and posterior to the paired nasal processes *(black arrows)* of the frontal bones.

TABLE 32–2. APERTURES AND TRANSCRANIAL PATHWAYS

APERTURE	LOCATION	CONTENTS AND TRANSMITTED STRUCTURE	CONNECTION
Cribriform plate	Midline–anterior cranial fossa	Olfactory nerve (cranial nerve [CN] I) Ethmoidal arteries	Anterior fossa to nasal cavity
Optic canal	Lesser wing of sphenoid bone	Optic nerve (CN II) Ophthalmic artery Subarachnoid space, cerebrospinal fluid, and dura around optic nerve	Orbit to middle cranial fossa
Superior orbital fissure	Between greater and lesser sphenoid wings	CNs III, IV, VI, and V₁ Superior ophthalmic vein	Orbit to middle cranial fossa
Foramen rotundum	Middle cranial fossa floor or anterior cavernous sinus	CN V₂ Emissary veins Artery of foramen rotundum	Meckel's cave to pterygopalatine fossa
Foramen ovale	Middle cranial fossa floor lateral to sella	CN V₃ Emissary veins Accessory meningeal artery	Meckel's cave to nasopharyngeal space
Foramen spinosum	Posterolateral to foramen ovale	Middle meningeal artery Recurrent (meningeal) branch of mandibular nerve	Middle cranial fossa to high masticator space (infratemporal fossa)
Foramen lacerum	Base of medial pterygoid plate at petrous apex	Meningeal branches of ascending pharyngeal artery (not internal carotid artery)	Not a true foramen; filled with fibrocartilage in life
Vidian (pterygoid) canal	In sphenoid bone below and medial to foramen rotundum	Vidian artery Nerve of the pterygoid canal	Foramen lacerum to pterygopalatine fossa
Carotid canal	Within petrous temporal bone	Internal carotid artery Sympathetic plexus	Carotid space to cavernous sinus
Jugular foramen	Posterolateral to carotid canal, between petrous temporal bone and occipital bone	Pars nervosa; inferior petrosal sinus (CN IX and Jacobson's nerve) Pars vascularis; internal jugular vein, CNs X and XI, nerve of Arnold, small meningeal branches of ascending pharyngeal and occipital arteries	Posterior fossa to nasopharyngeal carotid space (poststyloid parapharyngeal space)
Stylomastoid foramen	Behind styloid process	CN VII	Parotid space to middle ear
Hypoglossal canal	Occipital condyle	CN XII	Foramen magnum to nasopharyngeal carotid space
Foramen magnum	Floor of posterior fossa	Medulla and meninges CN XI (spinal segment) Vertebral arteries and veins Anterior and posterior spinal arteries	Posterior fossa to cervical spinal canal

Modified from Osborn AG, Harnsberger HR, Smoker WRK: Base of skull imaging. Semin Ultrasound CT MR 7:91–106, 1986.

later regresses as the frontal plates and ethmoid bones unite, leaving behind a small ostium called the foramen cecum (see Fig. 32–1). The normal foramen cecum, identified just anterior to the crista galli, is an important location of congenital abnormalities of the anterior skull base.

NORMAL ANATOMY

The skull base is composed of five bones: the frontal, sphenoid, ethmoid, temporal, and occipital. The frontal, ethmoid, and sphenoid bones are pertinent to this section. The temporal and occipital bones are addressed later. The sphenoid bone makes up the foundation of the central skull base and consists of central body, paired wings extending laterally, and paired pterygoid plates extending inferiorly. In the midline anteriorly, the sphenoid body articulates with the cribriform plate of the ethmoid bone, localized on sagittal MR images by the anterior wall of the sphenoidal sinus. The lesser sphenoid wings articulate with the frontal bones laterally, and the greater sphenoid wings

articulate with the frontal, parietal, and temporal bones. Posteromedially, the body and greater wing of the sphenoid bone and the apex of the petrous temporal bone converge to form the boundaries of the foramen lacerum. Posteriorly, the body of the sphenoid borders the basiocciput along the spheno-occipital synchondrosis.

The anterior skull base is composed of the ethmoid bone and the paired frontal bones. The ethmoid bone contribution to the anterior skull base consists of the cribriform plate and the crista galli. The paired frontal bones form the roof of the ethmoidal sinuses (fovea ethmoidalis), bordering the cribriform plates and the roof of each orbit. The foramen cecum, located at the anterior aspect of the crista galli, demarcates the anterior boundary of the ethmoid bone.[16]

Numerous apertures exist at the base of the skull, offering a myriad of pathways of potential extension of disease between the intracranial and extracranial compartments. Some foramina such as the foramen ovale are frequent sites of disease spread, whereas others are rarely involved, primarily due to the location and traversing structures. Table 32–2 summarizes the

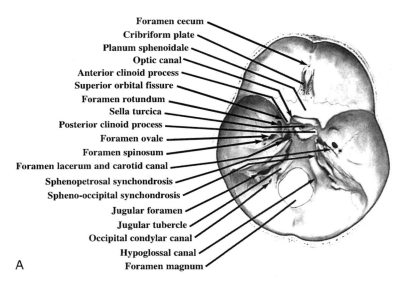

Foramen cecum
Cribriform plate
Planum sphenoidale
Optic canal
Anterior clinoid process
Superior orbital fissure
Foramen rotundum
Sella turcica
Posterior clinoid process
Foramen ovale
Foramen spinosum
Foramen lacerum and carotid canal
Sphenopetrosal synchondrosis
Spheno-occipital synchondrosis
Jugular foramen
Jugular tubercle
Occipital condylar canal
Hypoglossal canal
Foramen magnum

A

FIGURE 32–2. Important skull base apertures and pathology. *A,* Endocranial view of the skull base. *B,* Exocranial view of the skull base.

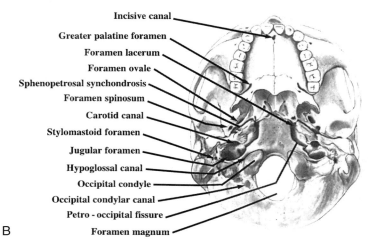

Incisive canal
Greater palatine foramen
Foramen lacerum
Foramen ovale
Sphenopetrosal synchondrosis
Foramen spinosum
Carotid canal
Stylomastoid foramen
Jugular foramen
Hypoglossal canal
Occipital condyle
Occipital condylar canal
Petro - occipital fissure
Foramen magnum

B

important apertures of the skull base. The major foramina and fissures of the skull base are shown in Figure 32–2.

CONGENITAL ABNORMALITIES

CEPHALOCELES

Congenital cephaloceles result from extracranial herniation of brain parenchyma or meninges through a midline defect in the skull and are classified by the site of the cranial defect through which the neural tissue protrudes. Most cephaloceles appear to be related to neural tube defects.[16] Meningocele refers to the herniation of meninges; an encephalocele contains both meninges and brain parenchyma. The frequency of cephalocele type varies with geographic location. Approximately 25% of cephaloceles in North America and Europe involve the anterior and central skull base and can be divided into sincipital (15%) and basal (10%) types.[19]

Sincipital or frontoethmoidal cephaloceles always present as a visible external mass along the nose or orbital margin of the forehead. The bony defect corresponds to a single ostium in the region of the foramen cecum in 90% of cases.[16] Frontoethmoidal cephaloceles are divided into nasofrontal, nasoethmoidal, and naso-orbital subtypes, depending on the involved suture. Basal or nasopharyngeal cephaloceles are usually divided into transethmoidal, sphenoethmoidal, transsphenoidal, and basioccipital subtypes.[20] Because of the absence of findings on physical examination, basal cephaloceles are typically clinically occult. Infants classically present with signs and symptoms of nasal obstruction. Adults may present with cerebrospinal fluid rhinorrhea, visual disturbance, or pituitary dysfunction. A basal cephalocele may appear as a nasal polyp on visual inspection of the nasal cavity. Herniation of the pituitary gland and optic chiasm can occur in sphenoidal cephaloceles.

Although CT is useful for examining the bony defect of a cephalocele, these malformations are optimally evaluated with MRI (Figs. 32–3 and 32–4). MRI better determines the contents within the herniated dural sac and the route of herniation, without the need for use

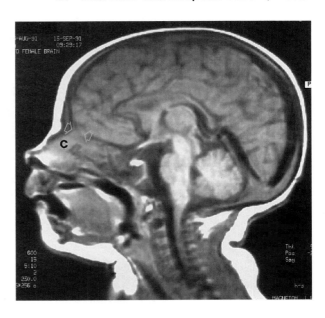

FIGURE 32–3. Frontoethmoidal encephalocele. T1-weighted sagittal MR image in a 2-month-old female infant who presented with widening of the dorsum of the nose. A soft tissue mass (C), in continuity with the right frontal lobe, extends through an enlarged foramen cecum *(arrows)* into the anterior nasal cavity. The location is consistent with a nasoethmoidal type of frontoethmoidal encephalocele. The unossified crista galli cannot be separated from brain tissue on this image. A nasofrontal type of frontoethmoidal encephalocele would be located at the position of the arrows.

of intrathecal contrast material. Imaging in the sagittal, coronal, and axial planes is recommended. Patients with cephaloceles have a high incidence of associated anomalies of the brain, including dysgenesis of the corpus callosum, intracranial lipomas, and dermoid tumors.[21] Therefore, it is important to carefully evaluate the entire intracranial contents (see also Chapter 16).

SKULL BASE DYSPLASIA

A variety of skeletal dysplasias can affect the cranial base. Fibrous dysplasia is the most common form of skeletal dysplasia to involve the skull base. Involvement of the skull base and facial bones may be present in up to 50% of patients with polyostotic fibrous dysplasia, whereas monostotic involvement is less common.[8] The sphenoid, frontal, maxillary, and ethmoid bones are most commonly involved, and the sclerotic type of fibrous dysplasia is most frequent. The MRI appearance is characterized by expansion of the marrow space with low to intermediate signal intensity on both T1- and T2-weighted sequences (Fig. 32–5). Marked enhancement is usually observed after gadolinium administration.

Skull base dysplasia can occur with neurofibromatosis type 1. These patients present with pulsating exophthalmos caused by abnormal development of the greater and lesser sphenoid wings.[22] Hypoplasia of the greater and lesser wings results in marked widening of the superior orbital fissure and protrusion of the temporal lobe and leptomeninges into the posterior orbit. This dysplasia may be unilateral or bilateral. The sphenoid ridge is elevated, and the foramen ovale and spinosum are absent. Other skeletal dysplasias affecting the skull base include achondroplasia, osteopetrosis, osteogenesis imperfecta, craniotubular dysplasias, and

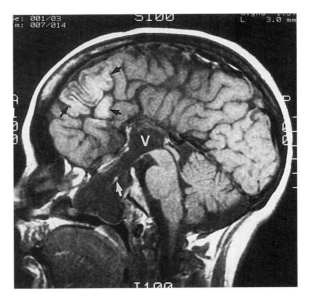

FIGURE 32–4. Transsphenoidal cephalocele. Sagittal T1-weighted MR image demonstrates a large defect within the sphenoid bone containing a fluid-filled sac that communicates with the third ventricle (V) and extends into the nasopharynx. The optic chiasm is displaced inferiorly *(white arrow)*. The patient underwent imaging to follow up a postpartum stroke of the left frontal lobe (note the subacute cortical hemorrhage *[black arrows]*). The cephalocele was clinically occult.

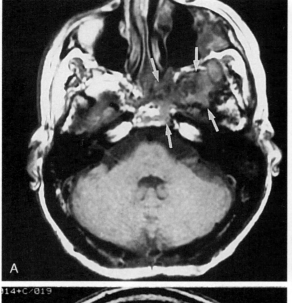

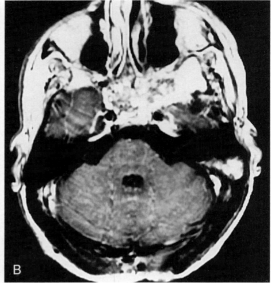

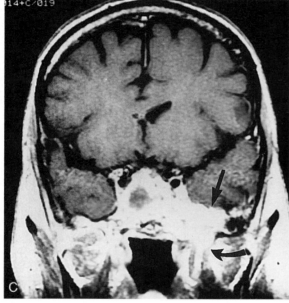

FIGURE 32–5. Fibrous dysplasia of the skull base. *A,* Axial T1-weighted MR image shows a mass of mixed signal intensity involving the central skull base and greater sphenoid wing *(arrows). B,* Contrast-enhanced image at the same level shows moderate to marked enhancement, delineating the actual margins of the lesion. *C,* Coronal contrast-enhanced image demonstrates expansion of the sphenoid wing *(straight arrow)* and extension into the parapharyngeal space *(curved arrow).* T2-weighted images revealed great variability in appearance with areas of hyperintensity intermixed with areas of intermediate signal intensity and marked hypointensity (not shown).

the mucopolysaccharidoses.[15] Marked thickening of the skull base with narrowing of the foramina and fissures is a prominent feature of the craniotubular dysplasias and osteopetrosis (Fig. 32–6).

NEOPLASTIC DISEASES

A number of tumors have the potential to involve the skull base, arising from the osteocartilaginous structures primarily or invading the base of skull secondarily from above or below. Aggressive skull base operative techniques require the radiologist to indicate precisely the extent of tumor and frequently to predict histology. Accurate identification of the site of origin is essential for predicting tumor histology. Once the tumor is accurately localized, a limited differential diagnosis is usually possible. Either CT or MRI can ade-

quately perform this function if the lesion is large; however, smaller lesions are more easily visualized with MRI. The second step in predicting tumor histology involves an analysis of tissue characteristics. MRI is superior to CT for soft tissue assessment. CT, on the other hand, is superior in assessing for bone changes and detecting calcification, an important factor in evaluating some skull base lesions and bony dysplasias. Finally, defining the extent of tumor in reference to the neurovascular structures traversing the skull base is crucial. The multiplanar imaging capabilities of MRI are of great advantage in assessing these relationships. Therefore, it is obvious that CT and MRI are complementary and that both techniques may be required for complete assessment, particularly with complex or unusual lesions. This section discusses the most common neoplastic lesions involving the anterior and central skull base. Tumors that primarily involve the posterolateral skull base are discussed in the section on the temporal bone.

MENINGIOMA

Meningiomas are the most common benign intracranial neoplasm, accounting for approximately 15% of all intracranial tumors.[23] They originate from meningothelial cells found in the arachnoid granulations. The sphenoid wing, cavernous sinus region, planum sphenoidale, and olfactory groove are common sites of anterior and central skull base involvement. Therefore, unlike most of the skull base tumors, meningioma may be in the differential diagnosis of a skull base mass, independent of location. Because of the relatively slow growth of this tumor, the symptoms tend to be more insidious in onset. Patients may present with headache, visual disturbance, anosmia, or other cranial nerve palsies. Symptoms may be minimal or entirely absent, despite the presence of obvious mass effect on imaging studies. However, skull base meningiomas tend to manifest themselves sooner than convexity lesions of similar size owing to compression of the adjacent brain stem and cranial nerves.

The most common cranial base location for a meningioma is the sphenoid ridge. Meningiomas of the sphenoid ridge can be subclassified into medial, middle, and lateral types.[24] The lateral (pterional) meningioma is frequently a hyperostosing en plaque lesion with considerable bone invasion and extension through the anterior fossa floor into the orbit. Reactive bone changes are best demonstrated with high-resolution CT but are also visible with MRI, particularly when there is osseous invasion. Transcranial foraminal extension through the foramen ovale can occur with tumors originating from the greater sphenoid wing or cavernous sinus dura (Fig. 32–7), producing foraminal

enlargement and remodeling that simulate a schwannoma; however, more destructive changes can also be seen. Meningiomas have also been reported to arise within the paranasal sinuses and within the sheaths of cranial nerves.[25] Therefore, meningioma should be kept in the differential diagnosis of transcranial anterior and central skull base mass lesions.

The imaging hallmark of the meningioma is a dura-based, well-circumscribed mass displacing the brain and adjacent structures. The majority of tumors are isointense or mildly hypointense relative to brain on T1-weighted images and isointense or mildly hyperintense with T2 weighting, depending on the histologic composition.[26] Focal or diffuse signal loss may also be observed on T2-weighted sequences secondary to susceptibility effects from intratumoral calcification. As a result, small tumors can be more difficult to detect on nonenhanced studies. Meningiomas lack a blood-brain barrier and thus typically enhance intensely and homogeneously after contrast medium administration. Psammomatous, nodular, or ring-like calcifications may be present in these tumors and appear as areas of hypointensity or signal void on T2-weighted images that fail to enhance. Occasionally, intratumoral or peritumoral cysts are seen (Fig. 32–8). Adjacent dural thickening and enhancement are common and may represent dural hypervascularity, expansion of the extracellular spaces, or extension of tumor. The "dural tail" sign has been reported to occur in 52% to 60% of meningiomas with a specificity of 92% to 100%.[27, 28] This sign can also rarely be seen with schwannomas and pituitary adenomas[29, 30] (see also Chapter 17).

ESTHESIONEUROBLASTOMA

Esthesioneuroblastoma, otherwise known as olfactory neuroblastoma, is an uncommon slow-growing ma-

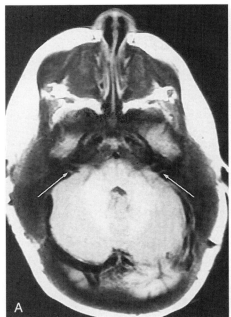
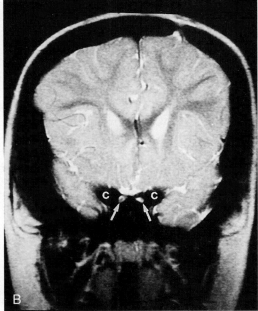

FIGURE 32–6. Osteopetrosis. *A,* Axial T1-weighted image at the level of the skull base shows marked thickening and hypointensity of the bony structures. Other than the small internal auditory canals *(arrows),* no landmarks are visible within the temporal bones. *B,* Coronal T2-weighted FSE image through the anterior clinoid processes shows small optic canals with atrophic appearing optic nerves *(arrows).* Magnetic susceptibility artifact related to the dense bone of the anterior clinoid processes (C) is present.

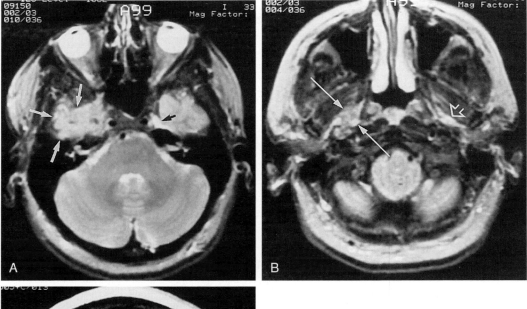

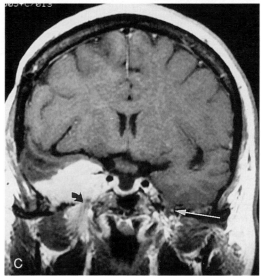

FIGURE 32–7. Meningioma with transcranial extension. *A,* Axial T2-weighted image. An isointense mass *(white arrows)* occupies the right middle cranial fossa with cavernous sinus involvement. Meckel's cave is normal on the left *(black arrow)* but invaded by tumor on the right. *B,* More inferiorly, the parapharyngeal space on the right contains a soft tissue mass *(solid arrows).* The parapharyngeal space fat on the left is normal *(open arrow). C,* Enhanced coronal image reveals transcranial extension of tumor through an enlarged foramen ovale *(black arrow)* into the parapharyngeal space. The foramen ovale on the left is normal *(white arrow).*

lignant neoplasm originating from the olfactory neuroepithelium of the upper nasal cavity, usually in the vicinity of the cribriform plate. This tumor can occur in any age group, but it has a predilection to occur in the second and sixth decades of life.[31] Clinical symptoms may include nasal obstruction, episodic epistaxis, hyposmia or anosmia, headaches, and visual disturbance. Histologically, these neoplasms demonstrate clusters of small round to ovoid cells, grouped by vascular septa, on a neurofibrillary background.[32] Small cell sarcoma or carcinoma, or lymphoma, may be difficult to exclude on a small or otherwise inadequate biopsy specimen. Esthesioneuroblastomas tend to grow slowly with submucosal extension and eventual invasion of the adjacent sinuses, orbits, intracranial cavity, and brain. Cerebrospinal fluid spread and remote metastases are seen in advanced cases.

The MRI signal characteristics of esthesioneuroblastoma are similar to those of other sinonasal neoplasms (Fig. 32–9). These masses tend to be relatively isoin-

tense relative to muscle and mucosa on T1-weighted images and hyperintense relative to muscle on T2-weighted images.[31] These tumors, like other sinonasal malignancies, are generally hypointense relative to mucosa on long-TR, long-TE images. Olfactory neuroblastomas reveal moderate, heterogeneous, or homogeneous enhancement after contrast medium administration.[31, 33] The degree of enhancement is less than that of mucosa, outlining the boundaries of the mass. Thus, when the tumor is small and confined to the high nasal cavity, the lesion is defined by the extent of nasal mucosal involvement. Although contrast-enhanced MRI and CT are probably equivalent for staging the sinonasal portion of the tumor, T2-weighted sequences are superior for differentiating sinonasal secretions from tumor.[34] MRI is also superior to CT for defining any intracranial extension because these tumors may extend through the cribriform plate without frank bone destruction. Inferior frontal lobe white matter edema is highly suggestive of brain invasion.

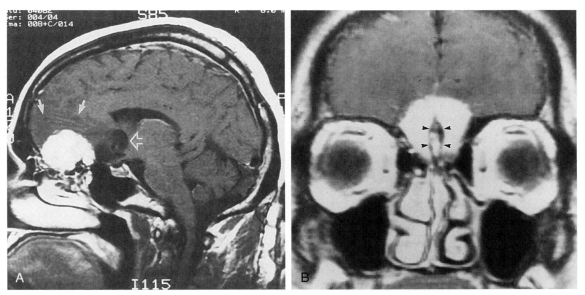

FIGURE 32–8. Meningioma of the anterior cranial fossa. *A,* Sagittal T1-weighted gadolinium-enhanced MR image shows an intensely enhancing mass arising from the cribriform plate with edema of the adjacent brain *(solid arrows).* Posterior to the mass there is nonenhancing cystic mass *(open arrow)* representing an acquired arachnoid cyst associated with the meningioma. *B,* Coronal gadolinium-enhanced image shows extension of the tumor into the depths of the anterior cranial fossa along the cribriform plate with preservation of the crista galli *(arrowheads).*

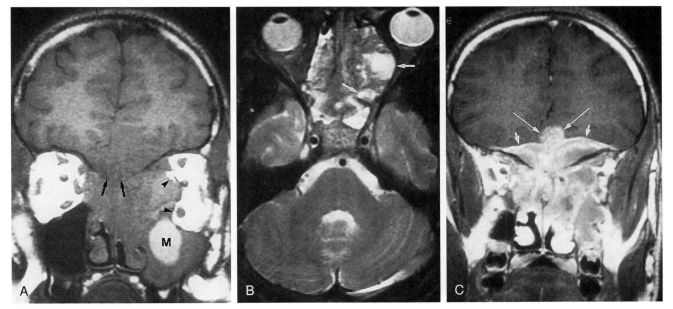

FIGURE 32–9. Esthesioneuroblastoma with intracranial extension. *A,* Coronal T1-weighted MR image. A large mass involves the ethmoidal sinuses and upper nasal cavity. The cribriform plate and fovea ethmoidalis are poorly seen *(arrows),* and the inferior frontal lobe gyri are not visible. There is extension into the left orbit with displacement of the medial rectus; however, the mass is contained by the periorbita *(arrowheads).* High signal intensity within the maxillary sinus (M) indicates inspissated secretions secondary to chronic obstruction. *B,* Axial T2-weighted image shows the tumor predominantly isointense relative to the pons with areas of hyperintensity *(arrows)* that could represent cyst formation, hemorrhage, or air cell obstruction. High signal intensity is present in both sphenoidal sinuses. *C,* Coronal T1-weighted contrast-enhanced image posterior to *A* confirms tumor extension into the anterior cranial fossa. Centrally, the tumor has penetrated the dura *(long arrows),* whereas more laterally the mass is contained by the dura *(short arrows).*

The differential diagnosis of a sinonasal mass with anterior skull base involvement in the pediatric age group includes lymphoma, rhabdomyosarcoma, and carcinoma. Squamous cell carcinoma, lymphoma, and metastatic disease are the primary considerations in the adult population. Esthesioneuroblastoma has also been reported to induce hyperostosis of adjacent bone, mimicking meningioma[35] (see also Fig. 33–10).

CHORDOMA

Chordomas are slow-growing, locally aggressive tumors of notochord origin that occur in virtually all age groups with a peak incidence between 20 and 50 years of age. Approximately 35% of chordomas arise in the spheno-occipital region.[36] Rare cases have been reported in the nasopharynx, paranasal sinuses, and intracranial dura.[37] Symptoms are secondary to local mass effect and bone destruction and include headache, diplopia (cranial nerve VI), facial pain and numbness (cranial nerve V), visual disturbance, dizziness, and ataxia. Although these tumors are histologically benign, metastases have been reported. Because of the degree of regional invasion usually seen at the time of presentation, prognosis is generally guarded.

Skull base chordomas usually arise in the midline, near the spheno-occipital synchondrosis (Fig. 32–10).

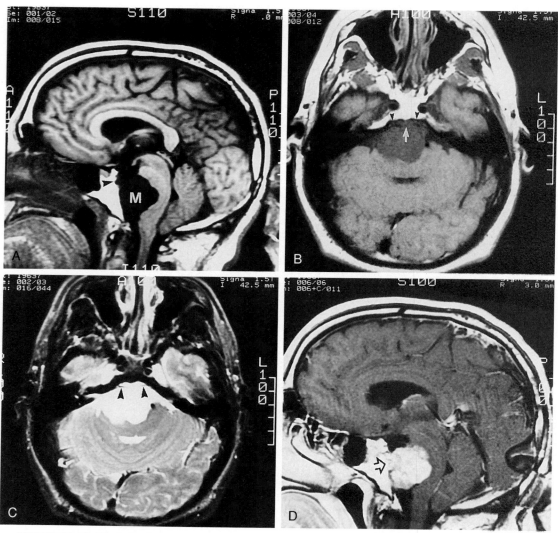

FIGURE 32–10. Clival chordoma. *A,* Sagittal T1-weighted inversion recovery image reveals a large hypointense mass (M) posterior to the clivus with marked brain stem compression. There is a small area of clival irregularity *(arrowhead). B,* Axial T1-weighted image. The mass is higher in signal intensity than cerebrospinal fluid but hypointense relative to the brain. There is a defect of the dura *(arrow)* along the clivus with extension of tumor between bone and dura *(arrowheads). C,* Marked hyperintensity is noted on the axial T2-weighted image. The tumor displays marked hyperintensity, and the dura is displaced away from the clivus *(arrowheads). D,* Contrast-enhanced sagittal image shows marked enhancement of the mass that is arising from a pedicle *(arrow)* along the posterior clivus. The manner of dural displacement suggests dural or cortical origin of this large exophytic chordoma.

Pathologically, chordomas contain nests of large mucin-containing cells referred to as physaliferous cells, surrounded by a myxoid matrix. Areas of recent or remote hemorrhage and areas of necrosis are common.[37] Intratumoral calcification is less common compared with chondroid tumors. Larger tumors frequently encase the internal carotid arteries, but luminal compromise is rare. There has been an ongoing debate regarding a variant of chordoma termed *chondroid chordoma*. This variant, which contains cartilaginous foci intermixed within the tumor matrix, was believed to actually be a myxoid chondrosarcoma by some authors.[38] More recently, immunohistochemical analysis has shown that these lesions are a true variant of chordoma.[39] Although some believe that chondroid chordoma carries a better prognosis than conventional chordoma,[36] this has been refuted by others.[40]

MRI features of chordomas reflect the myxoid and mucinous matrix found in these masses. The appearance ranges from isointensity to marked hypointensity on T1-weighted images and moderate to marked hyperintensity with T2 weighting[41] (see Fig. 32–10). The internal architecture of chordomas is frequently heterogeneous. Internal septa can be observed on both T1- and T2-weighted images. Foci of hyperintensity are not uncommon on T1-weighted images, representing areas of hemorrhage or proteinaceous content within the tumor. Areas of hypointensity on T2-weighted images may also reflect blood degradation products, calcification, or bone fragments. Most chordomas show heterogeneous, moderate to marked enhancement after gadolinium injection. Enhancement features are much more easily appreciated by MRI, compared with CT. Most authors report no significant difference in T2 relaxation times or enhancement features between conventional and chondroid chordomas.[41, 42] Although MRI should be the primary imaging modality for chordoma, CT is a useful adjunct for depicting bone erosion and destruction and intratumoral calcification. Because intratumoral calcifications are less frequent in chordoma compared with chondrosarcoma, CT may be helpful in distinguishing between these two tumors.[37]

CHONDROSARCOMA AND CHONDROMA

Chondrosarcomas of the head and neck are slow-growing, malignant primary bone neoplasms that account for 5% to 12% of all reported chondrosarcomas.[43–45] These tumors may originate from cartilage, endochondral bone, or mesenchymal tissue associated with the cranial base and meninges. The most common sites of skull base involvement are the petro-occipital synchondrosis (petroclival junction), the sphenoethmoid junction, and the sphenoethmoid-vomer junction.[46] Although central skull base chondrosarcomas tend to be off midline at the synchondroses, they can arise in the midline. Chondrosarcoma arising from the skull base dura has also been reported.[47]

Conventional chondrosarcoma is the most common form involving the skull base and is pathologically graded from 1 through 4. Calcification, myxoid change, and even ossification may be present in these tumors. Myxoid chondrosarcoma may be difficult to differentiate pathologically from the chondroid type of chordoma.[48] Mesenchymal and dedifferentiated chondrosarcomas are less common, are more aggressive, and have a poorer prognosis.[48]

As with the chordoma, optimal imaging of skull base chondrosarcoma requires the use of MRI and CT. CT is superior in demonstrating the characteristic bone destruction, present in almost all cases, and in showing tumoral calcification, which is reported to be present in up to 60% of tumors.[49] It may be difficult in some cases to differentiate between bone fragments related to destructive changes and tumoral calcification. Prominent enhancement is usually seen in the soft tissue portion of the tumor. MRI is superior to CT in depicting the soft tissue component of these lesions. The ease of multiplanar imaging with MRI enables more accurate assessment of the relationship of the tumor to critical neural and vascular structures. MR angiography can noninvasively evaluate the internal carotid artery for tumoral constriction and gives a unique 3D assessment, possibly obviating the need for catheter angiography.

Chondrosarcomas are generally low to intermediate in signal intensity on T1-weighted images (Fig. 32–11). Most tumors show marked hyperintensity on T2-weighted images.[50] Some heterogeneity may be present, depending on the degree of calcification and bone destruction (Fig. 32–12). Intratumoral hemorrhage can occur, but it is less common compared with chordomas. Enhancement after contrast medium administration, although prominent, is usually in a heterogeneous pattern.[50] Fat suppression techniques can be helpful in defining tumor margins when there is extension into the parapharyngeal space. As mentioned earlier, chordoma and chondrosarcoma can appear similar with both MRI and CT. The location of the mass is probably the best differentiating feature because chordomas usually arise from the clivus in the midline and chondrosarcomas usually arise more laterally from the petroclival fissure.

Chondroma of the skull base is much less common than chondrosarcoma. It may be difficult to differentiate chondroma from low-grade chondrosarcoma both radiographically and pathologically. In my limited experience, chondromas contain more calcification and are therefore more heterogeneous in appearance with MRI (Fig. 32–13). Enhancement features may be similar between the two tumors and are better depicted with MRI compared with CT, owing to intratumoral calcification. Treatment is similar for both lesions.

PITUITARY ADENOMA AND CRANIOPHARYNGIOMA

Pituitary adenoma is a common lesion affecting the central skull base, representing more than half of all sellar and parasellar masses.[51] These benign tumors arise from the anterior pituitary lobe. Microadenomas are usually detected as a result of endocrine dysfunc-

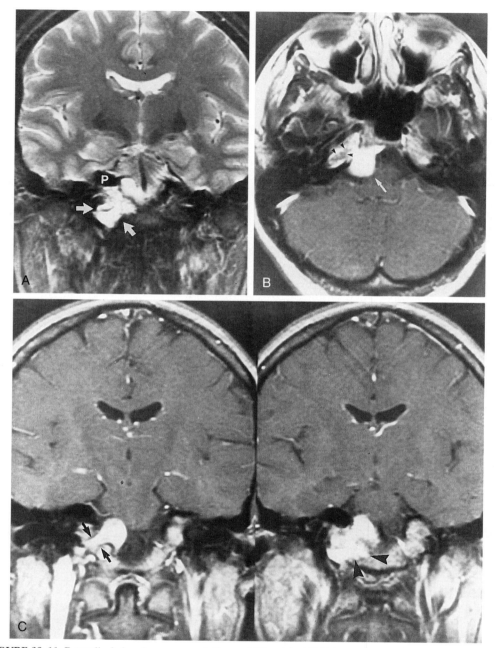

FIGURE 32–11. Petroclival chondrosarcoma. *A*, Coronal T2-weighted MR image shows replacement of the low-signal-intensity bone marrow of the clivus on the right by a hyperintense mass *(arrows)*. The petrous apex (P) above the tumor is aerated. *B*, Axial gadolinium-enhanced image reveals intense enhancement of the tumor with indentation of the ventral medulla *(arrow)*. The segment of tumor extending along the internal carotid artery anteriorly enhances less homogeneously *(arrowheads)*. *C*, Contiguous contrast-enhanced coronal images through the tumor show involvement of the hypoglossal canal *(arrows)* and a narrow zone of transition with the clival bone marrow *(arrowheads)*.

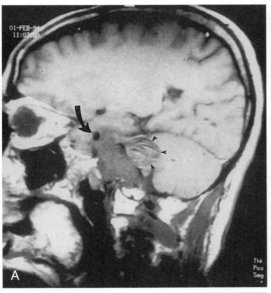

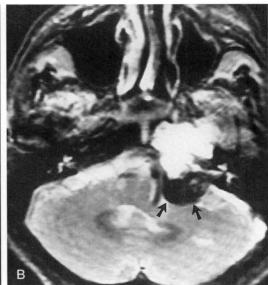

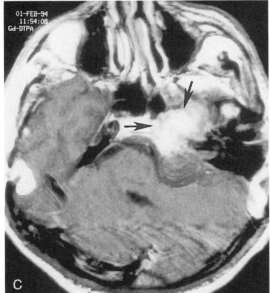

FIGURE 32–12. Large chondrosarcoma. *A,* T1-weighted parasagittal image reveals a large hypointense skull base mass, displacing the internal carotid artery *(arrow)*. A second component compressing the cerebellum is heterogeneous in signal intensity *(arrowheads)*. *B,* Axial T2-weighted image. The mass is predominantly hyperintense except for the markedly hypointense posterior aspect *(arrows)*. *C,* Axial contrast-enhanced image shows intense enhancement anteriorly *(arrows)* and absent enhancement posteriorly. A CT scan of the skull base (not shown) revealed acute hemorrhage in the posterior aspect of the tumor, accounting for the signal intensity changes of deoxyhemoglobin and intracellular methemoglobin on the MR images and the clinical presentation of acute deficits involving cranial nerves V and VIII.

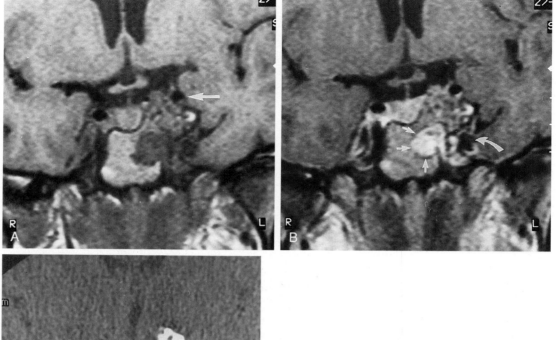

FIGURE 32–13. Chondroma. *A,* Coronal T1-weighted image of the sella shows a heterogeneous mass involving the sphenoid body and the left cavernous sinus with displacement of the cavernous carotid artery *(arrow). B,* Gadolinium-enhanced coronal image at the same level shows intense enhancement within the sphenoid *(straight arrows)* and mild, heterogeneous enhancement in the cavernous sinus. Areas of hypointensity, indicating calcification, are now more easily seen *(curved arrow). C,* Coronal nonenhanced CT scan shows extensive calcification. The extent of calcification is clearly underestimated by the T1-weighted sequences. The cartilaginous cap appeared as a signal void on T2-weighted images (not shown).

tion, whereas macroadenomas (tumors greater than 1 cm) are diagnosed when local mass effect from the tumor compromises adjacent structures. Pituitary macroadenomas are usually isointense on T1-weighted images and mild or moderately hyperintense relative to gray matter on T2-weighted images. Macroadenomas typically show strong homogeneous enhancement; however, larger adenomas can undergo internal hemorrhage and cystic degeneration, resulting in some heterogeneity on postcontrast images.

Although suprasellar extension is the earliest and most frequent direction of macroadenoma spread, involvement of the cavernous sinuses and bone erosion and destruction of the sellar floor are also common. Cavernous sinus invasion can be confidently seen with MRI only when there is actual encasement of the internal carotid artery or invasion of the temporal lobe.[52] Early invasion of the cavernous sinus is difficult to

detect by MRI owing to the lack of an easily identifiable landmark for the medial wall of the cavernous sinus. Gadolinium administration is not particularly helpful because of the similar degree of enhancement of the tumor and the cavernous sinus. Thus, the sensitivity for diagnosing cavernous sinus invasion with MRI, reported to be 55% in the pre-MRI contrast era,[52] has probably not significantly changed despite advances in imaging techniques and pulse sequences. Skull base invasion into the ethmoidal and sphenoidal sinuses and the clivus can be observed with large tumors. Rarely, this pattern of skull base involvement is present without suprasellar extension, making differentiation from primary sphenoidal sinus carcinoma, invasive nasopharyngeal carcinoma, or chordoma difficult (Fig. 32–14).

Craniopharyngiomas, in contrast, are more commonly seen in children, although a second, smaller peak occurs in middle-aged adults.[53] This benign lesion is usually centered in the suprasellar region, but frequently it involves the sella and, when large, may erode the central skull base. The MRI appearance of this tumor is more variable than that of the pituitary adenoma, and mixed, complex signal patterns are typical. Tumor calcification, present in 90% of cases, is best appreciated with CT. The majority of lesions have some cystic component that may be hypointense or hyperintense on T1-weighted images. Solid components of the tumor are hyperintense on T2-weighted images and enhance moderately (see also Chapter 18).

SCHWANNOMA

Schwannomas of the central skull base are rare, compared with more familiar acoustic schwannomas, which are subsequently discussed in the temporal bone section. Trigeminal schwannomas, the most common type encountered, usually arise from the region of the gasserian ganglion and less frequently from the preganglionic cisternal segment or postganglionic branches.[54] Patients typically present with numbness, paresthesias, and weakness involving the muscles of mastication. The majority do not have neurofibro-

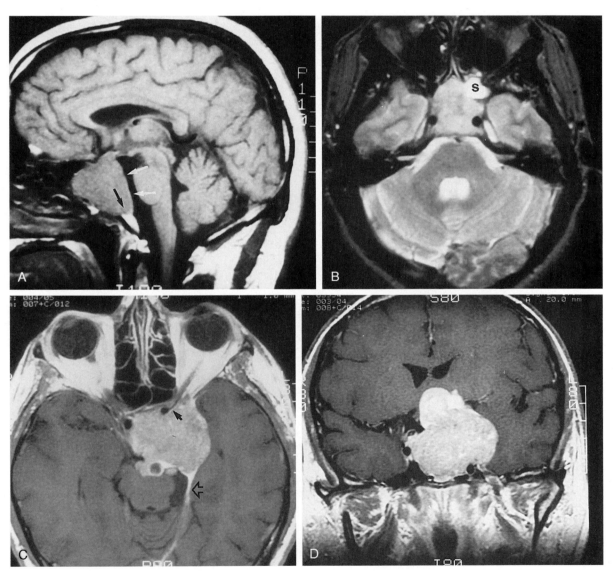

FIGURE 32–14. Invasive pituitary adenoma. *A,* T1-weighted midline sagittal image shows a large isointense mass occupying the entire sella and sphenoidal sinus with replacement of the normal marrow of the sphenoid body and invasion of the basiocciput *(black arrow)*. There is posterior expansion of the clival cortex *(white arrows)*. *B,* Axial T2-weighted image. The mass is mildly hyperintense. An obstructed lateral sphenoidal air cell (S) is noted on the left. The dural margins of the cavernous sinuses are straightened, but the internal carotid arteries do not appear encased. *C* and *D,* Contrast-enhanced axial *(C)* and coronal *(D)* images in another patient show marked homogeneous enhancement with carotid artery encasement on the left at the origin of the ophthalmic artery *(solid arrow)*. A "dural tail" is also observed *(open arrow, C)*. Although the dural tail sign is highly suggestive of meningioma, it has also been reported with pituitary adenomas and schwannomas.

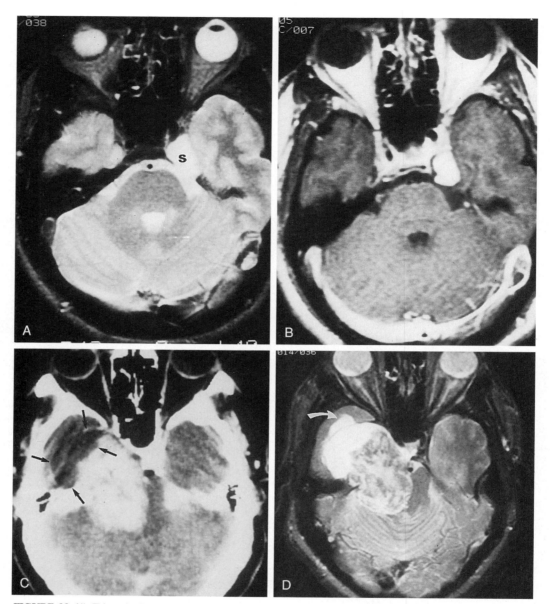

FIGURE 32–15. Trigeminal schwannoma. *A,* Axial T2-weighted image reveals a mass (S) centered at Meckel's cave. The signal intensity is similar to that of cerebrospinal fluid. *B,* Contrast-enhanced image at the same level shows intense homogeneous enhancement of the mass with extension into the prepontine cistern and mild displacement of the medial temporal lobe. *C,* Axial contrast-enhanced CT scan in a different patient shows a large extra-axial mass with erosion of the sphenoid body and petrous apex and marked compression of the brain stem. There is a cystic component in the middle cranial fossa *(arrows). D,* T2-weighted MR image shows mixed signal intensity within the tumor. The cystic component of the tumor is better delineated on the MRI study. There is also a small peritumoral arachnoid cyst *(arrow).*

matosis type 1. These tumors are slow growing and may be quite large at the time of diagnosis, with cranial neuropathy involving cranial nerves III through VIII. Primary schwannomas of cranial nerves III, IV, and VI are exceedingly unusual.[51]

Schwannomas are hypointense on T1-weighted images and hyperintense on long-TR, long-TE sequences (Fig. 32–15). Internal heterogeneity on T2-weighted images is common in the larger lesions as the result of internal degeneration and hemorrhage. Homogeneous or heterogeneous enhancement after contrast medium administration is a constant feature of all schwannomas. Bone erosion of the sphenoid and pe-

trous apex is common with larger lesions. Enlargement of the foramen ovale and foramen rotundum occurs when the tumor arises in the postganglionic segments of the trigeminal nerve (see also Chapter 19).

TEMPORAL BONE AND POSTEROLATERAL SKULL BASE ANATOMY

NORMAL ANATOMY

Detailed imaging of the temporal bone has historically fallen into the realm of high-resolution CT. For many disease processes, other than those affecting the internal auditory canal, CT remains the study of choice. More recently, high-resolution gradient-echo and FSE techniques and MR angiography have made MRI much more competitive regarding temporal bone imaging. This section reviews the pertinent anatomy of the petrous temporal bone and the jugular foramen, relative to skull base diseases, focusing on structures visible with MRI.

The MRI appearance of the petrous temporal bone is quite varied, as a result of variable pneumatization, and is frequently asymmetric. Dense bone and aerated spaces are similarly black on both T1- and T2-weighted sequences. Fatty marrow is easily recognized on T1-weighted images but may present problems with interpretation on non–fat-suppressed, gadolinium-enhanced T1-weighted and FSE sequences. On the other hand, the cerebrospinal fluid signal intensity within the internal auditory canal is a constant finding, lo-

cated on the posterior aspect of the petrous pyramid. The anteriorly located facial nerve and the more posterior vestibulocochlear nerve can be routinely identified on high-resolution T2-weighted FSE images (Fig. 32–16). The membranous labyrinth is also exquisitely demonstrated on axial and coronal FSE images, as a result of the hyperintensity of the endolymph and perilymph within these structures (see Fig. 32–16). Even greater resolution is afforded with surface coil imaging (Fig. 32–17). T1-weighted 3D gradient-echo imaging provides an additional technique for imaging the membranous labyrinth, allowing higher resolution and multiplanar reconstructions from a single acquisition at the expense of lower signal intensity from the labyrinth. In my experience, thin-section FSE using a routine head coil is most convenient and usually adequate.

The normal anatomic appearance of the jugular foramen with MRI has been described in detail.[55, 56]

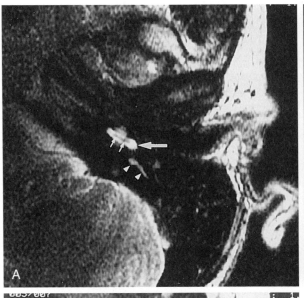

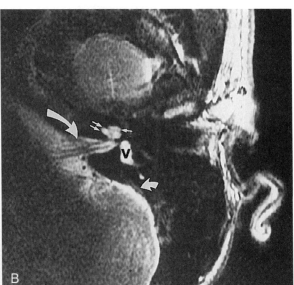

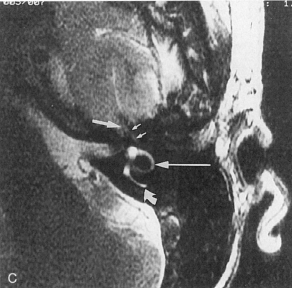

FIGURE 32–16. Temporal bone normal anatomy, axial plane. FSE images (TR/TE = 4000/120 effective) from inferior to superior. *A,* Image inferior to the internal auditory canal shows the basal turn of the cochlea *(large arrow)* and a portion of the posterior semicircular canal *(arrowheads).* The osseous spiral lamina is visible within the cochlea *(small arrows).* *B,* At the level of the internal auditory canal, two divisions of the vestibulocochlear nerve are visible within the canal. A vascular loop is present anteromedially *(long curved arrow).* The middle *(double arrows)* and apical *(single arrow)* turns of the cochlea are anteromedial to the vestibule (v). The endolymphatic sac *(short curved arrow)* is posterior to the posterior semicircular canal. *C,* Above the cochlea lies the geniculate ganglion *(large arrow)* and the tympanic segment of the facial nerve *(small arrows).* The lateral *(long arrow)* and posterior *(curved arrow)* semicircular canals are observed posteriorly.

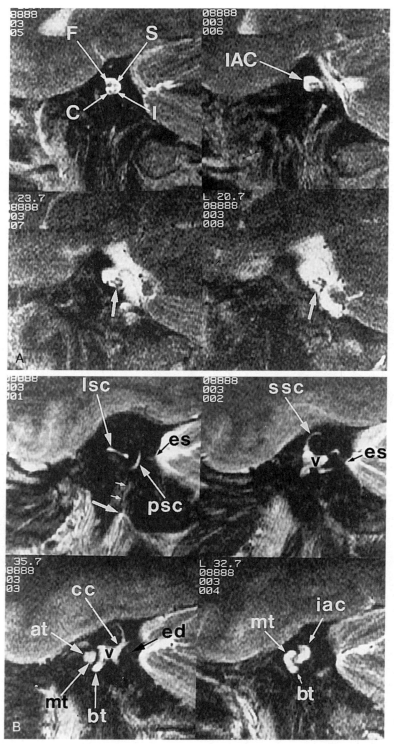

FIGURE 32–17. Temporal bone normal anatomy, sagittal plane. FSE images (TR/TE = 4000/120 effective) from medial to lateral. *A,* Set of four images of the internal auditory canal *(top row)* and cerebellopontine angle cistern *(bottom row)* reveals separation of the three main components of the vestibulocochlear nerve in the cistern and porus acusticus *(arrows)*. The facial (F), cochlear (C), superior vestibular (S), and inferior vestibular (I) nerves are clearly visualized in the internal auditory canal. The point of separation of the vestibulocochlear nerve in the cerebellopontine angle or internal auditory canal is variable. *B,* Set of four images through the membranous labyrinth from lateral *(top row)* to medial *(bottom row)*. Medially, the basal (bt) and middle (mt) turns of the cochlea are observed anterior to the internal auditory canal (iac). The endolymphatic duct (ed) is faintly visible at the level of the vestibule (v) and common crus (cc). Laterally *(top row)*, the endolymphatic sac (es) is posterior to the posterior (psc), lateral (lsc), and superior (ssc) semicircular canals. The mastoid segment of the facial nerve *(small arrows)* can be seen extending to the stylomastoid foramen *(large arrow)*.

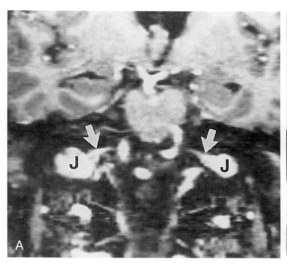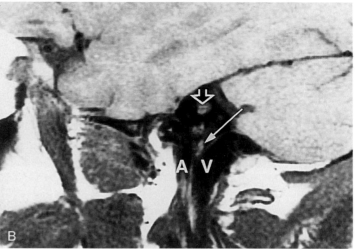

FIGURE 32–18. Anatomy of the jugular foramen. *A,* 3D T1-weighted gradient-echo coronal image demonstrates hyperintensity in the jugular bulbs (J) bilaterally from flowing blood. The inferior petrosal sinuses are visible medially *(arrows).* *B,* Sagittal T1-weighted image through the jugular foramen. The jugular vein (V) is located posterior to the internal carotid artery (A). The glossopharyngeal and vagus nerves are visible between the two structures *(solid arrow).* The internal auditory canal and vestibulocochlear nerve complex is visible superiorly *(open arrow).*

Briefly, this foramen is situated below and slightly posterior to the internal auditory canal. It is bounded anterolaterally by the petrous bone and posteromedially by the occipital bone (Fig. 32–18). The foramen is divided into the smaller pars nervosa anteromedially and the larger pars vascularis posterolaterally. The pars nervosa contains the glossopharyngeal nerve (cranial nerve IX), Jacobson's nerve (inferior tympanic branch of cranial nerve IX, sensory to the tympanic cavity), and the inferior petrosal sinus, which travels from the cavernous sinus along the petro-occipital (petroclival) fissure to the jugular vein. The pars vascularis contains the vagus nerve (cranial nerve X), the spinal accessory nerve (cranial nerve XI), Arnold's nerve (auricular branch of cranial nerve X, sensory to a portion of the external ear via the facial nerve), the jugular bulb, and small meningeal arterial branches from the external carotid system. On the endocranial aspect of the jugular foramen there is a dural septum that separates cranial nerve IX from cranial nerves X and XI. The bony carotid canal, containing the vertical segment of the petrous internal carotid artery, lies immediately anterior to the exocranial opening of the jugular foramen and is separated from the latter structure by the carotid spine. The genu of the petrous internal carotid artery, joining the vertical and horizontal segments, is located more superiorly, at the level of the hypotympanum.

VASCULAR VARIANTS

Several vascular variants found in the temporal bone and jugular foramen can simulate pathologic processes. These variants are often found in patients who are being evaluated for pulsatile tinnitus, but they may also be an incidental finding. The aberrant internal carotid artery is a rare developmental anomaly in which the internal carotid artery courses lateral to the vestibule, looping through the middle ear cavity, before joining the horizontal segment of the petrous internal carotid artery through a defect in the bony partition between the carotid canal and the middle ear cavity. The vascular retrotympanic mass produced by this anomaly simulates a glomus tumor on otoscopy.[57] The aberrant internal carotid artery has a characteristic appearance with CT and MR angiography (Fig. 32–19), thereby obviating the need for conventional angiography in establishing the diagnosis.

Jugular bulb variants can also present with pulsatile tinnitus and simulate paragangliomas, both on imaging studies and physical examination.[58] The high-riding jugular bulb (also called the jugular megabulb deformity) extends above the level of the external auditory canal, and the margins of the enlarged jugular bulb are smooth and normally corticated. The dehiscent jugular bulb occurs when the bony plate separating the enlarged jugular bulb from the middle ear cavity is absent, resulting in protrusion of the bulb into the middle ear cavity. A bluish retrotympanic mass is visible on otoscopy with a dehiscent jugular bulb. A jugular bulb diverticulum is a small extension of the jugular bulb superomedially, behind the internal auditory canal.[59] The jugular megabulb deformity and the jugular bulb diverticulum are best demonstrated and differentiated from other lesions with flow-sensitive gradient-echo techniques in the coronal plane (Fig. 32–20). CT is required to distinguish the dehiscent from the nondehiscent jugular bulb with imaging. It is important to recognize these arterial and venous vascular anomalies and alert the clinician to their presence to avoid biopsy and potential catastrophe.

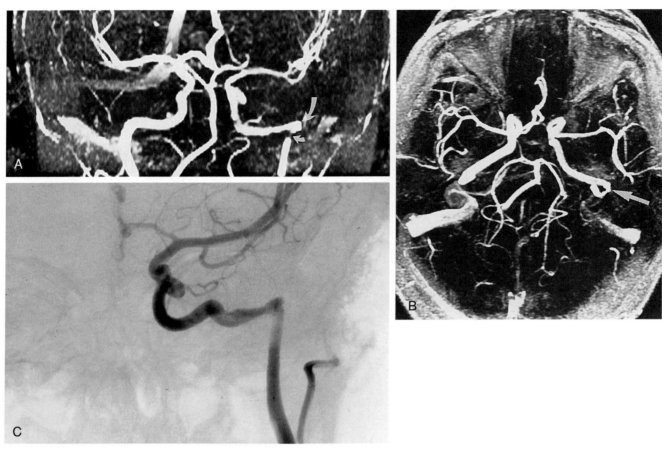

FIGURE 32–19. Aberrant internal carotid artery. *A*, 3D TOF MR angiogram, anteroposterior view, in a patient with pulsatile tinnitus shows a decrease in the caliber of the left internal carotid artery with lateral deviation at the junction of the vertical and horizontal intrapetrous segments *(large arrow)*. There is a focal high-grade stenosis just below the genu *(small arrow)*. *B*, Collapsed view MR angiogram again shows typical lateral displacement at the level of the middle ear *(arrow)*. *C*, Conventional contrast arteriogram in a different patient demonstrates the typical "figure 7" appearance of an aberrant internal carotid artery. (*A* and *B* courtesy of H. Ric Harnsberger, MD, Salt Lake City, UT.)

NEOPLASTIC DISEASE

Many of the neoplastic processes that affect the anterior and central skull base can also occur primarily in the temporal bone and posterolateral cranial base or involve this region by direct extension. Conversely, tumors common to the temporal bone may occasionally show direct invasion of the central skull base and adjacent bony structures. This section will highlight the more common tumors arising primarily within the posterolateral cranial base, including the lesions of the jugular foramen. Although epidermoidomas and cholesterol granulomas of the petrous apex are not true neoplasms, they are included in this section because their clinical presentation and radiographic appearance mimic neoplastic disease. Acquired cholesteatomas and other petrous temporal bone inflammatory processes are discussed in the section on inflammatory disease and infection (see also Chapter 19).

SCHWANNOMA

The schwannoma is the most common tumor involving the internal auditory canal and the second most common mass arising within the jugular foramen.[37] These benign lesions originate from Schwann cells and arise eccentrically from the parent nerve. Pathologically, they are encapsulated tumors containing both tightly compacted, cellular (Antoni's type A) and spongy, myxoid (Antoni's type B) elements.[60] The vascularity of schwannomas varies from minimal to moderate in degree. Temporal bone involvement can be seen with tumors arising from cranial nerves V through XII. This section discusses primarily those tumors arising from cranial nerves VII through X.

The MRI features of intracranial (cranial nerve) and skull base schwannomas are consistent, regardless of the nerve of origin. These tumors are sharply circumscribed masses with smooth borders. Smaller schwannomas are usually fairly homogeneous, whereas larger lesions tend to be more heterogeneous. They are hypointense (67%) or isointense (33%) on T1-weighted images.[61] Medium to large masses are mildly to moderately hyperintense on proton density– and T2-weighted images; however, smaller lesions can be isointense or only mildly hyperintense on T2-weighted sequences (Fig. 32–21). Tumor signal intensity is lower on T2-weighted sequences when FSE techniques are

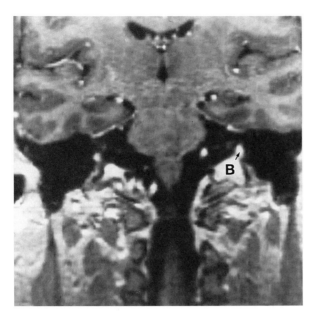

FIGURE 32–20. Jugular bulb diverticulum. Coronal T1-weighted gradient-echo image reveals a high-riding jugular bulb (B) with a diverticulum *(arrow)* projecting superiorly into the petrous temporal bone.

used. Intense enhancement after contrast agent administration is a constant feature of nearly all schwannomas. Homogeneous enhancement is present in two thirds of schwannomas, the remainder showing varying degrees of heterogeneity.[61] Larger tumors tend to show a greater degree of heterogeneity after contrast medium administration and may also contain areas of subacute or chronic hemorrhage (Fig. 32–22).

Acoustic schwannomas are the most common tumors involving the internal auditory canal, the vast majority arising from the superior or inferior vestibular nerves (giving rise to the term *vestibular schwannoma*). The salient clinical feature is progressive sensorineural hearing loss, although 15% of patients present with acute sensorineural hearing loss, probably secondary to intratumoral hemorrhage.[62] Other symptoms include tinnitus, vertigo, ataxia, and headaches. Vertigo, as the initial presenting symptom, in the absence of sensorineural hearing loss, is rare. The age at presentation is variable; however, most tumors present in the fifth to seventh decades of life. Cystic changes are observed in 10% to 15%, and 5% have an associated arachnoid cyst.[62] Meningioma of the cerebellopontine angle can mimic an acoustic schwannoma. A broad-based dural origin and dural "tail" strongly favor the diagnosis of meningioma,[27, 28] whereas extension of tumor into the internal auditory canal strongly supports the diagnosis of acoustic schwannoma.

The facial nerve (cranial nerve VII) is the third most common site of the posterolateral skull base schwannomas. Although the geniculate ganglion is the most frequent location, any of the intrapetrous facial nerve segments can be involved and involvement of multiple segments is common (Fig. 32–23). Tumors isolated to the internal auditory canal are rare. Facial nerve palsy is present in 40% to 50% of cases.[63] Lacrimation (via the superficial petrosal nerve) and taste may also be affected. Nevertheless, only 5% to 6% of facial nerve palsies are due to facial nerve schwannomas.[64, 65] Bell's palsy accounts for 50% to 80% of cases of peripheral facial nerve paralysis. Other causes include herpes zoster (Ramsay Hunt syndrome), trauma, otitis media with or without cholesteatoma, Lyme disease, and other tumors, including perineural metastasis to the facial nerve.

Schwannomas arising within the jugular foramen are

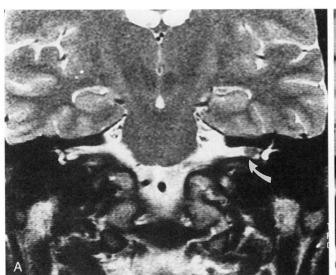

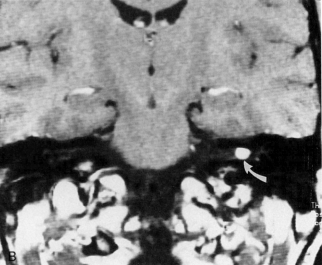

FIGURE 32–21. Intracanalicular acoustic schwannoma. *A,* Coronal T2-weighted FSE image shows a small well-circumscribed lesion *(arrow)* within the left internal auditory canal that is isointense relative to white matter. A small amount of cerebrospinal fluid is visible lateral to the mass within the fundus of the internal auditory canal. The right internal auditory canal is normal. *B,* Intense enhancement of the schwannoma *(arrow)* is noted after gadolinium administration.

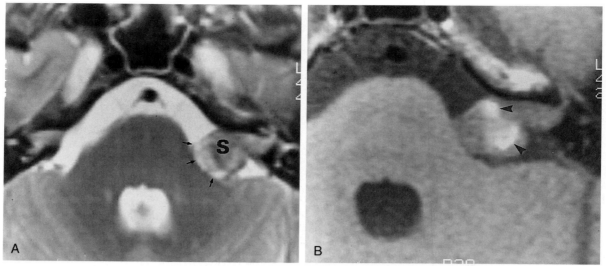

FIGURE 32–22. Acoustic schwannoma, moderate sized. *A,* Axial T2-weighted FSE image shows a moderate-sized acoustic schwannoma (S) that completely fills the internal auditory canal and extends into the cerebello-pontine angle cistern. The signal intensity of the cisternal component is heterogeneous *(arrows). B,* Axial T1-weighted nonenhanced image at the same level reveals areas of hyperintensity *(arrowheads),* consistent with subacute hemorrhage. FSE imaging is less sensitive than standard SE imaging to the magnetic susceptibility effects of breakdown products of blood.

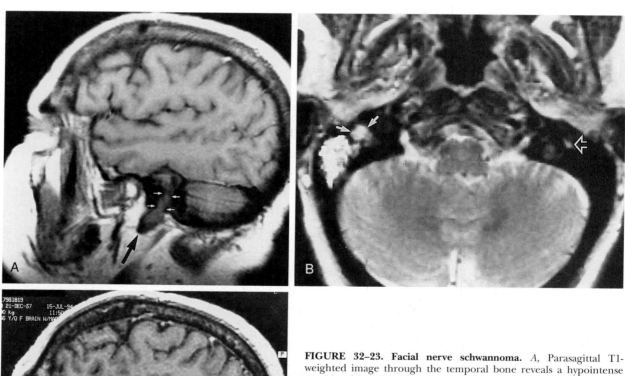

FIGURE 32–23. Facial nerve schwannoma. *A,* Parasagittal T1-weighted image through the temporal bone reveals a hypointense mass involving the descending facial nerve canal and stylomastoid foramen *(white arrows)* with extension into the parotid gland. The inferior pole of the mass within the parotid gland is even lower in signal intensity *(black arrow). B,* Axial T2-weighted image demonstrates hyperintensity within the mass in the descending facial nerve canal *(solid arrows)* and fluid in the right mastoid. The normal left facial nerve is visible for comparison *(open arrow). C,* Oblique sagittal T1-weighted 3D gradient-echo image after contrast medium administration shows abnormal enhancement extending from the geniculate ganglion *(white arrow)* to the stylomastoid foramen *(black arrow).* The nonenhancing cystic component at the inferior pole of the schwannoma *(open arrow)* within the parotid gland is clearly visible.

relatively infrequent lesions, most commonly arising from the vagus nerve (cranial nerve X).[66] These tumors may be foraminal, cisternal, or predominantly extracranial with only a small component in the jugular foramen (Fig. 32–24). Symptoms reflect cranial neuropathy involving cranial nerves IX through XI. When the mass is cisternal, brain stem compression or vestibulocochlear nerve dysfunction may be the presenting symptom complex.[59] Postcontrast sagittal and coronal sequences can be particularly helpful in confirming the location and demonstrating the extent of the mass. Unlike paragangliomas, jugular foramen schwannomas rarely extend into the middle ear. If the mass is small (<2 to 2.5 cm), it may be difficult to distinguish a schwannoma from a paraganglioma with MRI. High-resolution, bone-detail CT of the jugular foramen can be helpful in this instance. The cortex of the foramen is usually scalloped but intact with a schwannoma and is more likely to be irregular or indistinct and eroded with a paraganglioma.[59] Neurofibromas arising within

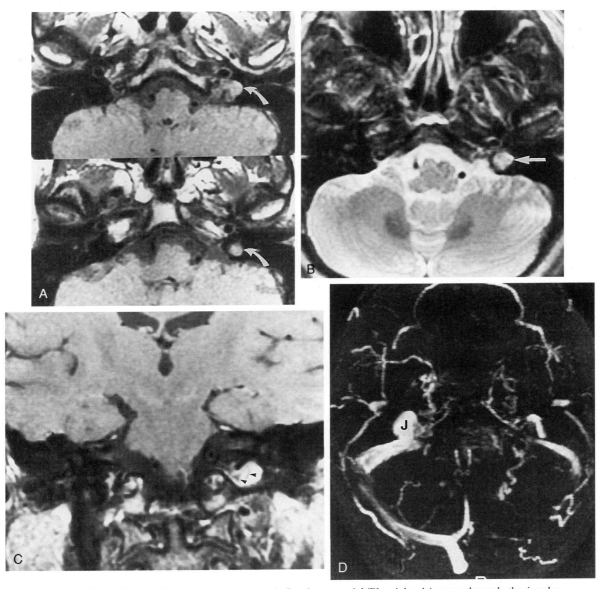

FIGURE 32–24. Jugular foramen schwannoma. *A,* Contiguous axial T1-weighted images through the jugular bulb reveal mixed signal intensity *(arrows)* that could represent slow flow or a soft tissue mass. *B,* Axial T2-weighted image also shows mixed signal intensity with the jugular bulb *(arrow). C,* Gadolinium-enhanced coronal image reveals intense enhancement of the mildly enlarged left jugular bulb. Triangular and curvilinear areas *(arrowheads)* of lower signal intensity still raise the question of flow artifact in the jugular bulb. *D,* 2D TOF MR venogram demonstrates flow in the large right jugular foramen (J) but absent flow on the left. A vagal schwannoma was found at surgery. MR angiography can be useful in difficult cases when there is a question of complex flow in an enlarged jugular bulb versus a soft tissue mass.

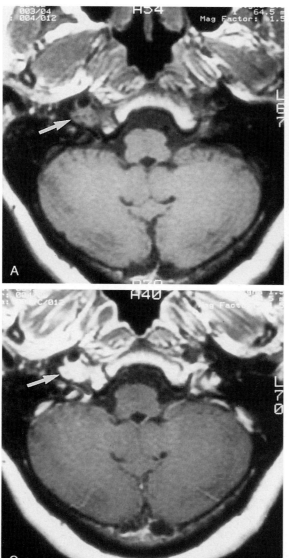

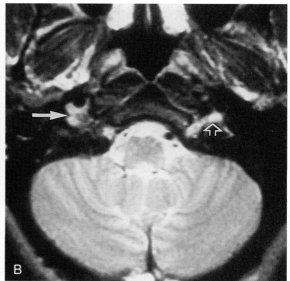

FIGURE 32–25. Small jugular foramen paraganglioma (glomus jugulare). *A,* Axial T1-weighted image at the level of the jugular foramen shows an isointense mass within the left jugular foramen *(arrow)* containing multiple small flow voids. The lesion partially encircles the internal carotid artery. *B,* T2-weighted image at the same level shows areas of hypointensity and hyperintensity within the mass *(solid arrow).* High signal intensity on the left side represents slow flow within the jugular bulb *(open arrow). C,* Contrast-enhanced MR image demonstrates intense homogeneous enhancement of the small jugular foramen paraganglioma *(arrow).*

the jugular foramen are not distinguishable from schwannomas with CT or MRI.

PARAGANGLIOMA

Paragangliomas, or glomus tumors, are benign neoplasms that arise from neural crest origin chemoreceptor cells associated with the autonomic nervous system of the head and neck. These cells, known as paraganglia or glomus bodies, are associated with the jugular bulb adventitia and branches of the vagus and glossopharyngeal nerves that innervate the middle ear.[59, 62] Jugular paragangliomas (glomus jugulare tumors) originate from the jugular foramen. They are designated glomus jugulotympanicum tumors if they also extend into the middle ear cavity. Tympanicum paragangliomas arise in the middle ear cavity along the cochlear promontory. Vagal paragangliomas arise from

the nodose ganglion of the vagus nerve just below the level of the jugular foramen and usually extend inferiorly along the carotid sheath. Glomus tumors most commonly occur in middle-aged women. Metastases are rare, and multicentricity is present in approximately 10% of cases.[59, 62, 67] The following discussion highlights features and characteristics of glomus jugulare tumors.

Jugular paragangliomas typically present with pulse-synchronous tinnitus and lower cranial neuropathy.[57] Cranial nerves IX through XI are most commonly involved; however, cranial nerves VII, VIII, and XII may also be affected, depending on the size and direction of invasion. A vascular retrotympanic mass is visible if the middle ear cavity has been invaded. There is some debate among experts on preferred initial imaging modality in the patient with a possible glomus jugulare tumor. I prefer MRI rather than CT for several reasons: 1) the ease of imaging the jugular foramen in multiple planes, 2) superior assessment of intratumoral vascularity, 3) superior ability to assess relationships with the brain stem and cerebellum when there is posterior fossa invasion, and 4) the availability of MR angiography for characterizing arterial and venous structures should there be questions of vascular patency, the presence of a vascular variant, or the presence of a dural arteriovenous fistula.

Paragangliomas are usually isointense on T1-weighted images and mild to moderately hyperintense relative to cerebellar white matter on T2-weighted images. Small flow voids are typically seen in larger lesions, producing a "salt-and-pepper" appearance, but they may be absent in smaller tumors.[68] After gadolinium administration, there is intense enhancement, with or without visible vascular flow voids. The margins of larger tumors are irregular and infiltrating, in contrast to the smoother margins of schwannomas and meningiomas (Fig. 32–25). However, smaller paragangliomas of the jugular foramen can be difficult to distinguish from schwannomas and meningiomas (Fig. 32–26).

Radiation therapy is being used with increasing frequency at many institutions as an alternative to surgical resection in the treatment of paragangliomas. Selective external carotid angiography may be necessary in selected instances when the diagnosis is in question. Mild reduction in size, reduction in T2-weighted signal intensity, decreased enhancement, and decreased flow voids have been reported after primary radiation treatment of glomus tumors. These MRI findings were observed in 50% to 60% of cases.[69]

CONGENITAL CHOLESTEATOMA AND CHOLESTEROL GRANULOMA

Despite their similar names, congenital cholesteatoma and cholesterol granuloma are unrelated lesions that can occur both in the petrous apex and in the mastoid and middle ear and are thus discussed together. The cholesterol granuloma (also known as cholesterol cyst, giant cholesterol cyst, or chocolate cyst) is a cyst of inflammatory origin and is the most common primary lesion encountered in the petrous apex. It arises when the air cells of the pneumatized petrous apex become chronically obstructed. Repeated hemorrhage occurs from the vascular granulation tissue that lines the obstructed air spaces. These cysts have a fibrous capsule composed of the granulation tissue and yield a yellowish brown fluid containing blood breakdown products and cholesterol crystals. Multinucleate giant cells and hemosiderin-laden macrophages are present within the solid component of the lesion.

Small cholesterol granulomas are often incidental findings on MR studies. Larger lesions can produce retro-orbital pain secondary to cranial nerve V_2 irritation or diplopia due to cranial nerve VI compression in Dorello's canal. Conductive and sensorineural hearing loss occurs as a result of middle ear and inner ear or internal auditory canal involvement, respectively.[70] These cysts demonstrate high signal intensity on T1-weighted images (Fig. 32–27). T2-weighted images show areas of both hyperintensity and marked hypointensity owing to the presence of old blood breakdown products and hemosiderin deposition.[71] The margins

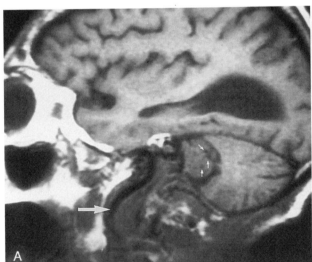

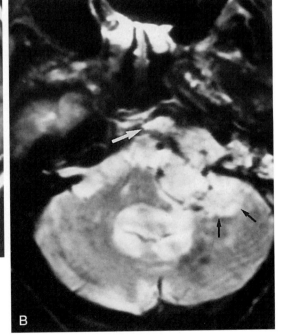

FIGURE 32–26. Paraganglioma with posterior fossa extension. *A,* T1-weighted parasagittal image reveals a large hypointense mass extending from the jugular foramen into both the posterior fossa and the nasopharyngeal carotid space with displacement of the internal carotid artery *(large arrow).* Multiple flow voids are present in the posterior fossa component *(small arrows). B,* T2-weighted axial image. There is mass effect on the brain stem and invasion of the clivus medially *(white arrow).* Old postoperative changes are present in the cerebellum *(black arrows),* and fluid or inflammatory debris is noted in the middle ear and mastoid. Local bone invasion helps distinguish this tumor from a schwannoma.

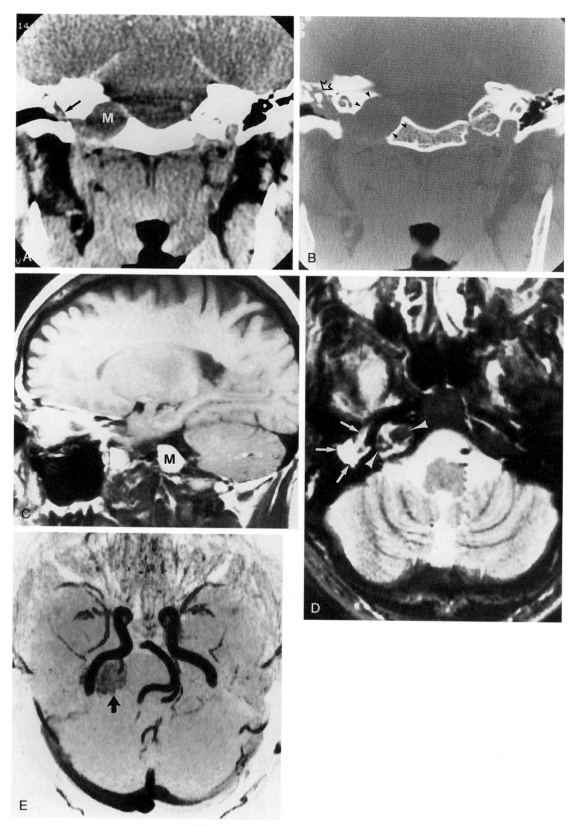

FIGURE 32–27 *See legend on opposite page*

may be smooth or irregular, depending on the extent of the cyst. Although rare, aneurysms of the horizontal segment of the petrous internal carotid artery can show similar signal characteristics if there is partial thrombosis of the lumen. MR angiography, using phase-contrast or 2D TOF technique, reveals high signal intensity within the lumen of the internal carotid artery aneurysm, differentiating it from a cholesterol cyst or tumor.

The congenital cholesteatoma, or primary epidermoid cyst, develops as a result of embryonic epithelial inclusion. These lesions can occur essentially anywhere in the body. There are five general sites of occurrence within the temporal bone: the petrous apex, the mastoid, the middle ear, the external auditory canal, and the squamous portion of the temporal bone.[72, 72a] When these lesions occur in the petrous apex, the clinical presentation may be similar to that of the cholesterol granuloma.[70] The lesions are usually both cystic and solid and contain a white, cheese-like material composed of keratin debris. Epidermoid cysts of the petrous apex are slow-growing lesions that usually remain asymptomatic, slowly eroding bone, until they erode into the internal auditory canal, facial nerve canal, or otic capsule. Erosion into the middle ear cavity can produce the appearance of a typical congenital or acquired middle ear cholesteatoma to the unknowing otologist. The actual extent of the mass becomes obvious only after an imaging study is obtained.

The MRI appearance reflects the histologic characteristic of this lesion (Fig. 32–28). In contrast to the cholesterol granuloma, T1-weighted sequences demonstrate low signal intensity that may be similar to cerebrospinal fluid. Thin, curvilinear stranding is sometimes visible within the cyst. On T2-weighted images, the cholesteatoma is hyperintense, again similar to cerebrospinal fluid signal intensity, and some mild heterogeneity can be observed within the mass. No central enhancement occurs after intravenous administration of gadolinium, although a thin rim of peripheral enhancement is sometimes present.[72]

Treatment of both congenital cholesteatoma and cholesterol granuloma requires surgical removal and drainage to prevent further destruction and compromise of cochlear, vestibular, and facial nerve function. Complete removal of large cholesteatomas can be challenging to the surgeon. Incomplete removal generally indicates recurrence. Evacuation of a cholesterol granuloma may include placement of a Silastic drain. Postoperative imaging shows collapse of the lesion, although imaging in the early postoperative period is difficult because residual fluid and blood products can mimic the initial lesion.

LOCAL TUMOR EXTENSION AND METASTATIC DISEASE

Metastatic disease can involve any portion of the skull base, from local extension of regional neoplasms, from perineural extension of head and neck tumors, or from hematogenous spread of a primary malignancy occurring elsewhere in the body. Local extension is more commonly seen with malignancies of the deep face and nasopharynx than with intracranial neoplasms. A variety of tumors, both benign and malignant, may extend rostrally from the paranasal sinuses and the deep face to involve the cranial base. In most cases, the differential diagnosis can be limited if the space or region of origin can be determined. For other malignancies, the primary tumor is more distant and the skull base involvement is secondary to perineural extension. Therefore, from an imaging standpoint, it is crucial to include the suprahyoid neck and oral cavity for any patient with symptoms referable to cranial nerves V, VII, and IX through XII if an obvious lesion is not identified at the level of the skull base (see also Chapters 33 to 35).

JUVENILE ANGIOFIBROMA

Juvenile angiofibroma is a highly vascular mass that originates in the posterior nasal cavity of young males, with a mean age of 15 years at the time of detection.[73] It is the most common benign mass in the nasopharyngeal region. Patients typically present with nasal obstruction and recurrent epistaxis. Unlike most benign tumors, juvenile angiofibromas can be highly aggressive and locally invasive. Invasion into the retroantral fat pad, nasopharyngeal masticator space, and sphenoidal sinus is common. Once the mass gains access to the pterygopalatine fossa, it can easily spread into the orbit and cavernous sinus region. Intracranial extension occurs in 5% to 20% of cases.[74]

Juvenile angiofibromas show intermediate signal intensity on T1-weighted images and are mild to moderately hyperintense with T2 weighting. Enlarged vessels are frequently visible on nonenhanced images. After contrast medium administration, prominent enhance-

---

FIGURE 32–27. Cholesterol granuloma. *A,* Coronal contrast-enhanced CT scan shows a large, nonenhancing soft tissue mass (M) within the petrous apex, extending into the middle ear cavity *(arrow). B,* Bone-window CT scan shows smooth erosion of the bony margins *(arrowheads).* The middle ear component of the lesion engulfs the ossicles *(arrow). C,* Parasagittal T1-weighted MR image demonstrates homogeneous hyperintensity within the expansile mass (M). *D,* Axial T2-weighted image reveals hyperintensity within the middle ear and mastoid component *(arrows)* of the lesion and mixed hyperintensity and hypointensity in the petrous apex portion of the lesion. The hypointense areas *(arrowheads)* are probably secondary hemosiderin deposition. *E,* 3D TOF MR angiogram, collapsed view, shows an apparent "vascular blush" within the mass *(arrow).* The vascular blush on the MR angiogram is a result of the T1-shortening effect of the chronic breakdown products of blood within the lesion and represents a potential pitfall in interpretation.

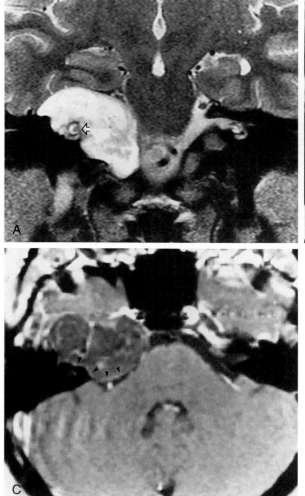

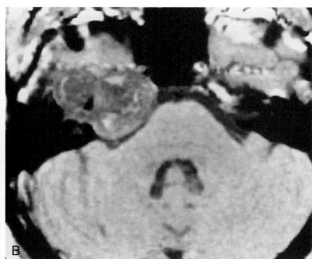

FIGURE 32–28. Congenital cholesteatoma (epidermoid cyst) of the petrous apex. *A*, T2-weighted FSE coronal image reveals a large hyperintense mass within the petrous temporal bone with bone destruction and erosion into the cochlea *(arrow)*. *B* and *C*, T1-weighted axial images before *(B)* and after *(C)* gadolinium infusion show a predominantly hypointense, heterogeneous mass with erosion of the entire petrous apex and extension into the cerebellopontine angle as well as the middle cranial fossa. Note the thin rim of enhancement at the periphery or the mass *(arrowheads)* on the postcontrast image *(C)*.

ment occurs. With the advent of more aggressive surgical approaches to the juvenile angiofibroma, the multiplanar imaging capabilities of MRI make this technique particularly valuable in preoperative planning. Therefore, it important to precisely identify the extent of any tumor invasion into the orbit, cavernous sinus region, and middle cranial fossa. Identification of involvement of the internal carotid artery in the cavernous sinus is imperative, because preoperative balloon test occlusion would need to be performed in these cases should carotid sacrifice be necessary during surgery. The combination of CT and MRI is usually needed for complete staging of the juvenile angiofibroma when there is extensive spread.

NASOPHARYNGEAL CARCINOMA

Squamous cell carcinoma of the nasopharynx is the most common carcinoma to involve the base of skull.[23] Because of their site of origin, usually in the lateral pharyngeal recess of Rosenmüller, nasopharyngeal carcinomas often remain asymptomatic for some time,

accounting for the advanced stage of many tumors at the time of diagnosis. Direct extension to the central skull base is frequent and may be superior into the sphenoidal sinus, posterior into the clivus, or posterolateral into the foramen ovale, carotid canal, and the jugular foramen.[75] The eustachian tube can also act as a conduit for spread to the posterolateral skull base.[76] Perineural extension is most common along the V_2 and V_3 divisions of the trigeminal nerve, producing numbness of the face and atrophy of the muscles of mastication.[12, 77] Involvement of cranial nerves III, IV, and VI implies cavernous sinus or superior orbital fissure invasion. Because nasopharyngeal carcinoma is treated primarily by radiation therapy, MRI is usually the only imaging examination necessary for staging purposes.

Similar to squamous cell carcinoma occurring elsewhere in the head and neck, these tumors are isointense relative to mucosa on T1-weighted images. With T2-weighted sequences they become hyperintense, paralleling the signal intensities of mucosa and lymphoid tissue. As a result, superficial carcinomas may be difficult to detect with MRI. Contrast-enhanced sequences with fat suppression are particularly helpful for demonstrating extension into the parapharyngeal space and skull base. The axial plane is helpful in defining clival invasion. Coronal images are useful in demonstrating direct invasion into the sphenoidal sinus and foramen lacerum, as well as showing perineural extension through the foramen ovale into the cavernous sinus and middle cranial fossa dural invasion (Fig. 32–29). MRI is the preferred study for assessing recurrence after radiotherapy, because postradiation fibrosis demonstrates low signal intensity on both T1- and T2-weighted sequences.[75]

SINONASAL CARCINOMA

Carcinomas originating in the nasal cavity and paranasal sinuses are significantly less common than those arising in other areas of the upper aerodigestive tract. Tumors arising in the nasal cavity and the sinuses adjacent to the skull base account for less than 35% to 45% of sinonasal malignancies.[2] Squamous cell carcinoma is the primary cell type, with adenocarcinoma and undifferentiated carcinoma constituting the majority of other histologic types found. Sinonasal carcinomas have a strong tendency for bone destruction, and therefore they have the potential for direct skull base invasion. These tumors are isointense or hypointense on T1-weighted images and show moderate hyperintensity with T2 weighting. Because inflammatory mucosa and obstructed secretions have longer T2 relaxation times than carcinomas, T2-weighted images are most useful in determining local tumor extent. Routine intravenous gadolinium administration is gen-

erally not needed to evaluate the extent of disease in the nose and sinuses,[78] but it can be useful in detecting dural invasion or perineural tumor extension.[34] When there is extensive involvement of the ethmoid complex and skull base, it is generally not possible to differentiate sinonasal carcinoma from esthesioneuroblastoma by imaging criteria alone.

HEAD AND NECK SARCOMAS

Rhabdomyosarcoma is the most frequently encountered sarcoma in the head and neck,[64] and the orbit and nasopharynx are the most common sites of origin. The vast majority of these tumors occur in children, with a peak incidence at 2 to 5 years of age. Rhabdomyosarcomas are usually divided into three groups in the head and neck: 1) orbital, 2) parameningeal, and 3) other head and neck location. The parameningeal group, which includes the nasopharynx, paranasal sinuses, and middle ear, has the poorest prognosis, owing to its predilection for skull base destruction and intracranial spread.[79] These tumors are isointense to slightly hyperintense relative to muscle on T1-weighted images and hyperintense on T2-weighted images (Fig. 32–30). Variable enhancement occurs after gadolinium administration.[80] After initiation of chemotherapy, the central portion often shows a reduction in signal intensity on T2-weighted sequences with a reduction in enhancement. Although much less common, Ewing's sarcoma can also occur in the head and neck. Tumors originating in the body of the mandible can extend superiorly to directly invade the skull base. Depending on size and location, it may be difficult to distinguish

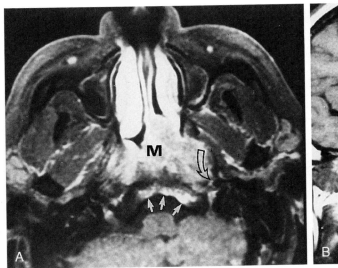
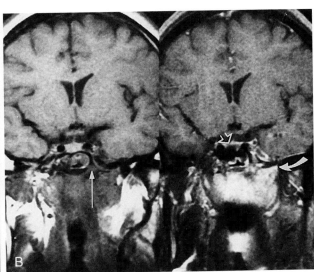

FIGURE 32–29. Nasopharyngeal carcinoma with central skull base invasion. *A,* Contrast-enhanced fat-suppressed T1-weighted axial image shows a large tumor (M) occupying the nasopharynx with anterior extension into the left nasal cavity. Hyperintense signal within the clivus *(solid arrows)* indicates bone marrow invasion, easily appreciated with the normal marrow signal suppressed. The tumor partially encases the left internal carotid artery *(open arrow). B,* T1-weighted precontrast *(left)* and postcontrast *(right)* coronal images show moderate enhancement of the tumor with bone invasion on the left *(solid long arrow)* and extension into the foramen spinosum *(solid curved arrow).* There is fat suppression susceptibility artifact within the sphenoidal sinus and sella, affecting pituitary gland visualization *(open arrow).* This artifact is more problematic when imaging in the coronal plane.

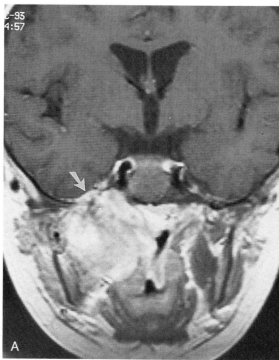

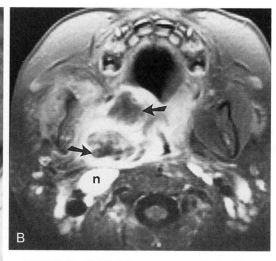

FIGURE 32–30. Rhabdomyosarcoma. *A,* Gadolinium-enhanced coronal image demonstrates a large enhancing mass within the deep face, displacing the nasopharyngeal airway. There is invasion of the sphenoid bone and extension along the middle cranial fossa dura *(arrow)*. *B,* Same patient after initial course of chemotherapy. Contrast-enhanced axial image with fat suppression reveals large areas of decreased enhancement centrally *(arrows)* consistent with tumor necrosis. A large retropharyngeal node is present posterior to the tumor (n). Central tumor necrosis is frequently seen in response to chemotherapy with rapidly growing childhood sarcomas.

Ewing's sarcoma from rhabdomyosarcoma with MRI. CT is helpful in demonstrating bone changes associated with Ewing's sarcoma. Craniofacial Ewing's sarcoma tends to occur in an older age group, and the prognosis is generally more favorable compared with that of those tumors arising elsewhere.

LYMPHOMA

Lymphoma is the second most common neoplasm to affect the head and neck, and the head and neck is the second most common site for extranodal disease after the gastrointestinal tract.[81] Extranodal disease involving the cranial base is almost always of the non-Hodgkin's type. Although most patients with non-Hodgkin's lymphoma of the head and neck have systemic disease, acquired immunodeficiency syndrome (AIDS)–related head and neck lymphoma may be isolated. Skull base involvement is usually secondary to extension from nasopharynx (Waldeyer's ring) or paranasal sinuses.

The reported MRI experience with non-Hodgkin's lymphoma involving the skull base is limited. The signal intensity of lymphoma is relatively homogeneous and similar to brain on both T1- and T2-weighted images.[82] Enhancement is typically homogeneous and intense, and juxtadural enhancement is common. Therefore, the MRI features of non-Hodgkin's lymphoma can mimic those of meningioma on both nonenhanced and enhanced images. Although bone involvement can occur with lymphoma, lack of significant bone erosion or destruction despite the appearance of tumor on both sides should raise a strong suspicion for lymphoma. Nasopharyngeal lymphoma can be indistinguishable from nasopharyngeal carcinoma with both CT and MRI. Aggressive local invasion with bone destruction, however, is more suggestive of carcinoma. Evaluation of the bony skull base with nonenhanced, high-resolution CT to look for hyperostosis (meningioma) and aggressive, lytic bone destruction (carcinoma) may be useful in difficult cases.

MRI is useful in evaluating for possible lymphoma in the paranasal sinuses. In patients with AIDS, who have a high frequency of inflammatory disease, MRI is superior to CT in differentiating inflammatory changes from tumor. T2-weighted sequences are the most useful in distinguishing tumor from sinus mucosa and inflammatory secretions.[2, 83] AIDS-related lymphomas, like non–AIDS-related lymphomas, are hypointense compared with mucosa and secretions on T2-weighted images. However, AIDS-related lymphomas may show only mild enhancement, in contrast to inflamed mucosa, after gadolinium administration. Nonenhanced and contrast-enhanced fat-suppressed T1-weighted images are helpful in determining invasion of the pterygopalatine fossa, superior orbital fissure, and cavernous sinus (Fig. 32–31).

METASTATIC DISEASE AND PERINEURAL TUMOR EXTENSION

Metastatic disease affecting the skull base is more common than primary neoplastic disease.[84] Hematogenous metastases from carcinoma of the breast, lung, and prostate are the most frequently encountered lesions. Although the disease may be limited to bone, a soft tissue component is often seen and may be responsible for the clinical symptoms such as cranial neuropathy that lead to the imaging examination.

Although CT is superior for depicting bone destruction, MRI has the advantages of better detection of early marrow infiltration and better definition of soft tissue extension. Cortical bone is hypointense on both T1- and T2-weighted sequences. The signal intensity of bone marrow, on the other hand, is age dependent. Marrow signal is usually symmetric from side to side and best assessed using short-TR, short-TE SE sequences. T1-weighted images show low signal intensity (isointense relative to muscle) of the clival bone marrow before 1 year of age in 89% of infants.[85] By age 10 years, most children show uniformly high signal intensity, indicating fatty conversion, with the majority showing some fatty conversion by 3 to 4 years of age.[85] Moderate or intense enhancement after gadolinium administration is common in children younger than 5 years.[86]

In the adult skull base, bone marrow signal follows fat signal; that is, it is hyperintense on T1-weighted images and hypointense on T2-weighted images. Some enhancement of the adult clivus can normally occur and was observed in 23% of patients in one study.[87] Metastatic disease results in T1 prolongation of marrow signal secondary to edema and increased cellularity[88] (Fig. 32–32). Standard SE T2-weighted images are more variable in appearance but generally show increased signal intensity. Because of the inherent increase in signal intensity of fat with FSE, this pulse sequence is less sensitive to marrow infiltration compared with standard SE sequences. After contrast agent infusion, marrow metastases may be rendered invisible on T1-weighted images unless fat suppression techniques are used. Careful comparison of precontrast and postcontrast images is necessary (Fig. 32–33). Conversely, the STIR sequence is sensitive to marrow edema and metastatic disease and offers another approach to imaging of bone marrow.

Perineural tumor spread can be seen with a number of tumors in the extracranial head and neck. Squamous cell carcinoma is the most common; however, adenoid cystic carcinoma has the greatest propensity for this type of metastatic spread. Other tumor types include lymphoma, melanoma, and mucoepidermoid carcinoma.[12] The exact mode of perineural tumor spread has been debated in the past. Presently, perineural metastasis is thought to represent direct microscopic extension from the primary lesion along the perineural and endoneural spaces, rather than embolic spread from perineural lymphatics.[89] Although any nerve can theoretically serve as a pathway for spread, cranial nerves V and VII are the most commonly involved nerves owing to their proximity to the upper aerodigestive tract mucosa (V), parotid gland (VII), and skin (V and VII). Recognition of perineural tumor extension to the skull base is critical. Demonstration of tumor spread through the skull base foramina usually changes the goal of therapy from curative to palliative, prohibiting complete surgical extirpation of disease in all but the most aggressive operations.

Perineural tumor involvement is observed as smooth thickening of the nerve with variable enlargement (Fig.

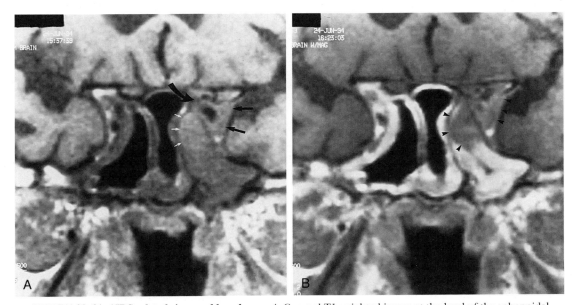

FIGURE 32–31. AIDS-related sinonasal lymphoma. *A,* Coronal T1-weighted image at the level of the sphenoidal sinus shows soft tissue of intermediate signal intensity filling the lateral air cell on the left. The signal intensity in the superior aspect is slightly higher *(white arrows),* and fat signal within the anterior cavernous sinus and anterior clinoid process has been replaced *(straight black arrows).* The inferior bony margin of the optic canal is indistinct *(curved black arrow). B,* After contrast medium administration, the sinus mucosa within the inferior aspect of the sinus enhances, whereas the mucosa superiorly and the soft tissue in the cavernous sinus *(arrowheads)* fail to enhance, suggesting invasive fungal infection. High-grade B cell lymphoma was found at biopsy. The presentation of progressive visual loss and ophthalmoplegia without fever favors lymphoma.

32–34). There may be mild enlargement of the associated skull base foramina.[77] Because perineural metastases enhance after gadolinium administration, contrast-enhanced, thin-section T1-weighted MRI in both axial and coronal planes affords the best chance of detecting perineural tumor spread. Fat within the spaces of the deep face poses a potential problem in the detection of perineural tumor. Fat suppression techniques are valuable after contrast medium administration to maximize the detection of abnormal nerve enhancement and enlargement. Unfortunately, these techniques are also more prone to susceptibility artifacts from air-bone and air–soft tissue interfaces in the paranasal sinuses and temporal bones.[5, 6] Therefore, it is recommended that at least one imaging plane include both T1-weighted pregadolinium and postgadolinium sequences without the use of fat suppression techniques. The coronal imaging plane is the most useful if perineural metastases of cranial nerves V_3 or VII are suspected. Postcontrast T1-weighted axial images, with or without fat suppression, are useful for

evaluating the cisternal segments and the brain stem, as well as the skull base and infratemporal fossa.

INFECTIOUS AND INFLAMMATORY DISEASE

MUCOCELE

Mucoceles are benign expansile lesions of the paranasal sinuses that most commonly arise as a complication of chronic inflammation and sinus obstruction. They can also develop as a result of sinus obstruction related to trauma or tumor. Pathologically, mucoceles are mucin-containing cyst-like structures lined by sinus mucosa. The frontal sinuses are the most frequent site of occurrence (60%), followed by the ethmoidal sinuses (30%), maxillary sinuses, and sphenoidal sinuses.[23] A variety of appearances have been described with MRI.[83, 90, 91] The expansile nature and varied ap-

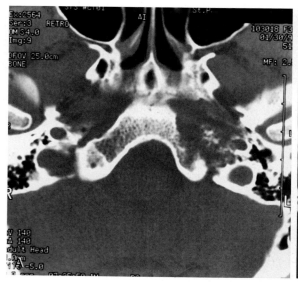

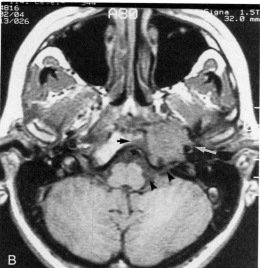

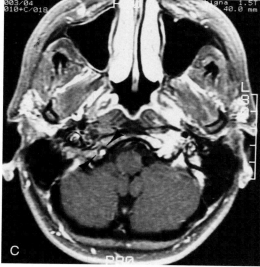

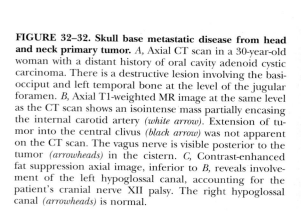

FIGURE 32–32. Skull base metastatic disease from head and neck primary tumor. *A,* Axial CT scan in a 30-year-old woman with a distant history of oral cavity adenoid cystic carcinoma. There is a destructive lesion involving the basi-occiput and left temporal bone at the level of the jugular foramen. *B,* Axial T1-weighted MR image at the same level as the CT scan shows an isointense mass partially encasing the internal carotid artery *(white arrow)*. Extension of tumor into the central clivus *(black arrow)* was not apparent on the CT scan. The vagus nerve is visible posterior to the tumor *(arrowheads)* in the cistern. *C,* Contrast-enhanced fat suppression axial image, inferior to *B,* reveals involvement of the left hypoglossal canal, accounting for the patient's cranial nerve XII palsy. The right hypoglossal canal *(arrowheads)* is normal.

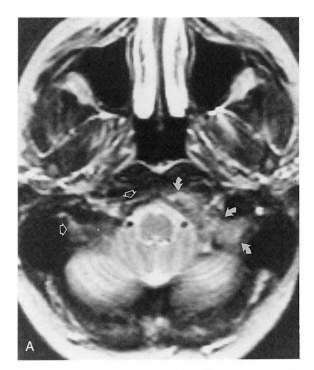

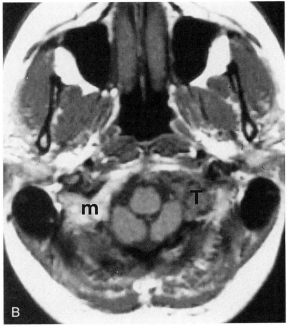

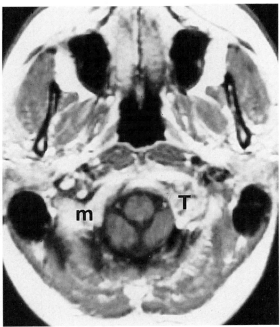

FIGURE 32–33. Hematogenous metastasis. *A,* Axial T2-weighted image shows a heterogeneous, predominantly isointense mass involving the left basiocciput and left occipital condyle *(solid arrows)*. There is no significant difference in signal intensity with the bone marrow on the right *(open arrows)*. *B,* T1-weighted axial precontrast *(left)* and postcontrast *(right)* images slightly caudal to *A* demonstrate heterogeneous enhancement of the tumor. Comparison with precontrast images or fat suppression techniques is necessary to differentiate enhancing tumor (T) from bone marrow (m).

pearance may, therefore, mimic other lesions, such as tumor or fibrous dysplasia.

The appearance of mucoceles on T1- and T2-weighted images varies according to the viscosity and protein concentration of the central mucin.[92] Subacute or early mucoceles are isointense to hypointense on T1-weighted images and hyperintense on T2-weighted images, reflecting a larger amount of unbound water protons. As the mucocele ages, the mucin contained within the lesion dehydrates and the viscosity and protein concentration increase. Increased signal intensity is present on T1-weighted images, reflecting the in-

crease in macromolecular "bound" water. A corresponding decrease in signal intensity with T2 weighting is seen (Fig. 32–35). Signal void can be observed, particularly on T2-weighted images, in chronic mucoceles, simulating an expanded, air-filled sinus.[93] This represents a potential pitfall in MRI of the chronic mucocele, compared with CT.

Variable signal intensity within a mucocele is not uncommon, making differentiation from a hemorrhagic lesion sometimes difficult. After gadolinium administration, rim enhancement is present, corresponding to the mucosal lining. Although, mucoceles can

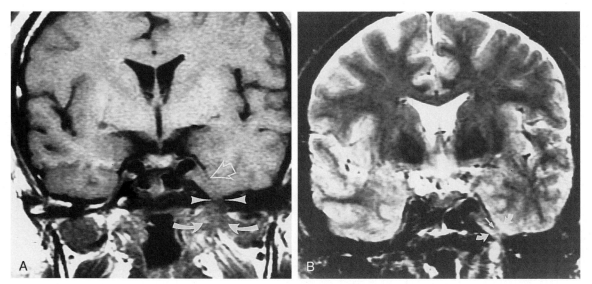

FIGURE 32–34. Perineural tumor spread. *A,* Coronal T1-weighted image demonstrates abnormal soft tissue in the left parapharyngeal space *(solid arrows)* with extension along cranial nerve V₃ through an enlarged foramen ovale *(arrowheads)* into the left cavernous sinus *(open arrow). B,* T2-weighted image at the same level shows hyperintense signal *(curved arrows)* surrounding the nerve *(straight arrow).* This patient had adenoid cystic carcinoma primary to the soft palate and also had cranial nerve V₂ involvement (not shown).

frequently be differentiated from a neoplasm on the basis of T1 and T2 signal characteristics alone,[2] contrast agent administration can be valuable in more difficult instances. MRI contrast agents are most valuable in evaluating cases in which there is a coexisting neoplasm to define the extent of the tumor relative to the mucocele[83] (see also Chapter 33).

FUNGAL INFECTION

Skull base mycotic infection, secondary to aspergillosis or mucomycosis, usually results as a complication of sinonasal infection in an immunocompromised host or diabetic patient. When these infections become invasive, direct extension to the orbital apex, cavernous

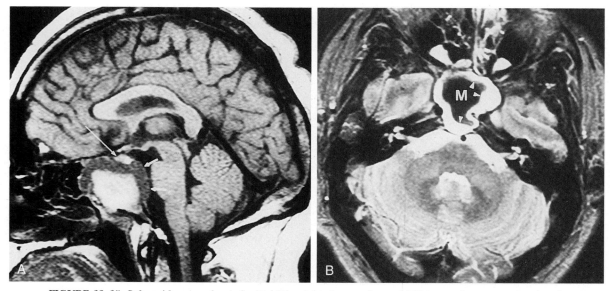

FIGURE 32–35. Sphenoid mucocele. *A,* Sagittal T1-weighted nonenhanced MR image demonstrates a sharply delineated mass of mixed signal intensity involving the sphenoid bone and basiocciput with expansion of the clivus *(short arrows)* and superior displacement of the sellar contents *(long arrow). B,* Axial T2-weighted image shows signal void centrally (M) corresponding to the region of hyperintensity on the T1-weighted image, representing viscous, proteinaceous content within the chronic mucocele. The hyperintense mucosa *(arrowheads)* is particularly thick. The signal void within the sphenoidal sinus could easily be mistaken for air when viewing the T2-weighted image alone.

sinus, and frontal lobes is the most common route of spread.[23] Orbital involvement results in ophthalmoplegia and visual loss. Proptosis is usually present and variable in severity. Extension into the cavernous sinus can lead to multiple cranial neuropathies and cavernous sinus thrombosis. Because these organisms have a propensity for angioinvasion, fungal arteritis develops, leading to thrombosis, infarction, and mycotic aneurysm formation.[94] The last complication is almost uniformly fatal. Direct extension through the cribriform plate results in cerebral abscess formation and parenchymal infarction (Fig. 32–36). Fungal meningitis occurs if there is extension into the subarachnoid space.

Radiologic differentiation from tumor is difficult, particularly with CT. Several authors have concluded that MRI is superior in differentiating neoplasm from infection and inflammatory disease in the sinonasal region.[2, 83] Inflamed, edematous mucosa in the paranasal sinuses is hyperintense with T2 weighting and enhances intensely after gadolinium infusion. Similar changes can be seen with invasive disease. However, invasive aspergillosis and mucormycosis can cause the mucosa to be hypointense on both T1- and T2-weighted sequences, probably secondary to angioinvasion and tissue infarction,[95] with little or absent enhancement of involved tissues. Meningeal and parenchymal enhancement occurs with further intracranial invasion (see also Chapter 33).

MALIGNANT OTITIS EXTERNA AND SKULL BASE OSTEOMYELITIS

Malignant otitis externa is a spectrum of diseases involving the external auditory canal, including soft tissue, cartilage, and, in the most severe cases, bone.[96] This disease usually occurs in diabetic or immunocompromised patients, and the responsible organism is almost always *Pseudomonas aeruginosa*. Some authors refer to the disease as necrotizing external otitis when it is limited to soft tissue and cartilage. When there is more generalized temporal bone and cranial base involvement, the disorder is called skull base osteomyelitis.[96] Necrotizing external otitis presents with severe otalgia, otorrhea, and swelling. Peripheral facial nerve palsy may be seen in 30% of cases.[97] Skull base osteomyelitis usually presents several weeks to months after initial treatment and apparent control of the disease. Deep temporo-occipital headache is the predominant symptom. Lower cranial nerve palsies from jugular foramen and hypoglossal canal involvement usually follow if the disease is left untreated. More advanced disease involving the central skull base can affect cranial nerves III through VI.[98, 99] Atypical skull base osteomyelitis occurs in the absence of preexisting necrotizing external otitis.[100, 101] Intractable headaches may be the only symptom. Imaging of atypical skull base osteomyelitis can be particularly frustrating and requires a high degree of suspicion.

CT changes reported with skull base osteomyelitis include areas of bone destruction and sclerosis, the presence of soft tissue inflammation and loss of normal fat planes in the high parapharyngeal space, middle ear and mastoid opacification, and meningeal enhancement.[97] However, more advanced disease is usually required to detect these changes with CT. MRI offers the possibility of earlier detection owing to the high sensitivity for marrow involvement on nonenhanced T1-weighted images. Gadolinium-enhanced imaging is more sensitive than CT for dural enhancement and abnormal marrow enhancement (Fig. 32–37). Furthermore, MRI offers more precise anatomic information as a result of the ease of multiplanar imaging. T2-weighted images may be insensitive, however, to early skull base osteomyelitis. Otogenic skull base osteomyelitis secondary to invasive *Aspergillus* infection has also been reported.[102] Loss of normal marrow signal on nonenhanced T1-weighted images and middle ear and mastoid effusion on T2-weighted images may be the sole manifestations of this process early in the disease course.

MRI should replace CT and nuclear medicine bone scanning in the diagnosis of most patients with skull base osteomyelitis. Most authors believe that gallium scanning is the most useful imaging modality for monitoring response to therapy.[96, 98] Indium-labeled white blood cell studies can also be used as an alternative to gallium scanning.[96] The exact role of MRI in monitoring the response to treatment of these patients remains uncertain; however, one report suggests that MRI is useful as an adjunctive modality.[102a]

APICAL PETROSITIS

Apical petrositis, or petrous apicitis, is an uncommon infectious process involving the apex of the petrous temporal bone. It is usually seen as a complication of otitis media and mastoiditis in the pneumatized petrous apex.[10] Patients classically present with otorrhea, deep facial pain (secondary to cranial nerve V involvement), and diplopia (secondary to cranial nerve VI involvement). This triad of clinical findings is referred to as Gradenigo's syndrome. MRI demonstrates intermediate signal intensity with T1-weighted images and high signal intensity on T2-weighted images. MRI contrast agents can be useful in differentiating petrous apicitis from early or atypical cholesterol granuloma or serous effusion in the petrous apex (Fig. 32–38). Bone enhancement and adjacent dura enhancement are indicators of more aggressive infection. More commonly, the petrous apex is involved as part of a more widespread skull base osteomyelitis, resulting from either sinonasal disease or otogenic infection such as necrotizing external otitis.

CHRONIC OTOMASTOIDITIS AND ACQUIRED CHOLESTEATOMA

Chronic middle ear inflammatory disease or chronic otomastoiditis and its complications result from eustachian tube dysfunction. Common manifestations in-

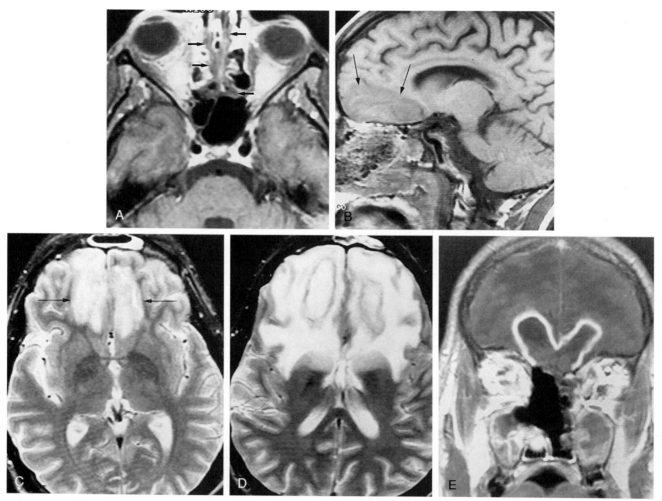

FIGURE 32–36. Fungal sinusitis with cerebral abscess. *A,* T1-weighted contrast-enhanced axial image in a 20-year-old diabetic man with mild proptosis and ophthalmoplegia shows some enlargement and loss of definition of the medial recti muscles bilaterally. There are areas of absent enhancement of the sinonasal mucosa *(arrows),* suggesting possible tissue infarction. *B* and *C,* T1-weighted sagittal *(B)* and T2-weighted axial *(C)* images obtained 3 days after *A* demonstrate abnormal signal intensity within the inferior frontal lobes *(arrows).* Postsurgical changes are present in the sinonasal cavity. *D* and *E,* T2-weighted axial *(D)* and T1-weighted contrast-enhanced coronal *(E)* images obtained 3 weeks after *A* reveal large bifrontal abscess cavities with extensive white matter edema. Biopsy of the brain revealed invasive mucormycosis.

clude middle ear and mastoid effusions, tympanic membrane retraction, granulation tissue, acquired cholesteatoma, and ossicular fixation and erosion.[59] When imaging is necessary, CT is generally recognized as the study of choice for evaluation of most patients with chronic otomastoiditis. This modality is ideal for evaluating the ossicular chain and identifying the bone erosion typical of cholesteatoma. However, inflammatory granulation tissue in the middle ear and mastoid is much more common than cholesteatoma, and CT is unable to consistently differentiate between granulation tissue and cholesteatoma.[103] Furthermore, these two entities may occur simultaneously. With MRI, both cholesteatoma and inflammatory granulation tissue are generally isointense relative to brain on T1-weighted images and hyperintense on T2-weighted images.[72] Granulation tissue demonstrates marked enhancement after gadolinium administration (Fig. 32–39), whereas cholesteatomas fail to show any enhancement[103] (Fig. 32–40). MRI is also useful in identifying cholesterol

granuloma in the middle ear and mastoid. The hyperintensity of the cholesterol granuloma on T1-weighted images distinguishes it from cholesteatoma and typical granulation tissue.[71] When abnormal soft tissue is present in the mastoidectomy cavity after mastoid surgery, CT cannot reliably differentiate granulation tissue from recurrent cholesteatoma. In addition, if the tegmen tympani is dehiscent, the possibility of brain herniation must be considered.[104] MRI is ideally suited to easily distinguish these three entities. Finally, MRI is superior to CT in the detection of meningeal enhancement or other intracranial disease secondary to middle ear and mastoid disease.

POSTOPERATIVE SKULL BASE

Imaging of the postoperative skull base can be challenging for the radiologist. Accurate interpretation requires knowledge of the type and location of the initial pathologic condition, an understanding of the procedure performed, and a familiarity of the normal postoperative appearance. Relatively little information is available in the literature regarding the imaging appearance with MRI or CT after major skull base surgery. Given the numerous surgical approaches to the cranial base, close communication between the surgeon and the radiologist is required to ensure accurate image interpretation.

The anterior skull base or craniofacial approach to tumors of the anterior cranial fossa permits resection of the ethmoid bone, the cribriform plate, and the medial orbital walls. These defects are typically reconstructed with a combination of dura, vascularized pericranium (from the frontal bones), and bone graft or titanium mesh.[105] Because the pericranium remains vascularized, persistent enhancement can be anticipated on follow-up imaging studies. Temporalis muscle flaps or rectus abdominis free flaps are commonly used for more complex resections involving the anterolateral skull base and middle cranial fossa. These grafts contain muscle, tendon, and fat tissue. Therefore, some atrophy will occur as part of the normal aging process of the graft. Viable tissue will continue to enhance after contrast agent administration. Recur-

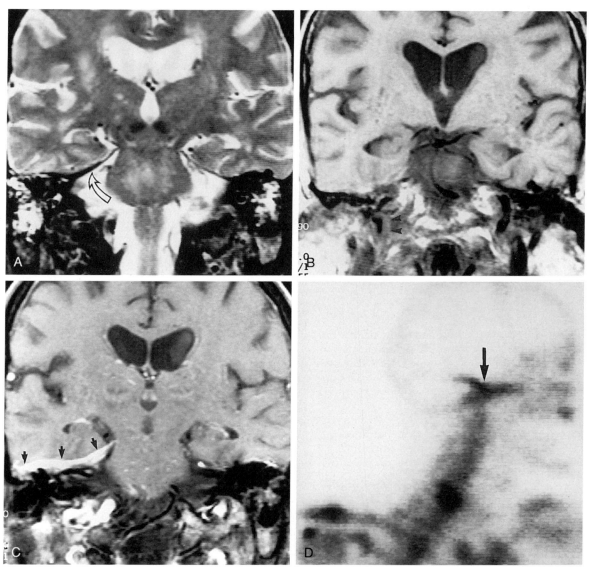

FIGURE 32–37. Skull base osteomyelitis with jugular foramen syndrome. *A,* Coronal T2-weighted image of the posterolateral skull base demonstrates inflammatory changes in the mastoid air cells bilaterally. There is tentorial thickening on the right side *(arrow). B,* Coronal T1-weighted image shows abnormal soft tissue in the region of the jugular fossa with thickening of the internal carotid artery wall *(arrowheads). C,* Gadolinium-enhanced coronal image reveals segmental dural enhancement along the petrous ridge and tentorium *(arrows)* and soft tissue enhancement in the jugular foramen region below. *D,* Technetium bone scan shows intense uptake within the right petrous temporal bone *(arrow).* At surgery, chronic inflammatory tissue was found but no organism was isolated.

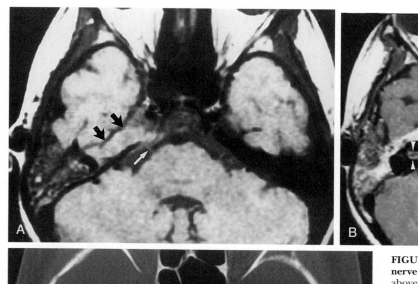

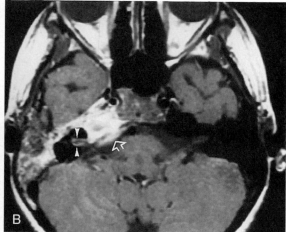

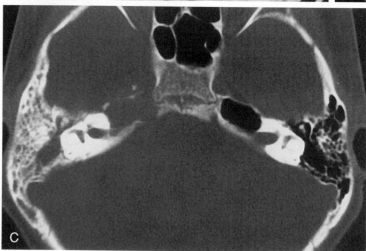

FIGURE 32–38. Petrous apicitis with abducens nerve palsy. *A,* Axial T1-weighted image just above the level of the internal auditory canal reveals abnormal signal *(black arrows)* within the right petrous apex extending to the clivus medially. The right abducens nerve *(white arrow)* travels into the lesion at Dorello's canal. Abnormal signal is also present within the right mastoid air cells. *B,* Gadolinium-enhanced axial image slightly inferior to *A* shows intense enhancement of the petrous apex inflammatory mass with extension into the posterior fossa *(arrow).* Note the dural enhancement within the right internal auditory canal *(arrowheads)* and enhancement within the mastoid air cells. (*B* reprinted with permission from Swartz JD, Harnsberger HR, Imaging of the Temporal Bone, 2nd ed, page 334, 1992, copyright Thieme Medical Publishers, Inc.) *C,* Axial CT scan at the same level as *B* demonstrates opacification and significant bone destruction of the right petrous apex air cell.

rent tumor tends to produce nodularity or infiltration of the tissues at the margins of the myocutaneous flap (Weissman JL, unpublished data, 1994). Because infection may be indistinguishable from tumor by imaging examination, CT-guided biopsy may be required if the clinical setting is uncertain.

The question often arises as to whether MRI or CT is the preferred modality for postoperative monitoring in patients with carcinoma of the head and neck. If only one modality has been used in the preoperative assessment, that same modality should be used for postoperative assessment. If both modalities have been used preoperatively (as is often the case), MRI is preferred for evaluation of postoperative tumor recurrence in most instances, particularly in the anterior cranial fossa where fat-containing reconstructive tissue grafts are not used. The addition of fat suppression techniques is recommended with postcontrast sequences if the myocutaneous graft contains a significant amount of adipose tissue. Fat suppression is also helpful in postoperative imaging of the patient with acoustic schwannoma when a translabyrinthine approach to the internal auditory canal has been performed and the bone defect has been packed with fat.

DIFFERENTIAL DIAGNOSIS

The spectrum and number of disease processes potentially involving the cranial base are extensive and include benign and malignant neoplasms, congenital malformations and bony dysplasias, and inflammatory and infectious processes. As previously stated, appropriate therapy is best achieved when the lesion is precisely localized and an accurate pretreatment imaging diagnosis or differential diagnosis is given. The multiplanar imaging capabilities of MRI enable the radiologist to accurately localize virtually all lesions involving the cranial base, with the possible exception of some processes isolated to the middle ear and mastoid region. Careful analysis of lesion characteristics with MRI, in conjunction with location, will provide an accurate differential diagnosis in most cases. CT and MRI should be thought of as adjunctive imaging studies when evaluating skull base disease, and in some instances CT will provide the information that leads to the correct diagnosis. It is incumbent on the radiologist who images the skull base to help guide the clinician to ensure appropriate yet cost-effective evaluation.

Therefore, it is essential to recognize when CT or MRI or both studies are necessary to accomplish this task.

Table 32–3 provides a comprehensive list of the common and uncommon lesions involving the anterior, central, and posterolateral skull base. The following discussion serves to highlight some of the more important issues regarding differential diagnosis of lesions affecting the base of skull.

When a locally invasive or destructive lesion is encountered in the anterior skull base, the main differential diagnosis in the adult patient includes squamous cell carcinoma, metastatic disease, lymphoma, and meningioma. In the pediatric patient, esthesioneuroblastoma is the primary tumor to consider, but this malignancy can also occur in the adult population. Sinonasal carcinoma arising within the ethmoidal sinuses has a vector of spread that is predominantly superior and lateral. This lesion can usually be differentiated from meningioma by the extent of bone destruction and enhancement characteristics. Carcinomas have a strong tendency to destroy bone. In contrast, meningiomas in the anterior cranial fossa are less destructive and may produce hyperostosis. Meningiomas usually enhance intensely, but enhancement patterns with carcinoma are more variable. Frontal lobe changes, dural enhancement, and peritumoral cyst formation can be seen with both tumors as well

as esthesioneuroblastoma. Metastatic disease and lymphoma can potentially mimic the appearance of either lesion, although bone destruction is usually less extensive with most lymphomas.

Analysis of T1- and T2-weighted imaging characteristics usually allows differentiation of tumor from inflammatory disease. Inflammatory tissue and obstructed secretions have a higher free water content, resulting in higher T2-weighted signal intensity. Gadolinium may be necessary for differentiation in difficult cases, or when both entities are present, to more accurately map the extent of tumor involvement. Mucoceles are readily identified by their expansile nature if the radiologist is knowledgeable regarding the change in T1- and T2-weighted signal characteristics with the chronicity of the lesion. Whereas fibrous dysplasia is easily identified by CT, it can mimic chronic mucocele formation with MRI. In the immunocompromised patient with cranial nerve symptoms, invasive aspergillosis and lymphoma are primary considerations. It should also be kept in mind that AIDS-related lymphoma may not adhere to the typical MRI appearance of lymphoma.

When approaching lesions of the central skull base, the radiologist should first determine whether the process or mass is midline, within the cavernous sinus, or more lateral. The next step is to determine the

TABLE 32–3. SKULL BASE MASSES AND LESIONS: DIFFERENTIAL DIAGNOSIS

ANTERIOR SKULL BASE

Common
Meningioma
Sinonasal carcinoma
Metastasis
Lymphoma

Uncommon
Cephalocele
Fibrous dysplasia
Mucocele
Extensive sinonasal polyposis
Sinusitis (fungal, epidural abscess)
Juvenile angiofibroma
Esthesioneuroblastoma
Chondrosarcoma

CENTRAL SKULL BASE AND CLIVUS

Common
Meningioma
Invasive pituitary adenoma
Nasopharyngeal carcinoma
Metastases
Lymphoma

Uncommon
Cephalocele
Fibrous dysplasia
Mucocele
Osteomyelitis
Fungal sinusitis
Juvenile angiofibroma
Sinonasal carcinoma
Craniopharyngioma
Chordoma
Chondrosarcoma
Sarcoma (Ewing's, rhabdomyosarcoma)
Myeloma

PETROUS APEX
Congenital cholesteatoma (epidermoidoma)
Cholesterol granuloma (giant cholesterol cyst)
Petrous apicitis or osteomyelitis
Chondrosarcoma
Chondroma
Metastasis
Rhabdomyosarcoma (pediatrics)
Internal carotid artery aneurysm

JUGULAR FORAMEN
Jugular megabulb deformity
Paraganglioma (glomus jugulare)
Schwannoma or neurofibroma
Meningioma
Chondrosarcoma
Metastasis

TEMPORAL BONE OR INTERNAL AUDITORY CANAL–CEREBELLOPONTINE ANGLE
Schwannoma (acoustic, facial nerve)
Meningioma
Cholesteatoma or epidermoid cyst
Malignant otitis externa or osteomyelitis
Metastasis
Malignant temporal bone tumors
Histiocytosis
Hemangioma

LESIONS AFFECTING ANY LOCATION OR DIFFUSE LESIONS
Fibrous dysplasia
Paget's disease
Langerhans' cell histiocytosis
Infection (osteomyelitis)
Meningioma
Metastases
Lymphoma
Myeloma

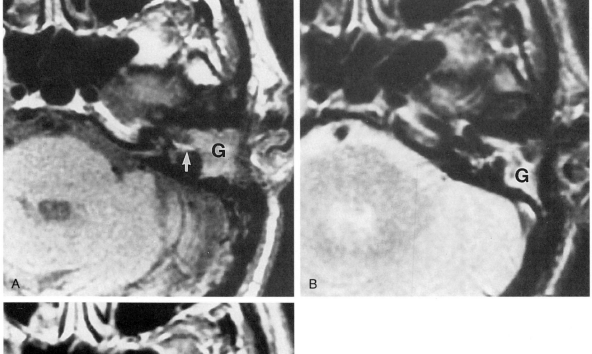

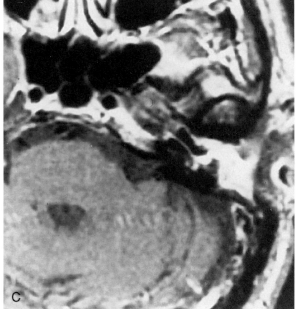

FIGURE 32–39. Granulation tissue in the middle ear and mastoid. *A,* Axial T1-weighted image at the level of the internal auditory canal shows isointense soft tissue within the mastoidectomy cavity (G) and a small crescent of hyperintense signal pattern adjacent to the lateral semicircular canal *(arrow). B,* The mastoid contents (G) are hyperintense with T2 weighting. *C,* Axial T1-weighted gadolinium-enhanced image shows marked enhancement of the granulation tissue. Enhancement with a cholesteatoma, if present, is limited to the periphery of the mass. Granulation tissue is frequently quite vascular and prone to hemorrhage, potentially leading to the formation of a cholesterol granuloma.

craniocaudal relationship to the skull base. Is the mass primarily above and extending inferiorly, predominantly within the bony structures, or infracranial and extending superiorly? When the lesion is infracranial with superior extension, is there direct bone invasion, transcranial spread via foramina and fissures, or both? Meningioma is by far the most common diagnosis of a mass laterally located along the greater sphenoid wing, followed by metastatic disease. Rarely, temporal lobe neoplasms, arachnoid cysts, and intracranial epidermoid tumors will cause bone erosion. Greater wing sphenoid dysplasia related to neurofibromatosis type 1 can also give the appearance of an expansile middle cranial fossa process. In the midline, masses that have a vector of extension from superior to inferior include

meningioma, pituitary adenoma, and craniopharyngioma. After contrast agent administration, both pituitary adenoma and meningioma typically show fairly homogeneous, intense enhancement. Meningiomas are generally less hyperintense than are adenomas on T2-weighted images. Craniopharyngiomas are more variable in appearance and enhance heterogeneously.

Intrinsic midline and paramedian masses include chordoma, chondrosarcoma, sphenoidal sinus malignancy, hematogenous metastasis, and invasive fungal infection. Although chordomas are classically midline whereas chondrosarcomas usually arise farther lateral along the petroclival fissure, these tumors are often quite large when detected and the exact site of origin may be difficult to determine. Both tumors are hypointense on T1-weighted images, are hyperintense with T2 weighting, and enhance, often intensely. Diffuse, marked hypointensity on T1-weighted images (myxoid matrix), intratumoral cyst formation, and intratumoral hemorrhage favor chordoma. Globular or linear calcifications favor chondrosarcoma (better delineated with CT). Invasive pituitary adenoma, meningioma, extensive nasopharyngeal carcinoma, and metastasis can all mimic chordoma and chondrosarcoma.

The differential diagnosis of the cavernous sinus mass depends largely on whether the lesion is unilateral or bilateral. Common and uncommon unilateral lesions include schwannoma, meningioma, vascular pathology, metastasis (perineural), lymphoma, and chordoma. When the process is bilateral, invasive pituitary adenoma, meningioma, metastasis, lymphoma,

and cavernous sinus thrombosis are the considerations. When there is enlargement or abnormal enhancement of the second or third divisions of the trigeminal nerve, imaging of the oral cavity and suprahyoid neck is necessary to search for the primary tumor.

Several tumors arising in the nasopharynx and deep face invade the skull base from below. The most common of these lesions is nasopharyngeal carcinoma. As previously stated, cranial base involvement may be the result of direct extension with bone destruction or from perineural tumor infiltration. Denervation atrophy of the muscles of mastication indicates cranial nerve V_3 invasion. If the tumor gains access to the cavernous sinus, neuropathies of cranial nerves III, IV, V_1, V_2, and VI may occur. The major advantage of MRI over CT in staging nasopharyngeal carcinoma is in the

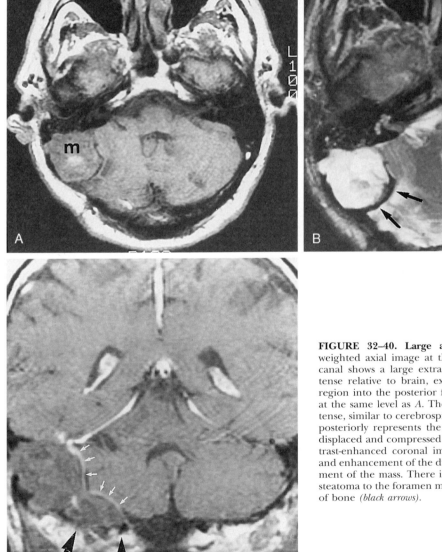

FIGURE 32–40. Large acquired cholesteatoma. *A*, T1-weighted axial image at the level of the internal auditory canal shows a large extradural mass (m), slightly hypointense relative to brain, extending from the right mastoid region into the posterior fossa. *B*, T2-weighted axial image at the same level as *A*. The mass is predominantly hyperintense, similar to cerebrospinal fluid. The dark linear border posteriorly represents the thickened dura of the medially displaced and compressed transverse sinus *(arrows)*. *C*, Contrast-enhanced coronal image shows abnormal thickening and enhancement of the dura *(white arrows)* but no enhancement of the mass. There is inferior extension of the cholesteatoma to the foramen magnum with considerable erosion of bone *(black arrows)*.

detection of perineural metastases and cavernous sinus invasion. Juvenile angiofibroma is one of the few benign processes that can aggressively invade the skull base. The imaging challenge with this lesion is not so much one of diagnosis but to accurately demonstrate the extent of the lesion relative to the cavernous sinus structures and posterior orbit, allowing appropriate preoperative surgical planning to take place. Rhabdomyosarcoma is the primary differential consideration in the pediatric population. Transcranial tumor extension portends a poorer prognosis in these patients. Finally, meningiomas can arise from meningothelial cells along the cranial nerves and may present as a primary deep facial mass with superior extension into the skull base or as a transforaminal mass centered at the level of the skull base foramina.

The jugular foramen normally varies considerably in size and shape. As a result, the radiologist is occasionally confronted with the sometimes difficult task of differentiating the enlarged jugular bulb (jugular megabulb deformity) as a normal variant from enlargement secondary to a pathologic process. Advances in MRI techniques, including MR angiography, have significantly improved our ability to distinguish normal variation from abnormal. The most common tumor arising in the jugular foramen is the paraganglioma (glomus jugulare tumor), followed by neural spectrum tumors (e.g., schwannoma, neurofibroma). Less common masses include meningioma, chondrosarcoma, and metastasis.

In patients with pulsatile tinnitus, paraganglioma, dural arteriovenous fistula, carotid artery stenosis, and arterial or venous vascular variants are the main diagnoses to consider. It is important to inquire as to the nature of the pulsatile tinnitus (i.e., objective versus subjective) and whether there is a concomitant vascular retrotympanic mass (vascular tympanic membrane) present. Carotid artery stenosis (atherosclerotic, fibromuscular dysplasia, arterial dissection) and dural arteriovenous fistula typically present with objective tinnitus, without a vascular tympanic membrane. The tinnitus is usually subjective with paragangliomas, and a vascular tympanic membrane is present with glomus tympanicum and jugulotympanicum tumors. A vascular retrotympanic mass and subjective pulse-synchronous tinnitus are the clinical findings in patients with an aberrant internal carotid artery and dehiscent jugular bulb. These patients can be effectively evaluated in a noninvasive manner with a combination of precontrast and postcontrast T1- and T2-weighted sequences along with MR angiography in both the arterial and venous phases. Sagittal nonenhanced images can be useful for determining the patency of the jugular bulb and upper jugular vein. 2D TOF MR angiography is superior to 3D TOF MR angiography in evaluating the arterial side for stenosis and enlarged arteries associated with dural arteriovenous fistula in my experience; however, phase-contrast MR angiography offers the advantage of evaluating both the arterial side and the venous side in one sequence and has advantages over TOF techniques in areas of turbulence or tortuous vascularity.

Acoustic schwannoma, meningioma, and epidermoid tumors constitute the differential diagnosis of masses in the cerebellopontine angle and internal auditory canal. Rarely, neuritis and hemangioma mimic the appearance of a small intracanalicular schwannoma. In the petrous temporal bone proper, infection and inflammatory disease, or their sequelae, predominate. When a cystic-appearing mass of the petrous apex is encountered, congenital cholesteatoma and giant cholesterol cyst (granuloma) can be distinguished by their signal characteristics on T1-weighted images. The cholesterol granuloma is hyperintense owing to the presence of hemoglobin breakdown products, whereas the cholesteatoma is hypointense, and neither lesion enhances. When a solid mass is present, considerations include metastatic disease (local extension or hematogenous), benign and malignant cartilaginous tumors, chordoma, and rhabdomyosarcoma (pediatrics). Malignant tumors of the mastoid portion of the temporal bone are rare, and most arise in the external auditory canal and extend medially and posteriorly. When there is a history of chronic otomastoiditis, most cholesteatomas are partially visible by otoscopy and CT is usually adequate for determining the extent of such lesions. MRI has been shown to be accurate in distinguishing inflammatory granulation tissue and cholesterol granuloma from cholesteatoma in the middle ear and mastoid. In the postmastoidectomy patient, MRI is the study of choice for differentiating recurrent cholesteatoma from granulation tissue or brain herniation. Finally, in the patient with malignant otitis externa, bone marrow changes and dural enhancement are important findings indicating progression to skull base osteomyelitis.

CONCLUSION

The skull base is a complex anatomic structure separating the intracranial compartment from the deep face and suprahyoid neck. A large number of pathologic processes have the potential to involve the cranial base. The numerous apertures of the cranial base provide a multitude of pathways for potential transcranial disease spread. As a result, the radiologist faces a tremendous challenge when imaging this area. Furthermore, conceptual and technical advances in cranial base surgery have placed more demand on the imager to interpret these imaging studies accurately and reliably. CT and MRI should be looked on as complementary studies in skull base imaging. Careful analysis of findings should give a fairly accurate preoperative diagnosis or a short list of differential considerations, allowing for appropriate treatment.

REFERENCES

1. Laine FJ, Nadel L, Braun IF: CT and MR imaging of the central skull base. Part I. Techniques, embryologic development, and anatomy. Radiographics 10:591–602, 1990.
2. Som PM, Shapiro MD, Biller HF, et al: Sinonasal tumors and inflamma-

tory tissues: differentiation with MR imaging. Radiology 167:803–808, 1988.

3. Zoarski GH, Mackey JK, Anzai Y, et al: Head and neck: initial experience with fast spin-echo MR imaging. Radiology 188:323–327, 1993.

4. Tien RD, Hesselink JR, Chu PK, Szumowski J: Improved detection and delineation of head and neck lesions with fat suppression spin-echo MR imaging. AJNR 12:19–24, 1991.

5. Barakos JA, Dillon WP, Chew WM: Orbit, skull base, and pharynx: contrast-enhanced fat suppression MR imaging. Radiology 179:191–198, 1991.

6. Anzai Y, Lufkin RB, Jabour BA, Hanafee WN: Fat-suppression failure artifacts simulating pathology on frequency-selective fat-suppression MR images of the head and neck. AJNR 13:879–884, 1992.

7. Brogan M, Chakeres DW, Schmalbrock P: High-resolution 3DFT MR imaging of the endolymphatic duct and soft tissues of the otic capsule. AJNR 12:1–11, 1991.

8. Casselman JW, De Jonge I, Neyt L, et al: MRI in craniofacial fibrous dysplasia. Neuroradiology 35:234–237, 1993.

9. Anderson CE, Saloner D, Lee RE, et al: Assessment of carotid artery stenosis by MR angiography: comparison with x-ray angiography and color-coded Doppler ultrasound. AJNR 13:989–1003, 1992.

10. Daniels DL: The jugular foramen and petrous apex lesions. In: Core Curriculum Course in Neuroradiology. Chicago: American Society of Neuroradiology, 1994, pp 135–143.

11. Rodgers GK, Applegate L, De la Cruz A, Lo W: Magnetic resonance angiography: analysis of vascular lesions of the temporal bone and skull base. Am J Otol 14:56–62, 1993.

12. Parker GD, Harnsberger HR: Clinical-radiologic issues in perineural tumor spread of malignant diseases of the extracranial head and neck. Radiographics 11:383–399, 1991.

13. Pernicone JR, Siebert JE, Laird TA, et al: Determination of blood flow direction using velocity-phase image display with 3-D phase-contrast MR angiography. AJNR 13:1435–1438, 1992.

14. Lustrin ES, Robertson RL, Tilak S: Normal anatomy of the skull base. Neuroimaging Clin North Am 4:465–478, 1994.

15. Koch BL, Ball WS Jr: Congenital malformations causing skull base changes. Neuroimaging Clin North Am 4:479–498, 1994.

16. Naidich TP, E OR, Bauer BS, et al: Embryology and congenital lesions of the midface. In: Som PM, Bergeron RT, eds. Head and Neck Imaging. 2nd ed. St. Louis: Mosby–Year Book, 1991, pp 1–50.

17. Ginsberg LE, Pruett SW, Chen MYM, Elster AD: Skull-base foramina of the middle cranial fossa: reassessment of normal variation with high-resolution CT. AJNR 15:283–291, 1994.

18. Kaplan SB, Kemp SS, Oh KS: Radiographic manifestations of congenital anomalies of the skull. Radiol Clin North Am 29:195–218, 1991.

19. Pollock JA, Newton TH, Hoyt WF: Transsphenoidal and transethmoidal encephaloceles: a review of clinical and Roentgen findings in eight cases. Radiology 90:442–453, 1968.

20. Nager GT: Cephaloceles. Laryngoscope 97:77–84, 1987.

21. Barkovich AJ, Vandermarck P, Edwards MSB, Cogen PH: Congenital nasal masses: CT and MR imaging features in 16 cases. AJNR 12:105–116, 1991.

22. Holt JF: Neurofibromatosis in children. AJR 130:615–639, 1978.

23. Hamlin JA, Hasso AN: Magnetic resonance imaging of the skull base. Top Magn Reson Imaging 6:183–201, 1994.

24. Ojemann RG: Meningiomas: clinical features and surgical management. In: Wilkins RH, Rengachary SS, eds. Neurosurgery. New York: McGraw-Hill, 1985, pp 635–654.

25. Hoye SJ, Hoar CS, Murray JE: Extracranial meningioma presenting as a tumor of the neck. Am J Surg 100:486, 1960.

26. Elster AD, Challa VR, Gilbert TH, et al: Meningiomas: MR and histopathologic features. Radiology 170:857–862, 1989.

27. Goldsher D, Litt AW, Pinto RS, et al: Dural "tail" associated with meningiomas on Gd-DTPA-enhanced MR images: characteristics, differential diagnostic value, and possible implications for treatment. Radiology 176:447–450, 1990.

28. Schorner W, Schubeus P, Henkes H, et al: "Meningeal sign": a characteristic finding of meningiomas on contrast-enhanced MR images. Neuroradiology 32:90–93, 1990.

29. Kutcher TJ, Brown DC, Maurer PK, Ghead VN: Dural tail adjacent to acoustic neuroma: MR features. J Comput Assist Tomogr 15:669–670, 1991.

30. Tien RD, Yang PJ, Chu PK: "Dural tail sign": a specific MR sign for meningioma? J Comput Assist Tomogr 15:64–66, 1991.

31. Li C, Yousem DM, Hayden RE, Doty RL: Olfactory neuroblastoma: MR evaluation. AJNR 14:1167–1171, 1993.

32. Mills SE, Frierson HF: Olfactory neuroblastoma: a clinicopathologic study of 21 cases. Am J Surg Pathol 9:317–327, 1985.

33. Derdeyn CP, Moran CJ, Wippold FJ, et al: MRI of esthesioneuroblastoma. J Comput Assist Tomogr 18:16–21, 1994.

34. Som PM, Dillon WP, Sze G, et al: Benign and malignant sinonasal lesions with intracranial extension: differentiation with MR imaging. Radiology 172:763–766, 1989.

35. Regenbogen VS, Zinreich SJ, Kim KS, et al: Hyperostotic esthesioneuroblastoma: CT and MR findings. J Comput Assist Tomogr 12:52–56, 1988.

36. Heffelfinger MJ, Dahlin DC, MacCarty CS, Beabout JW: Chordomas and cartilaginous tumors at the skull base. Cancer 32:410–414, 1973.

37. Weber AL, McKenna MJ: Radiologic evaluation of the jugular foramen. Neuroimaging Clin North Am 4:579–598, 1994.

38. Bourgouin PM, Tampieri D, Robitaille Y: Low-grade myxoid chondrosarcoma of the base of the skull: CT, MR, and histopathology. J Comput Assist Tomogr 16:268–273, 1992.

39. Rosenberg AE, Brown GA, Bhan AK, Lee JM: Chondroid chordoma—a variant of chordoma. A morphologic and immunohistochemical study. Am J Clin Pathol 101:36–41, 1994.

40. Forsyth PA, Cascino TL, Shaw EG, et al: Intracranial chordomas: a clinicopathological and prognostic study of 51 cases. J Neurosurg 78:741–747, 1993.

41. Meyers SP, Hirsch WL, Curtin HD: Chordomas of the skull base: MR features. AJNR 13:1627–1636, 1992.

42. Sze G, Uichanco LS III, Brant-Zawadzki MN, et al: Chordomas: MR imaging. Radiology 166:187–191, 1988.

43. Burke BB, Hoffman HT, Baker SR, et al: Chondrosarcoma of the head and neck. Laryngoscope 100:1301–1305, 1990.

44. Dahlin DC, MacCarty CS: Chordoma—a study of fifty-nine cases. Cancer 6:1170–1178, 1952.

45. Ruark DS, Schlenhaider UK, Shah JP: Chondrosarcomas of the head and neck. World J Surg 16:1010–1016, 1992.

46. Lee YY, Van Tassel PV: Craniofacial chondrosarcomas: imaging findings in 15 untreated cases. AJNR 10:165–170, 1989.

47. Lee YY, Van Tassel P, Raymond AK: Intracranial dural chondrosarcoma. AJNR 9:1189–1193, 1988.

48. Brown E, Hug EB, Weber AL: Chondrosarcoma of the skull base. Neuroimaging Clin North Am 4:529–541, 1994.

49. Grossman RI, Davis KR: Cranial computed tomographic assessment of chondrosarcoma of the base of the skull. Radiology 141:403–408, 1981.

50. Meyers SP, Hirsch WL Jr, Curtin HD, et al: Chondrosarcomas of the skull base: MR imaging features. Radiology 184:103–108, 1992.

51. Johnson DE, Woodruff WW, Allen IS, et al: MR imaging of the sellar and juxtasellar regions. Radiographics 11:727–758, 1991.

52. Scotti G, Tu C-Y, Dillon WP, et al: MR imaging of cavernous sinus involvement by pituitary adenomas. AJNR 9:657–664, 1998.

53. Russell DS, Rubenstein LJ: Pathology of Tumors of the Nervous System. 5th ed. Baltimore: Williams & Wilkins, 1989.

54. Felsberg GJ, Tien RD: Sellar and juxtrasellar lesion involving the skull base. Neuroimaging Clin North Am 4:543–560, 1994.

55. Daniels DL, Schenck JF, Foster T, et al: Magnetic resonance imaging of the jugular foramen. AJNR 6:699–703, 1985.

56. Daniels DL, Czervionke LF, Pech P, et al: Gradient recalled echo MR imaging of the jugular foramen. AJNR 9:675–678, 1988.

57. Remley KB, Harnsberger HR, Jacobs JM, Smoker WRK: Radiologic evaluation of pulsatile tinnitus and the vascular tympanic membrane. Semin Ultrasound CT MR 10:236–250, 1989.

58. Remley KB, Coit WE, Harnsberger HR, et al: Pulsatile tinnitus and the vascular tympanic membrane: CT, MR, and angiographic findings. Radiology 174:383–389, 1990.

59. Swartz JD, Harnsberger HR: Temporal bone vascular anatomy, anomalies, and diseases emphasizing the clinical-radiologic problem of pulsatile tinnitus. In: Imaging of the Temporal Bone. 2nd ed. New York: Thieme Medical Publishers, 1992, pp 154–191.

60. Burger PC, Scheithauer BW, Vogel FS: Surgical Pathology of the Nervous System and Its Coverings. 3rd ed. New York: Churchill Livingstone, 1991, pp 398–405.

61. Mulkens TH, Parizel PM, Martin JJ, et al: Acoustic schwannoma: MR findings in 84 tumors. AJR 160:395–398, 1993.

62. Harnsberger HR: Handbook of Head and Neck Imaging. 2nd ed. St. Louis: Mosby–Year Book, 1995, pp 522–542.

63. O'Donoghue GM, Brackman DE, House JW, Jackler RK: Neuromas of the facial nerve. Am J Otol 10:49–54, 1989.

64. Latack JT, Hutchinson RJ, Heyn RM: Imaging of rhabdomyosarcomas of the head and neck. AJNR 8:353–359, 1987.

65. May M: The Facial Nerve. New York: Thieme Medical Publishers, 1986.

66. Remley KB, Harnsberger HR, Smoker WRK, Osborn AG: CT and MRI in the evaluation of glossopharyngeal, vagal, and spinal accessory neuropathy. Semin Ultrasound CT MR 8:284–300, 1987.

67. Larson TC, Reese DF, Baker HL: Glomus tympanicum chemodectomas: radiographic and clinical characteristics. Radiology 163:801–806, 1987.

68. Olsen WL, Dillon WP, Kelly WM, et al: MR imaging of paragangliomas. AJNR 7:1039–1042, 1986.

69. Mukerju SK, Kasper ME, Tart RP, Mancuso AA: Irradiated paragangliomas of the head and neck: CT and MR appearance. AJNR 15:357–363, 1994.

70. Smith PG, Leonette JP, Kletzker GR: Differential clinical and radiographic features of cholesterol granulomas and cholesteatomas of the petrous apex. Ann Otol Rhinol Laryngol 97:599–604, 1988.

71. Martin N, Sterkers O, Mompoint D, et al: Cholesterol granulomas of the middle ear cavities: MR imaging. Radiology 172:521–525, 1989.

72. Mafee MF: MRI and CT in the evaluation of acquired and congenital cholesteatomas of the middle ear. J Otolaryngol 22:239–248, 1993.

72a. Robert Y, Carcasset S, Rocourt N, et al: Congenital cholesteatoma of the temporal bone: MR findings and comparison with CT. AJNR 16:755–762, 1995.

73. Neel HB III: Juvenile angiofibroma: review of 120 cases. Am J Surg 126:547–556, 1973.

74. Lloyd GAS, Phelps PD: Juvenile angiofibroma: imaging by magnetic resonance, CT and conventional techniques. Clin Otolaryngol 11:247–259, 1986.

75. Dillon WP: The pharynx and oral cavity. In: Som PM, Bergeron RT, eds. Head and Neck Imaging. 2nd ed. St. Louis: Mosby–Year Book, 1991, pp 407–466.

76. Teresi LM, Lufkin RB, Vinuela F, et al: MR imaging of the nasopharynx and floor of the middle cranial fossa. Part II. Malignant tumors. Radiology 164:817–821, 1987.

77. Laine FJ, Braun IF, Jensen ME, et al: Perineural tumor extension through the foramen ovale: evaluation with MR imaging. Radiology 174:65–71, 1990.

78. Som PM, Lawson W, Lidov MW: Simulated aggressive skull base erosion in response to benign sinonasal disease. Radiology 180:755–759, 1991.

79. Tefft M, Fernandez C, Donaldson M, et al: Incidence of meningeal involvement by rhabdomyosarcoma of the head and neck in children. Cancer 42:253–258, 1978.

80. Yousem DM, Lexa FJ, Bilaniuk LT, Zimmerman RI: Rhabdomyosarcomas in the head and neck: MR imaging evaluation. Radiology 177:683–686, 1990.

81. DePena CA, Van Tassel P, Lee YY: Lymphoma of the head and neck. Radiol Clin North Am 28:723–743, 1990.

82. Han MH, Chang KH, Kim IO, et al: Non-Hodgkin lymphoma of the central skull base: MR manifestations. J Comput Assist Tomogr 17:567–571, 1993.

83. Lanzieri CF, Shah M, Krauss D, Lavertu P: Use of gadolinium-enhanced MR imaging for differentiating mucoceles from neoplasms in the paranasal sinuses. Radiology 178:425–428, 1991.

84. Ginsberg LE: Neoplastic diseases affecting the central skull base: CT and MR imaging. AJR 159:581–589, 1992.

85. Okada Y, Aoki S, Barkovich AJ, et al: Cranial bone marrow in children: assessment of normal development with MR imaging. Radiology 171:161–164, 1989.

86. Applegate GR, Hirsch WL, Applegate LJ, Curtin HD: Variability in the enhancement of the normal central skull base in children. Neuroradiology 34:217–221, 1992.

87. Kimura F, Kim KS, Friedman H, et al: MR imaging of the normal and abnormal clivus. AJNR 11:1015–1021, 1990.

88. Vogler JB, Murphy WA: Bone marrow imaging. Radiology 168:679–693, 1988.

89. Batsakis JG: Nerves and neurotropic carcinomas. Ann Otol Rhinol Laryngol 94:426–427, 1985.

90. Ruelle A, Pisani R, Andrioli G: "Unusual" MRI appearance of sphenoid sinus mucocele. Neuroradiology 33:352–353, 1991.

91. Van Tassel P, Lee Y-Y, Jong BS, DePena CA: Mucoceles of the paranasal sinuses: MR imaging with CT correlation. AJNR 10:607–612, 1989.

92. Som PM, Dillon WP, Fullerton GD, et al: Chronically obstructed sinonasal secretions: observations on T1 and T2 shortening. Radiology 172:515–520, 1989.

93. Som PM, Dillon WP, Curtin HD, et al: Hypointense paranasal sinus foci: differential diagnosis with MRI and relation to CT findings. Radiology 176:777–781, 1990.

94. Press GA, Weindling SM, Hesselink JR, et al: Rhinocerebral mucormycosis: MR manifestations. J Comput Assist Tomogr 12:744–749, 1988.

95. Zinreich SJ, Kennedy DW, Malat J, et al: Fungal sinusitis: diagnosis with CT and MR imaging. Radiology 169:439–444, 1988.

96. Benecke JE Jr: Management of osteomyelitis of the skull base. Laryngoscope 99:1220–1223, 1989.

97. Murray ME, Britton J: Osteomyelitis of the skull base: the role of high resolution CT in diagnosis. Clin Radiol 49:408–411, 1994.

98. Chandler JR, Grobman L, Quencer R, Serafini A: Osteomyelitis of the base of the skull. Laryngoscope 96:245–251, 1986.

99. Malone DG, O'Boynick PL, Ziegler DK, et al: Osteomyelitis of the skull base. Neurosurgery 30:426–431, 1992.

100. Grobman LR, Ganz W, Casiano R, Goldberg S: Atypical osteomyelitis of the skull base. Laryngoscope 99:671–676, 1989.

101. Sie KCY, Glenn MG, Hillel AH, Cummings CW: Osteomyelitis of the skull base, etiology unknown. Otolaryngol Head Neck Surg 104:252–256, 1991.

102. Menachof MR, Jackler RK: Otogenic skull base osteomyelitis caused by invasive fungal infection. Otolaryngol Head Neck Surg 102:285–289, 1990.

102a. Grandis JR, Curtin HD, Yu VL: Necrotizing (malignant) external otitis: prospective comparison of CT and MR imaging in diagnosis and follow-up. Radiology 196:499–504, 1995.

103. Martin N, Sterkers O, Hahum H: Chronic inflammatory disease of the middle ear cavities: Gd-DTPA–enhanced MR imaging. Radiology 176:399–405, 1990.

104. Kaseff LG, Siedenwurm DJ, Nissen AH, et al: Endaural encephalocele: CT and MR imaging. Am J Otol 13:1–4, 1992.

105. Janecka IP: Surgical approaches to the skull base. Neuroimaging Clin North Am 4:639–656, 1994.

Paranasal Sinuses and Nasal Cavity

CHARLES F. LANZIERI

Diseases of the sinonasal tract include inflammatory and neoplastic processes, but for the most part sinonasal pathology takes the form of acute inflammatory diseases and seasonal allergies. The vast majority of these afflictions are well handled by the primary care physician. When patients present for consultation with head and neck surgeons for sinonasal complaints, and after unsuccessful medical therapy, imaging of the paranasal sinuses and nasal cavity may be undertaken.[1, 2] Traditionally, the initial examination of patients with sinonasal complaints consists of plain radiographs. In the era of low-cost spiral computed tomography (CT) it may not be long before the initial imaging evaluation of the paranasal sinuses becomes CT. CT is a mature modality in terms of the imaging physician's understanding of the findings seen by CT. Because we have relied on CT for so long and are familiar and comfortable with the CT manifestations of various pathologic conditions and normal variations, this remains the imaging modality of choice when first imaging patients with sinonasal complaints. Significant information is obtained with the initial imaging modality when it is properly performed and interpreted. CT of the paranasal sinuses remains the most cost-effective way to progress along the imaging algorithm.

In most instances no further imaging is necessary except for follow-up examination to gauge further medical therapy. CT continues to serve as the standard examination for the sinuses and is preferred by head and neck surgeons in the planning of functional endoscopic sinus surgery. In addition, stereotactic algorithms are based on CT of the paranasal sinuses. The intricate anatomy and minute structures that must be addressed during functional endoscopic sinus surgery continue to be best demonstrated by CT.

The role of magnetic resonance imaging (MRI) in the diagnosis and treatment of pathologic conditions of the sinonasal cavity can take one of several forms. One of the most important goals of MRI examination of the sinonasal cavity is to judge the extent of disease. Whereas CT can easily demonstrate opacification of the paranasal sinuses and erosion of underlying bone, MRI may show extension of inflammatory or neoplastic processes intracranially or into the soft tissues surrounding the paranasal sinuses. Changes in the marrow signal within the diploic space are also important findings for the staging of disease. Early staging by means of changes in the marrow signal is best achieved with MRI. Perineural extension of inflammatory or neoplastic processes is also best appreciated by MRI examination.

Apart from judging the extent of and staging diseases of the paranasal sinuses, tissue characterization can be performed through an analysis of relaxation characteristics as well as enhancement characteristics. For example, it is possible, with a reasonable degree of medical certainty, to identify neoplastic, inflammatory, or postoperative changes in the paranasal sinuses and nasal cavity through an analysis of the pulse sequences.

NORMAL ANATOMY AND ANATOMIC VARIATIONS[1–3]

Approximately 2 L of water is produced daily by the serous glands of the sinonasal cavity, which serve to moisturize and filter the air. The surface mucosa produces mucus, which traps larger particles. Cilia transport the mucus and particulate matter into the nasopharynx at approximately 1 cm/min. The nasal mucosa is a vascular pseudostratified ciliated columnar epithelium. The most superior portion of the nasal fossa is less well vascularized and nonciliated. This is the olfactory mucosa. It contains the efferent axons of the bipolar olfactory nerve fibers that transform the physical stimuli of odors into nerve impulses, which are then transmitted through the cribriform plate onto the olfactory gyri. A special lipoprotein is secreted by this mucosa. This lipoprotein is necessary for the dissolution of the odors so that they can be transmitted to the bipolar neurons. There is no ciliary action within the olfactory mucosa, so "sniffing" is necessary to bring the fragrance-bearing material to the olfactory recess.

The medial wall of each nasal cavity, the nasal sep-

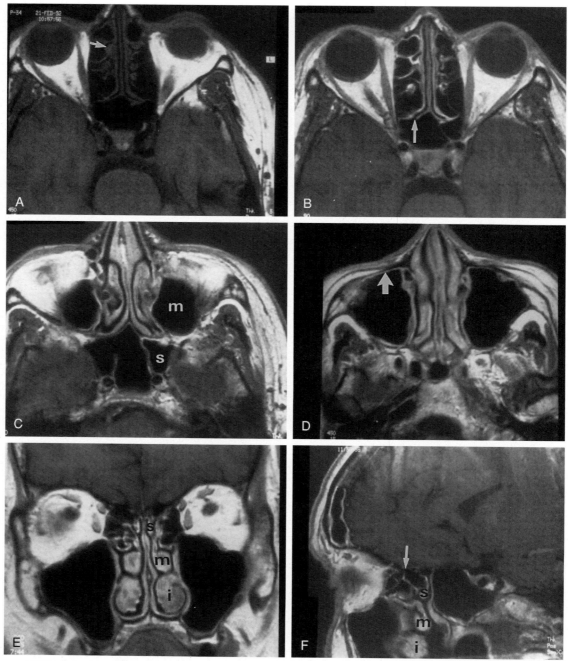

FIGURE 33–1. Normal anatomy. *A,* Non–contrast-enhanced axial image through the ethmoid air cells. The thin bony septa and covering mucosa are seen as curvilinear structures that are isointense relative to brain. Small retention cysts, polyps, or neoplasms are also isointense on T1-weighted images *(arrow). B,* Contrast-enhanced axial images through the ethmoid air cells. The mucoperiosteum is normally enhanced and exhibits a thin white line. Interruptions in this white line may represent sinus ostia. The natural ostium of the right sphenoid sinus is demonstrated *(arrow). C,* Axial contrast-enhanced image through the orbital floors. The maxillary sinus (m) and sphenoid sinus (s) can be seen. The thin mucoperiosteal white line of the maxillary sinus is not visualized when it abuts orbital fat laterally. The white line can be seen more medially. The mucoperiosteal white line of the sphenoid sinus is also obliterated anteriorly where it encounters marrow of the skull base, whereas more medially the thin enhanced white line can be seen. *D,* Contrast-enhanced axial image through the maxillary sinuses. The normal thin mucoperiosteal white line can be seen separated from the marrow fat by the inner table *(arrow).* Note the normal turbinate and septal enhancement seen within the nasal fossa here and in *E. E,* Contrast-enhanced coronal image through the nasal fossa and maxillary sinuses. The superior (s), middle (m), and inferior (i) turbinates are demonstrated. These are enhanced similarly to the right-sided turbinates. Some patients have alternate engorgement and disgorgement of blood from the turbinate submucosa. This may be visualized as alternate swelling and increased enhancement of the turbinates and should not be confused with a pathologic process. *F,* Oblique sagittal image through the paranasal sinuses and nasal fossa after injection of contrast material. The superior middle and inferior turbinates are labeled. The arrow indicates posterior ethmoid air cells that drain into the superior meatus between the superior and middle turbinates. Normal mucosal enhancement is visualized in the frontal sinus.

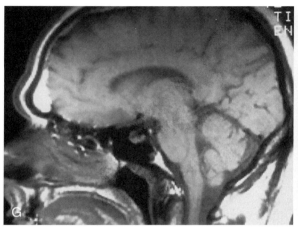
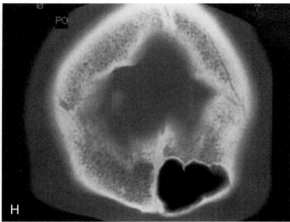

FIGURE 33–1 *Continued G,* This sagittal T1-weighted image through the brain demonstrates a normal variation of nonpneumatization of the frontal sinuses on the right side with replacement of the diploic space by fatty marrow. *H,* A coronal CT scan through the same patient's frontal bone confirms the presence of nonpneumatization and replacement of the diploic space by normal marrow.

tum, is partially bony, made up of the perpendicular plate of the ethmoid bone and the vomer. The more anterior inferior portion of the nasal septum is cartilaginous. On clinical examination of the nasal septum, this structure is nearly always in the midline, and if not in the midline it is considered contributory to obstructive symptoms in the ipsilateral nasal cavity. On imaging studies, on the other hand, deviation of the nasal septum is the rule rather than the exception. The junction of the bony nasal septum and cartilaginous nasal septum is often accompanied by a marked deviation from the midline toward one middle turbinate process or the other. This can result in narrowing of the ipsilateral middle meatus and secondary obstructive symptoms (Fig. 33–1). The lateral wall of the nasal fossa is extremely complex compared with the simple anatomy of the nasal septum. The ostium for each paranasal sinus opens into the nasal fossa along the lateral wall, which is separated into three or four fossae or meatus by three or four nasal turbinates or conchae. The nasal sinuses develop from outpouchings along the lateral nasal wall, which occur and extend laterally and superiorly in a predictable pattern. Therefore, the drainage pattern is also quite predictable. The frontal, anterior ethmoid, and maxillary sinuses nearly always drain between the middle and inferior nasal turbinates into the middle meatus. The posterior ethmoids most commonly drain between the superior and middle turbinates or superior meatus. The sphenoid sinus usually drains between the superior and supreme turbinates or the superior meatus, but it may also drain directly into the most superior and posterior portion of the nasal cavity, called the sphenoethmoidal recess.

In terms of functional endoscopic sinus surgery, it is most useful to think of each of these groupings of sinuses and their respective meatus as a single unit. The middle meatus, also called the ostiomeatal unit, is the grouping most frequently involved with inflammatory processes. This is largely due to the numerous anatomic variations that may affect the middle meatus and, therefore, the drainage of mucus from the fron-

tal, anterior ethmoid, and maxillary sinuses. Anatomic variations that affect the middle meatus include deviation of the nasal septum, as previously mentioned, and dilatation of the middle turbinate caused by pneumatization (concha bullosa). The middle turbinate itself may assume a reverse curve from its normal orientation. This configuration, an anatomic variant, is known as a paradoxical middle turbinate and may narrow the middle meatus. Anterior and inferiorly displaced ethmoid air cells may narrow the natural ostium of the maxillary sinus. These are known as agger nasi cells.

Although the normal pneumatization of the facial bones by the paranasal sinus outpouchings is predictable, it is not always identical in different individuals. Several anatomic variants are due to aberrant pneumatization of the facial bones by paranasal sinuses other than those that normally aerate these bones. For example, an anterior ethmoid air cell may extend superiorly into the frontal sinus. This configuration is easily recognized on both plain radiographs and CT scans and is known as a supraorbital ethmoid air cell. The agger nasi cell is another example of an aberrant paranasal sinus. In functional endoscopic sinus surgery, these changes are important when attempting to reestablish a normal drainage pattern through the nasal fossa.

In a large portion of the population (80% to 90%), there is an alternating pattern of increased production of nasal secretions and shunting of blood into the vascular mucosa of the inferior and middle turbinates. As this happens, the swelling of the turbinates and mucous secretions partly obstruct airflow through the nasal fossa. The nonfunctioning side of the nasal fossa retains secretions and the submucosa becomes edematous, while the functioning side carries the majority of inspired and expired air. The frequency of this nasal cycle varies between 30 minutes and several hours. It is important to bear in mind the existence of the nasal cycle in a large portion of the population when interpreting studies, especially MRI examinations, of the paranasal sinuses, because normally engorged turbinates can be mistaken for inflammatory or neoplastic processes.

The vascular supply to the nasal fossa and sinonasal tract involves branches of both the internal and external carotid arteries. The sphenopalatine division or the terminal branches of the internal maxillary artery, a branch of the external carotid artery, are the most important participants in the arterial supply to this region of the face. As the internal maxillary artery exits the pterygopalatine fossa, it divides into two primary parts. The posterolateral nasal branch gives rise to the nasal arteries, which ramify over the turbinates before providing collateral circulation to the paranasal sinuses. The posterior septal branch is commonly regarded as an extension of the sphenopalatine artery and extends medially along the roof of the nasal cavity, giving branches to the posterior portion of the nasal septum via the posterior septal arteries. These are terminal branches. The termination of the posterior septal arteries and the anterior portion of the nasal septum continues as the nasopalatine artery, which exits the incisive canal and anastomoses with the greater palatine artery.

The lymphatic drainage from the anterior portion of the sinuses and nasal cavity is into the anterior lymphatics within the face and finally into the submandibular group of lymph nodes (level I nodes). The posterior half of the sinonasal cavity and nasopharynx drain into the retropharyngeal and internal jugular lymph node chains (level II nodes).

The venous drainage from the sinonasal cavity is into the facial vein in the anterior portion of the face, which then anastomoses with the common facial vein and drains blood into the internal jugular vein. There is a good anastomosis with the ophthalmic vein, which drains into the pterygopalatine venous plexus and then to the cavernous sinus or into the cavernous sinus directly. Infection in the sinonasal cavity can rapidly gain access to the cavernous sinus and cranial cavity.

Supply from the internal carotid artery to the paranasal sinuses is via the ophthalmic artery. Anterior and posterior ethmoidal arteries extend superiorly and superomedially, sending branches through the cribriform plate to anastomose with the nasal branch of the sphenopalatine artery. An important anastomotic region known as Little's area or Kiesselbach's area is located anteriorly and inferiorly on the nasal septum. This is supplied by multiple branches of the facial artery, sphenopalatine artery, and greater palatine artery and is the site of the majority of epistaxes.

MRI PROTOCOL FOR THE PARANASAL SINUSES

Any protocol for MRI of the paranasal sinuses should include a pulse sequence that provides good contrast resolution between free water and bound water. At many sites, T2-weighted images serve this purpose. Because of bulk susceptibility artifact from adjacent osseous structures and dental amalgam, gradient-echo images are usually unsatisfactory for imaging

the paranasal sinuses. In the interest of saving scanner time, rapid-acquisition T2-weighted images or turbo T2-weighted images may be useful. These types of pulse sequences fill the k-space more rapidly than pulse sequences for normally reconstructed images and shorten imaging time.

A properly designed protocol should pay particular attention to the skull base and skull base foramina. Thin coronal sections through the orbits and sella as well as the cavernous sinus region are useful for evaluating invasion of these structures by paranasal sinus disease and for evaluating extension of disease from these structures into the paranasal sinuses.

Contrast-enhanced images have been shown to be quite useful in differentiating inflammatory from neoplastic processes within the paranasal sinuses, and acquisition of both non–contrast-enhanced and contrast-enhanced T1-weighted images in several planes is recommended.

In summary, a good examination of the paranasal sinuses includes T1- and T2-weighted images in multiple planes as well as contrast-enhanced T1-weighted images. Special attention must be paid to the skull base and basilar foramina.

PATHOLOGY

INFLAMMATORY PROCESSES[1, 3, 4]

The hallmark of inflammatory processes within the paranasal sinuses is increased sinonasal secretions (Fig. 33–2). The secretions formed within the paranasal sinuses are in equilibrium with interstitial fluids. About 95% of sinonasal secretions consists of water and 5% consists of macromolecular proteins, the majority being mucous glycoproteins. When sufficient sinonasal secretions accumulate in the paranasal sinuses, they are manifested as opacification of sinuses, which is of intermediate signal intensity on T1-weighted images and high signal intensity on T2-weighted images. As many as one third of all acute sinus processes become chronic processes. When sinonasal secretions remain trapped in one of the paranasal sinuses, dehydration occurs and there is a relative increase in the protein concentration. Thus, the secretions evolve from a primarily serous to a predominantly mucous composition. Ultimately, chronic secretions may become completely dehydrated. The change in free water content of chronic sinonasal secretions affects the signal characteristics (Table 33–1). In general, the more chronic the inflammatory process, the less well hydrated the secretions and the lower the signal intensity on T2-weighted images (Fig. 33–3). Although the signal changes associated with varying degrees of dehydration have been well demonstrated, it is not possible to predict with certainty how rapidly these changes occur in an individual sinus or individual patient.[5, 6]

The mucosa of the paranasal sinuses reacts to chronic inflammatory processes in a number of ways. In general, there is hypertrophy of the sinus mucosa with resulting polypoid mucosal thickening. Atrophic

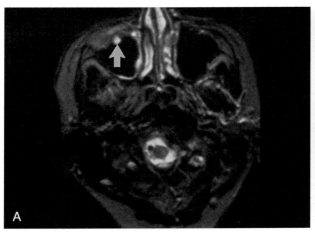
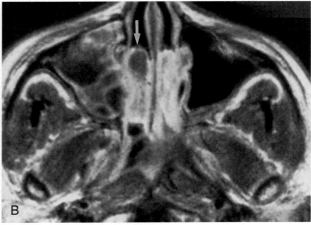
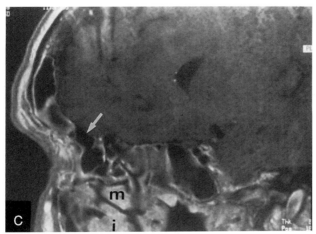

FIGURE 33–2. Inflammatory processes. *A,* T2-weighted axial image through the paranasal sinuses. A small retention cyst or polyp is present in the right maxillary sinus *(arrow).* Retention cysts, polyps, and sinus secretions are typically bright on T2-weighted images, matching cerebrospinal fluid. *B,* Contrast-enhanced axial image through the nasal fossa and maxillary sinuses. A nasal polyp is demonstrated within the right nasal cavity. This exhibits typical nonenhanced central stroma and curvilinear surface enhancement *(arrow).* The ipsilateral right maxillary sinus is filled with retention cysts or polyps. When these opacify, the maxillary sinus curvilinear enhanced mucosa meets and forms a network of lines within the maxillary sinus. *C,* Oblique sagittal image through the paranasal sinuses. The middle turbinate (m) and inferior turbinate (i) are labeled. The frontal sinus may drain either through the nasal frontal duct directly into the middle meatus or into an anterior ethmoid air cell *(arrow).* A retention cyst or polyp is identified within the dependent portion of the frontal sinus. The typical nonenhanced stroma and enhanced surface are visualized. This chronic inflammatory change may lead to obstruction of the frontal sinus.

sinus mucosa as well as fibrotic change may also coexist with areas of acutely inflamed sinus mucosa. Both the redundant mucosa, which forms intrasinus polyps, and the obstructed glands, which form intrasinus retention cysts, contain interstitial fluid. Polyps and retention cysts have the same bright signal on T2-weighted images and are indistinguishable. After contrast agent injection, T1-weighted images reveal linear enhancement on the surfaces of retention cysts or polyps. Acute

and chronically inflamed mucosa may be thickened with enhancement throughout. Although subtle bone changes accompany chronic sinus inflammation, these findings are difficult to appreciate on MR images. This clue to a chronic inflammatory process is much better appreciated with CT. Another pitfall of MRI of chronic inflammatory processes is related to inspissated secretions that have nearly completely lost their free water content. Because of the lack of free water, such secre-

TABLE 33–1. IMAGING CHARACTERISTICS OF OPACIFIED SINUSES

ENTITY	T1-WEIGHTED IMAGING	T2-WEIGHTED IMAGING	T1-WEIGHTED IMAGING WITH GADOLINIUM	CT	CT WITH CONTRAST AGENT
Secretions					
Acute	—	↑	—	↓	—
Subacute	↓	↑ ↑	—	—	—
Chronic	↓	↓	—	—‖—	—
Fungus	↓	↓ ↓	0	↑	0
Hemorrhage					
<24 h	↓	↓ ↓	0	—	0
>24 h	↑	↑	0	↑	0
Cyst	—	↑ ↑	+ linear	—	0
Polyp	—	↑ ↑	+ linear	—	0
Mucocele					
Acute	—	↑	+ linear	↓	0
Chronic	↑ ↓	↑ ↓	+ linear	↓	0
Mass	—	—	+ solid	—	+ solid

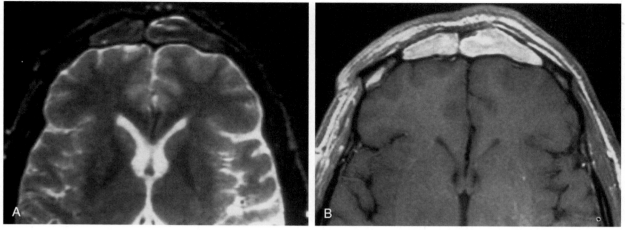

FIGURE 33–3. Retained sinus secretions. *A,* T2-weighted axial image through the frontal sinuses. The opacified frontal sinuses have decreased signal intensity, indicating the presence of dehydrated sinus secretions, hemorrhage, or fungal infection. *B,* Contrast-enhanced T1-weighted image. There is enhancement within the frontal sinuses bilaterally. This pattern of enhancement may be due to multiple small polyps, neoplasm, or a fibroosseous lesion with vascular stroma. In the present example, thick inflamed mucoperiosteum was found within the frontal sinuses at surgery.

tions may produce a signal void on both T1- and T2-weighted images and may be mistaken for a well-aerated paranasal sinus. Again, CT should be employed if there is any suspicion of intrasinus secretions with low signal intensity (Table 33–2).

It should be emphasized that although the MRI changes associated with acute and chronic inflammatory processes of the paranasal sinuses must be understood by the imaging physician, CT is probably the imaging modality of choice for first diagnosing and following inflammatory processes. The pitfalls of MRI, as well as the added expense of the modality and the contrast material, makes CT the imaging modality of choice.

Mucoceles[7]

When a chronically obstructed paranasal sinus becomes completely filled with hypertrophied mucosa and secretions, an impending mucocele may be present. Further elaboration of secretions and hypertrophy of mucosa eventually cause remodeling of the osseous walls of the paranasal sinuses. A secondary mass effect may affect the orbits, facial appearance, and intracranial contents. The majority of mucoceles occur in the frontal sinuses. The ethmoid and maxillary sinus mucoceles together constitute about one third of all mucoceles. A small percentage occur in the sphenoid sinuses. The signal characteristics of the contents of a mucocele are varied, again according to the protein concentration of the secretions. The role of MRI for

mucoceles is to assess the extension into orbital or intracranial structures and to evaluate for the presence of a neoplastic process. Mucoceles tend to be fairly bright on T1-weighted images compared with the adjacent brain and have decreased signal intensity on T2-weighted images compared with cerebrospinal fluid. Neoplastic processes tend to be isointense relative to brain on both T1- and T2-weighted images. Furthermore, when an intravenous contrast agent is given, mucoceles are enhanced on their periphery because of the remaining, active mucoperiosteum[8] (Fig. 33–4).

Fungal Disease[9]

One possible reason for failed antibiotic therapy in chronic sinus infection is superinfection with fungus. Fungal infections of the paranasal sinuses are more common in immunocompromised patients. Free intrasinus fluid resulting in air-fluid levels, although common in acute sinus infection, is uncommon in chronic infections and uncommon in superinfection with fungi. Reactive bone thickening and bone erosion are important clues to the presence of fungal infection. These findings and other bone changes are relatively difficult to appreciate by MRI examinations. With MRI, intrasinus fungal infections appear to be of low signal intensity on both T1- and T2-weighted images. This is due to the solid composition of fungal colonies and to the presence of manganese, which is paramagnetic and bound by many fungi. Fungal infections have a propensity for venous invasion, and if there is suspicion of fungal infection, attention should be paid to dural venous sinuses such as the superior sagittal sinus and cavernous sinus. Enhancement or lack of a signal void in these regions may indicate fungal thrombophlebitis, an ominous sign (see Table 33–2).

TABLE 33–2. SINUS WITH SIGNAL VOID (T1- AND/OR T2-WEIGHTED IMAGES)

Air	Fracture fragment
Fungus	Blood
Chronic secretions	Odontogenic tumor

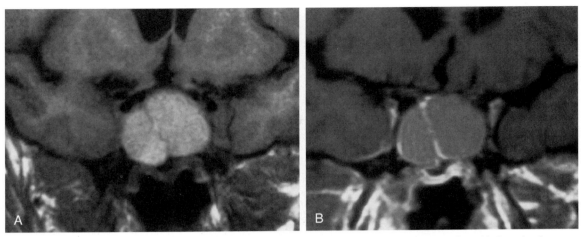

FIGURE 33–4. Mucocele. *A,* Non–contrast-enhanced T1-weighted image through the sphenoid sinus in the coronal plane. The sphenoid sinus is expanded by a mass that is bright on T1-weighted images and remained bright on T2-weighted images. This pattern of signal characteristics is consistent with a mucocele (see Table 33–1). *B,* Contrast-enhanced T1-weighted image through the sphenoid sinuses. There is mucosal enhancement. The secretions remain bright relative to the adjacent brain.

Granulomatous Diseases

The most commonly seen granulomatous process in North America is Wegener's disease. Sarcoidosis and tuberculosis, as well as nasal granulomas caused by cocaine abuse, are also seen in selected populations. On MRI examination, findings of chronic sinus infection are present. Bone destruction is seen out of proportion to the degree of mucosal involvement.

HEMORRHAGE[10, 11]

Hemorrhage into the paranasal sinuses may be secondary to trauma, vascular malformation, surgery, or neoplasm. In general, CT is employed for the traumatized patient, but one may encounter acute or chronic blood in the sinus. By using signal intensities observed on T1- and T2-weighted images, one can determine and accurately date hemorrhage within the sinus (see Table 33–1).

The same evolution of the hemoglobin molecule takes place in the sinus as in the brain, but the pace of degradation may be decelerated in the sinuses if they are not well aerated. As in the brain, intrasinus deoxyhemoglobin has a low signal intensity on both T1- and T2-weighted images. The signal intensity of intracellular methemoglobin is increased on T1- but decreased on T2-weighted images. That of extracellular methemoglobin is increased on T1- and on T2-weighted images (Fig. 33–5).

NEOPLASMS[12, 13]

Benign Lesions

Retention cysts and benign polyps are usually incidental findings in asymptomatic patients and cannot be differentiated from each other. Both are probably complications of allergic or inflammatory sinus infections in the past. These are most commonly seen in the maxillary sinuses. They are manifested as round masses that have low density on CT scans, are hypointense on T1-weighted images, and are hyperintense on T2-weighted images. There is no associated bone

FIGURE 33–5. Hemorrhage. *A,* T2-weighted axial image through the paranasal sinuses. A hemorrhage is seen in the left maxillary sinus. The peripheral bright signal represents edematous mucosa. The central bright signal represents extracellular methemoglobin. The intervening dark signal may represent the presence of deoxyhemoglobin, intracellular methemoglobin, or hemosiderin. *B,* Contrast-enhanced T1-weighted image. Peripheral enhancement of the mucosa is seen. The central bright signal has faded on T1-weighted images. This is therefore thought to represent deoxyhemoglobin and an acute sinus hemorrhage.

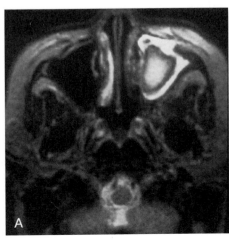
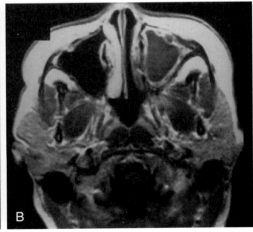

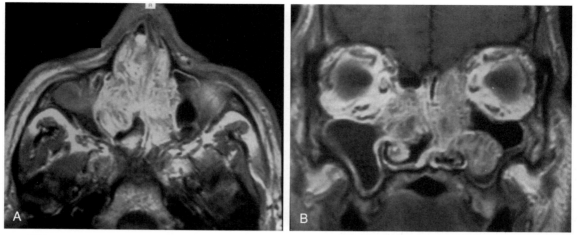

FIGURE 33–6. Inverted papilloma. Axial *(A)* and coronal *(B)* contrast-enhanced T1-weighted images through the nasal cavity and maxillary sinuses. There are bilateral enhanced masses in the nasal cavities with extension into the left maxillary sinus. The enhancement pattern is intricate with infolding of the mucosa typical of the enhancement pattern seen with inverted papilloma.

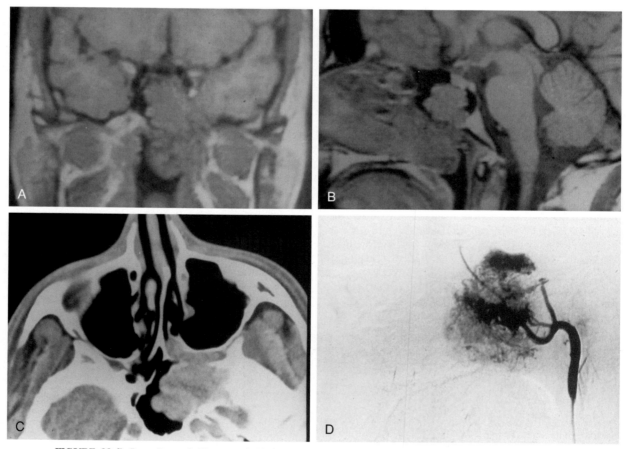

FIGURE 33–7. Juvenile angiofibroma. *A*, Non–contrast-enhanced, T1-weighted, coronal image through the nasopharynx showing a mass within the nasopharynx and right sphenoid sinus. The mass extends laterally into the skull base on the left side as well as into the lateral nasopharyngeal wall on the left side. *B*, Midline sagittal image. Again, an irregular mass is identified within the sphenoid sinus. *C*, Non–contrast-enhanced CT image through the paranasal sinuses. The left-sided sphenoid mass is again identified. The space between the maxillary sinus and pterygoid plate, the pterygopalatine fissure, is expanded by this soft tissue mass. This finding, in particular, is typical of a juvenile angiofibroma. *D*, Arterial phase from the left internal maxillary artery injection filmed in the lateral projection. The fine network of neovascularity is also typical of juvenile angiofibroma.

destruction. Polyps that are slightly hyperintense on T1-weighted images may be angiomatous polyps, and the hyperintensity is thought to represent slow flow in vascular channels. Alternatively, the fluid contents may be proteinaceous, increasing the signal intensity on T1-weighted images and slightly decreasing the intensity on T2-weighted images. Antrochoanal polyps are maxillary sinus polyps that extend through the natural ostia of the maxillary sinuses into the nasal cavity. These have homogeneous signal characteristics similar to those described for polyps. After contrast agent injection, surface enhancement of polyps is usually identified. Enhancement within the substance of the polyp itself indicates the presence of a vascular stroma and the possible presence of an angiomatous polyp. Note that internal enhancement is also one of the features of aggressive neoplastic processes or lymphoma of the paranasal sinuses. Multiple polyps are the most common expansile masses of the paranasal sinuses and nasal cavity. The term *polyposis* has been used to describe this syndrome. Skull base erosion and intracranial extension have been described. On T1- and T2-weighted images, sinonasal polyposis may mimic an aggressive inflammatory or neoplastic process. Injection of a contrast agent proves multiple polyps to be present. CT is also quite useful for demonstrating the expansile rather than destructive characteristics of the bone remodeling.

Papilloma

Epithelial papillomas of the nasal cavity are derived from the transitional epithelium of the lateral nasal wall or the nasal septum. A unilateral mass on the lateral nasal wall with an irregular surface may involve the maxillary and ethmoid sinuses. This mass is isointense on T1-weighted images and slightly hyperintense on T2-weighted images. Thick irregular enhancement is observed within papillomas (Fig. 33–6). The inverted papilloma on the lateral nasal wall is associated with degeneration into squamous cell carcinoma 10% to 15% of the time. The septal form, also known as fungiform papilloma, has no malignant potential.

Angiofibroma[3]

Angiofibroma is a common benign nasopharyngeal mass that occurs exclusively in adolescent males and presents with epistaxis, nasal obstruction, and facial deformity. It is most commonly identified in the region of the pterygopalatine fissure and may extend into the infratemporal fossa and adjacent paranasal sinuses as well as the intracranial fossa. The presence of a naso-

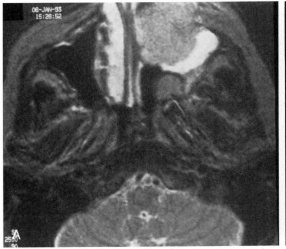
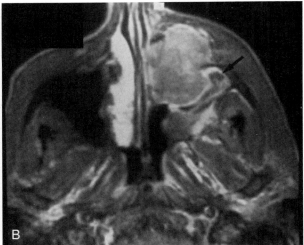
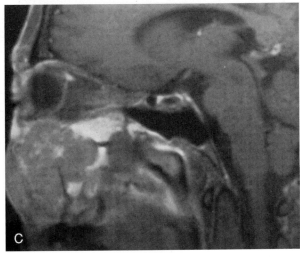

FIGURE 33–8. Squamous cell carcinoma. *A,* Axial T2-weighted image. In the left maxillary sinus is a mass that is isointense relative to the cerebellum adjacent to bright signal representing retained secretion or inflamed mucosa. Squamous cell carcinomas are typically isointense relative to brain on T2-weighted images and are thus separable from inflammatory changes. *B,* Contrast-enhanced axial image through the mass. Patchy enhancement is present in the mass itself, whereas the remaining portion of the maxillary sinus mucosa demonstrated normal mucosal enhancement *(arrow). C,* Sagittal contrast-enhanced T1-weighted image through the paranasal sinuses. Again, the mass is enhanced in a patchy pattern typical of squamous cell carcinoma. The mass can be seen extending superiorly into orbital structures.

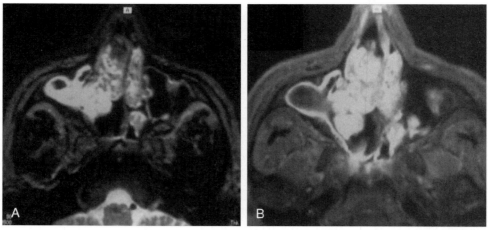

FIGURE 33–9. Adenoid cystic carcinoma. *A,* T2-weighted axial image through the nasal fossa and maxillary sinuses. The expanded inferior turbinate with a speckled bright signal represents a portion of an adenoid cystic carcinoma. The signal intensity of adenoid cystic carcinoma on T2-weighted images is increased compared with that of squamous cell carcinoma because of the mucoid secretions produced. *B,* Contrast-enhanced T1-weighted image. The normal linear enhancement of the right maxillary sinus can be seen. The solid polypoid bright enhancement of the adenoid cystic carcinoma is visualized in the right nasal cavity. This should be contrasted with the enhancement pattern of squamous cell carcinoma seen in Figure 33–8.

pharyngeal mass and widening of the pterygopalatine fossa in the presence of anterior bowing of the posterior wall of the maxillary sinus should alert the imaging physician to the presence of an angiofibroma. These lesions are inhomogeneous on T1- and T2-weighted images because of the varying velocities of blood flow within the vascular channels (Fig. 33–7; see also Fig. 34–22).

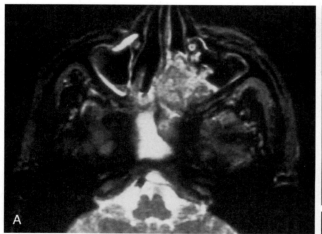

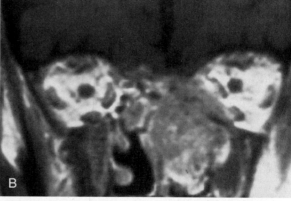

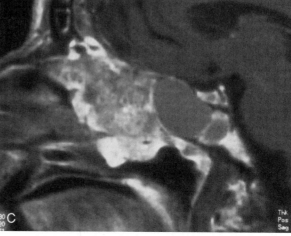

FIGURE 33–10. Olfactory neuroblastoma. *A,* T2-weighted axial image through the paranasal sinuses and nasopharynx. A nonhomogeneous mass with slightly increased signal intensity is identified within the left side of the nasal cavity. Extension is seen into the left maxillary sinus. The regions of increased signal within the mass suggest the presence of hemorrhage or a secreting tumor such as neuroblastoma or adenoid cystic carcinoma. Secondary obstruction of the right sphenoid sinus is also visualized. *B,* Coronal contrast-enhanced image through the paranasal sinuses. The patchy enhancement noted within the mass is typical of most neoplasms. There is extension toward the anterior cranial fossa with apparent violation of the anterior cranial fossa to the right of midline. Because olfactory neuroblastomas arise in the region of the olfactory mucosa, this finding is suggestive of the presence of an olfactory neuroblastoma. *C,* Contrast-enhanced sagittal image taken just to the left of midline. Again the mass is noted to be patchy in its enhancement quality. Extension to the skull base with secondary obstruction of the sphenoid sinus is seen.

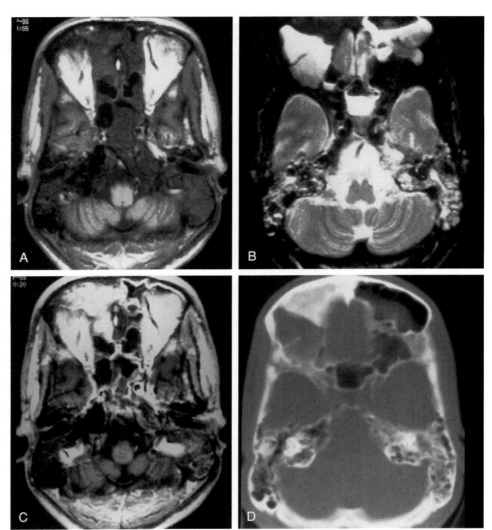

FIGURE 33–11. Fibrous dysplasia. *A,* Non–contrast-enhanced T1-weighted image. Soft tissue opacifies the right frontal sinus, both mastoid portions of the temporal bones, and the sphenoid sinus. *B,* T2-weighted axial image taken through the same levels. The mastoid and sphenoid sinuses reveal fluid within them. The right frontal sinus remains dark on T2-weighted images. This may suggest the presence of a fungal infection or neoplasm. *C,* After contrast agent injection, curvilinear enhancement is seen throughout the paranasal sinuses as well as mastoid sinuses, suggesting the presence of an inflammatory process. The right frontal sinus is enhanced in a homogeneous pattern. The summation of these findings suggests the presence of a neoplasm. *D,* Non–contrast-enhanced CT image taken through the paranasal sinuses at the same level in the axial plane. The right frontal sinus is opacified by bone. The findings illustrate the presence of fibrous dysplasia, which has decreased signal intensity on T2-weighted images and may be strongly enhanced by contrast agent injection because of the coarse network of vascular channels that is sometimes present. CT is necessary to confirm the presence of fibrous dysplasia.

Malignant Lesions[1, 3]

Squamous cell carcinoma is the most common malignancy of the sinonasal cavity. Clinical complaints include unilateral nasal obstruction and epistaxis, as well as facial pain, orbital pain, and headache. Eighty percent of squamous cell carcinomas occur in the maxillary sinus; occurrence in the sphenoid and frontal sinuses is considered rare. The hallmark of squamous cell carcinoma is bone destruction, which can be identified in 80% or more of imaging studies. Frank bone destruction as opposed to bone expansion is unusual for benign disease. Most squamous cell carcinomas are isointense relative to brain on both T1- and T2-weighted images (Fig. 33–8). After injection of a contrast agent, malignant tumors are enhanced in a salt-and-pepper pattern, reflecting alternating areas of rapid cell growth, neovascularity, and necrosis. Lymph node metastases are unusual; however, when a sinus malignancy is suspected, a thorough search should be made for lymphadenopathy in the retropharyngeal, submandibular, and high jugular lymph node chains.

Paranasal sinus malignancy may also arise from the glandular components of the mucosa. These account for approximately 10% of sinus malignancies and are best represented by the adenoid cystic carcinomas or minor salivary gland tumors (Fig. 33–9). This particular neoplasm has a propensity for perineural spread and a high recurrence rate. Other glandular-type carcinomas of the paranasal sinuses include adenocarcinoma, which is most common in the ethmoid air cells, mucoepidermoid carcinoma, and mixed tumors. Unlike squamous cell carcinomas, the glandular carcinomas have a high signal intensity on T2-weighted images and may be difficult to differentiate from benign inflammatory diseases.

Paranasal sinus lymphomas account for an additional 10% of sinus tumors. Extranodal lymphoma has increased in incidence within the paranasal sinuses with the epidemic of acquired immunodeficiency syndrome. These lesions are difficult to differentiate from squamous cell carcinomas. They tend to have a higher ratio of mass effect to bone destruction compared with the squamous cell carcinomas.

A unique malignancy of the sinonasal tract is the olfactory neuroblastoma or esthesioneuroblastoma (Fig. 33–10). This accounts for 3% of all sinonasal neoplasms and arises from the olfactory neuroepithelium at the level of the cribriform plate. There are two age peaks, with most tumors occurring between the ages of 10 and 40 years. A second peak occurs in the fifth and sixth decades. The location of a destructive mass should alert one to the presence of an esthesioneuroblastoma. Signal characteristics are similar to those of squamous cell carcinoma. Bone destruction is observed, and a moderate amount of vascularity may be manifested as a salt-and-pepper appearance on the T2-weighted images, again because of the varying velocities of blood flow within the internal vasculature (see also Chapter 32).

FIBRO-OSSEOUS LESIONS[14, 15]

Osteomas are benign bone tumors that occur most commonly in the frontal or ethmoid sinuses. These are usually incidental findings; however, spontaneous cerebrospinal fluid leakage may occur. These are difficult to identify on MR images because they produce a signal void similar to that of air. An internal marrow signal may sometimes be identified on T1-weighted images. This may lead to confusion with an intrasinus mass lesion (Fig. 33–11).

Fibrous dysplasia occurs in the paranasal sinuses. Classically, this produces a ground-glass, slightly expansile appearance on CT scans. Again, this may cause confusion and is a pitfall of MRI examination. The expansion and enhancement within the bone on MR images may raise suspicion of lymphoma or an expansile neoplastic or inflammatory mass.

REFERENCES

1. Lanzieri CF: CT/MRI of the sinonasal cavity. In: Haaga JR, Lanzieri CF, eds. CT and MR of the Entire Body. 2nd ed. New York: CV Mosby, 1994.
2. Weissman JL, Tabor EK, Curtin HD: MRI of the paranasal sinuses. Top Magn Reson Imaging 2(4):27–38, 1990.
3. Som PM: The sinonasal cavity. In: Som PM, Bergeron RT, eds. Head and Neck Imaging. 2nd ed. St. Louis: Mosby–Year Book, 1991, pp 51–277.
4. Som PM, Shaprio MD, Biller HF, et al: Sinonasal tumors and inflammatory tissues: differentiation with MR imaging. Radiology 167:803–808, 1988.
5. Som PM, Dillon WP, Fullerton GD, et al: Chronically obstructed sinonasal secretions: observations on T1 and T2 shortening. Radiology 172:515–520, 1989.
6. Dillon WP, Som PM, Fullerton GD: Hypointense MR signal in chronically inspissated sinonasal secretions. Radiology 174:73–78, 1990.
7. Van Tassel P, Lee Y-Y, Jing B-S, De Pena CA: Mucoceles of the paranasal sinuses: MR imaging with CT correlation. AJR 153:407–412, 1989.
8. Lanzieri CF, Shah M, Krauss D, Lavertu P: Use of gadolinium-enhanced MR imaging for differentiating mucoceles from neoplasms in the paranasal sinuses. Radiology 178:425–428, 1991.
9. Zinreich JS, Kennedy DW, Malat J, et al: Fungal sinusitis: diagnosis with MR and CT. Radiology 169:439–444, 1988.
10. Zimmerman RA, Bilaniuk LT, Hackney DB, et al: Paranasal sinus hemorrhage, evaluation with MRI. Radiology 162:499–503, 1987.
11. Som PM, Shugar JMA, Troy KM, et al: The use of MRI and CT in the management of a patient with intrasinus hemorrhage. Arch Otolaryngol Head Neck Surg 114:200–202, 1988.
12. Som PM, Dillon WP, Sze G, et al: Benign and malignant sinonasal lesions with intracranial extension: differentiation with MR imaging. Radiology 172:763–766, 1989.
13. Som PM, Lawson W, Lidov MW: Simulated aggressive skull base erosion in response to benign sinonasal disease. Radiology 180:755–759, 1991.
14. Han MH, Chang KH, Lee CH, et al: Sinonasal psammomatoid ossifying fibroma. AJNR 12:25–30, 1991.
15. Som PM, Dillon WP, Curtin HD, et al: Hypointense paranasal sinus foci: differential diagnosis with MR imaging and relation to CT findings. Radiology 176:777–781, 1990.

Nasopharynx and Deep Facial Compartments

ALEXANDER M. NORBASH

A great deal of overlap occurs when imaging issues in the face, head, and neck are discussed. The greatest overlaps are in sections dealing with the neck, the salivary glands, the skull base, the floor of the mouth and tongue, and the cervical lymph nodes. The reader is referred to Chapters 32, 33, 35, and 36 in this textbook for this complementary information.

This chapter is subdivided into five sections. Initially, the historical subdivisions of the deep face and nasopharynx are reviewed, followed by a discussion of the various modalities and techniques available to evaluate the head and neck region. A compartmentalized cross-sectional scheme is presented to categorize pathologic conditions in the nasopharynx and deep face. The final section focuses on sleep apnea, postoperative and postirradiation changes, and biopsy and interventional magnetic resonance imaging (MRI).

HISTORICAL SUBDIVISIONS

Historically, the suprahyoid head and neck have been subdivided into the nasopharynx and oropharynx (Fig. 34–1). The historical margins of the nasopharynx include the basisphenoid and clivus superiorly and the posterior horizontal continuation of the palate inferiorly, the cervical spine posteriorly, and the choanae anteriorly. The lateral boundaries of the nasopharynx are defined by the eustachian tube orifices and the lateral pharyngeal recess mucosa, including the fossa of Rosenmüller,[1] which are vertically oriented linear pockets of mucosa posterior to the eustachian tube orifices (Fig. 34–2).

The historical superior margin of the oropharynx includes the soft palate and its horizontal continuation. The inferior margin or floor of the historical oropharynx is defined by folds of tissue extending from the epiglottis to the posterior pharyngeal wall, and these structures also define the superior margin of the hypopharynx. These folds include the epiglottic folds anteroinferiorly, the continuing glossoepiglottic folds laterally, and the pharyngoepiglottic folds posteroinferiorly.

The anterior aspect of the historical oropharynx is defined by Waldeyer's ring, a semicoronal structure formed by the soft palate superiorly, the tonsillar pillars laterally, and the circumvallate papillae of the tongue inferiorly. The posterior aspect of the oropharynx is the superior and middle pharyngeal constrictors.

More recent schemes further subdivide the nasopharynx and deep face.[2] Although these schemes seem more complicated, they increase differential specificity in cross-sectional imaging, which is now the primary modality in radiologic work-up of this region. In describing the anatomy and pathology of the suprahyoid neck, a scheme is used that subdivides this region into eight discrete compartments with individualized contents and differential diagnoses. These eight compartments include the pharyngeal mucosal space, parapharyngeal space, masticator space, parotid space,

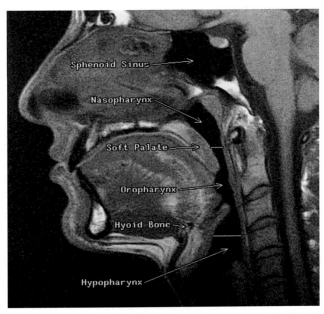

FIGURE 34–1. Sagittal midline T1-weighted image shows the historical divisions of the nasopharynx and oropharynx defined by the imaginary horizontal continuation of the soft palate.

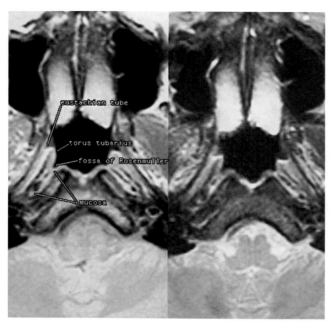

FIGURE 34–2. Proton density–weighted *(left)* and T2-weighted *(right)* cross-sectional axial images at the level of the eustachian tube orifices are shown. In this patient the apposed mucosa in the fossa of Rosenmüller is clearly demonstrated. The torus tubarius, which covers the levator palatini, is shown anterior to the fossa of Rosenmüller and posterior to the eustachian tube opening.

pterygopalatine space, retropharyngeal space, prevertebral space, and carotid space. In addition to assisting in diagnostic evaluation, this subcompartmentalization answers many staging questions that determine surgical and therapeutic options and approaches.

TECHNICAL CONSIDERATIONS

OVERVIEW OF MODALITIES

Four of the modalities used to evaluate disease in the suprahyoid neck include radiography, computed tomography (CT), MRI, and nuclear medicine. Radiographic methods include plain film imaging, plain film tomography, plain film contrast examinations, and videofluoroscopic evaluation such as swallowing studies and phonation studies. CT examinations include conventional cross-sectional imaging, three-dimensional reconstruction techniques, and newer spiral CT and CT angiographic techniques.[3]

Plain film imaging has most often been unreliable, superfluous, and underinformative when compared with cross-sectional modalities.[4] CT has replaced pluridirectional tomography in the evaluation of compact bone.[5] Some authors believe that CT and MRI are roughly comparable in evaluating the suprahyoid region; however, clear CT modality advantages include evaluating bony matrix destruction, showing soft tissue calcification and calculi, and extremely high resolution. Intravenous contrast material is essential in most cases of suprahyoid CT evaluation; at Stanford University Medical Center a 50-mL bolus of 60% contrast material is administered, followed by a 150-mL drip of 60% contrast material.

NUCLEAR MEDICINE

Nuclear medicine evaluates infection, inflammation, and tumor in the head and neck region with planar and tomographic radioisotope imaging, positron emission tomography (PET) scanning, and monoclonal antibody labeled scanning. Indium 111–labeled leukocytes are used to evaluate potential sites of head and neck infection. Leukocyte scanning may be falsely positive with increased uptake shown at nasogastric tube and tracheostomy sites.[6] Single photon emission CT with technetium 99m dimercaptosuccinic acid has been used to evaluate primary head and neck malignancies. A high false-negative rate was shown in one study; no abnormal isotope uptake was seen in 27 biopsy-proven pretreatment cases of malignancy, although there was some identification of cervical lymph node metastases.[7] ^{99m}Tc-methoxyisobutylisonitrile single photon emission CT has shown greater promise, with one study demonstrating increased radioisotope uptake in 70% of patients with nasopharyngeal carcinoma.[8] Interestingly, this same study did not demonstrate any relationship between methoxyisobutylisonitrile uptake and tumor size and differentiation. Serial thallium 201 scanning has been used to predict response of high-grade sarcomas to preoperative chemotherapy; responsive sarcomas show decreases in thallium uptake after therapy.[9]

PET has identified viable head and neck tumor after radiation therapy and has been used as a guide for biopsy of residual and recurrent tissue. Occasional advantages over MRI in identifying tumor tissue have been demonstrated with PET. In one study, PET with fluorodeoxyglucose demonstrated pretreatment malignant lymphadenopathy and the primary tumors in patients with normal MR images. PET has also demonstrated post-treatment disease persistence or recurrence in patients with unremarkable MR images.[10]

In differentiating post-therapy tumor and normal tissue, PET has shown decreased fluorodeoxyglucose uptake in head and neck tumors after treatment without concomitant decreases in normal head and neck tissue uptake.[11] Radiolabeled monoclonal antibodies allow additional opportunity for specific antigenic localization. As an example of poor tumoral specificity, lymphoma sites have been clearly visualized after injection of eosinophil peroxidase–directed radiolabeled murine monoclonal antibodies, although normal radiolabeled localization was also demonstrated in some patients' nasopharyngeal regions.[12]

MRI ADVANTAGES

The primary focus in this chapter is on the application of MRI in imaging the suprahyoid neck. Due to high soft tissue contrast, rapid yet subtle interval changes between studies may be appreciated, allowing heightened accuracy in differentiating between short-term inflammatory and longer term neoplastic changes.[13] In specific regard to staging head and neck tumors, head and neck imaging offers the opportunity to evaluate the presence and extent of poor prognostic factors. Poor prognostic factors in nasopharyngeal carcinomas include parapharyngeal spread, bone infiltration, cranial nerve involvement, bulky lymphadenopathy, and lymphadenopathy in the supraclavicular fossa, which are believed to be more reliably depicted with MRI than CT.[14] Demonstrated advantages of MRI over CT include the lack of ionizing radiation and associated risks, improved soft tissue contrast, clearer demonstration of mandible and cartilage infiltration,[15] and benefits of polyplanar imaging in demonstrating complex anatomy and pathology in the head and neck. In comparing CT and MRI of nasopharyngeal and parapharyngeal regions with receiver operating characteristic methodology, MRI has been superior to CT in evaluating soft tissue structures and larger bony structures, but CT has been superior to MRI in evaluating thin bony structures.[16] Various MRI techniques applied to the suprahyoid neck include conventional polyplanar MRI imaging, three-dimensional imaging, MR angiography, ultrafast dynamic MRI, and spectroscopy of head and neck tumors.

INTRAVASCULAR CONTRAST AGENTS

Debate continues regarding routine employment of intravenous tissue contrast agents.[2] Multicenter trials have evaluated the safety and efficacy of intravenous MRI contrast agents in imaging the head and neck. In one series, postinjection images altered the preinjection impressions in 37% of cases.[17] Another study showed improved anatomic depiction of subtle structures such as the pharyngobasilar fascia and palatini muscles, potentially altering staging and treatment approach, and improved appreciation of subtle infiltration with MRI.[18] In assessing presence or absence of malignancy, other studies have demonstrated greater than 86% accuracy by demonstration of lesion invasion of surrounding structures on T2-weighted images.[19]

Dynamic MRI contrast curve characteristics have been evaluated, and similar dynamic curve characteristics have been shown in metastatic and primary tumors, suggesting the potential value in evaluating tumor recurrence and metastasis.[19] Certain hypervascular lesions demonstrate specific dynamic patterns.[20] Glomus tumors show a reproducible dropout in dynamic enhancement in the early enhancement curve as a result of a paramagnetic phenomenon.[21]

When I employ intravenous tissue contrast agents in the head and neck region, I routinely use fat saturation techniques to better demonstrate and define areas of contrast enhancement. Suboptimal fat suppression techniques may create puzzling artifacts that mimic pathologic processes. Fat suppression failure artifacts may appear as relatively bright signals without geometric distortion, which may be dependent on surface coil design. These artifacts are independent of frequency or phase-encoding direction and are most often found in the high nasopharynx and low orbit.[22]

NEWER MRI TECHNIQUES

New developments include sequences such as T2-weighted fast spin-echo (FSE) and magnetization transfer imaging and new paramagnetic contrast agents that are being tested in the head and neck.

FSE techniques allow time savings and are often used in combination with fat suppression techniques. Studies have demonstrated better or equal FSE images compared with conventional T2-weighted images; more lesions may even be seen with FSE than with conventional T2 weighting.[23] FSE effective T2-weighted images show higher fat signal intensity than conventional T2-weighted images, which may mask pathologic processes or make diagnosis more difficult without appropriate application of fat saturation techniques. Lesion conspicuity and contrast are improved in T2-weighted FSE imaging with fat suppression compared with conventional contrast-enhanced T1-weighted spin-echo sequences with fat suppression. This comparison shows improved contrast between lesion and muscle, lesion and fat, and lesion and mucosa, which may potentially allow contrast savings.[24]

Three-dimensional imaging may be performed with reconstructions of three-dimensional sequences or with three-dimensional reconstructions of standard sequences. These formats define the relationship of lesions to the surrounding structures in a precise manner.[25] MR angiography allows evaluation of obstructions of larger vessels or deviations by masses and demonstration of vascular lesions such as aneurysms, pseudoaneurysms, and dissections.[25]

Ultrafast MRI has been investigated in the area of functional imaging of the upper airway. Evaluation of soft palate function has been helpful in patients with sleep apnea. In patients with cleft palates, changes in soft palate relationship to the airway and posterior pharyngeal wall were evaluated during phonation of specific sounds. The results of these evaluations were used to guide speech therapy and surgical planning.[26] Spectroscopy of head and neck tumors potentially allows evaluation of tissue characteristics in determining primary presentation of malignancy and possibly tumor recurrence.

NODE EVALUATION

Several schemes try to differentiate reactive from malignant lymphadenopathy. Metastatic head and neck primary lesions may primarily present with cervical, deep neck, and facial lymphadenopathy.[27] One study evaluated accuracy of absolute node size measurements, longitudinal-to-transverse node ratios, and necrotic centers and rim enhancement in accuracy of predicting malignant lymphadenopathy. Longitudinal-to-transverse node ratios less than 2 for nodes greater than 8 mm in length were 97% accurate for malignancy, minimal diameters greater than 8 mm were 88% accurate for malignancy, and necrotic centers and rim enhancement were 86% accurate for malignancy.[28] Exceptions to the absolute sizes include the jugulo-digastric and jugulo-omohyoid nodes, which are normally larger nodes.

At least one study showed no specific statistical advantage for contrast-enhanced fat-suppressed MRI over enhanced CT for evaluation of central nodal necrosis

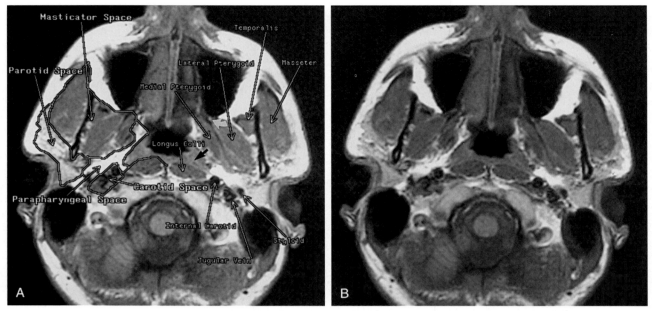

FIGURE 34–3. Labeled *(A)* and unlabeled *(B)* comparison axial T1-weighted MR images at the level of the nasopharynx. The masticator, parotid, parapharyngeal, and carotid spaces are shown. The left pterygopalatine space *(curved white arrow)* is seen posterior to the posterior margins of the maxillary sinuses. The pharyngeal mucosal space is indicated by a black arrow.

and extracapsular nodal spread.[29] Magnetization transfer imaging may help differentiate benign and malignant lymphadenopathy in patients with head and neck cancers.[30] This may be accomplished through evaluation of magnetization transfer ratios, presumably due to increased magnetization transfer with neoplastic infiltrated lymph nodes. Newer superparamagnetic contrast agents tested in the head and neck include BMS 180549, a dextran-coated superparamagnetic iron ox-

ide. Studies evaluating BMS 180549 for determination of malignant cervical lymphadenopathy show changes in lymph node signal intensity taking place after normal phagocytosis of this substance by the reticuloendothelial system. BMS 180549 should be phagocytosed by normal or reactive lymph nodes, resulting in signal drop on multiplanar gradient-recalled sequences due to increased node iron content. Malignant lymph nodes, however, which presumably lack functioning

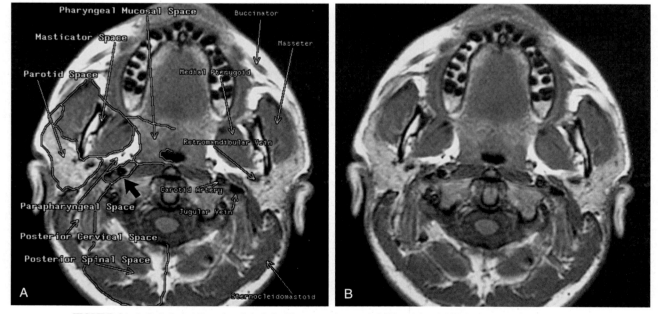

FIGURE 34–4. Labeled *(A)* and unlabeled *(B)* comparison axial T1-weighted MR images at the level of the soft palate. The masticator, parotid, parapharyngeal, and pharyngeal mucosal spaces are shown. The right carotid space is indicated by a black arrow.

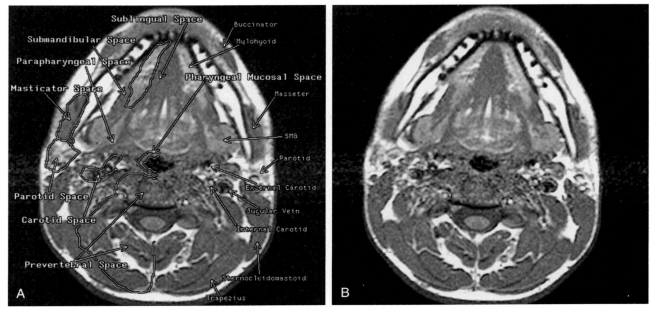

FIGURE 34–5. Labeled *(A)* and unlabeled *(B)* comparison axial T1-weighted MR images at the level of the floor of the mouth. The masticator, parotid, parapharyngeal, carotid, prevertebral, and pharyngeal mucosal spaces are shown. SMG indicates the left submandibular gland.

reticuloendothelial system cells, demonstrate either inhomogeneous uptake of contrast agent or greater signal intensity than is seen with benign or reactive lymph nodes.[31, 32]

ANATOMY

Cross-sectional axial reference T1-weighted MR images with and without annotations at the level of the nasopharynx are provided (Fig. 34–3), as are sections at the level of the soft palate (Fig. 34–4) and the floor of the mouth (Fig. 34–5). Also provided are similar reference coronal images in the plane of the foramen ovale (Fig. 34–6). These images are marked with anatomic compartments and major identified anatomic landmarks.

FASCIA

The deep face and nasopharynx can be subdivided into eight compartments, including the pharyngeal

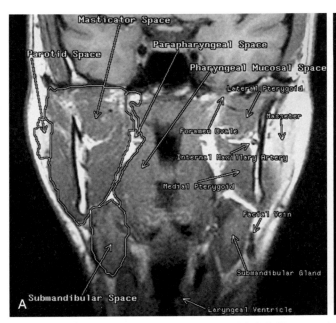
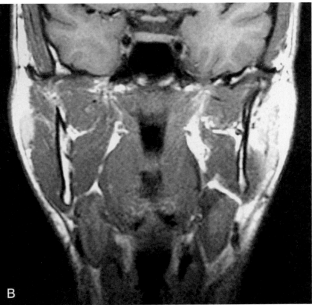

FIGURE 34–6. Labeled *(A)* and unlabeled *(B)* comparison coronal T1-weighted MR images at the level of the foramen ovale. The masticator, parotid, parapharyngeal, and pharyngeal mucosal spaces are shown. The left foramen ovale is indicated: note the medial position of the parapharyngeal space relative to the foramen and the inclusion of the foramen ovale in the masticator space.

mucosal space, parapharyngeal space, masticator space, parotid space, pterygopalatine space, retropharyngeal space, prevertebral space, and carotid space.

Many compartments of this region are defined by fascial planes. There are three major deep fascial compartments in the suprahyoid neck, not including the most superficial fascia, which is a single layer underlying the skin. The external deep fascia of the suprahyoid neck is "investing" fascia, the middle deep fascia is "visceral" fascia, and the internal deep fascia is "prevertebral" fascia. Two additional complex fascial layers include the pharyngobasilar and buccopharyngeal fascias.

The investing, or external, layer of deep cervical fascia underlies the platysma muscle and completely encircles the superficial neck structures. This fascial layer splits at the trapezius and sternocleidomastoid muscles to envelop each of them.

The visceral, or middle, layer of deep fascia encloses the "visceral" structures of the neck, including the trachea and esophagus.

The prevertebral, or internal, layer of deep fascia surrounds the deep muscles of the neck and the cervical vertebrae. The deep muscles include the scalenes, the longus colli and longus capitis, the levator scapulae, and the cervical erector spinae groups. The internal deep fascia also splits to envelop the carotid sheaths, which are lateral to the visceral compartment.

The thin buccopharyngeal fascia is a reflection of the visceral or middle deep cervical fascia, which incorporates the external investing layer of the superior pharyngeal constrictor and the buccinator muscles.

The dense pharyngobasilar fascia is part of the buccopharyngeal fascia, which is composed of the thicker aponeurosis of the superior pharyngeal constrictor and forms an elongated ring attaching superiorly to the skull base. The pharyngobasilar fascia contains the sinus of Morgagni, a perforation that transmits the levator veli palatini and eustachian tube from the skull base to the pharyngeal mucosal space. This perforation allows spread of tumor and inflammation between the skull base and the pharyngeal mucosal space.

Pharyngeal Mucosal Space

The pharyngeal mucosal space is not enclosed by fascia. The posterior boundaries of the pharyngeal mucosal space include the middle layer of deep cervical fascia and the retropharyngeal space. The medial boundary of the pharyngeal mucosal space is the airway, and the lateral margin is the parapharyngeal space.

The contents of the pharyngeal mucosal space include the mucosal lining of the nasopharyngeal and oropharyngeal airway and the contained minor salivary glands. The pharyngeal mucosal space has a rich lymphatic supply. The lingual and faucial tonsillar tissue and the adenoid glands are lymphatic tissue included in the parapharyngeal mucosal space. The medial carti-laginous semitubes of the eustachian tubes are also included in the pharyngeal mucosal space.

The muscles of the pharyngeal mucosal space include the levator palatini, the salpingopharyngeus, and the superior and middle pharyngeal constrictor muscles. The levator palatini forms the ridge also known as the torus tubarius, posterior to which is found the mucosal fold known as the fossa of Rosenmüller and which may occasionally be deep and "kissing" (see Fig. 34–2). The inferior continuation of the torus tubarius is the salpingopharyngeal fold, an elevated crease that covers the salpingopharyngeus muscle as it travels inferiorly and posteriorly.

The levator palatini originates from the medial eustachian tube cartilage, inserts on the palate aponeurosis, and raises the soft palate and opens the eustachian tube for middle ear pressure equalization. The salpingopharyngeus muscle originates from the inferior cartilaginous eustachian tube, inserts on the posterior thyroid cartilage, and acts to elevate the pharynx for swallowing. It also equalizes pressure in the eustachian tube. As discussed in the section on pharyngeal mucosal space pathology, it should be apparent that early submucosal neoplastic invasion may result in eustachian tube dysfunction or disordered swallowing.

The superior and middle pharyngeal constrictors are above the level of the hyoid bone. They originate from a superior ring, including the pterygoids, the mylohyoid line of the mandible, and the hyoid bone. They directly or indirectly insert on the posterior pharyngeal raphe and pull the posterior pharyngeal wall upward during swallowing to help close off the nasopharynx and propel a bolus into the esophagus.[33]

Parapharyngeal Space

The parapharyngeal space, like the pharyngeal mucosal space, is not enclosed by fascia. It is a centrally located fatty triangle contacting multiple suprahyoid compartments. The parapharyngeal space contacts the pharyngeal mucosal space medially, the masticator space anterolaterally, the parotid space laterally, and the carotid space posterolaterally.

The boundaries of the parapharyngeal space include the skull base superiorly and the hyoid bone inferiorly. It communicates freely with the submandibular space anteriorly. The posterior margin of the parapharyngeal space is defined by the anterior margin of the carotid sheath, and the lateral margin is defined by the superficial layer of the deep cervical fascia deep to the masticator and parotid spaces. The medial margin is defined by the visceral (middle deep) fascia as it sweeps laterally around the pharyngeal mucosal space.

The contents of the parapharyngeal space include fat and connective tissue. Other components include the proximal third (mandibular) branches of the trigeminal nerve, portions of the internal maxillary and ascending pharyngeal arteries, and the pharyngeal venous plexus, which may occasionally seem too prominent. The parapharyngeal space does not normally contain mucosa, muscle, bone, lymph nodes, or salivary glands.

MASTICATOR SPACE

The masticator space is partially defined by complex fascial anatomy. The superficial layer of the deep cervical fascia splits at the inferior margin of the mandible to form medial and lateral sublayers enclosing the masticator space. The medial fascial sublayer covers the pterygoid muscles. The lateral fascial sublayer covers the masseter muscle and then travels deep to the zygoma to cover the temporalis muscle.

The superior margins of the masticator space include the skull base medially and the temporalis muscle attachment laterally, where the suprazygomatic masticator space is formed. The inferior margin of the masticator space is the lower margin of the mandibular body.

The anterior margin is defined by the buccal space and maxilla, and the posterior margin is defined by the parotid space posterolaterally and the parapharyngeal space posteromedially.

The medial extent of the masticator space is formed by the medial enclosing layer of deep fascia bordering the parapharyngeal space and extends far medially, inserting on the skull base medial to the foramen ovale and allowing communication between the cavernous sinus/Meckel's cave and the masticator space (see Fig. 34–6). Note that the more medially positioned parapharyngeal space does not incorporate the foramen ovale. Intracranial involvement is therefore more commonly seen with masticator space than with parapharyngeal space processes. The lateral margin of the masticator space is defined by its border with the buccal space.

The contents of the masticator space include the body and posterior ramus of the mandible, several muscles of mastication, and traversing nerves and vessels. The muscles of mastication include the masseter, the temporalis, and the medial and lateral pterygoid muscles. The masseter originates from the lower and medial zygoma and inserts on the lateral ramus of the mandible acting to occlude the jaw. The temporalis originates from the dished lateral parietal bone and inserts on the mandibular coronoid process and anterior mandibular ramus, acting to elevate and retract the mandible. The medial and lateral pterygoids originate from the medial and lateral surfaces of the lateral pterygoid plate, respectively, inserting on the medial mandibular angle and neck of the mandible, respectively, acting to elevate and push the mandible forward. The inferior margin of the medial pterygoid plate serves as the site of attachment of the pharyngobasilar fascia.[34]

The nerves in the masticator space include motor elements of the mandibular nerve used for mastication and sensory elements of the mandibular nerve such as the inferior alveolar branch. Vessels include the inferior alveolar vein and artery. The parotid duct is not in the masticator space but courses superficial to the masseter muscle.

Because of the transmission of the trigeminal mandibular branch from the foramen ovale to the masticator space, intracranial spread of tumor is possible by perineural intracranial extension along the trigeminal mandibular branch. The trigeminal mandibular branch should therefore be followed from the root entry zone in the pons to the mental foramen of the mandible when excluding perineural spread of masticator space lesions.

PAROTID SPACE

The parotid space is the most lateral space in the suprahyoid space classification. The buccal space is lateral to the parotid space and is not technically considered one of the deep suprahyoid spaces. The parotid gland is divided into deep and superficial components separated by the facial nerve course. MRI detail allows visualization of parotid architecture such that portions of the ductal system may be seen as curvilinear areas of low T1-weighted signal intensity within the parotid gland.[35] Salivary gland lesions are described only briefly here; they are covered in greater detail in Chapter 35.

Dividing the parotid gland into separate deep and superficial components serves a therapeutic purpose; deep lobe lesions are most often treated with total parotidectomy with wide submandibular exposure, whereas superficial transfacial parotidectomy is usually performed for superficial masses. The surgical approach also differs for extracarotid and intracarotid space masses. If carotid space involvement is suspected, the proximal carotid and distal carotid are surgically exposed for appropriate control in case of bleeding.[36]

The anterior boundary of the parotid space is the mandibular ramus. The posterior boundaries of the parotid space are defined medially to laterally by the carotid space, the styloid process, and the posterior belly of the digastric muscle. The digastric muscle is a "dogleg" divided into posterior and anterior bellies joined by an "intermediate tendon." The intermediate tendon passes through a loop of fascia arising from the superior aspect of the hyoid bone, which acts as a sort of pulley. The posterior digastric belly originates from the medial aspect of the mastoid process and inserts on the intermediate tendon, and the anterior belly originates from the intermediate tendon and inserts on the body of the mandible. The digastric muscle depresses the mandible or elevates the hyoid bone. The medial boundary of the parotid space is the parapharyngeal space. Deep parotid lobe lesions may show widening of the stylomandibular notch.

The contents of the parotid space include the parotid gland and the intraparotid lymph nodes. The vessels contained in the parotid space include the retromandibular vein, which demarcates the posterior margin of the parotid gland on axial section, the second portion of the internal maxillary artery, and portions of the external carotid artery.

The facial nerve is also partially contained by the parotid space and occupies a position immediately lateral to an imaginary line connecting the lateral margin of the retromandibular vein to the stylomastoid foramen.

PTERYGOPALATINE SPACE

The pterygopalatine space is a small space defined by the pterygopalatine fossa and serves as a site of mutual communication among the nasal cavity, the suprazygomatic masticator space, the orbit, and the middle cranial fossa. The pterygopalatine space contains the pterygopalatine ganglion, which is one of the parasympathetic ganglia supplied by the trigeminal nerve.

The anterior margin of the pterygopalatine space is the posterior wall of the maxillary sinus, whereas the anterior superior margin is the inferior orbital fissure, which communicates with the orbit. The posterior margin is the pterygoid process of the sphenoid bone, which supports the pterygoid plates. The posterior and superior portions of the pterygopalatine space communicate with the middle cranial fossa through the foramen rotundum, which transmits the maxillary branch of the trigeminal nerve, and the vidian canal, which carries the vidian artery from the foramen lacerum to the pterygopalatine space. The medial margin of the pterygopalatine space is the nasal cavity, which is connected to the pterygopalatine space by means of the sphenopalatine foramen. The lateral margin of the pterygopalatine space is the suprazygomatic masticator space; the two spaces communicate through the pterygomaxillary fissure.

The pterygopalatine space includes the pterygopalatine ganglion, which is a parasympathetic ganglion associated with the trigeminal nerve, a portion of the main trunk of the mandibular branch of the trigeminal nerve, and a portion of the distal internal maxillary artery.

RETROPHARYNGEAL SPACE

The retropharyngeal space is a potential space that serves as a conduit to the mediastinum. The superior limit of the retropharyngeal space is the skull base. The anterior margin is the visceral (middle deep) cervical fascia and the pharyngeal mucosal space. The posterior margin is the prevertebral (deepest deep) cervical fascia and the prevertebral space. The lateral limit of the retropharyngeal space includes an anteriorly projecting slip of prevertebral (deepest deep) fascia and the carotid space.

The contents of the retropharyngeal space include lateral and medial retropharyngeal lymph nodes and retropharyngeal fat.

PREVERTEBRAL SPACE

The prevertebral space includes prevertebral and postvertebral portions. This space may be thought of as a ring encircling the vertebral column, incorporating much of the paraspinous musculature. The anterior margin of the prevertebral space is defined not only by the deep layer of the deep cervical fascia arching from the transverse process, anterior to the vertebral bodies to reach the contralateral transverse process, but also by the retropharyngeal space. The posterior margin of the prevertebral space is delineated by prevertebral (deepest deep) cervical fascia sweeping from the transverse process, posteriorly to the ligamentum nuchae. The ligamentum nuchae is a vertically aligned midline sagittal ligamentous sheet seen in the posterior neck, formed as a thickening of the supraspinous and interspinous ligaments in the cervical region, and originating from the seventh cervical vertebra to insert on the external occipital protuberance. The lateral extent of the prevertebral space is defined by the carotid space.

The contents of the anterior prevertebral space include the prevertebral, scalene, and paraspinal muscles. The prevertebral muscles include the longus cervicis and longus colli muscles arising, respectively, from cervical transverse processes and anterior middle to lower cervical vertebral bodies and inserting, respectively, on the basilar occiput and anterior superior vertebral bodies. These muscles act to flex the head and neck. The scalene muscles originate from the transverse processes and posterior tubercles of the cervical vertebrae and insert on the first and second ribs to elevate the first two ribs and to flex and rotate the cervical spine.[34]

Nerves in the anterior prevertebral space include the brachial plexus, the scalene nerve, and the phrenic nerve. Vascular contents include the vertebral arteries and vertebral veins. The vertebral bodies are also part of the anterior prevertebral space.

The posterior prevertebral space includes the posterior paraspinal muscles.

CAROTID SPACE

The carotid space is elongated and enclosed in fascia with the skull base as the superior boundary and the aortic arch as the inferior boundary. The contents of the carotid space include jugular chain lymph nodes, carotid sheath nerves, and internal jugular vein and carotid artery. The most superiorly positioned deep cervical chain lymph node in the carotid space is the jugulodigastric node found inferior to the angle of the mandible, slightly below the posterior belly of the digastric muscle. The jugulo-omohyoid is another large cervical chain lymph node found in the carotid chain at the chain's intersection with the omohyoid muscle, which extends from its origin at the superior border of the scapula to insert on the lateral border of the hyoid bone. The four cranial nerves found in the carotid space include the glossopharyngeal (IX), the vagus (X), the accessory (XI), and the hypoglossal (XII) nerves. The vagus nerve is located in the posterior caroticojugular notch, a groove formed by the adjoining carotid artery and jugular vein. The sympathetic chain plexus is found in the medial fascial wall of the carotid space.

PATHOLOGY

The pathologic processes involving the suprahyoid neck are addressed by examining each of the eight suprahyoid spaces discussed in the anatomy section. Table 34–1 shows characteristic, unusual but specific, and commonly seen lesions for each space. Table 34–2 specifically addresses "crossover lesions," which can exist in any of the discussed spaces; these lesions will not be discussed individually with each space's pathology.

PHARYNGEAL MUCOSAL SPACE

Major characteristic lesions of the pharyngeal mucosal space are listed in Table 34–1. The three major malignancies include epithelial carcinomas, tumors of

TABLE 34–1. PATHOLOGIC PROCESSES OF THE SUPRAHYOID NECK GROUPED BY SUPRAHYOID SPACES

PHARYNGEAL MUCOSAL SPACE
Malignancy
  Squamous cell
  Lymphoma
  Salivary gland origin
  Lymphoepithelioma
Inflammatory
  Tonsillitis
Congenital
  Pharyngeal adenoids
  Thornwaldt's cyst
Crossover lesions
PARAPHARYNGEAL SPACE
Malignancy
  Extension
    Other neck space primary
    Skull base tumor
  Salivary gland rest
  Plasmacytoma
  Amyloidoma
  Mesenchymal tumor
Masses
  Brain heterotopia
  Meningoencephalocele
  Ectopic paraganglioma
Congenital
  Second branchial cleft cyst
Crossover lesions
MASTICATOR SPACE
Malignancy
  Extension
    Intracranial primary
Inflammatory
  Odontogenic abscess
  Mandibular osteomyelitis
Congenital
  Ectopic parotid
Crossover lesions

PAROTID SPACE
Malignancy
  Mucoepidermoid
    carcinoma
  Adenoid cystic carcinoma
  Acinous cell carcinoma
  Malignant mixed tumor
Masses
  Pleomorphic adenoma
  Warthin's tumor
  Oncocytoma
  Lymphoepithelial cyst
Inflammatory
  Sarcoid
Crossover lesions
PTERYGOPALATINE SPACE
Masses
  Juvenile nasopharyngeal
    angiofibroma
Crossover lesions
RETROPHARYNGEAL SPACE
Infection
  Lymphadenitis
  Abscess
Crossover lesions
PREVERTEBRAL SPACE
Malignancy
  Lymphoma
  Chordoma
Infection
  Vertebral osteomyelitis
Crossover lesions
CAROTID SPACE
Masses
  Paraganglioma
  Neurofibroma
  Great vessel thrombosis
  Carotid pseudoaneurysm
Crossover lesions

TABLE 34–2. CROSSOVER LESIONS

Malignancy
  Direct extension from adjacent space
  Node metastasis from head and neck
  Distant metastasis
  Nerve sheath tumor
  Hemangioma
  Lymphangioma
Infection
  Cellulitis
  Abscess

gland origin, and lymphomas (most commonly non-Hodgkin's lymphoma). Head and neck lymphomas may demonstrate rapid growth and may violate fascial planes, resulting in large lesions with multicompartmental presentation (see Fig. 34–16). Up to 80% of malignancies in the pharyngeal mucosal space are squamous cell carcinomas.[37] All three malignancy groups may demonstrate a nearly identical appearance and may present with fluid in the middle ear due to either anatomic obstruction of the distal eustachian tube or functional interference with normal eustachian tube function. These patients may also present with disordered swallowing. When these malignancies metastasize to the lymph nodes of the head and neck, they tend to most often involve the spinal accessory or deep cervical lymph nodes.

Squamous cell carcinomas are often asymptomatic when limited to the pharyngeal mucosal space and therefore often present with invasion. They frequently occur in the fossa of Rosenmüller[38] and therefore may present with otitis related to drainage interference in the adjacent eustachian tube (Fig. 34–7). Some squamous neoplasms have abundant lymphoid infiltrate within the fibrous stroma; these lesions are known as lymphoepitheliomas[39] (Fig. 34–8).

The tonsil and tonsillar pillar represent the most common sites for oropharyngeal tumor presentation. These lesions spread rapidly to the soft palate and tongue base, and those with tongue base involvement have a worse prognosis. Lesions of the posterior tonsillar pillar often invade the parapharyngeal space (Fig. 34–9) and tend to involve the spinal accessory and posterior triangle lymph nodes. Lymph node involvement in tonsillar malignancy is associated with a 25% decrease in 5-year survival.[36]

Mesenchymal and neural sheath tumors may be found in the pharyngeal mucosal space. They can cause nasal cavity obstruction on epistaxis if the lesion is vascular. Lesion behavior may not necessarily correspond with the lesion's pathologic characteristics. Pathologically proven nasal septal neurinoma has been reported with aggressive features, including penetration of the nasal septum and extension into the contralateral nasal cavity.[40] Unusual mesenchymal tumors have also been reported in the nasal cavity, including a hairy teratoid polyp of the nasopharynx in a newborn presenting with respiratory distress and vomiting.[41]

Malignant amelanotic and melanotic melanomas may present in the nasopharynx with early invasion

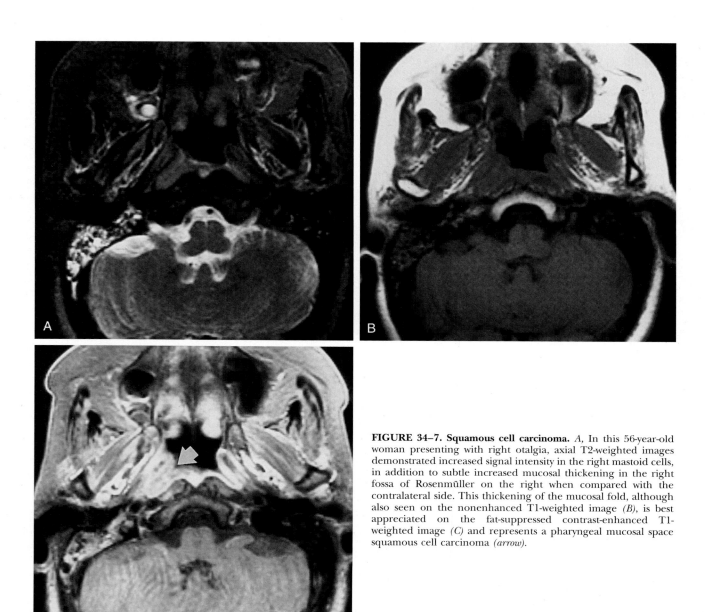

FIGURE 34–7. Squamous cell carcinoma. *A,* In this 56-year-old woman presenting with right otalgia, axial T2-weighted images demonstrated increased signal intensity in the right mastoid cells, in addition to subtle increased mucosal thickening in the right fossa of Rosenmüller on the right when compared with the contralateral side. This thickening of the mucosal fold, although also seen on the nonenhanced T1-weighted image *(B),* is best appreciated on the fat-suppressed contrast-enhanced T1-weighted image *(C)* and represents a pharyngeal mucosal space squamous cell carcinoma *(arrow).*

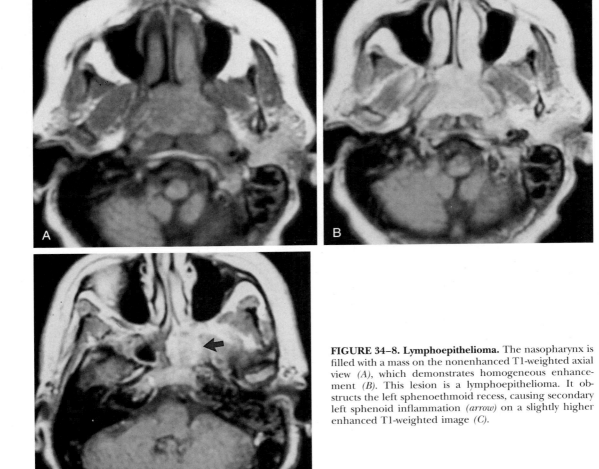

FIGURE 34–8. Lymphoepithelioma. The nasopharynx is filled with a mass on the nonenhanced T1-weighted axial view *(A)*, which demonstrates homogeneous enhancement *(B)*. This lesion is a lymphoepithelioma. It obstructs the left sphenoethmoid recess, causing secondary left sphenoid inflammation *(arrow)* on a slightly higher enhanced T1-weighted image *(C)*.

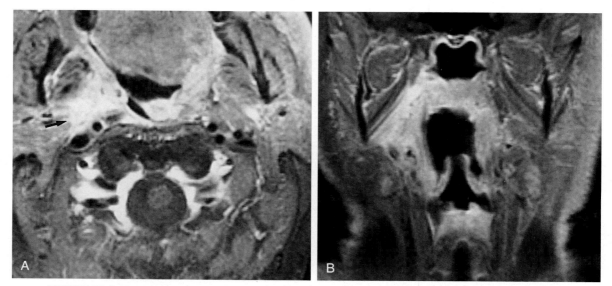

FIGURE 34–9. Tonsillar carcinoma. Enhanced T1-weighted axial *(A)* and coronal *(B)* images of a right tonsillar carcinoma are demonstrated in a 53-year-old man presenting with a chronic sore throat. Enhancing infiltration of the right parapharyngeal space is shown *(arrow)*. Note the medial position of the infiltrated parapharyngeal space relative to the uninvolved masticator space on the coronal image.

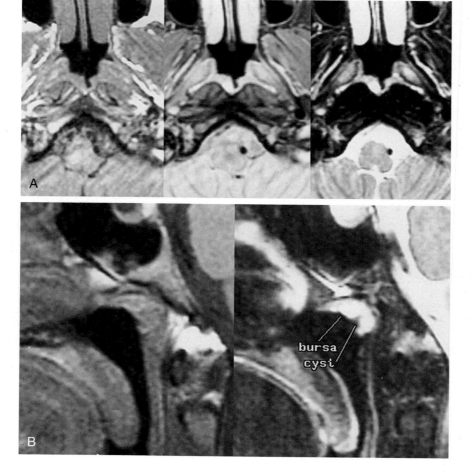

FIGURE 34–10. *A,* A nasopharyngeal adenoid, or tonsil, is demonstrated in the posterior nasopharynx. Three axial images at the level of the nasopharynx are shown (nonenhanced T1-weighted image is on the left; first-echo T2-weighted image, center; second-echo T2-weighted image, right) demonstrating a T1 isointense lesion with T2 hyperintensity. *B,* Sagittal midline T1-weighted *(left)* and T2-weighted *(right)* images show the prominent nasopharyngeal bursa or adenoid with T1 isointensity and T2 hyperintensity. The Thornwaldt cyst immediately below it shows slight hypointensity on the T1-weighted image.

and with lymph node metastasis.[42, 43] Imaging characteristics depend on the presence of melanin, hemosiderin, and products of hemorrhage, such as deoxyhemoglobin and methemoglobin. Histopathologic correlation suggests that the T1 shortening of melanomas is more often due to paramagnetic products of hemorrhage than of melanin.[44]

Benign tumors that involve the pharyngeal mucosal space include benign mixed tumors of minor salivary gland origin. These benign tumors may pedunculate into the upper airway.

The rich lymphatic and mucosal components of the pharyngeal mucosal space may become involved with inflammatory and immunologic responses. Nasopharyngeal obstruction secondary to isolated increased mucosal volume has been shown in guinea pig nasopharynx by MRI.[45] Inflammatory processes involving the pharyngeal mucosal space include tonsillitis and peritonsillar or submucosal abscesses. These inflammatory processes tend to extend rapidly to the parapharyngeal space. Inflammatory pharyngitis may be associated with infectious and radiation-induced causes. Postinflammatory sequelae may include retention cysts, which can be quite large, and occasional clump-like calcifications.

At the apex of the nasopharynx, a concavity may exist in the mucosa covering the bony roof, which is referred to as a *pharyngeal bursa*. This bursa may have sufficient peripheral lymphatic infiltration to form a pharyngeal tonsil or adenoid[36] (Fig. 34–10). Congenital lesions of the pharyngeal mucosal space include Thornwaldt's cysts, which are midline remnants of the cranial aspect of the primitive notochord.[36] They are seen in up to 20% of patients and demonstrate variable signal characteristics. Typically, Thornwaldt's cysts are nonenhancing areas of increased T2-weighted signal that most commonly have fluid signal characteristics. These lesions are usually in a midline or off-midline

position near the pharyngeal bursa (Fig. 34–11), and they may occasionally become infected, potentially presenting as superimposed cervical adenitis.[2, 46, 47]

Pharyngeal mucosal space pseudotumors, or normal variants, include adenoid tissue hypertrophy and normal asymmetry of the fossa of Rosenmüller. Suspicions of such conditions may be confirmed with direct visualization or can be further evaluated by imaging the changes seen with Valsalva's or Müller's maneuvers. Certain lesions may also appear to be of pharyngeal mucosal space origin, when in fact they may be arising outside the pharynx. An example of such an entity is the sphenochoanal polyp, which arises from the sphenoidal sinus and extends through the sphenoid ostium and sphenoethmoid recess into the nasopharynx and choanal region.[48]

PARAPHARYNGEAL SPACE

Major characteristic lesions of the parapharyngeal space are listed in Table 34–1. Lesions entirely contained within the parapharyngeal space should be surrounded by fat. The surgical approach chosen may be dependent on the presence of a lesion within the parapharyngeal space. Surgeons tend to approach parapharyngeal lesions from a submandibular or oral route rather than a transparotid route, thereby allowing greater control of the facial nerve. Such control may be helpful in addressing deep parotid lobe tumors as well.

Primary and secondary malignancies may involve the parapharyngeal space. Secondary malignancies include lesions spreading directly from adjoining spaces (Fig. 34–12). Such lesions include nasopharyngeal carcinomas, which can spread from the adjoining pharyngeal mucosal space. These lesions, which occur with greater frequency in Asia, are typically infiltrative and tend to

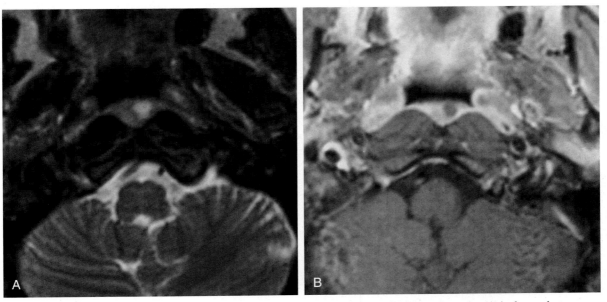

FIGURE 34–11. Thornwaldt's cyst. Focal posterior central nasopharyngeal T2 hyperintensity *(A)* is shown that corresponds with nonenhancement *(B)* on the enhanced fat-suppressed image.

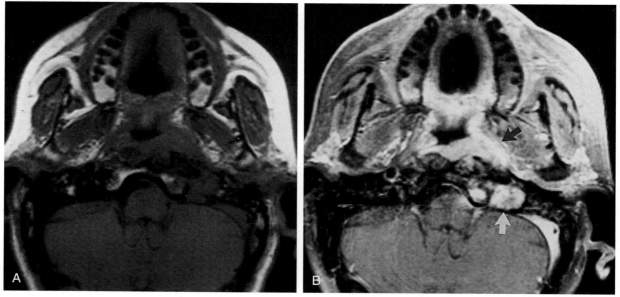

FIGURE 34–12. Squamous cell carcinoma. Axial nonenhanced *(A)* and enhanced fat-suppressed *(B)* images in this 50-year-old woman with cranial neuropathy show enhancing tumor in the region of the left fossa of Rosenmüller with submucosal invasion *(black arrow)* and abnormal enhancement of the left jugular fossa *(white arrow)*, which represented invasive squamous cell carcinoma.

be asymptomatic early in the disease course.[49] They may infiltrate the parapharyngeal space and from there spread to additional adjoining spaces. Nasopharyngeal primary lesions have been observed to extend into the posterior fossa through the jugular foramen, as seen in Figure 34–12.[50] Coronal images tend to show medial parapharyngeal tracking when tumor growth is in a superior direction. As we discussed in the sections on the parapharyngeal and masticator spaces, there is less of a tendency for parapharyngeal lesions to invade the foramen ovale than for masticator space lesions to do so (Fig. 34–13). Nasopharyngeal and other head and neck primary lesions may present initially as parapharyngeal space masses without apparent contiguous pharyngeal mucosal space disease (Fig. 34–14).

Primary parapharyngeal space malignancies such as malignant mixed tumors, mucoepidermoid carcinomas, and adenoid cystic carcinomas may arise from salivary rests. These malignancies may spread to surrounding spaces such as the skull base and produce bony erosion and infiltration.

Similarly, skull base neoplasms may spread to the contiguous and adjacent parapharyngeal space. Meningiomas, chordomas, and chondrosarcomas are traditionally thought of as neoplasms that can involve the parapharyngeal region from the juxtaclival skull base.

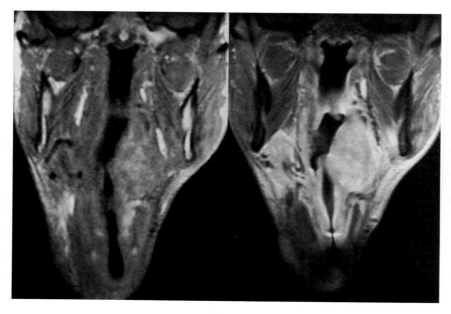

FIGURE 34–13. Squamous cell carcinoma. The medial location of the left parapharyngeal invading squamous cell carcinoma is demonstrated relative to the more lateral masticator space in these nonenhanced *(left)* and enhanced fat-suppressed *(right)* images in this 31-year-old man.

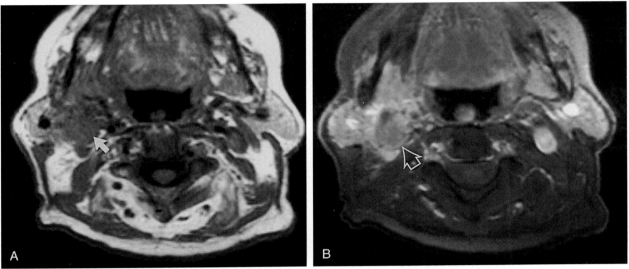

FIGURE 34–14. Squamous cell carcinoma. A right parapharyngeal lesion *(arrows)* was found in this 72-year-old man that demonstrated T1 isointensity *(A)* and enhancement *(B)*. Biopsy showed squamous cell carcinoma, although triple endoscopy did not demonstrate any abnormal focal mucosal-based lesions.

Retrospective reviews of chordoma series have shown low to intermediate T1 signal intensity, high and heterogeneous signal intensity in up to 79% of T2-weighted sequences, and predominantly heterogeneous T1-weighted contrast enhancement.[51] Chordomas also may demonstrate vessel displacement and encasement and direct adjacent extension into the nasopharynx, hypoglossal canal, and cavernous sinuses. Series have shown clival chordomas invading the upper cervical spinal canal and paravertebral fascial planes and eroding the petroclival region with extension into the parapharyngeal region. Although tumor calcification may not have been as easily seen as with CT in certain studies, MRI was believed to clearly demonstrate soft tissue extent, with multiplanar capability assisting in planning the treatment of the tumor.[52] Other parasellar and skull base–bordering lesions, such as craniopharyngiomas, which are not typically thought to involve the parapharyngeal space, have been shown to do so.[53] Ectopic infiltrative pituitary adenomas can rarely involve the clivus and parapharyngeal space,[54] with erosion of the floor of the middle cranial fossa and direct growth into the masticator space.[55] Primary bone tumors of the skull base may themselves grow to involve the compartments of the suprahyoid neck, as described in a review article, including discussion of parapharyngeal invasion by giant cell tumors of the sphenoid bone.[56]

Miscellaneous tumors found in the parapharyngeal region may include extramedullary plasmacytomas, which may represent up to 4% of nonepithelial lesions of the upper respiratory tract. These tumors may present as aggressive and locally destructive collections of neoplastic plasma cells and may rarely be associated with later development of multiple myeloma.[36, 57] Nasopharyngeal amyloidomas demonstrate variable T2 signal characteristics and may demonstrate a benign or destructive appearance. Amyloidomas have been re-

ported to demonstrate bony erosion at the skull base, while showing only moderate contrast enhancement and T2 isointensity or slight hyperintensity compared with muscle.[58] Amyloidomas of the skull base have been shown to demonstrate slightly high CT attenuation and homogeneous partial calcification. They may partially demonstrate decreased T2-weighted signal intensity due to diamagnetic susceptibility.[59] Decreased T2 signal intensity and susceptibility effects may also be seen with melanomas. Melanomas may be primarily or secondarily in the nasopharynx and may include melanotic and amelanotic subtypes.[42, 43] As discussed in the section on pathology of the pharyngeal mucosal space, variable paramagnetic effects may be seen in these tumors.[44]

Tumors of mesenchymal origin may be found in the parapharyngeal space, and they demonstrate variable signal characteristics. Rhabdomyosarcomas involve the head and neck region 30% of the time. The nasopharynx is among the four most common sites of head and neck involvement, with other sites including the orbit, the paranasal sinuses, and the middle ear. This tumor is most common in children younger than 6 years of age, although adult forms are not uncommon.[60] These are believed to arise from rhabdomyoblasts in one of the nasopharyngeal muscles. Various pathologic subtypes exist, with the pleomorphic subtype showing poorest survival rates.[61] Skull base invasion, recurrence, and distal metastasis are common, and MRI shows many similarities of rhabdomyosarcomas to squamous cell carcinoma. Variable enhancement is demonstrated with hypointense T1-weighted and hyperintense T2-weighted signal characteristics[38] (Fig. 34–15). Congenital nasopharyngeal teratomas have been seen in neonates and may be concurrently found with other central nervous system abnormalities.[62] Among more unusual mesenchymal tumors, malignant ectomesenchymomas are rare soft tissue tumors that have been

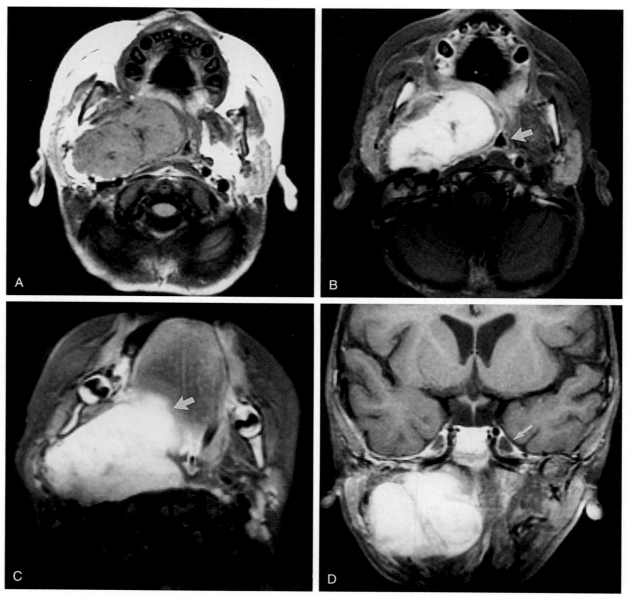

FIGURE 34–15. Rhabdomyosarcoma. *A*, This 20-month-old male infant with embryonal rhabdomyosarcoma presented with difficulty in breathing. A large lesion of the right parapharyngeal space is identified on an axial nonenhanced T1-weighted image with contained central hypointensities representing necrotic regions. *B*, An enhanced axial fat-suppressed image shows bright enhancement without appreciable contiguous skull-based infiltration, although there is significant mass effect and airway deviation *(arrow)*. *C*, A lower level enhanced axial fat-suppressed image shows invasion of the tongue *(arrow)*. *D*, Coronal enhanced fat-suppressed image at the level of Meckel's cave *(arrow)* shows that although this is a large parapharyngeal lesion there is predominant medial rather than superior growth into the skull base.

found in the parapharyngeal space. They arise from pluripotential migratory neural crest cells and include mesenchymal and neuroectodermal elements such as rhabdomyoma and neuroblastoma.[63]

Inflammatory lesions of the parapharyngeal space may also be found that manifest as large ill-defined masses showing adjacent skull base erosion and grossly invasive features. Although imaging features are highly suggestive of aggressive neoplastic infiltration, pathologic specimen and biopsy analysis may show only nonspecific inflammatory changes without evidence of malignancy.[64]

Benign tumors found in the parapharyngeal space include pleomorphic adenomas, which tend to be benign mixed tumors of minor salivary gland rest origin, schwannomas, and lipomas. Inflammation in the parapharyngeal space may result in cellulitis and abscess formation.

Unusual benign congenital lesions of the parapharyngeal space include brain tissue heterotopias. These are similar to brain heterotopias that may be found in the nose and are known as *nasal gliomas*. MRI may demonstrate persistent craniopharyngeal opening into the heterotopia; varied signal characteristics are found when comparing the heterotopia with brain tissue. Analysis for ectopic hypophysial tissue should be included in such cases so that potential removal of the sole functioning pituitary tissue is avoided.[65] Similarly, encephaloceles and meningoencephaloceles of the skull base have been reported as projecting into the parapharyngeal region. These lesions tend to demonstrate signal characteristics similar to those of the native brain substance and more commonly show broad-based transsphenoid attachments.[66] Primary paragangliomas may be seen in the parapharyngeal space; imaging characteristics are discussed in the section on pathology of the carotid space. Although these lesions primarily originate in the carotid space, more than 20 cases of primary parapharyngeal paragangliomas have been reported.[67]

Congenital lesions of the parapharyngeal space include second branchial cleft cysts. These cysts may contain variable amounts of cholesterol and may cause progressive medial bulging of the pharyngeal wall from desquamation of the epithelial lining.[2, 68] These cysts may be associated with branchial sinuses and drain through them, although they may also lie free in the neck anterior to the angle of the mandible. They may develop at any site anterior to the margin of the sternocleidomastoid muscle.[68] They occasionally extend to the skull base and may originate from the second branchial pouch or from endodermal cells disconnected from the inferior portion of the eustachian tube.[69] Imaging characteristics are variable depending on amount of cholesterol, lesion hydration, and superinfection. These lesions tend to be nonenhancing, with increased T2-weighted signal intensity, and show a T1-weighted signal pattern that is isointense relative to muscle.

The pharyngeal pterygoid venous plexus may normally be asymmetric and may therefore be misinterpreted as a tumor. This asymmetry can be recognized by keeping in mind the medial positioning of the pterygoid venous plexus in reference to the lateral pterygoids.

MASTICATOR SPACE

Major lesions of the masticator space are listed in Table 34–1. Masticator space malignancies may arise within the masticator space or may enter from an adjacent region. The masticator space adjoins the middle cranial fossa and communicates with Meckel's cave through the foramen ovale and from there to the intracranial space (Fig. 34–16). Therefore, intracranial and middle cranial fossa neoplasms may spread directly to the masticator space (Fig. 34–17) and may also involve the parapharyngeal space.[70] Such malignancies include those that are primarily considered of skull base origin. Malignancies found in the masticator space include sarcomas such as soft tissue sarcomas, chondrosarcomas, and osteosarcomas. Occasionally, large tumors of the suprasellar region have been reported to spread through the floor of the middle cranial fossa.[55] When the tumors are of possible pituitary origin, immunohistochemical evaluation may be of benefit in diagnosis. Squamous cell carcinomas in the masticator space may originate from the tonsillar or retromolar trigone region and may show perineural spread. Non-Hodgkin's lymphoma is also found within the masticator space. Malignant schwannoma, also known as neurogenic sarcoma, may be found in the masticator space; these are often of the tubular subtype. Primary or secondary mandibular tumors may also spread to the masticator space.

Benign masticator space tumors include leiomyomas, neurofibromas, and schwannomas. Inflammatory processes involving the masticator space include odontogenic abscess from the mandible and mandibular osteomyelitis. Congenital processes involving the mandible include hemangiomas and lymphangiomas.

Accessory parotid glands and benign masseteric hypertrophy may be misinterpreted as tumors and represent normal anatomic variants. Up to 21% of the population may possess accessory parotid tissue, which is most commonly identified by its location overlying the masseter muscle. Additional features of accessory parotid tissue include tissue intensity and enhancement characteristics similar to those of the parotid gland. Benign masseteric hypertrophy may be found unilaterally and may be seen with contralateral mandibular nerve (V_3) denervation atrophy. Unilateral masticator space muscle atrophy may be seen after functional denervation due to a lesion's mass effect or infiltration or may occur after therapy. In Figure 34–18, unilateral enhancing fatty pterygoid atrophy due to a trigeminal schwannoma with maxillary branch involvement is shown.

PAROTID SPACE

Major characteristic lesions of the parotid space are listed in Table 34–1. Parotid space pathology may be evaluated with sialography, CT, or MRI. Sialography is considered the most reliable method for evaluating small ductal calculi or stenoses and may therefore help evaluate parotid swelling that recurs with eating. CT evaluation of parotid pathology is often helpful for imaging calcification and calculi.

When MRI features of parotid space lesions are evaluated, malignancies tend to demonstrate less distinct margins than benign lesions. In one series of 116 patients, deep structure infiltration (parapharyngeal space, muscle, or bone) was believed to be the most reliable predictor of malignancy. When malignancy was differentiated from inflammatory and benign lesions, poor predictive values were shown for poor tumor margination, lesion homogeneity, signal intensity, and subcutaneous fat infiltration.[71] Mucoepidermoid carcinomas tend to be rock hard and arise from glandular ductal epithelium. Adenoid cystic carcinomas are infiltrating lesions arising from peripheral ducts and demonstrate perineural spread into the temporal bone. Other head and neck neoplasms demonstrating perineural spread include squamous cell carcinomas and lymphomas. Other malignancies found in the par-

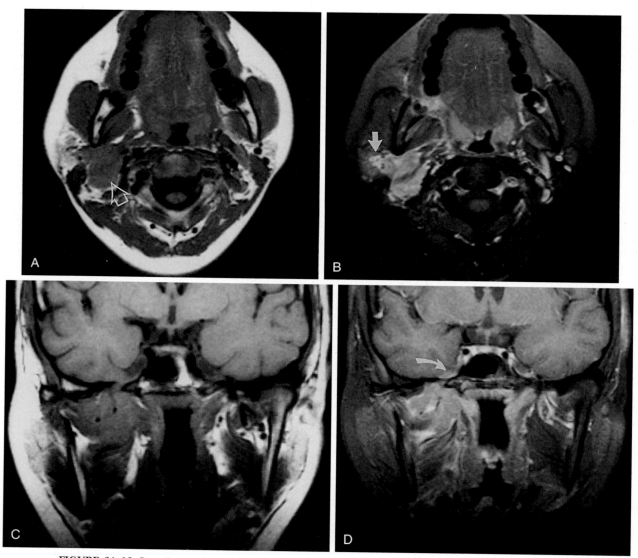

FIGURE 34–16. Lymphoma. This 15-year-old male lymphoma patient with multicompartment findings presented with right trismus. An axial nonenhanced T1-weighted image *(A)* shows a right parapharyngeal space mass *(open white arrow)* that demonstrated contrast enhancement *(B)* with apparent contiguous parotid enhancement *(white arrow).* Coronal images *(C and D)* show contrast enhancement extending to the skull base with involvement of the masticator space region and contiguous enhancement of the maxillary trigeminal branch above foramen ovale *(curved white arrow),* implying intracranial extension.

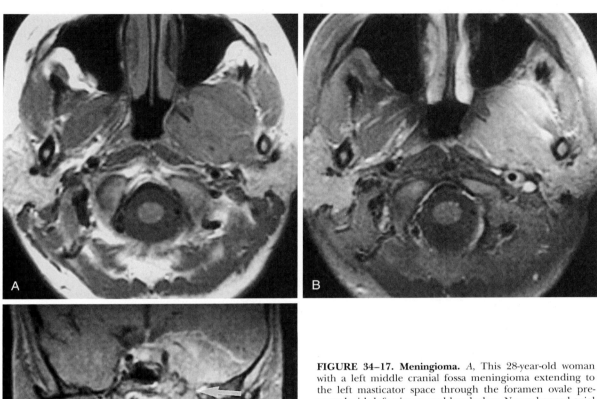

FIGURE 34–17. Meningioma. *A,* This 28-year-old woman with a left middle cranial fossa meningioma extending to the left masticator space through the foramen ovale presented with left trismus and headaches. Nonenhanced axial T1-weighted image shows left masticator space fullness with poor delineation of the lateral and medial pterygoids and with medial bowing of the pharyngeal mucosal surface. *B,* Enhanced fat-suppressed axial image corresponding with *A* shows diffuse enhancement throughout the left masticator space without easily identifiable left pterygoids. *C,* Coronal enhanced fat-suppressed image obtained at the level of the foramen ovale shows a large amount of tumor mass inferior to the foramen and a large amount of contiguous tumor above the level of the foramen, narrowing at the level of the foramen ovale *(arrow).*

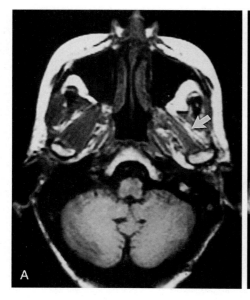

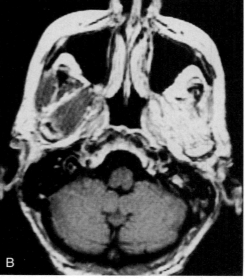

FIGURE 34–18. Schwannoma. In this 63-year-old woman with a trigeminal nerve schwannoma there is extensive atrophy of the left pterygoid muscles *(arrow)* on the nonenhanced axial T1-weighted image *(A)*, corresponding with marked contrast enhancement on the postcontrast image *(B)*.

otid space include acinous cell neoplasms, malignant mixed tumors (Fig. 34–19), lymphoma, and metastases (Fig. 34–20). Lesions metastatic to the parotid space often include other head and neck primary malignancies such as squamous cell carcinomas and melanomas.

Benign tumors in the parotid space include pleomorphic adenoma, Warthin's tumor of the parotid gland, lipoma (Fig. 34–21), and oncocytoma. Warthin's tumor of the parotid gland is a "papillary lymphadenoma adenomatosum," which arises from intraparotid heterotopic salivary gland tissue. Benign and usually multiple lymphoepithelial cysts may be found in the parotid gland and are are often associated with the acquired immunodeficiency syndrome.

Congenital parotid space lesions include first branchial cleft cysts, hemangiomas, and lymphangiomas. Warthin's tumors, metastases, and acquired immunodeficiency syndrome–associated benign lymph-

oepithelial cysts are lesions that may demonstrate multiplicity on presentation.

Parotid space inflammatory processes include cellulitis or abscess, reactive adenopathy, and sarcoid (see also Chapter 35).

PTERYGOPALATINE SPACE

Major characteristic lesions of the pterygopalatine space are listed in Table 34–1. The pterygopalatine space serves as a crossroads between the nasal cavity, the posterior palate, the suprazygomatic masticator space, and the orbit. This space may therefore become involved with inflammatory, infectious, and neoplastic processes from any of these spaces. Juvenile nasopharyngeal angiofibromas, as an example, are highly vascular lesions that are most commonly found in adoles-

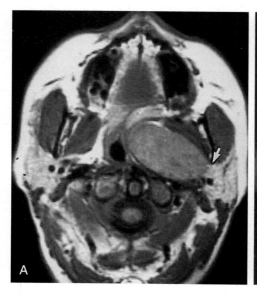

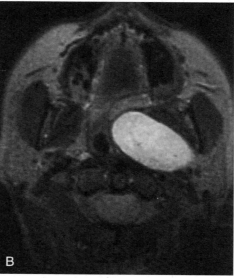

FIGURE 34–19. Parotid tumor. A left parapharyngeal region mass is found in this 43-year-old woman with left neck pain. This mass is inseparable from the deep lobe of the left parotid gland *(arrow)* on both axial nonenhanced T1-weighted *(A)* and T2-weighted *(B)* views. Surgical resection showed a malignant mixed tumor arising from the parotid gland.

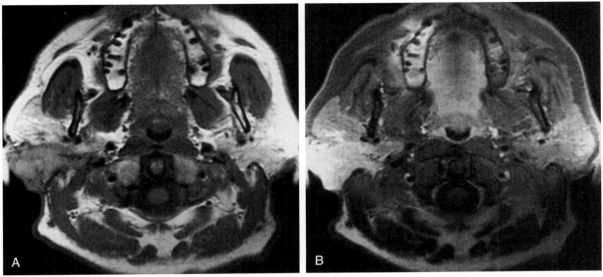

FIGURE 34-20. Metastasis. This example of renal cell carcinoma metastatic to the right parotid gland presented in a 61-year-old man with a palpable mass behind the right parotid. Nonenhanced (A) and enhanced fat-suppressed (B) axial T1-weighted images show a contiguous and enhancing mass approximately equal in cross-sectional size to the parotid gland.

FIGURE 34-21. Lipoma. A mass was felt anterior to the parotid in this 44-year-old man. The signal intensity of the mass is less on the T2-weighted image (right image, A) and much less on the enhanced fat-suppressed T1-weighted image (right image, B). Nonenhanced T1-weighted images (left image, A and B) show marked hyperintensity of the parotid margin lipoma (arrows).

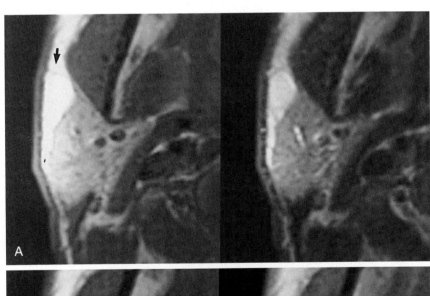

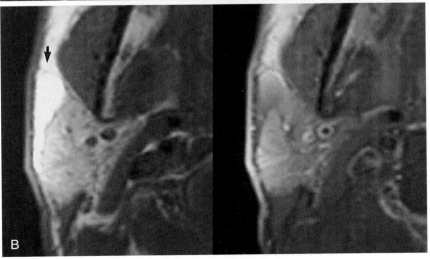

cent males. These patients present with a history of nasal obstruction associated with recurrent nosebleeds more than 80% of the time.[36, 72] Juvenile nasopharyngeal angiofibromas are primary nasal tumors that originate at the posterolateral wall of the nasal cavity where the pterygoid process of the sphenoid bone, the horizontal ala of the vomer, and the sphenoid process of the palatine bone meet, and they show early extension into the pterygopalatine space.[2, 36, 73] Staging depends on involvement of paranasal sinuses, extension into the pterygomaxillary fissure, forward displacement of the posterior wall of the maxillary sinus, invasion of the orbit, pterygomaxillary extension into the cheek and temporal fossa, and intracranial extension.[36] The appearance on MR images includes intermediate T1-weighted signal intensity, dense contrast enhancement often with contained flow voids, and T2-weighted signal hyperintensity (Fig. 34–22) (see also Fig. 33–7).

Retropharyngeal Space

Major characteristic lesions of the retropharyngeal space are listed in Table 34–1. Remember when differentiating retropharyngeal processes from prevertebral processes that retropharyngeal processes are found anterior to the prevertebral muscles.[1] Malignancies involving the retropharyngeal space include squamous cell carcinoma invading or metastasizing from adjoining spaces, nodal non-Hodgkin's lymphoma, and metastases to the lymph nodes of the retropharyngeal space. The lymph nodes of the retropharyngeal space have an unusual propensity for attracting metastases from head and neck melanoma and thyroid primary tumors.

The lateral retropharyngeal lymph nodes are found between the carotid artery and prevertebral muscles. The uppermost of these nodes, found anterior to the arch of C-1, are the nodes of Rouvière. These nodes can be identified in only 5.8% of the normal adult population, and identification is most easily made based on T2-weighted signal hyperintensity. Identification of these nodes should raise the question of reactive or malignant lymphadenopathy, both of which may demonstrate a similar appearance.[74]

Primary benign tumors of the retropharyngeal space include hemangiomas and lipomas. The inflammatory

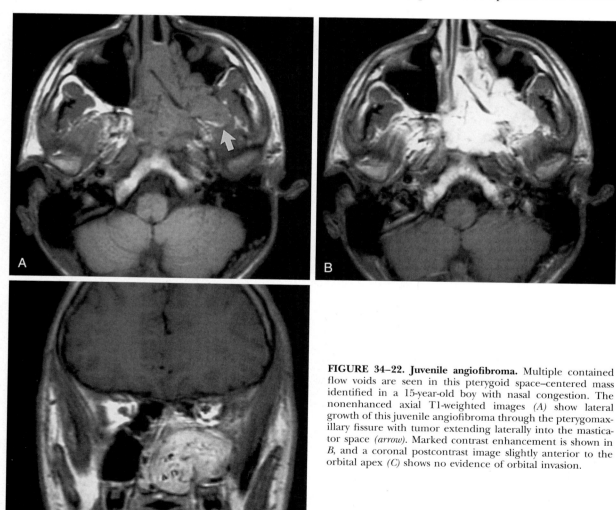

FIGURE 34–22. Juvenile angiofibroma. Multiple contained flow voids are seen in this pterygoid space–centered mass identified in a 15-year-old boy with nasal congestion. The nonenhanced axial T1-weighted images (A) show lateral growth of this juvenile angiofibroma through the pterygomaxillary fissure with tumor extending laterally into the masticator space (arrow). Marked contrast enhancement is shown in B, and a coronal postcontrast image slightly anterior to the orbital apex (C) shows no evidence of orbital invasion.

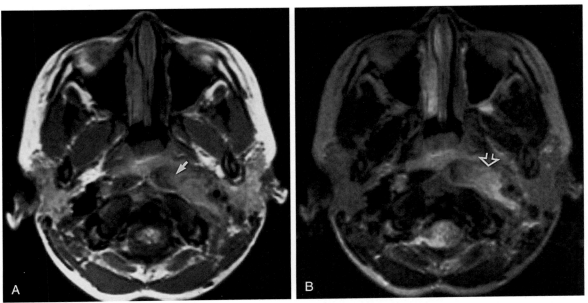

FIGURE 34–23. Cellulitis. This 8-year-old boy presented with left mastoiditis, left prevertebral cellulitis, and petrositis. Axial T1-weighted nonenhanced *(A)* and enhanced fat-suppressed *(B)* images show enlargement and lateral margin irregularity of the longus colli muscle *(solid white arrow)*, with heterogeneous enhancement most likely representing cellulitis *(open arrow)*.

processes that involve the retropharyngeal space include reactive adenopathy, cellulitis, and retropharyngeal abscess. Normal anatomic variants of the retropharyngeal space that may be mistaken as tumors include vascular ectasia and tissue edema or lymphedema secondary to venous or lymphatic obstruction.

PREVERTEBRAL SPACE

Major characteristic lesions of the prevertebral space are listed in Table 34–1. Because the prevertebral space includes bony vertebral structures, primary malignancies of the prevertebral space include vertebral primary lesions and vertebral and epidural metastases. Prevertebral processes tend to displace the prevertebral muscles anteriorly, as opposed to retropharyngeal processes, which ordinarily do not displace the prevertebral muscles.[1] Vertebral infiltration and metastasis are suggested not only in cases of diffuse decreased T1-weighted and increased T2-weighted signal infiltration but also with increased fat-suppressed marrow enhancement. Additional signs have been described that assist in positive and negative discrimination of metastasis. Increased central T1-weighted signal intensity of the lesion, denoted as a "bull's eye," indicates normal hematopoietic marrow with 95% sensitivity and 99.5% specificity, whereas a rim of increased T2-weighted signal intensity surrounding an osseous lesion, denoted as a "halo," suggests metastatic disease with 75% sensitivity and 99.5% specificity.[75] Primary malignancies of the prevertebral space include non-Hodgkin's lymphoma and chordomas. Chordomas are tumors of notochordal origin; more than 95% of chordomas are calcified. Chordomas either may arise

primarily within the cervical spine or may extend to the paravertebral fascial planes and upper cervical canal from primary involvement of the clivus and basion.[52] Benign lesions of the prevertebral space include neurofibromas and schwannomas. Squamous cell carcinomas from surrounding spaces may also invade the prevertebral space.

Osteomyelitis and cellulitis or abscess (Fig. 34–23) are examples of inflammatory processes involving the prevertebral space. The causative organism for osteomyelitis varies with the population of patients. Tuberculosis is seen in immunocompromised hosts and especially in children. *Staphylococcus* and *Enterobacter* are also causative organisms for osteomyelitis. One hazard of infection and inflammation in the prevertebral space is the danger of epidural spread. When osteomyelitis is evaluated, fat-suppressed contrast-enhanced MRI is significantly more sensitive than scintigraphy or nonenhanced MRI.[76] Benign lesions found in the prevertebral space include osteophytes and disk herniations.

CAROTID SPACE

Major characteristic lesions of the carotid space are listed in Table 34–1. Malignancies involving the carotid space include lymphomas primarily arising within carotid space lymph nodes, metastases to carotid space lymph nodes, and tumor extension from adjacent primary malignancies. Unusual mesenchymal tumors may present within the carotid space. Figures 34–24 and 34–25, respectively, illustrate spindle cell rhabdomyosarcoma and liposarcoma, with associated carotid space lymphadenopathy presenting in the carotid space in adults. An extensive list exists for causes of head and

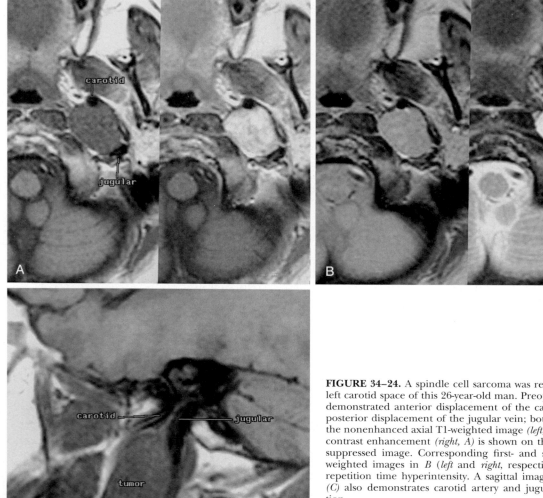

FIGURE 34–24. A spindle cell sarcoma was removed from the left carotid space of this 26-year-old man. Preoperative imaging demonstrated anterior displacement of the carotid artery and posterior displacement of the jugular vein; both are labeled in the nonenhanced axial T1-weighted image *(left, A)*, and marked contrast enhancement *(right, A)* is shown on the enhanced fat-suppressed image. Corresponding first- and second-echo T2-weighted images in *B (left* and *right*, respectively) show long repetition time hyperintensity. A sagittal image of this region *(C)* also demonstrates carotid artery and jugular vein separation.

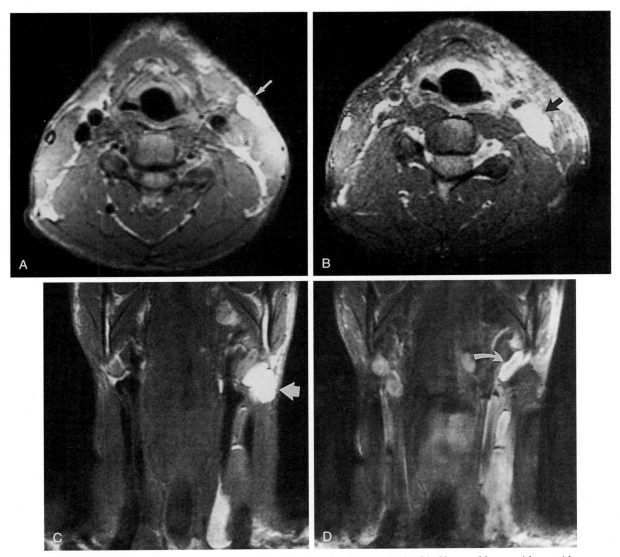

FIGURE 34–25. Liposarcoma. Nonenhanced axial T1-weighted image *(A)* in this 31-year-old man with carotid space liposarcoma and diffuse lymphadenopathy shows a superficial zone of fat-like hyperintensity *(thin white arrow)*. A corresponding fat-suppressed enhanced axial T1-weighted image *(B)* shows marked and unsuspected abnormal discrete enhancement in the left carotid sheath *(black arrow)*. T1 hyperintensity is shown on the nonenhanced *(C)* coronal image at the level of the middle ramus *(broad white arrow)*, which is suppressed on the corresponding enhanced fat-suppressed image *(D)*. Underlying this region, abnormal enhancement is shown *(curved white arrow)* that represents enhancing tumor.

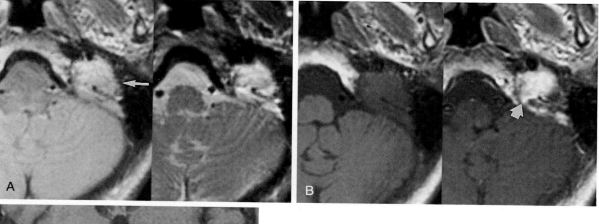

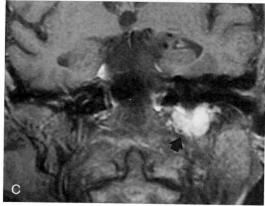

FIGURE 34–26. Glomus jugulare. *A*, A hyperintense lesion *(arrow)* with contained flow voids is demonstrated in the left jugular fossa on both first *(left)* and second *(right)* echoes of a T2-weighted sequence in this 76-year-old woman with a glomus jugulare who presented with tinnitus. *B*, Corresponding nonenhanced *(left)* and enhanced fat-suppressed *(right)* images show lesion *(arrow)* enhancement. *C*, A coronal enhanced fat-suppressed image at the level of the jugular bulb demonstrates the enhancing tumor mass *(arrow)* within the left jugular bulb.

neck lymphadenopathy, including massive lymphadenopathy associated with extranodal sinus histiocytosis.[77]

Benign tumors involving the carotid space include paragangliomas (Fig. 34–26), neurogenic tumors such as neurofibromas and schwannomas (Fig. 34–27), and second branchial cleft cysts (Fig. 34–28). When imaging features of neurogenic tumors and paragangliomas are compared, schwannomas tend to demonstrate distinctive bony scalloping (see also Chapter 32).

Paragangliomas may present with variable cranial neuropathy of cranial nerves IX, X, XI, and XII. They arise from hybrid neuromyocytic cells that are stretch receptors, and these tumors usually show slow growth characteristics.[39] The chromaffin paraganglioma subtype is a secretory tumor. Carotid body tumors are at the common carotid bifurcation and splay the internal and external carotid origins. Glomus tympanicum tumors overlie the cochlear promontory; glomus jugulare tumors involve the jugular fossa and cause erosion of the caroticojugular spine at the jugular foramen; and glomus vagale tumors are found adjacent to the course of the vagal nerve. Paragangliomas may be large and extend into adjoining spaces. Primary extracarotid space paragangliomas have also been separately reported, as discussed in the section on the pathology of the parapharyngeal space.[67] This family of tumors tends to demonstrate intense contrast enhancement and serpiginous flow voids. These lesions often possess a salt-and-pepper appearance due to a combination of hypointense flow voids and hyperintense subacute hemorrhage.[2] Combined use of MR

angiography and spin-echo imaging has been found to be useful in the evaluation of skull base paragangliomas. In one series, 16 of 18 tumors were identified correctly on the basis of spin-echo images alone, and four false-positive cases misinterpreted as paragangliomas due to slow-flowing venous enhancement were differentiated on the basis of separate arterial and venous MR angiographic sequences.[78] Second branchial cleft cysts may develop anterior to the margin of the sternocleidomastoid muscle; these lesions were discussed in the section on pathology of the parapharyngeal space. Lipomas and other nonspecific compartmental lesions may also be found in the carotid space (Fig. 34–29).

Carotid space inflammatory processes include cellulitis and abscess. Carotid space abscess should be considered a surgical emergency due to the potential for large artery involvement.

Additional vasculogenic differential considerations include jugular or carotid thromboses and aneurysms. Although masses may be correctly identified as being within the carotid space, unless peripheral MRI signal void or peripheral CT calcification or enhancement is sought, the operative approach may unexpectedly address a cervical carotid aneurysm with a potentially catastrophic outcome. Previous series have included patients with concomitant head and neck carcinomas with malignant lymphadenopathy and relatively asymptomatic patients with the erroneous presumptive preoperative diagnosis of neuroma.[79]

Entities that may mimic carotid space mass lesions

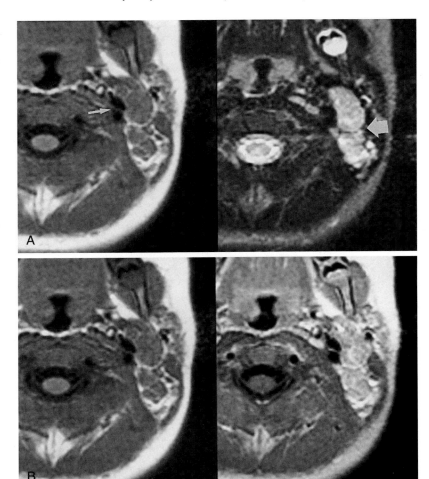

FIGURE 34–27. Neurofibromatosis. In this 18-month-old male infant with neurofibromatosis, multiple neurofibromas *(thick arrow)* are demonstrated superficial to the left carotid artery and jugular vein *(thin arrow)*. *A* contrasts the nonenhanced isointense T1-weighted *(left)* and hyperintense T2-weighted *(right)* appearance. *B* demonstrates contrast enhancement on the enhanced fat-suppressed image *(right)* compared with the nonenhanced T1-weighted image *(left)*.

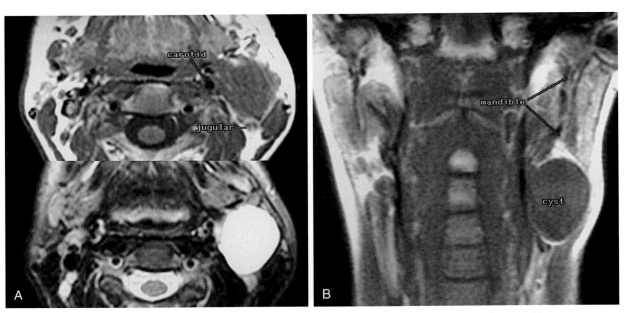

FIGURE 34–28. Branchial cleft cyst. *A,* A second branchial cleft cyst is shown separating the left carotid artery and jugular vein and displacing the jugular vein posteriorly in this 31-year-old woman presenting with a left neck mass. Nonenhanced axial T1-weighted *(top)* and T2-weighted *(bottom)* images show T1-weighted signal isointensity and T2-weighted signal hyperintensity. *B,* Coronal nonenhanced axial T1-weighted image shows the sharply marginated cyst located inferior to the left mandibular ramus.

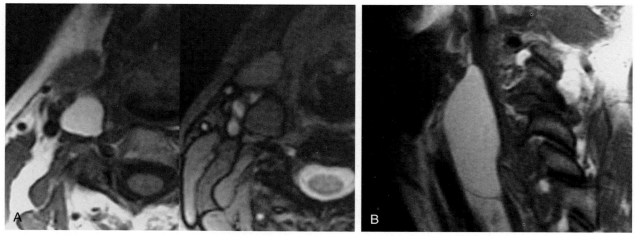

FIGURE 34–29. Lipoma. *A,* Conventional T1-weighted *(left)* and short-tau inversion recovery (STIR) *(right)* images show a lipoma in the right carotid sheath deep to the great vessels and sternocleidomastoid muscle, with decreased lipoma signal intensity on STIR. *B,* Sagittal T1-weighted image through the carotid sheath shows a thin capsule surrounding the lipoma that shows lateral displacement of the jugular vein.

include carotid space vascular thrombosis, normal variant vascular asymmetry, and normal variant ectasia of the jugular vein or carotid artery. Carotid space vascular thrombosis may be erroneously labeled as necrotic adenopathy, and it may be helpful to remember that adenopathy above the hard palate is not carotid space lymphadenopathy but rather lateral retropharyngeal lymphadenopathy.

MISCELLANEOUS

SLEEP APNEA

The role of imaging in evaluation of snoring- and sleep apnea–related disorders is being explored. MRI is being used to develop models to evaluate flow resistance and geometry in the human nasopharyngeal airway and to evaluate the flow-related effects of dimensional anatomic variabilities, local obstructions, and congestion.[80] Dynamic upper airway imaging has been performed in normal individuals by combining dynamic pneumotachygraphic air flow measurements with cine CT to evaluate level-specific changes in upper airway caliber throughout the breathing cycle. Such evaluations have suggested that dynamic respiratory upper airway changes are related to phase-dependent actions of the upper airway dilator muscles, positive intraluminal pressure, and negative intraluminal pressure.[81] Dynamic upper airway imaging has been employed to evaluate differences in breathing cycle changes taking place in the upper airway of normal individuals, snoring individuals, and individuals with mild sleep apnea and obstructive sleep apnea.[82] Patients with sleep apnea demonstrate circular or sagittally elongated pharyngeal airway cross sections, whereas normal populations demonstrate coronally elongated pharyngeal airway cross sections.[83] These findings have been confirmed through pharyngeal airway evaluation using ultrafast spoiled gradient-recalled

acquisition in the steady state (GRASS) MRI. When compared with dynamic CT evaluation of the upper airway, MRI is technically advantageous in demonstrating the sagittal plane and in allowing improved airway visualization in patients with metallic dental artifacts.[84] Three-dimensional reconstructions of the pharyngeal airway have been used to assess changes in volume measurements after operative reconstruction.[85]

POSTOPERATIVE AND POSTIRRADIATION CHANGES

Postoperative and postirradiation changes to the head and neck region may be extensive and difficult to evaluate. Combinations of surgery, radiation therapy, and chemotherapy are used to treat head and neck tumors, each causing various anatomic and signal-related changes in the treatment zone.[86] Treatment protocols for tumor locations with previously controversial treatment, such as the base of the tongue and tonsillar pillars, now demonstrate 5-year cause-specific survival rates as high as 77%.[87, 88] Surgical approaches may be heroic and elaborate, such as facial translocation and transoral surgery.[36, 89, 90] Approaches such as facial translocation were developed to allow exposure of the skull base, nasopharynx, infratemporal fossa, and superior orbital fissure for control of neurovascular structures.[89] Local relapse may be indicated clinically through progressive symptoms, new nasal or ear symptoms, cranial neuropathies, headaches, and neck node changes. Physical examination includes manual palpation, indirect mirror examination, and flexible and rigid endoscopy.[91] Difficulty in postoperative imaging evaluation may arise from changes in morphology as a result of tissue removal, tissue transfer, and tissue replacement. Difficulty can also be encountered in evaluating the changing tissue signal characteristics after irradiation and surgery, which must be distinguished from recurrent disease. Studies have demonstrated higher T2 values in patients with residual tumor than in patients with postirradiation fibrosis, although this finding is nonspecific in that high T2 values may also be seen with radiation edema and with infection.[92, 93] Studies have demonstrated up to 100% incidence of accompanying abnormal soft tissue masses in patients with recurrence. Therefore, combined increasing soft tissue mass in concert with hyperintense T2-weighted signal intensity is highly suggestive of tumor recurrence.[92]

Tissue removal may include large vessel resection, extensive resection of muscle and bone, and removal or denervation of neural components with concomitant changes. Denervated muscle shows short-tau inversion recovery (STIR) hyperintensity, conspicuous fatty infiltration on T1 weighting, and increased T2-weighted signal intensity.[94] Such changes are shown in Figure 34–30 in a patient with hemiatrophy of the left tongue with fat replacement occurring after invasion of the hypoglossal nerve from recurrent, previously treated primary squamous cell carcinoma of the pharyngeal mucosal space. Tissue transfers and replacement include myocutaneous flaps, free composite flaps, free jejunal grafts, and combination grafts. The most common sites of tumor recurrence after resection and flap reconstruction are in or near the reconstruction.[95] The demonstration of interval changes compared with a baseline study 4 to 6 weeks after therapy is critical in evaluating post-therapy recurrence. Recurrences typically underlie flaps or are at flap suture margins and present as solid or cystic-necrotic masses. Postsurgical recurrence after resection and flap reconstruction may manifest as isolated nodal disease.

In equivocal or uncertain MRI of recurrence, PET may be of value. PET has been of benefit in identifying primary head and neck tumors, malignant lymphadenopathy, and recurrent or residual head and neck tumors that were unappreciated by MRI.[10]

MRI is also of potential benefit in evaluating complications of therapy. MRI findings have been discussed in cases of radiation myelopathy. Long segment enlargement of the spinal cord may be seen, with low signal intensity on T1-weighted images and high signal intensity on T2-weighted images, corresponding geographically with the radiation port. These findings may manifest themselves up to 4 years after therapy and correspond well with the neurologically demonstrated deficit levels.[96]

BIOPSY AND INTERVENTIONAL MRI

MRI has been used to guide limited biopsy and intervention in the head and neck. Preoperative therapy and treatment planning of neoplasms in the head and neck have been assisted through percutaneous fine needle and core biopsy specimens obtained with more traditional CT, ultrasound, and fluoroscopic guidance.[97–99] These biopsy approaches have resulted in successful biopsies of the parapharyngeal and nasopharyngeal regions, the cervical and skull base lymph nodes, vertebral and paravertebral structures, intracranial lesions, and even Meckel's cave through the foramen ovale.[62, 100–102] Biopsy needles have been developed that contain high nickel alloy stainless steel, which changes magnetically susceptible α iron to less susceptible γ iron, allowing improved needle visualization without interfering artifact.[103] This allows opportunities for interventional MRI, including biopsy, MRI-compatible deep electrode implantation, and potential laser and interstitial therapy.[104, 105]

Transcoronoid, retromandibular, submastoid, and submalar biopsy approaches have been used successfully in the head and neck.[97] The transcoronoid approach is useful for biopsy of precarotid masses that are in the high parapharyngeal zone. This approach is undertaken with the patient's mouth closed on a bite block, and the needle is passed inferior to the zygomatic arch and superior to the partially opened mandibular coronoid notch. The retromandibular approach may be used to approach lesions situated in the parapharyngeal, prevertebral, and deep parotid spaces. One hazard of retromandibular approach is potential inadvertent carotid artery puncture. Submastoid approaches may occasionally be indicated for posterior carotid space masses that deviate the carotid sheath vessels anteriorly. Submastoid approaches are somewhat challenging owing to lack of tissue stability at this site and to the unusual cranial angulation that is usually demanded. Submalar approaches are directed under the malar eminence and involve a needle pass made parallel to the lateral wall of the maxillary sinus, allowing wide access to the skull base. Submalar approaches usually involve transgression of the pterygoid muscles and thereby allow stable and controlled needle placement, as contrasted to needle placement through looser areolar or fatty tissue.[97]

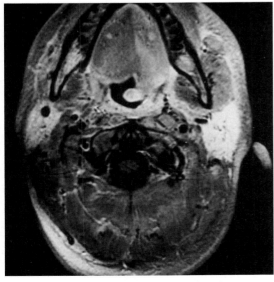

FIGURE 34–30. Fat-suppressed T1-weighted image in a 24-year-old man previously treated for pharyngeal mucosal space carcinoma shows abnormal increased left parapharyngeal enhancement from recurrence and left tongue fatty atrophy secondary to hypoglossal nerve involvement.

REFERENCES

1. Harnsberger H: Introduction to suprahyoid neck anatomy. Presented at the 26th Annual Meeting of the American Society of Head and Neck Radiology, Vancouver, 1993, abstract 1-11.
2. Harnsberger HR: Head and neck imaging. In: Osborne AG, Bragg DG, eds. Handbooks in Radiology. St. Louis: Mosby–Year Book, 1990.
3. Flanders A, Helinek G, Tom B, Rao V: Imaging of the nasopharynx. Crit Rev Diagn Imaging 31:357–411, 1991.
4. Waldron J, Kreel L, Metreweli C, Woo J, Van Hasselt C: Comparision of plain radiographs and computed tomographic scanning in nasopharyngeal carcinoma. Clin Radiol 45:404–406, 1992.
5. Vogl T, Dresel S: Diagnostic procedures in nasopharyngeal illness. Curr Opin Radiol 4:127–135, 1992.
6. Lalwani AK, Engelstad BL, Boles R: Significance of abnormal indium In 111–labeled leukocyte accumulation in the head and neck region. Arch Otolaryngol Head Neck Surg 117:1138–1143, 1991.
7. Kao C, Wang S, Wey S, et al: The detection of nasopharynx carcinoma in technetium-99m (V) dimercaptosuccinic acid SPECT imaging. Clin Nucl Med 18:321–323, 1993.
8. Kao C, Wang S, Lin W, et al: Detection of nasopharyngeal carcinoma using $^{99}Tc^m$-methoxyisobutylisonitrile SPECT. Nucl Med Commun 14:41–46, 1993.
9. Menendez LR, Fideler BM, Mirra J: Thallium-201 scanning for the evaluation of osteosarcoma and soft-tissue sarcoma: a study of the evaluation and predictability of the histological response to chemotherapy. J Bone Joint Surg 75:526–531, 1993.
10. Chaiken L, Rege S, Hoh C, et al: Positron emission tomography with fluorodeoxyglucose to evaluate tumor response and control after radiation therapy. Int J Radiat Oncol Biol Phys 27:455–464, 1993.
11. Rege SD, Chaiken L, Hoh CK, et al: Change induced by radiation therapy in FDG uptake in normal and malignant structures of the head and neck: quantitation with PET. Radiology 189:807–812, 1993.
12. Samoszuk M, Anderson A, Ramzi E, et al: Radioimmunodetection of Hodgkin's disease and non-Hodgkin's lymphomas with monoclonal antibody to eosinophil peroxidase. J Nucl Med 34:1246–1253, 1993.
13. Lanzieri C, Bangert B: Magnetic resonance imaging of the nasopharynx. Topics Magn Reson Imaging 2:39–47, 1990.
14. Tsao S, Chua E: Current problems in radiotherapy, chemotherapy, and staging of nasopharyngeal carcinoma (NPC). Ann Acad Med Singapore 20:649–655, 1991.
15. Castelijns J, van den Brekel M: Magnetic resonance imaging evaluation of extracranial head and neck tumors. Magn Reson Q 9:113–128, 1993.
16. Hunink M, de Slegte R, Gerritsen G, Speelman H: CT and MR assessment of tumors of the nose and paranasal sinuses, the nasopharynx and the parapharyngeal space using ROC methodology. Neuroradiology 32:220–225, 1990.
17. Hudgins P, Elster A, Runge V, et al: Efficacy and safety of gadopentetate dimeglumine in the evaluation of patients with a suspected tumor of the extracranial head and neck. J Magn Reson Imaging 3:345–349, 1993.
18. Vogl T, Dresel S, Bilaniuk L, et al: Tumors of the nasopharynx and adjacent areas: MR imaging with Gd-DTPA. AJR 154:585–592, 1990.
19. Takayashima S, Noguchi Y, Okumura T, et al: Dynamic MR imaging in the head and neck. Radiology 189:813–821, 1993.
20. Yousem D: Dynamic MR imaging of the head and neck: an idea whose time has come . . . and gone? Radiology 189:659–660, 1993.
21. Vogl TJ, Mack MG, Juergens M, et al: Skull base tumors: gadodiamide injection–enhanced MR imaging—drop-out effect in the early enhancement pattern of paraganglioma versus different tumors. Radiology 188:339–346, 1993.
22. Anzai Y, Lufkin RB, Jabour BA, Hanafee WN: Fat-suppression failure artifacts simulating pathology on frequency-selective fat-suppression MR images of the head and neck. AJNR 13:879–884, 1992.
23. Zoarski GH, Mackey JK, Anzai Y, et al: Head and neck: initial clinical experience with fast spin-echo MR imaging. Radiology 188:323–327, 1993.
24. Dubin MD, Teresi LM, Bradley WG, et al: Efficacy of T2-weighted fast spin echo imaging with fat saturation in the detection and characterization of head and neck lesions. Presented at the 32nd Annual Meeting of the American Society of Neuroradiology, Nashville, 1994, paper 133.
25. Vogl T, Dresel S: New developments in magnetic resonance imaging of the nasopharynx and face. Curr Opin Radiol 3:61–66, 1991.
26. McGowan J III, Hatabu H, Yousem D, et al: Evaluation of soft palate function with MRI: application to the cleft palate patient. J Comput Assist Tomogr 16:877–882, 1992.
27. Tart RP, Mukherji SK, Avino AJ, et al: Facial lymph nodes: normal and abnormal CT appearance. Radiology 188:695–700, 1993.
28. Steinkamp HJ, Hosten N, Richter C, et al: Enlarged cervical lymph nodes at helical CT. Radiology 191:795–798, 1994.
29. Yousem DM, Som PM, Hackney DB, et al: Central nodal necrosis and extracapsular neoplastic spread in cervical lymph nodes: MR imaging versus CT. Radiology 182:753–759, 1992.
30. Sheppard L, Yousem DM, Weinstein, G, et al: Magnetization transfer imaging of cervical lymphadenopathy. Presented at the 32nd Annual Meeting of the American Society of Neuroradiology, Nashville, 1994, paper 130.
31. Rogers JW, Sato Y, Yuh WTC, et al: Magnetic resonance evaluation of cervical adenopathy with an iron-based contrast agent. Presented at the 32nd Annual Meeting of the American Society of Neuroradiology, Nashville, 1994, paper 132.
32. Anzai Y, Lufkin RB, Blackwell K, et al: Clinical evaluation of Dextran covered superparamagnetic iron oxide (BMS 180549) for detection of metastatic lymph nodes in head and neck cancer. Presented at the 32nd Annual Meeting of the American Society of Neuroradiology, Nashville, 1994, paper 131.
33. Snell R: Clinical Anatomy. 2nd ed. Boston: Little, Brown & Co, 1981.
34. Gray H: Anatomy of the Human Body. 29th ed. Philadelphia: Lea & Febiger, 1973.
35. Thibault F, Halimi P, Bely N, et al: Internal architecture of the parotid gland at MR imaging: facial nerve or ductal system? Radiology 188:701–704, 1993.
36. Cummings C, Fredrickson J, Harker L, et al: Otolaryngology—Head and Neck Surgery. St. Louis: Mosby–Year Book, 1993.
37. Weber A: Computed tomography and magnetic resonance imaging of the nasopharynx. Isr J Med Sci 28:161–168, 1992.
38. Som P, Bergeron R, eds. Head and Neck Imaging. St. Louis: Mosby–Year Book, 1991.
39. Cotran R, Kumar V, Robbins S: Robbins Pathologic Basis of Disease. 4th ed. Philadelphia: WB Saunders, 1989.
40. Oi H, Watanabe Y, Shojaku H, Mizukoshi K: Nasal septal neurinoma. Acta Otolaryngol Suppl 504:151–154, 1993.
41. Kochanski S, Burton E, Seidel F, et al: Neonatal nasopharyngeal hairy polyp: CT and MR appearance. J Comput Assist Tomogr 14:1000–1001, 1990.
42. Ramos R, Som P, Solodnik P: Nasopharyngeal melanotic melanoma: MR characteristics. J Comput Assist Tomogr 14:997–999, 1990.
43. Crowley J, Lupetin A, Wang S: Primary nasal amelanotic melanoma: MR appearance. J Magn Reson Imaging 1:601–604, 1990.
44. Hammersmith S, Terk M, Jeffrey P, et al: Magnetic resonance imaging of nasopharyngeal and paranasal sinus melanoma. Magn Reson Imaging 8:245–253, 1990.
45. Sherwood J, Hutt D, Kreutner W, et al: A magnetic resonance imaging evaluation of histamine-mediated allergic response in the guinea pig nasopharynx. J Allergy Clin Immunol 92:435–441, 1993.
46. Battino RA, Khangure MS: Is that another Thornwaldt's cyst on M.R.I.? Australas Radiol 34:19–23, 1990.
47. Boucher RM, Hendrix RA, Guttenplan MD: The diagnosis of Thornwaldt's cyst. Trans Pa Acad Ophthalmol Otolaryngol 42:1026–1030, 1990.
48. Weissman J, Tabor E, Curtin H: Sphenochoanal polyps: evaluation with CT and MR imaging. Radiology 178:145–148, 1991.
49. Geist J, Chen F: Nasopharyngeal carcinoma: computed tomographic imaging in four cases. Oral Surg Oral Med Oral Pathol 75:759–766, 1993.
50. Mineura K, Kowada M, Tomura N: Perineural extension of nasopharyngeal carcinoma into the posterior cranial fossa detected by magnetic resonance imaging. Clin Imaging 15:172–175, 1991.
51. Meyers S, Hirsch W Jr, Curtin H, et al: Chordomas of the skull base: MR features. AJNR 13:1627–1636, 1992.
52. Schamschula R, Soo M: Clival chordomas. Aust Radiol 37:259–264, 1993.
53. Sener R: Giant craniopharyngioma extending to the anterior cranial fossa and nasopharynx. AJR 162:441–442, 1994.
54. Anand VK, Osborne CM, Harkey HL 3d: Infiltrative clival pituitary adenoma of ectopic origin. Otolaryngol Head Neck Surg 108:178–183, 1993.
55. Iwai Y, Hakuba A, Khosla V, et al: Giant basal prolactinoma extending into the nasal cavity. Surg Neurol 37:280–283, 1992.
56. Kioumehr F, Rooholamini S, Yaghmai I, et al: Giant-cell tumor of the sphenoid bone: a case report and review of the literature. Can Assoc Radiol J 41:155–157, 1990.
57. Wax M, Yun K, Omar R: Extramedullary plasmacytomas of the head and neck. Otolaryngol Head Neck Surg 109:877–885, 1993.
58. Hegarty J, Rao V: Amyloidoma of the nasopharynx: CT and MR findings. AJNR 14:215–218, 1993.
59. Gean-Marton A, Kirsch C, Vezina L, Weber A: Focal amyloidosis of the head and neck: evaluation with CT and MR. Radiology 181:521–525, 1991.
60. Kapadia SB, Meis JM, Frisman DM, et al: Adult rhabdomyoma of the head and neck: a clinicopathological and immunophenotypic study. Hum Pathol 24:608–617, 1993.
61. Kodet R, Newton WA Jr, Hamoudi AB, et al: Childhood rhabdomyosarcoma with anaplastic (pleomorphic) features: a report of the intergroup rhabdomyosarcoma study. Am J Surg Pathol 17:443–453, 1993.
62. Rybak L, Rapp M, McGrady M, et al: Obstructing nasopharyngeal teratoma in the neonate: a report of two cases. Arch Otolaryngol Head Neck Surg 117:1411–1415, 1991.
63. Matsko T, Schmidt R, Milam A, Orcutt J: Primary malignant ectomesenchymoma of the orbit. Br J Ophthalmol 76:438–441, 1992.
64. Esposito MB, Arrington JA, Murtagh FR, et al: Inflammatory lesions of the nasopharyngeal space which mimic invasive carcinoma. Presented at the Annual Meeting of the American Society of Neuroradiology, Nashville, 1994, paper 134.

65. Braun M, Boman F, Hascoet J, et al: Brain tissue heterotopia in the nasopharynx. Contribution of MRI to assessment of extension. J Neuroradiol 19:68–74, 1992.

66. Soyer P, Dobbelaere P, Reizine D, Ferquel C: Transalar sphenoidal meningoencephalocele associated with buccal angiomatosis: one case. J Neuroradiol 17:222–226, 1990.

67. Kanoh N, Nishimura Y, Nakamura M, et al: Primary nasopharyngeal paraganglioma: a case report. Auris Nasus Larynx 18:307–314, 1991.

68. Moore K: The Developing Human. Philadelphia: WB Saunders, 1988.

69. Shidara K, Urama T, Yasuoka Y, Kamei T: Two cases of nasopharyngeal branchial cyst. J Laryngol Otol 107:453–455, 1993.

70. Tryhus M, Smoker WR, Harnsberger H: The normal and diseased masticator space. Semin Ultrasound CT MRI 11:476–485, 1990.

71. Freling N, Molenaar W, Vermay A, et al: Malignant parotid tumors: clinical use of MR imaging and histologic correlation. Radiology 185:691–696, 1992.

72. Schuller D, Schleuning AI: Otolaryngology—Head and Neck Surgery. St. Louis: Mosby–Year Book, 1988.

73. Fowler S, Keller I: Nasopharyngeal angiofibroma: a case study. J Neurosci Nurs 25:208–211, 1993.

74. Ichimura K: Can Rouviere's lymph nodes in non-malignant subjects be identified with MRI? Auris Nasus Larynx 20:117–123, 1993.

75. Schweitzer ME, Levine C, Mitchell DG, et al: Bull's eyes and halos: useful MR discriminators of osseous metastases. Radiology 188:249–252, 1993.

76. Morrison WB, Schweitzer ME, Bock GW, et al: Diagnosis of osteomyelitis: utility of fat-suppressed contrast-enhanced MR imaging. Radiology 189:251–257, 1993.

77. Wenig B, Abbondanzo S, Childers E: Extranodal sinus histiocytosis with massive lymphadenopathy (Rosai-Dorfman disease) of the head and neck. Hum Pathol 24:483–492, 1993.

78. Vogl TJ, Juergens M, Balzer JO, et al: Glomus tumors of the skull base: combined use of MR angiography and spin-echo imaging. Radiology 192:103–110, 1994.

79. Weissman JL, Johnson JT, Snyderman CH, Steed DL: Thrombosed aneurysm of the cervical carotid artery: avoiding a retrospective diagnosis. Radiology 190:869–871, 1994.

80. Tan E, Chua S, Kwok R: Use of magnetic resonance imaging in the evaluation of nasopharyngeal cancer. Ann Acad Med Singapore 22:720–723, 1993.

81. Schwab R, Gefter W, Pack A, Hoffman E: Dynamic imaging of the upper airway during respiration in normal subjects. J Appl Physiol 74:1504–1514, 1993.

82. Schwab R, Gefter W, Hoffman E, et al: Dynamic upper airway imaging during awake respiration in normal subjects and patients with sleep disordered breathing. Am Rev Respir Dis 148:1385–1400, 1993.

83. Rodenstein D, Dooms G, Thomas Y, et al: Pharyngeal shape and dimension in health subjects, snorers, and patients with obstructive sleep apnea. Thorax 45:722–727, 1990.

84. Shellock FG, Schatz CJ, et al: Occlusion and narrowing of the pharyngeal airway in obstructive sleep apnea: evaluation by ultrafast spoiled GRASS MR imaging. AJR 158:1019–1024, 1992.

85. Metes A, Hoffstein V, Direnfeld V, et al: Three-dimensional CT reconstruction and volume measurements of the pharyngeal airway before and after maxillofacial surgery in obstructive sleep apnea. J Otolaryngol 22:261–264, 1993.

86. Bailet J, Mark R, Abemayor E, et al: Nasopharyngeal carcinoma: treatment results in primary radiation therapy. Laryngoscope 102:965–972, 1992.

87. Foote RL, Hilgenfeld RU, Kunselman SJ, et al: Radiation therapy for squamous cell carcinoma of the tonsil. Mayo Clin Proc 69:525–531, 1994.

88. McCaffrey TV: Treatment of tonsillar carcinoma. Mayo Clin Proc 69:603–604, 1994.

89. Janecka I, Nuss D, Sen C: Facial translocation approach to the cranial base. Acta Neurochir Suppl 53:193–198, 1991.

90. Makhmudov U, Tcherekayev V, Tanyashin S: Transoral approach to tumors of the clivus: report of two cases. J Craniofac Surg 3:35–38, 1992.

91. Sham J, Choy D, Wei W, Yau C: Value of clinical follow-up for local nasopharyngeal carcinoma relapse. Head Neck 14:208–217, 1992.

92. Gong Q, Zheng G, Zhu H: MRI differentiation of recurrent nasopharyngeal carcinoma from postradiation fibrosis. Comput Med Imaging Graphics 15:423–429, 1991.

93. Gong Q, Zhu H, Zheng G, et al: MRI-T2 values in the differentiation of recurrence and fibrosis after radiation of nasopharyngeal carcinoma. Chin Med J 105:135–138, 1992.

94. Fleckenstein J, Watumuli D, Conner K, et al: Denervated human skeletal muscle: MR imaging evaluation. Radiology 187:213–218, 1993.

95. Hudgins PA, Burson JG, Gussack GS, Grist WJ: CT and MR appearance of recurrent head and neck malignancy following resection and flap reconstruction. Presented at the 32nd Annual Meeting of the American Society of Neuroradiology, Nashville, 1994, paper 135.

96. Wang P, Shen W: Magnetic resonance imaging in two patients with radiation myelopathy. J Formosan Med Assoc 90:583–585, 1991.

97. Dillon WP: CT guided biopsies of the head and neck. Presented at the 24th Annual Meeting of the American Society of Head and Neck Radiology. Boston, 1991, abstract 141-146.

98. Siegert R, Kuppers P, Barreton G: Ultrasonographic fine-needle aspiration of pathological masses in the head and neck region. J Clin Ultrasound 20:315–320, 1992.

99. Dresel SHJ, Mackey JK, Lufkin RB, et al: Meckel cave lesions: percutaneous fine-needle-aspiration biopsy cytology. Radiology 179:579–581, 1991.

100. Geremia GK, Charletta DA, Granato DB, Raju S: Biopsy of vertebral and paravertebral structures with a new coaxial needle system. AJNR 13:169–171, 1991.

101. Borgstein RL, Moxon RA, Hately W, et al: Preliminary experience with the berger neurobiopsy device for ultrasound guided aspiration and biopsy of intracranial lesions. Clin Radiol 44:98–103, 1991.

102. Barakos JA, Dillon WP: Lesions of the foramen ovale: CT-guided fine-needle aspiration. Radiology 182:573–575, 1992.

103. Lufkin R, Teresi L, Hanafee W: New needle for MR-guided aspiration cytology of the head and neck. AJR 149:380–382, 1987.

104. Lufkin R: Interventional MRI. Presented at the 24th Annual Meeting of the American Society of Head and Neck Radiology, Boston, 1991, abstract 147-148.

105. Hathout G, Lufkin RB, Jabour B, et al: MR-guided aspiration cytology in the head and neck at high field strength. J Magn Reson Imaging 2:93–94, 1992.

Lower Face and Salivary Glands

WADE WONG

Imaging of the head and neck has developed significantly with the advent of computed tomography (CT) and magnetic resonance imaging (MRI). These modalities greatly complement the physical and endoscopic examinations by revealing possible blind areas, such as subtle extension of neoplasms from the lower face or salivary glands to deep spaces, nonpalpable adenopathy, bone marrow invasion, and distant metastasis.

MRI has several major advantages over CT. Superior soft tissue contrast is possible with MRI, leading to better delineation between tumor and adjacent musculature (Fig. 35–1), especially in the tongue and floor of mouth where relatively little fat is present between tissue planes. Multiplanar imaging can be extremely helpful in appreciating and confirming the extent of disease. Beam-hardening artifacts from dental fillings often plague CT examinations, but dental fillings cause only minimal susceptibility artifacts with MRI (Fig. 35–2). Nonremovable bridgework remains a problem for both techniques. In patients who cannot tolerate the

use of iodine as a contrast medium, MRI with gadolinium enhancement can still be considered.

However, MRI has some drawbacks compared with CT. Patients who are severely claustrophobic in a magnet usually tolerate the more open-spaced feeling a CT scanner offers. General contraindications to MRI such as cardiac pacemakers, ocular foreign bodies, aneurysm clips, and surgical ferromagnetic hardware would lead one to depend on CT rather than MRI. Evaluation of calcification for stones in the salivary duct is also more easily done with CT.

TECHNICAL CONSIDERATIONS

Significant problems with motion are frequently encountered when trying to image patients with oropharyngeal, oral cavity, and hypopharyngeal cancers because of secretions and gagging. Often, simple encouragement and coaching are all that is needed for such a patient to remain still. Steady, shallow abdomi-

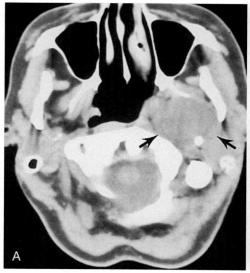
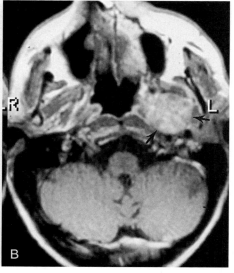

FIGURE 35–1. *A,* CT scan of a pleomorphic adenoma extending into the left parapharyngeal space. The mass *(arrows)* is isodense with the surrounding soft tissues and somewhat difficult to delineate. *B,* MR image (T1 weighted with gadolinium) demonstrates superb contrast resolution and clear delineation between the tumor *(arrows)* and the adjacent soft tissues.

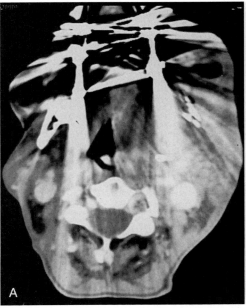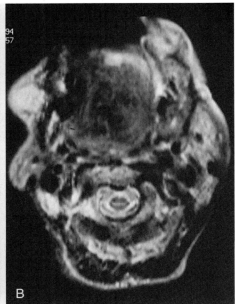

FIGURE 35-2. Imaging at the level of the oral cavity where the anterior mandible was resected owing to aggressive squamous cell carcinoma of the tongue and floor of the mouth that had invaded the mandible. *A*, CT scan demonstrates severe beam-hardening artifact from dental fillings. This makes it impossible to evaluate the oral cavity as well as the mandible. *B*, T2-weighted MR image is less affected by beam-hardening artifact. Only local susceptibility effects are seen in the region of the dental fillings. The mandibular resection is evident. The floor of the mouth and adjacent structures can be more optimally visualized.

nal breathing is helpful. In some cases, deep sedation may be necessary.

Speed of study is also important, because this limits the amount of motion degradation. Fast spin-echo sequences are helpful in this regard. Because fat remains bright on fast spin-echo T2-weighted sequences, fat saturation can be helpful in eliminating competing fat signal from the image, thereby making the pathologic process more conspicuous. Spin-echo T1-weighted gadolinium images and T2-weighted fast spin-echo images, both utilizing fat saturation, are the key means of evaluating tumors, because this optimizes the conspicuity of the tumor.

For fine detail, thin, 3- to 5-mm slices may be necessary, but when using thin slices, one may encounter signal drop-off. One trick for maintaining the signal is to use a larger field of view.

Although the axial plane is familiar to most who perform CT, the coronal plane is extremely beneficial with MRI, because it provides a vertical perspective from as far as the skull base to as low as the thoracic inlet. Often this plane is most helpful in evaluating tumor spread along important fascial spaces that are vertically oriented, such as the carotid space, the parapharyngeal space, the retropharyngeal space, and the prevertebral space. The coronal plane also provides side-to-side comparison, and it can assist in determining midline crossing. Also, the lymph node chains are nicely displayed on coronal images, and the round or oval lymph nodes are easily distinguished from the elongated muscles of the neck. For midline lesions such as those affecting the epiglottis or those invading the spine, the sagittal plane may be helpful.

Artifact suppression techniques such as flow compensation, cardiac gating, presaturation pulses, gradient moment nulling, and no phase wrap can improve image quality. Phase direction should be chosen so that any phase artifact is projected away from the area of interest. Most phase artifact is generated from carotid and jugular veins, and if the artifact is allowed to project along the transverse plane, there is a good chance that the prevertebral space may be obscured. Because this is a critical area for staging, I prefer to direct the phase direction along the anteroposterior plane.

THE LOWER FACE

ANATOMY

For purposes of this discussion, the lower face will include the oropharynx and the oral cavity, the hypopharynx, the adjacent deep structures, and the adjacent cutaneous and subcutaneous structures, particularly the lip.

Oropharynx

The oropharynx includes the posterior third of the tongue (or tongue base), the adjacent pharyngeal walls extending from the soft palate to the epiglottis, the palatine tonsils, the tonsillar fossa, and the vallecula. Because squamous epithelium lines the mucosal surfaces of the oropharynx, squamous cell carcinoma is common here. However, in addition to squamous epithelium, there are lymphoid tissue and minor salivary glands, so that lymphoma and salivary gland tumors can also arise in this area[1] (Fig. 35–3).

Oral Cavity

The oral cavity is situated anterior to the oropharynx. The oral cavity includes the anterior two thirds of the tongue (which is separated from the tongue base by the circumvallate papillae), the hard palate, the

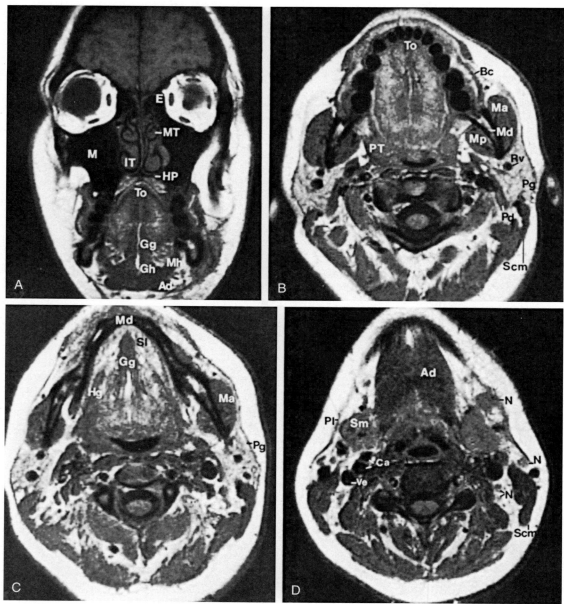

FIGURE 35–3. Normal oropharynx and salivary glands. *A,* Coronal image. *B* to *D,* Axial images. *B* is cephalad to *C,* which is cephalad to *D.* T1-weighted images (TR/TE = 800/17). *A* is through the oropharynx, maxillary sinuses, and nasal cavity. The intrinsic muscles of the tongue (To) can be seen separate from the extrinsic muscles: genioglossus (Gg); and the suprahyoid group, the geniohyoid (Gh), mylohyoid (Mh), and anterior belly of the digastric (Ad). Note also the hard palate (HP), the inferior turbinate (IT), and the middle turbinate (MT). The maxillary sinus (M) and ethmoidal air cells (E) are air containing and without signal. *B* shows the intrinsic muscles of the tongue (To); the palatine tonsils (PT); the medial pterygoid muscle (Mp); the masseter muscle (Ma); the mandible (Md), which contains marrow; and the parotid gland (Pg), which contains the retromandibular vein (Rv). The posterior belly of the digastric (Pd) is deep to the parotid gland, and the sternocleidomastoid muscle (Scm) is behind the parotid gland. The buccinator muscle (Bc) is lateral to the mandibular teeth. *C* is further caudad through the extrinsic muscles of the tongue, showing the mandible (Md), the genioglossus muscle (Gg), the hyoglossus muscle (Hg), the sublingual glands (Sl), the masseter muscle (Ma), and the tail or inferior portion of the parotid gland (Pg). *D* is a section through the submandibular gland (Sm), just above the hyoid bone at the level of the anterior belly of the digastric (Ad). The platysma muscle (Pl) is located superficially. The sternocleidomastoid muscle (Scm) is overlying the internal jugular vein (Ve) and the carotid artery (Ca). Lymph nodes (N) are present around the submandibular gland, superficial and deep to the sternocleidomastoid muscle.

mylohyoid muscle (which forms the floor of the mouth), and the buccal mucosa. Two additional spaces related to the oral cavity include the submandibular and sublingual spaces, which are separated by the mylohyoid muscle.[2]

Hypopharynx

The hypopharynx includes the piriform sinuses, the pharyngeal walls from the pharyngoesophageal junction to the vallecula, and the aryepiglottic folds.[1-3]

Adjacent Deep Spaces

Because malignant processes tend to invade neighboring spaces, a thorough understanding of the adjacent deep spaces is vitally important in evaluating pathologic change in the head and neck.[4-6]

The pharyngeal mucosal space represents the most superficial layer and includes the mucosa of the pharynx, Waldeyer's ring, the cartilaginous eustachian tube, the pharyngobasilar fascia, and the levator and constrictor muscles. Common tumors that arise in this space include squamous cell carcinoma, lymphoma, adenoid cystic carcinoma, and adenocarcinoma.

The parapharyngeal space is a vertical highway extending from the skull base to the hyoid bone. It contains fat, branches of the trigeminal nerve, and pterygoid veins. Lesions encountered in this space include metastatic carcinoma, especially squamous cell carcinoma that has penetrated deeply from the pharyngeal mucosal space and squamous cell carcinoma from the tongue base or tonsillar fossa. Pleomorphic adenomas, branchial cleft cysts, lipomas, and infections can also occur in this space.

Also called the infratemporal fossa, the masticator space contains the muscles of mastication, including the masseter, temporalis, and medial and lateral pterygoid muscles. This is another important space by which metastatic lesions, especially from squamous cell carcinoma, can spread vertically to reach the skull base. One should pay particular attention to tumor invasion intracranially from this space along certain routes that do not require skull base erosion or destruction. These routes include perineural spread along the third division of cranial nerve V (the nerve that activates the muscles of mastication) and along the pterygopalatine fossa, which leads to the inferior orbital fissure and orbital apex.[7] Common tumors found in this space include deeply invasive metastatic squamous cell carcinoma, adenoid cystic carcinomas, mucoepidermoid carcinomas, lymphomas, and rhabdomyosarcomas.[8]

The carotid space is another vertical highway for neoplasms to extend up to the skull base or down to the aortic arch. The contents of the space include not only the carotid artery but also the internal jugular vein, the internal jugular chain of nodes, and cranial nerves IX, X, and XI. Because of nodal drainage, metastases are frequently found in this space. Metastasis to this space can mean inoperability, particularly if there is carotid encasement[8a] that would require sacrifice of the carotid artery. Therefore, the carotid space is an extremely important space to consider in tumor staging.

The retropharyngeal space is a potential posterior midline space that can also provide a vertical highway, extending from the skull base to approximately the T-3 level. The retropharyngeal space includes primarily lymph nodes. Metastatic lesions, lymphomas, and infections[9-11] occur in this region (Fig. 35–4).

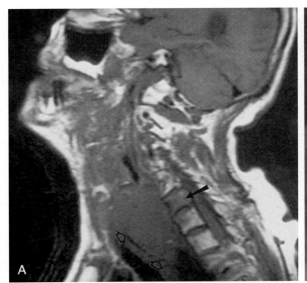
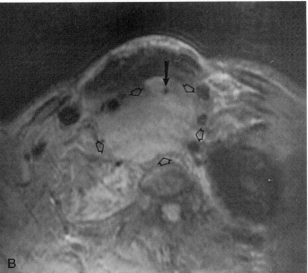

FIGURE 35–4. Squamous cell carcinoma of the tonsillar fossa with extension into the retropharyngeal and prevertebral space. *A,* Large retropharyngeal mass that displaces the esophagus *(open arrows)* anteriorly. The mass abuts the anterior aspect of the spine. There is also bone marrow replacement, as defined by low signal intensity at the C-3 vertebral body *(solid arrow)* on this T1-weighted image. *B,* Axial T2-weighted image shows narrowing of the esophagus *(solid arrow).* The mass has high signal intensity and is defined by open arrows. It pushes the carotid arteries and jugular veins laterally.

Lastly, along with the carotid space, the prevertebral space is another extremely important space when determining operability. The prevertebral space is enveloped by a deep layer of cervical fascia that attaches as far laterally as the transverse process and includes not only the longus colli muscles but also the paraspinous muscles, the vertebral artery and vein, the spinal cord, and the paraspinous muscles. Metastatic lesions to the prevertebral space can potentially determine inoperability, because the surgeon may be unable to find a tumor-free margin once tumor invades this space. Common tumors found in this space include metastatic lesions, particularly from squamous cell carcinoma. Chordomas can arise in this space, and infections from vertebral osteomyelitis or prevertebral abscesses may also be encountered in this region (see also Chapter 34).

Lymph Node Evaluation

Lymph nodes larger than 1.5 cm in diameter in the submandibular or internal jugular chain (jugulodigastric) should be considered abnormal. Nodes in all other areas of the neck exceeding 1 cm should also be considered abnormal.[3, 12] Also, benign reactive nodes tend to maintain their normal oval shape, whereas malignant nodes usually have a more rounded configuration. Nodes with necrosis should be considered potentially malignant provided there is no underlying history of tuberculosis or previous radiation therapy.[13] If metastatic disease is confined within a lymph node, a sharp border can be seen between the node and adjacent soft tissues. If the disease breaks out of

the nodal capsule, the margins of the node become ill defined and there may be infiltration in the surrounding fat planes. This is called *extracapsular extension*. Some investigators believe that evaluation of lymph nodes for extracapsular and central nodal necrosis is easier with CT than with MRI[14] (Figs. 35–5 and 35–6).

Abnormal supraclavicular lymph nodes may represent metastasis from anywhere, but particularly from lung, breast, and esophagus. Adenopathy along the inferior jugular chain may be due to metastatic disease from the subglottic larynx, esophagus, or thyroid. Tongue, pharynx, and supraglottic laryngeal cancers typically metastasize to the midjugular lymph node chain. Jugulodigastric nodes may be related to metastasis from the pharynx, tonsil, tongue, parotid gland, or supraglottic larynx. Submandibular adenopathy suggests metastasis from the adjacent skin (lip), submaxillary gland, or tongue. Posterior triangle nodes may show metastasis from tumors of the pharynx, tongue base, tonsil, or thyroid.[14–20]

PATHOLOGY

Malignant Tumors

Squamous Cell Carcinoma

Squamous epithelium lines the mucosal spaces of the oropharynx, the hypopharynx, and the oral cavity. Therefore, squamous cell carcinoma of the tongue, tonsillar fossa, hypopharynx, and oral cavity, including the lip, is quite prevalent. In the oropharynx, the most

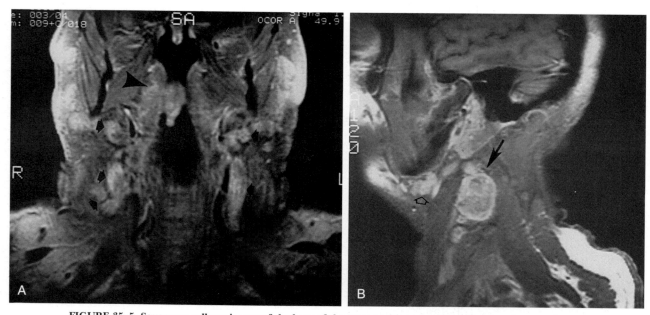

FIGURE 35–5. Squamous cell carcinoma of the base of the tongue with spread along the parapharyngeal space with associated extensive lymphadenopathy. *A,* Coronal T1-weighted gadolinium-enhanced image (with fat suppression) demonstrating enhancing tumor along the right parapharyngeal space extending across the uvula *(arrowhead).* There is extensive lymphadenopathy along the internal jugular chain of nodes bilaterally *(arrows).* *B,* Sagittal T1-weighted gadolinium-enhanced image (with fat suppression) demonstrates abnormally large lymph nodes in the high internal jugular chain *(solid arrow).* There is also abnormal lymphadenopathy in the submandibular space *(open arrow).*

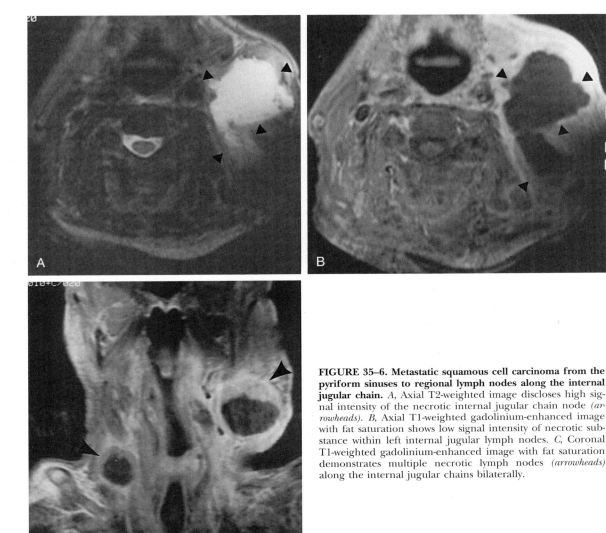

FIGURE 35–6. Metastatic squamous cell carcinoma from the pyriform sinuses to regional lymph nodes along the internal jugular chain. *A,* Axial T2-weighted image discloses high signal intensity of the necrotic internal jugular chain node *(arrowheads)*. *B,* Axial T1-weighted gadolinium-enhanced image with fat saturation shows low signal intensity of necrotic substance within left internal jugular lymph nodes. *C,* Coronal T1-weighted gadolinium-enhanced image with fat saturation demonstrates multiple necrotic lymph nodes *(arrowheads)* along the internal jugular chains bilaterally.

common site of origin of squamous cell carcinoma is the anterior tonsil.[2] Squamous cell carcinoma from this site can spread subtly and deeply beneath intact mucosa. It can spread to deep spaces through the superior constrictor muscles into the parapharyngeal and carotid spaces. The internal jugular chain of nodes is often affected, particularly in the jugulodigastric region. Because mucosal lesions are hard to evaluate by imaging, correlation and knowledge of the physical examination are essential for staging these lesions. Deep lesions, of course, are more accurately evaluated by imaging as opposed to physical examination.[2, 21–23]

The staging of oropharyngeal squamous cell carcinoma is based on the size of the tumor and invasion of adjacent structures.[1–3] Therefore, one needs to pay particular attention to tumor extension to deep spaces, especially to the parapharyngeal, carotid, and prevertebral spaces. Evaluation of adenopathy should be made accordingly, particularly in the carotid space.

Tongue base squamous cell carcinoma can also invade the adjacent deep spaces. Perineural spread is also a possibility. In addition, one should assess for midline crossing, because this can determine whether there can be a hemiglossectomy rather than total glossectomy (Fig. 35–7). Squamous cell carcinoma of the tongue base has the propensity to invade inferiorly into submandibular space and extend to the vallecula and pre-epiglottic space directly. In addition, any oropharyngeal or oral cavity carcinoma should be evaluated for mandibular invasion. Squamous cell carcinoma of the lip, particularly the lower lip, is the second most common site of squamous cell carcinoma of the head and neck, the skin being the most common. Squamous cell carcinoma of the lip can invade the buccal mucosa and the mandible as well as extend into deep spaces.[2, 24, 24a]

Squamous cell carcinoma of the hypopharynx most commonly involves the pyriform sinuses. Cancers that arise in this location tend to be silent and quite aggressive. They invade deep spaces early with numerous abnormal nodes. They can invade cartilage and even the larynx. Staging of squamous cell carcinoma of the

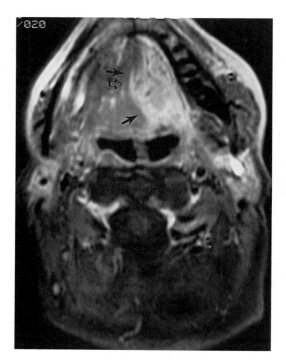

FIGURE 35–7. Squamous cell carcinoma of the tongue. Axial T1-weighted image with gadolinium enhancement and fat suppression clearly demonstrates an enhancing mass of the tongue *(solid arrows)* that remains unilateral and does not cross the midline *(open arrow* indicates medium raphe).

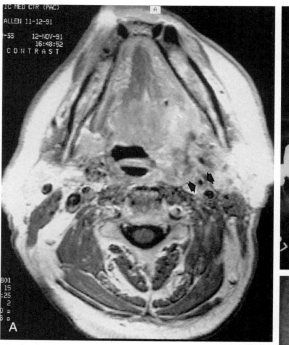

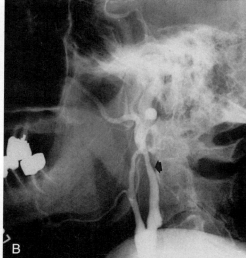

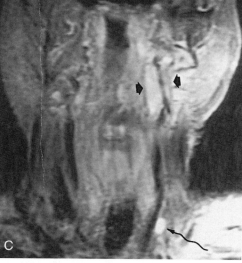

FIGURE 35-8. Squamous cell carcinoma of tonsillar fossa with spread to the floor of the mouth and tongue base as well as into the parapharyngeal space and carotid space. *A,* Axial T1-weighted image with gadolinium enhancement displays the neoplasm, centered at the tonsillar fossa with extension into the carotid space causing encasement of the carotid artery *(arrows).* There is also extension to the floor of the mouth. *B,* Lateral angiogram of common carotid demonstrates nonspecific narrowing of the internal and external carotid arteries *(arrow).* The nonspecific extent and nature of this narrowing on the angiogram makes it difficult to define the amount of involvement surrounding the arteries. *C,* T1-weighted coronal image after gadolinium enhancement reveals the extent of tumor encasement surrounding the left internal carotid artery *(arrows).* This is much more specific than the accompanying angiogram in *B,* which could have been seen with dissection and not necessarily tumor encasement. Also, note incidentally, a supraclavicular lymph node *(wavy arrow)* that had gone unnoticed on physical examination.

hypopharynx is based on location (number of subsites), fixation of the larynx, and invasion of local structures.[1-3]

For the deep structures, special attention should be given to invasion of the prevertebral space, because this could be an indication of inoperability. Violation of the deep cervical fascia, the longus colli muscles, or the spine itself with bone marrow replacement should be reported. Also, invasion of the carotid artery with encasement would be a prime concern in regard to resectability (Fig. 35–8). Some investigators believe that if tumor involvement of the carotid artery is less than 50%, the tumor likely can be dissected off the carotid. The likelihood of nonresectability increases markedly when the tumor encases more than 75% of the carotid.[2] Involvement of the masticator space can also occur with oropharyngeal or oral cavity cancers. Involvement of the masticator space should alert one to the possibility of skull base invasion, particularly through foramen ovale or along the pterygopalatine fossa. Other routes of skull base entry are along the carotid canal (Fig. 35–9), jugular foramen, and eustachian tube[25-27] (Fig. 35–10).

Lymphoma and Leukemia

Lymphoma and leukemia can arise from nodal tissue of the oropharynx, especially in the region of Waldeyer's ring (Fig. 35–11). These lesions are often bulky and also accompanied by large bulky lymph nodes. The most common form of lymphoma in the head and neck is non-Hodgkin's lymphoma. In fact, the head and neck region is the second most common site of non-Hodgkin's lymphoma (the first is the gastrointestinal tract).[2] If mediastinal nodes are also present, one may be dealing with Hodgkin's lymphoma rather than non-Hodgkin's lymphoma. Leukemia can present similarly with bulky lymph nodes and enlargement of Waldeyer's ring (Fig. 35–12).

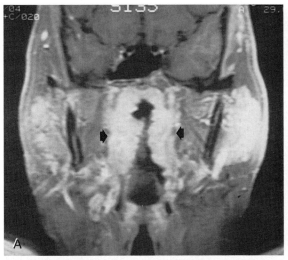

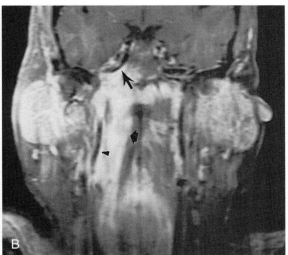

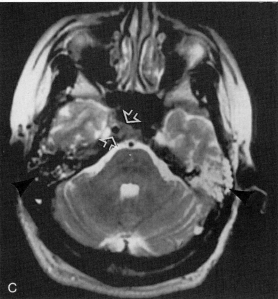

FIGURE 35–9. Squamous cell carcinoma of the tonsillar fossa with spread bilaterally along the pharyngeal mucosal space, the parapharyngeal space, and the left carotid space. Tumor extends to the base of the skull. *A,* Coronal T1-weighted gadolinium-enhanced image with fat saturation demonstrates the extent of this tumor vertically from the oropharynx crossing the nasopharynx and extending to the skull base. Extension into the parapharyngeal space is observed *(arrows). B,* T1-weighted coronal image with gadolinium enhancement and fat saturation also demonstrates the extent of tumor along the parapharyngeal mucosal space *(broad short arrow),* the parapharyngeal space, and the carotid space with abutment along the carotid artery *(arrowhead)* and extension to the foramen lacerum *(arrow). C,* Axial T2-weighted image discloses isointense tumor in the carotid space at the base of the skull *(open arrows).* The carotid artery at this level is encased by tumor. Arrowheads denote bilateral mastoiditis because the tumor has traversed from the oropharynx to the nasopharynx and occluded the eustachian tubes bilaterally.

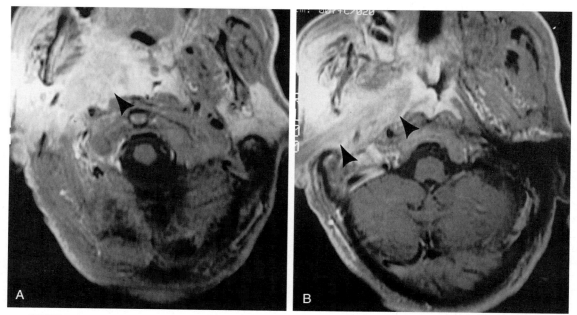

FIGURE 35–10. Squamous cell carcinoma in the tonsillar fossa. Axial T1-weighted images after gadolinium enhancement and fat saturation. *A*, Enhancing mass is evident in the tonsillar fossa with extension into the parapharyngeal and carotid spaces *(arrowhead)*. *B*, The tumor extends into the eustachian tube *(arrowheads)*.

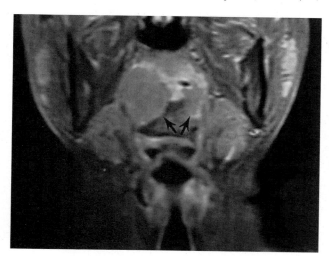

FIGURE 35–11. Non-Hodgkin's lymphoma. Coronal T1-weighted gadolinium-enhanced fat saturation image at the level of the tonsillar fossa demonstrates large bulky bilateral node masses *(arrows)* arising from lymphatic tissue of Waldeyer's ring.

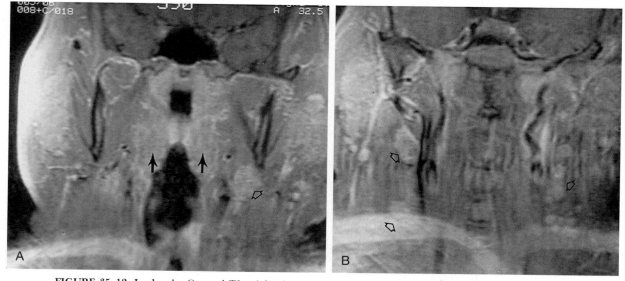

FIGURE 35–12. Leukemia. Coronal T1-weighted gadolinium-enhanced fat saturation image. *A*, Enlargement of nodal tissue at Waldeyer's ring *(solid arrows)* and bulky nodes *(open arrow)*. *B*, Multiple bulky lymph nodes *(open arrows)* along the internal jugular chains bilaterally. The findings may be similar with lymphoma.

Metastasis

A likely cause of metastatic disease is squamous cell carcinoma arising at other sites in the head and neck and spreading along the deep spaces such as the carotid or parapharyngeal space, the vertical highways. Popular hematogenous sources, however, include the lung, breast, colon, kidney, and thyroid. Naturally, the job of the diagnostic radiologist is not to try to guess the histology but rather to determine the extent of involvement.

Adjacent Masticator Space Lesions

Squamous cell carcinoma can invade deeply from the oropharynx or oral cavity and penetrate the muscles of mastication deeply. This is not at all uncom-

mon. Masses can arise within the masticator space and further invade the region of the oropharynx or oral cavity. In children, the rhabdomyosarcoma is the most common soft tissue sarcoma.[2, 3] The head and neck represent the second most common site of rhabdomyosarcomas, because approximately 40% occur in this region. There is propensity for skull base invasion, and coronal MRI is extremely helpful in this regard (Fig. 35–13). The embryonal type is more common in the head and neck, whereas the alveolar type is more often found in skeletal muscle. Other sarcomas that can arise in the masticator space include liposarcomas, which arise from lipoblasts and not preexisting lipomas. They contain some elements of fat but also sarcomatous elements. If they have more sarcomatous elements than fatty elements, their signal may not be predominantly that of fat on T1-weighted MR images (Fig.

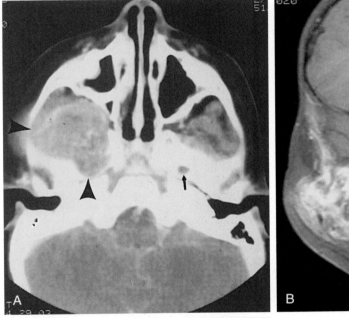

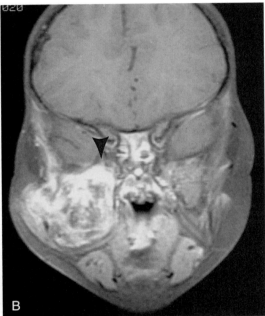

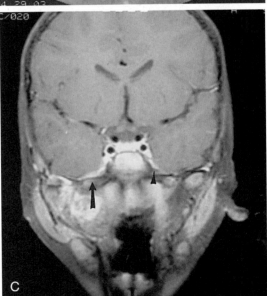

FIGURE 35–13. Rhabdomyosarcoma with apparent skull base invasion, but is there invasion to the brain? *A,* CT scan demonstrating large right masticator space mass *(arrowheads).* On this scan the right foramen ovale is not seen comparably to the left foramen ovale *(arrow).* This would suggest skull base invasion and obliteration. It is difficult on axial slices to determine if there is skull base invasion. Multiplanar imaging and improved soft tissue detail would be helpful. *B,* T1-weighted coronal image with gadolinium enhancement and fat saturation demonstrates enhancing mass *(arrowhead)* in the right masticator space that rises toward the temporal lobe but does not cross into the brain. *C,* Coronal T1-weighted image after gadolinium enhancement and fat saturation performed slightly more posteriorly reveals abnormal enhancement and thickening of the right third division of the fifth cranial nerve *(arrow)* as opposed to the normal left division *(arrowhead).* The findings reflect early perineural spread on the right.

35–14). Other sarcomas arising in this region may include osteosarcomas and chondrosarcomas. Metastatic lesions can also spread to the masticator space and to other parts of the lower face by hematogenous means.[25, 26]

Mandibular Lesions

Squamous cell carcinoma of the tongue or tonsillar fossa can invade the mandible. On MR images, one should look for signal drop-off in the bone marrow on T1-weighted images. High signal intensity may be seen on T1-weighted images with gadolinium enhancement and fat saturation.

Many of the primary mandibular lesions are cystic. Therefore, many appear bright on T2-weighted images and dark on T1-weighted images. Some may be hemorrhagic and hyperintense on both T1- and T2-weighted sequences. The most common odontogenic cystic mandibular lesion is the periapical cyst.[2, 28, 28a, 29] This lesion is associated with an infected tooth and can be located along the mandible or maxilla. It is usually detected on dental films and treated successfully, so it rarely needs evaluation by MRI (Fig. 35–15). Another common odontogenic lesion is the dentigerous cyst, which is a lytic unilocular lesion of the mandible. It is located adjacent to an unerupted tooth and has sclerotic borders; it may be better evaluated by radiographic techniques than by MRI. The ameloblastoma is another common mandibular lesion. This lesion tends to be multiloculated, lytic, and expansile; the bony cortex may be eroded.[30, 31] It can be associated with an underlying dentigerous cyst. Again, CT or Panorex films may be preferable to MRI for evaluation of cortical changes.

The malignant fibrous histiocytoma is a lesion that can appear to be similar to the ameloblastoma on Panorex films or CT scans in that it is lytic, is expansile, and causes cortical erosions. However, there is no underlying cystic characteristic of this lesion; rather, it is fibrous. Therefore, it can be characterized by MRI, which reveals it to be somewhat isodense with muscle on both T1- and T2-weighted imaging (Fig. 35–16).

Of the malignant tumors, metastasis from squamous cell carcinoma ranks high, particularly if there is an adjacent head and neck carcinoma. Other sources would include metastasis from other sites, such as breast or lung. Osteosarcomas of the mandible can occur, especially after radiation therapy for previous head and neck neoplasms. An aggressive periosteal reaction might be the prime differential finding, and this may be better appreciated with CT or Panorex films rather than with MRI. However, if it is necessary to define the extent of a soft tissue component related to a destructive mandibular mass, MRI can be helpful (Fig. 35–17). A host of other less common odontogenic and nonodontogenic tumors are often diagnosed satisfactorily by dental Panorex views and are never subjected to MRI for further evaluation.

Benign Cystic Lesions
Ranula

The ranula is a mucous retention cyst secondary to obstruction of a minor salivary gland or the sublingual gland. It is a unilocular cyst in the sublingual space (Fig. 35–18). One often sees the tail. It is considered simple if it is confined to the sublingual space. If the capsule breaks and there is extension from the sublingual space into the adjacent submandibular or

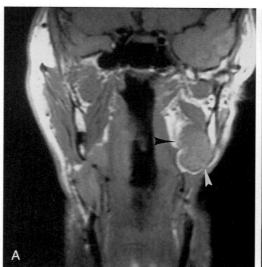
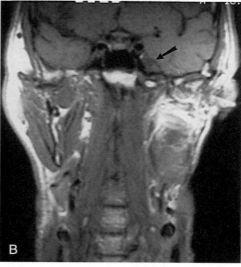

FIGURE 35–14. Liposarcoma. T1-weighted coronal images. *A,* Lobulated mass *(arrowheads)* in the masticator space that is isointense with muscle. Liposarcomas may have more sarcomatous elements than fatty elements and, therefore, may not exhibit predominant fat signal or brightness on T1-weighted images. *B,* Coronal T1-weighted image demonstrates abnormal enlargement of the left fifth nerve ganglion *(arrow)* at Meckel's cave when compared with the right. This reflects perineural spread to the ganglion from a masticator space mass. One should always be on the alert for perineural spread along the third division of cranial nerve V whenever there is a masticator space malignancy.

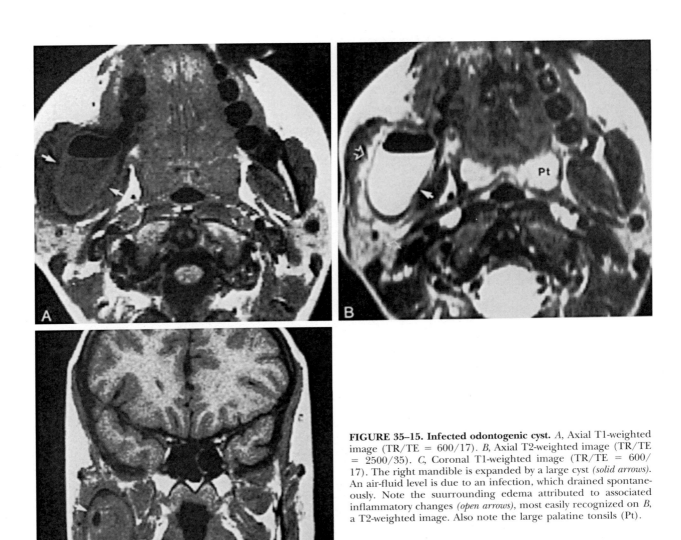

FIGURE 35–15. Infected odontogenic cyst. *A,* Axial T1-weighted image (TR/TE = 600/17). *B,* Axial T2-weighted image (TR/TE = 2500/35). *C,* Coronal T1-weighted image (TR/TE = 600/17). The right mandible is expanded by a large cyst *(solid arrows).* An air-fluid level is due to an infection, which drained spontaneously. Note the suurrounding edema attributed to associated inflammatory changes *(open arrows),* most easily recognized on *B,* a T2-weighted image. Also note the large palatine tonsils (Pt).

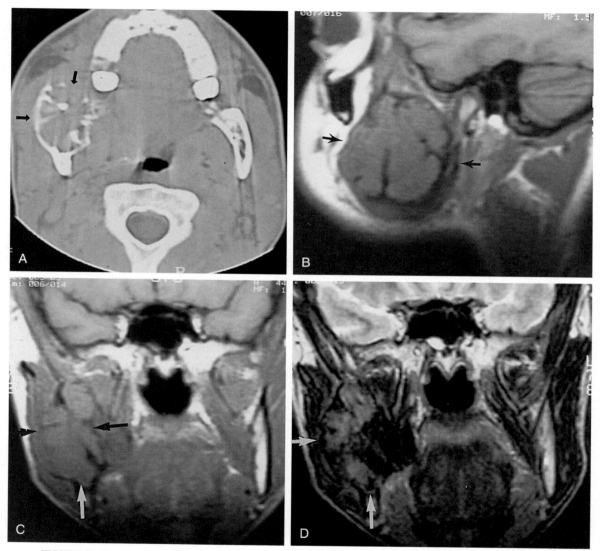

FIGURE 35–16. Malignant fibrous histiocytoma. *A*, CT scan of the mandible shows a lytic expansile destructive mass of the mandibular ramus *(arrows)*. *B* and *C*, T1-weighted sagittal and coronal images, respectively, disclose a lobulated soft tissue mass at the ramus of the mandible. This mass is isointense with muscle and is not cystic *(arrows)*. *D*, T2-weighted coronal image reveals no hyperintensity of the mandibular mass. It is isointense with muscle and has much more fibrous than water content *(arrows)*.

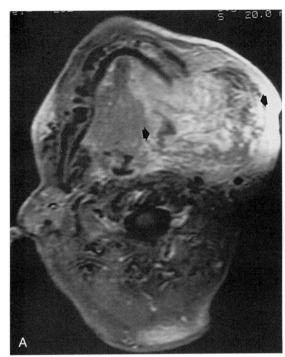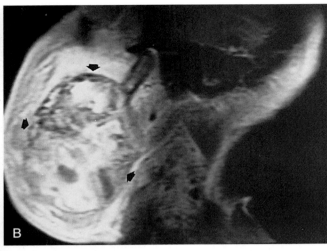

FIGURE 35–17. Osteogenic sarcoma. *A*, Axial T1-weighted image after gadolinium enhancement and fat saturation shows a large mass *(arrows)* arising from the mandible with invasion into the adjacent soft tissues, parapharyngeal space, carotid space, and floor of the mouth. *B*, Sagittal image showing the superior and inferior extent of this mass *(arrows)* and its relationship to the mandible.

parapharyngeal space, it is considered a diving or plunging ranula.[2, 3, 32–34]

Thyroglossal Duct Cyst

The thyroglossal duct cyst arises from a remnant of the thyroglossal duct that follows a course from the thyroid isthmus to the tongue base. Most of the thyroglossal duct cysts are in the midline, but approximately 25% may be paramedian. About 20% are suprahyoid[1–3] (Fig. 35–19) (see also Chapter 36).

Branchial Cleft Cyst

Approximately 95% of branchial cleft cysts arise from a remnant of a second branchial cleft that has failed to obliterate. They are usually found at the angle

of the mandible along the anterior border of the sternocleidomastoid, but their location can vary because the course of the second branchial cleft extends from the tonsillar fossa to the supraclavicular region.[35, 36] They are usually found in young adults and often present when they become infected. At this point they can have the appearance of an abscess. Like other cystic lesions, they tend to be bright on T2-weighted images and dark on T1-weighted images. If they are infected, they can have an enhancing rim when contrast medium is administered with T1-weighted imaging.

Cystic Hygroma and Lymphangioma

Cystic hygromas and lymphangiomas arise from lymphoid tissue. They tend to have cystic signal charac-

FIGURE 35–18. Ranula. T2-weighted axial image (TR/TE = 300/45). An obstructed sublingual gland *(arrow)* is evident as a fluid-containing cyst in the floor of the mouth. This is lateral to the genioglossus muscle (1) and above the hylohyoid muscle. Also note the palatine tonsils (2) and deep cervical nodes (3), which have a brighter signal on T2-weighted images, particularly with any degree of inflammatory change.

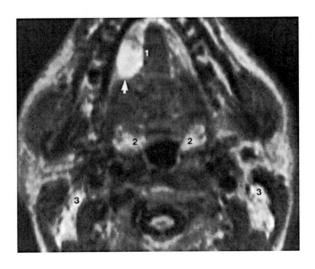

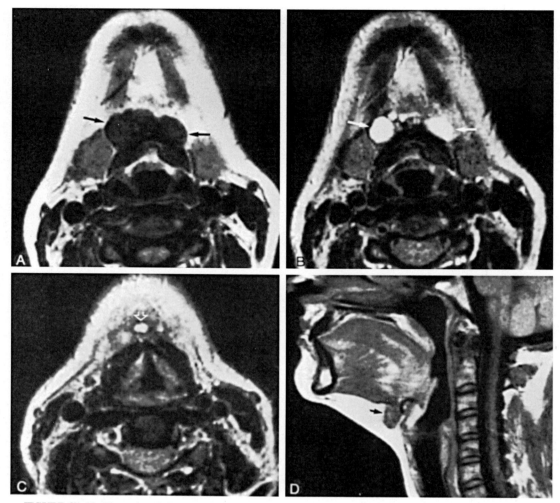

FIGURE 35–19. Thyroglossal duct cyst. *A*, Axial T1-weighted image (TR/TE = 500/40). *B* and *C*, Axial T2-weighted images (TR/TE = 1500/80). *D*, Sagittal T1-weighted image (TR/TE = 500/30). An atypical bilobed cyst extends from the prehyoid area *(closed arrows)* down to a small tract *(open arrow)* anterior to the thyroid cartilage. This proved to be a thyroglossal duct cyst containing a small colloid-producing carcinoma.

teristics and may present as tortuous cystic masses (Fig. 35–20). Intratumoral hemorrhage may occur. The posterior triangle tends to be a common site for these lesions[1-3] (see also Chapter 36).

Benign Tumors

Dermoid, Epidermoid, and Teratoma

Differential considerations of cystic lesions in the location of the tongue base and sublingual space should include epidermoid and dermoid tumors. These tumors are slow-growing cystic masses, usually located under the oral tongue. They tend to be unilocular. The dermoids tend to have mixed contents of fat and fluid as well as other substances and may be inhomogeneous in signal intensity on all sequences.[34, 36, 37] The epidermoids tend to be cystic and can be difficult to differentiate from a ranula. However, neither epidermoids nor dermoids tend to communicate with the parapharyngeal or sublingual space.[38]

Teratomas are congenital neoplasms that contain elements of all three germ layers. Therefore, a mixture of hair, bone, cartilage, water, and muscle may be encountered, which can lead to variable appearances that sometimes are quite complex and even bizarre (Fig. 35–21).

Lipomas

Lipomas often present as palpable masses. Both MRI and CT can be specific in evaluating the location and extent of these lesions as well as accurately characterizing them as fatty tumors. They are most common in obese women and have a tendency to occur in the posterior triangle, but they can be present anywhere (Fig. 35–22).

Vascular Lesions

Hemangiomas are common benign pediatric neoplasms. These tumors often extend from the superficial soft tissues to the deeper underlying tissues. They

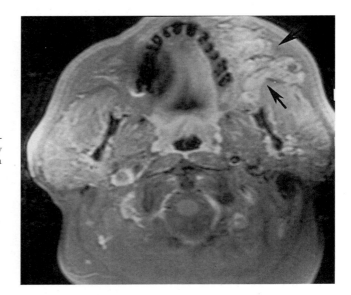

FIGURE 35–20. Lymphangioma. Axial T1-weighted gadolinium-enhanced image with fat saturation shows characteristic wavy, mildly enhancing serpentine spaces characteristic of a lymphangioma *(arrows).*

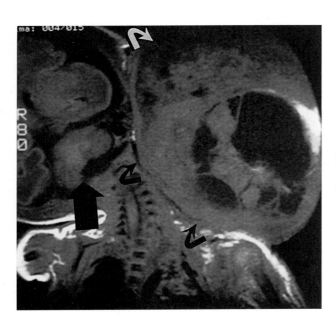

FIGURE 35–21. Teratoma. Coronal T1-weighted image of a newborn who on imaging appears to have two heads. The large arrow points to the true head, which contains dysplastic brain, while the curved arrows point to the teratoma, which has a mixture of muscle, fat, and fluid.

FIGURE 35–22. Lipoma. T1-weighted coronal image. Palpable mass at the angle of the mandible was suspected to be related to the parotid gland. However, MRI reveals that it has high signal intensity on a T1-weighted image consistent with fat. This represents a lipoma *(arrowheads),* which wrapped itself around the mandible and was not related to the parotid gland.

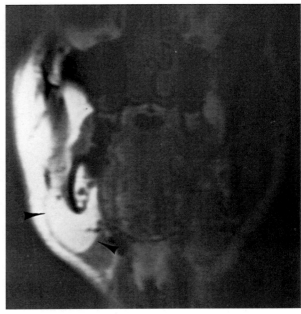

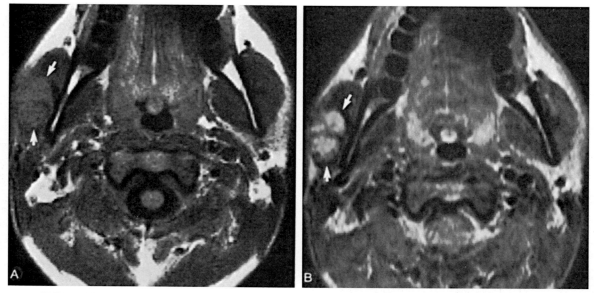

FIGURE 35–23. Hemangioma, masseter muscle. Axial images. *A,* T1-weighted image (TR/TE = 600/17). *B,* T2-weighted image (TR/TE = 2500/35). A mass *(arrows)* was felt by physical examination to be within the parotid gland but proved to be anterior to the parotid, within the masseter muscle. The signal is slightly brighter than muscle with T1 weighting *(A)* and much brighter with T2 weighting *(B).*

tend to be bright on T2-weighted images and even brighter on longer echo time images. When gadolinium is used, these lesions usually enhance brightly[1–3] (Fig. 35–23).

Arteriovenous malformations are uncommon abnormalities in the head and neck, but they can be seen as serpentine, tangled flow voids or areas of flow-related enhancement due to slow-flowing draining veins (Fig. 35–24). Phase artifact may be a tip-off, which can be accentuated with administration of gadolinium.

Infectious and Inflammatory Disease

Laryngitis and tonsillitis are the most common inflammatory lesions in the oral pharynx; however, usually no imaging is necessary because this area is amenable to direct visualization. If tonsillitis goes untreated and becomes complicated by peritonsillar abscess, which can spread to the parapharyngeal and lateral retropharyngeal spaces easily, MRI may be necessary to evaluate spread to the deep spaces. In children, a

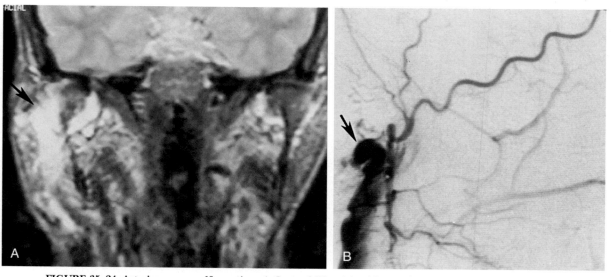

FIGURE 35–24. Arteriovenous malformation. *A,* Coronal T2-weighted image demonstrates tortuous serpentine tubular bright signal along the lateral aspect of the ramus of the mandible *(arrow).* This is consistent with a slow-flowing draining vein of the arteriovenous malformation, which is best demonstrated on *B. B,* Pre-embolization superselective angiogram of the superficial temporal artery. The vertically oriented draining vein can be seen *(arrow).*

retropharyngeal abscess can develop in response to an underlying inflammation usually from tonsillitis, but a traumatic perforation of the posterior pharyngeal wall can also be a cause. Masticator space infections are often due to dental infections that become complicated, but sometimes they can be due to otitis externa. Ludwig's angina, which is usually due to complicated *Streptococcus* or *Staphylococcus* infections, is often of dental origin. This represents an extensive infection of the floor of the mouth and can extend inferiorly along deep spaces to the mediastinum.[1-3]

On MR images, abscesses typically contain fluid centrally with a wall that enhances brightly when contrast medium is administered. A phlegmon, cellulitis, or fasciitis involves an area of soft tissue enhancement without fluid or gas formation.

In this age of intravenous drug abuse and the acquired immunodeficiency syndrome, one may find unusual abscesses often with multiple large nodes that can easily be mistaken for malignancy with metastatic lymphadenopathy. Clinical history of intravenous drug abuse and, in particular, attempted needle access to the jugular veins would be helpful in reaching a diagnosis[9-11, 13] (Fig. 35–25).

THE SALIVARY GLANDS

ANATOMY

The major salivary glands include the parotid, the submandibular, and the sublingual glands. The minor salivary glands are widely distributed over the mucosal surfaces of the oral cavity, the oropharynx, and the hypopharynx and, to a lesser extent, the nasopharynx, sinuses, and respiratory tract.[1-3]

The parotid space contains the parotid gland, the facial nerve, the external carotid artery, and the retromandibular vein. The parotid gland is divided into deep and superficial lobes, with the stylomandibular tunnel (which encloses the facial nerve) being the dividing line. Therefore, a portion of the parotid lies superficial to the mandibular ramus and another portion lies deep. The parotid gland is drained by Stensen's duct, which exits adjacent to the second maxillary molar.

The submandibular space contains the submandibular gland, submandibular nodes, a portion of the facial artery and vein, and a small segment of the cranial nerve XII. The submandibular gland is drained by Wharton's duct, which exits at the frenulum at the floor of the mouth.[39]

The sublingual space is a potential space that does not have a true fascial covering. It is located in the floor of the mouth superior and medial to the mylohyoid muscle. The sublingual gland is the smallest of the major salivary glands and may not be apparent by imaging. Compared with other major salivary glands, the sublingual gland tends to have the fewest lesions associated with it.[2, 40]

PATHOLOGY

Malignant Tumors
Mucoepidermoid Carcinoma

Mucoepidermoid carcinomas constitute about 30% of salivary gland malignancies. They are located most

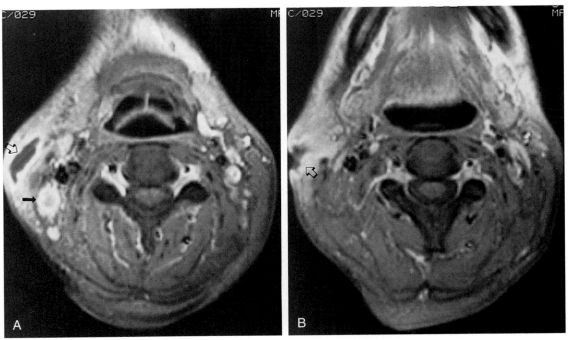

FIGURE 35–25. Neck abscess of an intravenous drug abuser seeking desperate intravenous access (the jugular vein). *A,* T1-weighted gadolinium-enhanced image with fat saturation. The abscess *(open arrow)* could easily have been mistaken for a necrotic malignancy with large necrotic lymph nodes *(solid arrow). B,* T1-weighted postgadolinium fat-saturated image shows an ulcerative lesion *(arrow)* on the skin surface related to the abscess. This could have easily been mistaken for a basal cell carcinoma or a superficial squamous cell carcinoma if important clinical history had been withheld.

often in the parotid; of parotid malignancies, they represent the most common malignancy. They are also the most common pediatric salivary tumor. Their appearance is extremely variable because the neoplasm can vary from high to low grade. The higher grade tumors tend to be extremely aggressive and infiltrating, whereas the low-grade tumors may be well encapsulated and appear similar to benign lesions, such as pleomorphic adenoma or Warthin's tumor (Fig. 35–26). The prognosis varies with the grade of the tumor.[41–43]

Adenoid Cystic Carcinoma

Adenoid cystic carcinomas are the most common salivary tumor of the minor salivary glands and also of the submandibular and sublingual glands. They tend to be slow growing but extremely persistent. They are known to have a high propensity for perineural spread, and one should look carefully for signs of perineural spread along the course of the facial nerve as well as of the third and second divisions of cranial nerve V, particularly on follow-up examinations for known adenoid cystic carcinoma.[2, 41 42]

Squamous Cell Carcinoma

Squamous cell carcinoma can be found in the salivary glands, often as the result of direct spread from an adjacent mucosal neoplasm or from metastasis to lymph nodes in the parotid or submandibular spaces. Therefore, one needs to search for a primary tumor whenever there is a diagnosis of squamous cell carcinoma in a salivary gland. Infrequently, squamous cell carcinoma can arise de novo, probably as the result of metaplasia of ductal columnar epithelium within the salivary gland. On MR images, these neoplasms tend to be hypointense on T2-weighted images, but they do enhance on T1-weighted images after gadolinium administration with fat suppression[1, 2, 41, 44] (Fig. 35–27).

Adenocarcinoma and Expleomorphic Carcinoma

Less commonly, adenocarcinoma involves the glandular tissue of the salivary glands, and it usually carries a poor prognosis. The signal intensity tends to be variable depending on whether the nature of the tumor is solid, mucinous, or cystic. Expleomorphic carcinoma may be the result of a pleomorphic adenoma that degenerates into a carcinoma. It is estimated that perhaps 20% of pleomorphic adenomas can do this. These malignancies can be aggressive with metastasis to the lungs and adjacent lymph nodes, in addition to extremely rapid growth of the primary tumor.[2, 3, 40, 42]

Lymphoma

Non-Hodgkin's lymphoma can affect almost any organ in the head and neck, and the salivary glands are not immune. These tumors tend to be quite bulky and are often associated with large bulky homogeneous lymph nodes. They can enlarge quite rapidly.

Benign Lesions

Pleomorphic Adenoma

Benign mixed cell or pleomorphic adenomas constitute about 80% of parotid neoplasms, making them the most common salivary gland neoplasms. They are usually solid, rounded, well-defined masses, most commonly found in the superficial lobe of the parotid. On T1-weighted images, they tend to be of low signal intensity relative to the gland, and they are generally of high signal intensity on T2-weighted images. There may be some fluid-containing spaces within the tumor. Unlike a typical cyst, however, with administration of contrast agent they tend to enhance rather brightly with some heterogeneity. Calcification may be evident within the tumor. A small number of these adenomas can degenerate into carcinomas.

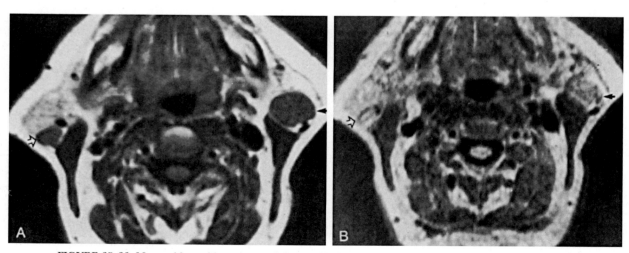

FIGURE 35–26. Mucoepidermoid carcinoma, left parotid gland. Axial images. *A*, T1-weighted image (TR/TE = 600/17). *B*, T2-weighted image (TR/TE = 3000/45). These show a sharply defined (*closed arrow*) tumor that looked benign but was found to be malignant. It has a low signal intensity in *A* but is isointense with the parotid in *B*. A sharply defined tumor (*open arrow*) is also present in the right parotid gland.

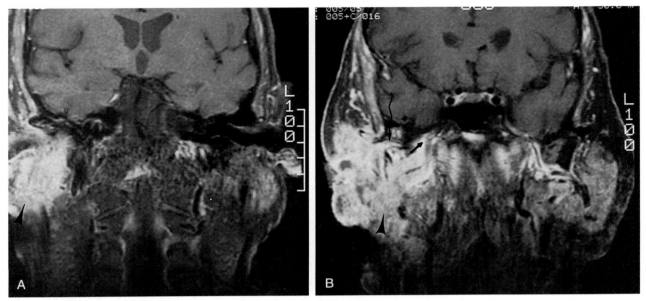

FIGURE 35–27. Malignancy of the parotid gland, squamous cell carcinoma. Regardless of the type of malignancy of the parotid, one of the characteristic features is skull base extension, particularly to the temporal bone. *A* and *B*, Coronal T1-weighted images after gadolinium enhancement and fat saturation. The image in *A* demonstrates the parotid mass *(arrow)* extending to the temporal bone, whereas in *B* there is additional extension of the mass into the adjacent soft tissues *(arrowhead)* as well as into the external auditory canal *(wavy arrow)* in addition to the carotid canal *(small straight arrow).*

Pleomorphic adenomas can arise from the deep lobe of the parotid and extend into the parapharyngeal space with an epicenter away from the parotid but well centered in the parapharyngeal space. At times, these lesions can be difficult to differentiate from other parapharyngeal and carotid space lesions such as schwannomas and glomus tumors. However, lesions that arise from the parotid tend to have a prestyloid location. They are separated from the carotid space by the tensor veli palatini fascia. Therefore, a mass extending into the parapharyngeal space that is of parotid origin will push the carotid artery and jugular vein posteriorly, whereas those that push the carotid anteriorly are more likely to be a schwannoma or glomus tumor[2, 21, 45–48] (Figs. 35–28 to 35–30).

Warthin's Tumor

Warthin's tumors are often bilateral and multicentric. Their imaging features resemble those of a pleomorphic adenoma in that they tend to have sharp borders. They also enhance with administration of contrast material, however, more centrally and less peripherally.[1, 2] They tend to be more common in males. They are not infiltrative and are usually limited to the gland.

Cystic Lesions

Of the cystic lesions, the lymphoepithelial cysts are being seen more often with the increase in imaging used for patients with the acquired immunodeficiency syndrome.[49] These cysts tend to be multiple and are often located in the parotid gland. They are often

associated with multiple cervical lymph nodes. They tend to have sharp borders and appear similar to adenomas on nonenhanced MR images but maintain cystic characteristics because they do not enhance.[1, 2, 3, 50]

The branchial cleft cyst can arise adjacent to the parotid gland, particularly if it is a second branchial cleft cyst, which has a propensity to arise near the

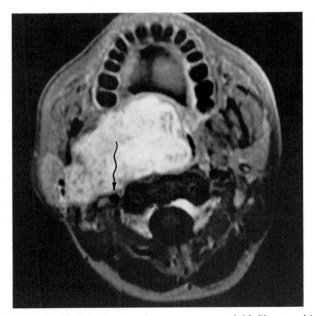

FIGURE 35–28. Parapharyngeal space mass prestyloid. Pleomorphic adenoma arises from the deep lobe of the parotid and grows into the parapharyngeal space anterior to the tensor veli palatini muscle tendon. It therefore situates itself anterior to the carotid artery *(arrow).*

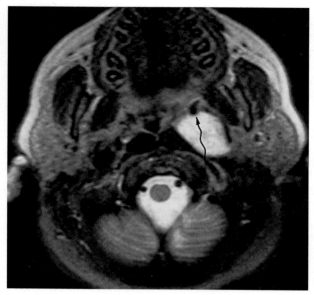

FIGURE 35–29. Schwannoma in the carotid/parapharyngeal space. Schwannoma arises from the 10th cranial nerve, which is located posterior to the carotid. Although this tumor appears to be similar to that shown in Figure 35–25 in that it abuts the deep lobe of the parotid, it can be differentiated from a prestyloid space mass (salivary gland tumor) because it is positioned posterior to the carotid artery and displaces the carotid anteriorly (arrow).

angle of the mandible. However, the first branchial cleft cyst is more likely to be found within the parotid, because the remnant first branchial cleft extends from the submandibular triangle to the external auditory canal. First branchial cleft cysts are often located at the inferior aspect of the parotid, either in the superficial or the deep lobe. They can also present as a mass at the external auditory canal. If branchial cleft cysts become infected, they can have an enhancing rim and mimic an abscess. They can also mimic Warthin's tumor or even a mucoepidermoid carcinoma with central necrosis.[2, 3, 21, 35]

As mentioned previously, potential cystic masses at the floor of the mouth in the vicinity of the sublingual gland and submandibular glands also include ranulas, plunging ranulas, dermoids, epidermoids, and thyroglossal duct cysts. Of these, the thyroglossal duct cyst can be paramedian, but it rarely has any communication with the sublingual or submandibular spaces. Retention cysts and simple congenital cysts may also be found in the salivary glands that are not associated with the branchial apparatus or other congenital remnants.[34]

Inflammatory Disease

Inflammatory lesions can also present as cystic abnormalities, including abscesses, some of which may be secondary to obstruction of the gland. Sialoadenitis may be the underlying cause and can present either with large abscesses or with multiple microabscesses. Inflammation of the peripheral salivary ducts may be related to an underlying autoimmune condition. An

example is Sjögren's disease, which is related to chronic sialoadenitis and results in a dry mouth from fibrous changes of the salivary glands (Fig. 35–31). It is often related to an underlying collagen-vascular disorder, such as rheumatoid arthritis or systemic lupus erythematosus.

A sialocele is a collection of saliva that is often located outside the gland or duct and is caused by leakage as the result of penetrating or blunt trauma.

Salivary gland calculi can cause obstruction of the glands. The diagnosis of calculi is made more easily and more accurately by radiographic techniques, such as CT or Panorex films, rather than MRI.[1–3, 21]

POSTSURGICAL AND POSTRADIATION CHANGE

After treatment by surgery or radiation therapy, the adjacent soft tissue changes and enhancement patterns can be confusing. After radiation therapy there tends to be a loss of the normal signal intensity in the adjacent subcutaneous fat. Loss of soft tissue planes also occurs, especially around the carotid sheath. The mucosa can thicken, especially at the epiglottis. Postsurgical edema can last for more than 8 weeks. Because there can be a recurrence of head and neck carcinoma

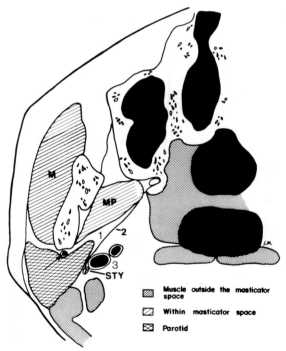

FIGURE 35–30. Diagram of prestyloid versus poststyloid parapharyngeal space compartments. Prestyloid space (1) is separated from poststyloid space (3) by tensor veli palatini (2). The deep lobe of the parotid gland extends into the prestyloid space. This permits masses of the parotid to be positioned anterior to the carotid artery (arrow). Cranial nerves run posterior to the carotid such that schwannomas and paragangliomas will push the carotid anteriorly. M = masseter muscle; Mp = medial pterygoid muscle; STY = styloid process. (From Tabor EK, Curtin HD: MR of the salivary glands. Radiol Clin North Am 27:379–392, 1989.)

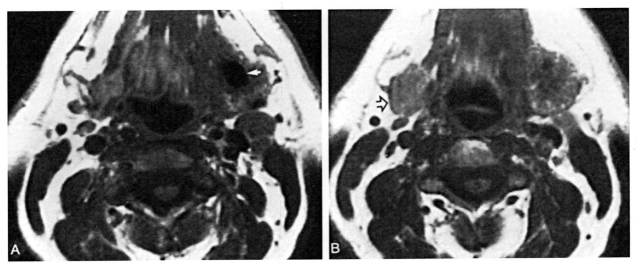

FIGURE 35–31. Sjögren's syndrome. *A*, T1-weighted axial image (TR/TE = 750/17). *B*, T2-weighted axial image (TR/TE = 3000/45). Bilateral sialadenitis with lymphoproliferative disease involving the salivary glands has resulted in mixed signal intensity bilaterally. Distention of the small peripheral ducts within the gland is due to lymphocytic infiltration.

in up to 90% in the first year, close follow-up, perhaps at 6-month intervals, is recommended. Some of the key concerns include an increase in the size or bulk of the original tumor mass, perineural spread, bone marrow changes suggesting a loss of bone marrow signal rather than simply radiation change, and increase in nodal size, but not necessarily necrosis, because radiation change can cause nodes to appear necrotic. Any changes that develop beyond the expected time intervals for radiation or surgical changes should draw suspicion, so that either close follow-up or biopsy can be directed to the area of concern.[2, 51, 52]

REFERENCES

1. Harnsberger HR: Head and Neck Imaging. Chicago: Year Book Medical Publishers, 1990.
2. Grossman RI, Yossem DM: Neuroradiology: The Requisites. St. Louis: Mosby–Year Book, 1994.
3. Som PM, Bergeron RT: Head and Neck Imaging. 2nd ed. St. Louis: Mosby–Year Book, 1991.
4. Harnsberger, HR, Osborn AG: Differential diagnosis of head and neck lesions based on their space of origin: the suprahyoid neck. AJR 157:147–154, 1991.
5. Smoker RK, Harnsberger HR: Differential diagnosis of head and neck lesions based on their space of origin. 2. The infrahyoid portion of the neck. AJR 157:155–159, 1991
6. Parker GD, Harnsberger HR: Radiographic evaluation of the normal and diseased posterior cervical space. AJR 157:161–165, 1991.
7. Laine FJ, Braun IF, Jensen ME, et al: Perineural tumor extension through the foramen ovale: evaluation with MR imaging. Radiology 174:65–71, 1990.
8. Feldman BA: Rhabdomyosarcoma of the head and neck. Laryngoscope 92:424–440, 1982.
8a. Yousem DM, Hatabu H, Hurst RW, et al: Carotid artery invasion by head and neck masses: prediction with MR imaging. Radiology 195:715–720, 1995.
9. Glasier CM, Stark JE, Jacobs RF, et al: CT and ultrasound imaging of retropharyngeal abscess in children. AJNR 13:1191–1195, 1992.
10. Davis WL, Harnsberger HR, et al: Retropharyngeal space: evaluation of normal anatomy and diseases with CT and MR imaging. Radiology 174:59–64, 1990.
11. Buckley AR, Moss EH, Blokmanis A: Diagnosis of peritonsillar abscess: value of intraoral sonography. AJR 162:961–964, 1994.
12. Som P: Lymph nodes of the neck. Radiology 165:593–600, 1987.
13. Reede DL, Bergeron RT: Cervical tuberculous adenitis: CT manifestations. Radiology 154:701–704, 1985.
14. Yossem D, Som PM, Hackney DB, et al: Central nodal necrosis and extracapsular neoplastic spread in cervical lymph nodes: MR imaging versus CT. Radiology 182:753–759, 1992.
15. Holliday RA: Neck nodes and masses. In: American Society of Head and Neck Radiology 26th Annual Conference and Postgraduate Course, May 13–16, 1993, pp 87–98.
16. Steinkamp HJ, Hosten N, Richter C, et al: Enlarged cervical lymph nodes at helical CT. Radiology 191:795–798, 1994.
17. Vassallo P, Wernecke K, Roos N, et al: Differentiation of benign from malignant superficial lymphadenopathy: the role of high-resolution U.S. Radiology 183:215–220, 1992.
18. Friedman M, Roberts N, Kirshenbaum GL, et al: Nodal size of metastatic squamous cell carcinoma of the neck. Laryngoscope 103:854–856, 1993.
19. Tart RP, Mukherji SK, Avino AJ, et al: Facial lymph nodes: normal and abnormal CT appearance. Radiology 188:695–700, 1993.
20. Chang DB, Yuan A, Yu CJ, et al: Differentiation of benign and malignant cervical lymph nodes with color Doppler sonography. AJR 162:965–968, 1994.
21. Lufkin RB, Bradley WG, Brant-Zwadzki M: MRI of the Head and Neck. New York: Raven Press, 1991.
22. Hudgins PA: The suprahyoid neck: normal anatomy. In: Ramsey R, ed. American Society of Neuroradiology Core Curriculum Course, May 1–2, 1994, pp 169–173.
23. Mancuso AA, Harnsberger HR: Diseases of the suprahyoid neck spaces. In: Ramsey R, ed. American Society of Neuroradiology Core Curriculum Course, May 1–2, 1994, pp 175–180.
24. Lufkin RB, Wortham DG, Dietrich RB: Tongue and oropharynx: findings on MR imaging. Radiology 161:69–75, 1986.
24a. Yasumoto M, Shibuya H, Takeda M, Korenaga T: Squamous cell carcinoma of the oral cavity: MR findings and value of T1-weighted fast spin-echo images. AJR 159:981–987, 1992.
25. Laine FJ, Nadel L, Braun IF: CT and MR imaging of the central skull base. Radiographics 10:797–821, 1990.
26. Ginsberg LE: Neoplastic diseases affecting the central skull base: CT and MR imaging. AJR 159:581–589, 1992.
27. Hutchins LG, Harnsberger HR, Jacobs JM: Trigeminal neuralgia (tic douloureux): MR imaging assessment. Radiology 175:837–841, 1990.
28. Abrahams JJ: Mandibular lesions and dental implants. In: American Society of Head and Neck Radiology 26th Annual Conference and Postgraduate Course, May 13–16, 1993, pp 63–71.
28a. Han MH, Chang KH, Lee CH, et al: Cystic expansile masses of the maxilla: differential diagnosis with CT and MR. AJNR 16:333–338, 1995.
29. Underhill TE, Katz JO, Pope TL, et al: Radiologic findings of diseases involving the maxilla and mandible. AJR 159:345–350, 1992.
30. Minami M, Kaneda T, Yamamoto H: Ameloblastoma in the maxillomandibular region: MR imaging. Radiology 184:389–393, 1992.
31. Weissman JL, Snyderman CH, Yossem SA, et al: Ameloblastoma of the maxilla: CT and MR appearance. AJNR 14:223–226, 1993.
32. Coit WE, Harnsberger HR, Osborn AG, et al: Ranulas and their mimics: CT evaluation. Radiology 163:211–216, 1987.

33. Batsakis JG, McClatcheg KD: Cervical ranula. Ann Otol Rhinol Laryngol 97:561–562, 1988.
34. Vogl TJ, Steger W, Ihrler S, et al: Cystic masses in the floor of the mouth: value of MR in planning surgery. AJR 161:183–186, 1993.
35. Salazar JE, Duke RA, Ellis JV: Second branchial cleft cyst: unusual location and a new CT diagnostic sign. AJR 145:965–966, 1985.
36. Miller MB, Rao VM, Tom BM: Cystic masses of the head and neck: pitfalls in CT and MR interpretation. AJR 159:601–607, 1992.
37. New GB, Erich JB: Dermoid cysts of the head and neck. Surg Gynecol Obstet 65:48–55, 1937.
38. Levegue H, Sarasew CA, Tang CK: Dermoid cysts of the floor of the mouth and lateral neck. Laryngoscope 89:296–305, 1979.
39. Thibault F, Halimi P, Bely N, et al: Internal architecture of the parotid gland at MR imaging: facial nerve or ductal system. Radiology 188:701–704, 1993.
40. Tabor EK, Curtain HD: MR of salivary glands. Radiol Clin North Am 27:379–392, 1989.
41. Vogl TJ, Dressel SH, Spath M, et al: Parotid gland: plain and gadolinium enhanced MR imaging. Radiology 177:667–674, 1990.
42. Schlakman BN, Yossem DM: MR of intraparotid masses. AJNR 14:1173–1180, 1993.
43. Casselman JW, Mancuso AA: Major salivary gland masses: comparison of MR and CT. Radiology 165:183–189, 1987.
44. Horowitz SW, Leonetti JP, Azar-kia B, et al: CT and MR of temporal bone malignancies primary and secondary to parotid carcinoma. AJNR 15:755–762, 1994.
45. Curtin HD: Separation of the masticator space from the parapharyngeal space. Radiology 163:195–204, 1987.
45a. Tabor EK, Curtin HD: MR of the salivary glands. Radiol Clin North Am 27:379–392, 1989.
46. Abramowitz J, Dion JE, Jensen MP, et al: Angiographic diagnosis and management of head and neck schwannomas. AJNR 12:977–984, 1991.
47. Van Gills AP, Vandenberg R, Falke TH: MR diagnosis of paraganglioma of the head and neck: value of contrast enhancement. AJR 162:147–153, 1994.
48. Vogl T, Bruning R, Schedel H, et al: Paragangliomas of jugular bulb and carotid body: MRI imaging with short sequences and Gd DTPA enhancement. AJNR 10:823–827, 1989.
49. Holliday RA, Cohen WA, Schinella RA, et al: Benign lymphoepithelial parotid cystic and hyperplastic cervical adenopathy in AIDS-risk patients: a new CT appearance. Radiology 168:439–441, 1988.
50. Minarmi M, Tanioka H, Oyama K: Warthin tumor of the parotid gland: MR-pathologic correlation. AJNR 14:209–214, 1993.
51. Som PM, Urken ML, Biller M, et al: Imaging the postoperative neck. Radiology 187:593–601, 1993.
52. Gussack GS, Hudgins PA: Imaging in recurrent head and neck tumors. Laryngoscope 101:119–124, 1991.

36

Neck

JANE L. WEISSMAN

TECHNIQUE

Magnetic resonance (MR) studies of the soft tissues of the anterior neck are readily tailored to the clinical question. For most studies except those of the brachial plexus, MR imaging (MRI) of the neck is best done with an anterior neck coil. To minimize motion artifacts, the patient should be instructed to breathe slowly and evenly, preferably from the abdomen, not to talk or cough, and to swallow rarely.

Saturation pulses help limit artifacts from large blood vessels in the neck. Most neck studies can be performed with the phase-encoding gradient oriented side to side. For evaluation of the larynx and hypopharynx, an anterior-posterior orientation of the phase-encoding gradient is helpful. The pulsation artifacts from vessels are then also oriented anterior-posterior and do not obscure the larynx.

Larynx and hypopharynx are best evaluated with axial T1-weighted sequences 3 mm thick, obtained with an interslice gap of 0.5 to 1 mm or with no interslice gap, and axial T2-weighted images. If the patient has a tumor, MRI may demonstrate submucosal extension of tumor around the laryngeal ventricle from false vocal cord to true vocal cord. Often, this is not apparent to the endoscopist. The best way to assess this transglottic spread is with coronal T1-weighted images 3 mm thick obtained perpendicular to the vocal cords and laryngeal ventricle.

Most squamous cell cancers are enhanced after gadolinium administration, which makes the tumors more conspicuous. However, tumor invasion of paraglottic or preepiglottic fat or the fatty marrow of ossified cartilage may be less conspicuous after gadolinium. In these instances, fat suppression techniques are helpful.

To assess the thyroid and parathyroid glands, lymph nodes, and neck masses, axial T1- and T2-weighted sequences 3 to 5 mm thick may be sufficient. Gadolinium is useful in identifying parathyroid adenomas, the enhanced septa of lymphangiomas, and the nonenhanced center of a necrotic lymph node. Except for tumors of the larynx, coronal images are rarely necessary for most processes involving the soft tissues of the neck.

The brachial plexus can be studied with a good body coil or a surface coil. The relationship of the components of the brachial plexus to anterior scalene muscle and subclavian artery is seen well on coronal and sagittal images. T1- and T2-weighted sequences can be obtained, and images may be 3 to 5 mm thick. Axial images also demonstrate brachial plexus; slices 4 to 5 mm thick may be obtained.

HYPOPHARYNX AND LARYNX

NORMAL ANATOMY

The hypopharynx begins at the hyoid bone. The hypopharynx is continuous with the oropharynx above the hyoid and with the cervical esophagus below the cricoid cartilage.[1]

The epiglottis is attached anteriorly by the median glossoepiglottic ligament (Fig. 36–1A) and laterally by the glossoepiglottic ligaments (one on each side). The base of the epiglottis is called the petiole. Anterior to the epiglottis are the valleculae (see Fig. 36–1A). The epiglottis is elastic cartilage.[2]

The paired arytenoepiglottic folds stretch from the epiglottis to the arytenoid cartilages. Each arytenoepiglottic fold creates a lateral recess, the pyriform sinus (Fig. 36–1B). The pyriform sinuses come together and continue inferiorly as the cervical esophagus. The pyriform sinuses are the largest division of the hypopharynx.[1]

The major laryngeal cartilages are the thyroid, cricoid, and paired arytenoid cartilages (Fig. 36–2). The thyroid cartilage has two alae. The cricoid cartilage is a complete ring. The paired arytenoid cartilages perch on the cricoid cartilage. One small corniculate cartilage sits on each arytenoid. The cuneiform cartilages are found within the arytenoepiglottic folds, along the lateral aspect of the corniculate cartilages. Between the greater cornu (horn) of the hyoid bone and the superior horn of the thyroid cartilage lies the triticeous cartilage.[2] Cuneiform, corniculate, and triticeous cartilages are usually not apparent on MR images.

Cricoid, thyroid, and arytenoid cartilages mineralize with age and often ossify.[3–5] Nonossified cartilage has intermediate signal intensity on spin-echo pulse sequences. The cortex of ossified laryngeal cartilage is a thin band of low signal intensity (Fig. 36–3A and B).

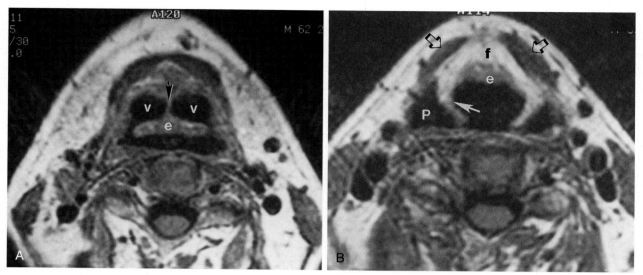

FIGURE 36–1. Normal hypopharynx. *A,* Axial T1-weighted image (repetition time/echo time/number of excitations = 783/20/2) shows the epiglottis (e), the median glossoepiglottic ligament *(arrow)*, and the valleculae (v). *B,* Slightly lower, the arytenoepiglottic folds *(white arrow)*, pyriform sinuses (P), petiole of the epiglottis (e), preepiglottic fat (f), and infrahyoid strap muscles *(open arrows)* are seen.

Fat in the marrow of ossified cartilage is hyperintense on T1-weighted images (see Fig. 36–3A).

The cartilaginous laryngeal skeleton supports several small muscles and a loose meshwork of fat and lymphatics.[5, 6] The fat is most conspicuous in the paraglottic and preepiglottic spaces[6] (see Fig. 36–1B).

Stratified squamous epithelium lines the hypopharynx (arytenoepiglottic folds, pyriform fossae) and true vocal cords.[2] Below the arytenoepiglottic folds and continuing down into trachea (except for true cords), the mucosa is pseudostratified ciliated columnar epithelium.[2] Normal mucosa is enhanced after gadolinium administration.

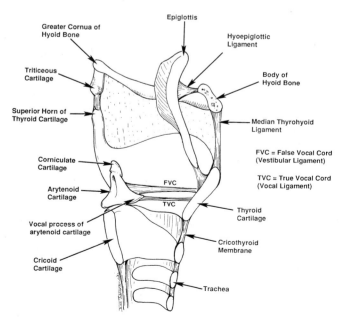

FIGURE 36–2. Larynx anatomy. Midsagittal diagram of the major cartilages and ligaments.

The false vocal cord stretches between the upper arytenoid cartilage and the thyroid cartilage (see Fig. 36–2). The false vocal cord, mostly fat and lymphatics, is the lower margin of the quadrangular membrane.[2] The superior edge of the quadrangular membrane is the arytenoepiglottic fold.

The true vocal cord extends from the vocal process of the arytenoid to the thyroid cartilage (see Fig. 36–2). The medial or free edge of the true cord is called the vocal ligament. The true cord is the upper margin of the conus elasticus (triangular membrane).[2]

Between the false cord (above) and the true cord (below) lies the laryngeal ventricle, an outpouching of the lumen lined by mucosa that bulges into the paraglottic (paralaryngeal) space.[1, 6] The false vocal cords, laryngeal ventricles, and petiole of the epiglottis constitute the supraglottic larynx.[1]

On axial images, the level of the false vocal cords is indicated by the upper arytenoid cartilage; the signal of the false cords is fat[4, 6] (see Fig. 36–3A). The true vocal cords are seen at the level of the vocal process of the arytenoid cartilage, where the thyroarytenoid muscle attaches. This muscle makes up most of the true vocal cord, so the signal representing the true cord is from muscle (see Fig. 36–3B). On axial images, the transition from the fat of the false vocal cord to muscle of the true vocal cord marks the location of the laryngeal ventricle. The ventricle itself is usually not apparent on axial images but can be seen on coronal images.[6] On coronal images, the fat of the false vocal cord is separated from the muscle of the true cord by the laryngeal ventricle, which may be only a slit.[6]

PATHOLOGY

Hypopharynx and Larynx Cancer

Most tumors of the hypopharynx are squamous cell cancers. These are classified by location[7]: pyriform si-

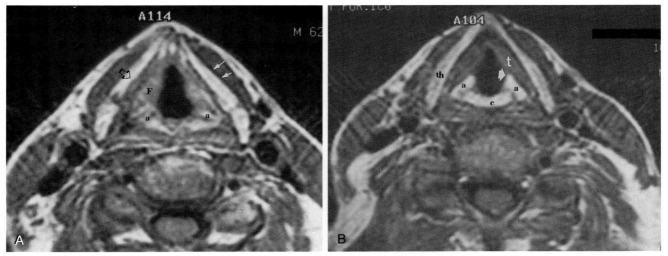

FIGURE 36–3. Normal larynx. *A,* Axial T1-weighted image (783/20/2) through the upper arytenoids (a) shows the fat signal of the false vocal cords (F). The thyroid alae are ossified and have fatty marrow in the medullary space *(open arrow)* and a hypointense cortex *(white arrows)*. *B,* Lower down, the signal of the true vocal cords is from muscle (t), reflecting the thyroarytenoid muscle that makes up most of the true cords. The articulation of the arytenoids (a) with the cricoid cartilage (c) is apparent. Arrow = vocal process of the arytenoid cartilage; th = thyroid cartilage.

nus (Fig. 36–4), posterior pharyngeal wall (Fig. 36–5*A* and *B*), and postcricoid or pharyngoesophageal junction. Some authors also describe a marginal area, the arytenoepiglottic folds[1] (Fig. 36–6*A* to *D*). Tumors of the marginal area may behave as pyriform sinus

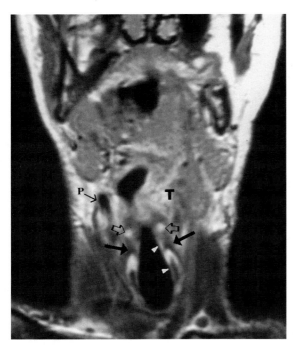

FIGURE 36–4. Hypopharynx tumor: pyriform sinus. A coronal T1-weighted image (516/15/2) after gadolinium administration demonstrates a left hypopharyngeal (pyriform sinus) tumor (T). The right pyriform sinus is normal (P). The fatty marrow of the arytenoid cartilages *(open arrows)* marks the level of the false cords; the true vocal cords have muscle signal *(solid arrows)*. Normal mucosa is thin and enhanced after gadolinium *(arrowheads)*.

tumors (hypopharynx) or as supraglottic larynx tumors.

Similarly, more than 90% of tumors of the larynx are squamous cell carcinomas.[6] Adenoid cystic carcinoma of the minor salivary glands, lymphoma, glomus tumor, and other neoplasms are seen much less frequently.

Coronal MR images and the great inherent tissue contrast of MR images have had a great impact on imaging tumors of the larynx.[4, 5] The primary tumor is usually apparent to the endoscopist. MRI provides important information about deep extension of tumor and invasion of laryngeal cartilage. Accurate delineation of the extent of tumor may allow a less radical, "voice-sparing" surgical resection instead of total laryngectomy.

A supraglottic tumor may infiltrate the paraglottic or preepiglottic fat. This is apparent on nonenhanced T1-weighted images and can also be appreciated on fat-suppressed gadolinium-enhanced T1-weighted images.

At the level of the true vocal cord, a deeply invasive tumor may be more difficult to detect on T1-weighted images, as the tumor and the thyroarytenoid muscle have similar signal intensities (Fig. 36–7*A*). Gadolinium-enhanced images (Fig. 36–7*B*) or T2-weighted sequences (Fig. 36–7*C*) are helpful. Tumor is hyperintense on T2-weighted sequences and is enhanced after gadolinium administration.

Normal laryngeal cartilage may mineralize or ossify irregularly. This can make the detection by computed tomography (CT) of tumor invading cartilage difficult.[4] MRI is the imaging study of choice to determine laryngeal cartilage involvement by tumor.[3] On pregadolinium T1-weighted images, tumor is hypointense with respect to fat in the cartilage marrow (see Fig.

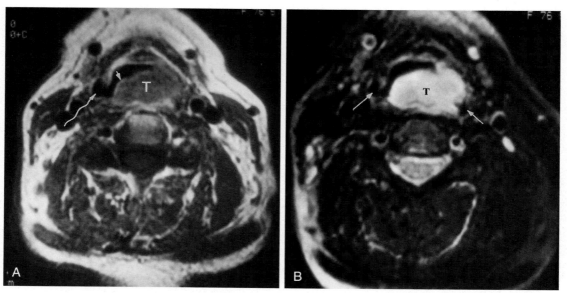

FIGURE 36–5. Hypopharynx tumor: posterior wall. *A*, Axial T1-weighted image (533/16/2) after gadolinium administration shows a tumor of the posterior wall of the hypopharynx (T). The tumor is minimally enhanced; the overlying mucosa is more intensely enhanced *(small arrow)*. The tumor encroaches on the left pyriform sinus; the right pyriform sinus *(wavy arrow)* is normal. *B*, On the T2-weighted image (3000/85/2), the tumor (T) is quite hyperintense. Arrows indicate pyriform sinuses.

36–7*A*). On conventional spin-echo T2-weighted images (or fast spin-echo T2-weighted images with fat suppression), the tumor is hyperintense with respect to the marrow fat (see Fig. 36–7*C*). After gadolinium, it may be difficult or impossible to distinguish enhanced tumor from uninvolved cartilage marrow unless fat suppression is used (see Fig. 36–7*B*).

Nonsurgical treatment (radiation therapy) is usually contraindicated if tumor invades cartilage, because there is a high incidence of chondronecrosis.[4] However, subtotal resection may be feasible.

The two major voice-sparing procedures are vertical hemilaryngectomy and supraglottic laryngectomy. A tumor confined to the true vocal cord may be amenable to a vertical laryngectomy.[8] Vertical hemilaryngectomy entails resection of the ipsilateral true and false vocal cords and thyroid ala, sometimes ipsilateral arytenoid cartilage, and, if the tumor crosses the midline slightly, a portion of the contralateral vocal cord and thyroid ala.

Subglottic tumor extending below the upper margin of the cricoid cartilage is a contraindication to vertical hemilaryngectomy. The conus elasticus, a thick membrane that stretches from vocal ligament (true vocal cord) to cricoid cartilage, separates an invasive mucosal tumor from the underlying cartilage. Below the inferior edge of the conus elasticus, an invasive tumor would come in contact with cartilage without the protection afforded the cartilage by the intervening conus. A relative contraindication to vertical hemilaryngectomy is tumor involving the cricoarytenoid joint, as this would necessitate resection of the cricoid cartilage.[8] The cricoid is the only complete ring of the cartilaginous skeleton of the larynx and provides important support. However, surgical advances have made partial resection of the cricoid possible.

The other voice-sparing procedure is supraglottic laryngectomy.[4] A tumor must be confined to the false vocal cord to be amenable to supraglottic laryngectomy. Deep (submucosal) extension of tumor around the ventricle into the true vocal cord is an absolute contraindication to supraglottic laryngectomy. Coronal MR images are the ideal way to look for this tumor extension (Fig. 36–8).

Laryngocele

The dilated saccule of the laryngeal ventricle is called a laryngocele or saccular cyst. A laryngocele forms when the orifice of the ventricle is obstructed.[9] A laryngocele may contain fluid or air[9] or both. Laryngoceles are benign. However, a small mucosal cancer may have obstructed the ventricle. The cancer may not be apparent on MR images (small mucosal lesions often are not). It is important to make the diagnosis of laryngocele to alert the clinician to the possibility of a mucosal lesion near the opening of the laryngeal ventricle. The endoscopist can then evaluate this area further.

Chondroid Lesions

Chondromas and chondrosarcomas of the larynx are rare tumors that most often arise from the cricoid cartilage.[10] The involved cartilage is expanded, has an inhomogeneous intermediate signal intensity on T1-weighted images (Fig. 36–9*A*), is enhanced after gadolinium administration (Fig. 36–9*B*), and has a hyperintense signal on T2-weighted images.[11] The calcified tumor matrix is more apparent on CT scans than on MR images (Fig. 36–9*C*).

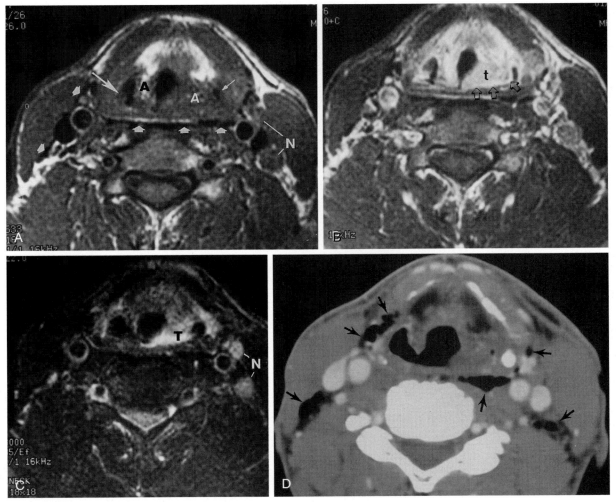

FIGURE 36–6. Hypopharynx tumor: arytenoepiglottic fold. *A,* Axial T1-weighted image (533/16/2) shows a tumor thickening the left arytenoepiglottic fold (white A) and encroaching on the pyriform sinus *(small arrow).* The arytenopiglottic fold (black A) and pyriform sinus *(long arrow)* are normal. There are enlarged zone II lymph nodes in the left spinal accessory chain (N). Air in the fascial planes *(short arrows)* from recent tracheostomy is quite subtle. *B,* Axial T1-weighted image (616/26/2) after gadolinium administration shows that the tumor (t) is enhanced slightly less than the overlying mucosa *(arrows).* Enhancement of the tumor makes it difficult to assess the extent of tumor infiltration into the paraglottic fat. *C,* On T2-weighted image (fast spin echo [FSE], 3000/85/1, with fat suppression), the arytenoepiglottic fold tumor (T) and the abnormal lymph node (N) are hyperintense. The interstitial emphysema is almost imperceptible. *D,* On an axial CT scan of the same patient on the same day, the cervical emphysema is much more conspicuous *(arrows).*

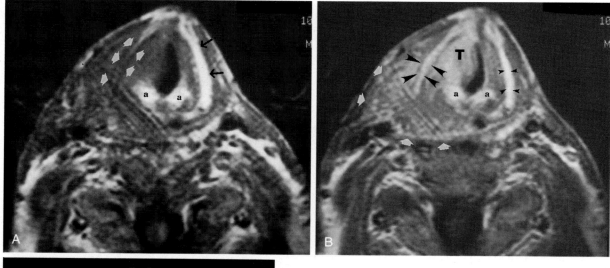

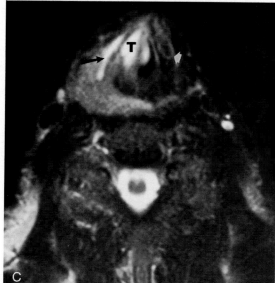

FIGURE 36–7. Larynx tumor. *A,* Axial T1-weighted image (611/11/2) shows a tumor of the right true vocal cord (unlabeled). The fatty marrow of the right thyroid ala *(white arrows)* is replaced by tumor or edema. The fat in the left ala is normal *(black arrows).* a = arytenoid cartilages. *B,* Axial T1-weighted image (70/11/2) shows enhancement of the true vocal cord tumor (T) and the involved cartilage *(large arrowheads).* Without fat suppression, it is difficult to distinguish normal fatty marrow *(small arrowheads)* from enhanced tumor in the marrow. The large tumor *(arrows)* extends between thyroid and arytenoid (a) cartilages, posterior and lateral to larynx. *C,* Axial T2-weighted image (6766/102/2 with fat suppression) allows the distinction between involved thyroid cartilage *(black arrow)* and normal cartilage *(white arrow).* T = true vocal cord tumor.

FIGURE 36–8. Transglottic tumor. Coronal T1-weighted image (600/20/2) shows the normal fat signal of the left false vocal cord (f) and muscle signal of the normal left true vocal cord (t). On the right, a large tumor (M) replaces the fat of the false cord and extends around the ventricle (V) into the true cord. T = thyroid cartilage; C = cricoid cartilage; P = pyriform sinus.

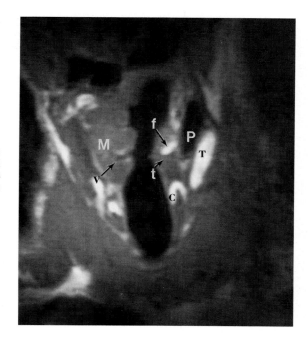

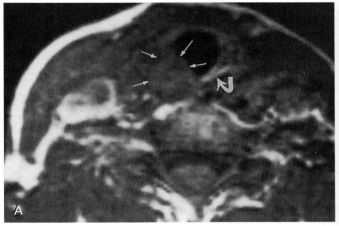

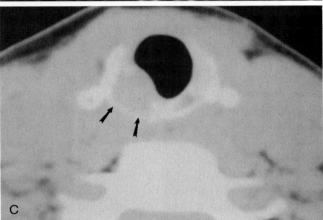

FIGURE 36–9. **Chondrosarcoma of the larynx.** *A,* Axial T1-weighted image shows that the right side of the cricoid cartilage is expanded *(straight arrows).* The normal fat signal of cricoid marrow *(curved arrow)* is replaced by tumor. *B,* Axial T1-weighted image with fat suppression and after gadolinium shows enhancement of the tumor *(arrows).* (Surrounding enhancement may be related to a recent biopsy.) *C,* Axial CT scan shows the expanded cricoid lamina *(arrows).*

Vocal Cord Paralysis

Vocal cord paralysis can be diagnosed clinically; imaging studies may identify the cause. Vocal cord paralysis results from damage to the recurrent laryngeal nerve, a branch of the vagus nerve. Imaging studies examine the nerve from its origin in the brain stem, through the jugular foramen where the vagus exits the skull base, down the neck in the carotid sheath, and into the upper mediastinum, where the right recurrent laryngeal nerve loops around the subclavian artery and the left recurrent nerve loops under the ligamentum arteriosum. The recurrent laryngeal nerves ascend through the neck in the tracheoesophageal groove to reach the larynx, where they innervate all the intrinsic muscles of the larynx except the cricothyroid muscle (innervated by the superior laryngeal nerve).

Trauma

MRI plays a larger role in assessing cervical spine trauma than in assessing trauma to the soft tissues of the anterior neck. Hematomas can be appreciated on MR images. Larynx trauma (cartilage fracture, cricoarytenoid subluxation or dislocation) is more easily evaluated with CT, especially in adults whose laryngeal cartilage has mineralized or ossified. In addition, cervical emphysema, an indirect finding suggesting disruption of the larynx, is more apparent on CT scans (see Fig. 36–6*A* to *D*).

LYMPH NODES

CLASSIFICATION

The many classifications of cervical lymph nodes have created some confusion. The six zones described by the American College of Otolaryngology–Head and Neck Surgery[12] are easy to understand and are clinically relevant.

Zone 1 includes submental and submandibular nodes. The hyoid bone is the inferior extent of zone 1; the mandible is the superior extent (Fig. 36–10).

Zone 2 nodes surround the upper one third of the jugular vein. Zone 2 extends from the skull base down to the hyoid bone (or carotid bifurcation) (see Fig. 36–10).

Zone 3 comprises the nodes around the middle third of the jugular vein, from hyoid bone down to omohyoid muscle. The anterior border is the lateral (posterior) edge of the sternohyoid (strap) muscle; the posterior border is the back of the sternocleidomastoid muscle (see Fig. 36–10).

Zone 4, or lower jugular, nodes lie between the omohyoid muscle and the clavicle (see Fig. 36–10).

Zone 5 is the posterior triangle and includes all nodes that lie behind the posterior edge of the sternocleidomastoid muscle. Supraclavicular nodes are part of zone 5 (see Fig. 36–10).

Zone 6 includes the pretracheal and peritracheal nodes and nodes along the recurrent laryngeal nerves.

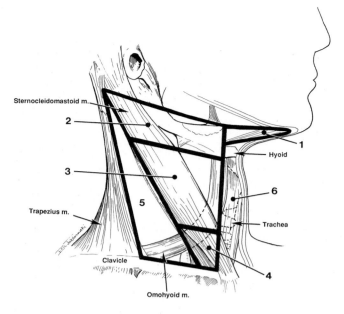

FIGURE 36–10. Lymph node classifcation. The six zones are indicated with respect to the landmarks that define them. (Redrawn from Robbins KT, Medina JE, Wolfe GT, et al: Standardizing neck dissection terminology. Official report of the Academy's Committee for Head and Neck Surgery and Oncology. Arch Otolaryngol Head Neck Surg 117:601–605, 1991. Copyright 1991, American Medical Association.)

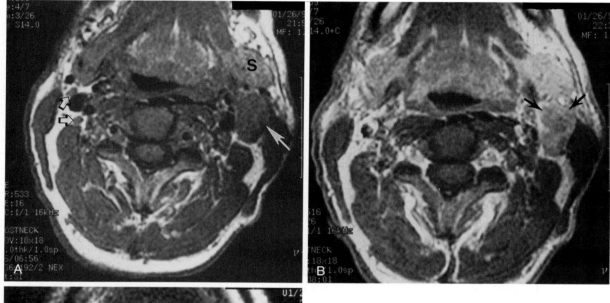

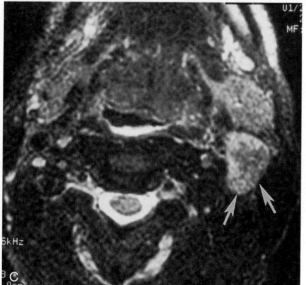

FIGURE 36–11. Lymphadenopathy. *A,* Axial T1-weighted image (533/16/2) shows an enlarged zone 2 (jugulodigastric) lymph node on the left *(white arrow).* The node is almost 2.5 cm in greatest diameter (centimeter scale at left) and is approximately isointense relative to muscle. There are normal lymph nodes on the right *(open arrows).* S = submandibular gland. *B,* Axial T1-weighted image (616/26/2) after gadolinium shows enhancement of the node *(arrows),* although the center is less intensely enhanced than the periphery. This could represent tumor or necrosis. *C,* Axial T2-weighted image (FSE, 2000/85/1, with fat suppression) shows that the node becomes hyperintense *(arrows),* although the central portion of the node is less hyperintense than the periphery.

Zone 6 extends from the hyoid bone to the suprasternal notch and back as far as the common carotid arteries (see Fig. 36–10).

ABNORMAL NODES

The size, signal intensity, and margins of a lymph node are all important in determining whether the node is abnormal.[13, 14] In the neck, lymph nodes larger than 1 cm are considered abnormal in all zones except zone 2 (jugulodigastric nodes), where 1.5 cm can be considered the upper limit of normal (Fig. 36–11A to C). Following these criteria decreases the number of prominent but normal lymph nodes inaccurately designated pathologically large.

A central low signal intensity on T1-weighted images (Fig. 36–12A and B) and hyperintense signal on T2-weighted images (Fig. 36–12C) of a lymph node are abnormal, regardless of the size of the node. It may be difficult or impossible to distinguish tumor from necrosis; both may be present[13, 14] (see Fig. 36–11A to C). Occasionally, necrotic nodes may mimic a cystic mass such as a lymphangioma (see Fig. 36–12A to C).

Irregular margins of the node and infiltration of adjacent structures or surrounding fat can suggest spread of metastatic tumor beyond the capsule of the node. This extracapsular spread of tumor (most often squamous cell carcinoma from a primary tumor of the upper aerodigestive tract) has a poor prognosis, and the patients usually receive radiation therapy after lymphadenectomy (neck dissection).

The many causes of cervical lymphadenopathy include infectious (bacterial, including granulomatous diseases and cat-scratch disease; viral, such as mononucleosis) and neoplastic (lymphomas as well as metastatic squamous cell and other primary carcinomas). A full differential diagnosis is beyond the province of this chapter. CT studies may be better than MRI when the etiology is metastatic thyroid cancer or granulomatous disease (especially tuberculosis), as calcifications in lymph nodes that may facilitate the diagnosis are often not apparent with MRI.

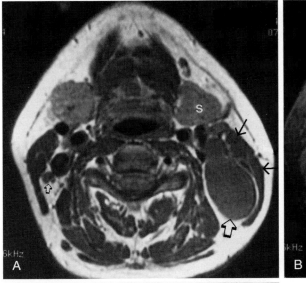

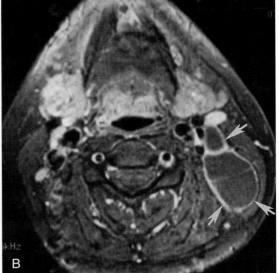

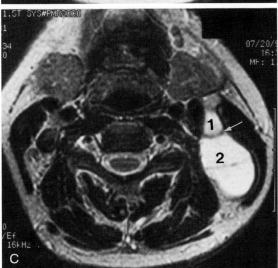

FIGURE 36–12. Necrotic lymphadenopathy. *A,* T1-weighted image (FSE, 666/17/2) shows a well-circumscribed mass *(large open arrow)* that is almost isointense relative to muscle. The mass lies behind the vessels, in the spinal accessory chain of zone 2. A normal node is seen in the same location on the right *(small open arrow).* Thin black arrows indicate sternocleidomastoid muscle; s = submandibular gland. *B,* A fat-suppressed T1-weighted image (FSE, 666/17/2) shows that the rim and internal septation of the nodes are enhanced *(arrows)* but the necrotic center is not. *C,* T2-weighted image (FSE, 3000/102/1) shows that the necrotic portion becomes quite hyperintense. The thicker septum *(arrow)* is probably the rim of a second, smaller node (1) that lies anterior to the larger node (2). The larger node has an internal septum.

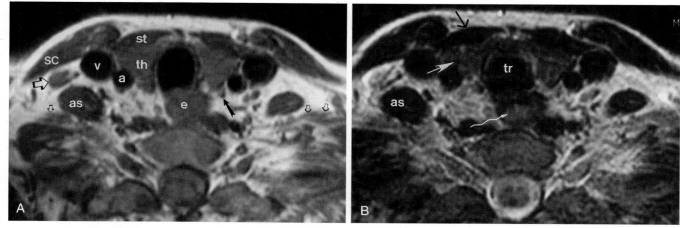

FIGURE 36–13. Normal thyroid gland. *A,* The signal of the thyroid gland (th) is slightly hyperintense relative to muscle and minimally inhomogeneous on a T1-weighted image (FSE, 666/17/2). e = esophagus; v = internal jugular vein; a = common carotid artery; solid arrow = minor neurovascular bundle; sc = sternocleidomastoid muscle; st = infrahyoid strap muscles; as = anterior scalene muscle; small open arrows = brachial plexus; large open arrow = small lymph node. *B,* On a T2-weighted image (FSE, 3000/102/1), the thyroid gland *(straight white arrow)* is slightly inhomogeneous and slightly hyperintense with respect to strap muscles *(black arrow).* The mucosa of the esophagus *(wavy white arrow)* is also slightly hyperintense. tr = trachea; as = anterior scalene muscle.

THYROID GLAND

NORMAL APPEARANCE

The normal thyroid gland has two lobes connected by an isthmus (Fig. 36–13A and B) and a small pyramidal process that is often not seen by MRI.[15] On T1-weighted images, the normal gland is approximately isointense relative to muscle[15] (see Fig. 36–13A). On T2-weighted images, normal thyroid is hyperintense relative to muscle[15] (see Fig. 36–13B). The normal thyroid is homogeneous or slightly inhomogeneous.[15]

The inferior thyroid artery and vein and the recurrent laryngeal nerve make up the lesser neurovascular bundle.[16] The vessels can be identified behind the lower pole of each thyroid lobe[15] (see Fig. 36–13A). Normal esophageal mucosa is hyperintense on T2-weighted images (see Fig. 36–13B) and is enhanced with gadolinium. Esophageal mucosa should not be mistaken for thyroid (or other) pathology.

PATHOLOGY

Focal and diffuse abnormalities of the thyroid gland are readily apparent on MR images.[15–17] However, it is usually not possible to make a specific histologic diagnosis or even to distinguish benign from malignant disorders based on MRI appearances.[16]

Benign Disease

Adenomas are round and well circumscribed[15] and usually clearly different from the surrounding gland.[17] On T1-weighted images, they may have a homogeneous or heterogeneous signal intensity,[15] sometimes with central hyperintensity resulting from prior hemor-

rhage.[15] Adenomas, like most thyroid pathology, are hyperintense on T2-weighted images.

A hemorrhagic cyst is hyperintense on T1- and T2-weighted images[15] (Fig. 36–14) and may have a hypointense rim, seen best on T2-weighted images.[15, 16] The rim is hemosiderin in macrophages. A hemorrhagic cyst presents with acute swelling and pain (see Fig. 36–14). A colloid cyst is also hyperintense on T1- and T2-weighted images[15] but lacks the hypointense rim of a hemorrhagic cyst.[16]

A functioning nodule is isointense relative to normal thyroid parenchyma on all pulse sequences.[15] A con-

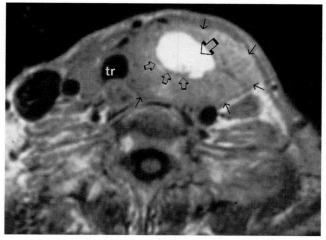

FIGURE 36–14. Hemorrhagic thyroid cyst. On a T1-weighted image (600/25/2), methemoglobin is hyperintense *(large open arrow).* There is a suggestion of a hypointense rim *(small open arrows),* which may help distinguish a hemorrhagic cyst from a colloid cyst. The entire left lobe is enlarged *(solid arrows),* displacing the trachea (tr) to the right. This young woman had experienced left neck swelling and pain. (Courtesy of Barbara Carter, MD, New England Medical Center, Boston, MA.)

tour bulge may be the only indication of the nodule, or the gland may look entirely normal.

Adenomatous multinodular goiter can affect the entire gland or portions of the gland. The signal is inhomogeneous on all pulse sequences, with hyperintense foci of prior hemorrhage.[15, 17] The interface between goitrous and normal gland may not be well defined. Calcifications may be subtle signal voids on MR images (Fig. 36–15A); they are more apparent on CT scans (Fig. 36–15B).

Malignant Tumors

Papillary carcinoma is the most frequent malignancy of the thyroid gland[18] and represents 50% to 60% of thyroid malignancy. Follicular carcinoma represents about 20%, medullary carcinoma (from parafollicular cells) 10%, anaplastic carcinoma 5%, and Hürthle cell carcinoma less than 5%.[18] Metastases to the thyroid gland and lymphoma may be indistinguishable from primary thyroid malignancies.

MRI can distinguish recurrence in the surgical bed from scar (Fig. 36–16A and B). Recurrent tumor is hyperintense on T2-weighted images and scar is hypointense.[16]

Some thyroid masses have a low-signal-intensity fibrous pseudocapsule at the interface between the tumor and normal parenchyma.[17] The pseudocapsule should not be mistaken for a chemical-shift artifact.[17] A discontinuous pseudocapsule is suggestive but not diagnostic of malignancy.

Autoimmune and Inflammatory Conditions

In Graves' disease, the gland may be enlarged. The signal is heterogeneous and hyperintense on all pulse sequences.[15, 16] There are usually no focal masses.[15] Hashimoto's thyroiditis also causes enlargement of the thyroid. The signal intensity on T1-weighted images is variable. Low-signal-intensity bands traverse the gland; these fibrous septa divide the gland into islands of parenchyma.[15] The vessels around the gland may be enlarged.[15]

Differential Features

In summary, almost all thyroid pathologic conditions have a hyperintense signal on T2-weighted images.[16] On T1-weighted images, hemorrhagic and colloid cysts are hyperintense but focal; in Graves' disease the gland appears hyperintense and diffuse. Adenomas, goiter, cancer, lymphoma, and some cysts have low signal intensity on T1-weighted images. It is apparent from this that MRI is of little value in differentiating benign from malignant lesions. MRI is superb at delineating the anatomic extent of a lesion.[16] Cervical lymphadenopathy, invasion of adjacent structures such as strap muscles, and distant metastases are evidence of malignancy. However, a high signal intensity of strap muscles on T2-weighted images could represent invasion by tumor or reactive edema.[16]

PARATHYROID GLANDS

EMBRYOLOGY AND ANATOMY

The parathyroid glands develop from endoderm of the pharyngeal pouches. The inferior pair of glands develops from the third pouches; the superior glands develop from the fourth pouches. Most people have four parathyroid glands, although as few as two and as many as eight glands have been described.[16]

The location of the glands may vary. Usually, the superior parathyroid glands lie behind the upper poles of the thyroid gland, and the inferior glands lie behind the lower poles. Normal parathyroid glands are usually not apparent on MR images.[16] The minor neurovascular bundle (inferior thyroid artery and vein, recurrent laryngeal nerve) is a useful landmark for the inferior parathyroid glands[16, 19] (see Fig. 36–13A). Parathyroid glands may also be found within the thyroid gland, in

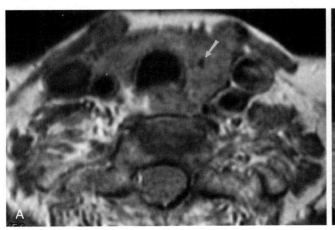
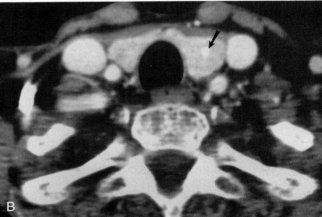

FIGURE 36–15. Thyroid calcification, presumed goiter. A, Axial proton density–weighted image (2000/17/1) demonstrates a focus of signal void within the left lobe *(arrow)*. B, Axial contrast-enhanced CT scan shows a calcification in the same location *(arrow)*. Thyroid parenchyma is inhomogeneous on both CT and MRI studies.

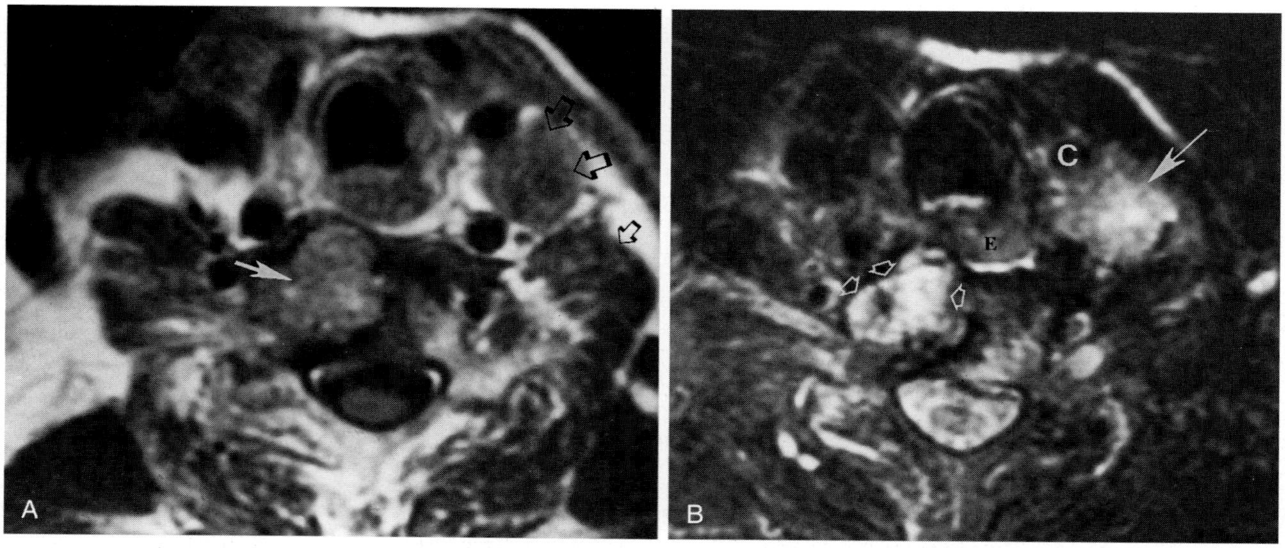

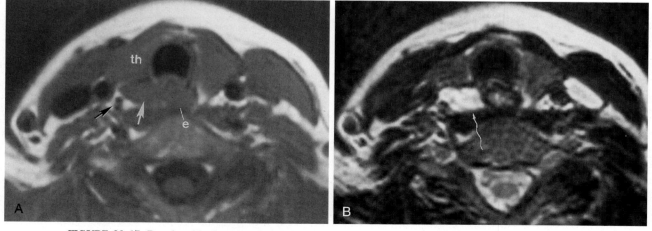

FIGURE 36–16. Recurrent follicular thyroid cancer. *A,* Axial T1-weighted image (500/13/3) shows a soft tissue mass *(large open arrows)* near the surgical site in a patient who previously underwent thyroidectomy. The mass is approximately isointense relative to the anterior scalene muscle *(small open arrow).* There is also a metastasis to the vertebral body *(solid arrow).* *B,* On the T2-weighted image (3400/90/2 with fat suppression), the recurrence *(solid arrow)* is hyperintense. The hyperintense signal is characteristic of a recurrence but not of scar. A metastasis to the vertebral body *(open arrows)* has the same signal intensity as the recurrence. E = esophagus; C = common carotid artery.

and around the thymus, behind the esophagus, and in the posterior mediastinum.[16]

PATHOLOGY

More than 85% of primary hyperparathyroidism is caused by a solitary parathyroid adenoma.[16] Diffuse hyperplasia accounts for about 10% of hyperparathyroidism.[16] Multiple adenomas are rare (4%), and parathyroid carcinoma accounts for about 1% of all cases of primary hyperparathyroidism.[16]

A parathyroid adenoma may be hypointense or hyperintense on T1-weighted images (Fig. 36–17A) and

hyperintense on T2-weighted images[16] (Fig. 36–17B). Parathyroid adenomas are enhanced after gadolinium administration. Parathyroid cancer may look the same as an adenoma.[16] In addition, thyroid disease may mimic parathyroid disease, because both appear hyperintense on T2-weighted images.

BRACHIAL PLEXUS

ANATOMY

Nerve roots C-5 through T-1 give rise to the brachial plexus. The roots coalesce to form trunks, the trunks

FIGURE 36–17. Parathyroid adenoma. *A,* Axial T1-weighted image (700/11/2) shows a nodule *(white arrow)* behind the upper pole of the right lobe of the thyroid gland (th). The nodule is isointense relative to thyroid. Black arrow indicates minor neurovascular bundle; e = esophagus. *B,* On the T2-weighted image (2800/152/2), the nodule becomes hyperintense *(arrow)* relative to thyroid gland.

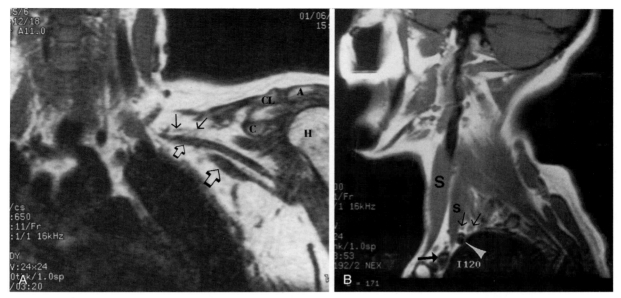

FIGURE 36–18. Normal brachial plexus. *A,* Coronal T1-weighted image (650/11/2) shows the subclavian and axillary artery *(small open arrow)* and vein *(large open arrow).* The brachial plexus *(solid arrows)* accompanies the artery. H = humerus; CL = clavicle; A = acromion; C = coracoid. *B,* Sagittal T1-weighted image (600/11/2). Components of the brachial plexus *(thin arrows)* run with the subclavian artery *(arrowhead).* The anterior scalene muscle (s) separates the artery from the subclavian vein *(thick arrow).* S = sternocleidomastoid muscle.

become divisions, and the divisions divide into cords, which continue as nerves.[20]

The brachial plexus runs with the subclavian artery between the anterior and middle scalene muscles (Figs. 36–18*A* and *B* and 36–19; see Fig. 36–13*A*). After passing between the muscles, the artery becomes the axillary artery (see Fig. 36–18*A*). The brachial plexus continues its course along the axillary artery.[21]

PATHOLOGY

The most frequent causes of brachial plexopathy are trauma and tumor.[22] Trauma may cause avulsion of

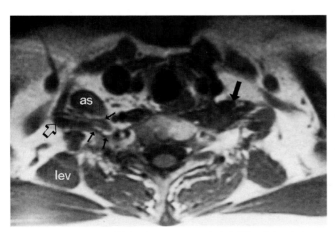

FIGURE 36–19. Brachial plexus mass. Axial T1-weighted image (650/13/2) shows the normal right brachial plexus *(small solid arrows)* running along the subclavian artery *(open arrow)* behind the anterior scalene muscle (as). lev = levator scapulae muscle. On the left, a mass near the neural foramen is in a location to impinge on the brachial plexus *(large solid arrow).*

cervical nerve roots. Tumors include primary neoplasms of the nerves, direct extension of tumor (from apex of lung, for example), and metastasis[20] (Fig. 36–20*A* and *B*; see Fig. 36–19). MRI is ideally suited for evaluation of the brachial plexus. Taking advantage of multiplanar imaging, MRI of the brachial plexus may include coronal and sagittal sequences as well as axial images.[20, 21]

NEUROGENIC TUMORS

NERVE SHEATH TUMORS

Neurofibromas contain axons and Schwann cells and do not have a capsule.[23] Neurofibromas may occur as solitary lesions. Multiple neurofibromas occur in neurofibromatosis type 1. The risk of malignant transformation is greater in neurofibromatosis than for solitary neurofibromas.[24] Neurilemomas are encapsulated benign tumors that contain Schwann cells and are therefore also called schwannomas.[23]

MRI has facilitated assessment of peripheral nerve sheath tumors. A neurofibroma grows by infiltrating normal nerve, causing diffuse enlargement of the nerve[25] (Fig. 36–21). A schwannoma (neurilemoma) is an eccentric, well-circumscribed mass protruding from the trunk of a nerve.[25]

Both neurofibromas and schwannomas have been found to have intermediate signal intensity on T1-weighted images, a moderately bright signal on proton density–weighted images, and a hyperintense signal on T2-weighted images and are often inhomogeneous on all sequences[24, 25] (see Fig. 36–21). A "target" appearance, with a central hypointense focus on T2-weighted images, has been described for some neurofibromas

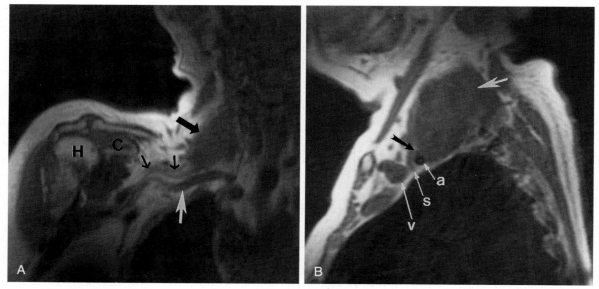

FIGURE 36–20. Brachial plexus mass. *A,* Coronal T1-weighted image (416/11/2) shows a mass *(large black arrow)* extending down from the neck to impinge on the brachial plexus *(small black arrows).* White arrow indicates subclavian artery; H = humerus; C = coracoid. *B,* Sagittal T1-weighted image (566/11/2) shows a large metastasis *(large white arrow)* extending from the lower neck down to the subclavian artery (a). The brachial plexus *(black arrow)* runs along the artery. v = subclavian vein; s = anterior scalene muscle.

but not for schwannomas or malignant nerve sheath tumors.[25] The low signal intensity corresponds to fibrosis on histologic examination.[25]

GLOMUS TUMORS

Paraganglia are derivatives of the neural crest. They accompany cranial nerves and their functions are

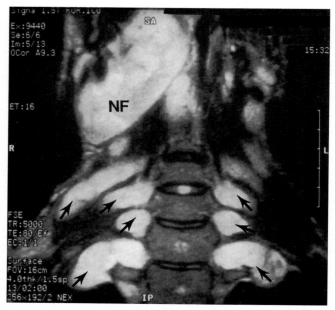

FIGURE 36–21. Neurofibromatosis type 1. Coronal T2-weighted image demonstrates an inhomogeneous, hyperintense neurofibroma (NF). There are many hyperintense masses in the neural foramina *(arrows);* these could be neurofibromas or meningoceles.

largely unknown, although carotid body paraganglia are chemoreceptors.

Tumors of paraganglia have a variety of names, including paraganglioma and chemodectoma. Glomus means ball and refers to the histologic appearance of these tumors; the characteristic findings at light microscopy are balls of cells or "Zellballen."[23] The paragangliomas of the head and neck are carotid body tumors, glomus vagale, glomus jugulare, glomus tympanicum, and the rare laryngeal glomus tumors.[26, 27] The paraganglioma most frequently encountered in the head and neck is the carotid body tumor.[23]

Paragangliomas have intermediate signal intensity on nonenhanced T1-weighted images, often with many punctate signal voids that represent tumor vessels[26] (Fig. 36–22A). After contrast agent administration, the tumor is intensely enhanced, giving a salt-and-pepper appearance[26] (Fig. 36–22B). The "salt" is the enhanced tumor stroma; the "pepper" is the punctate signal voids of tumor vessels (see Fig. 36–22B). Not all glomus tumors have this characteristic appearance, however, and other vascular tumors may have a similar appearance.[22] Paragangliomas have a hyperintense signal on T2-weighted images (Fig. 36–22C).

Glomus vagale tumors arise from the nodose ganglion of the vagus nerve, high in the neck beneath the skull base within the carotid sheath, in the poststyloid parapharyngeal space (also called the carotid space). Usually the tumor extends into the upper neck rather than intracranially.[22] As it grows, a glomus vagale tumor may extend between the internal carotid artery and the internal jugular vein. Like a carotid body tumor, a glomus vagale may also insinuate itself between internal and external carotid arteries; unlike a carotid body tumor, a glomus vagale does not arise from the bifurcation.[22]

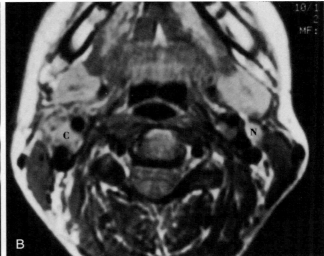

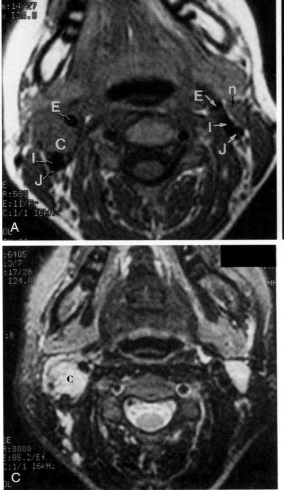

FIGURE 36–22. Carotid body tumor. *A,* Axial T1-weighted image (583/11/2) shows the carotid body tumor (C) interposed between the external (E) and internal (I) carotid arteries on the right. The tumor has a few hypointense foci that could represent vessels. A lymph node (n) on the left has signal similar to the tumor's but is lateral to the carotid bifurcation. J = internal jugular vein. *B,* Axial T1-weighted image (600/15/2) after gadolinium shows that the tumor (C) is intensely enhanced although a few hypointense foci persist, giving the tumor the salt-and-pepper appearance characteristic of glomus tumors. The lymph node on the left is also enhanced (N). *C,* Axial T2-weighted image (FSE, 3000/85/1) shows that the tumor (C) is quite hyperintense, almost isointense relative to cerebrospinal fluid.

CONGENITAL ANOMALIES

THYROGLOSSAL DUCT CYSTS

The thyroid originates at the foramen caecum at the base of the tongue, at the junction of the anterior two thirds and posterior one third of the tongue. As the embryo grows, the thyroid "descends" through the anterior neck, in front of the hyoid bone, the larynx, and the trachea. If the gland fails to descend, lingual thyroid results. Ectopic thyroid tissue may be encountered anywhere along the path of the descending gland. Remnants of the thyroglossal duct may fail to involute; the secretory mucosa lining these remnants eventually creates a thyroglossal duct cyst.[22]

Most thyroglossal duct cysts occur below the hyoid bone. The remainder occur either at the level of the hyoid or above the hyoid.[22] At and above the hyoid, thyroglossal duct cysts tend to be in the midline. Below the hyoid bone, thyroglossal duct cysts are more often slightly off the midline and embedded within the strap muscles.[22]

On T1-weighted images, the cyst is usually hyperintense[28] (Fig. 36–23A), probably because the cyst contents are similar to colloid and high in protein.[28] The cyst becomes increasingly hyperintense on progressively T2-weighted images (Fig. 36–23B and C). The location of a thyroglossal duct cyst is highly suggestive of the diagnosis.

BRANCHIAL CLEFT CYSTS

The embryo has six paired branchial (or pharyngeal) arches. Five pairs of branchial pouches separate the clefts; the pouches are lined by endoderm and extend out from the pharynx.[29] Similarly, five pairs of branchial clefts extend in from the surface; these are lined by ectoderm.[29] Epithelium is interposed between each cleft and pouch.[29]

Second branchial cleft cysts are the most frequent anomaly of the branchial apparatus.[22] These lie behind the submandibular gland, deep to the sternocleidomastoid muscle, and lateral to the carotid artery and internal jugular vein (Fig. 36–24A to C).

Cysts of the first branchial cleft are the next most frequent; these are found around the external auditory

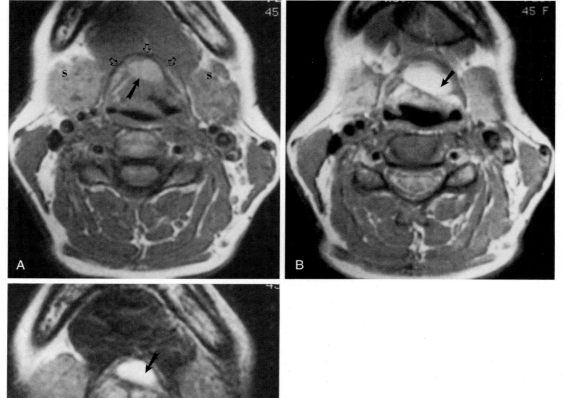

FIGURE 36–23. Thyroglossal duct cyst. *A*, Axial T1-weighted image (650/12/1) shows the hyperintense cyst *(solid arrow)* behind the hyoid bone *(open arrows)*. S = submandibular glands. *B*, Axial proton density–weighted image (FSE, 2000/17/1) shows that the cyst *(arrow)* becomes even more hyperintense with increased T2 weighting. *C*, Axial T2-weighted image (FSE, 3000/85/1) shows the markedly hyperintense cyst *(arrow)*.

canal, within or adjacent to the parotid gland.[30] Third and fourth branchial cleft cysts are rare.

The contents of an uncomplicated branchial cleft cyst vary from hypointense to slightly hyperintense on T1-weighted sequences and hyperintense on T2-weighted sequences[30] (see Fig. 36–24*A*). The cyst may have a thin, smooth rim. If a cyst has become infected or bled, the contents are not simple fluid and the rim may be thick and irregular and enhanced by contrast material.[30]

The differential diagnosis for an infected second branchial cleft cyst includes adenopathy and jugular vein thrombosis.[30] A first branchial cleft cyst within the parotid gland mimics a cystic Warthin tumor or the lymphoepithelial cysts of patients seropositive for the human immunodeficiency virus (although the lymphoepithelial cysts are usually multiple and bilateral). An infected first branchial cleft cyst could be mistaken for an infected parotid cyst or necrotic adenopathy.[30]

THYMIC CYSTS

The thymus develops from the third and fourth pharyngeal pouches that migrate down to the anterior mediastinum. Remnants of the right and left thymopharyngeal ducts are most often found in the lower neck, paramedian, anterior to the common carotid artery and internal jugular vein.[30]

LYMPHANGIOMAS AND HEMANGIOMAS

In the embryo, five sacs give rise to the lymphatic system: the paired jugular sacs (the largest sacs), the paired posterior sacs near the sciatic veins, and the unpaired retroperitoneal sac at the root of the mesentery.[31] Lymphangiomas form when the developing lymphatics fail to communicate with the developing veins. More than 75% of lymphangiomas occur in the neck.[30, 32]

There are three types of lymphangiomas. Cystic hygromas are collections of large lymphatic spaces that form when the developing lymph sac fails to communicate with the venous system.[33] Capillary (or simple) and cavernous lymphangiomas contain small lymphatic spaces and channels and develop from sequestered buds that would have formed terminal branches of the lymphatic system. The spaces of capillary lymphangiomas are smaller than the spaces of cavernous lymphangiomas, which in turn are smaller than the spaces of cystic hygromas.[33] All three histologic types may occur in the same lesion. Lymphangiomas have no malignant potential.[33]

Lymphangiomas are isointense relative to muscle on nonenhanced T1-weighted images and variably hyperintense on T2-weighted images.[31, 34] Hyperintense foci on T1-weighted images correspond to either fat (lipid, cholesterol) or methemoglobin.[31, 32] Occasion-

ally, fluid-fluid levels are seen[32, 33]; the supernatant is the hyperintense fluid.[32] T2-weighted images demonstrate the anatomic extent of the mass[34] and the internal septa. Cyst walls and the septa may be enhanced after gadolinium administration.[32]

Hemangiomas are characterized as capillary, cavernous, and mixed[34]; some authors also describe a juvenile or proliferative form.[30] Lymphangiomas that coexist with vascular malformations (hemangiomas) are called lymphangiohemangiomas.[33] Hemangiomas are enhanced by intravenous contrast medium (Fig. 36–25A and B). On MR images, a signal void within a hemangioma could represent a prominent vessel or a phlebolith. This distinction is easier in CT studies.

Lymphangiomas may be indistinguishable from hemangiomas on MR images,[34] and some lymphangiomas have hemangiomatous components. Some authors have not found gadolinium to be especially useful in MRI of lymphangiomas.[32]

DERMOID CYSTS AND TERATOMAS

Dermoid cysts contain ectoderm and mesoderm.[30] They usually occur in or near the midline and, unlike

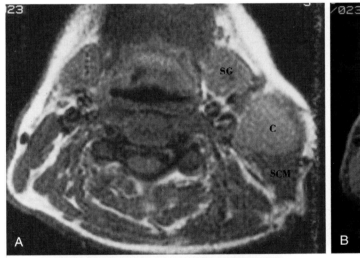

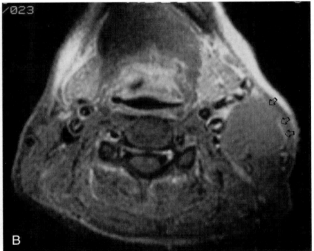

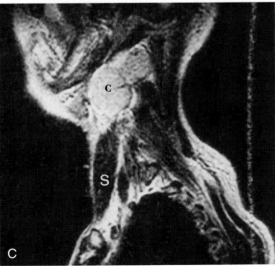

FIGURE 36–24. Second branchial cleft cyst. *A,* Axial T1-weighted image (400/11/2) shows the cyst (C), which is hyperintense with respect to cerebrospinal fluid. SCM = sternocleidomastoid muscle; SG = submandibular gland. *B,* Fat-suppressed axial T1-weighted image (650/11/2) after gadolinium shows enhancement of the cyst rim *(arrows)* but not the cyst contents. *C,* Sagittal T2-weighted image (FSE, 3400/119/2) shows the hyperintense, multilocular cyst (C). S = sternocleidomastoid muscle.

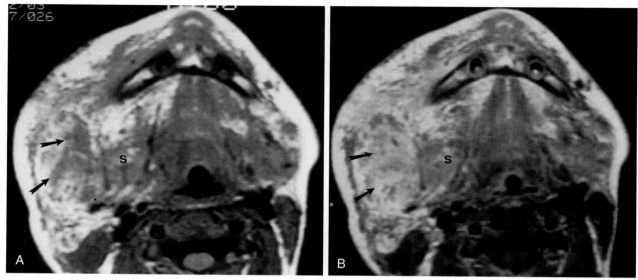

FIGURE 36–25. Hemangioma. *A,* T1-weighted image (500/20/4) shows diffuse infiltration of the subcutaneous fat *(arrows).* S = submandibular gland. *B,* After gadolinium administration (500/16/4), the hemangioma is so intensely enhanced that in some places it is isointense relative to fat *(arrows).* S = submandibular gland.

thyroglossal duct cysts, most occur above the level of the hyoid bone.[30] A dermoid cyst has a thin wall and may contain fat. Teratomas contain ectoderm, mesoderm, and endoderm and also occur in the midline. In addition to fat, they may contain calcium[30] and so may be better assessed by CT.

Acknowledgments

The author is grateful to Sabrina Jennings for her secretarial expertise and to Eric Jablonowski for assistance with the illustrations.

REFERENCES

1. Muntz H, Sessions DG: Surgery of laryngopharyngeal and subglottic cancer. In: Bailey BJ, Hiler HF, eds. Surgery of the Larynx. Philadelphia: WB Saunders, 1985, pp 293–315.
2. Graney DO, Flint PF: Anatomy (larynx). In: Cummings CW, ed. Otolaryngology—Head and Neck Surgery, Volume 3. St. Louis: Mosby–Year Book, 1993, pp 1693–1703.
3. Becker M, Zbaren P, Laeng H, et al: Neoplastic invasion of the laryngeal cartilage: comparison of MR imaging and CT with histopathologic correlation. Radiology 194:661–670, 1995.
4. Curtin HD: Imaging of the larynx: current concepts. Radiology 173:1–11, 1989.
5. Weissman JL, Curtin HD: The current approach to imaging the larynx. Curr Imaging 3:138–147, 1991.
6. Teresi LM, Lufkin RB, Hanafee WN: Magnetic resonance imaging of the larynx. Radiol Clin North Am 27:393–406, 1989.
7. Adams GL: Malignant neoplasms of the hypopharynx. In: Cummings CW, ed. Otolaryngology—Head and Neck Surgery, Volume 3. St. Louis: Mosby–Year Book, 1993, pp 1955–1980.
8. Olsen KD, DeSanto LW: Partial vertical laryngectomy—indications and surgical technique. Am J Otolaryngol 111:153–160, 1990.
9. Bastian RW: Benign mucosal and saccular disorders; benign laryngeal tumors. In: Cummings CW, ed. Otolaryngology—Head and Neck Surgery, Volume 3. St. Louis: Mosby–Year Book, 1993, pp 1897–1924.
10. Wippold FJ, Smirniotopoulos JG, Moran CJ, Glazer HS: Chondrosarcoma of the larynx: CT features. AJNR 14:453–459, 1993.
11. Mishell JH, Schild JA, Mafee MF: Chondrosarcoma of the larynx. Diagnosis with magnetic resonance imaging and computed tomography. Arch Otolaryngol Head Neck Surg 116:1338–1341, 1990.
12. Robbins KT: Pocket Guide to Neck Dissection Classification and TNM Staging of Head and Neck Cancer. Alexandria, VA: American Academy of Otolaryngology–Head and Neck Surgery Foundation, 1991.
13. Som PM: Detection of metastasis in cervical lymph nodes: CT and MR criteria and differential diagnosis. AJR 158:961–969, 1992.
14. Yousem DM, Som PM, Hackney DB, et al: Central nodal necrosis and extracapsular neoplastic spread in cervical lymph nodes. MR imaging vs. CT. Radiology 182:753–759, 1992.
15. Gefter WB, Spritzer CE, Eisenberg B, et al: Thyroid imaging with high-field-strength surface-coil MR. Radiology 164:483–490, 1987.
16. Higgins CB, Auffermann W: MR imaging of thyroid and parathyroid glands: a review of current status. AJR 151:1095–1106, 1988.
17. Noma S, Kanaoka M, Minami S, et al: Thyroid masses: MR imaging and pathologic correlation. Radiology 168:759–764, 1988.
18. Compagno J: Diseases of the thyroid. In: Barnes L, ed. Surgical Pathology of the Head and Neck. New York: Marcel Dekker, 1985, pp 1435–1486.
19. Babbel RW, Smoker WRK, Harnsberger HR: The visceral space: the unique infrahyoid space. Semin Ultrasound CT MR 12:204–223, 1991.
20. Posniak HV, Olson MC, Dudiak CM, et al: MR imaging of the brachial plexus. AJR 161:373–379, 1993.
21. Blair DN, Rapoport S, Sostman HD, Blair OC: Normal brachial plexus: MR imaging. Radiology 165:763–767, 1987.
22. Smoker WRK, Harnsberger HR, Reede DL, et al: The neck. In: Som PM, Bergeron RT, eds. Head and Neck Imaging. St. Louis: Mosby–Year Book, 1991, pp 497–592.
23. Barnes L, Peel RL, Verbin RS: Tumors of the nervous system. In: Barnes L, ed. Surgical Pathology of the Head and Neck. New York: Marcel Dekker, 1985, pp 659–724.
24. Stull MA, Moser RP Jr, Kransdorf MJ, et al: Magnetic resonance appearance of peripheral nerve sheath tumors. Skeletal Radiol 20:9–14, 1991.
25. Suh I-S, Abenoza P, Galloway HR, et al: Peripheral (extracranial) nerve tumors: correlation of MR imaging and histologic findings. Radiology 183:341–346, 1992.
26. Olsen WL, Dillon WP, Kelly WM, et al: MR imaging of paragangliomas. AJNR 7:1039–1042, 1986.
27. Bergeron RT, Lo WWM, Swartz JD, et al: The temporal bone. In: Som PM, Bergeron RT, eds. Head and Neck Imaging. St. Louis: Mosby–Year Book, 1991, pp 925–1115.
28. Blandino A, Salvi L, Scribano E, et al: MR findings in thyroglossal duct cysts: report of two cases. Eur J Radiol 11:207–211, 1990.
29. Cunningham MJ: The management of congenital neck masses. Am J Otolaryngol 13:78–92, 1992.
30. Faerber EN, Swartz JD: Imaging of neck masses in infants and children. Crit Rev Diagn Imaging 31:283–314, 1991.
31. Siegel MJ, Glazer HS, St Amour TE, Rosenthal DD: Lymphangiomas in children: MR imaging. Radiology 170:467–470, 1989.
32. Yuh WTC, Buehner LS, Kao SCS, et al: Magnetic resonance imaging of pediatric head and neck cystic hygromas. Ann Otol Rhinol Laryngol 100:737–742, 1991.
33. Zadvinskis DP, Benson MT, Kerr HH, et al: Congenital malformations of the cervicothoracic lymphatic system: embryology and pathogenesis. Radiographics 12:1175–1189, 1992.
34. Yonetsu K, Nakayama E, Hunihir M, et al: Magnetic resonance imaging of oral and maxillofacial angiomas. Oral Surg Oral Med Oral Pathol 16:783–789, 1993.

INDEX

Note: Page numbers in *italics* refer to illustrations; page numbers followed by t refer to tables.

Artifact(s) (Continued)
in musculoskeletal imaging, 1810–1812
presaturation method for, 73
prescanning adjustments for, 63
ringing, 71–72, *109*, 109–110
sources of, 88, *89*
specific absorption rate in, 67–68
susceptibility. See *Susceptibility artifact(s).*
third arm, 115, *116*
venetian blind, 140, *140*
wraparound, 113, *113–114*, 115
zebra-stripe, 312, *314*
Arytenoepiglottic fold(s), tumors in, 1135, *1137*
Arytenoid cartilage, 1133, *1135*
Ascites, 1325, *1326*, 1605–1606, *1606*
ASD (atrial septal defect). See *Atrial septal defect (ASD).*
ASE (asymmetric spin-echo) sequence(s). See *Asymmetric spin-echo (ASE) sequence(s).*
ASG (asialoglycoprotein). See *Asialoglycoprotein (ASG) receptors.*
Asialfetuin, in target-specific contrast agents, 209t, 210–211, *211*
Asialoglycoprotein (ASG) receptor(s), and contrast agents, 208–211, *210–211*
Askin tumor(s), of chest wall, 1674
Asplenia, 1579
Astrocytoma(s), 534–535, *536–537*
cerebellar, 618, *619*
epilepsy from, *715*, 716
giant cell, in tuberous sclerosis, 516, *517–518*
in suprasellar cistern, in neurofibromatosis type 1, *508*
of brain stem, 618, *620–621*, 621–622
of spinal cord, 1175, *1175*
scoliosis from, *1274*
pilocytic, of optic nerve, in children, 1002, *1004*, 1005
Asymmetric field of view imaging, musculoskeletal, 1800–1801, *1801*
Asymmetric sampling, 165
Asymmetric spin-echo (ASE) sequence(s), in brain activation studies, *263*, 263–264
sensitivity of, in cerebral hemorrhage, *225*, 225
Ataxia, Friedreich's, 920, *921*
Atelectasis, in children, 1333, *1334*
obstructive, vs. bronchogenic carcinoma, 1664, *1665*
Atherosclerosis, *775*, 777
in extremities, 1322–1323, *1323*
thoracic aortic aneurysms from, 1646
Atlas, occipitalization of, 1272
ATM (acute transverse myelopathy), 1185
Atom(s), group behavior of, in radiofrequency pulses, 6–7, *6–7*
ATP (adenosine triphosphate). See *Adenosine triphosphate (ATP).*
Atrial isomerism, left, dextrocardia from, *1693*, 1694
Atrial septal defect (ASD), 1693–1694, *1695*
in tricuspid atresia, 1698, *1700*
occluders for, compatibility with imaging systems, 416t–417t
Atrioventricular (AV) valve(s), anomalies of, 1697–1698, *1700*
Atrium (atria) (brain), plaques on, from multiple sclerosis, *858*, 858–859
Atrium (atria) (heart), metastatic disease in, *1620*

Attenuation curve(s), for diffusion, analysis of, *241*, 241–242
Attenuation factor (A(t)), in diffusion, 235–237
restricted, 239, *240*
of gadolinium-DTPA, 256, *256*
Auditory canal(s), internal, anatomy of, *1039*
schwannoma of, *1043–1044*
Auditory meatus, internal, axial view of, *477*
Auditory pathway, innervation of, 605
Autism, with cerebellar hypoplasia, 503, *504*
Autosomal dominant polycystic kidney disease, 1517, *1517–1518*
AV (atrioventricular) valve(s), anomalies of, 1697–1698, *1700*
Avascular necrosis, clinical staging of, 1941t
in children, 2131, 2133, *2133*
of bone marrow, 2087, *2087*
of carpal lunate, 1928–1929, *1928–1930*
of femoral head, 1941t, 1941–1942, *1942–1945*, 1944–1946, 2160–2161
of humeral head, 2164
of scaphoid, *1927*
of shoulder, 1871, *1871*
AVM(s) (arteriovenous malformations). See *Arteriovenous malformation(s) (AVMs).*
Axial compression fracture(s), 1296, *1297*, 1298
Axial plane, imaging in. See under specific body part, e.g., *Brain.*
Axonal injury, diffuse, 691, *692–694*

B_0 (main magnetic field), 146, *146*
B value, in diffusion imaging, 829
Bacterial meningitis, 627–629, *628, 630*
Balanced image(s). See *Proton density–weighted image(s).*
Band heterotopia, 725
Bandwidth, and signal-to-noise ratio, 76–77
and slice selection, 153
definition of, 10
in musculoskeletal imaging, 1809, *1809*
Bankart lesion(s), 1854, *1855*
Bankart repair, 1866, *1867*
Barium sulfate, 194, 1586
Barrier(s), physical, for safety, 55
Basal ganglia, abnormal signal in, etiology of, 884t
calcification of, in children, 882t, 882–883
in Creutzfeldt-Jakob disease, 915–916, *917*
in hepatic encephalopathy, 907, *907*
in Huntington's disease, 917, *917*
lesions of, with high signal intensity, in neurofibromatosis type 1, 505, *507*
Basal vein of Rosenthal, axial view of, *472, 480*
Basilar artery, axial view of, *470, 471, 476–479*
occlusion of, 806, 810, *810*
Basilar impression, 1271
Basilar tip, aneurysm of, impact zone of, 819, *822*
"Basilar tip" intracranial aneurysm, *742, 749*
Basiocciput, marrow of, axial view of, *476*
Basis pontis, axial view of, *471*

Behçet's disease, 780, *782*, 1655
"Bell clapper" deformity, and testicular torsion, 1417
Bellows, in respiration motion compensation, 74
Bell's palsy, 604
Benedikt's syndrome, 598
Berry aneurysm(s), with polycystic kidney disease, 737, 737–738
Biceps muscle, anatomy of, 1824
Biceps tendon, abnormalities of, 1850, *1852–1853*, 1853
anatomic variations in, 1833
anatomy of, 1830, *1832*
injuries of, 1887, 1890, *1890–1892*
Bicornuate uterus, *1447*, 1448, *1450*
Bicuspid valve(s), in aortic stenosis, 1703, *1705*
Bielschowsky's stain, for Pick's disease, 915
Bifurcation aneurysm(s), blood flow in, 735
of middle cerebral artery, 745
Bile, intraperitoneal, 1607
Bile duct(s), contrast agents for, 200, 201t, 202
excretion of contrast agents by, 186–188, *188–190*
obstruction of, from pancreatic carcinoma, *1573*
Biliary system, anatomy of, 1499
benign diseases of, 1500–1505, *1502–1505*
calculous, 1500, *1502, 1503*
cystic diseases of, 1505, *1506*
imaging of, techniques for, 1499–1500, *1501–1502*
infectious diseases of, 1505–1506, *1506*
malignant diseases of, 1506–1509, *1507–1509*
Binomial water-selective pulse sequence, 151–152, *152*
Biopsy, needles for, compatibility with imaging systems, 407t
of breast, imaging before, 1361–1365, *1362–1364*
magnetic resonance imaging–directed, 1378
stereotactic, 384–385, *385–386*
Black blood sequence, radiofrequency prepulses for, 163–164, *165*
Bladder, male, anatomy of, 1391–1392, *1393*
carcinoma of, 1393–1395, *1394–1395*
papillary, 1393–1394, *1394*
perivesicle fat invasion in, 1394, *1395*
staging of, 1394t, 1394–1395
imaging of, techniques for, 1393
urachus of, tumors of, 1395, *1396*
rupture of, 1607
Bleeding diathesis, brain hemorrhage from, 679–680, *680–681*
Bloch equation(s), 146
in spectroscopy, 353–356, *354–355*
Blood, and image contrast, 26–27
arterial, iron in, in hemorrhage, 222, *222*
bright, imaging sequence for, 72–73
dark, imaging sequence for, 73, 163–164, *165*
intraperitoneal, *1606*, 1606–1607
oxygenation of, in brain activation studies, 260–266, *261*
relaxivity of, in tissue, 183–184
viscosity of, 272